HEAD AND NECK SURGICAL PATHOLOGY

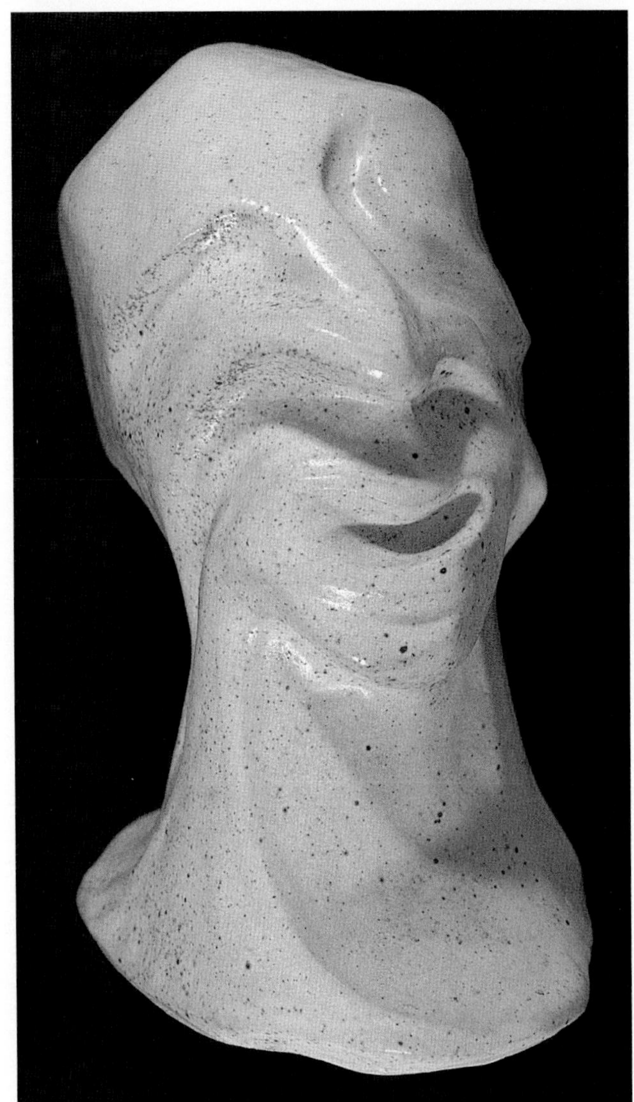

Sculpture by Debby Pilch

HEAD AND NECK SURGICAL PATHOLOGY

Edited by

BEN Z. PILCH

Associate Pathologist
Massachusetts General Hospital
Pathologist and Director of Otolaryngeal Pathology
Massachusetts Eye and Ear Infirmary
Associate Professor of Pathology
Harvard Medical School
Department of Pathology
Massachusetts General Hospital
Boston, Massachusetts

LIPPINCOTT WILLIAMS & WILKINS
PHILADELPHIA · NEW YORK · BALTIMORE

Acquisitions Editor: Ruth W. Weinberg
Developmental Editor: Anne Snyder
Production Editor: Robin E. Cook
Manufacturing Manager: Tim Reynolds
Cover Designer: David Levy
Compositor: Maryland Composition

530 Walnut St.
Philadelphia, PA 19106 USA
LWW.com

Printed in China

Library of Congress Cataloging-in-Publication Data
Head and neck surgical pathology / edited by Ben Z. Pilch
p. ; cm
Includes bibliographical references and index.
ISBN 0-397-51727-0
1. Head—Diseases—Diagnosis. 2. Neck—Diseases—Diagnosis. 3. Pathology, Surgical. I. Pilch, Ben Z.
[DNLM: 1. Head—pathology. 2. Head—surgery. 3. Neck—pathology. 4. Neck—surgery. 5. Pathology, Surgical—methods. WE 705 H4312 2000]
RC936.H434 2000
617.5′1—dc21

---

10 9 8 7 6 5 4 3 2 1

Dedication

This book is dedicated to Dr. Max L. Goodman, of blessed memory: teacher, mentor, colleague, and friend, without whom this work would not have come to pass, and who tragically did not live to shepherd it to completion.

". . . to reckon him who taught me this Art equally dear to me as my parents. . ." Oath of Hippocrates

and to my wife, Debby, whose unfailing love and support succored and sustained me during the course of this project.

"who can find a virtuous woman? for her price is far above rubies." *Prov 31:10.13*

Ben Z. Pich, M.D.

CONTENTS

Contributing Authors ix
Preface xi
Acknowledgments xiii

1. Congential Anomalies of the Head and Neck 1
Louis P. Dehner

2. Squamous Neoplasia of the Upper Aerodigestive Tract: Intraepithelial and Invasive Squamous Cell Carcinoma 34
John D. Crissman and Wael A. Sakr

3. The External Ear and Ear Canal, Middle Ear and Mastoid, Inner Ear, and Temporal Bone 53
Leslie Michaels

4. Nasal Cavity and Paranasal Sinuses: Embryology, Anatomy, Histology, and Pathology 80
Richard J. Zarbo, Frank X. Torres, and Jose Gomez

5. The Nasopharynx and Waldeyer's Ring 157
Ben Z. Pilch

6. Oral Cavity and Jaws: Common Odontogenic Lesions, Cysts of the Jaws, and Odontogenic Tumors 195
David G. Gardner

7. Larynx and Hypopharynx 230
Ben Z. Pilch

8. Salivary Glands 284
Mario A. Luna

9A. Pathology of the Thyroid 350
Maria J. Merino and Lavinia P. Middleton

9B. The Parathyroid Glands 379
Lavinia P. Middleton and Maria J. Merino

10. Soft Tissue Pathology of the Head and Neck 389
Suzanne B. Keel and Andrew E. Rosenberg

11. Pathology of Selected Diseases Affecting the Bones and Joints of the Head and Neck 438
G. Petur Nielsen, John X. O'Connell, and Andrew E. Rosenberg

12. Lymphoma and Lymphoid Hyperplasia in Head and Neck Sites 476
Judith A. Ferry and Nancy Lee Harris

13. Dermatopathology of the Head and Neck 534
Lyn M. Duncan

14. Cytopathology of the Head and Neck
A. Cytopathology of the Salivary Glands, Neck, Soft Tissue, and Skin 618
Teri L. Cooper
B. Cytopathology of the Eye, Orbit, Jaws, Oral Cavity, and Sinonasal Tract 663
Michele M. Weir
C. Cytopathology of the Thyroid Gland 686
William C. Faquin

Index 701

CONTRIBUTING AUTHORS

Teri L. Cooper, M.D. Instructor, Department of Pathology, Harvard Medical School, 25 Shattuck Street, Boston Massachusetts 02115, and Associate Director of Cytopathology, Department of Pathology, Massachusetts General Hospital, 55 Fruit Street, Warren 105B, Boston, Massachusetts 02114

John D. Crissman, M.D. Dean, School of Medicine, Wayne State University, 540 East Canfield Street, Room 1241, Detroit, Michigan 48201

Louis P. Dehner, M.D. Professor, Department of Pathology, Washington University School of Medicine, 660 South Euclid Avenue, Campus Box 8118, St. Louis, Missouri 63110, and Director of Anatomic Pathology and Surgical Pathology, Surgical Pathologist-in-Chief, Barnes Jewish Hosital, 1 Barnes Hospital Plaza, MS 90-23-357, St. Louis, Missouri 63110

Lyn M. Duncan, M.D. Director, Dermatopathology Training Program, Department of Pathology, Harvard Medical School, and Assistant Pathologist, Department of Pathology, Massachusetts General Hospital, Dermatopathology Unit WRN827, 55 Fruit Street, Boston, Massachusetts 02114

William C. Faquin, M.D., Ph.D. Clinical Instructor of Pathology, Harvard Medical School, and Assistant Pathologist, Department of Pathology, Massachusetts General Hospital, 55 Fruit Street, Warren 215, Boston, Massachusetts 02114

Judith A. Ferry, M.D. Associate Professor of Pathology, Department of Pathology, Harvard Medical School, 25 Shattuck Street, Boston, Massachusetts 02115, and Medical Director, Histology Laboratory, Department of Pathology, Massachusetts General Hospital, 55 Fruit Street, Boston, Massachusetts 02114

David G. Gardner, D.D.S., M.S.D. Professor Emeritus, Division of Oral Pathology and Oncology, University of Colorado School of Dentistry, 4200 East Ninth Avenue, Denver, Colorado 80262

Jose Gomez, M.D. Department of Pathology, Henry Ford Hospital, 2799 West Grand Boulevard, Detroit, Michigan 48202

Nancy Lee Harris, M.D. Professor of Pathology, Department of Pathology, Harvard Medical School, 25 Shattuck Street, Boston, Massachusetts 02215, and Director of Pathology Training Programs, Department of Pathology, Massachusetts General Hospital, 55 Fruit Street, Warren 2, Boston, Massachusetts 02114

Suzanne B. Keel, M.D. Connective Tissue Oncology Center, Department of Pathology, Harvard Medical School, Massachusetts General Hospital, 55 Fruit Street, Boston, Massachusetts 02114

Mario A. Luna, M.D. Professor of Pathology, Department of Pathology and Laboratory Medicine, Pathologist, Department of Anatomic Pathology, The University of Texas M.D. Anderson Cancer Center, 1515 Holcombe Boulevard, Box 85, Houston, Texas 77030

Maria J. Merino, M.D. National Cancer Institute, National Institutes of Health, Department of Pathology, Building 10, Room 2N212, Bethesda, Maryland 20892

Leslie Michaels, M.D. Professor Emeritus, Department of Histopathology, Royal Free and UCL Medical School, Rockefeller Building, University Street, London WC1E 6JJ, and Honorary Consultant, Royal National Throat, Nose, and Ear Hospital, Gray's Inn Road, London WCIX 8DA, United Kingdom

Lavinia P. Middleton, M.D. Assistant Professor, Department of Pathology, University of Texas M.D. Anderson Cancer Center, 1515 Holcombe Boulevard, Houston, Texas, 77030, and Adjunct Assistant Professor, Department of Pathology and Laboratory Medicine, University of Texas at Houston Medical School, 6431 Fannin Street, Houston, Texas 77030

G. Petur Nielsen, M.D. Assistant Pathologist, Department of Pathology, Massachusetts General Hospital, and Assistant Profesor, Department of Pathology, Harvard Medical School, 55 Fruit Street, Boston, Massachusetts 02114

John X. O'Connell, M.D. Consultant Pathologist, 13750 96th Avenue, Surrey, British Columbia, Canada V3V 1Z2

Ben Z. Pilch, M.D. Associate Pathologist, Massachusetts General Hospital, Pathologist and Director of Otolaryngeal Pathology, Massachusetts Eye & Ear Infirmary, Associate Professor of Medicine, Harvard Medical School, Department of Pathology, Massachusetts General Hospital, 55 Fruit Street, Boston, Massachusetts 02114

Andrew E. Rosenberg, M.D. Associate Professor, Department of Pathology, Harvard Medical School, and Associate Pathologist, Department of Pathology, Massachusetts General Hospital, 32 Fruit Street, Boston, Massachusetts 02114

Wael A. Sakr, M.D. Associate Professor, Department of Pathology, Wayne State University School of Medicine, 540 East Canfield, Detroit, Michigan 48201

Frank X. Torres, M.D. Senior Staff, Department of Pathology, Henry Ford Health System, 2799 West Grand Boulevard, Detroit, Michigan 48202

Michelle M. Weir, M.D., F.R.C.P. Lecturer, Department of Laboratory Medicine and Pathobiology, University of Toronto, and Staff Pathologist, Department of Pathology, University Health Network, 200 Elizabeth Street, Toronto, Ontario M56 2C4, Canada

Richard J. Zarbo, M.D., D.M.D. Professor, Department of Pathology, Case Western Reserve University School of Medicine, Henry Ford Health Sciences Campus, and Interim Chair, Department of Pathology, Henry Ford Hospital, 2799 West Grand Boulevard Detroit, Michigan 48202

PREFACE

Perhaps nowhere in the human body does such a rich and diverse variety of tissues and organs converge in such a compact area as in the head and neck. Consequently, a vast array of pathologic processes and disease entities can be found in this anatomic region. Indeed, a knowledge of the pathology of the head and neck presupposes a knowledge of much of the discipline of anatomic pathology in general, and, in this era of burgeoning medical knowledge and increasing subspecialization, head and neck pathology remains a bastion of general pathology.

With the foregoing perspective of the field in mind, we have assembled a group of contributors that reflects the varied areas of expertise that commingle in the study of the pathology of this region. It is hoped that this volume will provide a comprehensive, though not necessarily exhaustive or encyclopedic, discussion of the rich pathology of the head and neck. A chapter on diagnostic fine needle aspiration cytopathology of the head and neck is included, as this technique is increasingly utilized with productive and advantageous results.

The book is intended primarily as a text rather than an atlas, although illustrations are ample and varied. The aim is to provide a more than cursory discussion of the major entities covered. In general, the terminology used is that suggested by the World Health Organization (WHO), with variations as indicated. The content is meant to be practical as well as instructional, with a discussion of aids in differential diagnosis, often including helpful clinical information and data derived from ancillary studies such as immunohistochemistry. Various prevalent views regarding controversial issues are presented, with comments on generally accepted interpretations, as well as authors' opinions.

Head and Neck Surgical Pathology is intended primarily for trained pathologists and residents interested in diagnostic surgical pathology of the head and neck. It is hoped, however, that this work may prove useful and informative to nonpathologists involved in the diagnosis, treatment, and/or study of diseases of the head and neck, such as surgeons, radiologists, medical and radiation oncologists, and others.

I would like to express my deep and sincere appreciation and gratitude to all those involved in bringing this project to fruition. The contributors to this book have worked hard, faithfully, and enthusiastically. They brought their many talents and considerable expertise unreservedly to their tasks. The secretarial and photographic staffs of the Massachusetts General Hospital have been energetic and extremely competent and supportive in this endeavor. Lippincott Williams & Wilkins, throughout this long period of gestation, has remained unfailingly supportive, caring, patient (as Job), helpful, and enthusiastic.

Ben Z. Pilch, M.D.

PREFACE

ACKNOWLEDGMENTS

This work has been published due to the efforts of Dr. Max Goodman, my teacher, colleague, mentor, and friend. He was originally approached to undertake this project and generously asked me to participate. Max tragically died during the course of preparing this volume. I hope his fathomless knowledge, diagnostic acumen, and wisdom live on in these pages. Certainly his friendship, enthusiasm, and insightful teaching, as well as his great warmth, kindness, and humanity remain an indelible part of me. My debt to him is incalculable.

A special measure of thanks I give to my wife Debby, whose patience, support, and love have been sustaining and inspirational to me during the seemingly interminable course of this work.

I am very grateful not only to the excellent and hard working contributors to this manuscript, but also to the members of the pathology department of the Massachusetts General Hospital, and the otolaryngology department of the Massachusetts Eye and Ear Infirmary, both resident and staff, who provided support and encouragement during this project. Ms. Marlene Fairbanks, Carol Ann Gould, Chris Peters, and Maria Forcellati provided invaluable secretarial support. Mr. Stephen Conley and Ms. Michelle Forrestall were indefatigable stalwarts in the pathology department's photography lab at the Massachusetts General Hospital.

The following physicians are gratefully acknowledged for providing the material used in the following illustrations: Dr. Nancy Harris, Chapter 5, Fig. 5; Dr. Hugh Curtin, Chapter 5, Figs. 6 and 23; Dr. Antonio Perez-Atayde, Chapter 5, Figs. 20-22; Dr. Bruce Wenig, Chapter 5, Fig. 38; and Dr. Alfio Ferlito, Chapter 7, Fig. 38.

Ben Z. Pilch, M.D.

1

CONGENITAL ANOMALIES OF THE HEAD AND NECK

LOUIS P. DEHNER

The head and neck is the anatomic region with possibly the broadest array of developmental anomalies, resulting in numerous dysmorphogenetic syndromes with localized or systemic implications (1–3). One such example of the latter is the branchio-oto-renal syndrome with cystic dysplasia of the kidneys and focal segmental glomerulosclerosis (4,5). However, most developmental lesions of the head and neck region in children are not seen by the surgical pathologist, with the exception of those presenting as a mass lesion (6–9), and most children with these lesions do not have a defined syndrome.

Numerous embryologic events must be precisely coordinated in order for an organ to develop normally. In the head and neck region several organ systems are derived from the three embryonic cell layers, and any successful development must be precisely synchronized for the end result of such a complicated structure as the normal anatomy of the head and neck. A deviation may be so slight as to escape detection, to be judged clinically as inconsequential at one extreme, or to be devastatingly disfiguring at the other. Some deviations are in fact variations on normal development.

The pathologist becomes engaged in the diagnostic process when the clinical concern rises to the level of a biopsy or excision of a palpable mass or other lesion, which may represent a cyst or sinus tract, solid, or cystic mass in the soft tissues, or a polyploid lesion in the oral, nasal, or pharyngeal passages. Some of these tumefactions are the consequence of one or more dysembryonic events whose etiologies are unknown in many instances (Table 1). Some of the solid lesions are heterotopias or choristomas (otherwise normal tissue in an abnormal site) or hamartomas (disorganized growth of tissues native to the site). The pathogenesis and nosology of some lesions in the head and neck are unsettled, such as the hairy or teratoid polyp, salivary gland anlage tumor, and nasal chondromesenchymal hamartoma.

Some of the assumptions about pathogenesis enumerated in Table 1 may be arguable. In the category of tissue overgrowth with or without disorganization, there are examples of dysontogenetic neoplasms such as the teratoma and sialoblastoma. The nosology of the cystic lymphangioma, hemangioma, and fetal rhabdomyoma has been settled in the sense that they are considered soft tissue tumors, but their pathogenesis as a malformation or neoplasm remains open for discussion and disagreement.

Many of the lesions listed in Table 1 are congenital, as defined by their clinical detection before birth by ultrasonography or shortly after birth (10). However, a congenital or connatal mass presenting in the head and neck region is not necessarily a developmental aberration. Neuroblastoma, melanotic neuroectodermal tumor of infancy, fibromatosis colli, embryonal rhabdomyosarcoma, peripheral nerve sheath tumor, retinoblastoma, and malignant rhabdoid tumor represent an incomplete roster of neoplasms that we have seen in neonates in the last 25 years. Congenital tumors of the central nervous system should not be overlooked, although they are usually considered separately from the extracranial neoplasms of the head and neck region.

It is generally the case that most maldevelopmental lesions in the head and neck region in Table 1 come to clinical attention as a palpable cutaneous, subcutaneous, oral, nasal, or orbital mass whose midline or lateral location has relevance in the clinical, as well as the pathologic differential diagnosis (6,7,9,11). Those lesions in the nasal cavity or impinging upon the upper respiratory tract may be accompanied by symptoms and signs of airway obstruction, especially in an infant.

As a generalization, most tumefactive lesions of a developmental nature present clinically in childhood, but there is ample precedence for the initial presentation of a branchial cleft or thyroglossal duct cyst to be delayed into adulthood. A palpable mass in the head and neck region of a child has a greater than 50% likelihood of representing some type of congenital or developmental lesion; only 10% or so of cases are malignant, and the majority of these are Hodgkin's disease or non-Hodgkin lymphoma (12–15). On the other hand, Rapidis and co-workers reported that in a study of 1,007 head and neck tumors in children, only 17% were developmental anomalies or dysplasias (16). In adults, there is a substantial shift in the likelihood that a mass in the neck is not only neoplastic, but also malignant (17). Among 445 children who presented with a neck mass, Torsiglieri and associates reported that 55% of cases were congenital–developmental lesions; the branchial cleft and thyroglossal duct cysts together accounted for 62% of all congenital lesions and 34% of all neck masses in this series (18). Our own experience at the St. Louis Children's Hospital is coincidental to the latter observations from the Children's Hospital of Philadelphia. The clinical evaluation of a child with a mass in the

TABLE 1. PALPABLE MALDEVELOPMENTAL LESIONS OF THE HEAD AND NECK

Presumed Pathogenesis	Pathology
Anomalous surface ectoderm and neuroectoderm with or without a closure defect	Encephalocele
	Nasal "glioma" (nasal glial heterotopia)
	Heterotopic neuroglia
	Heterotopic meningocele
	Dermoid cyst or sinus
	Hairy polyp (teratoid)
Persistence of embryonic remnants	Branchial cleft cyst, sinus, and fistula
	Thyroglossal duct cyst
	Duplication cyst
	Cervical thymic cyst
	Parathyromatosis
	Lingual thyroid
Heterotopia	Salivary gland heterotopia
	Phakomatous choristoma
	Ectopic hamartomatous thymoma
Tissue overgrowth with or without organization	Teratoma
	Sialoblastoma
	Salivary gland anlage tumor
	Chondromesenchymal hamartoma
	Cherubism
	Fibrous dysplasia
	Hemangioma
	Lymphangioma (cystic hygroma)
	Fetal rhabdomyoma

head and neck region has been discussed by several researchers (12,13,15,18,19). There are overlapping diagnostic approaches to a head and neck mass whether the patient is a child or an adult.

One of the more widely applied techniques in the diagnosis of head and neck lesions, especially in a superficial location, is the fine-needle aspiration biopsy. Its utility has been well documented in numerous studies that have appeared in the literature over the past 10 to 15 years and is discussed in Chapter 14. Many head and neck masses in children are cystic and thus lend themselves to aspiration with a successful diagnostic outcome (Fig. 1).

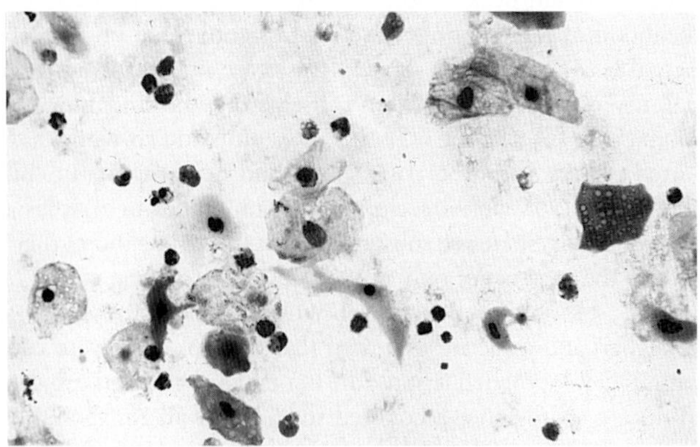

FIGURE 1. Fine-needle aspiration biopsy of a lateral neck mass in a child showing a mixture of squamous cells and neutrophils whose features were interpreted as an infected branchial cleft cyst that was confirmed after a resection.

ANOMALOUS DEVELOPMENT OF NEUROECTODERMAL AND SURFACE ECTODERM WITH OR WITHOUT CLOSURE DEFECT

The morphologic intricacies of craniofacial development have been appreciated from the earliest period of descriptive embryology with the recognition of a series of coordinated events that involve not only the neuroectoderm in its formation of the embryonic brain with neural tube closure and proliferation and the migration of neural crest cells, but the participation of the ectoderm, endoderm, and mesoderm in the genesis of the branchial apparatus. A separation occurs quite early between the neuroectoderm and the surface or integumental ectoderm (2). Other events in the period between the 4th and 6th weeks of embryonic life include the formation of the neurocranium as islands of membranous bone for the calvarium and foci of enchondral ossification for the base of the skull (20). By the 5th week of embryonic life, the branchial arches have made their appearance with their complex assortment of derivatives, which have been summarized by Gorlin and Cohen (1). As these events are transpiring into the 6th week, the earliest vestiges of a face are in evolution. Many small details in this period of early development must take place, such as the formation of foramina for cranial nerves and blood vessels, midline fusion of symmetrical anlage, and bony encasement of the craniospinal axis, while still allowing for growth of the brain and spinal cord and differential growth and migration of organs into their future definitive anatomic sites. There are countless successive events in this dynamic process that provide ample opportunities for one or more developmental missteps. It is not especially surprising under these circumstances that craniofacial anomalies are relatively common in the human population (1). A major or minor malformation or deformity in the head and neck region is found in 3% to 5% of the pediatric population (1,2). Studies confined to perinatal and neonatal autopsies yield an even higher incidence of congenital malformations of complex types, involving not only the craniofacial structures, but the central nervous system and not infrequently other major organ systems.

A distinction is made between a malformation that occurs in early embryonic life and represents an intrinsic perturbation in development and the appearance later in fetal life of a deformity resulting from an intrauterine event such as rupture of the amniotic sac. A single anomaly or malformation may initiate a series of secondary events whose morphologic manifestations are defined as a sequence (2). Insights into the mechanisms of a malformation have evolved from recent molecular genetic studies, with focus on the homeobox (*HOX*) and pair-box (*PAX*) genes as complex systems of integrated genes that control a substantial degree of the molecular events of embryogenesis (21). There are several excellent sources for more detailed discussions on the subject of the molecular genetics of craniofacial anomalies and syndromes (22–24). These basic studies may appear to be far removed from the daily activities of the surgical pathologist, but they provide some texture and even insight into our diagnostic activities.

Encephalocele

The encephalocele and meningocele are pathogenetic and nosologic examples of neural tube defects with an accompanying defect in the cranial bone or vertebra as a sequential anomaly. A disturbance in the separation of the surface ectoderm from the neuroectoderm in the later stages of neurulation is thought by some to be the principal pathogenetic mechanism in the occurrence of an encephalocele or meningocele, with or without demonstrable anatomic continuity with the underlying dura, brain, or spinal cord through a bony defect (25,26). When there is no anatomic connection with the underlying dura, brain, or spinal cord, and a bony defect is not detected in the course of diagnostic imaging studies, the heterotopic neural tissue can be regarded as a sequestered encephalocele, meningocele, meningoencephalocele, or meningomyelocele on the basis of the identifiable tissues found in microscopic examination of the focus. It has been estimated that an encephalocele occurs in approximately 0.5 to 1 per 1,000 to 4,000 live births (25,26).

Occipital encephaloceles comprise 75% to 80% of all such anomalies and infrequently require the services of the surgical pathologist, except when the pregnancy is terminated before 20 weeks' gestation, in which case the surgical specimen is submitted for fetopsy (25). Prenatal ultrasonography is the method by which most of these anomalies are detected (26). The very poor outcome of infants with an occipital encephalocele is the medical rationale for the interruption of the pregnancy (27,28). Most occipital encephaloceles are nonsyndromic, but there are several well-established associations, most notably the Meckel-Gruber syndrome, an autosomal recessive condition whose genetic abnormality has recently been mapped to chromosome 11q13 (29–33). In one case an infant with an occipital encephalocele also had a mediastinal enteric duplication cyst (34). Another neonate had an occipital encephalocele and a dermoid cyst (35). Ahdab-Barmada and Claassen have characterized the neuropathologic abnormalities in the Meckel-Gruber syndrome (36). Like all occipital encephaloceles, there is displacement of the segment of brain with the caudal third ventricle, cerebellar vermis, and fourth ventricle. In the case of the Meckel-Gruber syndrome, the displacement of the encephalocele occurs through the posterior fontanelle rather than through an occipital cranium bifidum. A strand of neural tissue connects the encephalocele with the intracranial portion of the brain with its additional anomalies.

Extraoccipital encephaloceles are more likely to come to the attention of the surgical pathologist because they present as an orbital, nasoorbital, frontoethmoidal, or intranasal mass that on biopsy shows the presence of mature neuroglial tissue (25,37). Anterior or frontal encephaloceles are typically seen at or before the age of 2 years (38). Males are affected more commonly than females, unlike the female predilection for occipital encephaloceles (25). The frequency of anterior encephaloceles in Southeast Asia is greater than in Europe and the United States for as yet unknown reasons (25). As in the case of the occipital encephalocele, there is a defect in the skull to accommodate the anatomic connection with the underlying brain. Grossly, the encephalocele is either a broad sessile or pedunculated lesion with a meningeal and mucosal or cutaneous covering. The amount of tissue submitted for histologic examination varies considerably from case to case. Smaller pedunculated encephaloceles may be excised *in toto,* whereas large encephaloceles are more problematic, especially in the presence of hydrocephalus. Large encephaloceles are often managed by craniofacial reconstruction, a procedure that may yield little if any tissue (37). The microscopic findings are generally restricted to nonspecific neuroglial tissue, but cortex and white matter with some retention of normal anatomic relationships are seen in some cases. Choroid plexus, glioneuronal heterotopias, ependyma, and dural–arachnoidal elements are identified in a minority of cases (25). Hirokawa and associates reported a case of a parietal encephalocele in an infant with microscopic areas resembling a giant cell fibroblastoma that likely represented meningothelial tissue (39).

Nasal Glial Heterotopia (Nasal "Glioma")

Nasal glial heterotopia (nasal "glioma") is one of several congenital mass lesions of the nose that are clinically detectable at birth or within the first 12 months of life (40–46). The estimated frequency of congenital nasal lesions of all pathologic types ranges from one case per 20,000 to 40,000 live births. The types and distribution of these various lesions, including nasal glioma, have been summarized from several series in the literature (Table 2). As noted from this review, nasal gliomas accounted for 6% of all congenital nasal lesions.

One recent estimate has placed the number of reported examples of nasal glioma in the literature at approximately 300 cases (47,48). There is a male predilection of 2 to 3:1. Virtually every researcher agrees that the designation of *glioma* is an unfortunate one, many preferring the term *nasal glial heterotopia,* which does not imply a malignant neoplasm as does *glioma.* The

TABLE 2. CONGENITAL NASAL LESIONS: LITERATURE REVIEW

	Bradley and Singh (41)	Morgan and Evans (42)	Barkovich et al. (44)	Paller et al. (46)	Total (%)
Nasal dermoid	67	20	7	36	130 (59)
Hemangioma	32	2	—	—	34 (15)
Encephalocele	2	2	8	9	21 (10)
Nasal glial heterotopia (nasal "glioma")	5	7	1	1	14 (6)
Neurofibroma	1	—	—	—	5 (1)
Hairy polyp	—	4	—		4 (1)
Cyst	—	2	—	—	2 (<1)
Fibroma	1	—	—	—	1 (<1)
Others	—	9	—	—	9 (2)
	108	50	16	46	220 (100)

term *nasal glioma,* however, dates to the earliest descriptions of this lesion in the mid-19th century according to Claros and associates (49). A distinction is made between the nasal glioma and encephalocele, although 15% to 20% of nasal gliomas have an anatomic connection with the intracranial contents (44,46,50). The pathogenetic and semantic issue is whether the nasal glioma should be considered a sequestered encephalocele or an unrelated heterotopia (51–53). Our purpose is not to resolve this dilemma, but to point out that the surgical pathology report or other means of communication should convey the possibility that the nasal glioma may be the proverbial tip of the iceberg, which is equally true for neuroglial heterotopias in the orbit, paranasal sinuses, middle ear, and nasopharynx.

Nasal gliomas are clinically apparent at or shortly after birth in the majority of cases as a firm to rubbery midline swelling or mass at the bridge of the nose or in the soft tissues adjacent to the medial canthus. Respiratory distress in the neonatal period has been reported in a minority of cases (54). Although most nasal gliomas are diagnosed in the first year of life, some cases do not come to clinical attention until later childhood, and rarely into adulthood (47). The presence of telangiectasias in the overlying skin may suggest a vascular lesion. Paradoxically, most nasal gliomas are, in fact, external to the nasal cavity (60% of cases) whereas 30% of cases present as a mass or polyp in the nasal cavity (49,50). The remaining 10% of lesions have an extra- and intranasal component.

The clinical distinction between a nasal glioma and encephalocele is ascertained mainly by imaging studies to determine whether a bony defect is present and whether anatomic continuity exists between the frontal lobe and the nasal mass. A minority of nasal gliomas have a fibrous cord or tract connecting to the intracranial contents without a demonstrable defect in the bone. The stalk of neuroglial or fibrous–meningothelial tissue extends beneath the nasal bone toward the cribriform plate (48).

A tannish-gray to yellowish mass measuring 1 to 3 cm in greatest dimension is well circumscribed but lacks a capsule (55,56). The consistency of the mass is determined by the amount of fibrous stroma relative to the softer neuroglial tissue. Microscopically, islands of mature or differentiated neuroglial tissue are separated by dense bundles of collagen, surrounded by skeletal muscle or present in the nasal stroma with glands (Fig. 2). The astrocytes may have fibrillary and gemistocytic features (Fig. 3). Neurons are found in a minority of cases. When the is-

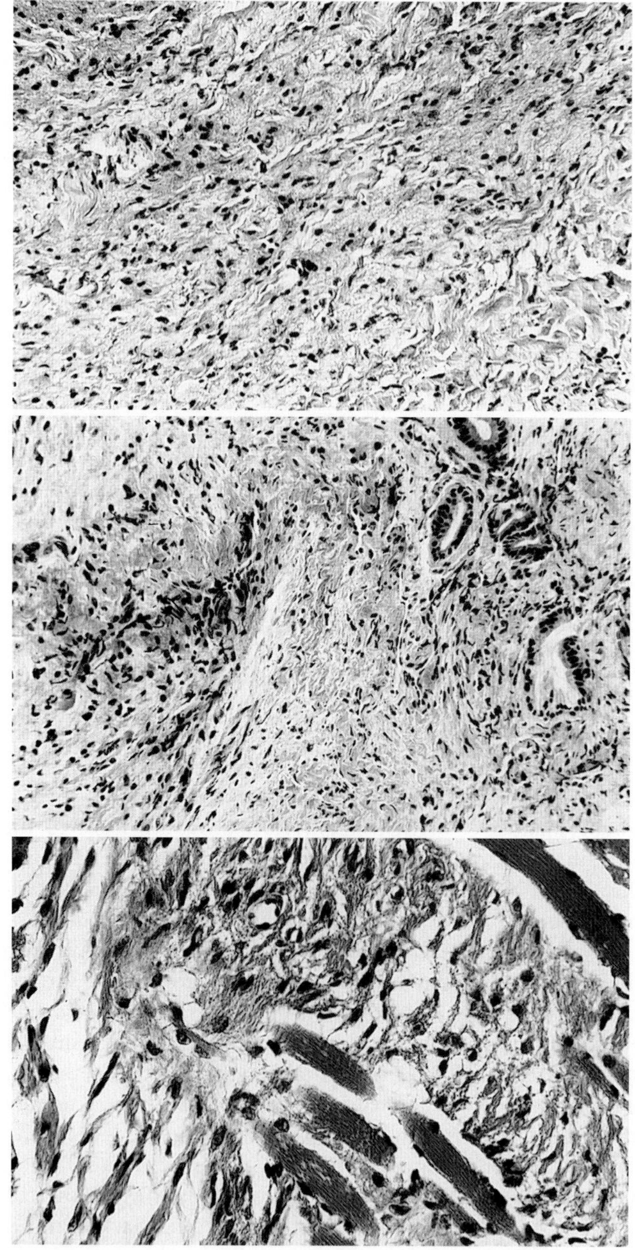

FIGURE 2. Nasal glioma showing ill-defined islands of fibrillary neuroglia within a loose fibrous stroma **(top)**, within the submucosa **(middle)**, and in skeletal muscle **(bottom)**.

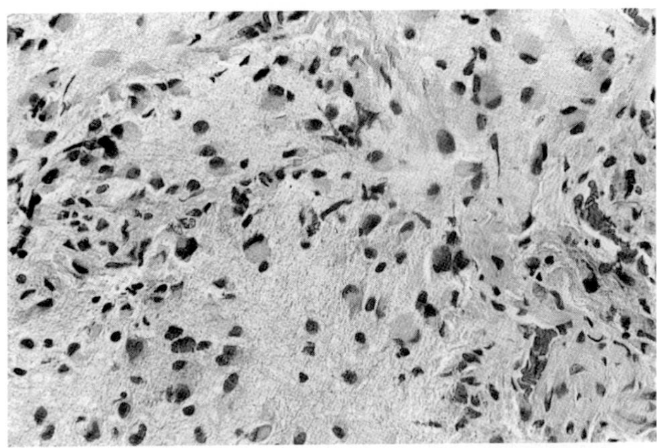

FIGURE 3. Nasal glioma showing both fibrillary and gemistocytic astrocytes, the latter with eccentric nuclei and abundant cytoplasm.

lands of neuroglial tissue are small and irregular rather then larger discrete nests, the predominantly fibrous mass may not be readily appreciated as a nasal glioma. Immunohistochemistry is a useful adjunct because the neuroglial islands are strongly positive for glial fibrillary acidic protein (57–59) (Fig. 4).

Because the nasal glioma is a maldevelopment, the rare "recurrence" is merely persistence of an incompletely excised lesion. Infectious complications may develop infrequently in those cases with an unappreciated tissue tract into the cranial cavity. Convincing examples of malignant degeneration have not been reported, but Chan and Lau reported an extraordinary case of a 34-year-old man who presented with nasal obstruction and had a mass that proved to be an astrocytoma of the frontal lobe with direct extension through the cribriform plate into the nasal cavity (60).

Extranasal Heterotopic Neuroglial Tissue

Elsewhere in the head and neck region, heterotopic neuroglia, exclusive of nasal gliomas, is rare as judged from our own experience and by examples in the literature. These lesions have been reported in the scalp, superficial and deep soft tissues of the face and neck, oral cavity (lip, tongue, soft palate), nasopharynx, and orbit (61–71). Multifocal heterotopias in the head and neck are rarer yet. Soft tissue gliomatosis or heterotopia is also known to occur in sites outside of the head and neck region (72). Most examples of neuroglial heterotopia in the head and neck present clinically in the first year of life, as early as the neonatal period, or as late as 10 years of age. A mass in the oral cavity or nasopharynx may result in feeding difficulties or respiratory distress in infants. Pasyk and associates have described a case of a disfiguring mass of heterotopic neuroglia in the upper lip of a neonate that was thought clinically to represent a hemangioma (61). Most extranasal neuroglial heterotopias do not have an anatomic connection to the brain or spinal cord, nor to an associated defect in the skull.

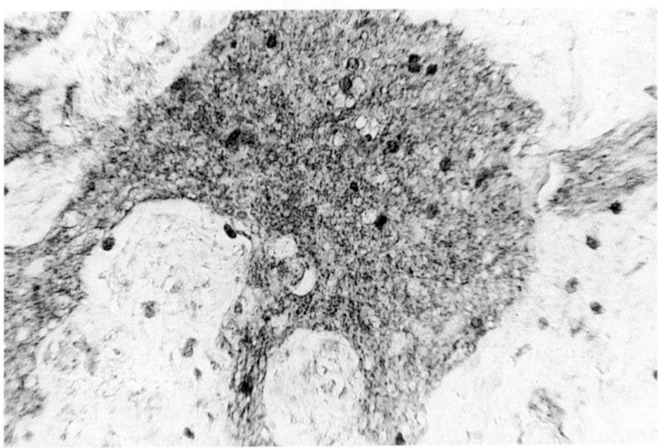

FIGURE 4. Nasal glioma demonstrating immunoreactivity for glial fibrillary acidic protein.

These tumefactions are seemingly well circumscribed on palpation, measure between 1 and 3 cm in greatest dimension, and have a firm consistency. The cut surface of the resected specimen has a white to grayish-tan appearance with indistinct borders from the surrounding tissues because the mass is often embedded in the soft tissues. Most tumors are solid, but on occasion may have intermingled cysts or a dominant cyst with or without identifiable papillary projections. The microscopic findings are virtually indistinguishable from those of the nasal glioma in that the neuroglia is differentiated or mature in most cases. In contrast, a teratoma of the head and neck in comparably aged infants is composed in part of immature cellular neuroepithelium with the formation of neural tubules. An intermixture of meningothelial elements is seen infrequently, and cysts if present are lined in part by choroid plexus. An intermixture of fat, smooth muscle, skeletal muscle, and fibrous tissue may raise the possibility of a teratoma, but the dominant neuroglial component favors the diagnosis of a heterotopia rather than a teratoma because these mesenchymal tissues are native to the location. Epithelial-lined cysts and tissues heterologous to the site are supportive of an interpretation of a mature teratoma. Like nasal gliomas, neuroglial heterotopias have a limited biologic potential, but there are isolated exceptions as in the case of an oligodendroglioma, which putatively arose in a heterotopia of the palate and nasopharynx in a 3-year-old girl (71).

Rudimentary Meningocele (Meningothelial Hamartoma)

The so-called rudimentary meningocele is an uncommon lesion that typically presents in the first year of life as a palpable pinkish nodule in the occipital scalp, although others sites of involvement in the head and neck and paraspinal regions are documented as well (73–81). Alopecia or tufted hairs in the overlying scalp have been reported in association with this lesion (82,83). A fibrous tract to the underlying central nervous system or a bony defect is identified in a minority of cases (84). Some researchers have proposed that the rudimentary meningocele is a variant of cutaneous meningioma (85–87). We have had the opportunity to study a case of an occipital mass in a 4-month-old boy with an encephalocele and an accompanying rudimentary meningocele (72).

A soft lobulated mass measuring 1 to 3.5 cm straddling the deep dermis and subcutis has a grayish-tan appearance. Focal

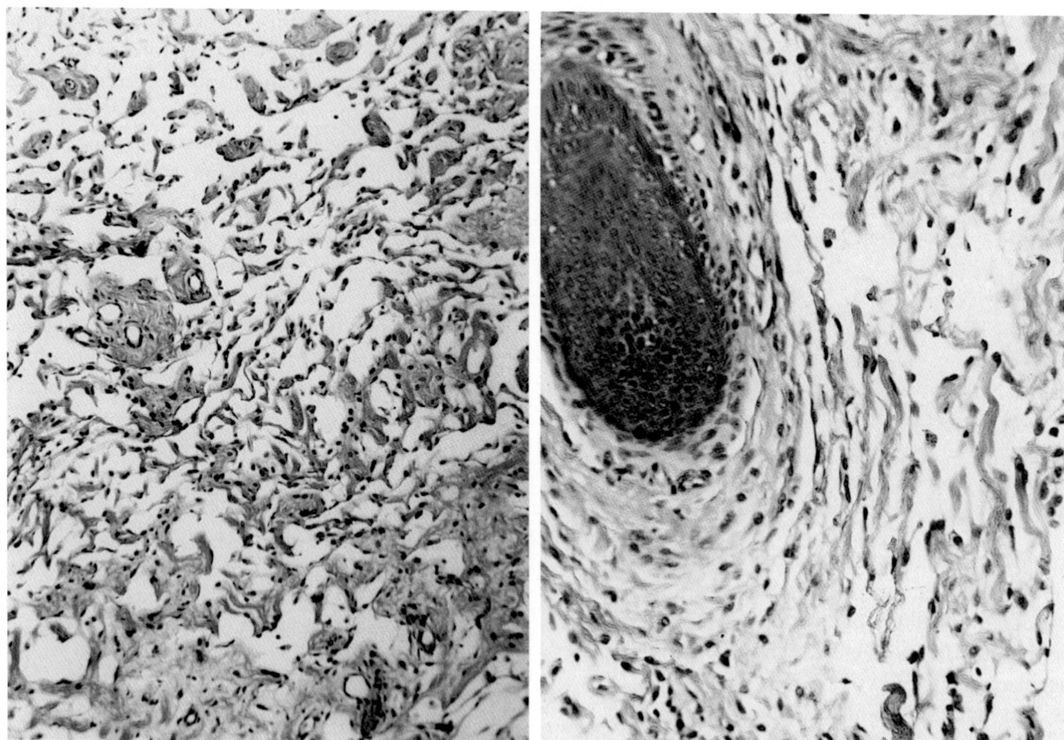

FIGURE 5. Rudimentary meningocele presenting in the occipital scalp of an infant and showing a sieve-like network of spaces in the subcutis (left) and spaces extending around a hair follicle (right).

hemorrhage may occur in these lesions. Microscopically, a sieve-like network of anastomosing spaces in a fibrotic stroma has a dissecting pattern of growth reminiscent of a vascular neoplasm (Fig. 5). The latter feature was emphasized in the report by Suster and Rosai (88). The channels or spaces are lined by flattened or plump cells and occasionally by multinucleated cells, which give this lesion some resemblance to giant cell fibroblastoma (Fig. 6). Although the major portion of growth is found in the subcutis, the reticulated channels may extend to the level of the superficial reticular dermis, and less often into the papillary dermis. The differentiation of a meningothelial from a vascular lesion is readily accomplished by immunohistochemistry, with the demonstrated coexpression of vimentin and epithelial membrane antigen in the rudimentary meningocele and one of the endothelial markers (Factor VIII–related antigen, *Ulex europaeus* lectin, CD31, or CD34) in the case of a vascular lesion (89) (Fig. 7). Because of the presence of giant cells in a rudimentary meningocele, a giant cell fibroblastoma can be effectively excluded by the absence of CD34 expression (90).

Dermoid Cyst and Dermoid

These cystic and solid maldevelopments originate from the surface ectoderm rather than from the neuroectoderm, although there are rare examples of combined lesions (91,92). The favored histogenesis of the dermoid cyst is invagination of surface ectoderm or displacement of embryonic skin, with the formation of an epidermal-lined cyst and accompanying hair follicles and supporting adnexa, in contrast to an epidermoid cyst without adnexal structures in the cyst wall (Fig. 8). Dermoids are not cystic structures but are solid masses, like the conjunctival dermoid or

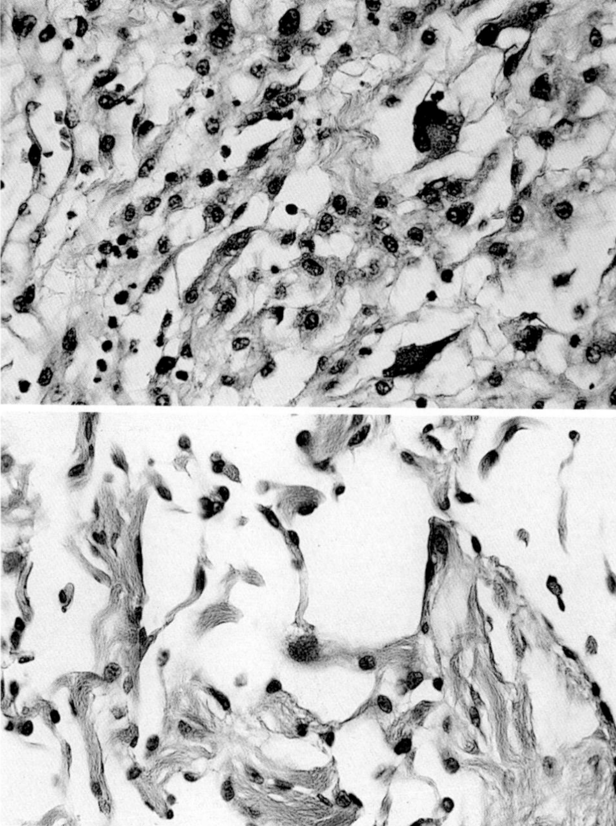

FIGURE 6. Rudimentary meningocele showing atypical multinucleated cells whose presence may suggest the diagnosis of a giant cell fibroblastoma (GCF) **(top)**. Dense bundles of collagen separate the angiectoid spaces in the GCF, but the stromal network of the rudimentary meningocele has a delicate, lacy appearance **(bottom)**.

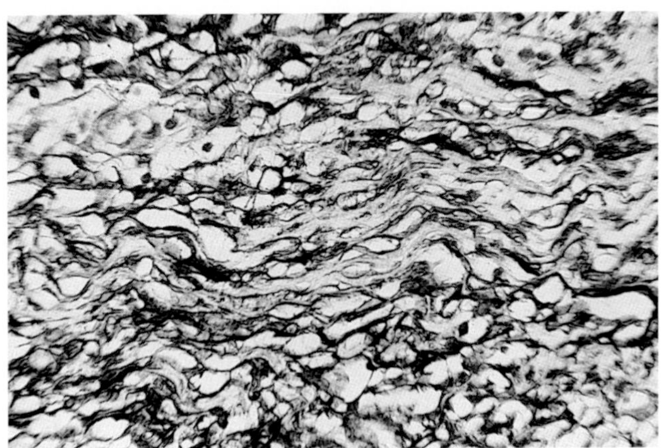

FIGURE 7. Rudimentary meningocele demonstrating immunoreactivity for epithelial membrane antigen and vimentin (not shown), which is characteristic of meningothelial tissue.

the pedunculated lesion of the nasopharynx and other sites in the upper aerodigestive tract known as a hairy or teratoid polyp (93–100). The dermoid cyst may or may not have a fistulous connection (dermoid sinus) into the central nervous system. Nasal dermoid cysts have contact with the dura in 5% to 35% of cases (101). Like other developmental anomalies of the head and neck, dermoid cysts tend to occur along the midline, but they may be found in the lateral neck, where distinguishing them from branchial cleft cysts can be problematic (102). Most dermoid cysts in the more superficial soft tissues are located along embryonic lines of fusion or fissures (103). One of the most common sites for the dermoid cyst is the lateral supraorbital ridge. Other sites include the anterior fontanelle, oral cavity (floor of mouth and tongue), nose, middle ear, orbit, and forehead (104–122). The dermoid cyst and sinus are the most common congenital lesions of the nose (Table 2). A nasal dermoid cyst has been reported in association with the Gorlin-Goltz or nevoid basal cell carcinoma syndrome (123). Dermoid and epidermoid cysts are also found in the cranial cavity (124–127). A common pathogenesis for the dermoid cyst and sinus and the encephalocele has been suggested when these lesions are found concurrently.

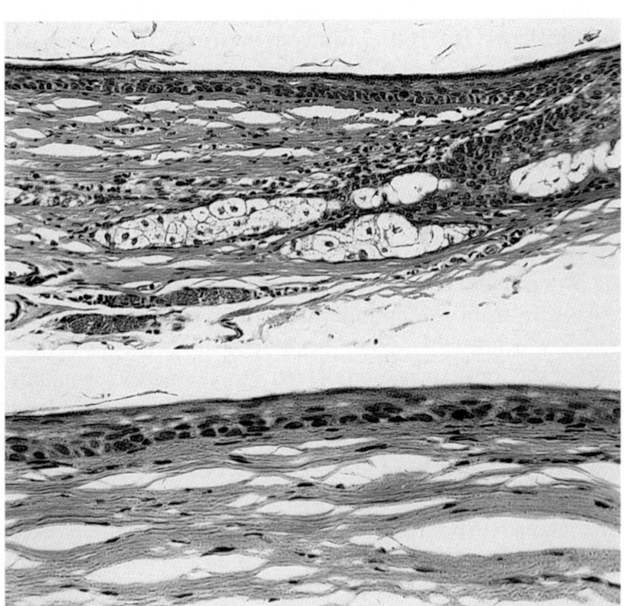

FIGURE 8. Dermoid cyst showing an attenuated keratinizing epidermis with sebaceous glands in the wall **(top)**. The distribution of adnexal structures in the cyst wall is somewhat haphazard, so an individual section may suggest the interpretation of an epidermal inclusion cyst **(bottom)**.

A *dermoid* arising on the conjunctiva or in the oro- or nasopharynx (hairy polyp) presents some unique clinical, pathologic, and therapeutic considerations. Epibulbar dermoids arise from the limbal or canthal portions of the conjunctiva, and most occur sporadically (128). However, they may be associated with a coloboma, epidermal nevus syndrome, or Goldenhar's syndrome (oculoauriculovertebral complex) in a minority of cases (129–132). A firm tan to white nodule measuring 0.3 to 1.5 cm extends to the superficial stroma. Microscopically, this lesion has an epithelial surface of keratinizing epidermis with hair follicles and sebaceous and sweat glands in a fibrous stroma resembling the dermis. Mature adipose tissue beneath the "dermis" in the "subcutis" is present in the conjunctival dermolipoma (133–135). Heterologous cartilage, bone, and neuroglia are present infrequently in these conjunctival lesions. When there are tissue types from the various embryonic germ layers, the question arises of differentiation between a teratoma and choristoma.

A *hairy (teratoid) polyp* or *dermoid* is a presumed developmental anomaly with the usual clinical presentation of a pedunculated mass in the oropharynx or nasopharynx of an infant (136–145). There is an unexplained female predilection of 6:1. Most children do not have other malformations, but there are individual reports of an associated cleft palate or multiple congenital anomalies, including the Dandy-Walker malformation in one neonate (146,147). In addition to the oropharynx and nasopharynx, the hairy polyp has been reported infrequently in the middle ear (148–151). The various theories of histogenesis have been discussed by Heffner and associates (152). The lateral wall of the nasopharynx, superior nasopharyngeal aspect of the soft palate, and tonsil are the sites of a broadly based or pedunculated polyp with a smooth, glistening mucosal surface. In common with dermoids elsewhere, the surface mucosa resembles epidermis with a delicate hyperkeratotic layer and pilosebaceous units in the "dermis" (Fig. 9). We had the opportunity to report the case of a neonate with hairy polyp with a rudimentary meningocele in the stroma (153) (Fig. 10). The hairy polyp is mainly differentiated from a teratoma by the limited variety of tissue types.

PERSISTENT EMBRYONIC REMNANTS

This pathogenetic category of developmental abnormalities accounts for the majority of neck masses in childhood, with the inclusion of the branchial cleft and thyroglossal duct cysts (6,7,12,18,154,155). However, the latter lesion is known to present in adults; as many as 30% to 35% of cases are diagnosed in patients over 20 years of age (19). Branchial cleft cysts more often than branchial cleft sinuses come to clinical attention after the age of 20 years. In children branchial cleft anomalies occur as often as thyroglossal duct cysts, but in adults the latter are twice to three times as common as branchial cleft cysts (6,7). A neck

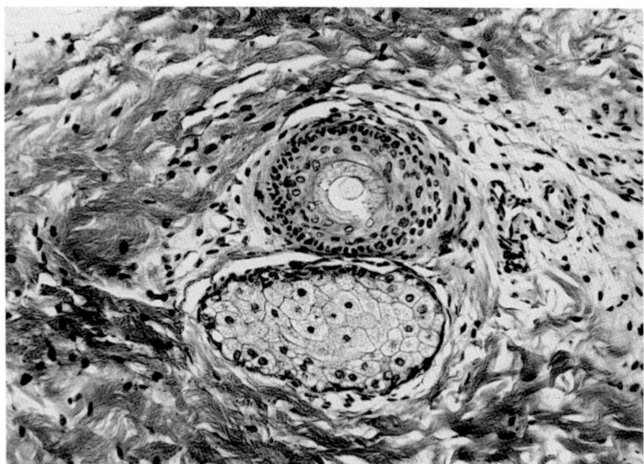

FIGURE 9. Hairy polyp of the oropharynx showing a hair follicle and sebaceous gland in the dense fibrous stroma.

mass in a child is considerably more likely to be a maldevelopment than a neoplasm, in contrast to adults (17).

Branchial Cleft Cysts and Sinuses

The branchial apparatus is a transient structure from which multiple anatomic structures or derivatives are formed after the 4th week of embryonic life (156–158). Six branchial arches of mesenchyme are formed from neural crest cells (neuroectoderm) and lateral mesoderm. Each of the branchial arches has a connecting vessel or aortic arch between the dorsal and ventral aorta. Between each branchial arch, there is an external groove or cleft of surface ectoderm and an internal pouch of endoderm. Thus, all three germ cell layers contribute to the formation of the branchial apparatus.

Most anomalies of the branchial apparatus of concern to the surgical pathologist present clinically as a cyst, fistula, or skin tag (12,13,154). Fistulas, sinuses, and skin tags present at a younger age than do the cysts (159). Branchial cleft cysts comprise approximately 75% to 80% of all branchial anomalies, and the fistulas and sinuses together account for 15% to 20% of all such malformations (160). Some series have reported that external fistulas, sinuses, and skin tags are more common than cysts (161–164).

The terms *branchial cleft cyst, sinus,* and *fistula* generally refer to anomalies of the second branchial cleft and pouch because these lesions account for the overwhelming majority of all such cases (155,158,160). Clinically a palpable mass or fistulous opening along the anterior border of the sternocleidomastoid muscle is the most common presentation. The cysts are usually positioned above the fistulas along the sternocleidomastoid muscle. The fistulous tract extends along the carotid sheath, where it exits in the region of the palatine tonsil (8). Embryologically, this tract is the remnant of the second branchial cleft or cervical sinus of His and the second branchial pouch, whose ultimate derivative is the palatine tonsil (156,158). Infrequently, branchial cleft cysts may present in the midline, just as a thyroglossal duct cyst may occur laterally, or as bilateral branchial cleft cysts (165). Fistulas tend to present in the first 2 years of life, whereas cysts

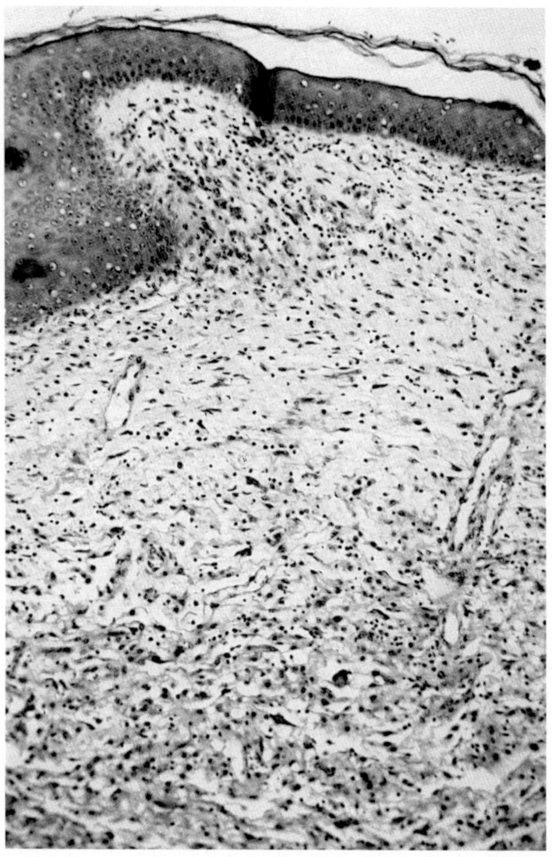

FIGURE 10. Hairy polyp of the oropharynx in an infant showing keratinizing squamous mucosa and a rudimentary meningocele in the stroma.

are diagnosed in later childhood and even into adulthood (160,163,164,166). Because of the opening to the skin, or oropharynx or nasopharynx, the cyst or fistulous tract may become infected (167,168). Most cysts present as a painless mass in the anterolateral cervical region, and although a fistula or sinus tract is not present in the majority of cases, a branchial cleft cyst may still become infected.

Most branchial cleft cysts of second branchial derivation are located near the bifurcation of the carotid artery (8,158). There is a preference for the left side. Despite the designation of these cysts as *branchial cleft cysts,* with the associated implication about the histogenesis, Regauer and associates have proposed that the cysts arise from the endodermally derived second branchial pouch, which would explain the presence of these cysts in the region of the tonsil or pharynx (169). An alternate explanation is that the cysts develop from cystic epithelial inclusions in lymph nodes. Golledge and Ellis have reviewed the various theories about the histogenesis of branchial cleft cysts (170).

The cysts measure from 1 to 10 cm in diameter (mean 4–5 cm). The external surface of the cyst has smooth contours, except when there is accompanying inflammation and fibrosis with mural thickening. Otherwise the cyst has a thin wall and mucoid or granular cheesy contents; the cysts may contain purulent material when infected. Two types of lining epithelium are found, and some cysts have both nonkeratinizing stratified squamous or a columnar ciliated respiratory-type epithelium (Fig. 11).

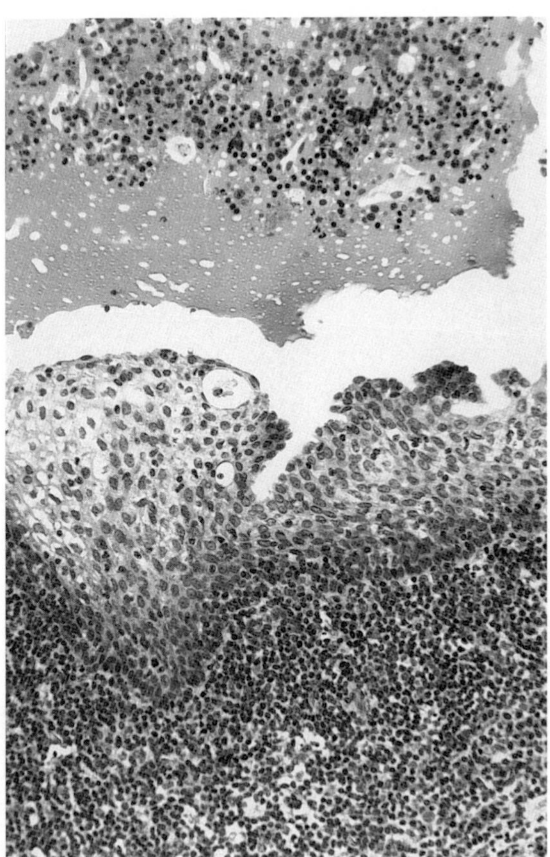

FIGURE 11. Branchial cleft cyst showing watery secretions with exfoliated cells in the lumen and a nonkeratinizing squamous mucosa and a dense lymphoid infiltrate in the wall.

Lymphoid aggregates with or without reactive germinal centers beneath the lining epithelium are found in a majority of cysts (75%–80% of cases) and typically are associated with a squamous epithelial-lined cyst (Fig. 12). It has been postulated by Regauer and associates that initially the cysts are lined by the endodermally derived pouch type or respiratory epithelium, which is replaced by squamous epithelium through an intermediate stage of pseudostratified transitional-type epithelium (169). This sequence, if correct, would explain those cysts with both types of epithelia. Acute and chronic inflammation, foreign body giant cell reaction, and fibrosis are the secondary microscopic findings in the wall of a cyst, fistula, or sinus with recent or past episodes of infection (Fig. 13). The epithelium may have reactive and atypical features in some cases to evoke momentary concern about the nature of the pathologic process (Fig. 14). A thymic cyst or cystic low-grade mucoepidermoid carcinoma with a prominent lymphoid reaction are considerations in the differential diagnosis of a branchial cleft cyst (Fig. 15).

Malignant transformation in a branchial cleft cyst or so-called branchiogenic carcinoma has received more than passing attention about its existence as an entity by proponents and opponents (171–176). It has been argued that most cases represent cystic metastatic squamous cell carcinoma in a cervical lymph node from an occult primary site in the head and neck, which coincides with our experience. Carroll and associates have reported a case of a putative branchiogenic carcinoma and have discussed the clinical and pathologic criteria for such a diagnosis (177). The differential diagnosis hinges on whether or not the lymphoid structure has the microanatomy of a lymph node. Discovery of a primary site in the head and neck region is not a requisite because it is widely recognized that small squamous carcinomas may escape detection despite thorough clinical and imaging studies. Thompson and Heffner reviewed 136 cases of cystic squamous cell carcinoma in the neck, and the most common primary sites were the lingual tonsil and the faucial tonsillar tissue in excess of 70% of cases (178).

The remaining anomalies of the branchial apparatus are those of first, third, and fourth branchial derivation. In aggregate, these anomalies account for 10% to 35% of all branchial-derived malformations because there is considerable variation in the proportion of branchial apparatus anomalies which are classified on the basis of their embryologic origin from the first through the fourth branchial clefts and pouches (158,160,164). In the series of Choi and Zalzal, 35% of branchial anomalies originated from the first, third, or fourth clefts or pouches, but 25% of cases were unclassifiable as to derivation (159). There were no examples of third and fourth branchial anomalies in the study of Agaton-Bonilla and Gay-Escoda (160), but rather, 25% and 75% of malformations originated from the first and second branchial clefts and pouches, respectively. On the other hand, Cunningham

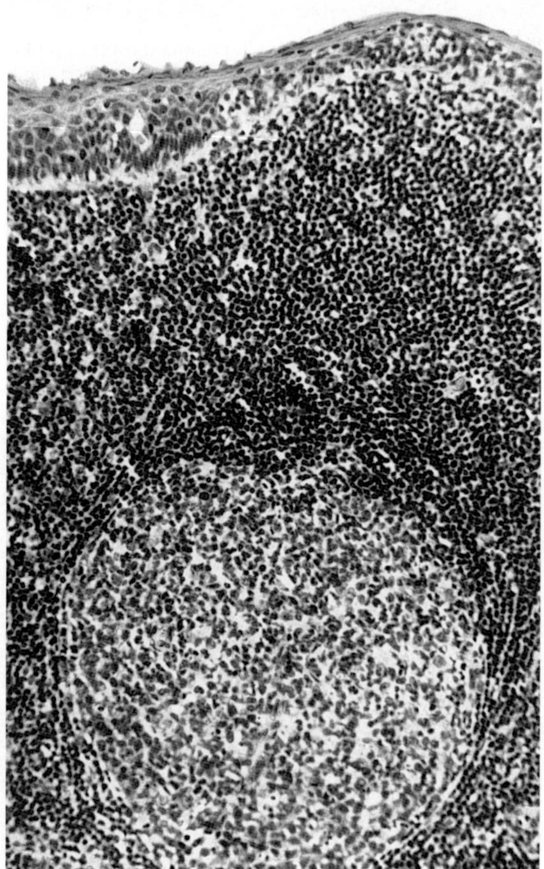

FIGURE 12. Branchial cleft cyst showing a focally attenuated squamous mucosa and a germinal center surrounded by small lymphocytes.

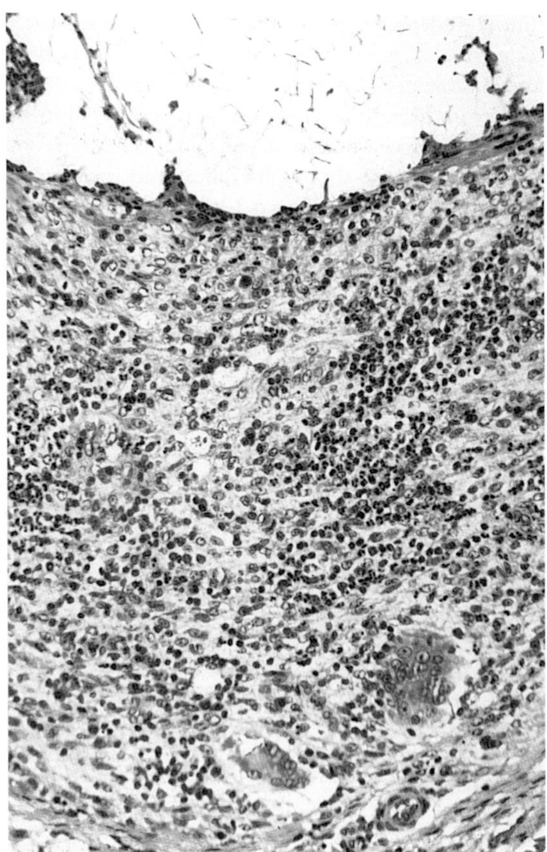

FIGURE 13. Branchial cleft cyst showing remnants of the epithelial lining and a mixed inflammatory infiltrate that has replaced the mantle of lymphocytes. Histiocytes, foreign-body giant cells, plasma cells, and some neutrophils near the surface are the features of an inflamed branchial cleft cyst.

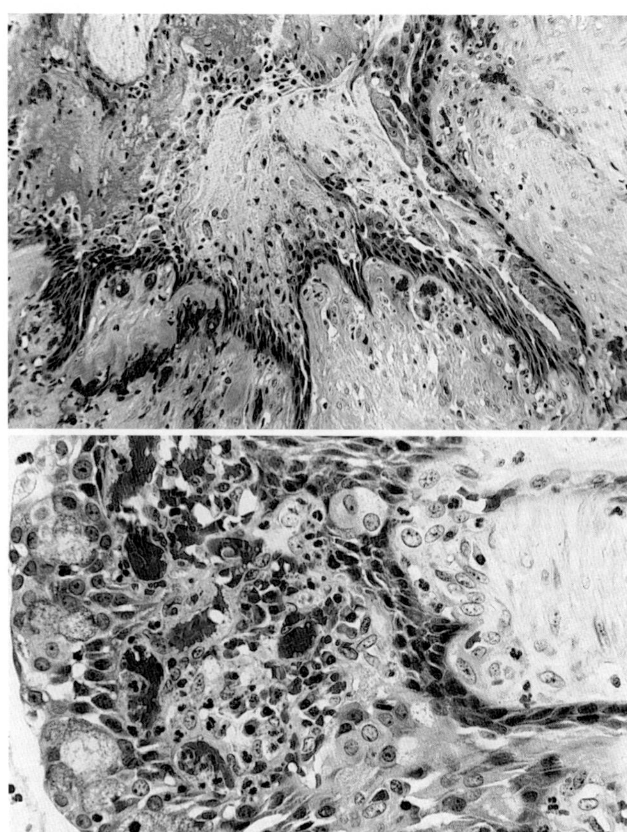

FIGURE 15. Low-grade mucoepidermoid carcinoma in a 13-year-old boy that presented as a cyst in the preauricular region thought to be a first branchial cleft cyst. A squamous-lined cyst (top) lacked an accompanying lymphoid infiltrate, and at higher magnification, mucinous cells were interspersed throughout the predominant squamous epithelium.

concluded that only 8% of branchial apparatus anomalies originated from the first cleft or pouch and the remaining cases all arose from the second cleft or pouch (179).

First branchial cleft cysts were more common than fistulas by a ratio of 3:1 in one study (160). The first branchial apparatus anomalies typically occur around the ear and parotid gland. The external auditory canal is the anatomic derivative of the first branchial cleft, and the eustachian tube, tympanic cavity, and mastoid air cells are the differentiated structures of the first branchial pouch (156,158). Often these anomalies present clinically as an infection (180–184). Triglia and associates have reviewed in detail the various types of first branchial cleft anomalies (185). Because of involvement of the parotid gland by a sinus or fistula, appropriate treatment may necessitate sacrificing the superficial lobe (184). A sinus or fistulous tract may parallel the external auditory canal and also may terminate at the chondroosseous junction of the external auditory canal (179). The histologic features of a first branchial cleft, sinus, or cyst may be obscured by the accompanying acute and chronic inflammation and fibrosis. When the cyst is intact, a keratinizing squamous epithelium or remnants of squamous epithelium are the microscopic findings. Cartilage and cutaneous adnexal structures are other microscopic findings (Fig. 16). Skin tags with or without cartilage around the ear are yet another morphologic manifestation of a first branchial anomaly (186). Similar appearing chondrocutaneous branchial remnants have been reported in the lateral neck, presumably as vestiges of the second branchial arch (187). Neither the fifth nor sixth branchial arches form clefts or pouches in humans (156).

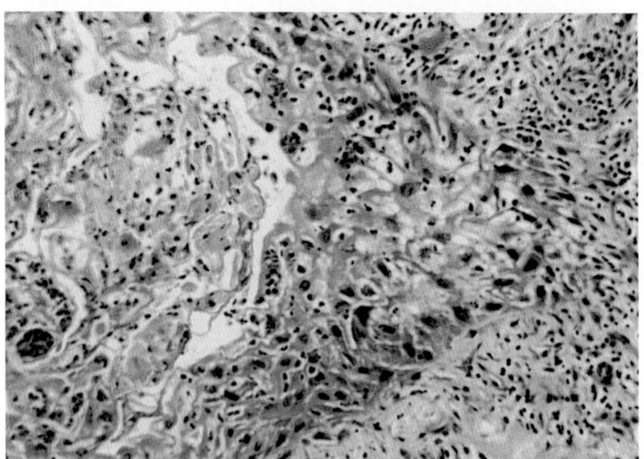

FIGURE 14. Branchial cleft cyst showing acute inflammation, keratotic debris, and atypical squamous epithelium with inflammatory and reactive features.

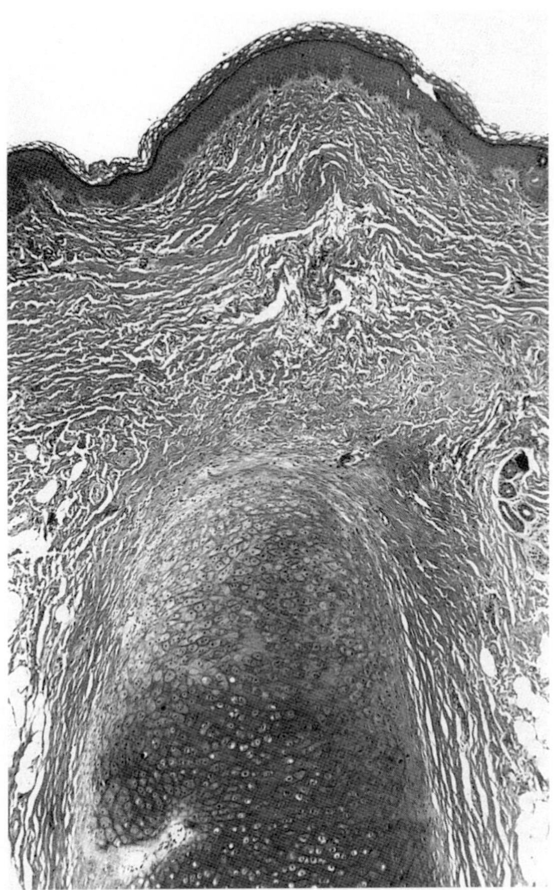

FIGURE 16. First branchial cleft remnant presenting as a preauricular skin tag showing a nodule of cartilage at the base of a pedunculated polyp with an accompanying sinus tract.

The *third* and *fourth branchial clefts* give rise to the cervical sinus of His (156). The third branchial pouch becomes the inferior parathyroid gland and thymus, and the fourth pouch is the progenitor of the superior parathyroid gland (158). Anomalies of the third and fourth branchial apparatus are rare and together account for less than 5% of all branchial cysts, sinuses, and fistulas (161,163,164). A fistula in the pyriform sinus is one of the more common manifestations of a third branchial anomaly (188,189). Recurrent infections of the left lower neck, including suppurative thyroiditis, and a fistulous tract into the pyriform sinus are the features of a fourth branchial cleft or pouch anomaly (190–195). Because of infection and the accompanying tissue reaction, it may be difficult to identify the cyst or sinus even after a thorough pathologic examination.

Branchial cleft cysts have been reported infrequently in the parotid, thyroid, parathyroid, floor of the mouth, tonsil, pharynx, and mediastinum (196–202). Many of these cysts have the microscopic features of lymphoepithelial cysts (Fig. 17). These cysts are regarded as developmental in origin, in contrast to the acquired lymphoepithelial cysts of the salivary glands in human immunodeficiency virus (HIV)-infected individuals (203–205).

Foregut duplication cysts (enteric or enterogenous cysts) are but one type of alimentary duplication that occur throughout the gastrointestinal tract (206). Duplications of the foregut include those lined by esophageal, gastric, and enteric mucosa or ciliated respiratory type epithelium (bronchogenic cyst). Both the tongue and sublingual region are sites for the rare duplication cysts of the oral cavity (207–212). Lipsett and associates have discussed the embryogenesis of lingual enteric duplication cysts (213). Similar appearing cysts have been described in the larynx (214,215). A distinction should be made from the equally rare mature cystic teratoma of the larynx.

Thyroglossal Duct Cyst and Ectopic Thyroid

Thyroglossal duct cyst (TDC) is typically a midline anomaly representing the cystic remnant(s) of the thyroid diverticulum, which originates from the floor or ventral aspect of the pharynx or tuberculum impar at the level of the second branchial arch (8,156,216). Among mass lesions of the neck in children, TDCs accounted for 16% of all cases and were slightly less common than branchial cleft cysts in one large series (18). Spinelli and associates reviewed their experience with neck masses in children and noted that 26 (17%) of 154 cases were TDCs, and branchial cleft cysts were less common (10 cases) (14). The thyroid gland is an endodermal derivative composed of two small lateral anlagen and the more substantial median anlage from the foramen cecum at the base of the tongue. Through elongated cephalad embryonic growth rather than active descent, the orthotopic pre-

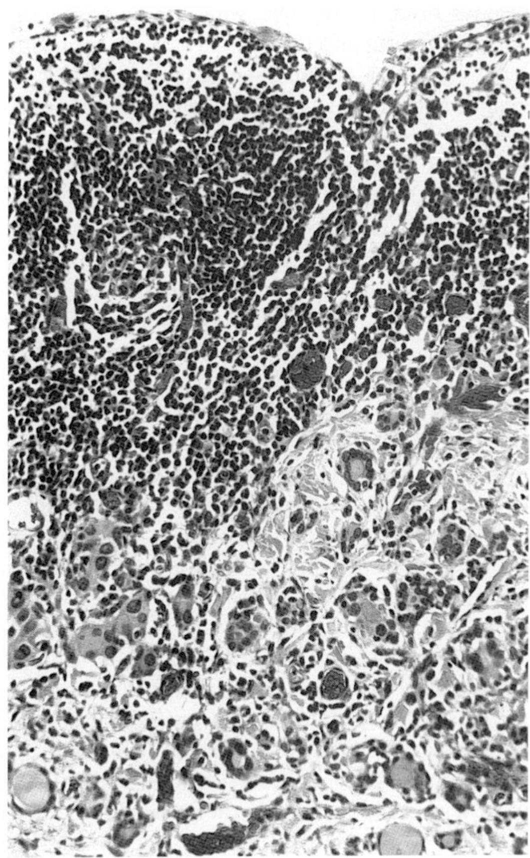

FIGURE 17. Branchial cleft or lymphoepithelial cyst of the thyroid showing an attenuated epithelial lining and a dense lymphoid infiltrate with scattered thyroid follicles.

tracheal location of the thyroid is caudal to the foramen cecum (156,217). The embryologic thyroglossal duct undergoes involution; however, remnants along its course are the source of the TDC. Because the duct passes anterior to the hyoid bone, the bone or a portion of it must be excised to avoid a recurrence or, more accurately, to avoid leaving behind a potential focus for another TDC (216,218–220). The cystic remnant is only rarely found within the bone itself (221). Gross visualization of the tract along its course in the anterior neck is usually not possible. Rarely, a sinus tract is found between the TDC and the pharynx.

A mobile midline mass in the anterior neck overlying the hyoid bone is the usual clinical presentation, and less frequently the cyst is present at the base of the tongue, floor of mouth, laterally in the neck, or within the thyroid itself (222). A cyst may become infected like the branchial cleft cyst. In the pediatric age group, most cysts are diagnosed in the first decade of life, and usually before 5 years of age (216,223). When all age groups are considered, approximately 20% to 50% of TDCs are seen in individuals over 20 years of age, and as many as 5% to 10% of cases are encountered in patients 60 years or older (224,225). North and associates reported the case of a 78-year-old man with an intrathyroidal TDC (226). Males and females are equally affected. Most TDCs occur sporadically, but there are familial examples with an apparent autosomal mode of inheritance and a female predilection (227). Surgical resection is the standard treatment, with excision of the mid-portion of the hyoid bone (Sistrunk procedure) and the foramen cecum to reduce the recurrence rate, which ranges from 4% to 30%, with a mean of 5% to 7.5% (228,229). Previously infected cysts recur more frequently than uninfected cysts. One cautionary note is the rare TDC and its coexistent ectopic thyroid as the only functioning thyroid tissue in the patient (230).

The TDC is infrequently a continuous structure in the soft tissues of the mid-anterior neck. A dominant cyst or cysts in the supra-, pre- or infrahyoid soft tissues may be accompanied by smaller and often imperceptible microcysts, because the thyroglossal duct is an arborizing structure near its origin from the foramen cecum (231,232). Most grossly visible cysts are located somewhat inferior to the hyoid bone. The cyst(s) range in size from 0.5 to 4 cm in diameter, and usually contain mucoid material if the cyst(s) is not infected, in which case mucopurulent material or pus is the nature of the cystic contents. Rarely, it is possible to identify reddish-tan tissue with a glistening surface in the soft tissues to indicate the presence of ectopic thyroid. Dense fibrosis in the surrounding soft tissues may imply past episodes of infection. One or more cystic spaces may be evident microscopically, although a solitary cyst is identified in the gross examination. The lining epithelium varies from one case to another, or within the same surgical specimen. A columnar to stratified cuboidal epithelium with cilia is the most common type of epithelial lining, found in 50% to 60% of cases (Fig. 18). In this respect, a TDC resembles the bronchogenic cyst, but without a muscularis, submucosal glands, and cartilage, although we have seen infrequently the presence of ectopic cartilage in TDCs. Tovi and associates have reported cartilage in a TDC from a child (233). Nonkeratinizing squamous epithelium is the second most frequent type of lining epithelium, found in 20% to 25% of cases. Other types of epithelia are also found

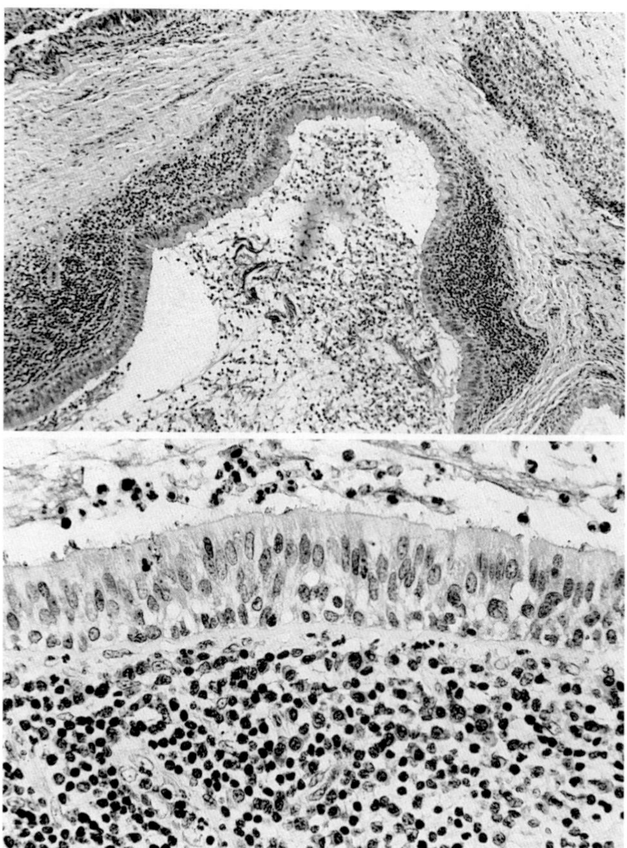

FIGURE 18. Thyroglossal duct cyst showing a cyst filled with cellular debris and an accompanying lymphoid infiltrate beneath the epithelial lining **(top)**. Portions of smaller cysts are seen at the periphery. A stratified ciliated columnar epithelium is seen at higher magnification **(bottom)**. Abundant neutrophils are indicative of an infected cyst.

(Fig. 19). It is not uncommon for the cysts to lack an intact epithelium (218). Those cysts with accompanying inflammation and fibrosis in the surrounding soft tissues often have a squamous epithelial lining, implying that this epithelial type may be metaplastic in nature. The lumina of the cysts may appear empty or contain a pale basophilic granular material. Histiocytes, cholesterol granulomas, and collections of neutrophils are the cystic contents in some cases (234) (Fig. 20). Lymphoid nodules in the wall of the cysts are found in 15% to 20% of cases, in contrast to their presence in 75% to 80% of all branchial cleft cysts (224). A TDC with a squamous epithelial lining and lymphoid nodules may be difficult to differentiate from a branchial cleft cyst. Immunoperoxidase staining for thyroglobulin may be helpful on occasion. Ectopic thyroid tissue is identified as collections of thyroid follicles in the soft tissues adjacent to the cyst in 3% to 20% of TDCs (Fig. 21), although these figures are related to some extent to the scrupulousness of tissue sampling and the extent of reactive and inflammatory changes in the surrounding soft tissues.

Hurthle cell adenomas and papillary carcinoma of the thyroid have been reported in less than 1% of TDCs (235–238). Yoo and associates found 115 cases of papillary carcinoma arising in TDCs in the literature, and most (96%) were reported in adults

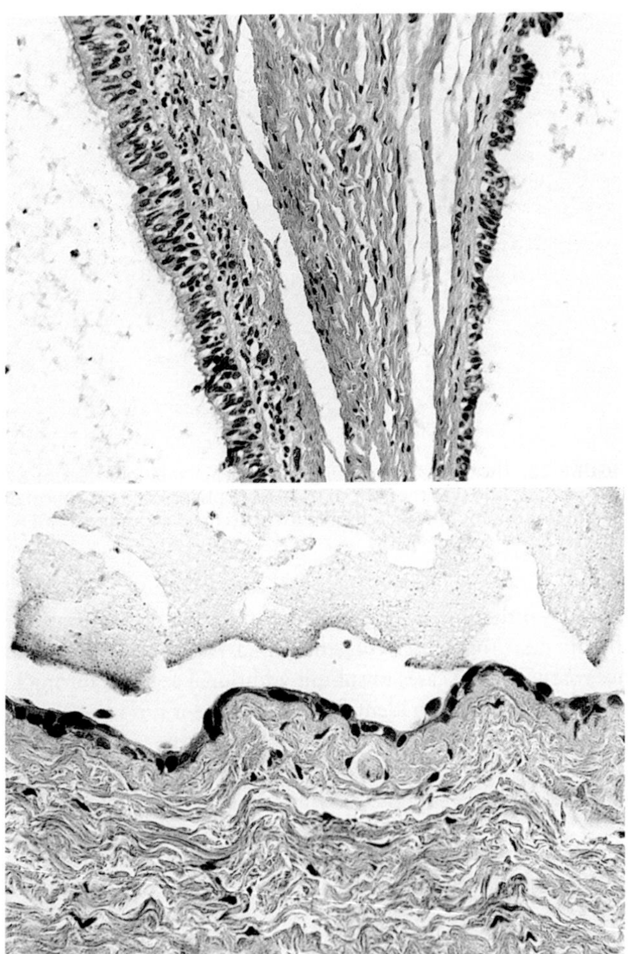

FIGURE 19. Thyroglossal duct cyst showing adjacent cysts, one lined by ciliated columnar epithelium **(top)** and the other by a cuboidal and flattened epithelium **(bottom)**.

(239). A few cases of papillary carcinoma in TDCs have been described in children (238,239). These tumors are typically intracystic papillary carcinomas. The thyroid gland itself is free of neoplastic involvement in most cases, although we have seen multifocal papillary carcinomas in the gland as well as in TDCs.

Some cysts may be difficult to classify because of an apparent discrepancy between the anatomic site of presentation and histologic features, indeterminate microscopic findings, loss of an intact epithelial lining, or a mixed histologic appearance, as in the case of a cyst that was reported by Tyson and Groff (240). The latter cyst presented in the lateral neck of a child and had mixed bronchogenic, branchial cleft, and thyroglossal duct features. When a final determination about the type of cyst is not possible, we have chosen to diagnose it as a "congenital or developmental cyst, indeterminate type."

Ectopic thyroid is defined by the gross or microscopic presence of thyroid tissue outside of the thyroid gland, most commonly from the base of the tongue (lingual thyroid) with or without cystic features to the mid-lower neck superior to the orthotopic thyroid (241–248). Thyroid tissue also has been reported in the heart, mediastinum, and several intraabdominal sites unrelated to the presence of a mature teratoma of the ovary. Batsakis and

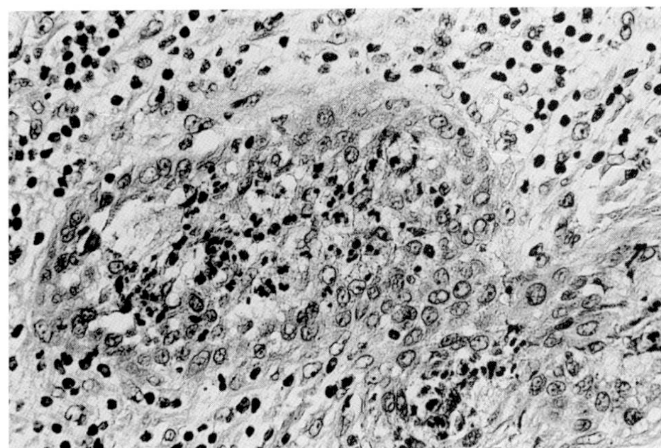

FIGURE 20. Thyroglossal duct cyst showing intense inflammatory reaction with near total obliteration of the epithelium and lumen by neutrophils. It may be difficult to identify the nature of the cyst in the presence of a dense inflammatory reaction.

associates noted a clinical prevalence of lingual thyroids of 1 in 10,000 individuals, but an autopsy prevalence of 1 in 10 (217). The ectopia may be complete or total, or, more commonly, associated with an orthotopic thyroid. Hypothyroidism is frequently found in patients with lingual thyroids (248). The follicles of ectopic thyroid tissue are often uniformly small, and the

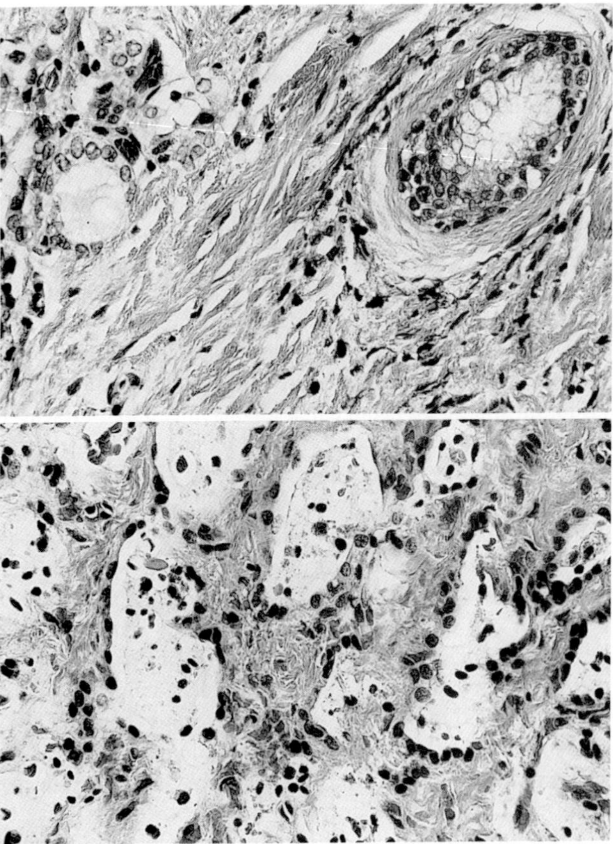

FIGURE 21. Thyroglossal duct cyst showing an isolated thyroid follicle adjacent to a small duct lined in part by mucinous epithelium **(top)**. Degenerative changes in the epithelium are common in thyroglossal cysts, which are seen in a focus of ectopic thyroid follicles.

microfollicles may contain minimal colloid. Skeletal muscle of the tongue may be interspersed among the follicles. We have seen at least one case of an alveolar soft part sarcoma in the base of the tongue of an infant that was initially thought to be lingual thyroid.

Lateral aberrant thyroid as a subset of ectopic thyroid is another of those issues in surgical pathology with its proponents and opponents in terms of its developmental or neoplastic pathogenesis (249–251). A distinction is made between the lateral aberrant thyroid and the sequestered adenomatous nodule and the hyperplastic follicles of Graves' disease. If the aberrant thyroid follicles are present in the sinuses of a cervical lymph node, carcinoma of the thyroid, particularly papillary carcinoma, is the pathologic diagnosis. An isolated nodule of non-neoplastic thyroid follicles in the anterolateral neck is likely a sequestered nodule from multinodular adenomatous hyperplasia.

Thymic cysts and *thymopharyngeal duct cysts* are generally considered maldevelopments of the thymus that present clinically as a mass in the lower anterolateral neck of a child from the neonatal period through adolescence. The mediastinum, rather than the cervical region, is the more common site for a thymic cyst in an adult.

Embryologically, the thymus develops as paired structures from the third branchial pouch at the 6th week (156). The endodermal primordium of the thymus has a ductal or luminal connection to the pouch that is known as the thymopharyngeal duct. Ventromedial and caudal growth of the respective thymic anlage eventuates in the separation of the thymus from the pharynx. The fragmented remnants of the solid thymopharyngeal duct are thought to be the progenitors of accessory parathyroid and thymic tissue in the neck (252). The inferior parathyroid glands also originate from the third pouch, and their descent with the thymus explains their localization relative to the superior parathyroids, which arise from the fourth branchial pouch. By the end of the 8th week, the lower poles of the thymic anlage approach each other, but do not fuse, at the level of the aortic arch (156). There is regression of the cephalad thymus, but remnants may persist in the neck as another source of ectopic thymic tissue.

Cervical thymic cyst is uncommon, with approximately 100 cases in children reported through 1995 (253). One thymic cyst was found among 244 congenital lesions in children presenting as a neck mass (18). Males are affected more commonly than females. There is a preference for the left side of the neck. Approximately 50% of thymic cysts initially present in the neck with or without a mediastinal component (254–262). A persistent thymopharyngeal duct is postulated as the anlage for the thymic cyst and thymopharyngeal duct cyst. A fibrous tract to the thymic cyst in approximately 50% of cases is thought to be the remnant of the thymopharyngeal duct. The cysts measure up to 10 to 15 cm in diameter and are uniloculated more often than multiloculated, but opinions vary on this point (Fig. 22). Clear watery fluid to a brownish gelatinous coagulum is the appearance of the cystic contents. If the uniloculated cyst represents the persistent thymopharyngeal duct, the multiloculated cyst may reflect the alternative theory of pathogenesis, which is cystic degeneration of the thymus. Microscopically, the lining epithelium has diverse epithelial cell types, as in branchial cleft and thyroglossal duct cysts (Fig. 23). Within the fibrous septa, islands of thymic epithelium with Hassall corpuscles differentiate the thymic cyst from other congenital pharyngeal cysts. It may be necessary in some cases to submit additional sections for microscopic examination to identify thymic tissue if it is not found after the initial histologic examination. Other aspects of the thymic cyst are the presence of secondary degenerative and inflammatory changes and cysts without an epithelial lining.

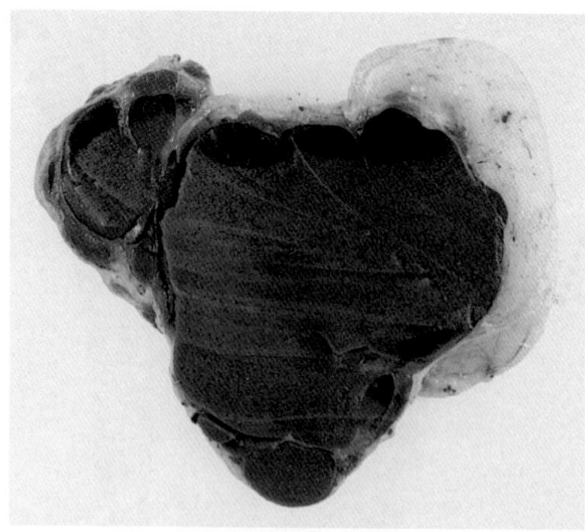

FIGURE 22. Thymic cyst presenting as a mass in the right neck of a 4-year-old boy who was thought to have a lymphangioma on clinical examination. This multiloculated circumscribed mass measured 4 × 4 × 3 cm.

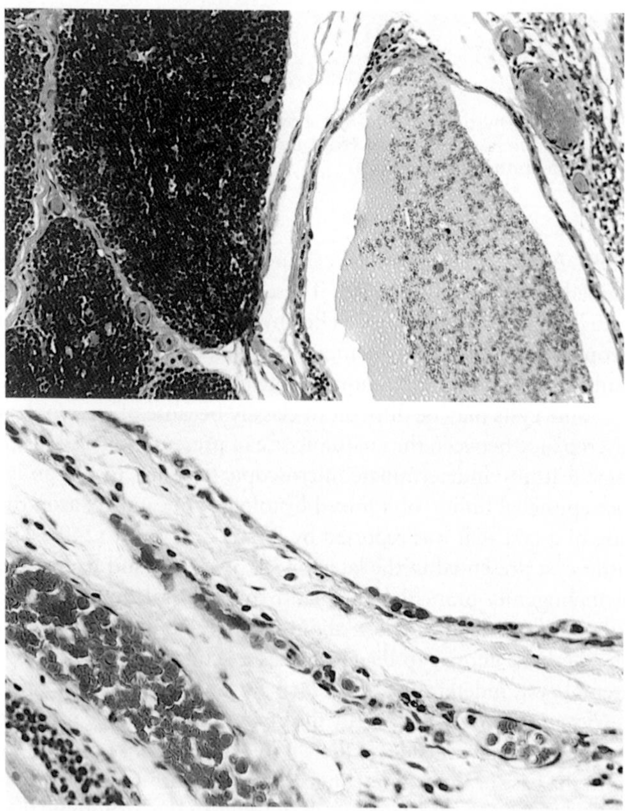

FIGURE 23. Thymic cyst as illustrated in Fig. 22 showing lobular thymic tissue adjacent to one of several cysts **(top)** that were lined by a flattened epithelium **(bottom)** and a compressed cord of thymic epithelium in the stroma.

Multiloculated thymic cysts have been reported in children with acquired immunodeficiency syndrome as presumably acquired lesions (263,264). The differential diagnosis includes the other congenital cysts of the neck, as well as the rare cystic presentation of Hodgkin's disease, thymoma, and germinoma. However, the latter three neoplasms are more likely to present in the anterior mediastinum.

The *persistent thymopharyngeal duct cyst* is a variant of the cervical thymic cyst, but is distinguished anatomically by the presence of a patent communication with the pharynx (265). Unlike the noncommunicating thymic cyst, the thymopharyngeal duct cyst, like the branchial cleft cyst, may present with clinical signs of an infection. Zarbo and associates reported just such a case in a 4-year-old boy whose cyst was accompanied by an undescended thymus–parathyroid complex of the third branchial pouch (266). These cysts are generally larger than the more common cervical thymic cysts because they occupy the embryologic route of descent of the thymus. The thymopharyngeal duct cyst is a single duct or cyst associated with inflammation and fibrosis, and fewer, if any, remnants of the thymus as compared with the cervical thymic cyst.

Ectopic thymus is a frequent incidental histologic finding in the examination of tissues from the neck (267). Small islands of thymic epithelium with thymocytes may be seen at the periphery of the thyroid or within the fatty soft tissues.

Parathyroids as noted earlier are embryologically derived from the third and fourth branchial pouches. The overwhelming majority (90%) of individuals have four parathyroids. The remainder have fewer than four or additional (supernumerary) parathyroids (156). It is estimated that 5% of individuals have supernumerary glands. Microscopic foci of parathyroid may be found as small islands of chief cells in the soft tissues of the neck or more commonly within the thymus (Fig. 24). These small islands of *heterotopic parathyroid* have been referred to as parathyromatosis (268).

Cysts of the parathyroid, like thymic cysts, have several morphologic features, including a persistent hollow tract with the third or fourth branchial pouch (269,270). It is estimated that 5% or less of neck cysts are parathyroid in origin. Few parathyroid cysts have been reported in childhood, implying that most are acquired, including the cystic parathyroid adenoma. True branchial cysts have been described in the parathyroid gland (159).

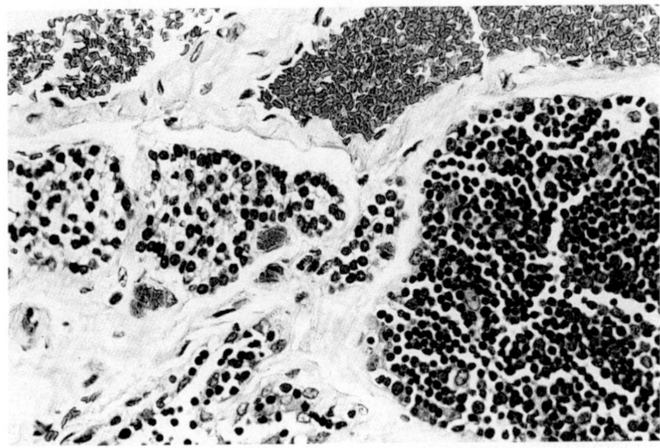

FIGURE 24. Ectopic parathyroid and thymus as an incidental microscopic finding in the soft tissues of the neck. These two tissues are derivatives of the third branchial pouch.

HETEROTOPIAS

The head and neck region may be the most common anatomic site for heterotopias of one type or another as judged from our own experience. Several examples of heterotopias have been discussed in preceding sections that mainly included examples of neural heterotopias. It is our impression that the various types of neural heterotopias are encountered with some frequency in a surgical pathology practice with a substantial proportion of pediatric cases. The non-neural heterotopias are the focus of discussion in this section.

Salivary Gland Heterotopias

Other than the infrequent heterotopias of salivary gland tissue in a variety of sites in the head and neck, there are few anomalies of the salivary glands, although individual cases of hamartomas, choristomas, vascular malformations, and cystic hygromas occur in the salivary gland.

Heterotopias of salivary gland tissue are probably more common than is generally documented when one considers the ubiquitous distribution of these tissues throughout the upper aerodigestive tract (271). Most salivary gland heterotopias that come to clinical attention are those that present as a mass in the neck with or without a draining sinus tract, oral cavity, middle ear, and mandible (272–286). Hiatt and Sauk have reviewed the development of the salivary glands as a localized surface epithelial proliferation of ectodermal (parotid gland) or endodermal (submandibular and sublingual gland) origin (287). Because the salivary glands do not migrate during development as do the parathyroid glands or thymus, it is suspected that most heterotopias of salivary glands arise *de novo* from the endoderm of the pharynx. As some support for this hypothesis, there are the rare examples of reported heterotopic salivary gland tissue in association with branchial cleft fistula (288,289). Salivary gland neoplasms have been reported in sites of heterotopic salivary glands (290–294). The recognition of a salivary gland as a heterotopia is based on the anatomic location of the tissue, and microscopically by the association and relationship to surrounding tissues. For instance, a salivary gland surrounded by skeletal muscle or in (extraparotid) lymph node is heterotopic.

Phakomatous Choristoma

This lesion presents as an enlarging mass on the medial aspect of the lower eyelid in an infant in the first few weeks or months of life (295–298). One case has been reported in the orbit of a 3-month-old infant (299). Zimmerman proposed that this lesion represented a "tumor of lenticular anlage" when he described it in 1971 (300). Because these lesions have a prominent fibrous stroma, they are firm on palpation and have a uniform grayish-white fibrous appearance on cross-section. Virtually all tumors

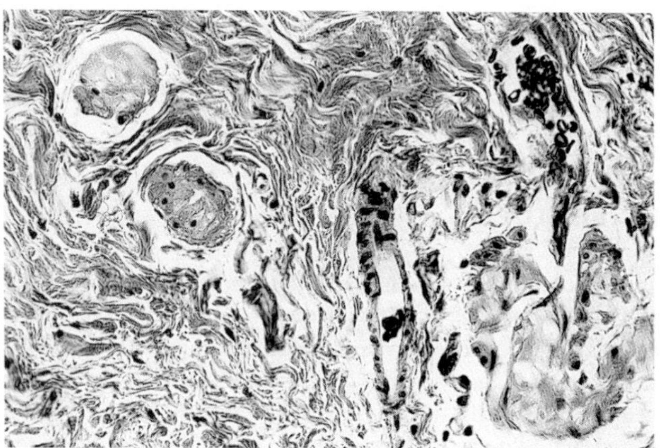

FIGURE 25. Phakomatous choristoma presenting as a small firm nodule inferior to the lower eyelid in a 1-year-old boy. Scattered nests of polygonal cells with abundant eosinophilic cytoplasm are present in dense fibrous stroma.

have measured less than 2 cm in diameter. Microscopically, the pale-staining epithelial component is arranged in nests, lobules, sheets, and tubules (Fig. 25). The individual cells have polygonal features with abundant, uniform, eosinophilic cytoplasm. Some nests are composed in part of degenerating cells, amorphous eosinophilic material, and dystrophic calcifications. Psammoma bodies are found in the stroma on occasion (301). The epithelial profiles may be difficult to distinguish from the surrounding fibrous stroma because of the eosinophilic quality of both components, but outlines of the nests are accentuated in a periodic acid-Schiff (PAS) stain with a delicate PAS-positive limiting membrane. Ultrastructural studies have supported the lenticular origin of the epithelial cells, and immunohistochemistry has demonstrated vimentin, S-100 protein, and neuron-specific enolase expression by these cells (295,302–304). Cytokeratin immunoreactivity is disputed, but the cells contain the lens-specific protein α-crystallin (303). Displacement of progenitor cells into the tarsal plate of the lower eyelid is the proposed histogenesis for these lesions. Excision is the treatment of choice, and recurrences are unknown.

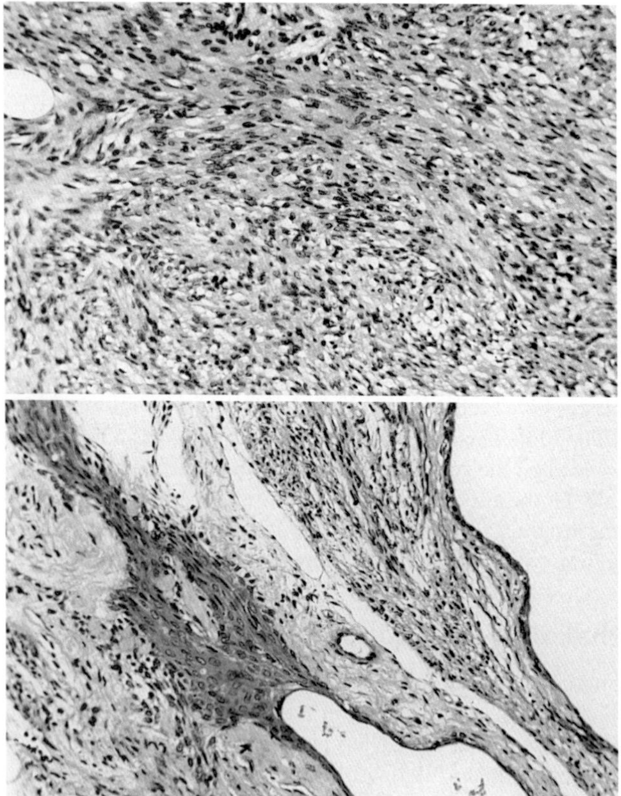

FIGURE 26. Ectopic hamartomatous thymoma presenting as a firm, painless mass near the sternal notch of a 30-year-old man. Fascicles of bland-appearing spindle cells **(top)** are accompanied by cysts and nests of epithelium, some with squamous features **(bottom)**.

Ectopic Hamartomatous Thymoma

This combined spindle cell and epithelial tumor presents as a soft tissue mass in the lower neck somewhat lateral to the sternal notch in the supraclavicular region. Virtually all cases to date

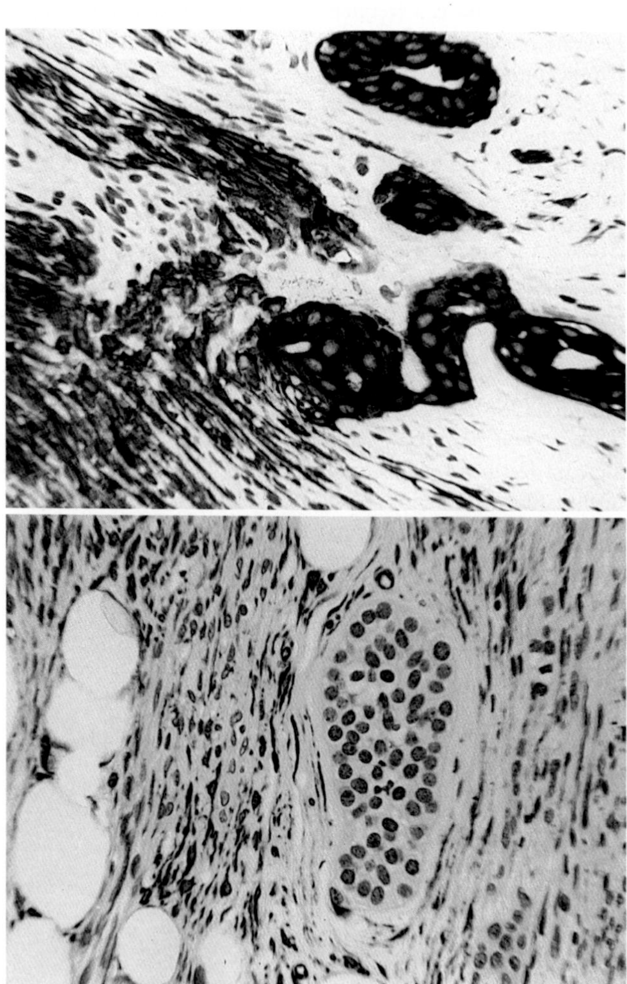

FIGURE 27. Ectopic hamartomatous thymoma demonstrating immunoreactivity for cytokeratin in the epithelial profiles and spindle cells **(top)** and for vimentin in the entrapped fat and stromal cells **(bottom)**. Note that the epithelial nest **(bottom)** is nonreactive for vimentin.

have presented in adults, and there is a male predilection (305–308). A circumscribed, nonencapsulated, firm mass measures 1 to 2.5 cm in diameter. Fascicles of bland-appearing spindle cells are accompanied by small epithelial islands and cysts among the spindle cells or toward the periphery (Fig. 26). The epithelial islands may have the lobulated contours of thymic epithelium, and a lymphocytic infiltrate is variable. Adipose tissue may be entrapped within the lesion, and myoid cells have been identified in a few cases (309,310). Michal and associates have reported several other unusual microscopic features (311). Ultrastructurally and immunohistochemically, the constituent cells have epithelial features and phenotype (Fig. 27). The differential diagnosis of this biphasic lesion includes synovial sarcoma, ectopic salivary gland tumor with a myoepithelial component, ectopic thymoma, teratoma, and a sweat gland neoplasm. The thyroid is the presenting site for a similar-appearing tumor, the spindle epithelial tumor with a thymus-like element (312–316) (see Chapter 9). Chan and Rosai have discussed the histogenesis of these various spindle cell tumors of the neck as possible derivatives of the third branchial pouch (317). On the other hand, Michal and associates noted salivary gland differentiation in the ectopic hamartomatous thymoma (311). The treatment of this tumor is excision, and recurrences are unusual. One caveat is the report of a case with putative carcinomatous transformation (318).

TISSUE OVERGROWTH WITH OR WITHOUT ORGANIZATION

The lesions in this heterogeneous group, like many of the other entities under discussion in this chapter, present as masses in most cases, but unlike the earlier lesions, there is uncertainty in some instances whether these tumors are the consequence of disordered development or a neoplastic process. It is clear that the teratoma and sialoblastoma are neoplasms, but the nosology of two other recently described entities, the salivary gland anlage tumor and the nasal chondromesenchymal hamartoma, is not entirely settled. The neurofibroma is a neoplasm whose diffuse and plexiform variants are manifestations of autosomal dominant neurofibromatosis. Fibrous dysplasia and giant cell granuloma are tumor-like lesions of the mandible and maxilla, which may have systemic or familial connotations in selected cases. Torsiglieri and associates included the hemangioma and lymphangioma or cystic hygroma as "congenital lesions" in their review of neck masses in children, yet the developmental versus neoplastic pathogenesis of these two common vascular lesions of childhood has not been resolved to everyone's satisfaction (18).

Teratomas

The head and neck region is an uncommon but well-documented site for germ cell neoplasms, with mature and immature teratomatous elements of ectodermal, endodermal, and mesodermal derivation, and rarely with the malignant patterns of endodermal sinus tumor and embryonal carcinoma (319,320). These tumors present in various locations in the head and neck and are diagnosed typically in children usually before the age of 5 years (319–323). Approximately 5% to 8% of all germ cell neoplasms in the pediatric age group occur in the head and neck region in the following sites: orbit, oronasopharynx, thyroid–anterior neck, mastoid–middle ear, and brain (324–332). These tumors are often quite large, disfiguring, and life threatening in neonates or young infants with airway obstruction, especially in the case of the pharyngeal (epignathus) and cervicothyroidal teratomas (333–335). Another manifestation of their size is the intracranial teratoma in the neonate with extensive basicranial and pharyngeal involvement (333,336–340). Most therapeutic options with an acceptable clinical outcome are precluded in these infants with heroic exceptions. The large intracranial teratomas are typically tumors of infancy, with the predominant histologic features of an immature teratoma that also characterize most extracranial head and neck teratomas in children of comparable age (339,341,342). Malignant germ cell neoplasms of the head and neck exclusive of central nervous system are rare in general (319,320,343–345).

Cervicothyroidal teratomas are the most common of the extracranial head and neck germ cell neoplasms in children (319–321,323). Byard and associates reported their experience with congenital teratomas of the head and neck: 14 of 18 tumors were in the neck and four in the nasopharynx (346). A smaller series by Carr and co-workers of nine cases revealed that five presented in the neck (325). These tumors have been detected prenatally by ultrasonographic examination (100,335,347). Overall, the teratoma is an uncommon cause of a neck mass in a child, as evidenced by a single case (0.2%) among 445 neck lesions in the pediatric population (18). If anything, teratomas of the head and neck in adults are rarer yet, but are more likely to be malignant, as documented in the study of Thompson et al. (348). In addition to a mass in the neck, severe respiratory distress, notably in the neonate, accelerates events to surgical resection (349–351). At least in the infant, the gross features of a cervicothyroidal teratoma have many similarities to the more common sacrococcygeal teratoma. The mass measures from 2 to 15 cm in greatest diameter and has a well- to poorly demarcated interface from the surrounding soft tissues. The mass fills the an-

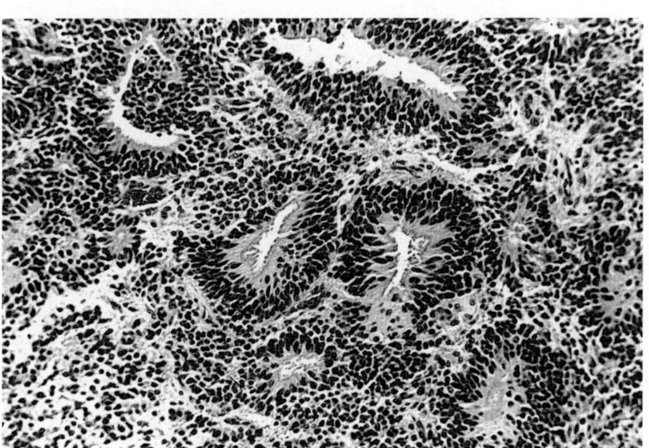

FIGURE 28. Cervicothyroidal teratoma in a neonate showing immature neuroepithelial rosettes or tubules. The presence of immature neural tissues in a teratoma in an infant, regardless of the primary site, is a common finding and is not indicative of malignancy.

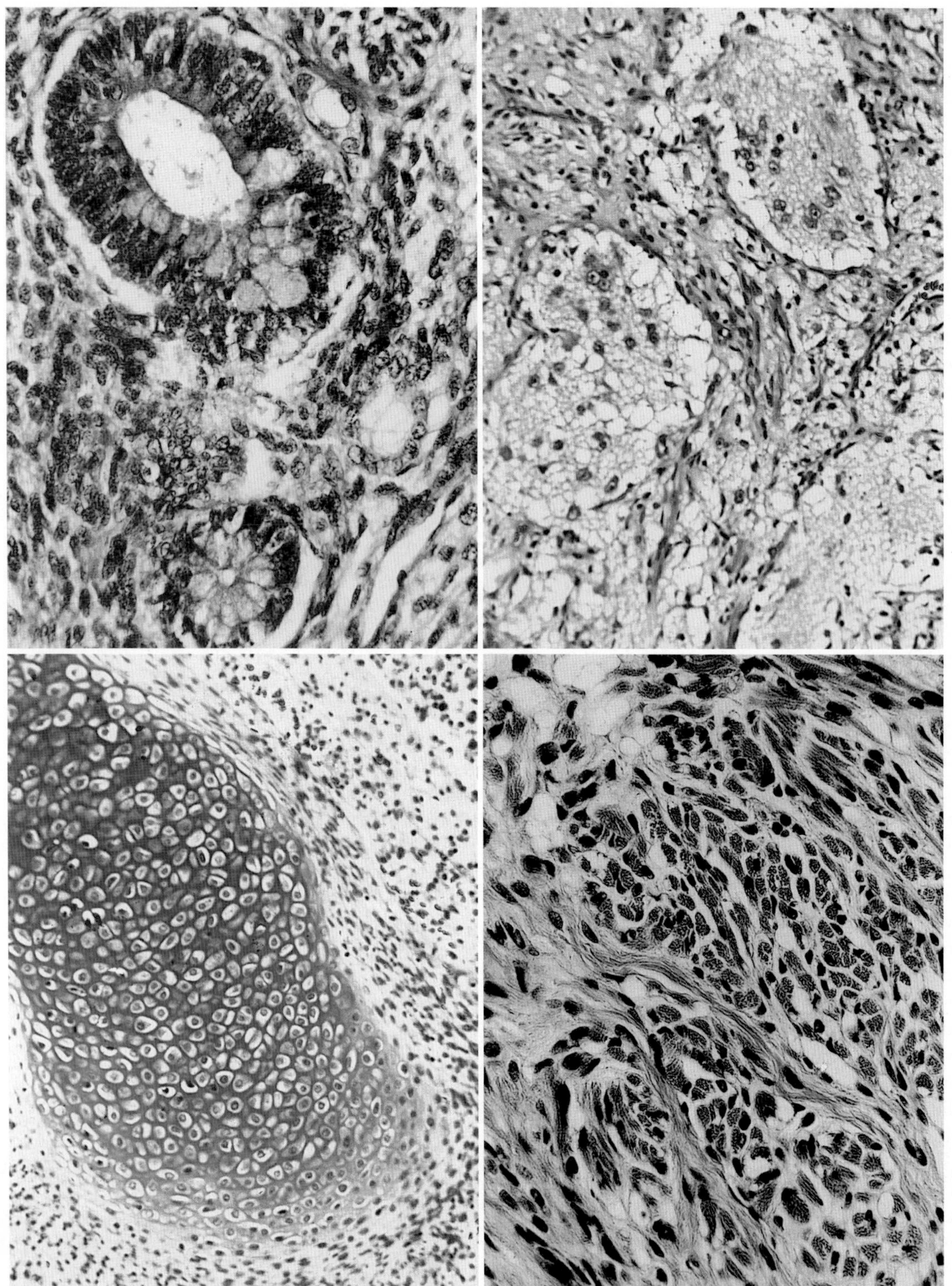

FIGURE 29. Cervicothyroidal teratoma in a neonate showing representative tissues from the three germ cell layers, including immature enteric tubules (**top**, left), ganglion cells in a fibrillary background (**top**, right), immature cartilage (**bottom**, left), and fetal-appearing skeletal muscle (**bottom**, right).

terior neck, with lateral expansion, especially in the infant. A plane between the mass and the adjacent soft tissues is a virtual one in many cases. Dense adherence to the contiguous soft tissue can complicate the surgical resection (352). These tumors have mixed solid and cystic features, with hemorrhage and necrosis in some cases, but without an implication of malignancy. The solid areas have a soft to friable grayish-white to tan appearance, with encephaloid qualities that reflect the often dominant immature and mature neuroepithelium. Residual thyroid parenchyma may be seen microscopically, if not grossly, when a tumor is small and confined to the thyroid. Histologically, the majority of tumors are composed of various immature and mature somatic tissues representing the three embryonic germ cell layers. Islands, tubules, and rosette-like profiles of immature neuroepithelium are consistently found to some extent in those tumors from infants through 12 months of age (Fig. 28). Nodules of developing cartilage, mature neuroglial tissues, and cysts lined by squamous, respiratory, and enteric-type mucosa are common features (Fig. 29). The stroma may have an embryonic appearance, and the skeletal muscle and fat may have an immature appearance (Fig. 30). Immaturity of the various constituent tissues in these tumors from infants does not impact on the otherwise favorable prognosis in most cases (353). On the other hand, one cannot be as sanguine about the immature teratoma in the neck of an older child or adult, which should be regarded as a malignancy (349). When the teratoma is composed exclusively of mature tissues, the prognosis is almost uniformly excellent. Foci of endodermal sinus tumor are extremely uncommon in these neoplasms in neonates and infants, and is evidence of malignancy (Fig. 31). In some cases mature and less often immature neuroepithelium is found in regional lymph nodes (Fig. 32) (354). These nodal deposits represent metastatic involvement; however, so-called nodal gliomatosis is not indicative of malignant biologic behavior. In fact, the favorable prognosis is unaffected by the presence of neuroglial tumor deposits in regional lymph nodes. A cervicothyroidal teratoma may recur in the neck of a child whose tumor was resected in infancy, but in most cases the recurrent tumor consists of mature neuroglial tissue. The primary tumors in these cases were often ones that had infiltrated into the soft tissues of the neck. The prognosis of the cervicothyroidal teratoma in the infant is excellent; however, this tumor has a more aggressive course with potentially lethal consequences in older children and adults when the tumor has immature teratomatous features or malignant elements such as endodermal sinus tumor or embryonal carcinoma (355). Among 30 teratomas of the thyroid, Thompson and associates reported that 14 tumors had immature features, 9 were malignant, and 7 had mature histology (348). All of the malignant teratomas occurred in adolescents or adults.

Oronasopharyngeal teratoma (epignathus) is typically a large disfiguring mass presenting in a neonate whose tumor has protruded from the oral cavity and has an attachment to the palate or base of the skull, or is contiguous with an intracranial component (330,337,356–364). These tumors may arise from the tonsil or paranasal sinus, in which case surgical resection may be more feasible. Most of these tumors are sporadic, but there is a report of one in a 24-week fetus with trisomy 13 (365). The pathologic features are those of a predominantly immature teratoma. Byard et al. reported a case of a cervicopharyngeal teratoma with mature features that was resected in the neonatal period and was followed later by an endodermal sinus tumor in the same site (366). This behavior is similar to the more common sacrococcygeal teratoma (367,368).

Orbital teratoma, like the cervicothyroid and oronasopharyngeal teratomas, is a neoplasm of the neonate who presents with congenital proptosis (329,369,370). Secondary orbital involvement by an intracranial teratoma may present in a similar manner (371). Most orbital teratomas are extraocular, but an intraocular teratoma in the neonate has been reported (372). These

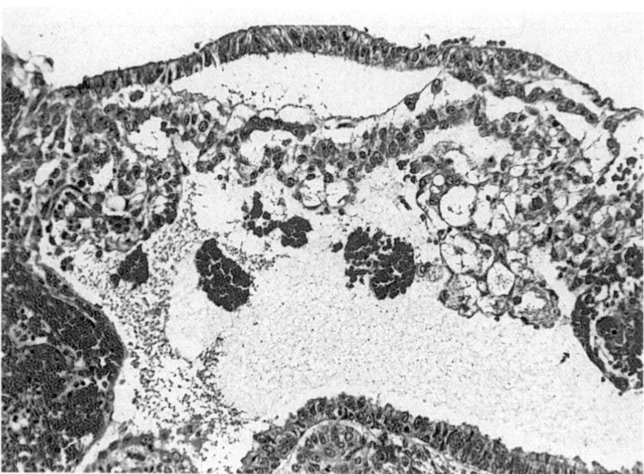

FIGURE 31. Cervicothyroidal teratoma in a neonate showing the reticulated–papillary pattern of endodermal sinus tumor.

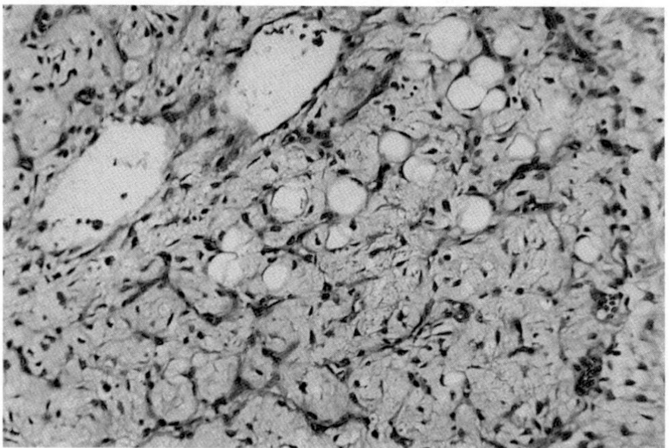

FIGURE 30. Cervicothyroidal teratoma showing immature fat resembling a lipoblastoma.

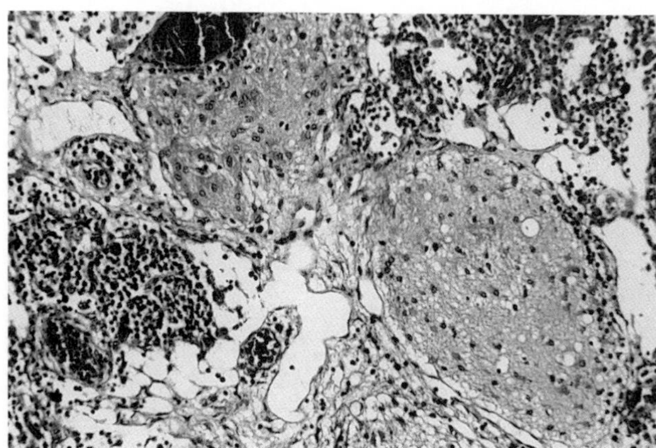

FIGURE 32. Cervical lymph node showing neuroglial tissue in the sinusoids. The lymph node was excised incidentally at the resection of a cervicothyroidal teratoma. The patient has remained disease free for 8 years following resection alone. Nodal gliomatosis appears to have the same prognostic significance as gliomatosis peritonei in a child with a solid teratoma of the ovary.

tumors tend to be more cystic than those in the preceding two sites, but the microscopic findings overlap with those of the cervicothyroidal and oronasopharyngeal teratomas. The prognosis is excellent, and prompt resection may result in the preservation of vision (373).

Germ cell neoplasms in other head and neck sites in aggregate are extremely rare (374–378). It is important to appreciate that malignant patterns of germ cell neoplasms may occur in the head and neck region. Endodermal sinus tumor may present as a soft tissue or orbital mass, principally in children and young adults (319,320,343). We have reported our experience with mixed schneiderian carcinoma–endodermal sinus tumor in two adults (379). Another very aggressive neoplasm of the paranasal sinuses with germ cell–like features is the rare teratocarcinosarcoma, which is more like a malignant mixed müllerian tumor than a germ cell neoplasm (380,381).

Sialoblastoma, Salivary Gland Anlage Tumor, and Other Dysontogenetic Lesions

These two lesions are dysembryonic tumors of the salivary gland, one with primitive features in the case of the sialoblastoma and the salivary gland anlage tumor with mixed epithelial–myoepithelial features. Both lesions present early in life, actually before the age of 2 years.

Sialoblastoma (Embryoma)

Sialoblastoma or embryoma presents as a firm mass in the cheek, where the origin of the tumor has been the parotid gland in all cases to date (382–388). The tumor is well circumscribed but nonencapsulated and measures 1 to 2 cm in diameter. Microscopically, the tumor has a monotonous pattern of solid nests of primitive-appearing small round basaloid cells with inapparent cellular borders (Fig. 33). Mitotic figures are readily identified. At the periphery of the cellular nests, duct-like structures may be appreciated. Unlike some of the malignant small cell tumors in the head and neck region, the formation of rounded nests in dense lobular groupings separated by fibrous bands is characteristic of the sialoblastoma and reminiscent of the appearance of a monomorphic basal cell adenoma (Fig. 34). Embryonal rhabdomyosarcoma and small cell carcinoma, although cytologically similar in some respects to a sialoblastoma, have an infiltrative growth into the adjacent salivary gland and surrounding soft tissues. The clinical behavior of the sialoblastoma is not aggressive in most cases, although mitotically active tumors should be viewed with caution.

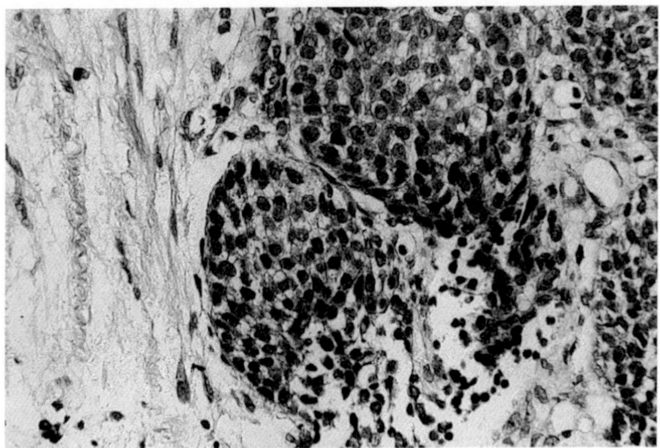

FIGURE 33. Sialoblastoma presenting as a mass in the parotid gland of a neonate showing solid, rounded nests of primitive-appearing cells.

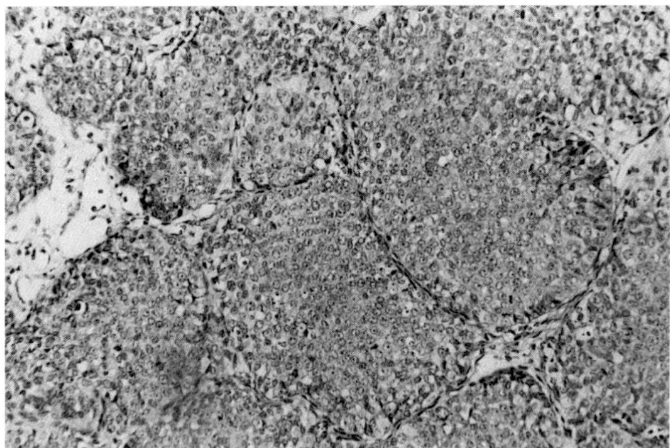

FIGURE 34. Sialoblastoma showing the multilobulated, well-demarcated nests of basophilic tumor cells, which differentiate this primitive tumor from the more infiltrative appearance of embryonal rhabdomyosarcoma or neuroblastoma.

Salivary Gland Anlage Tumor

Salivary gland anlage tumor (see also Chapter 5) or congenital pleomorphic adenoma is equally as rare as the sialoblastoma. A polyploid lesion in the midline of the nasopharynx with or without respiratory distress is the clinical presentation in a neonate within hours or days of life (389–391). A delicate pedicle connects the lesion to the posterior pharyngeal wall. The mass itself measures less than 3 cm and has a biphasic histologic pattern of squamous nests and duct-like structures that blend into the multinodular proliferation of stromal cells (Fig. 35). Extensive necrosis and cyst formation are present, with squamous metaplasia on occasion (389,392). The epithelial component is immunoreactive for cytokeratin, the stromal spindle cells are immunoreactive for vimentin and muscle-specific actin, and both the epithelial and stromal cells express salivary gland amylase (Fig. 36). Excision is curative in all cases to date without any known recurrences.

Other Dysontogenetic Lesions

The salivary gland, as noted from previous discussions in this chapter, may be the site for a branchial cleft cyst and teratoma and may be the constituent tissue of a choristoma. Seifert and associates reported an unusual tumor of the parotid gland in an 8-year-old girl that was composed of small cysts of keratinizing squamous epithelium and whose features were compared with a trichoadenoma (393). Another cystic choristoma was described by Tang and co-workers in the submandibular gland of a neonate (394).

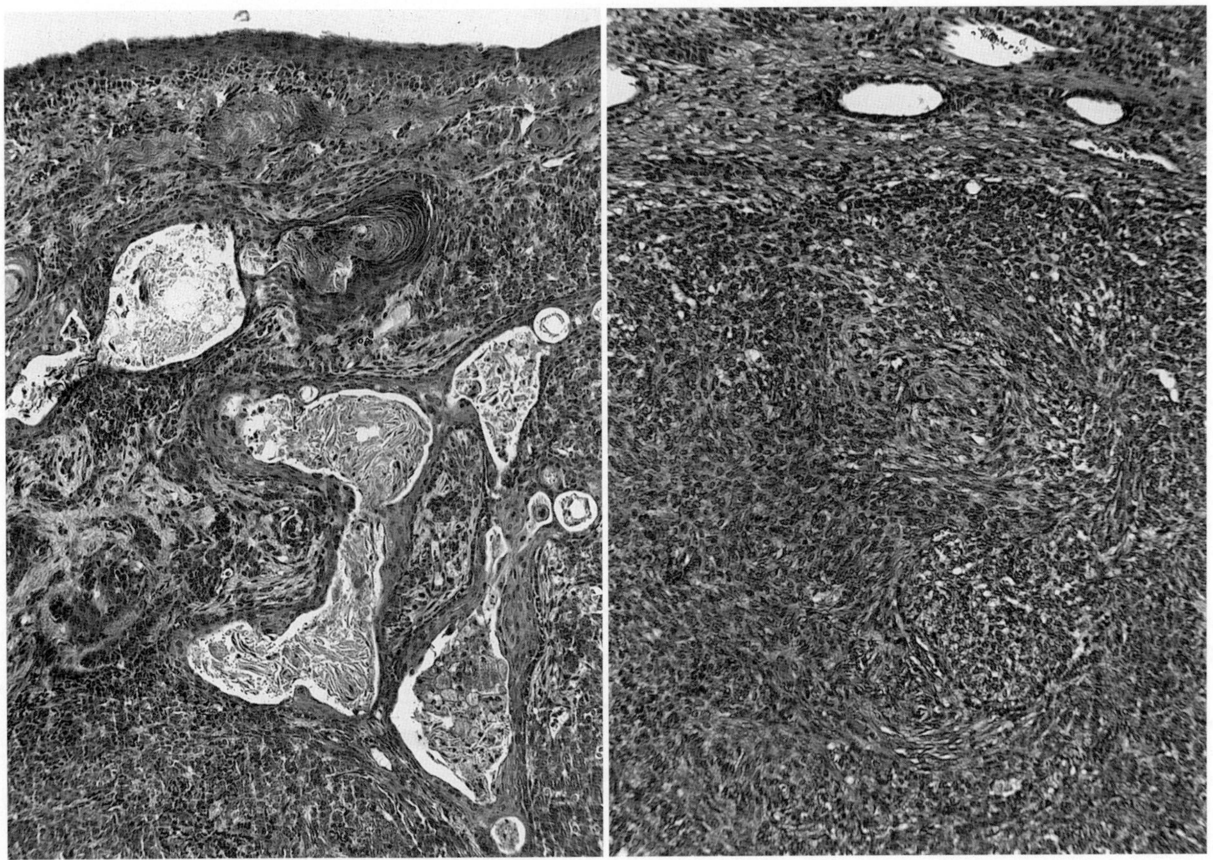

FIGURE 35. Salivary gland anlage tumor showing the peripheral aspects of the polyp with a complex network of branching tubular structures that are lined by squamous epithelium (left) and one of several central nodules of spindle cells with small ducts at the periphery (right)

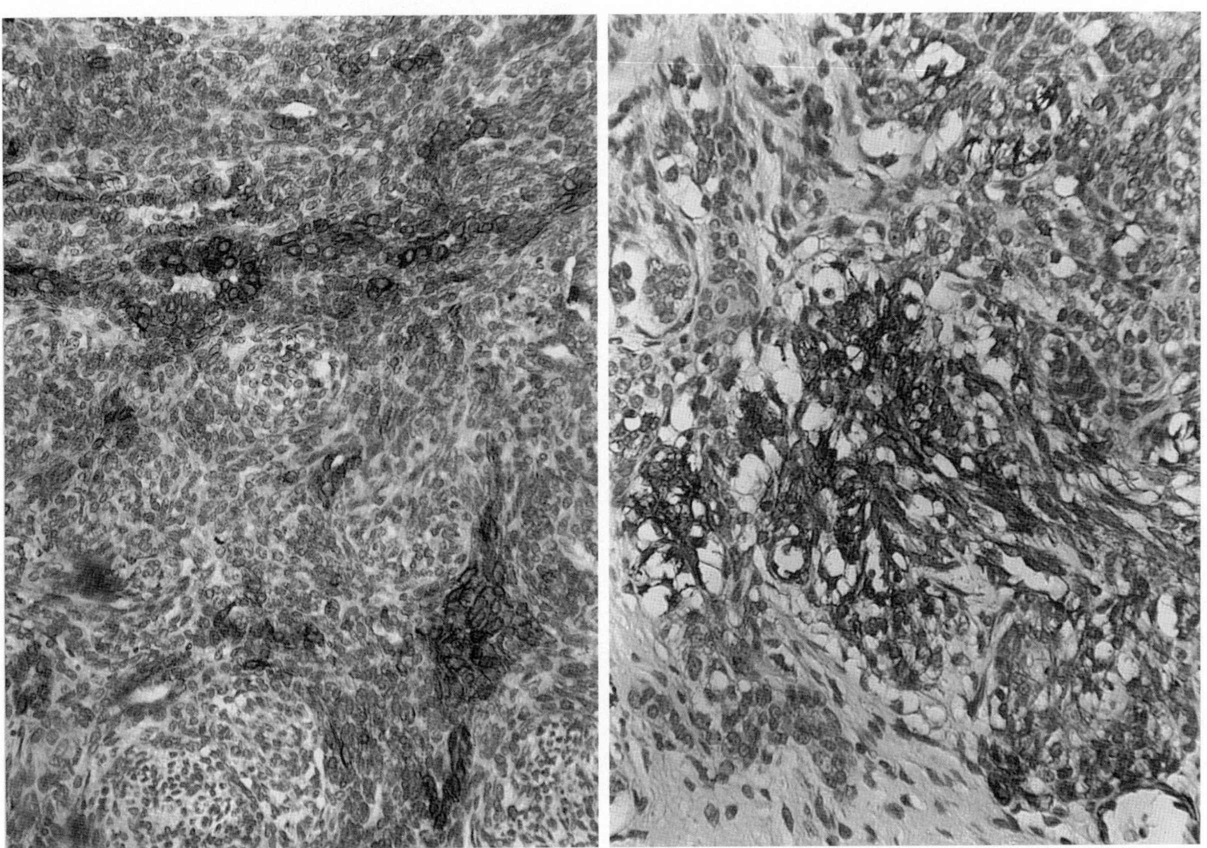

FIGURE 36. Salivary gland anlage tumor demonstrating immunoreactivity for cytokeratin in the tubular structures (left) and for muscle-specific actin in the spindle cell component (right).

Polycystic (dysgenetic) disease is a rare, tumor-like condition of the parotid gland and is possibly a maldevelopment in light of its familial occurrence in the limited number of cases (395,396). To date, the few cases of this predominantly bilateral disorder have been reported in females, with one exception (397–401). Pathologically, the cysts largely replace the acini, but the overall architecture is preserved. The ducts are either empty or contain secretions. It is thought that these cysts are derived from intercalated ducts.

Congenital basal cell adenoma, hamartoma, juvenile pleomorphic adenoma with embryonal features, and *embryonal carcinoma* distinct from the germ cell–derived neoplasm with the same appellation are some other rare lesions with dysontogenetic features (402–405). There are histologic similarities between the congenital basal cell adenoma and the sialoblastoma.

CHONDROMESENCHYMAL HAMARTOMA, GIANT CELL GRANULOMA, AND FIBROUS DYSPLASIA

These three lesions have in common their origin in bone or involvement of contiguous bony structures. The nosology of the giant cell granuloma, as a sporadic lesion or in association with cherubism, is an unsettled issue (see Chapter 11). A disturbance in the growth and organization is the generic abnormality in each of these lesions.

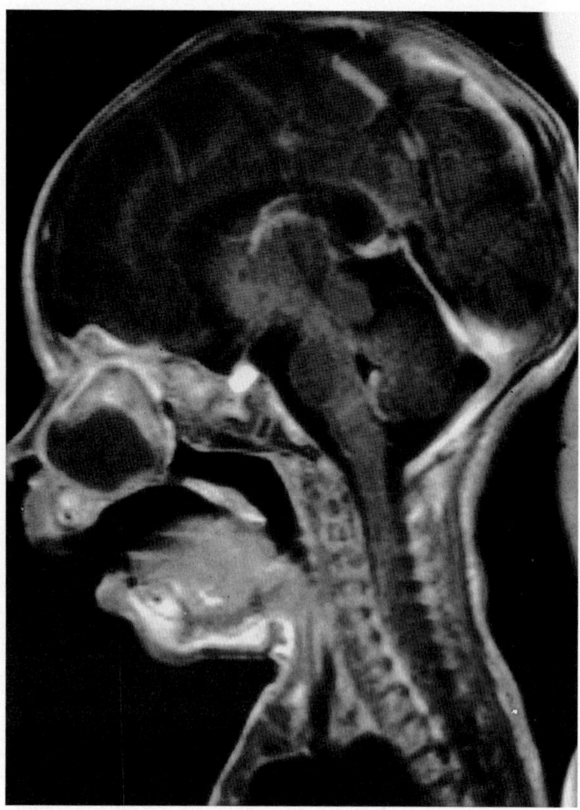

FIGURE 37. Nasal chondromesenchymal hamartoma presenting as an intranasal mass pushing against the cribriform plate.

Chondromesenchymal Hamartoma

This recently described entity of childhood presents as an intranasal mass in the first few weeks or months of life (406) (Fig. 37). Involvement of paranasal sinuses or orbit, and even erosion into the anterior cranial fossa are found in some cases. These lesions are removed in a piecemeal fashion, so a consistent gross characterization has been difficult to establish. The microscopic features include the presence of nodules of variably mature cartilage with an accompanying myxoid to spindle cell stroma, interspersed foci of dense collagenous bundles, and aneurysmal bone cyst–like areas (Fig. 38). Not all tumors have each of these patterns equally represented within a single lesion, or one or more of these patterns may dominate the overall histologic appearance. More than a single surgical resection may be necessary because of the extent of these lesions. Although we have designated this tumefaction as a hamartoma, we would regard the ultimate nature of this lesion as a discussion in progress.

Other types of hamartomas have been reported in and around the nasal fossa (407). Kuriloff has reported a cystic lesion in the nasolabial region that may represent a variant of a dermoid cyst (408). Another putative hamartoma of the nose has been described in a 46-year-old man in association with an inverted papilloma (409). An epithelial adenomatoid hamartoma of the nasal cavity and paranasal sinuses is a polyploid lesion with a prominent glandular component of respiratory-type epithelium (410). Mucinous metaplasia may give this lesion some features reminiscent of the nasal polyps in cystic fibrosis, but without the inspissation of mucin. Although this lesion has been interpreted as a hamartoma, most patients have not come to clinical attention until adulthood. Epithelial and mesenchymal hamartomas of the nasal cavity and nasopharynx have been reported by several investigators (411–414).

Giant Cell Granuloma and Fibrous Dysplasia

These lesions are discussed at length elsewhere (see Chapter 11), but it is worthwhile to acknowledge them as developmental and heredofamilial conditions in specific clinical settings.

Cherubism is an autosomal dominant disorder that presents in children usually before 6 years of age as enlargement of the four quadrants of the jaws by a giant cell lesion that has confusingly been referred to in the literature as "familial fibrous dysplasia" (415–421). Similar giant cell lesions in the jaws have been reported in Noonan's syndrome, Ramon's syndrome, and neurofibromatosis (422–425). There is eventual resolution of these lesions after substantial destruction of the periodontal and osseous tissues with loss of teeth. Microscopically, these lesions have the features of the sporadic central and peripheral giant cell granulomas (426,427).

Fibrous dysplasia is one of the more common tumor-like lesions of the mandible and maxilla in children (427,428). Multifocal craniofacial involvement may be present in a minority of cases. This lesion represents a disorganized overgrowth of woven bone with a spindle cell stroma (see Chapter 11).

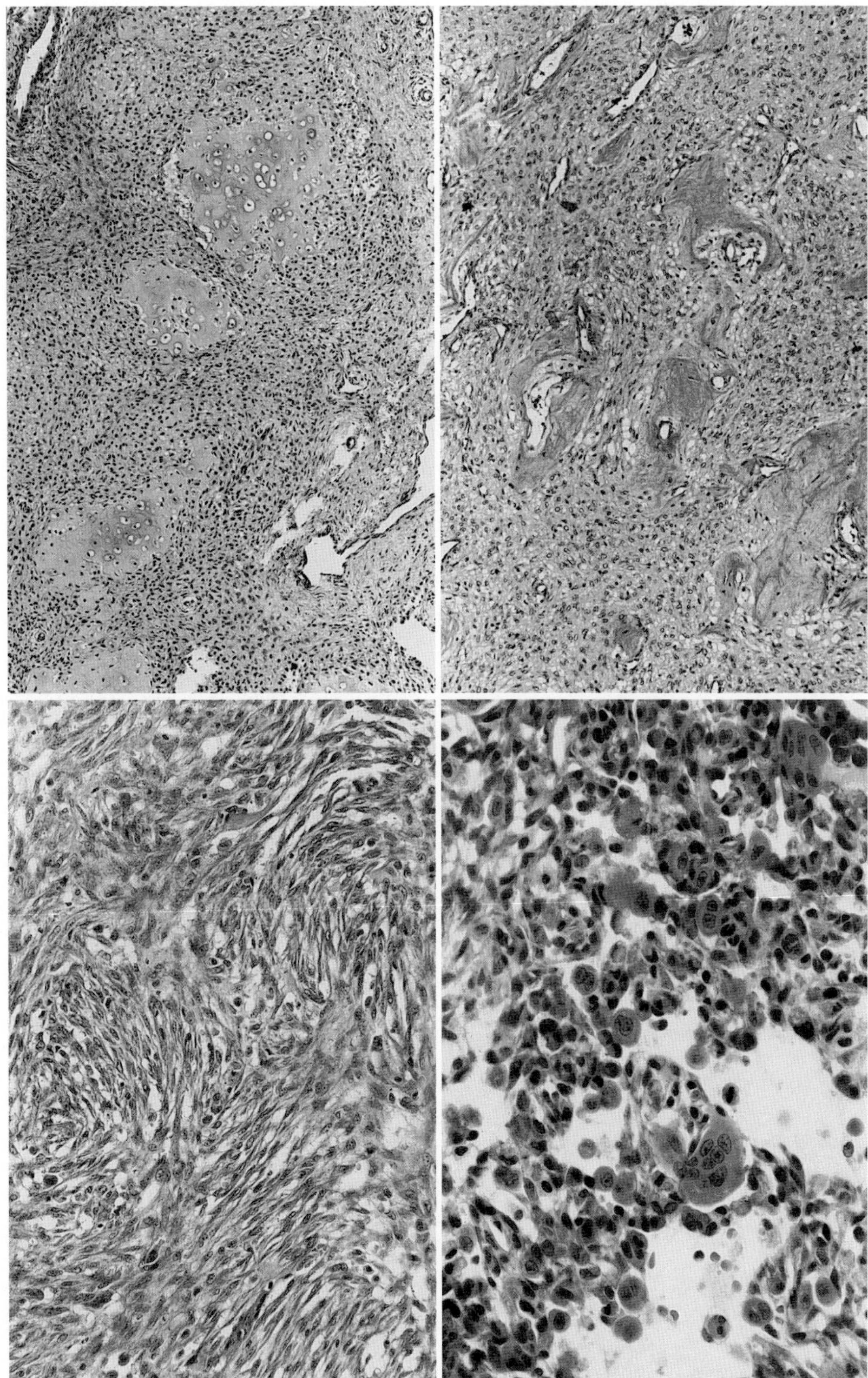

FIGURE 38. Nasal chondromesenchymal hamartoma showing several patterns: islands of cartilage in a spindle cell stroma (**top**, left); foci of hyalinization, often around small blood vessels, and the fibrous stroma (**top**, right); spindle cell stroma (**bottom**, left); and giant cells lining blood-containing tissue spaces (**bottom**, right).

SOFT TISSUE LESIONS

Hemangioma and Lymphangioma

Hemangioma and lymphangioma are the two most common tumor-like lesions of the soft tissue of the head and neck region. These lesions not only involve the soft tissues, but may infiltrate and involve the salivary glands, skeletal muscle, and lymph nodes (429–438). Torsiglieri and associates noted that 18% of congenital lesions of the neck with the clinical presentation of a mass were either a lymphangioma or hemangioma and together represented approximately 10% of all tumefaction of the neck in children (18). Both lesions have in common the formation of vascular spaces with a circumscribed or diffuse growth in the tissues. Like several other entities in this section, the pathogenesis as a vascular malformation or neoplasm is the subject of conjecture and discussion. The nuchal cystic hygroma is regarded by most clinicians as a malformation that is associated with several chromosomal abnormalities, including monosomy X and trisomies 13, 18, and 21 (439,440). Unlike the cervical cystic hygroma, which is composed of numerous lymphatic spaces within the soft tissue, the nuchal lesion is more often a solitary or uniloculated structure in the subcutaneous tissue. Neither of these lesions has a malignant potential, but certainly both may persist and recur.

Fetal Rhabdomyoma

This rare tumor has a predilection for the head and neck region, particularly around the ear, but other sites of involvement have been well documented (441–443). Kapadia and associates have reported their findings in 24 cases (444). An interesting association in a minority of cases is with the nevoid basal cell carcinoma syndrome (445,446). These lesions are possibly hamartomas, but there remains the occasionally difficult distinction from well-differentiated embryonal rhabdomyosarcoma (Fig. 39). In addition to this skeletal muscle lesion, a smooth muscle hamartoma in the oral cavity also has been reported (447).

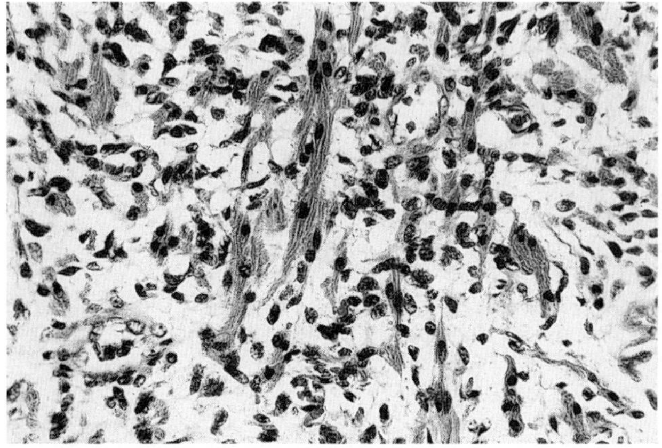

FIGURE 39. Fetal rhabdomyoma presenting as a parapharyngeal mass in a 12-year-old girl with the nevoid basal cell carcinoma syndrome. Note the alternating pattern of myotubes and immature myoblast-like cells. Mitotic activity was absent in this sizable mass. The patient has remained disease free 5 years after surgical resection alone.

Other Dysontogenetic Lesions

The quintessential dysontogenetic neoplasm of soft tissues is the embryonal rhabdomyosarcoma (see Chaper 10). Approximately 35% of rhabdomyosarcomas in children present in the head and neck region (448,449). The neck is the primary site of classic neuroblastoma, typically in cervical sympathetic chains, in 10% to 15% of cases in children, or as a lymph node metastasis from a primary abdominal tumor (450). Infrequently, the differential diagnosis of neuroblastoma in the neck is an immature teratoma. The melanotic neuroectodermal tumor of infancy has a predilection for the head and neck region, where it usually occurs in the anterior maxilla or cranium, and rarely in the soft tissues (451,452). Other immature tumors of the head and neck that present early in life, even as a congenital mass, are fibromatosis colli, infantile myofibromatosis, congenital granular cell tumor (epulis), lipoblastoma, and malignant extrarenal rhabdoid tumor (453–455).

REFERENCES

1. Gorlin RJ, Cohen MM Jr, Levin GS. *Syndromes of the head and neck,* 3rd ed. New York: Oxford University Press, 1990.
2. Stool SE, Post JC. Craniofacial growth, development, and malformations. In: Bluestone CD, Stool SE, Kenna MA, eds. *Pediatric otolaryngology,* 3rd ed. Philadelphia: WB Saunders, 1996:1–18.
3. Karmody CS. Developmental anomalies of the neck. In: Bluestone CD, Stool SE, Kenna MA, eds. *Pediatric otolaryngology,* 3rd ed. Philadelphia: WB Saunders, 1996:1497–1511.
4. Millman B, Gibson WS, Foster WP. Branchio-oto-renal syndrome. *Arch Otolaryngol Head Neck Surg* 1995;121:922–925.
5. Dumas R, Uziel A, Baldet P, et al. Glomerular lesions in the branchio-oto-renal (BOR) syndrome. *Int J Pediatr Nephrol* 1982;3:67–70.
6. Guarisco JL. Congenital head and neck masses in infants and children. Part I. *Ear Nose Throat J* 1991;70:40–47.
7. Guarisco JL. Congenital head and neck masses in infants and children. Part II. *Ear Nose Throat J* 1991;70:75–82.
8. Todd NW. Common congenital anomalies of the neck. Embryology and surgical anatomy. *Surg Clin North Am* 1993;73:599–610.
9. Marsot-Dupuch K, Levret N, Pharaboz C, et al. Congenital neck masses. Embryonic origin and diagnosis. Report of the CIREOL. *J Radiol* 1995;76:405–415.
10. Faerber EN, Swartz JD. Imaging of neck masses in infants and children. *Crit Rev Diagn Imaging* 1991;31:283–314.
11. Davenport M. Lumps and swelling of the head and neck. *BMJ* 1996; 312:368–371.
12. Telander RL, Filston HC. Review of head and neck lesions in infancy and childhood. *Surg Clin North Am* 1992;72:1429–1447.
13. Fallat ME. Neck. In: Oldham KT, Colombani PM, Foglia RP, eds. *Surgery of infants and children. Scientific principles and practice.* Philadelphia: Lippincott-Raven, 1997:835–855.
14. Spinelli C, Ricci E, Berti P, et al. Neck masses in childhood. Surgical experience in 154 cases. *Minerva Pediatr* 1990;42:169–172.
15. Clary RA, Lusk RP. Neck masses. In: Bluestone CD, Stool SE, Kenna MA, eds. *Pediatric otolaryngology,* 3rd ed. Philadelphia: WB Saunders, 1996:1488–1496.
16. Rapidis AD, Economidis J, Goumas PD, et al. Tumors of the head and neck in children. A clinicopathologic analysis of 1,007 cases. *J Craniomaxillofac Surg* 1988;16:279–286.
17. Otto RA, Bowes AK. Neck masses: benign or malignant? Sorting out the causes by age-group. *Postgrad Med* 1990;88:199–204.
18. Torsiglieri AJ Jr, Tom LWC, Ross AJ III, et al. Pediatric neck masses: guidelines for evaluation. *Int J Pediatr Otorhinolaryngol* 1988;16: 199–210.

19. Brown, RL, Azizkhan RG. Pediatric head and neck lesions. *Pediatr Clin North Am* 1998;45:889–905.
20. Siebert JR, Cohen MM Jr, Sulik KK, et al. *Holoprosencephaly. An overview and atlas of cases.* New York: Wiley-Liss, 1990:59–98.
21. Capecchi MR. Function of homeobox genes in skeletal development. *Ann N Y Acad Sci* 1996;785:34–37.
22. Vieille-Grosjean I, Hunt P, Gulisano M, et al. Branchial HOX gene expression and human craniofacial development. *Dev Biol* 1997; 183:49–60.
23. Whiting J. Craniofacial abnormalities induced by the ectopic expression of homeobox genes. *Mutat Res* 1997;396:97–112.
24. Cohen MM Jr. Genetics, syndromology, and craniofacial anomalies. In: Bluestone CD, Stool SE, Kenna MA, eds. *Pediatric otolaryngology,* 3rd ed. Philadelphia: WB Saunders, 1996:33–61.
25. Friede RL. *Developmental neuropathology,* 2nd revised and expanded ed. Berlin: Springer-Verlag, 1989:282–287.
26. Martinez-Lage JF, Poza M, Sola J, et al. The child with a cephalocele: etiology, neuroimaging, and outcome. *Childs Nerv Syst* 1996;12: 540–550.
27. Lorber J, Schofield JK. The prognosis of occipital encephalocele. *Z Kinderchir Grenzgeb* 1979;28:347–351.
28. Adetiloye VA, Dare FO, Oyelami OA. A ten-year review of encephalocele in a teaching hospital. *Int J Gynaecol Obstet* 1993;41: 241–249.
29. Salonen R. The Meckel syndrome: clinicopathological findings in 67 patients. *Am J Med Genet* 1984;18:671–689.
30. Paavola P, Salonen R, Baumer A, et al. Clinical and genetic heterogeneity in Meckel syndrome. *Hum Genet* 1997;101:88–92.
31. Salonen R, Paavola P. Meckel syndrome. *J Med Genet* 1998;35: 497–501.
32. Roume J, Ma HW, LeMerrer M, et al. Genetic heterogeneity of Meckel syndrome. *J Med Genet* 1997;34:1003–1006.
33. Genin RJ, Cormier-Daire V, Ma HW, et al. A gene for Meckel syndrome maps to chromosome 11q13. *Am J Hum Genet* 1998;63: 1095–1101.
34. Oruckaptan NH, Sennevsim O, Akalan N. Occipital encephalocele associated with mediastinal enteric duplication cyst. *Pediatr Neurosurg* 1997;27:214–217.
35. Martinez-Lage JF, Poza M, Ramos J, et al. Occipital encephalocele associated with a dermoid cyst. *J Child Neurol* 1992;7:427–430.
36. Ahdab-Barmada M, Claassen D. A distinctive triad of malformations of the central nervous system in the Meckel-Gruber syndrome. *J Neuropathol Exp Neurol* 1990;49:610–620.
37. Humphreys RP. Encephalocele and dermal sinuses. In: Cheer WR, ed. *Pediatric neurosurgery. Surgery of the developing nervous system,* 3rd ed. Philadelphia: WB Saunders, 1994:96–103.
38. Mahapatra AK, Tandon PN, Dhawan IK, et al. Anterior encephaloceles: a report of 30 cases. *Childs Nerv Syst* 1994;10:501–504.
39. Hirokawa M, Shimizu T, Manabe T, et al. Encephalocele with an area mimicking giant cell fibroblastoma. Case report. *APMIS* 1998;106: 647–650.
40. Hughes GB, Sharpino G, Hunt W, et al. Management of the congenital midline nasal mass: a review. *Head Neck Surg* 1980;2: 222–233.
41. Bradley PJ, Singh SD. Congenital nasal masses: diagnosis and management. *Clin Otolaryngol* 1982;7:87–97.
42. Morgan DW, Evans JNG. Developmental nasal anomalies. *J Laryngol Otol* 1990;104:394–403.
43. Kennard CD, Rasmussen JE. Congenital midline nasal masses: diagnosis and management. *J Dermatol Surg Oncol* 1990;16:1025–1036.
44. Barkovich AJ, Vandermarck P, Edwards MSB, et al. Congenital nasal masses: CT and MR imaging features in 16 cases. *Am J Neuroradiol* 1991;12:105–116.
45. Sweet RM. Lesions of the nasal radix in pediatric patients: diagnosis and management. *South Med J* 1992;85:164–169.
46. Paller AS, Pensler JM, Tomita T. Nasal midline masses in infants and children. *Arch Dermatol* 1991;127:362–366.
47. Pensler JM, Ivescu AS, Ciletti SJ, et al. Craniofacial gliomas. *Plast Reconstr Surg* 1996;98:27–30.
48. Magit AE. Tumors of the nose, paranasal sinuses, and nasopharynx. In: Bluestone CD, Stool SE, Kenna MA, eds. *Pediatric otolaryngology,* 3rd ed. Philadelphia: WB Saunders, 1996:893–904.
49. Claros P, Bandos A, Claros A Jr, et al. Nasal gliomas. Main features, management and report of five cases. *Int J Pediatr Otorhinolaryngol* 1998;46:15–20.
50. Swift AC, Singh SD. The presentation and management of the nasal glioma. *Int J Pediatr Otorhinolaryngol* 1985;10:253–261.
51. Younus M, Coode PE. Nasal glioma and encephalocele: two separate entities. Report of two cases. *J Neurosurg* 1986;64:516–519.
52. Bagger-Sjoback D, Bergstrand G, Edner G, et al. Nasal meningoencephalocele. A clinical problem. *Clin Otolaryngol* 1983;8:329–335.
53. Choudhury AR, Bandey SA, Haleem A, et al. Glial heterotopias of the nose. A report of two cases. *Childs Nerv Syst* 1996;12:43–47.
54. Puppala B, Mangurten HH, McFadden J, et al. Nasal glioma. Presenting as neonatal respiratory distress. *Clin Pediatr* 1990;29:49–52.
55. Fletcher CDM, Carpenter G, McKee PH. Nasal glioma. A rarity. *Am J Dermatopathol* 1986;8:341–346.
56. Patterson K, Kapur S, Chandra RS. "Nasal gliomas" and related brain heterotopias: a pathologist's perspective. *Pediatr Pathol* 1986;5: 353–362.
57. Dini M, Lo Russo G, Colafranceschi M. So-called nasal glioma: case report with immunohistochemical study. *Tumori* 1998;84:398–402.
58. Theaker JM, Fletcher CDM. Heterotopic glial nodules: a light microscopic and immunohistochemical study. *Histopathology* 1991;18: 255–260.
59. Tashiro Y, Sueishi K, Nakao K. Nasal glioma: an immunohistochemical and ultrastructural study. *Pathol Int* 1995;45:393–398.
60. Chan JKC, Lau W-H. Nasal astrocytoma or nasal glial heterotopia? *Arch Pathol Lab Med* 1989;113:943–945.
61. Pasyk KA, Argenta LC, Marks MW, et al. Heterotopic brain presenting as a lip lesion. *Cleft Palate J* 1988;25:48–52.
62. Seibert RW, Seibert JJ, Jimenez JF, et al. Nasopharyngeal brain heterotopia—a cause of upper airway obstruction in infancy. *Laryngoscope* 1984;94:818–819.
63. Hendrickson M, Faye-Petersen O, Johnson DG. Cystic and solid heterotopic brain in the face and neck: a review and report of an unusual case. *J Pediatr Surg* 1990;25:766–768.
64. Birrell JF, Tevendale J, Bain AD. Glioma of the nasopharynx. *J Laryngol Otol* 1966;80:1182–1186.
65. Madjidi A, Couly G. Heterotopic neuroglial tissue of the face. Report of six cases and review of the literature. *Oral Surg Oral Med Oral Pathol* 1993;76:284–288.
66. Morita N, Harada M, Sakamoto T. Congenital tumors of heterotopic central nervous system tissue in the oral cavity. Report of two cases. *J Oral Maxillofac Surg* 1993;51:1030–1033.
67. Van Geertruyden JP, Fourez TJ, Hansen P, Heimann PE, Brion J-P. Heterotopic brain tissue in the scalp. *Br J Plast Surg* 1995;48: 332–334.
68. Knox R, Pratt M, Garvin AJ, et al. Heterotopic lingual brain in the newborn. *Arch Otolaryngol Head Neck Surg* 1989;115:630–632.
69. Wilkins RB, Hofmann RJ, Byrd WA, et al. Heterotopic brain tissue in the orbit. *Arch Ophthalmol* 1987;105:390–392.
70. Yokoyama S, Nakayama I, Yamashita H, et al. Heterotopic brain of the tongue. *Acta Pathol Jpn* 1986;36:1397–1402.
71. Bossen EH, Hudson WR. Oligodendroglioma arising in heterotopic brain tissue of the soft palate and nasopharynx. *Am J Surg Pathol* 1987; 11:571–574.
72. McDermott MB, Glasner SD, Nielsen PL, et al. Soft tissue gliomatosis. Morphologic unity and histogenetic diversity. *Am J Surg Pathol* 1996;20:148–155.
73. Berry AD III, Patterson JW. Meningoceles, meningomyeloceles, and encephaloceles: a neuro-dermatopathologic study of 132 cases. *J Cutan Pathol* 1990;18:164–177.

74. Drapkin AJ. Rudimentary cephalocele or neural crest remnant? *Neurosurgery* 1990;26:667–674.
75. Imes RK, Hoyt WF, Brodsky MC. Meningocele or gliomatosis? *Ophthalmology* 199l;98:562.
76. Garrity JA, Trautmann JC, Bartley GB, et al. Optic nerve sheath meningoceles. Clinical and radiographic features in 13 cases with a review of the literature. *Ophthalmology* 1990;97:1519–1531.
77. Argenyi ZB. Cutaneous neural heterotopias and related tumors relevant for the dermatopathologist. *Semin Diagn Pathol* 1996;13:60–71.
78. Bale PM, Hughes L, de Silva M. Sequestrated meningoceles of scalp: extracranial meningeal heterotopia. *Hum Pathol* 1990;21:1156–1163.
79. Mihara Y, Miyamoto T, Hagari Y, Mihara M. Rudimentary meningocele of the scalp. *J Dermatol* 1997;24:606–610.
80. Yanagi T, Sato T, Fujiwara S, et al. A case of rudimentary meningocele. *J Dermatol* 1998;25:329–332.
81. Chan HH, Fung JW, Lam WM, et al. The clinical spectrum of rudimentary meningocele. *Pediatr Dermatol* 1998;15:388–389.
82. Khallouf R, Fetissof F, Machet MC, et al. Sequestrated meningocele of the scalp: diagnostic value of hair anomalies. *Pediatr Dermatol* 1994;11:315–318.
83. Stone MS, Walker PS, Kennard CD. Rudimentary meningocele presenting with a scalp hair tuft. Report of two cases. *Arch Dermatol* 1994;130:775–777.
84. Martinez-Lage JF, Sola J, Casas C, et al. Atretic cephalocele: the tip of the iceberg. *J Neurosurg* 1992;77:230–235.
85. Theaker JM, Fletcher CDM, Tudway AJ. Cutaneous heterotopic meningeal nodules. *Histopathology* 1990;16:475–479.
86. Miyamoto T, Mihara M, Hagari Y, et al. Primary cutaneous meningioma on the scalp: report of two siblings. *J Dermatol* 1995;22:611–619.
87. Sibley DA, Cooper PH. Rudimentary meningocele: a variant of "primary cutaneous meningioma." *J Cutan Pathol* 1989;16:72–80.
88. Suster S, Rosai J. Hamartoma of the scalp with ectopic meningothelial elements. A distinctive benign soft tissue lesion that may simulate angiosarcoma. *Am J Surg Pathol* 1990;14:1–11.
89. Marrogi AJ, Swanson PE, Kyriakos M, et al. Rudimentary meningocele of the skin. Clinicopathologic features and differential diagnosis. *J Cutan Pathol* 1991;18:178–188.
90. Harvell JB, Kilpatrick SE, White WL. Histogenetic relations between giant cell fibroblastoma and dermatofibrosarcoma protuberans. CD34 staining showing the spectrum and a simulator. *Am J Dermatopathol* 1998;20:339–345.
91. Pensler JM, Bauer BS, Naidich TP. Craniofacial dermoids. *Plast Reconstr Surg* 1988;82:953–958.
92. Peter JC, Sinclair-Smith C, de Villiers JC. Midline dermal sinuses and cysts and their relationship to the central nervous system. *Eur J Pediatr Surg* 1991;1:73–79.
93. Kayhan FT, Aydin YZ, Babalioglu M. A nasopharyngeal dermoid causing neonatal airway obstruction. *Int J Pediatr Otorhinolaryngol* 1997;40:195–201.
94. Emamy H, Ahmadian H. Limbal dermoid with ectopic brain tissue. Report of a case and review of the literature. *Arch Ophthalmol* 1977;95:2201–2202.
95. Oakman JH Jr, Lambert SR, Grossniklaus HE. Corneal dermoid: a case report and review of classification. *J Pediatr Ophthalmol Strabismus* 1993;30:388–391.
96. Felder H. Benign congenital neoplasms: dermoids and teratomas. *Arch Otolaryngol* 1975;101:333–334.
97. Holt GR, Holt JE, Weaver RG. Dermoids and teratomas of the head and neck. *Ear Nose Throat J* 1979;58:520–531.
98. Weinstein JM, Romano PE, O'Grady RB. Bone formation in association with a limbal dermoid. *Arch Ophthalmol* 1979:97:1121–1122.
99. McCollough ML, Glover AT, Grabski WJ, et al. Orbital dermoid cysts showing conjunctival epithelium. *Am J Dermatopathol* 1991;134:611–615.
100. Smirniotopoulos JG, Chiechi MV. Teratomas, dermoids, and epidermoids of the head and neck. *Radiographics* 1995;15:1437–1455.
101. Denoyelle F, Ducroz V, Roger G, et al. Nasal dermoid sinus cysts in children. *Laryngoscope* 1997;107:795–800.
102. Rosen D, Wirtschafter A, Rao VM, et al. Dermoid cyst of the lateral neck: a case report and literature review. *Ear Nose Throat J* 1998;125:129–132.
103. Bradley PJ. Nasal dermoids in children. *Int J Pediatr Otorhinol* 1981;3:63–70.
104. Reddy VS, Radhakrishna K, Rao PL. Lingual dermoid. *J Pediatr Surg* 1991;26:1389–1390.
105. Drucker C, Gerson CR. Sublingual contiguous thyroglossal and dermoid cysts in a neonate. *Int J Pediatr Otorhinolaryngol* 1992;23:181–186.
106. Cejas Mendez DL, de Serdio AJL, Goralsky FS. Choristoma of the salivary gland and dermoid cyst of the middle ear in a 3-year-old girl. Apropos of a case. *An Otorhinolaryngol Ibero Am* 1992;19:275–282.
107. Sinclair RD, Darley C, Dawber RP. Congenital inclusion dermoid cysts of the scalp. *Aust J Dermatol* 1992;33:135–140.
108. Hsu ST, Yu-Yun Lee J, Chao SC, et al. Congenital occipital dermal sinus with intracranial dermoid cyst complicated by recurrent *Escherichia coli* meningitis. *Br J Dermatol* 1998;139:922–924.
109. Takimoto T, Yoshizaki T, Tanaka S. Congenital dermoid cyst at the base of the tongue. *Auris Nasus Larynx* 1990;17:217–219.
110. Parizek J, Nemecek S, Nemeckova J, et al. Congenital dermoid cysts over the anterior fontanel. Report on 13 cases in Czechoslovak children. *Childs Nerv Syst* 1989;5:234–237.
111. Fujimaki T, Miyazaki S, Fukushima T, et al. Dermoid cyst of the frontal bone away from the anterior fontanel. *Childs Nerv Syst* 1995;11:424–427.
112. Quraishi HA, Ortiz O, Wax MK. Dermoid cyst of the floor of the mouth. *Otolaryngol Head Neck Surg* 1998;118:562–563.
113. Miles LP, Naidoo LC, Reddy J. Congenital dermoid cyst of the tongue. *J Laryngol Otol* 1997;111:1179–1182.
114. Walstad WR, Solomon JM, Schow SR, et al. Midline cystic lesion of the floor of the mouth. *J Oral Maxillofac Surg* 1998;56:70–74.
115. McAvoy JM, Zuckerbraun L. Dermoid cysts of the head and neck in children. *Arch Otolaryngol* 1976;102:529–531.
116. Reddy VS, Radhakrishna K, Rao PL. Lingual dermoid. *J Pediatr Surg* 1991;26:1389–1390.
117. Bonilla JA, Szeremeta W, Yellon RF, et al. Teratoid cyst of the floor of the mouth. *Int J Pediatr Otorhinolaryngol* 1996;5:71–75.
118. King RC, Smith BR, Burk JL. Dermoid cyst in the floor of the mouth. Review of the literature and case reports. *Oral Surg Oral Med Oral Pathol* 1994;78:567–576.
119. Glasauer FE, Levy LF, Auchterlonie WC. Congenital inclusion dermoid cyst of the anterior fontanel. *J Neurosurg* 1978;48:274–278.
120. Oygur T, Dursun A, Uluoglu O, et al. Oral congenital dermoid cyst in the floor of the mouth of a newborn. The significance of gastrointestine-type epithelium. *Oral Surg Oral Med Oral Pathol* 1992;74:627–630.
121. Berger S, Feinmesser R, Feinmesser M. Dermoid cyst of the submandibular area. *Ear Nose Throat J* 1990;59:659–660.
122. Shields JA, Kaden IH, Eagle RC Jr, et al. Orbital dermoid cysts: clinicopathologic correlations, classification, and management. The 1997 Josephine E. Schueler Lecture. *Ophthalmol Plast Reconstr Surg* 1997;13:265–276.
123. Pivnick EK, Walter AW, Lawrence MD, et al. Gorlin syndrome associated with midline nasal dermoid cyst. *J Med Genet* 1996;33:704–706.
124. Rubin G, Scienza R, Pasqualin A, et al. Craniocerebral epidermoids and dermoids. A review of 44 cases. *Acta Neurochir* 1989;97:1–16.
125. Gormley WB, Tomecek FJ, Qureshi N, et al. Craniocerebral epidermoid and dermoid tumours: a review of 32 cases. *Acta Neurochir* 1994;128:115–121.
126. Wardinsky TD, Pagon RA, Kropp RJ, et al. Nasal dermoid sinus cysts: association with intracranial extension and multiple malformations. *Cleft Palate Craniofac J* 1991;28:87–95.
127. Crawford R. Dermoid cyst of the scalp: intracranial extension. *J Pediatr Surg* 1990;25:294–295.
128. Spencer WH. Conjunctiva. In: Spencer WH, ed. *Ophthalmic pathology. An atlas and textbook,* 4th ed. Philadelphia: WB Saunders, 1996:48–56.

129. Cohen MM Jr, Rollnick BR, Kaye CI. Oculoauriculovertebral spectrum: an updated critique. *Cleft Palate J* 1989;26:276–286.
130. Ziavras E, Farber MG, Diamond GR. A pedunculated lipodermoid in oculoauriculovertebral dysplasia. *Arch Ophthalmol* 1990;108: 1032–1033.
131. Rollnick BR. Oculoauriculovertebral anomaly: variability and causal heterogeneity. *Am J Med Genet Suppl* 1988;4:41–53.
132. Johnson KA, Fairhurst J, Clarke NM. Oculoauriculovertebral spectrum: new manifestations. *Pediatr Radiol* 1995;25:446–448.
133. Mansour AM, Barber JC, Reinecke RD, et al. Ocular choristomas. *Surv Ophthalmol* 1989;33:339–358.
134. McNab AA, Wright JE, Caswell AG. Clinical features and surgical management of dermolipomas. *Aust N Z J Ophthalmol* 1990;18: 159–162.
135. Pokorny KS, Hyman BM, Jakobiec FA, et al. Epibulbar choristomas containing lacrimal tissue. Clinical distinction from dermoids and histologic evidence of an origin from the palpebral lobe. *Ophthalmology* 1987;94:1249–1257.
136. Kelly A, Bough ID Jr, Luft JD, et al. Hairy polyp of the oropharynx: case report and literature review. *J Pediatr Surg* 1996;31:704–706.
137. Walsh RM, Philip G, Salama NY. Hairy polyp of the oropharynx: an unusual cause of intermittent neonatal airway obstruction. *Int J Pediatr Otorhinolaryngol* 1996;34:129–134.
138. Mitchell TE, Girling AC. Hairy polyp of the tonsil. *J Laryngol Otol* 1996;110:101–103.
139. Cerezal L, Morales C, Abascal F, et al. Magnetic resonance features of nasopharyngeal teratoma (hairy polyp) in an adult. *Ann Otol Rhinol Laryngol* 1998;107:987–990.
140. Chaudhry AP, Lore JM Jr, Fisher JE, et al. So-called hairy polyps or teratoid tumors of the nasopharynx. *Arch Otolaryngol* 1978;104: 517–525.
141. McShane D, el Sherif I, Doyle-Kelly W, et al. Dermoids ("hairy polyps") of the oro-nasopharynx. *J Laryngol Otol* 1989;103:612–615.
142. Franco V, Florena AM, Lombardo F, et al. Bilateral hairy polyp of the oropharynx. *J Laryngol Otol* 1996;110:288–290.
143. Sexton M. Hairy polyp of the oropharynx. A case report with speculation on nosology. *Am J Dermatopathol* 1990;12:294–298.
144. Fried MP, Vernick DM. Dermoid cyst of the middle ear and mastoid. *Otolaryngol Head Neck Surg* 1984;92:594–596.
145. Mitchell TE, Girling AC. Hairy polyp of the tonsil. *J Laryngol Otol* 1996;110:101–103.
146. Aughton DJ, Sloan CT, Milad MP, et al. Nasopharyngeal teratoma ("hairy polyp"), Dandy-Walker malformation, diaphragmatic hernia, and other anomalies in a female infant. *J Med Genet* 1990;27: 788–790.
147. Haddad J Jr, Senders CW, Leach CS, et al. Congenital hairy polyp of the nasopharynx associated with cleft palate: report of two cases. *Int J Pediatr Otorhinolaryngol* 1990;20:127–135.
148. Kieff DA, Curtin HD, Limb CJ, et al. A hairy polyp presenting as a middle ear mass in a pediatric patient. *Am J Otolaryngol* 1998;19: 228–231.
149. Boedts D, Moerman M, Marquet J. A hairy polyp of the middle ear and mastoid cavity. *Acta Otorhinolaryngol Belg* 1992;46:397–400.
150. Nicklaus PJ, Forte V, Thorner PS. Hairy polyp of the eustachian tube. *J Otolaryngol* 1991;20:254–257.
151. Sichel JY, Dano I, Halperin D, et al. Dermoid cyst of the eustachian tube. *Int J Pediatr Otorhinolaryngol* 1999;48:77–81.
152. Heffner DK, Thompson LD, Schall DG, et al. Pharyngeal dermoids ("hairy polyps") as accessory auricles. *Ann Otol Rhinol Laryngol* 1996;105:819–824.
153. Olivares-Pakzad BA, Tazelaar HD, Dehner LP, et al. Oropharyngeal hairy polyp with meningothelial elements. *Oral Surg Oral Med Oral Pathol Oral Radiol Endod* 1996;79:462–468.
154. Smith CD. Cysts and sinuses of the neck. In: O'Neill JA, Rowe MI, Grosfeld JL, et al., eds. *Pediatric surgery,* 5th ed. St. Louis: CV Mosby, 1998:757–771.
155. Koeller KK, Alamo L, Adair CF, et al. Congenital cystic masses of the neck: radiologic-pathologic correlation. *Radiographics* 1999;19: 121–146.
156. Skandalakis JE, Gray SW, Todd NW. The pharynx and its derivatives. In: Skandalakis JE, Gray SW, eds. *Embryology for surgeons. The embryological basis for the treatment of congenital anomalies,* 2nd ed. Baltimore: Williams & Wilkins, 1994:17–64.
157. Wilson DB. Embryonic development of the head and neck. Part 2: The branchial region. *Head Neck Surg* 1979;2:59–66.
158. Benson MT, Dalen K, Mancuso AA, et al. Congenital anomalies of the branchial apparatus: embryology and pathologic anatomy. *Radiographics* 1992;12:943–960.
159. Choi SS, Zalzal GH. Branchial anomalies: a review of 52 cases. *Laryngoscope* 1995;105:909–913.
160. Agaton-Bonilla FC, Gay-Escoda C. Diagnosis and treatment of branchial cleft cysts and fistulae. A retrospective study of 183 patients. *Int J Oral Maxillofac Surg* 1996;25:449–452.
161. Doi O, Hutson JM, Myers NA, et al. Branchial remnants: a review of 58 cases. *J Pediatr Surg* 1988;23:789–792.
162. Takimoto T, Itoh M, Furukawa M, et al. Branchial cleft (pouch) anomalies: a review of 42 cases. *Auris Nasus Larynx* 1991;18:87–92.
163. McPhail N, Mustard RA. Branchial cleft anomalies: a review of 87 cases treated at the Toronto General Hospital. *Can Med Assoc J* 1966;94:174–179.
164. Kenealy JF, Torsiglieri AJ Jr, Tom LW. Branchial cleft anomalies: a five-year retrospective review. *Trans Pa Acad Ophthalmol Otolaryngol* 1990;42:1022–1025.
165. Ayache D, Ducroz V, Roger G, et al. Midline cervical cleft. *Int J Pediatr Otorhinolaryngol* 1997;40:189–193.
166. Vermeire VM, Daele JJ. Second branchial cleft-pouch set fistulae, sinuses and cysts in children. *Acta Otorhinolaryngol Belg* 1991;45: 437–442.
167. Papay FA, Kalucis C, Eliachar I, et al. Nasopharyngeal presentation of second branchial cleft cyst. *Otolaryngol Head Neck Surg* 1994;110: 232–234.
168. Paczona R, Jori J, Czigner J. Pharyngeal localizations of branchial cysts. *Eur Arch Otorhinolaryngol* 1998;255:379–381.
169. Regauer S, Gogg-Kamerer M, Braun H, et al. Lateral neck cysts-the branchial theory revisited. A critical review and clinicopathologic study of 97 cases with special emphasis on cytokeratin expression. *APMIS* 1997;105:623–630.
170. Golledge J, Ellis H. The aetiology of lateral cervical (branchial) cysts: past and present theories. *J Laryngol Otol* 1994;108:653–659.
171. Soh KB. Branchiogenic carcinomas: do they exist? *J R Coll Surg Edinb* 1998;43:1–5.
172. Krogdahl AS. Carcinoma occurring in branchial cleft cysts. *Acta Otolaryngol (Stockh)* 1979;88:289–295.
173. Browder JP, Wheeler MS, Henley JT Jr, et al. Mucoepidermoid carcinoma in a cervical cyst: a case of branchiogenic carcinoma? *Laryngoscope* 1984;94:107–112.
174. Batsakis JG. The pathology of head and neck tumors: the occult primary and metastases to the head and neck, Part 10. *Head Neck Surg* 1981;3:409–423.
175. Micheau C, Klijanienko J, Luboinski B, et al. So-called branchiogenic carcinoma is actually cystic metastases in the neck from a tonsillar primary. *Laryngoscope* 1990;100:878–883.
176. Park SS, Karmody CS. The first branchial cleft carcinoma. *Arch Otolaryngol Head Neck Surg* 1992;118:969–971.
177. Carroll WR, Zappia JJ, McClatchey KD. Branchiogenic carcinoma. *J Otolaryngol* 1993;22:26–28.
178. Thompson LD, Heffner DK. The clinical importance of cystic squamous cell carcinomas in the neck: a study of 136 cases. *Cancer* 1998;82:944–956.
179. Cunningham MJ. The management of congenital neck masses. *Am J Otolaryngol* 1992;13:78–92.
180. Finn DG, Buchalter IH, Sarti E, et al. First branchial cleft cysts: clinical update. *Laryngoscope* 1987:97:136–140.
181. Sichel JY, Halperin D, Dano I, et al. Clinical update on type II first branchial cleft cysts. *Laryngoscope* 1998;108:1524–1527.
182. Hickey SA, Scott GA, Traub P. Defects of the first branchial cleft. *J Laryngol Otol* 1994;108:240–243.
183. Arndal H, Bonding P. First branchial cleft anomaly. *Clin Otolaryngol* 1996;21:203–207.

184. Mounsey RA, Forte V, Friedberg J. First branchial cleft sinuses: an analysis of current management strategies and treatment outcomes. *J Otolaryngol* 1993;22:457–461.
185. Triglia JM, Nicollas R, Ducroz V, et al. First branchial cleft anomalies: a study of 39 cases and a review of the literature. *Arch Otolaryngol Head Neck Surg* 1998;124:291–295.
186. Nofsinger YC, Tom LW, LaRossa D, et al. Periauricular cysts and sinuses. *Laryngoscope* 1997;107:883–887.
187. Atlan G, Egerszegi EP, Brochu P, et al. Cervical chondrocutaneous branchial remnants. *Plast Reconstr Surg* 1997;100:32–39.
188. Edmonds JL, Girod DA, Woodroof JM, et al. Third branchial anomalies. Avoiding recurrences. *Arch Otolaryngol Head Neck Surg* 1997;123:438–441.
189. Lin JN, Wang KL. Persistent third branchial apparatus. *J Pediatr Surg* 1991;26:663–665.
190. Yang C, Cohen J, Everts E, et al. Fourth branchial arch sinus: clinical presentation, diagnostic workup, and surgical treatment. *Laryngoscope* 1999;109:442–446.
191. Murdoch MJ, Culham JA, Stringer DA. Infected fourth branchial pouch sinus with an extensive complicating cervical and mediastinal abscess and left-sided empyema. *Radiographics* 1995;15:1027–1030.
192. Hamoir M, Rombaux P, Cornu AS, et al. Congenital fistula of the fourth branchial pouch. *Eur Arch Otorhinolaryngol* 1998;255: 322–324.
193. Nicollas R, Ducroz NE, Garabedian EN, et al. Fourth branchial pouch anomalies: a study of six cases and review of the literature. *Int J Pediatr Otorhinolaryngol* 1998;44:5–10.
194. Rosenfeld RM, Biller HF. Fourth branchial pouch sinus: diagnosis and treatment. *Otolaryngol Head Neck Surg* 1991;105:44–50.
195. Bar-Ziv J, Slasky BSD, Sichel JY, et al. Branchial pouch sinus tract from the pyriform fossa causing acute suppurative thyroiditis, neck abscess, or both: CT appearance and the use of air as a contrast agent. *AJR* 1996;167:1569–1572.
196. Wyman A, Dunn LK, Talati VR, et al. Lympho-epithelial "branchial" cysts within the parotid gland. *Br J Surg* 1988;75:818–819.
197. Louis DN, Vickery AL Jr, Rosai J, et al. Multiple branchial cleft-like cysts in Hashimoto's thyroiditis. *Am J Surg Pathol* 1989;13:45–49.
198. Ryska A, Vokurka J, Michal M, et al. Intrathyroidal lymphoepithelial cyst. A report of two cases not associated with Hashimoto's thyroiditis. *Pathol Res Pract* 1997;193:777–781.
199. Apel RL, Asa SL, Chalvardjian A, et al. Intrathyroidal lymphoepithelial cysts of probable branchial origin. *Hum Pathol* 1994;25: 1238–1242.
200. Redleaf MI, Walker WP, Alt LP. Parathyroid adenoma associated with a branchial cleft cyst. *Arch Otolaryngol Head Neck Surg* 1995;121: 113–115.
201. Kumara GR, Gillgrass TJ, Bridgman JB. A lymphoepithelial cyst (branchial cyst) in the floor of the mouth. *N Z Dent J* 1995;91:14–15.
202. Chetty R. Branchial cysts in thyroid and parathyroid glands. *Hum Pathol* 1995;26:930.
203. Elliot JN, Oertel YC. Lymphoepithelial cysts of the salivary glands. Histologic and cytologic features. *Am J Clin Pathol* 1990;93:39–43.
204. Mandel L, Reich R. HIV parotid gland lymphoepithelial cysts. Review and case reports. *Oral Surg Oral Med Oral Pathol* 1992;74:273–278.
205. Maiorano E, Favia G, Viale G. Lymphoepithelial cysts of salivary glands: an immunohistochemical study of HIV-related and HIV-unrelated lesions. *Hum Pathol* 1998;29:260–265.
206. Bond SJ, Groff DB. Gastrointestinal duplications. In: O'Neill JA, Rowe MI, Grosfeld JL, et al., eds. *Pediatric surgery,* 5th ed. St. Louis: CV Mosby, 1998:1257–1267.
207. Boue DR, Smith GA, Krous HF. Lingual bronchogenic cyst in a child: an unusual site of presentation. *Pediatr Pathol* 1994;14:201–205.
208. Surana R, Losty P, Fitzgerald RJ. Heterotopic gastric cyst of the tongue in a newborn. *Eur J Pediatr Surg* 1993;3:110–111.
209. Ohbayashi Y, Miyake M, Nagahata S. Gastrointestinal cyst of the tongue: a possible duplication cyst of foregut origin. *J Oral Maxillofac Surg* 1997;55:626–630.
210. Willner A, Feghali J, Bassila M. An enteric duplication cyst occurring in the anterior two-thirds of the tongue. *Int J Pediatr Otorhinolaryngol* 1991;21:169–177.
211. Chen MK, Gross E, Lobe TE. Perinatal management of enteric duplication cysts of the tongue. *Am J Perinatal* 1997;14:161–163.
212. Mir R, Weitz J, Evans J, et al. Oral congenital cystic choristoma: a case report. *Pediatr Pathol* 1992;12:835–838.
213. Lipsett J, Sparnon AL, Byard RW. Embryogenesis of enterocystomas-enteric duplication cysts of the tongue. *Oral Surg Oral Med Oral Pathol* 1993;75:626–630.
214. Civantos FJ, Holinger LD. Laryngoceles and saccular cysts in infants and children. *Arch Otolaryngol Head Neck Surg* 1992;118:296–300.
215. Forte V, Warshawski J, Thorner P, et al. Unusual laryngeal cysts in the newborn. *Int J Pediatr Otorhinolaryngol* 1996;37:261–267.
216. Roback SA, Telander RL. Thyroglossal duct cysts and branchial cleft anomalies. *Semin Pediatr Surg* 1994;3:142–146.
217. Batsakis JG, El-Naggar AK, Luna MA. Thyroid gland ectopias. *Ann Otol Rhinol Laryngol* 1996;105:996–1000.
218. Soucy P, Penning J. The clinical relevance of certain observations on the histology of the thyroglossal tract. *J Pediatr Surg* 1984;19: 506–509.
219. Josephson GD, Spencer WR, Josephson JS. Thyroglossal duct cyst: the New York Eye and Ear Infirmary experience and a literature review. *Ear Nose Throat J* 1998;77:642–651.
220. Radkowski D, Arnold J, Healy GB, et al. Thyroglossal duct remnants. Preoperative evaluation and management. *Arch Otolaryngol Head Neck Surg* 1991;117:1378–1381.
221. Horisawa M, Sasaki J, Niinomi N, et al. Thyroglossal duct remnant penetrating the hyoid bone—a case report. *J Pediatr Surg* 1998; 33:725–726.
222. Sonnino RE, Spigland N, Laberge J-M, et al. Unusual patterns of congenital neck masses in children. *J Pediatr Surg* 1989;24:966–969.
223. deMello DE, Lima JA, Liapis H. Midline cervical cysts in children. *Arch Otolaryngol Head Neck Surg* 1987;113:418–420.
224. Verbin RS, Barnes L. Cysts and cyst-like lesions of the oral cavity, jaws, and neck. In: Barnes L, ed. *Surgical pathology of the head and neck.* New York: Marcel Dekker, 1985:1278–1295.
225. Katz AD, Hachigian M. Thyroglossal duct cysts. A thirty year experience with emphasis on occurrence in older patients. *Am J Surg* 1988;155:741–744.
226. North JH Jr, Foley AM, Hamill RL. Intrathyroid cysts of thyroglossal duct origin. *Am Surg* 1998;64:886–888.
227. Greinwald JH Jr, Leichtman LG, Simko EJ. Hereditary thyroglossal duct cysts. *Arch Otolaryngol Head Neck Surg* 1996;122:1094–1096.
228. Hoffman MA, Schuster SR. Thyroglossal duct remnants in infants and children: reevaluation of histopathology and methods for resection. *Ann Otol Rhinol Laryngol* 1988;97:483–486.
229. Ducic Y, Chou S, Drkulec J, et al. Recurrent thyroglossal duct cysts: a clinical and pathologic analysis. *Int J Pediatr Otorhinolaryngol* 1998;44:47–50.
230. al-Dousary S. Current management of thyroglossal-duct remnant. *J Otolaryngol* 1997;26:259–265.
231. Tovi F, Eyal A. Branched and polycystic thyroglossal duct anomaly. *J Laryngol Otol* 1985;99:1179–1182.
232. Horisawa M, Niinomi N, Ito T. What is the optimal depth for core-out toward the foramen cecum in a thyroglossal duct cyst operation? *J Pediatr Surg* 1992;27:710–713.
233. Tovi J, Barki Y, Maor E. Cartilage within a thyroglossal duct anomaly. *Int J Pediatr Otorhinolaryngol* 1988;15:205–210.
234. Aviel A, Segal M, Ostfeld E, et al. Cholesterol granuloma in a thyroglossal duct cyst. A case report. *J Laryngol Otol* 1983;97:379–381.
235. Yildiz K, Koksal H, Ozoran Y, et al. Papillary carcinoma in a thyroglossal duct remnant with normal thyroid gland. *J Laryngol Otol* 1993;107:1174–1176.
236. Grabowska H. Papillary carcinoma arising from ectopic thyroid gland in the wall of a thyroglossal duct cyst. *Pathol Res Pract* 1993;189: 1228–1232.
237. Tovi F, Fliss DM, Inbar-Yanai I. Hurthle cell adenoma of the thyroglossal duct. *Head Neck Surg* 1988;10:346–349.
238. Heshmati HM, Fatourechi V, van Heerden J, et al. Thyroglossal duct carcinoma: report of 12 cases. *Mayo Clin Proc* 1997;72:315–319.

239. Yoo KS, Chengazi VU, O'Mara RE. Thyroglossal duct cyst with papillary carcinoma in an 11-year-old girl. *J Pediatr Surg* 1998;33:745–746.
240. Tyson RW, Groff DB. An unusual lateral neck cyst with the combined features of a bronchogenic, thyroglossal, and branchial cleft origin. *Pediatr Pathol* 1993;13:567–572.
241. Di Benedetto V. Ectopic thyroid gland in the submandibular region simulating a thyroglossal duct cyst: a case report. *J Pediatr* Surg 1997;32:1745–1746.
242. Urao M, Teitelbaum DH, Miyano T. Lingual thyroglossal duct cyst: a unique surgical approach. *J Pediatr Surg* 1996;31:1574–1576.
243. Samuel M, Freeman NV, Sajwany MJ. Lingual thyroglossal duct cyst presenting in infancy. *J Pediatr Surg* 1993;28:891–893.
244. Dolata J. Thyroglossal duct cyst in the mouth floor: an unusual location. *Otolaryngol Head Neck Surg* 1994;110:580–583.
245. Damiano A, Glickman AB, Rubin JS, et al. Ectopic thyroid tissue presenting as a midline neck mass. *Int J Pediatr Otorhinolaryngol* 1996;34:141–148.
246. Kozol RA, Geelhoed GW, Flynn SD, et al. Management of ectopic thyroid nodules. *Surgery* 1993;114:1103–1107.
247. Sambola-Cabrer I, Fernandez-Real JM, Ricard W, et al. Ectopic thyroid tissue presenting as a submandibular mass. *Head Neck* 1996;18:87–90.
248. Strickland AL, Macfie JA, Van Wyk JJ, et al. Ectopic thyroid glands simulating thyroglossal duct cysts. Hypothyroidism following surgical excision. *JAMA* 1969;208:307–310.
249. De Jong SA, Demeter JG, Jarosz H, et al. Primary papillary thyroid carcinoma presenting as cervical lymphadenopathy: the operative approach to the "lateral aberrant thyroid." *Am Surg* 1993;59:172–176.
250. Rabinov CR, Ward PH, Pusheck T. Evolution and evaluation of lateral cystic neck masses containing thyroid tissue: "lateral aberrant thyroid" revisited. *Am J Otolaryngol* 1996;17:12–15.
251. Watson MG, Birchall JP, Soames JV. Is "lateral aberrant thyroid" always metastatic tumour? *J Laryngol Otol* 1992;106:376–378.
252. Hamilton WJ, Boyd JD, Mossman HW. *Human embryology.* Baltimore: Williams & Wilkins, 1962:220–226.
253. Burton EM, Mercado-Deane MG, Howell CG, et al. Cervical thymic cysts: CT appearance of two cases including a persistent thymopharyngeal duct cyst. *Pediatr Radiol* 1995;25:363–365.
254. Hendrickson M, Azarow K, Ein S, et al. Congenital thymic cysts in children—mostly misdiagnosed. *J Pediatr Surg* 1998;33:821–825.
255. Marra S, Hotaling AJ, Raslan W. Cervical thymic cyst. *Otolaryngol Head Neck Surg* 1995;112:338–340.
256. Miller MB, DeVito MA. Cervical thymic cyst. *Otolaryngol Head Neck Surg* 1995;112:586–588.
257. Lyons TJ, Dickson JAS, Variend S. Cervical thymic cysts. *J Pediatr Surg* 1989;24:241–243.
258. Dano I, Dangoor E, Eliasher R, et al. Thymic cyst mimicking a branchial cleft cyst. *J Otolaryngol* 1998;27:236–237.
259. Reiner M, Beck AR. Cervical thymic cysts in children. *Am J Surg* 1980;139:704–707.
260. Spigland N, Bensoussan AL, Blanchard H, et al. Aberrant cervical thymus in children: three case reports and review of the literature. *J Pediatr Surg* 1990;25:1196–1199.
261. Ozaki O, Sugimoto T, Suzuki A, et al. Cervical thymic cyst as a cause of acute suppurative thyroiditis. *Jpn J Surg* 1990;20:593–596.
262. Kelley DJ, Gerber ME, Willging JP. Cervicomediastinal thymic cysts. *Int J Pediatr Otorhinolaryngol* 1997;39:139–146.
263. Mishalani SH, Lones MA, Said JW. Multilocular thymic cyst. A novel thymic lesion associated with human immunodeficiency virus infection. *Arch Pathol Lab Med* 1995;119:467–470.
264. Shalaby-Rana E, Selby D, Ivy P, et al. Multilocular thymic cyst in a child with acquired immunodeficiency syndrome. *Pediatr Infect Dis J* 1996;15:83–86.
265. Vade A, Griffiths A, Hotaling A, et al. Thymopharyngeal duct cyst: MR imaging of a third branchial arch anomaly in a neonate. *J Magn Reson Imaging* 1994;4:614–616.
266. Zarbo RJ, McClatchey KD, Areen RG, et al. Thymopharyngeal duct cyst: a form of cervical thymus. *Ann Otol Rhinol Laryngol* 1983;92:284–289.
267. Bale PM, Sotelo-Avila C. Maldescent of the thymus: 34 necropsy and 10 surgical cases, including 7 thymuses medial to the mandible. *Pediatr Pathol* 1993;13:181–190.
268. DeLellis RA. *Tumors of the parathyroid gland.* Third series. Washington, DC: Armed Forces Institute of Pathology, 1993:1–10.
269. Rangnekar N, Bailer WJ, Ghani A, et al. Parathyroid cysts. Report of four cases and review of the literature. *Int Surg* 1996;81:412–414.
270. Alvi A, Myssiorek D, Wasserman P. Parathyroid cyst: current diagnostic and management principles. *Head Neck* 1996;18:370–373.
271. Batsakis JG. Heterotopic and accessory salivary tissues. *Ann Otol Rhinol Laryngol* 1986;95:434–435.
272. Cameselle-Teijeiro J, Varela-Duran J. Intrathyroid salivary gland-type tissue in multinodular goiter. *Virchows Arch* 1994;425:331–334.
273. Banerjee AR, Soames JV, Birchall JP, et al. Ectopic salivary gland tissue in the palatine and lingual tonsil. *Int J Pediatr Otorhinolaryngol* 1993;27:159–162.
274. Namdar I, Smoutha EE, Kane P. Salivary gland choristoma of the middle ear: role of intraoperative facial nerve monitoring. *Otolaryngol Head Neck Surg* 1995;112:616–620.
275. Brannon RB, Houston GD, Wampler HW. Gingival salivary gland choristoma. *Oral Surg Oral Med Oral Pathol* 1986;61:185–188.
276. Shinohara M, Harada T, Nakamura S, et al. Heterotopic salivary gland tissue in lymph nodes of the cervical region. *Int J Oral Maxillofac Surg* 1992;21:166–171.
277. Moore PJ, Benjamin BN, Kan AE. Salivary gland choristoma of the middle ear. *Int J Pediatr Otorhinolaryngol* 1984;8:91–95.
278. Joseph MP, Goodman ML, Pilch BZ, et al. Heterotopic cervical salivary gland tissue in a family with probable branchio-otorenal syndrome. *Head Neck Surg* 1986;8:456–462.
279. Ledesma-Montes C, Fernandez-Lopez R, Garces-Ortiz M, et al. Gingival salivary gland choristoma. A case report. *J Periodontal* 1998;69:1164–1166.
280. Lassaletta-Atienza L, Lopez-Rios F, Martin G, et al. Salivary gland heterotopia in the lower neck: a report of five cases. *Int J Pediatr Otorhinolaryngol* 1998;43:153–161.
281. Sevila A, Morell A, Navas J, et al. Orifices at the lower neck: heterotopic salivary glands. *Dermatology* 1997;194:360–361.
282. Hinni ML, Beatty CW. Salivary gland choristoma of the middle ear: report of a case and review of the literature. *Ear Nose Throat J* 1996:75:422–424.
283. Hwang SM, Ahn SK, Lee SH, et al. Heterotopic salivary glands simulating branchial cleft fistula in the lower neck. *J Dermatol* 1996;23:287–289.
284. Anderhuber W, Beham A, Walch C, et al. Choristoma of the middle ear. *Eur Arch Otorhinolaryngol* 1996;253:182–184.
285. Marshall JN, Soo G, Coakley FV. Ectopic salivary gland in the posterior triangle of the neck. *J Laryngol Otol* 1995;109:669–670.
286. Moon WK, Han MH, Kim IO, et al. Congenital fistula from ectopic accessory parotid gland: diagnosis with CT sialography and CT fistulography. *Am J Neuroradiol* 1995;16:997–999.
287. Hiatt JL, Sauk JJ. Embryology and anatomy of the salivary glands. In: Ellis GL, Auclair PL, Gnepp DR, eds. *Surgical pathology of the salivary glands.* Philadelphia: WB Saunders, 1991:2–9.
288. Shvero J, Hadar T, Avidor I, et al. Heterotopic salivary tissue and branchial sinuses. *J Laryngol Otol* 1986;100:243–246.
289. Takimoto T, Kato H. Branchial cleft fistula with heterotopic salivary gland tissue in the lower neck. *J Otorhinolaryngol Rel Spec* 1990;52:265–268.
290. Surana R, Moloney R, Fitzgerald RJ. Tumours of heterotopic salivary tissue in the upper cervical region in children. *Surg Oncol* 1993;2:133–136.
291. Rodgers GK, Felder H, Yunis EJ. Pleomorphic adenoma of cervical heterotopic salivary gland tissue: case report and review of neoplasms arising in cervical heterotopic salivary gland tissue. *Otolaryngol Head Neck Surg* 1991;104:533–536.
292. Evans MG, Rubin SZ. Pleomorphic adenoma arising in a salivary rest in childhood. *J Pediatr Surg* 1991;26:1314–1315.
293. Asai S, Tang X, Ohta Y, et al. Myoepithelial carcinoma in pleomorphic adenoma of salivary gland type, occurring in the mandible of an infant. *Pathol Int* 1995;45:677–683.

294. Tay HL, Howitt RJ. Heterotopic pleomorphic adenoma in the neck. *J Laryngol Otol* 1995;109:445–448.
295. Sinclair-Smith CC, Emms M, Morris HB. Phakomatous choristoma of the lower eyelid. A light and ultrastructural study. *Arch Pathol Lab Med* 1989;113:1175–1177.
296. Eustis HS, Karcioglu ZA, Dharma S, et al. Phakomatous choristoma: clinical, histopathologic, and ultrastructural findings in a 4-month-old boy. *J Pediatr Ophthalmol Strabismus* 1990;27:208–211.
297. Rosenbaum PS, Kress Y, Slamovits TL, Font RL. Phakomatous choristoma of the eyelid. Immunohistochemical and electron microscopic observations. *Ophthalmology* 1992;99:1779–1184.
298. Baggesen LH, Jensen OA. Phakomatous choristoma of lower eyelid. A lenticular anlage tumour. *Ophthalmologica* 1977;175:231–235.
299. Leatherbarrow B, Nerad JA, Carter KD, et al. Phakomatous choristoma of the orbit: a case report. *Br J Ophthalmol* 1992;76:507–508.
300. Zimmerman LE. Phakomatous choristoma of the eyelid, a tumor of lenticular anlage. *Am J Ophthalmol* 1971;71:169–177.
301. Tripathi RC, Tripathi BJ, Ringus J. Phakomatous choristoma of the lower eyelid with psammoma body formation: a light and electron microscopic study. *Ophthalmology* 1981;88:1198–1206.
302. McMahon RT, Font RL, McLean IW. Phakomatous choristoma of eyelid: electron microscopical confirmation of lenticular derivation. *Arch Ophthalmol* 1976;94:1778—1781.
303. Ellis FJ, Eagle RC Jr, Shields JA, et al. Phakomatous choristoma (Zimmerman's tumor). Immunohistochemical confirmation of lens-specific proteins. *Ophthalmology* 1993;100:955–960.
304. Kamada Y, Sakata A, Nakadomari S, et al. Phakomatous choristoma of the eyelid: immunohistochemical observation. *Jpn J Ophthalmol* 1998;42:41–45.
305. Rosai J, Limas C, Husband EM. Ectopic hamartomatous thymoma. A distinctive benign lesion of lower neck. *Am J Surg Pathol* 1984;8:501–513.
306. Mentzel T, Kriegsmann J, Kosmehl H, et al. Ectopic hamartomatous thymoma. Case report with special reference to differential diagnosis. *Pathologe* 1995;16:359–363.
307. Eulderink F, de Graaf PW. Ectopic hamartomatous thymoma located presternally. *Eur J Surg* 1998;164:629–630.
308. Fetsch JF, Weiss SW. Ectopic hamartomatous thymoma: clinicopathologic, immunohistochemical and histogenetic consideration in four new cases. *Hum Pathol* 1990;21:662–668.
309. Saeed IT, Fletcher CD. Ectopic hamartomatous thymoma containing myoid cells. *Histopathology* 1990;17:572–574.
310. Armour A, Williamson JM. Ectopic cervical hamartomatous thymoma showing extensive myoid differentiation. *J Laryngol Otol* 1993;107:155–158.
311. Michal M, Zamecnik M, Gogora M, et al. Pitfalls in the diagnosis of ectopic hamartomatous thymoma. *Histopathology* 1996;29:549–555.
312. Bradford CR, Devaney KO, Lee JI. Spindle epithelial tumor with thymus-like differentiation: a case report and review of the literature. *Otolaryngol Head Neck Surg* 1999;120:603–606.
313. Dorfman DM, Shahsafaei A, Miyauchi A. Intrathyroidal epithelial thymoma (ITET)/carcinoma showing thymus-like differentiation (CASTLE) exhibits CD5 immunoreactivity: new evidence for thymic differentiation. *Histopathology* 1998;32:104–109.
314. Su L, Beals T, Bernacki EG, et al. Spindle epithelial tumor with thymus-like differentiation: a case report with cytologic, histologic, immunohistologic, and ultrastructural findings. *Mod Pathol* 1997;10:510–514.
315. Chetty R, Goetsch S, Nayler S, et al. Spindle epithelial tumor with thymus-like element (SETTLE): the predominantly monophasic variant. *Histopathology* 1998;33:71–74.
316. Hofman P, Mainguene C, Michiels JF, et al. Thyroid spindle epithelial tumor with thymus-like differentiation (the "SETTLE" tumor). An immunohistochemical and electron microscopic study. *Eur Arch Otorhinolaryngol* 1995;252:316–320.
317. Chan JK, Rosai J. Tumors of the neck showing thymic or related branchial pouch differentiation: a unifying concept. *Hum Pathol* 1991;22:349–367.
318. Michal M, Neubauer L, Fakan F. Carcinoma arising in ectopic hamartomatous thymoma. An ultrastructural study. *Pathol Res Pract* 1996;192:610–618.
319. Lack EE. Extragonadal germ cell tumors of the head and neck region: review of 16 cases. *Hum Pathol* 1985;16:56–64.
320. Dehner LP, Mills A, Talerman A, et al. Germ cell neoplasms of head and neck soft tissues: a pathologic spectrum of teratomatous and endodermal sinus tumors. *Hum Pathol* 1990;21:309–318.
321. Kountakis SE, Minotti AM, Maillard A, et al. Teratomas of the head and neck. *Am J Otolaryngol* 1994;15:292–296.
322. April MM, Ward RF, Garelick JM. Diagnosis, management, and follow-up of congenital head and neck teratomas. *Laryngoscope* 1998;108:1398–1401.
323. Ward RF, April M. Teratomas of the head and neck. *Otolaryngol Clin North Am* 1989;22:621–629.
324. Wollner N, Ghavimi F, Wachtel A, et al. Germ cell tumors in children: gonadal and extragonadal. *Med Pediatr Oncol* 1991;19:228–239.
325. Carr MM, Thorner P, Phillips JH. Congenital teratomas of the head and neck. *J Otolaryngol* 1997;26:246–252.
326. Gobel U, Calaminus G, Engert J, et al. Teratomas in infancy and childhood. *Med Pediatr Oncol* 1998;31:8–15.
327. Washburne JF, Magann EF, Chauhan SP, et al. Massive congenital intracranial teratoma with skull rupture at delivery. *Am J Obstet Gynecol* 1995;173:226–228.
328. Naudin ten Cate L, Vermeij-Keers C, Smit DA, et al. Intracranial teratoma with multiple fetuses: pre- and post-natal appearance. *Hum Pathol* 1995;26:804–807.
329. Spinelli HM, Criscuolo GR, Tripps M, et al. Massive orbital teratoma in the newborn. *Ann Plast Surg* 1993;31:453–458.
330. Conran RM, Kent SG, Wargotz ES. Oropharyngeal teratomas: a clinicopathologic study of four cases. *Am J Perinatal* 1993;10:71–75.
331. Forrest AW, Carr SJ, Beckenham EJ. A middle ear teratoma causing acute airway obstruction. *Int J Pediatr Otorhinolaryngol* 1993;25:183–189.
332. Lalwani AK, Engel TL. Teratoma of the tongue: a case report and review of the literature. *Int J Pediatr Otorhinolaryngol* 1992;24:261–268.
333. Rybak LP, Rapp MF, McGrady MD, et al. Obstructing nasopharyngeal teratoma in the neonate. A report of two cases. *Arch Otolaryngol Head Neck Surg* 1991;117:1411–1415.
334. Williams LJ, Yankowitz J, Robinson RA, et al. Nasopharyngeal teratoma. Report of a case with prenatal diagnosis and postnatal management. *J Reprod Med* 1997;42:587–592.
335. Sherer DM, Woods JR Jr, Abramowicz JS, et al. Prenatal sonographic assessment of early, rapidly growing fetal cervical teratoma. *Prenat Diagn* 1993;13:1079–1084.
336. Fearon JA, Munro IR, Bruce DA, et al. Massive teratomas involving the cranial base: treatment and outcome—a two-center report. *Plast Reconstr Surg* 1993;91:223–228.
337. Candan S, Yilkiz K, Mocan H, et al. Nasopharyngeal teratoma as a respiratory emergency in the neonate. *J Otolaryngol* 1991;20:349–352.
338. Uchiyama M, Iwafuchi M, Naitoh S, et al. A huge immature cervical teratoma in a newborn: report of a case. *Surg Today* 1995;25:737–740.
339. Alagappan A, Shattuck KE, Rowe T, et al. Massive intracranial immature teratoma with extracranial extension into oral cavity, nose and neck. *Fetal Diagn Ther* 1998;13:321–324.
340. Smith NM, Chambers SE, Billson R, et al. Oral teratoma (epignathus) with intracranial extension: a report of two cases. *Prenat Diagn* 1993;13:945–952.
341. Raisanen JM, Davis RL. Congenital brain tumors. *Pathology* 1993;2:103–116.
342. Hunt SJ, Johnson PC, Coons SW, et al. Neonatal intracranial teratomas. *Surg Neurol* 1990;34:336–342.
343. Kusumakumari P, Geetha N, Chellam VG, et al. Endodermal sinus tumors in the head and neck region. *Med Pediatr Oncol* 1997;29:303–307.
344. Arezzo A, Gualco M, Bianchi C, et al. Immature malignant teratoma of the thyroid gland. *J Exp Clin Cancer Res* 1998;17:109–112.

345. Stephenson JA, Mayland DM, Kun LE, et al. Malignant germ cell tumors of the head and neck in childhood. *Laryngoscope* 1989;99: 732–735.
346. Byard RW, Jimenez CL, Carpenter BF, et al. Congenital teratomas of the neck and nasopharynx: a clinical and pathological study of 18 cases. *J Paediatr Child Health* 1990;26:12–16.
347. Kerner B, Flaum E, Mathews H, et al. Cervical teratoma: prenatal diagnosis and long-term follow-up. *Prenat Diagn* 1998;18:51–59.
348. Thompson RA, Frommel T, Rosai J, Heffess CS. Primary thyroid teratomas: a clinicopathological study of 30 cases [Abstract 396]. *Mod Pathol* 1999;12:70.
349. Jordan RB, Gauderer MW. Cervical teratomas: an analysis. Literature review and proposed classification. *J Pediatr Surg* 1988;23:583–591.
350. Jaarsma AS, Tamminga RY, de Langen ZJ, et al. Neonatal teratoma presenting as hygroma colli. *Eur J Pediatr* 1994;153:276–278.
351. Rothschild MA, Catalano P, Urken M, et al. Evaluation and management of congenital cervical teratoma. Case report and review. *Arch Otolaryngol Head Neck Surg* 1994;120:444–448.
352. Kuhel WI. Adherence of benign cervical teratomas to surrounding soft tissue. *Arch Otolaryngol Head Neck Surg* 1999;125:236–237.
353. Heifetz SA, Cushing B, Giller R, et al. Immature teratomas in children: pathologic considerations: a report from the combined Pediatric Oncology Group/Children's Cancer Group. *Am J Surg Pathol* 1998;22:1115–1124.
354. Touran T, Applebaum H, Frost DB, et al. Congenital metastatic cervical teratoma: diagnostic and management considerations. *J Pediatr Surg* 1989;24:21–23.
355. Azizkham RG, Haase GM, Applebaum H, et al. Diagnosis, management, and outcome of cervicofacial teratomas in neonates: a Children's Cancer Group study. *J Pediatr Surg* 1995;30:312–316.
356. Marras T, Poenaru D, Kamal I. Perinatal management of nasopharyngeal teratoma. *J Otolaryngol* 1995;24:310–312.
357. Tharrington CL, Bossen EH. Nasopharyngeal teratomas. *Arch Pathol Lab Med* 1992;116:165–167.
358. Uchida K, Urata H, Suzuki H. Teratoma of the tongue in neonates: report of a case and review of the literature. *Pediatr Surg Int* 1998; 14:79–81.
359. Zakaria MA. Epignathus (congenital teratoma of the hard palate): a case report. *Br J Oral Maxillofac Surg* 1986;24:272–276.
360. Valente A, Grant C, Orr JD, et al. Neonatal tonsillar teratoma. *J Pediatr Surg* 1988;23:364–366.
361. Ang AT, Ho NK, Ong CL. Giant epignathus with intracranial teratoma in a newborn infant. *Aust Radiol* 1990;34:358–360.
362. Holmgren G, Rydnert J. Male fetus with epignathus originating from the ethmoidal sinus. *Eur J Obstet Gynecol Reprod Biol* 1987;24:69–72.
363. Jaward AJ, Khattak A, al-Rabeeah A, et al. Congenital nasopharyngeal teratoma in newborn: case report and review of the literature. *Z Kinderchir* 1990;45:375–378.
364. Sciubba JJ, Younai F. Epipalatus: a rare intraoral teratoma. *Oral Surg Oral Med Oral Pathol* 1991;71:476–481.
365. Yapar EG, Ekici E, Gokmen O. Sonographic diagnosis of epignathus (oral teratoma), prosencephaly, meromelia and oligohydramnios in a fetus with trisomy 13. *Clin Dysmorphol* 1995;4:266–271.
366. Byard RW, Smith CR, Chan HS. Endodermal sinus tumor of the nasopharynx and previous mature congenital teratoma. *Pediatr Pathol* 1991;11:297–302.
367. Rescorla FJ, Sawin RS, Coran AG, et al. Long-term outcome for infants and children with sacrococcygeal teratoma: a report from the Children's Cancer Group. *J Pediatr Surg* 1998;33:171–176.
368. Schropp KP, Lobe TE, Rao B, et al. Sacrococcygeal teratoma: the experience of four decades. *J Pediatr Surg* 1992;27:1075–1078.
369. Kivela T, Tarkkanen A. Orbital germ cell tumors revisited: a clinicopathological approach to classification. *Surv Ophthalmol* 1994;38: 541–554.
370. Levin ML, Leone CR Jr, Kincaid MC. Congenital orbital teratomas. *Am J Ophthalmol* 1986;102:476–481.
371. Weiss AH, Greenwald MJ, Margo CE, et al. Primary and secondary orbital teratomas. *J Pediatr Ophthalmol Strabismus* 1989;26:44–49.
372. Kivela T, Merenmies L, Ilveskoski I, et al. Congenital intraocular teratoma. *Ophthalmology* 1993;100:782–791.
373. Bilgic S, Dayanir V, Kiratli H, et al. Congenital orbital teratoma: a clinicopathologic case report. *Ophthalmol Plast Reconstr Surg* 1997;13:142–146.
374. Cannon CR, Johns ME, Fechner RE. Immature teratoma of the larynx. *Otolaryngol Head Neck Surg* 1987;96:366–368.
375. Talmi YP, Sadov R, Dulitzky F, et al. Teratoma of the mastoid region in a newborn. *J Laryngol Otol* 1988;102:1033–1035.
376. Shaheen KW, Cohen SR, Muraszko K, et al. Massive teratoma of the sphenoid sinus in a premature infant. *J Craniofac Surg* 1991;2: 140–145.
377. Rose PE, Howard ER. Congenital teratoma of the submandibular gland. *J Pediatr Surg* 1982;17:414–416.
378. Parnes LS, Sun AH. Teratoma of the middle ear. *J Otolaryngol* 1995;24:165–167.
379. Manivel C, Wick MR, Dehner LP. Transitional (cylindric) cell carcinoma with endodermal sinus tumor-like features of the nasopharynx and paranasal sinuses. Clinicopathologic and immunohistochemical study of two cases. *Arch Pathol Lab Med* 1986;110:198–202.
380. Heffner DK, Hyams VJ. Teatocarcinosarcoma (malignant teratoma?) of the nasal cavity and paranasal sinuses. A clinicopathologic study of 20 cases. *Cancer* 1984;53:2140–2154.
381. Pai SA, Naresh KN, Masih K, et al. Teratocarcinosarcoma of the paranasal sinuses: a clinicopathologic and immunohistochemical study. *Hum Pathol* 1998;29:718–722.
382. Batsakis JG, Mackay B, Ryka AF, et al. Perinatal salivary gland tumours (embryomas). *J Laryngol Otol* 1988;102:1007–1011.
383. Taylor GP. Congenital epithelial tumor of the parotid-sialoblastoma. *Pediatr Pathol* 1988;8:447–452.
384. Batsakis JG, Frankenthaler R. Embryoma (sialoblastoma) of salivary glands. *Ann Otol Rhinol Laryngol* 1992;101:958–960.
385. Harris MD, McKeever P, Robertson JM. Congenital tumours of the salivary gland: a case report and review. *Histopathology* 1990;17: 155–157.
386. Som PA, Brandwein M, Silvers AR, et al. Sialoblastoma (embryoma): MR findings of a rare pediatric salivary gland tumor. *Am J Neuroradiol* 1997;18:847–850.
387. Hsueh C, Gonzalez-Crussi F. Sialoblastoma: a case report and review of the literature on congenital epithelial tumors of salivary gland origin. *Pediatr Pathol* 1992;12:205–214.
388. Bandwein M, Al-Naeif NS, Manwani D, et al. Sialoblastoma: clinicopathological immunohistochemical study. *Am J Surg Pathol* 1999; 23:342–348.
389. Dehner LP, Valbuena L, Perez-Atayde A, et al. Salivary gland anlage tumor ("congenital pleomorphic adenoma"). A clinicopathologic, immunohistochemical and ultrastructural study of nine cases. *Am J Surg Pathol* 1994;18:25–36.
390. Boccon-Gibod LA, Grangeponte MC, Boucheron S, et al. Salivary gland anlage tumor of the nasopharynx: a clinicopathologic and immunohistochemical study of three cases. *Pediatr Pathol Lab Med* 1996;16:973–983.
391. Bondeson L, Anderasson L, Olsson M, et al. Salivary gland anlage tumor: cytologic features in a case examined by fine-needle aspiration. *Diagn Cytopathol* 1997;16:518–521.
392. Michal M, Sokl L, Mukensnabl P. Salivary gland anlage tumor. A case with widespread necrosis and large cyst formation. *Pathology* 1996;28:128–130.
393. Seifert G, Donath K, Jautzke G. Unusual choristoma of the parotid gland in a girl. A possible trichoadenoma. *Virchows Arch* 1999;434: 355–359.
394. Tang TT, Glicklich M, Siegesmund KA, et al. Neonatal cystic choristoma in submandibular salivary gland simulating cystic hygroma. *Arch Pathol Lab Med* 1979;103:536–539.
395. Seifert G. Tumour-like lesions of the salivary glands. The new WHO classification. *Pathol Res Pract* 1992;188:836–846.
396. Smyth AG, Ward-Booth RP, High AS. Polycystic disease of the parotid glands: two familial cases. *Br J Oral Maxillofac Surg* 1993;31: 38–40.
397. Brown E, August M, Pilch BZ, et al. Polycystic disease of the parotid glands. *Am J Neuroradiol* 1995;16:1128–1131.

398. Ortiz-Hidalgo C, Cervantes J, de la Vega G. Unilateral polycystic (dysgenetic) disease of the parotid gland. *South Med J* 1995;88: 1173–1175.
399. Ficarra G, Sapp JP, Christensen RE, et al. Dysgenetic polycystic disease of the parotid gland: report of case. *J Oral Maxillofac Surg* 1996;54:1246–1249.
400. Seifert G, Thomsen S, Donath K. Bilateral dysgenetic polycystic parotid glands. Morphological analysis and differential diagnosis of a rare disease of the salivary gland. *Virchows Arch Pathol Anat* 1981;390: 273–288.
401. Warnock GR, Jensen JL, Kratochvil FJ. Developmental diseases. In: Ellis GL, Auclair PL, Gnepp DR, eds. *Surgical pathology of the salivary gland.* Philadelphia: WB Saunders, 1991:10–25.
402. Seifert G, Donath K. The congenital basal cell adenoma of salivary glands. Contribution to the differential diagnosis of congenital salivary gland tumours. *Virchows Arch* 1997;430:311–319.
403. Tsuda H, Morinaga S, Mukai K, et al. Hamartoma of the parotid gland: a case report with immunohistochemical and electron microscopic study. *Virchows Arch* 1987;411:473–478.
404. Seifert G, Donath K. Juvenile pleomorphic parotid adenoma of embryonal structure. *Pathologe* 1998;19:286–291.
405. Donath K, Seifert G, Lentrodt J. The embryonal carcinoma of the parotid gland. A rare example of an embryonal tumor. *Virchows Arch* 1984;403:425–440.
406. McDermott MB, Ponder TB, Dehner LP. Nasal chondromesenchymal hamartoma. An upper respiratory tract analogue of the chest wall mesenchymal hamartomas. *Am J Surg Pathol* 1998;22:425–433.
407. Kim DW, Low W, Billman G, et al. Chondroid hamartoma presenting as a neonatal nasal mass. *Int J Pediatr Otorhinolaryngol* 1999;15: 253–259.
408. Kuriloff DB. The nasolabial cyst-nasal hamartoma. *Otolaryngol Head Neck Surg* 1987;96:268–272.
409. Kaneko C, Inokuchi A, Kimitsuki T, et al. Huge hamartoma with inverted papilloma in the nasal cavity. *Eur Arch Otorhinolaryngol* 1999;256(suppl):33–37.
410. Wenig BM, Heffner DK. Respiratory epithelial adenomatoid hamartomas of the sinonasal tract and nasopharynx: a clinicopathologic study of 31 cases. *Ann Otol Rhinol Laryngol* 1995;104:639–645.
411. Chisin R, Ragozzino MW, Flexon PB, et al. MR assessment of a hamartoma of the nasal cavity. *AJR* 1989;149:1083–1084.
412. Majumder NK, Venkataramaniah NK, Gupta KR, et al. Hamartoma of nasopharynx. *J Laryngol Otol* 1977;91:723–727.
413. Mahindra S, Bazaz Malik G, Bais AS, et al. Vascular hamartoma of the paranasal sinuses. *Acta Otolaryngol (Stockh)* 1981;92:379–382.
414. Graeme-Cook F, Pilch BZ. Hamartomas of the nose and nasopharynx. *Head Neck* 1992;14:321–327.
415. Zohar Y, Grausbord R, Shabtai F, et al. Fibrous dysplasia and cherubism as an hereditary familial disease. Follow-up of four generations. *J Craniomaxillofac Surg* 1989;17:340–344.
416. Timosca GC. Cherubism: regression of the lesions and spontaneous bone regeneration. *Rev Stomatol Chir Maxillofac* 1996;97:172–177.
417. Peters WJ. Cherubism: a study of twenty cases from one family. *Oral Surg Oral Med Oral Pathol* 1979;47:307–311.
418. Kalantar Motamedi MH. Treatment of cherubism with locally aggressive behavior presenting in adulthood: report of four cases and a proposed new grading system. *J Oral Maxillofac Surg* 1998;56: 1336–1342.
419. Cannon ML, Spiegel RE, Cooley RO. Hereditary fibrous dysplasia of the jaws (cherubism): report of case. *J Dent Child* 1983;50:292–295.
420. Zachariads N, Papanicolaou S, Xypolyta A, et al. Cherubism. *Int J Oral Surg* 1985;14:138–145.
421. Ayoub AF, el-Mofty SS. Cherubism: report of an aggressive case and review of the literature. *J Oral Maxillofac Surg* 1993;51:702–705.
422. Betts NJ, Stewart JC, Fonseca RJ, et al. Multiple central giant cell lesions with a Noonan-like phenotype. *Oral Surg Oral Med Oral Pathol* 1993;76:601–607.
423. van Damme PA, Mooren RE. Differentiation of multiple giant cell lesions, Noonan-like syndrome, and (occult) hyperparathyroidism. Case report and review of the literature. *Int J Oral Maxillofac Surg* 1994;23:32–36.
424. Pina-Neto JM, Moreno AF, Silva LR, et al. Cherubism, gingival fibromatosis, epilepsy, and mental deficiency (Ramon syndrome) with juvenile rheumatoid arthritis. *Am J Med Genet* 1986;25:433–441.
425. Ruggieri M, Pavone V, Polizzi A, et al. Unusual form of recurrent giant cell granuloma of the mandible and lower extremities in a patient with neurofibromatosis type I. *Oral Surg Oral Med Oral Pathol Oral Radiol Endod* 1999;87:67–72.
426. Kaugars GE, Niamtu J 3rd, Svirsky JA. Cherubism: diagnosis, treatment and comparison with central giant cell granulomas and giant cell tumors. *Oral Surg Oral Med Oral Pathol* 1992;73:369–374.
427. Dehner LP. Tumors of the mandible and maxilla in children. I. Clinicopathologic study of 46 histologically benign lesions. *Cancer* 1973;31:364–384.
428. Sato M, Tanaka N, Sato T, et al. Oral and maxillofacial tumours in children: a review. *Br J Oral Maxillofac Surg* 1997;35:92–95.
429. Filston HC. Hemangiomas, cystic hygromas, and teratomas of the head and neck. *Semin Pediatr Surg* 1994;3:147–159.
430. Godin DA, Guarisco JL. Cystic hygromas of the head and neck. *J La State Med Soc* 1997;149:224–228.
431. Stal S, Hamilton S, Spira M. Hemangiomas, lymphangiomas, and vascular malformations of the head and neck. *Otolaryngol Clin North Am* 1986;19:769–796.
432. Premachandra DJ, Milton CM. Childhood haemangiomas of the head and neck. *Clin Otolaryngol* 1991;16:117–123.
433. Brock ME, Smith RJH, Parey SE, et al. Lymphangioma. An otolaryngologic perspective. *Int J Pediatr Otorhinolaryngol* 1987;14: 133–140.
434. Adeyemi SB. Management of cystic hygroma of the head and neck in Lagos, Nigeria; a 10-year experience. *Int J Pediatr Otorhinolaryngol* 1992;23:245–251.
435. Ricciardelli EJ, Richardson MA. Cervicofacial cystic hygroma. Patterns of recurrence and management of the difficult cases. *Arch Otolaryngol Head Neck Surg* 1991;117:546–553.
436. Osborne TE, Haller JA, Levin LS, et al. Submandibular cystic hygroma resembling a plunging ranula in a neonate. Review and report of a case. *Oral Surg Oral Med Oral Pathol* 1991;71:16–20.
437. Goshen S, Ophir D. Cystic hygroma of the parotid gland. *J Laryngol Otol* 1993;107:855–857.
438. Stenson KM, Mishell J, Toriumi DM. Cystic hygroma of the parotid gland. *Ann Otol Rhinol Laryngol* 1991;100:518–520.
439. Descamps P, Jourdain O, Paillet C, et al. Etiology, prognosis and management of nuchal cystic hygroma: 25 new cases and literature review. *Eur J Obstet Gynecol Reprod Biol* 1997;71:3–10.
440. Langer JC, Fitzgerald PG, Desa D, et al. Cervical cystic hygroma in the fetus: clinical spectrum and outcome. *J Pediatr Surg* 1990; 25:58–61.
441. Dehner LP, Enzinger FM, Font RL. Fetal rhabdomyoma. An analysis of nine cases. *Cancer* 1972;30:160–166.
442. Granich MS, Pilch BZ, Nadol JB, et al. Fetal rhabdomyoma of the larynx. *Arch Otolaryngol* 1983;109:821–826.
443. Bozic C. Fetal rhabdomyoma of the parotid gland in an infant: histological, immunohistochemical, and ultrastructural features. *Pediatr Pathol* 1986;6:139–144.
444. Kapadia SB, Meis JM, Frisman DM, et al. Fetal rhabdomyoma of the head and neck: a clinicopathologic and immunophenotypic study of 24 cases. *Hum Pathol* 1993;24:754–765.
445. Gorlin RJ. Nevoid basal-cell carcinoma syndrome. *Medicine (Baltimore)* 1987;66:98–113.
446. Klijanienko J, Caillaud JM, Micheau C, et al. Basal-cell nevomatosis associated with multifocal fetal rhabdomyoma. A case. *Presse Med* 1988;26:2247–2250.
447. Napier SS, Devine JC, Rennie JS, et al. Unusual leiomyomatous hamartoma of the hard palate: a case report. *Oral Surg Oral Med Oral Radiol Endod* 1996;82:305–307.
448. Wexler LH, Helman LJ. Rhabdomyosarcoma and the undifferentiated sarcomas. In: Pizzo PA, Poplack DG, eds. *Principles and practice*

of pediatric oncology, 3rd ed. Philadelphia: Lippincott-Raven, 1997: 799–829.

449. Lyos AT, Goepfert H, Luna MA, et al. Soft tissue sarcoma of the head and neck in children and adolescents. *Cancer* 1996;77:193–200.
450. Brodeur GM, Castleberry RP. Neuroblastoma. In: Pizzo PA, Poplack DG, eds. *Principles and practice of pediatric oncology,* 3rd ed, Philadelphia: Lippincott-Raven, 1997:761–797.
451. Pettinato G, Manivel JC, d'Amore ES, et al. Melanotic neuroectodermal tumor of infancy. A reexamination of a histogenetic problem based on immunohistochemical, flow cytometric, and ultrastructural study of 10 cases. *Am J Surg Pathol* 1991;15:233–245.
452. Kapadia SB, Frisman DM, Hitchcock CL, et al. Melanotic neuroectodermal tumor of infancy. Clinicopathological, immunohistochemical, and flow cytometric study. *Am J Surg Pathol* 1993;17:566–573.
453. Farrugia MK, Fearne C. Benign lipoblastoma arising in the neck. *Pediatr Surg Int* 1998;13:213–214.
454. White FV, Dehner LP, Belchis DA, et al. Congenital disseminated malignant rhabdoid tumor: a distinct clinicopathologic entity demonstrating abnormalities of chromosome 22q11. *Am J Surg Pathol* 1999;23:249–256.
455. Filie AC, Lage JM, Azumi N. Immunoreactivity of S-100 protein, alpha-1-antitrypsin, and CD68 in adult and congenital granular cell tumors. *Mod Pathol* 1996;9:888–892.

2

SQUAMOUS NEOPLASIA OF THE UPPER AERODIGESTIVE TRACT

INTRAEPITHELIAL AND INVASIVE SQUAMOUS CELL CARCINOMA

JOHN D. CRISSMAN
WAEL A. SAKR

EPIDEMIOLOGY

The major carcinogens clinically associated with the development of either intraepithelial or invasive squamous cell carcinoma (SCC) of the mucosa of the upper aerodigestive tract (UADT) include tobacco products, primarily cigarettes and oral tobacco products, and alcoholic beverages (1–3). The relative contributions of these two major groups of carcinogens vary depending on the carcinogen, the history of exposure, and the anatomic site in which the neoplastic transformation occurs. For example, the use of snuff and oral tobacco products invariably leads to extensive field changes in the squamous mucosa of the oral cavity, concentrated in the area of maximum contact with the carcinogen (4,5). Conversely, inhalation of tobacco smoke is a major cause of cancer in the laryngeal glottis, where high concentrations of carcinogens occur (6,7). However, cigarette smoke and alcoholic beverages affect essentially all of the UADT mucosa.

Other carcinogens have been associated with the development of squamous neoplasia in the UADT, including the oral use of betel quid (betel nuts), common in central and southeastern Asia (8). Peculiar cigarette smoking habits such as reverse smoking occurs in India and contributes to a high incidence of oral cancer (9). A great deal of interest in dietary factors and their association with the development of squamous neoplasia in the UADT is reflected in numerous current investigations (10,11). It appears that the most important role of nutrients is in their protective effect in preventing the development of head and neck cancers. Beta carotenes and other similar compounds are also being investigated as factors that result in the prevention of second tumors and as active agents in the reversal of intraepithelial neoplasia (12). The exact role of these various factors and nutrients is not well defined but does appear to involve enhancing the maturation of epithelial cell populations (13). Other putative carcinogens include previous radiation therapy for either benign or malignant diseases in which squamous mucosa in the UADT has been exposed to radiation. Higher incidence of neoplasia in the UADT has been associated with occupational exposure to wood products. The sites most affected by this exposure are the nasal and paranasal sinuses (14). Asbestos fiber inhalation has been well documented as a carcinogen with tobacco smoke in the lower respiratory tract and has been incriminated as an etiologic factor in the development of laryngeal cancer; however, critical analysis of the epidemiologic data does not seem to support the latter hypothesis (15,16). Alcohol-containing mouthwash has been associated with the development of oral cancer (17); however, this claim has not been substantiated, because mouthwash is commonly used to disguise the effects of smoking, alcohol ingestion, or poor oral hygiene, all known contributors to the development of oral cancers (18). Finally, there is a small minority of patients who develop squamous neoplasia with no apparent exposure to the carcinogens outlined above and who appear to have a normal dietary history. Why these patients develop squamous neoplasia of the UADT has not been defined.

As previously outlined, the two major carcinogens associated with UADT neoplasia in North America are tobacco products and alcohol (1–3). The two carcinogens appear to have a strong association with the development of upper aerodigestive cancers and are believed to have a synergistic effect, because when both are used the result is a much higher incidence of neoplasia than when either is used alone (19). Tobacco use in the form of snuff and other oral cavity tobacco products is typically associated with focal dysplastic or reactive changes in the mucosa where maximum contact with tobacco occurs. Although the tobacco-induced mucosal changes are usually most pronounced in the area of maximum contact, epithelial changes can occur throughout the adjacent mucosa (20,21). These mucosal alterations can take a variety of appearances, including leukoplakia or white patches, areas of verrucous or proliferative epithelial changes, and other mucosal alterations, including intraepithelial neoplasia (22). These clinical and histopathologic changes have been better defined recently, and a more detailed discussion of them will be provided in subsequent sections of this chapter. Generally, tobacco-related cancers can involve all sites of the UADT, with the larynx (both the glottis and supraglottic areas) and the hypopharynx being the most frequently affected areas (2,3). The oral cavity, lips, and oropharynx appear to be at lower risk, but tobacco use still results in multiples of relative risk above the nonsmoking population. The association with alcohol is considerably more variable and appears to be extremely sensitive to the amount of alcohol consumption and synergism with the coexisting use of tobacco products. The highest risk appears to be in the supraglottic and epiglottic portions of the larynx, the hypopharynx, and to a lesser extent the oral cavity (23). The association between exposure to these carcinogens and the development of squamous cancer has been the source of considerable epidemiologic study, with the general consensus clearly indicating that the overwhelming majority of cases of squamous neoplasia of the UADT result from exposure to both tobacco and alcohol products. In all instances the heavier the use of these carcinogens, the higher the risk for the subsequent development of squamous neoplasia.

MULTICENTRICITY

Squamous neoplasia of the UADT mucosa primarily results from two carcinogens, tobacco and alcohol. These carcinogens have direct contact with the overwhelming majority of the UADT mucosa. The long-term exposure to these carcinogens (discussed in the previous section) results in extensively damaged mucosa with numerous types of genetic alterations referred to as *field effect.* Although the genetic changes may be similar or different, the anatomic distribution of DNA damage is usually widespread. Not surprisingly, the extensive genetic damage believed to affect wide areas of the mucosal lining may lead to the development of multiple neoplasms. For many years the observation of multiple squamous carcinomas was a curiosity, and only in recent decades has this phenomenon been objectively addressed (24). Simultaneously presenting tumors or a second SCC occurring within 6 months of the initial tumor diagnosis are now recognized as common occurrences. This has resulted in careful endoscopic examination of the UADT in any patient presenting with a "new" cancer. Second neoplasms developing after 6 months of the diagnosis of the first cancer are referred to as metachronous cancers and are now also well recognized as common occurrences. The increased awareness of the high frequency of these second tumors in patients treated for SCC has resulted in the incorporation of efforts to detect them into the posttherapy clinical follow-up. The frequency of the development of second SCCs of the UADT varies, but series with rates of 17% (25), 20.9% (26), and 13% (27) have been reported, and many of the second neoplasms are synchronous: 57% (25), 30% (26), and 25% (27). Not surprisingly, the anatomic sites giving rise to these secondary neoplasms are the mucosa of the UADT, bronchi, and esophagus. The reported frequency of metachronous second neoplasms in the UADT is 33% (25) and 41% (26).

It is accepted that the high frequencies of simultaneous and metachronous SCCs are largely attributable to the extensive and diffuse DNA change created by years of tobacco and/or ethanol exposure, which results in widespread genetic damage or field effect to all of the lower respiratory and the upper digestive tract mucosa. Alcohol also appears to be an important carcinogen in the development of esophageal cancer.

CLINICAL PRESENTATION

Clinical and Gross Appearance of Precursor Mucosal Changes

The specific clinical symptoms and physical findings for neoplasms presenting in the various anatomic sites of the UADT are discussed in the specific chapters for each site. Nevertheless, a number of observations have been made regarding the appearances of premalignant, preinvasive, or intraepithelial neoplasia, and the presentation and appearances of invasive SCC (28). Intraepithelial neoplasia generally takes on two different appearances. One is associated with mucosal or epithelial proliferation leading to the hyperplasia associated with neoplastic transformation. These changes usually result in a thickened whitish appearing hyperkeratotic epithelium, which often gives the appearance of what is called leukoplakia in the oral cavity (29) or keratosis in the larynx (30,31). The epidemiology and clinical correlations of these changes are best documented in the oral cavity and larynx, where there is a variety of information correlating the gross appearance of intraepithelial neoplasia with the corresponding histologic changes. The second major epithelial alteration associated with neoplastic transformation is that of a thin mucosal lining in which immature cell proliferation replaces the full mucosal thickness but usually without hyperplasia of the epithelium (32). The epithelial changes associated with a thin epithelium are generally composed of markedly atypical cells with little cytoplasm or evidence of cell differentiation and with large pleomorphic, hyperchromatic nuclei. These high-grade forms of intraepithelial neoplasia or dysplasia are associated with submucosal inflammation and vascular dilatation or telangiectasis. These changes correlate with a reddish appearance of the mucosa that is fragile and easily traumatized, and they are referred to as erythroplakia or erythroplasia. Invariably, erythroplakic mucosal changes are associated with high-grade intraepithelial neoplasia or carcinoma *in situ* (CIS) and a high frequency of coexisting invasive carcinoma (33).

The gross appearance of intraepithelial neoplasia, however, is not always homogeneous, and it is recognized that speckled or mixed white and red mucosal lesions exist. The recognition of this admixture of mucosal appearances has clarified much of the confusion in the literature with respect to the biologic behavior of the two contrasting mucosal changes. The mucosal alterations of red or erythroplakic mucosa are invariably associated with high-grade intraepithelial neoplasia, CIS, or invasive SCC. White or leukoplakic mucosa is less likely to harbor dysplastic histology and is rarely associated with invasive cancer. It has been recognized that admixtures of these two distinctively different mucosal changes, which have been classified as speckled mucosa, exist (28). It appears that much of the older literature that have indicated a high association between homogeneous white mucosal patches and intraepithelial neoplasia and coexisting or subsequent carcinoma have indeed included the speckled mucosal patterns with white and erythroplakic alterations (Table 1).

Clinical Appearance of Invasive Carcinoma

Early invasive carcinomas may have the gross appearance of either leukoplakic patches or erythroplasia. The frequency of co-

TABLE 1. ORAL CAVITY HISTOLOGY, MUCOSAL APPEARANCE, AND CORRESPONDING HISTORY

Investigator	Reference	No. Patients	Dysplasia/CIS (%)	Invasive Carcinoma (%)
Leukoplakia				
Pindborg, 1963	35	150	5 (3)	1 (1)
Waldron, 1975	38	3,256	566 (17)	104 (3)
Bancozy, 1976	37	500	120 (24)	48 (10)
Mashberg, 1978	33	43	3 (7)	3 (7)
Silverman, 1984	34	107	2 (2)	7 (7)
Speckled				
Pindborg, 1963	35	35	18 (51)	5 (14)
Mashberg, 1978	33	58	6 (10)	33 (57)
Silverman, 1984	34	128	20 (16)	0 (23)
Erythroplakia				
Shafer, 1975	32	65	26 (40)	33 (51)
Mashberg, 1978	33	44	1 (2)	28 (64)

existing malignant transformation is most common in the erythroplakic red mucosal change (33). In general, as SCCs infiltrate and invade the underlying submucosal tissues, the mucosa becomes indurated or firm from the mass effect of the tumorous epithelium and the reactive desmoplasia. This finding is important in the physical examination of the area, because the indurated nodule is the most likely site to yield invasive cancer in a biopsy. As invasive neoplasia progresses and invades deeper into underlying tissues, ulceration commonly occurs. This is more apt to happen in advanced higher stage cancers and invasive carcinomas arising in thin, erythroplakic lesions. Induration and ulceration invariably should lead to a high degree of suspicion for invasive carcinoma, particularly with the mucosal changes described above. Invasive carcinomas arising in leukoplakic, hyperplastic epithelial mucosa often develop from the basal and suprabasal portions of the thick epithelium, especially in early or microinvasive SCC. These early or microinvasive cancers arising from the basal or suprabasal regions of high-grade squamous intraepithelial neoplasia (SIN) are often called "drop-off" neoplasms (28,34). The majority of the lining epithelium does not have the changes of SCC, but only the lower levels, giving the impression that the malignant tumors dropped off of the epithelium. This peculiar growth pattern makes it difficult to recognize and diagnose early cancer in hyperplastic white lesions by physical examination.

HISTOLOGIC FEATURES OF SQUAMOUS INTRAEPITHELIAL NEOPLASIA

When characterizing the microscopic changes associated with SIN, it is useful to contrast them with the histology of normal squamous epithelium. The latter has a matrix or mosaic type of nuclear pattern with increasing separation of the nuclei as increasing amounts of cytoplasm form during the cells' migration toward the surface. The increasing cytoplasm is due to accumulation of cytokeratin and normally is associated with smaller pyknotic nuclei or disorganized and fragmented nuclei (karyorrhexis). The basal cell layer—composed of cells with round nuclei and scant cytoplasm, and hence a high nuclear:cytoplasmic ratio—is thin in normal squamous mucosa, only a few cell layers in thickness (Fig. 1). The histologic characteristics of dysplasia or SIN represent a spectrum of features that vary from the thin atrophic erythroplakic change to the hyperplastic leukoplakic appearance (35–38). In their pure form, these two ends of the spectrum of SIN correlate with the gross mucosal changes discussed in the previous section on clinical appearance. Although the two ends of the histologic spectrum are easily defined, the majority of SIN cases encountered are represented by overlapping histologic changes. This unfortunately complicates the histologic definitions of SIN and represents the major obstacle in developing a simple definition of SIN in the UADT, where mixtures of these two histologic extremes are encountered.

The following histologic observations are extremely valuable in sorting out the complex observations in defining SIN.

1. Presence or absence of hyperplasia. Most changes of SIN, with the exception of pure erythroplakia, are preceded or accompanied by some degree of epithelial hyperplasia. This depends to some extent on the anatomic site, because the dor-

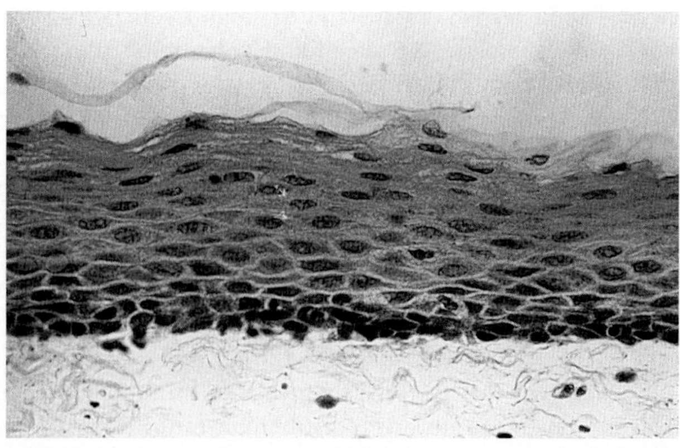

FIGURE 1. Normal, maturing squamous epithelium. There is a matrix or mosaic type of nuclear pattern with increasing separation of the nuclei as increasing amounts of cytoplasm form during cell migration toward the surface. The increasing cytoplasm is due to accumulation of cytokeratin and normally is associated with smaller pyknotic nuclei or disorganized and fragmented nuclei.

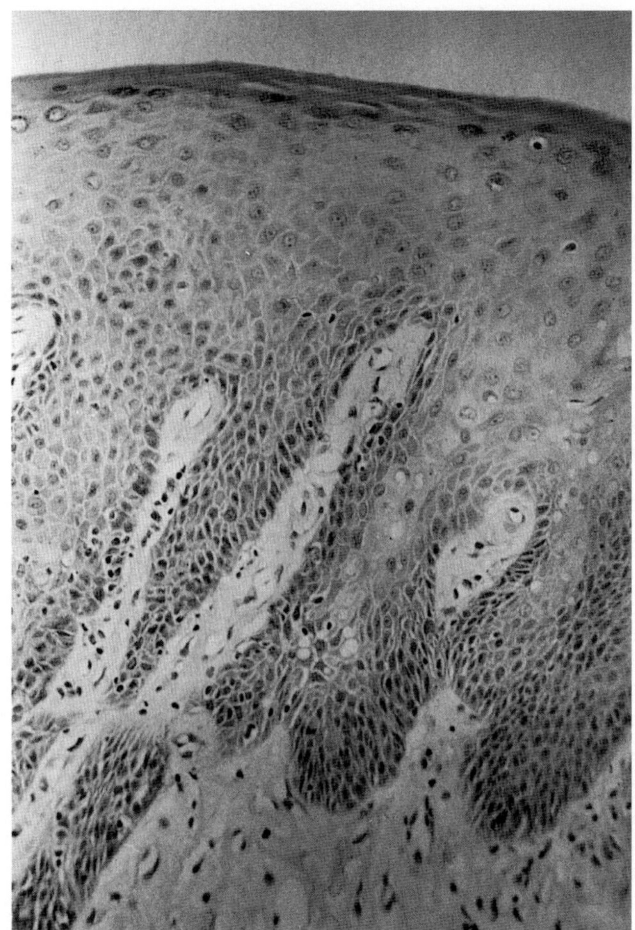

FIGURE 2. Hyperplasia can represent the earliest changes of squamous intraepithelial neoplasia. This benign, mature squamous lining shows increased thickness of the basal cell layer with elongated, sometimes anastomosing rete ridges.

sal tongue and alveolar and buccal mucosa have normally thick mucosa when compared with other sites (Fig. 2).

2. Distribution and abnormalities in nuclei. Basal cells have regular round nuclei with little cytoplasm and are referred to as immature or reserve cells. Normal maturation results in separation of nuclei as the cytoplasmic volume increases. Pyknosis, flattening, and eventual loss of the nuclei occur as surface cytoplasmic keratin develops in the process of surface maturation. The proliferation of immature or (more seriously) hyperchromatic pleomorphic nuclei into suprabasal and intermediate regions represents intraepithelial neoplastic transformation (Fig. 3).
3. Cytoplasmic keratin formation in the course of surface maturation is normal in hyperplasia and normally starts to predominate in the upper intermediate layers with loss of nuclei and extensive keratinization in the superficial layers. The premature keratinization of individual cells (dyskeratosis), groups of cells (pearl formation), or diffuse development of cytoplasmic keratin in the depths of the epithelium is abnormal and also indicative of SIN (Fig. 4).

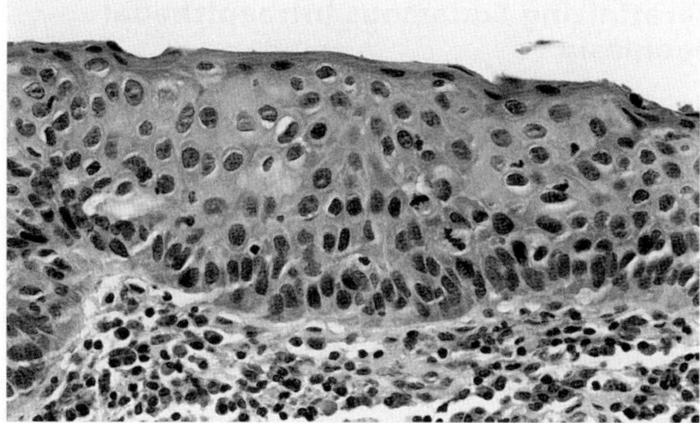

FIGURE 3. Nuclear abnormalities are a sign of squamous intraepithelial neoplasia. The presence of immature or hyperchromatic pleomorphic nuclei in the suprabasal and upper layers of the lining such as depicted here is believed to indicate a neoplastic intraepithelial transformation.

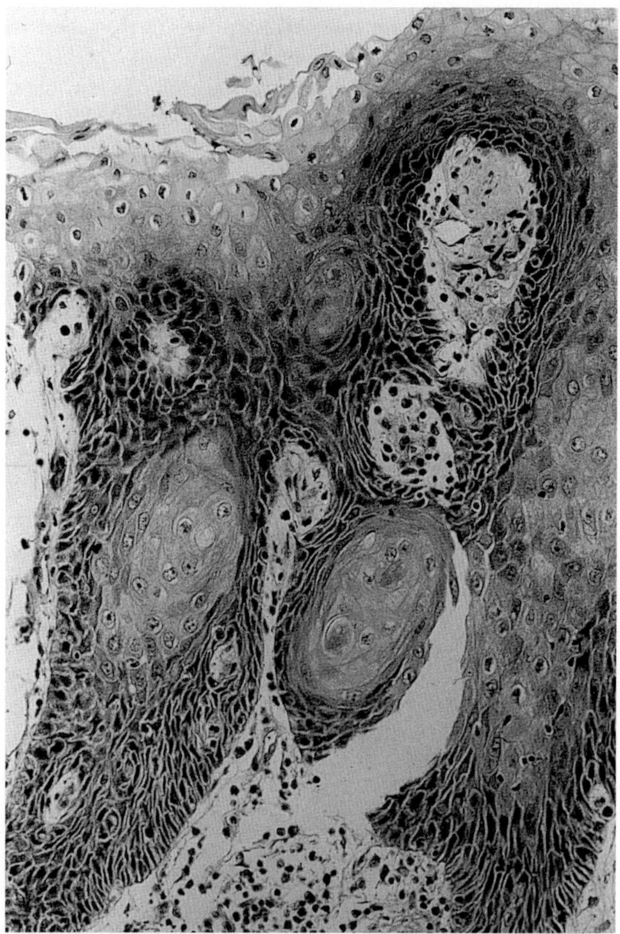

FIGURE 4. Abnormal intraepithelial cytoplasmic keratin formation is another sign of squamous intraepithelial neoplasia. Premature keratinization of individual cells (dyskeratosis), or of groups of cells (pearl formation) or diffuse development of cytoplasmic keratin in the depths of the epithelium is also indicative of intraepithelial transformation toward neoplasia.

Keratinizing Squamous Intraepithelial Neoplasia

Neoplastic transformation with hyperplasia results in a thickened mucosa, usually with evidence of surface maturation as expressed by extensive cytoplasmic keratinization. As mentioned before, this leads to the whitish gross appearance of these mucosal changes. Assessment of SIN in thickened mucosa depends on the degree of epithelial atypia (nuclear and cytoplasmic), which is prominent in the middle portions of the epithelium (34–37). The major controversy in grading epithelial changes in the UADT has been the result of applying criteria used to grade intraepithelial neoplasia in the uterine cervix, which is based on assessing the extent of immature cells found in the epithelium. However, it has been our experience that the presence of surface keratinization in hyperplastic SIN is common, and that evidence of surface maturation does not preclude a diagnosis of high-grade SIN (28,31). The most important feature is the degree of epithelial and cytologic changes in the lower two thirds of the mucosa (Fig. 5). Significant nuclear changes as characterized by nuclear hyperchromatism and pleomorphism in the suprabasal or intermediate epithelium and the distribution of nuclei within the mucosa are important parameters. Loss of the orderly mosaic nuclear distribution is also a significant alteration. The loss of the orderly mosaic pattern is clearly a sign of disordered or dysplastic growth. Conversely, the premature or early keratinization of cells in the lower levels of the epithelium is also a serious change (39,40). The presence of diffuse keratinization with or without nuclear changes is a serious form of intraepithelial neoplastic growth. Hellquist in 1981 (31) identified 12 cases of "well differentiated" severe dysplasia in which four patients progressed to invasive cancer and two patients developed recurrences. In reviewing the photomicrographs, "well differentiated" referred to prominent epithelial and surface keratinization. Other evidence that supports the serious nature of extensive epithelial keratinization is in the six examples of "moderate dysplasia" that we reported (41). DNA analyses of all six lesions revealed an aneuploid DNA content, which is a sign of neoplastic transformation. This maturation alteration clearly represents a serious form (high-grade) SIN and is not commonly recognized by the diagnostic surgical pathology community. In addition, when these changes are diffuse (i.e., involve all or most of a vocal cord), they constitute an ominous prognostic factor in which recurrence and progression to invasive SCC are more common (28,31,42).

Nonkeratinizing Squamous Intraepithelial Neoplasia

Intraepithelial neoplasia involving thin atrophic epithelium is characterized by a gross erythematous or red appearance (32,33). The mucosa is relatively thin and demonstrates little or no evidence of surface maturation. The histologic changes are more akin to the classic intraepithelial neoplastic alterations well described in the uterine cervix. Proliferation of small immature cells often with pleomorphic and hyperchromatic nuclei with little or no cytoplasm extending into the middle and upper epithelium are characteristic of this form of SIN (Fig. 6). In many instances, the immature pleomorphic cells may replace the entire thin epithelium, similar to classic CIS of the uterine cervix. One or two cell layers of surface keratinization should not preclude a diagnosis of high-grade SIN in the UADT.

Speckled mucosal change is not uncommon and is characterized by thickened hyperkeratotic epithelium with focal areas of epithelial atrophy, with little evidence of cell maturation in the focally thinned mucosa. The distinct histologic components account for the red and white speckled areas observed grossly. There has been considerable controversy in the literature as to

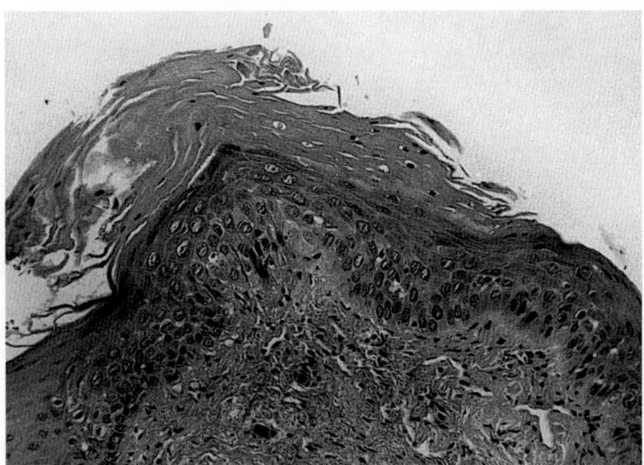

FIGURE 5. Keratinizing squamous intraepithelial neoplasia (SIN). Although most mucosal lesions appearing grossly as leukoplakia translate into benign, maturing epithelium, some represent keratinizing SIN. The degree of epithelial and cytologic changes in the lower half of the lining is the important factor in determining whether the lesion is a low-grade tumor as illustrated or a high-grade SIN with more significant changes.

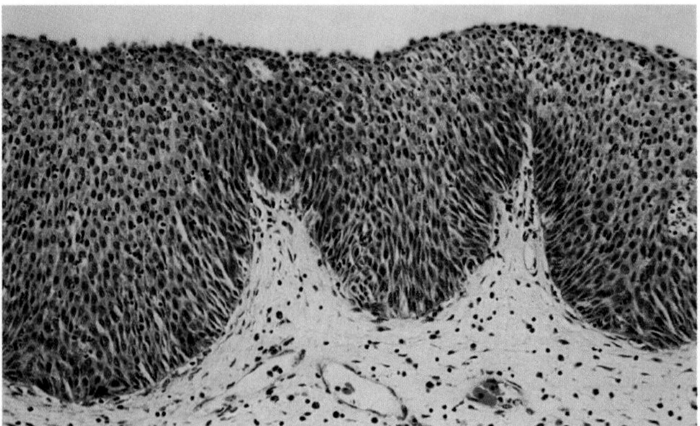

FIGURE 6. Nonkeratinizing squamous intraepithelial neoplasia. This form of intraepithelial neoplasia most often represents the microscopic translation of the gross lesion of erythroplakia. There is proliferation of small immature cells often with pleomorphic and hyperchromatic nuclei with little or no cytoplasm extending into the middle and upper layers of the epithelium. The appearance depicted here would correspond to the classic carcinoma in situ as described in the uterine cervix.

the propensity of leukoplakic patches without SIN to progress to invasive carcinoma. Much of the early literature observed a relatively high frequency of progression to invasive carcinoma that has not been observed when strict histologic criteria are used to establish the presence and the grade of the intraepithelial neoplastic change. It is our interpretation that many of these early studies that were grossly described as leukoplakic were lesions in which a speckled component representing the more ominous erythroplakic changes was present. This resulted in the erroneous opinion that leukoplakia had a high predisposition to the development of invasive cancer.

A more recently recognized form of intraepithelial neoplasia is that of verrucous change, which has been referred to as verrucous hyperplasia and more recently considered under the category of proliferative verrucous leukoplakia (39,43,44). In these mucosal changes the hyperplasia and thickening of the epithelium becomes extensive, with protrusion above the adjacent epithelium forming papillary projections resulting in a verrucoid or warty appearance. These forms of proliferative verrucous hyperplasia have a higher frequency of progression to invasive carcinoma than simple leukoplakia (39,40,43–45). One of the compounding issues in the evaluation and diagnosis of proliferative verrucous lesions is that one must surgically excise the exophytic raised mucosal lesion and examine it histologically to ensure that submucosal invasion by focal SCC has not occurred (40). This indicates that proliferative verrucous lesions need to be examined histologically to include (or exclude) the presence of submucosal invasion (verrucous carcinoma or a focus of invasive SCC). In addition, proliferative verrucous lesions commonly occur in mucosa with field effect genetic injuries that may harbor multiple foci of epithelial SIN or invasive carcinomas (40,45). Clearly proliferative verrucous lesions are commonly associated with separate synchronous and subsequent invasive cancers requiring careful patient evaluation and follow-up.

HISTOLOGIC GRADING OF SQUAMOUS INTRAEPITHELIAL NEOPLASIA

Our original studies defining SIN in the UADT used three grades analogous to the system then in place for the grading of uterine cervical dysplasia (28,30,39). Subsequently, we have elected to use a two-grade classification for SIN—high and low grade—to simplify a complex continuum of intraepithelial neoplastic transformation. However, we still recommend the use of the term *epithelial keratinizing hyperplasia without atypia or dysplasia.* This category is important for recognizing that reactive hyperplasia of the UADT mucosa is common and needs to be classified as such. Reactive keratinizing hyperplasia can be secondary to a number of reversible stimuli or alternatively to irreversible neoplastic influences. Only when significant atypia or dysplasia is identified can an unequivocal diagnosis of neoplastic transformation (SIN) be entertained and then graded to predict the risk for persistence and progression. The two-grade approach to classifying intraepithelial neoplasia is developing popularity and has been adopted for intraepithelial neoplasia of the uterine cervix, gastrointestinal tract, and prostate. It is our impression that simplifying the grading does not detract from signifying the biologic potential of the epithelial change. Low-grade lesions represent a neoplastic change but with low or minimal biologic consequences. In contrast, high-grade changes signify serious epithelial alterations that have a significant probability of progressing to invasive cancer. Having one major dividing line to separate complex histologic changes also simplifies the histologic grading and hopefully makes it more reproducible. In addition, we have deemphasized the diagnosis of CIS, because it only complicates the diagnostic schema for keratinizing proliferative SIN and does not have a more ominous prognosis than high-grade SIN. However, in our opinion, the diagnosis of CIS is still appropriate for the thin erythroplakic mucosa composed of immature and pleomorphic nuclei. We support this opinion because of the histologic appearance of the epithelial change and the high association of this specific histologic change with coexisting invasive cancer. Therefore, we believe that the diagnosis of CIS should be reserved for this specific nonkeratinizing epithelial change.

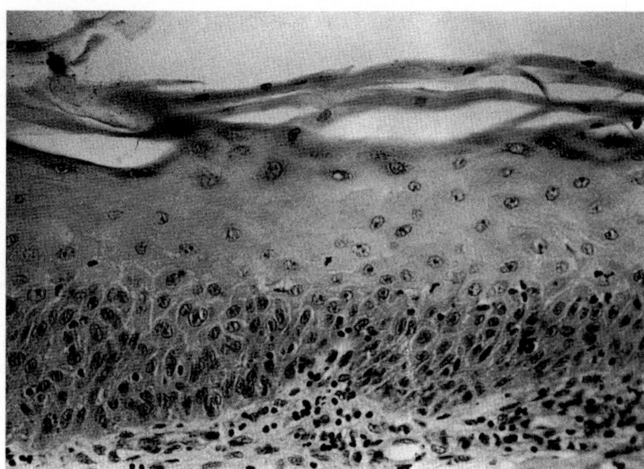

FIGURE 7. Low-grade squamous intraepithelial neoplasia. When the proliferation of basal-like or atypical cells remains limited to the lower half of the epithelium, the process is classified as low grade. The severity of intraepithelial neoplastic transformation can vary in both keratinizing and nonkeratinizing squamous intraepithelial neoplasia.

The separation of low- and high-grade SIN remains problematic. Proliferation of small regular basal-like cells limited to the lower half of the epithelium is classified as low grade. Similarly, widely separated, slightly enlarged nuclei in the keratinized surface layers of the upper half of the epithelium also are classified as low-grade SIN (Fig. 7). The major dividing line for high-grade SIN is the extension of the proliferation of the immature cells into the upper half of the epithelium, especially when nuclear crowding, pleomorphism, and hyperchromaticity are present (Fig. 8). The finding of diffuse cytoplasmic keratinization in the lower depths of a heavily keratinized epithelium, especially with coexisting nuclear enlargement, pleomorphism, and hyperchromatism, also signifies high-grade SIN (Tables 2–4).

TABLE 2. MICROSCOPIC FEATURES OF LOW- AND HIGH-GRADE SQUAMOUS INTRAEPITHELIAL NEOPLASIA

	Low-Grade Dysplasia/SIN	High-Grade Dysplasia/SIN
Atrophic (erythroplasia) mucosa	Hyperchromatic nuclei confined to basal or suprabasal areas	Hyperchromatic pleomorphic nuclei, all levels
	Evidence of cytoplasmic keratin (maturation in upper half)	Little or no evidence cytologic keratin
	Rare change	Common in erythroplasia
Intermediate	Minimal hyperchromasia and pleomorphism, usually lower epithelium; may have enlarged nuclei extending into upper epithelium	Pronounced nuclear pleomorphism and hyperchromasia in lower and middle epithelium, loss of orderly (mosaic) pattern
	Evidence of cytoplasmic keratinization or maturation in upper epithelium, occasional focal premature keratinization in lower epithelium	Superficial cytoplasmic keratin with maturation; keratinization may be pronounced and extend into middle and lower epithelium
Hyperplastic	Mild nuclear hyperchromatism and pleomorphism in basal and suprabasal regions; abnormal nuclei extending into middle epithelium	Marked nuclear pleomorphism and hyperchromasia, usually confined to lower epithelium; loss of orderly (mosaic) pattern, mitoses prominent
	Marked prominent upper and middle epithelial keratinization (maturation), often with hyperkeratosis with or without parakeratosis (often with enlarged nuclei)	Superficial keratin or maturation prominent with or without abnormal nuclei extending into areas of keratosis (abnormal parakeratosis); keratinization may be extensive, extending into lower epithelium, often with less nuclear abnormality

SIN, squamous intraepithelial neoplasia.

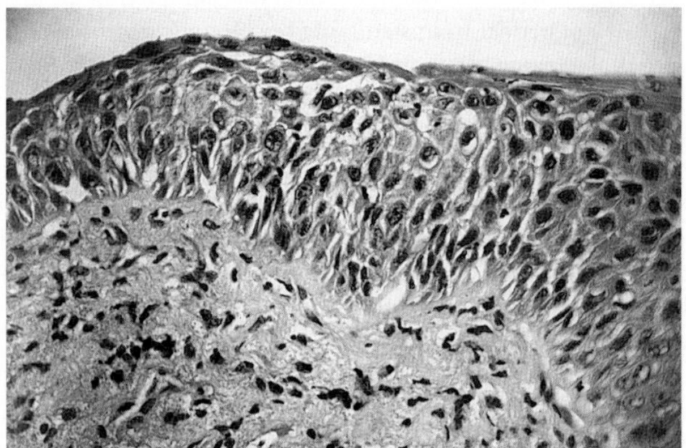

FIGURE 8. High-grade squamous intraepithelial neoplasia (SIN). More than half of the thickness of the squamous lining exhibits the nuclear or cytoplasmic abnormalities characteristic of SIN. The degree of these changes qualifies for high-grade SIN.

TABLE 3. HISTOLOGIC DYSPLASIA/SIN IN THE LARYNX AND FREQUENCY OF SUBSEQUENT INVASIVE CARCINOMA

	No. Patients	No. Cancers
Keratosis with or without slight atypia	362	5
Keratosis with moderate atypia	230	31
Keratosis with severe atypia/CIS	367	42

SIN, squamous intraepithelial neoplasia; CIS, carcinoma in situ.

TABLE 4. HISTOLOGIC GRADING OF DYSPLASIA/SIN OF THE UPPER AERODIGESTIVE TRACT

Hyperplasia without dysplasia	A thickened hyperplastic mucosa with normal maturation; immature cells confined to basal/suprabasal regions and surface keratinization
Dysplasia/SIN (low grade)	Invariably a hyperplastic mucosa with proliferation of "immature" basal cells into the lower and middle of the epithelium; little nuclear pleomorphism but commonly results in large nuclei found in superficial keratinized epithelium; may have thickened or minimal superficial keratinized layer
Hyperplastic dysplasia/SIN (high grade)	Generally hyperplastic epithelium with superficial keratinization; proliferation of "immature" basal cells into middle and occasionally upper layers; significant nuclear pleomorphism and hyperchromaticity; mitoses may be identified; hyperplastic epithelium invariably has some keratinization, which may be prominent; in some instances keratinization extends from the surface to the middle and lower epithelial zones, which may involve individual cells or cell groups, or be diffuse; all are evidence of disordered maturation, and the diffuse form may not have appreciable nuclear abnormalities
Atrophic (thin) dysplasia/SIN (high grade)	Comparable to "classic" CIS with little or no surface keratinization; most or all of the epithelium is replaced by "immature" basal cells, usually with some nuclear pleomorphism and hyperchromicity, this may be referred to as CIS in the old and current literature

SIN, squamous intraepithelial neoplasia; CIS, carcinoma in situ.

HISTOLOGIC FEATURES OF INVASIVE SQUAMOUS CELL CARCINOMA

Microinvasive Carcinoma

The concept of microinvasive carcinoma has not been well defined. This has resulted in less frequent diagnosis of this phase of squamous neoplasia, which represents, in our opinion, a real entity that does occur with some frequency in the UADT (28,46). The two most common problems in making this diagnosis are (a) careful histologic evaluation with properly oriented tissue sections to establish the presence of microinvasive foci and (b) the presence of normal submucosal tissue surrounding the invasive SCC, allowing assessment of the limits of the focus of microinvasive cancer. Quantifying the extent of the invasive SCC remains a problem, because there is little consensus on what constitutes microinvasion in contrast to invasive SCC not otherwise specified (NOS). This is often the case in hyperplastic keratinized forms of intraepithelial neoplasia in which the dysplasia is primarily found in the depths of the mucosa and small drop-off tumors are encountered (Fig. 9). The reference point for measurement of the extent of invasion should be the basement membrane, due to the great variation in epithelial thickness. This would seem to preclude measuring from the epithelial surface. The basement membrane, or basal lamina separating the epithelium from the underlying submucosal tissue, often becomes attenuated, and the epithelial–stromal interface blurred as intraepithelial neoplasia progresses to high-grade SIN (47). The first sign of invasive carcinoma occurs when this barrier, fully intact or attenuated, is broached by the invasive cells as they invade the underlying submucosa (Fig. 10). This change can be either broad based, characteristic of verrucous carcinoma, or it can manifest as focal infiltrative tongues or cords of neoplastic cells invading the underlying stroma. In the latter case, the recognition of invasive carcinoma is usually not difficult. Helpful histologic features suggesting that neoplastic cells have indeed penetrated the stroma include the presence of a reactive or desmoplastic stroma and the juxtaposition of large keratinized cells with stroma without the interposition of a layer of basaloid cells.

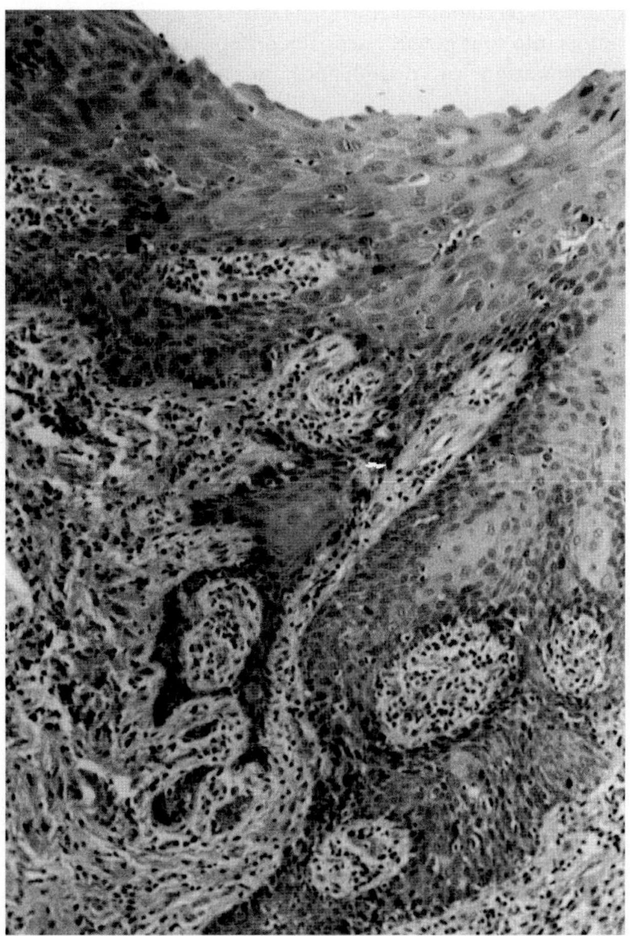

FIGURE 9. Drop-off tumors. These morphologic changes characterize areas of hyperplastic, usually keratinizing intraepithelial neoplasia in which the most severe changes of squamous intraepithelial neoplasia are primarily found in the depths of the mucosa. These often are associated with protrusion or extension of the neoplastic cells into the underlying stroma, representing microinvasion.

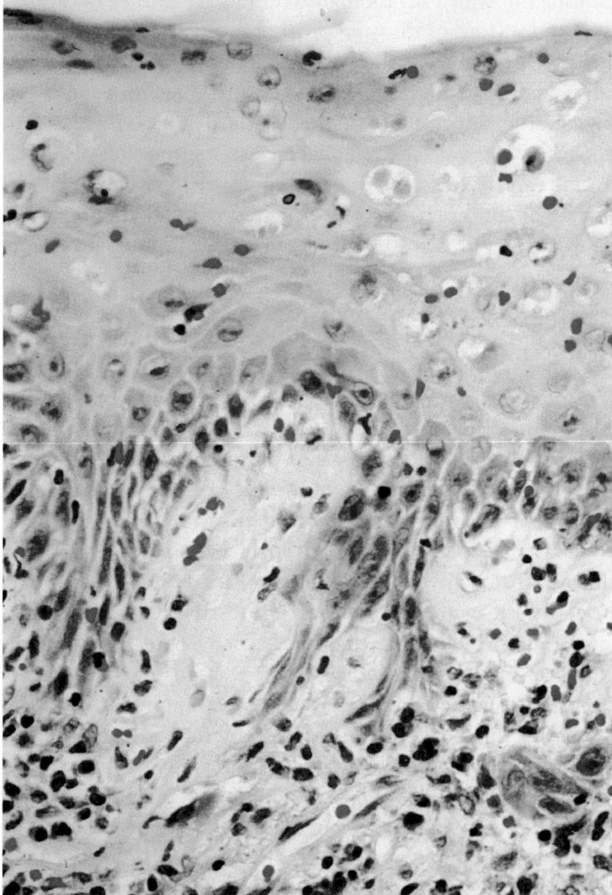

FIGURE 10. Microinvasive squamous cell carcinoma. Attenuation of the basement membrane that separates the epithelium from the underlying submucosal tissue and blurring of the epithelial–stromal interface constitute the first signs of invasiveness developing from intraepithelial neoplasia. Tumors limited to 2 mm from the basement membrane are considered microinvasive.

The separation of microinvasive from invasive SCC NOS is not well established. The best quantitative data defining microinvasive SCC have been described in cancers of the floor of the mouth in which 2 mm of invasion appears to be the dividing line for depths of invasion. There appears to be little or no metastatic potential for invasive carcinomas penetrating less than 2.0 mm and a substantially higher risk of metastases associated with more deeply invasive cancers in this site (46,48,49). The other site in which microinvasive carcinoma has been a topic of interest is in the laryngeal glottis. Early invasive carcinoma can occur in this site, although it is often difficult to diagnose because of the biopsy orientation. It is difficult to confirm that the only focus of invasion is restricted to 2 mm in thickness in many of the small randomly oriented biopsies characteristic of endoscopically generated biopsies. Therefore, the diagnosis of microinvasive carcinoma has to be established with a great deal of care, with the understanding that the specimen must be properly oriented and deeper levels obtained to account for any tangential sites of invasion deeper than the 2 mm, which seems to be the consensus for defining microinvasive cancers. In 1980 we published a study of floor of the mouth SCC in which significant vertical growth or tumor invasion was associated with a high rate of regional lymph node metastases (46). Since then, additional studies have been published in which invasion greater than 1.5 mm (48), 2.0 mm (49), and 4.0 mm (50) were predictive of either decreased survival or an increase in regional lymph node metastases. Subsequently we measured the depth of tumor invasion in our original study (46) and found that tumors with less than 2.0 mm of invasion did not have regional metastases (unpublished data). Overall, we feel that an isolated focus of invasive SCC with tongues or cords of tumor cells penetrating less than 2 mm from the existing epithelial stromal interface, in a properly orientated tissue section, meets the definition of microinvasion.

The pushing margins of invasion are a much more difficult process to evaluate, and many of the hyperplastic forms of intraepithelial neoplasia appear to have some pushing of the epithelial border into the submucosa. However, when the epithelial–submucosal interface is so well defined that a basal lamina appears to be present, one must assess the possibility of invasion with pushing borders with a great deal of caution. Perhaps the most classic example of this process is in verrucous carcinoma, in which the neoplastic proliferation grows in both directions (downward and upward), forming papillary projections above the surface of the epithelium, and the broad-based invasive components that are extremely well differentiated have easily delineated epithelial–submucosal borders. These well-documented borders must have penetrated into the submucosa impinging on or destroying normal structures in order to entertain a diagnosis of tumor invasion. It is our opinion that a conservative approach is appropriate when addressing the question of early invasion in epithelial proliferations with pushing borders. One of the reasons for assuming a conservative stance is that these well-defined pushing borders are incapable of penetrating blood or lymphatic capillaries, which is a requirement for the development of metastases.

Grading of Squamous Cell Carcinomas

Histologic grading of SCCs should ideally be an objective process. Quantitative criteria for grading have been described but not well delineated. The presence or absence of keratinization was the major criterion initially described by Broder in grading squamous carcinoma of the lip (51). Broder originally classified tumors into four grades essentially determined by the degree of differentiation or resemblance to the tissue of origin. Subsequently the majority of pathologists have simplified Broder's four grades into three groups: well-, moderately, and poorly differentiated tumors. The general histologic criteria for this classification are based on keratin formation and the degree of nuclear pleomorphism and chromatism. Neoplasms with abundant keratinization, often with keratin pearl formation in the central portions of the invading neoplasm, have nuclear changes that tend to be better differentiated or low grade (Fig. 11). The nonkeratinizing forms often have a high degree of nuclear pleomorphism, usually with a scanty amount of cytoplasm. These neoplasms are considered poorly differentiated or high-grade SCC (Fig. 12). The intermediate grades represent the tumors that are intermediate or share features or have a spectrum

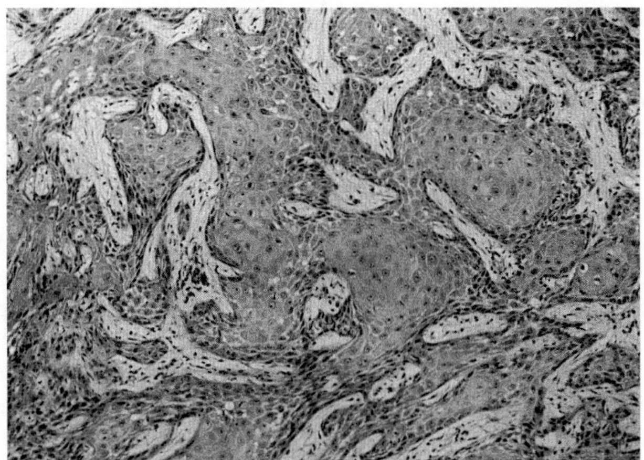

FIGURE 11. Low-grade, well-differentiated squamous cell carcinoma combines a cohesive growth pattern with larger tumor nests, lower nuclear grade, and often variable degrees of keratinization.

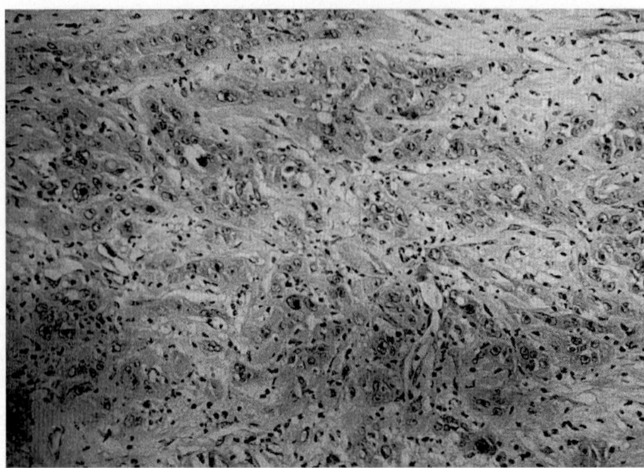

FIGURE 12. High-grade, poorly differentiated squamous cell carcinoma is characterized by a disassociated growth with invasion by smaller nests, clusters, and individual cells that have markedly abnormal nuclei, usually with minimal keratin.

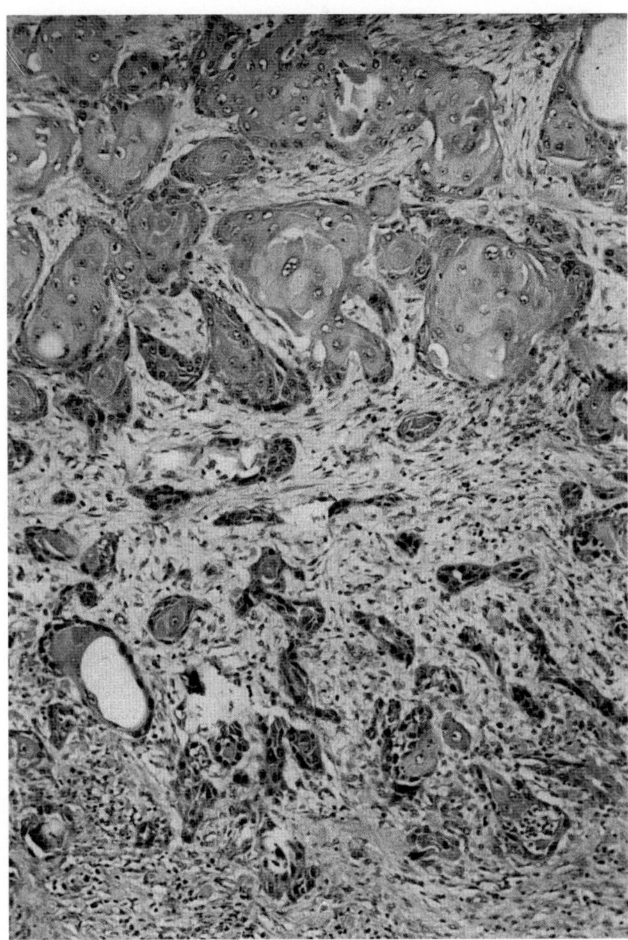

FIGURE 13. Intermediate grade squamous cell carcinoma shares features of both ends of the differentiation spectrum. This photomicrograph shows larger, keratinizing tumor nests adjacent to remarkably less differentiated, infiltrative squamous cell carcinoma.

of overlapping features of the low- and high-grade tumors (Fig. 13).

In 1973, Jakobsson (52) published a series of histologic observations that incorporated a number of parameters not traditionally included in determining histologic grade of SCC. These parameters can be classified into those that are intrinsic to the tumor:

1. Differentiation (primarily cytoplasmic keratin)
2. Nuclear pleomorphism (nuclear grade)
3. Mitoses (frequency and normality)
4. Structure (growth pattern, papillary, etc.) and parameters that represent host response:
5. Inflammatory response (lymphoplasmacytic or eosinophilic/neutrophilic infiltrates)
6. Stage of invasion (depth)
7. Pattern of tumor invasion into host stroma
8. Vascular invasion (blood and lymphatic)

Jakobsson evaluated a series of laryngeal SCCs using the above parameters and applied rigorous statistical evaluation, including regression analysis, to determine which parameters were statistically significant in predicting tumor stage, regional or distant metastases, local recurrence, and survival. Initially he assigned a point total determined by summing each individual parameter to quantify malignancy but also evaluated the individual parameters for statistical significance. He found the total point value, nuclear pleomorphism, and pattern of tumor invasion significant in predicting 5-year survival. This study was the first to statistically evaluate a variety of histologic observations to determine which tumor parameters were important in predicting clinically relevant end points. We found the same parameters, namely nuclear grade and pattern of invasion, to be strongly and significantly associated with DNA ploidy status of SCC of the UADT (53,54). Specifically, tumors with higher nuclear grade and a discohesive pattern of invasion composed of small cords and individual cells tended to be significantly more aneuploid.

Pattern of Invasion

It is our belief that pattern of invasion is an important prognostic parameter in the spectrum of histologic grading. The correlation between pattern of invasion and histologic grade is strong. The patterns of invasion vary from well-defined large aggregates of neoplastic cells in the submucosa or adjacent tissues with a broad, rounded tumor stromal interface to smaller aggregates of infiltrating cells ranging from large cohesive cords to thin trabeculae and single cells infiltrating into the adjacent host tissues. The former are generally well-differentiated tumors, and the latter less differentiated neoplasms. The large aggregates of invading SCC are less likely to penetrate or invade blood or lymphatic vessels with little opportunity to develop regional or distant metastases (Fig. 14). Conversely, SCCs infiltrating in thin irregular cords or individual cells are more likely to invade small vascular structures with an increased risk for formation of metastases (Fig. 15).

Vascular Invasion

The hallmark of malignant tumors is their ability to grow in an uncontrolled fashion with the ability to invade and destroy adja-

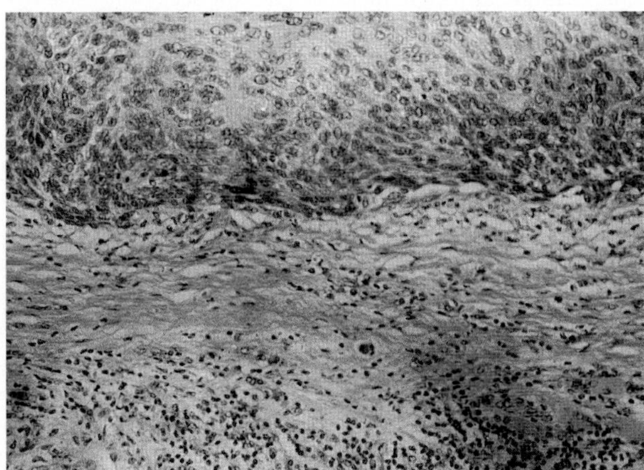

FIGURE 14. The pattern of tumor invasion is a good indicator of tumor differentiation. This figure depicts a squamous cell carcinoma with a broad, cohesive nest retaining a smooth tumor–stromal interface.

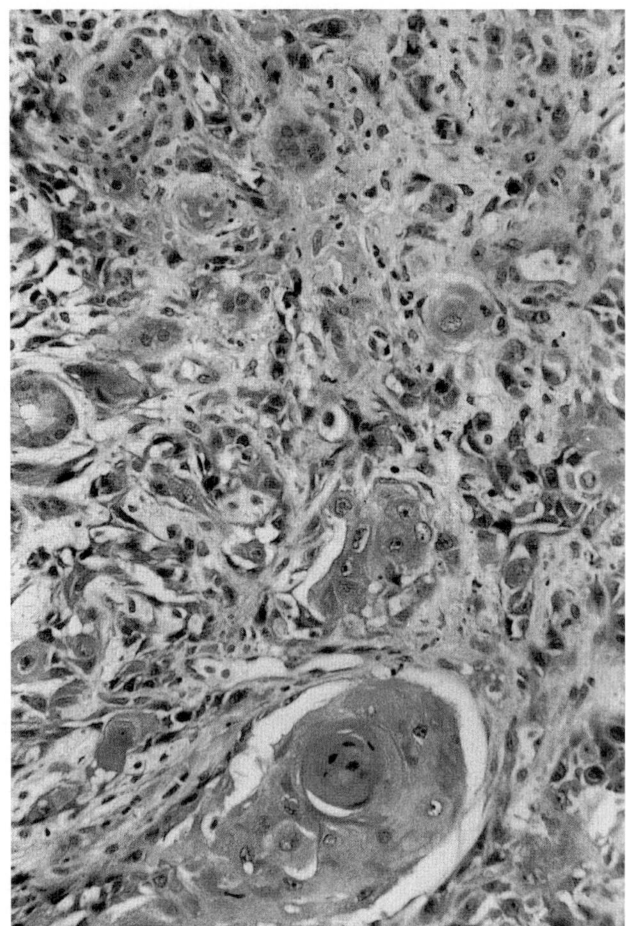

FIGURE 15. The tumor in this microscopic field invades in variably sized nests with a highly infiltrative growth.

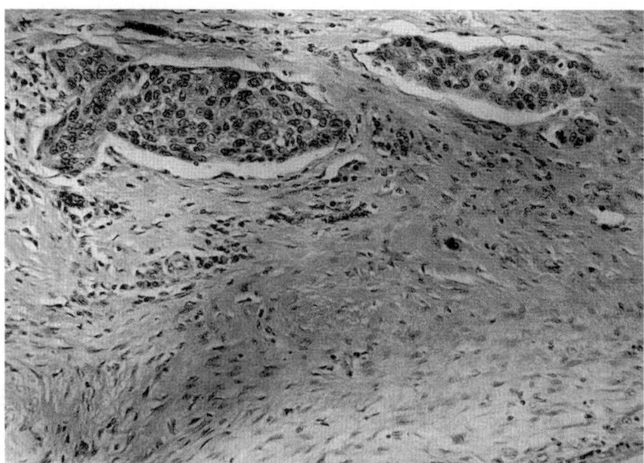

FIGURE 16. Vascular invasion is usually seen with the less differentiated, higher grade tumors and is associated with a higher rate of local metastases and recurrence. Lymphatic invasion is demonstrated in this figure.

cent tissue, often with associated penetration of blood or lymphatic vessels. The latter is a critical step in the metastatic cascade, which results in the development of regional or systemic metastases (55). In SCCs of the head and neck, vascular tumor invasion may be a prominent and destructive feature resulting in local recurrences (Fig. 16). Verrucous carcinoma is by far the classic example in which metastases do not occur and local invasion can be extremely destructive. In order for regional lymph node or distant metastasis to occur, penetration of vascular structures (either lymphatics or blood vessels) must occur (56). Well-differentiated neoplasms with pushing borders and well-defined epithelial–stromal interfaces generally do not have the capacity to penetrate the small vessels required to develop regional lymph node or distant metastasis. Conversely, single cells or small aggregates or cords of tumor invasion are most apt to have the capability to penetrate into these vascular structures and to be released into the circulation and extravasate, resulting in the development of metastatic foci. It is for these and other reasons that we feel the pattern of invasion and the presence (or absence) of vascular invasion are extremely important determinants of tumor grade. Pleomorphic malignant tumors invading as single cells or thin cords represent the greatest risk to develop regional or distant metastasis in our opinion and should be considered as aggressive neoplasms. A limited number of studies evaluating the importance of the presence of vascular invasion in the resected primary tumor have found such invasion to be associated with significant increases in regional lymph node metastases or decreased survival (53,56–59).

SPECIAL HISTOLOGIC SUBTYPES OF SQUAMOUS CELL CARCINOMA

Verrucous Carcinoma

The concept of verrucous carcinoma has been introduced in several of the previous sections of this chapter. It was originally grossly and histologically defined as a homogeneous proliferation of maturing squamous epithelium with growth patterns extending above the adjacent surface, often with extensive keratinization giving the typical verrucous or warty gross appearance (60,61). At the same time, the growth pattern extends or invades into the submucosal tissue with well-defined epithelial–submucosal borders that appear to push into the underlying normal tissues (Fig. 17). Clearly, the rigorous application of this histologic definition results in the identification of a neoplasm that cannot intravasate to small blood or lymphatic vessels and is unlikely to invade regional or distant metastasis. However, in advanced cases of verrucous carcinoma, extensive local destruction by the broad-based front of the tumor can occur.

One issue that has not been emphasized in much of the pathology literature about verrucous carcinoma is that in many instances the tumor can be associated with a variety of squamous mucosal changes ranging from leukoplakia to separate foci of verrucous and typical invasive squamous carcinomas. This is to be expected in mucosa that has been damaged by a variety of carcinogenic influences, especially chewing tobacco or snuff. Also many neoplasms initially classified as verrucous carcinoma may harbor foci of dedifferentiated typical invasive squamous carcinoma. In practice, this translates to the observation that patients with verrucous carcinomas, especially in the oral cavity, com-

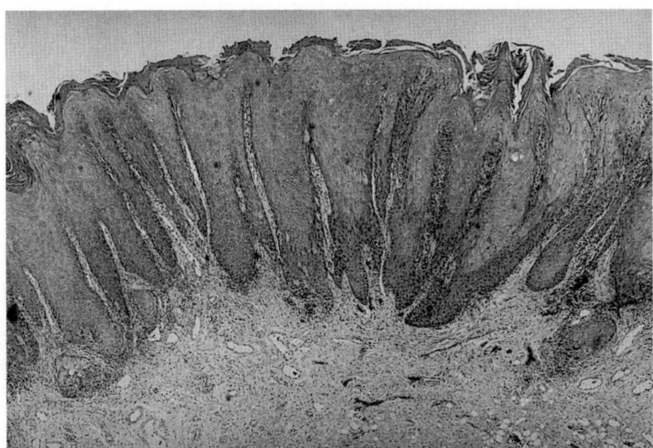

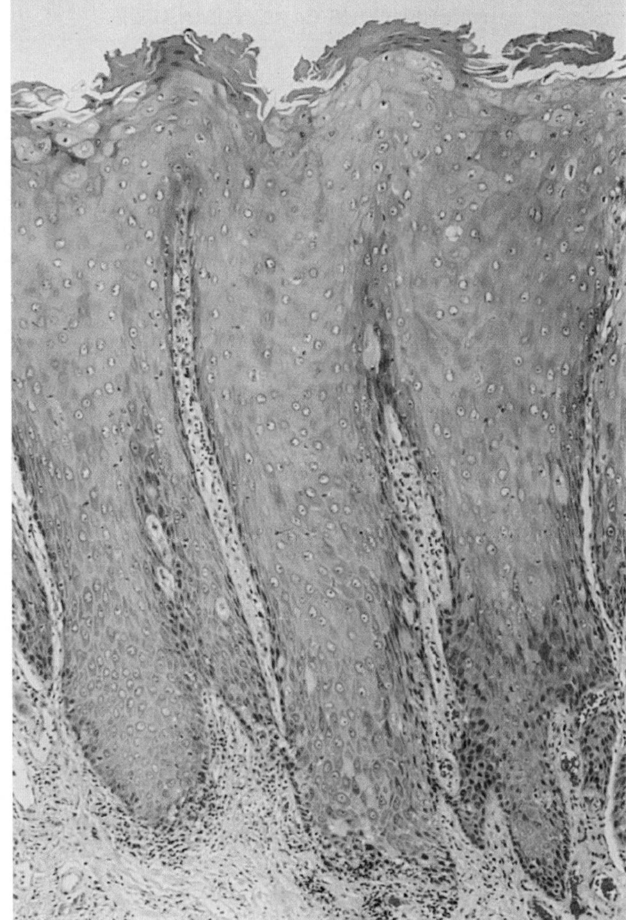

FIGURE 17. A and B: Verrucous carcinoma has a warty gross appearance with extensive keratinization. The growth pattern extends or invades into the submucosal tissue with well-defined epithelial submucosal borders that appear to push into the underlying normal tissues.

monly have a variety of other epithelial dysplasias and neoplasms. One of these epithelial proliferations is verrucous hyperplasia, now referred to as proliferative verrucous hyperplasia. Proliferative verrucous hyperplasia has the gross or surface appearance of a typical verrucous lesion. The differentiation between this category and verrucous carcinoma is the absence of invasion into the submucosa in the former lesion (43,44,62). This creates a problem in diagnosis because the gross appearance of verrucous hyperplasia and verrucous carcinoma are similar, especially in earlier stages of the latter. The surface is raised above the adjacent mucosa and has a rough pebbled or warty appearance (43,44). With similar gross or surface appearances, the only confident manner in which these two entities can be differentiated is by complete excision and histologic examination, and when one has to evaluate the presence or absence of underlying invasion, excisional biopsy must be performed (40). The same issue is encountered when one finds focal areas of typical SCC arising in a verrucous carcinoma. In one study 25% of the excised cases of verrucous carcinoma contained areas of dedifferentiation into typical invasive squamous neoplasia (63), the major point being that excision and careful histologic evaluation are required to make the diagnosis of hyperplasia or proliferative verrucous hyperplasia versus classic verrucous carcinoma or verrucous carcinoma with focal areas of SCC. In some proliferative verrucous hyperplasias, dysplasia or SIN changes may exist, which indicates a more advanced phase of transformation and therefore must be considered a more serious or ominous lesion. Clearly, the concept of proliferative verrucous hyperplasia has been developed because of the high frequent progression to invasive SCC (43,44,45) (Table 5).

One of the major difficulties in the diagnosis of this group of proliferative epithelial lesions, with or without submucosal invasion, is the inability to adequately sample the neoplasm by biopsy. Although excisional biopsy is often possible in the oral cavity, in other sites, particularly the larynx, forceps biopsy only allows for "nibbling," especially of the surface components of this thick proliferative epithelium, which results in the removal of small fragments of tissue. In these instances, the majority of the tissue contains strips of thickened keratinized mature epithelium in which the diagnosis of neoplasm is essentially impossible. Only when the clinical appearance of the neoplasm is characteristic of a verrucous carcinoma can correlation with these limited microscopic findings make the diagnosis of verrucous carcinoma possible. As previously mentioned, up to 25% of verrucous carcinomas harbor foci of dedifferentiated tumor or invasive SCC (63). These cases are from a patient series with a clinical appearance and biopsies consistent with verrucous carcinomas. After detailed histologic examination of the excised

TABLE 5. ASSOCIATED MUCOSAL PATHOLOGY IN CASES OF ORAL CAVITY VERRUCOUS CARCINOMA (VC)

	Total Patients	No. with Leukoplakia	Separate Foci of VC	Separate Foci of SCC in Oral Cavity	Separate Foci of SCC in UADT
Goethals, 1963 (61)	57	32	17	9	
Kraus, 1966 (64)	77	17	3	8	6
Burns, 1980 (65)	37	14	4	11	1
Medina, 1984 (63)	104			25	0

SCC, squamous cell carcinoma.

neoplasms, the foci of the invasive SCC were identified. This confirms the high frequency of dedifferentiation in verrucous carcinomas, and some examples of postradiation anaplastic transformation in cases of verrucous carcinoma may be related to this incomplete initial tumor sampling (64,65).

Papillary Squamous Cell Neoplasia

Papillary neoplasia in the UADT is not common and may be confused clinically with verrucous epithelial proliferations. For the purposes of this discussion, papillary is defined as gross proliferation above the adjacent mucosal surface that correlates with a specific histologic growth pattern of fronds or papillations with a central fibrovascular core covered by neoplastic squamous epithelium of varying thickness. The morphologic and cytologic features of the overlying epithelium differentiate papillomas from papillary carcinomas. These exophytic growth patterns are not to be confused with inverting papillomas, which occur primarily in the sinonasal mucosa (see Chapter 4). Papillary hyperplasia occurs primarily in the oral cavity. Most of these exophytic growths are fibroepithelial polyps occurring secondary to dental irritation and are not true papillomas (66,67). The histologic pattern of these reactive proliferations is a combination of submucosal fibrosis with inflammation and overlying epithelial hyperplasia, without SIN. Solitary papillomas are relatively common in the UADT, especially the oral cavity (68,69). These single papillomas are most common on the lips, tongue, palate, and buccal mucosa. The histology is of a typical papillary structure with a well-defined fibrovascular core covered by mature-appearing squamous epithelium. The squamous epithelium shows no cytologic atypia, although squamous carcinomas arising in solitary papillomas have been reported (70). The confusion regarding carcinoma arising in a papilloma and the development of papillomas in adults is the failure to realize that human papilloma virus (HPV)-associated papillomatosis can develop in adults and may present as a solitary papilloma (71,72).

The syndrome of papillomatosis associated with HPV occurs in all sites of the UADT and is most commonly encountered in the larynx and can occasionally extend into the lower respiratory tract (73,74) (see Chapter 7). This latter disease syndrome associated with exposure to HPV occurs primarily in children but can be present at any age. The peculiar interaction with the immune system and the exposure to HPV results in the development of multiple papillomas, many of which demonstrate koilocytotic atypia (Fig. 18) as well as increased DNA content with aneuploid profiles in some instances (72,75). The major consideration with this papillary neoplastic syndrome is that some cases may have sufficient epithelial atypia to be confused with papillary carcinoma (71,72). Recurrences of virally associated papillomas can extend into the lower respiratory tract (76) and result in death due to chronic obstruction with secondary pneumonia. This generally occurs in the juvenile age group, especially in patients with multiple recurrences. Occasional transformation to

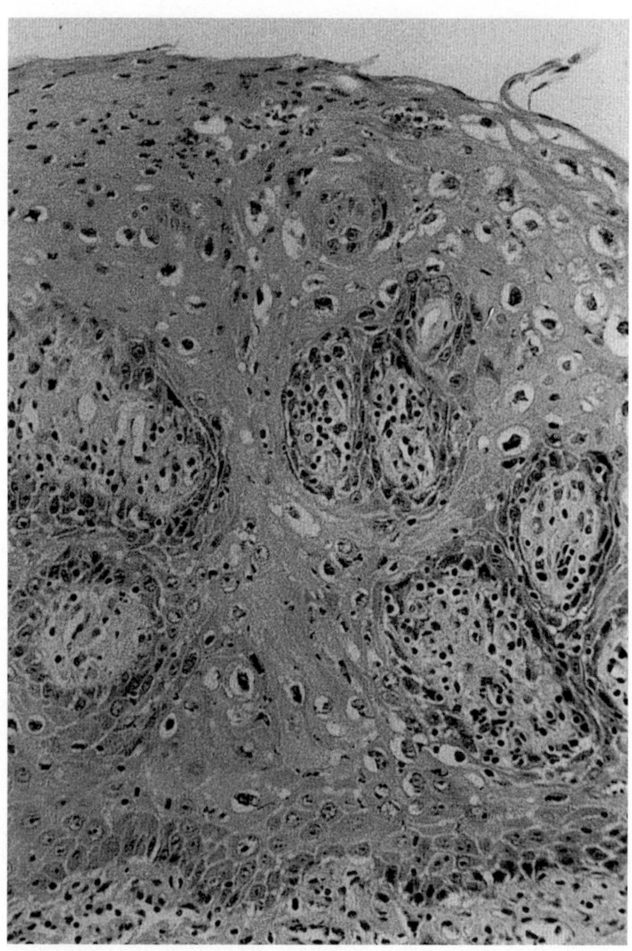

FIGURE 18. Squamous papillomas, particularly those occurring in the larynx in children and adolescents, are strongly associated with the human papilloma virus. Koilocytotic atypia evident in many keratinocytes represents the major morphologic effect of the infection.

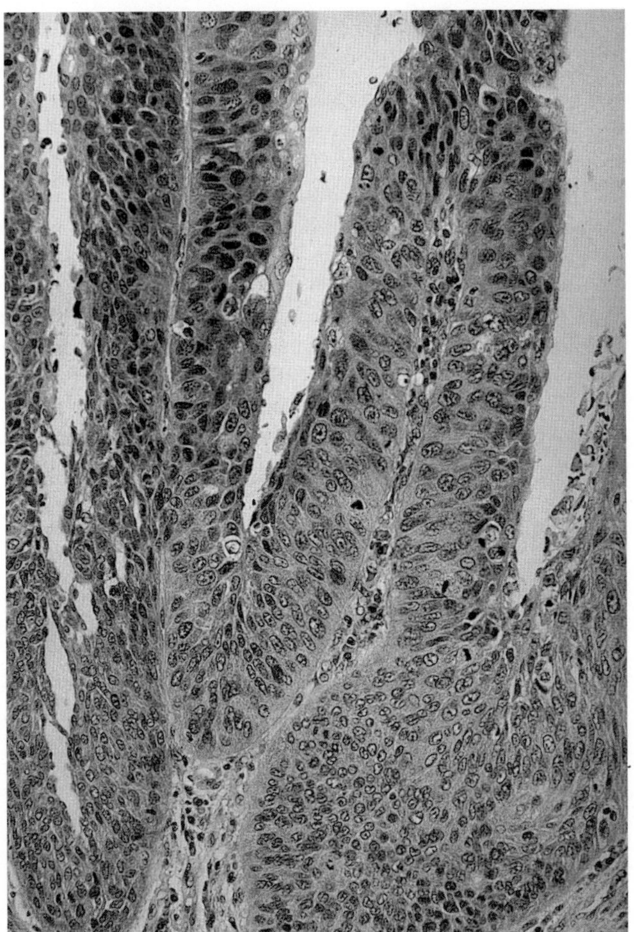

FIGURE 19. Papillary carcinoma shows the typical histology of papillary structures with well-defined fibrovascular cores covered by squamous epithelium. However, the lining exhibits variable degrees of architectural and mostly cytologic atypia.

typical squamous carcinomas have been described (76). The development of SCC in multiple HPV-associated papillomatosis is usually secondary to irradiation, which is no longer used as a therapy to relieve obstructive symptoms (77,78).

Papillary SCCs are relatively rare but do occur in the UADT and tend to be solitary (Fig. 19) (79). In many instances, papillary carcinomas have coexisting typical invasive SCCs, and the presence of the papillary component constitutes a morphologic interest rather than a prognostic component. Pure papillary carcinomas do not invade the submucosa and as a result are incapable of metastases.

Spindle Cell Carcinoma

Spindle cell carcinoma refers to an admixture of epithelial and mesenchymal-appearing malignant cells, referred to as spindle cell carcinoma in the UADT. The spindle cell or mesenchymal-appearing component is of unspecified histology, but malignant appearances reminiscent of virtually all sarcomas can occur (80) (Fig. 20). The most common types of mesenchymal-appearing components resemble fibrosarcoma or malignant fibrous histiocytoma, and more rarely chondrosarcoma or osteosarcoma. In some biopsy samples, the critical component of the epithelial malignancy may be difficult to identify, which makes the diagnosis hard to establish. However, in most instances, additional sections (or more tissue) will result in the identification of either squamous CIS or typical invasive carcinoma. In some instances, immunohistochemical identification of keratin intermediate filaments may be of value in documenting epithelial components in the poorly differentiated mesenchymal-appearing portion of the malignant tumor. In other cases, the common polypoid variant of this neoplasm has extensive areas of surface ulceration with loss of a large portion of the superficial squamous neoplastic component. Overall, spindle cell carcinomas are relatively rare tumors and account for approximately 0.59% of UADT neoplasms (80).

One of the most important aspects of spindle cell carcinoma is the confusion in nomenclature and the occasional difficulty in

A

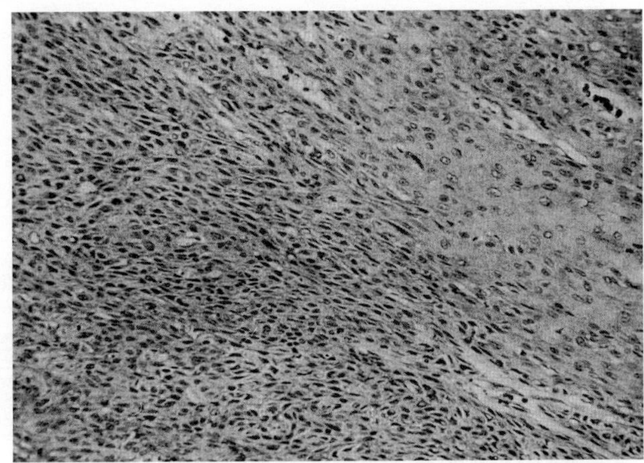

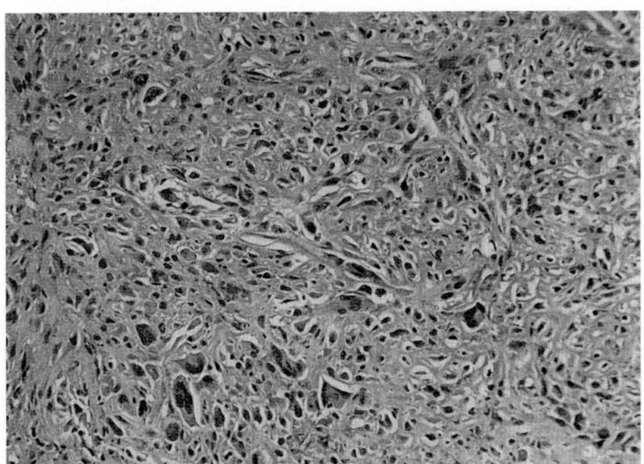

B

FIGURE 20. Spindle cell squamous carcinoma shows different proportions of an admixture of epithelial (**A**) and mesenchymal (**B**) malignant cells. Most tumors will have a component that can be recognized histologically as epithelial.

making an appropriate diagnosis. These neoplasms have been referred to as pseudosarcomas, pseudosarcomatous SCC, metaplastic carcinoma, carcinosarcoma, and spindle cell carcinoma (81–84). Spindle cell carcinomas can occur at all sites of the UADT but tend to be exophytic and polypoid when they occur in the larynx, the most common site. However, these neoplasms tend to be sessile and invasive when they are identified in the sinonasal or oral cavity mucosa; the latter site is relatively rare but results in highly aggressive tumors. The problem in diagnosis is biopsy sampling, because the malignant epithelial component tends to be focal and in some instances extremely difficult, if not impossible, to find. The spindle cell component varies greatly in its histologic grade, with high-grade tumors being in the minority and low-grade atypical spindle cell proliferation being most common. A biopsy of the spindle cell proliferation results in a difficult differential diagnosis, requiring the differentiation of atypical stromal reaction (especially postirradiation) versus spindle cell carcinoma versus sarcoma. Alternatively, the removal and subsequent careful histologic evaluation of laryngeal polypoid tumors allows for identification of the malignant epithelial component, therefore making it easier to establish the diagnosis. Sometimes in small biopsies of invasive or sessile spindle cell carcinomas, identification of both components is difficult.

The use of immunohistochemistry has improved our diagnostic accuracy in this relatively unusual tumor. Immunohistologic examination for keratin in the spindle cell population usually allows identification of some of the spindle cells as having epithelial differentiation (81). Although electron microscopy is occasionally helpful, the sampling error with the small tissue fragments inherent in electron microscopy evaluations do not really make this technology viable for routine diagnosis of spindle cell carcinoma (81).

The histiogenesis of these unusual neoplasms has been discussed extensively in the literature. Researchers have argued over the cell of origin with little concurrence. These are interesting discussions in light of the concept of metaplastic carcinoma (or matrix-producing carcinoma) of the breast and carcinosarcomas of other organ systems, which essentially have identical histologies but are accepted as derived from multipotential cells. Batsakis et al. (82) outlined several categories of cancers of the UADT with spindle cell proliferations. These categories serve as an appropriate differential diagnosis when encountering a tumor with spindle cell components:

1. A variant of SCC composed of a bimorphic epithelial and epithelial-derived spindle cell malignancy, producing metastases with a monophasic or mixed histologic pattern. (The term *epithelial-derived* remains controversial and may represent origin from a multipotential cell capable of differentiating in several directions.)
2. An SCC with an underlying benign pseudosarcomatous stromal reaction, resulting in only metastatic carcinoma.
3. An SCC with postirradiation stromal atypia, resulting in only metastatic carcinoma.
4. A carcinosarcoma composed of a true heterologous epithelial and mesenchymal malignancy, producing monophasic or mixed metastases (probably the same as no. 1 in this list).
5. A benign or malignant stromal tumor without the presence of carcinoma, which metastasizes as a sarcoma when malignant.
6. Spindle cell carcinoma without identifiable typical carcinoma, producing monomorphic or mixed metastases.

The growth patterns of these histologic mixed neoplasms is of paramount importance in predicting biologic behavior of the neoplasm. The most common growth pattern is the exophytic polypoid tumors that vary from 1 to 8 cm in diameter (83). These polypoid tumors are most common in the larynx and are often associated with limited invasion of the stalk and adjacent submucosa. An interesting phenomenon is that occasionally the stalks necrose, resulting in expectoration of the tumor, leaving little or no residual tumor. Sessile or flat spindle cell carcinomas tend to invade the underlying tissue and as a result are more likely to metastasize with a decreased survival. Sessile neoplasms are more common in sinonasal and oral cavity sites (84,85).

Basaloid Squamous Carcinoma

Basaloid squamous carcinoma is a recently described variant of SCC that occurs in numerous anatomic sites. Basaloid squamous carcinoma of the UADT represents a poorly differentiated SCC that behaves in an aggressive manner (86–90). This histologic variant was first reported in the UADT in 1986, and four major histologic cellular features were described (87):

1. Solid nests of poorly differentiated cells in a lobular configuration closely apposed to the surface mucosa
2. Small, crowded cells with little or scant cytoplasm
3. Dark, hyperchromatic nuclei without nucleoli
4. Small cystic spaces containing mucinlike material

In addition, other features include central areas of necrosis, sometimes extensive and sometimes small and comedo-like in appearance. Basaloid squamous carcinoma always has a squamous component manifested as areas of typical squamous carcinoma, SIN, or focal areas of typical squamous differentiation within the otherwise basaloid-appearing tumor (Figs. 21–23).

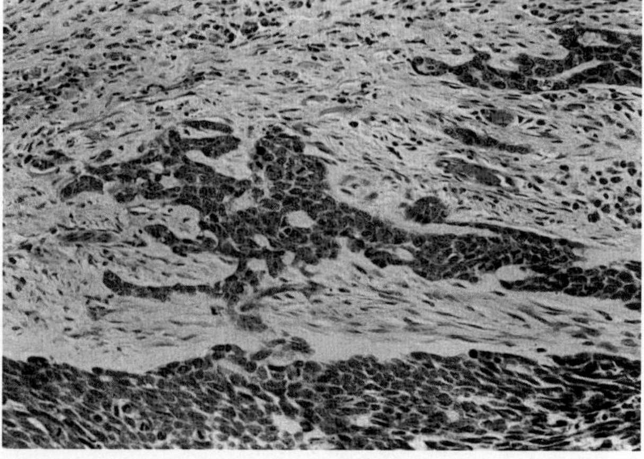

FIGURE 21. Basaloid squamous cell carcinoma exhibits a variety of growth patterns: basaloid squamous cell carcinoma growing in cords, trabeculae, and infiltrating individual cells arranged in single rows (lobular pattern).

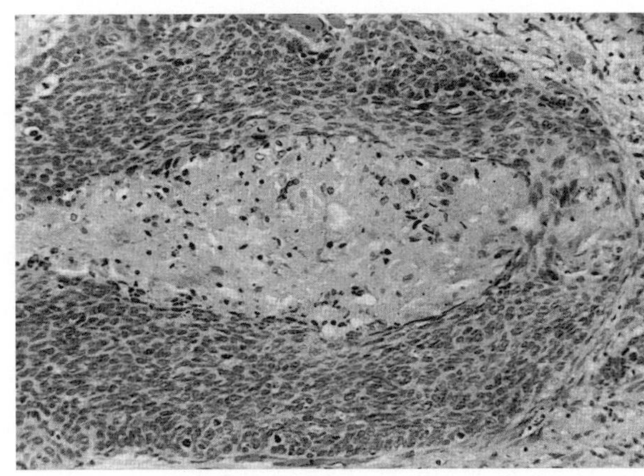
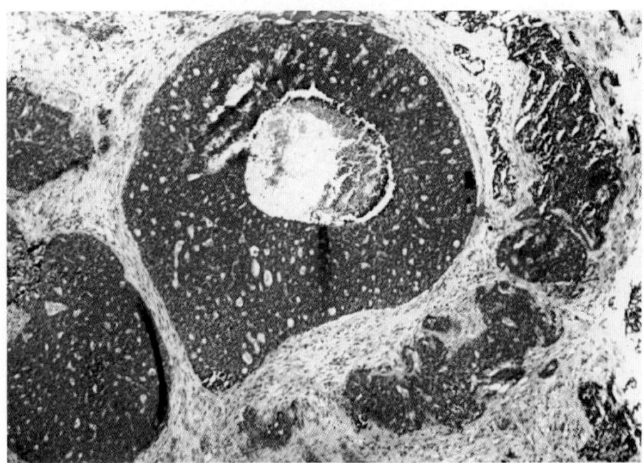

FIGURE 22. A and B: Basaloid squamous cell carcinoma often shows extensive central necrosis with a distinct comedo pattern of the larger tumor nests or involving wide areas of the tumor.

The histologic variants of this poorly differentiated SCC variant include:

1. A variety of growth patterns, including solid, lobular cords or single cell rows, cribriform and cystic or glandular
2. Necrosis with either large areas or comedo patterns, usually with solid growth patterns
3. Extensive hyaline or mucohyaline material, commonly seen with lobular cords or rows of single cells
4. Mucin-like material (periodic acid-Schiff and Alcian blue positive) in association with cystic or gland-like configurations

In addition, basaloid squamous carcinomas may rarely be associated with spindle cell variants of SCC (88,89). Some tumors also have prominent foci of SCC, often with obvious keratinization.

The differential diagnosis is generally not a problem, especially when adequate tissue is present to identify the characteristic histologic features. However, in small biopsy samples or when characteristic histologic features are not present, basaloid carcinoma can be confused with the following:

1. Adenoid cystic carcinoma, particularly the anaplastic variant when cribriform patterns and prominent hyaline or mucohyaline are present in the tumor. However, basaloid squamous carcinomas are S-100 protein and vimentin negative (88) and do not contain the prominent myoepithelial component of most adenoid cystic carcinomas. Furthermore, adenoid cystic carcinomas virtually never have squamous differentiation.
2. Neuroendocrine carcinoma. The lack of neuroendocrine markers should help to exclude this differential.
3. Adenocarcinoma or adenosquamous carcinoma. The cystic or glandular pattern may cause difficulties, but the admixture of small basaloid-like cells should help delineate this diagnosis.

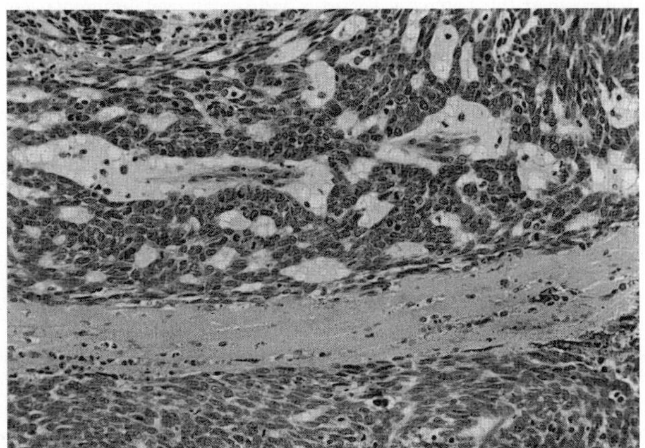

FIGURE 23. Basaloid squamous cell carcinoma can also grow in a pseudoglandular or adenoid pattern.

The most important rationale for recognizing basaloid squamous carcinoma is the advanced stage at the time of diagnosis and the poor prognosis. The neoplasm is quick to invade deeply, penetrating lymphatics and blood vessels with extensive regional lymph node metastases and commonly with distant metastases. In the largest published series (90), 40 patients were reported (35 men, 5 women, median age 62), 27 presented with regional metastases, and 15 developed distant disease. Unfortunately, the follow-up interval was less than 1 year. Clearly, basaloid squamous carcinoma is a highly aggressive, rapidly growing tumor with a significant associated incidence of mortality.

Nasopharyngeal Carcinoma and the Lymphoepithelioma Histology

Carcinomas arising in the nasopharynx have particular etiologic, epidemiologic, and morphologic features that are fairly distinct from the conventional SCCs of the rest of the UADT. Nasopharyngeal carcinomas are strongly linked to Epstein-Barr virus infection. The virus is implicated in the initiation phase of these neoplasms and can be demonstrated in tumor tissues by

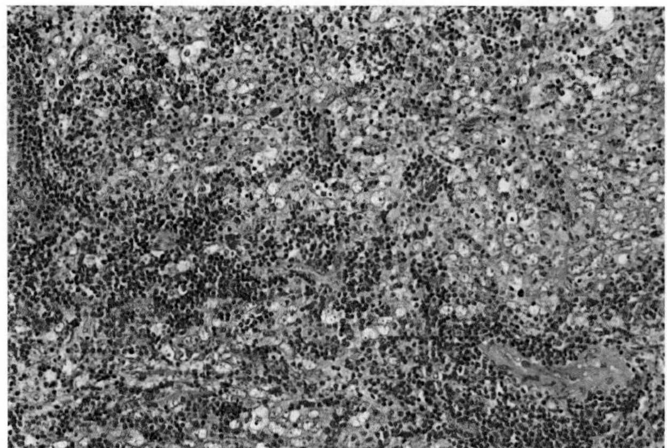

FIGURE 24. Lymphoepithelioma. This histologic type commonly associated with nasopharyngeal locations can occur in other locations in the head and neck region and other organ systems. The tumor exhibits a sheetlike growth of large cells with vesicular nuclei with prominent nucleoli reminiscent of large cell lymphoma. Typically, there is a heavy lymphoplasmacytic infiltrate.

means of immunohistochemistry, *in situ* hybridization, and various molecular techniques (91,92). These tumors are endemic in the Far East and are also common in parts of northern Africa (93,94) The pathologic features and clinical correlations of nasopharyngeal cancer are discussed in detail in Chapter 5.

Of interest are recent reports describing tumors with nasopharyngeal carcinoma-like or lymphoepithelioma histology occurring in locations in the head and neck region other than the nasopharynx. The common sites are the oropharynx, salivary gland, laryngohypopharynx, maxillary sinus/nasal cavity, and pyriform sinuses (95,96) (Fig. 24). The latter terminology describes a sheet-like growth pattern of large cells with vesicular nuclei with prominent nucleoli reminiscent of large cell lymphoma. Clearly, however, the neoplasm is of epithelial lineage and stains positively with epithelial markers like cytokeratin.

Similar to its nasopharyngeal counterpart, lymphoepithelioma of other sites within the UADT is reported to be responsive to radiation therapy (95).

REFERENCES

1. Cann CI, Fried MP, Rothman KJ. Epidemiology of squamous cell cancer of the head and neck. *Otolaryngol Clin North Am* 1985;18:1–22.
2. Decker J, Goldstein JC. Current concepts in otolaryngology. Risk factors in head and neck cancer. *N Engl J Med* 1982;306:1151–1156.
3. Blot WJ, McLaughlin JK, Winn DM, et al. Smoking and drinking in relation to oral and pharyngeal cancer. *Cancer Res* 1988;48:3282–3287.
4. Pindborg JJ, Reibel J, Roed-Petersen B, et al. Tobacco-induced changes in oral leukoplakic epithelium. *Cancer* 1980;45:2330–2336.
5. Anderson G, Bjornberg G, Curvall M. Oral mucosal changes and nicotine deposition in users of Swedish smokeless tobacco products: a comparative study. *J Oral Pathol Med* 1994;23:161–167.
6. Falk RT, Pickle LW, Brown LM, et al. Effect of smoking and alcohol consumption on laryngeal cancer risk in coastal Texas. *Cancer Res* 1989;49:4024–4029.
7. Raitiola HS, Pukander JS. Etiological factors of laryngeal cancer. *Acta Otolaryngol (Stockh)* 1997;529(suppl):215–217.
8. Singh AD, Von Essen CF. Buccal mucosa cancer in South India. Etiologic and clinical aspects. *Cancer* 1966;96:6–14.
9. Reddy CRRM, Raju MVS, Ramulu C, et al. Changes in the ducts of the glands of the hard palate in reverse smokers. *Cancer* 1972;30: 231–238.
10. Blot WJ, Hoover RN. Diet in the etiology of oral and pharyngeal cancer among women from Southern United States. *Cancer Res* 1984;44: 1216–1222.
11. Rao DN, Ganesh B, Rao RS, et al. Risk assessment of tobacco, alcohol and diet in oral cancer. *Int J Cancer* 1994;58:469–473.
12. Hong WK, Endicott J, Itri LM, et al. 13-CIS retinoic acid in the treatment of oral leukoplakia. *N Engl J Med* 1986;315:1501–1505.
13. Lipman SM, Hong WK. 13-cis-retinoic acid and cancer chemoprevention. *J Natl Cancer Inst Monogr* 1992;13:111–115.
14. Mohtashamipur E, Norpoth K, Luhmann F. Cancer epidemiology of woodworking. *J Cancer Res Clin Oncol* 1989;115:503–515.
15. Chan CK, Gee JB. Asbestos exposure and laryngeal cancer: an analysis of the epidemiologic evidence. *J Occup Med* 1988;30:23–27.
16. Muscat JE, Wynder EL. Tobacco, alcohol, asbestos and occupational risk factors for laryngeal cancer. *Cancer* 1992;69:2244–2251.
17. Winn DM, Blot WJ, McLaughlin JK. Mouthwash use and oral conditions in the risk of oral and pharyngeal cancer. *Cancer Res* 1991;51: 3044–3047.
18. Kabat GC, Hebert JR, Wynder EL. Risk factors for oral cancer in women. *Cancer Res* 1989;49:2803–2806.
19. Flanders WD, Rothman KJ. Interaction of alcohol and tobacco in laryngeal cancer. *Am J Epidemiol* 1982;115:371–379.
20. Salonen L, Axell T, Lellden L. Occurrence of oral mucosal lesions, the influence of tobacco habits and an estimate of treatment time in an adult Swedish population. *J Oral Pathol Med* 1990;19:170–176.
21. Kaugars GE, Mehailescu WL, Gunsolley JC. Smokeless tobacco use and oral epithelial dysplasia. *Cancer* 1989;64:1527–1530.
22. Shafer WG, Waldron CA. A clinical and histopathologic study of oral leukoplakia. *Surg Gynecol Obstet* 1961;112:411–420.
23. Brugere J, Guenel P, Leclerc A, et al. Differential effects of tobacco and alcohol in cancers of the larynx, pharynx and mouth. *Cancer* 1986; 57:391–395.
24. Moertel CG. Multiple primary malignant neoplasms: historical perspectives. *Cancer* 1977;40:1786–1792.
25. Cohn AM, Peppard SB. Multiple primary malignant tumors of the head and neck. *Am J Otolaryngol* 1980;1:411–417.
26. Gluckman JL, Crissman JD, Donegan JO. Multicentric squamous cell carcinoma of the upper aerodigestive tract. *Head Neck Surg* 1980;3: 90–96.
27. Shons LR, McQuarrie DG. Multiple primary epidermoid carcinomas of the upper aerodigestive tract. *Arch Surg* 1985;120:1007–1009.
28. Crissman JD, Zarbo RJ. Dysplasia, *in-situ* carcinoma and progression in squamous cell carcinoma of the upper aerodigestive tract. *Am J Surg Pathol* 1989;13(suppl 1):5–16.
29. Shafer WG, Waldron CA. A clinical and histopathologic study of oral leukoplakia. *Surg Gynecol Obstet* 1991;112:411–420.
30. Crissman JD. Laryngeal keratosis and subsequent carcinoma. *Head Neck Surg* 1979;1:386–391.
31. Hellquist H, Olofsson J, Grontoft O. Carcinoma in situ and severe dysplasia of the vocal cords. *Acta Otolaryngol* 1981;92:543–555.
32. Shafer WG, Waldron CA. Erythroplakia of the oral cavity. *Cancer* 1975;36:1021–1028.
33. Mashberg A. Erythroplasia: the earliest sign of asymptomatic oral cancer. *J Am Dent Assoc* 1978;96:615–620.
34. Silverman S, Gorsky M, Lozada F. Oral leukoplakia and malignant transformation. *Cancer* 1984;53:563–568.
35. Pindborg JJ, Renstrum G, Poulseu HE, et al. Studies in oral leukoplakias v. clinical and histologic signs of malignancy. *Acta Odontol Scand* 1963;21:404–414.
36. Silverman S, Rozen RD. Observations on the clinical characteristics and natural history of oral leukoplakia. *J Am Dent Assoc* 1968;76: 772–777.
37. Banoczy J, Ceiba A. Occurrence of epithelial dysplasia in oral leukoplakia. *Oral Surg Oral Med Oral Pathol* 1976;42:766–774.
38. Waldron CA, Shafer WG. Leukoplakia revisited. A clinicopathologic study of 3256 oral leukoplakias. *Cancer* 1975;36:1386–1392.

39. Crissman JD, Visscher DW, Sakr W. Premalignant lesions of the upper aerodigestive tract: pathologic classification. *J Cell Biochem* 1993;(suppl 17F):49–56.
40. Crissman JD, Gnepp DR, Goodman ML, et al. Precancerous lesions of the upper aerodigestive tract: histologic definitions and clinical applications (a symposium). *Pathol Annu* 1987;22(part 1):311–352.
41. Crissman JD, Zarbo RJ. Quantitation of DNA ploidy in squamous intraepithelial neoplasia of the laryngeal glottis. *Arch Otolaryngol Head Neck Surg* 1991;117:182–188.
42. Hellquist H, Lundgren J, Olofsson J. Hyperplasia, keratosis, dysplasia and carcinoma in situ of the vocal cords—a follow-up study. *Clin Otolaryngol* 1982;7:11–27.
43. Murrah VA, Batsakis JG. Proliferative verrucous leukoplakia and verrucous hyperplasia. *Ann Otol Rhinol Laryngol* 1994;103(part 1): 660–663.
44. Zakrzewska JM, Lopes V, Speight P, et al. Proliferative verrucous leukoplakia: a report of ten cases. *Oral Surg Oral Med Oral Pathol Oral Radiol Endod* 1996;82:396–401.
45. McDonald JS, Crissman JD, Gluckman JL. Verrucous carcinoma of the oral cavity. *Head Neck Surg* 1982;5:22–28.
46. Crissman JD, Gluckman JL, Whitely J, et al. Squamous cell carcinoma of the floor of the mouth. *Head Neck Surg* 1980;3:1–7.
47. Sakr WA, Zarbo RJ, Jacobs JR, et al. Distribution of basement membrane in squamous cell carcinoma of the head and neck. *Hum Pathol* 1987;18:1043–1050.
48. Mohit-Tabutab WH, Sobel HJ, Rush BG, et al. Relation of thickness of floor of mouth stage I and II cancers to regional metastasis. *Am J Surg* 1986;152:358–363.
49. Spiro FH, Huvos AG, Wong GY, et al. Predictive value of tumor thickness in squamous carcinoma confined to the tongue and floor of the mouth. *Am J Surg* 1986;152:345–350.
50. Asakage T, Yokose T, Mukai K, et al. Tumor thickness predicts cervical metastasis in patients with Stage I/II carcinoma of the tongue. *Cancer* 1998;82:1443–1448.
51. Broder AC. Squamous cell epithelioma of the lip. *JAMA* 1920;74: 656–664.
52. Jakobsson PA, Eneroth DM, Killander D, et al. Histologic classification and grading of malignancy in carcinoma of the larynx. *Acta Radiol Ther Phys Biol* 1973;12:1–8.
53. Crissman JD, Liu WY, Gluckman JL, et al. Prognostic value of histopathologic parameters in squamous cell carcinoma of the oropharynx. *Cancer* 1984;54:2995–3001.
54. Sakr W, Hussan M, Zarbo RJ, et al. DNA quantitation and histologic characteristics of squamous cell carcinoma of the upper aerodigestive tract. *Arch Pathol Lab Med* 1989;113:1009–1014.
55. Weiss L. A critical overview of the metastatic process. In: Honn KV, Power WE, Sloan BF, eds. *Mechanisms of cancer metastasis.* Boston: Martinus Nijhoff, 1986:23–52.
56. Poleksic S, Kalwaic HJ. Prognostic value of vascular invasion in squamous cell carcinoma of the head and neck. *Plast Reconstr Surg* 1978;61:234–240.
57. Woolgar JA, Scott J. Prediction of cervical lymph node metastasis in squamous cell carcinoma of the tongue/floor of mouth. *Head Neck* 1995;17:463–472.
58. Frierson HF, Cooper PH. Prognostic factors in squamous cell carcinoma of the lip. *Hum Pathol* 1986;17:346–354.
59. Close LG, Burns DK, Reisch J, et al. Microvascular invasion in cancer of the oral cavity and oropharynx. *Arch Otolaryngol Head Neck Surg* 1987;113:1191–1195.
60. Ackerman LV. Verrucous carcinoma of the oral cavity. *Surgery* 1948;23:670–678.
61. Goethals PO, Harrison EG, Devine KD. Verrucous squamous cell carcinoma of the oral cavity. *Am J Surg* 1963;106:845–851.
62. Shear M, Pindborg JJ. Verrucous hyperplasia of the oral cavity. *Cancer* 1980;46:1855–1862.
63. Medina JE, Dichtel W, Luna MA. Verrucous-squamous carcinomas of the oral cavity. A clinicopathologic study of 104 cases. *Arch Otolaryngol* 1984;110:431–440.
64. Kraus FT, Perez-Mesa C. Verrucous carcinoma. Clinical and pathological study of 105 cases involving oral cavity, larynx and genitalia. *Cancer* 1966;19:26–38.
65. Burns HP, van Nostrand AWP, Palmer JA. Verrucous carcinoma of the oral cavity: management by radiotherapy and surgery. *Can J Surg* 1980;23:19–25.
66. Bhaskar SN, Beasley JD, Cutright DE. Inflammatory papillary hyperplasia of the oral mucosa: report of 341 cases. *J Am Dent Assoc* 1970;81:949–952.
67. Yrastorza JA. Inflammatory papillary hyperplasia of the palate. *J Oral Surg* 1963;21:330–336.
68. Greer RO, Goldman HW. Oral papillomas: clinicopathologic evaluation and retrospective examination for dyskeratosis in 110 lesions. *Oral Surg* 1974;38:435–440.
69. Rose HP. Papillomas of the oral cavity. *Oral Surg* 1965;20:542–549.
70. Yoder MG, Batsakis JG. Squamous cell carcinoma in solitary laryngeal papilloma. *Otolaryngol Head Neck Surg* 1987;88:745–748.
71. Quick CA, Foucar E, Dehner LP. Frequency and significance of epithelial atypia in laryngeal papillomatosis. *Laryngoscope* 1979;89: 550–560.
72. Crissman JD, Kessis T, Shah KV, et al. Squamous papillary neoplasia of the adult upper aerodigestive tract. *Hum Pathol* 1988;19: 1387–1396.
73. Mounts P, Shah KV, Kashima H. Viral etiology of juvenile and adult onset squamous papilloma of the larynx. *Proc Natl Acad Sci U S A* 1982;79:5425–5429.
74. Mounts P, Kashima H. Association of human papilloma virus subtype and clinical course in respiratory papillomatosis. *Laryngoscope* 1984;94:28–33.
75. Olofsson J, Bielkenkrantz K, Grontoft O, et al. Juvenile laryngeal papilloma displaying malignant degeneration—a spectrophotometric investigation. *J Otolaryngol* 1978;7:353–365.
76. Runckel D, Kessler S. Bronchogenic squamous carcinoma in nonirradiated juvenile laryngotracheal papillomatosis. *Am J Surg Pathol* 1980;4:193–296.
77. Majoros M, Parkhill EM, Devine KD. Papilloma of the larynx in children. A clinicopathologic study. *Am J Surg* 1964;108:470–475.
78. Majoros M, Devine KD, Parkhill EM. Malignant transformation of benign laryngeal papillomas in children after radiation therapy. *Surg Clin North Am* 1963;43:1049–1061.
79. Ishiyama A, Eversole LR, Ross DA, et al. Papillary squamous neoplasms of the head and neck. *Laryngoscope* 1994;104:1446–1452.
80. Ferlito A. Histologic classification of larynx and hypopharynx cancers and their clinical implications. *Acta Otolaryngol Suppl* 1976;352:1–88.
81. Zarbo RJ, Crissman JD, Venkat H, et al. Spindle cell carcinoma of the upper aerodigestive tract mucosa. *Am J Surg Pathol* 1986;10:741–753.
82. Batsakis JG, Rice DH, Howard DR. The pathology of head and neck tumors: spindle cell lesions (sarcomatoid carcinomas, nodular fasciitis, and fibrosarcoma) of the aerodigestive tract, part 14. *Head Neck Surg* 1982;4:499–513.
83. Lambert PR, Ward PH, Berci G. Pseudosarcoma of the larynx. A comprehensive analysis. *Arch Otolaryngol* 1980;106:700–708.
84. Randall G, Alonso WA, Ogura JH. Spindle cell carcinoma (pseudosarcoma) of the larynx. *Arch Otolaryngol* 1975;101:63–66.
85. Hyams VJ. Spindle cell carcinoma of the larynx. In: Alberti PW, Bryce DP, eds. *Centennial conference on laryngeal carcinoma.* New York: Appleton-Century-Crofts, 1976:307—313.
86. Raslan WF, Barnes L, Krause JR, et al. Basaloid squamous cell carcinoma of the head and neck: a clinicopathologic and flow cytometric study of 10 new cases with review of the English literature. *Am J Otolaryngol* 1994;15:204–211.
87. Wain SL, Kier R, Volmer RT, et al. Basaloid-squamous carcinoma of the tongue, hypopharynx and larynx: report of 10 cases. *Hum Pathol* 1986;17:1158–1166.
88. Muller S, Barnes L. Basaloid squamous cell carcinoma of the head and neck with a spindle cell component. *Arch Pathol Lab Med* 1995;119:181–182.
89. Klijanicuko J, El-Naggar A, Ponzio-Prion A, et al. Basaloid squamous carcinoma of the head and neck. *Arch Otolaryngol Head Neck Surg* 1993;119:887–890.
90. Banks ER, Frierson HF, Mills SE, et al. Basaloid squamous cell carcinoma of the head and neck. A clinicopathologic and immunohistochemical study of 40 cases. *Am J Surg Pathol* 1992;16:939–946.

91. Alabashi DV, Levine PH, Prasad U, et al. Fourth international symposium on nasopharyngeal carcinoma application of field and laboratory studies to the control of NPC. *Cancer Res* 1983;43;2375–2378.
92. Ambinder RF, Mann RB. Detection and characterization of Epstein-Barr virus in clinical specimens. *Am J Pathol* 1994;145:239–252.
93. Brousset P, Butet V, Chittal S, et al. Comparison of *in situ* hybridization using different nonisotopic probes for detection of Epstein-Barr virus in nasopharyngeal carcinoma and immunohistochemical correlation with anti-latent membrane protein antibody. *Lab Invest* 1992;67:457–464.
94. Feinmesser R, Miyazaki I, Cheung R, et al. Diagnosis of nasopharyngeal carcinoma by DNA amplification of tissue obtained by fine needle aspiration. *N Engl J Med* 1992;326:17–21.
95. Dubey P, Ha CS, Ang KK, et al. Nonnasopharyngeal lymphoepithelioma of the head and neck. *Cancer* 1998;82:1556–1562.
96. Frank DK, Cheron F, Cho H, et al. Nonnasopharyngeal lymphoepitheliomas (undifferentiated carcinomas) of the upper aerodigestive tract. *Ann Otol Rhinol Laryngol* 1995;104:305–310.

3

THE EXTERNAL EAR AND EAR CANAL, MIDDLE EAR AND MASTOID, INNER EAR, AND TEMPORAL BONE

LESLIE MICHAELS

The ear is subject to a wide variety of pathologic conditions, many of which may be amenable to biopsy diagnosis. As in other parts, successful histologic diagnosis requires a knowledge of the normal anatomy and histology of the area, a summary of which is provided elsewhere (1).

Most surgical biopsy specimens taken from the ear are small. Many contain some bone for which brief decalcification is required. Resection specimens of the stapes superstructure or of the whole stapes should be oriented for embedding after decalcification so that the outline of the whole ossicle is revealed in the section; transverse sectioning is unsatisfactory. Care should be taken in orienting any skin or mucosal surface correctly in small biopsy samples during paraffin embedding so that sections will be cut at right angles to the epithelial surface.

Occasionally larger resection specimens are submitted, usually derived from the surgical treatment of squamous cell carcinoma of the external or middle ear. These include resection of the pinna and deep external auditory canal and "petrosectomy." The latter is far from being a resection of the whole petrous temporal bone, but consists of the external canal, tympanic membrane, middle ear contents, and sometimes part of the inner ear. The surviving normal anatomic structures should be identified in these specimens, and resection margins should be carefully sampled for evidence of tumor extension.

EXTERNAL EAR AND EAR CANAL

Non-neoplastic Lesions

Inflammatory Lesions

Some of the inflammatory lesions of the external ear are identical to those occurring elsewhere on the skin. Others are specific to or most common in the region of the external ear, and only these will be considered here.

Infections

Malignant Otitis Externa

Clinical Data. Malignant otitis externa was first described as a severe infection of the external auditory canal, usually in elderly diabetics, resulting in necrosis of cartilage, nerve, bone, and adjacent soft tissue, and extending to the ninth, tenth, eleventh, and twelfth cranial nerves, leading to meningitis and eventually death (2). It is likely that the inflammation reaches the jugular foramen region of the temporal bone via severe otitis media and osteomyelitis (3). The causative agent in all cases is said to be *Pseudomonas aeruginosa*.

Histologic Features. Tissues removed from the deep external canal to drain the inflammatory process show necrotic changes of external canal bone, accompanied by osteomyelitis with osteolytic and osteogenic reactions (4).

In Acquired Immunodeficiency Syndrome. In recent years several patients with the acquired immunodeficiency syndrome (AIDS) have been reported to have malignant otitis externa. In one of them acute osteomyelitis of the skull base was present, supporting the concept of osteomyelitis as the pathologic basis for the spread of the malignant otitis externa to the petrous apex (5).

Fungus Infections

Superficial pathogenic fungi, which occasionally infect the external ear, include *Trichophyton rubrum, Microphyton audouini,* and *Candida albicans.* The latter not uncommonly produces a low-grade infection after radical mastoidectomy. *Aspergillus fumigatus* and *A. nigrans* are also cultivated with some frequency from infected ear canals. Deep pathogenic fungus infections are more rare and include North American blastomycosis (*Blastomyces dermatitidis*), coccidioidomycosis (*Coccidioides immitis*), and cryptococcosis (*Cryptococcus neoformans*).

Virus Infections

Herpes Simplex

Both type 1 and type 2 herpes virus as well as herpes zoster virus may cause vesicles in the ear canal. Viral antigens may be detected in the epidermal cells by immunohistochemistry. The histologic appearance is characterized by intraepidermal vesicles produced by acantholysis of epidermal cells. Multinucleate keratinocytes in which the nuclei appear to be molded to each other, loss of cohesion, and rounding up of keratinocytes (acantholysis) are characteristic (6).

Herpes Zoster

Herpes zoster is caused by the virus of chicken pox (varicella-zoster virus), which travels from the nerve ganglia to the skin along nerves. When the geniculate ganglion is affected, a vesicular eruption of the pinna, ear canal, postauricular skin, uvula, palate, and anterior tongue is produced and facial palsy results. A combination of these features, with disturbances of hearing and balance due to involvement of the ganglia of the eighth nerve, is termed Ramsay Hunt syndrome. The skin lesions are histologically similar to those of herpes simplex.

Noninfectious Inflammatory Lesions

Starch Granuloma

Granulomatous inflammatory lesions in reaction to starch granules have been seen in the ear canal and middle ear. The starch was derived not from surgical glove powder but from insufflations of antibiotic, in which it was used as a vehicle to provide a mixture used in the treatment of external or middle ear otitis. Microscopically, there is an exudate of histiocytes and lymphocytes. Granules of starch are easily recognized as spherical or polyhedral basophilic bodies, 10 to 20 μm in diameter, often within histiocytes. The granules show a Maltese cross-birefringence and a brilliant red coloration after staining with periodic acid-Schiff (PAS) reagent (7).

Hair Granuloma

Biopsy sections taken from inflammatory lesions of the ear canal may show a granulomatous reaction with foreign body–type giant cells engulfing hair shafts. The hairs in hair granulomas of the ear canal are derived from the patient's own hair, possibly by ingrowth from those near the orifice of the canal, in the same fashion as occurs in cases of pilonidal sinus. In some instances the hair may enter the ear canal after hair cutting.

Inflammatory Lesions of Unknown Origin

Relapsing Polychondritis

Clinical Data. Relapsing polychondritis is a disease of adults characterized by recurring bouts of inflammation affecting cartilaginous structures, the eye, the myocardium, and the joints. Although the cartilage of the external ear is most frequently involved, it is the inflammation with destruction of the cartilages of the respiratory tract, particularly those of the larynx, that threatens life (8).

Gross Appearance. The lobule is usually normal. In the acute stage the auricle is erythematous. The anterior surface may develop a cobblestone appearance, and eventually the whole ear becomes atrophic.

In the larynx the epiglottic, thyroid, and cricoid cartilages are eroded and become fibrosed, leading to a loss of normal supporting skeleton, particularly in the cricoid region, which may cause laryngeal obstruction.

Histologic Features. The ground substance of the cartilage appears acidophilic (except for basophilia around some surviving lacunae) and shows deeper staining by the PAS method. There is invasion of altered cartilage by inflammatory tissue. At the interface with inflammatory tissue there is compression of cartilage lacunae, which often appear linear. Focal calcification and dystrophic ossification of the degenerated cartilage have been described (9). The early inflammatory exudate is composed of neutrophils. Later it is formed mainly by plasma cells and lymphocytes, with some histiocytes (Fig. 1). These cells invade the cartilage from the perichondrium. Fibroblasts multiply, and eventually a dense, poorly cellular scar results. A late stage of the disease displays cystic spaces containing gelatinous fluid in the degenerated cartilage (8).

Immunologic Findings. Autoantibodies to type II collagen have been found in cases of relapsing polychondritis (10). It is of interest, in view of the frequent occurrence of ocular inflammation in relapsing polychondritis, that type II collagen is a constituent of both eye and cartilage. Autoantibodies to cartilage (8) and cell-mediated immunity to cartilage have been described in lymphocytes in cases of relapsing polychondritis (11). The significance of these general immunologic findings specifically for relapsing polychondritis is doubtful. Autoantibodies to cartilage, for instance, may be detected in the serum of cases of rheumatoid arthritis and after infectious mononucleosis (8).

Keratosis Obturans, Keratosis of the Tympanic Membrane, and Keratin Implantation Granuloma

In keratosis obturans, the keratin produced by exfoliation from the skin of the tympanic membrane and external canal is retained on the epithelial surface, instead of being removed by auditory

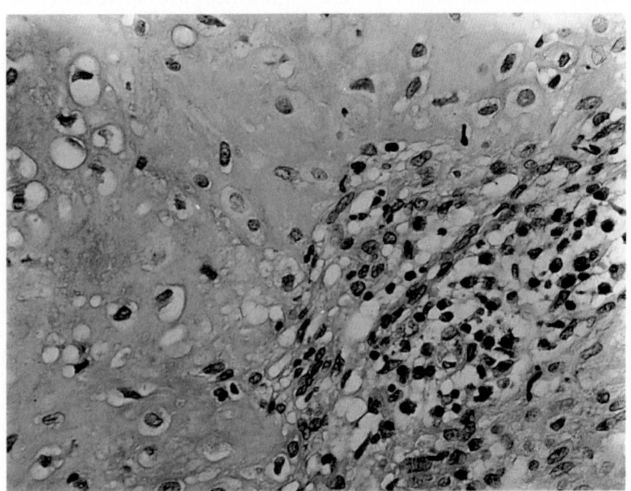

FIGURE 1. Cricoid cartilage in a case of relapsing polychondritis. The edge of the cartilage is eroded by plasma cells, lymphocytes, and macrophages. (Reprinted from Michaels L. *Ear, nose and throat histopathology.* London: Springer, 1987; with permission.)

epithelial migration, and forms a solid plug. This enlarges with erosion of the adjacent bony canal. The etiologic basis of keratosis obturans has been considered to be a defect of the migratory properties of the squamous epithelium of tympanic membrane and adjacent ear canal, which causes the accumulation of keratinous debris. Recent studies of the pattern of auditory epithelial migration in two cases of keratosis obturans showed that this was, indeed, abnormal in each case (12).

A condition of keratosis of the tympanic membrane in which deposits of keratin form on the eardrum and cause tinnitus also has been found to be associated with absent or defective auditory epithelial migration (13).

A granulomatous process in the external ear canal takes place when keratin squames become implanted into the deeper tissues following traumatic laceration (14). The granuloma contains foreign body–type giant cells, histiocytes, lymphocytes, plasma cells, and flakes of keratin. The latter are eosinophilic and birefringent in polarized light.

Metabolic Conditions

A number of metabolic conditions manifesting in the tissues of the ear may come to the attention of the pathologist.

Gout

The external ear is one of the most frequent places for gouty tophi in nonarticular tissues, and deposits may occur in the helix and antihelix. They may ulcerate, discharging a creamy white material within which needle-like crystals of sodium urate may be detected on microscopy.

Histologically the gouty tophus is composed of basophilic masses of amorphous material surrounded by foreign body giant cells and histiocytes. The sodium urate crystals are soluble in water and so are dissolved in the formaldehyde solution usually used for fixation. For this reason fixation in alcohol is preferred when a gouty tophus is suspected. A few crystals may then remain and possibly be identified as brownish, closely packed, needle-like structures that are birefringent (Fig. 2).

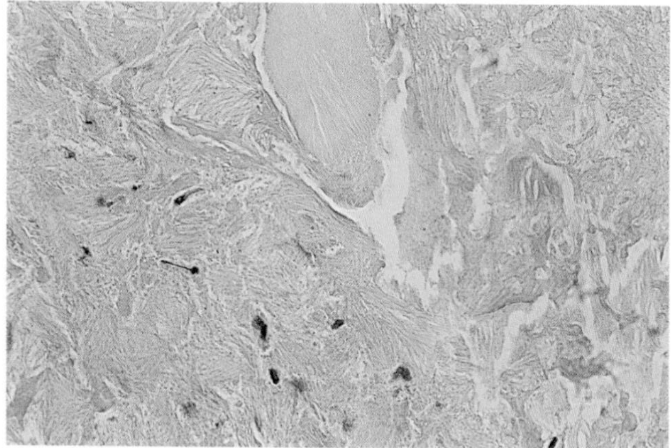

FIGURE 2. Gouty tophus from auricle. Note amorphous, basophilic material and crystalline structures. (Courtesy of Dr. B.Z. Pilch, Massachusetts Eye and Ear Infirmary.)

Ochronosis

Ochronosis (alkaptonuria) results in accumulation of homogentisic acid in a variety of places, but especially cartilage. The substance is colorless in the urine when first passed, but darkens to a black or brown polymer upon standing. The disease is inherited in an autosomal-recessive manner.

In the external ear there may be one or both of two manifestations: (a) dark color of the wax (when seen in a child, this may be the first manifestation of ochronosis); and (b) dark color of the aural cartilage due to the binding of the homogentisic acid to the cartilage ground substance.

Xanthoma Associated with Hyperlipoproteinemia

In rare cases of hyperlipoproteinemia, crystals of lipid with an associated histiocytic reaction may be found infiltrating bone trabeculae and marrow spaces of the mastoid (15). The appearances are similar to those of cholesterol granuloma, except that there is no trace of hemorrhage or hemosiderin in hyperlipoproteinemia, foam cells are more numerous than usual in cholesterol granuloma, and the lipid deposits and their cellular reaction mainly involve the bone itself and not the mucosa of the mastoid air cells in hyperlipoproteinemia (16) (Fig. 3).

Lesions Difficult to Classify

Several conditions may be found in the external ear that may show some similarity to neoplasms, but which are probably not.

Malakoplakia

This lesion, most characteristic of the urinary tract, may affect the external canal with involvement also of the tympanic cavity and mastoid (17,18). Microscopic examination shows

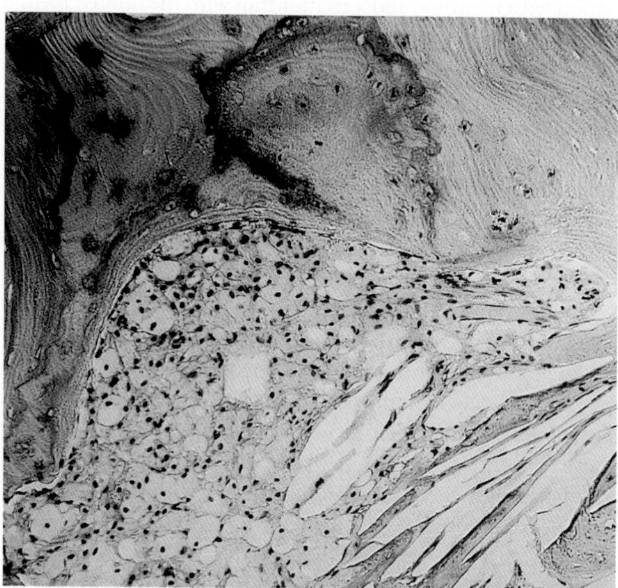

FIGURE 3. Xanthomatous deposit in mastoid bone in a patient with type V hyperlipoproteinemia. Foam cells and cholesterol clefts accompanied by foreign body–type giant cells infiltrate marrow spaces and bone trabeculae. (Reprinted from Michaels L. *Ear, nose and throat histopathology.* London: Springer, 1987; with permission.)

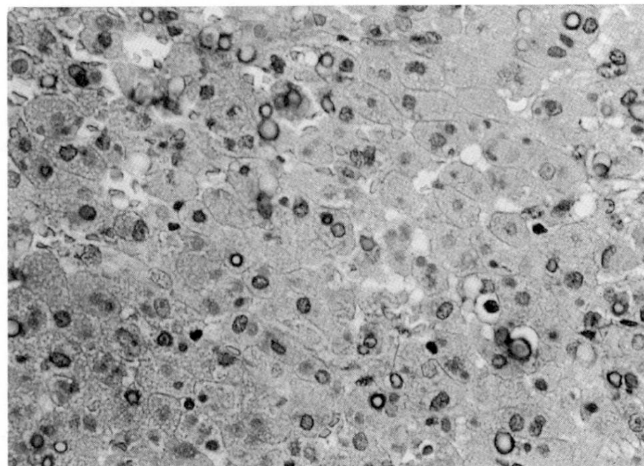

FIGURE 4. Malakoplakia of the ear. The tissue is composed of macrophages with abundant granular cytoplasm. Note also Michaelis-Gutmann bodies, often within macrophages. (Reprinted from Michaels L. *Ear, nose and throat histopathology.* London: Springer, 1987; with permission.)

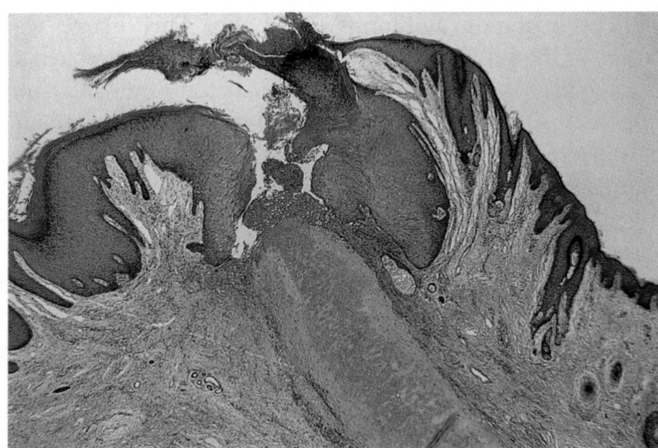

FIGURE 5. Chondrodermatitis nodularis chronica helicis. There is an ulcer extending down to the cartilage of the pinna and severe acanthosis. (Reprinted from Michaels L. The ear. In: Damjanov I, Linder J. *Anderson's pathology.* St. Louis: CV Mosby, 1996:2876–2900; with permission.)

macrophages with abundant cytoplasm containing diastase-resistant, PAS-positive granules (von Hansemann cells). Lamellated, calcified (Michaelis-Gutmann) bodies, often within macrophages, are also frequently present (Fig. 4).

Like the lesions in the urinary tract, those in the ear have been associated with a coliform infection.

Chondrodermatitis Nodularis Chronica Helicis

Clinical Data. In chondrodermatitis nodularis chronica helicis (Winkler's disease) (19), a small nodule forms, usually on the superior portion of the helix in a middle-aged man (20). Pain is severe. The literature both supports (19) and rejects (20) an association with frostbite, and a relationship with the limited form of systemic sclerosis also has been suggested (21). Obliteration via laser treatment is recommended (22,23).

Histologic Features. Histologically, the nodule shows ulceration with irregular acanthosis at its margins, a process that can sometimes be identified in the region of a hair follicle (24). The collagen locally shows increased eosinophilia and is often degenerated; there is also chronic inflammatory granulation tissue in skin and adjacent elastic cartilage (Fig. 5).

Spectacle Frame Acanthoma (Granuloma Fissuratum)

Spectacle frame acanthoma caused by irritation occurs behind the ear in the region of the postauricular groove. There is a raised pink nodule with a linear depression running through its center into which the frame fits exactly (25,26). Histologically there is acanthosis with chronic inflammation of the dermis and sometimes a shallow sulcus.

Epithelioid Hemangioma and Kimura's Disease

Epithelioid Hemangioma

Synonyms for this condition include benign angiomatous (nodules of the face and scalp, atypical pyogenic granuloma, and angiolymphoid hyperplasia with eosinophilia, among several others).

Clinical Data. Benign angiomatous nodules may occur anywhere in the skin, especially on the scalp and face, but there is a particular predilection for the external auricle and external auditory canal. It is a lesion of young and middle-aged individuals of both sexes and all races.

Gross Appearance. Grossly there are sessile or plaque-like red or reddish blue lesions 2 to 10 mm in diameter, which may coalesce to form large plaques that obstruct the ear canal. On transection the lesion is seen in the dermis and subcutaneous tissue.

Histologic Features. Microscopically, there is a mixture of two proliferated elements in the dermis: blood vessels and lymphoid tissue. The blood vessels are mainly capillaries lined by plump, often protruding (hobnailed), sometimes multilayered, endothelial cells (Fig. 6). Occasionally an artery or vein showing intimal

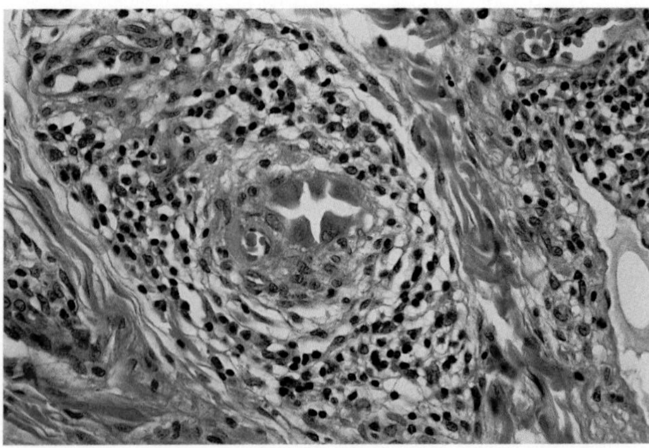

FIGURE 6. Subcutaneous tissue of skin near pinna from a patient with epithelioid hemangioma. Lymphoid tissue is present and a capillary lined by plump, hobnailed endothelial cells.

fibrous thickening is part of the vascular component. Solid clusters of cells, which are often vacuolated, show features intermediate between endothelial cells and histiocytes (27). The lymphoid tissue may possess germinal centers. Eosinophils (often extremely numerous), mast cells, and macrophages also may be prominent.

Kimura's Disease

Kimura's disease is thought to be a separate entity from epithelioid hemangioma. It is more common in Asians, mainly affecting young males. It involves the subcutaneous and deep soft tissues; lymph nodes are frequently affected. Microscopically, in Kimura's disease the main lesion is the lymphoid hyperplasia. Vascular proliferation is not marked (28) (see Chapter 12).

Both epithelioid hemangioma and Kimura's disease are benign entities. Both may show T-cell infiltration with B-cell clusters on immunohistochemical analysis (29). Recurrence is rare in the former, if completely excised, but more frequent in the latter, although eventually even in this condition the disease becomes stationary. A nephrotic syndrome may rarely occur in Kimura's disease.

Idiopathic Cystic Chondromalacia (Pseudocysts)

Clinical Data. Idiopathic cystic chondromalacia (pseudocysts) is an unusual lesion of the cartilage of the auricle (30,31). It occurs mainly in young and middle-aged adults. Its association with severe atopic eczema in four children (32) suggested that minor trauma from repeated rubbing of the auricle may play a part. Simple curettage will eliminate the lesion.

Gross Appearance. The gross appearance is one of a localized swelling of the auricular cartilage. The cut surface shows a well-defined cystic cavity in the cartilage, which is distended with yellowish watery fluid.

Histologic Features. Microscopically, the cyst is a simple space without an epithelial lining surrounded by degenerative or normal cartilage, hence a pseudocyst (33) (Fig. 7).

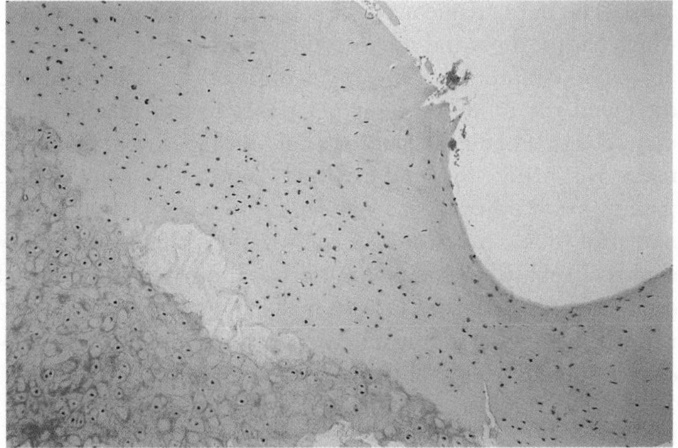

FIGURE 7. Cartilage of auricle showing a cyst of idiopathic cystic chondromalacia, which is lined by normal cartilage.

Keloid

Keloid, a common benign skin lesion, follows injury to the skin of the ear, often after piercing the earlobes to insert an earring, particularly in blacks. A lobulated swelling covered by normal skin shows microscopically a dermis enlarged by layered deposits of eosinophilic, poorly cellular collagen arranged in characteristic markedly thickened bundles.

Petrified Auricle

Petrified auricle is an uncommon condition in which the elastic cartilage of the auricle becomes calcified. This may be the result of ectopic calcification caused by local trauma or systemic diseases such as Addison's disease, hypopituitarism, thyroid or parathyroid disorders, or radiation therapy. Another form of petrified auricle is ectopic ossification in which the elastic cartilage is replaced by bone (34). The latter condition is usually preceded by severe acute hypothermia (frostbite). In neither form of petrified auricle is the cartilage of the superficial external canal affected.

Gross Appearance. In both forms the auricle is stony hard and moves as a rigid unit.

Histologic Features. Microscopically, in ectopic ossification the cartilage is replaced by bony trabeculae that may have haversian canals and marrow spaces.

NEOPLASMS

Epithelial

Basal Cell Carcinoma

Most malignant epithelial external ear neoplasms are basal cell carcinomas, a small number only being squamous cell carcinomas. Basal cell carcinomas arise mainly on the pinna and are usually slow-growing, but in a few cases may be recurrent and infiltrative. For a more complete discussion of basal cell carcinoma, the reader is referred to Chapter 13.

Squamous Cell Carcinoma

Squamous cell carcinoma of the external ear often arises within the external canal; if deeply situated, there is usually a concomitant origin from middle ear epithelium and dissolution of the tympanic membrane. Metastatic spread derived from squamous carcinoma of the pinna and external auditory meatus takes place in about 8% of cases (35). Tumors confined to the external ear usually have a good outlook after surgical therapy.

Verrucous Squamous Cell Carcinoma

The verrucous form of squamous cell carcinoma is encountered in the external canal (36–39). As is the case at other sites where this neoplasm occurs, the diagnosis may be delayed until several biopsies have been performed because of initial confusion with benign squamous papilloma or squamous cell hyperplasia secondary to inflammation. At initial presentation, measurement of the mean cell area in the malpighian cell region of the lesion (or, more simply, the mean cell diameter using an eyepiece micrometer) is a useful diagnostic aid. Verrucous squamous carcinomas have a mean cell area of greater than 300 μm^2 and a mean diameter of greater than 30 μm, whereas benign squamous lesions have a mean cell area of less than 250 μm squared and a mean diameter of less than 25 μm (40).

Neoplasms of Ceruminal Glands: Benign

Adenoma (Ceruminoma)

Clinical Data. Ceruminoma is a rare neoplasm that obstructs the lateral part of the external canal, producing deafness and discharge. An important part of the clinical investigation of all glandular neoplasms of the external canal is exclusion of an origin in the parotid gland or middle ear.

Gross Appearance. The tumor appears as a superficial gray mass, covered by skin.

Histologic Features. An adenoma has no definite capsule. Regular glands lined by bilayered epithelium, comprising glandular and myoepithelial cells, distinguish this neoplasm. The glandular cells show evidence of apocrine secretion into the lumen (Fig. 8). In some ceruminomas, acid-fast fluorescent pigment, similar to that of normal ceruminous glands (41,42), is present in the tumor cells.

Syringocystadenoma Papilliferum

Syringocystadenoma papilliferum, a benign lesion of apocrine cell origin, occasionally occurs in the external canal.

Cylindroma

Clinical Data. Cylindroma in the external ear may be present on the pinna or in the external canal. In these situations it may be part of a multiple turban tumor presentation of this neoplasm on the scalp.

Gross Appearance. A cylindroma forms a projecting smooth swelling beneath the skin.

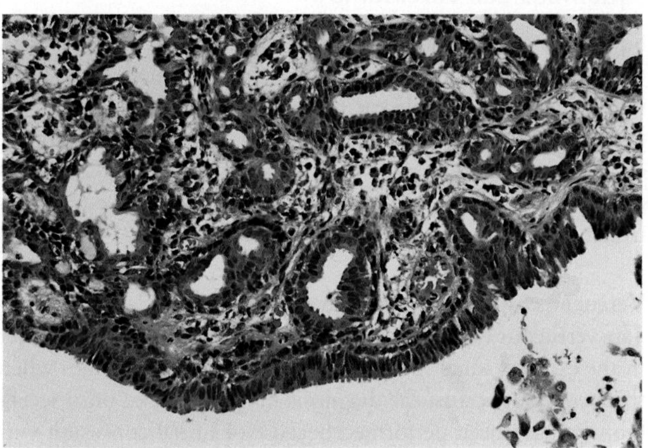

FIGURE 8. Ceruminoma of the external canal showing regular glands comprising glandular cells with apocrine secretion and myoepithelial cells.

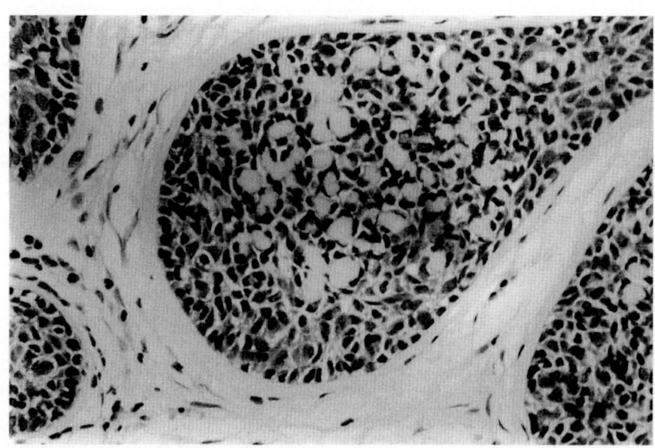

FIGURE 9. Cylindroma of the skin of the ear showing masses of small darkly stained cells within which are hyaline globules (pink- staining in the original). Similar hyaline material also surrounds the cellular masses.

Histologic Features. This neoplasm is composed of rounded masses of small, darkly staining cells in masses that seem to fit together in a jigsaw-like pattern and are surrounded by pink-staining hyaline material. Hyaline globules are often present in the cellular masses (Fig. 9), as are larger cells with vesicular nuclei.

Differential Diagnosis. A cylindroma, when it occurs in the external canal, may be confused with primary adenoid cystic carcinoma of this location. It differs from the latter in the absence of a cribriform structure, as well as in the presence of the larger cells with vesicular nuclei (43,44). Furthermore, the extensive tissue infiltration and perineural invasion characteristic of adenoid cystic carcinoma is not seen in a cylindroma.

Pleomorphic Adenoma

Pleomorphic adenoma is sometimes found in this location (45). It shows the same histologic features as pleomorphic adenoma of the parotid gland, which is what makes the exclusion of the latter origin so important (see Chapter 8).

Glandular Neoplasms: Malignant

Malignant glandular tumors are sometimes seen in the external canal. The most frequent of these is adenoid cystic carcinoma, which has the gross and microscopic features of the corresponding major or minor salivary gland neoplasms (Fig. 10), including their tendency to invade along nerve sheaths (see Chapter 8). It may sometimes be mistaken for a cylindroma. Relentless recurrence over many years and eventual bloodstream metastasis to the lungs and other organs are features of adenoid cystic carcinomas of the external canal, as with those arising from salivary glands. Primary mucoepidermoid carcinoma of the external canal has been described (46). A malignant glandular neoplasm without adenoid cystic or mucoepidermoid structure also may arise in the external canal.

Melanotic

Nevi are seen from time to time in the external canal, but they are distinctly rare on the pinna. Malignant melanotic neoplasms

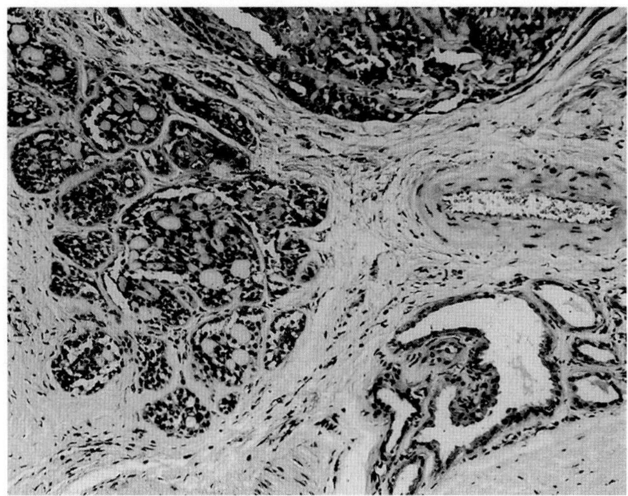

FIGURE 10. Adenoid cystic carcinoma of external canal showing cribriform pattern. Note normal apocrine (wax) glands at bottom right.

are uncommon in any part of the external ear. When they do occur in the ear they usually arise on the pinna, where they are often advanced, one third showing metastases to regional lymph nodes at their first visit (47) and the majority displaying Clark level IV invasion or more on histologic examination (48) (see Chapter 13).

Neoplasms of Connective Tissue and Bone

Myxoma

A syndrome of skin myxomas concomitant with myxoma of the left or right cardiac atrium, together with endocrine overactivity and skin lentigines, has been described (49). The skin myxomas mostly occurred in the lower eyelid, but the pinna and external auditory canal were involved in some cases. Histologically myxomas of the ear consist of an accumulation of basophilic ground substance in the dermis in which there are spindle mesenchymal cells staining negatively for S-100 protein immunohistochemically.

Benign Fibroosseous Lesion (Monostotic Fibrous Dysplasia or Ossifying Fibroma)

Clinical Data. A solitary lesion composed of woven bone and fibrous tissue occurring in the external ear is often difficult to diagnose within specific categories such as monostotic fibrous dysplasia or ossifying fibroma, and the term benign fibroosseous lesion is conveniently used to embrace such lesions. Most patients show obstruction of the external canal, often with computed tomographic (CT) evidence of involvement of the temporal bone (50).

Gross Appearance. Benign fibroosseous lesions show calcified tissue with a yellowish white appearance.

Histologic Features. Microscopically, irregular trabeculae of woven bone are embedded in a connective tissue stroma. Squamous epithelial-lined inclusions also may be found in the tumor. The reader is referred to Chapter 11 for a fuller discussion.

Biologic Behavior. The lesion grows slowly and is usually eliminated by curettage.

Osteoma and Exostosis

Two types of benign bony enlargement of the deeper bony portion of the external auditory meatus are recognized: osteoma and exostosis (51,52). Osteoma is a spherical mass projecting into the external ear, with a distinct bony pedicle. It is composed of lamellar bone and is covered by the normal stratified squamous epithelium of the external canal. Exostosis is a broad-based lesion, often bilateral and symmetrical (51). It is usually situated deeper in the ear canal than osteoma. In the bony portion of the normal external auditory canal there are no adnexal structures, and the distance between the epidermal surface and underlying bone is consequently small (1). This explains why exostoses may develop in this region in those who swim frequently in cold water. The latter enters the deep canal and exerts a cooling effect that stimulates the nearby periosteum to produce new bone. Troublesome bacterial or fungal infection may occur central to the bony obstruction and necessitate surgical removal of bone for drainage.

Reticuloendothelial Neoplasms

Langerhans' Cell Histiocytosis

Langerhans' cell histiocytosis (histiocytosis X, eosinophilic granuloma, Hand-Schüller-Christian disease) is a proliferative disorder of the reticuloendothelial system, which frequently affects bone. In the temporal bone, which sometimes is the first or only site affected, the disease is usually manifested as a bony lesion of the medial part of the external auditory meatus in children (53,54). In patients under 3 years of age, the disease process is more likely to be multifocal in the skull, and to have a worse prognostic outlook. Histologically the diagnosis is made by the presence of an accumulation of the characteristic Langerhans' cell macrophages. These display slit nuclei, express S-100 protein on immunochemistry, and show thin, elongated Birbeck granules in their cytoplasm on electron microscopy. Eosinophils and sometimes neutrophils are prominent in the exudate.

Malignant Lymphoma

Malignant lymphoma may appear in the external ear as part of a generalized process. Occasionally it may be primary in this situation, presenting as a B- or T-cell lymphoma of the skin of the pinna. A striking symmetry in the deposition of the lymphoid neoplasia has been described in some cases, each ear lobe or both earlobes and helices on each side being similarly affected (55). This can be explained either by migration from the circulation or by clonal proliferation, each of which would be programmed bilaterally and symmetrically on a site-specific basis.

MIDDLE EAR AND MASTOID

Non-neoplastic Lesions

Inflammatory Lesions

Otitis Media

Clinical Data. There are acute and chronic clinical forms of otitis media, and each often manifests its own appropriate pathologic changes, but intermediate or mixed pathologies are also frequent. The clinical features of acute otitis media are those of pain (particularly in the mastoid area), tenderness and swelling in the postauricular region, and edema of the posterosuperior wall of the external canal. The tympanic membrane is initially hyperemic and then bulges as more pus collects in the middle ear, until eventually it may burst.

In chronic otitis media perforation of the tympanic membrane may or may not be present. The major features of chronic otitis media with perforation are discharge from the middle ear and conductive hearing loss. Frequently polyps derived from middle ear mucosal inflammatory swelling over the promontory bulge out through a perforation, usually in the pars tensa region, and occlude the external canal. The middle ear inflammation, while often indolent, may at times spread to petrous bone, inner ear, meninges, and even brain, giving rise to serious complications and perhaps death. Chronic otitis media with an intact tympanic membrane (otitis media with effusion, serous otitis media, or glue ear) is a milder form. It is important to note that an advanced degree of otitis media may exist, but may remain undetected clinically and even may be undetectable (56).

Microbiology. In the acute phase, *Streptococcus pneumoniae* and *Haemophilus influenzae* are the most common causative organisms. *Staphylococcus aureus* and *Streptococcus pyogenes* are also possible etiologic agents (57). Infection with anaerobic organisms also may produce acute otitis media (58). Epidemiologic studies have indicated certain respiratory viruses—influenza viruses A and B, enterovirus, rhinovirus, parainfluenza virus, adenovirus, and respiratory syncytial virus—to be causative of acute otitis media in the early phases of the illness (59,60). In the chronic phase, gram-negative bacteria, particularly *Proteus* and *Pseudomonas*, are found, although *Staphylococcus pyogenes* and beta-hemolytic streptococci are sometimes isolated from the discharging pus of chronically inflamed ears. Anerobes may sometimes be grown at this stage, including anaerobic gram-positive cocci, *Bacteroides* species, and *Clostridium* species (61).

Although much less frequent than the above organisms, infection with *Mycobacterium tuberculosis* may give rise to chronic inflammation of the middle ear. In such cases the inflammatory reaction is distinctive.

Histologic Features. The sole biopsy material likely to be received by the pathologist in acute otitis media is the bone chips removed at mastoidectomy. These fragments feature congestion and edema of the mucosa of the mastoid air cells. The mucosa and air cells are filled with neutrophils. Pus destroys bone, the actual dissolution being achieved by osteoclasts. At the same time, new bone formation takes place, commencing as osteoid, later becoming woven and finally lamellar. Fibrosis also may be active even in the acute stage.

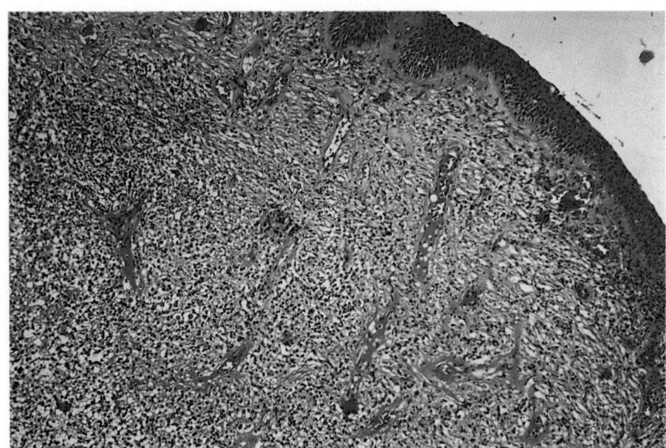

FIGURE 11. Aural polyp composed of inflammatory and granulation tissue. There is a covering of stratified squamous epithelium.

Chronic otitis media is characterized by various degrees of admixture of the following histologic features: (a) Chronic inflammation and chronic inflammatory granulation tissue formation in the mucosa; (b) glandular metaplasia of the middle ear epithelium; (c) cholesterol granuloma; (d) tympanosclerosis; and (e) bony sclerosis of mastoid bone.

a. The most characteristic feature of the pathology of chronic otitis media is the presence of inflammatory and granulation tissue. This cellular reaction has two components: inflammatory cells (lymphocytes, plasma cells, and macrophages) and granulation tissue (newly formed capillaries and fibroblasts). These two types of cellular reaction are seen together in aural polyps, which are usually covered by columnar epithelium, often ciliated. Sometimes the epithelium overlying aural polyps is of the stratified squamous type (Fig. 11). This may be produced by metaplasia from irritation, but its presence does not denote cholesteatoma of the middle ear. Goblet cells are greatly increased in the middle ear mucosa.

b. The mucosa in chronic otitis media indicates its kinship to the rest of the respiratory tract by the formation of glands via metaplasia of the lining mucosal epithelium. They each consist of a simple tubule of mucus-producing cells (Fig. 12). Glandular transformation may take place in the mastoid air cells as well as in the main middle ear cavity. The secretion derived from the glands is an important component of the aural discharge in chronic otitis media.

c. Yellow nodules are found in the tympanic cavity and mastoid in many cases of chronic otitis media. These are composed microscopically of crystals of cholesterol and its ester (dissolved away to leave empty clefts in paraffin-embedded histologic sections) surrounded by foreign body–type giant cells and other chronic inflammatory cells (Fig. 13). Such cholesterol deposits are almost always found in the midst of hemorrhage and are probably derived from breakdown of red blood corpuscles. Hemosiderin is often present among the inflammatory cells surrounding the cholesterol granuloma. Cholesterol granuloma in the mastoid air cells should be distinguished from lipid deposits of hyperlipoproteinemia (Fig. 3).

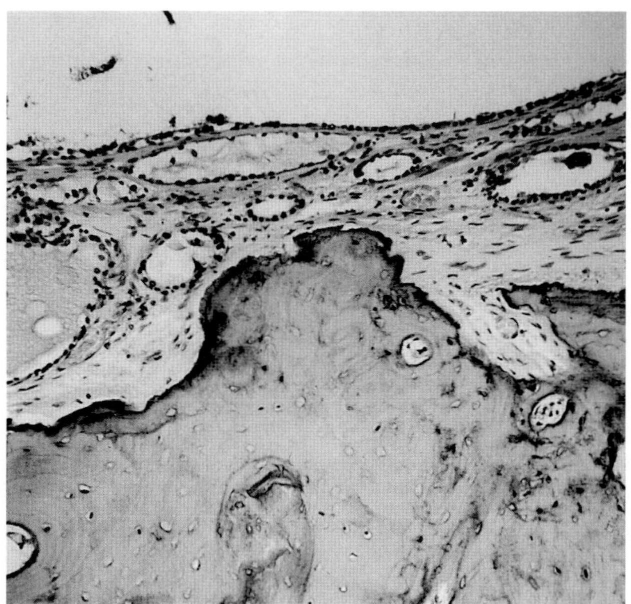

FIGURE 12. Mucosal middle ear surface of bone of promontory in chronic otitis media. Note glands in mucosa and irregular edge of bone. (Reprinted from Michaels L. *Ear, nose and throat histopathology.* London: Springer, 1987; with permission.)

d. Tympanosclerosis is a special form of fibrosis that is often encountered in chronic otitis media. Deposits of dense white tissue are laid down in the middle ear mucosa, not only on the tympanic side of the tympanic membrane (common in otitis media with effusion), but also following chronic suppurative otitis media, on the crura of the stapes, within the tympanic cavity, and sometimes in the mastoid air cells. On dissection, the tympanosclerotic deposit may show a lamellated onion skin–like structure. Microscopically, the material is composed of hyaline collagen deposited in the mucosa. Deposits of calcium salts, appearing as basophilic dust–like areas, are irregularly distributed through the collagen. A multilayered structure corresponding to the gross appearance of lamellation is frequently observed. Bone is also often present in tympanosclerotic plaques (Fig. 14).

e. The mastoid air cells show fibrosis, and their bony walls are markedly thickened. Cement lines in the lamellar bone are numerous and irregular, often forming a mosaic pattern. Osteoid seams may be present on the inner surface of air cell bone (Fig. 15). These changes indicate the recent active deposition and resorption of bone as a result of the inflammatory pro-

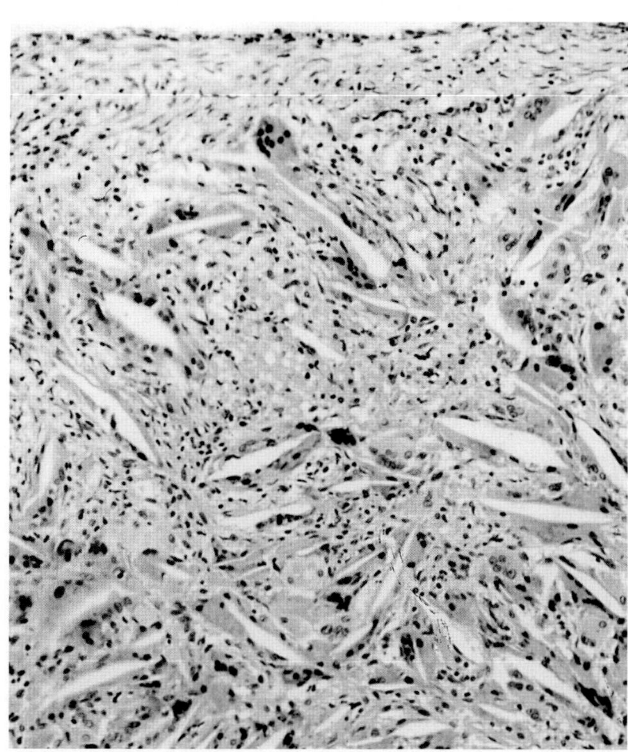

FIGURE 13. Cholesterol granuloma of middle ear surrounded by foreign body type giant cells and other chronic inflammatory cells. (Reprinted from Michaels L. *Ear, nose and throat histopathology.* London: Springer, 1987; with permission.)

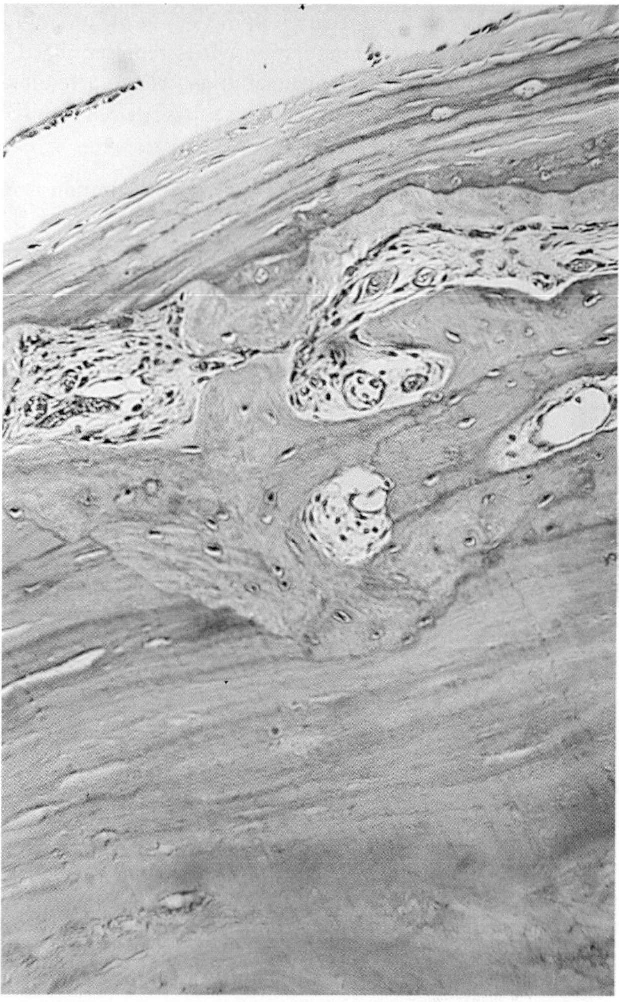

FIGURE 14. Tympanosclerosis from middle ear showing a plaque of multilayered, calcified, hyaline collagen with an area of bone.

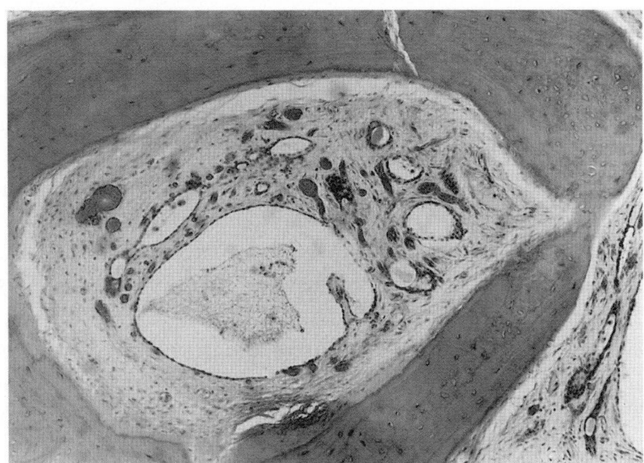

FIGURE 15. Low-grade otitis media with effusion from temporal bone taken from a patient with AIDS at autopsy. The middle ear mucosa is on the right and a mastoid air cell in the center. Note fibrinous exudate in mastoid air cell. The mucosa of middle ear and mastoid air cell is thickened by fibrous tissue within which are numerous glands. An osteoid seam lines the bone. (Reprinted from Michaels L, Soucek S, Liang J. The ear in the acquired immunodeficiency syndrome: I. Temporal bone histopathologic study. *Am J Otol* 1994;15:515–522; with permission.)

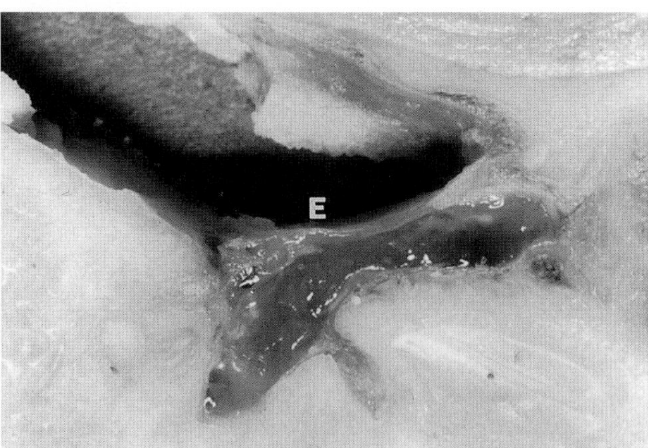

FIGURE 16. Gross photograph of microslice of temporal bone from a patient with AIDS, showing otitis media with effusion as manifested by gelatinous secretion (glue) in middle ear cavity. *E*, external canal. (Reprinted from Michaels L, Soucek S, Liang J. The ear in the acquired immunodeficiency syndrome: I. Temporal bone histopathologic study. *Am J Otol* 1994;15:515–522; with permission.)

cess. The product of these reparative processes in the mastoid is a patchy sclerosis with some cystic cavities representing distended air cells. Eradication of mastoid air cells as a result of chronic otitis media, with bony replacement, is referred to as secondary sclerosis.

In some ears the mastoid air cells lack pneumatization from an early age. This has been ascribed to inflammatory change, but such an interpretation has been doubted by others who have regarded the sclerosis as primary, perhaps due to genetic factors (62). The appearance of the mastoid in primary arrest of pneumatization is said to be unlike that following otitis media because in the former the mastoid air cell system is small and the bone is diffusely sclerotic.

Otitis Media with Effusion

Synonyms commonly in use for otitis media with effusion (OME) include secretory otitis media, serous otitis media, catarrhal otitis media, tubotympanitis, and glue ear. It is a common cause of hearing loss in children, but also may occur in adults. It is characterized by a glue-like effusion behind a nonperforated eardrum in the absence of frank symptoms of acute infection (Fig. 16). Few biopsy or autopsy temporal bone pathologic studies have been described. All the features of chronic otitis media may be present, including glandular metaplasia (Fig. 15), cholesterol granuloma, chronic inflammatory granulation tissue, ossicular destruction, and tympanosclerosis.

Obstruction of the eustachian tube at its nasopharyngeal end by adenoidal tissue is probably causative of OME in most children with this affection. The most prominent tympanic feature of the histopathology in childhood seems to be new formation of glands in the middle ear mucosa (63).

Otitis media with effusion also occurs in adults by a similar mechanism, but in this age group it is neoplasms of the nasopharynx, such as undifferentiated carcinoma, that occlude the nasopharyngeal orifice of the eustachian tube. Histopathologic examination of the middle ear mucosa in adult OME at autopsy in one study also showed glandular metaplasia, but there was more inflammatory infiltrate than in the childhood cases of OME (64).

Mycobacterial (Tuberculous) Otitis Media

Tuberculous otitis media is an unusual form of chronic otitis media, which is often, but not always, associated with active pulmonary tuberculosis. Complications, especially involvement of the facial nerve, are more frequent than in the more common form of chronic otitis media (65). The diagnosis is usually made at pathologic examination of biopsy material (66).

Histologic examination shows tuberculoid granulation tissue, composed of epithelioid cells and lymphocytes, often with Langhans' giant cells (Fig. 17) and areas of caseation situated in the middle ear mucosa. Bone destruction is pronounced. Acid-

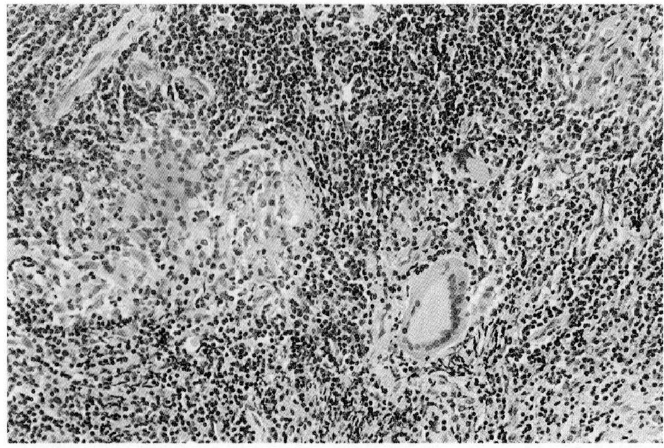

FIGURE 17. Tuberculous otitis media showing large numbers of lymphocytes, Langhans' giant cells, and a group of epithelioid histiocytes. Caseation was present in other parts of the specimen.

fast bacilli are normally found with difficulty in the granulomatous material, but culture of the middle ear inflammatory tissue usually produces tubercle bacilli.

Some exceptional cases of tuberculous otitis media have been encountered in which vast numbers of acid-fast bacilli were present in the granulomas, confirmed in each case as *Mycobacterium tuberculosis hominis* by culture (67). The patients were otherwise healthy men with little or no evidence of tuberculosis of the lung or other internal organs and no predisposing factors for human immunodeficiency virus infection or other causes of immunosuppression.

Sarcoidosis

Although rare, non-caseating tuberculoid granulomatous changes have been described in the middle ear in patients with manifestations of sarcoidosis in the lungs (68).

Actinomycosis

Actinomycosis of the middle ear, an uncommon infection caused by the anaerobic organism *Actinomyces israelii,* cannot usually be identified in the middle ear without open operation in order to obtain samples of tissue containing the organism (69,70).

AIDS Otitis Media

In a postmortem study of patients with AIDS, OME was found in 60% of 49 temporal bones (71), characterized by the extensive exudation of fibrin into the middle ear spaces, as well as the features of OME mentioned previously (Figs. 15 and 16). In one case, cytomegalovirus infection was present in the middle ear mucosa (Fig. 18). Changes of a more active otitis media with suppuration in the middle ear cleft were identified in 23%, a much higher proportion than was found in a large clinical study

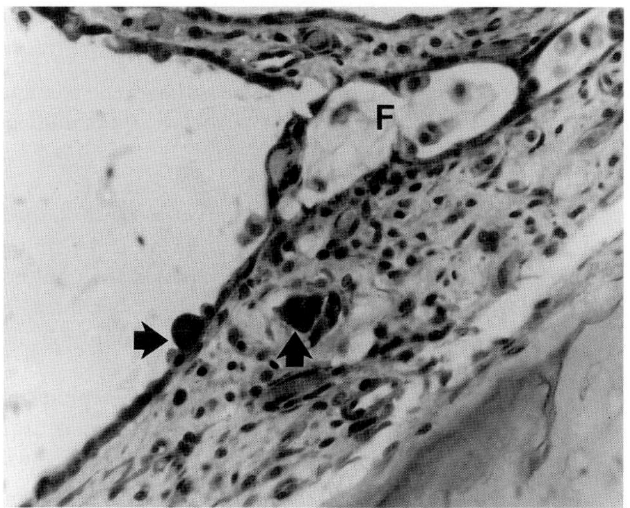

FIGURE 18. Middle ear mucosa with fibrous band from temporal bone taken from a patient with AIDS at autopsy. Groups of cytomegalic inclusion-bearing cells (*arrows*) are in epithelium and blood vessel. Note fibrin (*F*) between fibrous band and mucosa. (Reprinted from Michaels L, Soucek S, Liang J. The ear in the acquired immunodeficiency syndrome: I. Temporal bone histopathologic study. *Am J Otol* 1994;15:515–522; with permission.)

of patients with AIDS, suggesting that severe otitis media may occur frequently in the terminally sick patient with AIDS, perhaps at the site of a middle ear mucosa already weakened by OME.

Wegener's Granulomatosis

Wegener's granulomatosis is a systemic inflammatory condition affecting the kidneys, lungs, and often the nose and many other organs. An antineutrophil cytoplasmic antibody (ANCA), refined by the identification of a cytoplasmic (C) component, has been found in the serum of patients with Wegener's granulomatosis. However, this test yields many false-positive results if it is not executed meticulously. Unfortunately cases of otitis media without renal or pulmonary manifestations, or even histologic evidence of Wegener's such as angiitis, have been given the label of Wegener's on the basis only of a positive C-ANCA test result and apparent success in treating the condition with cyclophosphamide (72). Pathologists should be cautious in interpreting such cases as a locoregional form of Wegener's (73).

Lesions Difficult to Classify

Cholesteatoma

It is now certain that there is a congenital or primary form of cholesteatoma of the middle ear, situated behind an intact tympanic membrane, which is distinct from the acquired form manifesting a perforation of the tympanic membrane. The term *congenital cholesteatoma* is also applied to a squamous epithelial cyst arising at the apex of the petrous temporal bone.

Both acquired and congenital cholesteatoma may take one of the two forms presented in the older literature: (a) a closed, keratinous cyst, or (b) an open lesion, comprising multiple layers of keratinous squames, which is not entirely surrounded by living epidermis (74). In most cases of acquired cholesteatoma the lesion is open. The majority of cases of congenital cholesteatoma, on the other hand, present a closed cyst.

Acquired Cholesteatoma

Gross Appearance. Cholesteatoma appears as an open, pearly white mass. The matrix may be seen as a thin membrane. The cholesteatoma is usually situated in the upper and posterior part of the middle ear cleft and may extend through the aditus into the mastoid antrum and mastoid air cells. Frequently the outline of the cholesteatomatous matrix is adapted to that of normal structures such as ossicles. Inflammatory changes, including marked congestion and pockets of pus, are always present. In most cases at least one ossicle is seriously damaged, so interrupting the continuity of the ossicular chain. The scutum, the upper part of the bony ring of the tympanic opening, is eroded in most cholesteatomas. An eardrum perforation is present in most cases and is situated in the pars flaccida; in some cases it may be near the margin of the pars tensa of the tympanic membrane.

Histologic Features. The pearly material of the cholesteatoma consists of dead, anucleate, keratin squames, the corneal layer of stratified squamous epithelium. The matrix is composed of fully differentiated squamous epithelium similar to the epidermis of skin, but without adnexal structures, and rests on connective tis-

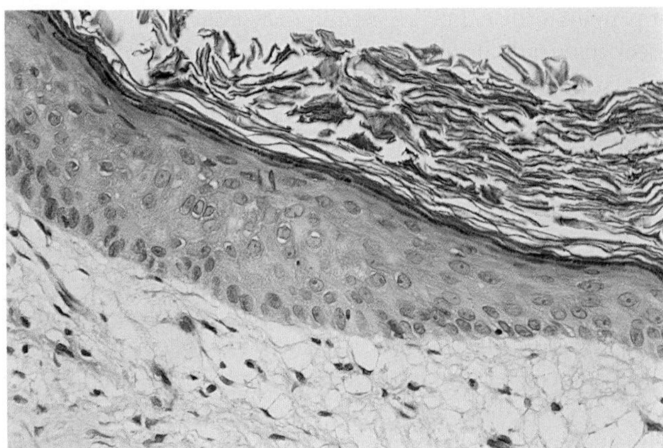

FIGURE 19. Cholesteatoma of the middle ear. Note the keratinous debris **(top)**, which constitutes most of the pathologic material of this lesion at surgery. The matrix **(bottom)** is the living epithelium, composed of regular cells with prominent eosinophilic nucleoli. Note also the mildly inflamed connective tissue deep to the matrix.

sue (Fig. 19). The sole irregularity in comparison with normal stratified squamous epithelium that can be identified in routinely stained sections is that the deeper layers of the epithelium of the cholesteatoma matrix often show evidence of activity in the form of downgrowths into the underlying connective tissue (Figs. 20).

The eroded ossicles may be invested by the squamous epithelial tissue of the cholesteatoma. Even in these circumstances, there is always a layer of chronic inflammatory granulation tissue in contact with the bone, and it seems likely that it is the chronic inflammatory covering, not the squamous epithelium, that produces the erosion.

Features Indicating Increased Proliferation. Recent studies have indicated that cholesteatomatous epithelium possesses innate features of a powerful growth activity that distinguishes it from normal skin epithelium. The techniques of immunohistochemistry and molecular biology have been useful in making this distinction.

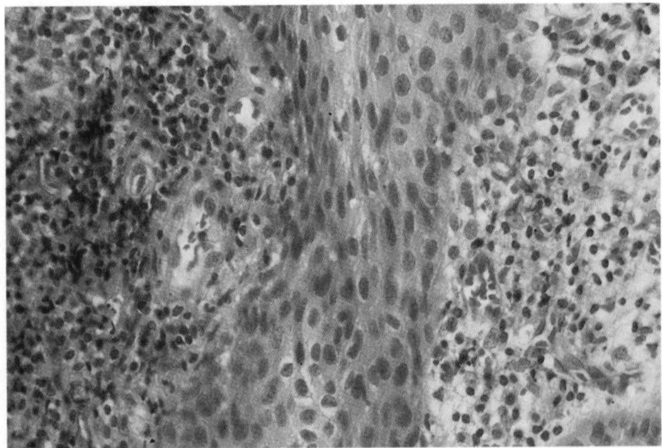

FIGURE 20. Downgrowth of stratified squamous epithelium from matrix of acquired cholesteatoma. Note marked inflammatory exudate.

The cytokeratin expression of simple (cuboidal) middle ear mucosal epithelium on the one hand and that of stratified squamous epithelium of the external canal on the other, has been compared with the cytokeratin expression of cholesteatomatous epithelium. In one such study (75), external ear and cholesteatoma epithelium both expressed cytokeratins characteristic of mature stratified squamous epithelium, but middle ear epithelium did not, expressing in contrast cytokeratins characteristic of simple epithelia. An unexpected finding in the immunohistochemical analysis of the cytokeratins of cholesteatoma, however, was the evidence that it provided for the strong growth activity of the cholesteatoma epithelium. Cytokeratin 16 (CK16) is a marker for hyperproliferative keratinocytes. The strong expression of CK16 by cholesteatoma, but its absence in normal middle ear epithelium and external ear epidermis, has been emphasized (76) and the powerful reproductive activity of cholesteatoma confirmed using antibodies against the antigen Ki-67, which is a marker of proliferative activity throughout most of the growth cycle in frozen sections (77), and against its paraffin section counterpart, MIB-1 (78). The site of the most concentrated expression of increased proliferative activity was found in the epithelial downgrowths of the cholesteatoma (79).

The number of argyrophilic nucleolar organizer regions (AgNORs) that are demonstrable in the cells of a particular tissue have been related to the proliferative activity of that tissue. In middle ear cholesteatoma the number of AgNORs is significantly higher than in normal external canal skin (80).

Pathogenesis. Four concepts of the pathogenesis of acquired cholesteatoma have been put forward:

1. From metaplasia of the epithelium of the middle ear
2. From invasion of canal and tympanic membrane epithelium into the middle ear
3. From invagination of tympanic membrane as a retraction pocket
4. From trauma such as blast injury or insertion of ventilation tubes into the eardrum

There is evidence to favor all of these pathogenetic concepts except the first, and in the following analysis a model unifying the latter three will be provided.

Cholesteatoma from Metaplasia. Islands of metaplastic squamous epithelium in the middle ear from which acquired cholesteatoma could originate have been reported (81), but not confirmed. The concept of metaplasia as a source of cholesteatoma must thus at present be considered unproven.

Cholesteatoma from Invasion. Stratified squamous epithelium may grow from the tympanic membrane or external canal through a perforation to reach the middle ear. Such an ingrowth frequently occurs in perforations, but does not usually produce a cholesteatoma (82). The entrance of stratified squamous epithelium into the middle ear from the external canal as the source of cholesteatoma often has been assumed to be the result of an aberration of the normal process of auditory epithelial migration.

Auditory Epithelial Migration. The cylinder of stratified squamous epithelium lining the outer surface of the tympanic membrane and the deep external canal as far as the junction with the superficial external canal is in constant lateral motion in the process of auditory epithelial migration. The purpose of this activity is to move keratinizing epithelium off the tympanic membrane so as to avoid the buildup of keratin there, which would be deleterious to audition.

The pathways of movement of auditory epithelial migration have been studied by observation of daubs of dye placed on the living eardrum. Observations of the development of this epithelium correlated with the pathways of its movement over the living human eardrum have shown that auditory epithelial migration is the persistence of fetal growth in the mature ear, the augmented epithelium being eliminated by apoptosis at the junction of the deep with the superficial external canal (83–86 and unpublished personal observations). The fetal origin of this growth activity would account for its vigor, and it seems likely that a disturbance of the control mechanisms regulating it could result in aberrant migration (i.e., middle ear cholesteatoma).

Experimental Observations. Penetration of stratified squamous epithelium through the intact tympanic membrane to the middle ear with production of cholesteatoma has been successfully induced in animals by the provocation of otitis media with chemical irritants (87,88) or bacteria (89) placed into the middle ear cavity. After the instillation of propylene glycol solution into the middle ears of chinchillas (90,91), destruction of the epithelium of both middle ear and lateral tympanic membrane surfaces was followed by reepithelialization with hyperplastic epidermal cells and their penetration through the thickened fibrous layer of the tympanic membrane to reach the middle ear cavity, leading to cholesteatoma. The invading stratified squamous epithelium often became necrotic, and perforations of the tympanic membrane with viable epidermal cells at their margins could result. Thus, eardrum perforation in cholesteatoma may be the result of necrosis of inwardly invading stratified squamous epithelium.

These experimental findings throw light on the pathogenesis of human acquired cholesteatoma. It seems possible that, as a result of severe otitis media with damage to the tympanic membrane, epithelium on the lateral surface of the eardrum, characterized by its powerful fetal-like growth potential, loses apoptotic and other local control mechanisms and may be diverted to enter the fibrous layer of the tympanic membrane and then the middle ear.

Cholesteatoma from Invagination (Retraction Pocket). A retraction pocket is an invagination of part of the tympanic membrane, usually in the pars flaccida, into the middle ear cavity. It frequently becomes adherent to the posterior wall of the middle ear in the region of the facial nerve, stapes, or promontory. Histologic sections of the wall of the retraction pocket show an absence of the normal tympanic membrane connective tissue, which may have been destroyed by inflammation. Histologic examination of 12 retraction pockets in postmortem temporal bones showed no evidence of obstruction of the mouth of a retraction pocket that could lead to the development of cholesteatoma (92). In two of the retraction pockets, however, small keratinizing epidermoid foci connected to the squamous epithelium of the retraction pocket by a band of stratified squamous epithelium with occasional foci of keratosis were seen on the malleus and incus within the middle ear (Fig. 21). Similar active downgrowths of pars flaccida epithelium have been described in eardrums not affected by retraction pocket (93,94) and are reminiscent of the incursive activity of regenerated epidermis described in the experimental situation (90). If retraction pocket gives rise to cholesteatoma, it may do so through such an invasive activity rather than by any failure of its drainage. Damage to apoptotic and other restraining mechanisms of tympanic membrane epithelium may be a feature of retraction pockets as a result of otitis media.

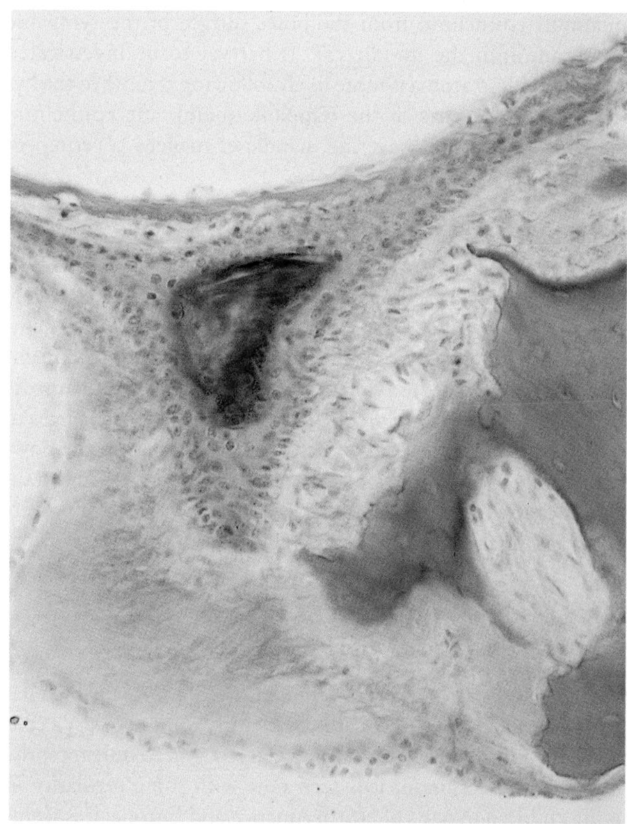

FIGURE 21. Surface of markedly eroded incus (at right) from temporal bone taken at autopsy containing retraction pocket of tympanic membrane. Passing across the incus, just below the middle ear surface, is a band of stratified squamous epithelium that had been traced in serial section from the epidermis of the fundus of the retraction pocket. There is a zone of darkly staining keratosis within a thickened portion of the epithelial band.

Cholesteatoma from Trauma (Blast Injury or Ventilation Tubes). Trauma would seem to be the prime factor in the induction of a few acquired cholesteatomas. Cholesteatoma is found at tympanoplasty up to 18 months after blast injury in 7.6% of ears that have sustained perforation of the tympanic membrane at the time of the injury. The incidence of cholesteatoma increases with the severity of the perforation so produced (95).

Cholesteatoma also has been seen deep to the site of application of a ventilation tube through the tympanic membrane (96). It seems likely that the trauma leads to the entry of stratified squamous epithelium from the outer surface of the tympanic membrane into the middle ear. It has yet to be investigated whether cholesteatoma is more likely following trauma to the hyperproliferative parts of the tympanic membrane epithelium (i.e., the pars flaccida covering, handle of malleus covering) or annulus areas.

Model for Pathogenesis of Acquired Cholesteatoma. Based on the findings described above, it is possible to suggest a model for the pathogenesis of acquired cholesteatoma (Table 1). Chronic otitis media may lead to sufficient damage to the tympanic membrane to cause loss of apoptotic and other growth control mechanisms. Damage to the tympanic membrane from otitis media also may produce retraction pockets (92) with similar changes to growth control mechanisms. These changes may affect the powerful fetal-type growth of auditory epithelial migration in certain regions of the tympanic membrane, resulting in entry of powerfully growing epidermis into the middle ear and cholesteatoma. A similar change may occur following trauma to the tympanic membrane.

Congenital Cholesteatoma

Clinical Data. In contrast to acquired cholesteatoma, which has been established as a clinicopathologic entity for more than a century, congenital cholesteatoma has been recognized only recently. Although not common, it is seen now with some regularity in young children in parts of North America and Europe; it is seemingly rare in some other parts of the world. Most patients present with a lesion in the anterosuperior part of the middle ear. In one quarter of patients the cholesteatoma occupies much of the tympanic cavity. In 3% of patients the congenital cholesteatoma is bilateral (97). Possible reasons for the greater recent frequency of diagnosis of this formerly rare entity include (a) the use of the operating microscope in diagnosis, (b) the improved lighting of otoscopes by the use of the halogen bulb, (c) the screening of tympanic membranes of normal young children by pediatricians, and (d) the possibility that the lesions of which many patients with congenital cholesteatoma formerly underwent "spontaneous abortion" following acute otitis media may now survive with the cure of the otitis in the early stages by antibiotics (97).

Gross Appearances and Appearances at Surgery. Congenital cholesteatoma is seen in most cases as a spherical, whitish object in the anterosuperior part of the tympanic cavity behind an intact tympanic membrane. In some cases the lesion may fill most of the tympanic cavity.

At operation the cholesteatoma is usually a cyst measuring 3 mm or more in diameter, which is situated in close relation to the tympanic membrane, tensor tympani tendon, neck of the malleus, and mouth of the eustachian tube. The cyst may have no firm attachments to the wall of the tympanic cavity (98) or there may be just a thin tenuous connection to the wall (97). Bone erosion is not present when the cholesteatoma is small, but in larger lesions some degree of this change is present (99), and eventually it may enlarge to involve the mastoid and even grow into the middle cranial fossa (100). It thus seems possible that in some cases of congenital cholesteatoma the lesion may enlarge to become indistinguishable from acquired cholesteatoma. In approximately 10% of cases the cholesteatoma is open (101).

Histologic Features. The microscopic appearances of the matrix of congenital cholesteatoma are those of epidermis, as with the acquired variety. The surface of dead, keratinous squames merges with the keratinous contents of the cyst, or lamellae in the case of the open type. In the epithelium of the congenital cholesteatoma in one investigation, there was a similar high degree of growth activity, as shown by the expression of CK16, to that present in acquired cholesteatoma (76).

TABLE 1. PATHOGENESIS OF ACQUIRED CHOLESTEATOMA

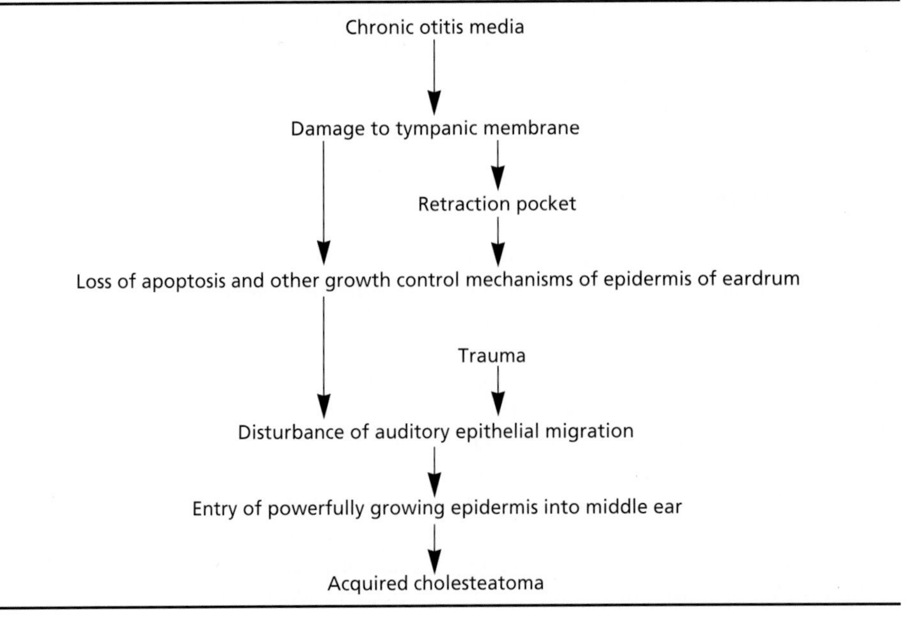

In opportune cases, a double layer of epithelium may be seen surrounding the keratin core. On the outside a single layer of middle ear epithelium is continuous with the epithelium covering the stalk of the cholesteatoma. Separated from the middle ear epithelium only by a thin and often markedly inflamed lamina propria is the basal layer of the stratified squamous epithelium of the congenital cholesteatoma (97).

Pathogenesis. It has been suggested that congenital cholesteatoma may arise from an epidermoid cell rest, which is formed during development in the middle ear epithelium. The discovery of such a cell rest in the anterior superior part of the middle ear in 1936 (102), its rediscovery in 1986 (103), and confirmation in 1987 (104) validated such an origin. This stratified squamous cell rest, the epidermoid formation, is frequently found in the middle ears of fetuses and young infants, always in the same position in the epithelium: at the junction of the eustachian tube with the middle ear, in the region of the anterior superior quadrant of the tympanic membrane, adjacent to the bony annulus (Fig. 22). A tube of epithelium is often present in the mucosa at the same position as the epidermoid formation. An epidermoid formation, often showing keratinization, is often seen in relation to the tube. A tubular structure in the early developing guinea pig middle ear has been shown in section to be derived from the fundus of the first branchial cleft (105).

The epidermoid formation is thus a cell rest found in the same position as the majority of congenital cholesteatomas and has now become generally accepted as the source of congenital cholesteatoma.

Developmental Tumor–like Anomalies

Choristoma

Choristomas, developmental anomalies derived from tissues foreign to the part, are occasionally seen in the middle ear and eustachian tube. They usually grow slowly and are first observed at imaging or surgery. Salivary gland choristomas consist of mixed mucous and serous elements (106) (Fig. 23). A case of primary pleomorphic adenoma of the middle ear was thought to have arisen from such a choristoma (107). Glial choristomas are composed largely of astrocytes, as confirmed by immunochemical staining for glial fibrillary acidic protein. When such masses are identified in biopsy material from the middle ear, a bony deficit with consequent herniation of brain tissue into the middle ear should be ruled out (108). A sebaceous choristoma has been reported, presenting as a mass in the hypotympanum (109).

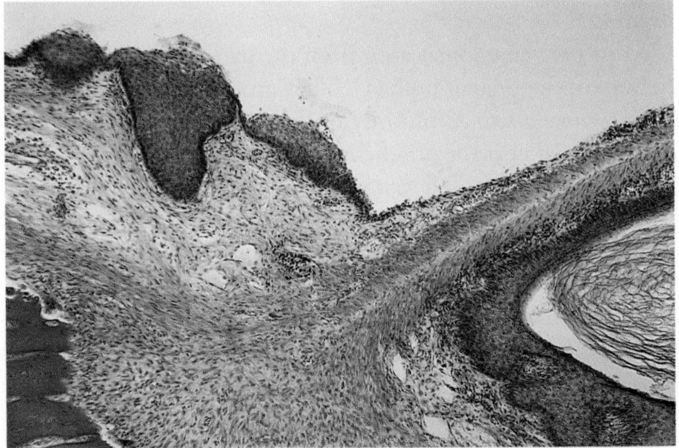

FIGURE 22. Epidermoid formation in a 32-week fetus, which appears as three mounds of stratified squamous epithelium at the junction of the eustachian tube with middle ear epithelium on the upper left. On serial section the mounds were found to merge, forming a single epidermoid mass. The anterior root of the tympanic membrane passes from near the center to the right edge. Below is the anteromedial end of the external canal. At the left lower edge the bony anterior limb of the annulus of the tympanic membrane can be seen.

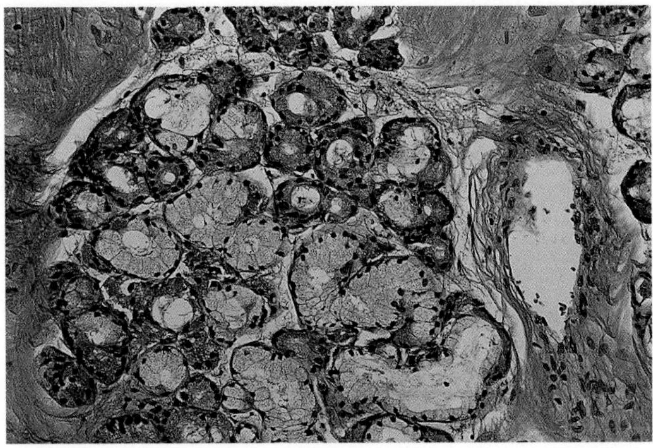

FIGURE 23. Salivary gland choristoma that presented as a mass in the middle ear cavity. It is composed of both mucous and serous elements.

Hamartoma

Hamartomas of the middle ear are rare, the sole representative being the hemangioma. In the few cases in which this has been seen, it was filling the middle ear; it also may arise from the region of the facial nerve or the eustachian tube (110).

True Neoplasms

Locally Arising

Adenoma

A benign glandular neoplasm confined to the middle ear and originating from its epithelium was first described in 1976 (111,112) and now is recognized as the most frequent epithelial neoplasm of the middle ear. The epithelium of the middle ear, although normally nonglandular, forms metaplastic glands even under mildly pathologic conditions. Adenoma is a benign neoplastic transformation of the same epithelial type.

Gross Appearance. The neoplasm may arise in the tympanic cavity or even on the middle ear surface of the tympanic membrane (113). Sometimes it may spread to the mastoid air spaces. Rarely, it extends through a perforation into the external canal (111) or may even penetrate through an apparently intact tympanic membrane (114). Recurrence after surgery has been reported in this condition (115,116), but only one case of metastasis of such a tumor has been reported in the literature (117).

The neoplasm appears white, gray, or reddish brown at operation and may sometimes be grossly vascular. It seems to peel off

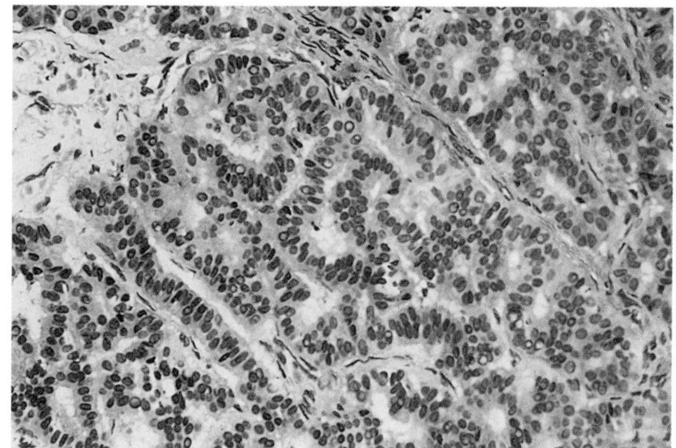

FIGURE 24. Adenoma of middle ear showing back-to-back arrangement of small glands with regular epithelial cells.

the bony walls of the middle ear, although ossicles may sometimes be entrapped in the tumor and may even show destruction.

Histologic Features. Microscopically, adenoma appears to be formed by closely apposed small glands with a "back-to-back" appearance (Fig. 24). In some places a solid or trabecular arrangement is present in which the glandular pattern appears to be lost. This appears to be related to the trauma of the biopsy procedure (Fig. 25). The cells are regular, cuboidal, or columnar, and there is no myoepithelial layer.

Special Studies. Mucous secretion may be present both in the gland lumina and in the cytoplasm of some of the tumor cells. The neoplasm is cytokeratin positive. Grimelius stain may reveal granules in the cytoplasm at the base of the cells (periphery of the acini) (118). Neuroendocrine-associated polypeptide substances (119) may be found by immunocytochemistry in many adenomas; the test result for neuron-specific enolase is most frequently positive, but those for chromogranin and other polypeptides less frequently so.

Electron microscopy may show a mucinous differentiation with microvilli projecting from the lumenal surfaces of the cells, desmosomes at points of contact with other cells at the base, and large electron-dense granules, probably secretory in character, in the cytoplasm of many cells (111). In an electron microscopic study (120) both mucinous and neuroendocrine differentiation was observed in each of the five adenomas studied, the former demonstrated by dark-appearing cells with apical microvilli and mucous granules and the latter by clear cells with basal neurosecretory granules.

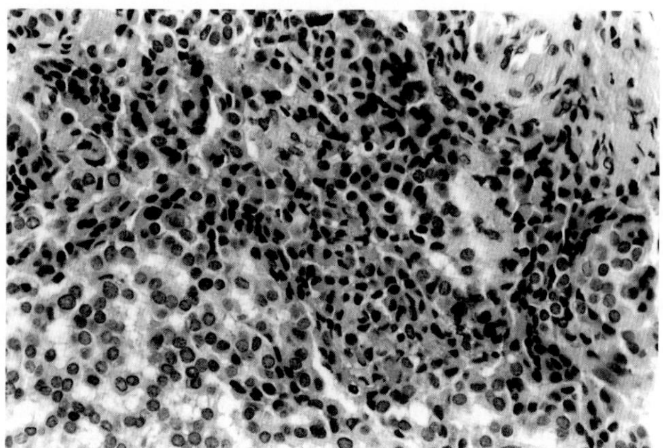

FIGURE 25. Adenoma of middle ear showing a solid cellular arrangement.

Differential Diagnosis. The label *carcinoid tumor* has been given to an adenomatous neoplasm of the middle ear with neuroendocrine features (121). There is, in fact, no difference in behavior between the latter neoplasms and those adenomas that do not display neuroendocrine features; both behave in a benign fashion. Nevertheless, the carcinoid designation has been held to be associated with "low-grade malignancy" in these neoplasms (121). Such a distinction within the group of glandular middle ear neoplasms is not justified. It is more likely that many, perhaps the majority of, adenomas, almost all benign in behavior, may differentiate in both directions (120).

Adenoma of the middle ear has been mistaken for jugulotympanic paraganglioma, and both the vascularity and the neuroendocrine features that the adenoma often exhibits may enhance this suspicion. The imaging techniques of magnetic resonance imaging (MRI) and CT may exclude jugular paraganglioma, because of the wide invasion of the latter through the apical portion of the temporal bone, which does not take place in adenoma of the middle ear. Tympanic paraganglioma is, like adenoma, confined to the middle ear. A distinction may be made on the positive expression of cytokeratin by adenoma, but its negativity by paraganglioma.

Paraganglioma

Clinical Data. Jugulotympanic paraganglioma (glomus jugulare tumor or chemodectoma) usually presents in the middle ear, more commonly in females (122), as a red vascular mass behind the intact tympanic membrane or sprouting through it. An attempt to examine this tumor via biopsy may result in severe bleeding.

Most paragangliomas arise from the paraganglion situated in the wall of the jugular bulb (1). They are therefore termed *jugular paragangliomas.* A minority of them arise from the paraganglion situated near the middle ear surface of the promontory (1); these tumors are called *tympanic paragangliomas.* The clinical distinction between jugular and tympanic paragangliomas can be made by imaging, the jugular neoplasm showing evidence of invasion of the petrous bone, the tympanic neoplasm being confined to the hypotympanum. A rare origin of paraganglioma from the fallopian canal, causing facial nerve symptoms, has been described (123).

Jugulotympanic paragangliomas may be multicentric or coexist with other tumor types. They may be bilateral in the same patient and coexist with carotid body paragangliomas, which may be bilateral (124). They also may coexist with adrenal gland pheochromocytomas, which can produce hypertension. A familial tendency to grow paragangliomas has been noted, particularly in patients with multiple tumors of this type. In such family groups of patients with head and neck (including jugulotympanic) paragangliomas, there is a preponderance for the male sex and inheritance is autosomal dominant, with an increase of the penetrance with age (125). There is evidence from molecular genetic studies that the gene underlying familial paragangliomas is located on chromosome 11q proximal to the tyrosinase gene locus (126).

Gross Appearance. Viewed from the external canal by otoscopy, the neoplasm is a reddish mass. In the jugular variety there is infiltration of the petrous temporal bone by a vascular neoplasm, which appears to arise in the wall of the jugular bulb at the apex of the bone and then to infiltrate the latter until it reaches the middle ear space, which it fills as far as the tympanic membrane (Fig. 26). In the tympanic variety the tumor occupies the lower half of the tympanic cavity. The bony labyrinth is rarely invaded by paraganglioma.

Histologic Features. The tumor resembles the carotid body tumor histologically. Epithelioid, uniform cells, often forming clusters or balls of cells (*Zellballen*), are separated by numerous capillary blood vessels (Fig. 27). In some areas the latter are closed down and their presence may be revealed only by special stains (e.g., reticulin). Nuclei are usually uniform and small (but see below and Fig. 29). Areas of fibrous tisue are often seen.

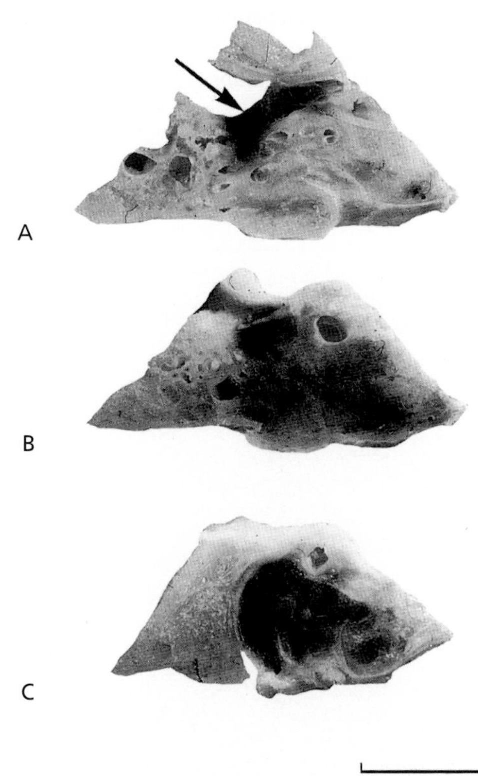

FIGURE 26. Microslices of temporal bone in a case of jugular paraganglioma. The tumor appears as dark areas, bright red in the original. **C:** Tumor is arising within the lumen and fills and extends from the jugular bulb. **B:** Tumor has reached the middle ear. **A:** Tumor fills middle ear and lies against but has not penetrated the tympanic membrane (*arrow*). (Reprinted from Michaels L. The ear. In: Damjanov I, Linder J. *Anderson's pathology.* St. Louis: CV Mosby, 1996:2876–2900; with permission.)

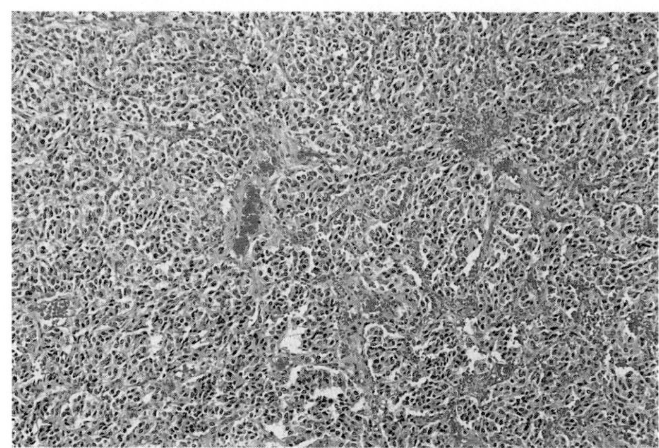

FIGURE 27. Jugulotympanic paraganglioma showing groups of small darkly staining cells arranged as *Zellballen* separated by capillary blood vessels.

Special Studies. Neuron-specific enolase and chromogranin, as demonstrated by immunoperoxidase immunohistochemistry, are usually present in the cells of this neoplasm. Cytokeratins are not usually expressed (127). Normal paraganglia contain two types of cells: chief or type I cells, which express neuroendocrine markers, and sustentacular or type II cells, which express S-100 protein. Jugulotympanic paragangliomas contain moderate numbers of the latter, sometimes at the periphery of the *Zellballen* (128) (Fig. 28). Electron microscopic examination of paraganglioma shows membrane-bound, electron-dense neurosecretory granules in the cytoplasm of the tumor cells.

Differential Diagnosis. The highly vascular nature of this neoplasm together with the compact groups of small neuroendocrine-positive cells usually indicates a definite diagnosis of paraganglioma. Diagnosis is sometimes made difficult by the presence of bizarre or multinucleate cells (Fig. 29). These do not denote malignant change if associated with the otherwise typical appearances of paraganglioma. Middle ear adenoma in

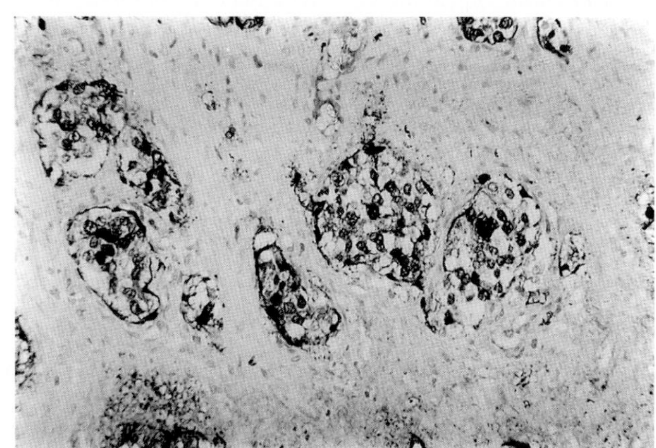

FIGURE 28. Biopsy of jugulotympanic paraganglioma from middle ear showing threadlike, S-100 protein–positive, sustentacular-type cells at periphery of *Zellballen.* Some of the inner tumor cells appear to be expressing the protein (immunoperoxidase stain for S-100 protein).

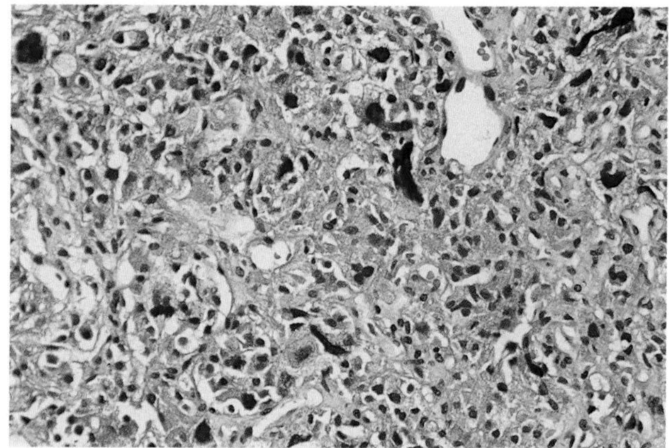

FIGURE 29. Jugulotympanic paraganglioma with bizarre cells containing enlarged darkly staining nuclei, but an otherwise typical pattern.

its solid phase may occasionally be mistaken for paraganglioma, and this error may be underscored by the positive expression of neuroendocrine markers that is so common in adenomas of the middle ear. The absence of back-to-back glandular acini and of staining for cytokeratins will usually rule out adenoma. Conversely paraganglioma may occasionally present spaces in the *Zellballen* that simulate glands so that a diagnosis of adenoma may be considered.

Biologic Behavior. This is a neoplasm of slow growth. The jugular variety infiltrates the petrous bone, but distant metastasis is reported to occur in only 2% of cases (128). Recurrence occurs in one third to one half of surgically treated cases, and the mortality rate is about 17% (129). Death usually results from spread of the tumor to the cranial cavity.

Every paraganglioma has a significant content of catecholamines (epinephrine and norepinephrine), but the incidence of clinically functioning paraganglioma is only 1% to 3% (130). Symptoms and signs are those of norepinephrine excess, particularly hypertension.

Squamous Cell Carcinoma

Clinical Data. Squamous cell carcinoma is uncommon but still is one of the more frequent of the neoplasms of the middle ear. Because aural discharge is present in all patients, it is often suggested that chronic otitis media is a precursor, but this has not been proven. Previous cholesteatoma has been found in some series (131) but not in others (132).

Gross Appearance. The tumor forms a whitish mass in the middle ear cavity, eroding the ossicles and extending into the mastoid air cells, extending through the tympanic membrane into the external canal and anteriorly into the eustachian tube.

Histologic Features. In microscopic sections the tumor is an epidermoid carcinoma arising from metaplastic squamous epithelium of the cubical or columnar epithelium in the middle ear. In some cases an origin of the tumor may be identified from the external as well as the middle ear epithelium. Severe dysplasia may be seen in some parts of the middle ear epithelium adjacent to the growth.

Differential Diagnosis. Concentrically laminated eosinophilic masses, known as middle ear corpuscles, may be confused with keratinized pearls of squamous carcinoma, particularly at frozen section (Fig. 30). Middle ear corpuscles are a normal feature of the aging middle ear. They are composed largely of collagen, and are formed, sometimes in considerable numbers, in bone-free mastoid air cell septa in the mastoid antrum (133).

Biologic Behavior. The carcinoma spreads widely from the middle ear. It soon grows into and erodes the thin bony plate in the medial wall of the eustachian tube and thence into the carotid canal (1). Penetration of posterior mastoid air cells by tumor leads to spread to the dura of the posterior surface of the temporal bone, from which growth may take place into the internal auditory canal and so into the membranous labyrinth. It causes death by intracranial extension (133,134). Lymph node metastasis is unusual, and spread by the bloodstream even more so.

Schneiderian-type Mucosal Papilloma

Benign epithelial tumors of the nose and paranasal sinuses with the appearances of everted stratified squamous, everted columnar, and inverted papilloma have been banded together under the designation of *papilloma* or *schneiderian papilloma* with the concept that that they are a single pathologic entity with histologic and etiologic links to each other (135). In a recent study of a large number of cases of nasal papilloma, this notion has been questioned by the finding that there were no intermediate forms between the three morphologic groups (136).

A report of five middle ear tumors, each with the histology of schneiderian papilloma, has brought this nasal problem into the middle ear (137). Scrutiny of the photographs of these middle ear lesions in the light of the text of this report, however, suggests

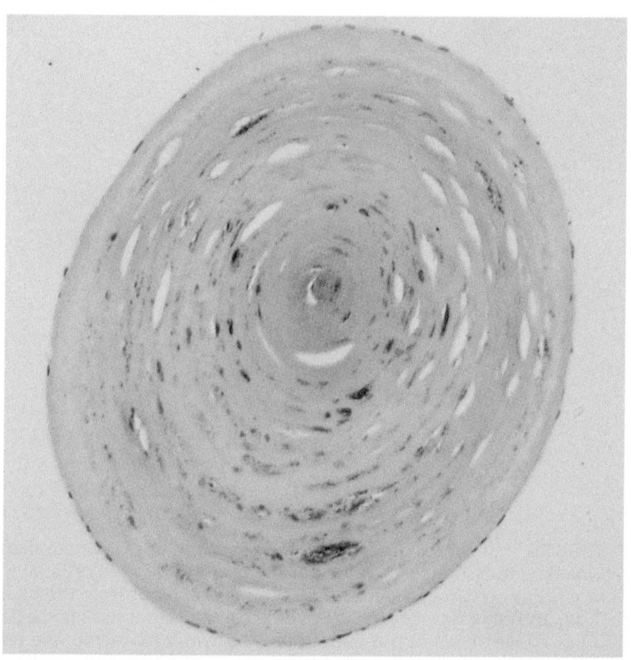

FIGURE 30. Middle ear corpuscle showing spherical structure with concentrically laminated bands of collagen.

that each of the five cases resembles the cylindric cell papilloma of the nose and paranasal sinuses, the supposedly inverted areas of stratified squamous epithelium being squamous metaplasia at the bases of the columnar epithelial papillae, which is often seen in cylindric cell papilloma. The neoplasms all behaved in a benign fashion similar to that of the latter neoplasm in the nose and paranasal sinuses.

A definitive opinion on the tissue of origin of these tumors and the validity of the claim that they are of the type found in the nose must await detailed study of further cases.

Papillary Adenocarcinoma

A primary papillary glandular malignant neoplasm of the middle ear has been described (138). It seems probable that this may be the same entity as that designated as low-grade adenocarcinoma of endolymphatic sac origin, and this problem will be discussed in a later section on the latter. Papillary adenocarcinoma, primary in the nasopharynx, may occasionally spread to the middle ear cavity by way of the eustachian tube.

Neural

A schwannoma of the facial nerve in its tympanic or extratympanic (descending) portion is occasionally seen. Histologically the features are those of a typical neurilemmoma.

Rhabdomyosarcoma

Rhabdomyosarcoma, usually of embryonal type, is seen occasionally in the middle and external ear of young children, where it forms a lobulated, dark red, hemorrhagic mass. It is highly malignant and spreads extensively into the cranial cavity, externally to the skin, or internally to the pharyngeal region. Lymph node and bloodstream metastases frequently develop (139,140) (see Chapter 10).

Neoplasms Extending from Other Sites

Meningioma

Meningiomas have been described as arising from a number of regions within the temporal bone itself, most commonly the middle ear cleft (141), but imaging techniques have revealed that they usually arise from outside the petrous bone, infiltrating the latter until the middle ear is reached.

Gross appearances are those of a granular or even gritty mass. Microscopically, the neoplasm takes the same forms as any of the intracranial types of meningioma (Fig. 31). Most of the immunocytochemical markers are negative, including those for cytokeratins, but those for vimentin and epithelial membrane antigen are said to be positive in the majority (142).

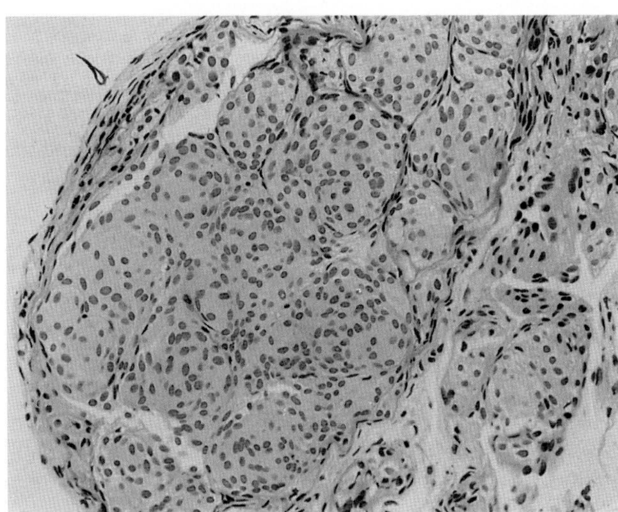

FIGURE 31. Meningioma presenting in middle ear. The tumor cells form regular epithelioid groups with a whorled arrangement of component cells.

Jugular Paraganglioma

The jugular variety of paragangliomas presenting in the middle ear cavity does not arise there, but in the jugular bulb. The neoplasm then invades through the petrous bone to reach and fill the middle ear cavity.

Yolk Sac Tumor

Endodermal sinus tumors (yolk sac tumors) are malignant germ cell tumors that usually arise in the gonads. They are characterized by the presence of glomeruloid structures (Schiller-Duval bodies) and extracellular round hyaline bodies. In a single report of this neoplasm in the ear, the tumor was present in a developmentally delayed child with an abnormal temporal bone and exhibited histopathologic and immunocytochemical features identical to those of endodermal sinus tumors of gonadal origin (143).

Metastatic Neoplasms

Metastasis of malignant neoplasms to the middle ear region of the temporal bone is not uncommon. The breast, lung, kidney, stomach, and larynx are possible primary sources of metastatic tumors (144), as is malignant melanoma (145).

INNER EAR AND TEMPORAL BONE

Inner Ear

Surgical intervention in the inner ear is required mainly for the treatment of neoplasms in this region. Neoplasms of the inner ear are infrequent. Most of those that do occur are found in the internal auditory canal or in the jugular foramen region. From each of those sites expansion to the cerebellopontine angle is prone to take place.

Neoplasms

Internal Auditory Canal and Cerebellopontine Angle Tumors

Tumors occurring in the internal auditory canal are the solitary vestibular schwannoma, the bilateral vestibular schwannoma (neurofibromatosis 2), usually accompanied in this situation by neoplasm-like masses of meningioma and neurofibroma, and lipoma. These tumors, on enlargement, extend into the cerebellopontine angle.

Vestibular Schwannoma (Acoustic Neuroma)

Clinical Data. Vestibular schwannoma arises on the eighth cranial nerve. It is usually unilateral, but 9% are bilateral (146) (i.e., a manifestation of neurofibromatosis 2). The neoplasm may grow slowly for years without causing symptoms and may be first diagnosed only at postmortem examination, where it has been found in about 1 in 220 consecutive adults (147). Although it arises on the vestibular branch of the eighth cranial nerve, hearing loss and tinnitus are early symptoms produced by involvement of the cochlear division of the nerve; in the later stages vertigo and abnormal caloric and electronystagmographic responses develop from damage to the vestibular division itself.

Gross Appearance. The neoplasm is stated to arise most commonly at the glial–neurilemmal junction of the eighth nerve, which is usually near the opening of the internal auditory canal (1) (Fig. 32). In most cases it arises from the vestibular division of the nerve. Growth takes place from its origin, both centrally out of the canal and into the region of the cerebellopontine angle, and peripherally along the canal. The tumor may rarely arise in the vestibule (148) or the cochlea.

The neoplasm is of variable size and of round or oval shape. The larger tumors often have a mushroom shape with two components: the stalk (an elongated part in the canal) and an expanded part in the region of the cerebellopontine angle. The bone of the internal auditory canal is widened funnelwise as the neoplasm grows. The tumor surface is smooth and lobulated. The cut surface is yellowish, often with areas of hemorrhage and cysts. The vestibular division of the eighth nerve may be identified on the surface of the tumor.

Histologic Findings. Acoustic neuroma has the features of a neoplasm of Schwann cells showing Antoni A and Antoni B types. Antoni A areas display the spindle cells closely packed together with palisading of nuclei (Fig. 33). Verocay bodies, which

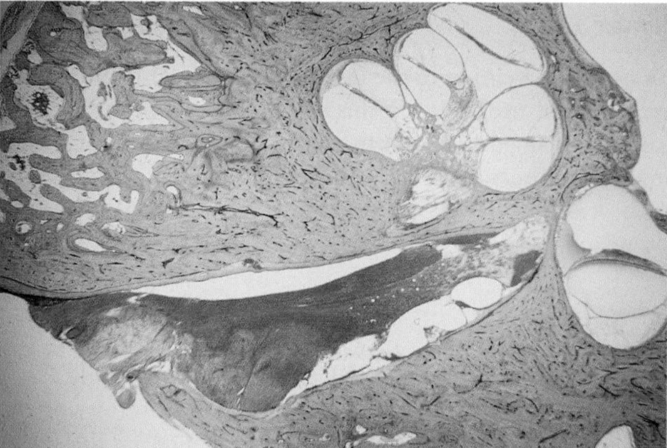

FIGURE 32. Autopsy temporal bone showing a small vestibular schwannoma in the internal canal near its opening. There is a slight concavity of the adjacent bone caused by the neoplasm, but no general widening of the canal. There is also no eosinophilic fluid in the spaces of the cochlea and vestibule. Both of these features are present in larger vestibular schwannomas.

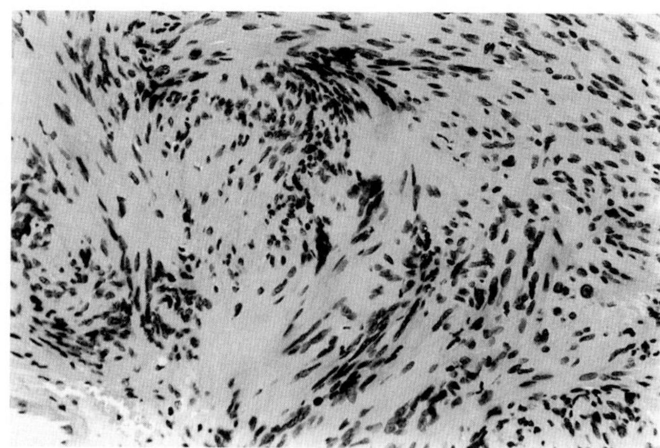

FIGURE 33. Vestibular schwannoma showing palisading of nuclei (Antoni type A appearance).

may be present in the Antoni A areas, are whorled formations of palisaded tumor cells resembling tactile corpuscles (Fig. 34). The spindle cells of the tumor may lack palisading and Verocay bodies, however. The degree of cellularity of the neoplasm can be high or low. The spindle cells frequently are moderately pleomorphic, but mitotic figures are rare. The presence of pleomorphism does not denote a malignant tendency. Antoni B areas, probably a degenerated form of the Antoni A pattern, show a loose reticular pattern, sometimes with histiocytic proliferation (Fig. 35). Thrombosis and necrosis may be present in some parts of the neoplasm.

A mild degree of invasion of modiolus or vestibule along cochlear or vestibular nerve branches may be present even in solitary vestibular schwannomas. Granular or homogeneous fluid exudate is usually present in the perilymphatic spaces of the cochlea and vestibule. This may arise as a result of pressure by the neoplasm on veins draining the cochlea and vestibule in the internal auditory meatus. Hydrops of the endolymphatic system may occur, and in larger tumors there is atrophy of spiral ganglion cells and nerve fibers in the basilar membrane (149).

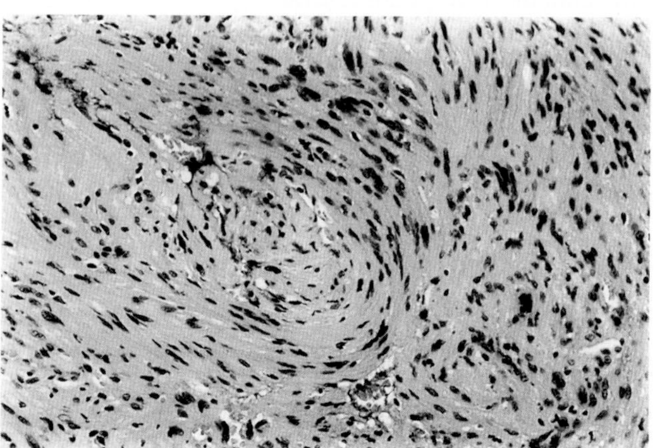

FIGURE 34. Vestibular schwannoma showing whorled arrangement (Verocay body).

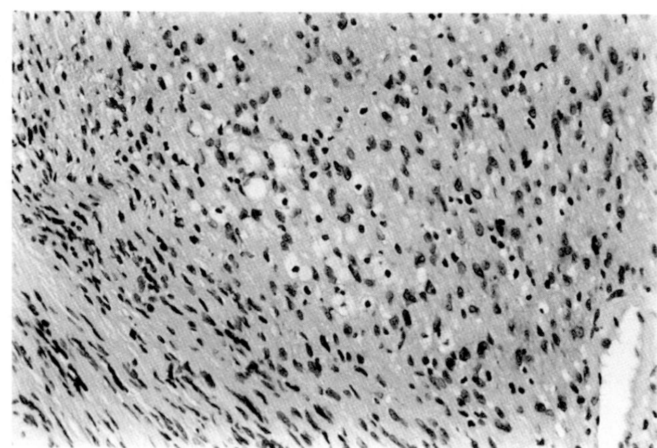

FIGURE 35. Vestibular schwannoma showing loose pattern with round cells and histiocytes (Antoni B).

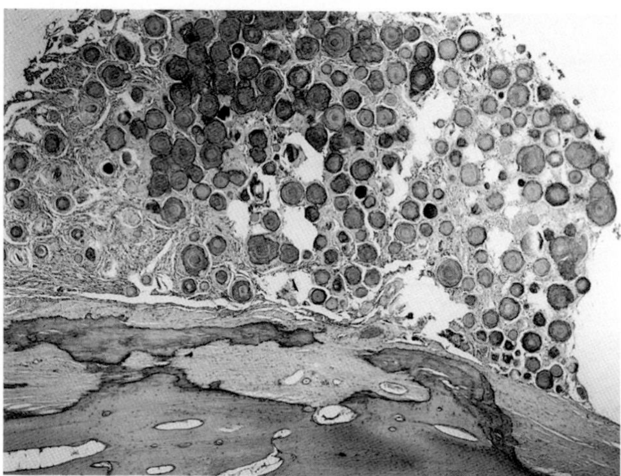

FIGURE 36. Meningioma-like mass composed of psammoma bodies arising from the posterior surface of the temporal bone in a case of neurofibromatosis 2. (Reprinted from Michaels L. *Ear, nose and throat histopathology.* London: Springer, 1987; with permission.)

Biologic Behavior. The tumor is benign and usually grows slowly. Serious symptoms and even death may occur, however, due to damage to cerebral structures if the neoplasm grows to a large size.

Neurofibromatosis 2 (Bilateral Acoustic Neuromas)

Bilateral acoustic neuroma (neurofibromatosis 2), unlike neurofibromatosis 1 (von Recklinghausen's disease), is not associated with large numbers of cutaneous neurofibromas and café au lait spots, but the temporal bone locality of the neural tumor and its bilaterality are inherited as an autosomal dominant trait (150). This condition has been related to a gene localized near the center of the long arm of chromosome 22 (151).

At autopsy of cases of neurofibromatosis 2, neural neoplasms are present in both eighth nerves and other central nerves. There are often many small schwannomas and collections of cells of neurofibromatous and meningiomatous appearance growing on cranial nerves and on the meninges in the vicinity of the vestibular schwannomas and sometimes even intermixed with them (Fig. 36). The neurofibromatosis 2 tumors are histologically similar to those of the single tumors except that the former have more Verocay bodies and more foci of high cellularity (152). The neurofibromatosis 2 tumors are more invasive, however, tending to infiltrate the cochlea and vestibule more deeply (149,153).

Lipoma

Lipomas of the internal auditory canal and cerebellopontine angle are rare tumors that may be confused clinically with the more common vestibular schwannoma. On MRI, however, this tumor displays characteristics of adipose tissue rather than those of schwannoma. There may be erosion of the walls of the internal auditory canal as with vestibular schwannoma, and lipoma may be grossly similar to the latter at operation. Because the seventh and eighth cranial nerves may pass through the lesion and their integrity may be damaged by removal of the tumor, it is recommended that diagnosis be made whenever the possibility of this neoplasm is suspected by intraoperative examination of frozen sections. If a diagnosis of lipoma is made in this way, it should not be resected, because its further growth does not constitute a threat to vital structures (154).

Apex of Petrous Temporal Bone and Cerebellopontine Angle Tumors

A variety of neoplasms and tumor-like lesions may present at the apex of the petrous temporal bone. These include jugular paraganglioma, jugular foramen schwannoma usually arising from the vagus nerve, low-grade adenocarcinoma of probable endolymphatic sac origin, cholesteatoma (epidermoid cyst), and cholesterol granuloma. Such lesions, on enlargement, may extend into the cerebellopontine angle.

Low-grade Adenocarcinoma of Probable Endolymphatic Sac Origin. There is evidence of the existence of a rare epithelial neoplasm of the endolymphatic system, mainly in the endolymphatic sac (3,155–157). Although of benign glandular histologic appearance and of slow growth, the neoplasm seems to have considerable invasive capacity. Therefore, the term *low-grade adenocarcinoma of probable endolymphatic sac origin* has been applied (157). Some patients have presented with bilateral neoplasms of the same type, and some neoplasms have been associated with von Hippel-Lindau disease (158).

The course of the tumor's growth may extend over many years. Tinnitus or vertigo, similar or identical to the symptoms of Meniere's disease, are present in about one third of patients. It is presumed that early obstruction of the endolymphatic sac leads to hydrops of the endolymphatic system of the labyrinth and also to Meniere's symptoms. Imaging reveals a lytic temporal bone lesion, appearing to originate from the region between the internal auditory canal and sigmoid sinus (which is the approximate position of the endolymphatic sac). There is usually prominent extension into the posterior cranial cavity and invasion of the middle ear.

In most cases the tumor has a papillary–glandular appearance, the papillary proliferation being lined by a single row of low

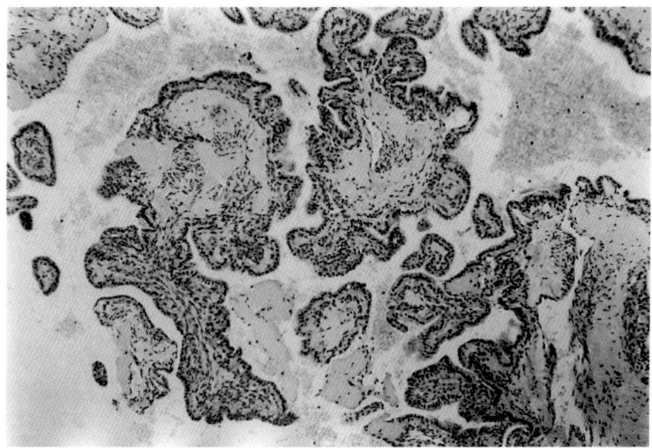

FIGURE 37. Middle ear biopsy in a case of low-grade adenocarcinoma of the endolymphatic sac showing papillae lined by low cuboidal cells.

cuboidal cells (Fig. 37). The vascular nature of the papillae in some cases has given the tumor a histologic resemblance to choroid plexus papilloma. In some cases the tumor also shows areas of dilated glands containing a secretion that has some resemblance to colloid, and under these circumstances the lesion may resemble papillary adenocarcinoma of the thyroid. Such thyroid-like areas may even dominate the histologic pattern. A few cases show a clear cell predominance resembling carcinoma of the kidney. On immunocytochemistry the epithelial cells of this neoplasm contain antigens of cytokeratins. Some tumors contain glial fibrillary acidic protein. Thyroglobulin is always absent.

It seems possible that the so-called aggressive papillary middle ear tumor (138) may be low-grade adenocarcinoma of endolymphatic sac origin with extension of neoplasm to the middle ear. The argument that the lumen of the endolymphatic sac in a described case appeared to be tumor free (although the wall of that structure was involved) together with the nonspecific ultrastructural and immunohistochemical features found in that case lent little support for the authors' contention that the origin of that tumor was the mucosa of the pneumatic spaces (middle ear) surrounding the jugular bulb rather than the endolymphatic sac (159).

The histologic appearances of low-grade adenocarcinomas of probable endolymphatic sac origin are indeed in keeping with the normal histologic structure of the endolymphatic sac, which is lined by a papillary columnar epithelial layer. The development of the endolymphatic sac is characterized by a stage in which the epithelium is closely associated with a network of capillaries to give rise to the endolymphatic glomerulus (160,161). This may account for an appearance similar to that of the choroid plexus papilloma displayed by some of the low-grade adenocarcinomas of the endolymphatic sac.

Cholesteatoma (Epidermoid Cyst). This lesion usually presents owing to symptoms relating to its involvement of the seventh and eighth cranial nerves in the cerebellopontine angle (162). The histologic appearance is similar to that of middle ear cholesteatoma. It is probably of congenital origin, but no cell rest has been discovered from which it might arise.

Cholesterol Granuloma. A lesion of the petrous apex, with the typical features of cholesterol granuloma as seen in the middle ear and mastoid in chronic otitis media, has been shown via MRI in recent years with increasing frequency. At operation it appears cystic, the contents being altered blood and cholesterol clefts with a foreign body giant cell reaction. Microscopic examination shows nonspecific granulation tissue and hemosiderin deposits in its wall (Fig. 38). It is believed to result from an inflammatory response to an obstruction of the pneumatized air cells at the apex of the temporal bone. Hemorrhage into the air cells breaks down to hemosiderin and cholesterol with a foreign body reaction and progressive granuloma formation. As the process develops, bone is eroded by this expansile lesion, often involving the petrous apex, the cerebellopontine angle, and the middle ear (163,164).

Metastatic Tumors

The temporal bone is frequently the site of blood-borne metastasis for carcinomas originating in the following organs: breast, kidney, lung, stomach, larynx, prostate, and thyroid. The internal auditory meatus is a common location for such growth. Once deposited, further spread into the cochlea and vestibule may take place through the foramina for branches of the eighth nerve (165).

Kaposi's Sarcoma

Kaposi's sarcoma may be found deposited in many parts of the body in patients with AIDS, most commonly in the lungs and skin, including that of the external ear (166). In the inner ear a deposit has been described in the eighth nerve in the internal auditory meatus (71).

Temporal Bone

Otosclerosis

Otosclerosis is a common focal lesion of the otic capsule of unknown etiology, which is found principally in relation to the cochlea and footplate of the stapes.

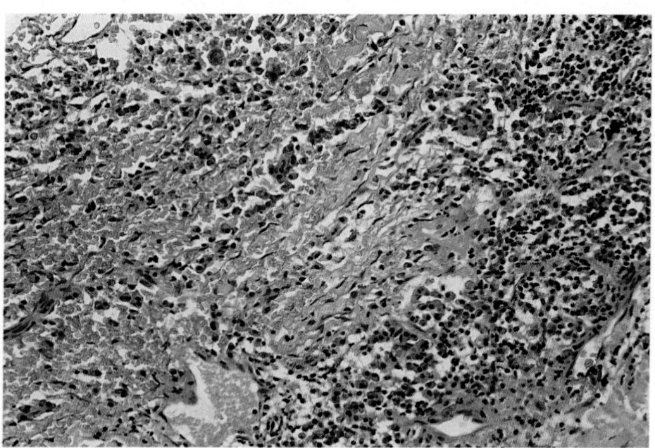

FIGURE 38. Wall of cholesterol granuloma of petrous apex showing fibrous and inflammatory granulation tissue and hemosiderin deposition. The center of the lesion was composed of cholesterol clefts with foreign body–type giant cells and hemorrhagic material.

Clinical Data. Approximately 50% of patients with histologic otosclerosis have the symptom of conductive hearing loss. This is the result of the extension of the otosclerotic lesion to involve the stapes footplate, which leads to its fixation and hence its inability to transmit sound vibrations. A sensorineural loss of varying degree also may be present, and this is the result of spread of the otosclerotic process to the edge of the scalae of the cochlea (167). The lesions of otosclerosis may be appreciated at CT as sclerosis or spongiosis of varying degree in the temporal bone near the stapes footplate.

Gross Appearance. Otosclerotic deposits not associated with hearing loss have been described in 10% to 12.75% of adult temporal bones at autopsy of white people in the United States (168,169). The deposits are found mainly in the otic capsule bone anterior to the oval window (footplate of the stapes), where they may be demonstrated as well-demarcated pink, vascular patches on the cut surface of the bone (Fig. 39). In patients with prominent otosclerotic involvement of the otic capsule and conductive deafness, the lesion may be seen at operation on the middle ear as a pink swelling of the promontory, and this may sometimes even be detected clinically through a particularly transparent tympanic membrane. When manipulated at surgery or at autopsy, the stapes are rigidly fixed and clearly unable to vibrate.

Histologic Findings. Under low-power, patches of otosclerosis are sharply demarcated and basophilic in contrast to the eosinophilic staining of the normal otic capsule (1). The characteristic feature of otosclerosis is the presence of trabeculae of woven bone with abundant osteoblasts and osteocytes (Fig. 40). Osteoclasts may be present and are accompanied by evidence of bone resorption. Blood vessels are always numerous and prominent. Lamellar bone may be deposited later in otosclerosis.

The surgical treatment of otosclerosis is stapedectomy with replacement of the natural stapes by a prosthesis to restore the continuity of the ossicular chain. In most cases only the head or crura of the stapes are removed, leaving the footplate behind. Because the otosclerotic process involves only the footplate and not the head and crura, when the latter only are available for histologic examination following the stapedectomy operation, as is usually the case, no otosclerosis will be seen in the specimen. In the unusual event of the whole stapes being removed, the otosclerotic process, if it is present in the specimen, will be in the footplate only. Even under these circumstances otosclerosis may not be found at all, because the stapes is often fixed by pressure of an otosclerotic mass in the otic capsule without its actual invasion by the disease process.

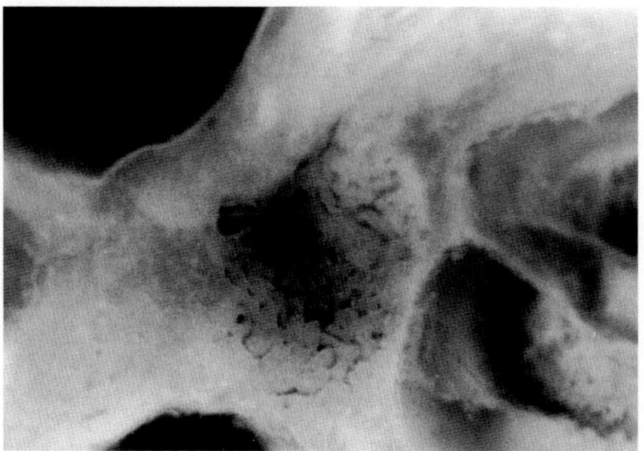

FIGURE 39. Microsliced temporal bone taken at autopsy showing a focus of otosclerosis (pink in the original) near the cochlea (at right), but not extending to the footplate of the stapes. Note the vascularity and well-demarcated nature of the lesion. (Reprinted from Michaels L. *Ear, nose and throat histopathology.* London: Springer, 1987; with permission.)

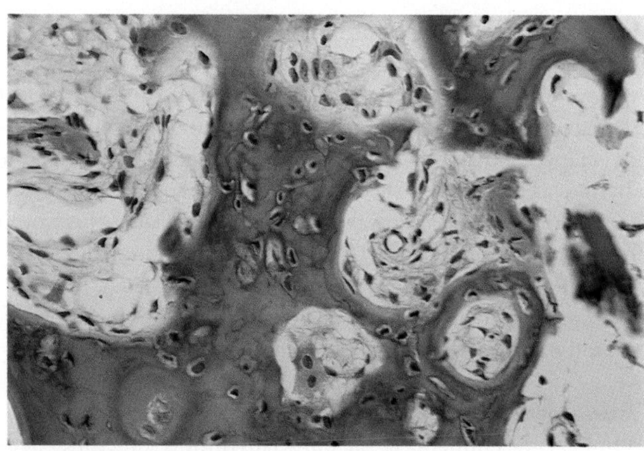

FIGURE 40. Otosclerotic focus affecting the footplate of the stapes. The lesion is composed of woven bone with numerous osteocytes and osteoblasts. (Reprinted from Michaels L. The ear. In: Damjanov I, Linder J. *Anderson's pathology.* St. Louis: CV Mosby, 1996:2876–2900; with permission.)

Pathogenesis. Because otosclerosis has some histologic similarity to Paget's disease of bone and there is mounting evidence of a viral basis for Paget's disease (170), it was natural that otosclerosis should also be investigated for possible virus infection. Transmission electron microscopy of surgically removed stapes footplate fragments with active otosclerosis have revealed structures morphologically identical to measles virus nucleocapsid in osteoblasts, and immunocytochemical studies of the same material have indicated the presence of the same nucleocapsid antigen in active lesions (171). By use of the polymerase chain reaction, measles virus RNA sequences were detected in 13 of 14 specimens of bone fragments from surgically removed stapides of patients suffering from otosclerosis. Furthermore, immunoglobulin G anti–measles virus antibodies were detected in the perilymph of six patients (172). These findings suggest that measles virus is implicated in the pathogenesis of otosclerosis.

Congenital Stapes Fixation: "Gushers" and "Oozers" of Cerebrospinal Fluid

Fixation of the footplate to the surrounding otic capsule bone may occur as a congenital condition. A prosthesis may be inserted surgically in such cases to restore ossicular vibration. In some cases there is an associated congenital communication of the vestibule with the subarachnoid space, and as soon as the stapes has been released surgically from the oval window, a strong flow of cerebrospinal fluid occurs (gushers); sometimes there may be a relentless slow ooze only (oozers) (173,174).

Communication between cerebrospinal fluid and middle ear associated with meningitis may take place spontaneously without stapedectomy in cases with a congenitally defective labyrinth. The stapes in such cases and in the spontaneous gushers and oozers shows a central defect in the footplate. This would normally be covered by the mucosa of the middle ear and by the lining of the vestibule. In the presence of otitis media, however, these coverings may rupture, so allowing a direct connection between the subarachnoid space and middle ear (175).

Osteogenesis Imperfecta

In osteogenesis imperfecta the bony labyrinth is sometimes deficient, but the membranous structures of the inner ear are usually normal. The stapes footplate is frequently fixed by new bone at the same site as otosclerosis, but the nature of this bony tissue is problematic. Some claim that it is conventional otosclerotic bone, others that it is a specific bone reaction of osteogenesis imperfecta (176,177).

REFERENCES

1. Michaels L. The ear. In: Sternberg S, ed. *Histology for pathologists,* 2nd ed. New York: Lippincott-Raven, 1997:337–366.
2. Chandler JR. Malignant external otitis. *Laryngoscope* 1968;78: 1257–1294.
3. Schuknecht HF. *Pathology of the ear,* 2nd ed. Philadelphia: Lea & Febiger, 1993.
4. Ostfeld E, Segal M, Czernobilsky B. External otitis: early histopathologic changes and pathogenic mechanism. *Laryngoscope* 1982;91: 965–970.
5. Weinroth SE, Schessel D, Tuazon CU. Malignant otitis externa in AIDS patients: case report and review of the literature. *Ear Nose Throat J* 1992;73:772–774.
6. Solomon AR. Nonneoplastic diseases of the skin. In: Sternberg SS, ed. *Diagnostic surgical pathology,* 2nd ed. New York: Raven, 1994:1–56.
7. Michaels L, Shah N. Dangers of corn starch powder [Letter]. *BMJ* 1973;2:714.
8. Hughes RA, Berry CL, Seifert M, et al. Relapsing polychondritis. Three cases with a clinicopathological study and literature review. *Q J Med* 1972;41:363–380.
9. Verity MA, Larson WM, Madden SC. Relapsing polychondritis. Report of two necropsied cases with histochemical investigation of the cartilage lesion. *Am J Pathol* 1963;42:251–269.
10. Foidart JM, Abe S, Martin GR, et al. Antibodies to type II collagen in relapsing polychondritis. *N Engl J Med* 1978;299:1203–1207.
11. Rajapakse DA, Bywaters EG. Cell mediated immunity to cartilage proteoglycan in relapsing polychondritis. *Clin Exp Immunol* 1974;16:497–502.
12. Corbridge RJ, Michaels L, Wright A. Epithelial migration in keratosis obturans. *Am J Otolaryngol* 1996;17:411–414.
13. Soucek S, Michaels L. Keratosis of the tympanic membrane and deep external canal: a defect of auditory epithelial migration. *Eur Arch Otorhinolaryngol* 1993;250:140–142.
14. Hawke M, Jahn AF. Keratin implantation granuloma in external ear canal. *Arch Otolaryngol* 1974;100:317–318.
15. Koch HJ, Lewis JJ. Hyperlipemic xanthomatosis with associated osseous granulomas. A clinical report. *N Engl J Med* 1956;255:387–393.
16. Emery PS, Gore M. An extensive solitary xanthoma of the temporal bone associated with hyperlipoproteinaemia. *J Laryngol Otol* 1982;96:451–457.
17. Azadeh B, Ardehali S. Malakoplakia of middle ear: a case report. *Histopathology* 1983;7:129–134.
18. Azadeh B, Dabiri S, Mosfegh M. Malakoplakia of the middle-ear. *Histopathology* 1991;19:276–278.
19. Winkler M. Knotchenformige Erkrankung am Helix (Chondermatitis Nodularis Chronica Helicis). *Arch Dermatol Syph* 1915;12:278–285.
20. Metzger SA, Goodman ML. Chondermatitis helicis. A clinical re-evaluation and pathological review. *Laryngoscope* 1976;86:1402–1412.
21. Bottomley WW, Goodfield MD. Chondrodermatitis nodularis helicis occurring with systemic sclerosis—an under-reported association? *Clin Exp Dermatol* 1994;19:219–220.
22. Hesse G, Schmoeckel C, Wichmann-Hesse A. Argon laser therapy of chondrodermatitis nodularis chronica helicis. *Hautarzt* 1994;45: 222–224.
23. Taylor MB. Chondrodermatitis nodularis chronica helicis. Successful treatment with the carbon dioxide laser. *J Dermatol Surg Oncol* 1991;17:862–864.
24. Hurwitz RM. Painful papule of the ear: a follicular disorder. *J Dermatol Surg Oncol* 1987;13:270–274.
25. Barnes HM, Calman CD, Sarkany I. Spectacle frame acanthoma (granuloma fissuratum). *Trans St Johns Hosp Dermatol Soc* 1974; 60:99–102.
26. Tennstedt D, Lachapelle JM. Acanthome fissure. Revue de la littérature et diagnostic histopathologique differentiel avec le nodule douloureux de l'oreille. *Ann Dermatol Venereol* 1979;106:219–225.
27. Barnes L, Koss W, Nieland ML. Angiolymphoid hyperplasia: a disease that may be confused with malignancy. *Head Neck Surg* 1980;2: 425–434.
28. Chan JK, Hui PK, Ng CS, et al. Epithelioid haemangioma (angiolymphoid hyperplasia with eosinophilia) and Kimura's disease in Chinese. *Histopathology* 1989;15:557–574.
29. Helander SD, Peters MS, Kuo TT, et al. Kimura's disease and angiolymphoid hyperplasia with eosinophilia—new observations from immunohistochemical studies of lymphocyte markers, endothelial antigens, and granulocyte proteins. *J Cutan Pathol* 1995;22:319–326.
30. Hansen JE. Pseudocysts of the auricle in Caucasians. *Arch Otolaryngol* 1967;85:13–14.
31. Santos VB, Pilisar IA, Ruffy ML. Bilateral pseudocysts in a female. *Ann Otol Rhinol Laryngol* 1974;83:9–11.
32. Devlin J, Harrison CJ, Whitby DJ, et al. Cartilaginous pseudocyst of the external auricle in children with atopic eczema. *Br J Dermatol* 1990;122:699–704.
33. Heffner DK, Hyams VJ. Cystic chondromalacia (enchondral pseudocysts) of the auricle. *Arch Pathol Lab Med* 1986;110:740–743.
34. DiBartolomeo JR. The petrified auricle: comments on ossification, calcification and exostoses of the external ear. *Laryngoscope* 1985; 95:566–576.
35. Metcalf PB Jr. Carcinoma of the pinna. *N Engl J Med* 1954;251: 91–95.
36. Woodson GE, Jurco S III, Alford BR, et al. Verrucous carcinoma of the middle ear. *Arch Otolaryngol* 1981;107:63–65.
37. Proops DW, Hawke WM, Van Nostrand AWP, et al. Verrucous carcinoma of the ear. Case report. *Ann Otol Rhinol Laryngol* 1984;93: 385–388.
38. Edelstein DR, Smouha E, Sacks SH, et al. Verrucous carcinoma of the temporal bone. *Ann Otol Rhinol Laryngol* 1986;95:447–453.
39. Stafford ND, Frootko NJ. Verrucous carcinoma in the external auditory canal. *Am J Otol* 1986;7:443–445.
40. Cooper JR, Hellquist HB, Michaels L. Image analysis in the discrimination of verrucous carcinoma and squamous papilloma. *J Pathol* 1992;166:383–387.
41. Cankar V, Crowley H. Tumors of ceruminous glands: a clinicopathological study of seven cases. *Cancer* 1964;17:67–75.
42. Wetli CV, Pardo V, Millard M, et al. Tumors of ceruminous glands. *Cancer* 1972;29:1169–1178.
43. Wilson RS, Johnson JT. Benign eccrine cylindroma of the external auditory canal. *Laryngoscope* 1980;90:379–382.
44. Sharma HS, Meorkamal MZ, Zainol H, et al. Eccrine cylindroma of the ear canal—report of a case. *J Laryngol Otol* 1994;108:706–709.
45. Haraguchi H, Hentona H, Tanaka H, et al. Pleomorphic adenoma of the external auditory canal: a case report and review of the literature. *J Laryngol Otol* 1996;110:52–56.

46. Pulec JL. Glandular tumors of the external auditory canal. *Laryngoscope* 1977;87:1601–1612.
47. Pack GT, Conley J, Oropega R. Melanoma of the external ear. *Arch Otolaryngol* 1970;92:106–113.
48. Davidsson A, Hellquist HB, Villman K, et al. Malignant melanoma of the ear. *J Laryngol Otol* 1993;107:798–802.
49. Carney JA, Gordon H, Carpenter PC, et al. The complex of myxomas, spotty pigmentation and endocrine overactivity. *Medicine* 1985;64:270–283.
50. Nager GT, Kennedy DW, Kopstein E. Fibrous dysplasia: a review of the disease and its manifestations in the temporal bone. *Ann Otol Rhinol Laryngol* 1982;92(suppl):1–52.
51. Sheehey JH. Diffuse exostosis and osteomata of the external auditory canal: a report of 100 operations. *Otolaryngol Head Neck Surg* 1982; 90:337–342.
52. Graham M. Osteomas and exostosis of the external auditory canal. A clinical, histopathological and scanning electron microscopic study. *Ann Otol Rhinol Laryngol* 1979;88:566–572.
53. Tos M. A survey of Hand-Schüller-Christian disease in otolaryngology. *Acta Otolaryngol (Scand)* 1966;62:217–228.
54. Quesada P, Navarrete ML, Perrello E. Eosinophilic granuloma of the temporal bone. *Eur Arch Otorhinolaryngol* 1990;247:194–195.
55. Goudie RB, Soukop M, Dagg JH, et al. Hypothesis: symmetrical cutaneous lymphoma. *Lancet* 1990;1:316–318.
56. Paparella MM, Kimberley BP, Alleva M. The concept of silent otitis media. Its importance and implications. *Otolaryngol Clin North Am* 1991;24:763–773.
57. Sugita R, Fujimaki Y, Deguchi K. Bacteriological features and chemotherapy of adult acute purulent otitis media. *J Laryngol Otol* 1985;99:629–635.
58. Brook I, Anthony BF, Finegold SM. Aerobic and anaerobic bacteriology of acute otitis media in children. *J Pediatr* 1978;92:13–16.
59. Chonmaitree T, Howie VM, Truant AL. Presence of respiratory viruses in middle ear fluids and nasal wash specimens from children with acute otitis media. *Pediatrics* 1986;77:698–702.
60. Buchman CA, Doyle WJ, Skoner DP, et al. Influenza A virus–induced acute otitis media. *J Infect Dis* 1995;172:1348–1351.
61. Brook I. Chronic otitis media in children. Microbiological studies. *Am J Dis Child* 1980;134:564–566.
62. Albrecht W. Pneumatisation und Konstitution. *Z Hals Nasen Ohrenheilkunde* 1924;10:51–55.
63. Tos M. Pathogenesis and pathology of chronic secretory otitis media. *Ann Otol Laryngol* 1980;89(suppl 68):91–97.
64. Ishii T, Toriyama M, Suzuki J-I. Histopathological study of otitis media with effusion. *Ann Otol Rhinol Laryngol* 1980;89(suppl 68): 83–86.
65. Ramages LJ, Gertler R. Aural tuberculosis: a series of 25 patients. *J Laryngol Otol* 1985;99:1073–1080.
66. Odetoyinbo O. Early diagnosis of tuberculous otitis media. *J Laryngol Otol* 1988;102:133–135.
67. Buchanan G, Rainer EH. Tuberculous mastoiditis. *J Laryngol Otol* 1988;102:440–446.
68. Tyndel FJ, Davidson GS, Birman H, et al. Sarcoidosis of the middle ear. *Chest* 1994;105:1582–1583.
69. Olsen TS, Seid AB, Pransky SM. Actinomycosis of the middle ear. *Int J Pediatr Otorhinolaryngol* 1989;17:51–55.
70. Tarabichi M. Actinomycosis otomycosis. *Arch Otolaryngol Head Neck Surg* 1993;119:561–562.
71. Michaels L, Soucek S, Liang J. The ear in the acquired immunodeficiency syndrome: I. Temporal bone histopathologic study. *Am J Otol* 1994;15:515–522.
72. Macias JD, Wackym PA, McCabe BF. Early diagnosis of otologic Wegener's granulomatosis using the serologic marker C-ANCA. *Ann Otol Rhinol Laryngol* 1993;102:337–341.
73. Fauci AS, Wolff SM. Wegener's granulomatosis: studies in eighteen patients with a review of the literature. *Medicine (Baltimore)* 1973; 52:535–561.
74. Politzer A. Das Cholesteatom des Gehürgans vom anatomischen und klinischen Standpunkte. *Wiener Medizinische Wochenschr* 1891;8: 329–333.
75. Van Blitterswijk CA, Grote JJ, Lutgert RW, et al. Cytokeratin patterns of tissues related to cholesteatoma pathogenesis. *Ann Otol Rhinol Laryngol* 1989;98:635–640.
76. Broekaert D, Couke P, Leperque S, et al. Immunohistochemical analysis of the cytokeratin expression in middle ear cholesteatoma and related epithelial tissues. *Ann Otol Rhinol Laryngol* 1992;101:931–938.
77. Bajia J, Schilling V, Holly A, et al. Hyperproliferation-associated expression in human middle ear cholesteatoma. *Acta Otolaryngol* 1993; 113:364–368.
78. Sudhoff H, Bujia J, Fisselereckhoff A, et al. Expression of a cell-cycle-associated nuclear antigen (MIB1) in cholesteatoma and auditory meatal skin. *Laryngoscope* 1995;105:1227–1231.
79. Maigot D, Bene MC, Perrin C, et al. Restricted expression of Ki-67 in cholesteatoma epithelium. *Arch Otolaryngol Head Neck Surg* 1993;119:656–658.
80. Sudhoff H, Fisseler-Eckhoff A, Stark F, et al. Agyrophilic nucleolar organizer regions (AgNORs) in auditory meatal skin and middle ear cholesteatoma. *Clin Otolaryngol* 1997;22:545–548.
81. Sadé J, Berco E, Buyanover D, et al. Ossicular damage in chronic middle ear inflammation. In: Sadé J, ed. *Cholesteatoma and mastoid surgery.* Proceedings of the second international conference. Amsterdam: Kugler, 1982:347–358.
82. Palva T, Karma P, Makinen J. The invasion theory. In: Sadé J, ed. *Cholesteatoma in mastoid surgery.* Proceedings of the second international conference. Amsterdam: Kugler, 1982:249–264.
83. Michaels L, Soucek S. Development of the stratified squamous epithelium of the human tympanic membrane and external canal: the origin of auditory epithelial migration. *Am J Anat* 1989;184: 334–344.
84. Michaels L, Soucek S. Auditory epithelial migration. III. Development of the stratified squamous epithelium of the tympanic membrane and external canal in the mouse. *Am J Anat* 1991;191: 280–292.
85. Michaels L, Soucek S. Stratified squamous epithelium in relation to the tympanic membrane: its development and kinetics. *Int J Pediatr Otolaryngol* 1991;22:135–149.
86. Michaels L, Soucek S. Auditory epithelial migration. II. The existence of two discrete pathways and their embryologic significance. *Am J Anat* 1990;189:189–200.
87. Ruedi L. Pathogenesis and treatment of cholesteatoma in chronic suppuration of the temporal bone. *Ann Otol Rhinol Laryngol* 1957;66: 283.
88. Fernandez C, Lindsay JR. Aural cholesteatoma: experimental observations. *Laryngoscope* 1960;70:1119–1141.
89. Friedmann I. Epidermoid cholesteatoma and cholesterol granuloma, experimental and human. *Ann Otol Rhinol Laryngol* 1959;68:57–59.
90. Wright CG, Meyerhoff WL, Burns DK. Middle ear cholesteatoma: an animal model. *Am J Otolaryngol* 1985;6:327–341.
91. Masaki M, Wright CG, Lee DH, et al. Experimental cholesteatoma. Epidermal ingrowth through tympanic membrane following middle ear application of propylene glycol. *Acta Otolaryngol (Stockh)* 1989; 108:113–121.
92. Wells MD, Michaels L. Role of retraction pockets in cholesteatoma formation. *Clin Otolaryngol* 1983;8:39–45.
93. Ruedi L. Pathogenesis and treatment of cholesteatoma in chronic suppuration of the temporal bone. *Ann Otol Rhinol Laryngol* 1957;66: 283–304.
94. Palva T, Johnsson L. Findings in a pair of temporal bones from a patient with secretory otitis media and chronic middle ear infection. *Acta Otolaryngol* 1984;98:208–220.
95. Kronenberg J, Ben-Shoshan J, Modam M, et al. Blast injury and cholesteatoma. *Am J Otol* 1988;9:127–130.
96. Suzuki M, Kodera K. Long term follow-up of secretory otitis media in children: the effects of adenotonsillectomy with insertion of a ventilation tube. *Auris Nasus Larynx* 1985;12(suppl 1):237–238.
97. Friedberg J. Congenital cholesteatoma. *Laryngoscope* 1994;104 (suppl):1–24.
98. Derlacki EL, Clemis JD. Congenital cholesteatoma of the middle ear and mastoid. *Ann Otol Rhinol Laryngol* 1965;74:707–727.

99. McGill TJ, Merchant S, Healy GB, et al. Congenital cholesteatoma of the middle ear in children: a clinical and histopathological report. *Laryngoscope* 1991;101:606–613.
100. Grundfast KM, Ahuja GS, Parisier SC, et al. Delayed diagnosis and fate of congenital cholesteatoma (keratoma). *Arch Otolaryngol Head Neck Surg* 1995;121:903–907.
101. Cohen D. Locations of primary cholesteatoma. *Am J Otol* 1987;8: 61–65.
102. Teed RW. Cholesteatoma verum tympani. Its relationship to the first epibranchial placode. *Arch Otolaryngol* 1936;24:455–474.
103. Michaels L. An epidermoid formation in the developing middle ear; possible source of cholesteatoma. *J Otolaryngol* 1986;15:169–174.
104. Wang RG, Hawke M, Kwok P. The epidermoid formation (Michaels' structure) in the developing middle ear. *J Otolaryngol* 1987;16: 337–380.
105. Rabl H. Die Entwicklung der Derivate des Kiernendarmes beim Meerschweinschen. *Arch Mikr Anat* 1913;82:79; cited by Teed RW. Cholesteatoma verum tympani (its relationship to the first epibranchial placode). *Arch Otolaryngol* 1936;24:455–474.
106. Kartush JM, Graham MD. Salivary gland choristoma of the middle ear: a case report and review of the literature. *Laryngoscope* 1984;94:228–230.
107. Peters BR, Maddox HE 3rd, Batsakis JG. Pleomorphic adenoma of the middle ear and mastoid with posterior fossa extension. *Arch Otolaryngol Head Neck Surg* 1988;114:676–678.
108. Kamerer DB, Caparosa RJ. Temporal bone encephalocele—diagnosis and treatment. *Laryngoscope* 1982;92:878–881.
109. Nelson EG, Kratz RC. Sebaceous choristoma of the middle ear, *Otolaryngol Head Neck Surg* 1993;108:372–373.
110. Jackson CG, Levine SC, McKennan KX. Hemangioma of the middle ear. *Am J Otol* 1987;8:131–132.
111. Hyams VJ, Michaels L. Benign adenomatous neoplasms (adenoma) of the middle ear. *Clin Otolaryngol* 1976;1:17–26.
112. Derlacki EL, Barney PL. Adenomatous tumors of the middle ear and mastoid. *Laryngoscope* 1976;86:1123–1135.
113. Arnold B, Zietz C. Adenoma of the middle ear mucosa. *Eur Arch Otorhinolaryngol* 1996;253:65–68.
114. Jahrdoerfer RA, Fechner RE, Selman JW, et al. Adenoma of the middle ear. *Laryngoscope* 1983;93:1041–1044.
115. Mills SE, Fechner RE. Middle ear adenoma. A cytologically uniform neoplasm displaying a variety of architectural patterns. *Am J Surg Pathol* 1984;8:677–685.
116. Stanley MW, Horwitz J, Levinson RM, et al. Carcinoid tumors of the middle ear. *Am J Clin Pathol* 1987;87:592–600.
117. Mooney EE, Dodd LG, Oury TD, et al. Middle ear carcinoid: an indolent tumor with metastatic potential. *Head Neck* 1999;21: 72–77.
118. Hale RJ, McMahon RF, Whittaker JS. Middle ear adenoma: tumour of mixed mucinous and neuroendocrine differentiation. *J Clin Pathol* 1991;44:652–654.
119. Polak JM, Bloom SR. *Endocrine tumours.* Edinburgh: Churchill Livingstone, 1985.
120. Wassef M, Panagiotis K, Polivka M, et al. Middle ear adenoma. A tumor displaying mucinous and neuroendocrine differentiation. *Am J Surg Pathol* 1989;13:838–847.
121. Krouse JH, Nadol JB, Goodman ML. Carcinoid tumors of the middle ear. *Ann Otol Rhinol Laryngol* 1990;99:547–552.
122. Alford BR, Guilford FR. A comprehensive study of tumors of the glomus jugulare. *Laryngoscope* 1962;72:765–785.
123. Bartels LJ, Pennington J, Kamerer DB, et al. Primary fallopian canal glomus tumors. *Otolaryngol Head Neck Surg* 1990;102:85–88.
124. Ophir D. Familial multicentric paragangliomas in a child. *J Laryngol Otol* 1991;105:376–380.
125. van Baars FM, Cremers CW, van den Broek P, et al. Familial nonchromaffinic paragangliomas (glomus tumors). Clinical and genetic aspects (abridged). *Acta Otolaryngol (Stockh)* 1981;91:589–593.
126. Mariman EC, van Beersum SE, Cremers CW, et al. Analysis of a second family with hereditary non-chromaffin paragangliomas locates the underlying gene at the proximal region of chromosome 11q. *Hum Genet* 1993;91:357–361.
127. Martinez-Madrigal F, Bosq J, Micheau C, et al. Paragangliomas of the head and neck. Immunohistochemical analysis of 16 cases in comparison with neuro-endocrine carcinomas. *Pathol Res Pract* 1991;187: 814–823.
128. Kliewer KE, Duan-Ren W, Pasquale A, et al. Paragangliomas: Assessment of prognosis by histologic, immunohistochemical and ultrastructural techniques. *Hum Pathol* 1989;20:29–39.
129. Rosenwasser H. Long-term results of therapy of glomus jugulare tumors. *Arch Otolaryngol* 1973;97:49–54.
130. Schwaber MK, Glasscock ME, Jackson CG, et al. Diagnosis and management of catecholamine secreting glomus tumors. *Laryngoscope* 1984;94:1008–1015.
131. Hahn SS, Kim JA, Goodchild N, et al. Carcinoma of the middle ear and external auditory canal. *Int J Radiat Oncol Biol Phys* 1983;9: 1003–1007.
132. Michaels L, Wells M. Squamous cell carcinoma of the middle ear. *Clin Otolaryngol* 1980;5:235–248.
133. Michaels L, Liang J. Origin and structure of middle ear corpuscles. *Clin Otolaryngol* 1993;18:257–262.
134. Phelps PD, Lloyd GA. The radiology of carcinoma of the ear. *Br J Radiol* 1981;54:103–109.
135. Hyams VJ, Batsakis J, Michaels L. Tumors of the upper respiratory tract and ear. *Fascicle of tumor pathology,* 2nd series. Washington, DC: Armed Forces Institute of Pathology, 1988.
136. Michaels L, Young M. Histogenesis of papillomas of the nose and paranasal sinuses. *Arch Pathol Lab Med* 1995;119:821–826.
137. Wenig BM. Schneiderian-type mucosal papilloma of the middle ear and mastoid. *Ann Otol Rhinol Laryngol* 1996;105:226–233.
138. Gaffey MJ, Mills ES, Fechner RE, et al. Aggressive papillary middle-ear tumor. A clinico-pathologic entity distinct from middle-ear adenoma. *Am J Surg Pathol* 1988;12:790–797.
139. Castillo M, Pillsbury HC 3rd. Rhabdomyosarcoma of the middle ear: imaging features in two children. *AJNR* 1993;14:730–733.
140. Wiatrak BJ, Pensak ML. Rhabdomyosarcoma of the ear and temporal bone. *Laryngoscope* 1989;99:1188–1192.
141. Nager GT. *Meningiomas involving the temporal bone.* Springfield, IL: Charles C Thomas, 1963.
142. Shanmugaratnam K, ed. *Histological typing of upper respiratory tract tumours,* 2nd ed. Berlin: Springer, 1991.
143. Stanley RJ, Scheithauer BW, Thompson EI, et al. Endodermal sinus tumor (yolk sac tumor) of the ear. *Arch Otolaryngol Head Neck Surg* 1987;113:200–203.
144. Hill BA, Kohut RI. Metastatic adenocarcinomas of the temporal bone. *Arch Otolaryngol* 1976;102:568–571.
145. Jahn AF, Farkashidy J, Berman JM. Metastatic tumors in the temporal bone—a pathophysiologic study. *J Otolaryngol* 1979;8:85–95.
146. Erickson LS, Sorenson GD, McGavran MH. A review of 140 acoustic neurinomas (neurilemmoma). *Laryngoscope* 1965;75:601–627.
147. Leonard J, Talbot M. Asymptomatic acoustic neurilemmoma. *Arch Otolaryngol* 1970;91:117–124.
148. Wanamaker WH. Acoustic neuroma: primary arising in the vestibule. *Laryngoscope* 1972;82:1040–1044.
149. Sidek D, Michaels L, Wright A. Changes in the inner ear in vestibular schwannoma. In: Iurato S, Veldman JE, eds. *Progress in human auditory and vestibular histopathology.* Amsterdam: Kugler Publications, 1996:95–101.
150. Young DF, Eldridge R, Gardner WJ. Bilateral acoustic neuroma in a large kindred. *JAMA* 1970;214:347–353.
151. Wertelecki W, Rouleau GA, Superneau MD, et al. Neurofibromatosis 2: clinical linkage studies of a large kindred. *N Engl J Med* 1988;5:278–283.
152. Sobel RA. Vestibular (acoustic) schwannomas: histologic features in neurofibromatosis 2 and in unilateral cases. *J Neuropathol Exp Neurol* 1993;52:106–113.
153. Igarashi M, Jerger J, Alford BR, et al. Functional and histological findings in acoustic tumor. *Arch Otolaryngol* 1974;99:379–384.
154. Singh SP, Cottingham SL, Slone W, et al. Lipomas of the internal auditory canal. *Arch Pathol Lab Med* 1996;120:681–683.
155. Gussen R. Meniere's disease: new temporal bone findings in two cases. *Laryngoscope* 1971;81:1695–1707.

156. Hassard AD, Boudreau SF, Cron CC. Adenoma of the endolymphatic sac. *J Otolaryngol* 1984;13:213–216.
157. Heffner DK. Low-grade adenocarcinoma of probable endolymphatic sac origin. A clinicopathologic study of 20 cases. *Cancer* 1989; 64:2292–2302.
158. Poe DE, Tarlov EC, Thomas CB, et al. Aggressive papillary tumors of temporal bone. *Otolaryngol Head Neck Surg* 1993;108:80–86.
159. Pollak A, Bohmer A, Spycher M, et al. Are papillary adenomas endolymphatic sac tumors? *Ann Otol Rhinol Laryngol* 1995;104: 613–619.
160. Kronenberg J, Leventon G. Histology of the endolymphatic sac of the rat ear and its relationship to surrounding blood vessels: the "endolymphatic glomerulus." *Am J Otol* 1986;7:130–133.
161. Kronenberg J, Rickenbacher J. The vascular pattern of the endolymphatic sac in the human embryo. *Am J Otol* 1986;7:326–329.
162. de Souza CE, Sperling NM, da Costa SS, et al. Congenital cholesteatomas of the cerebellopontine angle. *Am J Otol* 1989;10: 358–363.
163. Henick DH, Feghali JG. Bilateral cholesterol granuloma: an unusual presentation as an intradural mass. *J Otolaryngol* 1994;23:15–18.
164. Amedee RG, Marks HW, Lyons GD. Cholesterol granuloma of the petrous apex. *Am J Otol* 1987;8:48–55.
165. Nelson EG, Hinojosa R. Histopathology of metastatic temporal bone tumors. *Arch Otolaryngol Head Neck Surg* 1991;117:189–193.
166. Gnepp DR, Chandler W, Hyams V. Primary Kaposi's sarcoma of the head and neck. *Ann Intern Med* 1984;100:107–114.
167. Linthicum FH Jr. Histopathology of otosclerosis. *Otolaryngol Clin North Am* 1993;26:335–352.
168. Guild SR. Histologic otosclerosis. *Ann Otol Rhinol Laryngol* 1944; 53:246–266.
169. Hueb MM, Giycoolea MV, Paparella MM, et al. Otosclerosis: the University of Minnesota temporal bone collection. *Otolaryngol Head Neck Surg* 1991;105:395–405.
170. Mills BG, Singer FR, Weiner LP, et al. Evidence for both respiratory syncytial virus and measles virus antigens in the osteoclasts of patients with Paget's disease of bone. *Clin Orthop* 1984;183:303–311.
171. McKenna MJ, Mills BG, Galey FR, et al. Filamentous structures morphologically similar to viral nucleocapsids in otosclerotic lesions in two patients. *Am J Otol* 1986;7:25–28.
172. Niedermeyer HP, Arnold W. Otosclerosis: a measles virus associated inflammatory disease. *Acta Otolaryngol (Stockh)* 1995;115:300–303.
173. Phelps PD. Congenital cerebrospinal fluid fistulae of the petrous temporal bone. *Clin Otolaryngol* 1986;11:79–92.
174. Schuknecht HF, Reisser C. The morphologic basis for gushers and oozers. *Adv Otorhinolaryngol* 1988;39:1–12.
175. Phelps PD, King A, Michaels L. Cochlear dysplasia and meningitis. *Am J Otol* 1993;15:551–557.
176. Igarashi M, King AI, Schwenzfeier CW, et al. Inner ear pathology in osteogenesis imperfecta congenita. *J Laryngol Otol* 1980;94:697–705.
177. Marion MS, Hinojosa R. Osteogenesis imperfecta. *Am J Otolaryngol* 1993;14:137–138.

4

NASAL CAVITY AND PARANASAL SINUSES

EMBRYOLOGY, ANATOMY, HISTOLOGY, AND PATHOLOGY

RICHARD J. ZARBO
FRANK X. TORRES
JOSE GOMEZ

EMBRYOLOGY

The development of the face begins early in the 4th week of gestation, and results from the participation of five facial primordia that surround the primitive mouth: the frontonasal prominence (unpaired) from mesenchyme ventral to the primitive brain, the maxillary prominences (paired) from the first branchial arch, and the mandibular prominences (paired), also originating from the first branchial arch. Toward the end of the 4th week, two oval-shaped thickenings of surface ectodermal origin, the nasal placodes, develop on either side of the lower frontonasal prominence. These structures represent the primordia of the lining of the nasal cavity and the external nose. The epithelial lining of the sinonasal cavities is thus of surface ectodermal origin. The olfactory mucosa is also derived from the surface ectoderm; however, around the 7th week of embryonic life, the tissue begins to show evidence of specialization characteristic for this region of the nasal cavity. The maxillary prominences participate indirectly in the successive development of the external nose, and directly, together with the frontonasal prominence derivatives, participate in the formation of portions of the nasal cavity floor (palate), nasal septum, and craniofacial bones. Formation of the paranasal sinuses occurs late in fetal life; they are represented by small diverticula in the lateral nasal walls. Throughout childhood and adolescence, the sinuses display steady progression to the eventual adult form and size. Similar to the nasal cavity, the associated nasolacrimal duct and lacrimal sac develop from surface ectoderm (1).

ANATOMY

The roughly pyramid-shaped nasal cavity is divided into right and left halves by the septum. The narrower apical portion is located superiorly along the cribriform plate of the ethmoid bones. The wider base corresponds to the floor of the nasal cavity and is structurally formed by the palatine processes of the maxillary bones and the horizontal processes of the ethmoid bones. The relatively flat medial surface of each half of the nasal cavity is formed by the septal cartilage, vomer, and perpendicular plate of the ethmoid bone. Within the lateral surfaces of the nasal cavity, formed by the maxillary bones, inferior conchal bones, and ethmoid bones, are three curled delicate bony ridges that correspond to the superior, medial, and inferior turbinates or conchae. When present, the fourth ridge is at the uppermost portion of the lateral nasal wall and represents the supreme turbinate. The surface of the lateral nasal cavity walls are further marked by the superior, medial, and inferior meatuses, located under each of the corresponding turbinates. These openings within the osseous framework of the nasal cavity are the passageways for communication between the paranasal sinuses and the nasal cavity. Each of the paranasal cavities (maxillary, ethmoid, frontal, and sphenoid sinuses) is enclosed by its corresponding craniofacial bone. Despite the short distance between the paranasal sinuses and the nasal cavity, the narrowness of the meatus creates an anatomic bottleneck for the drainage of the secretory contents of the sinuses, which is further compounded by the inflammation and edema that accompanies many infectious and allergic processes. The nasal cavity ends posteriorly at the choanae, which permit passage of inspired air and secretions to the nasopharynx and eventually the oropharynx (2,3).

LYMPHATIC DRAINAGE

Nose

Lymphatic drainage for the vestibular region of the nose goes to the submandibular lymph node chain. The floor of the nasal cavity and portions of the lower aspects of the inferior turbinates drain to the internal jugular lymph node chain. The upper portions of the inferior and middle turbinates have lymphatic drainage to retropharyngeal nodes and to the internal jugular lymph node chain. The superior turbinates and uppermost aspects of the nasal cavity drain to the retropharyngeal and deep cervical lymph nodes in the vicinity of the digastric muscle. There are lymphatic communications between the olfactory region of the nasal fossae and the subarachnoid space of the brain, which constitute a potential pathway for infectious agents to gain access to the meninges.

Paranasal Sinuses

The lymphatic drainage for the frontal, maxillary, and the anterior and medial group of ethmoid sinuses is to the submandibular nodes. The posterior ethmoid group and sphenoid sinuses drain to the retropharyngeal nodes.

CLINICAL RELEVANCE

The clinical signs and symptoms commonly associated with diseases of the sinonasal tract are secondary to, or greatly influenced by (a) the location of the sinonasal tract with its involvement as a conduit for air in the breathing process; (b) the interconnection of the nasal cavity with the various paranasal sinuses; (c) the enclosure of the sinonasal spaces within a relatively rigid boundary, represented by the craniofacial bones; and (d) the close proximity or intimate association of various cranial sensory–motor nerve branches, which provide innervation not only to the sinonasal tract, but also to portions of the oral cavity, face, and ocular regions. All of these factors contribute to a greater or lesser degree in the clinical manifestations that are commonly expressed by patients with diseases of the sinonasal tract: nasal stuffiness, congestion, rhinorrhea, epistaxis, sensation of facial fullness, and local and referred pain.

The anatomy of the nasal and paranasal sinuses can be both an advantage and a disadvantage, particularly in reference to neoplasms. The bony shell surrounding the airways acts as a relatively strong barrier to tumor spread; however, many of the tumors are discovered in relatively late stages, due to the availability of space for growth within the airways themselves and compounded by secondary infections masking the underlying neoplasm. Furthermore, sinonasal tumors may clinically mimic a non-neoplastic process. The osseous barrier is effective only when the inherent biologic nature of the tumor is not one of an aggressive–destructive neoplasm. The interconnectedness of the contiguous air spaces also provides an avenue for tumor extension to areas of least resistance, with consequent tumor spread and increased clinical stage at the time of diagnosis. Numerous vital structures are separated by the collectively strong, but individually tenuous bony structures comprising the osseous framework of the sinuses and nose. This creates problems of cranial nerve palsies, ocular disturbances, and possible intracranial extension of the neoplasm. The anatomic location of the sinonasal tract makes resectability of advanced tumors difficult if not impossible.

HISTOLOGY

External Nose

The supporting framework is predominantly composed of hyaline cartilage and scant bone represented by the nasal bones proper, the nasal portion of the frontal bone, and the frontal processes of the maxillae. There is scant skeletal muscle and overlying connective tissue. The skin covering the external nose has abundant sebaceous glands and small hairs.

Nasal Cavity

The external nares are continuous with the skin and share similar histology. The adjacent nasal vestibule is also lined by stratified squamous epithelium. The limen nasi separates the vestibule from the nasal cavity proper; it corresponds to a ridge on the lateral nasal wall, formed by the lower end of the lateral nasal cartilage (2). Within the vestibular region, there are abundant stiff hairs that are felt to represent a rough primary filtration system for inspired air. Approximately at the level of the limen nasi is the transition point where the lining of the nasal cavity loses similarity to the skin. It is initially composed of squamous epithelial mucosa and gradually changes into nonciliated cuboidal or columnar epithelium. Farther into the nasal cavity, this transitional epithelium is continuous with the pseudostratified ciliated columnar epithelium, which corresponds to the respiratory epithelium that normally lines most of the nasal cavity and all of the contiguous paranasal sinuses. Interspersed within the surface respiratory epithelium are scattered goblet cells, and along the base of the epithelial lining are small basophilic cells. The lamina propria is thin and continuous with the periosteum and perichondrium of the skeletal and cartilaginous framework of the nose and paranasal sinuses. Within the lamina propria are numerous seromucous glands and scattered lymphocytes and plasma cells. The glands are more abundant in the nasal cavity and tend to be sparse in the thin connective tissue layer underlying the lining epithelium of the paranasal sinuses. The nasal cavity has an extensive vascular supply, particularly in the form of large venous plexuses in the lower part of the septum and in the middle and inferior turbinates. These vessels have prominent perivascular smooth muscle cuffs that are believed to alter the blood flow through the nasal cavity, therefore assisting in regulating the conditions of the inspired air as it passes through the upper airways (e.g., humidifying and warming the air). The closely packed vessels with their muscular walls have been referred to as pseudoerectile tissue as opposed to the true erectile tissue of the penis, for example, whose veins have valves, unlike the large veins of the turbinate.

The outline of the olfactory mucosa is irregular; however, it is usually limited to the upper surface of the superior conchae, nasal surface of the cribriform plate, and the most superior aspect of the nasal septum. Microscopically the olfactory membrane is mainly lined by nonciliated sustentacular cells. Intermingled within these tall, slender supporting cells are bipolar sensory neurons and a few scattered small basal cells (Fig. 1). Each sensory cell has dendritic processes in the form of long and slender cilia that project above the surface of the epithelium and lie parallel to the olfactory membrane surface within the secretory products of Bowman's serous glands, which are present in the tenuous lamina propria of the olfactory mucosa. The cilia function as the receptors for detection of odorants. Each sensory cell also gives off a basal axon, which joins the other sensory cell axons in the lamina propria and eventually forms the filia olfactoria, which pass

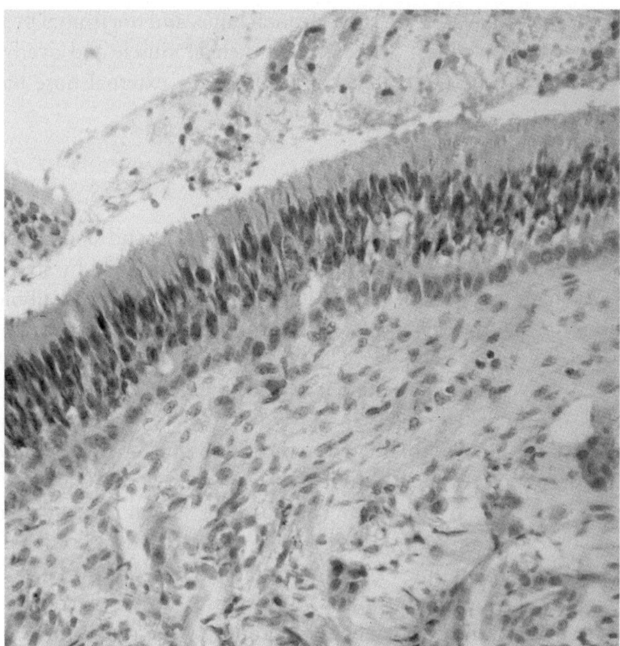

FIGURE 1. Olfactory mucosa. Tall sustentacular cells mixed with bipolar sensory neurons and small basal cells.

through the cribriform plates of the ethmoid bone. It is believed that the basal cells represent undifferentiated stem cells that can give rise to both sustentacular cells and sensory cells. This theory has not been proven in humans; in mice, however, basal cells can generate new olfactory receptor neurons. This would be an exceptional method of replacement of sensory neurons, not described elsewhere in the body. Moreover, it would explain the ability to retain the sense of smell throughout a lifetime of exposure to various airborne noxious elements (4–6).

SINUSITIS

The nasal cavity and adjacent paranasal sinuses are normally sterile. The region is supplied with a relatively efficient defense system against the numerous potential environmental pathogens. The defense mechanisms include the mucus secreted by the submucosal glands, with its contents of specific antimicrobial factors represented by secretory immunoglobulin A (IgA) and IgM, serum-derived IgG, and nonspecific antimicrobial factors, such as lysozyme and lactoferrin (7). The cilia present on the luminal surface of the lining epithelium further enhance the effectiveness of the mucus substance. The continuous movement of the cilia, assisted by gravity, drives the mucus and entrapped foreign substances posteriorly toward the nasopharynx, removing potential pathogens from the upper airways. Although the mucociliary system is an effective preventive method of infection control, there are many points of weakness within the defense mechanism. Defects in any of the components of the mucociliary system may result in the development of an inflammatory or infectious process, but establishment of sinusitis is most likely multifactorial, the result of an aggregate of deficiencies within the constituents of the mucociliary defense mechanism.

Acute Sinusitis

Clinical Data

Most cases of acute sinusitis arise after a recent bout of viral or allergic rhinitis. Both predisposing conditions are characterized by excessive thin mucus production, congestion, and edema (8).

Clinical symptoms include nasal congestion, purulent nasal discharge, postnasal drip and sore throat, halitosis, facial pain (particularly when stooping forward), low-grade fever, and systemic malaise. The most common pathogens in acute sinusitis are *Hemophilus influenzae,* pneumococci, streptococci and *Moraxella catarrhalis* (9).

The unfortunate increase of human immunodeficiency virus (HIV)-infected individuals has altered the list of common diseases associated with acute sinusitis. Individuals in this immunocompromised population tend to have severe, refractory, or recurrent disease with multiple sinus involvement that often progresses to chronic sinusitis (10,11). The infectious agents responsible for sinusitis in severely immunocompromised individuals include both common and uncommon pathogens such as cytomegalovirus (12).

Radiologic Findings

The radiologic hallmark is an air–fluid level in the affected sinus. Nonetheless, most of the imaging findings are nonspecific, showing smooth or nodular thickening of the mucosa and opacification of the sinus. Children do not have clearly visible sinuses on radiographs because pneumatization of the sinuses is not completed until puberty (13).

Histopathologic Features

The pathologist rarely, if ever, receives specimens from patients suffering from acute sinusitis, because it is usually treated medically. The histologic findings are nonspecific and include prominent congestion and edema. Within the subepithelial stroma there is a mixed inflammatory infiltrate dominated by neutrophils. Unless there is a history of recurrent sinusitis, with the exception of a hyalinized basement membrane, there are usually no histologic indicators of chronicity, such as stromal fibrosis.

Chronic Sinusitis

Clinical Data

Chronic sinusitis is a common disease that affects all age groups. In a survey performed in 1994 in the United States (14), it was estimated that close to 35 million individuals suffered from this disease. It also appears to be more common in individuals under 45 years of age, with a 1.3:1 female predominance in this same age group. Patients with chronic sinusitis can have varied symptoms, including usually frontal headaches, facial pain, nasal congestion, and nasal discharge. Similar to acute sinusitis, there can be a remote history of viral or allergic rhinitis. However, as previously discussed, other contributing factors, particularly obstruction to the ostia of the paranasal sinuses, are usually necessary for progression to chronicity. Chronic sinusitis is a good example of multifactorial promotion of upper airway infection. The usual common denominator is stasis of mucus within a cavity, which is an appropriate growth medium for microorganisms. A key role is played by the peculiar regional anatomy of the sinonasal region, characterized by relatively small ostia and narrow passages draining paranasal sinuses. It is not necessary to have a gross anatomic defect in the area, because obstruction can be produced by simple edema of the mucosa lining these delicate openings. Common colds, allergies, or poorly managed acute sinusitis can all produce edema in these narrow passages (15–18). It should be noted that contributing factors are not limited to primary mechanical obstruction to the ostia, but also may involve primary defects in the cilia (immotile cilia syndrome) (19,20), increased viscosity of mucus (cystic fibrosis) (21,22), and immunologic (secretory IgA) deficiencies (23). Other causes of obstruction include nasal septum deviation, concha bullosa, obstructing hypertrophied adenoids, and infectious processes extrinsic to the sinonasal tract, such as dental infections with direct extension into the maxillary sinus (16).

The inflammatory response releases antimicrobial substances that also unfortunately cause tissue damage, with concurrent release of cytokines and other factors such as interleukin 4 (IL-4) and IL-5, which promote more inflammation, as well as recruitment of eosinophils. Eosinophils have highly toxic granules and contribute to the overall tissue destruction within the affected sinus (7,24). The microorganisms most frequently involved include anaerobes, *Staphylococcus aureus,* and enteric gram-negative bacteria. However, chronic sinusitis in most instances is a polymicrobial infection (9).

Radiologic Findings

The radiologic findings are nonspecific. Computed tomography (CT) imaging studies suggestive of chronic sinusitis include mucosal thickening, sinus opacification, evidence of reactive bone thickening, and presence of polyps (13).

Histopathologic Features

In contrast to acute sinusitis, it is fairly common to receive mucosal fragments from patients with persistent or recurrent bouts of chronic sinusitis. Many of the specimens are submitted after functional endoscopic sinus surgery has been performed in an effort to alleviate obstructions and to remove devitalized or nonfunctional mucosa (25).

Histologically, the respiratory mucosa can show a wide range of inflammatory changes. The inflammatory cells commonly present include lymphocytes, plasma cells, eosinophils, and neutrophils. The predominant inflammatory cell within the infiltrate will vary from case to case, and on the degree of active inflammation; however, plasma cells and lymphocytes usually dominate. The presence of eosinophils does not necessarily reflect an allergic process, but is part of the overall chronic inflammatory response, recruited by locally produced cytokines, as previously discussed. Depending on the degree of tissue destruction and chronicity of the process, there will be stromal fibrosis and, in some cases, polypoid hyperplasia of the mucosa (Fig. 2) or hyperplasia of the seromucous glands normally present within the respiratory mucosa (Fig. 3). Scarred and thinned mucosa associated with reactive sclerotic bone is occasionally seen. These latter findings are often accentuated in a mucocele. In the most severe or extensive cases, the accompanying bone can be involved by the inflammatory process with secondary chronic osteitis. Inflammatory polyps frequently accompany the tissue submitted for pathologic examination.

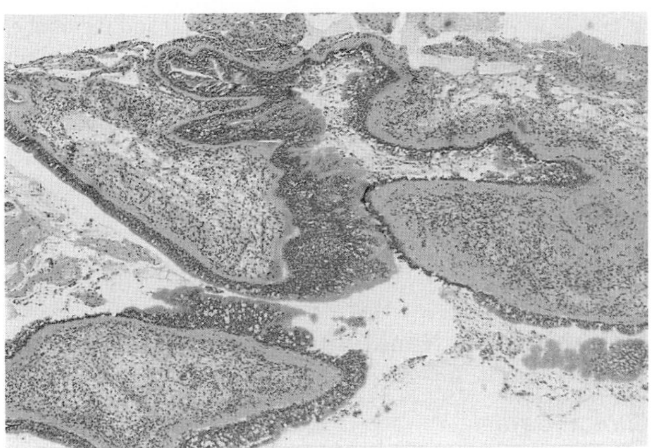

FIGURE 2. Chronic sinusitis. Polypoid hyperplastic respiratory mucosa. The presence of thickened basement membrane and lack of inversion distinguish this from inverted papilloma.

Treatment and Complications

In the majority of cases, treatment of acute and chronic sinusitis will be medical, with antibiotics and local or systemic substances that promote drainage of obstructed sinuses. Currently, functional endoscopic sinus surgery is used in recurrent disease or disease unresponsive to initial medical management (25). In children, the possibility of cystic fibrosis or selective immunodeficiencies should be investigated. Complications of untreated

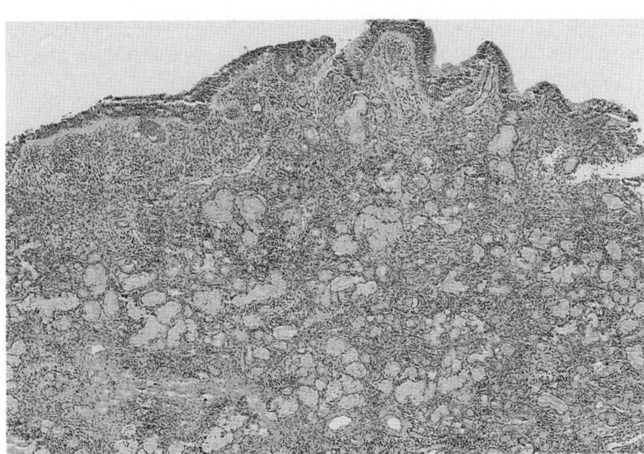

FIGURE 3. Chronic sinusitis. Hyperplasia of seromucous glands. The preserved lobular architecture at low power distinguishes this from low-grade adenocarcinoma.

or poorly treated chronic sinusitis include local and regional extension of the infectious process through the thin nasal and paranasal sinus bones. This can result in chronic osteitis, osteomyelitis in the case of the marrow-containing frontal bone, orbital cellulitis and periorbital abscess formation, direct extension into the cranial cavity, and retrograde venous extension of the infection, causing septic cavernous sinus thrombophlebitis and brain abscesses (26,27).

Inflammatory Nasal and Antrochoanal Polyps

Clinical Data

These lesions are polypoid outfoldings of the respiratory mucosa rather than neoplasms. There has been much discussion of their association with allergic conditions, aspirin intolerance, infectious processes, cystic fibrosis, and Kartagener's syndrome (19,28–30). In a review by Settipane (31), nasal polyps were found in approximately 36% of patients with aspirin intolerance and in 7% with a history of asthma. The peak incidence was at age 50. Only 0.1% of asthmatic children presented with nasal polyps. However, polyps were found in 20% of children with cystic fibrosis. Because of this association with cystic fibrosis, finding nasal polyps in children (particularly in children under 16 years of age) (32) should initiate the exclusion of underlying cystic fibrosis. This is particularly important in a child with a history of recurrent sinonasal tract infections, in view of the fact that sinonasal tract disease may be the initial presentation of cystic fibrosis (22). An interesting finding is the low frequency of nasal polyps in allergic rhinitis (1.5%) found in a review of 6,037 patients (33). Despite these known or suspected associations, the precise etiology is still currently unknown, the morphologic findings are nonspecific, so inflammatory polyps may represent a common lesion resulting from a variety of unrelated conditions.

The overall incidence of nasal polyps is unknown; males and females appear to be equally affected (33). The most common clinical complaint is nasal stuffiness. On physical examination a soft glistening, semitranslucent, smooth round, or pear-shaped polypoid mass (or masses) is found (34), usually originating from the lateral nasal mucosa in the region of the middle meatus, near or within the ethmoidal or maxillary ostia. Nasal polyps are frequently bilateral and multiple (35).

Antrochoanal polyps are not commonly associated with allergic processes. Chronic sinusitis is present in about 25% of the affected individuals (36), but it is not clear whether this represents a secondary or an etiologic process. The age of presentation ranges from late childhood to 70 years (36). The polyps are usually solitary and unilateral and arise from the maxillary antrum, projecting through the sinus ostia into the posterior nasal cavity and nasopharynx, through the choana. Frequently the antral portion of the polyp is cystic. Berg et al. suggest that antrochoanal polyps may actually represent expanding cysts that eventually protrude into the nasal cavity (37). However, a discrete epithelial lining surrounding the pseudocystic fluid-filled region of an antrochoanal polyp is virtually never seen.

Gross Appearance

The macroscopic appearance of both inflammatory and antrochoanal polyps is similar. If most of the antrochoanal polyp has been resected, a definite stalk can be grossly identified. In contrast, nasal inflammatory polyps will appear broad based. Both types of polyps will have a smooth surface. The cut surface is usually glistening and edematous in appearance. However, a few of these lesions will have variable fibrotic areas possibly secondary to trauma or chronic inflammation.

Histologic Features

Distinction between an antrochoanal and an inflammatory nasal polyp is primarily accomplished clinically. As mentioned above, an antrochoanal polyp can be suspected in a polyp with a narrow and well-defined stalk; however, there are no specific distinguishing microscopic features that permit an unequivocal diagnosis of inflammatory or antrochoanal polyp. Both types of polyps have analogous histologic characteristics and represent polypoid outgrowths of the respiratory mucosa, mainly as a result of an expanded lamina propria. The polyps are lined by respiratory epithelium, which can focally display respiratory basal cell hyperplasia or squamous metaplasia. The basement membrane is variably thickened and in some instances has underlying areas of stromal hyalinization. The bulk of the lesion is represented by edematous subepithelial stroma with variable inflammation and occasional fibrosis (Fig. 4). The inflammatory infiltrate is composed of a mixture of neutrophils, eosinophils, lymphocytes, and plasma cells. Some polyps can display a prominent eosinophilic infiltrate; however, this does not necessarily imply an allergic etiology. Possibly due to expansion of the respiratory mucosa, there

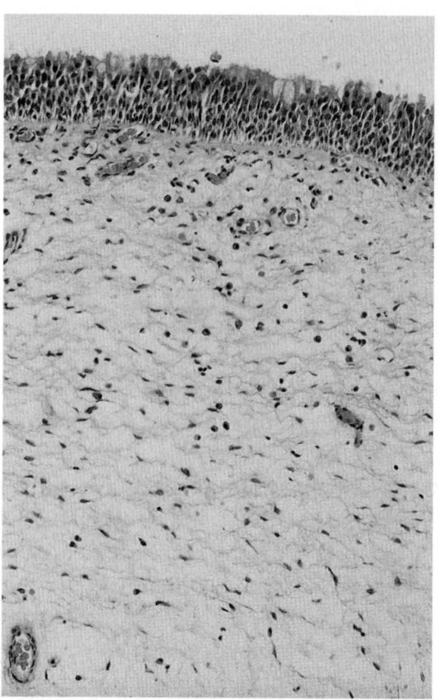

FIGURE 4. Inflammatory nasal polyp. Edematous stroma devoid of seromucous glands with variable inflammation forms a polypoid outfolding of respiratory mucosa.

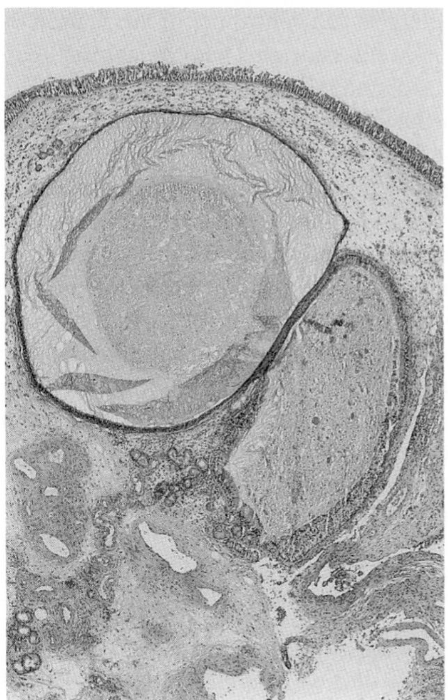

FIGURE 5. Inflammatory nasal polyp. Polyp with submucosal dilated ductal retention cysts.

appears to be a decrease in the number of seromucous glands. In approximately 5% of inflammatory polyps, there is hyperplasia of mucous glands within the polyp (38). Also occasionally seen are cystically dilated glands and ducts (Fig. 5).

It is reported that polyps arising in association with cystic fibrosis have a distinct histopathology, permitting their separation from ordinary inflammatory polyps (39) (Fig. 6). Polyps in cystic fibrosis allegedly do not display a thickened basement membrane or hyalinization of the underlying stroma, a feature commonly seen in ordinary inflammatory polyps. In addition, histochemical stains using the Alcian blue–periodic acid-Schiff (PAS) stain should demonstrate the presence of acid mucin within glands and the mucus covering the surface epithelium. In both areas the mucin should be predominantly neutral in patients who do not have cystic fibrosis. However, others report no significant histologic differences between polyps associated with cystic fibrosis and those not associated with cystic fibrosis (40). More recently, Batsakis and El-Naggar stated that the polyps arising within cystic fibrosis are of an inflammatory nature, and therefore are probably not distinguishable from polyps presenting in patients without cystic fibrosis (30). From a practical point of view, children and adolescents with recurrent sinus infections and inflammatory polyps should be clinically evaluated for the presence of underlying cystic fibrosis.

Differential Diagnosis

Stromal cell atypia within inflammatory nasal polyps is a well-known finding (41,42); however, the true frequency of this finding is unknown. Stromal cell atypia is more commonly seen in younger individuals with a mean age of 10 years (41). The atypical stromal cells have bizarre, enlarged, and hyperchromatic nuclei; however, the nuclear to cytoplasmic ratio is not enlarged. The nuclei of these atypical cells frequently have an angulated contour, giving them a slightly stellate appearance (Fig. 7). Increased mitoses or atypical mitoses are not seen. The atypical stromal cells are haphazardly distributed, an important microscopic feature, because one of the major differential diagnoses is botryoid embryonal rhabdomyosarcoma. In this type of polypoid rhabdomyosarcoma the neoplastic cells tend to create a hypercellular cambium layer beneath the surface epithelium.

It should be noted that the surface epithelium of inflammatory nasal polyps is not exempt from developing dysplasia or malignancy. Further still, inflammatory polyps may accompany schneiderian papillomas. Therefore, some maintain that all tissue from sinonasal curettage should be submitted for histopathologic examination (43).

Biologic Behavior

Treatment consists of controlling, if possible, any underlying or associated conditions that may contribute to the formation of in-

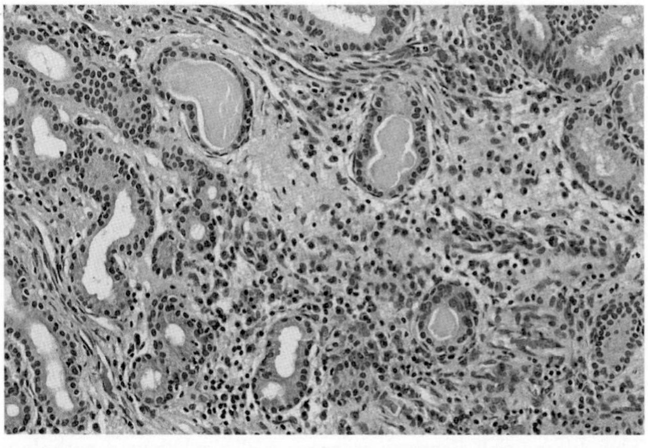

FIGURE 6. Nasal polyp–cystic fibrosis. Inspissated secretions in mucoserous glands are common in but not pathognomonic of mucoviscidosis.

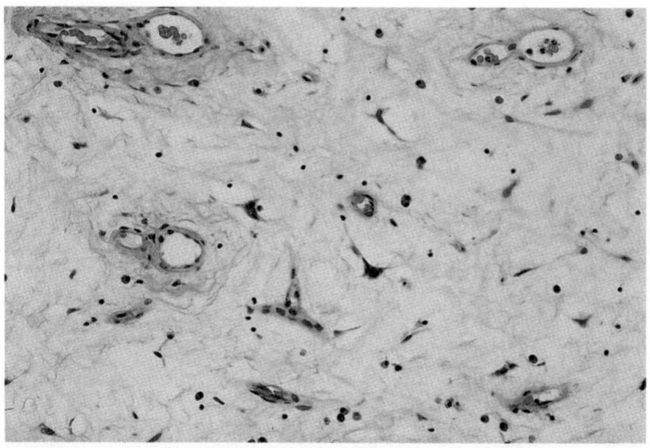

FIGURE 7. Nasal polyp–stromal cell atypia. Haphazardly distributed benign atypical stromal cells with enlarged, hyperchromatic nuclei and stellate contours.

flammatory nasal polyps. This treatment strategy is important because recurrences are common. Topical steroids for limited disease, antibiotics to resolve accompanying infections, and systemic steroids combined with surgical removal of the lesions in severe cases are some of the current therapeutic choices for management of inflammatory polyps (44).

Mucocele

Clinical Data

Mucocele is a benign non-neoplastic condition characterized by cystic expansion of a paranasal sinus by retained mucoid secretions. The wall of the mucocele is represented by the mucosal, submucosal and osseous components of the affected sinus (Fig. 8). In a retrospective study of 112 patients with mucoceles, Natvig and Larsen (45) report that the most frequently involved sinuses are frontal (77%), frontal and ethmoid combined (16%), ethmoid (7%), and maxillary (3%). Mucoceles are created by occlusion of the ostia draining the affected sinus (46). It is hypothesized that continued mucus production accumulates within a sinus that has partial or complete lack of drainage, causing secondary expansion of the sinus. The continuous expansile growth of the mucocele can lead to eventual involvement of neighboring sinuses or extrasinusoidal structures, and in this way, there can be orbital, intranasal, subdural, and even intracranial involvement (47). Expansion of the sinus cavity and extension into extrinsic structures is the result of bone erosion or destruction. The most likely mechanism for bone destruction is simple, but continuous, mechanical pressure with secondary ischemia, bone necrosis, and eventual resorption. However, the presence of osteolytic cytokines within mucoceles has been reported (48), and these preliminary data provide an alternate explanation for bone destruction by the mucocele. Sudden rapid expansion of a relatively slow growing mucocele can be a sign of secondary infection. When the mucocele content is predominantly purulent material it is commonly known as a pyocele. Bacteriologic studies performed on the mucopurulent contents most frequently show the presence of *Staphylococcus* species, *Streptococcus pneumoniae,* and *Haemophilus influenzae* (49).

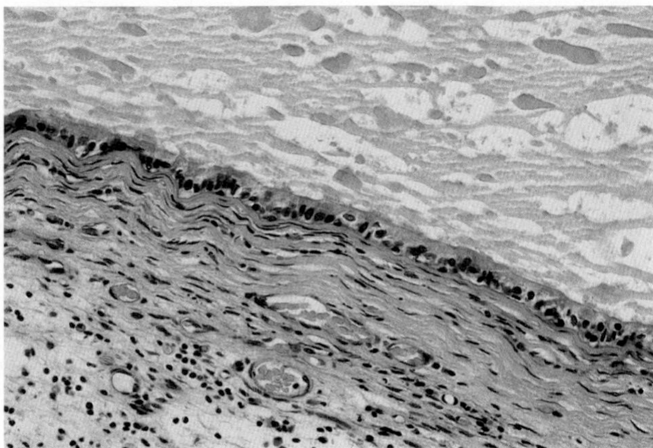

FIGURE 8. Mucocele. Mucoid secretions expand the paranasal sinus and attenuate the respiratory epithelium.

Conditions that can contribute to mechanical obstruction of ostia are commonly associated with mucoceles. Association with chronic sinusitis and inflammatory nasal polyps, allergic rhinitis, trauma or prior sinonasal surgery, and benign or malignant neoplasms have been described (45,50,51).

Mucoceles tend to involve a single paranasal sinus and can occur in any age group, but they are more common in individuals over 30 years of age and affect men and women equally (45,51). Related symptoms and signs include visible or palpable periorbital swelling; visual changes secondary to orbital involvement and proptosis, with blurred vision, conjunctivitis, epiphora, and local periorbital or frontal pain; and symptoms of nasal obstruction, with nasal congestion and swelling in the area of the mucocele, and in some cases the presence of nasal polyps (51). Drainage of the lesion will produce characteristic thick, tenacious, greenish mucus.

Radiologic Studies

Radiographic studies demonstrate the expanded sinus and show evidence of bone destruction and of nonspecific sinus inflammation with opacification. On CT scan a mucocele appears as a nonspecific hypodense, nonenhancing mass that fills and expands the sinus cavity (13). CT studies can provide the best evidence of the extent of bone involvement. Magnetic resonance imaging (MRI) studies can provide valuable information regarding the status of surrounding soft tissue, and add additional information regarding the nature of the cyst contents. This can provide valuable imaging evidence to assist in distinguishing a mucocele from a possible neoplasm (47).

Gross Appearance

The specimen obtained from the excision of these lesions is usually fragmented and, with the exception of the greenish tenacious mucoid substance described above, does not display specific gross findings.

Histologic Features

Microscopically, the cyst wall fragments show a lining composed of respiratory epithelium, with variable flattening and attenuation of the pseudostratified columnar epithelium, scattered remnant goblet cells, and varying degrees of epithelial hyperplasia and squamous metaplasia of the mucocele lining. There may be submucosal fibrosis, at times dense and focally keloid-like, and evidence of chronic inflammation, with an infiltrate of lymphocytes, plasma cells and variable numbers of eosinophils. Acute inflammation will be seen with a coexistent secondary infection. The accompanying bone fragments can display evidence of remodeling, woven bone formation, osteoblastic activity, increased vascularization, and foci of active bone destruction (51).

Differential Diagnosis

The differential diagnosis is more a clinical than a pathologic problem, because this locally destructive lesion can simulate a malignant neoplasm. Many of the histopathologic findings are nonspecific inflammatory changes that acquire more significance with an appropriate clinical history.

Biologic Behavior

Untreated, the natural course of the disease process is that of continued growth and expansion, with possible local and regional infections, such as periorbital abscess formation, meningitis, or brain abscess (27).

The objectives of treatment include correction of any underlying conditions, decompression of the mucocele by providing appropriate drainage and aeration to the affected sinus (47), and, in some instances, complete surgical excision of the lesion (49,50). Despite adequate surgical treatment, long-term follow-up is necessary in view of the possible recurrence of the lesion months or years after its initial excision (51). It is postulated that entrapped remnant mucocele tissue in the surgical site can be a cause of recurrence (50).

Myospherulosis

Clinical Data

Myospherulosis is an interesting foreign body granulomatous inflammatory process caused by interaction of the oil of oil-based hemostatic packing materials with blood present in a postsurgical wound bed. It may be an asymptomatic incidental finding, or, conversely, may be the source of sinusitis-associated symptoms.

The iatrogenic inflammatory process forms fungus-like spherular structures and was initially described as a soft tissue lesion. The term *myospherulosis* is a reflection of these structures, resembling an endospore-bearing fungal organism, and the prior description of a very similar, if not identical, lesion in skeletal muscle in Africans (52,53). Kyriakos reported the occurrence of myospherulosis in the paranasal sinuses and middle ear and suggested that it represented an iatrogenic disease linked to the petrolatum-based ointments present in hemostatic packing materials (52).

The most common antecedent surgical procedure was a Caldwell-Luc operation, and consequently, the maxillary sinus was the most frequently affected site (52,54,55). Subsequently, it was demonstrated that the funguslike structures were actually degenerating erythrocytes produced by interaction of red blood cells with the ointments commonly present in wound packing materials (56).

Gross Appearance

At the time of surgery there may be mucosal thickening of the affected paranasal sinus, inflammatory polyps, or a rubbery to firm mass composed of dense fibrous tissue (52).

Histologic Features

Myospherulosis is characterized by the presence of submucosal cyst-like spaces of varied size that can be up to 1.0 mm in diameter. The spaces are located within a mildly to moderately inflamed fibrous stroma and do not involve the overlying lining epithelium. The cyst-like structures may be surrounded by histiocytes and foreign body giant cells. The tissue spaces may be empty, contain cellular debris, or have sac-like structures of varied size that may be attached to the walls of the tissue spaces or lie freely within the lumen of these spaces. The sacs have a thin membranous wall and may have a double-layered appearance. Within the sacs are a few to several hundred relatively uniform-sized, empty-appearing, round structures that are degenerating erythrocytes, originally thought to represent endospores (Fig. 9). On hematoxylin and eosin–stained sections, the sacs and degenerating erythrocytes have a light to dark brown hue. Some of the degenerating erythrocytes may retain their concave contour. However, they also have a brownish discoloration. A few of the degenerated erythrocytes, together with smaller, densely staining round structures, which may represent collapsed erythrocytes, can be seen within the fibrous stroma outside of the tissue spaces (52).

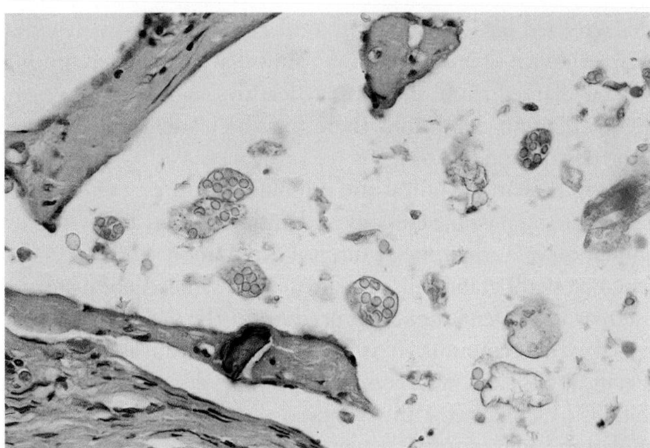

FIGURE 9. Myospherulosis. Fungus-like structures with degenerating erythrocytes that mimic endospores, produced by interaction with oil-based hemostatic packing materials. (Courtesy Dr. M. Kyriakos.)

Differential Diagnosis

Confusion with rhinosporidiosis or coccidioidomycosis may occur, but distinction can be readily accomplished on morphologic grounds and by the lack of positivity for Grocott's methenamine silver (GMS) and PAS stains. In addition, histochemical stains for hemoglobin and lipofuscin will stain the so-called spherules, providing further support for a diagnosis of myospherulosis (56).

Biologic Behavior

Treatment is probably limited to symptomatic cases and consists of debridement of the tissue containing the foreign body granulomatous process.

Sinonasal Cholesterol Granuloma and Cholesteatoma (Rhinitis Caseosa)

Clinical Data

Cholesterol granulomas and sinonasal cholesteatoma, also known as rhinitis caseosa (57), are two similar clinical conditions characterized by long-standing local pain, together with radiologic evidence of a mass within a sinus cavity, most commonly the maxillary antrum, that display features suggestive of a cystic lesion. In both conditions there may be evidence of localized bone destruction (58,59).

Despite sharing clinical and radiologic features, there are dissimilarities in possible etiology and in the findings at physical examination or at the time of surgical exploration.

Cholesterol granulomas usually have an antecedent history of trauma or a recent surgical procedure in the vicinity of the affected paranasal sinus. It is believed that extravasated blood, specifically the cell wall components of erythrocytes, contribute the basic elements for the formation of cholesterol. Similar to cholesterol granulomas frequently seen in the middle ear and temporal bone, it appears that hemorrhage into a relatively enclosed anatomic space with poor aeration and lymphatic drainage greatly contributes to the pathogenesis of the lesion (60).

Sinonasal cholesteatoma, on the other hand, has a more obscure pathogenesis and is possibly linked to trauma or a prior infectious or inflammatory process (58).

On physical examination, cholesterol granulomas are typically submucosal bluish to green-appearing lesions, that may fill the entire sinus cavity (61). Sinonasal cholesteatoma is characterized by the presence of a cystic lesion with a malodorous grumous content, which explains the other designation for this process: rhinitis caseosa (58).

Histologic Features

Histologically, cholesterol granuloma is characterized by granulation tissue formation, presence of hemosiderin, histiocytes, and most importantly by the presence of fusiform clefts, representing the sites where cholesterol was present prior to removal by tissue processing. These so-called cholesterol clefts may be extracellular or present within multinucleated giant cells, and for this reason this pathologic process is known as cholesterol granuloma (Fig. 10) (57).

The microscopic hallmark of sinonasal cholesteatoma, on the other hand, is the presence of keratinous debris and fragments of benign keratinizing stratified squamous epithelium, which is the source of the grumous material seen at gross examination (57). In other words, the morphology is akin to that of an epidermal inclusion cyst or a cholesteatoma of the middle ear (see Chapter 3).

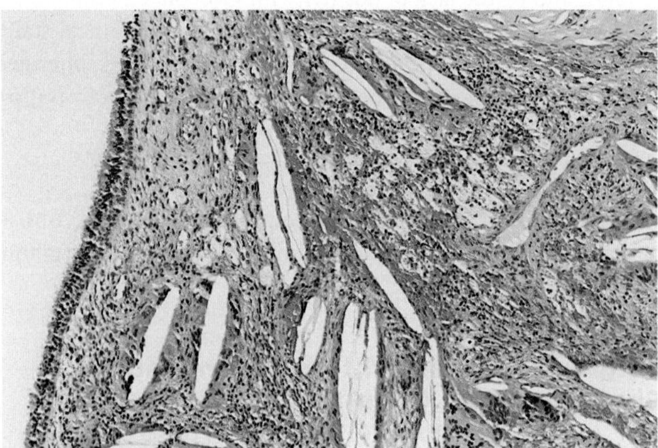

FIGURE 10. Cholesterol granuloma. Hemorrhage into an enclosed space with poor aeration and drainage may produce this mass lesion. Note the characteristic cholesterol clefts.

In both conditions, the accompanying sinonasal mucosa may show varying degrees of chronic inflammation.

Differential Diagnosis

The clinical and pathologic features of both diseases are relatively characteristic and are not usually a source of diagnostic confusion. However, the presence of multinucleated giant cells in a cholesterol granuloma may elicit the investigation of an underlying granulomatous infection.

Biologic Behavior

Both disease processes are managed surgically by complete excision and are not associated with recurrence of the lesion (58,60,61).

FUNGAL DISEASES OF THE SINONASAL TRACT

In general, fungal diseases of the sinonasal tract are divided into two broad groups, namely noninvasive and tissue-invasive fungal infections. However, this division does not entirely take into account the probable mechanisms by which fungi elicit sinonasal disease.

If the partially understood mechanisms of disease are considered, sinonasal mycotic processes can be further subdivided into (a) noninvasive colonization of paranasal sinuses, also illustratively designated as "fungus ball"; (b) noninvasive hypersensitivity reaction to fungi or allergic fungal sinusitis; (c) invasive indolent chronic sinusitis; and (d) invasive fulminant fungal rhinosinusitis (62). The basic disease processes in the first three conditions may differ, but some of their clinical and histologic characteristics can have overlapping features, and consequently they will be discussed jointly. Invasive fulminant fungal rhinosinusitis has a different clinical presentation and course. It also tends to occur in a distinct clinical population and therefore will be discussed separately.

Chronic Fungal Diseases

Clinical Data

The clinical history of patients with noninvasive or invasive indolent chronic fungal diseases will range from minor upper respiratory tract complaints to a clinical picture of marked chronic sinusitis, recalcitrant to conventional medical treatment that is not infrequently directed against the "usual suspects" (i.e., bacterial organisms). A detailed description of the numerous fungal organisms involved in chronic sinonasal tract disease is beyond the scope of this chapter; numerous excellent publications are available for a more extensive and detailed review (62–64). The most frequently cited culprits are members of the *Aspergillus* species, and more recently, in cases of allergic fungal sinusitis, dematiaceous fungi (65). Some reports find dematiaceous fungi, such as *Curvularia, Alternaria,* and *Bipolaris* species, to be the predominant pathogenic agents in allergic fungal sinusitis (66) rather than *Aspergillus,* as originally described for this condition (67). Accordingly, *allergic* Aspergillus *sinusitis* is now more appropriately designated *allergic fungal sinusitis.* In a review of publications on allergic fungal sinusitis (67–73), Hartwick and Batsakis summarize the findings on 32 patients (74) and report that all cases had more than one sinus involved. The maxillary antrum was the most frequently affected sinus, followed by the ethmoid, sphenoid, and frontal paranasal sinuses. In Bent and Kuhn's review of allergic fungal sinusitis (66), they describe multiple sinus involvement, with a tendency for unilateral presentation.

Individuals with a so-called fungus ball, can be relatively asymptomatic, have a vague sensation of facial fullness, or have another clinically dominating disease of the sinonasal tract, with the fungus ball representing an incidental finding. Examples of this latter instance are patients suffering from cystic fibrosis or individuals that are known to have a mucocele. A fungus ball can represent saprophytic colonization of the sinus in a case of bacterial sinusitis. Parenthetically, a fungus ball can be an incidental finding in chronic invasive fungal sinusitis. The fungus ball represents a relatively inert mycotic colony that produces minimal accompanying tissue reaction and is usually a colony of one of the *Aspergillus* species (75).

Invasive indolent chronic sinusitis generally displays more pronounced clinical manifestations. Commonly, there are variable symptoms of chronic sinusitis, punctuated by repeated exacerbations of acute rhinosinusitis. Symptomatology may include nasal congestion and obstruction, a sensation of facial fullness and pain, nasal and postnasal discharge, purulent nasal discharge, and variable fever, particularly if there is a superimposed bacterial infection. Physical examination reveals evidence of upper airway inflammation, with congestion, edema, and frequently inflammatory polyps. Paranasal sinus involvement in indolent chronic fungal sinusitis is variable, with multiple or single sinus involvement described (76).

Allergic and indolent chronic sinusitis can present over a wide age range from children through the elderly, with predominance in young to middle-aged adults. There appears to be a slight tendency for chronic fungal sinus diseases to arise within the male population. Individuals afflicted by either allergic or indolent chronic sinusitis are usually immunocompetent, in contrast to patients with fulminant rhinocerebral fungal infection, in which a concurrent immunologic impairment is commonly present. The frequent association of allergic fungal sinusitis and history of atopy or asthma cannot be used as a clinical discriminating factor, because either form of sinusitis can arise in the presence or absence of a history of atopy.

Radiologic Studies

Analogous to the extent of disease involvement, imaging studies also vary from showing minimal to extensive involvement.

In cases of a clinically uncomplicated fungus ball, plain films may not have any significant findings, or they may display slight expansion of the sinus lumen. With superimposed bacterial infections or in cases of mild noninvasive allergic fungal sinusitis or invasive indolent chronic fungal sinusitis, there may be opacification of multiple sinuses and mucosal thickening, suggestive of acute inflammation. However, air–fluid levels are uncommon in fungal sinusitis without superimposed bacterial infections (77). On CT scan, there may be changes compatible with chronic sinusitis, hypointense sinus cavities, and serpiginous areas of high attenuation, described as secondary to release of ferromagnetic elements by fungi (78). In addition, in cases of allergic and indolent chronic sinusitis, there may be changes compatible with bone destruction. In Hartwick and Batsakis' accumulated data (74), radiographic evidence of sinus expansion and bone erosion was present in 28% of cases. Therefore, it appears that osseous changes are not limited to invasive fungal disease. Despite these findings, in the most severe cases, usually associated with invasive chronic fungal sinusitis, there may be extensive bone destruction and evidence of extension into the nasal cavity or adjacent soft tissue (77). In cases of allergic fungal sinusitis, radiographs can show a mass in the sinus simulating a neoplasm.

Gross Appearance

A fungus ball is usually fragmented when received in the pathology laboratory and can have a varied gross appearance, from grayish white and cottonlike, to dark brown debris resembling decaying wood. If secondary retention of secretions is associated with the fungus ball, tenacious, greenish mucus also can accompany the clumps of fungal organisms.

In cases of noninvasive allergic fungal sinusitis or invasive chronic fungal sinusitis, there may be fragments of sinus mucosa, bone particles, edematous inflammatory polyps, and occasional collections of amorphous debris similar to that described for the fungus ball. Most frequently associated with allergic fungal sinusitis is the presence of collections of thick mucus, illustratively described by Wenig as "snotoma" (79). The color of the mucoid material varies according to the type of fungal or superimposed bacterial organisms present in the inspissated mucoid material, from tan-white to yellowish to green to a dark brown pastelike appearance. The allergic mucin of allergic fungal sinusitis is characteristically extremely thick and tenaceous and may actually resemble soft tissue.

Histologic Features

Microscopic examination of a fungus ball reveals a characteristic collection of matted hyphae with a layered or radiated appearance, and it most commonly is composed of organisms with the morphology of *Aspergillus* species (i.e., septate hyphae with acute angle branching). Occasionally, conidiophores or fruiting bodies may be seen in the fungus ball. The accompanying sinus mucosa may have variable nonspecific chronic inflammation. In view of the sheer bulk of fungi present, identification of the offending organisms is relatively easy, and the rationale behind using special stains for fungi is to exclude the remote possibility of an indolent tissue-invasive fungal infection.

In allergic fungal sinusitis, one of the most characteristic features appreciated at microscopic examination, particularly at low

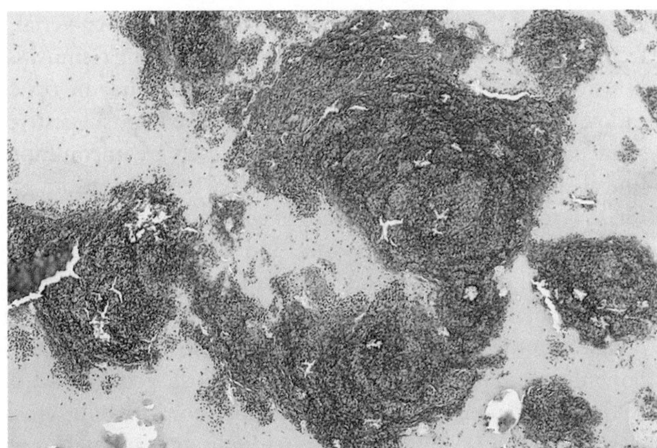

A

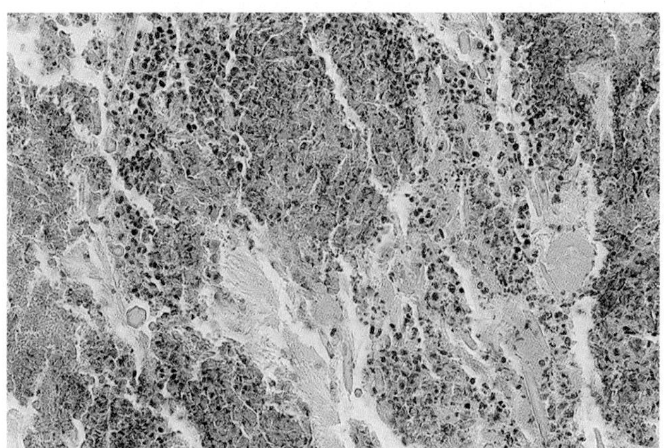

B

FIGURE 11. A: Allergic mucin. Eosinophilic mucin containing layered clumps of degenerated basophilic inflammatory cells that can be misinterpreted as neoplastic. **B:** Inset shows Charcot-Leyden crystals, hexagonal in cross-section.

magnification, is the layered or laminated aspect of clumped basophilic cells within the eosinophilic allergic mucin. At higher magnification, the clumped basophilic cells have the appearance of degenerated inflammatory cells, predominantly eosinophils, with poorly defined eosinophilic cytoplasmic borders and slightly smudged intensely basophilic chromatin (Fig. 11). On rare occasions, particularly in the absence of appropriate clinical history, these degenerating cells may be overinterpreted as neoplastic cells. The majority of the degenerated cells represent degranulated eosinophils, admixed with other types of inflammatory cells and sloughed sinus epithelial cells. Within the allergic mucin, there will be variable numbers of fungal hyphae and scattered roughly rhomboid structures, that correspond to Charcot-Leyden crystals, by-products of eosinophil degranulation. Hyphae in the allergic mucin may not be very abundant, and a special stain (e.g., GMS) may be necessary to demonstrate the presence of fungi within this characteristic mucus.

The fragments of sinus mucosa and polyps commonly show mixed acute and chronic inflammatory cell infiltrates, including variable numbers of eosinophils. The surface epithelium can have extensive areas of erosion or ulceration with underlying necrosis, granulation tissue formation, and vascular congestion. Some of the seromucous glands can display a moderate degree of cystic dilatation and in addition may contain fungal hyphae within the eosinophilic glandular content. It is particularly important not to overinterpret the areas of erosion and necrosis, or presence of fungi within the cystically dilated glands as histologic proof of an invasive fungal disease. Fungi must be present within the sinus mucosa to confirm the existence of an invasive fungal infection.

The respiratory mucosa of some cases of invasive chronic fungal sinusitis may display histologic features similar to those described above. However, special stains will assist in the identification of fungi within the submucosa or other accompanying soft tissue or bone fragments. In more established cases of invasive chronic fungal sinusitis, there will be fibrosis and variable acute and chronic inflammation of the sinus mucosa, including collections of plasma cells and eosinophils. A distinctive histologic feature is the presence of granulomas without necrosis or with focal areas of necrosis within the granulomas and extensive fibrinoid necrosis in the submucosal tissue, postulated to occur secondary to toxins produced by some of the fungi (62).

Finally, chronic fungal infections are not restricted to organisms that are characterized by hyphal morphology. Reports have been published of fungi that invade in yeast form, for example, in cryptococcal sinusitis (80).

Differential Diagnosis

The differential diagnosis includes not only diseases of nonfungal origin, such as seasonal or perennial allergic rhinosinusitis and common bacterial sinusitis, but also other types of chronic fungal sinonasal disease.

The diagnosis of an uncomplicated fungus ball is relatively straightforward. However, accompanying mucosal tissue and bone fragments, if present, within the material submitted to pathology, should be examined. It is of prime importance to rule out invasive fungal infection by thorough microscopic examination of histologic sections appropriately stained for fungal organisms.

Descriptions of "allergic sinusitis" with allergic mucin in which fungal organisms cannot be identified have been cited (66,81). Hypothetically, it is possible that other allergens, not exclusively fungi, can generate an identical tissue response. Tentatively, in the right histologic background, it can be inferred that some of the findings can correspond to a hypersensitivity reaction to an unknown allergen, but even in the absence of positive microbiologic cultures, the presence of fungal disease cannot be definitively ruled out. In the same manner, distinction between noninvasive allergic fungal sinusitis, in which the fungus acts as an allergen rather than an infectious pathogen, and invasive chronic fungal sinusitis, in which a significant chronic tissue reaction has not been developed, is only attained with a careful and thorough microscopic examination of all the material submitted. It should also be underlined that histologic evidence of invasive fungi can be very focal and missed if tissue is randomly sampled and a cursory microscopic examination has been performed.

Other diseases associated with retained or inspissated mucus should be considered not only within the differential diagnosis, but as a possible contributing cause of fungal infections. These include mucoceles, cystic fibrosis, and Kartagener's syndrome. In cases of granulomatous inflammation, other common causes associated with this type of inflammation should be considered, including tuberculosis, leprosy, Wegener's granulomatosis, sarcoidosis, Churg-Strauss disease, and malignant lymphoma. Finally, myospherulosis, characterized by yeast-like structures actually related to erythrocytes associated with the use of intranasal petrolatum-based substances, should not be forgotten in the differential diagnosis (52,56).

Biologic Behavior

Treatment consists of removal of the saprophytic fungus ball, simultaneously addressing any contributing or underlying conditions. Establishment of appropriate drainage and aeration to the sinus harboring the colonizing fungi can assist in preventing recurrent colonization. Management of noninvasive allergic fungal sinusitis is difficult, particularly due to the ubiquitous nature of the hypersensitivity-producing agents. Treatment is directed at the control of the accompanying chronic sinusitis, excision of inflammatory polyps to improve breathing, and use of either topical steroids or short courses of systemic steroids. However, recurrences are very common. In view of the difficult, if not impossible, task of completely eliminating the source of the immune reaction, interest has developed in using allergy desensitization as an alternative treatment modality (66). The importance of excluding invasive fungal sinusitis becomes obvious, because part of the treatment arsenal for allergic fungal sinusitis includes use of steroidal agents with consequent attenuation of the natural immune reaction. Treatment of invasive chronic fungal sinusitis includes some of the measures described above as well as the use of antifungal agents. In addition, it is frequently necessary to remove all grossly devitalized tissue, because it can harbor and promote growth of fungi.

Complications include exacerbation of any of the chronic fungal diseases by a bacterial superinfection and progression of an allergic form of fungal sinusitis to an invasive chronic fungal sinusitis. In the latter case, there may be eventual involvement of neighboring structures, such as orbital or intracranial contents.

Fulminant Invasive Fungal Sinusitis

Clinical Data

Unlike the three types of the chronic fungal diseases previously discussed, fulminant invasive fungal infections arise almost exclusively in immunocompromised individuals or in patients with severe metabolic alterations. This condition is commonly referred to as mucormycosis, in view of the frequent isolation of *Mucor* species. But other members of the class of Phycomycetes, which includes the order of Mucorales, can be involved in this acute fungal infection. Therefore, the broader term *phycomycosis* is more accurate. Due to the frequent orbital and intracranial extension of fulminant fungal sinusitis, this process is also additionally known as rhinoorbital or rhinocerebral mucormycosis. In a review of 224 cases of mucormycosis conducted by Anand et al., orbital and intracranial involvement was encountered in 84% and 55% of cases, respectively (82). Rarely, *Aspergillus* species may cause fulminant invasive fungal sinusitis.

Blitzer and Lawson found only 4% of cases with no underlying disease in their series of 179 cases of rhinocerebral mucormycosis (63). In general, the common denominators are conditions that favor fungal growth, or that do not permit an adequate inflammatory response to the invading pathogen. A good example illustrating both situations is observed in diabetic ketoacidosis, in which low systemic pH promotes fungal growth and also appears to cause a sluggish inflammatory response. In the series by Anand et al., diabetes mellitus was present in 63% of 224 patients (82). Hematologic malignancies, especially leukemias, are also frequent predisposing conditions of fulminant fungal infections. However, the basic mechanism in these conditions is loss of the functional cell population responsible for restriction and elimination of the offending fungal organisms. Organ transplant recipients subject to immunosuppression represent another large patient group at risk for fulminant sinonasal fungal infections. Numerous other factors are probably involved in eliciting and promoting fulminant fungal sinusitis, but thorough analysis is beyond the scope of this chapter. Interestingly, it appears that HIV-related immunosuppression does not predispose to acute invasive fungal sinusitis (66).

The common clinical presentation is that of nasal obstruction, headache, facial pain, cranial nerve deficit, facial swelling, ulceration of the palate, proptosis, and visual loss. Physical examination of the nasal cavity may show deeply erythematous or black areas along the nasal turbinates (63). This rapidly progresses, in a matter of hours or a few days, to coma and stupor, and is therefore appropriately designated fulminant fungal sinusitis, an unquestionable medical emergency.

Radiologic Studies

Radiographic findings range from nonspecific inflammatory changes of the sinus mucosa (e.g., clouding of multiple sinuses and mucosal thickening) to bone erosion. CT scans may show changes compatible with disease progression, with evidence of soft tissue invasion and necrosis, early bone erosion, and cavernous sinus thrombosis. MRI appears to be helpful in the assessment of intracranial extension and early changes.

Histopathologic Features

Primary and secondary vascular changes are the most prominent microscopic features of fulminant invasive fungal sinusitis. The tendency of fungi to invade blood vessels causes direct damage to the vascular wall with necrosis, mixed acute and chronic inflammation, congestion, hemorrhage, and thrombosis. Thrombosis of arteries leads to ischemia and infarction of dependent areas downstream to the occlusion, whereas venous thrombosis causes marked vascular congestion. In smaller biopsy specimens, the finding of large geographic areas of ischemic necrosis should always raise the suspicion of an underlying fungal infection. The most commonly identified species are of the order Mucorales, characterized by branching, broad empty-appearing hyphae. The

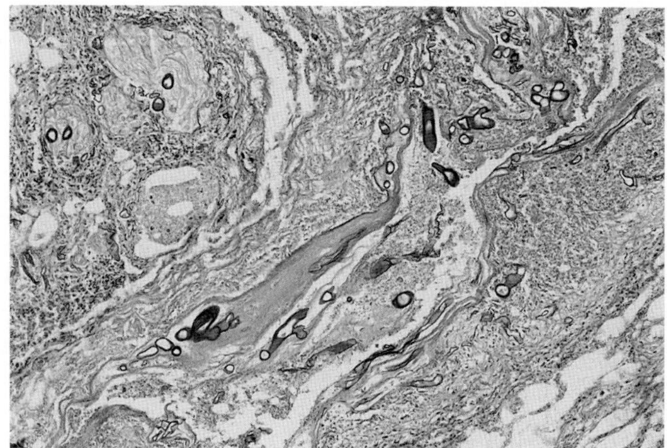

FIGURE 12. Mucormycosis. Infarcted tissue with intravascular and tissue invasion by characteristic broad nonseptate branching hyphae.

hyphae are very irregular and are devoid of septae (Fig. 12). *Aspergillus* species are also frequently present in this clinical setting. However, in contrast to the relatively ordered pattern of radiating hyphae observed in an *Aspergillus* fungus ball, the organisms in fulminant invasive fungal sinusitis are present more in the affected tissue, primarily in vascular structures (62).

Differential Diagnosis

The clinical background of predisposing systemic conditions, rapid onset and progression of acute fungal sinusitis, help to distinguish it from indolent fungal diseases or other conditions associated with a mid-facial destructive behavior. Histologically, prominent tissue necrosis and fungal invasion of blood vessels are present; these features generally are lacking in nonfulminant fungal sinus disease.

Biologic Behavior

Spread of the fulminant fungal infection to the cranial cavity and other important structures can occur by (a) direct invasion, (b) mycotic emboli, (c) perineural invasion of cranial nerves, and (d) through the cribriform plate of the ethmoid bone. Therefore, complications can be secondary to mycotic embolization or direct invasion (e.g., brain abscess, meningitis, or brain infarcts).

Survival rates are variable; however, this is a life-threatening and potentially lethal disease. In Blitzer and Lawson's series, overall survival for patients without predisposing conditions was 75%. Patients with diabetes mellitus had an overall survival of 60%, and individuals afflicted with other systemic disorders had the poorest survival rate of 20% (63,83). Therefore, the main factor influencing outcome appears to be the underlying systemic disease. Patients with systemic metabolic derangements that are amenable to medical treatment (e.g., diabetic ketoacidosis) fare better than individuals who have a disorder that is not readily controllable (e.g., leukemia).

In general, treatment includes administration of systemic antifungal medication, hyperbaric oxygen therapy, and, most importantly, debridement of any necrotic tissue, which may at times necessitate radical extirpation of tissue as for a neoplasm. The objectives of surgical debridement are multiple and include the removal of nonvital tissue harboring fungi, elimination of any necrotic tissue that because of low pH promotes fungal growth, and excision of thrombosed and ischemic tissue, in an effort to eliminate areas sequestered from the reach of systemic antifungal agents (82).

MID-FACIAL NECROTIZING LESIONS

Mid-facial necrotizing lesions are infiltrative and variably destructive disease processes involving the upper aerodigestive tract. *Mid-facial necrotizing lesion* is a clinical diagnosis used to direct attention toward numerous possible diseases that have been linked to necrosis of facial structures, including infectious, idiopathic inflammatory, and neoplastic conditions. It is for this reason, that the term *mid-facial necrotizing lesion* should not be used as a pathologic diagnosis. The older term *lethal midline granuloma* has been used to describe this clinical syndrome of mid-facial necrosis; it is not a specific diagnostic term and is, appropriately, little used in current literature.

From the clinical standpoint, mid-facial necrotizing lesions may be complicated disease processes, not only because of the long list of possible etiologies, but also because of the frequent nonspecific histologic findings in biopsy material. This may be a reflection of poor biopsy site selection and the inherently limited size of the biopsy specimen. These problems are magnified if a significant clinical history does not accompany the biopsy material. Further complicating matters is the fact that many of the diseases linked to a mid-facial necrotizing lesion are characterized by a gradual onset of signs and symptoms that initially may be subtle but with time show a relentless disease progression. As a reflection of this clinical behavior, it is obvious that the microscopic features will not have a static appearance, and therefore, the histopathologic picture will be a complex array of microscopic findings associated with early, established, and resolving lesions that will range from nonspecific histologic features to the rare classic histopathologic picture. These introductory remarks highlight the importance of biopsy site selection, which should be directed to areas thought to contain active disease, avoiding superficial, obviously necrotic or scarred areas. Furthermore, and if at all possible, samples from various affected sites may provide a greater diagnostic yield.

The disease entities most frequently linked to mid-facial necrotizing lesions are Wegener's granulomatosis, malignant lymphomas (particularly angiocentric lymphomas), and the diagnostically unsatisfying idiopathic midline granuloma (84,85) (Table 1).

The majority of conditions associated with mid-facial necrotizing lesions have common clinical features. Some are relatively nonspecific, such as malaise, fever, weight loss, arthralgias, and myalgias. Frequent upper aerodigestive tract symptomatology includes facial and sinus-related pain, nasal obstruction, rhinorrhea, postnasal discharge, and occasional bloody or purulent nasal discharge, which may be malodorous. Physical examination may show variable mucosal thickening and ulceration, mucosal friability, and crusting along the nasal passages. Advanced cases can display perforation of the septum and nasal deformities

TABLE 1. HISTOLOGIC FEATURES OF MID-FACIAL NECROTIZING LESIONS

Wegener's granulomatosis	Necrotizing vasculitis involving arteries or veins of various sizes Granulomatous vasculitis Fibrinoid degeneration of collagen Vascular and extravascular scarring Geographic degeneration of collagen with epithelioid histiocytic rimming Microabscesses
Churg-Strauss syndrome	Eosinophilic infiltrate Eosinophilic microabscesses Focal necrotizing granulomas with palisading histiocytes No vasculitis (in nasal biopsy)
Sarcoidosis	Tight, compact granulomas Multinucleated giant cells (Langhans type) Occasional punctate necrosis in granulomas No vasculitis Secondary scar formation
Tuberculosis	Necrotizing granulatous inflammation Caseous necrosis Multinucleated giant cells (Langhans type, occasionally with asteroid or Schaumann bodies) Acid-fast bacilli
Leprosy (lepromatous)	Mixed inflammatory cell infiltrate (macrophage predominant) Acid-fast bacilli, particularly within macrophages
Rhinoscleroma	Exudative phase Mixed inflammation and edema Supurative necrosis Squamous metaplasia Proliferative phase Mikulicz's cells containing bacilli Giemsa/Warthin-Starry stain Fibrotic stage Scarring Chronic inflammation Rare to absent Mikulicz's cells
Rhinosporidiosis	Sporangia in subepithelial stroma Ruptured sporangia with acute inflammation No granulomas
Cocaine abuse	Nonspecific inflammation Ulcers Granulation tissue Bone necrosis and remodeling Foreign body granulomas with polarizable foreign material
Angiocentric lymphoma	Polymorphous to monomorphous atypical lymphoid infiltrate Perivascular and vascular invasion Zonal coagulative necrosis No granulomas

such as the saddle nose deformity. Beyond the sinonasal tract there can be disease manifestations in the oral cavity, with mucosal inflammatory changes and ulcerations; eustachian tube involvement with secondary otitis media and mastoiditis; and proptosis secondary to periorbital soft tissue disease.

Some of the clinical manifestations of mid-facial necrotizing lesions may be closely associated with a few of the causative diseases. Examples include ocular or thoracic manifestations of sarcoidosis (86), renal and pulmonary signs and symptoms in patients with Wegener's granulomatosis (87), known history of pulmonary tuberculosis in patients with suspected nasal tuberculosis (88), and a history of asthma in individuals with suspicion of Churg-Strauss syndrome (89). However, despite these known associations, the final diagnosis in practically all instances of mid-facial necrotizing lesions will be highly dependent on a comprehensive clinicopathologic correlation.

Wegener's Granulomatosis

Clinical Data

Wegener's granulomatosis is a chronic systemic disease of unknown etiology. It is characterized by a clinicopathologic complex of necrotizing granulomatous vasculitis of the upper and lower respiratory tract, glomerulonephritis, and small vessel vasculitis (90).

In a study of 158 patients with Wegener's granulomatosis, 90% of the subjects sought initial medical attention for symptoms related to upper and lower respiratory disease. The upper airways alone represented the reason for medical consultation in 73% of the patients. Overall, upper airway involvement was eventually present in 92% of cases (87). The average age of presentation is from the late thirties to mid-forties, but may range from childhood to old age (87,90). Both men and women are afflicted by Wegener's granulomatosis, with some studies showing male predominance (90).

Many of the systemic and head and neck signs and symptoms described in the introduction to mid-facial necrotizing lesions can be present in Wegener's granulomatosis. Frequently at presentation there is nasal obstruction, sinusitis, and rhinorrhea. This progresses to purulent and rarely bloody nasal discharge. A relatively constant finding within the nasal mucosa is granulation tissue formation with associated large, greenish, foul-smelling mucosal crusts that on removal reveal a highly friable surface. Eventually cartilage or bone involvement can be seen, causing saddle nose deformity (91). Pulmonary symptomatology, such as cough, hemoptysis, pleuritis, and renal manifestations of the disease can be present at initial presentation or may eventually arise in the course of the disease. In 30% of the cases, pulmonary and renal symptomatology may be absent, causing further delay in final diagnosis (87).

Clinical laboratory tests may yield valuable information in cases with a high index of suspicion. These include evidence of microhematuria in urinalysis and an elevated erythrocyte sedimentation rate. Currently, assay of antineutrophil cytoplasmic antibodies (C-ANCA), is frequently used in patients suspected of having the disease. However, a negative C-ANCA does not exclude Wegener's granulomatosis. Nonetheless, it can provide valuable clinical follow-up information because it appears to closely correlate with the presence of active vasculitis (92). ANCA positivity is more common in generalized Wegener's granulomatosis than in cases of so-called limited Wegener's granulomatosis, where the disease is restricted to the head and neck. Cases of limited disease have been seen that present in the orbit rather than the sinonasal tract (93).

Radiologic Studies

Radiographs of the paranasal sinuses will show nonspecific inflammatory changes consisting mainly of mucosal thickening and sinus opacification. Chest radiographic findings are also nonspecific and may include nodular infiltrates and cavities. Despite the nonspecific results of the imaging studies, the findings provide valuable pieces in the complex diagnostic puzzle.

Histologic Features

Wegener's granulomatosis shows a constellation of histologic findings that include, in addition to mucosal ulcerations, both vascular and extravascular changes (94,95). Vascular involvement may include evidence of granulomatous inflammation, varying degrees of acute and chronic inflammation, and fibrinoid necrosis (Fig. 13). Scarring of blood vessels, presumably after resolution of the active phase of vasculitis, may be present and consists of intimal fibrosis, concentric fibrosis of the vascular wall, and fibrous obliteration of the lumen. Within the parenchyma, foci of extravascular fibrinoid degeneration of collagen (at times extensive and geographic), poorly formed granulomas, scattered giant cells, microabscesses with and without granulomatous change, and variable inflammatory cell infiltrates can be seen. The inflammatory cell infiltrates are composed of plasma cells, lymphocytes, neutrophils, occasional multinucleated giant cells, and few eosinophils, although Devaney et al. found moderate to numerous eosinophils within 15% and 4% of their cases, respectively (94).

The frequency with which the previously described histologic features appear within nasal or paranasal sinus biopsies is variable from case to case, and not all of the microscopic changes should be expected to be present in any given biopsy. In a review of 58 biopsy specimens performed by Colby et al. (which included 30 cases from Del Buono et al.), evidence of vasculitis was present in 48% of biopsy samples, necrosis in 53%, giant cells in 52%, and eosinophils in 67% of cases (95,96). Some microscopic features may appear to be more strongly associated with Wegener's granulomatosis (e.g., vasculitis); however, despite the close association, none of these findings in and of themselves are sufficiently specific to make a diagnosis of Wegener's granulomatosis with certainty. As a reflection of this lack of diagnostic specificity, and also taking into account the systemic nature of this disease process, Devaney et al. developed a series of criteria for the diagnosis of Wegener's granulomatosis (94). Application of

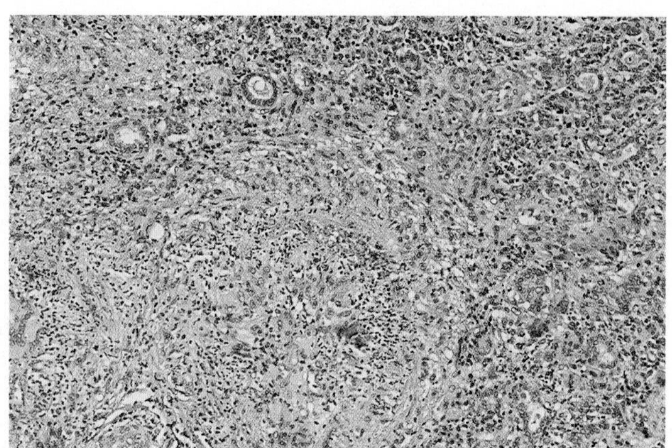

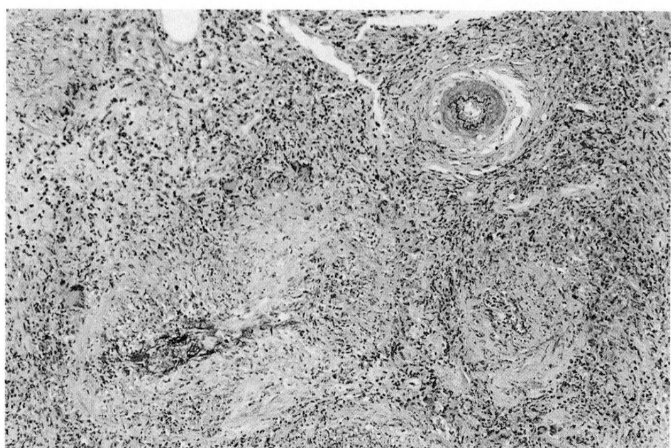

FIGURE 13. Wegener's granulomatosis. **A:** Nasal biopsy with characteristic necrotizing granulomatous vasculitis. **B:** Elastichrome stain showing inflamed, sclerotic collapsed vessels with fragmented elastica.

these criteria resulted in five categories: diagnostic, probable, suggestive, suspicious, and nonspecific. To meet the criteria of "diagnostic" for Wegener's granulomatosis, granulomatous inflammation, necrosis, and vasculitis all must be present in the biopsy material. In addition, there must be evidence of lung or kidney disease for a diagnosis of systemic Wegener's granulomatosis to be rendered. Alternatively, to meet the criteria of the diagnostic category for systemic disease, two of the histologic features plus lung and kidney involvement must be present. The "probable" category includes two of the above histologic criteria plus involvement of one of the extranasal sites (lung or kidney). The "suggestive" category is represented by one of the histologic features plus evidence of lung and kidney involvement. The "suspicious" category is defined by one histologic criterion with one extranasal site of involvement. Finally, the "nonspecific" category does not show any of the three required histologic features, despite evidence of lung or kidney involvement.

Differential Diagnosis

The differential diagnosis of Wegener's granulomatosis includes infectious processes, particularly those that can cause granulomatous inflammation, including fungi, tuberculosis, and leprosy. Special stains and, if at all possible, cultures should be performed to exclude an infectious etiology.

Sarcoidosis represents another entity that has a granulomatous appearance; however, in contrast to the poorly formed granulomas found in Wegener's granulomatosis, sarcoidal granulomas are well defined, distinct, and compact. The granulomas also have a tendency to be confluent. Rarely, sarcoidosis may have foci of necrosis, which if seen are within the granulomas, and not in the intervening stroma, as opposed to what is seen in Wegener's granulomatosis.

So-called idiopathic mid-facial necrotizing lesion, if this is truly a distinct disease entity, is extraordinarily difficult to prove (97). It is characterized by a markedly destructive mid-facial lesion that histologically may show some of the features associated with Wegener's granulomatosis. However, definitive evidence of vasculitis, including fibrinoid necrosis of blood vessels, is lacking. In addition, idiopathic mid-facial necrotizing lesions do not display systemic manifestations.

The differential diagnosis also includes the polymorphic reticulosis–angiocentric lymphoma group of diseases. The key point in the differential diagnosis is lack of atypical lymphoid cells, particularly in an angiocentric arrangement, in Wegener's granulomatosis. Despite the polymorphous nature of some of the malignant lymphomas affecting the sinonasal region, granulomatous inflammation is not a histologic feature of these lymphomas.

Allergic angiitis and granulomatosis, also known as Churg-Strauss syndrome, can have nasal manifestations in approximately 70% of cases (94). Characteristically, there is an antecedent history of asthma, pulmonary infiltrates, peripheral eosinophilia, and systemic vasculitis (89,98). Churg-Strauss syndrome is histologically characterized by abundant eosinophils, sometimes forming eosinophilic microabscesses, and focal necrotizing granulomas with palisading histiocytes. In a review of 32 patients with Churg-Strauss syndrome, vasculitis was not seen in any of the nasal biopsies (99). Therefore, the presence of vasculitis would favor a diagnosis of Wegener's granulomatosis.

Biologic Behavior

The currently accepted treatment for Wegener's granulomatosis includes long-term administration of cyclophosphamide or glucocorticoids, and usually involves concurrent use of both medications. In a large study of patients with Wegener's granulomatosis, most patients displayed marked clinical improvement or remission when they received both medications; however, it was occasionally necessary for individuals to be treated for up to 4 to 6 years to attain clinical remission (87). In this same study, approximately 50% of patients in remission had at least one incidence of recurrence, sometimes many years after having achieved remission. A 20% overall mortality rate was reported, with 13% of deaths attributed to active Wegener's granulomatosis (87). Other causes of death can be secondary to treatment complications or complications of the disease process, such as renal failure.

Sarcoidosis

Clinical Data

Sarcoidosis is a chronic granulomatous inflammatory disease of unknown etiology. It can involve multiple organs within the body; however, it has an affinity for the respiratory tract, and the sinonasal tract may be involved. In general, sarcoidosis tends to follow a slowly progressive and indolent clinical course. However, it also can present as a rapidly progressive, widespread granulomatous process. The estimated overall incidence of sarcoidosis is 6 to 10 individuals per 100,000 (100).

A review of 2,319 patients with sarcoidosis demonstrated involvement of the head and neck region in 9% of cases. The most commonly affected sites were eyes and lacrimal glands (40%), skin (26%), and nose (13%). In this same study, the peak age of affliction with nasal sarcoidosis was between 40 and 60 years, although the disease was seen in adolescent through elderly age groups (86). It appears that sarcoidosis has a tendency to present in female patients, with a male:female ratio of 1:3 (86,100). Symptoms related to nasal involvement include nasal obstruction, epistaxis, nasal pain, and anosmia. On physical examination, patients may present with nasal crusting, yellowish submucosal nodules, nonspecific mucosal thickening, and nasal polyps. Therefore, it should not be surprising to encounter patients that have been treated for common chronic sinusitis, particularly in cases in which nasal involvement by sarcoidosis is the first manifestation of the disease. Because of easy access to the upper airway mucosa, a nasal biopsy also may be performed for signs and symptoms related to involvement of less readily accessible sites, as in patients with radiologic evidence of hilar lymphadenopathy or pulmonary infiltrates. Laboratory findings of elevated serum and urine calcium levels, or high serum levels of angiotensin-converting enzyme, are commonly increased in patients with sarcoidosis (100).

Disease progression may cause prominent nasal crusting, epistaxis, intranasal synechiae with stenosis, cartilage destruction, saddle nose deformity, and occasionally nasal cutaneous fistulization (101).

Radiologic Studies

Similar to other inflammatory diseases that affect the sinonasal tract, radiologic findings are usually nonspecific, consisting of mucosal thickening and sinus opacification.

Histologic Features

The primary histopathologic finding in sarcoidosis is the presence of granulomas (Fig. 14). These consist of tight aggregates of epithelioid histiocytes accompanied by variable numbers of Langhans' type multinucleated giant cells. Some of the giant cells may contain several types of nonspecific inclusion bodies such as asteroid and Schaumann bodies. Occasionally present within the granulomas are small foci of fibrinoid necrosis. Notably absent are extensive caseous necrosis and vasculitis. Secondary scar tissue and mild nonspecific chronic inflammation may be seen in the background. If the biopsy sample is from deeper lesional tissue, granulomatous inflammation may be seen eroding the cartilage.

Differential Diagnosis

Despite the distinctive appearance of the granulomatous inflammation seen in sarcoidosis, this is a diagnosis reached by exclusion. Foremost on the list of diseases to exclude are fungal infections and tuberculosis, which can be addressed with the appropriate special stains for fungal and acid-fast microorganisms, respectively. Use of special stains for microorganisms is a relatively crude and insensitive method of bacteriologic investigation; therefore, negative results do not necessarily exclude the possibility of infection. If possible, material should be harvested for a more sensitive assessment through microbiologic cultures.

Other diseases to consider in the differential diagnosis are other potential mid-facial destructive diseases, including Wegener's granulomatosis, Churg-Strauss syndrome, and angiocentric lymphomas. Sarcoidosis does not show the granulomatous vasculitis and stromal fibrinoid degeneration of collagen characteristic of Wegener's granulomatosis. Conversely, Wegener's granulomatosis does not exhibit the well-defined and occasionally confluent granulomas characteristic of sarcoidosis. Additional helpful clinical information for differential diagnosis would be the existence of the necrotizing glomerulonephritis seen in Wegener's granulomatosis. Prominent eosinophilia, necrotizing granulomas, and vasculitis, together with the history of asthma and systemic eosinophilic vasculitis seen in Churg-Strauss disease, are not characteristic of sarcoidosis and assist in distinguishing these conditions. The prominent polymorphous cellular infiltrate, including atypical cells with angiocentric arrangement, and the locally aggressive behavior seen in polymorphous reticulosis–angiocentric lymphomas, are important features that distinguish this disease group from sarcoidosis.

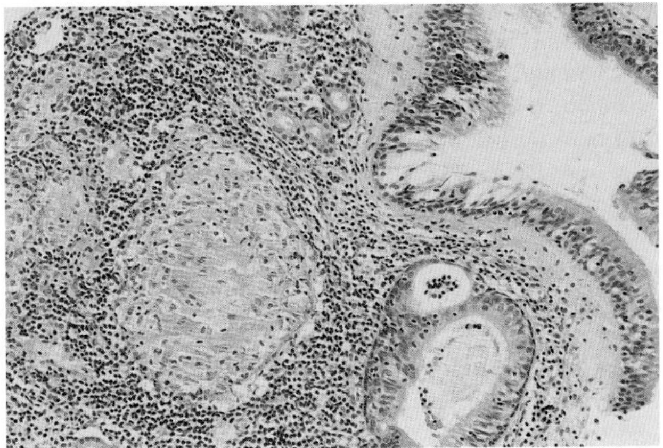

FIGURE 14. Sarcoidosis. Sinus mucosa containing compact epithelioid granuloma with peripheral rim of lymphocytes.

Biologic Behavior

Untreated, sarcoidosis may remain relatively stable or show slow, unrelenting destruction of sinonasal structures with deformity of external and internal anatomic landmarks. Treatment is tailored to the severity of disease and can range from observation or topical steroid medications in low-grade disease to local injection or systemic administration of steroidal agents. Surgery is sometimes necessary to alleviate some of the airway obstruction caused by the sequelae of the granulomatous inflammation (100).

Tuberculosis

Clinical Data

Nasal tuberculosis is a chronic granulomatous infection caused by the bacillus *Mycobacterium tuberculosis.* Occurrence in the nose can be either primary or secondary to disease elsewhere in the body. Primary infection is probably secondary to inhalation of bacilli-bearing droplets or dust particles.

The disease is most frequently seen in middle-aged and elderly individuals. Clinical presentation of nasal infection is characterized by painless unilateral or bilateral nasal obstruction, mucopurulent rhinorrhea, and postnasal discharge. Occasionally epistaxis is seen, and the patients may complain of nasal itching and sneezing (88).

On physical examination, the lesion may consist of a small shallow mucosal ulceration that occasionally has a roughly granular edge, or a small nodule with a pale red granular surface that tends to bleed easily on manipulation. Foul-smelling crusts may accumulate on the mucosal surfaces. The most frequent site of involvement within the nasal cavity is the cartilaginous septum, which may result in septal perforation; the septal bone is infrequently involved (88). The turbinates and floor of the nose are other frequently affected sites. The so-called lupus variant of tuberculosis is caused by regional spread of the infection to the facial and nasal skin.

Histologic Features

Biopsy samples from the grossly observed lesions will demonstrate granulomatous inflammation with areas of necrosis. The granulomas are predominantly composed of epithelioid histiocytes, with scattered multinucleated giant cells, usually of Langhans' type.

Differential Diagnosis

Regardless of the appearance of the granulomas, it is always necessary to perform special stains, such as a Ziehl-Neelsen, to highlight the acid-fast bacilli that are otherwise undetected with conventional stains. The quantity of bacilli is highly variable; however, in morphologically suspicious cases, a thorough search for acid-fast microorganisms should be performed to satisfactorily confirm or fail to confirm their presence. On limited material, it may be difficult to exclude the possibility of Wegener's granulomatosis, particularly if systemic manifestations of tuberculosis are not present. Wegener's granulomatosis is not characterized by formation of well-defined granulomas or tubercles with Langhans' type giant cells. Necrotizing granulomatous inflammation may be prominent in both tuberculosis and Wegener's granulomatosis; however, finding histologic areas with serpiginous fibrinoid degeneration surrounded by epithelioid histiocytes would favor the presence of Wegener's granulomatosis. Prominent eosinophilia and atypical lymphocytes are not seen; therefore, their absence assists in microscopically excluding Churg-Strauss syndrome and polymorphic reticulosis–malignant lymphoma. Sarcoidosis is another disease process included in the differential diagnosis of tuberculosis. The quality of the granulomas is similar; however, necrosis is less frequently seen in sarcoidosis. Despite the presence or absence of necrosis, special stains or microbiologic cultures are sometimes necessary to distinguish between these morphologically similar conditions. Other infectious conditions to consider, albeit rare, include leprosy, syphilis, rhinoscleroma, and invasive fungal infections.

Biologic Behavior

Treatment consists of antituberculous therapy. Due to the presence of drug-resistant strains of *Mycobacterium tuberculosis,* it is usually necessary to use a combination of antimycobacterial agents. The course of untreated nasal tuberculosis is that of a protracted and continuously destructive disease with eventual involvement of cartilage, bone, and regional extension of the infectious process.

Leprosy

Clinical Data

Leprosy is a chronic infectious granulomatous disease, produced by the bacillus *Mycobacterium leprae.* It occurs mainly in tropical countries; however, it is endemically present in certain locations of the United States, including Texas, Louisiana, Florida, California, Hawaii, and New York (102). As a consequence of increased global travel and immigration, sporadic cases of leprosy may present in patients living in nonendemic areas or locations not commonly associated with this exotic infectious disease. It is therefore important not to dismiss the remote possibility of leprosy and to include it in the differential diagnosis of mid-facial necrotizing lesions.

Leprosy has an affinity for peripheral nerves and skin. The classification of leprosy is in reality a reflection of the clinical manifestation of the disease at the poles of a disease spectrum. At one end of the spectrum is tuberculoid leprosy, in which there is a high endogenous resistance to the pathogen. In general, its clinical manifestations are associated with neural involvement of the trigeminal and facial nerves. At the other extreme, lepromatous leprosy is characterized by low immunologic resistance. It commonly affects the nasal mucosa, which may be one of the first manifestations of disease (102). Symptoms include hyposmia, crusting, obstruction, and bloody nasal discharge. A pale plaque-like nodule may be seen on the nasal mucosa, most commonly on the anterior portion of the inferior turbinate. With disease progression there is pronounced obstruction, mucosal ulceration, and septal perforation. Other areas of involvement in the head and neck include the face, external ears, mouth, oropharynx, larynx, and rarely the palate and free edge of the epiglottis (102). Borderline leprosy may show features of both tuberculoid and lepromatous leprosy.

Radiologic Studies

There are few characteristic radiologic changes. In the lepromatous variant of the disease, there may be loss of the anterior nasal spine and eventual nasal collapse secondary to periostitis (102).

Histologic Features

The acid-fast bacilli can be demonstrated with a Fite stain or Ziehl-Neelsen stain for mycobacteria. In tuberculoid leprosy rare bacilli may be identified, in contrast to the exuberant presence of bacilli in the lepromatous variant of the disease. Bacilli can be found free within the lumina of seromucous glands and ducts, acini, vascular spaces, endothelial cells, perivascular histiocytes, and so-called Virchow cells, which represent bacilli-laden macrophages. There is also a polymorphic inflammatory cell infiltrate, including epithelioid and giant cells. Plasma cells can be numerous in some patients (103). Discrete granulomas are more characteristic of tuberculoid than lepromatous leprosy.

Differential Diagnosis

It is obvious that leprosy, particularly the lepromatous variant, should be included in the long list of diseases that may cause mid-facial necrotizing lesions. The polymorphous inflammatory infiltrate together with the presence of epithelioid giant cells requires distinction from Wegener's granulomatosis. However, despite the presence of bacilli within endothelial cells, vasculitis and areas of stromal fibrinoid degeneration are not features of leprosy. Frequent involvement of peripheral nerve branches by granulomatous inflammation may provide a hint as to the true nature of the underlying inflammatory process. Atypical lymphoid or epithelial cells are not a feature of leprosy and therefore usually are not a source of difficulty in the differential diagnosis of leprosy and neoplasms, at least from the pathologic point of view.

Biologic Behavior

The treatment of choice is dapsone combined with other medications (e.g., rifampin), particularly in light of the existence of medication-resistant *Mycobacterium leprae* strains. Long-term treatment, sometimes for life, is recommended for lepromatous leprosy (102).

Rhinoscleroma

Clinical Data

Rhinoscleroma is a chronic granulomatous inflammatory disease caused by the gram-negative coccobacillus *Klebsiella rhinoscleromatis.* It displays a predilection for upper airway involvement, frequently affecting the nasal cavity. However, it also can involve any portion of the respiratory tract, and is therefore also known simply as scleroma (104). Nevertheless, it is difficult to give up the term *rhinoscleroma* for this disease, even in instances in which nasal cavity involvement is slight (105).

The infectious disease is probably transmitted from person to person via airborne droplets, but does not appear to be very contagious, because it requires prolonged intimate contact for disease transmission. Contributing factors also include low socioeconomic conditions, poor hygiene, and a crowded living environment. Rhinoscleroma is endemic throughout much of the world, including eastern and central Europe, Mexico, Central and South America, Africa, India, and Indonesia. In the United States, it is a rare condition, with sporadic cases usually afflicting individuals that have immigrated from one of the known endemic regions (106). Growth of the immigrant population from endemic regions has generated concern that rhinoscleroma may be increasingly identified in the United States (106,107).

Rhinoscleroma is a slowly progressive disease that can destroy nasal cartilage and bone, eventually producing nasal deformity. It can spread locally to the paranasal sinuses, nasopharynx, orbit, palate, oral cavity, and soft tissues of the lip. As a consequence of the scarring process produced by the granulomatous disease, there is development of stenosis of the affected air passages. A recent review of 11 patients from an endemic region showed an equal involvement of male and female patients. Their ages ranged from 16 to 60 years (108). However, it appears that rhinoscleroma becomes clinically apparent most frequently in the second and third decades of life (106).

Rhinoscleroma has been divided into three stages: exudative, proliferative, and fibrotic or cicatricial, in view of the dominating clinical and pathologic features commonly recognized in the evolution of the disease (104,109,110).

In the exudative phase the disease manifestations are secondary to a nonspecific active chronic inflammation and include unilateral or bilateral nasal obstruction, mucosal edema, congestion, crusting, and discharge of purulent and malodorous secretions (104,106). Disease progression into the proliferative phase presents slightly more characteristic features, such as epistaxis, progressive nasal deformity, and labial edema. In this stage, manifestations of disease extension into adjacent structures may appear, producing sinus symptomatology, anosmia, and anesthesia of the soft palate. Physical examination shows rubbery bluish red granulomatous lesions that eventually evolve into a pale indurated granulomatous mass (106). Disease progression may lead to destruction of cartilage and bone, hence the inclusion of rhinoscleroma in the group of mid-facial destructive lesions (104). The clinical manifestations of the scarring or cicatricial stage are characterized by increased anatomic distortion and stenosis of affected regions, with indurated and fibrotic-appearing granulomatous lesions (106).

Histologic Features

The exudative phase of rhinoscleroma displays an acute and chronic inflammatory reaction, together with edema, congestion, suppurative necrosis, and squamous metaplasia of the mucosal surface epithelium. The degree of inflammation may obscure the infective organisms (104), underscoring the importance of clinical history, because many of the early histologic findings are nonspecific. The proliferative phase will show histologic features that are more closely associated with rhinoscleroma (Fig. 15). Leading the list of microscopic findings are Mikulicz's cells, which are large histiocytes (100–200 μm in diameter) with a single nucleus and prominent, finely vacuolated cytoplasm. Mikulicz's cells are arranged in clusters or sheets beneath the basement membrane of the surface epithelium. When sufficient numbers of bacilli are present, they can be visible within the cytoplasmic vacuoles of Mikulicz's cells and free within the mucosal tissue on conventional hematoxylin and eosin–stained sections. If necessary, PAS (Fig. 16), Giemsa, or Warthin-Starry special stains can be performed to identify the microorganisms. An immunohistochemical stain is available that employs an antibody directed against a capsular antigen of

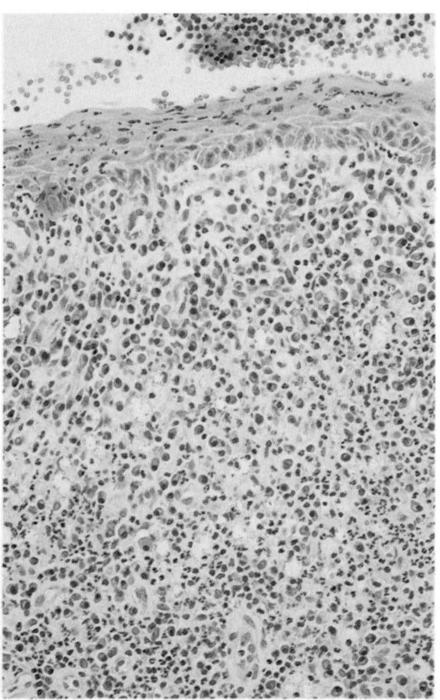

FIGURE 15. Rhinoscleroma. Mucosa displays a marked acute and chronic inflammatory reaction with occasional scattered larger vacuolated histiocytes (Mikulicz's cells) containing bacillary microorganisms. Note the abundance of plasma cells.

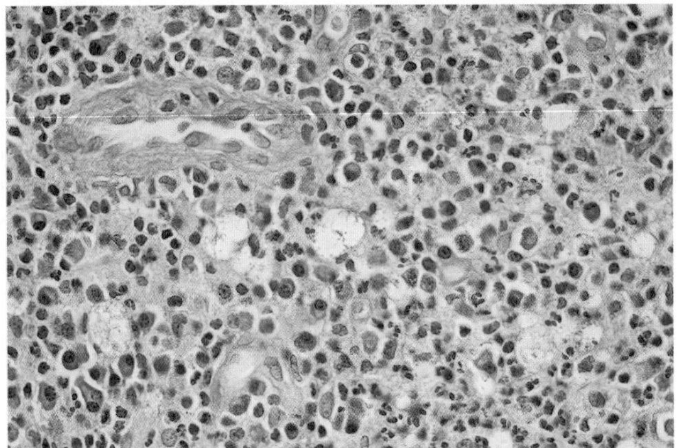

FIGURE 16. Rhinoscleroma. Periodic acid-Schiff stain accentuates the small bacilli present within the cytoplasmic vacuoles of the histiocytes and free within the tissue.

Klebsiella rhinoscleromatis (111). However, because of the current rarity of this disease in the United States, and with the exception of very specialized laboratories, it does not appear to be a practical component in the arsenal of diagnostic immunohistochemical stains of most institutions. Additional histologic features of the proliferative stage include pseudoepitheliomatous hyperplasia and chronic inflammation, including numerous plasma cells with Russell bodies.

The fibrotic stage of rhinoscleroma is characterized by prominent scarring, with fibrosis and mild chronic inflammation. Few if any Mikulicz's cells or microorganisms can be seen.

Differential Diagnosis

The differential diagnosis includes other mid-facial destructive lesions, such as other infectious granulomatous processes. Due to the presence of large vacuolated histiocytes, a main differential diagnosis is leprosy. In this situation, special stains for acid-fast microorganisms will distinguish leprosy (acid-fast positive) from rhinoscleroma (acid-fast negative). The causative organism of rhinoscleroma is, unfortunately, very difficult to culture. The other major bacterial granulomatous infection, tuberculosis, evinces caseous necrosis and has well-defined epithelioid granulomas. Other major mid-facial destructive diseases [e.g., Wegener's granulomatosis, Churg-Strauss syndrome, and nasal/nasal–type T-cell/natural killer (NK) cell lymphomas] can be readily distinguished because of granulomatous vasculitis and other systemic manifestations of disease (Wegener's), eosinophilic infiltrates, vasculitis, a history of asthma (Churg-Strauss syndrome), or atypical lymphoid infiltrates with an angiocentric arrangement (nasal angiocentric lymphomas).

Biologic Behavior

Untreated rhinoscleroma is characterized by a continuous course of active inflammation followed by a prominently deforming scarring process. The ensuing sequelae are both aesthetic and functional, with stenosis of affected airways. This infectious disease is difficult to treat and characterized by multiple relapses. Currently, combined antimicrobial therapy is used. The treatment regimen can be prolonged, lasting months to years and includes the use of surgery for cosmetic reasons and improvement of airflow function (106).

Rhinosporidiosis

Clinical Aspects

Rhinosporidiosis is a chronic infectious disease caused by the fungus *Rhinosporidium seeberi.* It is rarely seen in the United States, where it sporadically presents in individuals originally from one of the known endemic regions, mainly India, Sri Lanka, Eastern Africa, Indonesia, and Brazil (113). However, recently cases of rhinosporidiosis arising in individuals that have not traveled outside of the United States have been reported (114).

The exact mode of transmission of the disease is unknown, and it is suspected that exposure to contaminated water from swimming or bathing in stagnant ponds or urban exposure to dust particles containing spores may be the source of infection (113).

The nasal cavity is the primary site of involvement, although the nasopharynx, oropharynx, larynx, conjunctivae, and lacrimal sacs also can be affected (104).

Clinically, the nasal manifestations of rhinosporidiosis are characterized by formation of one or multiple sessile or pedunculated masses, which can involve one or both sides, and usually the floor of the nasal cavity, inferior turbinates, and nasal septum (115). Patients with rhinosporidiosis complain of nasal obstruction, epistaxis, and rhinorrhea.

Histopathologic Features

Within the subepithelial stroma of the polypoid masses are varying numbers of sporangia, 10 to 300 μm in diameter, with thick double-layered walls. The sporangia contain numerous endospores and both can be identified with a conventional hematoxylin and eosin stain or with special stains for fungal organisms (Fig. 17). Some of the sporangia rupture and release their con-

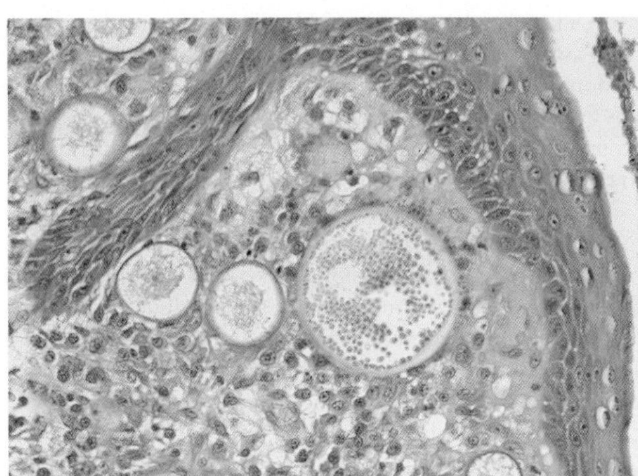

FIGURE 17. Rhinosporidiosis. Sporangia containing numerous endospores of *Rhinosporidium seeberi* readily identified in hematoxylin and eosin stain.

tents into the adjacent tissue, causing an acute inflammatory reaction. An important finding for differential diagnostic purposes is the absence of distinct granulomatous inflammation (79).

Differential Diagnosis

The main differential diagnosis of rhinosporidiosis is coccidioidomycosis. This fungal infection is native to the southwestern United States and therefore, more commonly seen than rhinosporidiosis. Both infectious fungal organisms have endospores contained within sporangia. However, the endospores of rhinosporidiosis attain a larger diameter. More importantly, there is a lack of appreciable granulomatous inflammation, a common feature of coccidioidomycosis.

Biologic Behavior

Treatment is surgical excision of the polypoid nasal lesions. Recurrence is seen in approximately 10% of cases (79).

Cocaine Abuse

Clinical Data

The acute toxic effects of cocaine abuse, particularly the cardiovascular and neurologic medical complications, are well known (116,117). In addition, chronic and heavy use of cocaine, via nasal insufflation (snorting), can produce very destructive lesions of the sinonasal tract that may require distinction from other causes of mid-facial necrotizing lesions (118–121). This may be particularly challenging in small biopsy specimens obtained from patients who deny cocaine abuse.

The incidence of destructive mid-facial lesions secondary to prolonged nasal insufflation of cocaine is unknown. The number of sinonasal tract destructive lesions associated with cocaine abuse has probably diminished as a result of a shift in type of drug presentation from the commonly insufflated powder form of cocaine hydrochloride to the currently preferred freebase and crack cocaine, which are predominantly smoked and cause pulmonary morbidity (116,117).

In a large study evaluating 233 patients with medical conditions associated with cocaine abuse, there was an overall male predominance, with a male:female ratio of 3.2:1. The age range was from 16 to 51 years, with a mean of 29.5 years. In this study group, only 8.2% of patients had symptomatology attributable to the head and neck region (117).

The clinical manifestations of sinonasal destruction produced by chronic cocaine abuse are similar to those of other mid-facial necrotizing lesions described in this section. Frequently described symptoms and signs include nasal congestion, rhinorrhea, occasional epistaxis, anosmia, nasal quality of speech, nasal deformity, mucosal crusting, and stenosis of nasal passages. Initially, there may be septal perforation, and with continued cocaine abuse, there may be widespread destruction of the nasal septum, turbinates, adjacent paranasal sinus structures, and perforation of the palate (118–121). These pronounced anatomic alterations are the result of some of the local pharmacologic effects of cocaine, which include pronounced vasoconstriction with consequent ischemia, and anesthesia followed by unperceived damage from repeated minor trauma. Some of the adulterants almost invariably added to cocaine (lidocaine, lactose, plaster, talcum power, quinine, etc.) may have a local irritant effect on the sinonasal structures, amplifying the destructive effect of cocaine. The overall end results of the chemical and pharmacologic effects of the insufflated powdery mixture are mucosal ulceration, ischemic damage, and osteocartilaginous necrosis, frequently with superimposed bacterial infections (119).

Radiologic Studies

Computed tomography scans demonstrate varying degrees of cartilage destruction of the nasal septum and osseous destruction of the nasal turbinates, adjacent ethmoid and maxillary paranasal sinuses, nasal cavity floor, and underlying palate. In addition, secondary to superimposed infection, there may be nonspecific opacification of paranasal sinuses (119,120).

Histologic Features

In contrast to the dramatic clinical appearance of this disease process, the histologic findings are nonspecific and are characterized by acute and chronic inflammation, with a variable mixture of neutrophils, lymphocytes, plasma cells, and histiocytes. Evidence of ulceration and granulation tissue may be seen, and if present in the biopsy material, bone tissue can show reactive remodeling changes, inflammation, and necrosis.

The most important differential feature of microscopic examination is the absence of granulomatous inflammation and vasculitis. It is important to note that scattered foreign body giant cells may be present in the inflamed mucosal tissue, and foreign particles may be identifiable under polarized light.

Differential Diagnosis

The differential diagnosis includes a variety of infectious processes, such as tuberculosis, leprosy, syphilis, rhinoscleroma, fungal infections, and other exotic infectious causes such as mucocutaneous leishmaniasis (122). Appropriate special stains and microbiologic methods to exclude these possibilities should be included in the initial diagnostic workup.

Wegener's granulomatosis is another entity that is included in the differential diagnosis. The absence of vasculitis, zonal fibrinoid degeneration, and systemic manifestations of Wegener's granulomatosis assist in distinguishing the destructive lesions of cocaine abuse.

Low grade nasal T-cell/NK-cell lymphoma, previously known as polymorphic reticulosis, is also included in the differential diagnosis, and may be extraordinarily difficult to distinguish from the effects of chronic cocaine abuse. In this situation, clinical history is extraordinarily important. If present, the suggestion of angiocentricity or evidence of vascular wall infiltration by atypical cells will favor a nasal T-cell/NK-cell lymphoma. Unfortunately, these angiocentric features are infrequently seen in small biopsy specimens, and the pathologist is frequently compelled to provide a diagnosis of nonspecific inflammation.

In the future, use of *in situ* hybridization for detection of Epstein-Barr virus (EBV) genomic material may provide a method to distinguish borderline low-grade nasal T-cell/NK-cell lymphomas (123).

Despite the shortcomings of histologic evaluation, particularly in the clinical setting of a mid-facial destructive lesion, the suspicion of a lesion associated with cocaine abuse should be communicated to the clinician.

Biologic Behavior

The course of this disease process is obviously related to the continued use of cocaine. In addition to appropriate substance abuse counseling, management includes antibiotic treatment of secondary infections and irrigation to remove crusts and promote healing. If long-term cessation of drug abuse is successful, reconstructive surgery of nasal deformities is appropriate not only for cosmetic reasons but to improve respiratory function.

Malignant Lymphomas

Clinical Data

The sinonasal tract is an uncommon site for primary non-Hodgkin's lymphomas in the United States and other Western countries, and when all sites are considered, it is estimated to harbor 1.5% of cases (124,125). Primary sinonasal lymphomas are more frequently observed in Asian countries. In a large retrospective series from the Chinese population of Hong Kong, primary sinonasal lymphomas were found to represent 3% of all non-Hodgkin's lymphomas (126). More interesting observations from the geographic point of view are the patent immunophenotypic and morphologic differences that exist between sinonasal lymphomas arising in Western and Asian countries. Studies have shown that European and American population groups, with some regional exceptions in Latin America (127), are predominantly afflicted with nasal malignant lymphomas of B-cell lineage. An immunophenotypic analysis of a group of cases from the United States found B-cell lineage in 84% of sinonasal lymphoid neoplasms (125). A more recent study performed on Northern European patients found 61% of sinonasal cases displaying a B-cell immunophenotype (123).

In sinonasal lymphomas presenting in Western countries, there is a great variety of morphologic subtypes that range from low- to high-grade morphology (124). By contrast, in Asian countries there is a marked preponderance of non B-cell tumors with a peculiar tendency for a polymorphous tumor cell population, an angiocentric growth pattern (128), and a close link to EBV infection (123,129). These intriguing nasal lymphoproliferative lesions that have a polymorphous cellular composition are angiocentric and angioinfiltrative, and they are frequently associated with extensive tissue necrosis, whether occurring in Asians or Westerners. They have been described using several diagnostic terms, including Stewart's granuloma, polymorphic reticulosis, malignant midline reticulosis, and angiocentric immunoproliferative lesions. Recent advances in the immunohistochemistry and molecular biology of these lesions have shown that they represent malignant lymphomas of a cell type that shares features with T cells and NK cells. They can occur in other sites, but are typically found in the sinonasal tract, and they are currently termed, in the Revised European-American Classification of Lymphoid Neoplasms (or REAL classification), nasal/nasal–type T-cell/NK-cell lymphomas (130). These lesions are discussed further in Chapter 12.

In general, lymphomas of the sinonasal tract are more common in men, with a male:female ratio of 2:1. The age at presentation ranges from the second to the eighth decades of life, with a mean age in the late forties to early fifties (124,126,128,131). The most common initial manifestations of sinonasal lymphoma are nasal obstruction, unilateral facial or nasal swelling, diplopia, headache, and epistaxis. Systemic symptoms, so-called B symptoms, and cervical lymphadenopathy are infrequent initial disease manifestations (126,128,131). Physical examination may show changes that range from nonspecific mucosal edema and inflammation, to granular-appearing nasal mucosa and ulcerations. Bulky disease (>10 cm) is not very common and was only seen in 11 of 100 patients with nasal lymphoma (126). Evidence of extensive necrosis is seen in T-cell/NK-cell lymphoma and may include perforation of the nasal septum and palate (123). Because of this destructive behavior, which is probably related to angiocentricity, T-cell/NK-cell sinonasal lymphoma is included within the group of mid-facial necrotizing lesions. In a study of 18 T-cell/NK-cell sinonasal lymphomas, with the exception of one patient with stage IV disease at presentation, all had tumors of early stage, with the majority initially involving the nasal cavity (131). Patients with Western variants (B cell) of sinonasal lymphoma also show a trend for early stage (I–II) at presentation (125). However, in addition to nasal involvement, there is frequently a tumor within an adjacent paranasal sinus cavity (124).

Radiologic Studies

Imaging studies display evidence of a mass in the majority of cases, as well as opacification of sinuses and evidence of bone erosion (124).

Histologic Features

Nasal lymphomas of the Western type can show a variety of morphologic subtypes, but are predominantly intermediate- to high-grade non-Hodgkin's lymphomas (125) (see Chapter 12). The histologic description here will be focused on lymphomas of postulated T-cell/NK-cell lineage, which have a distinct affinity for sinonasal tract involvement and are presently designated nasal type T/NK cell lymphomas in the REAL classification scheme.

Regarding the nasal T-cell/NK-cell lymphomas, the current understanding of this disease process recognizes the theoretical existence of a spectrum of morphologic features that range from low- to high-grade angiocentric lymphoma. At the low-grade end of the morphologic spectrum are cases that probably were previously classified as polymorphic reticulosis. Progression along the spectrum toward high-grade morphology is attained through an increase in the number of large atypical lymphoid cells or incremental cytologic atypia. This spectrum has been previously classified as polymorphic reticulosis, polymorphic reticulosis–like lymphoma, and lymphoma with conventional morphology (e.g., diffuse large cell) (128). Regardless of the preferred terminology, it is important to recognize the existence of this quantitative and qualitative spectrum of cytologic atypia. Moreover, it is particularly important to critically study cases with the appearance of low-grade lesions in which there is a clinical history of a mid-facial necrotizing lesion. It is conceivable that at an early stage, angiocentric lymphomas may not be histologically recognizable and theoretically may correspond to the so-called idiopathic midline destructive disease (97), a perhaps questionable and unsatisfying nosologic category. Cases that have advanced along the spectrum from low- to high-grade histology have been described (123).

The histologic hallmark of this morphologically variable disease process is the presence of angiocentric and angiodestructive atypical lymphoid infiltrates. The extensive areas of coagulative necrosis commonly associated with this entity have a geographic pattern of distribution and are probably secondary to vascular involvement by lymphoma. Lack of microscopic evidence of vascular involvement may represent a sampling problem. Occasionally, the only viable tissue in the section will consist of the atypical perivascular lymphoid infiltrate (132). To consider a lesion angiocentric, tumor cells must preferentially be concentrated around and within blood vessels (Fig. 18), and not simply represent blood vessels entrapped in a sea of tumor cells (133).

The cellular elements of the tumor can be heterogeneous and may include a polymorphous mixture of lymphocytes, plasma cells, immunoblasts, histiocytes, and variable numbers of atypical lymphoid cells. The atypical cells can be represented by small, medium-sized, or large cells. The nuclei also can have a heterogeneous appearance, with elongated and irregular nuclear outlines, rounded open nuclei with one or more small nucleoli, hyperchromatic nuclei, and large cells characterized by frequent nuclear folding (128). In addition, there may be predominance of one cell type, or a mixture of the various types of atypical cells. The number and type of atypical cells are the focus of diagnostic difficulty. The most difficult cases to recognize, particularly in small nasal biopsy specimens obtained via limited sampling, are neoplasms composed of sparse small to medium-sized atypical cells that have a prominent mixed inflammatory cell infiltrate in the background. It is this type of case that is frequently mistaken for an inflammatory process (133), and is highly dependent on appropriate clinical history as well as ancillary studies for diagnostic guidance (see Chapter 12).

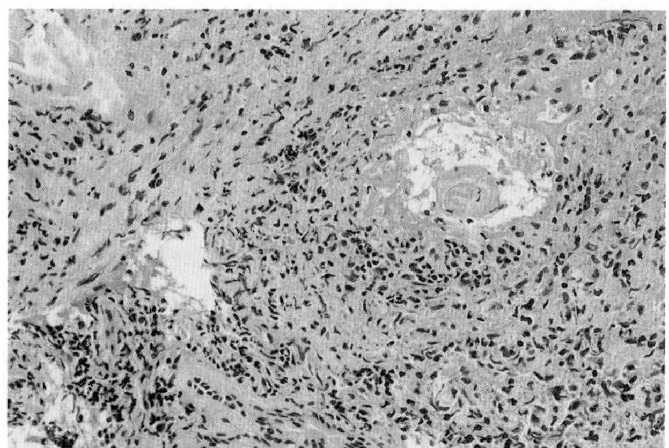

FIGURE 18. Sinonasal angiocentric lymphoma. Necrotic vessel with mural infiltrate of cytologically atypical lymphoid cells.

Differential Diagnosis

The differential diagnosis of sinonasal angiocentric lymphoma includes inflammatory diseases with an exuberant inflammatory infiltrate. Wegener's granulomatosis should be considered, particularly if the biopsy material demonstrates evidence of vasculitis. Presence of a granulomatous type of vasculitis, giant cells and the peculiar serpiginous zonal fibrinoid degeneration of collagen bordered by granulomatous inflammation, favor a diagnosis of Wegener's granulomatosis.

The infectious processes that have been previously discussed are also entities that should be included in the differential diagnosis, particularly if extensive necrosis is the dominating histologic feature. Attention should be directed at excluding mycobacterial and fungal infections with the appropriate special stains or other microbiologic methods.

Churg-Strauss syndrome can have vasculitis and necrosis; however, the inflammatory infiltrate in the typical case is primarily composed of eosinophils; more importantly, the cellular infiltrate lacks the atypical lymphoid cells associated with sinonasal angiocentric lymphoma.

In the clinical setting of a destructive mid-facial lesion, nonhematolymphoid malignancies also enter into the differential diagnosis of this entity, especially if the angiocentric lymphoma is at the high-grade end of the morphologic spectrum. The angiocentric character of the neoplastic infiltrate, prominent irregularity of nuclear outlines, and geographic areas of coagulative necrosis are features that favor an angiocentric lymphoma. It should be noted that despite the well-known and prominent association of sinonasal lymphoma of probable T-cell/NK-cell lineage and Asian ethnic groups, this entity is not restricted to Asian geographic regions, because similar neoplasms arising in Western countries have been reported (134). On the other hand, in the Western hemisphere, conventional B-cell type non-Hodgkin's lymphoma should be considered as a more likely diagnosis, particularly if there is no evidence of a predominantly angiocentric atypical lymphoid infiltrate. Performing a panel of immunohistochemical stains for B- and T-cell markers will further confirm the true cell lineage of the malignant lymphoid neoplasm in most cases.

Biologic Behavior

Sinonasal angiocentric lymphoma is characterized by secondary spread to local anatomic structures, skin, subcutaneous tissue, gastrointestinal tract, and testis (133). It infrequently disseminates to lymph nodes. Bone marrow involvement is not characteristic of this disease process (131). Radiation therapy and chemotherapy are the usual treatment modalities. However, despite having an early clinical stage at presentation, outcome is poor, with a median disease-free survival of 9 months and median survival of only 12 months reported (131). Death is usually secondary to local dissemination of disease.

There is limited information to correlate histologic features to biologic behavior and prognosis. Extrapolating data from an earlier study that included the histologic spectrum of polymorphic reticulosis, polymorphic reticulosis–like lymphoma, and conventional lymphoma, it would appear that morphologically low-grade sinonasal angiocentric lymphoma is associated with a better long-term survival, with 68% of patients showing 5-year disease-free survival. This compares to 58% survival of patients with polymorphic reticulosis–like lymphoma and no survival of patients with conventional lymphoma, corresponding to the high-grade end of the spectrum of sinonasal angiocentric lymphoma (128).

In contrast, Western-type malignant lymphoma, most commonly of B-cell lineage, is clinically characterized by frequent dissemination to lymph nodes and also secondary spread to brain, kidneys, and bone (124).

In a published report of 100 patients with nasal lymphoma, which included B- and T-cell lymphomas, of which 24 cases corresponded to angiocentric lymphomas, it was found by multivariate analysis of a series of possible prognostic factors that clinical stage I disease was the only significant independent prognostic factor. Gender, histologic subtype, immunophenotype, features of angiocentricity, and bulky disease (>10 cm) did not adversely affect clinical outcome (126).

HAMARTOMATOUS AND TERATOID NEOPLASMS

Hamartoma

Clinical Data

The term *hamartoma* comes from the Greek roots *hamartia* (defect, error, or sin) and *oma* (tumor-like growth, apparently adapted from *onkoma,* or *onkos,* meaning mass). It was coined by Albrecht in 1904 and further characterized by Willis in the 1950s (135–138). Strictly defined, a hamartoma corresponds to a non-neoplastic developmental malformation composed of an admixture of mature cells and tissues indigenous to the anatomic area of occurrence, often with one element predominating. This definition allows us to discriminate hamartomas from other non-hamartomatous lesions of the nasal and paranasal region such as choristomas, teratomas, and dermoids, which are composed of either mature or immature tissues nonindigenous to the anatomic location. The pathogenesis of hamartomas in general and that of sinonasal hamartomas remains speculative. Inflammation may act as an inducing or potentiating mechanism, so lesions classified as sinonasal hamartomas may not be strictly congenital malformations (139).

Hamartomas are exceedingly rare in the sinonasal region. The most common location in the nasal cavity is the nasal septum, but the lateral wall, middle meatus, and inferior turbinate are also affected (139). Paranasal sinus locations (i.e., ethmoid, frontal, maxillary) have been described (139,140). Nasopharyngeal hamartomas also have been documented (135,141–144). The clinical presentation usually consists of nonspecific obstructive or infectious symptoms, generally in early life, sometimes with proptosis or fullness of cheeks (140), although the course may be asymptomatic. Additional symptoms such as respiratory distress, choking sensation, paroxysmal nocturnal dyspnea, cough, nasal or postnasal discharge, obstruction and epistaxis can be due to superimposed rhinosinusitis, septal nasal deformity, or obstruction by the mass (139,145).

Radiologic Studies

Hamartomas are usually found incidentally on radiography (138). Displacement of the turbinates or opacification of the sinuses may be observed on roentgenographs (145) to complex solid and cystic masses with erosion of the surrounding bone with intracranial extension (146). CT scan may show a spectrum of features ranging from masses of uniform attenuation filling the nasal cavity and the sinuses and mucus retention without bone destruction (147).

Gross Appearance

Hamartomas may present as discrete pedunculated polypoid masses or diffuse submucosal expansions (135,140,145).

Histologic Features

Histogenically, hamartomatous tissues are derived from any one of the germ cell layers (endoderm, ectoderm, and more commonly the mesoderm) (138) and are better classified according to the predominant element, be it epithelial or mesenchymal.

The most common type is that in which a mesenchymal element predominates. The described cases are lipomas, fibrolipomas, chondromas, neurofibromas, and angiomas (135). Classifying these lesions as hamartomas is debatable. Recently, a nasal chondromesenchymal hamartoma with features analogous to the chest wall mesenchymal hamartoma has been described (146) (see Chapter 11).

The more uncommon second type, with an epithelial component predominating, is composed of a spectrum of squamous and cuboidal epithelial ducts and occasionally dilated serous or mucinous exocrine glands that in areas may impose a polypoid appearance to the lesion, usually associated with various stromal elements (Fig. 19). Continuity with the surface epithelium might be present. Cilia are often present, but cribriforming is not observed. Stromal hyalinization may be seen (135,139). Lymphoplasmacytic or polymorphous inflammatory infiltrates (more frequently subepithelial in location), prominent vascularity, and cystic dilatations of the glandular epithelial components may be present (139,145). Foci of cartilage or bone formation due to stromal metaplasia are acceptable in this setting (135). No skin appendages are present in contrast to dermoids (148). No specific anatomic location is favored by hamartomas with epithelial elements. The growth pattern, overall architecture, absence of significant atypia and expansile growth of tissues are features that support the diagnosis of hamartoma (145). Dysplasia is usually not present (139). Some researchers consider the presence of seromucous glands as a reactive phenomenon and restrict the epithelial component to respiratory epithelium, acknowledging that seromucous gland hamartomas occur, albeit uncommonly (139).

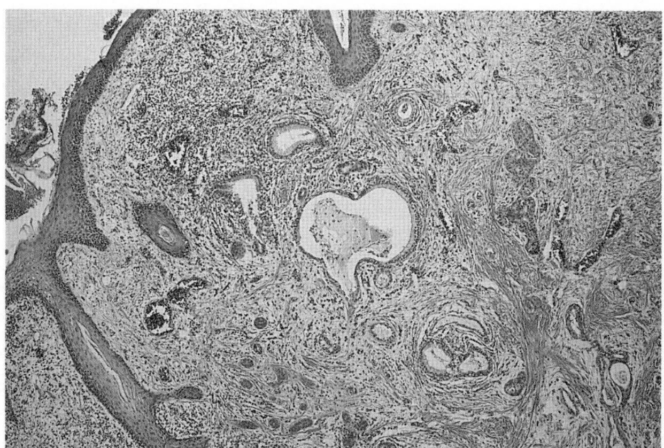

FIGURE 19. Hamartoma. Epithelial type is a loose edematous soft tissue mass containing numerous epithelial-lined ducts extending from the surface and disorganized cystic ducts, some with a mucinous lining.

Differential Diagnosis

Clinical differential diagnoses of a nasal mass in infants and children includes encephalocele, nasal dermoid cyst, nasal glial heterotopia, nasolabial (nasoalveolar) cyst, teratoma, hemangioma, rhabdomyosarcoma, neurofibroma, and nasolacrimal duct cyst (149). Although diagnosis is histologically straightforward once the possibility of hamartoma is contemplated, sometimes hamartomas may be histologically indistinguishable from teratomas. Neoplastic and inflammatory processes also must be included in the differential diagnosis. Inverted schneiderian papillomas and adenocarcinomas are among the most frequent diagnostic difficulties. Differentiation is crucial because both of these entities have different biologic potential. Inverted papillomas are characterized by infoldings and invaginations of the mucosal epithelium, not associated with glandular proliferations. Low-grade adenocarcinomas show crowded glandular proliferations and varying degrees of cytologic atypia. The solitary tumor-like nature of the lesion, and more epithelial proliferation than is usually seen in inflammatory polyps, help distinguish hamartomas from this latter lesion.

Biologic Behavior

Hamartomas exhibit self-limited growth as the tissue components reach maturity and cease to reproduce. They may present at birth or manifest later as the individual matures (135). Lack of follow-up information on reported cases prevents evaluation of recurrence potential, although recurrences appear to be uncommon in the reported cases (139,146). Total surgical removal is the treatment of choice.

Nasolabial (Nasoalveolar) Cyst–Hamartoma

Clinical Data

The nasolabial cyst–hamartoma was first described by Zuckerkandl in 1892 and further defined by Rao in 1955 (150,151). It is a cyst of the soft tissues at the junction of the premaxilla and the alveolar processes of the maxilla, with a predominance in females, blacks, and Hispanics (mean age 51 years) (138,150). Facial deformity with protrusion of the upper lip, elevation of the ala nasi, and effacement of the nasolabial fold is the common complaint. There may be partial nasal obstruction if the cyst is large, and infection also can occur (138).

Radiologic Studies

Roentgenographs usually reveal no bony erosion or dental disease.

Gross Appearance

Grossly, cysts are gray-blue with mucoid or yellow, sometimes hemorrhagic, or mucopurulent contents (150).

Histologic Features

These fibrous walled cysts may be lined by respiratory-type epithelium with abundant goblet cells, low cuboidal, or squamous epithelium.

Differential Diagnosis

The differential diagnosis includes globulomaxillary and radicular cysts, which are usually associated with bony changes on radiography. Other cysts in consideration are midline in location and are also associated with radiologic changes (e.g., dermoids, medial alveolar cysts, incisive canal cysts, and median palatal cysts) (see Chapter 6).

Biologic Behavior

Excision is curative. Malignancy has been reported in one case (138).

Dermoid and Hairy Polyp

Clinical Data

Dermoids of the nose are thought to arise in epithelial deposits entrapped during embryonal development. They comprise 3% of all dermoids, and 5.5% to 12% of those of the head and neck region (152–154). They may be cystic or polypoid. The cystic type has a lining that recapitulates skin histology, has cheesy, yellow-white contents, and is generally associated with a sinus tract. Polypoid dermoids are lined on the outside by skin and adnexal structures and are thus also referred to as hairy polyps. The latter have been more commonly described in the nasopharynx (see Chapter 5) (155), and some researchers favor their separate classification as choristomas (148). Although a male predominance has been described for cystic dermoids, earlier reports of hairy polyps indicate a female predominance (155,156). Cystic dermoids usually present as a small mass, subcutaneous to the bridge of the nose, and always in the midline. Unusually they may be located in the glabella, nasal tip, or columella and associated with a small dimple (58,154). They may cause broadening of the nasal bridge and on occasion may present with cellulitis or purulent discharge. According to Reuter, Ford described the first hairy polyp in 1784 (155). Hairy polyps are pedunculated, usually attached to the hard and soft palate, filling the nares or the oral cavity and presenting with intermittent symptoms of obstruction. Other anomalies, especially cleft palate, have been described in association with them. Both types of dermoids generally present at birth (see Chapter 1).

Radiologic Studies

Radiologic exploration is essential because nearly half of dermoids extend deeply to the nasal bones and have potential intracranial or frontal sinus involvement (154,156). Contrast studies are generally recommended to rule out the frequently occurring fistulous tracts or sinuses. On radiographs, hairy polyps present as soft tissue opacities within the nasal cavities (157).

Gross Appearance

Although cystic dermoids are skin-lined cysts containing yellow, cheesy material, hairy polyps are skin-covered, with fine hair and irregular firm, cartilaginous consistency.

Histologic Features

Dermoid cysts are composed of elements of the ectodermal layer, recapitulating the structure of the skin with squamous epithelium and adnexa, and lack an endodermal component. Occasional mesodermal tissue (such as cartilage) may be found (148). Minor salivary glands, found on occasion, may have been secondarily incorporated. Hairy polyps may be covered by skin with fine hair, or columnar epithelium associated with skin appendages, and may contain cartilage, smooth muscle, adipose tissue, bone, and sebaceous and mucus glands (see Chapter 5) (154,156,157).

Differential Diagnosis

Dermoid cysts should be clinically differentiated from encephalocele, which occurs in the same anatomic area (see Chapter 1). Epidermal inclusion cysts may resemble cystic dermoids but do not contain adnexa and are more frequent in adults, in contrast to dermoids, which present in children and young adults (148).

Biologic Behavior

Due to the frequent association of sinus tracts, inadequate excision of dermoid cysts may be associated with recurrence, infection, and additional facial deformity. One fourth to one half of patients give a history of one or more attempts to eradicate these lesions (158).

Teratoma

Clinical Data

Teratomas are rare in the nasopharynx and sinuses. They are true neoplasms composed of all three germinal layers (mesoderm, ectoderm, and endoderm) with histologic components not limited to the native tissue of the originating organ and with mature or immature differentiation (138,154). Multiple theories of origin and suggested classification schemes have been elegantly proposed (159).

Teratomas may arise in any body area but usually do so close to the midline or in the gonads. They most commonly occur in children (1 in 4,000 births) and mainly in females. The preferred locations are the sacrococcyx (in children), ovaries (in adults), testes, anterior mediastinum, and retroperitoneum (154). A small proportion (1.7%) of teratomas occur in the head and neck region, presenting more frequently in the neonatal period and rarely beyond 2 years of age. They are rare in the nasopharyngeal area, where they have a female preponderance of 6:1 (154,156,159). Nasopharyngeal teratomas usually arise in the midline or the lateral wall of the nasopharynx. They are associated with obstructive symptoms such as dysphagia, respiratory stridor or distress, nasal hypersecretion, or oral or pharyngeal mass. Polyhydramnios due to upper alimentary tract obstruction also can be seen (160). Teratomas may frequently be associated with other skull deformities, anencephalia, hemicrania, and palatal fissures (see Chapter 1) (156).

Radiologic Studies

Radiologic studies may reveal calcification, ossification, or radiodensities within the tumor mass and disclose associated anomalies such as vertebral deformities, cleft palate, or secondary displacement of normal structures (159). Radiologic studies also may help to determine if the tumor is primary or consists of an extension from an intracranial or extracranial teratoma.

Gross Appearance

Teratomas may be solid or cystic. These gross features do not correlate well with tissue types (148). Although the gross appearance of teratomas is varied, a particular variant of teratoma (although extremely rare) is worth mentioning. Epignathi were initially described by Ahlfeld in 1875 and classified by Arnold in 1888 and Schwalbe in 1907. They are teratomas that have differentiated, well-formed organs and limbs of a parasitic fetus and are usually found attached to the sphenoid bone (156,157,160,161). The more highly developed these tumors are, the greater the chance of a stillbirth (156). The term *epignathus* is subject to debate because it means "upon the jaw." *Episphenoid* and *epipalati* have been postulated as alternative terms (160).

Histologic Features

Teratomas are composed of varied admixtures of mature or immature skin, skin appendages, fat, glial tissue, smooth muscle, cartilage, bone, minor salivary gland, and respiratory or gastrointestinal epithelium. Neuroectodermal and neural tissues may be seen more often in teratomas of the nose and paranasal sinuses (156). Immature neuroectodermal tissues may resemble neuroblastoma, retinoblastoma, or embryonic medullary plate, whereas immature mesenchymal tissues may consist of metanephric blastema, fetal mesenchyme, or rhabdomyoblasts (148). One or more of the tissue components may undergo malignant transformation with locally aggressive and metastatic behavior. The association of choriocarcinoma or endodermal sinus tumor is unusual in head and neck teratomas but has been described (154,162).

Differential Diagnosis

Although the variegated histologic appearance of teratomas is usually diagnostic, nasal glial heterotopia may be considered in the differential diagnosis.

Biologic Behavior

Truly malignant degeneration of nasopharyngeal teratomas has not been reported in children (154). Gonzalez-Crussi has established several prognostic determinants of behavior, mainly, the age of presentation, the technical complexity of the surgical removal and the nature of the tissues composing the teratoma. The presence of choriocarcinoma or endodermal sinus tumor worsens the prognosis, so extensive sampling (i.e., one section per centimeter with a minimum of 10 slides per tumor) is recommended (154).

Teratocarcinosarcoma

Teratocarcinosarcomas of the nose and paranasal sinuses are extremely rare neoplasms presenting most commonly in men at a median age of 60 years (163). They are aggressive tumors that usually present after a short course of nasal obstruction and epistaxis and are evident on radiography as nasal cavity masses, with opacification of the sinuses and bone destruction (164). Histologically, they are composed of mature, often clear squamous epithelium, immature intestinal and respiratory epithelium, neuroepithelial rosettes, pseudorosettes, or neurofibrillary matrix, cartilage, smooth muscle, occasionally skeletal muscle, or immature fibroblastic stroma with frequent prominent mitotic figures, primitive undifferentiated carcinoma-like tissue, and occasionally hepatic cells with bile-containing ductules (163–166). No seminoma, embryonal carcinoma, or choriocarcinoma components are present. Immunohistochemistry shows occasional weak positivity for human chorionic gonadotropin and α-fetoprotein (163). Thirty-five percent of these tumors develop metastasis, and 60% of patients are generally dead with disease within 3 years (163).

SCHNEIDERIAN (SINONASAL) PAPILLOMAS

The respiratory epithelial lining of the nasal cavity and paranasal sinuses is unique and differs from the endoderm or foregut-derived pharyngotracheobronchial mucosa. The nasal cavity and paranasal sinus mucosa is derived from an invagination of ectoderm associated with the olfactory placode (167,168). This mucosa of the nasal cavity and paranasal sinuses is referred to as the schneiderian membrane in honor of Victor Conrad Schneider, a 17th century anatomist (169). Ewing was the first to use the term *schneiderian papilloma* to identify these sinonasal tumors (170). The term *schneiderian papilloma* is becoming increasingly popular and is qualified when identifying the three histomorphologic variants: fungiform (exophytic), inverted (endophytic), and columnar cell (cylindrical cell or oncocytic) types. This separate designation implies a different biologic behavior from papillomas arising in other anatomic sites in the upper aerodigestive tract. Sinonasal papillomas with a fungiform growth pattern occur most frequently on the nasal septum (171,172), and inverted and cylindrical cell papillomas preferentially involve the lateral nasal wall and paranasal sinuses. The differences in the two growth patterns of these papillomas may be due to inherent differences in the submucosal tissues at the two sites (171).

Clinical Data

Schneiderian papillomas are rare and account for 0.4% to 4.7% of sinonasal tumors (171). A reliable population incidence is not known, but one report of 3 new cases per 1.5 million population per year would translate into an incidence rate of 0.2 per 100,000 per year (173). In comparison, inflammatory or allergic nasal polyps, which are distinct from schneiderian papillomas, are 25 to 50 times more frequent in occurrence and in many instances may coexist with papillomas (174,175).

Schneiderian papillomas are not associated with papillomas elsewhere in the upper or lower aerodigestive tract, including multifocal papillomatosis occurring in squamous and respiratory epithelium. They occur over a wide age range from the second to the seventh decades of life, with a mean age of 49 years at diagnosis (176). Schneiderian papillomas (except for the cylindrical cell type) display a male predominance, whereas the usual types of nasal polyps have no sex predilection (171). Sinonasal papillomas are usually unilateral, whereas the usual allergic or reactive nasal polyps are bilateral (171,174,175).

Many sinonasal papillomas are asymptomatic, although they can cause symptoms of nasal obstruction with epistaxis, followed by the patient's perception of a nasal mass, occasionally with facial pain (171,176). Cranial or orbital symptoms are not common and may indicate the evolution of malignant transformation of a preexisting papilloma (171). Symptoms of allergic or chronic inflammatory nasal disease are distinctly unusual and indicate two separate diseases when present. These nonspecific symptoms do not distinguish schneiderian papillomas from nasal or antrochoanal polyps or other benign and malignant tumors of the nasal cavity and paranasal sinuses.

The etiologic stimulus of these rare and unusual tumors is unknown. There is no apparent association with smoking, allergy, presence or history of nasal polyps, or other forms of chronic inflammation (171,174). Nasal papillomas and carcinomas have been induced in hamsters by the carcinogen diethylnitrosamine, but chemical or occupational exposures in humans have not been associated with schneiderian papillomas (177). More recently, polymerase chain reaction and *in situ* hybridization techniques have been used, suggesting human papillomaviruses (HPVs) in the pathogenesis of some sinonasal papillomas. Gaffey and colleagues report detecting HPV types 6 or 11 consistently in fungiform papillomas, HPV types 11 or 16 in a minority of inverted papillomas, and no HPV in cylindrical cell papillomas (178). Furthermore, no EBV was detected within the papillomas proper but within stromal lymphocytes of a few cases, contradicting earlier reports of a potential etiologic role for EBV (179).

Gross Appearance

The clinical appearance of schneiderian papillomas varies from a discrete cauliflower-like growth with a narrow or sessile base to a diffuse irregular studding of the entire mucosa by small sessile elevated single nodules that range from 0.5 to 1 cm in size (180). The fungiform or exophytic papillomas (common to the nasal septum) appear as verrucous-like firm and rubbery, pale gray to reddish gray opaque growths. Papillomas from the lateral nasal wall and paranasal sinus characteristically have an inverted growth pattern on histologic examination but have a polypoid, often bulky clinical appearance (Fig. 20). The inverted papillomas are also firm, with increased vascularity and lack the translucency of the more common inflammatory or allergic nasal polyps (Fig. 21). The cylindrical cell type of papillomas involve the same lateral nasal wall and sinus sites as the inverted papillomas, but are distinctly papillary and ragged in appearance with a beefy red color (171).

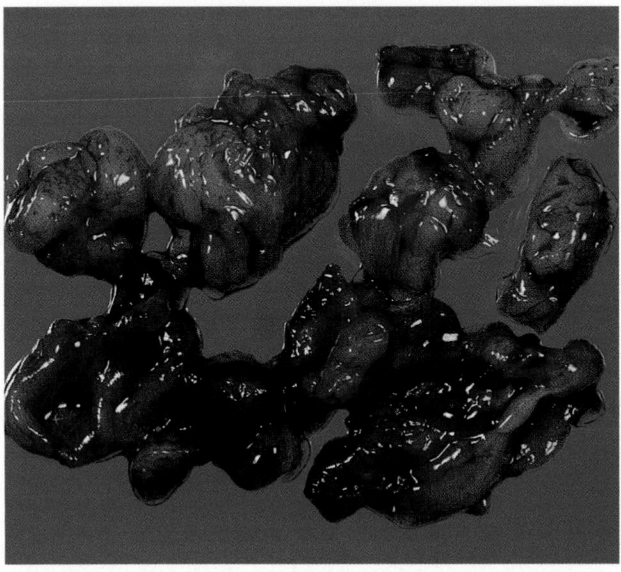

FIGURE 21. Inverted papilloma. Reddish tan polypoid fragments of inverted papilloma lack the translucency of inflammatory nasal polyps.

Radiologic Studies

The most common radiographic findings are a unilateral mass in either the nasal fossa or paranasal sinus. The latter appear clouded, usually with opacification of the involved sinus. Thinning or erosion of the bone of the sinus walls is not unusual and is attributed to pressure erosion by the expanding papilloma. Periosteal soft tissue also may be noted, suggesting an expanding mucosal mass. Displacement, thinning, or actual destruction of the lateral wall of the nasal fossa or medial wall of the maxillary sinus or orbit may occur with advanced aggressive papillomas in the absence of overt malignancy (181–183) (Fig. 22).

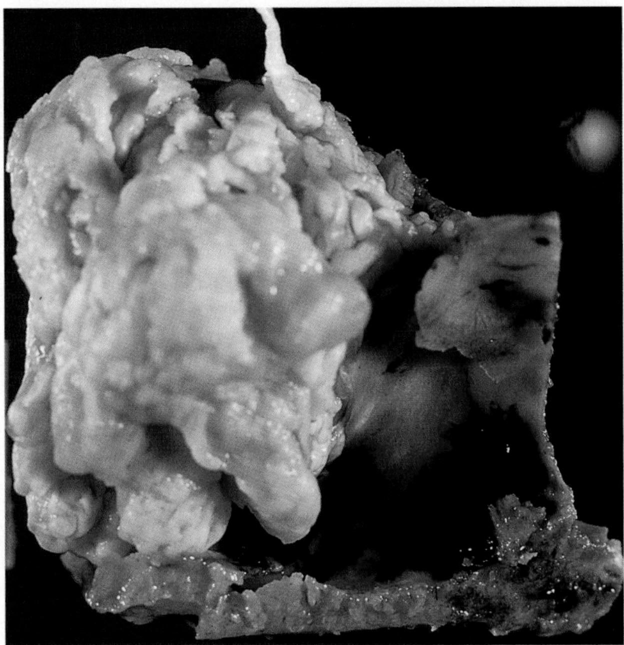

FIGURE 20. Inverted papilloma. Gross appearance of bulky, polypoid inverted papilloma involving maxillary antrum.

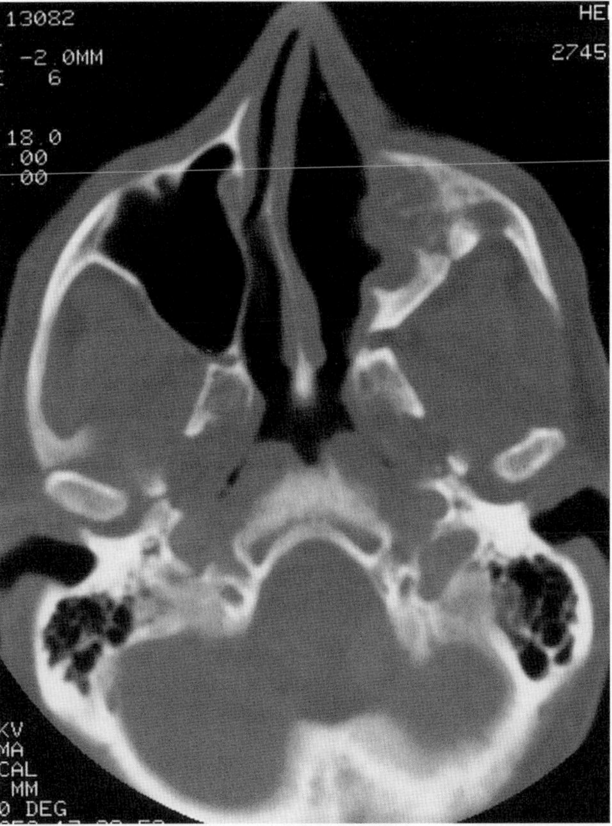

FIGURE 22. Inverted papilloma. Computed tomography view of inverted papilloma filling the left maxillary sinus. This film was taken following a previous surgical procedure, accounting for the reduced size of the left maxillary sinus.

TABLE 2. MORPHOLOGIC AND CLINICAL CHARACTERISTICS OF SCHNEIDERIAN PAPILLOMAS

Papilloma Type	Architecture	Favored Site	Recurrence	Carcinoma
Fungiform	Exophytic	Septum	22%–42%	<0.5%
Inverted	Endophytic/ exophytic	Lateral nasal wall	45%–74%[a]	10%–15%
		Maxillary sinus	0–13%	
Columnar (cylindrical) cell	Endophytic/ exophytic	Lateral nasal wall Maxillary sinus	36%	10%–15%

[a] Recurrence rate depends on extent of surgical removal, conservative excision (45%–74%) versus lateral rhinotomy (0–13%).

Histologic Features

Sinonasal papillomas composed of histologically similar epithelium have been subdivided by growth patterns into fungiform (exophytic) and inverted (endophytic) types. A special oncocytic histologic variant that shares clinicopathologic features of inverted papilloma is designated columnar cell (cylindrical cell or oncocytic) papilloma and usually displays a mixed exophytic and inverted growth pattern. In practice, there is great overlap in growth patterns of the sinonasal papillomas, although they tend to fall into these three major categories. The specific clinical, histopathologic, and biologic features of each variant are discussed in detail below and summarized in Table 2.

Schneiderian Papilloma, Fungiform Type

Clinical Data

Schneiderian papillomas with a fungiform or exophytic growth pattern account for 50% of all sinonasal papillomas in the largest series reported (171). Although they typically arise on the septum, our review of the literature revealed that 20% of 142 reported exophytic papillomas were purely nonseptal, arising in the nasal floor, lateral nasal walls, maxillary sinus, or nasopharynx (171,172,176). In contrast to the diffuse and often bilateral nature of chronic sinusitis, fungiform papillomas are usually solitary but have a less than 5% frequency of multifocality and are rarely bilateral (172,176). Fungiform papillomas are rarely associated with carcinoma (Table 2).

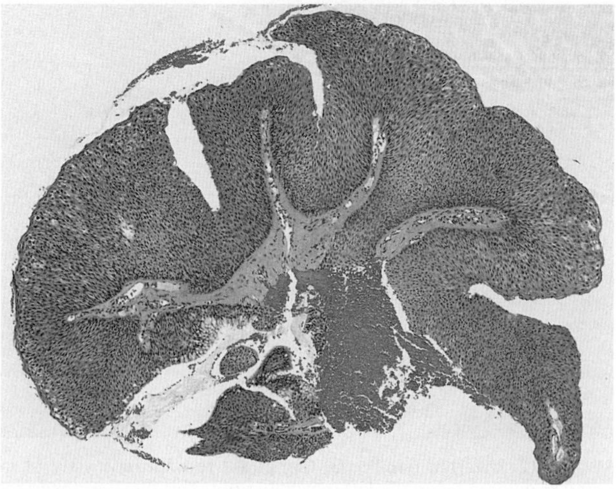

FIGURE 23. Fungiform papilloma. Proliferative, exophytic respiratory epithelium forms this papilloma of the nasal septum.

Histologic Features

Microscopically, fungiform papillomas have branching fibrovascular stalks covered by hyperplastic nonkeratinizing squamous to transitional type epithelium that averages 20 to 30 cell layers in thickness (172) (Fig. 23). Few papillomas display areas of surface keratinization with an underlying granular cell layer (171), and keratinization when present is often minimal and focal (172). Occasionally, a single layer of columnar ciliated respiratory epithelial cells lines the surface of hyperplastic transitional cells. Intraepithelial goblet cells and small mucous cysts (microcysts) are present, identical to the strictly inverted type of papillomas (Fig. 24). Mitotic figures, if present, are located in the basal and lower zones of the epithelium. Excessive and atypical mitoses are not features of fungiform papillomas and should raise the possibility of nonkeratinizing or papillary squamous cell carcinoma (SCC).

Differential Diagnosis

Overlapping and mixed exophytic and endophytic growth patterns composed of the same epithelium exist in schneiderian papillomas, including those located solely on the nasal septum

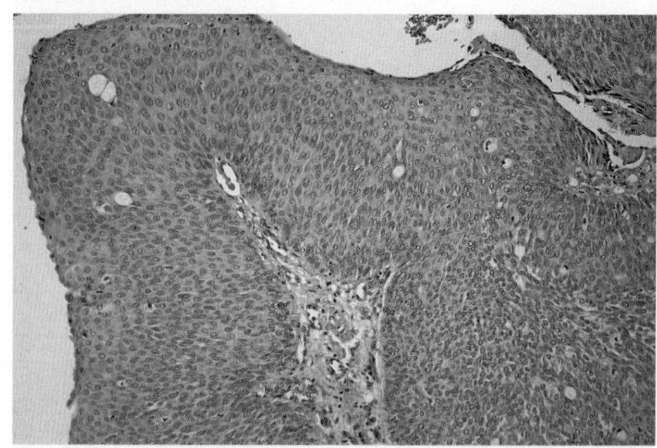

FIGURE 24. Fungiform papilloma. High-power view of proliferative transitional-type epithelium containing intraepithelial mucinous microcysts.

(184), indicative of the close relationship between fungiform and inverted papillomas.

An exuberant polypoid or papillary sinusitis may exhibit some degree of hyperplasia of the surface respiratory epithelium, thereby mimicking fungiform papilloma. In exophytic papillomas, there is a diffuse hyperplastic surface lining epithelium, the basement membrane zone is intact and not thickened, and the underlying stroma contains few mucoserous glands or inflammatory cells in contrast to papillary sinusitis.

Some exophytic papillomas arising in the vestibule and nostrils are not derived from the schneiderian mucosa and correspond to typical cutaneous verruca vulgaris or seborrheic keratosis. The more common verruca is distinguished by papillomatosis and hyperkeratosis with a prominent granular cell layer and by lack of ciliated respiratory lining cells and intermediate-type epithelium or included mucous goblet cells, which are characteristic of the schneiderian membrane.

Papillary SCC of the sinonasal tract may have the same growth pattern as the fungiform papilloma. Although papillomas may display atypical changes, the cytologic atypia in carcinoma is marked and meets the criteria as defined for carcinoma *in situ* elsewhere in the upper aerodigestive tract (see Chapter 2). The sine qua non for the diagnosis of malignancy in a papillary neoplasm is the demonstration of stromal invasion. Whether fungiform papilloma serves as a precursor of papillary squamous carcinoma is unproved. In review, only 1 of 214 reported fungiform papillomas has been associated with invasive carcinoma (171,172,176). This was invasive SCC adjacent to the fifth recurrence of the papilloma (172).

Biologic Behavior

Fungiform papillomas display a significant propensity for recurrence, with a reported range of 22% to 42% of cases. Multiple recurrences, up to six per case, have been recorded (171). No histologic differences between nonrecurrent and recurrent papillomas or histologic features indicative of the potential to recur have been found (171,172). Although the great majority of fungiform papillomas arise on the nasal septum, no one location appears more prone to recurrence (172). Hyams has found that recurrences can be expected to occur in the same anatomic site of the initially removed papilloma (171). This suggests that recurrences are due to the inadequate surgical removal of involved adjacent epithelium. However, multifocality with recurrences in different locations is also documented (184) and supports the concept that much of the mucosa is predisposed to papillomatosis.

A pure fungiform type of papilloma in a septal location might be expected to have a significant recurrence rate if inadequately excised, but would have a negligible association with malignancy. From our review of 214 cases in the literature, the incidence of malignancy associated with fungiform papilloma is less than 0.5% (171,172,176). This low association with malignancy distinctly contrasts with that of inverted papillomas. This, in part, may be related to location rather than growth pattern and explained by the rare occurrence of SCCs of the nasal septum compared with the more common lateral nasal wall and paranasal sinus primary sites of carcinoma.

Schneiderian Papilloma, Inverted Type

Clinical Data

Forty-seven percent of sinonasal papillomas exhibit an inverted or endophytic growth pattern with an invagination of the epithelial layer pushing into the underlying stroma. In marked contrast to the fungiform papillomas, 92% of inverted papillomas arise in nonseptal sites, with only 8% arising from the nasal septum (169,171,175,176,184–187). The most common site of origin is the lateral nasal wall in the region of the middle turbinate or ethmoid recess (185). Often there is contiguous extension to the maxillary or ethmoid sinuses. Primary origin in the maxillary sinus without nasal involvement is far more common than origin in the ethmoid or frontal sinuses (171), and rarely is the sphenoid sinus involved. Not uncommonly, large papillomas fill the nose and extend posteriorly into the nasopharynx (185). Involvement of the nasolacrimal duct and sac via adjoining anterior ethmoidal cells (185) is reported but unusual (171). There is a 3% incidence of bilaterality in nonseptal sites. Inverted papillomas arising in the nasal septum have a similarly low incidence of bilaterality (0.7%) as fungiform papillomas of the nasal septum (169,171,175,176,184–187). Inverted papillomas have a significant recurrence rate that is dependent on extent of surgical removal (Table 2) and an association with coincident or subsequent carcinoma in the same anatomic site of about 13% (171).

Histologic Features

Although inverted papillomas often have a grossly polypoid appearance, they differ from common nasal polyps and are recognized by the diffuse multilayered hyperplasia of the lining epithelium. Some inverted papillomas will exhibit varying degrees of a mixed endophytic and papillary growth pattern (176) (Fig. 25). Like the fungiform papillomas, the lining epithelium of inverted papillomas most often is a nonkeratinizing stratified squamous type (Fig. 26). Other microscopic types of the hyperplastic epithelium include pseudostratified or stratified ciliated columnar (Fig. 27) and transitional type epithelium (Fig. 28). We also have seen a mucous cell–rich variant. Gradations

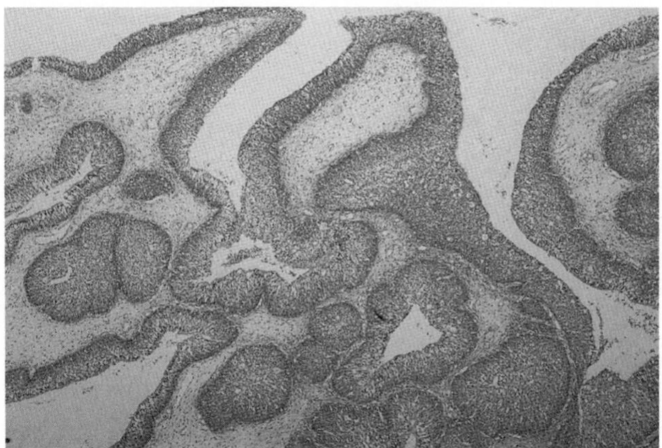

FIGURE 25. Inverted papilloma. An inverted growth is diagnostic, but an exophytic papillary component also may be seen.

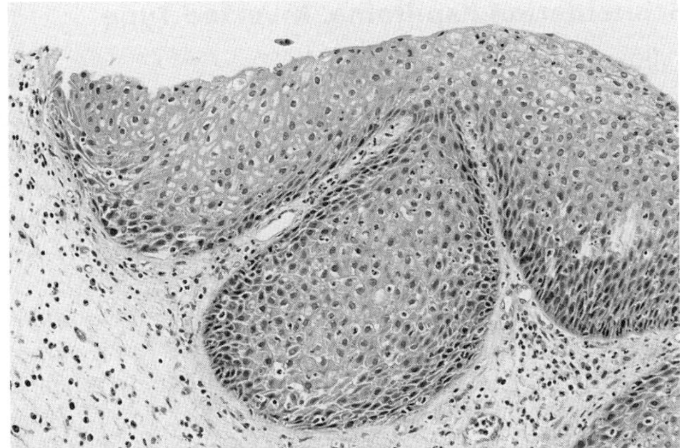

FIGURE 26. Inverted papilloma. Nonkeratinized stratified squamous epithelial lining.

of all three histologic types of epithelium may be present in the same tumor. Kramer and Som have suggested that these epithelial types represent metaplastic changes due to local environmental differences, including pressure and secondary infection (180). The purely eosinophilic oncocytic cylindrical–respiratory type of epithelium is unusual and is classified as a distinct histomorphologic entity: columnar or cylindrical cell papilloma. In about 10% of cases, there is surface keratinization with an underlying granular cell layer (171) (Fig. 29). But an inverted proliferation composed of abundant squamous epithelium is atypical for an inverted papilloma and should raise the possibility of malignancy. Surface keratinization often accompanies malignant transformation, and all tissue should therefore be examined microscopically in this setting. Focal zones of clear cell change in the epithelium are attributed to cytoplasmic glycogen, although these areas are sometimes reminiscent of koilocytotic change. Mucous intraepithelial microcysts are characteristic of sinonasal papillomas but may be so sparse as to require mucin stains for visualization. They probably represent entrapment of normal mucous cells of the respiratory mucosa. Intraepithelial neutrophils are also common. A single layer of ciliated columnar epithelium overlying the hyperplastic epidermoid cells is often present on the surface and in the invaginations extending into the stroma.

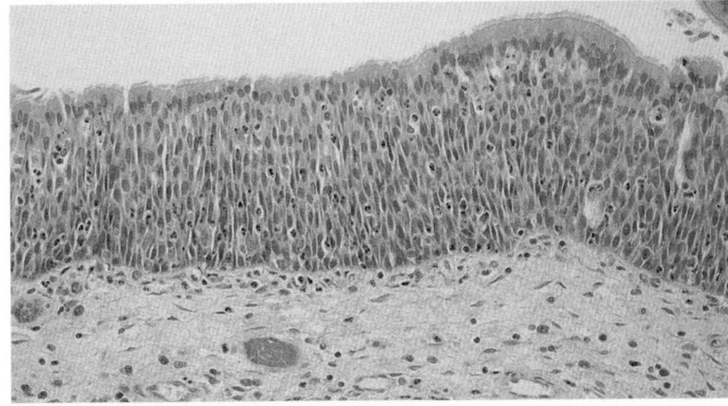

FIGURE 27. Inverted papilloma. Stratified ciliated columnar epithelial lining.

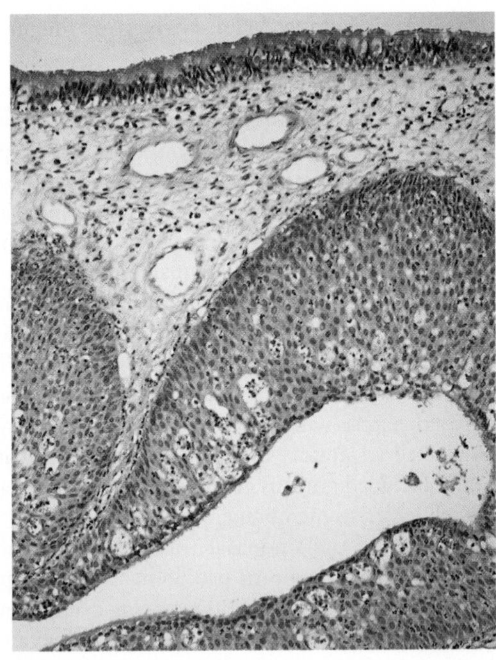

FIGURE 28. Inverted papilloma. Compare normal surface respiratory epithelium with transitional-type epithelium of the inverted papilloma. Note prominent intraepithelial microcysts containing neutrophils.

The individual epidermoid cells of the hyperplastic epithelium are uniform, with distinct cell borders and appreciable intercellular bridges. The cells maintain a degree of polarity, and the nuclei often appear monotonous, especially if the epithelium is tangentially sectioned. This stratified appearance of basaloid cells should not be mistaken for carcinoma *in situ*. Tangential sections also may isolate circumscribed nests of epithelium within the stroma, simulating invasion. Occasional mitotic figures are present in the basal and lower layers of the epithelium. Basal cells may exhibit polarization, and if the nuclei in the peripheral palisade are polarized away from the basement membrane this will lend a pseudoadamantine (pseudoameloblastic) appearance to the proliferation. This is a nonspecific feature

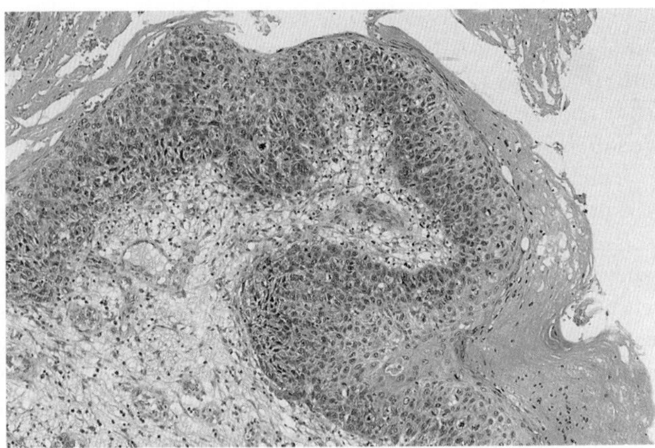

FIGURE 29. Inverted papilloma. Surface keratinization and marked cytologic atypia indicative of malignant transformation.

shared by benign and malignant basaloid tumors. The stroma of inverted papillomas varies from edematous to fibrous, but mucoserous glands are sparse and an inflammatory component is variable but usually minimal. Marked inflammation may be associated with ulceration.

The inverting epithelium, even in locally aggressive papillomas, exhibits a distinct basement membrane. Some of the ribbons of papilloma extending into the stroma represent the preexisting accessory ductal glandular units used as a scaffolding by the papilloma. The extension of the papillomatous proliferation is thought to occur by metaplasia of the adjacent mucosa. This would account for the appearance of the hyperplastic epithelium growing along the basement membrane and leaving the overlying adjacent normal respiratory epithelium intact. Multiple foci of basal cell hyperplasia due to a neoplastic mucosal field effect also may contribute to multicentricity and growth of the papilloma. Secondary involvement of underlying mucoserous glands is more likely the case than primary origin in submucosal mucoserous gland ducts and acini as proposed by Oberman (175). Ringertz had proposed that inverted papillomas develop by metaplastic transformation and proliferation of the surface epithelium of nasal polyps, but the clinical and pathologic differences already reviewed make this sequence of events unlikely (188). This type of horizontal mucosal spread would also account for extension through ostia to involve contiguous sinuses. However, with progressive inverted growth, erosion and even destruction of bone by histologically benign inverted proliferations (Fig. 30) would argue at the least that normal structures used as scaffoldings are grossly expanded or that the blunt border represents actual stromal invasion. Just where the histologic demarcation exists for invasion and atypia indicative of a well-differentiated nonkeratinizing carcinoma is not easy to define histologically in some cases (180).

Malignant transformation within an inverted papilloma may take on the histologic appearance of all grades of SCC and variants. Most of these infiltrative malignant inverted papillomas invade as either broad nests or dissociated irregular cords of carcinoma (Fig. 31).

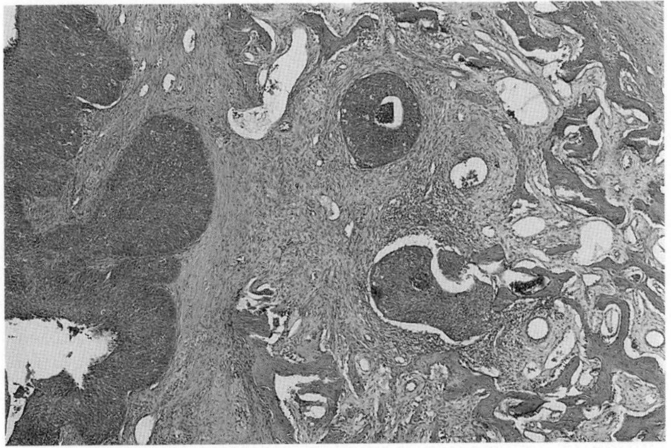

FIGURE 30. Inverted papilloma. Extension down to the level of underlying bone.

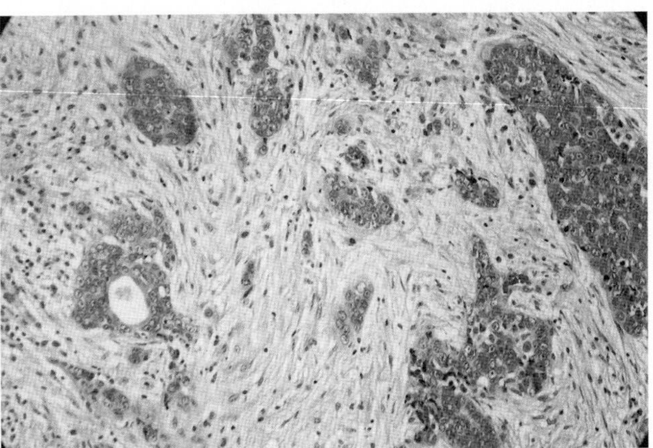

FIGURE 31. Malignant inverted papilloma. Infiltrating cords of carcinoma arising from an inverted papilloma with associated stromal desmoplasia.

Differential Diagnosis

The most common simulant of a schneiderian papilloma is a sinonasal polyp with epithelial hyperplasia. Although polyps of the sinonasal tract may exhibit hyperplasia of the surface respiratory epithelium, there is no expansive inversion of this hyperplastic epithelium into the underlying stroma. Unlike inverted papilloma, eosinophils and basement membrane thickening are characteristic of sinonasal polyps.

Schneiderian carcinomas with an invasive nonkeratinizing squamous cell histology can mimic inverted papilloma by exhibiting similar growth patterns with polypoid exophytic growths and endophytic invasive ribbon-like bands. This also may be the histologic appearance of malignant transformation of inverted papilloma. The distinction between the two malignancies becomes problematic when small areas resembling benign papilloma are associated with abundant carcinoma. However, very few schneiderian carcinomas can be proven to have arisen in precursor schneiderian papillomas. These nonkeratinizing carcinomas within the nasal cavity have been designated the transitional variant of nonkeratinizing carcinoma by the World Health Organization (WHO) (189). Obviously, the term *transitional* is not entirely precise, because this epithelium only resembles that of urothelium and lacks ultrastructural similarity (169) (see later section on Squamous Cell Carcinoma).

Schneiderian Papilloma, Columnar (Cylindrical, Oncocytic) Cell Type

Schneiderian papillomas composed of multilayered eosinophilic, columnar (cylindrical) epithelial cells were designated as cylindrical cell papillomas by Hyams. They are also referred to as oncocytic schneiderian papillomas because of the cytoplasmic accumulation of mitochondria and as columnar cell papillomas in the WHO classification (189). They account for 3% of all schneiderian papillomas and display similar age and sex parameters, sites of involvement, recurrence rate (36%), and association with carcinoma (10%–15%) as the inverted type of papillomas (190). No instance of origin from the nasal septum or bilaterality is yet reported. These rare papillomas are deserving of distinction as a histomorphologic entity to facilitate their identification and the unique differential diagnosis often considered.

Histopathologic Features

The clinical and histologic growth pattern of columnar cell papilloma may display abundant exophytic papillary fronds in addition to inversions into the stroma (Fig. 32). The proliferating epithelium varies from several columnar cells to multiple layers of cells in thickness. A squamoid component is minimal or absent. The individual cells have well-defined cytoplasmic borders and are unique in containing eosinophilic and granular cytoplasm. Some of these columnar cells are decorated by numerous surface cilia, indicating that they are modified respiratory epithelial cells. The nuclei are uniform, round, and darkly staining with rare mitotic figures. Within the epithelium there are numerous intraepithelial cysts containing inspissated mucin or neutrophils (Fig. 33). Intraepithelial eosinophilic globules are also found in these papillomas and correspond to intracellular lumina by electron microscopy.

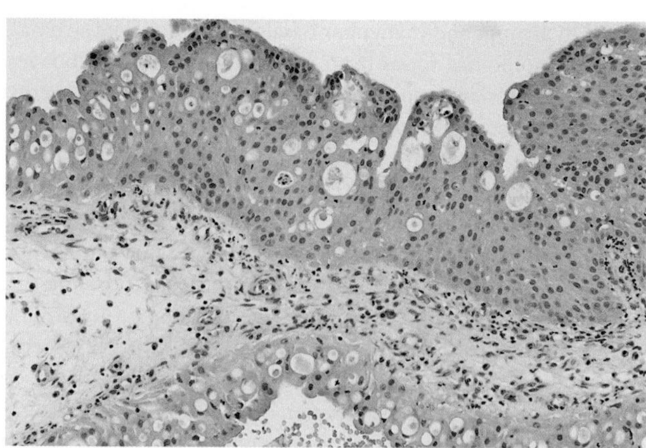

FIGURE 33. Columnar (cylindrical) cell papilloma. Cells with eosinophilic granular cytoplasm containing numerous intraepithelial microcysts with inspissated mucin and focal neutrophils.

Special Studies

Histochemical Stains

This oncocytic transformation of epithelial cells is not considered a degenerative process but rather a mitochondrial hyperplasia compensating for a functional enzyme defect (191). Not all cases of columnar cell papilloma can be shown to stain for mitochondria with the phosphotungstic acid hematoxylin stain (192,193), but histochemical stains may be negative in the face of characteristic ultrastructural findings (191). Barnes and Beditti (193) have correlated by immunohistochemical means large quantities of the mitochondrial oxidative enzyme cytochrome oxidase with electron microscopic findings in a series of columnar cell papillomas. Of interest were the presence of transitional forms between respiratory epithelial cells and typical oncocytic cells. We also have noted that histologically typical inverted papillomas with a surface layer of ciliated respiratory epithelial cells may have numerous mitochondria in these scattered surface cells. All of these findings confirm that columnar cell papillomas arise from the surface schneiderian epithelium and can be considered oncocytic variants of schneiderian papilloma with inverted and exophytic growth.

Electron Microscopy

Electron microscopic studies have clearly shown that the eosinophilic granular cytoplasmic character of columnar cell papilloma is due to the presence of numerous mitochondria (193,194). This feature is seen throughout the epithelium, from the surface ciliated respiratory and microvillous lined transitional surface cells, to the mid-zone polygonal and basal cells (Fig. 34). This confirmation of mitochondria-rich cytoplasm has prompted Barnes and Bedetti to suggest the term *oncocytic schneiderian papilloma* for this histologic subtype of sinonasal papilloma (193). At the ultrastructural level, the intraepithelial mucous microcysts are lumina formed by multiple oncocytic epithelial cells lined by microvilli that contain a few small cytoplasmic secretion granules. Intracytoplasmic lumina filled with peripheral microvillous processes and electron-dense

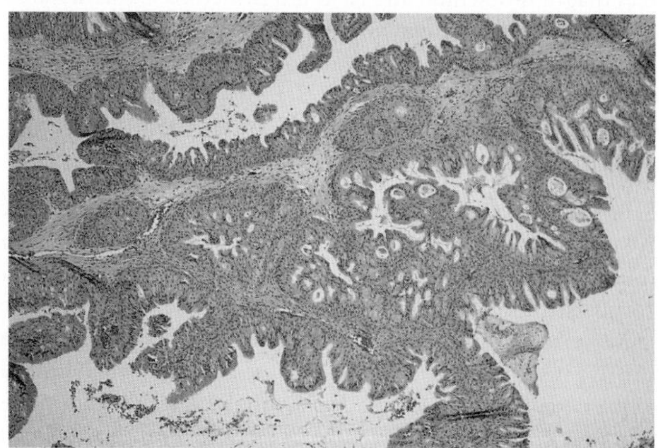

FIGURE 32. Columnar (cylindrical) cell papilloma. Exophytic and inverted growth of oncocytic respiratory epithelium.

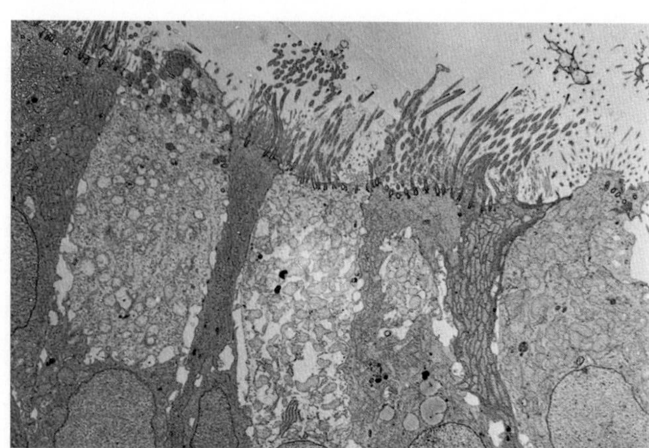

FIGURE 34. Columnar (cylindrical) cell papilloma. Ultrastructure shows mitochondria-rich cytoplasm here demonstrated in surface ciliated epithelium.

inspissated secretions appear as eosinophilic globules by light microscopy.

Differential Diagnosis

The intramucosal cysts of the papilloma may be mistaken for the cyst-like sporangia of the endosporulating fungus *Rhinosporidium seeberi.* The cyst-like sporangia (10–200 μm) and free spores (2–4 μm) of rhinosporidiosis are predominantly submucosal and not intraepithelial in location but can focally invade the epithelium, causing microabscesses. The sporangia are of similar size as the mucinous cysts and contain spores that take silver stains and homogeneous eosinophilic material that will also stain with mucicarmine. This chronic infection causing a vascularized papillomatous proliferation of the mucous membranes of the nose and pharynx is extremely rare in North America but endemic in India and Sri Lanka (195).

The papillary surface architecture and numerous small intraepithelial cysts can be confused for glandular proliferations of a low-grade oncocytoid papillary adenocarcinoma. The sinonasal tract mucosa is believed to give rise to glandular neoplasms distinct from those arising in submucosal ductuloacinar elements (salivary gland type). Many of these surface glandular proliferations are so well differentiated that they might be considered adenomas.

Some of the low-grade sinonasal adenocarcinoma variants display papillary patterns with uniform, sometimes oncocytoid cytologic features and uniform glandular architecture. These features are readily confused with the columnar cell variant of schneiderian papilloma. The epithelium in most of these low-grade adenocarcinomas is of single cell thickness with rare mitoses and is devoid of surface cilia. Most display intra- and extracellular mucin production. Both the papillomas and low-grade adenocarcinomas are cytologically bland in appearance, but the biologic behavior of the adenocarcinomas includes local destructiveness, aggressive recurrences, and the capability of metastasis. The features that help to distinguish columnar cell papilloma from these low-grade adenocarcinomas are the multilayered epithelium, surface ciliated columnar cells, intraepithelial microcysts, intracellular eosinophilic globule lumina in the papillomas, and the inverted growth pattern in the papillomas. In comparison, the low-grade adenocarcinomas are likely to display true glandular proliferations in the stroma that are lined by a single layer of epithelial cells and display an infiltrative growth pattern (196).

Dysplasia and Malignancy in Schneiderian Papillomas

Epithelial atypia in schneiderian papillomas is not uncommon, occurring in 45% of cases studied by Snyder and Perzin (174). However, this does not appear to have any clinical significance, because following complete surgical removal, even cases with carcinoma *in situ* and small foci of invasive carcinoma treated adequately follow a benign clinical course (197). Severe epithelial atypias with histologic progression to invasive carcinoma are documented and support the concept that some carcinomas do evolve from preexisting benign papillomas (174,176,197). Snyder and Perzin have demonstrated that 63% (5 of 8) of benign papillomas associated with carcinoma displayed significant epithelial atypia compared with significant atypia in 16% (5 of 31) of papillomas not associated with carcinoma. The majority of carcinomas associated with papillomas coexist in the same anatomic site as the papilloma with no histologic evidence of transition or occur less commonly in the same site following previous surgical resection of the papilloma. Snyder and Perzin's data in conjunction with the different clinical settings of carcinoma associated with inverted papilloma make a strong case for considering these papillomas premalignant "soil" or precursors of malignancy. It can be argued, however, that the coexistence of papilloma and carcinoma in the same anatomic site is coincidental, and it also can be argued that when histologically benign and malignant areas coexist within the same tumor, the papilloma is a malignancy from inception, only possessing well-differentiated areas that appear benign (186).

Our literature review of 589 papillomas by histologic type reveals associations with invasive carcinoma similar to those found by Hyams in his review of 315 papillomas. With the exception of one case of carcinoma associated with a fungiform papilloma, 10% to 15% of inverted papillomas and cylindrical cell papillomas have been associated with invasive carcinoma. Clearly, there is a small but significant association between sinonasal papillomas and carcinoma.

Regardless, no histologic changes in schneiderian papillomas have been found that will predict which will develop or be associated with coincident or subsequent malignancy. It is our impression and that of others (197) that surface keratinization in a papilloma often accompanies malignant transformation, but its value as a predictor is uncertain. Interval to recurrence and number of recurrences of papillomas do not appear related to the subsequent development of associated malignancy (171). Neither have clinical findings, including presentation with facial pain or bone erosion, been able to predict malignant transformation (185).

The histologic types of malignancy associated with or arising in inverted papillomas are many and include the more common keratinizing squamous and nonkeratinizing transitional cell carcinomas, but also reported are sarcomatoid (spindle cell) squamous carcinoma, undifferentiated (nasopharyngeal type) carcinoma (176), verrucous carcinoma (197), mucoepidermoid carcinoma (174), clear cell carcinoma (175), and adenocarcinoma (181). In the three reported cases of malignancy associated with cylindrical cell papillomas, four were SCCs (171,190,192) and one a mucoepidermoid (193) type of carcinoma. In the two cases reported by Ward and colleagues, there was continuity of carcinoma with dysplastic surface epithelium, indicating that the carcinomas originated from malignant transformation of the oncocytic papilloma (190). There is only one reported case of an invasive SCC occurring in the same anatomic region of multiple previously excised recurrences of fungiform papillomas involving the anterior septum, nasal floor, and inferior turbinate (172).

The biologic behavior of carcinomas associated with schneiderian papilloma has varied from incidental findings cured by resection of the papilloma to aggressive local disease, at times productive of regional and distant metastases.

Biologic Behavior

Recurrence of schneiderian papillomas is a major clinical problem that must be addressed in light of the biologic behavior of the neoplasm and the surgical approaches to complete excision. Most recurrences occur within 1 to 2 years of treatment but may be multiple and even delayed as late as after 23 years (169). Histologic features of these papillomas, including degree of atypia and pattern of growth, are not predictive of recurrence (169).

A number of intrinsic factors, including multicentricity, diffuse mucosal extension into neighboring cavities, and a possible field change in clinically uninvolved mucosa, probably contribute to these recurrences. In addition, incomplete removal of tumor with adjacent areas of predisposed mucosa has been shown to have a marked influence on rate of recurrence. The tendency of recurrences to occur in areas of surgical inaccessibility also has suggested that many cases are not recurrent but represent regrowth because of inadequate initial excision (171). As early as 1938, Ringertz had identified incomplete removal as the most important factor contributing to recurrence (188). For this reason, comparisons of recurrence rates over the decades are greatly influenced by surgical management.

Recurrence rates of 45% to 74% after conservative intranasal or Caldwell-Luc removal (169,174,187,198,199) have been significantly reduced to 0 to 13% recurrence with the lateral rhinotomy approach (185,187,197,198). For adequate exposure of papillomas involving the lateral nasal wall and paranasal sinuses, this external lateral rhinotomy procedure uses a modified Weber-Fergusson incision through the upper lip, around the base of the ala to the inner aspect of the brow with reflection of a cheek flap to remove the nasal bone, paper plate of ethmoid, and adjacent anterior wall of the maxillary sinus. This allows en bloc resection of the lateral nasal wall and removal or electrocoagulation of all mucosa lining the ethmoid, maxillary, frontal, and sphenoid sinuses (185). Depending on the location of the papilloma and extent of involvement, more conservative intranasal wide local excision of nasal septal papillomas, with coagulation of the mucosal margins and Caldwell-Luc procedures for isolated papillomas of the maxillary antrum, are possible (185). Total extirpation of extensive papillomas may require maxillectomy. Possible excision in selected cases using endoscopic sinus surgical techniques is a currently controversial topic.

Radiation therapy plays no role in the primary treatment of these radioresistant schneiderian papillomas or as an adjunct to surgery to prevent recurrences (174). Furthermore, the possibility of irradiation-induced malignancy has been suggested (174,200). At present, radiation therapy is reserved for documented malignancy associated with sinonasal papillomas.

The manner in which the schneiderian papillomas are most effectively managed focuses on a biologic behavior that includes significant local invasiveness and destruction and capacity for recurrence. Their increased association with malignancy and range of dysplastic epithelial changes has suggested to some that these neoplasms are premalignant. Their aggressiveness, even when cytologically benign, is not inconsistent with the modifiers *borderline tumor* or *low-grade malignancy* and calls into question their designation as papillomas. Regarding biologic behavior, Willis had stated that "no sharp distinction can be made between benign papillomas and papillary carcinoma" (201). We have seen a rare example of an inverted papilloma that appeared to superficially invade bone, and a similar finding has been described by others (174). Histologically, benign papillomas can exhibit significant local invasion with extension beyond the nose and paranasal sinuses to involve the orbit, pharynx, or brain. In many instances this local aggressiveness is seen in recurrences and may be enhanced by the surgical disruption of natural hard and soft tissue barriers. The case of a well-differentiated inverted sinonasal papilloma that metastasized to cervical lymph nodes a year following resection of the primary tumor calls into question our present understanding of these sinonasal proliferations (202).

These features of inverted papillomas are not unlike those of odontogenic jaw tumors, such as ameloblastomas, that are also cytologically benign but locally aggressive tumors that rarely metastasize (see Chapter 6). Schneiderian papillomas, however, are unique in that uninvolved adjacent mucosa also appears to be at risk to proliferate and result in recurrence of papilloma or malignant transformation. In the presently accepted surgical management of schneiderian papillomas, they are best considered potentially aggressive benign neoplasms for initial therapeutic purposes to mitigate the morbidity associated with treating recurrent disease and to avoid the low but significant chance of carcinoma occurring in the same anatomic site.

GLANDULAR NEOPLASMS

Glandular neoplasms of the sinonasal region can be characterized as those that resemble benign and malignant salivary gland neoplasms and those that do not. Both categories are believed by some to arise *de novo* from the respiratory mucosal lining epithelium (203). The nonsalivary type adenocarcinomas have been referred to as intestinal mucous membrane, papillary, mucinous, simple, nonspecific, enteric, intestinal, or colonic type, and low-grade adenocarcinoma (204). In aggregate, adenocarcinomas comprise less than 1% of all malignancies and 10% to 20% of all primary malignant neoplasms of the nasal cavity and paranasal sinuses (204,205).

Salivary-type Glandular Neoplasms

Pleomorphic Adenoma (Benign Mixed Tumor)

Clinical Data

Pleomorphic adenomas are the most common benign salivary-type neoplasms of the sinonasal tract. Roughly three fourths arise in the nasal septum, and the remaining tumors arise in the lateral nasal cavity wall or turbinate. Although mixed tumors may rarely arise in the paranasal sinuses, it is more common for them to secondarily extend into the maxillary sinus (206–212).

Pleomorphic adenomas predominantly affect whites 20 to 60 years of age, with approximately equal sex distribution (58,206). Patients usually complain of nasal obstruction, mass sensation, or epistaxis, generally of less than 1 year in duration (206).

Radiologic Studies

Roentgenograms usually reveal an expanding intranasal soft tissue lesion, generally larger than clinically expected and associated with bone destruction (206).

Gross Appearance

Tumors occasionally are pedunculated, but most are broad-based, polypoid, well-demarcated, lobular masses, covered by a translucent mucosa or membrane, suggestive of pseudoencapsulation. On cut surface they are gray, moist to mucoid, translucent, rubbery to fleshy, and granular to friable. Rarely, cystic or hemorrhagic changes are noted. Median size for the lesions is approximately 2.6 cm (206).

Histologic Features

Histologically, sinonasal pleomorphic adenomas are well-demarcated lesions with a biphasic appearance consisting of epithelial and mesenchymal components in variable ratios, similar to the analagous tumors of the salivary glands (see Chapter 8). Mixed tumors of the sinonasal tract tend to be more cellular than those of the major salivary glands, with a preponderance of epithelial elements and in some cases little to absent myxochondroid stroma. Virtually no atypical mitoses or anaplasia are noted. The epithelial element consists of sheets of disorganized but uniform cells, mostly with ductal morphology surrounded by an outer layer of cuboidal to spindle myoepithelial cells. The mesenchymal component is usually cartilaginous or myxomatous in appearance.

Histologic variants in which only the epithelial element is present are designated cellular pleomorphic adenoma, or variants of basal cell (or monomorphic) adenoma. A rare dermal analogue variant of basal cell adenoma resembling dermal eccrine cylindroma has been described arising in the nasal cavity in association with the salivary gland–skin adnexal tumor diathesis (see Chapter 8) (213) (Fig. 35). An additional variant composed of uniform spindle-shaped cells immunoreactive for S-100 protein and smooth muscle actin, and devoid of pleomorphism or mitoses, is designated myoepithelioma (214).

Differential Diagnosis

Given the spindle cell, mesenchymal, and epithelial components of pleomorphic adenomas and their varied appearances, many entities can be considered in the differential diagnosis. These include chondroma, chondromyxoid fibroma, hemangiopericytoma, low-grade fibrosarcoma, mucoepidermoid carcinoma, adenoid cystic carcinoma, malignant mixed tumor, and rhabdomyosarcoma. The consistent presence of benign features and discriminatory immunohistochemical stains such as cytokeratin, S-100 protein, glial fibrillary acidic protein (GFAP) and smooth muscle–specific proteins such as calponin aid in the identification of pleomorphic adenomas (215–217).

Biologic Behavior

A recurrence rate of up to 10% is reported in some series (206,218). It has been hypothesized that intraoperative spillage with consequent reseeding may occur, especially of the myxoid component (206). If the tumor recurs, additional conservative but complete removal is usually curative (207).

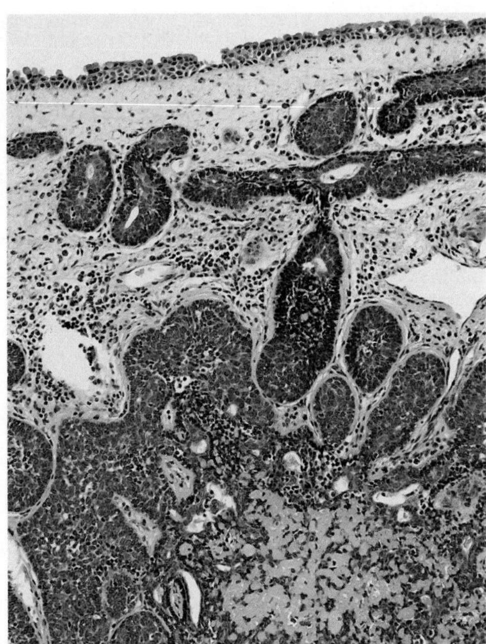

FIGURE 35. Benign salivary-type adenoma. Basal cell (monomorphic) adenoma of dermal analogue type in nasal cavity resembles dermal eccrine cylindroma with prominent accumulation of reduplicated basal lamina.

Adenoid Cystic Carcinoma

Clinical Data

Adenoid cystic carcinoma is the most frequent malignant salivary-type glandular neoplasm of the sinonasal area (219,220). Spies, in his defining monograph of 1930, listed three cases in the antrum and two in the nose (221). Although 40% of sinonasal adenoid cystic carcinomas occur in the nasal cavity, the most frequently involved sinus is the maxillary antrum (30%) followed by the ethmoid, sphenoid, and frontal sinuses and combinations of all (58,207,222,223).

Adenoid cystic carcinoma affects both sexes between 30 and 50 years of age, with a slight male predominance (58,207). Although adenoid cystic carcinomas may present as slow-growing, asymptomatic masses, they may be associated with nasal obstruction, epistaxis, symptoms of chronic sinusitis, facial pain, or neuralgia. Symptom duration is 1 year on average (207,221,222). Involvement of the cheek, palate, or orbit with ocular symptoms is also possible (217,222,224).

Radiologic Studies

The radiographic appearance of adenoid cystic carcinoma may be that of opacification of the sinus associated with bone loss (224).

Gross Appearance

Adenoid cystic carcinomas are usually infiltrating masses generally more than 2 cm in greatest dimension (58,207).

Histologic Features

Adenoid cystic carcinomas are unencapsulated tumors that infiltrate in and around nerves, along tissue planes, and into the bone, generally without bony destruction (unless the tumor is large) or

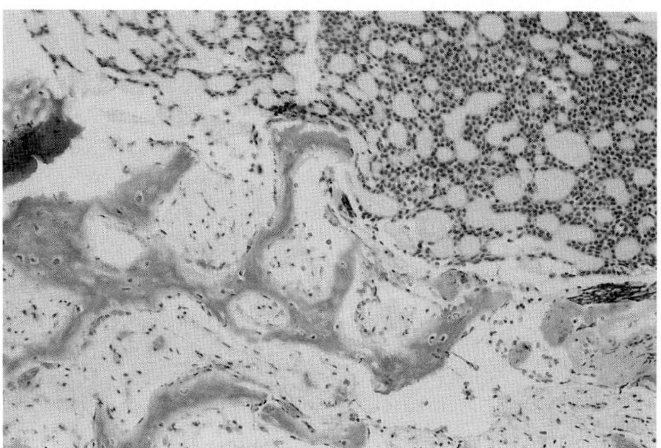

FIGURE 36. Adenoid cystic carcinoma. Bone of maxillary sinus infiltrated by adenoid cystic carcinoma.

reactive new bone formation (224) (Fig. 36). They are composed of small, hyperchromatic, round to oval cells with little amphophilic cytoplasm, angulated nuclei, and rare mitoses. Ductal-type cells with eosinophilic cytoplasm and larger ovoid nuclei are also present. Cribriform and solid patterns are more common in the upper respiratory tract (225). The tumors resemble the analagous neoplasms in the salivary glands (see Chapter 8).

The cribriform pattern consists of gland-like (actually pseudoglandular; see Chapter 8) spaces of variable size, irregularly arranged in a sieve-like fashion, containing mucin or eosinophilic hyaline-like material, and lined by poorly oriented neoplastic cells (Fig. 37). The basaloid or anaplastic patterns also may coexist within the same lesion, and display small or large areas of coagulative necrosis. The basaloid pattern consists of tiny cystic spaces lined by a basaloid arrangement of small cells with dark nuclei and inconspicuous nucleoli. Cells in the anaplastic pattern tend to have larger vesicular nuclei and distinct nucleoli (224). Perineural invasion is almost a constant feature in all variants.

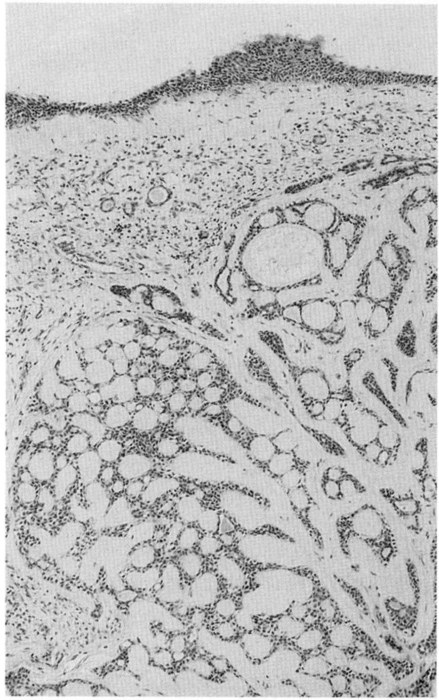

FIGURE 37. Adenoid cystic carcinoma. Tumor of maxillary sinus with cribriform pattern.

Differential Diagnosis

Adenocarcinoma not otherwise specified (NOS) can be considered in the differential diagnosis, although larger nuclei and abundant cytoplasm are usually distinguishing features. Distinction is sometimes impossible, and a diagnosis of adenocarcinoma with adenoid cystic features may be justified (207). Pleomorphic adenoma is a worthy consideration, especially in the scenario of fragmented surgical specimens. Basal cell (monomorphic) adenoma and polymorphous low-grade adenocarcinoma are extremely rare in the sinonasal tract to offer a common diagnostic difficulty.

Biologic Behavior

The best prognostic indicator is the extent of tumor at the time of discovery rather than morphology (226). However, solid areas with anaplastic or basaloid patterns are associated with more rapid progression (224). Adenoid cystic carcinomas are prone to recur locally or as distant metastases (generally late in their course), even after radical surgery (223,227). Other factors adding to poor prognosis include extensive growth before discovery, positive margins of resection, and closeness to vital structures, such as the brain. Seventy-five percent of the tumors relapse, 50% with local recurrence (222). Survival rates vary in different series from 7% to 33% at 10 years (207,228) to 25% at 15 years (58). Treatment with combined surgery and external beam radiotherapy offers the best chance for local control and probably improves survival (222). Fast neutron radiotherapy plays an important role in the management of adenoid cystic carcinomas, providing high locoregional control and survival rates for patients with locally advanced, unresectable tumors (229–231).

Adenocarcinoma Not Otherwise Specified

Clinical Data

The antrum, ethmoid, and nasal cavity are the most common locations for adenocarcinoma NOS after the accessory seromucous glands of the palate (232). These tumors usually present with nasal obstruction and facial pain.

Radiologic Studies

On radiologic examination, adenocarcinomas are usually sizable tumors involving the adjacent bone.

Histologic Features

Many histologic patterns have been described. These are a histologically diverse group of adenocarcinomas of intermediate and high nuclear grades, including mucinous, papillary, trabecular, clear cell, apocrine, papillary with focal clear cell change, and tubulocystic types (232,233).

Differential Diagnosis

A specific tumor should not be forced into one of the recognized salivary-type neoplasm diagnostic categories. It is often reasonable to withhold a salivary gland-type diagnosis for most high-grade, poorly differentiated adenocarcinomas of the sinonasal tract (207).

Biologic Behavior
Staging and grading are more prognostically significant than the extent of the surgery. Cure rates are 21%, 15% and 10% at 5, 10, and 15 years respectively, according to one series (232).

Mucoepidermoid Carcinoma

Mucoepidermoid carcinoma is a rare tumor in the sinonasal area. In some series it has developed after nasal cosmetic surgery (207).

Histologic Features
Mucoepidermoid carcinoma is generally a low-grade infiltrative neoplasm composed of mucous cells, intermediate cells, and bland, epidermoid cells, arranged in a multicystic growth pattern (see Chapter 8) (234). It may originate from surface epithelium in the sinonasal tract despite similarities with salivary mucoepidermoid carcinoma (207).

Differential Diagnosis
Low-grade mucoepidermoid carcinomas can be confused with necrotizing sialometaplasia and with mucus retention cysts showing squamous metaplasia and mucous cell hyperplasia. High-grade tumors may be difficult to distinguish from SCCs with mucus cell production, and the distinction may be a moot point.

Biologic Behavior
The most important prognostic factors are tumor size and stage, histologic grade, and presence of tumor at the resection margins (234). Low-grade mucoepidermoid carcinomas have a good prognosis after surgery, whereas high-grade ones have the same treatment and prognosis as SCC of comparable stage (58,218).

Polymorphous Low-grade Adenocarcinoma

Polymorphous low-grade adenocarcinoma is primarily a minor salivary gland neoplasm characterized by variable architecture, uniform cytology, and an infiltrating growth pattern. The most common variant is also known as terminal duct carcinoma of minor salivary glands (235). Rarely described in the sinonasal or nasopharyngeal tract, its immunohistochemical and ultrastructural features have been elegantly reviewed by Dardick and Wenig and colleagues (112,236).

Carcinoma Ex Pleomorphic Adenoma (Malignant Mixed Tumor)

Carcinoma ex pleomorphic adenoma (malignant mixed tumor) arises from the malignant transformation of the epithelial component in a benign pleomorphic adenoma. The incidence in the sinonasal tract is not known, but is probably less than that of major salivary glands (207). The literature reflects a paucity of cases (218). Teratocarcinasarcoma can be considered in the differential diagnosis.

Acinic Cell Carcinoma

A small series of predominantly serous acinic cell carcinomas of the nasal cavity has been described (58). These presented in adults, with equal involvement of men and women. No follow-up data are available. Diagnosis may be confirmed by immunoperoxidase stain for amylase and electron microscopy for the identification of secretory granules (237,238).

Oncocytic Neoplasms

These are rare, small septal lesions or extensive paranasal sinus masses associated with bony erosion and formed by solid nests, cords, tubules or sheet-like arrangements of oncocytes, apparently derived from the surface epithelium (196,239). Oncocytic metaplasia with hyperplasia, columnar (oncocytic) cell papillomas, and granular cell ameloblastomas are in the differential diagnosis. It is noteworthy that pleomorphic adenomas and mucoepidermoid carcinomas can have areas of oncocytic differentiation, at times extensive. Large oncocytic neoplasms have the potential for aggressive behavior, and some may represent low-grade adenocarcinomas (196,240). Therefore, conservative, but complete surgical removal is the treatment of choice (196,239,240).

Nonsalivary-Type Adenocarcinomas

Clinical Data

In 1903, Citelli and Calamida recognized nasal cavity adenocarcinomas of the nonsalivary gland type for the first time. Masson and Martin reported Kulchitsky's cells in some of these lesions in 1928 (241), and Ringertz described the papillary morphology seen in some of these lesions in 1938. Major interest in nonsalivary sinonasal adenocarcinomas, however, was sparked in 1965 by Macbeth's report of Hadfield's observation of an increase in ethmoid adenocarcinoma among English woodworkers (242).

The risk of nasal adenocarcinoma is significantly increased with exposure to wood dust, paints, varnishes, lacquers, glues, and adhesives, apparently in a dose-response relationship (204,205,243–245). It also increases in women exposed to textile dust (246). The very strong association with wood dust (70–500 times more risk than in nonwoodworkers) has obscured the role of formaldehyde in the genesis of sinonasal adenocarcinoma, but some studies suggest that exposure to wood dust and formaldehyde may increase the risk of sinonasal adenocarcinoma when compared with exposure to wood dust alone (204,243). Inhaled dust particles 5 μm or larger, especially from hardwood, beech, and oak, concentrate in the anterior part of the nasal septum and posterior end of the middle turbinate, inducing cuboidal or squamous metaplasia with consequent impairment of mucociliary clearance and prolonged mucosal contact with a putative carcinogen. The average length of exposure is 40 to 43 years (204,247).

Leather and flour dust have been implicated by some investigators, although these particles also share an association with increased incidence of sinonasal SCC. Smoking and allergic associations also have been reported (204).

Nonsalivary adenocarcinomas may affect any age group, but overall there is a greater incidence in middle-aged and older men. Clinical differences between well-differentiated and poorly differentiated adenocarcinomas are to be noted.

The well-differentiated adenocarcinomas present in the nasal cavity as polypoid or papillomatous tumors. Destructive manifestations may predominate in the sinuses where the tumors fill or obliterate the nasal cavity as a secondary phenomenon. The more common presenting symptoms are unilateral nasal obstruction, epistaxis, and pain, usually of a few months' duration. There may be clear or purulent rhinorrhea. These well-differentiated lesions preferentially involve the ethmoid, nasoethmoid, and nasal cavities, and less frequently the nasal septum, multiple combined sinuses, or maxillary and nasomaxillary regions. Patients tend to be younger than those with poorly differentiated adenocarcinomas (median 54 years), and women and men tend to be equally affected (196,204,242,248,249).

Poorly differentiated adenocarcinomas also present with nasal obstruction and epistaxis, but associated pain and facial deformity are more frequent than with the better differentiated lesions, as is a shorter duration of the symptomatic period. The maxillary and nasomaxillary cavities are preferentially involved, followed by multiple combined sinuses, and the ethmoid, nasoethmoid, and nasal cavities in decreasing order of frequency. Involvement of the maxillary sinus may present as a soft-tissue mass of the cheek associated with exophthalmos. Trismus, paralysis of the buccal branch of the facial nerve, and bleeding oral ulcers secondary to tumoral involvement have been described. There is a definite male predominance, with a median age of 63 years (196,204,242,248,249).

Radiologic Studies

Radiologic findings include soft tissue density within the nasal cavity or maxillary and ethmoid sinuses, cloudiness or opacification of one or more of the ipsilateral sinuses and bone destruction (204).

Gross Appearance

Tumors tend to be firm, gray-white to dark red raspberry-like polyps, papillary, nodular, or fungating masses, some of which may be friable, ulcerated, or hemorrhagic and mucoid on occasion. Tumors involving the sinuses also have a polypoid appearance at surgery (204,248).

Histologic Features

Many nonsalivary adenocarcinomas appear to arise from the surface epithelium because there is frequently a demonstrable area of transition between the normal mucosa and the neoplasm (196). The papillary type is thought to arise from the surface epithelium, the colonic type from the surface epithelium and from the accessory mucoserous gland ducts, and the mucinous type from the seromucous glands. Multidirectional differentiation of a common stem cell could account for the variety of cells (Paneth, endocrine, goblet, absorptive) encountered in these neoplasms (204,220,250).

Low-grade sinonasal adenocarcinomas should be regarded as a separate clinicopathologic category, given their differences in clinical presentation and better prognosis (196). Distinction of low- from high-grade sinonasal adenocarcinomas is based on simple histopathologic features, mainly their uniform glandular architecture and bland cytologic characteristics. Most are composed of small uniform glands lined by a single layer of cuboidal to columnar cells. A "back-to-back" glandular arrangement without intervening stroma may be prominent (196). Large, irregular cystic spaces and papillary formations may be present. Encapsulation is not evident. Significant nuclear pleomorphism is absent, nuclear uniformity being striking. Mitoses are usually scarce. Calcospherules and calcification may be present. Several histologic subgroups have been described (196). The acinic cell variant is characterized by small nests and acini of rounded polyhedral cells with granular basophilic cytoplasm. Oncocytic (Fig. 38), papillary (Fig. 39), cystadenocarcinomatous, clear cell (Fig. 40), and nonspecific subtypes have been documented.

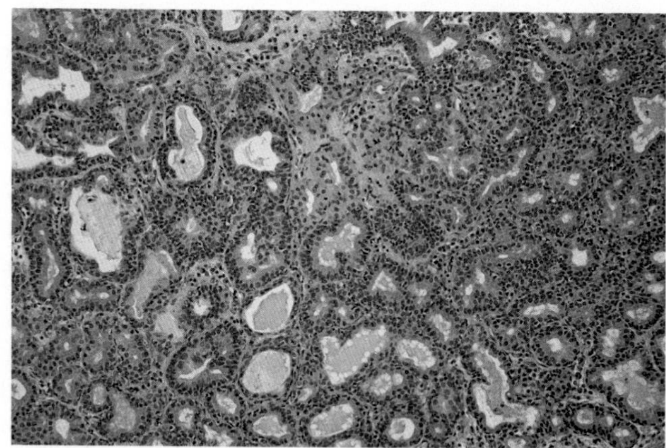

FIGURE 38. Sinonasal low-grade adenocarcinoma. Oncocytoid cytologic variant with uniform glandular architecture and glands of single cell thickness.

Five additional major histologic types of nonsalivary adenocarcinoma are recognized. In general, these are higher grade tumors that may be associated with necrosis, inflammation, hemorrhage, and perineural invasion. Some may have a mucin-producing papillary cystadenomatous pattern, the epithelial component similar to colloid or mucinous carcinoma of the intestine or breast. These tend to be associated with the woodworking industry (204). Wood dust associated adenocarcinoma is generally of the papillary or colonic types, whereas in the spo-

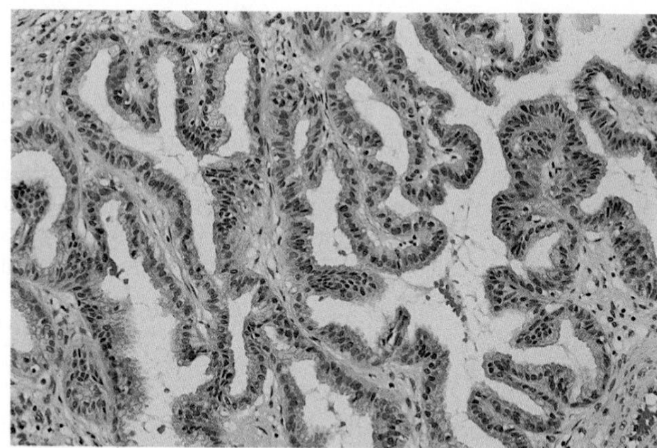

FIGURE 39. Sinonasal low-grade adenocarcinoma. Papillary variant. (Courtesy Dr. J.D. Crissman.)

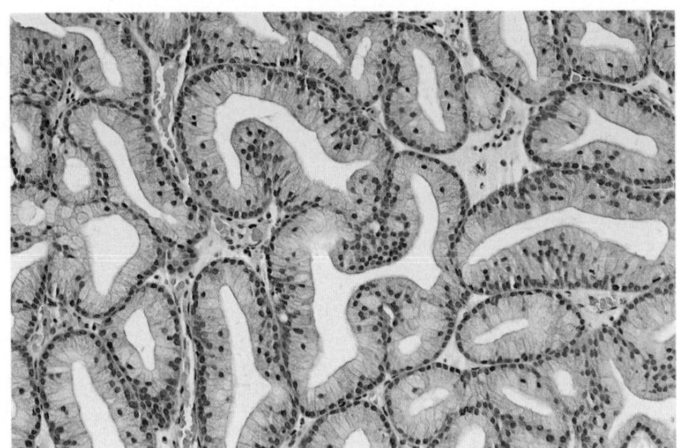

FIGURE 40. Sinonasal low-grade adenocarcinoma. Clear cell variant with closely packed neoplastic glands composed of ample faint staining cytoplasm.

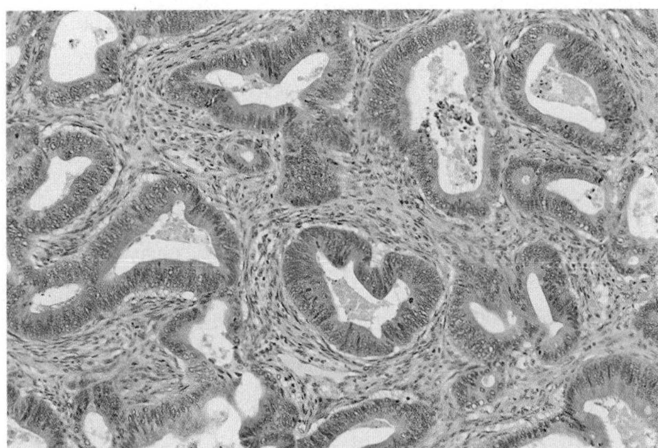

FIGURE 41. Sinonasal adenocarcinoma. Colonic-type adenocarcinoma histologically similar to colorectal adenocarcinoma.

radic cases, although papillary and colonic types predominate, the other types are also relatively increased (204). These adenocarcinomas are graded according to the degree of differentiation (204,242).

Papillary Type

This variant is characterized by elongated, exophytic, occasionally branching fronds similar to those of villous adenoma of the colon, with loose, edematous, and myxoid to compact and fibrous fibrovascular cores. The papillae are lined by stratified, nonciliated columnar cells variably admixed with goblet cells in a polarized fashion, but may well be crowded and disorganized. The cytoplasm is pink, and nuclei are round to elongated with smooth, slightly indented nuclear membranes. The nuclear appearance varies from hyperchromatic to vesicular, with uniform chromatin distribution showing one to three basophilic nucleoli.

Colonic Type

Colonic type adenocarcinoma is composed of well- to moderately differentiated glands histologically similar to those of typical colorectal adenocarcinoma. Glands and cystic gland–like spaces are lined by pseudostratified columnar epithelium (242) (Fig. 41). Cells are larger than those of the papillary variant and have a pink cytoplasm with occasional mucin droplets. Nuclei are large and round to irregular, with a vesicular chromatin pattern having one to three small eosinophilic nucleoli. Goblet cells are rare to absent. Paneth, argentaffin, and absorptive intestinal type cells also can be seen (250). Interestingly, an aggressive nasal tumor resembling normal intestinal mucosa has been described (250).

Solid Type

The solid variant is cytologically identical to the colonic type, but with minimal gland formation. Cytoplasmic mucin droplets are present, but typical goblet cells are scarce to absent.

Mucinous Type

Two different patterns have been described. The first consists of compact tumor clusters with small glands or short papillary structures with or without fibrovascular cores, lying in pools of mucin or nesting in a mucomyxoid matrix (Fig. 42). Some have prominent goblet or columnar cells. Intracytoplasmic mucin droplets can be seen occasionally, giving an almost signet ring appearance in some cases. Most nuclei are small, round, and hyperchromatic, with occasional large ones displaying a vesicular texture and prominent nucleoli.

The second pattern is represented by large, mucus-distended glands, some of them occasionally ruptured and eliciting a brisk inflammatory and granulation tissue response.

Mixed Types

This term is used to describe those adenocarcinomas exhibiting two or more of the previously described patterns, in approximately similar proportions, without predominance of any.

Special Studies

Groupings of argyrophilic and neuroendocrine cells, histologically similar to those seen in adenocarcinomas of the gastroin-

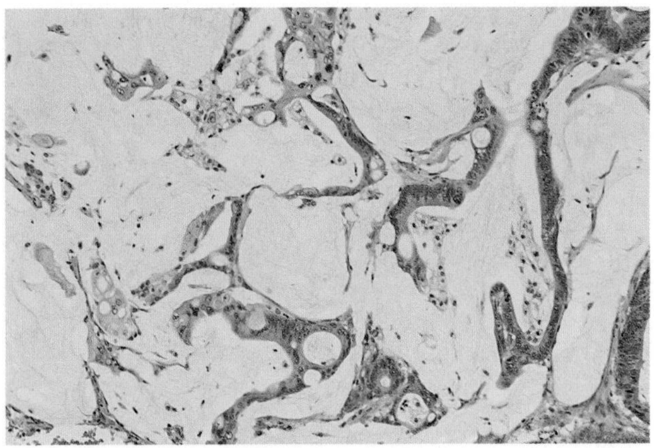

FIGURE 42. Sinonasal adenocarcinoma. Mucinous-type adenocarcinoma with pools of mucin containing strands of neoplastic glandular epithelium.

testinal tract, have been demonstrated in some of the enteric types. These adenocarcinomas also may show immunoreactivity to gastrointestinal type hormones: gastrin, glucagon, serotonin, cholecystokinin, somatostatin, and leu-enkephalin (248). Histochemical stains for mucin are useful to identify mucopolysaccharide-containing secretions.

Ultrastructural features such as straight microvilli with filamentous core rootlets, and aggregates of glycocalyx-associated, Paneth, and mid-gut argentaffin cell-like granules are in keeping with an intestinal type of cell differentiation (248).

Differential Diagnosis

The markedly edematous inflammatory stroma in papillary sinusitis may be confused with mucinous material from the papillary or colonic type of sinonasal adenocarcinoma. Papillary sinusitis, however, is generally bilateral, exhibits no cellular pleomorphism, mitoses, or necrosis, and is characterized by a rather myxoid, eosinophil-rich stroma with persistence of the epithelial cilia (204).

Low-grade, well-differentiated adenocarcinomas with oncocytoid cytologic features and uniform glandular architecture should be differentiated from cylindrical cell (oncocytic) papillomas and hyperplasia of mucoserous glands. The epithelium in most of these low-grade adenocarcinomas is of single cell thickness with rare mitoses and devoid of surface cilia. The schneiderian oncocytic papillomas have a bimorphic endophytic–exophytic architecture with an oncocytic cytoplasmic character (204). These latter proliferations tend to have a more abundant and myxomatous stroma, stratified rather than a simple lining epithelium, intraepithelial microcysts as opposed to glands, surface ciliated columnar cells, and an inverted pushing rather than infiltrative growth pattern (196).

The possibility of metastasis from distant regions should always be considered. Carcinomas from the kidney, prostate (Fig. 43), lung, breast, gastrointestinal tract (stomach, colon, and rectum), testis, uterus, adrenal, pancreas, thyroid, and cutaneous melanoma have all been reported to metastasize to the nasal cavity and paranasal sinuses (204,251,252). Although enteric-type sinonasal adenocarcinoma resembles metastatic colorectal carcinoma, the latter is exceedingly rare and tends to be associated with large areas of dirty necrosis with neutrophilic infiltrate. However, sinonasal involvement has been described as the first presentation of a colonic primary tumor (196,204,242). The cavities more frequently involved by metastases, in order of decreasing frequency, are maxillary, ethmoid, frontal, and nasal (253).

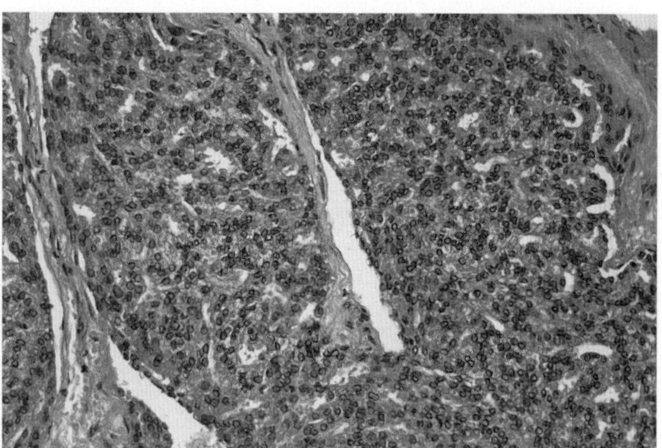

FIGURE 43. Metastatic adenocarcinoma. Prostate adenocarcinoma metastatic to sphenoid sinus simulating low-grade sinonasal adenocarcinoma.

Biologic Behavior

The prognosis of high-grade sinonasal adenocarcinoma is generally poor: two thirds of patients are dead from disease within 3 years (196,204). However, low-grade adenocarcinomas carry a better prognosis in general (196,254). Some series report a 5-year survival rate of 78%, although grading is not mentioned (255).

All grades of sinonasal adenocarcinoma tend to be locally aggressive, and invasion of the base of the skull or orbits is not uncommon (250). Distant metastases are rare, even in advanced cases. Cervical lymph nodes, lungs, liver, and vertebral bodies are the preferred sites. Metastasis to the breast, although rare, also has been reported (204,242,256). The adenocarcinomas associated with wood dust exposure predominantly involve the nasal and ethmoid cavities in men and have a better prognosis than the sporadic cases that tend to present in women and preferentially involve the maxillary sinus. The papillary type has the best prognosis but, nevertheless, behaves in a smoldering, locally destructive fashion (204,254). Alveolar goblet cell predominant adenocarcinomas also appear to carry a better prognosis (254).

Complete surgical removal with clear margins is the treatment of choice. Postoperative radiation and chemotherapy have been of little apparent success, although this is difficult to assess in view of the lack of standardized regimens. Elective neck dissection is not warranted (242).

SQUAMOUS CELL CARCINOMA

Clinical Data

Carcinoma of the nasal cavity and paranasal cavities accounts for 3% of head and neck malignancies (257). Most of these carcinomas are SCCs, with 70% occurring in the maxillary sinus, 12% in the nasal cavity, 10% in the other sinuses, and 7% in the nasal vestibule (228,258–260). We will focus on the diverse histopathology of the common variants of SCCs, as well as some of the more unusual histologic variants arising in this region.

Site-specific etiologic associations of SCC are recognized that include cigarette smoking for cancer in the nasal vestibule; cigarette smoking and industrial nickel exposure for cancer in the nasal cavity (261–263); and industrial exposure to chromium, mustard gas, isopropyl alcohol, radium (264) and the medical radionuclide Thorotrast in SCC in the maxillary sinuses (265). Nickel-induced nasal SCC may exhibit a latency period of 25 to 32 years after exposure and usually arises from the middle turbinate (263,266), whereas Thorotrast-associated carcinomas may show a latency of 12 to 24 years. Other possible predispositions include chronic inflammatory conditions inducing squamous metaplasia, such as chronic rhinosinusitis, oroantral fistula, and rhinoscleroma. Less strong associations are also noted for nose picking and snuff use (264,267–269). Rare cases associated with radiation and chemotherapy have been reported (261,270). The roughly 10% to 15% risk for development of synchronous or metachronous carcinoma with schneiderian papillomas of the inverted and cylindrical cell type is addressed elsewhere in this chapter. Although human papillomaviruses have been detected in sinonasal SCCs, an etiologic role is unproven (271).

Squamous cell carcinomas in all sinonasal sites arise most commonly in men 55 to 65 years of age (272,273). Symptoms may range from a nasal ulcer or mass with nasal obstruction, rhinorrhea, epistaxis, or pain. Sinus tumors may present as chronic sinusitis, facial asymmetry, or intraoral tumor bulge with referred oral, ocular, and neurologic symptoms due to tumor extension. Roughly 15% of nasal carcinomas present bilaterally secondary to septal perforation, and 15% may be associated with a synchronous or metachronous second primary malignancy. Of these second primary cancers, 40% involve the head and neck and 60% the lungs, gastrointestinal tract, or breasts (272). Five percent of maxillary sinus SCCs are associated with a second primary cancer in the contralateral antrum, but no increased risk for distant second primary cancers is noted (274).

Histopathologic Features

The diverse histologic appearances of most sinonasal SCCs can be classified as a spectrum of differentiation of two basic histomorphologic types: conventional keratinizing SCC (epidermoid carcinoma) and nonkeratinizing carcinoma (transitional cell carcinoma, papillary carcinoma, cylindrical or columnar cell carcinoma, intermediate cell carcinoma, schneiderian carcinoma, and Ringertz's carcinoma). Sinonasal anaplastic or undifferentiated carcinomas will be discussed under a separate heading because they are not considered to be variants of SCC.

Other special types of SCC that arise less commonly in the sinonasal tract include sarcomatoid (spindle cell) squamous carcinoma (275,276), verrucous carcinoma (277), adenosquamous carcinoma (278), and basaloid SCC (279). These entities are more common in other head and neck mucosal sites and are addressed in more detail in other chapters on the oral cavity and larynx. An extremely unusual carcinoma in the sinonasal region has been described by Manivel and colleagues as transitional cell carcinoma with endodermal sinus tumor–like areas. Frierson et al. have reported a difficult to classify small cell neoplasm with mixed epithelial, neural, and myogenous antigens following radiation therapy for bilateral retinoblastomas (280,281).

The two main histomorphologic types of SCC can be distinguished as follows.

Keratinizing Squamous Cell Carcinoma

This is the conventional SCC that shows a spectrum of nuclear cytologic differentiation, cytoplasmic keratinization, keratin pearl formation, and various patterns of stromal invasion from broad pushing fronts, thick nests, ragged thin cords to sprays of single infiltrative cells. A tripartite well-moderate-poor or four-part Broders' scheme may be applied for grading, factoring degrees of nuclear pleomorphism, cytoplasmic differentiation, and mitotic rate (Figs. 44 and 45) (see Chapter 2).

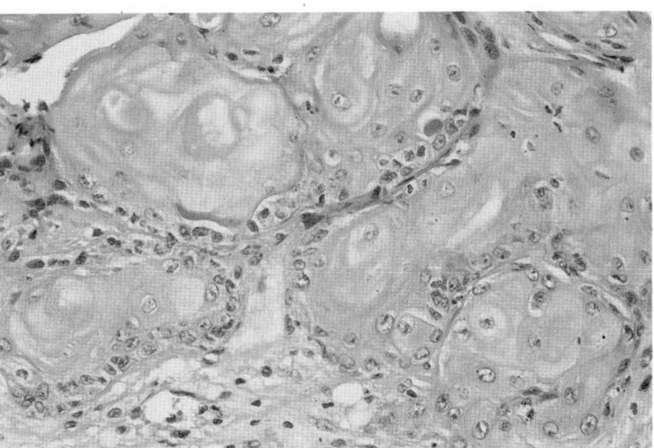

FIGURE 44. Keratinizing squamous cell carcinoma. Well-differentiated squamous cell carcinoma of maxillary sinus with prominent cytoplasmic keratinization.

Nonkeratinizing Carcinoma

The unusual and distinctive histologic appearance of this form of carcinoma in the sinonasal tract is reflected in the profusion of names applied to it. However, similar appearing nonkeratinizing SCCs arise in the nasopharynx, base of tongue, tonsil, and hypopharynx. Again, a spectrum of differentiation marks these carcinomas, all of which share a pushing or plexiform invasive growth pattern of anastomosing garlands, ribbons, and festoons of neoplastic epithelium delimited by a persistent basement membrane. Although this carcinoma is identified as nonkeratinizing, there are often small keratin pearls interspersed within the proliferation, and some may form surface keratin that fills cystic spaces. Rarely, extensive squamous metaplasia will create a histologic overlap indistinguishable from keratinizing SCC. Comedo necrosis also may be noted. Most nonkeratinizing car-

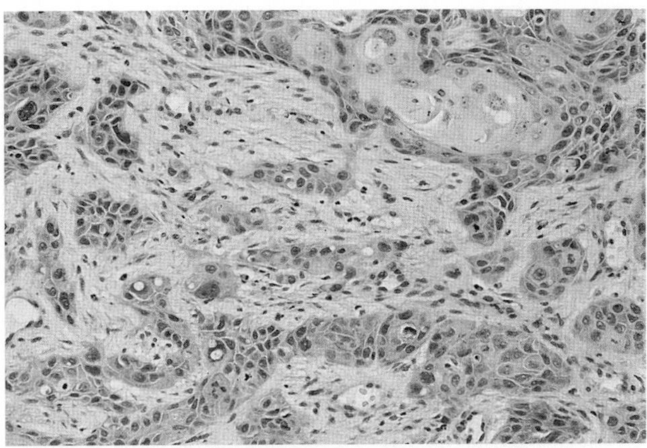

FIGURE 45. Keratinizing squamous cell carcinoma. Moderately differentiated keratinizing squamous cell carcinoma with more marked nuclear pleomorphism, infiltrating in pattern of thin irregular cords.

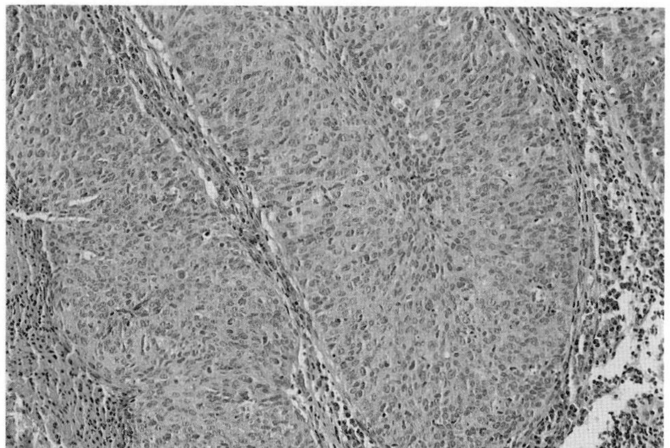

FIGURE 46. Nonkeratinizing carcinoma. Well-differentiated carcinoma with anastomosing ribbons resembling transitional epithelium.

cinomas are well differentiated, resembling transitional epithelium (Fig. 46) reminiscent of urothelium; some are poorly differentiated, composed of layers of disordered small anaplastic cells (Fig. 47); and yet others bear pseudostratified tall cylindric cells with a basal palisade of columnar cells. A papillary surface component also may be present as well as foci of small cell carcinoma or high-grade adenocarcinoma (282,283).

Differential Diagnosis

At times the ribbon-like invasive architecture and monomorphic nuclear cytology of nonkeratinizing SCC may mimic inverted papilloma. Thus, Osborn called inverted papillomas *transitional papillomas* and sinonasal nonkeratinizing carcinomas *transitional carcinomas* (284). However, the focal keratin pearl formation, increased mitotic activity (including the presence of mitoses high in the epithelial layer), and nuclear pleomorphism distinguish the nonkeratinizing SCC.

It may be impossible to discriminate nonkeratinizing SCC from a carcinoma ex inverted papilloma (malignant inverted papilloma) characterized by diffuse dysplasia of the epithelium unless there is residual, better differentiated underlying inverted papilloma present.

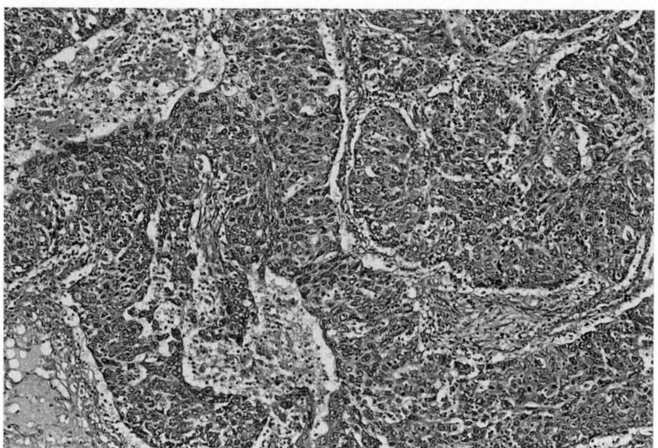

FIGURE 47. Nonkeratinizing carcinoma. Poorly differentiated variant with ribbons lined by disordered small anaplastic cells.

Ameloblastomas arising in the maxilla may extend into and present in the maxillary sinus or nasal cavity. These maxillary odontogenic tumors tend to be more densely cellular than the mandibular tumors and may form keratin pearls in the acanthomatous variant, and therefore can be confused with carcinoma. Both the benign ameloblastoma and cytologically malignant ameloblastic carcinoma are distinguished by cell nests, strands or sheets lined at the periphery by a layer of palisaded columnar cells with nuclei polarized away from the basement membrane, and an edematous stellate reticulum-like zone in the epithelium. However, a prominent stratified basal layer can be seen in some nonkeratinizing SCCs, lending an adamantinoid or pseudoameloblastic appearance. In some cases radiographic evidence of a maxillary alveolus-based tumor is helpful in discriminating the ameloblastoma (see Chapter 6).

Poorly differentiated SCC may be difficult to distinguish from basaloid SCC. However, the distinctive pseudoglandular spaces, peripheral palisading of nuclei in nests, and accumulation of basement membrane–type material resembling adenoid cystic carcinoma as well as zones of accompanying conventional SCC are diagnostic of basaloid SCC.

Small cell carcinomas may simulate poorly differentiated keratinizing and nonkeratinizing SCC. Focal squamous differentiation may be common to all entities. However, a combination of diffusely dispersed nuclear chromatin, minimal cytoplasm, nuclear molding, and crush artifact usually identify small cell carcinoma. Immunohistochemical demonstration of neuroendocrine antigens, chromogranin, and synaptophysin also serve to distinguish small cell carcinoma from SCC.

Biologic Behavior

Biologic behavior differs by both site of involvement and histologic type. Nasal carcinomas have a more favorable outcome than those in paranasal sinuses for all carcinoma types. Also, nonkeratinizing carcinomas of both nasal and paranasal sinus sites, which have less of a tendency to metastasize, have more favorable 3- and 5-year survival rates compared with squamous cell and undifferentiated carcinomas (284). This biologic difference based on histology also applied at 3 years to tumors treated by radical surgery and radiation as well as those treated primarily by irradiation (284). A TNM staging classification for extent of tumor spread exists only for carcinoma of the maxillary sinus. The classification of primary tumor extent (T stage) is based on Ohngren's line, a theoretical plane joining the medial canthus of the eye with the angle of the mandible, used to divide the maxillary antrum into the anteroinferior infrastructure and the superoposterior suprastructure (Fig. 48). T1 tumors are those limited to the antral mucosa, with no erosion or destruction of bone; T2 tumors erode or destroy the infrastructure, including the hard palate and/or the middle nasal meatus; T3 tumors invade the skin of the cheek, posterior wall of the maxillary sinus, floor or medial wall of the orbit, or anterior ethmoid sinus; and T4 tumors invade orbital contents and/or the cribriform plate, posterior ethmoid or sphenoid sinuses, nasopharynx, soft palate, pterygomaxillary or temporal fossae, or base of the skull. Most carcinomas of the paranasal sinuses present as advanced T3 and T4 lesions with destruction of bone (285).

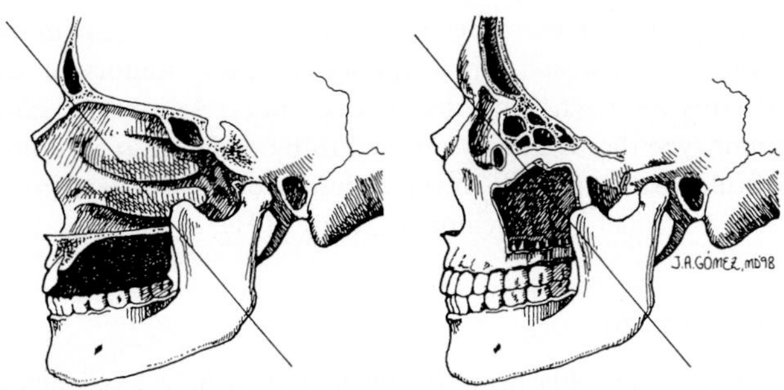

FIGURE 48. Diagram of Ohngren's line demarcating boundary for tumor staging of maxillary sinus carcinomas.

The TNM assessment of regional cervical lymph nodes is the same as for laryngeal carcinomas (286). Only roughly 10% of patients with carcinoma of the nasal cavity and paranasal sinuses have metastatic disease in the neck at presentation, arguing against the need for routine neck dissection and irradiation (287–289).

Nasal Vestibule

Squamous cell carcinomas of the nasal vestibule have overall 3- and 5-year survival rates of 76% and 74%, respectively. This is probably based on easier recognition at an earlier stage and ease of removal of bulky disease. The usual treatment is excision and radiation therapy. Those with localized disease appear to have a good prognosis, despite close or positive margins (273).

Nasal Cavity

Surgery or radiation therapy as well as radium seeds are the potential treatment modalities for SCCs of the nasal cavity, depending on the stage of disease. The average 5-year survival rate for all stages and nasal sites of involvement is 62% (range 4%–80%) (272). Local uncontrolled or recurrent disease is responsible for most deaths.

Maxillary Sinus

Surgery and pre- or postoperative irradiation appears most effective in the treatment of SCCs of the maxillary sinus with 5-year survival rates of 12% to 58% compared with 0 to 28% survival for irradiation alone (272). A 5-year survival rate of 75% has been reported for T3 tumors treated by surgery and postoperative irradiation, with 33% survival in T4 lesions subjected to combined therapy (290). Therapeutic failures are usually due to locally recurrent disease, often of rapid onset (median 4 months) (290). Metastatic disease to cervical lymph nodes is uncommon when the carcinoma is confined within the bony walls of the sinus. Lymph node involvement is more common when there is invasion of regional soft tissues of the pterygopalatine fossa, oral cavity, face, and skin with their associated lymphatics.

Basaloid Squamous Cell Carcinoma

Clinical Data

Basaloid SCC is a histopathologic variant of SCC. It arises more commonly in the base of the tongue, tonsil, larynx, and hypopharynx and is rare in the nasal cavity and nasopharynx (see Chapter 7). In the largest series of 40 cases, 2 were primary in the nasal cavity and nasopharynx (279). Overall, patients presenting with basaloid SCC have a median age of 62 years (range 27–88 years). There is a marked male predominance, and nearly all affected individuals are smokers and drinkers (279).

Histopathologic Features

The features that characterize basaloid SCC from conventional poorly differentiated SCC are the small, anaplastic basaloid cells forming lobules, nests and cribriform patterns, commonly with foci of abrupt squamous differentiation within the nests (Fig. 49). The basaloid cells at the periphery of the nests may exhibit nuclear palisading. Comedo necrosis and single cell necrosis are common in larger nests. Basaloid SCC is usually accompanied by areas of conventional keratinizing SCC or SCC *in situ* of the overlying mucosa. The basaloid cells with scant cytoplasm are anaplastic with moderately pleomorphic nuclei characterized by either densely hyperchromatic or vesicular nuclei and prominent nucleoli. Mitotic figures are numerous. The variable presence of pseudoglandular spaces, reduplicated hyalinized eosinophilic basement membrane material, and myxoid-appearing stroma may mimic adenoid cystic carcinoma (see Chapter 7).

Differential Diagnosis

Poorly differentiated SCC may at times be difficult to distinguish from basaloid SCC. However, the distinctive pseudoglandular spaces, peripheral pallisading of nuclei in nests, and accumulation of basement membrane–type material are more consistent with basaloid SCC.

Sinonasal adenoid cystic carcinomas, even of the solid, high-grade type, lack the degree of nuclear pleomorphism, squamous differentiation, and surface carcinoma *in situ* seen in basaloid SCC. Only the cribriform and pseudoglandular spaces with basement membrane–type material are common to both neoplasms. Again, the tubule formation in adenoid cystic carcinoma is characteristically a double cell layer.

Adenosquamous carcinoma, another rare accessory mucoserous gland carcinoma, is similar to basaloid SCC because of

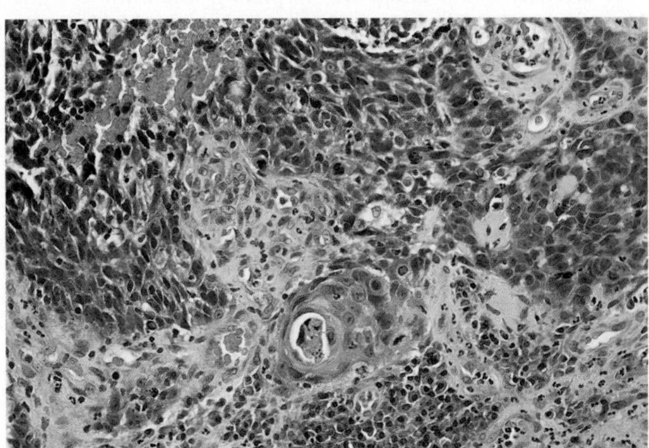

FIGURE 49. Basaloid squamous cell carcinoma. Nests of anaplastic basaloid cells with focal abrupt squamous differentiation.

the presence of surface carcinoma *in situ*, infiltrative conventional SCC, and basaloid cell nests forming gland-like spaces containing mucous cells. However, its histologic appearance more closely mimics mucoepidermoid carcinoma and has a true glandular component (278).

Small cell carcinomas may show focal squamous or glandular differentiation and rosette formation, simulating basaloid SCC. They usually lack surface carcinoma *in situ* and do not demonstrate cribriform patterns with basement membrane–type material. Immunohistochemical demonstration of neuroendocrine antigens, chromogranin, and synaptophysin also serve to distinguish small cell neuroendocrine carcinoma from basaloid carcinoma (279).

Biologic Behavior

There are too few cases of basaloid SCC of the nasal cavity or nasopharynx to assess site-specific biologic behavior. In general, basaloid SCCs of the head and neck are frequently associated with cervical lymph node metastases and present in higher stages III and IV. When corrected for stage of disease, behavior and treatment of basaloid SCC are similar to that of conventional SCC of the head and neck.

NEUROENDOCRINE, NEURAL, AND NEUROECTODERMAL TUMORS

Olfactory Neuroepithelial Neoplasms: Olfactory Neuroblastoma and Neuroendocrine Carcinoma

Tumors arising from the region of the olfactory mucosa constitute a fascinating and diverse group of neoplasms, and the various names applied to members of this group reflect its heterogeneity: olfactory neuroblastoma, neuroendocrine carcinoma, esthesioneuroblastoma, esthesioneurocytoma, esthesioneuroepithelioma, and perhaps even so-called sinonasal undifferentiated carcinoma. Basically, these tumors exhibit a range of neural and epithelial differentiation, from the virtually purely neural to the predominantly epithelial (Fig. 50). This diversity is not altogether surprising when one considers the unique nature of the olfactory mucosa, which contains sensory receptor neurons, epithelial sustentacular cells, and, significantly, basal cells thought to be able to differentiate toward either of the other two types. Thus, the term *neuroendocrine carcinoma,* when applied to these tumors of the olfactory mucosa, most likely does not refer to the same tumor type that is usually referred to by this term (i.e. tumors of Kulchitsky type cells of the diffuse endocrine system in the carcinoid/small cell carcinoma group) (291).

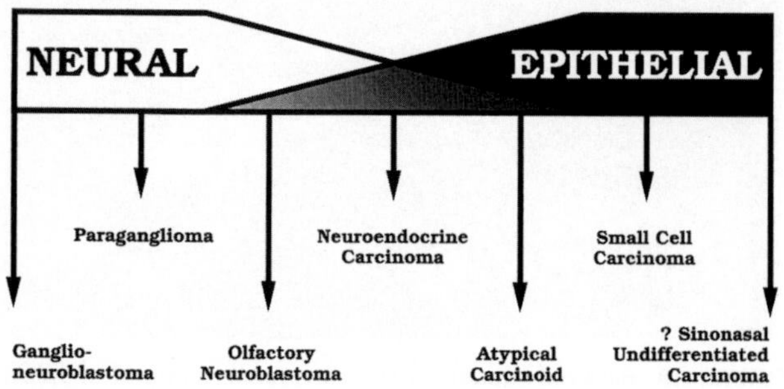

FIGURE 50. Phenotypic spectrum of neuroepithelial neoplasms in the sinonasal tract.

Clinical Data

Olfactory neuroblastoma is considered to be a nasal neural tumor that originates from the olfactory neuroectoderm, as originally suggested by Berger and colleagues in 1924 (292). The olfactory apparatus arises from a neuroectodermal thickening, the olfactory placode, which eventually lines the medial and lateral walls in the upper fifth of the nasal cavity. The neuroectoderm differentiates into the olfactory nerve receptor cells, whose cell bodies remain in the olfactory epithelium and whose nerve fibers penetrate the cribriform plate then enter and synapse with the secondary nerve cells in the olfactory bulb region of the cerebral hemisphere. The olfactory epithelium consists of the ciliated bipolar receptor neurons surrounded by epithelial columnar supporting (or sustentacular) cells with nuclei located at the microvillous cell apex. Both of these cell types lie on a basal cell layer, and it is postulated that this stem cell, the esthesioneuroblast, renews the cell populations (293,294).

Olfactory neuroblastomas occur in all age groups, but display a bimodal peak incidence in the second (16.8%) and sixth (22.8%) decades of life (295,296). They are almost equally distributed in males and females (297), whereas some series report a slightly increased incidence in women (54%) (295,296,298). There is no apparent racial predilection.

The presenting symptoms are most often nasal obstruction and epistaxis. Less frequently there are other rhinologic and ophthalmologic symptoms or facial pain and swelling related to involvement by the nasal tumor (298). These symptoms are progressive and may be present for years.

No predisposing carcinogen is known for olfactory neuroblastomas occurring in humans. Olfactory neuroepithelial tumors with neurosecretory granules, Homer Wright rosettes and Flexner-Wintersteiner rosettes have been induced in rats and hamsters by the administration of nitrosamines (299,300).

Some researchers have proposed classifying olfactory neuroblastoma with the Ewing's sarcoma/peripheral neuroectodermal tumor (PNET) family of tumors based on the finding of chromosome 11:22 reciprocal translocations and *c-myc* but not *N-myc* oncogene expression as well as molecular genetic demonstration of fusion of EWS and FLI1 genomic sequences. This remains controversial, however, because other investigators have found no evidence of the chimeric EWS/FLI1 transcript or the MIC2 antigen (CD 99) characteristic of Ewing's sarcoma (301–304).

Radiologic Studies

Radiographically, the tumors appear as a unilateral soft tissue density within the nose and paranasal sinus and may display focal calcifications, mucosal thickening, or opacification of the sinus or bony destruction of the nasoantral or orbital walls (305).

TABLE 3. HYAMS HISTOLOGIC GRADING SYSTEM FOR OLFACTORY NEUROBLASTOMA

	Grade I	Grade II	Grade III	Grade IV
Cytoarchitecture	Lobular	Lobular	± Lobular	± Lobular
Mitotic rate	0	Low	Moderate	High
Nuclear pleomorphism	None	Slight	Moderate	Marked
Fibrillary matrix	Prominent	Present	Slight	None
Rosettes	± Homer Wright	± Homer Wright	Flexner	None
Necrosis	None	None	Mild	Frequent

±, may or may not be present.

Gross Appearance

Clinically, these tumors are often unilateral, smooth polypoid to fungating, and friable bleeding tumors that vary from soft to hard in consistency and from gray to deep red in color (306). They usually fill the upper nasal cavity in the distribution of the olfactory epithelium along the upper superior turbinate and upper nasal septum and cribriform plate regions. When small, they may involve just the medial or lateral nasal walls (306), but often involve the adjacent paranasal sinuses.

Histologic Features

The variation in histologic appearance of olfactory neural tumors originally resulted in the distinction of three microscopic types that were designated olfactory esthesioneuroepithelioma (292), olfactory esthesioneurocytoma (307), and esthesioneuroblastoma (308). This purely histologic division reflected well-differentiated to poorly differentiated neoplasms with Flexner-Wintersteiner rosettes, Homer Wright rosettes, and no rosettes, respectively. The grading scheme proposed by Hyams is a useful framework to demonstrate the histologic spectrum of these tumors encompassed by the present single designation of olfactory neuroblastoma (Table 3) (295).

Grade I Olfactory Neuroblastoma

The most differentiated tumors display a lobular architecture, with fibrous septa, no necrosis, and variable amounts of calcification (Fig. 51). The tumor cells are small and have uniform round to vesicular nuclei without nucleoli or mitoses. Nuclear chromaticity varies. Cytoplasmic borders are indistinct, and the cells are set in a neurofibrillary matrix (Fig. 52). Neurofibrils in this stroma can sometimes be appreciated in hematoxylin and eosin stains and can be enhanced with silver stains for neuronal processes. With Grimelius stain, black-brown neurosecretory granules can be seen in the cytoplasm. Homer Wright rosettes may or may not be evident. These rosettes are defined as a collar of cells surrounding a central area filled with eosinophilic neurofibrillary material. At times, the stroma can be extremely vascular and edematous to the point of mimicking a vascular neoplasm or a hemangiopericytoma. The vascularity, no doubt, leads to the common clinical symptom of epistaxis.

Grade II Olfactory Neuroblastoma

These tumors retain a lobular architecture, but larger sheets of tumor cells are often present, as are circumscribed tumor nests. There is increased nuclear pleomorphism and hyperchromaticity. Occasional mitotic figures can be identified. A neurofibrillary background is less evident, and occasionally cells have a rim of clear cytoplasm with distinct borders. Similar to grade I tumors, calcification and Homer Wright rosettes may be present and there is no necrosis. Careful observation of circumscribed nests may reveal peripheral encircling nuclei that belong to sustentacular Schwann cells (Fig. 53). These Schwann cells, verified

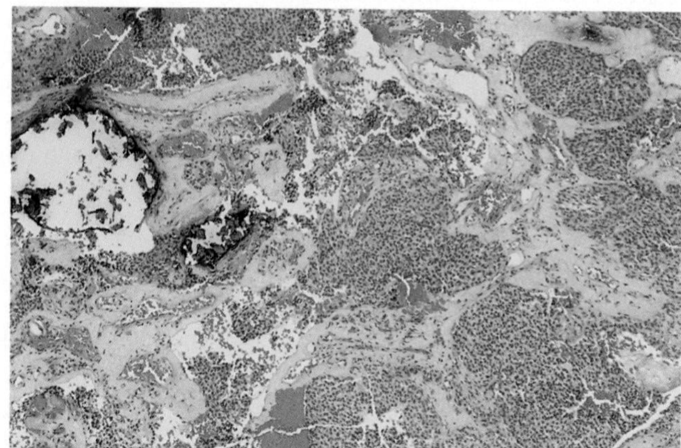

FIGURE 51. Olfactory neuroblastoma. Low-grade tumor with lobular architecture, highly vascular stroma, and calcifications.

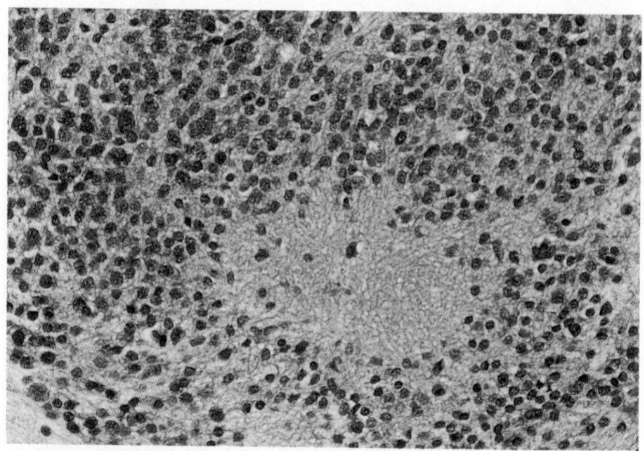

FIGURE 52. Olfactory neuroblastoma. Grade I tumor consists of small cells with relatively bland nuclei in a neurofibrillary matrix.

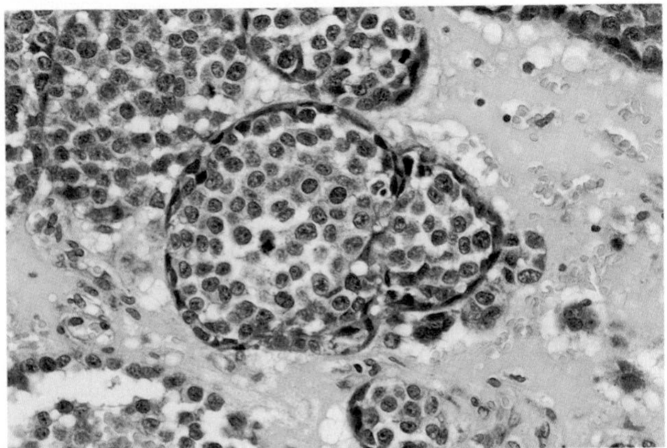

FIGURE 53. Olfactory neuroblastoma. Unusually prominent sustentacular Schwann cells encircle this nest of a cytologic grade II olfactory neuroblastoma.

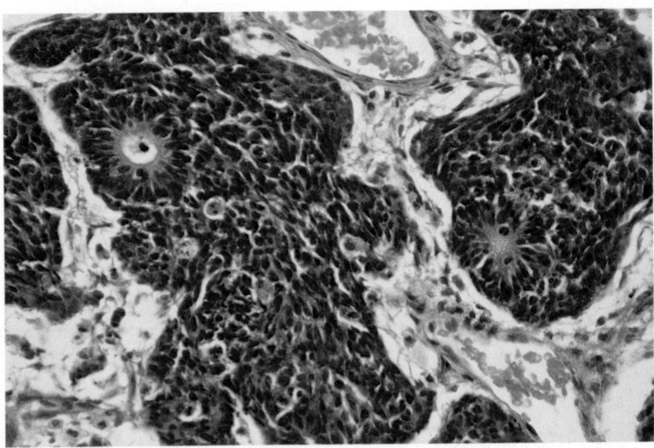

FIGURE 55. Olfactory neuroblastoma. Grade III tumor distinguished by true neural (Flexner-Wintersteiner) rosette on left and more densely hyperchromatic nuclei. Note Homer Wright rosette on right.

by immunoelectron microscopy (309), can be demonstrated with immunohistochemical stains for S-100 protein both at the periphery of cell nests and scattered within sheets of tumor cells (Fig. 54) (309–311). Some tumor nests surround or trap ductal structures of submucosal glands. This occurs most commonly just beneath the mucosal surface, and this appearance of gland-like structures may evoke consideration of a poorly differentiated adenocarcinoma. This intimate association of neuroepithelial tumor cells in the olfactory neuroblastoma family with glands was described by Silva et al. in tumors without a clear neurofibrillary background that they referred to as neuroendocrine carcinomas (312). These ducts can be demonstrated with immunohistochemical stains to cytokeratin. Grade I and II tumors have been designated olfactory esthesioneurocytoma in the older literature (313).

Grade III Olfactory Neuroblastoma

This is a hypercellular tumor with a suggestion of lobular architecture. Nuclei are densely hyperchromatic with readily identifiable mitotic figures. A neurofibrillary matrix is not usually appreciated, and neuronal processes cannot be demonstrated by histochemical stains. Flexner-Wintersteiner rosettes distinguish this tumor from the other variants (Fig. 55). This rosette is defined as a radial array of single nonciliated columnar cells with a basal nucleus forming a true lumen with a cuticular border (297). They are reminiscent of ependymal-type rosettes, but cilia have not been demonstrated by electron microscopic examination. These rosettes also may result in an erroneous diagnosis of adenocarcinoma if mistaken for gland lumina. Calcifications are not seen, but necrosis may be present. Occasionally olfactory neuroblastomas can have true epithelial olfactory rosettes recapitulating the olfactory sense organ (291,312,314).

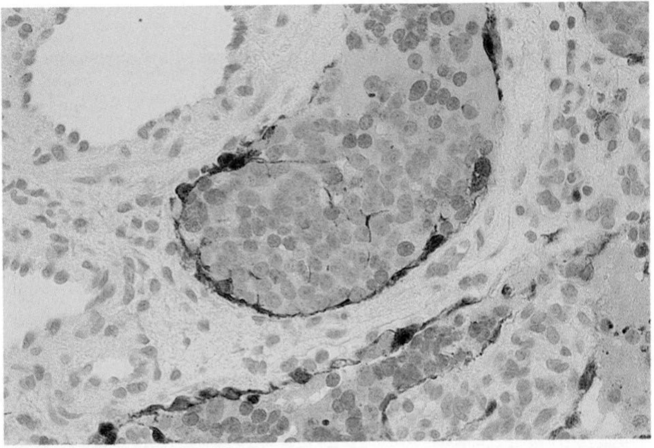

FIGURE 54. Olfactory neuroblastoma. S-100 protein immunostaining accentuates sustentacular cells and dendritic processes at the periphery and within tumor cell nests.

Grade IV Olfactory Neuroblastoma

These are undifferentiated malignancies composed of small to medium-sized cells with hyperchromatic nuclei and a prominent mitotic rate. A lobular architecture may be preserved, but differentiating features such as the neurofibrillary matrix or rosettes are absent. No axons are demonstrable. Necrosis is commonly encountered. In fact, with the exception of a proper anatomic site of involvement, there are no histologic features that confirm olfactory or neural differentiation. This may well be a "grab bag" of poorly differentiated and clinically aggressive malignant neoplasms that are presently difficult to define despite ancillary immunohistochemical and electron microscopic studies (see later section on Biologic Behavior). Perhaps some cases of the so-called sinonasal undifferentiated carcinoma belong among this group of tumors (315).

Unusual Histologic Features

Rare cases of olfactory neuroblastoma have been reported with unusual histologic features that include melanotic pigment (316), foci of adenocarcinoma, ganglioneuroblastoma, and squamous differentiation in a poorly differentiated small cell carcinoma–like component (317).

Special Studies

Immunohistochemistry

Olfactory neuroblastoma, although morphologically distinct from paraganglioma, closely resembles its immunophenotype (Table 4). The use of immunohistochemical profiles may be of some value in differential diagnosis, especially with use of leukocyte common antigen for lymphoma; monotypic cytoplasmic kappa and lambda immunoglobulin light chains for plasmacytoma; desmin, myoglobin, or muscle-specific actin for rhabdomyosarcoma; S-100 protein and HMB-45 for melanoma; and cytokeratins in carcinoma. However, it appears that small cell (undifferentiated) carcinoma may share many neuroendocrine antigens with olfactory neuroblastomas [neurofilament, chromogranin, neuron-specific enolase (NSE)] (310), including several reports of cytokeratin in olfactory neuroblastoma and in olfactory rosettes of neuroblastoma (311,318–320). This may reflect a component of epithelial differentiation in these olfactory neural (or neuroepithelial) tumors, hence Silva and colleagues' subgroup of neuroendocrine carcinoma (312). Distinct immunocytochemical markers to distinguish olfactory neuroblastoma from the nasal neuroendocrine carcinoma described by Silva et al. (312) do not exist, including S-100–positive cells in a supporting Schwann cell distribution (311). The overlap in immunologic antigen-detected profiles of olfactory neuroblastoma and this form of nasal neuroendocrine carcinoma described by Silva et al. may indicate that this separation is arbitrary. In our experience, in small cell carcinomas of the head, neck, and lung, one can consistently demonstrate diffuse low molecular weight cytokeratin immunoreactivity in contrast to our experience with olfactory neuroblastoma (321). The possible cytokeratin peptide immunoprofile in relation to degrees of differentiation in olfactory neuroblastoma is not known at this time and will undoubtedly require confirmation by immunoblot experiments. At present, the presence of an organized rim of S-100 protein–positive supporting cells in lower grades of olfactory neuroblastoma in conjunction with synaptophysin positivity and negative staining for CD99 (MIC-2 gene product) detected by antibodies 12E7, HBA71, or ON13 may help in the distinction from pediatric neuroblastomas, small cell carcinoma, peripheral neuroepithelioma, rhabdomyosarcoma, lymphoma, and Ewing's sarcoma (319,322–324). These differentiating features may not apply in grade IV olfactory neuroblastomas, and discrimination from small cell (undifferentiated) carcinoma may not be possible because even electron microscopic demonstration of cytoplasmic neurosecretory granules may not resolve difficult cases.

A single study has suggested that a higher incidence of S-100 protein–positive cells and a low Ki-67 labeling index of less than 10% may correlate with survival (320).

Electron Microscopy

Ultrastructural examination of olfactory neuroblastomas with prominent neural differentiation reveals tumor cells with neuritic processes, microtubules, neurofilaments, and dense core granules (100–200 nm) located in the cell body and neuritic processes (Fig. 56) (325). An acinar space containing a bulbous expansion resembling the terminal end of an immature olfactory vesicle with microvilli has been reported as a feature supporting olfactory receptor differentiation in some cases (314,318). This may correspond to the presence of olfactory rosettes seen on light microscopy in some cases. True olfactory vesicles, however, display surface olfactory cilia (293). Curiously, Schwann cells are consistently noted at the periphery of cell nests by EM and with immunohistochemical stains for S-100 protein in the better differentiated tumors. The presence of S-100 protein–positive Schwann cells forming a continuous peripheral network around clusters of tumor cells in olfactory neuroblastoma is similar to the presence of supporting Schwann cells in normal paraganglia and paragangliomas (309).

Differential Diagnosis

The histologic features of olfactory neuroblastomas of grades I to III are sufficiently characteristic to be diagnostic without ancillary studies. Immunohistochemistry or electron microscopy is usually necessary to differentiate a primitive olfactory neuroblastoma from the more common poorly differentiated SCC or adenocarcinoma, lymphoma, plasmacytoma, amelanotic melanoma, and the more rare rhabdomyosarcoma and Ewing's sarcoma (Table 4). Careful attention to the nature of the rosettes and involvement of entrapped minor salivary gland ducts is useful in discriminating olfactory neuroblastoma from adenocarcinoma.

Biologic Behavior

Olfactory neuroblastoma is a locally aggressive tumor that most commonly invades the paranasal sinuses, orbit, base of the skull, and cranial cavity. Using the Kadish staging system, our review of the literature found that 30% of tumors were confined to the nasal cavity (stage A), 42% had involvement of one or more paranasal sinuses (stage B), and 28% had local extension into other surrounding structures or cervical lymph node metastasis at presentation (stage C).

Distant blood-borne metastatic disease accounted for only 1.3% of the reviewed cases at presentation. Unusual distant sites of metastasis have been reported (298), but the most common are cervical lymph nodes, bone, and lungs (297,306). Multiple local recurrences are not uncommon and may relate to either inadequate surgical excision or multicentricity (326). Some tumor recurrences are rapid and lethal, whereas others are slow and progressive with patients surviving for many years. Fifty percent to seventy percent of patients develop local recurrence, and 20% to 30% eventually develop distant metastasis (296). Local recurrences have been reported with disease-free intervals up to 17 years (326), and 10-year intervals to metastasis also have been reported (327). Prolonged follow-up is required because of the possibility of late recurrence and metastasis even after 5 years. Seventy-six percent of patients dying of disease do so within the first 3 years, resulting in a 5-year determinate survival of 90%, 70.8%, and 46.7% for Kadish stages A, B, and C, respectively.

The survival rates of the 20 patients with nasal neuroendocrine carcinomas reported by Silva and colleagues were 100% at 5 years, 88% at 7 years, and 67% at 10 years. Recurrences and

TABLE 4. IMMUNOHISTOCHEMICAL DIFFERENTIAL DIAGNOSIS OF SINONASAL TUMORS (FORMALIN FIXED, PARAFIN EMBEDDED TISSUES)

Tumor Type	CK/EMA	Vimentin	GFAP	S-100	HMB-45	Synapto	Chromog	Desmin	Mus actin	CD99	Factor 8	CD34	LCA	Monotypic Ig
Undifferentiated carcinoma														
Small cell carcinoma														
Olfactory neuroblastoma		S	S	S										
Paraganglioma			S	S										
Pituitary tumor														
Melanoma														
Ewing's sarcoma/PNET														
Rhabdomyosarcoma														
Angiosarcoma														
Hemangiopericytoma														
Solitary fibrous tumor														
Fibrous histiocytoma														
Fibrosarcoma														
Nerve sheath tumor														
Synovial sarcoma														
Meningioma	EMA													
Lymphoma										*				
Plasmacytoma														

CK/EMA, cytokeratin/epithelial membrane antigen; GFAP, glial fibrillary acidic protein; Synapto, Synaptophysin; Chromog, chromogranin; Mus actin, muscle actin; LCA, leucocyte common antigen; Ig, immunoglobulin; S, sustentacular cells; *, lymphoblastic lymphoma.
Dark box, characteristic, strong staining; light box, weak, focal or <10% staining.

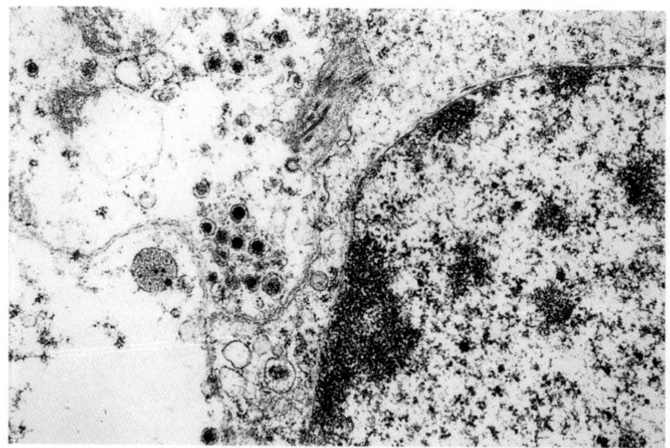

FIGURE 56. Olfactory neuroblastoma. In addition to neuritic processes and microtubules, dense core granules (100–200 nm) are seen on ultrastructural examination. (Courtesy Dr. H. Battifora.)

metastasis in 70% of the patients occurred later than the third year. This is similar to the clinical course of olfactory neuroblastoma, which these cases resemble morphologically.

Many studies of olfactory neuroblastoma, all with fewer than 30 tumors, have shown that histologic features of olfactory neural tumors do not appear to be significant in predicting prognosis. Examination of the limited data presented in 1983 by Hyams assessing 46 tumors from the Armed Forces Institute of Pathology (AFIP) Registry shows an apparent correlation of tumor grade with prognosis. In that analysis of patients treated by surgical excision and radiation therapy, none of six patients with grade I tumors died of disease, 3 of 25 (12%) of those with grade II tumors, 6 of 11 (55%) with grade III, and all 4 patients with grade IV tumors died of disease (295). However, in 1993, investigators from the Mayo Clinic documented no significant survival differences among patients with grade I, II, or III tumors (328). Hyams' original data and the more recent study of 49 tumors from the Mayo Clinic reveal that only the grade IV tumors are associated with a uniformly poor prognosis that supersedes the significance of tumor stage (295,328). The fact that these undifferentiated grade IV tumors are exceedingly difficult to distinguish from other small cell malignancies of the region should not be lost on the reader. Because most olfactory neuroblastomas are of the readily recognizable histologic types, there does not appear to be much value for grade in predicting outcome, with the exception of identifying the anaplastic grade IV malignancies.

Craniofacial resection is presently the preferred surgical therapy (329). Surgery alone appears to be effective for low-grade, low-stage tumors when free margins are obtainable. Postoperative adjuvant radiation therapy is considered in low-grade tumors with close margins and for residual or recurrent disease, and has been shown capable of improving local control, especially in high-grade, high stage tumors (328,330). Because of the overall 5-year survival rate of approximately 50% and difficulty in local control, addition of adjuvant chemotherapy for advanced stages and metastatic disease has been attempted, with some complete and partial remissions reported (328,331,332).

Small Cell Carcinoma and Allied Tumors

Clinical Data

Oat cell-like small cell undifferentiated carcinoma arising in the paranasal sinuses was first described by Raychoudhuri in 1965. Other cases exhibiting a spectrum of neuroendocrine differentiation from classic small (oat) cell, intermediate cell, and large cell (atypical carcinoid-like) tumors have since been reported arising in the nose and paranasal sinuses (333–337). Summarizing the demographic data from these studies, there was an equal gender distribution with an age range of 26 to 82 years at diagnosis. The mean age of involvement was similar for nasal tumors (45 years) and for paranasal tumors (50 years). Some of these tumors are believed to be derived from submucosal accessory mucoserous glands from diverse sites in the nasal cavity and paranasal sinuses. Although there is a significant association of cigarette smoking with laryngeal small cell carcinomas, little is known of the predisposing factors for these neuroendocrine malignancies of the nasal cavity and paranasal sinuses.

Histologic Features

The small cell carcinoma/atypical carcinoid group of the upper respiratory tract is a morphologically heterogeneous group of tumors composed of a spectrum of cell types. A minority are capable of divergent differentiation and have composite features with foci of SCC or adenocarcinoma admixed with the undifferentiated component. Histologically, these are submucosal proliferations that grow as sheets, nests, and ribbons of carcinoma. The histologic variants of neuroendocrine carcinoma are similar to the small (oat) cell, intermediate cell, and atypical carcinoid-type carcinomas of the lower respiratory tract. Those with the smaller oat-like cells have round to ovoid nuclei with minimal cytoplasm and nuclei with dispersed chromatin. The nuclear features of an individual case are influenced by tissue preservation and fixation, and tumor nuclei in less than optimally fixed or preserved specimens may appear more hyperchromatic. In general, the chromatin is finely dispersed and nucleoli are absent in these small cell variants. Sheets of tumor composed of spindled cells are not uncommon. In some of the intermediate cell variants, the tumor cells are larger and the nuclei have stippled to coarse chromatin and occasional small nucleoli. These intermediate cells have a small amount of cytoplasm. In both variants, tumor necrosis, individual cell necrosis, and mitotic figures are frequent (Fig. 57A). The atypical carcinoid-like proliferations are composed of larger cells with a range of nuclear pleomorphism and nucleolar size. They have a moderate amount of granular cytoplasm with ill-defined borders and are arranged in solid nests with fibrovascular stroma forming alveolar structures.

Special Studies

Immunohistochemistry

Neurosecretory granules can rarely be demonstrated in any variant with argyrophil or argentaffin stains. Although all of these carcinomas should contain cytokeratin (Fig. 57B), immunohistochemical markers of neuroendocrine differentiation such as

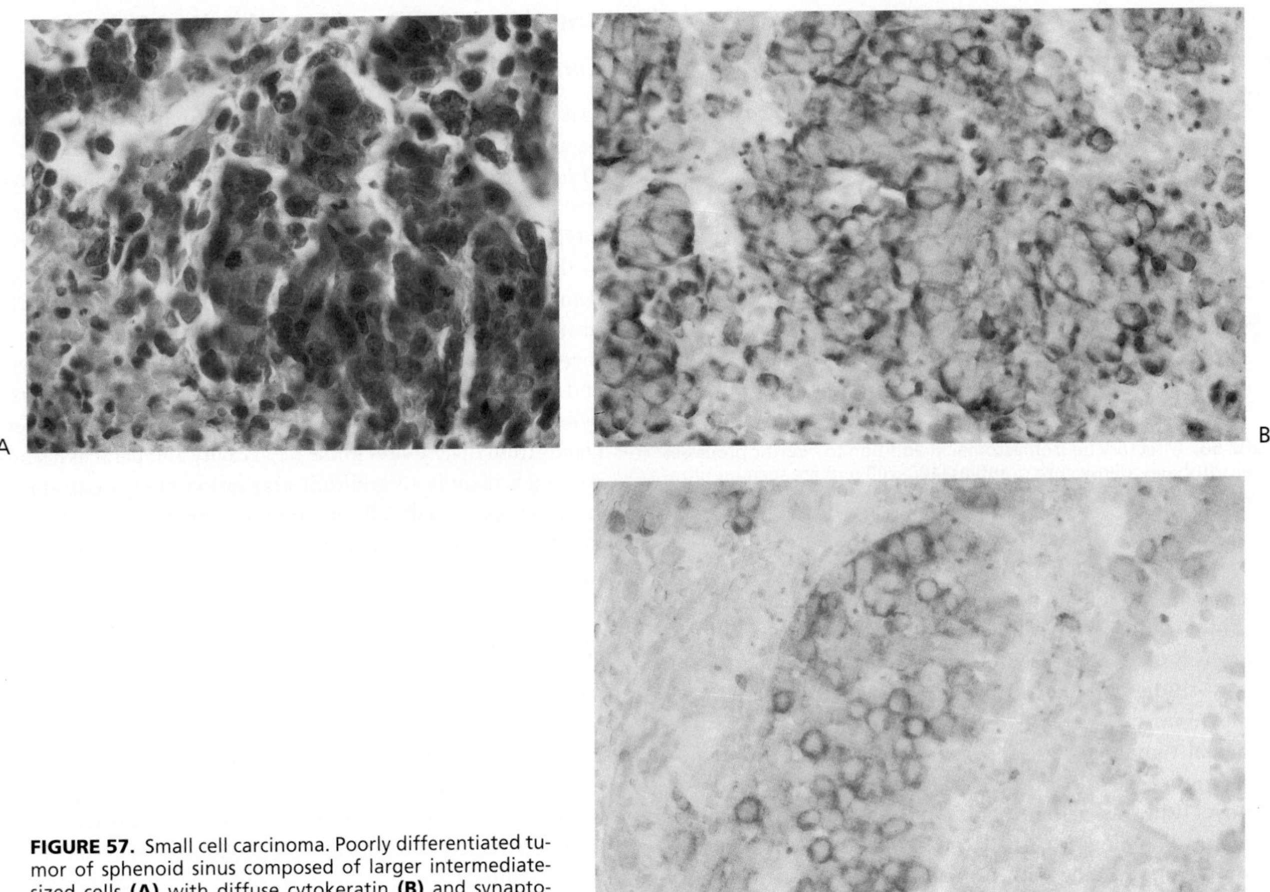

FIGURE 57. Small cell carcinoma. Poorly differentiated tumor of sphenoid sinus composed of larger intermediate-sized cells **(A)** with diffuse cytokeratin **(B)** and synaptophysin immunoreactivity **(C)**.

chromogranin or synaptophysin (Fig. 57C) are often negative in the small cell variants.

Electron Microscopy

By electron microscopy the majority of these neuroendocrine carcinomas contain dense core neurosecretory granules, detected more readily in the tumors bearing more cytoplasm. The characteristic dense core neurosecretory granules range in size from 100 to 380 nm. However, not all small cell carcinomas can be shown to contain neurosecretory granules by ultrastructural examination. Even in the prototypic pulmonary small cell carcinomas, neurosecretory granules are absent in roughly 11% of cases (338). Ultrastructurally, small cell carcinomas with neuroendocrine differentiation also may have small primitive intercellular junctions, dispersed cytoplasmic filaments, and rare bundles of tonofilaments. Some cells may have squamous features with well-formed desmosomes, intracytoplasmic tonofilaments, and even tripartite glandular, squamous, and neuroendocrine differentiation within the same cell (339–341).

Differential Diagnosis

The histologic typing of neuroendocrine carcinomas can be extremely difficult. These diagnoses are often made only after extensive use of the ancillary diagnostic techniques of immunohistochemistry and electron microscopy. The morphologic differential diagnosis usually includes poorly differentiated SCC or adenocarcinoma, olfactory neuroblastoma, and malignant paraganglioma.

The discrimination of small cell undifferentiated carcinoma from poorly differentiated SCC or adenocarcinoma can be extremely difficult, if not impossible, especially in composite carcinomas with mixed squamous and glandular phenotypic differentiation at the ultrastructural level. Demonstration of a morphologically characteristic small cell component with or without neuroendocrine differentiation by immunohistochemical staining or by electron microscopy is imperative.

Small cell carcinomas may infrequently form rosettes and may be difficult to distinguish from poorly differentiated olfactory neuroblastomas (grade IV). The high-grade neuroblastomas usually lack S-100 protein–positive Schwann cells and a fibrillary neuropil stroma and may have moderately pleomorphic cells, similar to small cell undifferentiated carcinoma. Common to both are the presence of neuroendocrine markers, which are therefore not helpful in the discrimination of the neural differentiation of olfactory neuroblastoma from the neuroendocrine differentiation of small cell undifferentiated carcinoma. Theoretically, all carcinomas should contain cytokeratin filaments, but some olfactory neural tumors are also reported to stain for cytokeratin. This is not our experience, however, and we would interpret a small cell malignant neoplasm with appropriate nuclear features and diffuse, strong cytokeratin immunoreactivity to be a small cell undifferentiated carcinoma, regardless of the lack of neuroendocrine marker differentiation by immunohistochemistry or electron microscopy.

Sinonasal paragangliomas exhibit the characteristic prominent *Zellballen* arrangement of polygonal to spindled cells without significant pleomorphism that is rimmed by S-100 protein–containing sustentacular cells. However, malignant paragangliomas demonstrating locally destructive, recurrent, and metastatic disease show weak or absent staining for neuroendocrine markers such as NSE and chromogranin and a marked reduction to absent S-100 protein staining of sustentacular cells (342). Therefore, these malignant tumors may be exceedingly difficult to discriminate from sinonasal neuroendocrine carcinomas because both demonstrate neurosecretory granules by electron microscopy. The great majority of paragangliomas are keratin negative immunohistochemically, and this feature may be a helpful differential diagnostic aid.

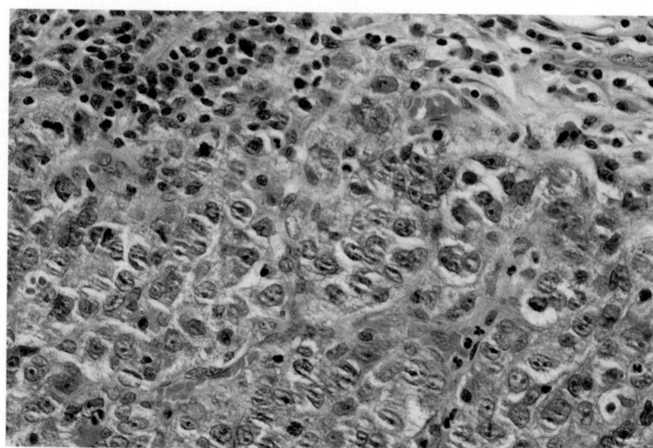

FIGURE 58. Undifferentiated carcinoma. Sheets of polygonal cells with marked nuclear pleomorphism and prominent nucleoli lacking squamous or glandular differentiation.

Biologic Behavior

Neuroendocrine carcinomas of the nasal cavity and paranasal sinuses appear to have a more favorable prognosis than morphologically similar laryngeal and pulmonary carcinomas. However, based on the relatively few reports of these tumors, there does not appear to be any significant value in discriminating the histologic neuroendocrine carcinoma variants (e.g., small cell from carcinoid-like) of the sinonasal region because all types have exhibited locally aggressive and metastatic behavior (333–337).

There is a propensity for multiple recurrences, and some carcinomas are capable of both early and late, often widespread metastases. Many patients have died of disease in less than 1 year, although some have died in 6 to 10 years after suffering numerous recurrences (333,335,337). Most deaths are due to local failure and intracranial extension. Complete surgical excision in conjunction with chemotherapy and radiation therapy is the recommended treatment (333).

Undifferentiated (Anaplastic) Carcinoma

Clinical Data

Sinonasal undifferentiated or anaplastic carcinomas are uncommon, highly aggressive neoplasms that are often difficult to diagnose and likely related to the previously described neuroendocrine carcinomas. They arise over a broad age range of 20 to 82 years, with a slight female predilection. The symptom duration is usually short, typically with swelling of the nasal cavity or face, proptosis, diplopia, paresthesia, and cervical lymphadenopathy. Most patients present in advanced stages with erosion of bone and invasion of adjacent structures, such as the paranasal sinuses, nasopharynx, orbit, and cranial cavity (343–345).

Histopathologic Features

These tumors are composed of medium-sized polygonal cells with moderate to marked nuclear pleomorphism and prominent nucleoli (Fig. 58). Growth patterns include nests, trabeculae, ribbons, and sheets with a vague organoid pattern but rare cord-like patterns of infiltration (281,344). Mitoses are readily identified but are rarely numerous. No mucin but cytoplasmic glycogen may be demonstrated. Tumor necrosis, apoptosis, and vascular invasion are common. The stroma is fibrous, and a prominent lymphoid reaction is not seen. Nearly all undifferentiated carcinomas stain for cytokeratin or epithelial membrane antigen (EMA) (343,345). Some undifferentiated carcinomas may have a neuroendocrine phenotype, reacting with antibodies to NSE and showing rare, single dense core granules by electron microscopy (281).

Differential Diagnosis

Because of the undifferentiated nature of this carcinoma, the differential diagnosis may be broad. It is most often confused with poorly differentiated SCC, but adenocarcinoma, undifferentiated carcinoma of the nasopharyngeal type (lymphoepithelioma), small cell carcinoma, lymphoma, melanoma, rhabdomyosarcoma, olfactory neuroblastoma, and neuroendocrine carcinoma also may be considered. Pertinent negative light microscopic findings are helpful in the differential diagnosis and include lack of even focal squamous or glandular differentiation, the syncytia and uniform vesicular nuclei of lymphoepithelioma, melanin pigment of melanoma, rosettes and fibrillary intercellular matrix of olfactory neuroblastoma, and the uniform small densely hyperchromatic or diffuse nuclei and indiscernible nucleoli of small cell carcinoma. An immunohistochemical battery of stains is most appropriate for this entity to exclude many of the other undifferentiated mimics listed above. One can anticipate that future studies will show overlap with those tumors capable of a neuroepithelial phenotype (Table 4).

Biologic Behavior

Sinonasal undifferentiated carcinoma has an extremely poor prognosis with a median survival of 4 months to 1 year and a crude 5-year survival rate of 15.5% (343–345). It is rarely resectable because of the advanced stages at presentation and is therefore treated by radiation therapy or chemotherapy. A worse prognosis is associated with paranasal sinus rather than nasal-based primary sites, and a positive neck or orbital invasion at presentation (343,344).

Paraganglioma

Clinical Data

Paragangliomas arising in the nasal cavity and paranasal sinuses are rare. It has been postulated that these neuroectodermal tumors arise from the nodose ganglion of the vagus nerve at the skull base or from paraganglionic tissue in the pterygopalatine fossa (346). But this does not explain the origin of these tumors in the middle turbinates and ethmoid sinuses.

Incomplete demographic data accompany the 23 cases reported to date, so there is little to summarize clinically. The 12 benign nasal cavity and 11 paranasal sinus–based paragangliomas have occurred over a wide age range of 8 to 89 years, affecting females slightly more than males (1.5:1) (347–349). Symptoms have included pulsating nasal mass, airway obstruction, epistaxis, and frontal headache. One case of Cushing's syndrome resulting from ectopic adrenocorticotrophic hormone production by a paraganglioma of the sinuses has been reported (350).

Nasal tumors have arisen commonly from the middle turbinate–lateral nasal wall or the high nasal vault (347,351,352). They have ranged from 1.5 to 4 cm in greatest dimension (352,353). Paranasal sinus tumors have arisen most often in the ethmoid sinuses but also in the maxillary and sphenoid sinuses (347).

Gross Appearance

Nasal paragangliomas have been described as polypoid vascularized masses, one noted to be broad based (352,353). They are spongy on section with lobules separated by thin connective tissue septa. One of the malignant paragangliomas was locally aggressive, invading bone and soft tissue (354).

Histopathologic Features

All sinonasal paragangliomas have been characterized by the typical *Zellballen* small groupings of uniform rounded to spindled cells separated by a delicate fibrovascular framework (Fig. 59). The benign nasal tumors have shown no significant pleomorphism. Malignant paranasal cavity tumors have been described as both cytologically bland and pleomorphic (347,354). As in paragangliomas in other body sites, the presence of nuclear atypia and mitotic activity are not consistent indicators of malignancy, although morphologically, malignant paragangliomas of the head and neck tend to show mitotic figures, foci of necrosis, and vascular invasion (352). Diagnosis of malignant sinonasal paraganglioma is best reserved for tumors that demonstrate invasion of bone or distant metastases.

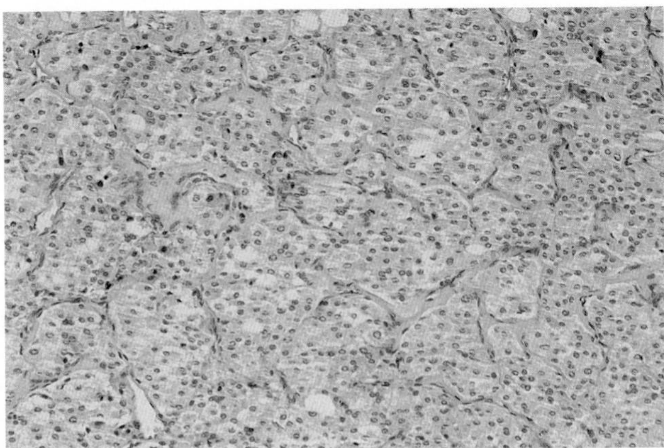

FIGURE 59. Paraganglioma. Typical small *Zellballen* groupings of uniform rounded to spindled cells in a delicate fibrovascular framework.

Special Studies

The neuroendocrine nature of the tumor is evident in cytoplasmic silver staining of argyrophilic granules and ultrastructural demonstration of dense core neurosecretory granules ranging in diameter from 120 to 200 nm (352). In our experience, the chief cells consistently immunostain for NSE, synaptophysin, and chromogranin. Cytokeratin has been detected in 10% of paragangliomas from other head and neck sites but as yet is not described in sinonasal paragangliomas (355).

In the benign tumors, chief cell nests are typically rimmed by S-100 protein and GFAP-containing sustentacular cells. However, malignant and aggressive recurrent paragangliomas show weak or absence of staining for neuroendocrine markers such as NSE and chromogranin and a marked reduction to absence of S-100 protein staining of sustentacular cells (342). These malignant paragangliomas may be exceedingly difficult to discriminate from sinonasal neuroendocrine carcinomas because both demonstrate neurosecretory granules by electron microscopy. Immunohistochemical staining for keratin may be helpful.

Differential Diagnosis

The round to spindle cell morphology, highly vascular nature, and sinonasal location of these tumors raises a broad histologic differential diagnosis, including olfactory neuroblastoma, meningioma, hemangiopericytoma, angiosarcoma, spindle cell sarcoma, and poorly differentiated SCC. With the exception of olfactory neuroblastoma, a neuroendocrine phenotype, demonstrable immunologically even in distorted biopsy samples, distinguishes paraganglioma. Although olfactory neuroblastoma and paraganglioma have a similar immunophenotype (i.e., NSE, synaptophysin, and chromogranin-positive chief cells and S-100 protein–positive sustentacular cells), the morphologic growth patterns of the variants of olfactory neuroblastoma with larger tumor nests, neuropil, and rosettes are distinct, as detailed previously.

Biologic Behavior

Of the 12 nasal paragangliomas that we have reviewed, all have been benign and never metastasized, although some have recurred, one of them up to six times (342,352). Three of eleven paranasal sinus paragangliomas have been malignant. Two tumors metastasized to brain and one metastasized to numerous skeletal bones after a prolonged clinical course requiring numerous surgeries for recurrences (347,351,354). One of these tumors was also locally aggressive, recurring, despite medial maxillectomy, to invade the floor of the orbit and soft tissue of the cheek as well (354). All three malignant sinus-based paragangliomas have been fatal.

The primary treatment of sinonasal paraganglioma is complete surgical excision. This may be difficult because of the location and vascular nature of the tumor. However, incomplete removal contributes to local recurrence. Radiation therapy may play a role in slowing tumor growth and rate of recurrence (356). Chemotherapy has been ineffective (347).

Malignant Melanoma

Clinical Data

Primary malignant melanoma of the sinonasal tract is rare, accounting for approximately 1% of all malignant melanomas and representing 18% of the noncarcinomatous malignancies of the region in the Birmingham Regional Cancer Registry (258,357,358). Metastatic melanoma to the sinonasal region is even more rarely seen as a consequence of disseminated disease, originating in a variety of cutaneous sites, at 5.5 years after initial diagnosis on average (359,360).

Malignant melanoma more commonly arises in the nasal cavity than in the paranasal sinuses, where it comprises 2.4% of all nasal malignancies (258). In the sinonasal tract, the anatomic sites of origin in descending order of frequency are nasal septum, lateral nasal wall, middle and inferior turbinates, nasal vestibule, maxillary sinus, and ethmoid sinus (361,362). Malignant melanoma involving the frontal and sphenoid sinuses is seen more commonly as a direct extension rather than as a primary site of origin (363–365).

The age range of onset is broad, without sex predilection. Most cases arise in the fifth to seventh decades of life (358,362). Nasal obstruction, epistaxis, or a black nasal discharge are the usual complaints.

Gross Appearance

The usual appearance is that of a sessile or polypoid mass, often grossly necrotic or hemorrhagic. The gross presence of melanin pigment is variable and often not evident on clinical examination (366).

Histologic Features

As in melanomas from other sites, there may be considerable histologic diversity (367). Cell types observed in sinonasal melanomas are small blue, spindle shaped, epithelioid, and pleomorphic (368) (Fig. 60A). A botryoid variant with myxoid stroma also has been described in this site (369). The majority of melanomas from this region have cytologic melanin pigment, making for a ready morphologic diagnosis (358,368). Unlike melanomas from cutaneous sites, other morphologic clues in the case of amelanotic melanoma are seldom found. These are large, ulcerated tumors at presentation, so junctional involvement is seen only in about one third of cases (368).

Special Studies

The same histochemical and immunohistochemical approach to the undifferentiated malignant neoplasm of any site applies in the case of amelanotic malignant melanoma arising in this region. Fontana-Masson argentaffin silver stain may demonstrate melanin pigment. This technique has largely been replaced by the immunohistochemical demonstration of S-100 protein and melanoma-associated antigen detected by antibody HMB-45 (Fig. 60B). Spindled melanomas are more apt to be negative for both of these markers. Melanomas should stain very strongly for vimentin; some also may demonstrate cytokeratin staining, but usually not to the same degree as carcinomas (370). Cases with

A
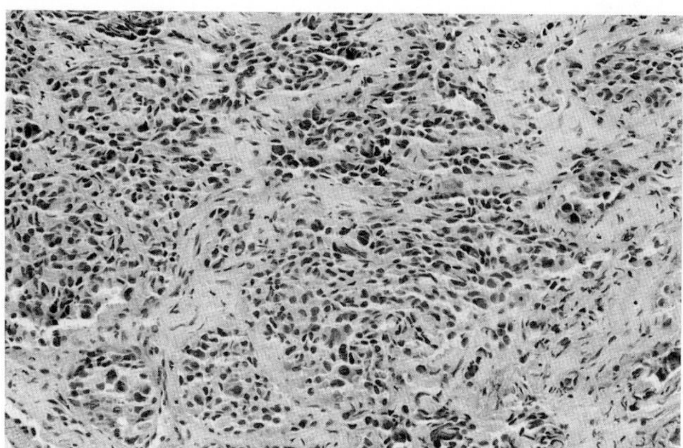

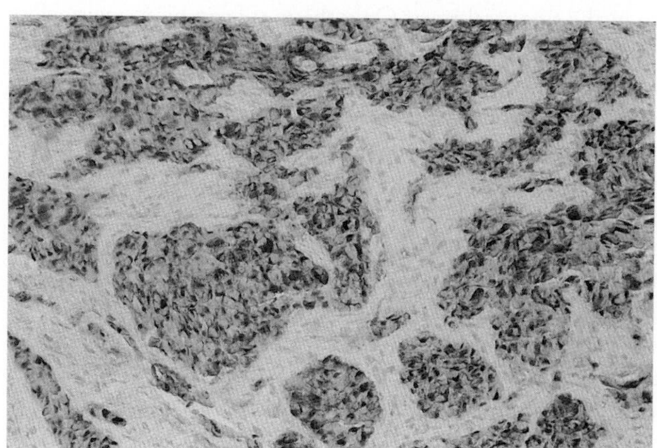
B

FIGURE 60. Malignant melanoma. **A:** Epithelioid malignant melanoma of nasal cavity. **B:** Immunohistochemical demonstration of melanoma-associated antigen detected by antibody HMB-45 (more specific but less sensitive than S-100 protein).

anomalous staining may be diagnosed by ultrastructural demonstration of premelanosomes, even when tissue is retrieved from paraffin blocks.

Differential Diagnosis

The diverse histomorphology, especially when the tumor is amelanotic, raises the usual broad differential of carcinoma, lymphoma, and sarcoma. In this region, the small cell variant evokes the possibility of olfactory neuroblastoma and rhabdomyosarcoma. The myxoid botryoid variant also mimics embryonal rhabdomyosarcoma. This wide differential may be resolved with an immunohistochemical battery of stains (Table 4). In the cases of olfactory neuroblastoma and paraganglioma it is worthy to note that the S-100 protein immunoreactivity is present in the sustentacular cells at the periphery of tumor cell nests and not in the tumor chief cells proper.

Biologic Behavior

These are highly aggressive neoplasms even when detected at an early clinical stage, with a very poor 5-year disease-free survival rate of 25% and a median survival of 18.5 months to 2 years (365,368,371). Nasal and sinus cavity tumors have a high recurrence rate of 40% (361). Aggressive surgical resection is the primary treatment, but despite clear margins, both local recurrence and distant metastasis may occur late in the course of disease (371). Sites of regional spread include the orbit, infratemporal space, parotid gland, and intracranial cavity (361). Immunotherapy, radiation therapy, and chemotherapy are used as palliative measures for disseminated disease with no significant impact on survival. One study has shown a correlation between tumor thickness of less than 7 mm and 3-year disease-free survival, but in general, neither depth of invasion nor size have been shown to be helpful prognosticators (371).

MESENCHYMAL TUMORS

A great number of benign and malignant soft tissue tumors may arise in the sinonasal tract. Only the more common, regionally unique, or diagnostically challenging tumors are addressed in detail in this chapter.

We will only mention that the following benign soft tissue tumors can occur in the sinonasal tract: leiomyoma arising in nasal polyps (372), lipoma of the maxillary sinus (373), chondroma of the nasal septum (374,375), ivory osteoma of the frontal and ethmoid sinus (376–380), and chordoma (a malignant neoplasm) (381–383). The benign skeletal muscle tumor, rhabdomyoma, of both the fetal and adult types, has been reported in the nasopharynx (384). The craniofacial bones of the sinonasal tract are also involved by fibrous dysplasia, ossifying fibroma, giant cell tumor, and osteoblastoma, described further in Chapter 11 (376,385–391).

The sarcomas that can arise in the sinonasal tract, not further detailed in this chapter, include leiomyosarcoma (372,392), synovial sarcoma (393), malignant schwannoma (394,395), liposarcoma (373), chondrosarcoma (374), and osteosarcoma (376) (see Chapters 10 and 11).

Vascular Tumors

The complete range of vascular proliferations, from developmental malformations and hamartomas to benign, borderline, and malignant tumors, can involve the sinonasal tract.

Angiomatous hamartomas (arteriovenous anomaly) and diffuse congenital angiomatosis rarely involve the sinonasal tract (396). They occur most often in bone, especially in the maxillary sinus. Hemangiomas of the cavernous and venous type are less common than the lobular capillary hemangiomas of the septum; tend to involve the turbinates, as well as the maxillary and sphenoid sinuses; and may be invasive within bone (396,397). Angiofibromas involve the nasopharynx and are discussed in Chapter 5. Glomus tumors may rarely present in the nasal cavity, especially on the septum (396,398). Kaposi's sarcoma in the head and neck rarely occurs in the sinonasal tract (399), more commonly involving the oral and oropharyngeal mucosa. Angiosarcoma is likewise rare in the sinonasal tract (397,400,401). Lobular capillary hemangioma and low-grade hemangiopericytoma (hemangiopericytoma-like tumor) are two distinct but often problematic vascular lesions of the sinonasal tract that are addressed here in detail.

Lobular Capillary Hemangioma (Pyogenic Granuloma)

Clinical Data

Lobular capillary hemangioma, the underlying proliferation of pyogenic granuloma, may involve the nasal cavity, usually the anterior nasal septum, followed by the turbinates and nasal vestibule. Typical clinical associations are male predilection (82%) when it arises in those under 18 years of age and pregnancy (granuloma gravidarum), skewing the demographics to a female predilection (86%) in the reproductive years (402). A bleeding episode is the usual presentation.

Gross Appearance

This is a raised or polypoid mucosal mass, often with surface ulceration.

Histologic Features

Biopsy sampling and age of the lesion influence the histologic appearance. The underlying process is that of a capillary hemangioma with a lobular architectural pattern with larger feeding vessels often in the center of the lobules (Fig. 61). The proliferation may be either cellular packed endothelial and spindled cells with minimal vascular lumen formation or more dilated typical capillary spaces or a mixture of both. Mitotic figures may be common, but atypical mitoses are not seen. Surface ulceration results in granulation tissue, edema, and acute inflammation. Larger vascular spaces may undergo organization of thrombi at times in the pattern of papillary endothelial hyperplasia. Older lesions may show sclerosis of the stroma with a less pronounced lobular vascular proliferation (Fig. 62).

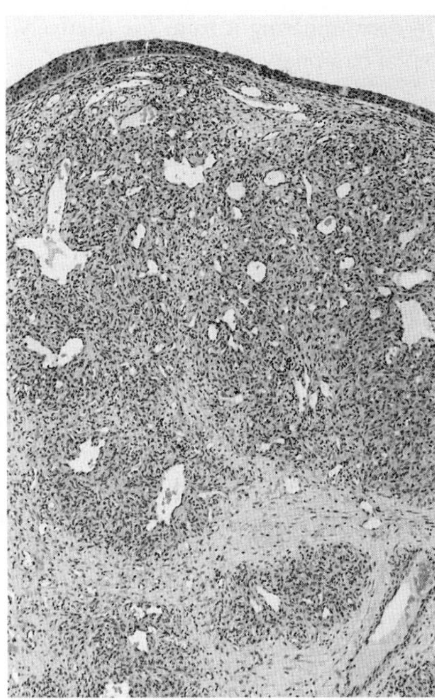

FIGURE 61. Lobular capillary hemangioma. Low-power demonstration of the lobular architectural proliferation of small capillary spaces in this nasal lesion.

Special Studies

Immunohistochemistry is usually not indicated for diagnosis. Much of the cellular proliferation will mark with vascular-associated antigens, Factor VIII, CD31, and CD34. The spindled cells stain for muscle-specific actin, reflecting their pericytic nature (403).

Differential Diagnosis

The marked cellularity and mitotic activity may raise the specter of angiosarcoma. But the lobular pattern of this capillary hemangioma, appreciated best at low power, and lack of anaplasia or abnormal mitoses are key clues. Sclerotic variants of lobular capillary hemangioma may be confused with nasopharyngeal angiofibroma, chiefly because of the nasal involvement, but the septal origin of capillary hemangioma rather than the far posterior nasal cavity–nasopharyngeal origin excludes that possibility. Clinical correlation in this regard is critical.

Biologic Behavior

The treatment of lobular capillary hemangioma–pyogenic granuloma is simple excision. Recurrence is rare. When pregnancy is associated, postpartum lesional regression may occur.

Hemangiopericytoma

Clinical Data

Hemangiopericytomas are rare vascular neoplasms, 10% to 30% of which arise in the head and neck (404). They most often affect adults of either sex in the fifth and sixth decades of life. They may arise in the nasal cavity or the paranasal sinuses (405). The presentation may be that of nasal obstruction, watery rhinorrhea, or epistaxis.

Gross Appearance

These tumors may appear as reddish tan polypoid submucosal masses high in the nasal cavity that bleed readily on manipulation (406).

Histologic Features

Hemangiopericytoma is characterized by a growth pattern of numerous dilated, branching, vascular spaces, often in a characteristic stag-horn arrangement. This vascular pattern may be common to several soft tissue tumors, including smooth muscle tumors, mesenchymal chondrosarcoma and synovial sarcoma, all of which should be excluded by careful sampling.

A hemangiopericytoma in this site is usually a histologically low-grade, well-differentiated tumor that some have termed a hemangiopericytoma-like tumor because of its generally fairly benign clinical behavior (405–407). The tumor is a densely cellular proliferation of uniform oval to spindled cells, usually devoid of much intervening collagenous stroma arranged around characteristic irregular dilated vascular spaces (Fig. 63). Nasal he-

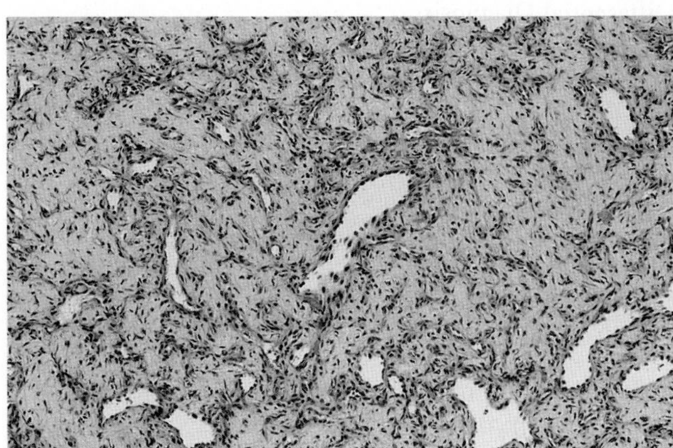

FIGURE 62. Lobular capillary hemangioma. Sclerosis of stroma and less pronounced lobular vascular proliferation is characteristic of this older lesion and may lead to confusion with nasopharyngeal angiofibroma.

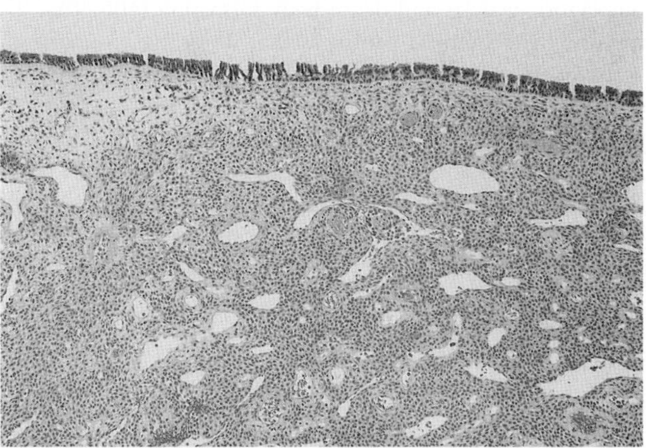

FIGURE 63. Hemangiopericytoma. Irregular dilated stag-horn vascular space surrounded by densely cellular proliferation of uniform oval cells without intervening collagen.

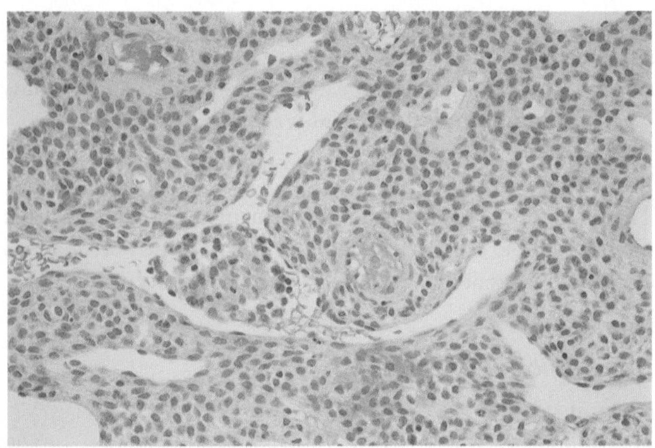

FIGURE 64. Hemangiopericytoma. Bland, small round to only slightly fusiform tumor cells characterize these nasal type tumors.

mangiopericytomas differ from those in other sites by having characteristically bland small round to only slightly fusiform tumor cells, as opposed to the more spindled cells of lesions in other areas (Fig. 64). Also, the vessels tend to be rounder or oblong and less stag-horn than is true in other sites. Fibrosis and focal myxoid stromal change are secondary features that may obscure the diagnosis. With the exception of superficial changes secondary to ulceration, there is no hemorrhage or necrosis, and mitotic figures are rare.

Higher grade hemangiopericytomas also may arise and are characterized by significant cytologic atypia, high mitotic rate, and tumor necrosis.

Special Studies

Reticulin stains may be used to define the relationship of the cellular proliferation to the vasculature and outline the fine, connective tissue deposits around individual cells, indiscernible by conventional hematoxylin and eosin microscopy. Electron microscopic evaluation has confirmed the hemangiopericytic nature of the proliferation, showing tumor cells with tapered processes, partially invested by basal lamina completely separating tumor cells from endothelial cells. Tumor cells also contain cytoplasmic intermediate-sized filaments and show occasional pinocytotic vesicles and dense body formation (405,408). The immunohistochemical profile is that of strong vimentin and variable, often weak, smooth muscle actin staining, with negative staining for desmin and cytokeratin. Occasional staining for CD34 and Factor XIIIA has been reported. Immunohistochemistry may be helpful in excluding some of the potential mimics such as smooth muscle tumors (muscle actin and desmin positive), peripheral nerve sheath tumors (S-100 positive), and synovial sarcoma (cytokeratin and EMA positive).

Differential Diagnosis

Hemangiopericytoma is a diagnosis reached after other soft tissue entities such as leiomyosarcoma, malignant fibrous histiocytoma, mesenchymal chondrosarcoma, synovial sarcoma, and peripheral nerve sheath tumor (described in detail elsewhere) have been excluded through complete histologic sampling and special studies. The degree of cellularity in hemangiopericytoma is a useful clue in discriminating it from the relatively paucicellular angiofibroma, of nasopharyngeal origin.

Biologic Behavior

Malignancy in hemangiopericytomas from other sites has been associated with nuclear atypia, tumor size, mitotic activity, and the presence of tumor necrosis, but confident prediction of biologic behavior from histology is not possible. Sinonasal hemangiopericytomas usually follow a benign course and remain localized despite incomplete excision, with only rare cases resulting in metastasis (405). In the more recent literature, a significant recurrence rate of 40% to 50% is documented (405). Recurrences have been noted on prolonged follow-up intervals of 10 to 20 years, with the mean interval to first recurrence at 6.5 years and one case recurring 17.5 years after presentation (405,409). Although the recurrence rate of these sinonasal hemangiopericytomas is akin to similar tumors arising in other sites, the metastasis and mortality rates are lower (405).

Fibrous Tumors

Fibroma

Clinical Data

Fibromas of the nasal cavity are small asymptomatic benign mucosal nodules analogous to traumatic or irritation fibromas of the oral cavity. In Fu and Perzin's series they arose from the posterior nasal vestibule, floor of the nasal cavity and nasal septum in patients 32 to 59 years of age. Discovery is incidental (410).

Gross Appearance

These are small, localized, slightly raised, smooth-surfaced mucosal nodules measuring 1 cm or less.

Histologic Features

Fibromas are localized lumps composed of mature, paucicellular fibrous connective tissue surfaced by benign epithelium. The fibroblasts may be plump and stellate shaped or even multinucleate. The histologic appearance is similar to that of the fibrous papule of nasal skin.

Differential Diagnosis

Lack of infiltrative growth excludes a sparsely cellular fibromatosis. The possibility exists that fibromas represent other lesions, such as minute polyps that are fibrosed. Fu and Perzin believe that they represent a reparative process rather than a true neoplasm (410).

Biologic Behavior

Fibromas are treated by conservative simple surgical excision with no expectation of recurrence.

Inflammatory Pseudotumor (Tumefactive Fibroinflammatory Lesion)

Clinical Data

Inflammatory pseudotumor arising in the nasal region and maxillary sinus was described in 1983 by Wold and Weiland as tumefactive fibroinflammatory lesion (411). Both of their patients were women, ages 33 and 47, respectively. The patient with a nasal tumor had a history of inflammatory myxomatous nasal polyps, and the one with a sinus lesion had experienced multiple operations due to her presentation with facial pain. A destructive pseudotumor of the maxillary sinus was subsequently reported in 1988 by Weisman and Osguthorpe (412). These are extremely rare lesions in the sinonasal tract.

Gross Appearance

The lesions are firm, gray-tan, and well circumscribed but not encapsulated.

Histologic Features

The histologic appearance is similar to that of sclerosing mediastinitis, Reidel's thyroiditis, and retroperitoneal fibrosis. It is composed of mature hypocellular fibrous tissue with variable collagenization or hyalinization admixed with an inflammatory infiltrate composed of lymphocytes and polymorphonuclear leukocytes (Fig. 65). The lesion invades adjacent tissue structures at its periphery.

Differential Diagnosis

The main histologic diagnostic consideration is fibromatosis, which is also infiltrative but usually more cellular with fibroblasts arranged in bundles and fascicles without the inflammatory infiltrate. Nodular fasciitis, although containing lymphocytic infiltrates, is more cellular, neovascularized, and less collagenized, and often contains mitotic figures (see Chapter 10). Sarcomatoid SCCs dominated by the spindle cell element may rarely have hypocellular areas with a prominent fibromyxoid stroma and may focally lack prominent significant atypia. An appropriate immunohistochemical profile of cytokeratin and vimentin, and occasionally muscle actin, may be discriminating (275,413).

Biologic Behavior

Neither of Wold and Weiland's sinonasal lesions recurred after excision, although recurrence of inflammatory pseudotumors of other head and neck sites despite multiple surgeries has been described. The patient with the nasal cavity lesion developed SCC of the nasal cavity 3 years after excision of the lesion and died from it (411). The pseudotumor described by Weisman and Osguthorpe destroyed the lateral wall of the maxillary sinus and extended into the infratemporal region and orbit, thereby simulating malignancy (412).

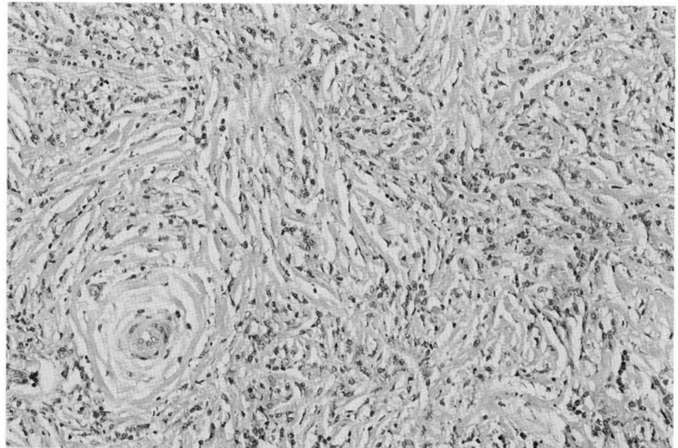

FIGURE 65. Inflammatory pseudotumor (tumefactive fibroinflammatory lesion). Maxillary sinus lesion with wiry, hyalinized collagen fibers admixed with a mononuclear inflammatory cell infiltrate.

Eosinophilic Angiocentric Fibrosis

Clinical Data

Eosinophilic angiocentric fibrosis of the upper respiratory tract, a non-neoplastic fibrous proliferation, was first described by Roberts and McCann in 1985 (414). This entity is extremely rare, with one additional case involving the nasal cavity reported in 1997 (415). Nasal cavity lesions have involved the lateral nasal wall and nasal septum. Additional cases have been reported in the subglottic region. All cases have occurred in women 25 to 59 years of age. Eosinophilic angiocentric fibrosis results in progressive stenosis of the nasal cavity with airway obstruction. An allergic etiology has been proposed.

Gross Appearance

The mucosa is thickened with the formation of a polypoid soft tissue mass.

Histologic Features

This is a non-neoplastic proliferation of fibrous connective tissue and blood vessels with a characteristic angiocentric whorling of the collagen bundles. An admixed inflammatory cell infiltrate composed of lymphocytes, plasma cells, neutrophils, and numerous eosinophils is also characteristic. Migration of eosinophils through the walls of small vessels with swollen endothelium is compatible with a small vessel vasculitis. Inflammatory and fibrotic zones within the same biopsy have suggested an evolving inflammatory process with small vessel vasculitis and secondary stromal response.

Differential Diagnosis

The angiocentric whorling fibrosis is unique to this entity and serves to distinguish it from inflammatory pseudotumor, also characterized by mixed cellular inflammatory infiltrates and fibrosis. It also has been suggested that the eosinophilic angiocentric fibrosis represents a mucosal variant of granuloma faciale; however, the fibrosis in that entity lacks angiocentric whorling. Kimura's disease also lacks angiocentric whorling fibrosis and contains prominent lymphoid aggregates with germinal centers. Likewise, angiolymphoid hyperplasia with eosinophilia lacks the distinctive fibrosis.

Fibromatosis

Presentation of fibromatosis in this region has been documented over a wide age range, 2 to 61 years, affecting both males and females. Symptoms have included nasal obstruction, epistaxis, maxillary mass, facial pain, and a nonhealing tooth extraction site (410). These lesions have centered on the turbinates and maxillary sinuses, sometimes in combination and occasionally with bilateral involvement (410). A syndromic case of multiple maxillofacial, cranial, vertebral, and skeletal lesions has been described (410). Fibromatosis infiltrates into adjacent normal structures and therefore the pathologist should attempt to document margin status in resection specimens, because a positive margin is predictive of future recurrence (see Chapter 10).

Solitary Fibrous Tumor

Clinical Data

Solitary fibrous tumor in the nasal cavity is a rare entity, nine cases having been reported (416–418). Some tumors have extended into the nasopharynx, perforated the septum or eroded bone, and extended into the adjacent paranasal sinuses. All of those affected were between 30 and 64 years of age, with no sex predilection. All presented with nasal symptoms of obstruction, congestion, or occasional epistaxis.

Gross Appearance

These tumors present as rubbery, gray-white polypoid intranasal masses that may have a stalk attachment.

Histologic Features

The solitary fibrous tumors of the nasal cavities are histologically identical to the tumors of the same name arising in the pleura earlier called, inappropriately, benign fibrous mesothelioma. They are composed of an unencapsulated proliferation of plump spindled cells with bland nuclei in a haphazard or patternless arrangement. There is variable cellularity with zones of hypo- and hypercellularity and generally inconspicuous mitoses (Fig. 66). The stroma is variably collagenized, often thick and keloid-like. The vascularity is prominent, with numerous thin, dilated blood vessels that may focally have a hemangiopericytoma pattern.

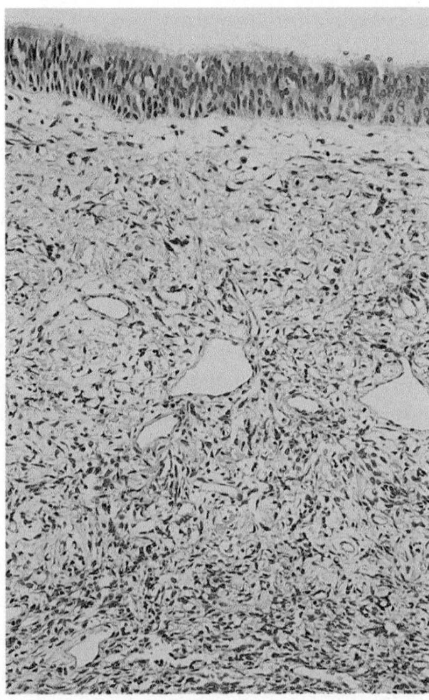

FIGURE 66. Solitary fibrous tumor. Lesion with a patternless fibroblastic proliferation of variable cellularity and collagenization with prominent thin dilated blood vessels. (Courtesy of Dr. B. Pilch.)

Notably absent are giant cells, necrosis, hemorrhage, ulceration, and invasion of bone (see Chapter 10).

Special Studies

The fibroblasts stain only for vimentin and are negative for cytokeratin, S-100 protein, desmin, muscle actins, myoglobin, Factor VIII, and neurofilaments. Diffuse, strong positive CD34 immunostaining obtained in a study of one nasal tumor is identical to that of solitary fibrous tumors of pleural and other nonpleural sites and may be helpful in differential diagnosis (Table 4) (418).

Differential Diagnosis

Solitary fibrous tumor most closely simulates hemangiopericytoma. However, hemangiopericytomas of this region are more diffusely cellular, less collagenized, and have a more diffuse branching, stag-horn vascular pattern. Their recurrence rate is also significant, an assessment yet to be made on long-term observation of the solitary fibrous tumors. Other differential diagnostic considerations would include peripheral nerve sheath tumor (palisading and S-100 protein positivity), fibrous histiocytoma (storiform pattern with histiocytes), fibrosarcoma (herringbone pattern, malignant histology), and nasopharyngeal angiofibroma. The latter is seen in adolescent boys, arises from the nasopharynx, and is less cellular, with parallel collagen fibers and a vasculature consisting of both thick and thin vessels.

Biologic Behavior

All of the sinonasal lesions have behaved in a benign fashion after local excision or lateral rhinotomy and maxillectomy. All patients but one were alive with no evidence of disease, and the latter had persistent stable disease 4 years after local resection and tumor embolization. No metastases have been documented. However, follow-up intervals for this rare entity have been relatively short, from 3 months to 12 years (median 2 years).

Myxoma

Clinical Data

Sinonasal myxomas are benign but locally aggressive tumors that appear to arise within facial bones, more commonly the mandible than the maxilla. When based in the maxilla they frequently extend into the nasal cavity, sinuses, and soft tissues. Clinical symptoms include facial and maxillary swelling, headache, nasal stuffiness, and earache (419). Nasal myxomas often occur in children.

Radiologic Studies

The typical radiographic appearance is that of a mass lesion of soft tissue density in the maxilla, destroying bone and extending to fill the maxillary sinus most commonly and the nasal cavity less often. More extensive lesions may erode the bone of the orbit and base of the skull (419).

Gross Appearance

Myxomas appear as firm, gray to white, gelatinous multinodular masses. The interface with adjacent tissue is usually well defined, but there is no capsule (419).

Histologic Features

Myxomas are paucicellular tumors composed largely of myxoid stroma with inconspicuous vascularity. Within this stroma lie scattered stellate and spindled cells with small, dark, benign nuclei and elongated cytoplasmic tails. Focally there may be zones of increased cellularity, fibrosis, or odontogenic epithelium, leading to other terms being used to describe this tumor such as fibromyxoma, myxofibroma, and odontogenic myxoma. It is doubtful that many of these maxillary–sinonasal myxomas are of odontogenic origin because they lack odontogenic epithelium and are not associated with tooth-bearing areas of the maxilla. Nasal myxomas infiltrate with a sharply demarcated margin, as opposed to intramuscular myxomas, replacing osseous tissue with minimal reactive bone formation.

Differential Diagnosis

Myxoma is a diagnosis reached after other neoplasms with myxomatous stroma, such as myxoid peripheral nerve sheath tumors, fibromatosis, fibrosarcoma, rhabdomyosarcoma, myxoid liposarcoma, and chondroblastic tumors, are excluded. Myxoid change in the latter tumors is often focal, with other characteristic areas establishing the microscopic diagnosis. The myxoid appearance of dental pulp from impacted teeth or odontomas and the mucopolysaccharide-rich dental follicle also may be confused with myxoma (see Chapter 6). This can readily be excluded by clinical history, radiography, and the presence of odontogenic epithelium or dental hard tissues. The stroma of nasal polyps may superficially simulate myxoma because of the marked edema (Fig. 4).

Biologic Behavior

The lesion is benign. Metastatic behavior is not reported (419).

Fibrosarcoma

Clinical Data

With the advent of immunohistochemistry and the ability to classify soft tissue tumors more accurately, the diagnosis of fibrosarcoma has been used less frequently. This diagnosis, however, has enjoyed a resurgence of late, at least in the sinonasal region (395). Fibrosarcomas arise in the nasal cavity and paranasal sinuses over a wide age range, 10 to 77 years. Nasal or maxillary mass and swelling, nasal polyps, obstructive nasal symptoms, epistaxis, peripheral nerve symptoms of pain or hypoesthesia, headache, and chronic sinusitis have all been associated with the presentation of this tumor (410).

Radiologic Studies

The characteristic radiographic appearance is that of a mass lesion with destruction of adjacent bone.

Gross Appearance

These are homogeneous, firm, white tumors that may project into the nasal cavity or sinuses as polypoid masses. They destroy bone by expansion or invasion. The tumor borders may be circumscribed but are microscopically unencapsulated (410).

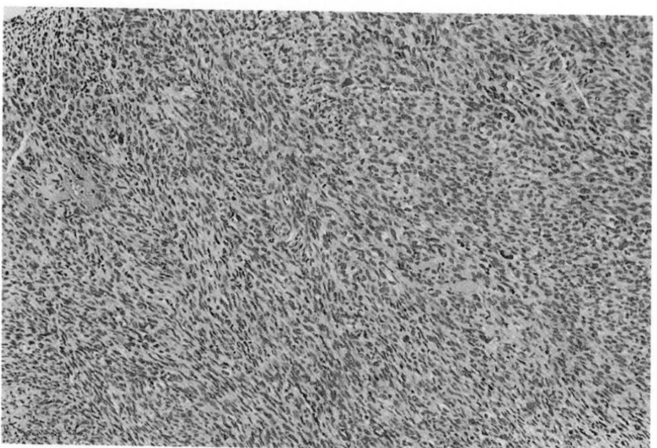

FIGURE 67. Fibrosarcoma. Densely hypercellular, atypical fibroblastic proliferation arranged in fascicles.

Histologic Features

In contrast to the preceding fibroblastic proliferations, fibrosarcomas are usually densely cellular and cytologically atypical (Fig. 67). The fibroblastic proliferation is uniform and arranged in fascicles that often assume a herringbone pattern. More collagenized, less cellular areas may be encountered, but the more highly cellular fields predominate. Mitoses are readily recognized and may be atypical (Fig. 68). Hemangiopericytoma-like patterns may be encountered (410). Again, margin assessment of resection specimens should be performed.

Differential Diagnosis

The cellular fibrosarcomatous herringbone pattern may be common to numerous sarcomas, including leiomyosarcoma, malignant fibrous histiocytoma, malignant peripheral nerve sheath tumor, synovial sarcoma, osteosarcoma, and chondrosarcoma. Therefore, a diagnosis of fibrosarcoma is partially one of exclusion. A herringbone pattern is usually focal in the other sarcomas, which can be diagnosed by a combination of adequate sampling, attention to more characteristic growth patterns, nuclear shape, presence of pleomorphic, multinucleate

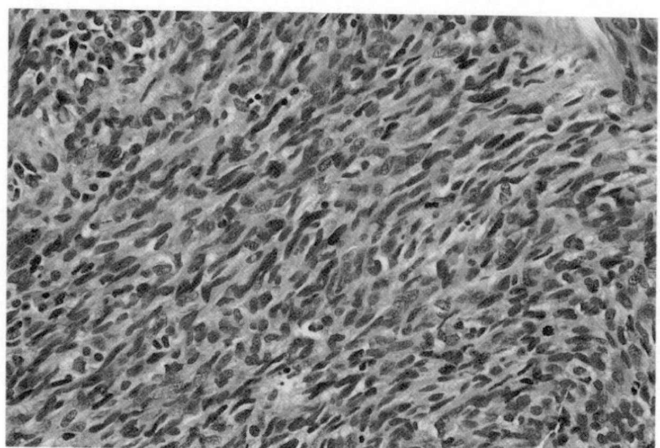

FIGURE 68. Fibrosarcoma. Spindled cells with hyperchromatic, mitotically active nuclei in this fibrosarcoma of the nasal cavity.

cells, production of malignant extracellular osteoid or chondroid matrix, and use of immunohistochemistry and ultrastructure (see Chapter 10).

In this site, other more common spindle cell malignancies to consider, but which do not have a herringbone pattern, are sarcomatoid carcinoma and amelanotic melanoma. Fibrosarcoma should contain only the intermediate filament vimentin. Some of the other tumors are well characterized by the presence of muscle proteins, cytokeratins and EMA, S-100 protein, and melanosome-associated antigens (Table 4). Spindle cell carcinoma, however, may evince little if any keratin immunohistochemical positivity (see Chapter 7) (275).

Biologic Behavior

Fibrosarcomas are more slowly growing, less infiltrative, and less metastatic than other sarcomas of this region and therefore tend to have a better prognosis. Locally aggressive disease is responsible for most deaths, although fibrosarcoma is capable of metastasis, with a frequency of roughly 10% (410). Fibrosarcomas treated by limited local excision are prone to recurrence, and wide en bloc resection with clear margins is recommended (410).

Fibrohistiocytic Tumors

Clinical Data

The age range of sinonasal fibrohistiocytic tumors is very broad, from newborn to 82 years of age without sex predilection (420). Among sinonasal sites of 31 fibrohistiocytic tumors reviewed by Daou et al., the maxillary sinus predominated, followed by the nasal cavity, ethmoid, and frontal and sphenoid sinuses (421). Symptoms have included mass or swelling, nasal obstruction, epistaxis, loose teeth, and facial pain (420). Malignant fibrous histiocytomas can arise in this region as a result of previous radiation therapy after a long latent period (422).

Radiologic Studies

Radiographic findings include soft tissue mass lesion, destruction of bone, and sinus opacification (420).

Gross Appearance

The gross appearances have varied from mass lesions with polypoid expansion into the nasal cavity to small polypoid nasal tumors than can be locally excised (420).

Histologic Features

These fibrohistiocytic tumors range from cytologically bland to malignant proliferations. Features such as anaplasia and mitotic activity, especially abnormal mitoses, are likely to result in a malignant diagnosis.

The diagnosis is based on the presence of spindle-shaped fibroblasts forming storiform patterns (Fig. 69) with or without the presence of multinucleated histiocyte-like tumor giant cells or xanthoma cells. Myxoid stromal change (Fig. 70) and fascicular and focal hemangiopericytoma patterns may be encountered. Most are classified as the malignant storiform–pleomorphic type, but a rare inflammatory variant may present in the head and neck (see Chapter 10) (423).

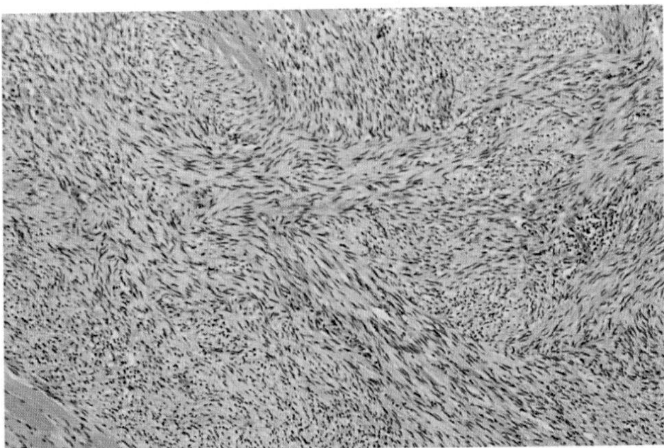

FIGURE 69. Malignant fibrous histiocytoma. Destructive cellular spindle cell proliferation of maxillary sinus with storiform pattern.

Differential Diagnosis

Differential histologic considerations of low-grade or benign fibrous histiocytomas include the non-neoplastic inflammatory pseudotumor and benign spindle cell tumors, most often fibromatosis, peripheral nerve sheath tumor, smooth muscle tumor, myxoma, and hemangiopericytoma. Malignant fibrous histiocytoma may be a pattern common to a number of high-grade sarcomas (424). As previously mentioned, complete histologic sampling and judicious use of immunohistochemistry and electron microscopy are helpful in differentiating these entities.

Biologic Behavior

Fibrohistiocytic tumors are infiltrative neoplasms and therefore have a propensity to recur if incompletely excised. This behavior includes low-grade fibrohistiocytic tumors with bland cytologic features that might be designated benign fibrous histiocytoma. Because of tumor heterogeneity that may bias small biopsy samples, caution should be exercised in this assessment. The malignant fibrous histiocytomas, so designated because of varying degrees of nuclear atypia, pleomorphic giant cells, and mitotic activity, are regarded as malignant neoplasms capable of metastasis, although the metastatic rate in the series of 21 tumors re-

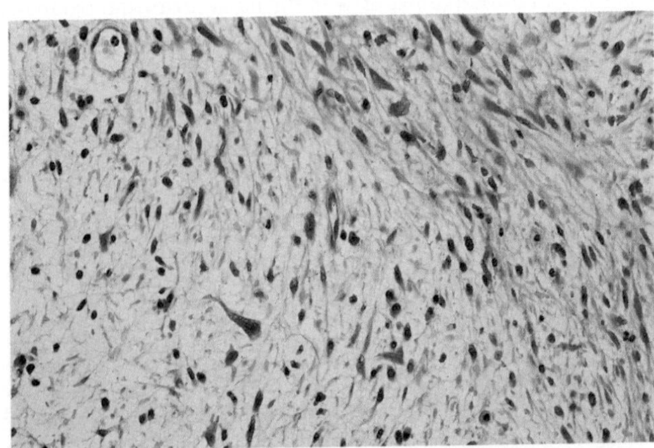

FIGURE 70. Malignant fibrous histiocytoma. High-power photomicrograph of myxoid-appearing area of same tumor as in Fig. 69.

ported and reviewed by Perzin and Fu was 19%. Malignant fibrous histiocytomas of this region have metastasized to bone, lung, and cervical and paraaortic lymph nodes (420). Small polypoid nonatypical tumors have been treated by polypectomy, but the follow-up interval is short at 2 years and limited to one tumor in Perzin and Fu's study (420). Surgical excisions have ranged from local to radical resections, varying with the location and extent of tumor. Because of the infiltrative nature of all fibrous histiocytomas, common sense would dictate that clear margins should be attained as in the fibromatosis–fibrosarcoma spectrum of tumors.

Peripheral Nerve Sheath Tumors

Clinical Data

Roughly 25% to 45% of peripheral nerve sheath tumors involve the head and neck region, with less than 4% arising in the nasal cavity and paranasal sinuses (425). Less than 70 cases have been reported to date (426). There is a broad age distribution, most arising in adults of middle age. The maxillary and ethmoid sinuses and nasal cavity are the most commonly involved (425–428). Typical nasal symptoms of obstruction, epistaxis, rhinorrhea, or paranasal sinus mass–related symptoms of facial–orbital swelling and pain may be encountered (394). Most cases of neurofibroma have not been associated with von Recklinghausen's disease (394,425). It is postulated that sinonasal peripheral nerve sheath tumors may arise from the ophthalmic or maxillary branches of the trigeminal nerve.

Radiologic Studies

Imaging studies show soft tissue density mass lesions. Bone erosion and destruction may be seen in both benign and malignant peripheral nerve sheath tumors with the potential for intracranial extension (394,425–427).

Gross Appearance

Both benign and malignant neoplasms may simulate nasal polyps because of an intracavitary polypoid configuration (394,395).

Histologic Features

Schwannomas and neurofibromas (Fig. 71) usually have distinctive histologic features, but there may be some histologic overlap. Myxoid Antoni B changes, characteristic of schwannoma, also can be seen in neurofibroma, but nuclear palisading is usually a feature of schwannoma (Fig. 72) (see Chapter 10). Interestingly, although schwannomas are typically known as well-encapsulated tumors, often a discriminating feature from neurofibromas, this does not appear to be the case in the sinonasal tract (426).

Tumors compatible with the cellular variant of schwannoma have been described in the sinonasal tract (426). These tumors are more likely to be misdiagnosed as malignant because of the predominance of the hypercellular Antoni A pattern in long fascicles, with mitotic activity and rare focal necrosis. The lack of encapsulation makes this diagnosis even more problematic in this region.

Malignant peripheral nerve sheath tumors (malignant schwannomas) are usually composed of densely cellular,

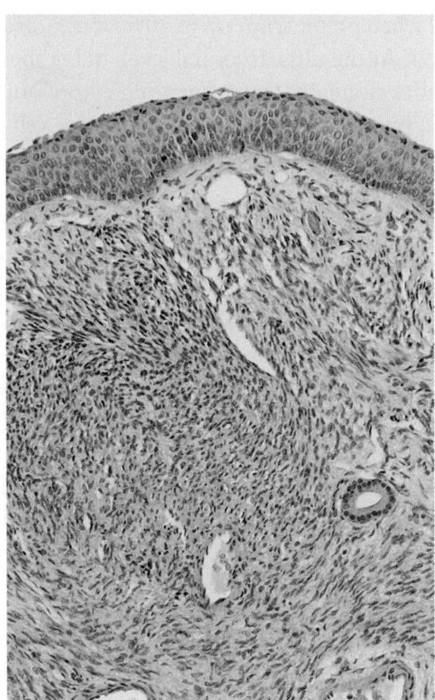

FIGURE 71. Peripheral nerve sheath tumor. Unencapsulated peripheral nerve sheath tumor involving nasal cavity with cellular Antoni A area.

monotonous spindle cells with serpentine nuclei forming densely packed fascicular patterns. The growth pattern may resemble that of fibrosarcoma or monophasic synovial sarcoma; therefore, special studies may be required for diagnosis. Mitotic activity in sinonasal malignant schwannoma can be extremely variable, and many tumors have a low mitotic rate (395). The designation of malignant triton tumor may be applied to malignant schwannomas showing foci of skeletal muscle differentiation (394,395).

Special Studies

Schwannomas stain for S-100 protein more intensely than neurofibromas, reflecting the higher relative density of Schwann cells. S-100 protein staining in malignant schwannomas is diagnosti-

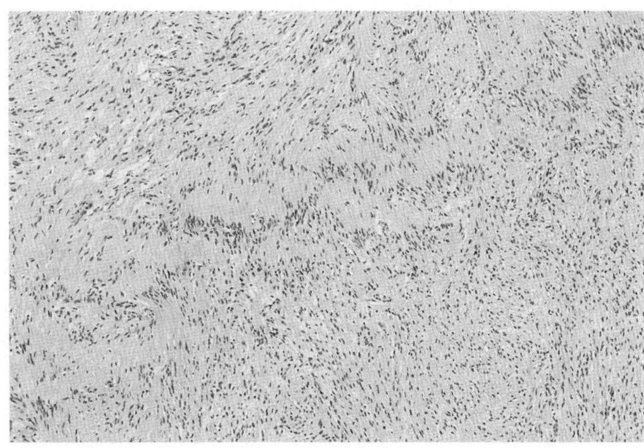

FIGURE 72. Schwannoma. Tumor of nasal cavity with characteristic nuclear pallisading.

cally helpful when present, but up to 40% of tumors may be nonreactive (429). At the ultrastructural level, nerve sheath differentiation includes elongated, interdigitating cytoplasmic processes, basal lamina, pinocytotic vesicles, and primitive cell junctions.

Differential Diagnosis

The lack of encapsulation, spindle cell morphology, and variable cellularity of peripheral nerve sheath tumors of the sinonasal tract raises a broad differential diagnosis of fibrous lesions (solitary fibrous tumor, fibromatosis, fibrosarcoma), fibrous histiocytoma, myxoma, hemangiopericytoma, smooth muscle tumors, meningioma, spindle cell melanoma, and synovial sarcoma. Of these, fibrous histiocytoma and fibrosarcoma are the most likely histologic simulants. Careful attention to histologic features described in previous sections of this chapter and a panel of distinguishing immunomarkers (Table 4) are useful in excluding these diagnostic possibilities.

Biologic Behavior

Both benign and malignant peripheral nerve sheath tumors should be completely excised to avoid local recurrence. The nature of the resection is dictated by the location and extent of tumor. The addition of radiation and chemotherapy is usually considered in high-grade malignant schwannomas. Neither erosion of bone nor intracranial extension, although commonly seen in malignant schwannoma, are absolute indicators of malignancy of peripheral nerve sheath tumors in this region (394,426).

Most sinonasal malignant schwannomas have been considered to be both histologically and biologically low grade, analogous in behavior to locally aggressive sinonasal fibrosarcomas (395). However, even low-grade tumors have metastasized. The most common sites of metastasis are lungs, bone, and liver (395).

Overall, 22% of patients with malignant tumors died of disease, with increased risk of death associated with higher mitotic rate (greater than 4 mitoses per 50 high-power fields), increased tumor cellularity, and male sex (395).

Rhabdomyosarcoma

Clinical Data

Rhabdomyosarcomas in children have a predilection for head and neck sites in the following order of frequency: the orbit, nasal cavity, nasopharynx, ear and ear canal, paranasal cavities, soft tissues of the face and neck, and oral cavity (430). Most arise in the first decade of life, but rare cases occur in adults (384,431). Presentations include mass lesion, epistaxis, nasal obstruction, ear pain, headache, recurrent nasal polyps, rhinorrhea, proptosis, and visual disturbances (384).

Radiologic Studies

The typical radiographic appearance is that of a tumor mass that may show cloudiness of multiple sinuses, destruction of bone, extension into the skull base, nasopharynx, and sphenoid region (384).

Gross Appearance

The tumors are firm, gray or red-gray, infiltrative masses. Those presenting in the nasal alae and nasal vestibule may be recognized at an earlier stage as small, red, smooth-surfaced nodules, in contrast to the usual mass lesions that occlude the nasal passages. The presentation as multiple sinonasal polyps has corresponded to the grape-like botryoid variant of embryonal rhabdomyosarcoma (384).

Histologic Features

The histology of the vast majority of rhabdomyosarcomas of the sinonasal tract is that of the embryonal variant, and a minority of these present the polypoid growth pattern of sarcoma botryoides. Rarely do the alveolar and spindle cell variants occur in this region (384,432). The embryonal rhabdomyosarcoma is a primitive diffuse cellular proliferation of round to spindled cells with hyperchromatic nuclei and scant cytoplasm. Occasional cells may have a small amount of eccentric or elongated eosinophilic cytoplasm, but cross-striations are difficult to visualize. There are variable numbers of mitotic figures. Zones of hypocellularity and myxoid stroma are frequent. There may be a cellular zone of undifferentiated cells just below the mucosa of the polypoid myxomatous tumor masses (cambium layer) (see Chapter 10). Chemotherapy or radiation therapy may induce a curious finding of cytologic differentiation in primitive rhabdomyosarcoma, with populations of cells containing abundant eosinophilic cytoplasm (433).

Special Studies

The diagnosis is most rapidly and reliably confirmed by immunohistochemical demonstration of one or more muscle antigens. The more sensitive markers in classic embryonal rhabdomyosarcoma are the intermediate filament desmin (100%), myogenic regulatory proteins MyoD1 (92%) and myogenin (88%), and muscle-specific actin antibody HHF-35 (88%) (434). Electron microscopy, although presently less popular, is a proven diagnostic technique to discriminate rhabdomyosarcoma from the other undifferentiated sarcomas (435). The former demonstrate both thick and thin myofilaments and occasionally primitive Z-band formation.

Differential Diagnosis

The usual suspects in any primitive small blue cell tumor encountered in the sinonasal tract should be considered and excluded by immunohistochemistry, electron microscopy, and microscopic evaluation of resected tissues. In addition to rhabdomyosarcoma, this would include malignant lymphoma, Ewing's sarcoma/PNET, olfactory neuroblastoma, mesenchymal chondrosarcoma, and undifferentiated carcinoma. The distinctive immunoprofiles of these entities are detailed in Table 4 and the histologic appearances of the sarcomas discussed in depth in Chapter 10. The myxoid stroma and polypoid configuration of some rhabdomyosarcomas might also be mistaken for nasal polyps or myxoma, where careful search for a primitive cell population with a muscle phenotype is important. More differentiated varieties of rhabdomyosarcoma might be confused with fetal (cellular or myxoid type) rhabdomyoma, which is distinguished by its circumscription and lack of atypia and mitotic activity. Also, leiomyosarcoma enters into the differential diagnosis of the rare spindle cell variant of embryonal rhabdomyosarcoma.

Biologic Behavior

Treatment of rhabdomyosarcoma is largely conservative surgery with multiagent chemotherapy and radiotherapy. Although compared with other head and neck sites, sinonasal rhabdomyosarcoma is not prognostically favorable, there has been an improvement in the 5-year survival rate to 44% with current combined chemotherapy and radiation treatment modalities (431,436).

TUMORS FROM ADJACENT STRUCTURES

Odontogenic Tumors

Numerous odontogenic cysts and tumors arise in the maxilla and may extend into the maxillary sinus. These proliferations arise by unknown stimulus from the epithelium of the tooth-forming apparatus in the jaws, and some are histologically reminiscent of stages in tooth development. As a group, they are often problematic lesions for general pathologists and may be confused with benign and malignant salivary gland tumors and more importantly SCC. Because of this potential for misdiagnosis and the implementation of inappropriate therapy, we will mention in this chapter the most common and several of the morphologically unique odontogenic tumors that may be encountered as sinonasal masses. A more complete description of the odontogenic cysts and tumors may be found in Chapter 6.

Ameloblastoma

Clinical Data

Ameloblastoma is the most common odontogenic tumor. Roughly 15% of these benign, painless, slow-growing, yet locally invasive tumors arise in the maxilla, usually the posterior regions, and may extend into and present in the maxillary sinus or nasal cavity. They affect a broad age range without sex predilection but are predominantly encountered in patients 35 to 45 years of age. Roughly 86% of ameloblastomas are the conventional solid, multicystic type, 13% are unicystic, and 1% are peripheral, arising in the gingival tissues. Malignant ameloblastoma, presenting at a mean age of 30 years, is morphologically indistinguishable from benign ameloblastoma except for the presence of metastatic disease. Ameloblastic carcinoma, on the other hand, again presenting at a mean age of 30 years, is a histologically malignant primary ameloblastoma that exhibits rapid and destructive growth. Both of these malignant varieties are rare, favor the mandible, and have a poor outcome (437).

Radiologic Studies

The conventional solid ameloblastomas are characteristically multilocular radiolucencies that may expand the cortex and resorb the roots of teeth. Solid ameloblastomas also may present as unilocular radiolucent defects and may mimic a dentigerous cyst when associated with an impacted tooth. The unicystic ameloblastomas are purely unicystic lucencies that are associated with an unerupted tooth in half the cases.

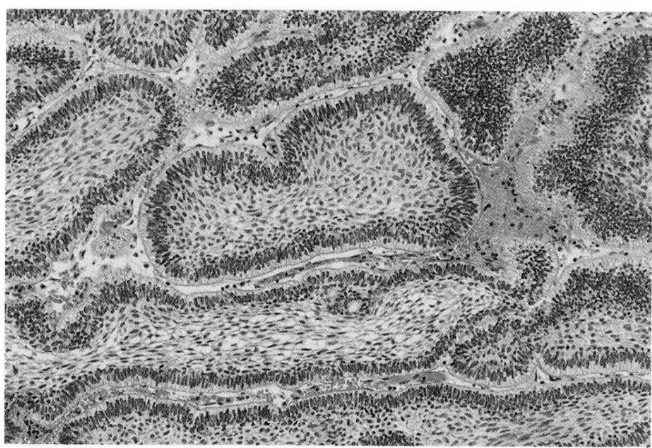

FIGURE 73. Ameloblastoma. Follicular nests of maxillary ameloblastoma lined by a peripheral palisade of columnar cells with nuclei polarized away from the basement membrane and the central edematous spindled epithelium resembling stellate reticulum.

Histologic Features

The histologic criterion for all ameloblastomas is a well-differentiated columnar epithelium with minimal atypia arranged as a peripheral palisade of cells with nuclei polarized away from the basement membrane (so-called reverse polarization). Central to this basal layer is an edematous, spindled epithelium resembling the stellate reticulum of the enamel organ (Fig. 73). The various growth patterns include follicular nests, strands, plexiform networks, and cyst linings. Typically there is budding of epithelium from nests. Within the stellate reticulum–like areas, the epithelium may keratinize or undergo granular cell change

Numerous histologic types of solid ameloblastoma are recognized but, with the exception of the unicystic ameloblastoma, do not bear any relationship to biologic behavior (see Chapter 6). The ameloblastic carcinoma is usually a solid proliferation of tumor cells with an ameloblastomatous architectural pattern composed of cells with cytologically malignant enlarged, hyperchromatic, vesicular nuclei bearing prominent nucleoli, having increased and abnormal mitoses, and showing necrosis and calcification.

Differential Diagnosis

A biopsy sample of ameloblastoma when received as a maxillary sinus or nasal mass may be confused with basal cell neoplasms of salivary gland origin, most often variants of basal cell (monomorphic) adenoma, adenoid cystic carcinoma, and basal cell adenocarcinoma. Careful attention to the ameloblastomatous differentiation of the columnar cells and formation of stellate reticulum–like zones are important clues to diagnosis, as is recognition of the capability of ameloblastomas to keratinize and show granular cell change.

Maxillary ameloblastomas tend to be more densely cellular than the mandibular tumors, and when interpreted in the context of an infiltrative tumor forming keratin pearls, may be readily confused with carcinoma. Both the benign ameloblastoma and cytologically malignant ameloblastic carcinoma are distinguished by cell nests, strands, or sheets lined at the periphery by a layer of palisaded columnar cells with nuclei polarized away from the basement membrane and an inner edematous stellate reticulum–like zone. A prominent stratified basal layer, however, can be seen in some nonkeratinizing SCCs, lending an adamantinoid (ameloblastomatous) appearance. In some cases, radiographic evidence of a maxillary bony tumor is helpful in discriminating the ameloblastoma. Again, the ameloblastomatous character of the peripheral palisaded cells, low-grade cytologic nuclear features, and rarity of mitoses lead to the correct diagnosis.

Biologic Behavior

Conventional solid ameloblastoma is best treated by resection with 1-cm margins. The recurrence rate for this type of excision is virtually nil, but cannot always be accomplished in the maxilla. With lesser extents of removal, higher recurrence rates can be expected: 50% to 90% for curettage and 15% for simple surgical excision. Pure unicystic ameloblastoma can be treated by enucleation and curettage rather than resection. The prognosis of the malignant variants of ameloblastoma is poor, with 50% of patients dying of disease (437).

Calcifying Epithelial Odontogenic Tumor

Clinical Data

Calcifying epithelial odontogenic tumor (CEOT), also known as the Pindborg tumor, is an uncommon benign but infiltrative odontogenic tumor. It presents over a broad age range (mean 40 years) as a slowly enlarging, painless mass. Most CEOTs are in the posterior mandible and are frequently associated with an impacted tooth (437). Only about one third of cases occur in the maxilla.

Radiologic Studies

The radiographic appearance is that of a multilocular or unilocular radiolucent defect that may contain opacities of variable size and radiodensity.

Histologic Features

Calcifying epithelial odontogenic tumor presents a unique histology of large polygonal epithelial cells with abundant eosinophilic cytoplasm, forming sheets, nests, and strands in a homogeneous eosinophilic stroma. The cells have distinct cell borders with intercellular bridges and may show considerable nuclear pleomorphism but rare mitoses. Foci of clear cells may be encountered. The extracellular eosinophilic matrix is an amyloid-like substance that contains concentric calcific deposits known as Liesegang rings that correspond to the radiopacities. The proliferating epithelium may surround this matrix in a cribriform pattern (see Chapter 6).

Special Studies

The hyalin matrix stains like amyloid with Congo red and thioflavin T.

Differential Diagnosis

Familiarity with the benign CEOT is necessary to avoid serious overcalls of malignancy. Most often CEOT is misdiagnosed as SCC because of the large polygonal cells, nuclear pleomorphism,

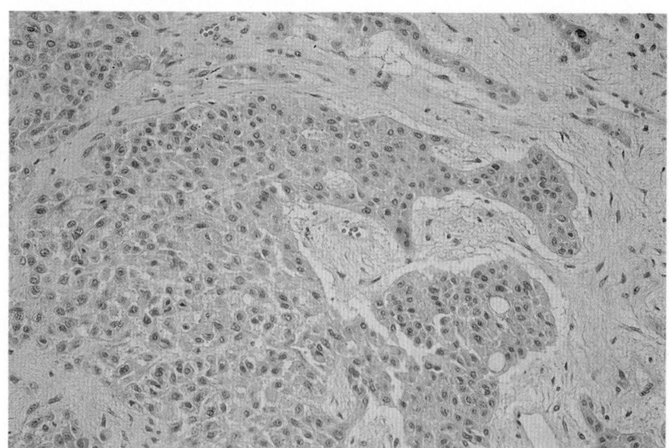

FIGURE 74. Calcifying epithelial odontogenic tumor (Pindborg tumor). Sheets and strands of large polygonal cells with distinct cell borders, intercellular bridges, and nuclear pleomorphism simulate squamous cell carcinoma.

distinct cell borders, and intercellular bridges (Fig. 74). The epithelial strands, globules of extracellular amyloid matrix, and cribriform patterns (Fig. 75) also may raise the remote possibility of metastatic medullary thyroid carcinoma or adenoid cystic carcinoma. The former is excluded by lack of calcitonin immunoreactivity in CEOT and the latter by lack of a basaloid cell proliferation with outer myoepithelial cell layer characteristic of adenoid cystic carcinoma.

Biologic Behavior

Calcifying epithelial odontogenic tumor is less aggressive than ameloblastoma, with a recurrence rate of less than 20%. Therapy is conservative resection with a free margin (437).

Adenomatoid Odontogenic Tumor

Clinical Data

Adenomatoid odontogenic tumor (AOT), formerly known as adenoameloblastoma, is a unique odontogenic tumor that is

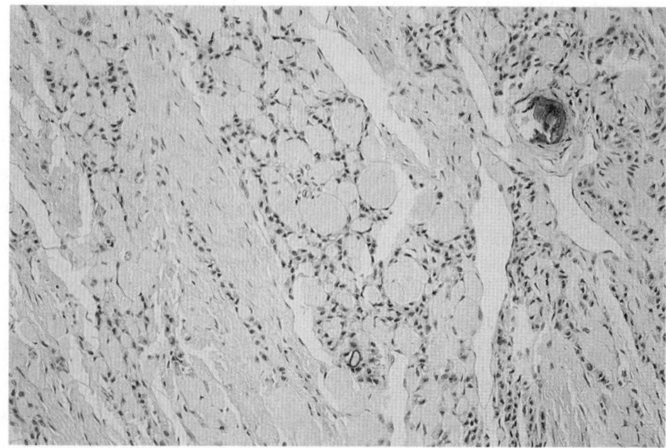

FIGURE 75. Calcifying epithelial odontogenic tumor (Pindborg tumor). Extracellular amyloid matrix and epithelial strands in cribriform patterns, which may simulate medullary thyroid carcinoma or adenoid cystic carcinoma. Note the Liesegang ring calcific deposit.

clinically and morphologically distinctive. This benign tumor is most common in adolescents, especially girls, and preferentially involves the anterior maxilla. Unfamiliarity with the histology can lead to a potentially disastrous diagnostic error.

Radiologic Studies

The radiographic appearance is that of a radiolucency usually associated with an impacted tooth that often contains fine calcifications.

Histologic Features

The tumor is an encapsulated cyst with a solid cellular proliferation of cytologically bland polyhedral and spindled epithelial cells. Unique to this odontogenic tumor, and variably present, are columnar cells forming distinctive rosettes and gland-like or duct-like structures. The nuclei of these cells are polarized away from the luminal space. The tumor also produces calcified hard tissues. Small calcifications are believed to be abortive enamel (enameloid), whereas larger matrix deposits that calcify are interpreted as dentinoid. These calcifications scattered throughout the epithelial proliferation are responsible for the opacities seen on radiography (see Chapter 6).

Differential Diagnosis

Adenomatoid odontogenic tumor may be confused with the more aggressive ameloblastoma. But the distinctive gland-like or duct-like structures and enameloid calcifications serve to distinguish AOT. The more ominous mistake is to misinterpret the rosettes, glands, and ducts of AOT as adenocarcinoma. Remembering that AOT usually arises in adolescent girls who are unlikely to have an adenocarcinoma, observing a lack of anaplasia and correlating the radiographic appearance with the distinctive epithelial and hard tissue morphology leads to the correct diagnosis.

Biologic Behavior

Treatment of this benign tumor is conservative enucleation. Recurrences are rare.

CENTRAL NERVOUS SYSTEM HETEROTOPIAS AND RELATED LESIONS

Nasal Glial Heterotopia (Nasal Glioma)

Clinical Data

Nasal glial heterotopia, also inappropriately referred to as nasal glioma or ganglioglioma, consists of congenital rests of central nervous system tissue embryologically misplaced in the nasal bridge area; as the developing neural tube detaches from the surface ectoderm, parts of this neural tissue become isolated from the intracranial contents. A thin strand of fibrous tissue may extend from the mass to the cribriform plate of the skull, or the heterotopic neural tissue might be associated with a connection to the intracranial space through a bony defect (148,438) (see Chapter 1).

These lesions are generally present at birth and exhibit slow and sustained growth. They may rarely be found in the frontal and maxillary sinuses, tongue, palate, and tonsillar region. There is a male predominance of 3:1 (148). Sixty percent of heterotopias present as extranasal, subcutaneous, small, firm masses of tissue on the bridge of the nose, 30% as submucosal, occasionally polypoid masses in the superior portion of the nasal cavity and 10% as lesions at both locations (438,439). Cases have been described in the nasopharynx, one of these with consequent development of oligodendroglioma (440,441).

Obstruction of the affected nasal cavity with associated breathing or feeding difficulty is the most prominent symptom. Cerebrospinal fluid leak, epistaxis, anosmia, and deformity also have been described (438).

Radiologic Studies

Radiographs are valuable to assess bony defects when intracranial extension is suspected.

Gross Appearance

Grossly, lesions are smooth, soft, light tan to gray, and range from 1 to 3 cm in dimension. They appear encephaloid and rarely cystic, and when intranasal, polypoid and mucosa-covered (148).

Histologic Features

Nasal glial heterotopias usually consist of unencapsulated brain tissue with evenly spaced astrocytes, oligodendroglia, microglia, fibrillar glial tissue, and rare to absent neurons, all compartmentalized by fibrous tissue bands (Fig. 76). Mitoses are rare. Glial tissue may show focal fibrosis and increased vascularity. Gemistocytic astrocyte forms may occasionally be present (442). The presence of choroid plexus and ependymal and pigmented cells with retinal differentiation also have been described (148,443).

Special Studies

S-100 protein, NSE, and GFAP immunoreactivity are the rule. Electron microscopy aids in the identification of astrocytes, myelin, and glial and axonal processes (443).

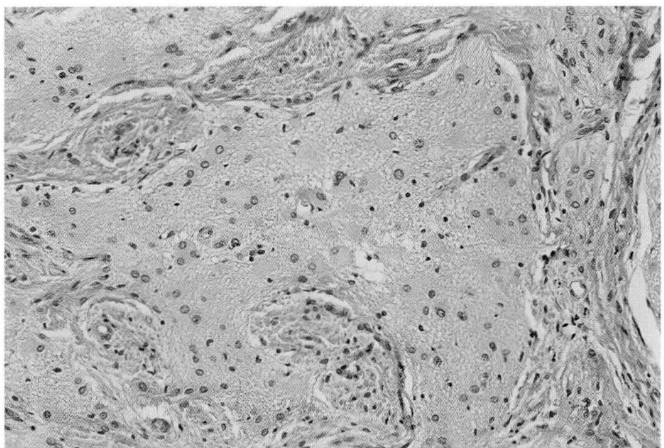

FIGURE 76. Nasal glial heterotopia. Unencapsulated brain tissue compartmentalized by fibrous tissue bands contains numerous gemistocytic astrocytes and no neurons. (Courtesy Dr. K-L. Ho.)

Differential Diagnosis

Dermoid cysts of the bridge of the nose share a similar clinical appearance to that of nasal glioma. Meningocele and myelomeningocele should also be considered in the differential diagnosis. It is important to remember that S-100, NSE, and GFAP immunoreactivity will be present in both nasal glioma and encephalocele and will not aid in distinguishing between them. Nasal glial heterotopias are firmer than nasal polyps, the latter also being extremely rare in childhood.

Biologic Behavior

Simple excision for uncomplicated cases is generally curative, although a recurrence rate of 4% to 10% has been reported (148,443). Intracranial connection must be ruled out before surgery and addressed surgically if present to avoid meningitis and cerebrospinal fluid rhinorrhea. Thus, it is crucial to distinguish glial heterotopias from inflammatory nasal polyps.

Encephalocele

Meningocele and meningoencephalocele (encephalocele) are congenital (rarely trauma induced) lesions associated in roughly one third of cases with other midline facial malformations (148). They usually present on the nasal bridge or superior nasal cavity and consist of a normal meningeal (dura or arachnoid) sac with or without normal brain tissue contents (Fig. 77). The discrimination between brain tissue heterotopia is based on the absence of fibrous compartments and the prominent presence of neurons and meninges in encephalocele. Recognition is important because of the potential to develop meningitis and cerebrospinal fluid leak (see Chapter 1) (438,444).

Meningioma

Clinical Data

Meningiomas of the sinonasal tract may invade directly from the central nervous system or originate *de novo* from embryologically misplaced arachnoid tissue either associated with nerve fibers or trapped outside of the skull after the fusion of the cranial bones (445). The sinonasal tract is an uncommon place for extracranial meningiomas, which are more commonly seen in the orbit, skin, and ear (446).

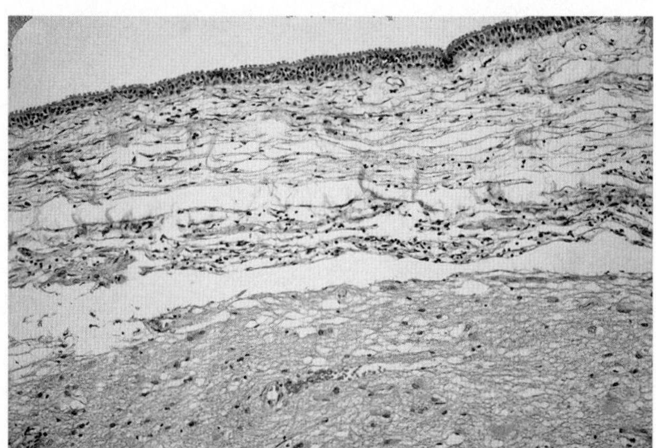

FIGURE 77. Encephalocele. Nasal cavity extension of neuron containing brain tissue enclosed within a meningeal sac.

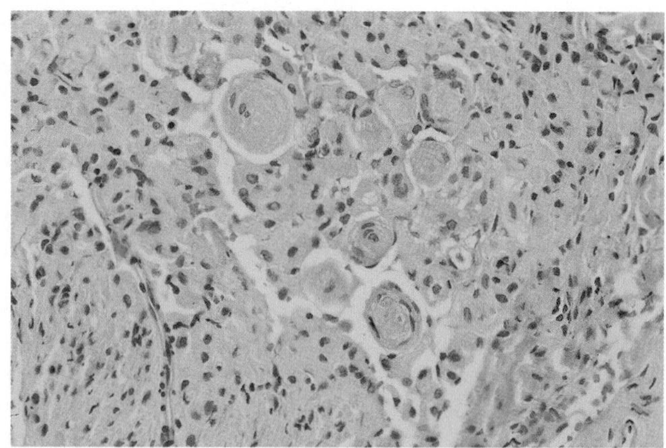

FIGURE 78. Meningioma. Ethmoid sinus tumor with whorled pattern of meningothelial variant.

Sinonasal meningiomas are slowly growing masses that occur in younger patients (median age 28 years) than those with intracranial meningioma (median age 45 years) (446). Although Hyams described no sex predilection in his series from the AFIP, Ho reported a slight male tendency (58,446). The incidence is increased in patients with neurofibromatosis, especially neurofibromatosis type II (58). Clinical presentation is nonspecific and might be related to involvement or compression of the orbit or facial deformity.

Radiologic Appearance

Sclerosis of adjacent bone, tumor calcification, bony destruction and extensive sinus involvement are usually observed on radiography (447,448).

Gross Appearance

Lesions usually consist of mucosa-covered polypoid masses that are firmer than common inflammatory polyps.

Histologic Features

The histology is identical to that of primary intracranial meningiomas. The meningothelial variant is the most common, with meningothelial cells arranged in whorled patterns occasionally associated with psammoma bodies (445,446) (Fig. 78). Mixed (transitional) and psammomatous variants also have been described in the paranasal sinuses (446). However, none of the other benign or malignant variants of intracranial meningioma have been reported.

Special Studies

Most meningiomas are immunoreactive for vimentin and EMA and less commonly for cytokeratin and S-100 protein (449).

Differential Diagnosis

Fibrous histiocytoma may mimic meningioma, but the absence of psammoma bodies and the presence of spindle and giant cells may aid in the differential diagnosis. Neurilemmoma and neurofibroma will exhibit palisading of S-100 protein–positive spindle cells within a myxoid stroma and should be EMA negative. Myoepithelioma is cytokeratin positive and usually does not present a whorling pattern or psammoma bodies. Amelanotic malignant melanoma and olfactory neuroblastoma have distinctive morphologic and immunohistochemical profiles. Psammomatous ossifying fibroma might also be considered in the differential diagnosis (see Chapter 11).

Biologic Behavior

Complete resection is curative, but recurrence may follow incomplete excision.

Pituitary Adenoma

Clinical Data

Pituitary adenomas of the paranasal sinuses can be primary entities or extensions from intrasellar tumors. Roughly 2% of pituitary adenomas will invade beyond the sella turcica and extend into the sphenoid sinus, posterior nasal cavity, or superior nasopharynx, presenting as upper respiratory polypoid lesions or space-occupying masses (450–452). Uncommonly, pituitary adenomas may be primary sinonasal lesions associated with normal pituitary glands and generally reported in the nasal cavity, sphenoid sinus (Fig. 79), nasopharynx, sphenoidal wing, and petrous temporal bone (453–458). It is theorized that the primary tumors arise from the small nests of normally occurring nasopharyngeal pituitary tissue (see Chapter 5) or from ectopic pituitary tissue misplaced during the migration of the anterior pituitary cells from Rathke's pouch (450,453). Intracranial dissemination of adenomatous cells during pituitary surgery is also postulated as a pathophysiologic mechanism (457).

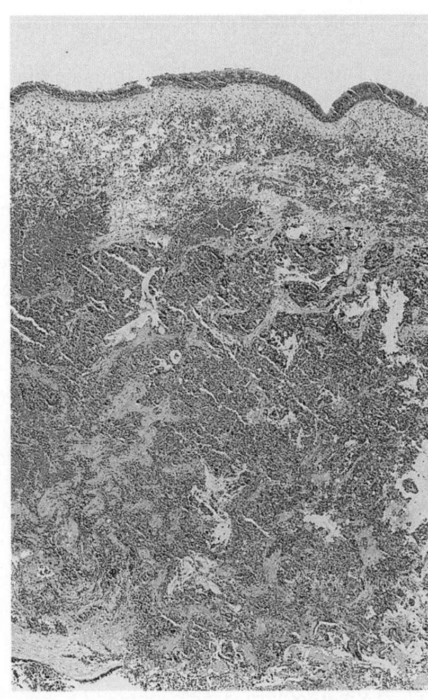

FIGURE 79. Pituitary adenoma. Cellular tumor of sphenoid sinus; such specimens may be diagnostically challenging in small fragmented biopsy samples. (Courtesy of Dr. K-L. Ho.)

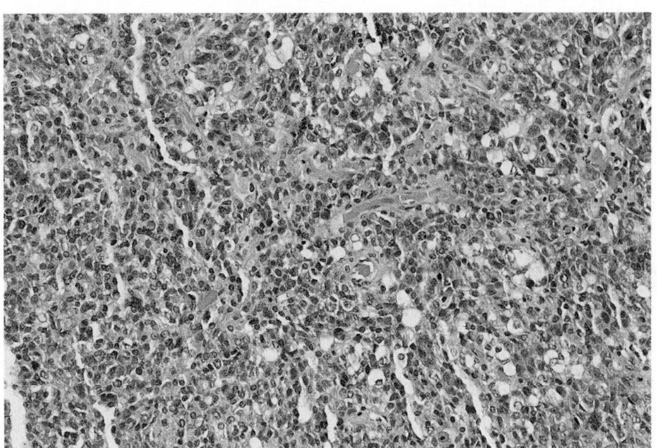

FIGURE 80. Pituitary adenoma. Nested epithelial pattern of cells with abundant cytoplasm with coarse granules is histologically identical to lesions of the sella. (Courtesy of Dr. K-L. Ho.)

These tumors may be functional through production of prolactin, thyroid stimulating hormone, and adrenal corticotrophic hormone, sometimes with consequent Cushing's syndrome (454,456,457). Headache, sinonasal pain, nasal obstruction, and visual symptoms may be some of the presenting symptoms.

Radiologic Studies

Radiography and computed axial tomography may aid in the differentiation of ectopic adenoma from the extracranial extension of a pituitary adenoma.

Histologic Features

Pituitary adenomas in this region are histologically identical to those within the sella, consisting of nests and cords of cells with a nested epithelial pattern, moderate degree of pleomorphism, mild mitotic activity, and abundant cytoplasm with coarse or fine granules (Fig. 80). Nuclei may be eccentric, imparting a plasmacytoid appearance to the lesion.

Special Studies

Pituitary adenomas have a cytokeratin intermediate filament skeleton and neuroendocrine granules that stain for synaptophysin and chromogranin.

Differential Diagnosis

The differential diagnosis of pituitary adenomas may be challenging, especially in small fragmented biopsy samples. Undifferentiated carcinoma, plasmacytoma, and paraganglioma may be among the diagnostic considerations. Confusion with olfactory neuroblastoma and paraganglioma may be avoided if a fibrillary background in olfactory neuroblastoma and larger cell nests with S-100 protein–positive sustentacular cells in both olfactory neuroblastoma and paraganglioma are detected. Immunohistochemical detection of pituitary hormones also may be helpful in the identification and differential diagnosis (315). The distinctive immunoprofiles of these entities are shown in Table 4.

Biologic Behavior

The biologic behavior of sinonasal pituitary adenomas may be locally aggressive and destructive.

METASTATIC TUMORS

When a morphologically unusual tumor, especially a glandular neoplasm, is encountered in the nasal cavity and paranasal sinuses, the possibility of metastatic disease should be considered and excluded clinically. Metastases are encountered in order of decreasing frequency, in the maxillary, ethmoid, and frontal sinuses followed by the nasal cavity (253).

The most common source of metastatic malignancy is renal cell adenocarcinoma followed by carcinomas of lung, breast, testis, and gastrointestinal tract (253). Metastases from the prostate, stomach, uterus, adrenal, pancreas, and thyroid have all been reported to metastasize to the nasal cavity and paranasal sinuses. Melanoma is only rarely metastatic to this region (359). There also may be involvement by direct extension from cutaneous basal cell carcinoma. Leukemic and lymphomatous infiltrates of the sinonasal tract may be encountered as a component of systemic dissemination.

Occasionally tissue-specific markers such as prostate specific antigen and prostatic acid phosphatase (in the prostate); gross cystic disease fluid protein (GCDFP-15), estrogen, and progesterone receptors (in the breast); villin, CK7, and CK20 (in the colon); and surfactant (in the lung) may be helpful in defining a distant primary site for some glandular neoplasms (459,460).

REFERENCES

1. Moore KL. *The developing human,* 2nd ed. Philadelphia: WB Saunders, 1977:168–175.
2. Hollinshead WH. The nose and paranasal sinuses. In: *Anatomy for surgeons: the head and neck,* 3rd ed. Philadelphia. Harper & Row, 1982:223–267.
3. Williams PL, Bannister LH, Berry MM, et al. In: Bannister L, ed. *Gray's anatomy: the anatomical basis of medicine and surgery,* 38th ed. New York: Churchill Livingstone, 1995:1631–1637.
4. Cormack DH. *Ham's histology,* 9th ed. Philadelphia: JB Lippincott, 1987:544–546.
5. Harding J, Graziadei PPC, Monti-Graziadei GA, et al. Denervation in the primary olfactory pathway of mice. IV. Biochemical and morphological evidence for neuronal replacement following nerve section. *Brain Res* 1977;132:11–28.
6. Graziadei PPC, Monti-Graziadei GA. Development of sensory systems: continuous nerve cell renewal in the olfactory system. In: Jacobson M, ed. *Handbook of sensory physiology.* New York: Springer-Verlag, 1978:55.
7. Brandtzaeg P. Immunocompetent cells of the upper airway: functions in normal and diseased mucosa. *Eur Arch Otorhinolaryngol* 1995;252(suppl):8–21.
8. Gwaltney JM. Rhinovirus infection of the normal human airway. *Am J Respir Crit Care Med* 1995;152(suppl):36–39.
9. Simon HB. Infectious disease, bacterial infections of the upper respiratory tract. In: Dale DC, Federman DD, eds. *Scientific American medicine.* New York: Scientific American, 1978–1997:1–12.
10. Zurlo JJ, Feuerstein IM, Lebovics R, et al. Sinusitis in HIV-1 infection. *Am J Med* 1992;93:157–162.
11. Godofsky EW, Zinreich J, Armstrong M, et al. Sinusitis in HIV infected patients: a clinical and radiographic review. *Am J Med* 1992;93:163–170.
12. Marks SC, Upadhyay S, Crane L. Cytomegalovirus sinusitis. A new manifestation of AIDS. *Arch Otolaryngol Head Neck Surg* 1996;122: 787–791.
13. Oliverio PJ, Benson ML, Zinreich SJ. Update on imaging for functional endoscopic sinus surgery. *Otolaryngol Clin North Am* 1995; 28:585–608.
14. Adams PF, Marano MA. Current estimates from the National Health Interview Survey. *Vital Health Stat* 1994;10:83–84.
15. Parsons DS, Wald ER. Otitis media and sinusitis. *Otolaryngol Clin North Am* 1994;29:11–25.
16. Melen I. Chronic sinusitis: clinical and pathophysiologic aspects. *Acta Otolaryngol* 1994;515:45–48.
17. Parsons DS. Chronic sinusitis. A medical or surgical disease? *Otolaryngol Clin North Am* 1996;29:1–9.
18. Karlsson G, Holmberg K. Does allergic rhinitis predispose to sinusitis? *Acta Otolaryngol* 1994;515(suppl):26–29.
19. Teknos TN, Metson R, Chasse T, et al. New developments in the diagnosis of Kartagener's syndrome. *Otolaryngol Head Neck Surg* 1997; 116:68–74.
20. de Longh RU, Rutland J. Ciliary defects in healthy subjects, bronchiectasis, and primary ciliary dyskinesia. *Am J Respir Crit Care Med* 1995;151:1559–1567.
21. Nishioka GJ, Cook PR. Paranasal sinus disease in patients with cystic fibrosis. *Otolaryngol Clin North Am* 1996;29:193–205.
22. Wiatrak BJ, Myer CM, Cotton RT. Cystic fibrosis presenting with sinus disease in children. *Am J Dis Child* 1993;147:258–260.
23. Strober W, Sneller MD. IgA deficiency. *Ann Allergy* 1991;66: 363–375.
24. Brandtzaeg P, Jahnsen FL, Farstad IN. Immune functions and immunopathology of the mucosa of the upper respiratory pathways. *Acta Otolaryngol* 1996;116:146–159.
25. Kennedy DW, Senior BA. Endoscopic sinus surgery: a review. *Otolaryngol Clin North Am* 1997;30:313–330.
26. Rice DH, Fishman SM, Barton RT, et al. Cranial complications of frontal sinusitis. *American Family Physician* 1980;22:145–149.
27. Yamasoba T, Kikuchi S. Intracranial complications resulting from frontal pyocele: case presentation and review of experience in Japan. *Head Neck* 1993;15:450–454.
28. Larsen K. The clinical relationship of nasal polyps to asthma. *Allergy Asthma Proc* 1996;17:243–249.
29. Stierna PLE. Nasal polyps: relationship to infection and inflammation. *Allergy Asthma Proc* 1996;17:251–257.
30. Batsakis JG, El-Naggar AK. Cystic fibrosis and the sinonasal tract. *Ann Otol Rhinol Laryngol* 1996;105:329–330.
31. Settipane GA. Epidemiology of nasal polyps. *Allergy Asthma Proc* 1996;17:231–236.
32. Settipane GA. Nasal polyps: epidemiology, pathology, immunology and treatment. *Am J Rhinol* 1987;1:119–126.
33. Settipane G, Chafee FH. Nasal polyps in asthma and rhinitis: a review of 6,037 patients. *J Allergy Clin Immunol* 1977;59:17–21.
34. Sullivan WB, Linehan AT, Hilman BC, et al. Flexible fiberoptic rhinoscopy in the diagnosis of nasal polyps in cystic fibrosis. *Allergy Asthma Proc* 1996;17:287–292.
35. Larsen PL, Tos M. Origin of nasal polyps. *Laryngoscope* 1991;101: 305–312.

36. Batsakis JG, Sneige N. Choanal and angiomatous polyps of the sinonasal tract. *Laryngology* 1992;101:623–625.
37. Berg O, Carenfelt C, Silfversward C, et al. Origin of the choanal polyp. *Arch Otolaryngol Head Neck Surg* 1988;114:1270–1271.
38. Hellquist HB. Nasal polyps update. Histopathology. *Allergy Asthma Proc* 1996;17:237–242.
39. Oppenheimer EH, Rosenstein BJ. Differential pathology of nasal polyps in cystic fibrosis and atopy. *Lab Invest* 1979;40:445–449.
40. Tos M, Mogensen C, Thomsen J. Nasal polyps in cystic fibrosis. *J Laryngol Otol* 1977;91:827–835.
41. Compagno J, Hyams VJ, Lepore ML. Nasal polyposis with stromal atypia. *Arch Pathol Lab Med* 1976;100:224–226.
42. Kindblom LG, Angerwall L. Nasal polyps with atypical stromal cells. *Acta Pathol Microbiol Immunol Scand* 1984;92:65–72.
43. De La Cruz-Mera A, Sanchez-Lopez MJ, Merino-Royo E, et al. Premalignant changes in nasal and sinus polyps: a retrospective 10 year study. *J Laryngol Otol* 1990;104:210–212.
44. Mygind N, Lildholdt T. Nasal polyps treatment: medical management. *Allergy Asthma Proc* 1996;17:275–282.
45. Natvig K, Larsen TE. Mucocele of the paranasal sinuses: a retrospective clinical and histological study. *J Laryngol Otol* 1982;92: 1075–1082.
46. Wolfowitz BL, Solomon A. Mucoceles of the frontal and ethmoid sinuses. *J Laryngol Otol* 1972;86:79–82.
47. Benninger MS, Marks S. The endoscopic management of sphenoid and ethmoid mucoceles with orbital and intranasal extension. *Rhinology* 1995;33:157–161.
48. Lund VJ, Henderson B, Song Y. Involvement of cytokines and vascular adhesion receptors in the pathology of fronto-ethmoidal mucoceles. *Acta Otolaryngol* 1993;113:540–546.
49. Evans C. Aetiology and treatment of fronto-ethmoidal mucocele. *J Laryngol Otol* 1981;95:361–375.
50. Marks SC, Latoni JD, Mathog RH. Mucoceles of the maxillary sinus. *Otolaryngol Head Neck Surg* 1997;117:18–21.
51. Canalis RF, Zajtchuk JT, Jenkins HA. Ethmoidal mucoceles. *Arch Otolaryngol* 1978;104:286–291.
52. Kyriakos M. Myospherulosis of the paranasal sinuses, nose and middle ear: a possible iatrogenic disease. *Am J Clin Pathol* 1977;67: 118–130.
53. McClatchie S, Warambo M, Bremner A. Myospherulosis. A previously unreported disease? *Am J Clin Pathol* 1969;51:699–704.
54. DeSchryver-Kecskemeti K, Kyriakos M. Myospherulosis: an electron microscopic study of a human case. *Am J Clin Pathol* 1977;67: 555–561.
55. Wheeler TM, Sessions RB, McGavran MH. Myospherulosis: a preventable iatrogenic nasal and paranasal entity. *Arch Otolaryngol* 1980;106:272–274.
56. Rosai J. The nature of myospherulosis of the upper respiratory tract. *Am J Clin Pathol* 1978;69:475–481.
57. Hyams V, Batsakis J, Michaels L. Tumors simulating neoplasia or of questionable neoplastic classification. In: *Tumors of the upper respiratory tract and ear.* Washington, DC: Armed Forces Institute of Pathology, 1988:28–30.
58. Hyams VJ. Pathology of the nose and paranasal sinuses. In: English GM, ed. *Otolaryngology.* Philadelphia: Harper & Row, 1987:1–95.
59. Tzerbos FH, Mavrogeorgis A, Kavantzas NG, et al. A cholesterol granuloma in the maxillary sinus: report of case. *J Oral Maxillofac Surg* 1994;52:1205–1207.
60. Erpek G, Ustun H. Cholesterol granuloma in the maxillary sinus. *Eur Arch Otorhinolaryngol* 1994;251:246–247.
61. Marks SC, Smith DM. Endoscopic treatment of maxillary sinus cholesterol granuloma. *Laryngoscope* 1995;105:551–552.
62. Brandwein M. Histopathology of sinonasal fungal disease. *Otolaryngol Clin North Am* 1993;26:949–981.
63. Blitzer A, Lawson W. Fungal infections of the nose and paranasal sinuses. *Otolaryngol Clin North Am* 1993;26:1007–1035.
64. Lawson W, Blitzer A. Fungal infections of the nose and paranasal sinuses. Part II. *Otolaryngol Clin North Am* 1993;26:1037–1068.
65. Zieske L, Kopke R, Hamill R. Dematiaceous fungal sinusitis. *Otolaryngol Head Neck Surg* 1991;105:567–577.
66. Bent JP, Kuhn FA. Allergic fungal sinusitis/polyposis. *Allergy Asthma Proc* 1996;17:259–268.
67. Katzenstein A, Sale S, Greenberger P. Pathologic findings in allergic aspergillus sinusitis: a newly recognized form of sinusitis. *Am J Surg Pathol* 1983;7:439–443.
68. Goldstein MF, Atkins PC, Cogen FC, et al. Allergic aspergillus sinusitis. *J Allergy Clin Immunol* 1985;76:515–524.
69. Jonathan D, Lund V, Milroy C. Allergic aspergillus sinusitis—an overlooked diagnosis? *J Laryngol Otol* 1989;103:1181–1183.
70. Waxman JE, Spector JG, Sale SR, et al. Allergic aspergillus sinusitis: concepts in diagnosis and treatment of a new clinical entity. *Laryngoscope* 1987;97:261–266.
71. Jackson IT, Schmitt E, Carpenter HA. Allergic aspergillus sinusitis. *Plast Reconstr Surg* 1986;79:804–808.
72. Philip G, Keen CE. Allergic fungal sinusitis. *Histopathology* 1984;14:222–224.
73. Manning SC, Vuitch F, Weinberg AG, et al. Allergic aspergillosis: a newly recognized form of sinusitis in the pediatric population. *Laryngoscope* 1989;99:681–685.
74. Hartwick RW, Batsakis JG. Sinus aspergillosis and allergic fungal sinusitis. *Ann Otol Rhinol Laryngol* 1991;100:427–430.
75. Stammberger J, Jakse R, Beaufort F. Aspergillosis of the paranasal sinuses x-ray diagnosis, histopathology, and clinical aspects. *Ann Otol Rhinol Laryngol* 1984;93:251–256.
76. Chakrabarti A, Sharma SC, Chander J. Epidemiology and pathogenesis of paranasal sinus mycosis. *Otolaryngol Head Neck Surg* 1992; 107:745–750.
77. Som PM. Imaging of paranasal sinus fungal disease. *Otolaryngol Clin North Am* 1993;26:983–994.
78. Yoo GH, Francis HW, Zinreich SJ. Imaging quiz case: non-invasive aspergillus sinusitis. *Arch Otol* 1993;119:123–124.
79. Wenig B. *Atlas of head and neck pathology.* Philadelphia: WB Saunders, 1993:16.
80. Choi SS, Lawson W, Bottone E, et al. Cryptococcal sinusitis: a case report and review of the literature. *Otolaryngol Head Neck Surg* 1988;99:414–418.
81. Corey J. Fungal diseases of the sinuses. *Otolaryngol Head Neck Surg* 1990;103:1012–1015.
82. Anand V, Alemar G, Griswold J. Intracranial complications of mucormycosis: an experimental model and clinical review. *Laryngoscope* 1992;102:656–662.
83. Blitzer A, Lawson W, Meyers B. Patient survival factors in paranasal sinus mucormycosis. *Laryngoscope* 1980;90:635–648.
84. Mills S, Fechner R. The nose, paranasal sinuses, and nasopharynx. In: Sternberg S, ed. *Diagnostic surgical pathology.* New York: Raven, 1987:851–891.
85. Batsakis J, Luna M. Midfacial necrotizing lesions. *Semin Diagn Pathol* 1987;4:90–116.
86. McCaffrey T, McDonald T. Sarcoidosis of the nose and paranasal sinuses. *Laryngoscope* 1983;93:1281–1284.
87. Hoffman G, Kerr G, Leavitt R, et al. Wegener's granulomatosis: an analysis of 158 patients. *Ann Intern Med* 1992;116:488–498.
88. Waldman S, Levine H, Sebek B, et al. Nasal tuberculosis: a forgotten entity. *Laryngoscope* 1981;91:11–16.
89. Churg J, Strauss L. Allergic granulomatosis, allergic angiitis, and periarteritis nodosa. *Am J Pathol* 1951;27:277–301.
90. Leavitt R, Fauci A, Bloch D, et al. The American College of Rheumatology 1990 criteria for the classification of Wegener's Granulomatosis. *Arthritis Rheumatism* 1990;33:1101–1107.
91. McDonald T, DeRemee R, Kern E, et al. Nasal manifestations of Wegener's granulomatosis. *Laryngoscope* 1974;84:2101–2112.
92. Specks U, Homburger H. Anti-neutrophil cytoplasmic antibodies. *Mayo Clin Proc* 1994;69:1197–1198.
93. Kirby RE, Fechner FP, Pilch BZ. Orbital Wegener's granulomatosis: a clinicopathologic study of 13 cases [Abstract]. *Mod Pathol* 1998; 11:120A.
94. Devaney K, Travis W, Hoffman G, et al. Interpretation of head and neck biopsies in Wegener's granulomatosis: a pathologic study of 126 biopsies in 70 patients. *Am J Surg Pathol* 1990;14:555–564.

95. Del-Buono E, Flint A. Diagnostic usefulness of nasal biopsy in Wegener's granulomatosis. *Hum Pathol* 1991;22:107–110.
96. Colby T, Tazelaar H, Specks U, et al. Nasal biopsy in Wegener's granulomatosis. *Hum Pathol* 1991;22:101–104.
97. Tsokos M, Fauci A, Costa J. Idiopathic midline destructive disease (IMDD): a subgroup of patients with the "midline granuloma" syndrome. *Am J Clin Pathol* 1982;77:162–168.
98. Chumbley L, Harrison E, DeRemee R. Allergic granulomatosis and angiitis (Churg-Strauss syndrome): report and analysis of 30 cases. *Mayo Clin Proc* 1977;52:477–484.
99. Olsen K, Neel H, DeRemee R, et al. Nasal manifestations of allergic granulomatosis and angiitis (Churg-Strauss syndrome). *Otolaryngol Head Neck Surg* 1980;88:85–89.
100. Krespi Y, Kuriloff D, Aner M. Sarcoidosis of the sinonasal tract: a new staging system. *Otolaryngol Head Neck Surg* 1995;112:221–227.
101. Fischer R, Kennedy K. Sarcoidosis presenting as chronic sinusitis with facial fistulization. *Am J Rhinol* 1991;5:67–70.
102. Pollack J, Pincus R, Lucente F. Leprosy of the head and neck. *Otolaryngol Head Neck Surg* 1987;97:93–96.
103. McDougall A, Rees R, Weddell A, et al. The histopathology of lepromatous leprosy in the nose. *J Pathol* 1975;115:215–226.
104. Batsakis J, El-Naggar A. Pathology consultation: rhinoscleroma and rhinosporidiosis. *Ann Otol Rhinol Laryngol* 1992;101:879–882.
105. Alfaro-Monge J, Fernandez-Espinosa J, Soda-Merhy A. Scleroma of the lower respiratory tract: case report and review of literature. *J Laryngol Otol* 1994;108:161–163.
106. Andraca R, Edson R, Kern E. Rhinoscleroma: a growing concern in the United States? Mayo Clinic experience. *Mayo Clin Proc* 1993; 68:1151–1157.
107. Toohill R: Editorial: Rhinoscleroma in perspective. *Mayo Clin Proc* 1993;68:1219.
108. Sedano H, Carlos R, Koutlas I: Respiratory scleroma: a clinicopathologic and ultrastructural study. *Oral Surg Oral Med Oral Pathol Oral Radiol Endod* 1996;81:665–671.
109. Shum T, Whitaker C, Meyer P. Clinical update on rhinoscleroma. *Laryngoscope* 1982;92:1149–1153.
110. Lenis A, Ruff T, Diaz J, et al. Rhinoscleroma. *South Med J* 1988; 81:1580–1582.
111. Meyer P, Shum T, Becker T, et al. Scleroma (rhinoscleroma). A histologic immunohistochemical study with bacteriologic correlates. *Arch Pathol Lab Med* 1983;107:377–383.
112. Wenig BM, Harpaz N, DelBridge C. Polymorphous low-grade adenocarcinoma of seromucous glands of the nasopharynx. A report of a case and a discussion of the morphologic and immunohistochemical features. *Am J Clin Pathol* 1989;92:104–109.
113. Ratnaker C, Madhavan M, Sankaran V, et al. Rhinosporidiosis in Pondicherry. *J Trop Med Hygiene* 1995;95:280–283.
114. Gaines J, Clay J, Chandler F, et al. Rhinosporidiosis: three domestic cases. *South Med J* 1996;89:65–67.
115. Von-Haacke N, Mugliston T. Rhinosporidiosis. *J Laryngol Otol* 1982;96:743–750.
116. Warner E. Cocaine abuse. *Ann Intern Med* 1993;119:226–235.
117. Brody S, Slovis C, Wrenn K. Cocaine-related medical problems: consecutive series of 233 patients. *Am J Med* 1990;88:325–331.
118. Deutsch H, Millard R. A new cocaine abuse complex: involvement of nose, septum, palate, and pharynx. *Arch Otolaryngol Head Neck Surg* 1989;115:235–237.
119. Kuriloff D, Kimmelman C. Osteocartilaginous necrosis of the sinonasal tract following cocaine abuse. *Laryngoscope* 1989;99: 918–924.
120. Sercarz J, Strasnick B, Newman A, et al. Midline nasal destruction in cocaine abusers. *Otolaryngol Head Neck Surg* 1991;105:694–701.
121. Sevinsky L, Woscoff A, Jaimovich L, et al. Nasal cocaine abuse mimicking midline granuloma. *J Am Acad Dermatol* 1995;32:286–287.
122. Zajtchuk J, Casler J, Netto E, et al. Mucosal leishmaniasis in Brazil. *Laryngoscope* 1989;99:925–939.
123. Dictor M, Cervin A, Kalm O, et al. Sinonasal T-cell lymphoma in the differential diagnosis of lethal midline granuloma using in situ hybridization for Epstein-Barr virus RNA. *Mod Pathol* 1996; 9:7–14.
124. Frierson H, Mills S, Innes D. Non-Hodgkin's lymphomas of the sinonasal region: histologic subtypes and their clinicopathologic features. *Am J Clin Pathol* 1984;81:721–727.
125. Frierson H, Innes D, Mills S, et al. Immunophenotypic analysis of sinonasal non-Hodgkin's lymphomas. *Hum Pathol* 1989;20: 636–642.
126. Liang R, Todd D, Chan T, et al. Treatment outcome and prognostic factors for primary nasal lymphoma. *J Clin Oncol* 1995;13:666–670.
127. Arber D, Weiss L, Albujar P, et al. Nasal lymphomas in Peru, high incidence of T-cell immunophenotype and Epstein-Barr virus infection. *Am J Surg Pathol* 1993;17:392–399.
128. Ho F, Choy D, Loke S, et al. Polymorphic reticulosis and conventional lymphomas of the nose and upper aerodigestive tract: a clinicopathologic study of 70 cases, and immunophenotypic studies of 16 cases. *Hum Pathol* 1990;21:1041–1050.
129. Chan J, Yip T, Tsang W, et al. Detection of Epstein-Barr viral RNA in malignant lymphomas of the upper aerodigestive tract. *Am J Surg Pathol* 1994;18:938–946.
130. Harris NL, Jaffe ES, Stein H, et al. A revised European-American classification of lymphoid neoplasms: a proposal from the International Lymphoma Study Group. *Blood* 1994;84:1361–1392.
131. Kwong Y, Chan A, Liang R, et al. $CD56^+$ NK lymphomas: clinicopathological features and prognosis. *Br J Haematol* 1997;97: 821–829.
132. Jaffe E. Post-thymic T-cell lymphomas. In: Jaffe E, ed. *Surgical pathology of the lymph nodes and related organs.* Philadelphia: WB Saunders, 1995:344–389.
133. Jaffe E, Chan JKC, Su I-J, et al. Report of the workshop on nasal and related extranodal angiocentric T/natural killer cell lymphomas. *Am J Surg Pathol* 1996;20:103–111.
134. Ferry J, Sklar J, Zukerberg K, et al. Nasal lymphoma: a clinicopathologic study with immunophenotypic and genotypic analysis. *Am J Surg Pathol* 1991;15:268–279.
135. Zarbo RJ, McClatchey KD. Nasopharyngeal hamartoma: report of a case and review of the literature. *Laryngoscope* 1983;93:494–497.
136. Kacker SK, Dasgupta G. Hamartomas of ear and nose. *J Laryngol Otol* 1973;87:801–805.
137. Majumder NK, Venkataramiah NK, Gupta KR, et al. Clinical records: hamartoma of nasopharynx. *J Laryngol Otol* 1977;91: 723–727.
138. Day LH, Arnold GE. Rare tumors of the ear nose and throat. *Laryngoscope* 1971;81:1138–1174.
139. Wenig BM, Heffner DK. Respiratory epithelial adenomatoid hamartomas of the sinonasal tract and nasopharynx: a clinicopathologic study of 31 cases. *Ann Otol Rhinol Laryngol* 1995;104:639–645.
140. Mahindra S, Malik GB, Bais AS, et al. Vascular hamartoma of the paranasal sinuses. *Acta Otolaryngol* 1981;92:379–382.
141. Brandenburg JH, Finch WW, Lloyd R. Cystic hamartoma of the nasopharynx. *Trans Am Acad Ophthalmol Otol* 1977;84:152–153.
142. Birt BD, Knight-Jones EB. Respiratory distress due to nasopharyngeal hamartoma. *BMJ* 1969;3:281–282.
143. Baillie EE, Batsakis JG. Glandular (seromucinous) hamartoma of the nasopharynx. *Oral Surg* 1974;38:760–762.
144. Ladapo AA. A case of benign congenital hamartoma of the nasopharynx. *J Laryngol Otol* 1978;92:1141–1145.
145. Graeme-Cook F, Pilch BZ. Hamartomas of the nose and nasopharynx. *Head Neck* 1992;14:321–327.
146. McDermott MB, Ponder TB, Dehner LP. Nasal chondromesenchymal hamartoma. An upper respiratory tract analogue of the chest wall mesenchymal hamartoma. *Am J Surg Pathol* 1998;22:425–433.
147. Chisin R, Ragozzino MW, Flexon PB, et al. MR assessment of a hamartoma of the nasal cavity [Letter]. *Am J Radiol* 1987;149: 1083–1084.
148. Kapadia SB, Popek EJ, Barnes L. Pediatric otorhinolaryngic pathology: diagnosis of selected lesions. *Pathol Annu* 1994;29:159–209.
149. Reilly JR, Koopman CF, Cotton R. Nasal mass in a pediatric patient. *Head Neck* 1992;1:415–418.
150. Kuriloff DB. The nasolabial cyst-nasal hamartoma. *Otolaryngol Head Neck Surg* 1987;96:268–272.
151. Rao RV. Nasolabial cyst. *J Laryngol Otol* 1955;69:352–354.

152. Frodel JL, Larrabee WF, Raisis J. The nasal dermoid. *Otolaryngol Head Neck Surg* 1989;101:392–396.
153. Ward RF, April M. Teratomas of head and neck. *Otolaryngol Clin North Am* 1989;22:621–629.
154. Gnepp DR. Teratoid neoplasms of the head and neck. In: Barnes L, ed. *Surgical pathology of the head and neck.* New York: Marcel Dekker, 1985:1411–1433.
155. Kelly AB. Hairy or dermoid polypi of the pharynx and nasopharynx. *J Laryngol Rhinol Otol* 1918;33:65–70.
156. Batsakis JG. Teratomas of the head and neck. In: Batsakis MD, ed. *Tumors of the head and neck.* Baltimore: Williams & Wilkins, 1979:226–232.
157. Bicknell MR. Hairy polyp of the nasopharynx. *J Laryngol Otol* 1967;81:1045–1048.
158. Taylor BW, Erich JB. Dermoid cysts of the nose. *Mayo Clin Proc* 1967;42:488.
159. Gonzalez-Crussi F. Teratomas of head (extracranial). *Extragonadal teratomas.* Washington, DC: Armed Forces Institute of Pathology, 1982:109–117.
160. Ehrich WE. Teratoid parasites of the mouth (episphenoids, epipalati [epurani], epignathi). *Am J Orthodont Oral Surg* 1945;31:650–659.
161. Willis RA. Some unusual developmental heterotopias. *BMJ* 1968;3:267–272.
162. Lack EE. Extragonadal germ cell tumors of the head and neck region: review of 16 cases. *Hum Pathol* 1985;16:56–64.
163. Heffner DK, Hyams VJ. Teratocarcinosarcoma (malignant teratoma?) of the nasal cavity and paranasal sinuses. A clinicopathologic study of 20 cases. *Cancer* 1984;53:2140–2154.
164. Patchefsky A, Sundmaker W, Marden PA. Malignant teratoma of the ethmoid sinus. Report of a case. *Cancer* 1968;21:714–721.
165. Dicke TE, Gates GA. Malignant teratoma of the paranasal sinuses. Report of a case. *Arch Otolaryngol* 1970;91:391–394.
166. Abt AB, Toker C. Malignant teratoma of the paranasal sinuses. *Arch Pathol* 1970;90:176–180.
167. Hamilton WJ, Mossman HW. *Human embryology,* 4th ed. Baltimore: Williams & Wilkins, 1972:293–299.
168. Geschickter CF. Tumors of the nasal and paranasal cavities. *Am J Cancer* 1935;24:637–660.
169. Ridolfi RL, Lieberman PH, Erlandson RA, et al. Schneiderian papillomas: a clinicopathologic study of 30 cases. *Am J Surg Pathol* 1977; 1:43—53.
170. Ewing J. Some phases of intraoral tumors, with special reference to therapy by radiation. *Radiology* 1927;4:359–370.
171. Hyams VJ. Papillomas of the nasal cavity and paranasal sinuses. *Ann Otol Rhinol Laryngol* 1971;80:192–206.
172. Norris HJ. Papillary lesions of the nasal cavity and paranasal sinuses. Part II. Exophytic (squamous) papillomas. A study of 28 cases. *Laryngoscope* 1962;72:1784–1797.
173. Henriksson NG. Papillomas of the nose: a clinical survey and contribution to our knowledge of these tumors. *Acta Otolaryngol* 1952; 42:18–29.
174. Snyder RN, Perzin KH. Papillomatosis of nasal cavity and paranasal sinuses (inverted papilloma, squamous papilloma). A clinicopathologic study. *Cancer* 1972;30:668–690.
175. Oberman HA. Papillomas of the nose and paranasal sinuses. *Am J Clin Pathol* 1964;42:245–258.
176. Christensen WN, Smith RRL. Schneiderian papillomas: a clinicopathologic study of 67 cases. *Hum Pathol* 1986;17:393–400.
177. Herrold KM. Epithelial papillomas of the nasal cavity. *Arch Pathol* 1964;78:189–195.
178. Gaffey MJ, Frierson JF, Weiss LM, et al. Human papillomavirus and Epstein-Barr virus in sinonasal schneiderian papillomas. *Am J Clin Pathol* 1996;106:475–482.
179. MacDonald MR, Le KT, Freeman J, et al. A majority of inverted sinonasal papillomas carries Epstein-Barr virus genomes. *Cancer* 1995;75:2307–2312.
180. Kramer R, Som ML. True papilloma of the nasal cavity. *Arch Otolaryngol* 1935;22:22–43.
181. Momose KJ, Weber AL, Goodman M, et al. Radiological aspects of inverted papilloma. *Radiology* 1980;134:73–79.
182. Skolnik EM, Loewy A, Friedman JE. Inverted papilloma of the nasal cavity. *Arch Otolaryngol* 1966;84:83–89.
183. Mainzer F, Stargardter FL, Connolly ES, et al. Inverted papilloma of the nose and paranasal sinuses. *Radiology* 1969;92:964–968.
184. Kelly JH, Joseph M, Carroll E, et al. Inverted papilloma of the nasal septum. *Arch Otolaryngol* 1980;106:767–771.
185. Vrabec DP. The inverted schneiderian papilloma: a clinical and pathological study. *Laryngoscope* 1975;85:186–220.
186. Norris HJ. Papillary lesions of the nasal cavity and paranasal sinuses. Part III: Inverting papillomas, a study of 29 cases. *Laryngoscope* 1963;73:1–17.
187. Suh KW, Facer GW, Devine KD, et al. Inverting papilloma of the nose and paranasal sinuses. *Laryngoscope* 1977;87:35–46.
188. Ringertz N. Pathology of malignant tumors arising in nasal and paranasal cavities. *Acta Otolaryngol* 1938;27:31–42.
189. Shanmugaratnam K, Sobin L. Histological typing of upper respiratory tract tumours. In: *International histological classification of tumours,* 2nd ed. Geneva, Switzerland: World Health Organization, 1991: 31–32.
190. Ward BE, Fechner RE, Mills SE. Carcinoma arising in oncocytic Schneiderian papilloma. *Am J Surg Pathol* 1990;14:364–369.
191. Batsakis JG. Tumors of the head and neck. *Clinical and pathological considerations,* 2nd ed. Baltimore: Williams & Wilkins, 1979:58.
192. Fechner RE. Cylindrical cell papilloma (pathologic quiz, case 2). *Arch Otolaryngol* 1981;107:454–457.
193. Barnes L, Bedetti C. Oncocytic Schneiderian papilloma: a reappraisal of cylindrical cell papilloma of the sinonasal tract. *Hum Pathol* 1984;15:344–351.
194. DeBoom GW, Jensen JL, Wuerker RB. Cylindrical cell papilloma. *Oral Surg* 1986;61:607–610.
195. Jimenez JF, Young DE, Hough AJ. Rhinosporidiosis. A report of two cases from Arkansas. *Am J Clin Pathol* 1984;82:611–615.
196. Heffner DK, Hyams VJ, Hauck KW, et al. Low-grade adenocarcinoma of the nasal cavity and paranasal sinuses. *Cancer* 1982;50: 312–322.
197. Myers EN, Schramm VL Jr, Barnes EL. Management of inverted papilloma of the nose and paranasal sinuses. *Laryngoscope* 1981;91: 2071–2084.
198. Trible WM, Lekagul S. Inverting papilloma of the nose and paranasal sinuses: report of 30 cases. *Laryngoscope* 1971;81:663–668.
199. Cummings CW, Goodman ML. Inverted papillomas of the nose and paranasal sinuses. *Arch Otolaryngol* 1970;92:445–449.
200. Lampertico P, Russel WO, MacComb WS. Squamous papilloma of upper respiratory epithelium. *Arch Pathol* 1963;75:81–90.
201. Willis RA. *Pathology of tumors,* 3rd ed. Washington, DC: Butterworth, 1960.
202. Schoub L, Timme AH, Usy CJ. A well differentiated inverted papilloma of the nasal space associated with lymph node metastases. *S Afr Med J* 1973;47:1663–1665.
203. Gnepp DR, Heffner DK. Mucosal origin of sinonasal tract adenomatous neoplasms. *Mod Pathol* 1989;2:365–371.
204. Barnes L. Intestinal-type adenocarcinoma of the nasal cavity and paranasal sinuses. *Am J Surg Pathol* 1986;10:192–202.
205. Moran CA, Wenig BM, Mullick FG. Primary adenocarcinoma of the nasal cavity and paranasal sinuses. *Ear Nose Throat J* 1990;70: 821–828.
206. Compagno J, Wong RT. Intranasal mixed tumors (pleomorphic adenomas). A clinicopathologic study of 40 cases. *Am J Clin Pathol* 1977;68:213–218.
207. Heffner DK. Sinonasal and laryngeal salivary gland lesions. In: Ellis GL, Auclair PL, Gnepp DR, ed. *Surgical pathology of the salivary glands.* Philadelphia: WB Saunders, 1991:544–559.
208. Stevenson HN. Mixed tumor of the nasal septum. *Ann Otol Rhinol Laryngol* 1932;41:563–570.
209. Baer S, Alexander CM. Mixed tumor of salivary gland type in the nose. *NY State J Med* 1950;50:2206.
210. Gabriel GE. A case of mixed salivary tumour of the nasal septum. *J Laryngol Otol* 1952;66:329–330.
211. Ersner MS, Saltzman M. A mixed tumor of the nasal septum. Report of a case. *Laryngoscope* 1944;54:287–296.

212. Sooy FA. Primary tumors of the nasal septum. *Laryngoscope* 1950;60:964–992.
213. Zarbo RJ, Ricci A, Kowalczyk PDH, et al. Intranasal dermal analogue tumor (membranous basal cell adenoma). *Arch Otolaryngol* 1985;111:333–337.
214. Bégin LR, Rochon L, Frenkiel S. Spindle cell myoepithelioma of the nasal cavity. *Am J Surg Pathol* 1991;15:184–190.
215. Zarbo RJ, Regezi JA, Batsakis JG. S-100 protein in salivary gland tumors: an immunohistochemical study of 129 cases. *Head Neck Surg* 1986;8:268–275.
216. Zarbo RJ, Hatfield JS, Trojanowski JQ, et al. Immunoreactive glial fibrillary acidic protein in normal and neoplastic salivary glands: a combined immunohistochemical and immunoblot study. *Surg Pathol* 1988;1:55–63.
217. Savera AT, Gown AM, Zarbo RJ. Immunolocalization of three novel smooth muscle-specific proteins in salivary gland pleomorphic adenoma: assessment of the morphogenetic role of myoepithelium. *Mod Pathol* 1997;10:1093–1100.
218. Rafla S. Mucous gland tumors of paranasal sinuses. *Cancer* 1969;24: 683–691.
219. Goepfert H, Luna MA, Lindberg RD. Malignant salivary gland tumors of the paranasal sinuses and nasal cavity. *Arch Otolaryngol* 1983;109:662–668.
220. Batsakis JG, Holtz F, Sueper RH. Adenocarcinoma of nasal and paranasal cavities. *Arch Otolaryngol* 1963;77:625–633.
221. Spies JW. Adenoid cystic carcinoma. Generalized metastases in three cases of basal cell type. *Arch Surg* 1930;21:365–404.
222. Tran L, Sidrys J, Horton D, et al. Malignant salivary gland tumors of the paranasal sinuses and nasal cavity. The UCLA experience. *Am J Clin Oncol* 1989;12:387–392.
223. Mesara BW, Batsakis JG. Glandular tumors of the upper respiratory tract. A clinicopathologic assessment. *Arch Surg* 1966;92:872–878.
224. Eby LS, Johnson DS, Baker HW. Adenoid cystic carcinoma of the head and neck. *Cancer* 1972;29:1160–1168.
225. Perzin KH, Gullane P, Clairmont AC. Adenoid cystic carcinomas arising in salivary glands. A correlation of histologic features and clinical course. *Cancer* 1978;42:265–282.
226. Kadish SP, Goodman ML, Wang CC. Treatment of minor salivary gland malignancies of upper food and air passage epithelium. A review of 87 cases. *Cancer* 1972;29:1021–1026.
227. Batsakis JG. Salivary gland neoplasia: an outcome of modified morphogenesis and cytodifferentiation. *Oral Surg* 1980;49:229–232.
228. Parsons JT, Mendenhall WM, Mancuso AA, et al. Malignant tumors of the nasal cavity and ethmoid and sphenoid sinuses. *J Radiat Oncol Biol Phys* 1988;14:11–22.
229. Douglas JG, Laramore GE, Austin-Seymour M, et al. Neutron radiotherapy for adenoid cystic carcinoma of minor salivary glands. *Int J Radiat Oncol Biol Phys* 1996;36:87–93.
230. Buchholz TA, Shimotakahara SG, Weymuller EA, et al. Neutron radiotherapy for adenoid cystic carcinoma of the head and neck. *Arch Otolaryngol Head Neck Surg* 1993;119:747–752.
231. Prott FJ, Haverkamp U, Willich N, et al. Ten years of fast neutron therapy in Munster. *Bull Cancer Radiother* 1996;83(suppl):115–121.
232. Spiro RH, Huvos AG, Strong EW. Adenocarcinoma of salivary origin. Clinicopathologic study of 204 patients. *Am J Surg* 1982;144: 423–431.
233. Robinson RA. Tubulocystic adenocarcinoma arising in the nasal cavity. *J Laryngol Otol* 1987;101:607–610.
234. Healey WV. Mucoepidermoid cancer of salivary gland origin. *Cancer* 1970;26:368–388.
235. Frierson HF. Pathologic quiz case 1. *Arch Otolaryngol Head Neck Surg* 1986;112:568–570.
236. Dardick I, van Nostrand AWP. Polymorphous low-grade adenocarcinoma: a case report with ultrastructural findings. *Oral Surg Oral Med Oral Pathol* 1988;66:459–465.
237. Perzin KH, Cantor JO, Johannessen JV. Acinic cell carcinoma arising in nasal cavity: report of a case with ultrastructural observations. *Cancer* 1981;47:1818–1822.
238. Ordonez NG, Batsakis JG. Acinic cell carcinoma of the nasal cavity: electron-optic and immunohistochemical observations. *J Laryngol Otol* 1986;100:345–349.
239. Cohen MA, Batsakis JG. Oncocytic tumors (oncocytomas) of minor salivary glands. *Arch Otolaryngol* 1968;88:97–99.
240. Handler SD, Ward PH. Oncocytoma of the maxillary sinus. *Laryngoscope* 1979;89:372–376.
241. Sanchez-Casis G, Devine KD, Weiland LH. Nasal adenocarcinomas that closely simulate colonic carcinomas. *Cancer* 1971;28:714–720.
242. Alessi DM, Trapp TK, Fu YS, et al. Nonsalivary sinonasal adenocarcinoma. *Arch Otolaryngol Head Neck Surg* 1988;114:996–999.
243. Luce D, Gerin M, Leclerc A, et al. Sinonasal cancer and occupational exposure to formaldehyde and other substances. *Int J Cancer* 1993;53:224–231.
244. Engzell U, Englund A, Westerholm P. Nasal cancer associated with occupational exposure to organic dust. *Acta Otolaryngol* 1978;86: 437–442.
245. Klintenberg C, Olofsson J, Hellquist H, et al. Adenocarcinoma of the ethmoid sinuses. A review of 28 cases with special reference to wood dust exposure. *Cancer* 1984;54:482–488.
246. Brinton LA, Blot WJ, Becker JA, et al. A case-control study of cancers of the nasal cavity and paranasal sinuses. *Am J Epidemiol* 1984;119: 896–906.
247. Wilhelmsson B, Hellquist H, Olofsson J, et al. Nasal cuboidal metaplasia with dysplasia. Precursor to adenocarcinoma in wood-dust-exposed workers. *Acta Otolaryngol* 1985;99:641–648.
248. Batsakis JG, Mackay B, Ordonez NG. Enteric-type adenocarcinoma of the nasal cavity. An electron microscopic and immunocytochemical study. *Cancer* 1984;54:855–860.
249. Kleinsasser O. Terminal tubular adenocarcinoma of the nasal seromucous glands. A specific entity. *Arch Otorhinolaryngol* 1985;241: 183–193.
250. Mills SE, Fechner RE, Cantrell RW. Aggressive sinonasal lesion resembling normal intestinal mucosa. *Am J Surg Pathol* 1982;6: 803–809.
251. Fortson JK, Bezmalinovic ZL, Moseley DL. Bilateral ethmoid sinusitis with unilateral proptosis as an initial manifestation of metastatic prostate carcinoma. *J Natl Med Assoc* 1994;86:945–948.
252. Gilmore JR, Gillespie CA, Hudson WR. Adenocarcinoma of the nose and paranasal sinuses [Letter]. *Ear Nose Throat J* 1987;66:56–58.
253. Bernstein JM, Montgomery WW, Balogh K. Metastatic tumors to the maxilla, nose and paranasal sinuses. *Laryngoscope* 1966;76:621–650.
254. Franquemont DW, Fechner RE, Mills SE. Histologic classification of sinonasal intestinal-type adenocarcinoma. *Am J Surg Pathol* 1991; 15:368–375.
255. Bridger GP, Mendelsohn MS, Baldwin M, et al. Paranasal sinus cancer. *Aust N Z J Surg* 1991;61:290–294.
256. Vizel M, Oster MW. Ethmoid sinus adenocarcinoma metastatic to breast. *J Surg Oncol* 1981;18:257–260.
257. Majumdar B, Kent S. Malignant neoplasms of the nose and paranasal sinuses. A survey of cases treated in a regional centre. *Clin Otolaryngol* 1983;8:97–102.
258. Robin PE, Powell DJ, Stansbie JM. Carcinoma of the nasal cavity and paranasal sinuses: incidence and presentation of different histological types. *Clin Otolaryngol* 1979;4:432–456.
259. Weber AL, Stanton AC. Malignant tumors of the paranasal sinuses: radiological, clinical, and histopathologic evaluation of 200 cases. *Head Neck Surg* 1984;6:761–776.
260. Gadeberg CC, Hjelm-Hansen M, Sogaard H, et al. Malignant tumors of the paranasal sinuses and nasal cavity. A series of 180 patients. *Acta Radiol Oncol* 1984;23:181–187.
261. Beatty CW, Pearson BW, Kern EB. Carcinoma of the nasal septum: experience with 85 cases. *Otolaryngol Head Neck Surg* 1982;90: 90–94.
262. Bosch A, Vallecillo L, Frias Z. Cancer of the nasal cavity. *Cancer* 1976;37:1458–1463.
263. Virtue JA. The relationship between the refining of nickel and cancer of the nasal cavity. *Can J Otolaryngol* 1972;1:37–42.
264. Rousch GC. Epidemiology of cancer of the nose and paranasal sinuses: current concepts. *Head Neck Surg* 1979;2:3–11.

265. Goren AD, Harley N, Eisenbud L, et al. Clinical and radiobiologic features of Thorotrast-induced carcinoma of the maxillary sinus. A case report. *Oral Surg Oral Med Oral Pathol* 1980;49:237–242.
266. Torjusson W, Solberg LA, Hogetveit AC. Histopathologic changes of nasal mucosa in nickel workers. A pilot study. *Cancer* 1979;44: 963–974.
267. Badib AD, Kurohara SS, Webster JH, et al. Treatment of cancer of the nasal cavity. *Am J Roentgenol Radiat Ther Nucl Med* 1969;106: 824–830.
268. Boone MLM, Harle TS, Higholt HW, et al. Malignant diseases of the paranasal sinuses and nasal cavity. *Am J Roentgenol Radiat Ther Nucl Med* 1968;102:627–636.
269. MacComb WS, Martin HE. Cancer of the nasal cavity. *Am J Roentgenol Radiat Ther* 1942;47:11–23.
270. Perzin KH, Lefkowitch JH, Hui RM. Bilateral nasal squamous carcinoma arising in papillomatosis. Report of a case developing after chemotherapy for leukemia. *Cancer* 1981;48:2375–2382.
271. Furuta Y, Takasu T, Asai T, et al. Detection of human papillomavirus DNA in carcinomas of the nasal cavities and paranasal sinuses by the polymerase chain reaction. *Cancer* 1992;69:353–357.
272. Barnes L, Verbin RS, Gnepp DR. Diseases of the nose, paranasal sinuses, and nasopharynx. In: Barnes L, ed. *Surgical pathology of the head and neck.* New York: Marcel Dekker, 1985:403–451.
273. Taxy JB. Squamous carcinoma of the nasal vestibule. An analysis of five cases and literature review. *Am J Clin Pathol* 1997;107:698–703.
274. Shibuya H, Amagasa T, Hanai A, et al. Second primary carcinomas in patients with squamous cell carcinoma of the maxillary sinus. *Cancer* 1986;58:1122–1125.
275. Zarbo RJ, Crissman JD, Venkat H, et al. Spindle-cell carcinoma of the upper aerodigestive tract mucosa. *Am J Surg Pathol* 1986;10:741–753.
276. Piscioli F, Aldovini D, Bondi A, et al. Squamous cell carcinoma with sarcoma-like stroma of the nose and paranasal sinuses: report of two cases. *Histopathology* 1984;8:633–639.
277. Hanna GS, Ali MH. Verrucous carcinoma of the nasal septum. *J Laryngol Otol* 1987;101:184–187.
278. Gerughty RM, Hennigar GR, Brown FM. Adenosquamous carcinoma of the nasal, oral and laryngeal cavities. A clinicopathologic survey of ten cases. *Cancer* 1968;22:1140–1155.
279. Banks ER, Frierson HF, Mills SE, et al. Basaloid squamous cell carcinoma of the head and neck. A clinicopathologic and immunohistochemical study of 40 cases. *Am J Surg Pathol* 1992;16:939–946.
280. Manivel C, Wick MR, Dehner LP. Transitional (cylindric) cell carcinoma with endodermal sinus tumor-like features of the nasopharynx and paranasal sinuses. Clinicopathologic and immunohistochemical study of two cases. *Arch Pathol Lab Med* 1986;110:198–202.
281. Frierson HF, Ross GW, Stewart FM, et al. Unusual sinonasal small-cell neoplasms following radiotherapy for bilateral retinoblastomas. *Am J Surg Pathol* 1989;13:947–954.
282. Crissman JD, Kessis T, Shah KV, et al. Squamous papillary neoplasia of the adult upper aerodigestive tract. *Hum Pathol* 1988;19: 1387–1396.
283. Shanmugaratnam K. World Health Organization. *Histologyical typing of tumors of the upper respiratory tract and ear,* 2nd ed. Berlin: Springer-Verlag, 1991:31–32.
284. Osborn DA. Nature and behavior of transitional tumors in the upper respiratory tract. *Cancer* 1970;25:50–60.
285. Cheng VST, Wang CC. Carcinomas of the paranasal sinuses. A study of sixty six cases. *Cancer* 1977;40:3038–3041.
286. American Joint Committee on Cancer. Paranasal sinuses. In: Fleming ID, et al., eds. *Cancer staging manual,* 5th ed. Philadelphia: Lippincott-Raven, 1997:47–52.
287. Lund VJ. Malignant tumors of the nasal cavity and paranasal sinuses. *Otol Rhinol Laryngol* 1983;45:1—12.
288. Hopkin N, McNicholl W, Dalley VM, et al. Cancer of the paranasal sinuses and nasal cavities. Part I. Clinical features. *J Laryngol Otol* 1984;98:585–595.
289. Robin PE, Powel DJ. Regional node involvement and distant metastases in carcinoma of the nasal cavity and paranasal sinuses. *J Laryngol Otol* 1980;94:301–309.
290. Ahmad K, Cordoba RB, Fayos JV. Squamous cell carcinoma of the maxillary sinus. *Arch Otolaryngol* 1981;107:48–51.
291. Ordonez NG, MacKay B. Neuroendocrine tumors of the nasal cavity. Part II. *Pathol Annu* 1993;28:77–111.
292. Berger L. L'esthesioneuroepitheliome olfactif. *Bull Cancer* 1924; 13:410–421.
293. Naessen R. The "receptor surface" of the olfactory organ (epithelium) of man and guinea pig. A descriptive and experimental study. *Acta Otolaryngol* 1971;71:335–348.
294. Dibble PA, Brown AK. Esthesioneuroepithelioma. *Laryngoscope* 1961;71:192–199.
295. Hyams VJ. Olfactory neuroblastoma (case 6). In: Batsakis JG, Hyams VJ, Morales AR, eds. *Special tumors of the head and neck.* Chicago: ASCP Press, 1982:24–29.
296. Elkon D, Hightower SI, Lim ML, et al. Esthesioneuroblastoma. *Cancer* 1979;44:1087–1094.
297. Skolnik EM, Massari FS, Tenta LT. Olfactory neuroepithelioma: review of the world literature and presentation of two cases. *Arch Otolaryngol* 1966;84:644–653.
298. Mills SE, Frierson HF. Olfactory neuroblastoma. A clinicopathologic study of 21 cases. *Am J Surg Pathol* 1985;9:317–327.
299. Herrold KM. Induction of olfactory neuroepithelial tumors in Syrian hamsters by diethylnitrosamine. *Cancer* 1964;17:114–121.
300. Vollrath M, Altmannsberger M, Weber K, et al. Chemically induced tumors of rat olfactory epithelium: a model for human esthesioneuroepithelioma. *J Natl Cancer Inst* 1986;76:1205–1215.
301. Sorensen PHB, Wu JK, Berean KW, et al. Olfactory neuroblastoma is a peripheral primitive neuroectodermal tumor related to Ewing sarcoma. *Proc Natl Acad Sci U S A* 1996;93:1038–1043.
302. Cavazzana AO, Navarro S, Noguera R, et al. Olfactory neuroblastoma is not a neuroblastoma but is related to primitive neuroectodermal tumor (PNET). *Adv Neuroblast Res* 1988;2:463–473.
303. Whang-Peng J, Freter CE, Knutsen T, et al. Translocation t(11;22) in esthesioneuroblastoma. *Cancer Genet Cytogenet* 1987;29:155–157.
304. Argani P, Perez-Ordonez B, Caruana SM, et al. Olfactory neuroblastoma is not related to the Ewing family of tumors. Absence of EWS/FLI1 gene fusion and MIC2 expression. *Am J Surg Pathol* 1998;22:391–398.
305. Kadish S, Goodman M, Wang CC. Olfactory neuroblastoma: a critical analysis of 17 cases. *Cancer* 1976;37:1571–1576.
306. Mendeloff J. The olfactory neuroepithelial tumors: a review of the literature and report of six additional cases. *Cancer* 1957;10:944–956.
307. Berger L, Coutard H. L'esthesioneurocytome olfactif. *Bull Cancer* 1926;15:404–414.
308. Portmann BM. Sur un cas de tumeur nerveuse des fosses nasales (esthesioneuroblastome). *Acta Otolaryngol (Stockh)* 1928;13:52–57.
309. Choi H-S, Anderson PJ. Olfactory neuroblastoma: an immunoelectron microscopic study of S-100 protein–positive cells. *J Neuropathol Exp Neurol* 1986;45:576–587.
310. Dayal Y, DeLellis RA, Tischler AS, et al. Olfactory neuroblastoma: an ultrastructural and immunohistochemical study [Abstract]. *Lab Invest* 1985;52:17–18.
311. Taxy JB, Bharani NK, Mills SE, et al. The spectrum of olfactory neural tumors. A light-microscopic immunohistochemical and ultrastructural analysis. *Am J Surg Pathol* 1986;10:687–695.
312. Silva EG, Butler JJ, MacKay B, et al. Neuroblastomas and neuroendocrine carcinomas of the nasal cavity. A proposed new classification. *Cancer* 1982;50:2388–2405.
313. Gerard-Marchant R, Micheau C. Microscopical diagnosis of olfactory esthesioneuromas: general review and report of five cases. *J Natl Cancer Inst* 1965;35:75–82.
314. Mackay B, Luna MA, Butler JJ. Adult neuroblastoma. Electron microscopic observations in nine cases. *Cancer* 1976;37:1334–1351.
315. Mills SE, Fechner RE. "Undifferentiated" neoplasms of the sinonasal region: differential diagnosis based on clinical, light microscopic, immunohistochemical and ultrastructural features. *Semin Diagn Pathol* 1989;6:316–328.
316. Curtis JL, Rubinstein LJ. Pigmented olfactory neuroblastoma. A new example of melanotic neuroepithelial neoplasm. *Cancer* 1982;49: 2136–2143.

317. Miller DC, Goodman ML, Pilch BZ, et al. Mixed olfactory neuroblastoma and carcinoma. A report of two cases. *Cancer* 1984:54: 2019–2028.
318. Silva E, Battifora H. Immunoreactivity for keratin and neuron-specific enolase in neuroblastomas and neuroendocrine carcinomas of the nasal cavity [Abstract]. *Lab Invest* 1985;52:62–63.
319. Devaney K, Wenig BM, Abbondanzo SL. Olfactory neuroblastoma and other round cell lesions of the sinonasal region. *Mod Pathol* 1996;9:658–663.
320. Hirose T, Scheithauer BW, Lopes MB, et al. Olfactory neuroblastoma. An immunohistochemical, ultrastructural, and flow cytometric study. *Cancer* 1995;76:4–19.
321. Schmidt JL, Zarbo RJ, Clark JL. Olfactory neuroblastoma: clinicopathologic and immunohistochemical characterization of four representative cases. *Laryngoscope* 1990;100:1052–1058.
322. Nakajima T, Watanabe S, Sato Y, et al. An immunoperoxidase study of S-100 protein distribution in normal and neoplastic tissues. *Am J Surg Pathol* 1982;6:715–727.
323. Hashimoto H, Enjoji M, Nakajima T, et al. Malignant neuroepithelioma (peripheral neuroblastoma). A clinicopathologic study of 15 cases. *Am J Surg Pathol* 1983;7:309–318.
324. Nelson RS, Perlman EJ, Askin FB. Is esthesioneuroblastoma a peripheral neuroectodermal tumor? *Hum Pathol* 1995;26:639–641.
325. Kahn L. Esthesioneuroblastoma: a light and electron microscopical study. *Hum Pathol* 1974;5:364–371.
326. Shah JP, Feghai J. Esthesioneuroblastoma. *CA Cancer J Clin* 1983; 33:154–159.
327. Olsen KD, DeSanto LW. Olfactory neuroblastoma. Biologic and clinical behavior. *Arch Otolaryngol* 1983;109:797–802.
328. Morita A, Ebersold MJ, Olsen KD, et al. Esthesioneuroblastoma: prognosis and management. *Neurosurgery* 1993;32:706–715.
329. Levine PA, McLean WC, Cantrell RW. Esthesioneuroblastoma: the University of Virginia experience. *Laryngoscope* 1986;96:742–746.
330. Foote RL, Morita A, Ebersold MJ, et al. Esthesioneuroblastoma: the role of adjuvant radiation therapy. *Int J Radiat Oncol Biol Phys* 1993;27:835–842.
331. Wade PM, Smith RE, Johns ME. Response of esthesioneuroblastoma to chemotherapy. Report of five cases and review of the literature. *Cancer* 1984;53:1036–1041.
332. Walters TR, Pushparaj N, Ghander AZ. Olfactory neuroblastoma: response to combination chemotherapy. *Arch Otolaryngol* 1980;106: 242–243.
333. Rejowski JE, Campanella RS, Block LJ. Small cell carcinoma of the nose and paranasal sinuses. *Otolaryngol Head Neck Surg* 1982;90: 516–517.
334. Weiss MD, DeFries HO, Taxy JB, et al. Primary small cell carcinoma of the paranasal sinuses. *Arch Otolaryngol* 1983;109:341–343.
335. Koss LG, Spiro RH, Hajdu S. Small cell (oat cell) carcinoma of minor salivary gland origin. *Cancer* 1972;30:737–741.
336. Kameya T, Shimosato Y, Adachi I, et al. Neuroendocrine carcinoma of the paranasal sinus. A morphological and endocrinological study. *Cancer* 1980;45:330–339.
337. Lloreta-Trull J, Mackay B, Troncoso P, et al. Neuroendocrine tumors of the nasal cavity: an ultrastructural and morphometric study of 24 cases. *Ultrastruc Pathol* 1992;16:165–175.
338. Vollmer RT, Shelburne JD, Iglehart JD. Intercellular junctions and tumor stage in small cell carcinoma of the lung. *Hum Pathol* 1986;18:22–27.
339. Mills SE, Cooper PH, Garland TA, et al. Small cell undifferentiated carcinoma of the larynx. Report of two patients and review of 13 additional cases. *Cancer* 1983;51:116–120.
340. Hayashi Y, Nagamine S, Yanagawa T, et al. Small cell undifferentiated carcinoma of the minor salivary gland containing exocrine, neuroendocrine, and squamous cells. *Cancer* 1987;60:1583–1588.
341. Sun C-C, Hall-Craggs M, Adler B. Oat cell carcinoma of larynx. *Arch Otolaryngol* 1981;107:506–509.
342. Kliewer KE, Cochran AJ, Wen D-R, et al. An immunohistochemical study of 37 paragangliomas. *Med Sci Res* 1987;15:87–88.
343. Gallo O, Graziani P, Fini-Storchi O. Undifferentiated carcinoma of the nose and paranasal sinuses. An immunohistochemical and clinical study. *Ear Nose Throat J* 1993;72:588–595.
344. Helliwell TR, Yeoh LH, Stell PM. Anaplastic carcinoma of the nose and paranasal sinuses. Light microscopy, immunohistochemistry and clinical correlation. *Cancer* 1986;58:2038–2045.
345. Frierson HF, Mills SE, Fechner RE, et al. Sinonasal undifferentiated carcinoma. An aggressive neoplasm derived from Schneiderian epithelium and distinct from olfactory neuroblastoma. *Am J Surg Pathol* 1986;10:1986.
346. House JM, Goodman ML, Gacek RR, et al. Chemodectomas of the nasopharynx. *Arch Otolaryngol* 1972;96:138–141.
347. Nguyen QA, Gibbs PM, Rice DH. Malignant nasal paraganglioma: a case report and review of the literature. *Otolaryngol Head Neck Surg* 1995;113:157–161.
348. Parisier SC, Sinclair GM. Glomus tumor of the nasal cavity. *Laryngoscope* 1968;78:2013–2024.
349. Gosavi DK, Mohidekar AT. Chemodectoma of the nose and sphenoid sinus. *J Laryngol Otol* 1978;92:813–816.
350. Apple D, Kreines K. Case report. Cushing's syndrome due to ectopic ACTH production by a nasal paraganglioma. *Am J Med Sci* 1982;283:32–35.
351. Volkov YN, Schechking VN. Chemodectoma of the nose and of the accessory sinuses. *Vestn Otorhinolaringol* 1976;4:56–59.
352. Lack EE, Cubilla AL, Woodruff JM. Paragangliomas of the head and neck region. A pathologic study of tumors from 71 patients. *Hum Pathol* 1979;10:191–218.
353. Moran TE. Nonchromaffin paraganglioma of the nasal cavity. *Laryngoscope* 1962;72:201–206.
354. Branham GH, Gnepp DR, O'McMenomey S, et al. Malignant paraganglioma: a case report and literature review. *Otolaryngol Head Neck Surg* 1989;101:99–103.
355. Johnson TJ, Zarbo RJ, Lloyd RV, et al. Paragangliomas of the head and neck: Immunohistochemical neuroendocrine and intermediate filament typing. *Mod Pathol* 1988;1:216–223.
356. Spector GJ, Campagno J, Perez CA, et al. Effects of radiotherapy. *Cancer* 1975;35:1316–1321.
357. Moore ES, Martin H. Melanoma of the upper respiratory tract and oral cavity. *Cancer* 1955;8:1167–1176.
358. Holdcraft JH, Gallagher JC. Malignant melanomas of the nasal and paranasal sinus mucosa. *Ann Otol Rhinol Laryngol* 1969;78:5–20.
359. Bizon JG, Newman RK. Metastatic melanoma to the ethmoid sinus. *Arch Otolaryngol Head Neck Surg* 1986;112:664–667.
360. Billings KR, Wang MB, Sercarz JA, et al. Clinical and pathologic distinction between primary and metastatic mucosal melanoma of the head and neck. *Otolaryngol Head Neck Surg* 1995;112:700–706.
361. Conley J, Pack GT. Melanoma of the mucous membranes of the head and neck. *Arch Otolaryngol Head Neck Surg* 1974;99:315–319.
362. Lund V. Malignant melanoma of the nasal cavity and paranasal sinuses. *J Laryngol Otol* 1982;96:347–355.
363. Freedman HM, DeSanto LW, Devine KD, et al. Malignant melanoma of the nasal cavity and paranasal sinuses. *Arch Otolaryngol* 1973;97:322–325.
364. Harrison DFN. Malignant melanomata of the nasal cavity. *Proc R Soc Med* 1968;61:13–18.
365. Gallagher JC. Upper respiratory melanoma: pathology and growth rate. *Ann Otol Rhinol Laryngol* 1970;79:551–556.
366. Snow GB, Van der Waal I. Mucosal melanomas of the head and neck. *Otolaryngol Clin North Am* 1986;19:537–547.
367. Nakhleh RE, Wick MR, Rocamora A, et al. Morphologic diversity in malignant melanomas. *Am J Clin Pathol* 1990;93:731–740.
368. Franquemont DW, Mills SE. Sinonasal malignant melanoma. A clinicopathologic and immunohistochemical study of 14 cases. *Am J Clin Pathol* 1991;96:689–697.
369. Chetty R, Slavin JL, Pitson GA, et al. Melanoma botryoides: a distinctive myxoid pattern of sino-nasal malignant melanoma. *Histopathology* 1994;24:377–379.
370. Zarbo RJ, Gown AM, Nagle RB, et al. Anomalous cytokeratin expression in malignant melanoma: one and two dimensional Western

blot analysis and immunohistochemical survey of 100 melanomas. *Mod Pathol* 1990;3:494–501.

371. Trapp TK, Fu Y-S, Calcaterra TC. Melanoma of the nasal and paranasal sinus mucosa. *Arch Otolaryngol Head Neck Surg* 1987;113: 1086–1089.
372. Fu Y-S, Perzin KH. Nonepithelial tumors of the nasal cavity, paranasal sinuses, and nasopharynx: a clinicopathologic study. IV. Smooth muscle tumors (leiomyoma, leiomyosarcoma). *Cancer* 1975;35:1300–1308.
373. Fu Y-S, Perzin KH. Non-epithelial tumors of the nasal cavity, paranasal sinuses, and nasopharynx: a clinicopathologic study. VIII. Adipose tissue tumors (lipoma and liposarcoma). *Cancer* 1977;40: 1314–1317.
374. Fu Y-S, Perzin KH. Non-epithelial tumors of the nasal cavity, paranasal sinuses, and nasopharynx: a clinicopathologic study III. Cartilaginous tumors (chondroma, chondrosarcoma). *Cancer* 1974;34:453–463.
375. Kildy D, Ambegaokar AG. The nasal chondroma. *J Laryngol Otol* 1977;91:415–426.
376. Fu Y-S, Perzin KH. Non-epithelial tumors of the nasal cavity, paranasal sinuses and nasopharynx: a clinicopathologic study. II. Osseous and fibro-osseous lesions, including osteoma, fibrous dysplasia, ossifying fibroma, osteoblastoma, giant cell tumor and osteosarcoma. *Cancer* 1974;33:1289–1305.
377. Atallah N, Jay MM. Osteomas of the paranasal sinuses. *J Laryngol Otol* 1981;95:291–304.
378. Broniatowski M. Osteomas of the frontal sinuses. *Ear Nose Throat J* 1984;1:267–271.
379. Boysen M. Osteomas of the paranasal sinuses. *J Otolaryngol* 1978;7:366–370.
380. Earwaker J. Paranasal sinus osteomas: a review of 46 cases. *Skel Radiol* 1993;22:417–423.
381. Perzin KH, Pushparaj N. Nonepithelial tumors of the nasal cavity, paranasal sinuses, and nasopharynx: a clinicopathologic study. XIV. Chordomas. *Cancer* 1986;57:784–796.
382. Campbell WM, McDonald TJ, Unni KK, et al. Nasal and paranasal presentations of chordomas. *Laryngoscope* 1980;90:612–618.
383. Shugar JMA, Som PM, Krespi YP, et al. Primary chordoma of the maxillary sinus. *Laryngoscope* 1980;90:1825–1830.
384. Fu Y-S, Perzin KH. Nonepithelial tumors of the nasal cavity, paranasal sinuses, and nasopharynx: a clinicopathologic study. V. Skeletal muscle tumors (rhabdomyoma and rhabdomyosarcoma). *Cancer* 1976;37:364–376.
385. Shapeero LG, Vanel D, Ackerman LV, et al. Aggressive fibrous dysplasia of the maxillary sinus. *Skel Radiol* 1993;22:563–568.
386. Slootweg PJ, Panders AK, Koopmans R, et al. Juvenile ossifying fibroma. An analysis of 33 cases with emphasis on histopathological aspects. *J Oral Pathol Med* 1994;23:385–388.
387. Johnson LC, Yousefi M, Vinh TN, et al. Juvenile active ossifying fibroma. Its nature, dynamics and origin. *Acta Otolaryngol* 1991;(suppl 488):1–40.
388. Fechner RE. Problematic lesions of the craniofacial bones. *Am J Surg Pathol* 1989;13:17–30.
389. Wolfe JT, Scheithauer BW, Dahlin DC. Giant-cell tumor of the sphenoid bone. Review of ten cases. *J Neurosurg* 1983;59:322–327.
390. Boysen ME, Olving JH, Vaten K, et al. Fibro-osseous lesions of the cranio-facial bones. *J Laryngol Otol* 1979;93:793–807.
391. Marvel JB, Marsh MA, Catlan FI. Ossifying fibroma of the mid-face and paranasal sinuses: diagnostic and therapeutic considerations. *Otolaryngol Head Neck Surg* 1991;104:803–808.
392. Kuruvilla A, Wenig BM, Humphrey DM, et al. Leiomyosarcoma of the sinonasal tract. A clinicopathologic study of nine cases. *Arch Otolaryngol Head Neck Surg* 1990;116:1278–1286.
393. Moore DM, Berke GS. Synovial sarcoma of the head and neck. *Arch Otolaryngol Head Neck Surg* 1987;113:311–313.
394. Perzin KH, Panyu H, Wechter S. Non-epithelial tumors of the nasal cavity, paranasal sinuses and nasopharynx: a clinicopathologic study. XII. Schwann cell tumors (neurilemmoma, neurofibroma, malignant schwannoma). *Cancer* 1982;50:2193–2202.
395. Heffner DK, Gnepp DR. Sinonasal fibrosarcomas, malignant schwannomas, and "triton" tumors. A clinicopathologic study of 67 cases. *Cancer* 1992;70:2912–2928.
396. Fu Y-S, Perzin KH. Non-epithelial tumors of the nasal cavity, paranasal sinuses and nasopharynx: a clinicopathologic study. I. General features and vascular tumor. *Cancer* 1974;33:1275–1288.
397. Yasuoka T, Okumura Y, Okuda T, et al. Hemangioma and malignant hemangioendothelioma of the maxillary sinus: case reports and clinical consideration. *J Oral Maxillofac Surg* 1990;48:877–881.
398. Potter AJ, Khatib G, Pepard SB. Intranasal glomus tumor. *Arch Otolaryngol* 1984;110:755–756.
399. Lemlich G, Schwam L, Lebwohl M. Kaposi's sarcoma and acquired immunodeficiency syndromes: postmortem findings in 24 cases. *J Am Acad Dermatol* 1987;16:319–325.
400. Zakrzewska JM. Angiosarcoma of the maxilla–a case report and review of the literature including angiosarcoma of maxillary sinus. *Br J Oral Maxillofac Surg* 1986;24:286–292.
401. Bankaci M, Myers EN, Barnes L, et al. Angiosarcoma of the maxillary sinus: literature review and case report. *Head Neck Surg* 1979;1: 274–280.
402. Mills SE, Cooper PH, Fechner RE. Lobular capillary hemangioma: the underlying lesion of pyogenic granuloma. A study of 73 cases from the oral and nasal mucous membranes. *Am J Surg Pathol* 1980; 4:471–479.
403. Nichols GE, Gaffey MJ, Mills SE, et al. Lobular capillary hemangioma. An immunohistochemical study including steroid hormone receptor status. *Am J Clin Pathol* 1992;97:770–775.
404. Gorenstein A, Facer GW, Weiland LH. Hemangiopericytoma of the nasal cavity. *ORL J Otorhinolaryngol Rel Spec* 1978;86:405–415.
405. Eichhorn JH, Dickerson GR, Bhan AK, et al. Sinonasal hemangiopericytoma: a reassessment with electron microscopy, immunohistochemistry and long term follow-up. *Am J Surg Pathol* 1990;14: 856–866.
406. Compagno J. Hemangiopericytoma-like tumors of the nasal cavity: a comparison with hemangiopericytoma of soft tissues. *Laryngoscope* 1978;88:460–469.
407. Compagno J, Hyams VJ. Hemangiopericytoma-like intranasal tumors. A clinicopathologic study of 23 cases. *Am J Clin Pathol* 1976;66: 672–683.
408. Batsakis JG, Jacobs JB, Templeton AC. Hemangiopericytoma of the nasal cavity: electron-optic study and clinical correlations. *J Laryngol Otol* 1983;97:361–368.
409. El-Naggar AK, Batsakis JG, Garcia GM, et al. Sinonasal hemangiopericytomas. A clinicopathologic and DNA content study. *Arch Otolaryngol Head Neck Surg* 1992;188:134–137.
410. Fu Y-S, Perzin KH. Nonepithelial tumors of the nasal cavity, paranasal sinuses, and nasopharynx. A clinicopathologic study. VI. Fibrous tissue tumors (fibroma, fibromatosis, fibrosarcoma). *Cancer* 1976;37:2912–2928.
411. Wold LE, Weiland LH. Tumefactive fibro-inflammatory lesions of the head and neck. *Am J Surg Pathol* 1983;7:477–482.
412. Weisman RA, Osguthorpe JD. Pseudotumor of the head and neck masquerading as neoplasia. *Laryngoscope* 1988;98:610–614.
413. Nakhleh RE, Zarbo RJ, Ewing S, et al. Myogenic differentiation in spindle cell (sarcomatoid) carcinoma of the upper aerodigestive tract. *Appl Immunohistochem* 1993;1:58–68.
414. Roberts PF, McCann BG. Eosinophilic angiocentric fibrosis of the upper respiratory tract: a mucosal variant of granuloma faciale? A report of three cases. *Histopathology* 1985;9:1217–1225.
415. Altemani AM, Pilch BZ, Sakano E, et al. Eosinophilic angiocentric fibrosis of the nasal cavity. *Mod Pathol* 1997;10:391–393.
416. Zukerberg LR, Rosenberg AE, Randolph G, et al. Solitary fibrous tumor of the nasal cavity and paranasal sinuses. *Am J Surg Pathol* 1991;15:126–130.
417. Witkin GB, Rosai J. Solitary fibrous tumor of the upper respiratory tract. A report of six cases. *Am J Surg Pathol* 1991;15:842–848.
418. Fukunaga M, Ushigome S, Nomura K, et al. Solitary fibrous tumor of the nasal cavity and orbit. *Pathol Int* 1995;45:952–957.

419. Fu Y-S, Perzin KH. Non-epithelial tumors of the nasal cavity, paranasal sinuses and nasopharynx: a clinicopathologic study. VII. Myxomas. *Cancer* 1977;39:195–203.
420. Perzin KH, Fu Y-S. Non-epithelial tumors of the nasal cavity, paranasal sinuses and nasopharynx: a clinico-pathologic study XI. Fibrous histiocytomas. *Cancer* 1980;45:2616–2626.
421. Daou RA, Attia EL, Viloria JB. Malignant fibrous histiocytomas of the head and neck. *J Otolaryngol* 1983;12:383–388.
422. Amendola BE, Amendola MA, McClatchey KD, et al. Radiation-associated sarcoma: a review of 23 patients with post radiation sarcoma over a 50-year period. *Am J Clin Oncol* 1989;12:411–415.
423. Barnes L, Kanbour A. Malignant fibrous histiocytoma of the head and neck. A report of 12 cases. *Arch Otolaryngol Head Neck Surg* 1988;114:1149–1156.
424. Fletcher CDM. Soft tissue tumors. In: Fletcher CDM, ed. *Diagnostic histopathology of tumors.* New York: Churchill Livingstone, 1995: 1043–1096.
425. Hillstrom RP, Zarbo RJ, Jacobs JR. Nerve sheath tumors of the paranasal sinuses: electron microscopy and histopathologic diagnosis. *Otolaryngol Head Neck Surg* 1990;102:257–263.
426. Hasegawa SL, Mentzel T, Fletcher CDM. Schwannomas of the sinonasal tract and nasopharynx. *Mod Pathol* 1997;10:777–784.
427. Shugar JMA, Som PM, Biller HF, et al. Peripheral nerve sheath tumors of the paranasal sinuses. *Head Neck Surg* 1981;4:72–76.
428. Robitaille Y, Seemayer TA, El Deiry A. Peripheral nerve tumors involving paranasal sinuses: a case report and review of the literature. *Cancer* 1975;35:1254–1258.
429. Johnson TL, Lee MW, Meis JM, et al. Immunohistochemical characterization of malignant peripheral nerve sheath tumors. *Surg Pathol* 1991;4:121–135.
430. Enzinger FM, Weiss SW. *Soft tissue tumors,* 3rd ed. Chapter 22. St. Louis: CV Mosby, 1995:559–577.
431. Sutow WW, Lindberg RD, Gehan EA, et al. Three-year relapse-free survival rates in childhood rhabdomyosarcoma of the head and neck. Report from the intergroup rhabdomyosarcoma study. *Cancer* 1982;49:2217–2221.
432. Cavazzana AO, Schmidt D, Ninfo V, et al. Spindle cell rhabdomyosarcoma. A prognostically favorable variant of rhabdomyosarcoma. *Am J Surg Pathol* 1992;16:229–235.
433. Molenaar WM, Oosterhuis JW, Kamps WA. Cytologic "differentiation" in childhood rhabdomyosarcomas following polychemotherapy. *Hum Pathol* 1984;15:973–979.
434. Wang NP, Marx J, McNutt MA, et al. Expression of myogenic regulatory proteins (myogenin and MyoD1) in small blue round cell tumors of childhood. *Am J Pathol* 1995;147:1799–1810.
435. Erlandson RA. The ultrastructural distinction between rhabdomyosarcoma and other undifferentiated "sarcomas." *Ultrastruct Pathol* 1987;11:83–101.
436. Callender RA, Weber RS, Janjan N, et al. Rhabdomyosarcoma of the nose and paranasal sinuses in adults and children. *Otolaryngol Head Neck Surg* 1995;112:252–257.
437. Waldron CA. Odontogenic cysts and tumors. In: Neville BW, Damm DD, Allen CM, Bouquot JE, ed. *Oral and maxillofacial pathology.* Philadelphia: WB Saunders, 1995:493–538.
438. Karma P, Rasanen O, Karja J. Nasal gliomas. A review and report of two cases. *Laryngoscope* 1977;87:1169–1179.
439. Enfors B, Herngren L. Nasal glioma. *J Laryngol Otol* 1975;89: 863–868.
440. Seibert RW, Seibert JJ, Jimenez JF, et al. Nasopharyngeal brain heterotopia—a cause of upper airway obstruction in infancy. *Laryngoscope* 1984;94:818–819.
441. Bossen EH, Hudson WR. Oligodendroglioma arising in heterotopic brain tissue of the soft palate and nasopharynx. *Am J Surg Pathol* 1987;11:571–574.
442. Mirra SS, Pearl GS, Hoffman JC, et al. Nasal "glioma" with prominent neuronal component. Report of a case. *Arch Pathol Lab Med* 1981;105:540–541.
443. Patterson K, Kapur S, Chandra RS. "Nasal gliomas" and related brain heterotopias: a pathologist's perspective. *Pediatr Pathol* 1986;5: 353–362.
444. Fletcher CDM, Carpenter G, McKee PH. Nasal glioma, a rarity. *Am J Dermatopathol* 1986;8:341–346.
445. Perzin KH, Pushparaj N. Nonepithelial tumors of the nasal cavity, paranasal sinuses, and nasopharynx. A clinicopathologic study. XIII: Meningiomas. *Cancer* 1984;54:1860–1869.
446. Ho KL. Primary meningioma of the nasal cavity and paranasal sinuses. *Cancer* 1980;46:1442–1447.
447. Persky MS, Som ML. Olfactory groove meningioma with paranasal sinus and nasal cavity extension: a combined approach. *Trans Am Acad Ophthalmol Otolaryngol* 1978;86:714–720.
448. Taxy JB. Meningioma of the paranasal sinuses. A report of two cases. *Am J Surg Pathol* 1990;14:82–86.
449. Artlich A, Schmidt D. Immunohistochemical profile of meningiomas and their histological subtypes. *Hum Pathol* 1990;21:843–849.
450. Kay S, Lees JK, Stout AP. Pituitary chromophobe tumors of the nasal cavity. *Cancer* 1950;3:695–704.
451. Jefferson G. Extrasellar extensions of pituitary adenomas. *Proc R Soc Med* 1940;33:433–458.
452. Cole IE, Keene M. Nasal obstruction in pituitary tumours. *J Laryngol Otol* 1981;95:183–189.
453. Rasmussen P, Lindholm T. Ectopic pituitary adenomas. *Clin Endocrinol* 1979;11:69–74.
454. Kammer H, George R. Cushing's disease in a patient with ectopic pituitary adenoma. *JAMA* 1981;246:2722–2724.
455. Davis JM, Weber AL. Pituitary adenoma presenting as a sphenoid sinus lesion. *Ann Otol Rhinol Laryngol* 1980;89:483–484.
456. Lloyd RV, Chandler WF, Kovacs K, et al. Ectopic pituitary adenomas with normal anterior pituitary glands. *Am J Surg Pathol* 1986;10: 546–552.
457. Gillespie CA, Walker JS, Burch WM, et al. Cushing's syndrome secondary to ectopic pituitary adenoma in the sphenoid sinus. *Otolaryngol Head Neck Surg* 1987;96:569–572.
458. Chessin H, Urdaneta N, Smith H, et al. Chromophobe adenoma manifesting as a nasopharyngeal mass. *Arch Otolaryngol* 1976;102: 631–633.
459. Langel DJ, Zarbo RJ, Savera AT, et al. Monoclonal antibodies (MAbs) to surfactant apoprotein-A can distinguish between pulmonary and nonpulmonary adenocarcinoma [Abstract]. *Mod Pathol* 1996;8:159.
460. Savera AT, Torres FX, Linden MD, et al. Primary versus metastatic pulmonary adenocarcinoma: an immunohistochemical study using villin and cytokeratins 7 and 20. *Appl Immunohistochem* 1996;4: 86–94.

5

THE NASOPHARYNX AND WALDEYER'S RING

BEN Z. PILCH

NASOPHARYNX

Anatomic Considerations

The nasopharynx (rhinopharynx) is the uppermost of the three regions of the pharynx, the other two being the oropharynx and the hypopharynx or laryngopharynx. It is continuous anteriorly with the nasal cavities at the choanae and inferiorly with the oropharynx at the level of the soft palate; thus, the superior surface of the soft palate is nasopharyngeal and lined by respiratory epithelium, and its inferior surface is oropharyngeal and lined by stratified squamous epithelium. The superior extent of the nasopharynx is bounded by the sphenoid bone: the floor of the sphenoid sinus anteriorly and the floor of the sella turcica more posteriorly. Posteriorly it is bounded by the basiocciput superiorly and the arch of the atlas inferiorly.

The orifices of the auditory or eustachian tubes are in the lateral walls of the nasopharynx, and each is bounded superiorly and posteriorly by a mound of tissue, the torus tubarius. Above and behind the torus tubarius is a pharyngeal recess, the fossa of Rosenmüller, which is a common site of origin of nasopharyngeal carcinoma. Its rather inconspicuous location helps account for the elusiveness of small carcinomas to the examining clinician. The proximity of Rosenmüller's fossa to the eustachian tubes leads to the tube's blockage by a mass in the fossa; thus, a unilateral serous otitis media in an adult is a worrisome indicator of a possible nasopharyngeal carcinoma.

In the posterosuperior wall of the nasopharynx in the midline is the pharyngeal tonsil, or adenoid, a part of Waldeyer's ring that is differentiated histologically from the palatine or faucial tonsils by the fact that it is lined in children and at least in part in adults by respiratory rather than squamous mucosa. It should be remembered, however, that the lining of some palatine tonsillar crypts may occasionally consist of respiratory mucosa, perhaps as a result of metaplasia or as an anatomic variant. The pharyngeal tonsil does not have a discrete fibrous capsule, as does the palatine tonsil. A lesser known and smaller collection of lymphoid tonsillar tissue is present in the area of the torus tubarius, eustachian tube, and fossa of Rosenmüller bilaterally. These are known as tubal tonsils (1) and are components of Waldeyer's ring. They may represent lateral extensions of the pharyngeal tonsil. A swelling of the pharyngeal or tubal tonsils, resulting from lymphoid hyperplasia, can cause obstruction of the eustachian tube and lead to serous otitis media. This is more common in children than in adults, as children's tonsils are larger and generally more prone to lymphoid hyperplasia.

A recess in the posterior wall of the nasopharynx in the midline, in the area of the pharyngeal tonsil, is present in most individuals and is known as the pharyngeal bursa (2,3). It represents the remnant of the pharyngeal component of an embryologic communication between the posterior pharynx and the primitive notochord. This bursa can become obstructed and develop into a cyst (Tornwaldt's cyst) (2) that is commonly infected and may produce clinical disease (see below).

Anteriorly in the roof of the nasopharynx in the midline, at the junction of the posterosuperior edge of the vomer bone of the nasal septum with the sphenoid bone, lies a collection of adenohypophyseal tissue, the pharyngeal hypophysis (4,5). This structure contains a complement of hormone-secreting endocrine tissue similar to the sellar anterior pituitary, has a vascular connection to the pituitary portal system, and is a normal structure, present in virtually every individual, rather than representing a heterotopic focus of pituitary in the nasopharynx. This finding is plausible embryologically because the adenohypophysis develops from Rathke's pouch, a cranial extension of the primitive embryonic oral cavity or stomodeum, which passes through the area of the future pharyngeal hypophysis. Thus, occasional pituitary lesions may be entirely nasopharyngeal and not connected to the sella. Craniopharyngiomas (4,6–9) and pituitary adenomas involving the nasopharynx, sphenoid sinus, and/or clival area have been reported in patients with normal sellar pituitary glands (4,6–9). These lesions likely arise from the pharyngeal hypophysis.

The mucosal lining of the nasopharynx is predominantly respiratory, but areas of squamous mucosa are present and may well increase in area with the age of the individual.

Congenital Anomalies

Congenital anomalies of the nasopharynx are rare. These include choanal atresia, pharyngeal stenosis, heterotopic brain, branchial pouch cysts or sinuses, and various teratomatous masses.

Choanal Atresia

Choanal atresia represents an obstruction or discontinuity between the nasal cavity and nasopharynx at the choana caused by tissue covering the normal choanal opening. This obstruction can be partial or complete, unilateral or bilateral, and osseous or only membranous. Generally girls with the anomaly outnumber boys (10), and osseous atresia is more common than only membranous.

The primary symptom of significant atresia is acute respiratory distress at birth. Because neonates are obligate nose breathers (11), bilateral complete atresia is life threatening. There are usually no external nasal malformations, and so the diagnosis is not immediately obvious, and maneuvers such as attempting to pass a tube through the nose into the pharynx are usually required to establish the diagnosis.

Interestingly, choanal atresia has been found to be accompanied often by one or more associated anomalies embracing various organ systems, referred to by the mnemonic, the CHARGE association (10,11). These include coloboma or other ocular anomalies (C), congenital heart disease (H), atresia choanae (A), retarded growth and development (R), genital abnormalities in boys but not girls (G), and external ear malformations with or without associated deafness (E). Thus, if choanal atresia is found, it is important to evaluate the child for other abnormalities, some of which (i.e., congenital heart disease) can be potentially fatal.

The pathogenesis of choanal atresia was traditionally considered to be a defect in the normal breakdown of the embryonic buccopharyngeal membrane at about the 45th day of gestation. More recently, however, it has been proposed that the CHARGE association may be related to abnormalities involving neural crest tissue, including its cephalic migration (11).

Histologically, on examination of specimens of resection of the choanal atresia plate or membrane, one sees lamellar bone of varying thickness, at times with prominent areas of ligamentous insertion (Sharpey's fibers) and mucosal soft tissue, at times fibrotic.

Pharyngeal Stenosis

Congenital stenosis involving the nasopharynx can cause significant dyspnea, especially during sleep. Such stenosis is usually the result of various craniofacial anomalies such as mandibular hypoplasia, as in the Pierre-Robin syndrome, or craniofacial dysostosis, in which the maxillary complex fails to grow adequately, as in Crouzon's or Apert's syndrome (10). Occasionally, nasopharyngeal stenosis may involve the presence of abnormal pharyngeal bands of tissue, thought to be fetal remnants of palatal arches. Such tissue bands histologically have been composed of a squamous mucosa overlying skeletal muscle (10).

Heterotopic Brain

Glial heterotopia is well described in the nose (see Chapter 1), often associated with bony defects in the cranial base, but ectopic central nervous system (CNS) tissue in the nasopharynx is much less common. When it occurs, as with most nasopharyngeal anomalies, it is associated with respiratory obstruction, occasionally resulting in death (12,13). Nasopharyngeal CNS heterotopia is thought to be caused, as in nasal cases, by abnormalities of closure of the craniofacial base, with incomplete closure resulting in herniation or ill-timed closure resulting in trapping of CNS tissue (13). Hence, it is important to evaluate for the presence of associated bony defects and intracranial connections in cases of nasopharyngeal as well as nasal glial heterotopia. Some nasopharyngeal cases have been associated with cleft palate (12).

Heterotopic CNS tissue in the nasopharynx always contains glial tissue, usually astrocytes, and about half of such cases have neurons. Most contain ependymal or choroid plexus tissue, as opposed to nasal glial heterotopias, most of which do not (12). In addition, rare cases have been reported containing retina-like structures, and a focus of oligodendroglioma (12) in heterotopic pharyngeal brain has been described.

Dermoids and Teratomas

Tumorous masses composed of several tissue types foreign to the location of the mass are uncommon in the head and neck. In the pharyngeal region (nasopharynx and/or oropharynx) they occur almost exclusively in neonates and infants. Such lesions have traditionally been classified as dermoids, teratoids, teratomas, and epignathi (14–18), but they are currently usually grouped as dermoids and teratomas.

Dermoids

Pharyngeal dermoids are pedunculated or sessile polypoid masses covered by skin with its appendages, including hairs; hence, its commonly used synonymous term "hairy polyp" (19–21). They are present at birth and usually present clinically in the neonatal period or in infancy, although an exceptional case may not be recognized until adulthood (20). Pharyngeal dermoids are commonly elongated finger-like masses that hang down from the nasopharynx and/or project into the oropharynx. They may produce symptoms of respiratory obstruction if they block the airway and may have the potential to cause suffocation (20). Most (about 60%) arise from the nasopharynx, usually the lateral wall or superior surface of the soft palate, and most if not all of the others arise from the oropharynx, commonly the tonsillar area (19). Girls are more commonly affected than boys. The lesions are uncommon, with about 120 cases reported in the literature by 1989 (20). They are usually not associated with other congenital anomalies.

Grossly, dermoids are polypoid elongated sausage- or finger-shaped masses. They are commonly pedunculated and occasionally sessile, with the grayish-white external appearance of skin. Fine surface hairs may be appreciated. Their size has been reported as ranging from 0.5 to 6 cm (19). On cut section they are solid with a core of fatty or fibrofatty tissue and occasionally with the presence of a central cartilage plate (Fig. 1). This polypoid configuration is in contrast to the cystic nature of analogous lesions in other locations such as the neck or ovary, accounting for the use of the term "dermoid" and not "dermoid cyst."

Microscopically the polyps are lined with normal-appearing skin with hair follicles, arrector pili muscles, sebaceous glands, and sweat glands (Fig. 2). The fatty/fibrofatty core commonly contains cartilage and may also contain muscles, nerves, minor

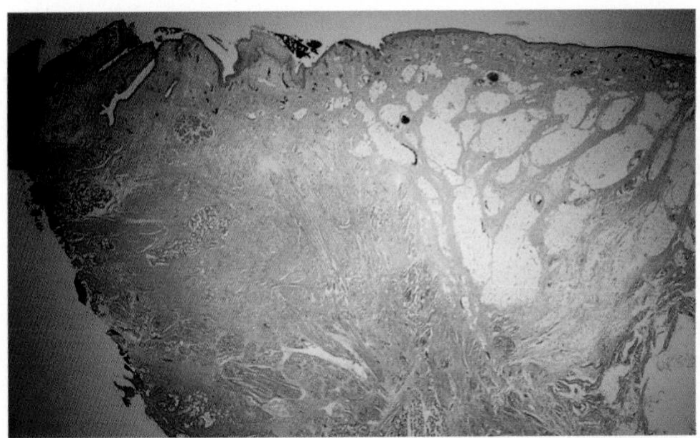

FIGURE 1. Nasopharyngeal dermoid. The protuberant lesion is covered by skin with subcutaneous fat, on the **right,** and is continuous with nasopharyngeal mucosa, on the **left.**

salivary glands, or lymph nodes (19). The cutaneous lining tissue often reverts to the normal pharyngeal mucosal lining in the area of the pedicle or base of the polyp.

These lesions are bigerminal in that they contain tissues arising from ectoderm and mesoderm but not endoderm, as opposed to teratomas, which generally contain tissue from all three germ layers. Pharyngeal dermoids are generally considered congenital malformations rather than true neoplasms (19,21) and are invariably benign and usually cured by complete excision.

Teratoma

Teratomas (also see Chapter 1) are fascinating growths that, especially in the nasopharyngeal area, blur the distinction between neoplasms and congenital malformations (15). They are generally considered to represent neoplasms containing tissues from all three germ layers, some foreign to the site of the tumor's origin, arranged in a more or less disorganized fashion (the word teratoma is derived from the Greek *"teras"* or *"teratos,"* meaning "monster"). So-called "teratoids" were originally considered to contain less well organized trigerminal tissue than "teratomas," but this distinction appears rather artificial (14), and the term is not widely used today. Nasopharyngeal or basicranial teratomas tend to be larger than dermoids, at times presenting at birth as obvious masses protruding through the mouth and/or nares (14,15,22). They may attain considerable size and in very rare instances occur as huge masses with recognizable limbs or other structures emanating from a newborn's mouth, at times giving somewhat the impression of a grossly malformed parasitic twin. Such a lesion has been termed an "epignathus," as it was thought to arise from the upper jaw, although it is considered actually to arise from the cranial base in the base of sphenoid area. Epignathi are extremely rare. They are usually incompatible with life but may occasionally be successfully surgically removed (22).

Less dramatic, more conventional teratomas in the nasopharyngeal area are also rather rare, with 28 cases reported in a review of the literature in 1992. They are often associated with other anomalies of the skull. Teratomas in general are about five to six times more common in girls than boys (14,18). The principal and most serious clinical symptoms relate to respiratory obstruction.

As may be expected, teratomas vary markedly in gross appearance, being lobular, ill-formed masses that may be solid or variably cystic. Recognizable tissue types (e.g., fat, hair, teeth) may at times be grossly appreciated. Histologically tissues from all three germ layers may be found in a more or less disorganized fashion (Fig. 3; also see cervical teratoma, Chapter 1). The nasopharyngeal teratomas tend to have a significant amount of CNS tissue (Fig. 3D), the tissues are virtually always mature for age, and the tumors in infants have thus far all been benign.

The etiology and pathogenesis of dermoids and teratomas have been the subject of much speculation and debate and are still not definitely known (23). Probably the most generally held current opinion is that, at least in extragonadal locations, such as the head and neck, these lesions are a result of a sequestration of multipotent embryonal or stem cells that have escaped or become dissociated from normal regulatory influences (14,15,19,24). It is intriguing to speculate that nasopharyngeal dermoids may be an anomaly of branchial development, with the cutaneous component representing anomalous tissue of ectodermal first or second branchial groove origin and the cartilaginous component representing anomalous tissue of mesodermal first or second branchial arch origin. This notion is

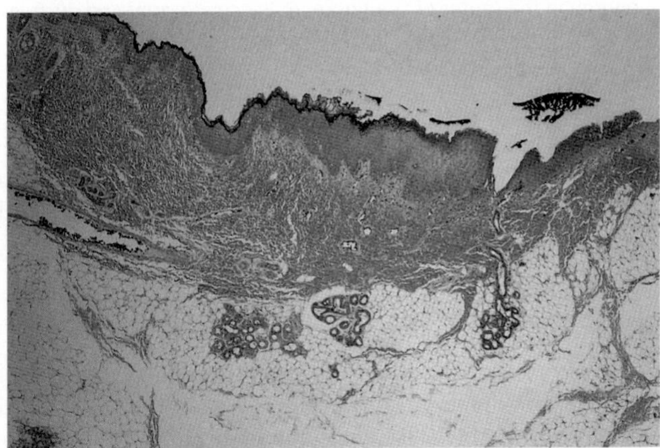

A

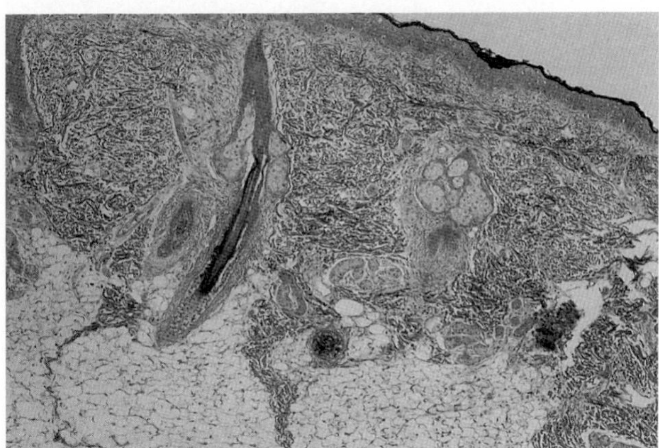

B

FIGURE 2. Nasopharyngeal dermoid. **A:** The polyp is lined by skin with epidermis, dermis, and sweat glands. Subcutaneous fat is deep. **B:** The skin contains hair follicles and sebaceous glands ("hairy polyp").

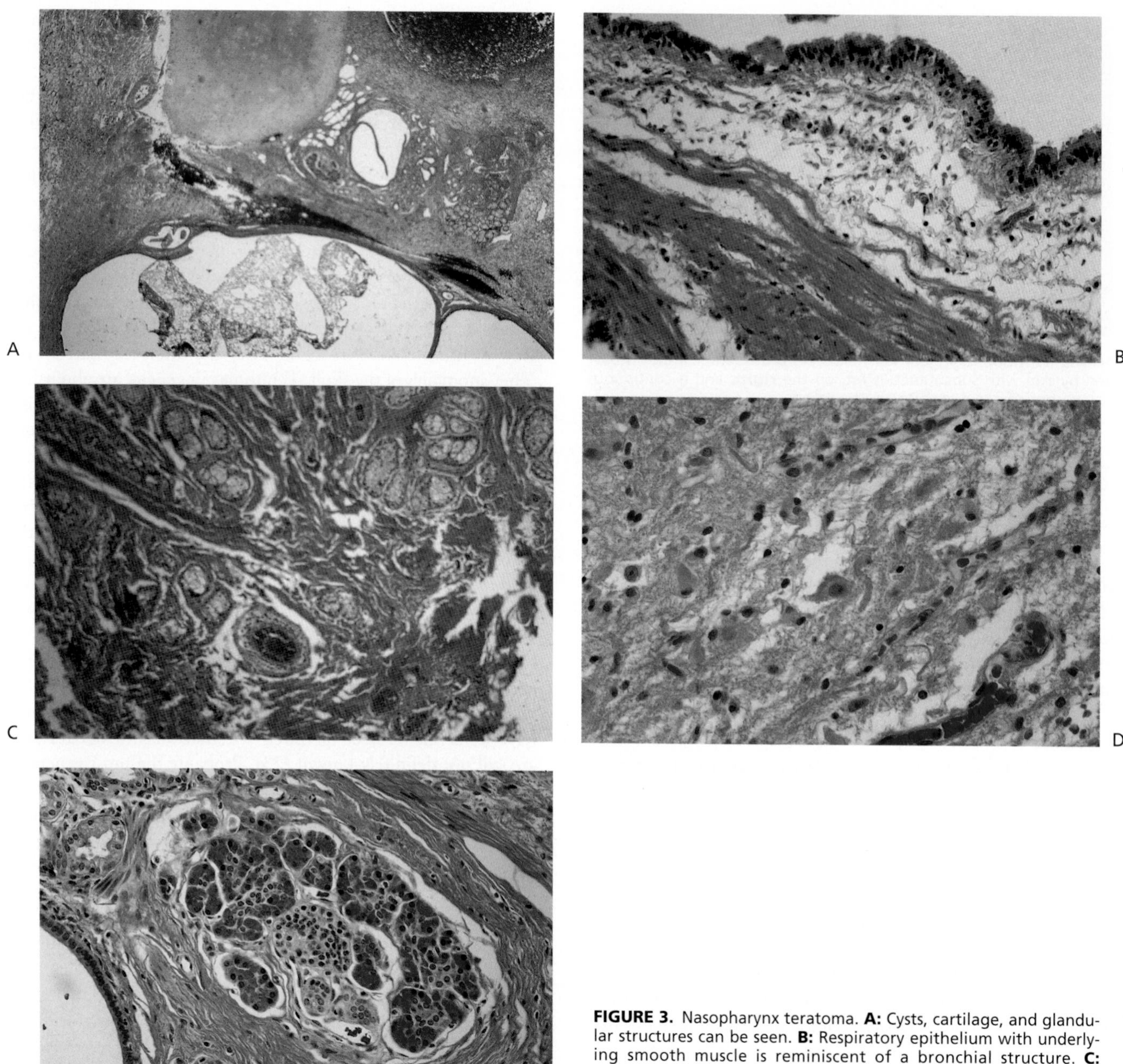

FIGURE 3. Nasopharynx teratoma. **A:** Cysts, cartilage, and glandular structures can be seen. **B:** Respiratory epithelium with underlying smooth muscle is reminiscent of a bronchial structure. **C:** Cutaneous appendages are present. **D:** Glial tissue with a prominent neuron in the center of the figure. **E:** Pancreatic acini and ductules surround a central islet of Langerhans.

supported by the occasional report of a pharyngeal dermoid resembling an auricle (24a).

Branchial Cyst

Occasional rare cases of laterally placed nasopharyngeal cysts of presumed congenital branchial origin have been reported (25–27). Such cysts arise laterally in the nasopharynx and may be asymptomatic or, if large, may produce nasal obstruction (27). Their relatively silent clinical nature usually leads to their discovery during adulthood. Most are thought to be derived from the second branchial pouch (26) and are lined, as are most branchial cysts, by squamous, columnar ciliated, or a mixture or intermediate form of these epithelia. They may or may not have mural lymphoid tissue. They are separated from Tornwaldt's cysts by their lateral as opposed to midline location.

Inflammatory Lesions

The nasopharynx responds to infection primarily by means of lymphoid hyperplasia of the pharyngeal tonsil. Such reactive lymphoid hyperplasia is quite common in children and less so in adults. Adenoidal hyperplasia can contribute to breathing difficulties and occasionally sleep apnea in children as well as to hy-

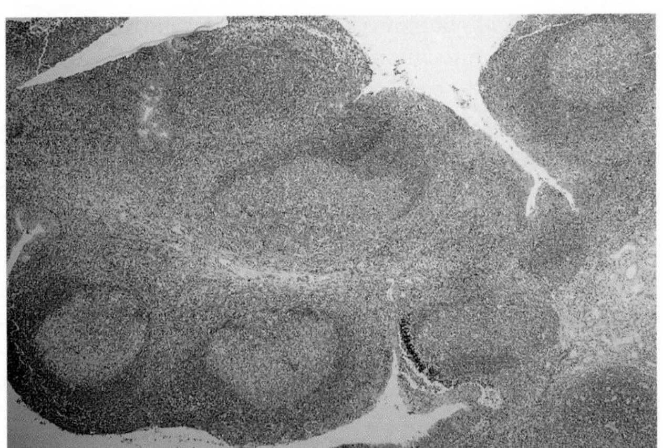

FIGURE 4. Nasopharynx: adenoids with follicular lymphoid hyperplasia in an 11-year-old.

ponasal speech. The overwhelming majority of adenoidal enlargements in children are benign, and the lymphoid hyperplasia appears histologically as a follicular hyperplasia, with germinal centers at times attaining considerable size. The classic features of benign follicular lymphoid hyperplasia are seen with discrete, enlarged, round to oval, occasionally curved or hourglass-shaped germinal centers surrounded by a distinct dark mantle zone of small lymphocytes (Fig. 4). The germinal centers at times exhibit zonation of large round cells to one side of the follicle and small cleaved cells to the other and typically have many tingible body macrophages and mitotic figures. The differentiation from malignant lymphoma is rarely a problem in children in whom follicular lymphomas are exceedingly rare. An important exception is that benign infection with Epstein-Barr virus (EBV), as in infectious mononucleosis, can lead to a histologic picture that may mimic Hodgkin's disease or other lymphomas (28–31). One may see a somewhat polymorphous proliferation of lymphoid cells, including many large immunoblasts with very prominent nucleoli, at times binucleated, that can closely resemble Reed-Sternberg cells (Fig. 5A). Obviously, correlation with clinical data is important in these cases, with serologic testing for mononucleosis at times offering some reassurance. Further, the Reed-Sternberg cells in Hodgkin's disease of Waldeyer's ring, as in nodal Hodgkin's disease, usually stain immunohistochemically with CD15 (Leu M1) and/or CD30 (Ber-H2) (32), whereas the Reed-Sternberg–like cells of infectious mononucleosis should be CD15 negative (Fig. 5B). It should also be remembered that Hodgkin's disease involving Waldeyer's ring is uncommon, especially as a primary site, although it does occur (32–34).

It is common to find small aggregates of mature plasma cells superficially located near the mucosal epithelium in nasopharyngeal biopsies with lymphoid hyperplasia. Occasionally, I have even found intranuclear material reminiscent of Dutcher bodies in a rare plasma cell. This is usually nonproblematic, as the plasma cells do not form a mass lesion, and plasmacytoid lymphomas and lymphomas of mucosa-associated lymphoid tissues (MALT) or marginal zone lymphomas are rare in the nasopharynx (see Chapter 12).

In adults, the differentiation of nasopharyngeal follicular lymphoid hyperplasia and follicular lymphoma may at times be problematic (29). The criteria for distinguishing these conditions in lymph nodes may be applied to extranodal sites, including the nasopharynx. Briefly, follicular lymphomas have less distinct follicles with less well defined mantle zones, absence of zonation of large round and small cleaved cells, fewer tingible bodies and mitoses, and at times (but not always) a more uniform intrafollicular cell population than follicular hyperplasia. Also, the abnormal lymphomatous cells in follicular lymphoma tend to extend into interfollicular areas. When in doubt, immunophenotypic studies for monotypic surface immunoglobin are usually quite helpful.

Rare examples of more unusual infections such as tuberculosis of the nasopharynx are reported, but these are quite uncommon currently in industrialized nations (35).

A

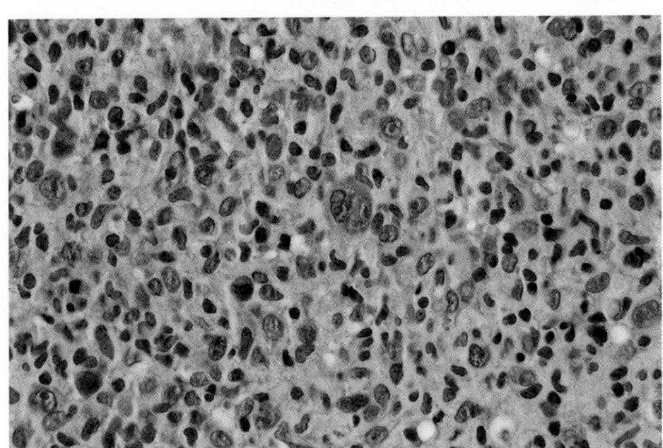

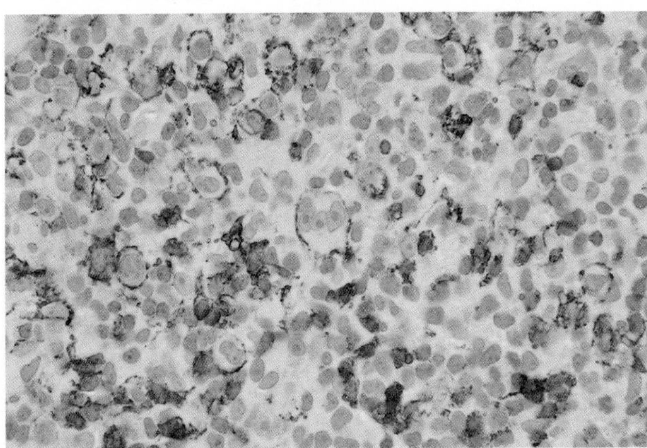

B

FIGURE 5. Nasopharynx: infectious mononucleosis in a 6-year-old. **A:** Lymphoid proliferation containing large immunoblastic cells with a Reed-Sternberg–like cell in the center of the field. **B:** An immunohistochemical stain for CD20 (L26), a B-cell marker, shows staining of the immunoblastic cells, including the central Reed-Sternberg–like cell. True Reed-Sternberg cells in Hodgkin's disease (except in the lymphocyte-predominant subtype) do not stain with B-cell markers. (Case courtesy of Dr. Nancy L. Harris.)

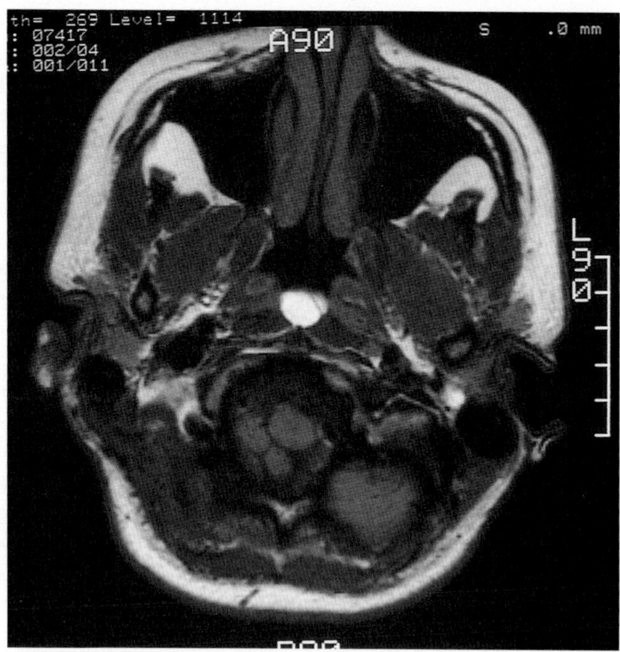

FIGURE 6. Nasopharynx: Tornwaldt cyst. A T_1-weighted MR radiologic image demonstrates the midline bright-appearing cyst in the nasopharyngeal region.

Nonneoplastic Tumorous Conditions

Cysts

Tornwaldt's Cyst

A Tornwaldt cyst is a cystic dilation of the pharyngeal bursa, a structure present in about 3% to 4% of adults that represents the remnant of an embryologic connection between the notochord and the nasopharynx (2,36,37). It is located in the posterior wall of the nasopharynx superiorally in the midline, above the superior pharyngeal constrictor muscles (37). If the bursal orifice becomes obstructed, a cyst may develop that may produce symptoms or be asymptomatic. It occasionally becomes infected, resulting in an abscess. When symptomatic, the lesion may produce a complex of symptoms known as Tornwaldt's disease (36). Such clinical manifestations include nasopharyngeal drainage, occipital headaches, bad breath, fullness or pain in the ears, or neck muscle pain or stiffness (the pharyngeal bursa runs between the two longus capitis muscles).

On endoscopy, the lesion appears as a bulging cystic mass generally covered by normal-appearing mucosa, high in the posterior nasopharynx in the midline, at times presenting superior to the adenoidal pad (2). If it is infected, purulent material may be expressed through a midline orifice on exertion of pressure on the cyst.

Radiologic studies are helpful in differentiating Tornwaldt's cyst from a branchial pouch cyst, which is more laterally located (Fig. 6). A Rathke's pouch cyst, or remnant of Rathke's pouch (see Anatomic Considerations) would be superior and anterior to the location of a Tornwaldt cyst (37). Histologically, a Tornwaldt cyst is lined by respiratory, squamous, intermediate, or transitional epithelium or a combination thereof. Some reports note that the lining of a Tornwaldt cyst is devoid of significant lymphoid tissue (2,36), whereas other authors state that lymphoid tissue with germinal centers is a common if not characteristic finding (3). The pharyngeal bursa is in close proximity to the pharyngeal tonsil, and thus, it is not surprising that tonsillar lymphoid tissue should be present in the vicinity of a Tornwaldt cyst. The amount of lymphoid tissue in the nasopharynx tends to decrease with age and is rather variable, so a variation in the amount of lymphoid tissue in the wall of a Tornwaldt cyst might not be unexpected. A small cyst might appear histologically quite similar to a cyst arising from a dilated tonsillar crypt, and the two may be virtually impossible to distinguish. Thus, the lining of Tornwaldt's cysts is nonspecific histologically; and a Tornwaldt cyst is a clinicopathologic diagnosis. Cysts of the nasopharynx lined by respiratory epithelium and not definitely clinically categorized as Tornwaldt's cysts occur (Figs. 7 and 8).

Branchial Cysts

Branchial cysts, though presumably congenital in origin, are frequently clinically silent and often present in adulthood. They are described under congenital anomalies.

A

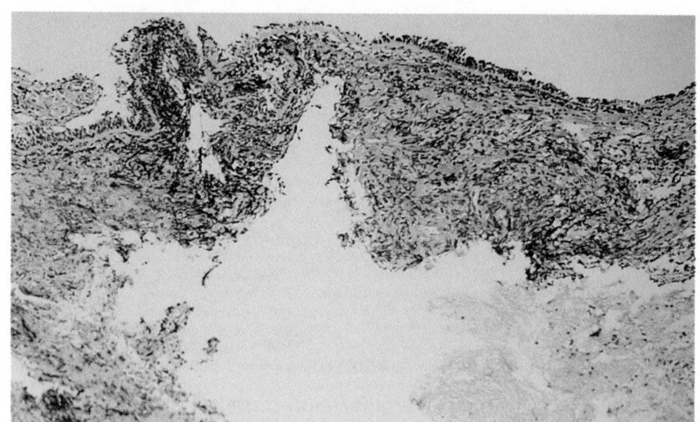

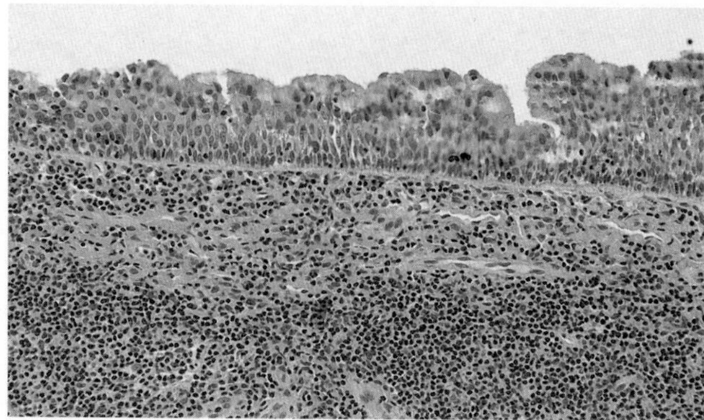

B

FIGURE 7. Nasopharynx: cyst thought clinically to be a Tornwaldt cyst. **A:** In this example, a columnar epithelial lining overlies a fibrous wall with a slight to moderate quantity of lymphocytes. **B:** In this example, a thickened columnar epithelial lining covers tissue with an abundant lymphoid component.

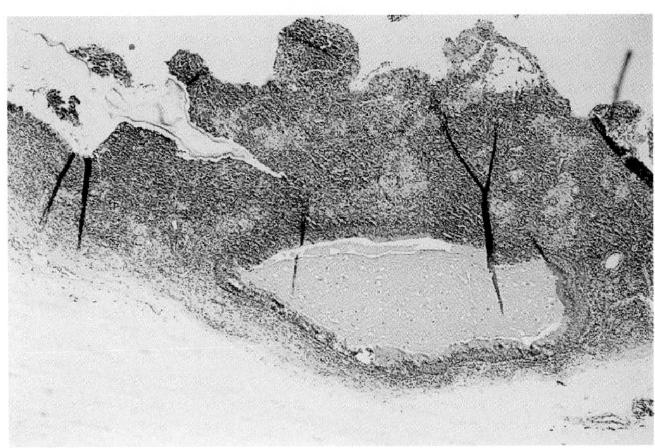

FIGURE 8. Nasopharynx: cyst. An irregular cyst lining overlies a smaller cystic structure that may represent an invagination of the large cystic cavity.

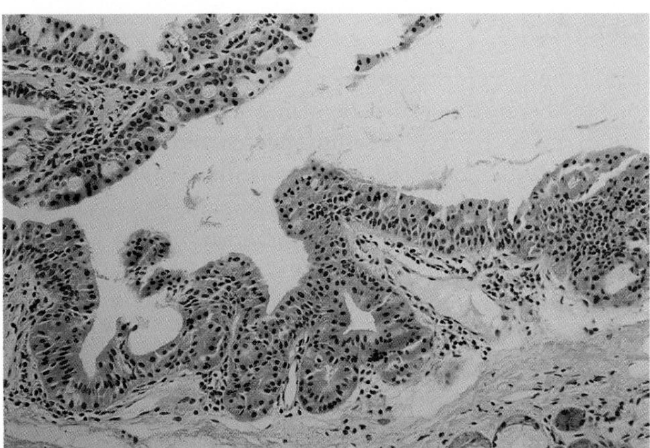

FIGURE 10. Nasopharynx: oncocytic cyst. The cyst is lined by a hyperplastic double-layered oncocytic epithelium thrown up into papillary folds, not unlike the epithelium in a Warthin's tumor.

Glandular Retention Cysts

These cysts arise from dilation of seromucinous gland ducts in the nasopharynx. They are frequently small and encountered incidentally on histologic examination of a nasopharyngeal specimen, but they may become large enough to present clinically as a nasopharyngeal mass. If infected, they may be painful. Histologically, one sees dilation of ducts, frequently multiple, of seromucinous glands (36). The dilated duct structures are filled with mucinous material and lined by cuboidal ductal epithelium (Fig. 9). Occasionally, the lining epithelium may be oncocytic and associated with oncocytic metaplasia and/or hyperplasia of glandular tissue. Such lesions are analogous to the oncocytic cysts seen in the larynx (Chapter 7) (38). Such lesions, if located near the torus tubarius, may produce eustachian tube dysfunction with otitis media (38,39). If oncocytic metaplasia, manifested as cells with ample granular pink cytoplasm representing a greatly increased number of cytoplasmic mitochondria, is prominent, then the designation oncocytic cyst is appropriate (Fig. 10); otherwise the term "duct retention cyst" may be used.

Oncocytic cysts with oncocytic metaplasia and hyperplasia are not uncommonly encountered as an incidental finding in the nasopharynx of older individuals and may possibly represent a degenerative change (Fig. 11). Three intriguing cases with melanin deposition in the oncocytic epithelium have recently been published (39,40).

Encephalocele

Glial heterotopia with or without associated encephalocele is more commonly encountered in the nasal region than in the nasopharynx (see Chapter 1); nonetheless, it is important to exclude an intracranial connection of any nasopharyngeal cyst, especially one in the midline, as meningitis may complicate manipulation of an unrecognized encephalocele.

Rathke's Cleft Cyst

A Rathke's cleft cyst, representing a dilated remnant of the embryologic Rathke's pouch (see Anatomic Considerations), has occasionally been reported in the suprasellar area and may possibly be located in the sphenoid sinus, but it is rarely, if at all, encountered in the nasopharynx. Such a cyst if present should be located anterior and superior to the location of a Tornwaldt cyst.

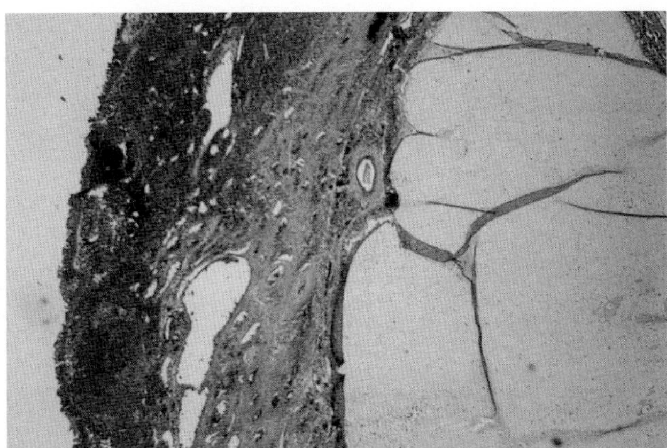

FIGURE 9. Nasopharynx. A glandular retention cyst is filled with mucin.

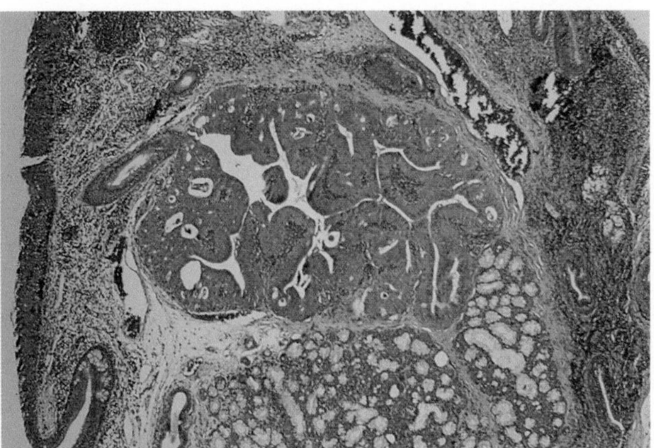

FIGURE 11. Nasopharynx: oncocytic metaplasia and hyperplasia resulting in a small cystic cavity.

Hamartomas

Hamartomas are disorganized proliferations of tissues indigenous to the area in which they arise. They have self-limited growth potential and are thus not considered neoplasms. Although Willis considered them to represent a developmental defect, usually present at birth, the exact pathogenesis of various lesions conventionally designated as hamartomas is not always clear (41,42).

Such lesions are rare in the nasopharyngeal region, and until recently, only scattered case reports had appeared in the literature (43–45). Recently, several series of cases have been reported (41,42,46). The recently reported cases have involved adults, ranging in age from 24 to 81 years (41,42,45). The lesions are usually single polypoid growths generally occurring in the posterior nasal cavity, often along the posterior septum and/or involving the nasopharynx. Occasionally two masses occur bilaterally, and a few are reported in paranasal sinuses (42). Symptoms usually include nasal stuffiness or obstruction and occasionally epistaxis or nasal discharge.

Grossly, nasal/nasopharyngeal hamartomas are polypoid masses (Fig. 12), generally firmer than most inflammatory polyps (42). They range in size from about 1 cm to about 5 cm in diameter. Histologically, most of the hamartomas exhibit a proliferation of epithelial elements. The surface at times has a subtle lobulated or leaf-like pattern, reminiscent of that of a phyllodes tumor of the breast (Fig. 13). There is frequently ingrowth of surface respiratory epithelium into the stroma, creating prominent gland-like spaces lined by pseudostratified ciliated epithelium (42) (Fig. 14). I have, however, seen similar gland-like ciliated surface invaginations in lesions clinically and pathologically consistent with chronic polypoid rhinosinusitis (see Chapter 4), although in such cases they are generally less prominent than in harmatomas. These spaces are sometimes cystically dilated and may contain a mucinous secretion. Cyst linings are sometimes attenuated to a flattened epithelium (Fig. 15), and there may be focal squamous metaplasia of the lining epithelium.

Some authors describe an associated disorganized proliferation of seromucinous glands, sometimes closely associated with

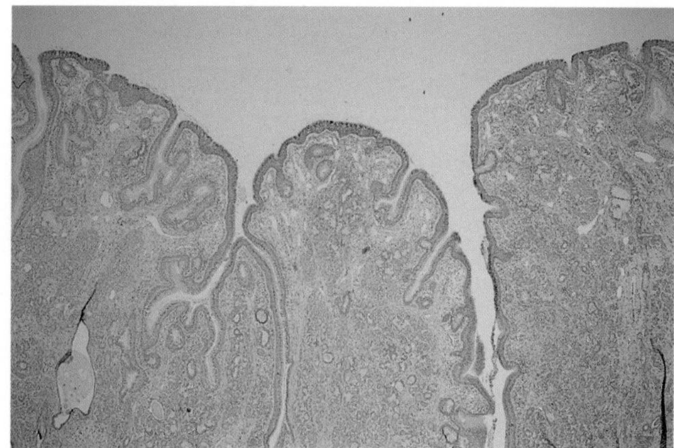

FIGURE 13. Nasopharynx: hamartoma. Leaf-like (phyllodes tumor-like) surface.

the respiratory epithelial-lined cystic structures. The fibroblastic stroma is at times cellular and may contain prominent blood vessels somewhat reminiscent of a juvenile angiofibroma (Fig. 16). Inflammation, though usually present, is not especially prominent and is less than that seen in many inflammatory polyps.

Although a second type of mesenchymal hamartoma has been described in the literature (45), those have usually represented unilateral overgrowth of a single mesenchymal element and may well be considered benign mesenchymal neoplasms rather than hamartomas (e.g., lipoma, angioma, neurofibroma, chondroma). One case that we consider a true mesenchymal hamartoma was a polypoid structure that had the phyllodes-like leafy pattern but no glandular proliferation; there was a subepithelial proliferation of loose fibrous tissue with spindled to stellate cells, a fibrillar background with prominent blood vessels, a lymphoplasmacytic infiltrate, and scattered disorganized skeletal muscle fibers (41) (Fig. 17). A recent report of combined mesenchymal and epithelial sinonasal/nasopharyngeal hamartomas, in this case chondroosseous and epithelial, has appeared in the literature (46).

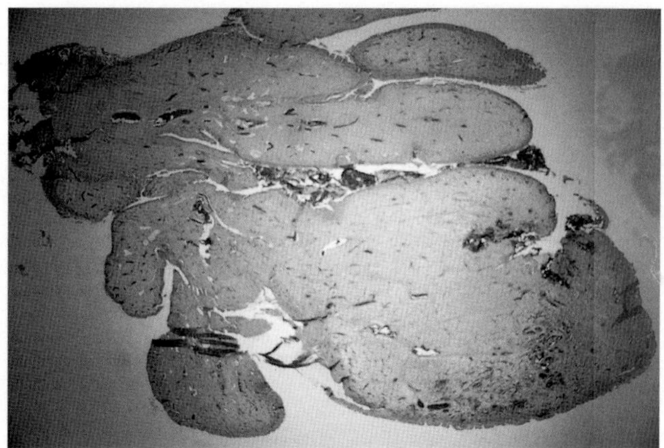

FIGURE 12. Anterior nasopharyngeal hamartoma with polypoid appearance and irregular surface.

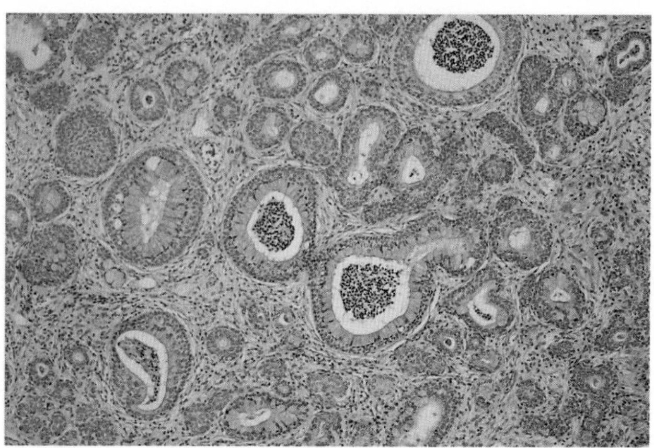

FIGURE 14. Nasopharynx: hamartoma. Gland-like spaces lined by respiratory epithelium.

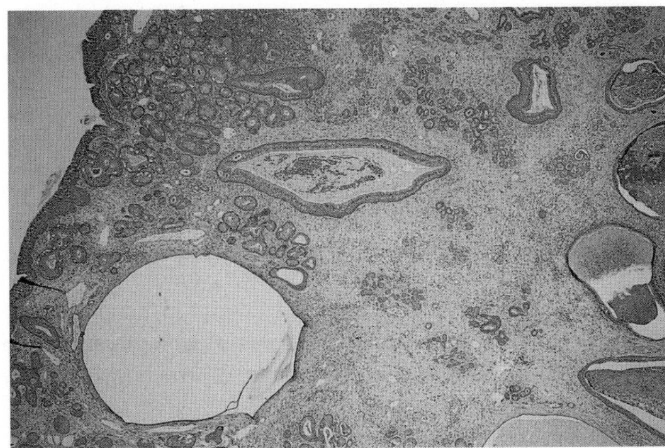
A

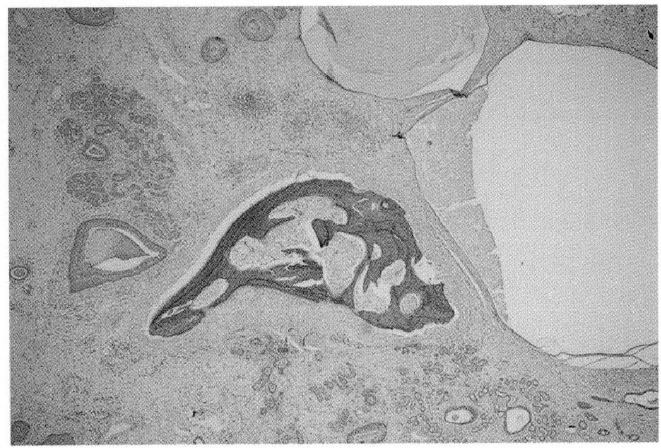
B

FIGURE 15. Nasopharynx: hamartoma. **A:** Cystic spaces focally with an attenuated epithelial lining. **B:** Cystic spaces with adjacent bone—a mesenchymal component to the hamartoma.

The most important differential diagnostic consideration is an adenocarcinoma. Hamartomas do not infiltrate surrounding normal tissues but are self-contained. Their cells do not exhibit pleomorphism or cytologic atypicality. Although rare low-grade adenocarcinomas of the nasopharyngeal region may be cytologically bland, they often feature more solid packed back-to-back glands, and their glandular components do not recapitulate normally present seromucinous glands as closely as do those of hamartomas. Inflammatory polyps are often multiple, more edematous and inflammatory, lack the leafy phyllodes-like structure, and their components tend to be less haphazardly arranged than in a hamartoma. It should be mentioned that surface invagination of ciliated epithelium into underlying stroma can be seen in inflammatory polyps/polypoid rhinosinusitis and that the presence of a clinically discrete mass is desirable for a firm diagnosis of hamartoma. The distinction between a mesenchymal hamartoma and a benign mesenchymoma may be somewhat semantic, but we would consider a mesenchymoma to represent a proliferation of multiple immature mesenchymal tissues without an epithelial component. Inverted papillomas show the characteristic proliferative schneiderian epithelium that is absent in hamartomas (see Chapter 4).

Amyloid Deposition

Localized amyloid deposition rarely occurs in the nasopharynx, the most common site of localized upper respiratory amyloid deposition being the larynx (see Chapter 7). Most instances of amyloid causing significant symptoms in the upper respiratory tract appear to be caused by localized deposition rather than systemic amyloidosis (47). The few reported localized nasopharyngeal cases have been associated with symptoms such as nasal obstruction and discharge and otitis media (48–51).

Histologically, the amyloid appears similar to that in other sites (see Chapter 7); briefly, deposition of a homogeneous eosinophilic amorphous extracellular substance is present, infiltrating the tissue, in vessel walls, surrounding and/or replacing seromucinous gland structures, or in interstitial areas (Fig. 18). The amyloid exhibits a light green birefringence when stained with Congo Red and viewed under polarized light. A chronic inflammatory infiltrate, often including a prominent component of plasma cells, is often present (Fig. 19), and foreign-body–type giant cells may be scattered in relation to the amyloid material. Rarely, calcification or even ossification of the amyloid may occur (52).

FIGURE 16. Nasopharynx: hamartoma. Fibrous stroma with large vascular space on the left of the figure.

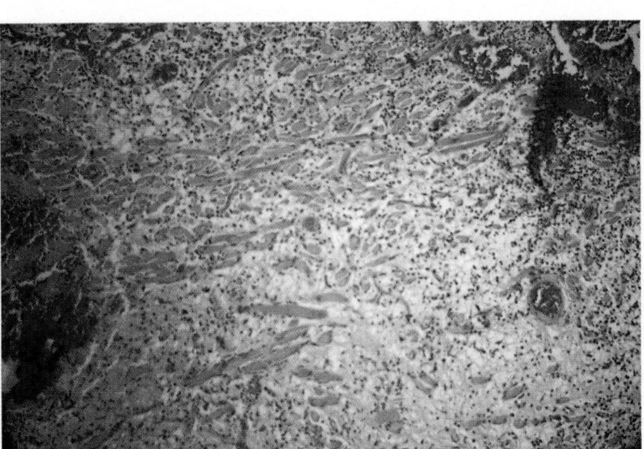

FIGURE 17. Anterior nasopharyngeal hamartoma (soft palate area): disorganized skeletal muscle.

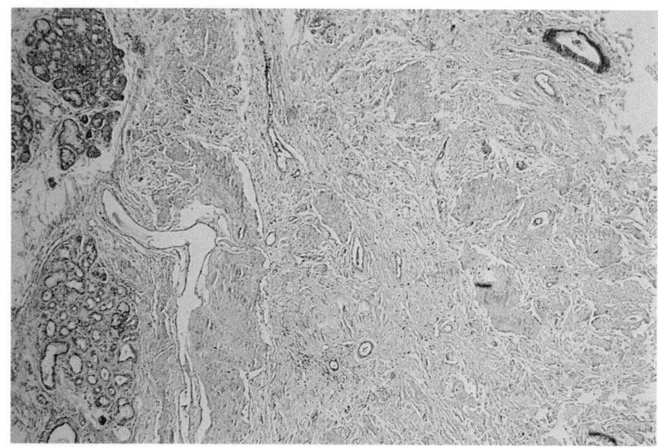

FIGURE 18. Nasopharynx: amyloid deposition. Extracellular masses of homogeneous eosinophilic amyloid.

Amyloid may be produced in association with plasmacytomas, of which neoplasm of the nasopharynx is a prominent extraosseous site, and Michaels and Hyams (52) reported finding significant deposits of amyloid in 7 of 12 cases of nasopharyngeal plasmacytoma. In one case of nasal amyloidosis not associated with plasmacytoma, the amyloid protein was identified as amyloid immunoglobulin light chain (AL), λ (49). Interestingly, in this case the associated plasmacytic infiltrate showed a significant excess of cytoplasmic λ light chain (the λ:κ ratio being about 10:1), consistent with the notion of the localized amyloid being produced by an oligoclonal population of plasma cells.

Others

An unusual case of actinomycosis with abscess formation following a dental procedure that presented as a nasopharyngeal/paranasopharyngeal mass has recently been reported (53).

Benign Neoplasms

Benign epithelial neoplasms of the nasopharynx are extremely uncommon. Some small nasopharyngeal tumors reported as oncocytomas or oncocytic cystadenomas may in fact represent oncocytic metaplasia and hyperplasia with or without oncocytic cysts.

Salivary Gland Anlage Tumor

A very rare and interesting nasopharyngeal tumor seen in neonates and babies (the oldest reported patient was 3 ½ months old at presentation) is the so-called salivary gland anlage tumor (SGAT) (54). This nasopharyngeal mass lesion presents, usually in the neonatal period, with respiratory obstruction and/or feeding difficulties. The mass is often midline.

Grossly, the tumors have ranged from 1.3 to 3 cm in greatest dimension (54). They are reported as being firm and smooth surfaced, at times bosselated. Histologically, one sees a biphasic neoplasm composed of epithelial and small fusiform stromal-type cells. The surface of the tumor is lined by stratified squamous epithelium. Duct-like structures, at times with a component of squamous metaplasia, are present near the surface, disposed in a rather loose stroma, and at times connect with the surface epithelium (Fig. 20). Nodules of densely cellular stromal tissue composed of small fusiform compact cells with bland-appearing ovoid nuclei are present, generally in a central location (Fig. 21). Circular gland-like structures, lined by cells similar to the stromal cells, are intimately admixed with the stromal nodules (Fig. 22). Hemorrhage and focal necrosis may occasionally be seen. Rarely, this epithelioid component may focally assume a papillary configuration. The resemblance of this tumor to the embryonic developing salivary gland has been noted and has prompted the appellation "salivary gland anlage tumor." An earlier example was reported under the designation of congenital pleomorphic adenoma (55). Immunohistochemically, the cells (gland-like, squamous, and stromal) stain for cytokeratin and epithelial membrane antigen, and the stromal cells stain for vimentin and muscle-specific actin. All groups of tumor cells generally stain for salivary gland amylase (54). This profile is consistent with differentiation along epithelial and myoepithelial lines, and ultrastructural observations have confirmed this impression (54).

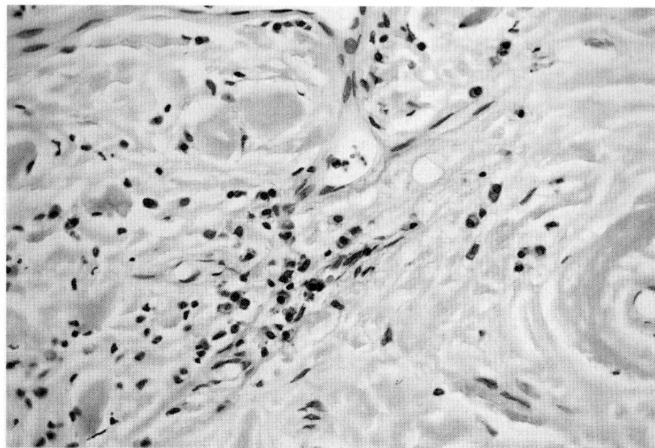

FIGURE 19. Nasopharynx: amyloid deposition. A mononuclear infiltrate rich in plasma cells is associated with the amyloid.

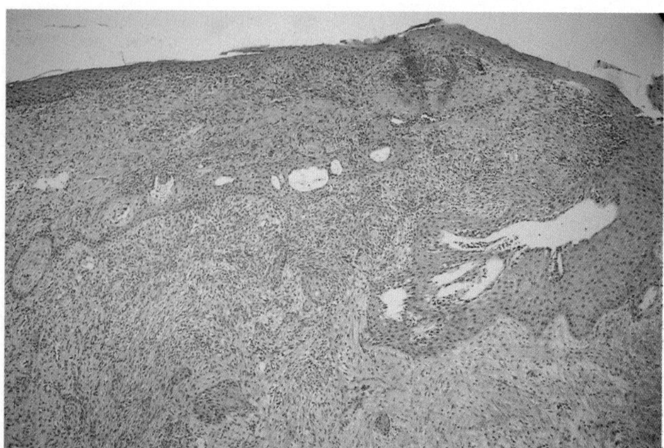

FIGURE 20. Nasopharynx: salivary gland anlage tumor (SGAT). A squamous epithelial-lined surface overlies duct-like structures, at times with squamous metaplasia, and underlying fusiform stromal-type tissue.

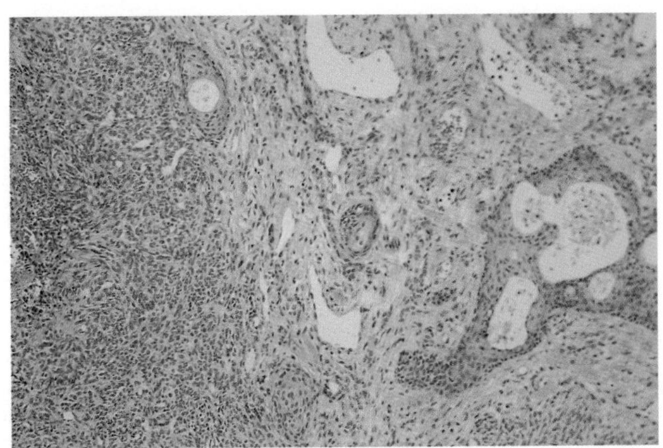

FIGURE 21. Nasopharynx: salivary gland anlage tumor (SGAT). Junction of peripheral duct-like structures and more central fusiform cellular stromal component.

Rare cases of similar tumors have been reported in major salivary glands of neonates under the rubric of salivary embryomas or sialoblastomas (56,57) (see Chapter 8). These have also been reminiscent of the developing salivary gland anlage. Interestingly, a single report of parotid gland tumors in adults (seventh and eighth decades) describes tumors that bear some resemblance to SGAT. They have prompted the somewhat cumbersome designation of "basal cell adenoma with myoepithelial cell-derived 'stroma'" (58).

All of the SGATs reported to date have behaved in a benign fashion, as have the analogous adult parotid tumors. Most of the infantile sialoblastomas of major salivary glands have also been benign, but an exceptionally rare case of neonatal basaloid carcinoma of major salivary gland origin is encountered (56,57).

SGATs are sufficiently distinctive histologically to preclude differential diagnostic dilemmas, with rare exceptions. Synovial sarcomas, though known to occur in the head and neck region of young individuals (see Chapter 10), are exceedingly rare in newborns. A distinguishing feature of SGATs is the budding-off appearance of epithelial elements from the surface mucosa and its absence in synovial sarcomas. Abundant mast cells, often present in synovial sarcomas, are not reported in SGATs (54), and Dehner et al. (54) have found the stromal cells in synovial sarcomas generally to have a more sweeping, fibrosarcoma-like pattern than in SGATs. A case of a lesion termed "nasal blastoma" has been reported (59), occurring in the posterior nasal cavity of an adult of 38, that also consists of epithelial and primitive mesenchymal elements. The mesenchymal elements in nasal blastoma have the characteristics of myofibroblasts rather than myoepithelial cells, however, and the pattern of the spindle cells appears (in an accompanying photomicrograph) more fascicular than in SGAT. Finally, a single case of a blastoma involving the nasopharynx and sinonasal tract was reported in a 62-year-old (60), much of which appeared benign and possibly hamartomatous, but with areas of histologically atypical mitotically active mesenchymal tissue surrounding islands of epithelial-appearing tissue, at times forming gland-like spaces.

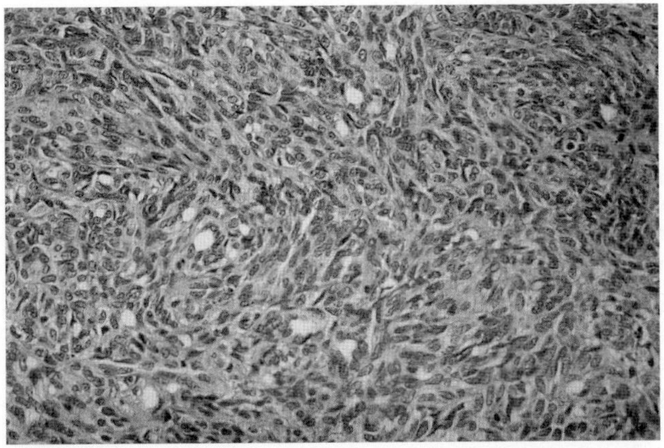

FIGURE 22. Nasopharynx: salivary gland anlage tumor (SGAT). Stromal nodule containing scattered duct-like spaces lined by stroma-like cells.

Juvenile Angiofibroma

Juvenile angiofibroma is an intriguing tumor that, although uncommon, has prompted a considerable literature as well as some controversy. It is a benign but potentially locally aggressive vascular and fibrous tumor occurring almost exclusively in adolescent boys, with rare cases being reported in boys as young as 7 years and in young men. An exceptionally rare case in an older man has been published (61). The patients in multiple published series have been exclusively male (62–68), although in exceptionally rare cases a female patient has been reported (69–71). Alleged cases in female patients should be viewed with a healthy skepticism. The lesions generally present with symptoms of nasal obstruction and/or epistaxis, which may be quite severe. On examination, a rounded lobulated mass of spongy to firm to scirrhous consistency, depending on the relative amounts of vascular and fibrous tissue present in the lesion, is encountered. The tumor is present in the posterior nasal cavity(ies) and nasopharynx and not infrequently extends to adjacent structures (see below). Tumors may be quite large and extensive, and in such cases one may observe a mass in the cheek or in the orbit displacing the globe or causing exophthalmos.

Radiographs are characteristic and show a mass lesion involving the nose and nasopharynx with frequent bowing of the posterior wall of the maxillary sinus anteriorly (63,66) (Fig. 23). Erosion of the base of the medial pterygoid plate is virtually a constant finding (66). Most patients have radiographic evidence of invasion of adjacent structures, most commonly maxillary, sphenoid, or ethmoid sinuses (63), and extension to the pterygomaxillary and infratemporal fossae is not uncommon. Angiography produces a typical vascular tumor blush, with the internal maxillary artery being the principal feeding vessel in most cases (66).

Despite the widely used nomenclature of "nasopharyngeal" juvenile angiofibroma, careful study and observation of numerous cases have shown the actual point of origin of these lesions to be not in the nasopharynx proper but rather in the posterior lateral roof of the nasal cavity in the area of the sphenopalatine foramen (63,66). From this point, the tumor grows along the poste-

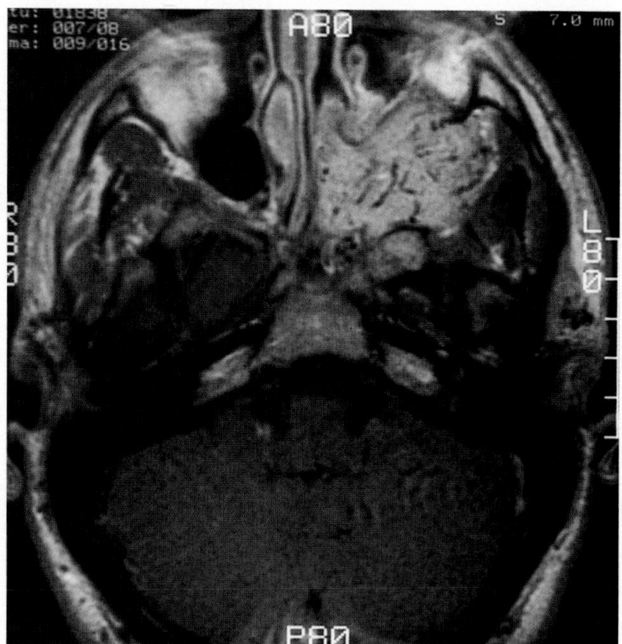

FIGURE 23. Nasopharynx: juvenile angiofibroma (JAF). A T_2-weighted MR imaging study after gadolinium injection shows the large tumor in the nasopharynx and left nasal cavity, extending through the pterygopalatine fossa into the infratemporal fossa. A flow void delineates the prominent blood vessels traversing the lesion.

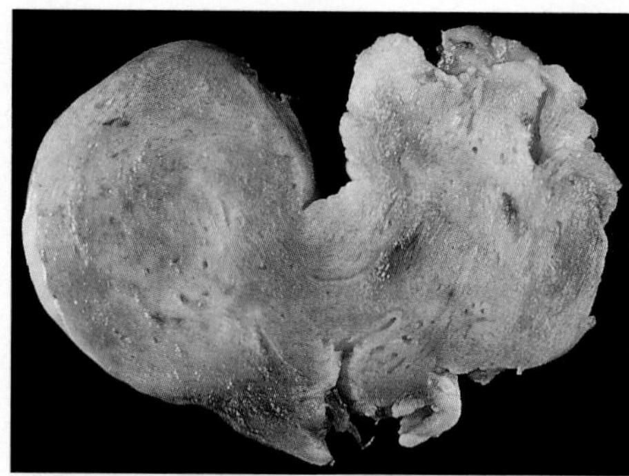

FIGURE 24. Nasopharynx: juvenile angiofibroma (JAF). A gross cut section of the tumor shows a solid polypoid mass containing somewhat prominent vascular spaces. (From Goodman ML, Pilch BZ. Tumors of the upper respiratory tract. In: Fletcher CDM, ed. *Diagnostic histopathology of tumors.* Edinburgh: Churchill Livingstone, 1995:82.)

rior border of the nasal septum and into the nasopharynx and nasal cavity(ies). From here the tumor may extend through the sphenopalatine foramen to enter the ptergopalatine fossa. Destruction of the posterior wall of the maxillary sinus and the floor of the sphenoid sinus leads to invasion of these structures, and lateral extension through the pterygomaxillary fissure leads to invasion of the infratemporal fossa, producing the characteristic swelling of the cheek of advanced lesions (63). Invasion of the orbit can occur through the inferior orbital fissure causing proptosis (63,65), and further growth can lead to invasion of the middle cranial fossa.

Grossly, the tumors are lobulated and firm gray-tan masses. On cut section, one may appreciate numerous vessels traversing the fibrous stroma, imparting a somewhat spongy quality to the more vascular lesions (Fig. 24). Histologically, the findings are characteristic. The tumor is unencapsulated and consists of numerous blood vessels of varying caliber coursing through a fibrous tissue stroma (Fig. 25). A zonal arrangement to the vasculature has been described in the literature (62,72), with a generally narrow superficial or peripheral area of small capillary-sized vessels close to the surface epithelium and a predominant more central zone of large vessels in more collagenous fibrous tissue. The lumina of the prominent large, at times somewhat tortuous, vessels are often lined by little more than an endothelial layer. Some vessels are lined by muscular walls of varying thickness. A distinguishing feature of juvenile angiofibromas is the nonuniformity of the thickness of the muscular coat of individual vessels, with thick muscular walls around an individual vessel suddenly becoming thin or virtually nonexistent (62,72), reminiscent of the normal structure of the adrenal vein (Fig. 26). Elastic fibers are lacking in the vascular walls. These features (nonuniform muscle walls and absence of elastic fibers) contribute to the marked tendency for these tumors to bleed, and biopsy or resection of an angiofibroma without good control of the vascular supply can result in severe, potentially exsanguinating hemorrhage.

The fibrous component varies in amount and in cellularity. Generally, plump fibroblasts with ample ovoid but cytologically bland nuclei are dispersed in collagenous tissue that may contain a scattering (usually not many) of inflammatory cells. The stromal cells may at times assume a stellate configuration, and these can have darker, more hyperchromatic nuclei. Occasionally, the stroma may become cellular, populated by large dark nuclei, and can superficially resemble a sarcoma; however, mitoses are generally not prominent, and the atypicality has a somewhat degenerative appearance, reminiscent of that seen in an ancient schwannoma (62).

Arterial embolization of an angiofibroma is sometimes performed before surgery to reduce operative bleeding, and this procedure frequently achieves this result. Histologically, one can see intravascular embolic material, be it gelfoam, polyvinyl alcohol, or other material, in specimens of successfully embolized cases (Fig. 27). Fibrin thrombi are often associated with this material. Such embolization rarely induces frank infarction of the richly vascular angiofibroma, however.

Juvenile angiofibroma is a distinctive-appearing lesion and usually does not present a significant differential diagnostic problem. Inflammatory polyps may occasionally be quite vascular, but they are usually more edematous and inflamed than angiofibromas. Angiofibromas do not have an epithelial glandular component, as hamartomas or inflammatory polypoid lesions may. Pyogenic granulomas do not have such large gaping vessels nor such prominent collagenous stroma; the vessels of hemangiopericytomas do not have the variable muscular walls of angiofibromas, and their stroma is much more cellular. A biopsy of a schwannoma may at times pose a troublesome differential problem, for they often have large, thick-walled vessels and a stroma of varying cellularity; however, the palisading spindled cells and Verocay bodies of the Antoni A–type areas should distinguish these tumors from angiofibromas.

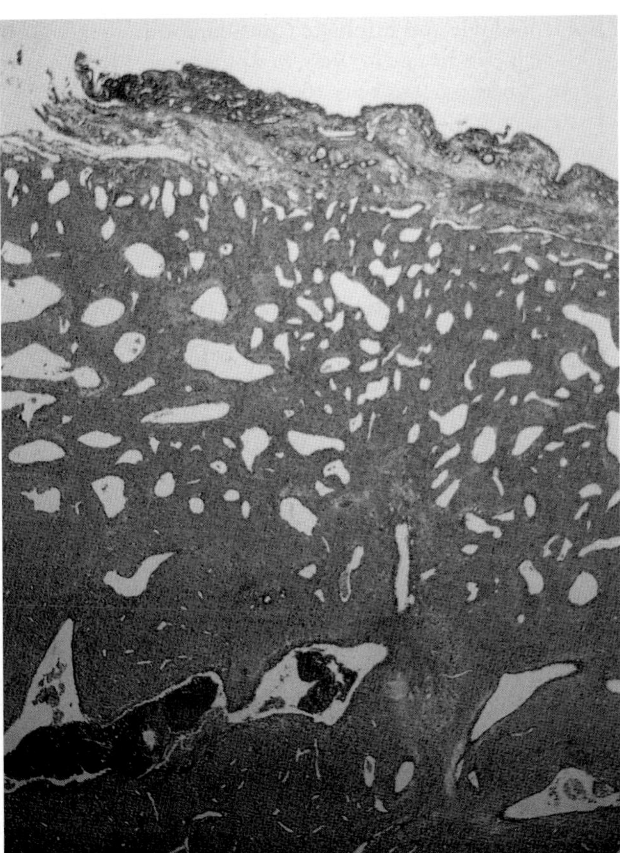

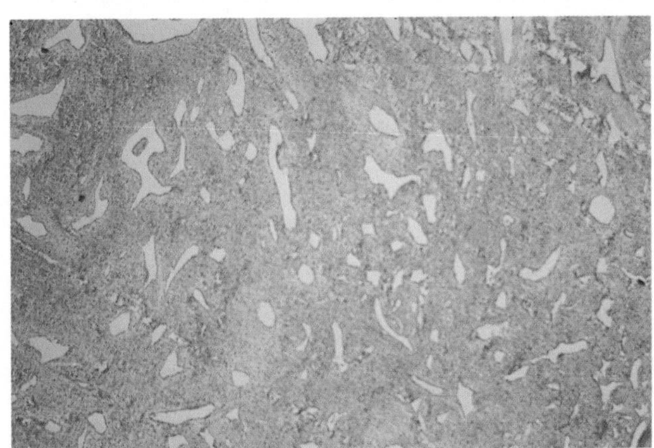

FIGURE 25. Nasopharynx: juvenile angiofibroma (JAF). **A:** A low-power photomicrograph shows numerous large and tortuous vessels disposed in fibrous tissue. **B:** A higher-power view of the prominent vessels lying in a moderately cellular fibrous tissue.

Juvenile angiofibromas are unusual tumors in that there are two types of proliferating tissue—vascular and fibrous—that are both thought to be intrinsic components of the tumor (62). It is probably most useful to view the lesion as a benign yet locally aggressive neoplasm that can invade adjacent structures and continue to enlarge but not metastasize. Reports in the earlier literature have referred to occasional spontaneous regression; however, although, interestingly, tumor regression after incomplete surgical removal has been noted, spontaneous regression without any treatment has not been observed in a large series of 120 cases (63).

Both surgery and radiation therapy have been used as therapeutic modalities (73). Most current opinion seems to favor surgery as the optimal initial therapy for most cases. Rare cases of malignant transformation of juvenile angiofibromas have been reported, almost always following irradiation therapy (74–77); a single case report in the contemporary literature of malignant transformation in a nonirradiated patient exists (78). The malig-

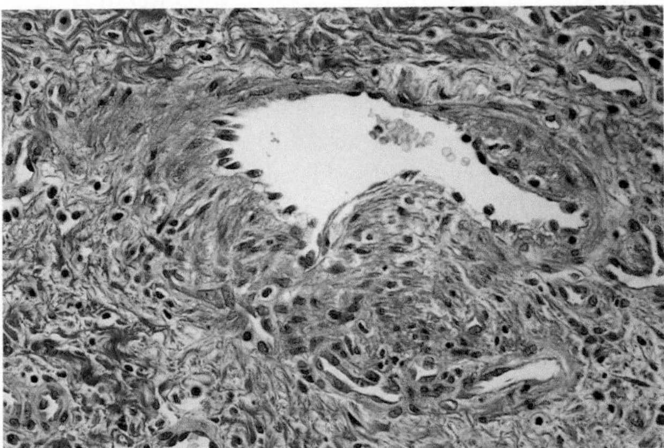

FIGURE 26. Nasopharynx: juvenile angiofibroma (JAF). The muscular wall of this large vessel varies in thickness from thick to very thin (Trichrome stain).

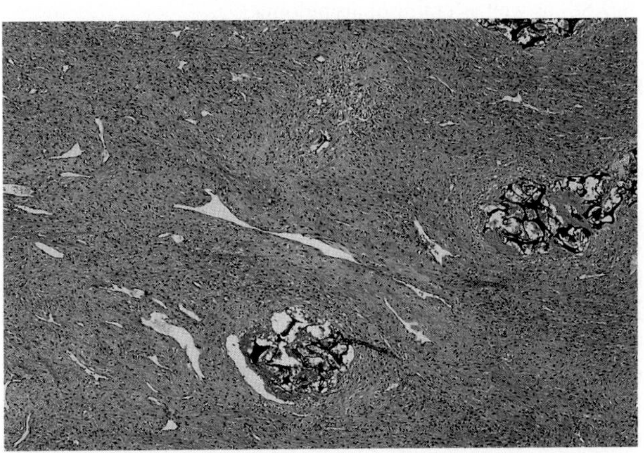

FIGURE 27. Nasopharynx: juvenile angiofibroma (JAF). Several vessels contain therapeutic gelfoam emboli.

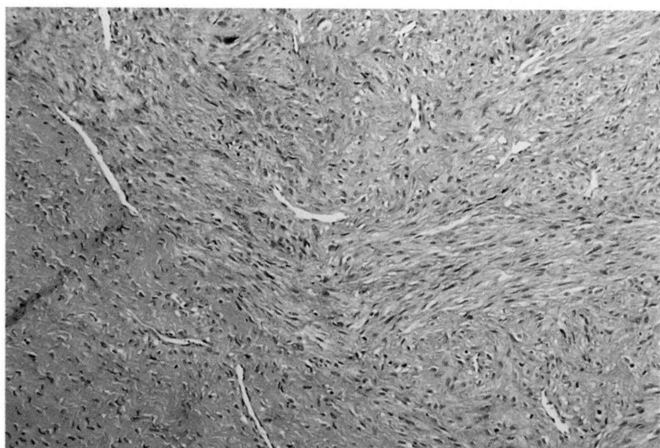

FIGURE 28. Nasopharynx: juvenile angiofibroma (JAF) with sarcomatous transformation following irradiation. The residual angiofibroma is seen at the **lower left** of the figure with the more cellular and pleomorphic sarcomatous component on the **right-hand side.** The sarcomatous region retains a vascular component to the lesion.

nant component in these cases has been the fibromatous portion, and the sarcomas resembled fibrosarcomas or, in one case, a malignant fibrous histiocytoma (76). A case in our institution in a patient (who had been irradiated) as well as that reported by Makek et al. (77) still maintained the vascular component amid the fibrosarcomatous tissue (Fig. 28). Although metastases have not been reported in these cases, the sarcoma has on occasion been fatal (74,76).

Rarities

Benign tumors that have been reported as very rarely occurring in the nasopharynx include rhabdomyoma (79,80), juvenile capillary hemangioma (81), chondroma (82), paraganglioma (83–85), and solitary fibrous tumor (see Chapter 10) (86,87). In addition, pituitary tumors may rarely involve the nasopharynx either by direct extension from the sella or as extrasellar lesions involving the nasopharynx and/or basicranium without demonstrated connection to the sella, possibly as a result of origin in the pharyngeal hypophysis or Rathke's pouch remnant (see Anatomic Considerations). These include pituitary adenoma (8,9,88) as well as crainopharyngioma (7).

Malignant Tumors

Nasopharyngeal Carcinoma

Nasopharyngeal carcinoma (NPC), although a rare tumor in the general population, has striking and characteristic epidemiologic, virologic, etiologic, and pathologic characteristics that have made it the object of great interest and intense investigation. The term NPC as used here and in most publications refers to conventional squamous cell carcinomas and to nonkeratinizing or undifferentiated carcinomas arising from the surface or tonsillar crypt epithelium of the nasopharynx, the latter group considered to be variants of squamous cell carcinoma (see below). Unless otherwise specified, NPC does not refer to the much rarer adenocarcinomas or to other malignant neoplasms arising in the nasopharynx.

Epidemiologic and Etiologic Considerations

Although NPC is rare in Western whites, generally with an incidence of between 0 to 1 per 100,000 population (89), it is much more common among Chinese in the southern portion of China, especially Guangdong province, and among Chinese in Taiwan.

The incidence of NPC in Southern Chinese has been reported as about 10 to 20 per 100,000 population in men and 5 to 10 in women (89–92). The tumor is also common among Chinese in Hong Kong and Singapore and among Alaskan, Canadian, and Greenland Eskimos (89,91,93,94). Interestingly, first-generation Chinese immigrants to other countries maintain a high incidence of NPC, but the incidence decreases among second- and third-generation Chinese in nonendemic areas, although this rate is still higher than that of whites (89,91). In most countries investigated, including China, the incidence of NPC in men is about twice that in women (89). These epidemiologic data suggest an etiologic role for both genetic and environmental factors in NPC.

The nonkeratinizing or undifferentiated forms of NPC, which account for the vast majority of tumors in Chinese and other populations with a high incidence of the disease, are intimately related to Epstein-Barr virus (EBV). Thus, certain anti-EBV antibodies, particularly the IgA antibody to viral capsid antigen (VCA) and the IgG antibody to early antigen (EA), are significantly high in NPC patients, both Chinese, Western, and Alaskan Eskimo (90,94–97). The titers are high in patients with occult primary tumors and metastatic cervical lymph nodes and tend to increase in patients with increase in tumor burden, at times even before the appearance of clinical evidence of metastases (95,97). In addition, levels of antibody-dependent cellular cytotoxicity have been correlated with prognosis in NPC patients; that is, patients with high levels tend to do better than those with low titers (98). Furthermore, EBV-encoded RNA (EBER1) has been found in NPC cells as well as in "preinvasive" nasopharyngeal epithelial cells (dysplastic cells or cells of carcinoma *in situ*) (99–101). These latter studies have also provided evidence that the malignant or premalignant epithelial cells are clonal and that the lesions arose from a single EBV-infected cell. Although it was originally thought that the differentiated or keratinizing form of nasopharyngeal squamous cell carcinoma was not associated with EBV, more recent studies utilizing molecular biological techniques have identified EBV DNA (102) and EBV-encoded RNA (EBER) (103) in differentiated nasopharyngeal carcinoma; however, EBER expression was less abundant, and EBV DNA was detected in lower copy number in differentiated than in undifferentiated NPC (102,103).

There has also been work linking NPC to certain histocompatability antigen patterns (90) and to environmental factors such as ingestion of nitrosamine-containing salted fish (89,104,105).

Clinical Data

In endemic Oriental populations, NPC occurs most commonly between the ages of 30 and 69 (91,106). Interestingly, in non-Oriental populations, including in the United States, there is a higher frequency among younger patients, mainly adolescents,

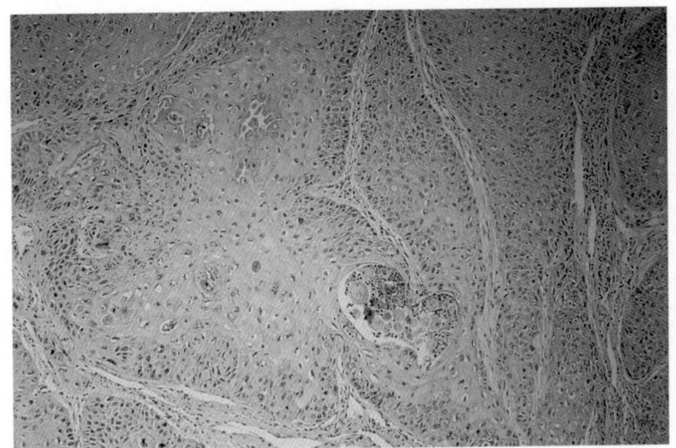

FIGURE 29. Nasopharynx: keratinizing squamous cell carcinoma. Nests of keratinizing large eosinophilic epidermoid cells infiltrate a fibrotic stroma.

so that in some areas there is a somewhat bimodal distribution of tumor incidence, with a small peak among adolescents and a large one in middle age (90,106). This more common incidence in adolescence is especially noted in African countries and among black Americans. Male patients outnumber female patients by about 2 to 1 in all patient populations.

Presenting symptoms are most commonly related to a neck mass, secondary to metastatic disease, followed in incidence by aural symptoms such as hearing loss or otitis media, especially unilateral, secondary to eustachian tube involvement (91,92,106). Thus, unilateral otitis media in an adult should arouse suspicion of a possible NPC, and NPC is a prime candidate for the primary site of a metastatic cervical carcinoma whose origin is not obvious, especially if the tumor is "undifferentiated" or a poorly differentiated squamous cell carcinoma. Nasal obstruction or bleeding may also occur, but pain or cranial nerve palsies are uncommon presenting symptoms, often indicative of advanced disease. Most NPCs are located in the lateral walls of the nasopharynx, in the area of the fossa of Rosenmüller, or in the nasopharyngeal vault. Although a large proportion of NPCs are exophytic on clinical examination (91), a significant number of tumors that have already produced nodal metastases may be difficult to visualize clinically because of their small size or deep infiltrating nature underneath normal appearing mucosa. For this reason, even if a distinct tumor is not visualized on endoscopic search for an "unknown" primary site of metastatic neck disease, random or "blind" nasopharyngeal biopsies are often taken.

Histopathology of NPC

The most prevalent form of NPC has an unusual, striking, and potentially confusing morphology that has prompted several classification schemes over the years. Since the 1970s, the World Health Organization (WHO) (107) has proposed a classification system, recently revised (108), that has been generally internationally adopted. The revised WHO classification is described here, with references to other systems and/or nomenclature when appropriate.

Squamous Cell Carcinoma (Keratinizing Squamous Cell Carcinoma)

This type of NPC is essentially identical to squamous cell carcinomas occurring elsewhere in the head and neck (see Chapter 2). It is composed of epithelial cells showing definite light microscopic evidence of squamous differentiation: the presence of extracellular keratin or intracellular keratinization and/or the presence of intercellular cytoplasmic "bridges." The better differentiated examples characteristically have cells with ample eosinophilic cytoplasm arranged in a mosaic-like pattern, often in a desmoplastic stroma (Fig. 29). Surface carcinoma *in situ* is often present. This histologically recognizable squamous differentiation must encompass most of the tumor to qualify as the squamous cell carcinoma subtype of NPC. Although squamous cell carcinoma is by far the most common type of mucosal malignancy in the head and neck area, it is the rarest type of NPC, is quite uncommon in endemic areas, and is not as strongly associated with EBV infection as other types of NPC. It corresponds to the former WHO type I category of NPC (107) (see Table 1). In 1995, three cases of basaloid-squamous carcinoma, a variant of squamous cell carcinoma, were reported in the nasopharynx in a paper from Hong Kong (109). Interestingly, all three cases were associated with EBV RNA.

Nonkeratinizing Carcinoma

The other, much more common type of NPC is the nonkeratinizing carcinoma. This is the type that is prevalent in endemic areas, is closely related to EBV infection, and has the character-

TABLE 1. HISTOLOGIC TYPES OF NASOPHARYNGEAL CARCINOMA

WHO 1978 (107)	WHO 1991 (108)	"Lymphoepithelioma"	EBV-Associated	Endemic in South China
Squamous cell carcinoma (keratinizing squamous cell carcinoma), type I	Squamous cell carcinoma (keratinizing squamous cell carcinoma)	No	Yes (less strongly expressed)	No
Nonkeratinizing carcinoma, type II	Nonkeratinizing carcinoma Differentiated	When admixed with lymphocytes	Yes	Yes
Undifferentiated carcinoma (undifferentiated carcinoma of NP type), type III	Undifferentiated (undifferentiated carcinoma of nasopharyngeal type)	When admixed with lymphocytes	Yes	Yes

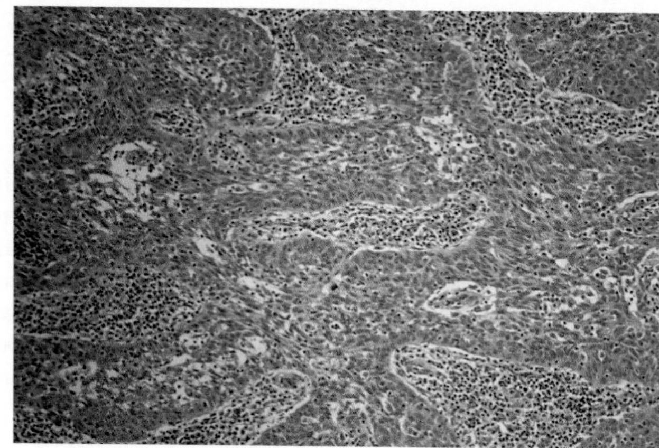

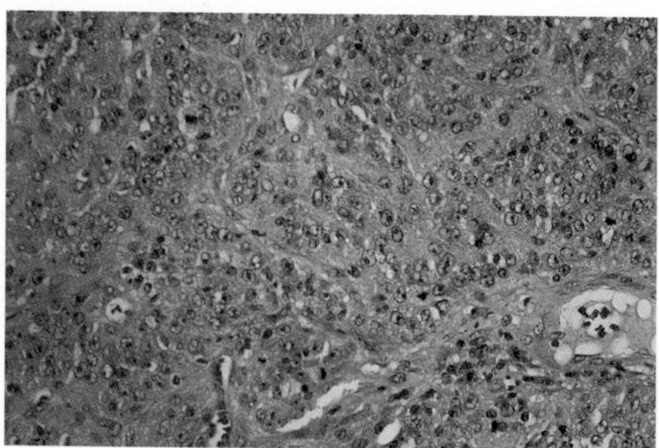

FIGURE 30. Nasopharynx: nonkeratinizing carcinoma, differentiated. **A:** A plexiform arrangement of well-defined strands or ribbons of carcinoma that does not exhibit keratinization. **B:** Nests of malignant squamoid epithelial cells in a mosaic-like arrangement but nonkeratinizing.

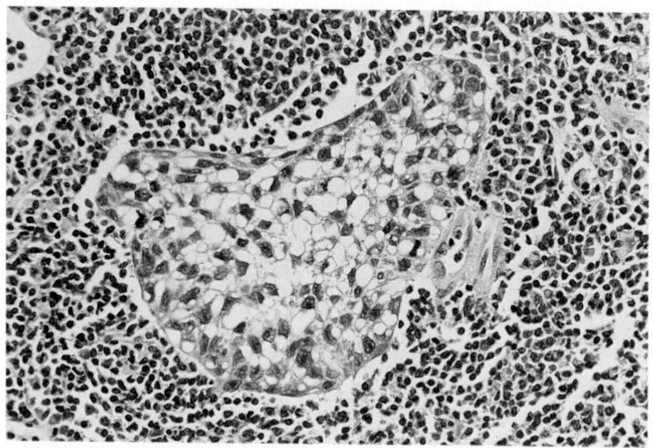

FIGURE 31. Nasopharynx: carcinoma (NPC). Rarely, nests of nasopharyngeal carcinoma can assume a clear cell pattern, as illustrated in this figure. This has been described in association with the differentiated nonkeratinizing type of NPC. In the particular case illustrated here, keratinization was present elsewhere.

istic, potentially diagnostically challenging morphology associated with NPC. Its histologic hallmark is a poorly differentiated or undifferentiated malignant appearance with very sparse or absent keratinization. Two subtypes are recognized by the WHO.

Differentiated nonkeratinizing carcinoma (NPC, nonkeratinizing, differentiated) has a recognizably epithelial pattern, often with a plexiform or ribbon-like architecture of stratified or pseudostratified cells (Fig. 30). Individual cell borders can generally be appreciated. The appearance is not unlike the "transitional-type" carcinoma of the sinonasal tract. Keratinization is very sparse or absent, and a desmoplastic stroma is generally absent or not prominent. This subtype corresponds to the former WHO type II of NPC. Rarely, one may see nests of clear cells in NPC (Fig. 31).

Undifferentiated carcinoma (NPC, nonkeratinizing, undifferentiated) is the subtype classically most closely associated with NPC. Light microscopic evidence of squamous differentiation is totally or almost completely absent. The cells are arranged in a

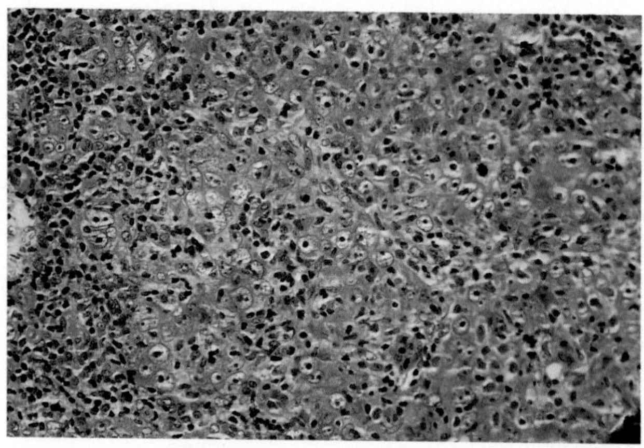

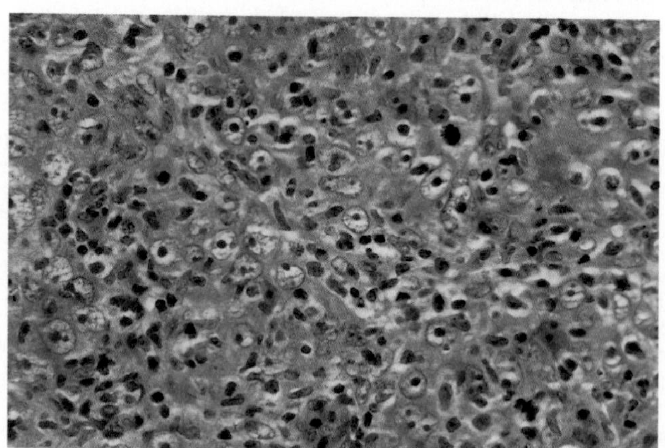

FIGURE 32. Nasopharynx: carcinoma (NPC), nonkeratinizing, undifferentiated. **A:** A large nest of malignant epithelial cells in a syncytial arrangement intimately admixed with lymphoid cells (so-called "lymphoepithelioma"). **B:** The individual carcinoma cells have vesicular nuclei with prominent central generally single nucleoli.

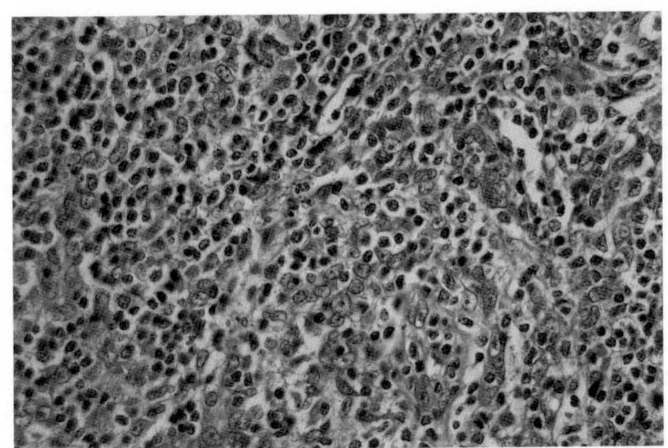

FIGURE 33. Nasopharynx: carcinoma (NPC), nonkeratinizing, undifferentiated. The malignant cells are individually dispersed in a lymphoid background, without formation of a distinct tumor cell nest (so-called Schminke pattern).

syncytial pattern, with indistinct cell borders. Nuclei are large and vesicular, and nucleoli are prominent, central, and generally solitary (Fig. 32). The tumor cells may be arranged in nests (so-called Regaud pattern) or sprinkled individually among the lymphoid cells of the nasopharynx (so-called Schmincke pattern) (Fig. 33) (100). Tumor cells may at times be fusiform or spindled (Fig. 34). A desmoplastic stromal response is generally but not universally lacking. Surface carcinoma *in situ* may not be observed. In children and adolescents especially, a significant number of eosinophils may be present (Fig. 35). This subtype corresponds to the former WHO type III of NPC. These two subtypes of nonkeratinizing carcinoma frequently are present to varying degrees in the same tumor. If one subtype predominates, it is appropriate to use its name for the tumor; if neither type clearly predominates, the more general term "nonkeratinizing carcinoma" is appropriate. Both subtypes are associated with EBV infection and are characteristically seen in endemic areas. Either subtype, but especially the undifferentiated carcinoma, can be intimately associated with lymphocytes in and among the epithelial tumor cells. This appearance is common and is historically referred to as "lymphoepithelioma." These tumor-associated lymphocytes are benign nonneoplastic accompanying or "passenger" cells. Division into Regaud and Schmincke subtypes, though of historical interest, is not considered meaningful and is currently little used.

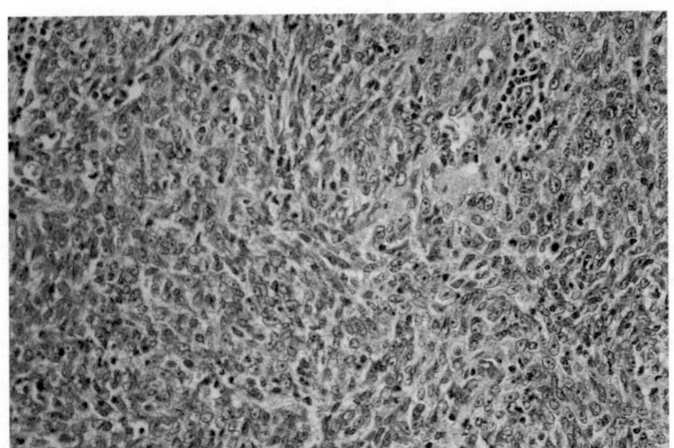

FIGURE 34. Nasopharynx: carcinoma (NPC), nonkeratinizing. The tumor cells are focally spindled.

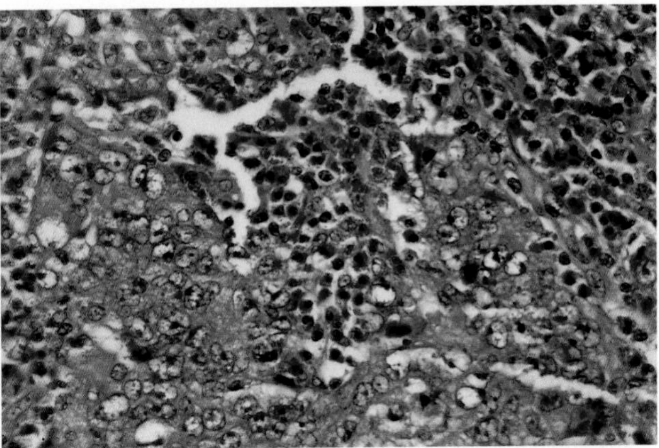

FIGURE 35. Nasopharynx: carcinoma (NPC), nonkeratinizing. The tumor in this 12-year-old patient is associated with numerous eosinophils.

NPC is said to arise from surface or tonsillar crypt epithelium and, even the undifferentiated type, is generally considered a variant of squamous cell carcinoma. Electron microscopic examinations have repeatedly shown evidence of squamous differentiation, such as the presence of desmosomes and tonofilaments (108,110,111). Interestingly, the cells of the undifferentiated lymphoepitheliomatous type of NPC have been shown to share certain characteristics with tonsillar crypt epithelium (112). This would certainly correspond to the histologic similarity of lymphoepithelial carcinoma to tonsillar crypt epithelium, which is poorly differentiated and intimately associated with lymphocytes.

The application of immunohistochemical techniques to diagnostic surgical pathology has been of great benefit in the diagnosis of NPC because this tumor is often so poorly differentiated and can simulate other neoplasms, particularly large-cell lymphoma, but also malignant melanoma and olfactory neuroblastoma. NPCs stain strongly for epithelial markers such as keratin proteins (e.g., AE1/AE3) and epithelial membrane antigen (EMA) (111,113,114). Stains for vimentin, leucocyte common antigen, S-100 protein, HMB45, and synaptophysin are negative (114).

The histomorphology of metastatic NPC in cervical lymph nodes mimics that in the primary site. Thus, the characteristic appearance of nonkeratinizing carcinoma with features of the undifferentiated or lymphoepitheliomatous type in metastatic cervical nodes where the primary site is unknown strongly suggests a nasopharyngeal origin for the tumor. An intriguing finding in some lymph nodes containing metastatic NPC is the presence of epithelioid granulomas, which may or may not be caseating, mimicking tuberculosis or sarcoidosis (115). These granulomas may be quite prominent and tend to obscure the underlying NPC, which must be diligently sought. Some metastatic NPC cells in lymph nodes may closely simulate Reed-Sternberg cells, and such nodes may contain eosinophils as well, and so Hodgkin's disease may be a differential diagnostic consideration in cases of metastatic NPC (116). The use of immunohistochemistry greatly facilitates the evaluation of such troublesome cases. In biopsies of metastatic neck nodes as well as fine needle aspiration biopsies of neck nodes harboring metastatic NPC, it has been possible to demonstrate the presence of EBV nucleic acid by polymerase chain reaction in fine needle aspirates (117) and by *in situ* hybridization in nodal biopsy specimens (118), providing a useful diagnostic tool for evaluating metastatic poorly differentiated carcinomas in cervical nodes. Recently, EBV-encoded RNA was also found in distant metastases of nonkeratinizing NPC (119) as well as in primary tumors and lymph node metastases (120).

Although the distinctive appearance of the lymphoepitheliomatous type of carcinoma is most closely associated with NPC, carcinomas at other sites may have a lymphoepitheliomatous appearance. Perhaps not surprisingly, carcinomas arising elsewhere in Waldeyer's ring, such as the palatine tonsils, may have an appearance virtually identical to that of NPC. In addition, a rare type of lymphoepitheliomatous carcinoma of the salivary glands seen especially in Eskimos of North America and Greenland (121–123) and also to a lesser extent in Southern Chinese (124) bears a striking resemblance to undifferentiated NPC. These tumors may be familial (125), and they have been shown to be associated with EBV (123,126,127) (see Chapter 8). Other sites where lymphoepithelioma-like carcinomas have been reported include the thymus, lung, stomach, urinary bladder, skin, uterine cervix, breast, and larynx (100,128,129). Interestingly, EBV genomic material has been found in lymphoepitheliomatous lung tumors in Asians but not Western patients (130–132). EBV viral DNA has also been found in a lymphoepitheliomatous thymic carcinoma in a Hispanic man (133) and in lymphoepitheliomatous gastric carcinoma, primarily in Asians (134). Interestingly, however, three lymphoepitheliomas of the palatine tonsil in white patients have been negative for EBV genomic material (130). Lymphoepitheliomatous carcinomas of the skin (135), uterine cervix, breast (136), and urinary bladder (100) have also been negative for EBV nucleic acid. Finally, EBV is not necessarily associated exclusively with those carcinomas of lymphoepitheliomatous or nasopharynx-like type, for association with EVB has been found in typical gastric adenocarcinomas (137) and in a sinonasal intestinal-type adenocarcinoma in a Chinese patient (138).

Differential Diagnosis

Keratinizing squamous cell NPC poses little differential diagnostic difficulty; however, undifferentiated NPC may be difficult to diagnose and must be differentiated from other poorly differentiated malignant round or polygonal cell neoplasms. One of the most difficult differential diagnoses can be between NPC and *diffuse large-cell lymphoma,* for which the nasopharynx is a not uncommon extranodal location. If the NPC is nested, this may be a clue to the correct diagnosis. Both lesions (especially the immunoblastic type of large-cell lymphoma) may have large vesicular nuclei with prominent single central nucleoli. Fortunately, immunohistochemistry provides an excellent means of differentiating the two diseases, with lymphomas being keratin negative and leukocyte common antigen positive and NPCs evincing the opposite staining profile. *Plasmacytomas* can be distinguished by their characteristic cytologic features of eccentric clock-faced nuclei with a perinuclear hof or clear zone. If there is doubt, immunohistochemistry will be useful, with plasmacytomas staining keratin negative and having cytoplasmic staining for monotypic immunoglobulin and often for epithelial membrane antigen (EMA).

Malignant melanomas may closely mimic undifferentiated carcinomas. Cytoplasmic melanin pigment may be sought, perhaps with the aid of its positivity with the Fontana-Masson stain, and is most helpful when found. Melanoma cells are often "plasmacytoid" with eccentric nuclei. Immunohistochemically, they are keratin negative, S-100 positive, and frequently HMB45 positive. *Olfactory neuroblastomas* may at times be poorly differentiated with little intercellular fibrillary neuropil-like material. They may occasionally be keratin positive. They will, however, almost always stain for neuroendocrine markers such as neuron-specific enolase (not in itself a particularly specific marker for neuroendocrine differentiation), chromogranin, or especially synaptophysin, and ultrastructural examination will disclose the characteristic neurosecretory-type granules.

Rhabdomyosarcomas, like NPC, may occur in the nasopharynx of adolescents. They may have spindly "strap" cells, brightly eosinophilic cytoplasm, or, rarely, distinctly visible cross striations. In difficult cases, ancillary studies again are most useful, with rhabdomyosarcomas staining keratin negative (usually), vimentin positive, and positive for muscle markers such as desmin, muscle-specific actin, or myoglobin. Electron microscopy should show the presence of the diagnostic combination of thick and thin myofilaments. *Pituitary adenomas* may involve the nasopharynx either by direct extension from the sella or by arising from pharyngeal pituitary tissue. An organoid or endocrine arrangement of the tumor cells may suggest this diagnosis, and immunohistochemical staining for pituitary hormones should provide confirmation. Ultrastructural examination will show secretory granules in these cases. In general, ultrastructural demonstration of squamous differentiation, such as the presence of tonofilaments and desmosomes, should greatly aid in differentiating undifferentiated NPC from its mimics.

Biological Behavior and Therapy

Nonkeratinizing NPC appears to be more radiosensitive than keratinizing squamous cell NPC, and patients with this type have a better prognosis (92). Thus, one series reported only 30% of patients with squamous cell NPC to survive 3 years and fewer than 20% to survive 5 years (92). The corresponding figures for patients with nonkeratinizing NPC were 70% and 59%, respectively. For all histologic types, survival after conventional radiotherapy was 60% at 3 years and 50% at 5 years (92). As may be expected, patients with disease limited to the nasopharynx fare substantially better than those with more advanced disease.

The mainstay of treatment for NPC is irradiation therapy. Recent evidence suggests that combined radiation and chemotherapy may be advantageous for patients with advanced disease. Although traditionally a nonsurgical area, recent advances in skull base surgery have allowed selected patients with cases of recalcitrant NPC to be possible candidates for surgical resection.

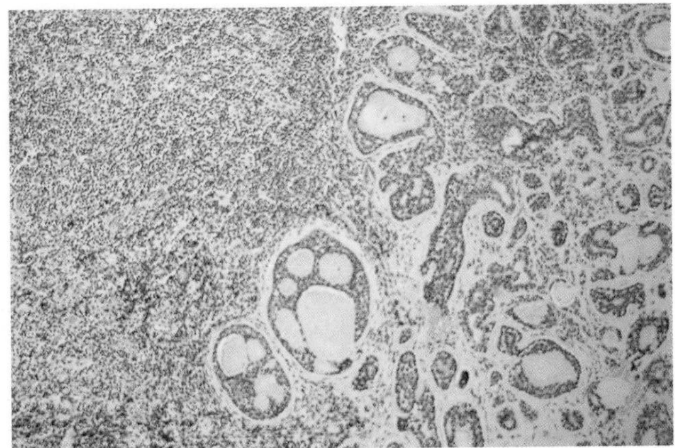
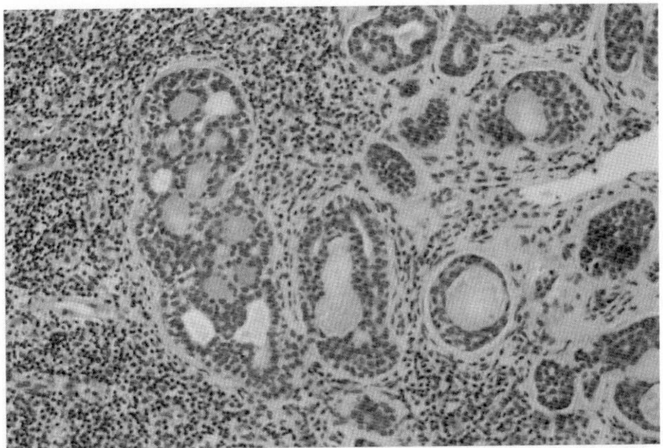

FIGURE 36. Nasopharynx: adenoid cystic carcinoma. **A:** Nasopharyngeal lymphoid tissue is on the left, and adenoid cystic carcinoma with cribriform and tubular patterns is on the right. **B:** Higher-power view of adenoid cystic carcinoma.

Adenocarcinoma

Adenocarcinomas of the nasopharynx are extremely rare lesions. They include salivary gland–type neoplasms such as adenoid cystic carcinomas and polymorphous low-grade adenocarcinoma and an adenocarcinoma of putative surface mucosal origin, nasopharyngeal papillary adenocarcinoma.

Adenoid cystic carcinomas of the nasopharynx are uncommon neoplasms, with about 38 cases reported in the literature up to 1985 (139,140). These appear to be tumors of adults, with a median age of 51 years and a range of 37 to 64 years, according to published cases with available demographic data (139). Symptoms appear insidiously and frequently include facial pain along the fifth cranial nerve distribution, epistaxis, diplopia, and hearing loss (139). The tumor may present as either a large nasopharyngeal mass or a smaller submucosal swelling. The histomorphology of these lesions is essentially identical to that of the much more common adenoid cystic carcinoma of salivary gland (Fig. 36) (see Chapter 8). The biological behavior of this tumor in the nasopharynx is also similar to that of its counterpart in the salivary glands: slow relentless local progression, high recurrence rate, and usual eventual distant metastasis (139). Because of its nasopharyngeal location, surgery is usually not a practicable therapeutic option, although it has been utilized (140). Radiation therapy often provides temporary relief of symptoms, but the long-term prognosis is grim (139).

A case of *polymorphous low-grade adenocarcinoma* apparently arising in the nasopharynx has been reported in a 44-year-old woman (141); it had a histomorphology analogous to that of its salivary gland counterpart (see Chapter 8) (Fig. 37).

An uncommon glandular nasopharyngeal neoplasm thought to arise from surface mucosal epithelium has been reported under the designation of *nasopharyngeal papillary adenocarcinoma* (142). Patients ranged in age from 22 to 64 years. The most common presenting symptom was nasal or airway obstruction. Histologically these tumors are composed of papillary and glandular patterns with an infiltrating border (Fig. 38). The tumors are cellular with little intervening stroma. Occasionally one may appreciate foamy histiocytes in papillary cores, similar to those seen in papillary renal cell carcinomas (Fig. 38D). Psammoma

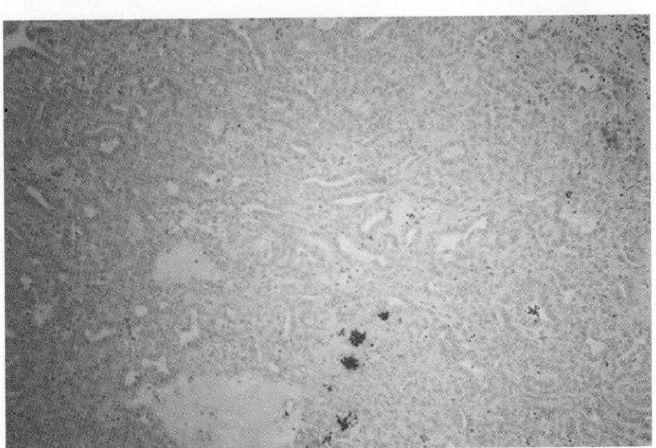
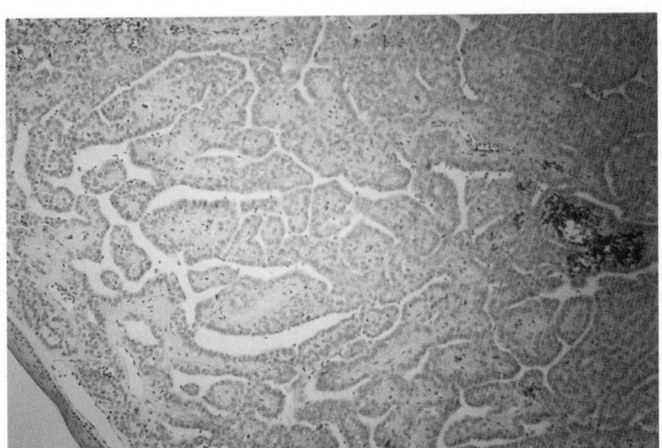

FIGURE 37. Nasopharynx: polymorphous low-grade carcinoma. **A:** Adenocarcinoma with tubular, glandular, and more solid patterns. **B:** Focal papillary architectural pattern.

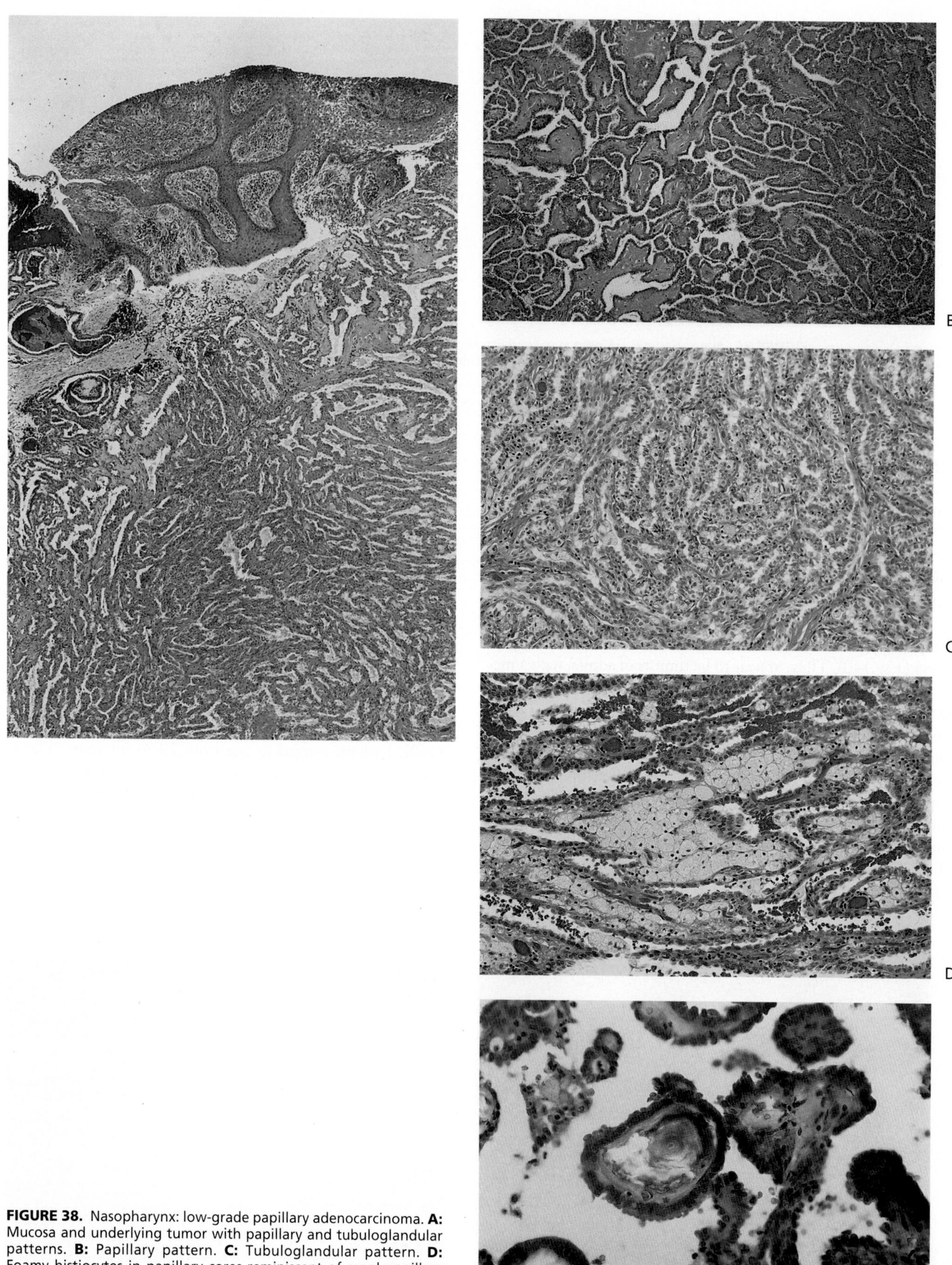

FIGURE 38. Nasopharynx: low-grade papillary adenocarcinoma. **A:** Mucosa and underlying tumor with papillary and tubuloglandular patterns. **B:** Papillary pattern. **C:** Tubuloglandular pattern. **D:** Foamy histiocytes in papillary cores reminiscent of renal papillary carcinomas. **E:** Psammoma body. Note the bland cytology. (Cases courtesy of Dr. Bruce M. Wenig.)

bodies are rarely found (Fig. 38E). Tumor cells have bland cytologic features. Nuclei are vesicular and at times somewhat clear. Mitoses and necrosis are uncommonly found (142). The clear nuclei and papillary architecture may cause confusion with papillary thyroid carcinoma, but Weing et al. (142) emphasize a transition and continuity between normal surface mucosa and neoplastic glandular epithelium, and immunohistochemical staining for thyroglobulin should resolve this differential diagnostic problem. This is a low-grade neoplasm with an excellent prognosis with only one report of a local recurrence following irradiation. Surgical therapy appears to afford excellent results, and all of the patients of Weing et al. were alive and free of disease at follow-up intervals ranging from 1 to 14 years (142). Perhaps these tumors are related to the low-grade adenocarcinomas of the sinonasal tract (see Chapter 4).

Sarcomas

Sarcomas of the nasopharynx are quite rare. Among these, the most common is probably *rhabdomyosarcoma.*

Nasopharyngeal rhabdomyosarcomas occur almost exclusively in young children. The head and neck are frequent sites of pediatric rhabdomyosarcomas, and it is estimated that about 18% of these occur in the nasopharynx (143). The most common symptom is nasal obstruction, followed by otitis media. The usual gross appearance is that of a firm smooth mass filling the nasopharynx. A botryoid or polypoid configuration is less common (143). The histologic appearance seems generally to be that of an embryonal rhabdomyosarcoma (143), as described in Chapter 10 (Fig. 39). These tumors, as do most other rhabdomyosarcomas, tend to grow rapidly and invade neighboring structures. Metastases are common, and sites include lung, bone, and occasionally lymph nodes (143). The disease, if untreated or treated with surgery alone, is virtually uniformly fatal. Fortunately, current therapy combining chemotherapy and radiation has significantly improved the prognosis of this disease.

Other primary nasopharyngeal tumors are extremely rare curiosities. *Malignant fibrous histiocytoma* (144), *malignant schwannoma* (malignant peripheral nerve sheath tumor) (145), and *ossifying fibromyxoid tumor, nonossifying variant* (146), have been reported.

Chordomas

Chordomas are malignant neoplasms derived from rests of notochordal tissue, most commonly occurring in the sacral and sphenooccipital or basicranial locations. The characteristic location for cranial chordomas is the clivus, but the proximity of the nasopharynx to this region accounts for the presence of a mass in the nasopharynx or nasal area in a substantial number of patients (147,148). The patients with nasopharyngeal involvement by chordoma reported by Richter et al. (147) presented at 11 to 69 years of age (mean 53 years). Symptoms typically related to abnormalities of cranial nerves and vision and to headaches. Masses

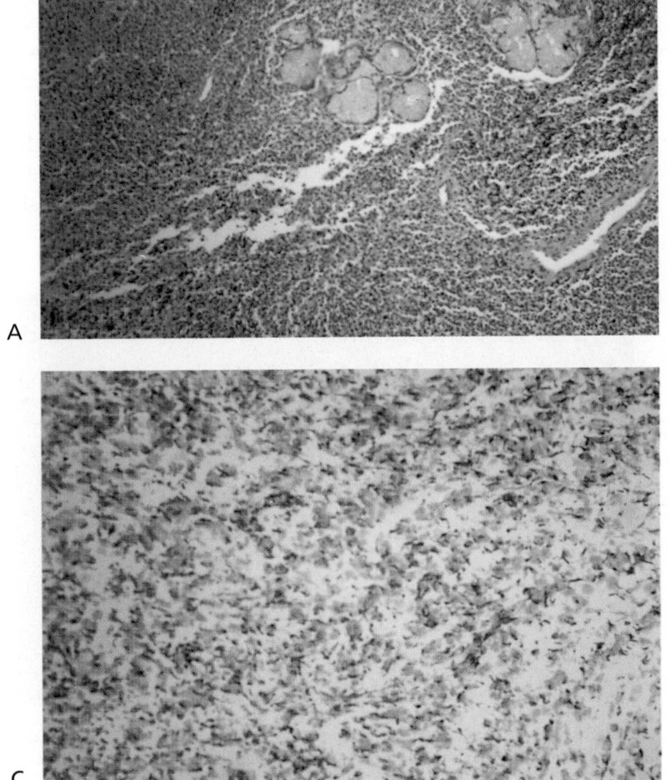

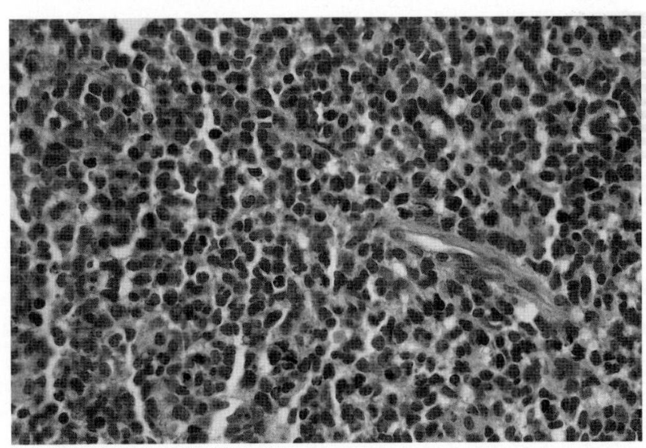

FIGURE 39. Nasopharynx: embryonal rhabdomyosarcoma. **A:** A neoplastic cellular infiltrate surrounds nasopharyngeal glands. **B:** The neoplasm is composed of small dark round cells. **C:** Immunohistochemical stain for desmin (frozen tissue) is strongly positive.

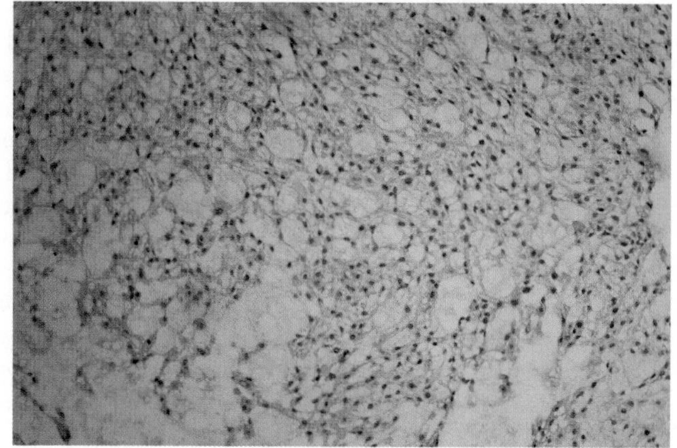

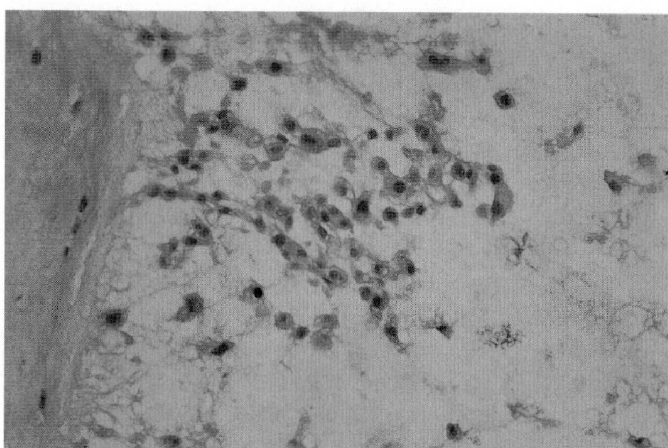

FIGURE 40. Nasopharynx: chordoma. **A:** Nests and cords of epithelial cells are disposed in a myxoid stroma. **B:** High-power view of epithelial cords.

extending into the nasopharynx from the clivus and skull base are seen radiographically. The histopathology of chordomas is described in some detail in Chapter 11. Briefly, nests and cords of plump, usually eosinophilic cells are dispersed in a myxoid, occasionally chondroid stroma (Fig. 40). Some tumor cells may evince a vacuolated, bubbly, or "physaliferous" cytoplasm, although in our experience this is often not as prominent a feature as is often stressed in the literature. The presence of a distinctive subtype of "chondroid chordoma" associated with a better prognosis than classical chordoma is somewhat controversial, but this histologic subtype is recognized in our department (149) (see Chapter 11). The previous grim prognosis of clival chordomas has been improved by the utilization of new modes of therapy, such as proton radiotherapy (150). If surgical debulking is employed as a therapeutic modality, recurrence along lines of surgical resection may occur, possibly as a result of seeding during surgical excision. These cases have tended to have a poor prognosis, in our experience.

Metastases

Metastases to the nasopharynx from primary neoplasms at other sites are extremely uncommon, with only about 17 cases reported by 1989 (151). Most have been malignant melanomas (Fig. 41), with examples of renal cell carcinoma, bronchogenic carcinoma, breast carcinomas, Wilms' tumor, and colon and cervix cancer also being reported (151). Obviously, appropriate prior history will greatly aid in making the correct diagnosis in such cases.

Extramedullary Plasmacytoma

Extramedullary plasmacytomas (EMP) are neoplasms of plasma cells that arise in the extraosseous soft tissue. Although both patients with solitary plasmacytomas of bone and those with primary EMP may progress to multiple myeloma, this association is stronger among patients with plasmacytoma of bone (152,153).

The majority of EMPs, 80% in some series, present in the head and neck (152,154,155), and the nasopharynx is a common site for such lesions (152,154). In contrast, solitary plasmacytomas of bone rarely present in the head and neck (155). Patients with nasopharyngeal plasmacytoma tend to be middle-aged to elderly men. Symptoms generally relate to the presence of a soft tissue mass or swelling, including nasal airway obstruction. Epistaxis occasionally occurs (152,153). The tumor presents on examination as a solid soft tissue mass, occasionally pedunculated, generally several centimeters in diameter.

Histologically, the tumors manifest as cellular masses composed almost exclusively of plasma cells with little intercellular stroma (Fig. 42). Some of the plasma cells may be mature, but often many are larger and less mature appearing than normal plasma cells, and atypical forms with more vesicular nuclei than normal as well as multinucleated forms may be present. Amyloid deposition may occasionally be present (52). The differential diagnosis includes nasopharyngeal carcinoma, malignant melanoma, neuroblastoma, and lymphoma. The diagnosis is greatly facilitated by the application of immunohistochemistry, as plasmacytomas will exhibit monotypic staining of intracellular immunoglobulin on paraffin sections and will not stain for keratin, neural markers, S-100 protein, or HMB45. Plasmacytomas often stain, however, for epithelial membrane

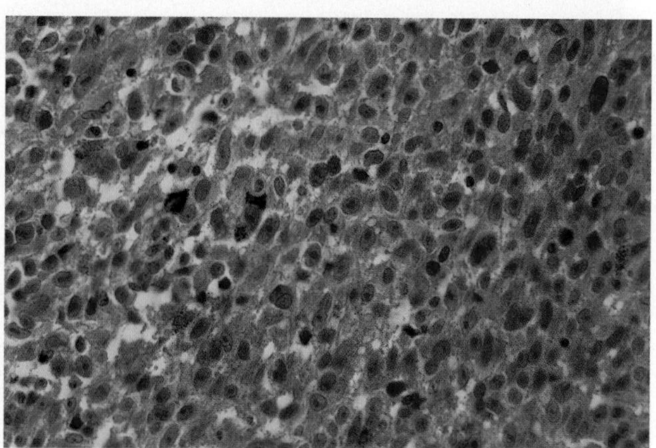

FIGURE 41. Nasopharynx: metastatic malignant melanoma. Poorly differentiated epithelioid malignant neoplasm with focal intracellular brown pigment.

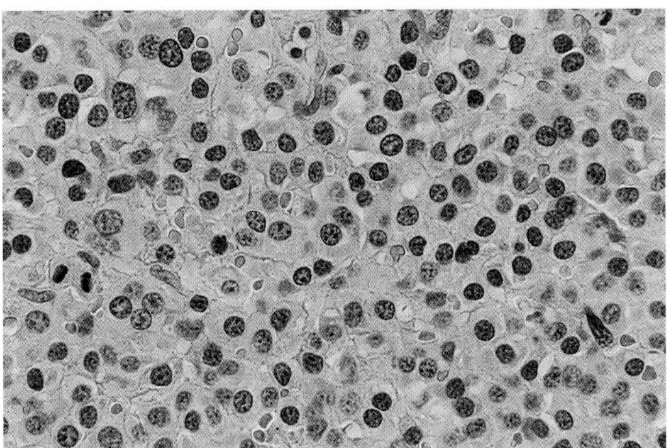

FIGURE 42. Nasopharynx: plasmacytoma. The tumor is composed of plasma cells, some larger and less mature appearing. A mitotic figure is seen on the far left.

antigen (EMA). The differential diagnosis between plasmacytomas and lymphoma with plasmacytoid differentiation is more problematic (see Chapter 12).

EMP is a malignant neoplasm, and local recurrence, spread to regional lymph nodes or other soft tissue sites, or dissemination and progression to multiple myeloma may occur. At presentation, the patient with EMP should be evaluated for the presence of other lesions or evidence of multiple myeloma (153). Patients with solitary EMP generally do not have Bence-Jones proteinuria, serum monoclonal gammopathy, or plasmacytosis of the bone marrow. Nasopharyngeal plasmacytomas are very radiosensitive lesions. Local control is generally good, although a substantial number of patients (about 30%–40%) may develop disseminated disease or multiple myeloma (152,155), and so it is recommended that patients with EMP be followed for life (153).

Malignant Lymphoma

This is more fully described in the section on Waldeyer's ring.

Rarities

Tumors that are more common elsewhere but very rarely reported in the nasopharynx include paraganglioma (83,156) and yolk sac tumors, the latter occurring alone or in association with other nasopharyngeal neoplasms (157,158).

THE TONSILS OF WALDEYER'S RING

A tonsil is a small round mound of tissue. The term is used most commonly to refer to a mound or protuberance of lymphoid tissue. Waldeyer's ring refers to a discontinuous ring of lymphoid tonsillar tissue located in the pharyngeal region, the principal components of which are the pharyngeal tonsil or adenoid (discussed with the nasopharynx), the palatine or faucial tonsils, and the lingual tonsils. There are often minor components to Waldeyer's ring, such as the tubal tonsils of the torus tubarius (see nasopharynx) and the lateral pharyngeal bands, minor structures situated in the posterolateral oropharyngeal wall, just behind the posterior tonsillar pillars (1). I have seen small tonsillar structures in the pyriform sinus area that I believe may also be part of Waldeyer's ring. These are at times biopsied when a clinically subtle lesion (e.g., an inapparent primary site for a metastatic cervical squamous cell carcinoma) is being sought. The lingual tonsils are a group of small tonsils at the base of the tongue. When used alone without a further descriptive term, tonsil generally refers to the palatine or faucial tonsils. These are bilateral lymphoid structures located in the oropharynx, between the palatoglossal fold (or anterior tonsillar pillar) and palatopharyngeal fold (or posterior tonsillar pillar).

The lymphoid tissue of the palatine tonsil (hereafter "tonsil") is intimately associated with the overlying mucosal squamous epithelium, which penetrates deeply into the tonsils, forming crypts that extend to the deepest juxtacapsular region of the tonsil. This lymphoepithelial crypt mucosa does not mature and flatten as does the typical stratified squamous mucosal epithelium of the oral cavity and thus appears different and less mature. Combined with the crypts' penetration into the tonsil, this feature may cause crypt epithelium to appear worrisome in a small biopsy specimen of tonsil, and care should be taken not to overinterpret this normal crypt epithelium as carcinoma (29). Although palatine tonsillar crypt epithelium is characteristically squamous, occasional foci of ciliated columnar epithelium may at times be seen. Aggregates of oral flora often collect in the tonsillar crypts, at times forming so-called sulfur granules, clumps of oral flora rich in *Actinomyces* and *Actinomyces*-like organisms (Fig. 43). Such a finding is innocuous if the organisms are confined to the crypt. The tonsillar lymphoid tissue contains follicles with germinal centers, as in lymph nodes. Adjacent to the palatine tonsils are mucous minor salivary glands termed Weber's glands. These are thought to be a reservoir for bacteria and provide a source for the causative organisms of peritonsillar abscesses. Hence, they are generally removed during tonsillectomy.

Occasionally one finds small foci of cartilage in the area of the fibrous capsular tissue of the tonsil, just adjacent to the lymphoid tissue (Fig. 44). Rarely, bone is found as well. The source of this

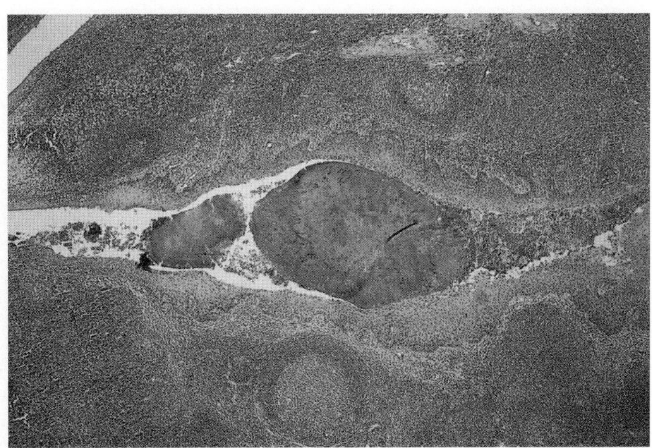

FIGURE 43. Tonsil: sulfur granules. Several nodular aggregates of matted oral flora containing *Actinomyces*-like organisms are present in a tonsillar crypt.

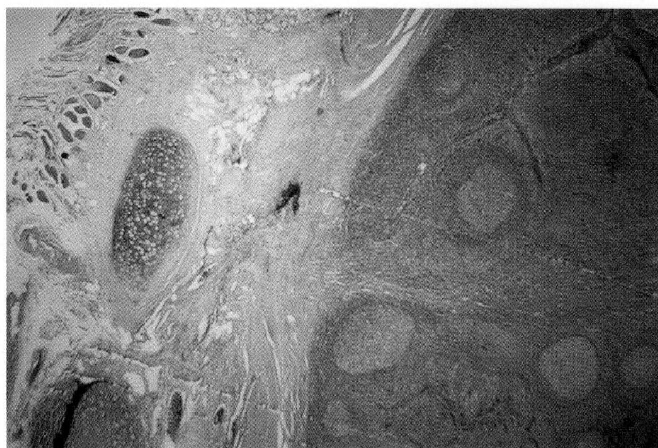
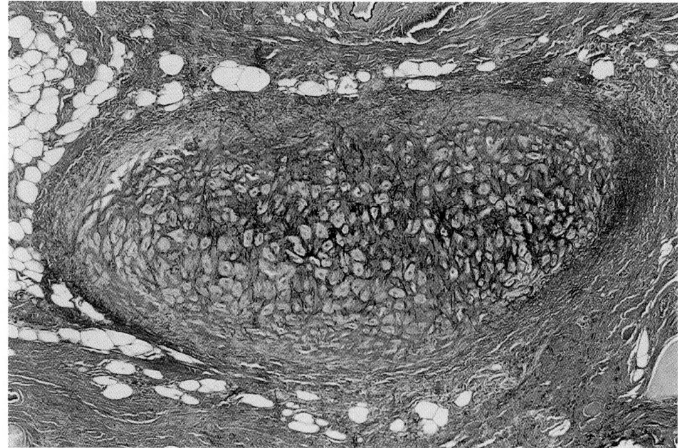

FIGURE 44. Tonsil: cartilage. **A:** Capsular location of a fragment of elastic cartilage. **B:** An elastic tissue stain demonstrates the black staining of elastic fibers in this peritonsillar cartilage fragment.

tissue is somewhat controversial. A popular notion is that such cartilage and/or bone represents metaplasia secondary to previous bouts of tonsillitis (29,159). An argument that has been offered in support of this hypothesis is that such cartilage or bony tissue is seen more frequently in adult tonsillectomy specimens (159). In my experience, however, such cartilaginous foci are always found in the same location (fibrous tissue adjacent to lymphoid tissue) and are always composed of elastic cartilage as opposed to hyaline cartilage (Fig. 44B). Elastic cartilage was also found in all of 15 operated cases of cervical chondrocutaneous branchial remnants, as described by Atlan et al., and was thought most probably to arise from the second branchial arch (160). The tonsil originates from the corresponding second branchial pouch. Thus, I favor the alternative theory that such tissue represents embryologic branchial arch remnants (29).

Tonsillitis

Tonsillitis is one of the most common afflictions of children and young adults. "Sore throat," tonsillitis, or enlarged tonsils have prompted innumerable visits to the doctor. Tonsillectomy is one of the most common surgical procedures, and before the establishment of definite guidelines and stringent indications for tonsillectomy, the procedure was even more widespread, and it was indeed uncommon to come across an individual in a non–medically deprived region of the United States who had not had his or her tonsils out.

Actually, most cases of tonsillitis are viral and largely innocuous. More serious are repeated bouts of tonsillitis caused by group A β-hemolytic streptococci, which raise the threat of the development of poststreptococcal glomerulonephritis or rheumatic fever. Also of concern is the development of peritonsillar abscess (Fig. 45), which may lead to infection of the deep spaces of the neck or, by direct extension, to mediastinitis. Although this complication is much less common in the current antibiotic era than previously, it still can be fraught with danger. Such occurrences of peritonsillar abscess, repeated streptococcal infections, and hyperplasia of the lymphoid tissue of Waldeyer's ring sufficient to induce significant respiratory obstruction are currently the principal indications for tonsillectomy.

A 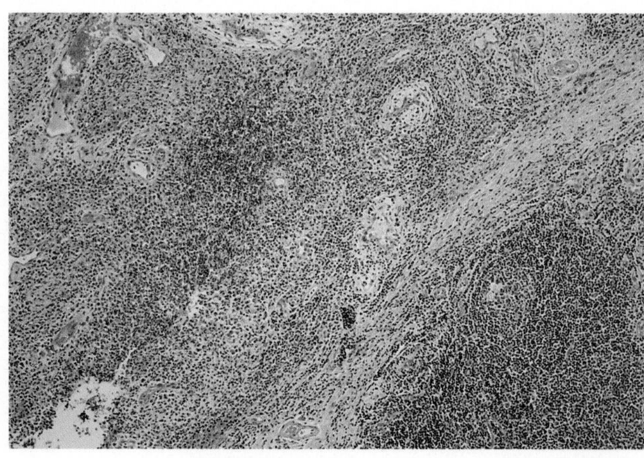
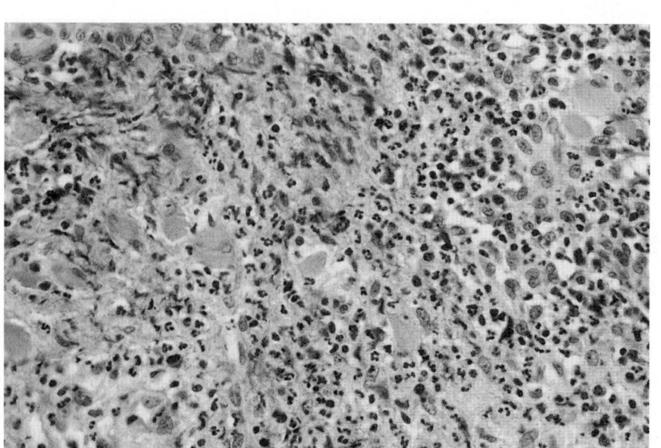 B

FIGURE 45. Peritonsillar abscess. **A:** A phlegmonous inflammatory mass is present in peritonsillar tissue, at the left of the figure. The tonsil is at the lower right. **B:** Acute cellulitis of peritonsillar skeletal muscle.

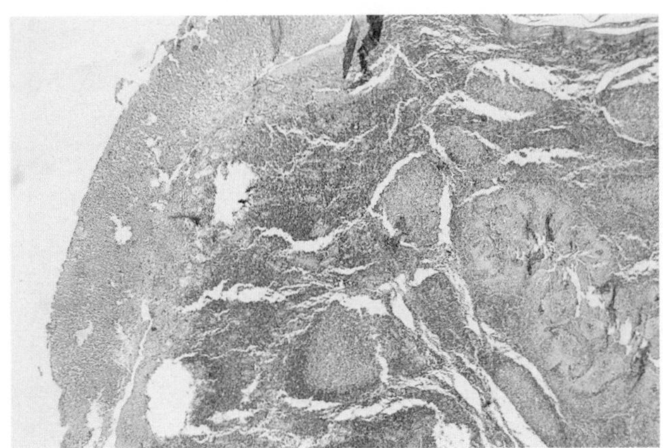

FIGURE 46. Tonsil: diphtheria. The fibrinous diphtheritic membrane at the left of the figure directly overlies tonsillar lymphoid tissue. There is no surface mucosal epithelium in this area.

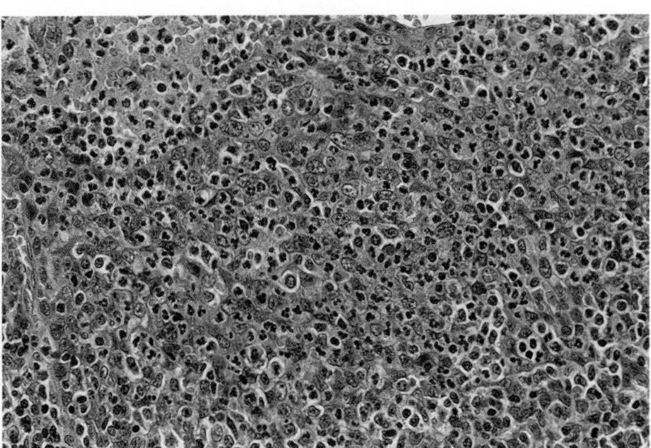

FIGURE 47. Acute tonsillitis. A neutrophilic inflammatory infiltrate is present in tonsillar epithelium.

Gross Appearance

Hyperplastic tonsils can become quite large, especially in the proportionately smaller throats of children, even to the point of touching each other in the midline ("kissing" tonsils). When acutely inflamed, they may appear erythematous, and streptococcal infection may induce a punctate purulent tonsillar exudate to appear. Infectious mononucleosis can lead to a white membrane forming on the tonsillar surface. When this is peeled off the patient's tonsils, the generally intact underlying mucosa will be exposed, and bleeding should not occur. This is in contrast to the tonsillar membrane of diphtheria (fortunately very seldom seen today), which often causes an ulcerative tonsillar surface. The diphtheritic membrane lies adjacent to granulation tissue, thus prompting bleeding when it is clinically stripped off the tonsil (Fig. 46). Occasionally in the normal or diseased tonsil, one can appreciate a small dot of yellowish or white material at the mouth of the tonsillar crypt. This is a small sulfur granule, a matted mass of oral flora usually containing a prominent component of *Actinomyces*-like organisms, not uncommonly encountered in the tonsils.

Histologic Features

Tonsils are seldom surgically excised during active bouts of acute tonsillitis, except for the occasional "quinsy" tonsillectomy performed for an acute peritonsillar abscess. Specimens of acute tonsillitis will frequently contain hyperplastic germinal centers (often markedly hyperplastic in children) and an acute cryptitis, with collections of neutrophils in crypts and infiltrating crypt epithelium (Fig. 47).

Chronic tonsillitis, despite its frequent occurrence, is a rather ill-defined pathologic entity. Tonsils removed for chronic tonsillitis have lymphoid germinal centers with reactive hyperplasia. Such germinal centers may be quite large (especially in children). There will often be fibrosis in the tonsil, with increased prominence of tonsillar fibrous bands, especially in adults with recurring bouts of tonsillitis (Fig. 48). Skeletal muscle of the pharyngeal wall is often pulled up into the tonsil proper, probably as a result of repeated scarring from previous infections. Neutrophils may or may not accumulate in crypts, and a plasmacytic infiltrate may involve crypt epithelium. Frequently the crypt epithelium will be thrown up into small papillary folds, assuming a papillomatous appearance in cases of chronic tonsillitis.

Tonsillectomy specimens will often include minor salivary gland tissue (so-called Weber's gland, a putative reservoir for pathologic bacteria). In cases of peritonsillar cellulitis or abscess, the peritonsillar skeletal muscle is chronically inflamed, often with fibrosis, granulation tissue, and histiocytic infiltration. A neutrophilic infiltrate may be present in more acute cases, at times with frank abscess formation.

One may occasionally encounter examples of follicle lysis (i.e., ingrowth of mantle zone lymphocytes into germinal centers, partially subdividing them) in reactive tonsils. Although this finding is described in association with human immunodeficiency virus (HIV)-related lymphadenopathy, it is by no means specific, and, in and of itself, should not arouse a suspicion of HIV infection. The changes in tonsils and adenoids that are associated with HIV infection have recently been described (161,162) and reflect those encountered in cases of

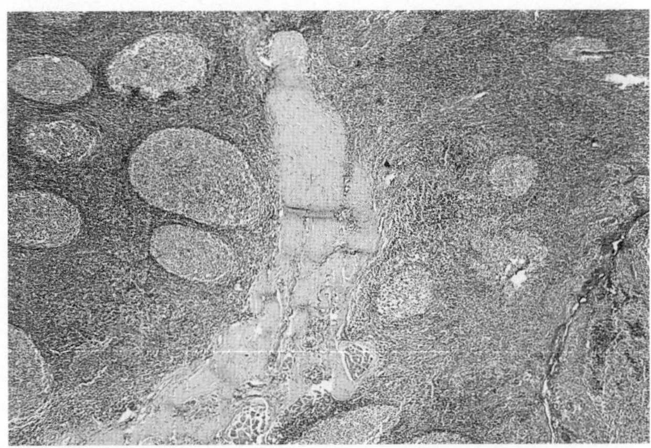

FIGURE 48. Chronic tonsillitis. There is follicular lymphoid hyperplasia and a thickened band of fibrosis.

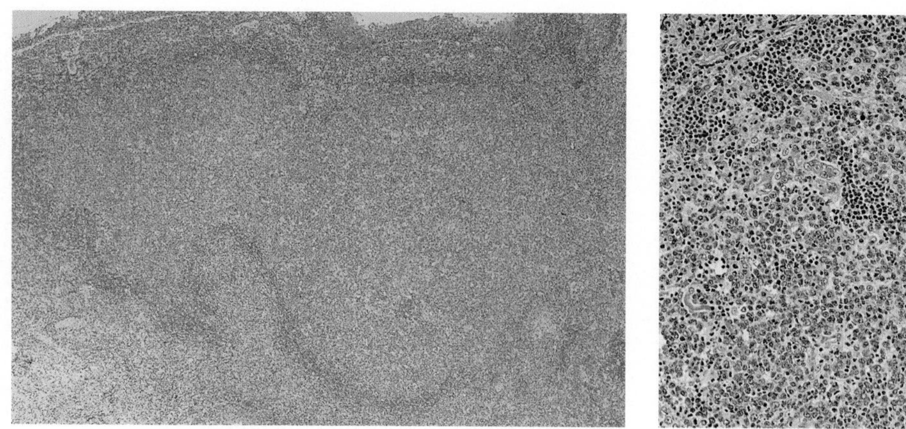

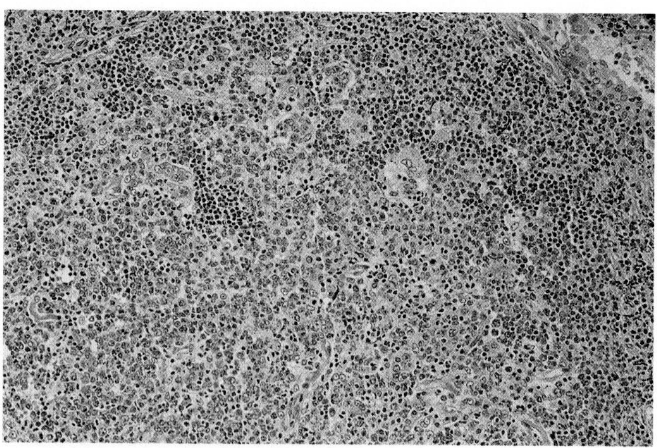

FIGURE 49. Nasopharynx: HIV-positive patient. **A:** A very large hyperplastic germinal center is surrounded by an attenuated mantle zone. **B:** Follicle lysis, with small lymphocytes infiltrating into and "breaking up" a germinal center.

HIV-associated persistent generalized lymphadenopathy: marked follicular hyperplasia, mantle zone depletion, and follicle lysis (Fig. 49). At times marked involution of follicles may occur associated with interfollicular proliferation of immunoblast-like cells (Fig. 50). Weing et al. (161) describe the presence of multinucleated giant cells as a prominent HIV-associated finding; although I have occasionally encountered the presence of rare multinucleated histiocytic giant cells adjacent to tonsillar crypts in patients without known HIV infection, possibly representing a foreign body–type reaction to material extravasated from crypts, the giant cells associated with HIV infection are more prominent (Fig. 51).

The tonsils in cases of infectious mononucleosis (IM) often show proliferation of atypical-appearing enlarged immunoblastic cells, at times in sheets, as well as cells that may strikingly resemble Reed-Sternberg cells (28). These findings may simu-

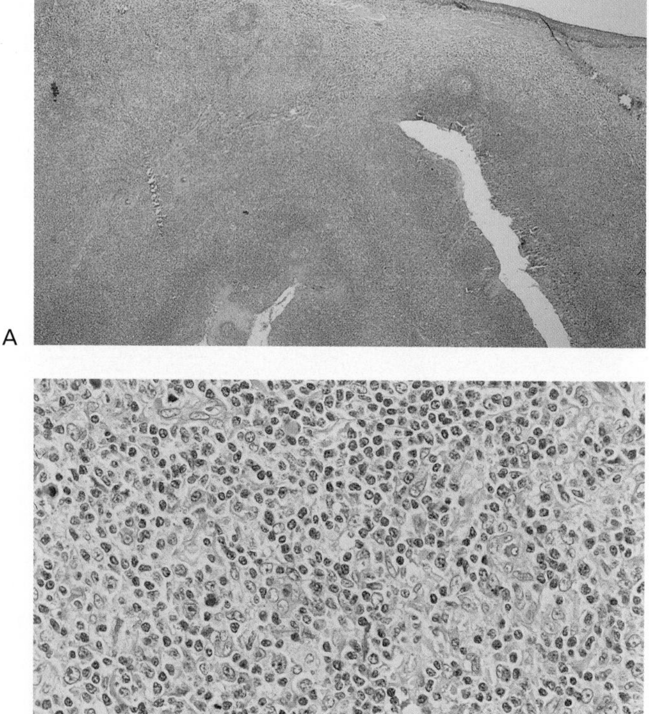

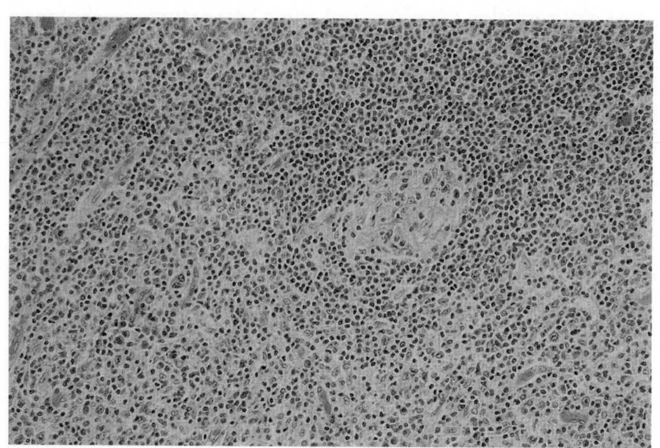

FIGURE 50. Tonsil: HIV-positive patient. **A:** There is diffuse interfollicular lymphoid hyperplasia, but the follicles are involuted. **B:** An involuted follicle. **C:** Interfollicular proliferation of large immunoblastic cells.

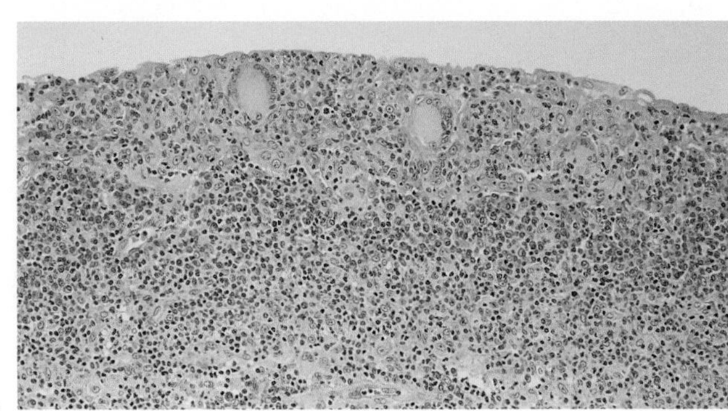

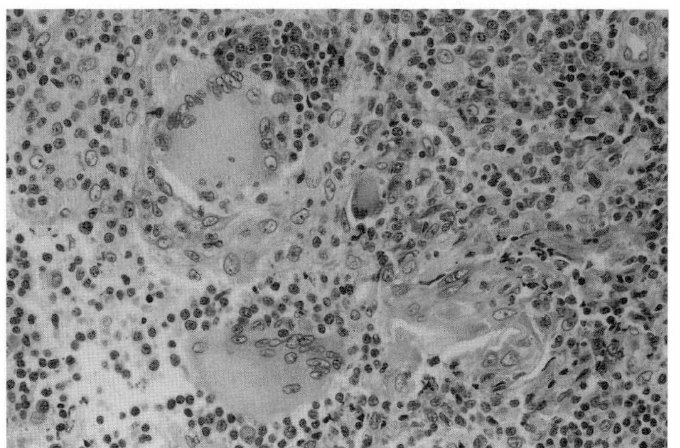

FIGURE 51. Nasopharynx: HIV-positive patient. **A:** Several multinucleated histiocytic giant cells are present in the epithelium. **B:** Higher-power view of giant cells.

late Hodgkin's or non-Hodgkin's lymphoma. Hodgkin's disease rarely occurs in the tonsils (see below), and recognizing the reactive background cells of IM rather than the cellular background characteristic of Hodgkin's disease may help in this distinction (28). The presence of recognizable reactive germinal centers, a "mottled" paracortical lymphoid expansion seen in IM, and the presence of a reticulum architecture of the tonsil that is intact helps to separate IM from Hodgkin's lymphoma (28,31).

Occasionally noncaseating granulomas have been noted in tonsils removed for tonsillitis (163,164) (Fig. 52). The tonsil may be involved in sarcoidosis, albeit uncommonly (165,166). Also, involvement of the tonsils in tuberculosis is now encountered only very rarely (159). In my experience, such tonsillar noncaseating granulomas are usually seen in germinal centers. Some may possibly represent follicular histiocytes acquiring the appearance of epithelioid histiocytes. At any rate, the presence of such granulomas, if isolated in the tonsils, has generally proven to be an innocuous finding (164).

Nonneoplastic Masses

Small cystic lesions are often encountered in tonsils, often in the base of the tongue in the area of the lingual tonsils. These consist of small cystic spaces lined by squamous epithelium containing keratinous or amorphous debris, characteristically surrounded intimately by benign lymphoid tissue, often with one or more germinal centers. These are for the most part innocuous lesions, termed *lymphoepithelial cysts* (Fig. 53); some may represent cystic dilation of lingual tonsillar crypts.

Lymphangiomatous tonsillar polyps (*lymphangiectatic fibrous polyps*) are rare polypoid masses, generally arising from a pedicle attached to the tonsil and projecting into the oropharynx (29,167–169). They are found incidentally on examination or present with symptoms of the presence of a mass or sensation of a foreign body; occasionally such a polyp may be partially swallowed (167). These lesions have been reported in adults and children. They are lined by squamous epithelium and consist of fibrous tissue, variably loose or more dense, usually containing

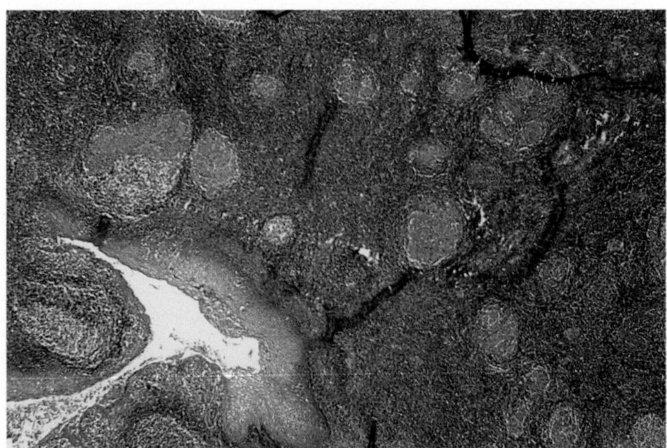

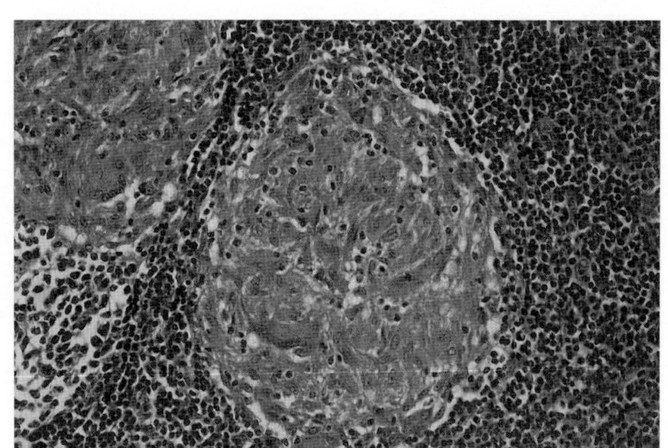

FIGURE 52. Tonsil: granulomas. **A:** Multiple granulomatous structures are present in the tonsil; most appear located in germinal centers. **B:** Higher-power view of a tonsillar sarcoid-like noncaseating granuloma.

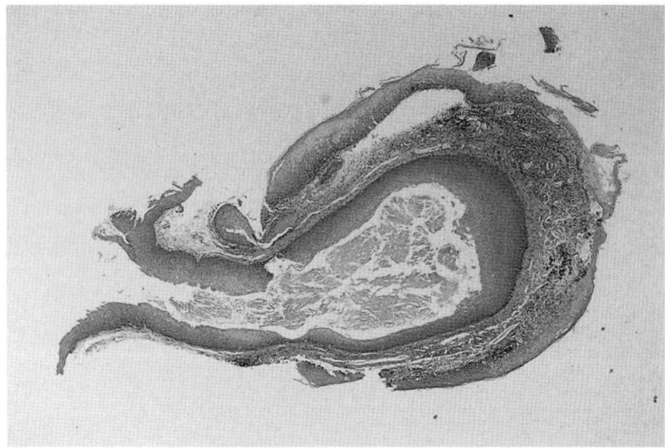
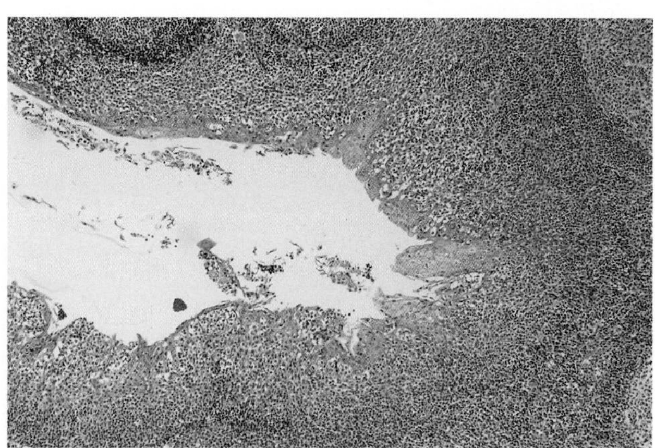

FIGURE 53. Vallecula: lymphoepithelial cyst. **A:** A small squamous-lined cyst containing amorphous-appearing debris is surrounded by lymphocytes. **B:** A cystically dilated lingual tonsillar crypt.

dilated lymphatic channels and a variable component of lymphoid tissue (Fig. 54). Depending on the relative amount of their constituent parts, they have been termed lymphangiectatic fibrous polyps (167), lymphangiomatous polyps (29,169), or fibrous polyps (29). These are benign lesions generally assumed to be hamartomatous in nature. A possible pathogenesis may involve inflammatory obstruction to lymphatic channels leading to lymphangiectasia and edema (167).

An extremely rare possibly related lesion has been reported by Carillo-Farga et al. (170) as lymphoid papillary hyperplasia of the tonsils. In this case, both tonsils of a 9-year-old girl were enlarged by multiple small to medium-sized polypoid protrusions consisting of a squamous epithelial mucosa overlying benign hyperplastic lymphoid tissue.

Dermoids or *hairy polyps* of the pharynx occur most commonly in the nasopharynx (see above), but a few have been reported in the oropharynx attached to or near the tonsil (21,24a,171). These occur in neonates or infants, are generally attached to the tonsil or pharynx by a pedicle, and may cause respiratory or feeding difficulties, possibly of potentially life-threatening seriousness. As in the nasopharynx, they are generally oblong or sausage-shaped, although one report describes an oropharyngeal lesion bearing a striking similarity to an auricle (24a). They are polypoid masses lined by skin containing hair and appendages with a fatty core, often containing a cartilage plate as well as skeletal muscle and neurovascular structures, corresponding to their nasopharyngeal counterparts. The striking auricle-like example lends credence to the hypothesis that these lesions may represent a proliferative anomaly of the first and/or second branchial apparatus.

Other nonneoplastic tumorous masses of the tonsil are occasionally encountered as rarities or isolated cases. Localized deposits of amyloid are rare in Waldeyer's ring. They occasionally occur in the nasopharynx (see above), and exceptional cases are reported to involve the tonsils (172,173) or the tissues of Waldeyer's ring in general, including the tonsil, nasopharynx, and base of tongue (174). Interestingly, a tonsillar amyloidoma described by Amado et al. (173) was associated with a monotypic (IgG-κ) population of plasma cells. An exceptional case of *malakoplakia,* an unusual histiocytic reaction to infection, usually to *Escherchia coli* and usually occurring in the urinary tract, has been reported as presenting as a tumorous mass

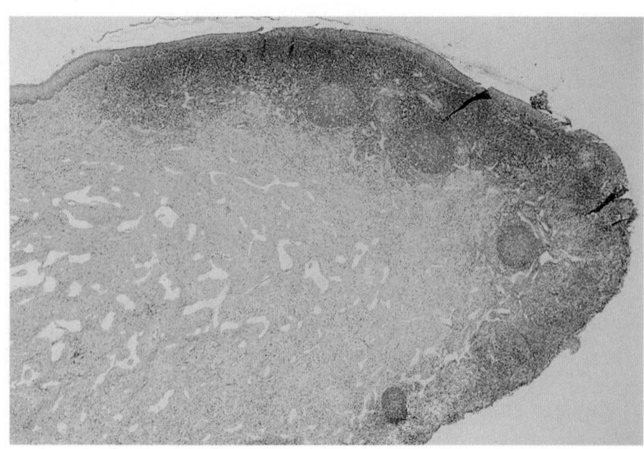
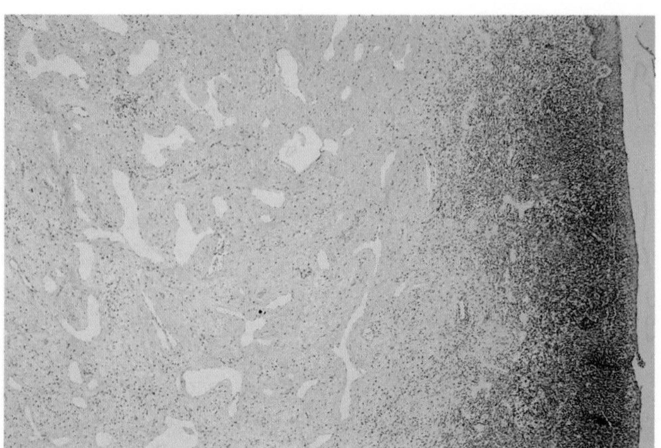

FIGURE 54. Tonsil: lymphangiectatic fibrous polyp. A polypoid protrusion from the tonsil has a core of fibrous tissue with multiple dilated lymphatics with peripheral lymphoid tissue. **A:** Low power. **B:** Higher power.

of the tonsil (175). A case of so-called *"inflammatory pseudotumor"* of the tonsil has been reported (176), analogous to similar lesions occurring in other sites (e.g., lung and orbit), composed of an inflammatory infiltrate rich in plasma cells with focal fibrosis. Interestingly, this patient had a history of retroperitoneal fibrosis, adding some support to the theory that such plasma cell–containing fibrosing lesions occurring in various locations (e.g., Riedel's struma of the thyroid, sclerosing mediastinitis, inflammatory orbital pseudotumor, and sclerosing cholangitis) may be related (177). The term *multifocal idiopathic fibrosclerosis* has been suggested for these related conditions (178).

Neoplasms: Benign

Squamous papillomas represent 75% of the benign tonsillar masses collected in the Armed Forces Institute of Pathology (AFIP) Otolaryngic Pathology Registry from 1945 to 1976 (179). They are usually small innocuous papillary mucosal lesions occurring mainly in the tonsillar area but occasionally on the uvula or soft palate. Rarely, larger tonsillar squamous papillomas, up to several centimeters in size, may be encountered *(unpublished observation).* They are usually discovered incidentally or, if palatal, may produce an unpleasant sensation in the throat.

Histologically, tonsillar squamous papillomas are composed of well-differentiated benign-appearing squamous epithelial papillae on thin fibrovascular stalks (Fig. 55A). Invasion below the level of the mucosa as seen in verrucous carcinoma does not occur. The vast majority of such lesions do not manifest the viral-associated koilocytotic changes of human papillomavirus (HPV)-associated laryngeal papillomas (Fig. 55B). They are generally easily differentiated from papillary squamous cell carcinomas by their cytologic blandness and lack of invasive properties (29).

Rarely, a lesion with koilocytotic change suggestive of HPV infection occurs, at times in association with papillomas in other locations in the head and neck *(unpublished observations)* (Fig. 56).

Neoplasms: Malignant

Squamous Cell Carcinoma

Epidemiologic and Clinical Data

Cancer of the pharynx, including the tonsil and base of tongue, is less common than that of the oral cavity, occurring only about one third as often (180). In 1998, 8,600 new cancers of the pharynx were estimated to have occurred in the United States (180). Squamous cell carcinoma is by far the most common malignant neoplasm of the tonsil and base of tongue. This tumor type comprises about three fourths of the malignant neoplasms of the tonsil collected in the AFIP Otolaryngic Pathology Registry from 1945 to 1976 (179). The disease is more common (about three times greater incidence) in men than in women (180) and occurs most frequently in patients older than 45 years (181). As with most squamous cell carcinomas in the head and neck, there is a strong association with smoking and alcohol abuse, with alcohol being particularly associated with oropharyngeal cancer as compared with cancer of other sites in the head and neck (181). The most common presenting symptom is pain in the throat, with otalgia, a foreign body sensation, or bleeding also reported (180,181). Enlarged cervical lymph nodes are often present when the disease is diagnosed, probably related both to the rich lymphatics in Waldeyer's ring as well as to the generally relatively late presentation of the disease, the base of tongue in particular being a rather difficult site to examine clinically. The jugulodigastric nodes are most commonly affected, and lesions of the tongue base not uncommonly metastasize to bilateral cervical nodes. When tonsillar carcinomas progress and invade the parapharyngeal space, they may cause trismus via involvement of the pterygoid muscles and, with deeper invasion to the carotid sheath region, may extend superiorly to the skull base or inferiorly to the mediastinum (181).

The tumor may be seen clinically as an ulcerated mass with raised edges. Larger tumors may be fungating and exophytic; alternatively, tonsillar cancers may be deeply penetrating ulceroinfiltrative lesions with but a small surface component. Carcinomas arising deep in tonsillar crypts may be notoriously difficult to identify clinically, and tonsillar (both faucial and lingual) cancers may present as an enlarged neck node with an "un-

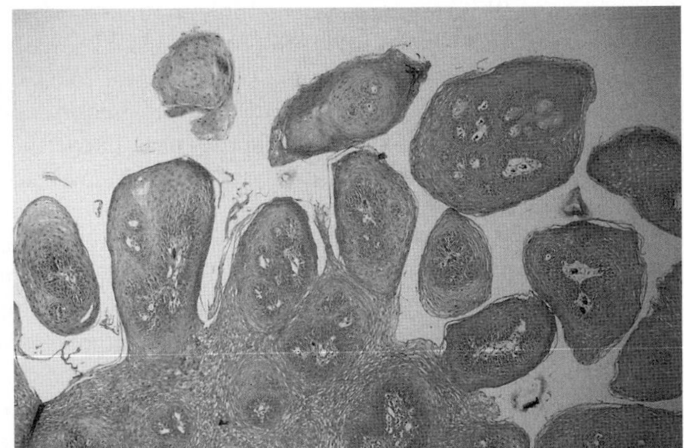
A

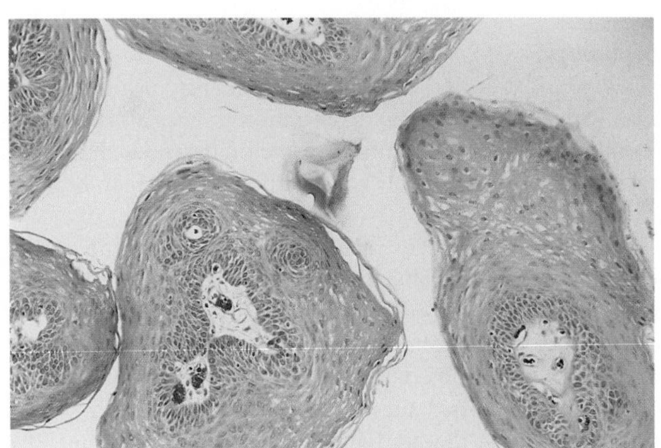
B

FIGURE 55. Tonsil: squamous papilloma. **A:** Squamous epithelium lines fibrovascular papillary cores. **B:** Absence of viral-associated koilocytosis.

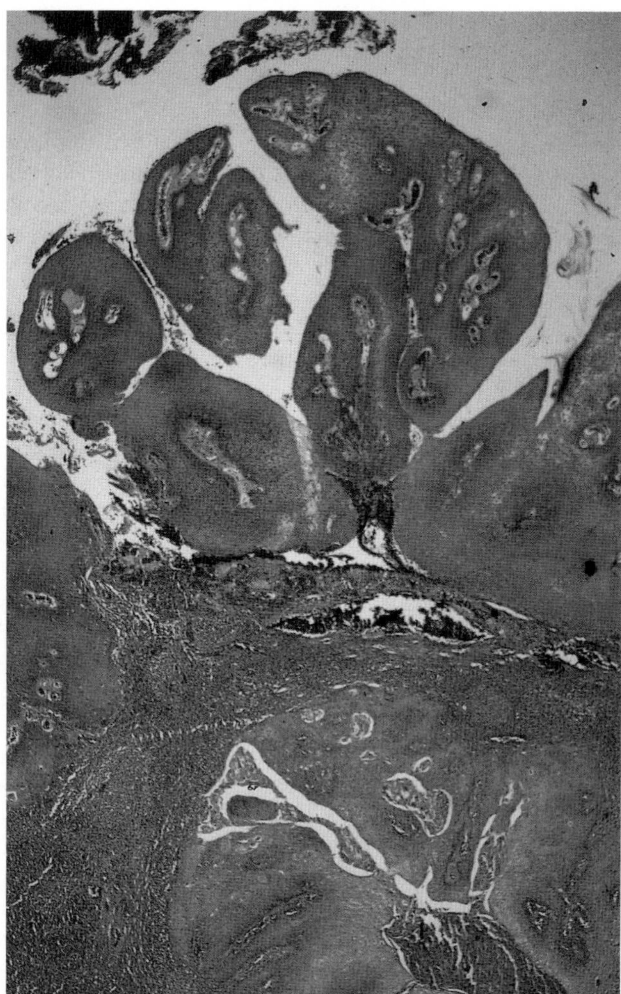

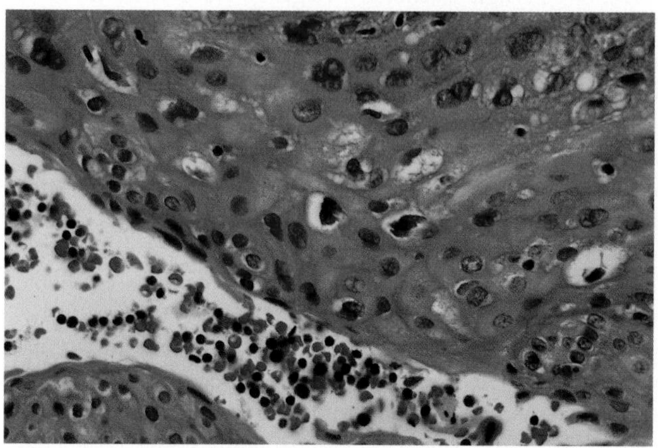

FIGURE 56. Tonsil: large squamous papilloma. **A:** The papilloma is present on the surface and appears to be involving crypt epithelium. **B:** Koilocytosis with hyperchromatic wrinkled nuclei surrounded by perinuclear cytoplasmic clearing. Several multinucleated epithelial cells can be seen.

known" primary site (Fig. 57). Because cervical nodal metastases of head and neck squamous cell carcinomas are often cystic, they may erroneously simulate the excruciatingly rare entity of primary branchial cleft carcinoma (182). The tonsil may be a primary site for these metastatic nodes with undiscovered primaries (along with the base of tongue, pyriform sinus, and nasopharynx) and should be thoroughly evaluated in such cases (29).

Morphology

Grossly, tonsillar cancers are generally firm, gritty, whitish solid masses with occasional cystic degeneration or necrosis that may be exophytic or ulceroinfiltrative. Less well-differentiated tumors with less keratin production and sclerotic stroma may be less hard and gritty appearing.

Histologically, most squamous cell carcinomas of the tonsil and base of tongue resemble those in other head and neck locations (see Chapter 2). In general, the majority of them tend to be moderately or poorly differentiated rather than well differentiated (179,181) (Fig. 58). The bases of tongue and tonsil are the most common reported sites of occurrence of basaloid–squamous carcinoma in the head and neck (183) (see Chapter 7). Nonkeratinizing carcinoma of the "transitional" (179) or "sinonasal type" (see Chapter 4) is another poorly differentiated variant of squamous cell carcinoma seen in the tonsillar region. Undifferentiated or lymphoepithelial carcinoma of nasopharyngeal type also occurs in the oropharyngeal region, although much more rarely than in the nasopharynx (see above) (184). Despite the morphologic similarity of these tumors to their nasopharyngeal counterparts, and in striking contrast to them, three tonsillar lymphoepitheliomatous carcinomas have been found to be negative for EBV genomic material (130), and thus a relationship between such cancers in the oropharynx and EBV has not been convincingly demonstrated. Oropharyngeal NPC-type lymphoepitheliomatous carcinomas are quite radiosensitive, like their nasopharyngeal counterparts, and thus have a better prognosis than other oropharyngeal squamous cell carcinomas (184). Interestingly, although EBV has not been associated with tonsillar carcinoma, a recent study has found human papillomavirus (HPV) DNA in 9 of 15 (60%) squamous cell carcinomas of the tonsillar fossa (185), a rate much higher than was found in other head and neck sites in this study. Another study, although with results less dramatic, also found HPV more frequently in oropharyngeal squamous cell carcinoma than in other locations (186). Although the oral cavity is the most common site for verrucous carcinomas in the head and neck, such tumors are quite rare in the oropharynx. Spindle-cell or sarcomatoid variants of

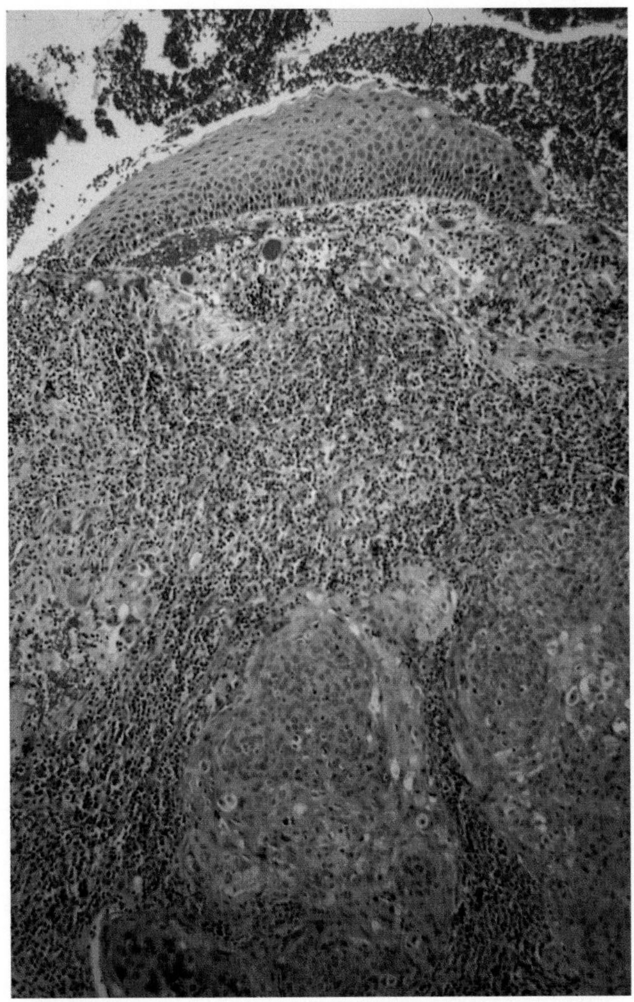

FIGURE 57. Lateral pharyngeal wall: squamous cell carcinoma. Nests of carcinoma are present in the lower half of the figure, in lymphoid tissue deep to an intact surface mucosal epithelial layer. This lesion was found on search for a primary site of a metastatic cervical lymph node.

squamous cell carcinomas are also very rare in the tonsillar region (187,188).

Differential Diagnosis

Two problems in histopathologic differential diagnosis relate to tonsillar squamous cell carcinomas. One involves the histologic appearance of tonsillar crypt epithelium. This epithelium is infiltrated by lymphocytes to a significant extent and shows less maturation to mature flattened squamous cells than the usual surface mucosal squamous epithelium. The crypt epithelium also invaginates deeply into the tonsillar tissue. These factors might make benign crypt epithelium in a small biopsy specimen resemble an infiltrating squamous cell carcinoma (29). Careful attention to the bland cytologic appearance of the epithelial cells as well as to the preserved noninvasive crypt architecture may help to prevent such errors in interpretation.

A second major differential diagnostic problem involves the distinction of poorly differentiated or lymphoepitheliomatous carcinomas from malignant lymphomas. As with similar tumors in the nasopharynx (see above), immunohistochemical stains are extremely helpful in distinguishing these conditions, with carcinomas staining for epithelial markers (keratin proteins) and lymphomas generally staining negative for keratin and positive for lymphoid markers (e.g., leukocyte common antigen, B-cell or T-cell markers).

Biological Behavior

Squamous cell carcinomas of the oropharynx, especially of the infiltrative variety, are biologically aggressive lesions that are often encountered when relatively advanced, often with cervical lymph node metastases present at diagnosis (see above). Radiation therapy, surgical excision, or various combinations of the two with or without adjuvant chemotherapy have been utilized as therapy. Patients with predominantly exophytic lesions that are not deeply invasive tend to do well (181). For tonsillar lesions, early-stage lesions tend to do well, although 5-year cure rates decrease to 60% and 38% for the two highest clinical stages (181). For base of tongue cancers, 5-year survival rates of 64% for stage III and 59% for stage IV have been reported (181).

Minor salivary gland carcinomas occur rarely in the oropharyngeal region. These types of tumors are discussed in Chapter 8.

Malignant Lymphomas

Malignant lymphomas are the second most common type of malignant neoplasm of Waldeyer's ring, after squamous cell carcinoma (179). The faucial tonsils are the predominant site of involvement, followed by the nasopharynx and lingual tonsils (177–180). The age range at presentation is wide, though most patients appear to present in their fifties and sixties (189–194). Symptoms relate mainly to a mass or sore throat in tonsillar cases (Fig. 59) or to nasal obstruction and/or otitic symptoms in nasopharyngeal cases (189).

The vast majority of Waldeyer's ring lymphomas are non-Hodgkin's large B-cell lymphomas, and most are diffuse (Fig. 60). Hodgkin's disease of Waldeyer's ring is very uncommon (179,189,192). A few of the nasopharyngeal lymphomas (more so in parts of Asia) are of the T–natural killer (NK) cell variety, classified currently in the Revised European American Lymphoma (or REAL) Classification (195) as sinonasal type T-NK lymphomas and previously known by such terms as angiocentric lymphoma, polymorphic reticulosis, or lethal midline granuloma (196–200). See Chapter 12 for a further discussion of these lesions as well as for a discussion of the morphology of lymphomas of the head and neck.

One interesting topic worthy of brief mention here is the relationship of Waldeyer's ring lymphomas to marginal zone lymphomas or so-called lymphomas of mucosa-associated lymphoid tissue (MALT). MALT lymphomas were originally described in the stomach and are common in the GI tract, and analogous lesions of essentially the same morphology and biological behavior are found in the head and neck, notably in the parotid gland, orbit, and thyroid gland (see Chapter 12). Inasmuch as the lymphoid tissue of Waldeyer's ring is intimately associated with mucosal epithelium, this location might also be expected to be the site of MALT lymphomas. Lymphomas of classic MALT type,

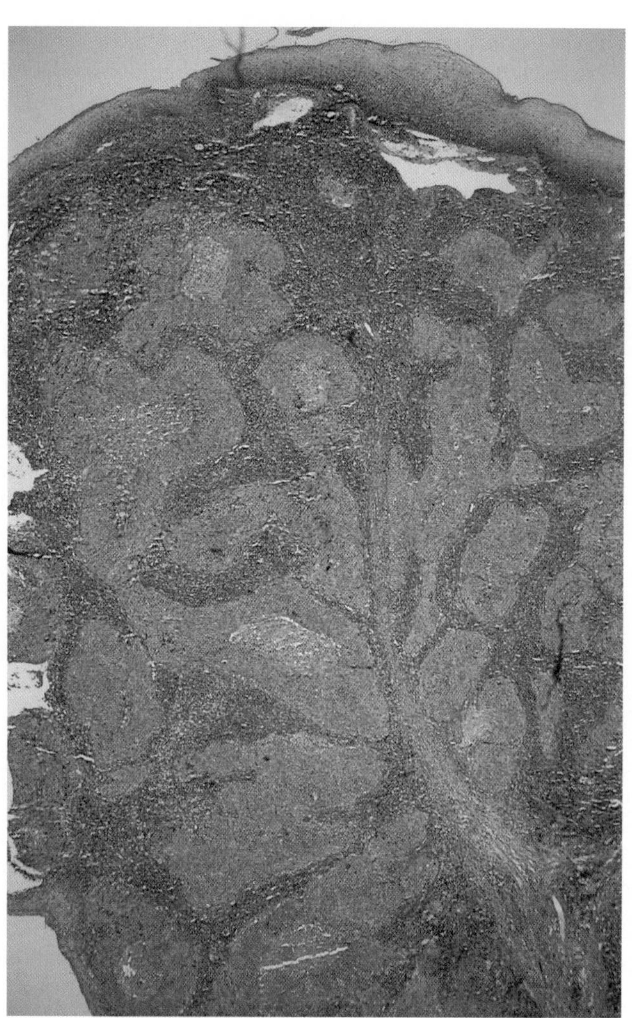

A

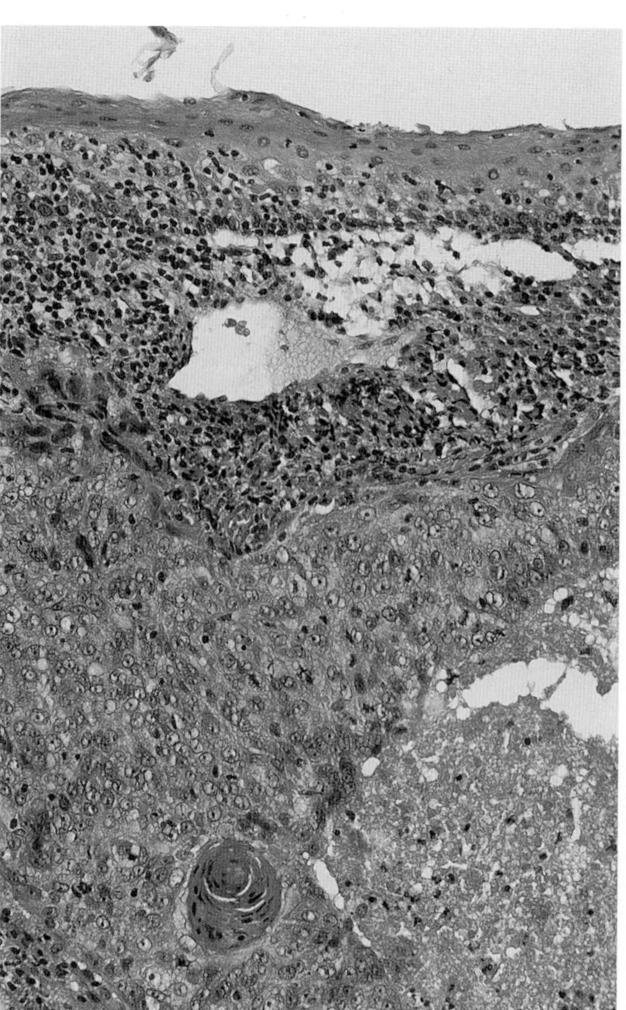

B

FIGURE 58. Base of tongue: squamous cell carcinoma. **A:** Ribbons of poorly differentiated squamous cell carcinoma infiltrate submucosal lymphoid tissue. The mucosal epithelium appears intact in this figure. **B:** Focal keratinization is present in the tumor.

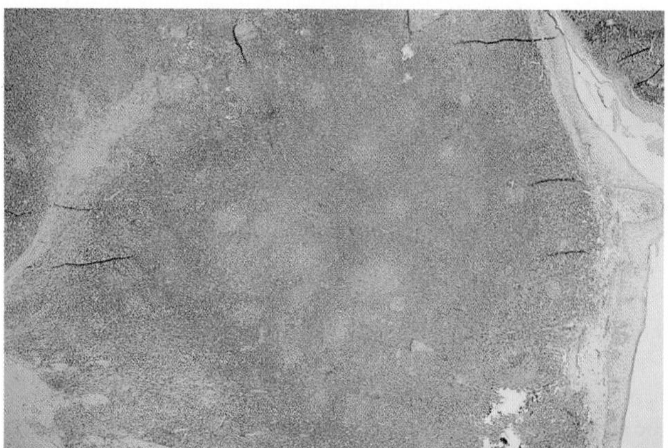

FIGURE 59. Tonsil: chronic lymphocytic leukemia/small lymphocytic lymphoma. A mass of small lymphocytes underlies the mucosa. The paler areas represent proliferation centers (or "pseudogerminal" centers) seen in this condition.

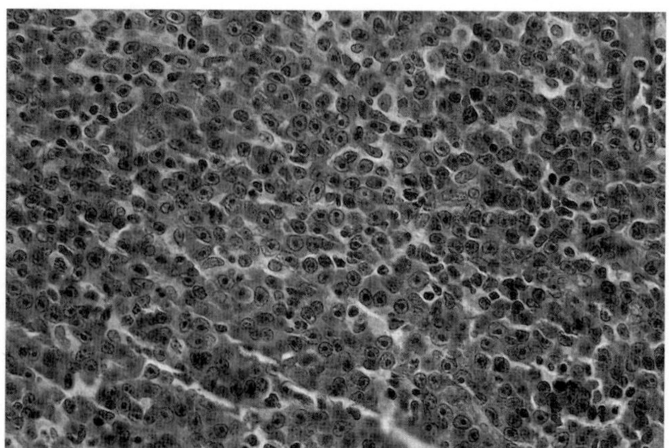

FIGURE 60. Nasopharynx: diffuse large B-cell lymphoma. A neoplastic sheet of immunoblasts (immunoblastic lymphoma) is seen.

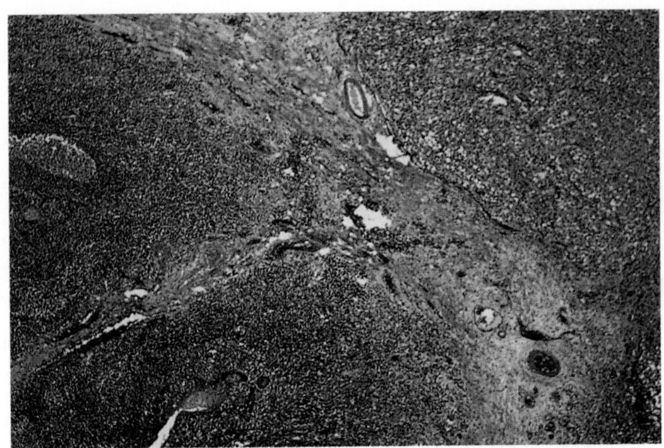
A

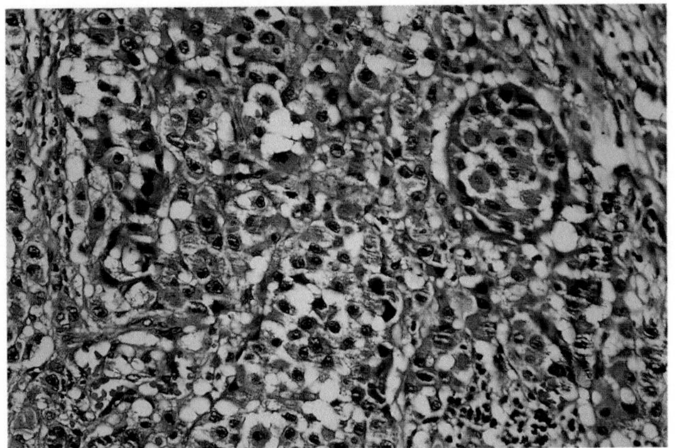
B

FIGURE 61. Tonsil: metastatic malignant melanoma. **A:** The metastasis is on the right of the figure; tonsillar tissue is on the left. **B:** A higher-power view of the malignant nevomelanocytic cells.

however, are very rare in Waldeyer's ring and in fact have only recently been definitely identified in this location (201). MALT lymphomas are characteristically low-grade B-cell lymphomas of small lymphoid cells, whereas Waldeyer's ring (WR) lymphomas are most often of large-cell type. Although cells of WR lymphoma infiltrate epithelium, the characteristic destructive lymphoepithelial lesions of MALT lymphomas as seen in the stomach and elsewhere are not observed (201,202). Nonetheless, several features are shared by WR lymphomas and MALT lymphomas. Interestingly, a high proportion of WR lymphomas relapse in the gastrointestinal tract, particularly the stomach, a prime site for MALT lymphomas (189,190,193,194). Also, WR lymphomas, as well as MALT lymphomas, tend to show a lower incidence of bcl-2 expression (a proliferation marker) than do nodal lymphomas, the value for WR lymphomas being intermediate between those for nodal lymphomas and MALT lymphomas (192,202), and both WR and MALT lymphomas showed a lower stage and better survival than nodal lymphomas in the study by Menarguez et al. (192). Could most WR lymphomas represent a high-grade variant of MALT lymphoma? Clearly, the relationship between WR and MALT lymphomas needs additional study and clarification.

Therapy for WR lymphomas consists of irradiation for small, low-stage lesions, often combined with chemotherapy for higher-stage lesions. Some authors advocate combined irradiation and chemotherapy for low-stage lesions as well (203). Recent 5-year survival rates reported for WR lymphomas have been 51.4% (190) and 65% (192); patients with stage II disease fare worse than those with stage I disease.

Extramedullary plasmacytomas are relatively common in the nasopharynx (see above) but are rare in the palatine tonsils.

Other primary neoplasms of the tonsils are extremely rare. A case of a primary meningioma of the tonsil has been reported (204), and we have seen a case of Kaposi's sarcoma involving the tonsil in an HIV-positive patient.

Metastatic Neoplasms

Metastatic neoplasms to the palatine tonsil are quite rare but well documented. Renal cell carcinoma, malignant melanoma, and carcinomas of the lung and breast have been reported to metastasize to the tonsil (Fig. 61) (205). Isolated cases of tonsillar metastases of prostate, rectal, and pancreatic carcinomas, Wilms' tumor, and choriocarcinoma have also been reported (206).

Other Conditions

Two examples of involvement of the lymphoid tissue of Waldeyer's ring in systemic noninfectious disease are Tangier disease and primary immune deficiency of childhood such as severe combined immunodeficiency disease (SCID).

Tangier disease is an extremely rare incompletely understood familial metabolic disease of plasma lipid transport characterized by low plasma cholesterol levels, very low levels or absence of plasma high-density lipoproteins, and accumulation of cholesterol esters in macrophages in various sites as well as in Schwann cells and nonvascular smooth muscle (207,208). Interestingly, the tonsils are a prime site for accumulation of lipid-filled macrophages, and patients characteristically have enlarged tonsils with prominent and characteristic yellow to yellow-orange streaks. In fact, the combination of enlarged yellowish tonsils and low plasma cholesterol is thought to be pathognomonic of the disease (208). Histologically, prominent accumulations of large foamy macrophages are present in the tonsils, mainly in perifollicular areas, though some are present in follicles as well (207,208).

In *severe combined immunodeficiency disease* (SCID), the tonsils as well as lymph nodes are small and rudimentary. Tonsils are markedly depleted of lymphoid cells in both B-cell and T-cell regions. The underlying reticular framework and tonsillar crypts remain (209).

REFERENCES

1. Dolen WK, Spofford B, Selner JC. The hidden tonsils of Waldeyer's ring. *Ann Allergy* 1990;65:244–248.
2. Miyahara H, Matsunaga T. Tornwaldt's disease. *Acta Otolaryngol (Stockh) [Suppl]* 1994;517:36–39.
3. Ash JE, Raum M. *An atlas of otolaryngic pathology.* Washington DC: Armed Forces Institute of Pathology, 1956:212–214.

4. Lewin R, Ruffolo E, Saraceno C. Craniopharyngioma arising in the pharyngeal hypophysis. *South Med J* 1984;77:1519–1523.
5. Fuller GN, Batsakis JG. Pharyngeal hypophysis. *Ann Otol Rhinol Laryngol* 1996;105:671–672.
6. Gili AB, Garcia BG. Craneofaringioma de nasofaringe. A propósito de un caso. *Acta Otorrinolaring Esp* 1991;42:269–272.
7. Graziani N, Donnet A, Bugha TN, et al. Ectopic basisphenoidal craniopharyngioma: case report and review of the literature. *Neurosurgery* 1994;34:346–349.
8. Anand VK, Osborne CM, Harkey HL III. Infiltrative clival pituitary adenoma of ectopic origin. *Orolaryngol Head Neck Surg* 1993;108:178–183.
9. Chessin H, Urdaneta N, Smith H, et al. Chromophobe adenoma manifesting as a nasopharyngeal mass. *Arch Otolaryngol* 1976;102:631–633.
10. Kawashiro N, Koga K, Tsuchihashi N, et al. Choanal atresia and congenital pharyngeal stenosis. *Acta Otolaryngol (Stockh) [Suppl]* 1994;517:27–32.
11. Kaplan LG. The CHARGE association: Choanal atresia and multiple congenital anomalies. *Otolaryngol Clin North Am* 1989;22:661–672.
12. Bossen EH, Hudson WR. Oligodendroglioma arising in heterotopic brain tissue of the soft palate and nasopharynx. *Am J Surg Pathol* 1987;11:571–574.
13. Ruff T, Diaz JA. Heterotopic brain in the nasopharynx. *Orolaryngol Head Neck Surg* 1986;94:254–256.
14. Hjertaas RJ, Morrison MD, Murray RB. Teratomas of the nasopharynx. *J Otolaryngol* 1979;8:411–416.
15. Dekelboum AM. Teratoma of the nasopharynx in the newborn. *Orolaryngol Head Neck Surg* 1979;87:628–634.
16. Rowe LD. Neonatal airway obstruction secondary to nasopharyngeal teratoma. *Orolaryngol Head Neck Surg* 1980;88:221–226.
17. Ward RF, April M. Teratomas of the head and neck. *Otolaryngol Clin North Am* 1989;22:621–629.
18. Tharrington CL, Bossen EH. Nasopharyngeal teratomas. *Arch Pathol Lab Med* 1992;116:165–167.
19. Chaudhry AP, Loré JM Jr, Fisher JE, et al. So-called hairy polyps or teratoid tumors of the nasopharynx. *Arch Otolaryngol* 1978;104:517–525.
20. McShane D, El Sherif I, Doyle-Kelly W, et al. Dermoids ("hairy polyps") of the oro-nasopharynx. *J Laryngol Otol* 1989;103:612–615.
21. Walsh RW, Philip G, Salama NY. Hairy polpy of the oropharynx: an unusual cause of intermittent neonatal airway obstruction. *Int J Pediatr Otorhinolaryngol* 1996;34:129–134.
22. Hatzihaberis F, Stamatis D, Staurinos D. Giant epignathus. *J Pediatr Surg* 1978;13:517–518.
23. Gonzalez-Crussi F. *Extragonadal teratomas. Atlas of tumor pathology, 2nd ser.* Washington DC: Armed Forces Institute of Pathology, 1982:9–24.
24. Kountakis SE, Minotti AM, Maillard A, et al. Teratomas of the head and neck. *Am J Otolaryngol* 1994;15:292–296.
24a. Kanzaki S, Yamada K, Fujimoto M, et al. So-called hairy polyp resembling an auricle. *Otolaryngol Head Neck Surg* 1988;99:424–426.
25. Shaheen OH. Two cases of bilateral branchiogenic cysts of the nasopharynx. *J Laryngol Otol* 1961;75:182–186.
26. Shidara K, Uruma T, Yasuoka Y, et al. Two cases of nasopharyngeal branchial cyst. *J Laryngol Otol* 1993;107:453–455.
27. Tamagawa Y, Kitamura K, Miyata M. Branchial cyst of the nasopharynx: resection via the endonasal approach. *J Laryngol Otol* 1995;109:139–141.
28. Childs CC, Parham DM, Berard CW. Infectious mononucleosis. The spectrum of morphologic changes simulating lymphoma in lymph nodes and tonsils. *Am J Surg Pathol* 1987;11:122–132.
29. Heffner DK. Pathology of the tonsils and adenoids. *Otolaryngol Clin North Am* 1987;20:279–286.
30. Shin SS, Berry GJ, Weiss LM. Infectious mononucleosis. Diagnosis by *in situ* hybridization in two cases with atypical features. *Am J Surg Pathol* 1991;15:625–631.
31. Strickler JG, Fedeli F, Horwitz CA, et al. Infectious mononucleosis in lymphoid tissue. Histopathology *in situ* hybridization, and differential diagnosis. *Arch Pathol Lab Med* 1993;117:269–278.
32. Kapadia SB, Roman LN, Kingma DW, et al. Hodgkin's disease of Waldeyer's ring. Clinical and histoimmunophenotypic findings and association with Epstein-Barr virus in 16 cases. *Am J Surg Pathol* 1995;19:1431–1439.
33. Eavey RD, Goodman ML. Hodgkin's disease of the nasopharynx. *Am J Otolaryngol* 1982;3:417–421.
34. O'Reilly BM, Kershaw JB. Hodgkin's disease of the nasopharynx. *J Laryngol Otol* 1987;101:506–507.
35. Goodman RS, Mattel S, Kaufman D, et al. Tuberculoma of the nasopharynx. *Laryngoscope* 1981;91:794–797.
36. Miller RH, Sneed WF. Tornwaldt's bursa. *Clin Otolaryngol* 1985;10:21–25.
37. Weissman JL. Thornwaldt cysts. *Am J Otolaryngol* 1992;13:381–385.
38. Morin GV, Shank EC, Burgess LPA, et al. Oncocytic metaplasia of the pharynx. *Orolaryngol Head Neck Surg* 1991;105:86–91.
39. Shek TWH, Luk ISC, Nicholls JM, et al. Melanotic oncocytic metaplasia of the nasopharynx. *Histopathology* 1995;26:273–275.
40. Kurihara K, Nakagawa K. Pigmented variant of benign oncocytic lesion of the pharynx. *Pathol Int* 1997;47:315–317.
41. Graeme-Cook F, Pilch BZ. Hamartomas of the nose and nasopharynx. *Head Neck* 1992;14:321–327.
42. Wenig BM, Heffner DK. Respiratory epithelial adenomatoid hamartomas of the sinonasal tract and nasopharynx: a clinicopathologic study of 31 cases. *Ann Otol Rhinol Laryngol* 1995;104:639–645.
43. Baillie EE, Batsakis JB. Glandular (seromucinous) hamartoma of the nasopharynx. *Oral Surg* 1974;38:760–762.
44. Brandenburg JH, Finch WW, Lloyd R. Cystic hamartoma of the nasopharynx. *Trans Am Acad Ophtholmol Otolaryngol* 1977;84:152–153.
45. Zarbo RJ, McClatchey KD. Nasopharyngeal hamartoma: report of a case and review of the literature. *Laryngoscope* 1983;93:494–497.
46. Adair CF, Thompson LDR, Wenig BM, et al. Chondro-osseous and respiratory epithelial hamartomas of the sinonasal tract and nasopharynx. *Mod Pathol* 1996;9:100A.
47. Lewis JE, Olsen KD, Kurtin PJ, et al. Laryngeal amyloidosis: a clinicopathologic and immunohistochemical review. *Orolaryngol Head Neck Surg* 1992;106:372–377.
48. Simpson GT II, Skinner M, Strong MS, et al. Localized amyloidosis of the head and neck and upper aerodigestive and lower respiratory tracts. *Ann Otol Rhinol Laryngol* 1984;93:374–379.
49. Mufarrij AA, Busaba NY, Zaytoun GM, et al. Primary localized amyloidosis of the nose and paranasal sinuses. A case report with immunohistochemical observations and a review of the literature. *Am J Surg Pathol* 1990;14:379–383.
50. Strunski V, Goin M, Guillem I, et al. Amylose du cavum. A propos d'une observation. *Ann Oto-Laryng (Paris)* 1991;108:49–51.
51. Dominguez S, Weinberg P, Clarós A, et al. Primary localized nasopharyngeal amyloidosis. A case report. *Int J Pediatr Otorhinolaryngol* 1996;36:61–67.
52. Michaels L, Hyams VJ. Amyloid in localised deposits and plasmacytomas of the respiratory tract. *J Pathol* 1979;128:29–38.
53. Scott A, Stansbie JM. Actinomycosis presenting as a nasopharyngeal tumour: a case report. *J Laryngol Otol* 1997;111:163–169.
54. Dehner LP, Valbuena L, Perez-Atayde A, et al. Salivary gland anlage tumor ("congenital pleomorphic adenoma"). A clinicopathologic, immunohistochemical and ultrastructural study of nine cases. *Am J Surg Pathol* 1994;18:25–36.
55. Har-El G, Zirkin HY, Tovi F, et al. Congenital pleomorphic adenoma of the nasopharynx. Report of a case. *J Laryngol Otol* 1985;99:1281–1287.
56. Batsakis JG, MacKay B, Ryka AF, et al. Perinatal salivary gland tumours (embryomas). *J Laryngol Otol* 1988;102:1007–1011.
57. Batsakis JG, Frankenthaler R. Embryoma (sialoblastoma) of salivary glands. *Ann Otol Rhinol Laryngol* 1992;101:958–960.
58. Dardick I, Daley TD, van Nostrand AWP. Basal cell adenoma with myoepithelial cell-derived "stroma": a new major salivary gland tumor entity. *Head Neck Surg* 1986;8:257–267.
59. Patterson SD, Ballard RW. Nasal blastoma: a light and electron microscopic study. *Ultrastruct Pathol* 1980;1:487–494.

60. Meinecke R, Bauer F, Skouras J, et al. Blastomatous tumors of the respiratory tract. *Cancer* 1976;38:818–823.
61. Pradillo JA, Rodriguez HA, Arroyo JF. Nasopharyngeal angiofibroma in the elderly: report of a case. *Laryngoscope* 1975;85:1063–1065.
62. Sternberg SS. Pathology of juvenile nasopharyngeal angiofibroma—a lesion of adolescent males. *Cancer* 1954;7:15–28.
63. Neel HB III, Whicker JH, Devine KD, et al. Juvenile angiofibroma. Review of 120 cases. *Am J Surg* 1973;126:547–556.
64. Waldman SR, Levine HL, Astor F, et al. Surgical experience with nasopharyngeal angiofibroma. *Arch Otolaryngol* 1981;107:677–682.
65. Duval AJ III, Moreano AE. Juvenile nasopharyngeal angiofibroma: diagnosis and treatment. *Otolaryngol Head Neck Surg* 1987;97: 534–540.
66. Harrison DFN. The natural history, pathogenesis, and treatment of juvenile angiofibroma. *Arch Otolaryngol Head Neck Surg* 1987;113: 936–942.
67. Jacobsson M, Petruson B, Svendsen P, et al. Juvenile nasopharyngeal angiofibroma. A report of eighteen cases. *Acta Otolaryngeol (Stockh)* 1988;105:132–139.
68. Beham A, Fletcher CDM, Kainz J, et al. Nasopharyngeal angiofibroma: an immunohistochemical study of 32 cases. *Virchows Arch A Pathol Anat* 1993;423:281–285.
69. Finerman WB. Juvenile nasopharyngeal angiofibroma in the female. *Arch Otolaryngol Head Neck Surg* 1951;54:620–623.
70. Osborn DA, Sokolovski A. Juvenile nasopharyngeal angiofibroma in a female. *Arch Otolaryngol Head Neck Surg* 1965;92:629–632.
71. Ewing AJ, Shively EH. Angiofibroma: a rare case in an elderly female. *Otolaryngol Head Neck Surg* 1981;89:602–603.
72. Stiller D, Küttner K. Growth patterns of juvenile nasopharyngeal angiofibromas. Histologic analysis of 40 cases. *Zentralbl Allg Pathol Pathol Anat* 1988;134:409–422.
73. Cummings BJ, Blend R, Fitzpatrick P, et al. Primary radiation therapy for juvenile nasopharyngeal angiofibroma. *Laryngoscope* 1984; 94:1599–1605.
74. Gisselsson L, Lindgren M, Stenram U. Sarcomatous transformation of a juvenile, nasopharyngeal angiofibroma. *Acta Pathol Microbiol Scand* 1958;42:305–312.
75. Chen KTK, Bauer FW. Sarcomatous transformation of nasopharyngeal angiofibroma. *Cancer* 1982;49:369–371.
76. Spagnolo DV, Papadimitriou JM, Archer M. Postirradiation malignant fibrous histiocytoma arising in juvenile nasopharyngeal angiofibroma and producing alpha-1-antitrypsin. *Histopathology* 1984;8: 339–352.
77. Makek MS, Andrews JC, Fisch U. Malignant transformation of a nasopharyngeal angiofibroma. *Laryngoscope* 1989;99:1088–1092.
78. Donald PJ. Sarcomatous degeneration in a nasopharyngeal angiofibroma. *Otolaryngol Head Neck Surg* 1979;87:42–46.
79. Fu Y-S, Perzin KH. Nonepithelial tumors of the nasal cavity, paranasal sinuses, and nasopharynx. A clinicopathologic study. V. Skeletal muscle tumors (rhabdomyoma and rhabdomyosarcoma). *Cancer* 1976;37:364–376.
80. Kapadia SB, Meis JM, Frisman DM, et al. Adult rhabdomyoma of the head and neck: a clinicopathologic and immunophenotypic study. *Hum Pathol* 1993;24:608–617.
81. Strauss M, Widome MD, Roland PS. Nasopharyngeal hemangioma causing airway obstruction in infancy. *Laryngoscope* 1981;91: 1365–1368.
82. Fu Y-S, Perzin KH. Non-epithelial tumors of the nasal cavity, paranasal sinuses and nasopharynx: a clinicopathologic study. III. Cartilaginous tumors (chondroma, chondrosarcoma). *Cancer* 1974;34:453–463.
83. House JM, Goodman ML, Gacek RR, et al. Chemodectomas of the nasopharynx. *Arch Otolaryngol* 1972;96:138–141.
84. Chambers EF, Norman D, Dedo HH, et al. Primary nasopharyngeal chemodectoma. *Neuroradiology* 1982;23:285–288.
85. Schuller DE, Lucas JG. Nasopharyngeal paraganglioma. Report of a case and review of the literature. *Arch Otolaryngol* 1982;108: 667–670.
86. Job A, Walter N, David TM. Solitary fibrous tumour of the nasopharynx. *J Laryngol Otol* 1991;105:213–214.
87. Witkin GB, Rosai J. Solitary fibrous tumor of the upper respiratory tract. A report of six cases. *Am J Surg Pathol* 1991;15:842–848.
88. van Der Mey AGL, van Krieken JHJM, van Dulken H, et al. Large pituitary adenomas with extension into the nasopharynx. Report of three cases with a review of the literature. *Ann Otol Rhinol Laryngol* 1989;98:618–624.
89. Hirayama T. Descriptive and analytical epidemiology of nasopharyngeal cancer. In: De-Thé G, Ito Y, eds. *Nasopharyngeal carcinoma: etiology and control.* Lyons: International Agency for Research on Cancer, 1978:167–189.
90. Batsakis JG, Solomon AR, Rice DH. The pathology of head and neck tumors: carcinoma of the nasopharynx, part 11. *Head Neck Surg* 1981;3:511–524.
91. Dickson RI. Nasopharyngeal carcinoma: an evaluation of 209 patients. *Laryngoscope* 1981;91:333–354.
92. Neel HB III. Nasopharyngeal carcinoma. Clinical presentation, diagnosis, treatment, and prognosis. *Otolaryngol Clin North Am* 1985;18: 479–490.
93. Nielsen NH, Mikkelsen F, Hansen JPH. Nasopharyngeal cancer in Greenland. The incidence in an Arctic Eskimo population. *Acta Pathol Microbiol Scand A* 1977;85:850–858.
94. Lanier A, Bender T, Talbot M, et al. Nasopharyngeal carcinoma in Alaskan Eskimos, Indians, and Aleuts: a review of cases and study of Epstein-Barr virus, HLA, and environmental risk factors. *Cancer* 1980;46:2100–2106.
95. Neel HB III, Pearson GR, Weiland LH, et al. Anti-EBV serologic tests for nasopharyngeal carcinoma. *Laryngoscope* 1980;90:1981–1990.
96. Neel HB III, Pearson GR, Weiland LH, et al. Application of Epstein-Barr virus serology to the diagnosis and staging of North American patients with nasopharyngeal carcinoma. *Otolaryngol Head Neck Surg* 1983;91:255–262.
97. Pearson GR, Weiland LH, Neel HB III, et al. Application of Epstein-Barr virus (EBC) serology to the diagnosis of North American nasopharyngeal carcinoma. *Cancer* 1983;51:260–268.
98. Pearson GR, Neel HB III, Weiland LH, et al. Antibody-dependent cellular cytotoxicity and disease course in North American patients with nasopharyngeal carcinoma: a prospective study. *Int J Cancer* 1984;33:777–782.
99. Raab-Traub N, Flynn K. The structure of the termini of the Epstein-Barr virus as a marker of colonal cellular proliferation. *Cell* 1986;47:883–889.
100. Gulley ML, Amin MB, Nicholls JM, et al. Epstein-Barr virus is detected in undifferentiated nasopharyngeal carcinoma but not in lymphoepithelioma-like carcinoma of the urinary bladder. *Hum Pathol* 1995;26:1207–1214.
101. Pathmanathan R, Prasad U, Sadler R, et al. Clonal proliferations of cells infected with Epstein-Barr virus in preinvasive lesions related to nasopharyngeal carcinoma. *N Engl J Med* 1995;333:693–698.
102. Raab-Traub N, Flynn K, Pearson G, et al. The differentiated form of nasopharyngeal carcinoma contains Epstein-Barr virus DNA. *Int J Cancer* 1987;39:25–29.
103. Pathmanathan R, Prasad U, Chandrika G, et al. Undifferentiated, nonkeratinizing, and squamous cell carcinoma of the nasopharnx. Variants of Epstein-Barr virus-infected neoplasia. *Am J Pathol* 1995;146:1355–1367.
104. Anderson EN Jr, Anderson ML, Ho HC. Environmental backgrounds of young Chinese nasopharyngeal carcinoma patients. In: De-Thé G, Ito Y, eds. *Nasopharyngeal carcinoma: etiology and control.* Lyons: International Agency for Research on Cancer, 1978:231–239.
105. Henderson BE, Louie E. Discussion of risk factors for nasopharyngeal carcinoma. In: De-Thé G, Ito Y, eds. *Nasopharyngeal carcinoma: etiology and control.* Lyons: International Agency for Research on Cancer, 1978:251–260.
106. Baker SR. Malignant tumors of the nasopharynx. *J Surg Oncol* 1981; 17:25–32.
107. Shanmugaratnam K, Sobin LH. *International histological classification of tumours, no. 19: Histological typing of upper respiratory tract tumours.* Geneva: World Health Organization, 1978.
108. Shanmugaratnam K. *Histological typing of tumours of the upper respiratory tract and ear.* Berlin: Springer-Verlag, 1991.

109. Wan S-K, Chan JKC, Lau W-H, et al. Basaloid–squamous carcinoma of the nasopharynx. An Epstein-Barr virus-associated neoplasm compared with morphologically identical tumors occurring in other sites. *Cancer* 1995;76:1689–1693.
110. Weiland LH. The histopathological spectrum of nasopharyngeal carcinoma. In: De-Thé G, Ito Y, eds. *Nasopharyngeal carcinoma: etiology and control.* Lyons: International Agency for Research on Cancer, 1978:41–50.
111. Taxy JB, Hidvegi DF, Battifora H. Nasopharyngeal carcinoma: Antikeratin immunohistochemistry and electron microscopy. *Am J Clin Pathol* 1985;83:320–325.
112. Möller P, Wirbel R, Hofmann W, et al. Lymphoepithelial carcinoma (Schmincke type) as a derivate of the tonsillar crypt epithelium. *Virchows Arch [Pathol Anat]* 1984;405:85–93.
113. Shi S-R, Goodman ML, Bhan AK, et al. Immunohistochemical study of nasopharyngeal carcinoma using monoclonal keratin antibodies. *Am J Pathol* 1984;117:53–63.
114. Wick MR, Stanley SJ, Swanson PE. Immunohistochemical diagnosis of sinonasal melanoma, carcinoma, and neuroblastoma with monoclonal antibodies HMB-45 and anti-synaptophysin. *Arch Pathol Lab Med* 1988;112:616–620.
115. Lennert K, Kaiserling E, Mazzanti T. Diagnosis and differential diagnosis of lymphoepithelial carcinoma in lymph nodes: histological, cytological and electron-microscopic findings. In: De-Thé G, Ito Y, eds. *Nasopharyngeal carcinoma: etiology and control.* Lyons: International Agency for Research on Cancer, 1978;51–64.
116. Carbone A, Micheau C. Pitfalls in microscopic diagnosis of undifferentiated carcinoma of nasopharyngeal type (lymphoepithelioma). *Cancer* 1982;50:1344–1351.
117. Macdonald MR, Freeman JL, Hui MF, et al. Role of Epstein-Barr virus in fine-needle aspirates of metastatic neck nodes in the diagnosis of nasopharyngeal carcinoma. *Head Neck* 1995;17:487–493.
118. Dictor M, Sivén M, Tennvall J, et al. Determination of nonendemic nasopharyngeal carcinoma by *in situ* hybridization for Epstein-Barr virus EBER1 RNA: sensitivity and specificity in cervical node metastases. *Laryngoscope* 1995;105:407–412.
119. Chao T-Y, Chow K-C, Chang J-Y, et al. Expression of Epstein-Barr virus-encoded RNAs as a marker for metastatic undifferentiated nasopharyngeal carcinoma. *Cancer* 1996;78:24–29.
120. Tsai S-T, Jin Y-T, Su I-J. Expression of EBER1 in primary and metastatic nasopharyngeal carcinoma tissues using *in situ* hybridization. A correlation with WHO histologic subtypes. *Cancer* 1996; 77:231–236.
121. Nielsen NH, Mikkelsen F, Hansen JPH. Incidence of salivary gland neoplasms in Greenland with special reference to an anaplastic carcinoma. *Acta Pathol Microbiol Scand [A]* 1978;86:185–193.
122. Povah WB, Beecroft W, Hodson I, et al. Malignant lympho-epithelial lesion—the Manitoba experience. *J Otolaryngol* 1984;13:153–159.
123. Krishnamurthy S, Lanier AP, Dohan P, et al. Salivary gland cancer in Alaskan natives, 1966–1980. *Hum Pathol* 1987;18:986–996.
124. Hanji D, Gohao L. Malignant lymphoepithelial lesions of the salivary glands with anaplastic carcinomatous change. Report of nine cases and review of the literature. *Cancer* 1983;52:2245–2252.
125. Merrick Y, Albeck H, Nielsen H, et al. Familial clustering of salivary gland carcinoma in Greenland. *Cancer* 1986;57:2097–2102.
126. Hamilton-Dutoit SJ, Therkildsen MH, Nielsen NH, et al. Undifferentiated carcinoma of the salivary gland in Greenlandic Eskimos: Demonstration of Epstein-Barr virus DNA by *in situ* nucleic acid hybridization. *Hum Pathol* 1991;22:811–815.
127. Leung SY, Chung LP, Yuen ST, et al. Lymphoepithelial carcinoma of the salivary gland: *in situ* detection of Epstein-Barr virus. *J Clin Pathol* 1995;48:1022–1027.
128. Micheau C, Luboninski B, Schwaab G, et al. Lymphoepitheliomas of the larynx (undifferentiated carcinomas of nasopharyngeal type). *Clin Otolaryngol* 1979;4:43–48.
129. Ferlito A, Weiss LM, Rinaldo A, et al. Lymphoepithelial carcinoma of the larynx, hypopharynx, and trachea. *Ann Otol Rhinol Laryngol* 1997; 106:437–444.
130. Weiss LM, Movahed LA, Butler AE, et al. Analysis of lymphoepithelioma and lymphoepithelioma-like carcinomas for Epstein-Barr viral genomes by *in situ* hybridization. *Am J Surg Pathol* 1989;13: 625–631.
131. Pittaluga S, Wong MP, Chung LP, et al. Clonal Epstein-Barr virus in lymphoepithelioma-like carcinoma of the lung. *Am J Surg Pathol* 1993;17:678–682.
132. Chan JKC, Hui P-K, Tsang WYW, et al. Primary lymphoepithelioma-like carcinoma of the lung. A clinicopathologic study of 11 cases. *Cancer* 1995;76:413–422.
133. Leyvraz S, Henle W, Chahinian AP, et al. Association of Epstein-Barr virus with thymic carcinoma. *N Engl J Med* 1985;312: 1296–1299.
134. Min K-W, Holmquist S, Peiper SC, et al. Poorly differentiated adenocarcinoma with lymphoid stroma (lymphoepithelioma-like carcinomas) of the stomach. *Am J Clin Pathol* 1991;96:219–227.
135. Carr KA, Bulengo S, Weiss LM, et al. Lymphoepitheliomalike carcinoma of the skin. A case report with immunophenotypic analysis and *in situ* hybridization for Epstein-Barr viral genome. *Am J Surg Pathol* 1992;16:909–913.
136. Kumar S, Kumar D. Lymphoepithelioma-like carcinoma of the breast. *Mod Pathol* 1994;7:129–131.
137. Shibata D, Weiss LM. Epstein-Barr virus-associated gastric adenocarcinoma. *Am J Pathol* 1992;140:769–774.
138. Leung SY, Yuen ST, Chung LP, et al. Epstein-Barr virus is present in a wide histological spectrum of sinonasal carcinomas. *Am J Surg Pathol* 1995;19:994–1001.
139. Lee D-J, Smith RRL, Spaziani JT, et al. Adenoid cystic carcinoma of the nasopharynx. Case reports and literature review. *Ann Otol Rhinol Laryngol* 1985;94:269–272.
140. Sofferman RA, Heisse JW Jr. Adenoid cystic carcinoma of the nasopharynx after previous adenoid irradiation. *Laryngoscope* 1985; 95:458–461.
141. Wenig BM, Harpaz N, DelBridge C. Polymorphous low-grade adenocarcinoma of seromucous glands of the nasopharynx. A report of a case and a discussion of the morphologic and immunohistochemical features. *Am J Clin Pathol* 1989;92:104–109.
142. Wenig BM, Hyams VJ, Heffner DK. Nasopharyngeal papillary adenocarcinoma. A clinicopathologic study of a low-grade carcinoma. *Am J Surg Pathol* 1988;12:946–953.
143. Canalis RF, Jenkins HA, Hemenway WG, et al. Nasopharyngeal rhabdomyosarcoma. A clinical perspective. *Arch Otolaryngol* 1978; 104:122–126.
144. O'Reilly BJ, Ryan J, Reynard J, et al. Malignant fibrous histiocytoma of the nasopharynx. *J Laryngol Otol* 1989;103:1076–1079.
145. Imoto K, Yamazaki Y, Kawahara E, et al. Malignant melanocytic schwannoma of the nasopharynx. *Otorhinolaryngology* 1991;53: 48–51.
146. Thompson J, Castillo M, Reddick RL, et al. Nasopharyngeal nonossifying variant of ossifying fibromyxoid tumor: CT and MR findings. *Am J Neuroradiol* 1995;16:1132–1134.
147. Richter HJ, Batsakis JG, Boles R. Chordomas: nasopharyngeal presentation and atypical long survival. *Ann Otol* 1975;84:327–332.
148. Campbell WM, McDonald TJ, Unni KK, et al. Nasal and paranasal presentations of chordomas. *Laryngoscope* 1980;90:612–618.
149. Rosenberg AE, Brown GA, Bhan AK, et al. Chondroid chordoma—a variant of chordoma. A morphologic and immunohistochemical study. *Am J Clin Pathol* 1994;101:36–41.
150. Austin-Seymour M, Munzenrider J, Goitein M, et al. Fractionated proton radiation therapy of chordoma and low-grade chondrosarcoma of the base of the skull. *J Neurosurg* 1989;70:13–17.
151. McKay MJ, Carr PJ, Jaworski R, et al. Cancer of distant primary site relapsing in the nasopharynx: a report of two cases and review of the literature. *Head Neck* 1989;11:534–537.
152. Kapadia SB, Desai U, Cheng VS. Extramedullary plasmacytoma of the head and neck. A clinicopathologic study of 20 cases. *Medicine* 1982;61:317–329.
153. Wax MK, Yun JK, Omar RA. Extramedullary plasmacytomas of the head and neck. *Otolaryngol Head Neck Surg* 1993;109:877–885.

154. Fu Y-S, Perzin KH. Nonepithelial tumors of the nasal cavity, paranasal sinuses and nasopharynx. A clinicopathologic study. IX. Plasmacytomas. *Cancer* 1978;42:2399–2406.
155. Batsakis JG. Plasma cell tumors of the head and neck. *Ann Otol Rhinol Laryngol* 1983;92:311–313.
156. Scoppa J, Tonkin JP. Non-chromaffin paraganglioma of the nasopharynx. *J Laryngol Otol* 1975;89:653–656.
157. Manivel C, Wick MR, Dehner LP. Transitional (cylindric) cell carcinoma with endodermal sinus tumor-like features of the nasopharynx and paranasal sinuses. Clinicopathologic and immunohistochemical study of two cases. *Arch Pathol Lab Med* 1986;110:198–202.
158. Devaney KO, Ferlito A. Yolk sac tumors (endodermal sinus tumors) of the extracranial head and neck regions. *Ann Otol Rhinol Laryngol* 1997;106:254–260.
159. Nicoucar R, Schrago R. Considérations sur les résultats de l'examen anatomo-pathologique systématique des amygdales opérées au cours des 16 derinères années à la clinique universitaire d'oto-rhino-laryngologie de Genève. *Pract Otorhinolaryngol* 1969;31:188–192.
160. Atlan G, Egerszegi P, Brochu P, et al. Cervical chrondrocutaneous branchial remnants. *Plast Reconstr Surg* 1997;100:32–39.
161. Wenig BM, Thompson LDR, Frankel SS, et al. Lymphoid changes of the nasopharyngeal and palatine tonsils that are indicative of human immunodeficiency virus infection. A clinicopathologic study of 12 cases. *Am J Surg Pathol* 1996;20:572–587.
162. Frankel SS, Wenig BM, Ferlito A. Human immunodeficiency virus-1 infection of the lymphoid tissues of Waldeyer's ring. *Ann Otol Rhinol Laryngol* 1997;106:611–618.
163. Erwin SA. Unsuspected sarcoidosis of the tonsil. *Otolaryngol Head Neck Surg* 1989;100:245–247.
164. Taxy JB. Granulomatous tonsillitis. An unusual host response with benign clinical evolution. *Int J Surg Pathol* 1995;3:23–28.
165. Miglets AW, Barton CL. Sarcoid of the tonsil. Response to local steroid injection. *Arch Otolaryngol* 1970;92:516–517.
166. Somers K. Random biopsies in the diagnosis of sarcoid. *Eye Ear Nose Throat Mon* 1973;52:369–373.
167. Hiraide F, Inouye T, Tanaka E. Lymphangiectatic fibrous polyp of the palatine tonsil. A report of three cases. *J Laryngol Otol* 1985;99:403–409.
168. Abu Shara KA, Al-Muhana AA, Al-Shennawy M. Harmartomatous tonsillar polyp. *J Laryngol Otol* 1991;105:1089–1090.
169. Roth M. Lymphangiomatous polyp of the palatine tonsil. *Otolaryngol Head Neck Surg* 1996;115:172–173.
170. Carillo-Farga J, Abbud-Neme F, Deutsch E. Lymphoid papillary hyperplasia of the palatine tonsils. *Am J Surg Pathol* 1983;7:579–582.
171. Mitchell TE, Girling AC. Hairy polyp of the tonsil. *J Laryngol Otol* 1996;110:101–103.
172. Eriksen HE. A case of primary localized amyloidosis in both tonsils. *J Laryngol Otol* 1970;84:525–531.
173. Amado ML, Patino MJL, Blanco GL, et al. Giant primary amyloidoma of the tonsil. *J Laryngol Otol* 1996;110:613–615.
174. Beiser M, Messer G, Samuel J, et al. Amyloidosis of Waldeyer's ring. A clinical and ultrastructural report. *Acta Otolaryngol* 1980;89:562–569.
175. Kalfayan B, Seager GM. Malakoplakia of palatine tonsil. *Am J Clin Pathol* 1982;78:390–394.
176. Newman JP, Shinn JB. Inflammatory pseudotumor of the tonsil. *Otolaryngol Head Neck Surg* 1995;113:798–801.
177. Malotte MJ, Chonkich GD, Zuppan CW. Riedel's thyroiditis. *Arch Otolaryngol Head Neck Surg* 1991;117:214–217.
178. Nielsen HK. Multifocal idiopathic fibrosclerosis. Two cases with simultaneous occurrence of retroperitoneal fibrosis and Riedel's thyroiditis. *Acta Med Scand* 1980;208:119–123.
179. Hyams VJ. Differential diagnosis of neoplasia of the palatine tonsil. *Clin Otolaryngol* 1978;3:117–126.
180. Landis SH, Murray T, Bolden S, et al. Cancer statistics, 1998. *CA Cancer J Clin* 1998;48:6–29.
181. Civantos FJ, Goodwin WJ Jr. Cancer of the oropharynx. In: Myers EN, Suen JY, eds. *Cancer of the head and neck.* Philadelphia: WB Saunders, 1996:361–380.
182. Thompson LDR, Heffner DK. The clinical importance of cystic squamous cell carcinomas in the neck. A study of 136 cases. *Cancer* 1998;82:944–956.
183. Banks ER, Frierson HF Jr, Mills SE, et al. Basaloid squamous cell carcinoma of the head and neck: a clinicopathologic and immunohistochemical study of 40 cases. *Am J Surg Pathol* 1992;16:939–946.
184. Bansberg SF, Olsen KD, Gaffey TA. Lymphoepithelioma of the oropharynx. *Otolaryngol Head Neck Surg* 1989;100:303–307.
185. Paz IB, Cook N, Odom-Maryon T, et al. Human papillomavirus (HPV) in head and heck cancer. An association of HPV 16 with squamous cell carcinoma of Waldeyer's tonsillar ring. *Cancer* 1997;79:595–604.
186. Fouret P, Monceaux G, Temam S, et al. Human papillomavirus in head and neck squamous cell carcinomas in nonsmokers. *Arch Otolaryngol Head Neck Surg* 1997;123:513–516.
187. Zarbo RJ, Crissman JD, Venkat H, et al. Spindle-cell carcinoma of the upper aerodigestive tract mucosa. An immunohistologic and ultrastructural study of 18 biphasic tumors and comparison with seven monophasic spindle-cell tumors. *Am J Surg Pathol* 1986;10:741–753.
188. Ellis GL, Langloss JM, Heffner DK, et al. Spindle-cell carcinoma of the aerodigestive tract. An immunohistochemical analysis of 21 cases. *Am J Surg Pathol* 1987;11:335–342.
189. Saul SH, Kapadia SB. Primary lymphoma of Waldeyer's ring. Clinicopathologic study of 68 cases. *Cancer* 1985;56:157–166.
190. Economopoulos T, Asprou N, Stathakis N, et al. Primary extranodal non-Hodgkin's lymphoma of the head and neck. *Oncology* 1992;49:484–488.
191. Kojima M, Tamaki Y, Nakamura S, et al. Malignant lymphoma of Waldeyer's ring. A histological and immunohistochemical study. *APMIS* 1993;101:537–544.
192. Menárguez J, Mollejo M, Carrión R, et al. Waldeyer ring lymphomas. A clinicopathological study of 79 cases. *Histopathology* 1994;24:13–22.
193. Barton JH, Osborne BM, Butler JJ, et al. Non-Hodgkin's lymphoma of the tonsil. A clinicopathologic study of 65 cases. *Cancer* 1984;53:86–95.
194. Shimm DS, Dosoretz DE, Harris NL, et al. Radiation therapy of Waldeyer's ring lymphoma. *Cancer* 1984;54:426–431.
195. Harris NL, Jaffe ES, Stein H, et al. A revised European-American classification of lymphoid neoplasms: a proposal from the International Lymphoma Study Group. *Blood* 1994;84:1361–1392.
196. Chan JKC, Ng CS, Lau WH, et al. Most nasal/nasopharyngeal lymphomas are peripheral T-cell neoplasms. *Am J Surg Pathol* 1987;11:418–429.
197. Ferry JA, Sklar J, Zukerberg LR, et al. Nasal lymphoma. A clinicopathologic study with immunophenotypic and genotypic analysis. *Am J Surg Pathol* 1991;15:268–279.
198. Ohguro S, Himi T, Harabuchi Y, et al. Adult T-cell leukaemia-lymphoma in Waldeyer's ring: a report of three cases. *J Laryngol Otol* 1993;107:960–962.
199. Davison SP, Habermann TM, Strickler JG, et al. Nasal and nasopharyngeal angiocentric T-cell lymphomas. *Laryngoscope* 1996;106:139–143.
200. Petrella T, Delfau-Larue M-H, Caillot D, et al. Nasopharyngeal lymphomas: further evidence for a natural killer cell origin. *Hum Pathol* 1996;27:827–833.
201. Paulsen J, Lennert K. Low-grade B-cell lymphoma of mucosa-associated lymphoid tissue type in Waldeyer's ring. *Histopathology* 1994;24:1–11.
202. Wright DH. Lymphomas of Waldeyer's ring. *Histopathology* 1994;24:97–99.
203. Uematsu M, Kondo M, Kiramatsu H, et al. Stage IA non-Hodgkin's lymphoma of the Waldeyer's ring. Limited chemotherapy and radiation therapy versus radiation therapy alone. *Acta Oncol* 1993;32:675–678.

204. Kaur A, Shetty SC, Prasad D, et al. Primary ectopic meningioma of the palatine tonsil—a case report. *J Laryngol Otol* 1997;111:179–181.
205. Sellars SL. Metastatic tumours of the tonsil. *J Laryngol Otol* 1971;85:289–292.
206. Moar E, Tovi F, Sacks M. Carcinoma of the pancreas presenting with bilateral tonsillar metastases. *Ann Otol Rhinol Laryngol* 1983;92: 192–195.
207. Bale PM, Clifton-Bligh P, Benjamin BNP, et al. Pathology of Tangier disease. *J Clin Pathol* 1971;24:609–616.
208. Ferrans VJ, Fredrickson DS. The pathology of Tangier disease. A light and electron microscopic study. *Am J Pathol* 1975;78:101–158.
209. Abramowsky CR. Immunodeficiency disorders. In: Stocker JT, Dehner LP, eds. *Pediatric pathology.* Philadelphia: JB Lippincott, 1992:355–384.

6

ORAL CAVITY AND JAWS

COMMON ODONTOGENIC LESIONS, CYSTS OF THE JAWS, AND ODONTOGENIC TUMORS

DAVID G. GARDNER

The most common odontogenic lesions reviewed by surgical pathologists who receive tissue from oral and maxillofacial surgeons and other dentists are the periapical lesions and dental follicles. The first part of this chapter is concerned with these relatively straightforward specimens.

The cysts of the jaws are divided into two groups, namely those that are derived from odontogenic epithelium (the odontogenic cysts) and those that are not. Until fairly recently, the latter cysts were referred to as fissural cysts because they were thought to be caused by the entrapment of epithelium in embryonal fissures of the orofacial complex. This explanation is no longer accepted, and consequently, these cysts are now referred to simply as nonodontogenic developmental cysts of the jaws (1). The five putative lesions that had been included under "fissural cysts" were the nasopalatine duct (incisive canal) cyst, the nasolabial cyst, the median palatal cyst, the globulomaxillary cyst, and the median mandibular cyst (Fig. 1). Of these, only two, the nasopalatine duct cyst and the nasolabial cyst, are currently accepted as being pathologic entities. The "median palatal cyst" is now recognized as representing a large nasopalatine duct cyst that has extended posteriorly (1), whereas the "globulomaxillary" and "median mandibular" cysts really represent examples of various odontogenic cysts, such as the radicular cyst, odontogenic keratocyst, lateral periodontal cyst, and glandular odontogenic cyst, which happen to be located in the globulomaxillary or median mandibular regions, respectively (2–6). The globulomaxillary fissure was thought to occur between the maxillary lateral incisor and canine teeth, and the so-called globulomaxillary cyst exhibited a characteristic inverted-pear-shaped radiolucency between these two teeth (Fig. 2). However, this radiographic appearance can be caused by various lesions, including odontogenic cysts, certain odontogenic tumors, and giant-cell granulomas.

Apart from the radicular cyst, which is a periapical lesion, the most common and important odontogenic cysts are the dentigerous cyst and odontogenic keratocyst. It is imperative that the latter be correctly diagnosed because it is a destructive lesion, tends to recur, and is the cyst found in the nevoid basal cell carcinoma syndrome. The less common odontogenic cysts are then discussed.

Finally, the odontogenic tumors are described. This is a specialized area, and often it is advisable to consult with an oral and maxillofacial pathologist when attempting to reach the correct diagnosis. The only common odontogenic tumor is the odontoma. Even the ameloblastoma, which is an important lesion and the best-known of the odontogenic tumors, is quite uncommon; the remainder are rare. The classical intraosseous ameloblastoma is a slow-growing invasive tumor that can be quite destructive. It exhibits a high rate of recurrence if not adequately treated and occasionally may kill the patient by direct extension into the cranium. Consequently, considerable emphasis is placed on the biological behavior and differential diagnosis of this tumor. The other odontogenic tumors and related lesions are then described, with care being taken to indicate diagnostic pitfalls.

DENTAL FOLLICLES

Dental follicles are the normal fibrous connective tissue sacs that surround the crowns of unerupted teeth. When an unerupted tooth, frequently a third molar (wisdom tooth), is removed, the surgeon may submit the follicle for pathologic examination, either still attached to the tooth at the cervical line or separately.

The fibrous connective tissue of dental follicles varies somewhat in density. Often present is a considerable amount of ground substance, which stains blue-gray with hematoxylin and eosin (Fig. 3). The sacs may be lined with low columnar cells or cuboidal cells, which represent ameloblasts and other epithelial cells of the enamel organ that have served their function and have become less differentiated (the reduced enamel epithelium) (Fig. 4), or a thin layer of stratified squamous epithelium (7). However, many examples exhibit no epithelial lining, it presumably having remained attached to the enamel of the tooth.

Dental follicles are simple structures. However, several questions may arise. The surgeon may make the clinical diagnosis of dentigerous cyst. The distinction between a dentigerous cyst and a dental follicle is one of size. Dentigerous cysts are derived from dental follicles and therefore have the same microscopic appearance as those follicles that have epithelial linings. If, at gross examination, the lesion is obviously a large sac, the diagnosis of

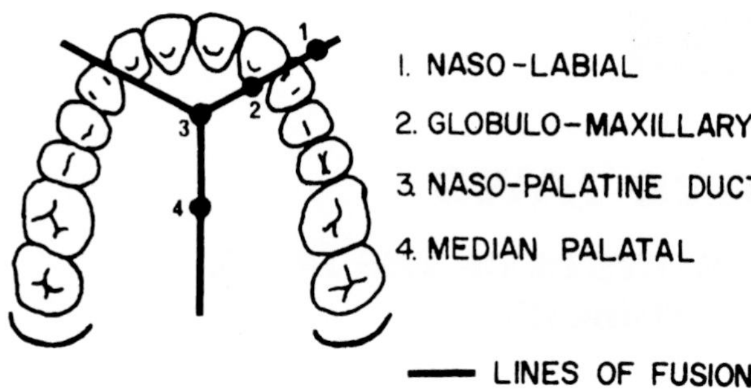

FIGURE 1. Locations of the traditionally described "fissural" cysts of the maxilla. (From Gardner DG, Sapp JP, Wysocki GP. Epithelial cysts of the jaws. *Int Pathol* 1976;17:6–22.)

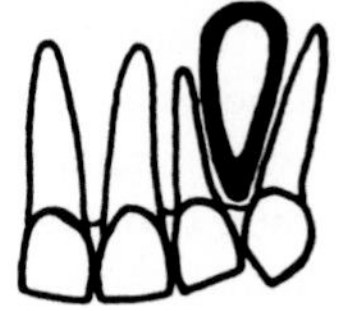

FIGURE 2. The classical pear-shaped appearance of the so-called globulomaxillary cyst. (From Gardner DG, Sapp JP, Wysocki GP. Epithelial cysts of the jaws. *Int Pathol* 1976;17:6–22.)

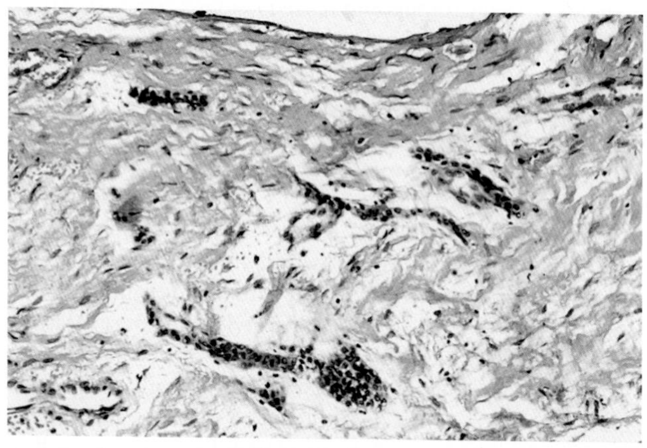

FIGURE 3. Dental follicle. This typical example is composed of loosely arranged connective tissue, a moderate amount of ground substance, and a few rests of odontogenic epithelium.

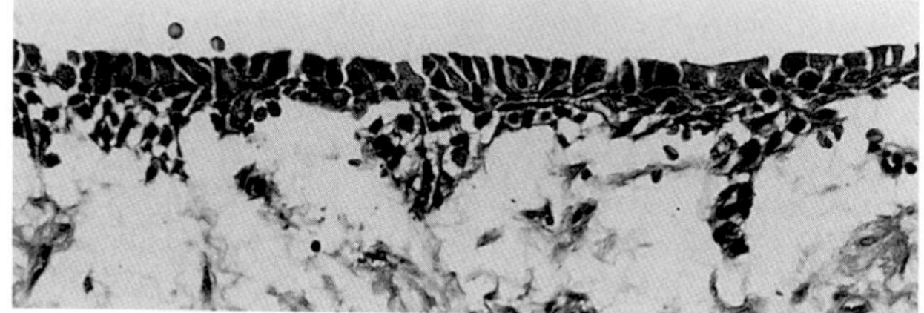

FIGURE 4. Dental follicle. This example is lined with eosinophilic, low cuboidal cells—the reduced enamel epithelium.

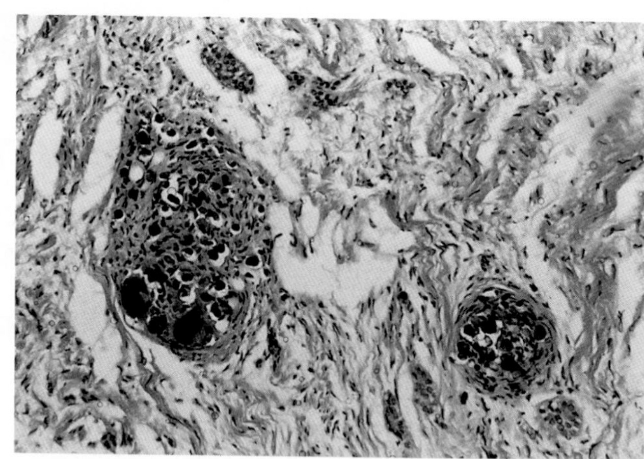

FIGURE 5. Hyperplastic dental follicle of regional odontodysplasia: characteristic whorled structures containing calcifications.

dentigerous cyst is appropriate. However, if the submitted tissue is fragmented or small, then a diagnosis of "consistent with dentigerous cyst or dental follicle" is indicated. The clinician will have to make the definitive diagnosis, based on the clinical and radiologic findings.

Rather uncommonly, the fibrous connective tissue of a dental follicle may become hyperplastic (8). The resulting thickened follicle is apparent radiologically as a radiolucent band around the crown of the tooth, but this appearance is indistinguishable from that of a small dentigerous cyst. Such a lesion is not cystic but exhibits the same microscopic appearance as a normal follicle except that it is enlarged. One problem is the tendency for pathologists to diagnose these hyperplastic follicles as odontogenic fibromas, which are very rare tumors. Histologically they are similar, but odontogenic fibromas are considerably larger lesions than hyperplastic follicles and do not appear as narrow radiolucent bands around the crowns of teeth.

Dental follicles often exhibit a few dormant rests of odontogenic epithelium. Moreover, they sometimes contain a wide variety of other odontogenic structures (7,9) such as numerous or enlarged epithelial rests, calcifications that may be nondescript or resemble cementum, or material that stains positively for amyloid. All of these are simply remnants of odontogenesis. It is important that the examining pathologist not be trapped into mistaking them for an odontogenic tumor. In particular, enlarged or proliferating epithelial rests should not be confused with ameloblastoma.

The dental follicles of a rare developmental condition of teeth, regional odontodysplasia, are often enlarged and exhibit numerous characteristic calcifications (Fig. 5) (10,11). A similar appearance may occur rarely in the follicles of unerupted teeth that are not affected by regional odontodysplasia (12).

PERIAPICAL LESIONS

The three common periapical lesions that the surgical pathologist will encounter are the periapical granuloma, the radicular cyst, including the residual radicular cyst, and the apical scar. Any one of these lesions can also exhibit microscopic evidence of a concomitant abscess.

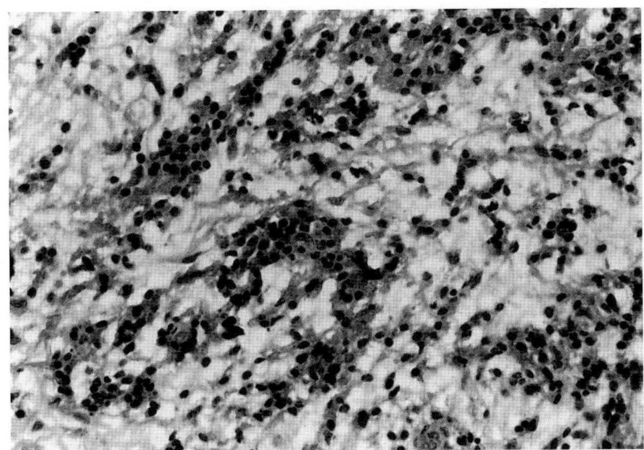

FIGURE 6. Periapical granuloma. Chronically inflamed connective tissue. Some examples are more fibrous.

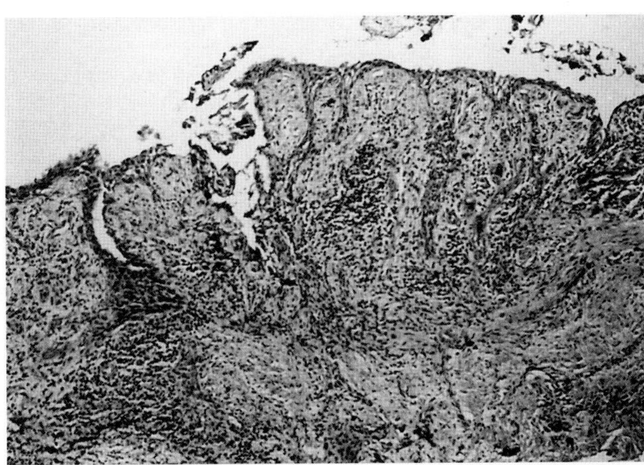

FIGURE 7. Radicular cyst. The epithelial lining is nonkeratinized stratified squamous epithelium with irregular rete ridges. There is an intense chronic inflammatory cell infiltrate in the connective tissue wall of the cyst.

Periapical Granuloma

A periapical granuloma is a mass of chronically inflamed immature connective tissue (Fig. 6) that develops at the apex of a nonvital tooth in reaction to toxins emanating from the pulp canal. Both the periapical granuloma and the radicular cyst *(q.v.)* may be submitted for pathologic examination, either attached to the root of a tooth or separately if the lesion was curetted out or enucleated. Microscopically, it is a simple lesion. Some examples exhibit a relatively dense fibrous connective tissue capsule around the lesional connective tissue, which in turn tends to become more collagenous with time. The inflammatory cell infiltrate consists chiefly of plasma cells and lymphocytes, but some neutrophils and macrophages may be present. Russell bodies are frequently found. Inconstant features include hemosiderin, cholesterol crystal clefts, and epithelium that is derived from odontogenic rests of the periodontal ligament (the rests of Malassez). The epithelium quite commonly proliferates within the granuloma, but the diagnosis of radicular cyst should be made only if an epithelial-lined lumen is present. Some granulomas are curetted out during the surgical removal of the apex of a tooth (apicoectomy), in which case small pieces of dentin or bone fragments may be present. Dark brown granular deposits may also be found. They represent either dental amalgam or root canal sealer, both of which are used in endodontic procedures. A periapical granuloma that has been removed requires no further treatment.

Radicular Cyst (Periapical Cyst)

Radicular cysts develop from periapical granulomas, and, consequently, the two lesions share many microscopic features. A cyst occurs when the inflammatory process stimulates the epithelium within a granuloma to proliferate and the central part of that epithelial proliferation subsequently degenerates.

At gross examination it is often apparent that the lesion is a cyst, but this is not true if a small cyst is included within a granuloma or if the tissue is submitted in fragments. A mature radicular cyst consists of a fibrous connective tissue wall surrounding a central lumen, which is lined by stratified squamous epithelium; the wall of the cyst usually exhibits a chronic inflammatory cell infiltrate. Characteristically, the epithelial lining is irregular (Fig. 7) and, in inflamed areas, may have proliferated quite markedly. It is important that this irregular epithelial proliferation not be mistaken for a plexiform ameloblastoma *(q.v.)*, as has occasionally occurred. A flat epithelial–connective tissue interface may also occur in radicular cysts, usually in longstanding lesions in which there is no longer any inflammation present (Fig. 8). Cholesterol crystal clefts with associated multinucleated giant cells are common (Fig. 9). Rushton (hyaline) bodies are eosinophilic, hyalinized structures that occur quite frequently as incidental findings in the epithelial lining of radicular cysts (Fig. 10); their origin is controversial. Less frequently, mucous cells and/or ciliated epithelium may be present, illustrating the potential of odontogenic epithelium to form a wide variety of structures; they do not affect the diagnosis or biological behavior.

Sometimes it may be difficult to decide whether a specific specimen represents an incipient radicular cyst or a periapical granuloma exhibiting epithelial proliferation. It is better to confine the diagnosis of radicular cyst to those lesions that exhibit cystic lumina. Clinicians like to know whether they were dealing with a radicular cyst or a periapical granuloma. However, once the lesion has been removed, this distinction is not important because no further treatment is indicated.

Residual Cyst (Residual Radicular Cyst)

The term *residual cyst* theoretically could apply to any cyst that remains in the jaw after the surgical removal of the associated

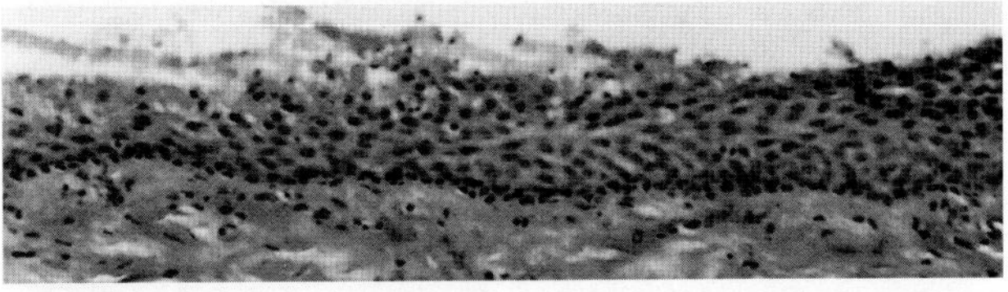

FIGURE 8. Radicular cyst. This example exhibits no inflammation, and consequently the interface of the epithelium and connective tissue is flat. See also Fig. 12.

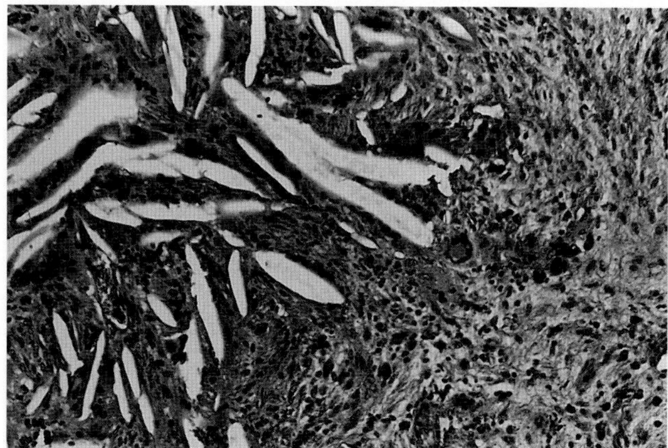

FIGURE 9. Radicular cyst. Cholesterol crystal clefts with associated multinucleated giant cells. This feature also occurs in periapical granulomas.

tooth, but in practice, it refers to a residual radicular cyst. Consequently, its microscopic features are those of that lesion. In longstanding examples, the inflammatory cell infiltrate may be much less intense than in most radicular cysts, and the epithelial–connective tissue interface consequently flat.

Lateral Radicular Cyst (Lateral Granuloma)

Lesions that are microscopically identical to periapical cysts and granulomas sometimes occur on the lateral surfaces of the roots of nonvital teeth. They originate from the openings of accessory pulp canals.

Apical Scar

After an apicoectomy (the surgical removal of the apical portion of a tooth that has had its root canal obliterated therapeutically), the resulting bony defect is usually replaced by new bone. However, sometimes the defect remains as a periapical radiolucency. Clinicians tend to reoperate in this situation, even if the patient is symptomless. The resulting tissue may represent a radicular cyst or periapical granuloma if the original root canal therapy was unsuccessful. However, more often it consists of scar tissue (Fig. 11), which may exhibit a few chronic inflammatory cells and perhaps brownish granular material that represents amalgam or root canal sealer used in the apicoectomy. These lesions should be diagnosed as apical scars.

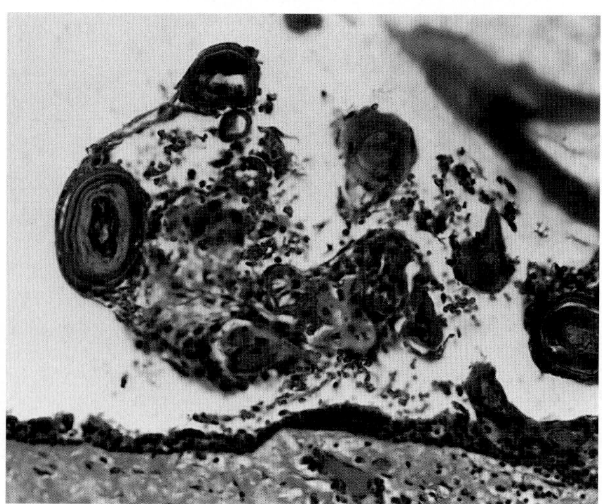

FIGURE 10. Radicular cyst. Rushton (hyaline) bodies.

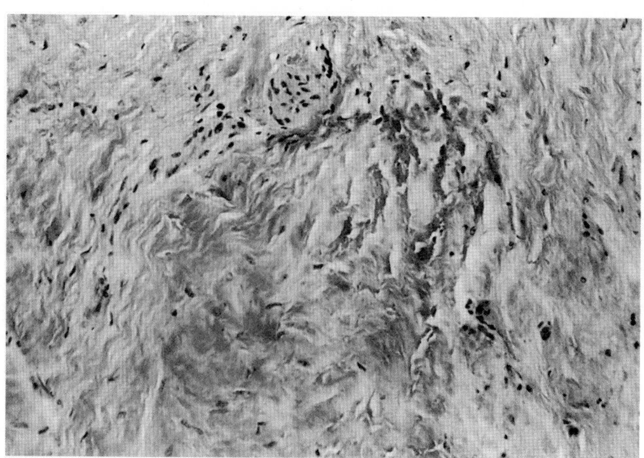

FIGURE 11. Apical scar. Dense fibrous connective tissue.

Three Other Pertinent Conditions

There are three other inflammatory lesions with which the surgical pathologist who receives tissue from dentists should be familiar because they are closely related to the disorders of the teeth and supporting structures. Moreover, they enter into the differential diagnosis of the lesions just discussed. They are pericoronitis, gingivitis and periodontitis, and the parulis.

Pericoronitis

Pericoronitis is inflammation of the flap of tissue that partially covers the crown of an incompletely erupted tooth, most commonly a mandibular third molar. Patients in their late teens and early twenties frequently have these teeth removed because of

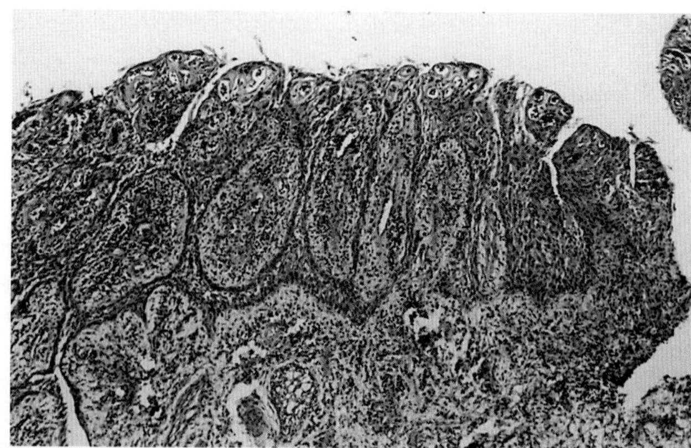

FIGURE 12. Pericoronitis. Stratified squamous epithelium with irregular rete ridges and chronically inflamed connective tissue. This appearance also occurs in radicular cysts, inflamed developmental cysts such as dentigerous cysts, gingivitis, and periodontitis.

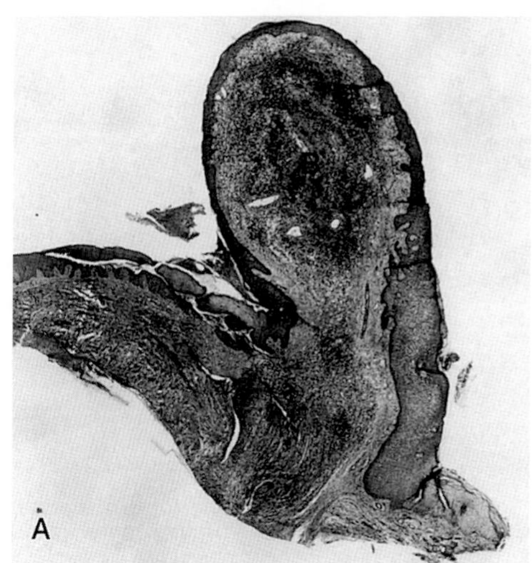

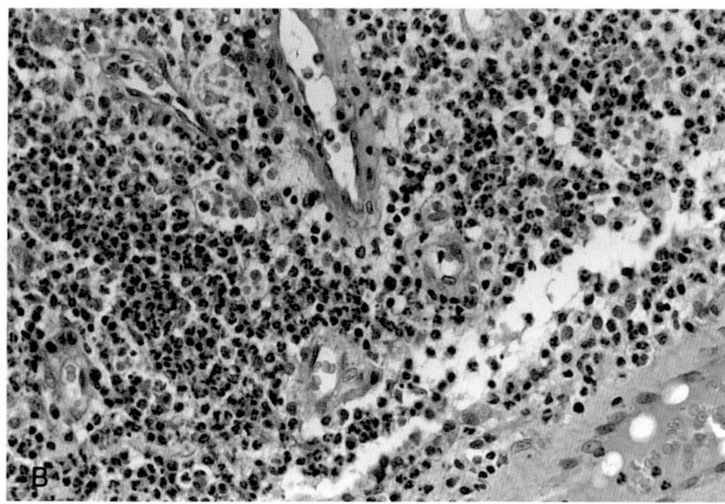

FIGURE 13. Parulis. **A:** A typical example, although the sinus tract (fistula) is not as evident as is sometimes the case. **B:** The area marked *B* in **A** illustrates the intense inflammatory cell infiltrate.

pericoronitis, and the resulting soft tissue may be submitted for pathologic examination. Pericoronitis is really an inflamed dental follicle, and its microscopic appearance is therefore identical to that of a small inflamed dentigerous cyst (Fig. 12), except that often the overlying mucosal epithelium is also present.

Gingivitis and Periodontitis

The distinction between gingivitis and periodontitis is a clinical one. *Gingivitis* refers to inflammation that is confined to the gingiva, whereas *periodontitis* is used when the alveolar bone, periodontal ligament, or cementum is also involved. Sometimes inflamed gingiva is submitted for pathologic examination, but there is little one can do but confirm the clinician's diagnosis. Pathologists should not make the diagnosis of the more advanced lesion, periodontitis, because they do not know if the extent of the lesion justifies it. Tissue curetted from a periodontal pocket consists of delicate epithelium (the crevicular epithelium) and inflamed connective tissue. Consequently, it exhibits the same histologic features as fragments of radicular cysts, inflamed dentigerous cysts, and pericoronitis. The inflammatory cell infiltrate is usually chronic, originates near the crevicular epithelium, and varies in intensity. The cells are lymphocytes and plasma cells with occasional neutrophils near the crevicular epithelium. Some examples exhibit a very intense plasma cell infiltrate, which superficially resembles plasmacytoma. On close examination this infiltrate will be found to be mixed. Immunocytochemistry can be used to demonstrate its polyclonal nature but is rarely necessary. A dense plasma cell infiltrate may also be associated with the specific entity *plasma cell gingivitis* (13), which clinically appears as an erythematous gingivostomatitis and is associated with hypersensitivity to various agents found in chewing gums, toothpaste, and so on. Cinnamon is a major offender. The clinical findings of severe erythema and the history aid in the differential diagnosis. Quite commonly, gingival specimens exhibit odontogenic rests, dystrophic calcifications, and other products of odontogenesis. These are simply incidental findings.

Parulis

This lesion, which is the layman's gum boil, represents the opening of a sinus tract originating from an infected tooth or a periodontal pocket, surrounded by a small elevated mass of inflamed granulation tissue (Fig. 13). It is occasionally submitted for pathologic examination if the clinician does not recognize it. A central sinus tract is sometimes evident microscopically, establishing the diagnosis. It is seldom lined by epithelium, but that part adjacent to the orifice rarely may be. In many examples no real tract is evident microscopically at the time of examination. Similar lesions may occur on the facial skin if an odontogenic infection points percutaneously, although that situation is uncommon.

NONODONTOGENIC DEVELOPMENTAL CYSTS OF THE JAWS

These are the cysts that were formerly referred to as "fissural cysts." As discussed at the beginning of this chapter, that term is no longer considered appropriate.

Nasopalatine Duct (Incisive Canal) Cyst

Nasopalatine duct cysts (14,15) are quite common lesions that appear as well-circumscribed round, oval, or heart-shaped radi-

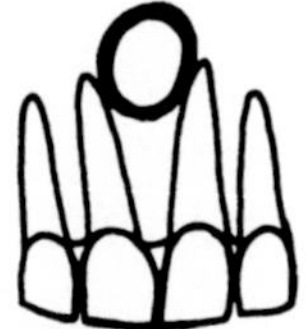

NASO-PALATINE DUCT CYST

FIGURE 14. The typical location of the nasopalatine duct cyst. (From Gardner DG, Sapp JP, Wysocki GP. Epithelial cysts of the jaws. *Int Pathol* 1976;17:6–22.)

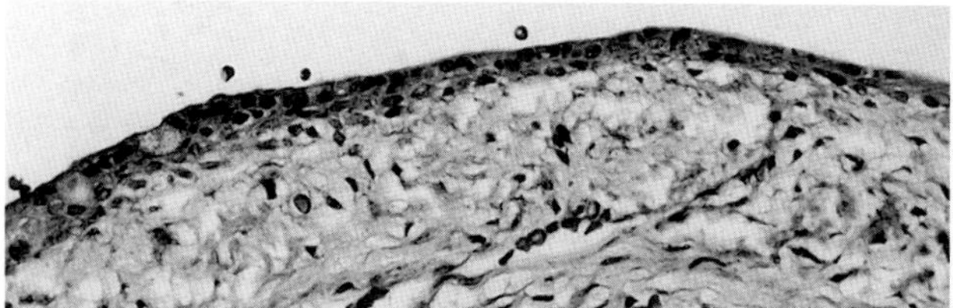

FIGURE 15. Nasopalatine duct cyst. This field exhibits a double layer of cuboidal epithelium with an occasional mucous cell.

olucencies between the apices of the permanent maxillary central incisors (Fig. 14). Their development is related to the persistence within the incisive canals of remnants of the paired embryonic nasopalatine ducts that normally become obliterated during embryogenesis. Many are asymptomatic, being discovered on routine radiographic examination, but most are associated with pain and swelling of the anterior palate. They are somewhat more common in men than in women, and, although they occur over a wide age range, they are most common in the fourth to sixth decades.

A few nasopalatine duct cysts occur completely within the soft tissue around the incisive papilla, a soft tissue elevation located immediately palatal to the maxillary central incisors. They appear as inflammatory swellings of that region, are not evident radiographically, and are referred to as cysts of the incisive papilla.

Nasopalatine duct cysts are generally received in the pathology laboratory in fragments. They are lined by stratified squamous, cuboidal, or pseudostratified columnar epithelium or, commonly, some combination of these types (Fig. 15). Mucous cells are common in the lining (Fig. 16). Most are inflamed. Characteristically, mucous glands and relatively large blood vessels and nerves, representing the contents of the incisive canal, are present within the connective tissue (Fig. 17). An embryologic cartilaginous rest, a common structure in this region, may also be present and should not be mistaken for a tumor.

One lesion that may have to be distinguished microscopically from the nasopalatine duct cyst is the radicular cyst. The latter does not exhibit the blood vessels, nerves, and mucous glands that are present in many nasopalatine duct cysts. The epithelial lining of the two cysts also usually differs. The radicular cyst is

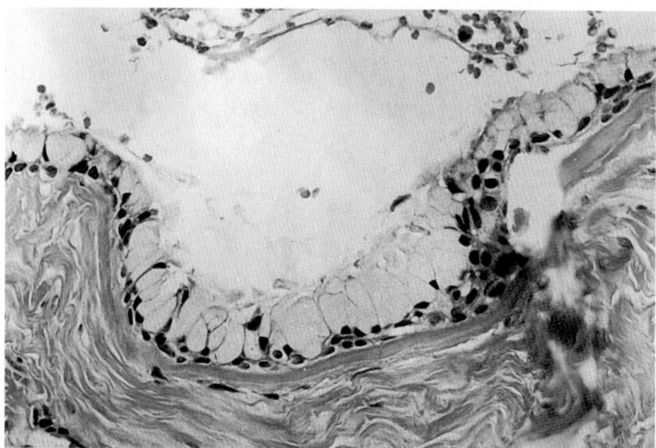

FIGURE 16. Nasopalatine duct cyst. The lining in this field consists predominantly of mucous cells.

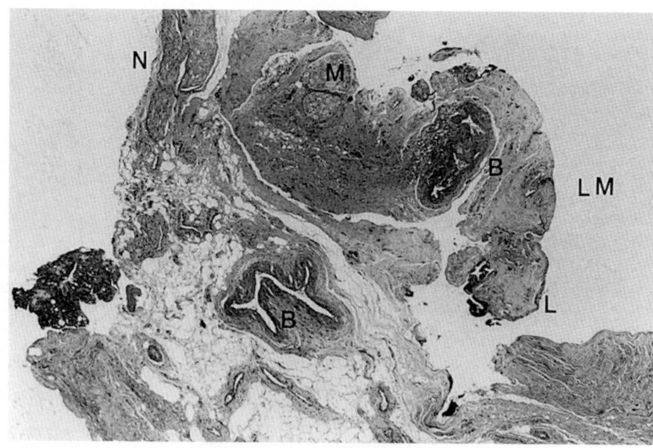

FIGURE 17. Nasopalatine duct cyst showing some of the anatomic features found variably in specimens of this cyst. *B*, prominent blood vessels; *M*, mucous glands; *N*, prominent nerve; *LM*, lumen; *L*, epithelial lining.

lined by stratified squamous epithelium with irregular rete ridges. It may exhibit mucous cells within the lining but not true glands within the connective tissue.

There are also certain clinical features that help to distinguish between the two cysts. The pulps of the central incisors adjacent to a nasopalatine duct cyst are usually vital, whereas the pulp of a tooth that is associated with a radicular cyst is not. Moreover, changing the angulation at which the periapical radiographs are taken can demonstrate that a nasopalatine duct cyst is not intimately associated with the apex of a tooth, as in the case of a radicular cyst.

Nasopalatine duct cysts are usually curetted because they are difficult to enucleate. They seldom recur.

Nasolabial (Nasoalveolar) Cyst

Nasolabial cysts (16) (Fig. 18) occur as soft tissue swellings below and lateral to the ala of the nose and may partially obliterate the nasolabial fossa, distorting the nostril. They are rare, more common in women than in men, and most occur in the fourth and fifth decades of life. They probably arise from the inferior part of the nasolacrimal duct. The synonym, nasoalveolar cyst, is inappropriate because these cysts do not involve the alveolar process.

They are most commonly lined by pseudostratified columnar epithelium, often with mucous cells and cilia (Fig. 19), but stratified squamous or cuboidal epithelium may be present.

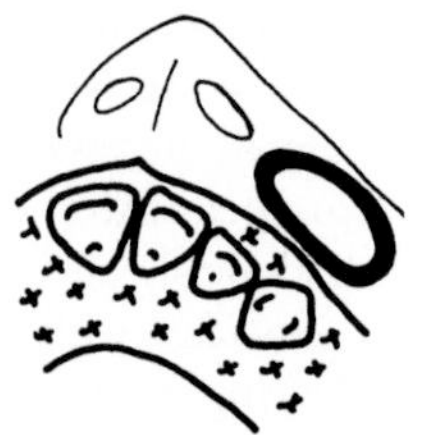

FIGURE 18. The typical location of the nasolabial cyst. (From Gardner DG, Sapp JP, Wysocki GP. Epithelial cysts of the jaws. *Int Pathol* 1976; 17:6–22.)

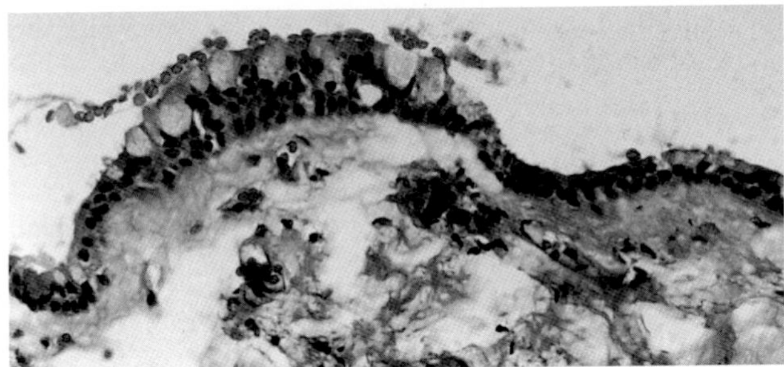

FIGURE 19. Nasolabial cyst. Pseudostratified columnar epithelium with mucous cells.

Inflammation is variable, depending on whether the cyst has become infected.

Nasolabial cysts are usually enucleated from an intraoral approach; they seldom recur.

ODONTOGENIC CYSTS

This is the correct term for the group of cysts that arise from odontogenic epithelium. However, errors in nomenclature occur, as in the use of *dentigerous cyst* and *dental cyst* as synonyms for *odontogenic cyst. Dentigerous cyst* is the most common designation for a specific odontogenic cyst, and *dental cyst* is a synonym for radicular cyst.

The odontogenic cysts (1,17–19) are all true cysts; that is, they are pathologic cavities that are lined by epithelium. As can be seen from the 1992 World Health Organization's classification of epithelial cysts of the jaws (Table 1), they are divided into developmental and inflammatory cysts. The most common inflammatory cyst, the radicular cyst and its variants, has already been discussed. This section therefore concentrates on the developmental odontogenic cysts and the two remaining inflammatory odontogenic cysts.

TABLE 1. THE 1992 WORLD HEALTH ORGANIZATION'S HISTOLOGIC TYPING OF CYSTS OF THE JAWS

Developmental
Odontogenic
"Gingival cysts" of infants (Epstein pearls)
Odontogenic keratocyst (primordial cyst)
Dentigerous (follicular) cyst
Eruption cyst
Lateral periodontal cyst
Gingival cyst of adults
Glandular odontogenic cyst; sialo-odontogenic cyst
Nonodontogenic
Nasopalatine duct (incisive canal) cyst
Nasolabial (nasoalveolar) cyst
Inflammatory
Radicular cyst
Apical and lateral
Residual
Paradental (inflammatory collateral, mandibular infected buccal) cyst

Source: Kramer IRH, Pindborg JJ, Shear M. *Histological typing of odontogenic tumours, 2nd ed.* Berlin: Springer-Verlag, 1992.

As a group, cysts of the jaw are common lesions, but the prevalence of the separate entities varies greatly, from the very common radicular and dentigerous cysts to such rare entities as the developmental lateral periodontal cyst and the glandular odontogenic cyst. Their accurate diagnosis is important because of the significant differences in their clinical behaviors. It is especially important to identify the quite common odontogenic keratocyst because it can destroy a significant amount of bone, frequently recurs, and is a component of the nevoid basal cell carcinoma syndrome. Similarly, the glandular odontogenic cyst must be diagnosed accurately because of its destructive nature and marked tendency to recur. However, it is a very rare lesion.

Some cysts of the jaw are sufficiently characteristic, microscopically, to permit their diagnosis on that basis alone. This is true of the odontogenic keratocyst and the glandular odontogenic cyst. In general, however, it is important to consider the clinical and especially the radiologic findings before making a definitive diagnosis. In this connection, the exact location of the cyst within the jaws and its relationship to the teeth is most important (Fig. 20). The radiographs that give the most detailed information are periapical and occlusal films. Panoramic radiographs are superior to the standard head plates for providing examination of the jaws from one temporomandibular joint to the other, although they provide less detail than do the intraoral films.

Inflammatory Odontogenic Cysts

Of the inflammatory odontogenic cysts, only the paradental cyst remains to be discussed. There is a possibility of confusion in terminology here. The lesion described below as the *inflammatory lateral periodontal cyst* coincides with the lesion listed in the WHO classification as the *paradental cyst.* However, the lesion described here as *Craig's paradental cyst* is the one that many workers refer to simply as the *paradental cyst.* This latter cyst is discussed in the WHO classification as a variant of paradental cyst.

Inflammatory Lateral Periodontal Cyst

An inflammatory cyst similar in all respects to the lateral radicular cyst occurs rather uncommonly in the periodontal ligament of a vital tooth. It arises from a periodontal pocket and is usually located near the cervical line of the tooth. In contrast, the lateral radicular cyst generally occurs closer to the apex of a tooth but can occur at any level of the periodontal ligament. The inflammatory lateral periodontal cyst should not be confused with the developmental lateral periodontal cyst *(q.v.).*

Craig's Paradental Cyst (Paradental Cyst)

This term has been used for an uncommon inflammatory cyst (20,21) that exhibits the same microscopic features as a radicular cyst but that occurs on the buccal or distal surface of a partially erupted mandibular third molar. It appears to be an extension of pericoronitis, but it could be considered a variant of dentigerous cyst. The mandibular infected buccal cyst (22) mentioned in the

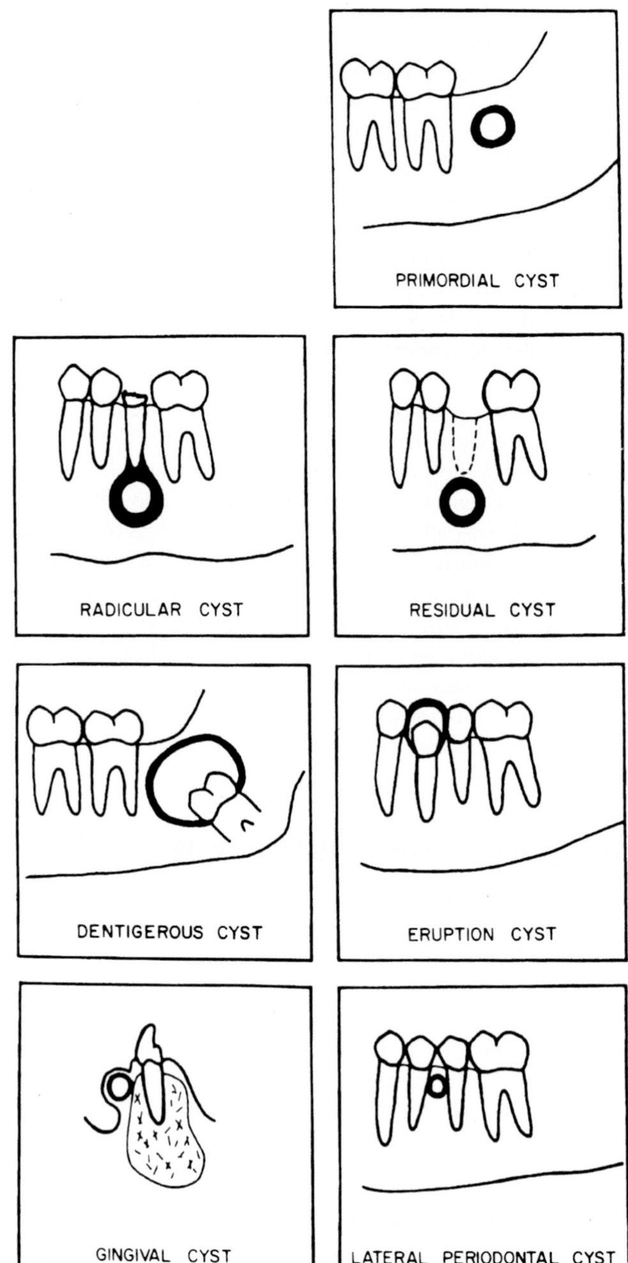

FIGURE 20. Diagrams illustrating typical locations of odontogenic cysts. That of the primordial cyst illustrates the original concept of its forming instead of a tooth. (From Gardner DG, Sapp JP, Wysocki GP. Epithelial cysts of the jaws. *Int Pathol* 1976;17:6–22.)

WHO classification (1) is a similar lesion that occurs on the buccal surfaces of the mandibular first molars in children aged 6 to 8 years. It is not widely recognized.

Developmental Odontogenic Cysts

One way to discuss these cysts would be to follow the list in the WHO classification (Table 1) (1). However, two of these, the dentigerous cyst and the odontogenic keratocyst, are far more important than the others because of their frequency and their biological behavior and will therefore be discussed first.

Dentigerous (Follicular) Cyst

The dentigerous cyst, the most common of the developmental odontogenic cysts, develops by the accumulation of fluid within the follicular space of an unerupted tooth after its crown has fully formed. Consequently, it is always attached to the cervical line of the tooth, that is, where the enamel of the crown joins the cementum of the root (Fig. 20). This association is referred to as the dentigerous relationship in discussions of the anatomic relationship of any tumor or cyst to a specific tooth.

Dentigerous cysts occur almost exclusively in the permanent dentition, most commonly in association with mandibular and maxillary third molars (the wisdom teeth), the maxillary canines, and the mandibular premolars, these teeth being the ones that most frequently fail to erupt. This failure to erupt is often because the involved tooth is also impacted, that is, physically prevented from erupting, possibly by an adjacent tooth. Dentigerous cysts usually occur in the second or third decades and are found in both sexes. Small cysts usually exhibit no clinical symptoms, but the less common larger ones cause bony expansion. Radiographically, dentigerous cysts appear as well-circumscribed, usually unilocular, radiolucencies that surround the crowns of the unerupted teeth and demonstrate the dentigerous relationship. The unerupted tooth is often displaced markedly within the jaw by the cyst. This radiographic appearance is not pathognomic of dentigerous cysts, although they are by far the most common lesions to exhibit it; the odontogenic keratocyst and certain odontogenic tumors may have a similar appearance.

A dentigerous cyst may be submitted to the pathology service as a membranous sac or in fragments. If the involved tooth is also submitted, the dentigerous relationship of the cyst to the tooth's cervical line will be readily apparent. One reason for submitting an apparent dentigerous cyst for pathologic examination is to rule out the presence of a unicystic ameloblastoma, and it is therefore important that any nodule that extends into the lumen be examined microscopically; otherwise, representative sections of the cyst should be taken.

Dentigerous cysts are typically lined by nonkeratinizing stratified squamous epithelium, which varies in thickness (Fig. 21); in noninflamed examples, it may be only two or three cells thick. The interface of the epithelium and the connective tissue is flat unless inflammation causes the epithelium to proliferate as irreg-

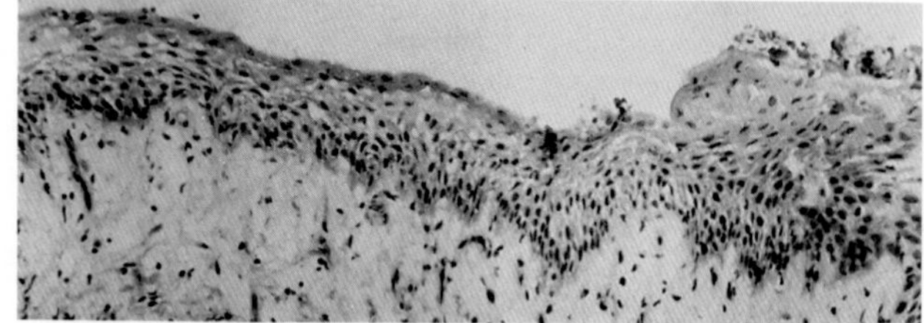

FIGURE 21. Dentigerous cyst. Typical lining consisting of nonkeratinized stratified squamous epithelium.

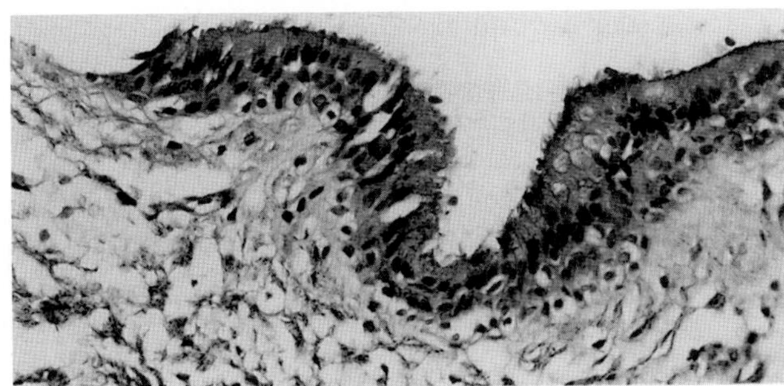

FIGURE 22. Dentigerous cyst. Occasionally dentigerous cysts may be lined partially or wholly by pseudostratified columnar epithelium with cilia and mucous cells.

ular rete ridges. When this happens, the microscopic appearance is similar to that of a radicular cyst. The fibrous connective tissue resembles that of a dental follicle in that it often exhibits abundant ground substance. Mucous cells occur quite commonly in the epithelial lining, with ciliated and sebaceous cells being less common histologic variants (Fig. 22). As in dental follicles, various remnants of odontogenesis such as calcifications (Fig. 23), amyloid-like material, enamel matrix, and reduced enamel epithelium may sometimes occur within the fibrous capsules of dentigerous cysts. Rarely a nodule that resembles adenomatoid odontogenic tumor *(q.v.)* occurs within the epithelial lining. It is debatable whether it should be considered an incipient tumor or an incidental finding.

One potentially important diagnostic problem concerns the presence of rests of odontogenic epithelium within the fibrous capsule (Fig. 24). These structures occur commonly as an incidental finding. However, they may become hyperplastic, and it is then important not to diagnose them as ameloblastoma *(q.v.)*. It is best to be cautious in this regard and, if there is any doubt, to seek consultation with a pathologist who is experienced with odontogenic lesions.

The diagnosis of a dentigerous cyst depends on both the clinical and microscopic findings. The relationship of the cyst lining to the cervical line of the tooth is all-important. Clinicians tend to submit unenlarged dental follicles for pathologic examination with the clinical diagnosis of dentigerous cyst. If an epithelial lining is present, the only way of distinguishing between the two is by size, a dentigerous cyst being a cyst of a dental follicle.

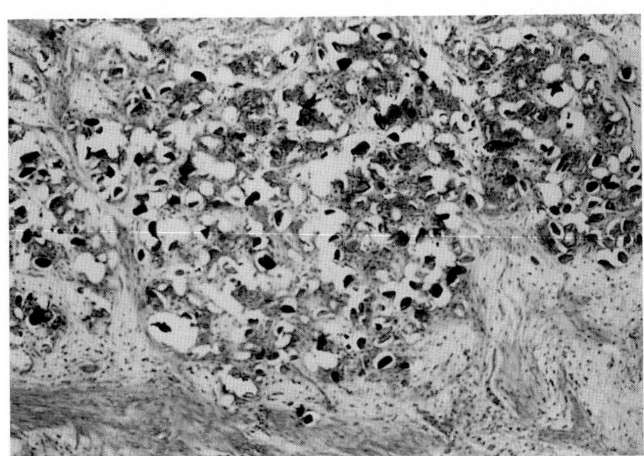

FIGURE 23. Calcifications in the wall of a dentigerous cyst.

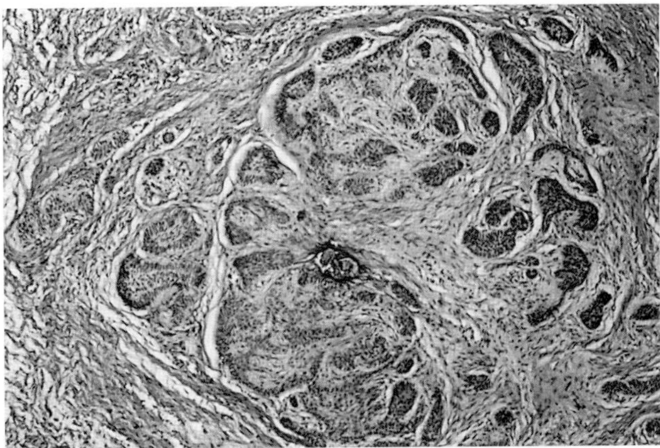

FIGURE 24. An unusually florid example of epithelial rests within the wall of a dentigerous cyst. A small calcification is also present.

The distinction microscopically between a dentigerous cyst and an odontogenic keratocyst, while important, is not usually difficult because the latter has a pathognomic microscopic appearance. Dentigerous cysts seldom exhibit keratinization. When they do (Fig. 25), they should be diagnosed as such, not as odontogenic keratocysts. It has been suggested that the very rare squamous cell carcinomas that occur in dentigerous cysts (Fig. 26) are found mainly in those examples that exhibit keratinization, but this hypothesis has yet to be confirmed.

An important lesion that must be distinguished from a dentigerous cyst is the relatively uncommon unicystic ameloblastoma *(q.v.)*. Although it is often stated that ameloblastomas may arise in preexisting dentigerous cysts, it is possible that some or even all unicystic ameloblastomas are really neoplastic from inception. This is an unsolved academic question. Of more significance, all putative dentigerous cysts should be examined microscopically for the presence of ameloblastoma *(q.v.)*.

The major significance of dentigerous cysts is that they may be quite destructive and displace teeth. They are usually treated by curettage or enucleation, sometimes after so-called marsupialization, and seldom recur. The presence of unicystic ameloblastoma in putative dentigerous cysts and the development of squamous cell carcinoma have already been mentioned. Both are rare. One possible explanation for the source of the rare intraosseous mucoepidermoid carcinoma is the presence of mucous cells in the lining of some dentigerous cysts.

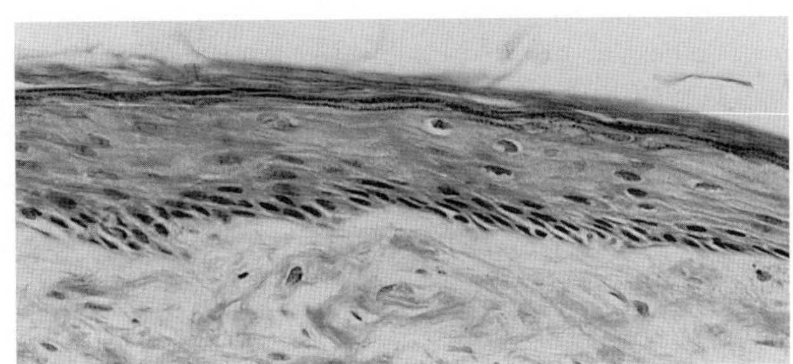

FIGURE 25. Dentigerous cyst lined by orthokeratin.

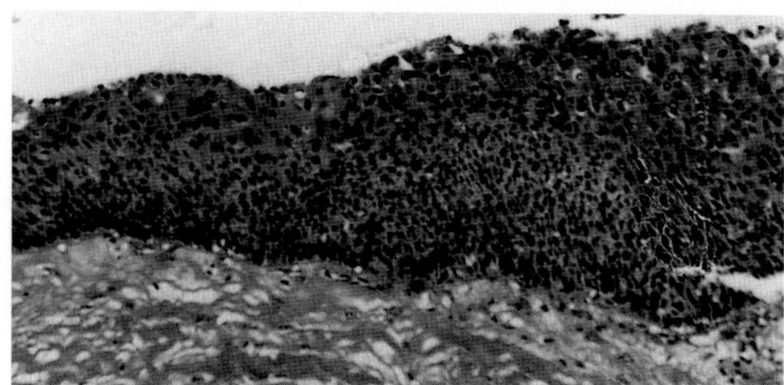

FIGURE 26. Dentigerous cyst exhibiting epithelial dysplasia.

Eruption Cyst

The eruption cyst (Fig. 20) is a variant of dentigerous cyst that is caused by the accumulation of fluid within the follicle of an erupting tooth that is having difficulty breaking through the overlying connective tissue. It is therefore found only in children and adolescents and generally appears as a bluish, fluctuant swelling over the crown of the involved tooth. Some examples contain blood and are termed eruption hematomas. These cysts require no treatment because the involved teeth gradually erupt through them; occasionally the clinician lances them to expedite the process.

Eruption cysts are seldom submitted for pathologic examination. When they are, it is usually only the roof of the cyst that is received. The microscopic appearance of such specimens consists of stratified squamous epithelium from the oral mucosa, a generally inflamed lamina propria, and, at the deep surface of the specimen, a cystic lining similar to that of any dentigerous cyst.

Odontogenic Keratocyst

This quite common lesion (23–26), with its distinctive microscopic features, is important because it can be very destructive, tends to recur, and is a basic component of the nevoid basal cell carcinoma syndrome. Unfortunately, there has been considerable confusion as to the relationship between odontogenic keratocysts (OKC) and the so-called primordial cyst.

The original concept of a primordial cyst was of a developmental odontogenic cyst that arose from degeneration of the enamel organ before any dental hard tissues had formed; it was, therefore, believed to develop instead of a tooth. Consequently, this diagnosis was made whenever a cyst occurred in a region of the jaws where a tooth was developmentally missing, frequently in the mandibular third molar region (Fig. 20). Some clinicians still use the term *primordial cyst* in this manner.

In 1956, the term *odontogenic keratocyst* was introduced for any odontogenic cyst that exhibited keratinization, but it was soon restricted to those cysts that exhibited the specific microscopic features described below. There has been some reluctance to drop the designation *primordial cyst,* and some workers have continued to use it as a synonym for OKC. It is used in this manner in the 1992 WHO classification (1), although there OKC is considered the preferred term. This continued use of "primordial cyst" has been justified because the OKC is believed to originate from the dental lamina, which, in turn, is the primordium of teeth.

The situation can be summarized as follows:

- Not all OKCs develop instead of a tooth.
- Cysts that arise in the developmental absence of a tooth, in my experience, exhibit the microscopic features of OKCs (27).
- There is no justification for considering the primordial cyst to be a pathologic entity distinct from OKC, and the term "primordial cyst" should consequently be abandoned.
- An odontogenic cyst that merely exhibits keratinization is not necessarily an OKC; the specific microscopic features of that lesion have to be present to justify that diagnosis.

This last point is important because it addresses an area where there has been considerable confusion. The OKC is a specific pathologic entity with specific microscopic features (Fig. 27) and specific biological behavior. Certain odontogenic cysts, notably the dentigerous cyst and the radicular cyst, may occasionally exhibit foci of keratinization. This does not, however, justify their being diagnosed as OKCs.

Odontogenic keratocysts are somewhat less common than dentigerous cysts and much less so than radicular cysts. They occur over a wide age range, with a peak incidence in the second and third decades, and are rather more common in men than women. Although they occur in any part of the jaws, they are approximately twice as common in the mandible than the maxilla. The single most common site is the posterior part of the mandible, including the ascending ramus. They are usually solitary lesions. The nevoid basal cell carcinoma syndrome should be considered seriously if the patient has multiple OKCs, either concurrently or over the years, or if there is a familial history of cysts of the jaws. Odontogenic keratocysts are usually symptomless, partly because they tend to grow anteroposteriorly rather than causing expansion of the jaws. An important point is that radiographically they may mimic any other cyst of the jaws, including the appearance that is associated with the lesions previously called "globulomaxillary" and "median mandibular" cysts.

An intact OKC is a typical sac, but the specimen may be submitted to the pathology laboratory in fragments, mainly because the lining of OKCs is often very thin and consequently tears readily. A clue at surgery, or at gross examination, that the lesion may be an OKC is the presence within the lumen of abundant caseous material, which on microscopic examination proves to be keratin. In those OKCs that resemble dentigerous cysts clinically or radiologically, the cyst is generally not attached to the tooth in the dentigerous relationship. Instead, it surrounds the

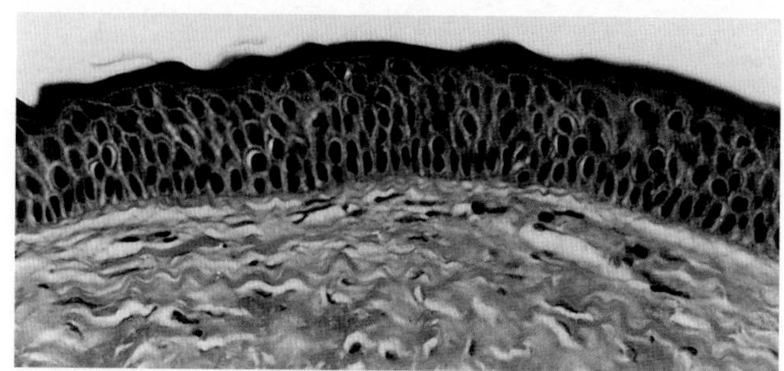

FIGURE 27. Typical odontogenic keratocyst exhibiting a corrugated parakeratinized surface. In some examples the nuclei of the basal cells are more markedly hyperchromatic.

crown of the tooth without actually being attached to it. The microscopic features of the OKC are characteristic (Fig. 27), although they can be altered by inflammation if the cyst is infected (Fig. 28). They consist of (a) a lining of stratified squamous epithelium, six to eight cells thick, that exhibits a flat interface with the underlying connective tissue, (b) a prominent cuboidal basal cell layer with hyperchromatic nuclei, (c) a corrugated (undulated) surface layer of parakeratin, (d) a thin connective tissue wall, especially in the larger cysts, and (e) an uninflamed connective tissue wall, unless the cyst has become infected.

These microscopic features are so characteristic that the diagnosis of a typical OKC should not be a problem. Two aspects that may cause difficulty, however, are the so-called orthokeratinized variant (28) and the presence of epithelial proliferation that superficially resembles ameloblastoma. In addition to exhibiting orthokeratinization, the "orthokeratinized variant" lacks the prominent basal cell layer that is characteristic of OKCs. Moreover, it is less destructive, does not tend to recur, and is not found in the nevoid basal cell carcinoma syndrome. There is no general agreement, but it is probably best to consider this lesion as a nonspecific one, that is, as an odontogenic cyst that happens to exhibit an orthokeratinized lining rather than as an OKC, which is a pathologic entity. Most of the former are probably dentigerous cysts; a few appear to be radicular or residual cysts. The second potential diagnostic problem is that some OKCs exhibit focal proliferation of the lining epithelium into the underlying connective tissue (referred to as "budding") whereas others exhibit microcysts (daughter cysts) (Fig. 29), which are often keratinized, within the wall. It is important not to mistake these histologic variations for ameloblastoma. Authentic ameloblastomas have been reported in OKCs, but exceedingly rarely.

The definitive diagnosis of an OKC is established by microscopic examination. However, two tests have been advocated for the preoperative evaluation of suspected OKCs, although they are not widely used. The first is electrophoresis of the cystic fluid, because that of OKC contains considerably less protein than those of other cysts of the jaws. The second involves the cytologic examination of smears obtained from the cystic fluid: the presence of epithelial squames is strongly suggestive of OKC.

Odontogenic keratocysts may destroy a considerable amount of bone, although some remain quite small. They may be unilocular or multilocular and rarely may extend into the adjacent soft tissues. Treatment is basically enucleation, but some extensive examples may require resection of part of the jaw. They have a marked tendency to recur, the rate varying in different series. The recurrence rate appears to be decreasing as surgeons modify their treatment based on increased recognition of the biological behavior of these cysts. A reasonable estimate of the recurrence rate at present is 30%. Recurrence is thought to be caused by the proliferation of rests of dental lamina adjacent to the original cyst. Moreover, remnants of the original cyst may remain after curettage because the lining is often friable and therefore difficult to remove completely. Many surgeons now advocate the use of cautery of the surgical cavity, especially with Carnoy's fluid, or removal of bone from that site with a burr (peripheral ostectomy) in an attempt to avoid recurrence. Long-term follow-up of the surgical site, for at least 5 years, is advisable.

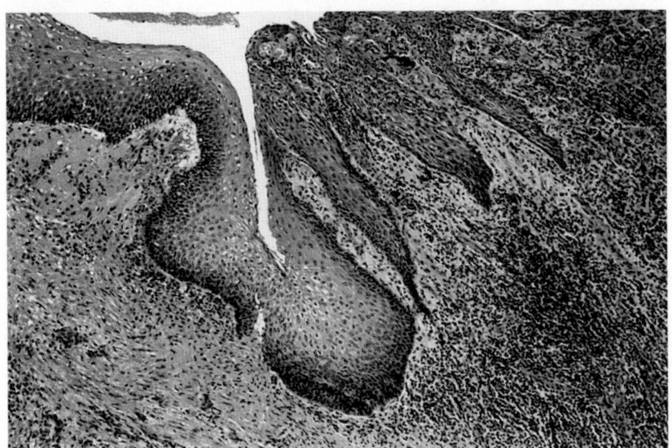

FIGURE 28. Odontogenic keratocyst. The typical microscopic features have been altered by inflammation.

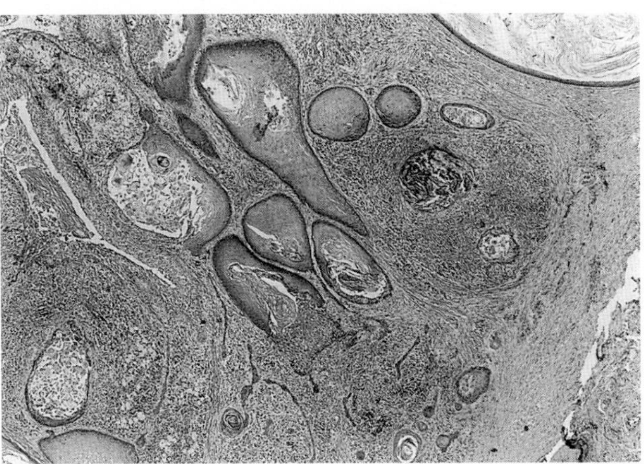

FIGURE 29. Odontogenic keratocyst. This type of epithelial proliferation in the wall of odontogenic keratocysts has sometimes been misdiagnosed as ameloblastoma. It is referred to as daughter cysts.

Nevoid Basal Cell Carcinoma Syndrome (Basal Cell Nevus Syndrome)

Most OKCs occur as single lesions. However, some patients exhibit several cysts, either concurrently or throughout life. When this happens, the patient and the family should be investigated for the nevoid basal cell carcinoma syndrome because multiple OKCs are characteristic of this disorder.

The syndrome (29) has four basic features:

1. Multiple OKCs. These cysts are true odontogenic keratocysts, although sometimes in the medical literature they have been referred to erroneously as dentigerous cysts.
2. Multiple basal cell carcinomas. These tend to occur first around puberty and are not confined to the regions of the body exposed to actinic radiation. They may become very numerous, and some are clinically aggressive.
3. Various skeletal anomalies, of which a bifid rib is the most common.
4. Autosomal dominant inheritance.

There are also a number of other features that occur less constantly. One relatively common skeletal feature is prominence of the frontal and temporal regions, hypertelorism, and a slightly prognathic mandible. In addition, medulloblastoma, a malignant brain tumor of early childhood, occurs more frequently than usual in families with this syndrome.

This relatively uncommon syndrome is important because the oral findings may lead to the diagnosis of the entire complex, including the basal cell carcinomas and familial tendency to development of medulloblastoma.

Gingival Cysts

Two different pathologic entities are included under this designation, the gingival cyst of the newborn and the gingival cyst of the adult (Fig. 20). Both are small innocuous lesions. The gingival cyst of the newborn is poorly named because it is really a cyst of the alveolar mucosa; gingiva is the tissue surrounding the neck of an erupted tooth.

Gingival Cyst of the Newborn

These relatively uncommon cysts (30) occur as fluid-filled, soft tissue swellings of the alveolar ridges of newborn infants. They may be multiple, are caused by the degeneration of remnants of odontogenic epithelium, and are of no clinical consequence in that they soon exfoliate into the oral cavity. Microscopically, they are lined by stratified squamous epithelium and often contain keratinous debris (Fig. 30). They are not, however, odontogenic keratocysts because they lack the specific microscopic features of those lesions. Similar cysts, which are not of odontogenic origin, occur along the median palatal raphe of some newborns; they too are harmless and are often called Epstein's pearls. A problem in terminology exists in this area. Originally, the terms *Epstein's pearls* and *Bohn's nodules* referred to these palatal lesions, but currently they are often also used for gingival cysts of the newborn. Consequently, these eponyms are best avoided. Surgical pathologists will rarely be called on to examine any of these cysts.

Gingival Cyst of the Adult

Gingival cysts of the adult (Fig. 20) are uncommon lesions that occur mainly on the mandibular gingiva in the premolar region in adults of both sexes over the age of 40. They are fluctuant, often bluish, and seldom more than 1 cm in diameter. Suspected examples should be excised for cosmetic reasons and to confirm the diagnosis microscopically; they seldom recur. These cysts probably arise from rests of the dental lamina. Their microscopic appearance is characteristic and consists of a thin layer of nonkeratinized, often cuboidal epithelium surrounding a central lumen; the epithelial–connective tissue interface is flat, and the cysts are generally not inflamed (Fig. 31A). Many of the epithelial cells are vacuolated (Fig. 31B), and these vacuolated cells, which contain glycogen, often form focal thickenings (Fig. 31B) in the epithelial lining. Less frequently, the focal thickenings are composed of nonvacuolated cells (Fig. 32).

In addition to these specific gingival cysts, small cysts are a fairly common microscopic finding in gingivectomy specimens. These microcysts are not evident clinically and are often keratinized, similar to gingival cysts of the newborn. They represent cystic degeneration of dental lamina rests and are of no consequence.

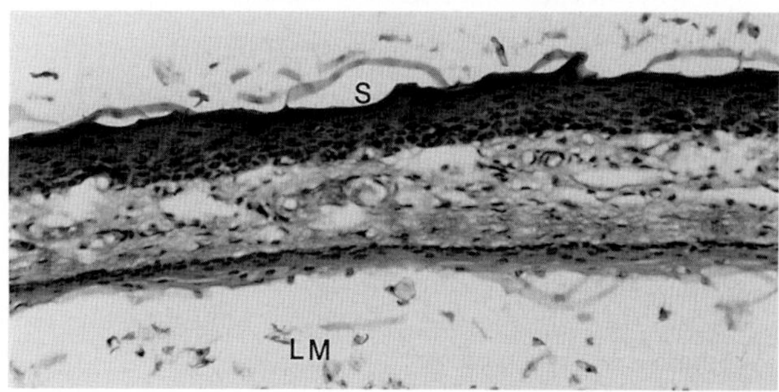

FIGURE 30. Gingival cyst of the newborn lined by stratified squamous epithelium. *LM,* lumen; *S,* surface epithelium of alveolar mucosa.

The Developmental Lateral Periodontal Cyst (Lateral Periodontal Cyst)

This uncommon cyst (31,32) (Fig. 20) is the intraosseous counterpart of the gingival cyst of the adult, occurring as a small, well-circumscribed radiolucency of the alveolar bone between the roots of adjacent teeth. It exhibits the same histologic appearance as the gingival cyst of the adult (Figs. 31 and 32) and, like that lesion, occurs mainly in the mandibular premolar region of adults over the age of 40. Moreover, at surgery, many developmental lateral periodontal cysts are found to lie partly within the gingiva, there being a defect within the cortical plate. Developmental lateral periodontal cysts seldom exceed 1 cm in diameter and do not recur once removed. However, a very rare multilocular variant, the botryoid odontogenic cyst, tends to recur (33).

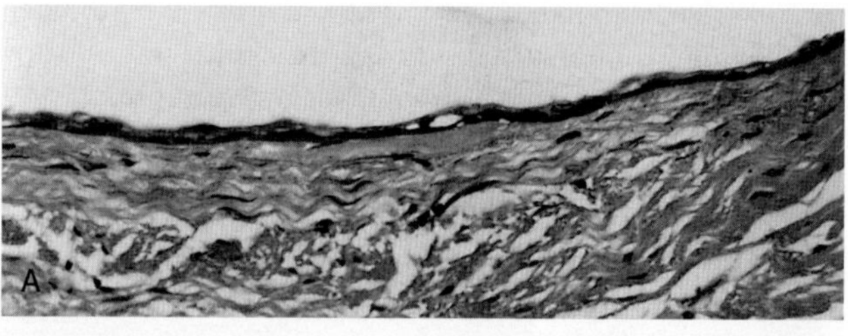

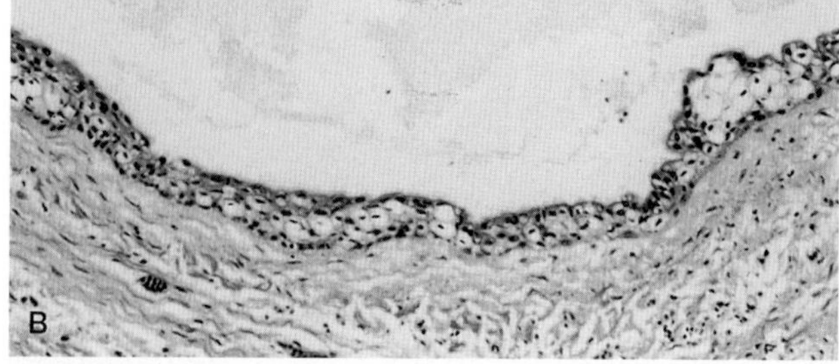

FIGURE 31. Gingival cyst of the adult. **A:** The epithelial lining in this example is very thin. **B:** Here, the epithelial cells are vacuolated, and there is one focal thickening of these vacuolated cells present.

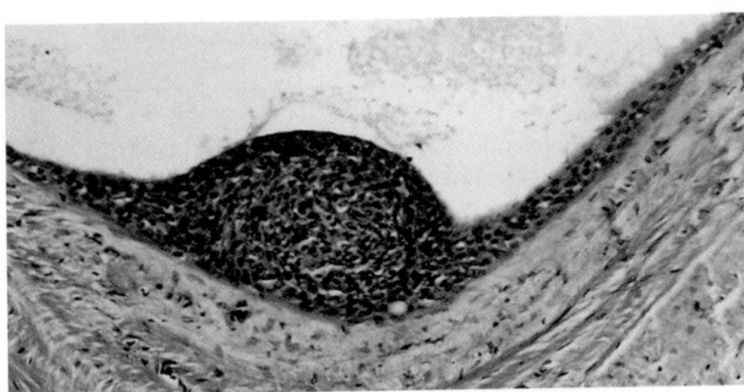

FIGURE 32. Gingival cyst of the adult. A well-formed focal thickening of nonvacuolated epithelial cells.

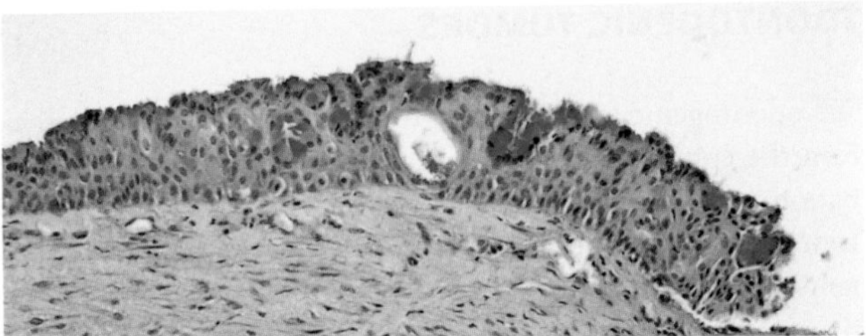

FIGURE 34. Glandular odontogenic cyst. The crypts contain mucinocarminophilic material; isolated mucous cells may be present within the epithelium. Mucicarmine stain.

The Glandular Odontogenic Cyst

This rare lesion (34), which is sometimes referred to as the mucoepidermoid odontogenic cyst or as the sialodontogenic cyst, is the most recently described odontogenic cyst. The synonyms are inappropriate because this cyst is not related to salivary glands, and *mucoepidermoid odontogenic cyst* invites confusion with mucoepidermoid carcinoma. It is important because it can become quite large and tends to recur if treated by curettage or enucleation. Approximately 20 examples have been reported so far, but more are being diagnosed now that it has been recognized as a pathologic entity. The glandular odontogenic cyst occurs over a wide age range (19–85 years in one review) (35) and in both sexes, but there appears to be a predilection for the fifth and sixth decades of life. It can occur in various locations in the jaw, but approximately half of the reported examples have been in the incisor region of the mandible. Most have exhibited a multilocular appearance, but unilocular examples have occurred.

The microscopic features are characteristic (Fig. 33). The lining of the cyst consists of stratified squamous epithelium of varying thickness, which exhibits a flat interface with the underlying connective tissue; the latter tissue is not usually inflamed. The basal cells are prominent, usually cuboidal, and may be vacuolated. The superficial epithelial cells are an important feature. They are eosinophilic, cuboidal, and may be ciliated. Equally important are the crypts within the epithelium. They generally contain mucinocarminophilic material (Fig. 34) and are lined by eosinophilic cuboidal cells similar to those on the surface; mucous cells may also be apparent. Other characteristic, if inconstant, features are spherical epithelial structures that may protrude from the surface of the epithelium, giving it a papillary appearance (Fig. 35). Foci of calcified material may occur directly beneath the epithelium but are not present in all examples.

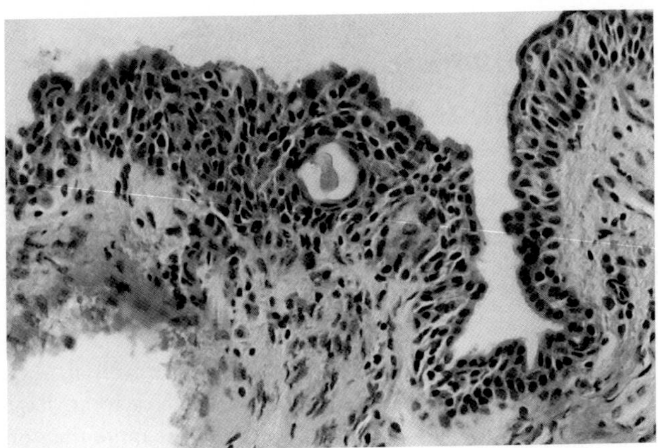

FIGURE 33. Glandular odontogenic cyst. The superficial epithelial cells are eosinophilic, cuboidal, and may exhibit cilia. Crypts lined by similar eosinophilic cells occur within the epithelium.

There are two other lesions that must be considered in the differential diagnosis. The first is intraosseous low-grade mucoepidermoid carcinoma, some examples of which exhibit foci that are similar to this cyst. It is also possible that some lesions that have been diagnosed previously as mucoepidermoid carcinoma were in fact examples of glandular odontogenic cyst. The only way to solve this problem is to study multiple sections of the lesions in question, being especially cautious of those that suggest tumor clinically, rather than cyst.

The other diagnostic pitfall is confusing other odontogenic cysts, especially dentigerous cysts that exhibit mucous cells in their lining, with this lesion. The problem is solved if the cyst exhibits the typical anatomic relationship of a dentigerous cyst, that is, is attached to a tooth at its cervical line. Mucous cells are not unusual in the lining of odontogenic cysts, and the diagnosis of glandular odontogenic cyst requires identification of the other microscopic features of that lesion, not just the presence of mucous cells.

Calcifying Odontogenic Cyst

This lesion is not a simple cyst and therefore is discussed in the section on odontogenic tumors.

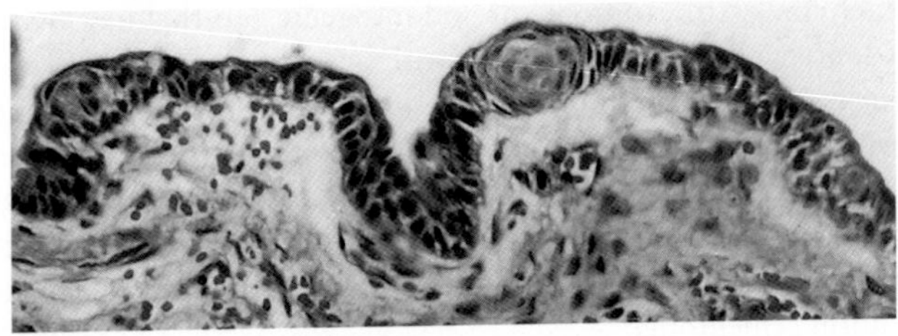

FIGURE 35. Glandular odontogenic cyst. Spherical epithelial structure.

ODONTOGENIC TUMORS

The odontogenic tumors are a group of lesions that are derived from the epithelium and connective tissue involved in the formation of teeth, that is, from the enamel organ. Some arise from tissues of the functional enamel organ, others from remnants of that structure after the tooth has formed. Tooth formation is complicated, and it is therefore not surprising that there exists a correspondingly complicated group of odontogenic tumors and that their microscopic features are complex. The group of lesions that have traditionally been considered as odontogenic tumors contain some that are true neoplasms (e.g., ameloblastomas), some that are hamartomas (e.g., odontomas), and some that are really dysplastic conditions (e.g., periapical cemental dysplasia and florid osseous dysplasia). It is a mark of progress that these dysplastic conditions, which have generally been included in the category of cementomas, are incorporated in the 1992 WHO classification (1) under the designation of neoplasms and lesions related to bone, not as odontogenic tumors. This altered designation also illustrates an important point, namely, the lack of need to separate cementum from bone and the consequent simplification of the differential diagnosis of certain lesions of the jaws. In many situations, it is not possible to distinguish microscopically between bone and cementum, the latter being only a modified form of bone. Only when the tissue occurs in its normal anatomic location—covering the root of a tooth—can it confidently be designated as cementum. In other situations one pathologist may interpret a focus of collagenous matrix as osteoid, and another may consider it to be cementum.

Most odontogenic tumors are benign. Some, however, are locally invasive. They infiltrate between the trabeculae of the bone of the jaws and therefore require wider excision than the others if recurrence is to be avoided. The locally invasive odontogenic tumors are the typical intraosseous ameloblastoma, the odontogenic myxoma, and the calcifying epithelial odontogenic tumor. A few truly malignant odontogenic tumors exist. They are extremely rare and may be either carcinomas or sarcomas.

For practical purposes the benign odontogenic tumors may be separated into three basic groups: (a) epithelial tumors, (b) mesenchymal tumors, and (c) tumors exhibiting both epithelial and mesenchymal components.

This simple classification (Table 2) may be more useful to the surgical pathologist than the more complicated terminology used in the 1992 WHO classification (1) (Table 3). In that publication, the benign odontogenic tumors are divided into (a) tumors of odontogenic epithelium without odontogenic ectomesenchyme, (b) tumors of odontogenic epithelium with odontogenic ectomesenchyme, with or without dental hard tissue formation, and (c) tumors of odontogenic ectomesenchyme with or without included odontogenic epithelium.

In the 1971 WHO classification (36), four lesions were listed as types of cementoma: (a) benign cementoblastoma, (b) cementifying fibroma, (c) periapical cemental dysplasia, and (d) gigantiform cementoma.

In the 1992 WHO classification (1), all but the benign cementoblastoma were included in a category entitled "neoplasms and lesions related to bone," and the classification in Tables 2 and 3 reflects this change. However, the concept of four types of cementoma is firmly entrenched in oral pathology and clinical dentistry, and the surgical pathologist may encounter this usage.

Finally, most odontogenic tumors are intraosseous lesions. A few occur on the gingiva or alveolar process and do not involve the underlying bone. They are referred to as peripheral odontogenic tumors and resemble their intraosseous counterparts microscopically. However, their prognosis is much better because they do not invade bone and are readily excised. Occasionally, an odontogenic tumor, such as an ameloblastoma, is diagnosed microscopically in the soft tissues of the oral cavity other than the gingiva or alveolar process. Such diagnoses are almost invariably erroneous.

TABLE 2. A CLASSIFICATION OF ODONTOGENIC TUMORS

- Benign
  - Epithelial odontogenic tumors
    - Ameloblastoma
    - Squamous odontogenic tumor
    - Adenomatoid odontogenic tumor
    - Calcifying epithelial odontogenic tumor
    - Calcifying odontogenic cyst
  - Mesenchymal odontogenic tumors
    - Odontogenic myxoma
    - Odontogenic fibroma
    - Granular cell odontogenic tumor
    - Cementoblastoma
  - Mixed odontogenic tumors
    - Odontoma
      - Complex
      - Compound
    - Ameloblastic fibroma
    - Ameloblastic fibroodontoma
    - Odontoameloblastoma
- Malignant
  - Odontogenic carcinomas
  - Odontogenic sarcomas
    - Ameloblastic fibrosarcoma

Ameloblastoma

The ameloblastoma is the best-known and, excepting the odontoma, most frequently encountered odontogenic tumor, but nevertheless, it is not common. It is said to represent 1% of all oral tumors, but there is little accurate information available concerning its prevalence. A Swedish study estimated an incidence of 0.6 cases per 1 million people per year (37). It is a true neoplasm that has a bad reputation for destruction and recurrence; moreover, it can become very large. It has become a cliche to state that the treatment of ameloblastoma is controversial, but in fact the principles are well understood, although each case has to be assessed individually, and sometimes there is more than one appropriate approach to its treatment. The term *adamantinoma* is an obsolete synonym for ameloblastoma.

There are three types of ameloblastoma (38): (a) the solid or multicystic ameloblastoma, (b) the unicystic ameloblastoma,

TABLE 3. THE 1992 WORLD HEALTH ORGANIZATION'S HISTOLOGIC TYPING OF NEOPLASMS AND OTHER TUMORS RELATED TO THE ODONTOGENIC APPARATUS

Benign
- Odontogenic epithelium without odontogenic ectomesenchyme
- Ameloblastoma
- Squamous odontogenic tumor
- Calcifying epithelial odontogenic tumor (Pindborg tumor)
- Clear cell odontogenic tumor
  - Odontogenic epithelium with odontogenic ectomesenchyme, with or without dental hard tissue formation
  - Ameloblastic fibroma
  - Ameloblastic fibrodentinoma (dentinoma) and ameloblastic fibro-odontoma
  - Odontoameloblastoma
  - Adenomatoid odontogenic tumor
  - Calcifying odontogenic cyst
  - Complex odontoma
  - Compound odontoma
- Odontogenic ectomesenchyme with or without included odontogenic epithelium
  - Odontogenic fibroma
  - Myxoma (odontogenic myxoma, myxofibroma)
  - Benign cementoblastoma (cementoblastoma, true cementoma)

Malignant
- Odontogenic carcinomas
  - Malignant ameloblastoma
  - Primary intraosseous carcinoma
  - Malignant variants of other odontogenic epithelial tumors
  - Malignant changes in odontogenic cysts
- Odontogenic sarcomas
  - Ameloblastic fibrosarcoma (ameloblastic sarcoma)
  - Ameloblastic fibrodentinosarcoma and ameloblastic fibro-odontosarcoma
  - Odontogenic carcinosarcoma

Source: Kramer IRH, Pindborg JJ, Shear M. *Histological typing of odontogenic tumours, 2nd ed.* Berlin: Springer-Verlag, 1992.

and (c) the peripheral ameloblastoma. They are considered separately because their clinical features and biological behavior, and hence their treatment, differ. It is far more important to categorize ameloblastomas into one of these three types than into one of the many histopathologic patterns that are described.

Solid or Multicystic Ameloblastoma

This is the most common type (perhaps 80% of cases) and is the one that comes to mind when ameloblastoma is mentioned. Its unwieldy name reflects that it may be a solid lesion or, as in many epithelial tumors, it may undergo cystic degeneration, a feature that may be apparent at surgery. When this happens, the term *cystic ameloblastoma* is sometimes used. However, this designation has no clinical significance and tends to be confused with unicystic ameloblastoma. The solid or multicystic ameloblastoma is often referred to as the *classical intraosseous ameloblastoma.*

The solid or multicystic ameloblastoma occurs approximately equally in both sexes and over a wide age range. However, most examples are diagnosed between 30 and 60 years of age. This type of ameloblastoma is seldom found before the age of 20, unlike the unicystic ameloblastoma, adenomatoid odontogenic tumor, and ameloblastic fibroma, all of which may be confused with it microscopically. It is rare in the first decade. Interestingly, ameloblastomas appear to be more common in blacks in Africa than in other populations. Larger tumors are seen there than in the industrialized world, presumably reflecting less accessibility to health care. This tumor has a marked predilection for the posterior part of the mandible, although it can occur anywhere in the jaws. About 80% arise in the mandible. Most of the maxillary lesions arise in the posterior region and tend to involve the maxillary sinus. The tumor may be detected radiographically, or it may cause enlargement of the jaw.

Ameloblastomas can become very large. One example in a white patient reportedly weighed 1.5 kg (39). However, really large examples are seldom encountered nowadays in the industrialized nations because they are treated before they can attain such a size. Ameloblastomas grow very slowly, a feature that is important in planning treatment and follow-up examinations.

The solid or multicystic ameloblastoma may be a unilocular or multilocular radiolucent lesion. Its borders are usually well defined and may exhibit sclerosis reflecting its slow growth. The multilocular appearance is considered typical and is sometimes referred to as resembling soap bubbles or a honeycomb.

There are basically two histopathologic patterns of solid or multicystic ameloblastoma, the follicular and the plexiform, although many others have been described. Their importance lies in the pathologist's recognizing them as ameloblastoma; there is no clinical significance in distinguishing between them.

The follicular pattern is the more common. It consists of islands of odontogenic epithelium within a mature connective tissue stroma (Fig. 36). The basal cells of these islands typically ex-

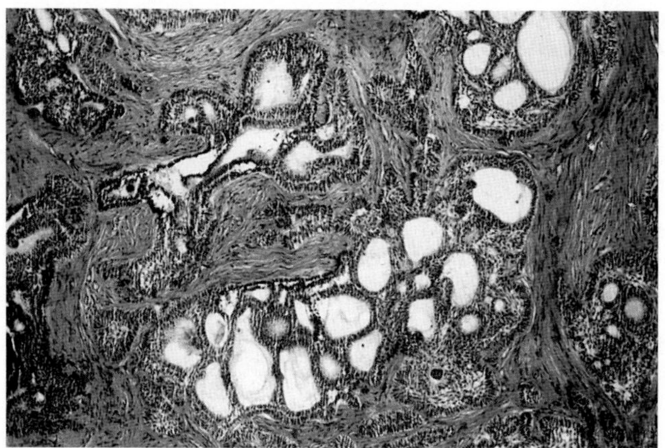

FIGURE 36. Solid or multicystic ameloblastoma. (Classical intraosseous ameloblastoma.) Follicular pattern. This pattern consists of islands of odontogenic epithelium within a mature connective tissue stroma. In this example there has been considerable cystic degeneration of the stellate reticulum—a common finding.

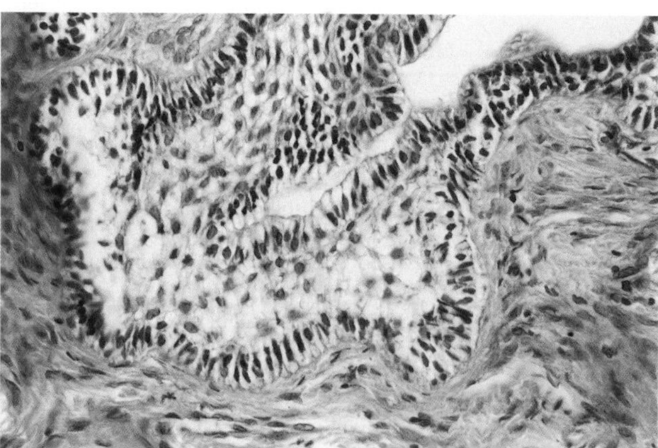

FIGURE 37. Ameloblastoma, follicular pattern. In this classical example the basal cells are palisaded, columnar, and exhibit cytoplasmic vacuolation and hyperchromatic nuclei, which are located at the distal ends of the cells, that is, away from the basement membrane (reverse polarization). The inner cells are loosely arranged and resemble stellate reticulum of the enamel organ.

hibit hyperchromatic nuclei, are columnar, and are palisaded like a picket fence (Fig. 37). Moreover, their cytoplasm is generally vacuolated, and their nuclei are located at the distal ends of the cells, away from the basement membrane. This last feature is termed reverse polarization and is similar to that of the cells of the inner enamel epithelium of the enamel organ before enamel is produced. It is characteristic of ameloblastomas, but some examples exhibit it less prominently than others. In some cases the basal cells are simply hyperchromatic. The central cells of the epithelial islands are loosely arranged and resemble the stellate reticulum of the enamel organ (Fig. 37). These inner areas quite often undergo cystic degeneration.

The inner cells of the typical follicular pattern may become modified in various ways. If they become squamous, the term *acanthomatous ameloblastoma* is often used (Fig. 38). The importance of this variant is twofold. If the stellate reticulum is completely replaced by squamous cells, the tumor may be mistaken for squamous cell carcinoma, although the epithelium of the ameloblastoma is not dysplastic as in a carcinoma. Moreover, a carcinoma does not exhibit the typical basal cells of ameloblastoma. Secondly, the so-called acanthomatous ameloblastoma may be confused microscopically with the squamous odontogenic tumor *(q.v.),* but that tumor also lacks the typical basal cell pattern of the ameloblastoma. If the inner cells are spindle shaped (Fig. 39), granular, resembling the cells of the granular cell tumor *(q.v.)* (Fig. 40), or basaloid, the terms *spindle cell ameloblastoma, granular cell ameloblastoma,* and *basal cell ameloblastoma* may be used, respectively. An important diagnostic pitfall lies in misdiagnosing the basaloid pattern of adenoid cystic carcinoma as ameloblastoma or vice versa. This error occurs occasionally, especially in the posterior maxilla–maxillary sinus region. The separation of the follicular pattern into these various subtypes, besides having no clinical significance, is somewhat artificial because an individual ameloblastoma may exhibit two or more of these patterns in different parts of the tumor.

The second major pattern (Fig. 41), the plexiform pattern, is quite different. The polarized basal cells are arranged in a network of anastomosing strands, and little stellate reticulum is present. Moreover, the generally delicate stroma between the strands tends to degenerate markedly; it sometimes becomes sufficiently vascular to suggest the term *hemangioameloblastoma.* However, this is not a separate entity.

Recently, a ghost-cell ameloblastoma (40,41), which shares some microscopic features with the calcifying odontogenic cyst, has been described. In this rare lesion, ghost cells and calcifications are prominent features; abnormal dentin (dentinoid) may also be present. The so-called ghost cells are squamous cells that have degenerated and lost their nuclei but have maintained a faint outline of their cellular and nuclear membranes.

This "ghost-cell ameloblastoma" is the same lesion as the "dentinogenic ghost-cell tumor" (40), which has previously been included within the type 2 (neoplastic) category of calcifying odontogenic cysts (COC) (42) *(q.v.).* The concepts and terminology concerning this neoplastic type of COC are not yet settled. However, several workers (41–44), including me, believe

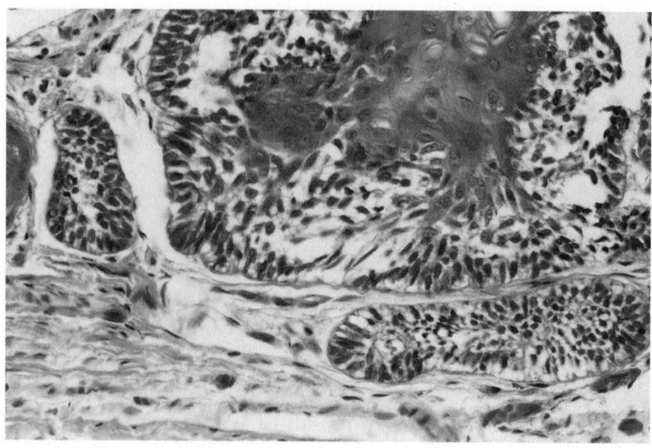

FIGURE 38. Ameloblastoma, acanthomatous pattern. The stellate reticulum region has been partially replaced by squamous cells. This feature may be more extensive than in this example.

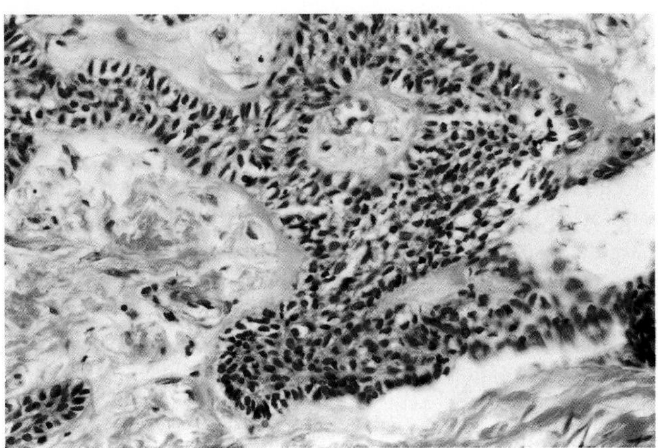

FIGURE 39. Ameloblastoma, spindle cell pattern. The stellate reticulum region has been replaced by spindle cells; the basaloid pattern is very similar.

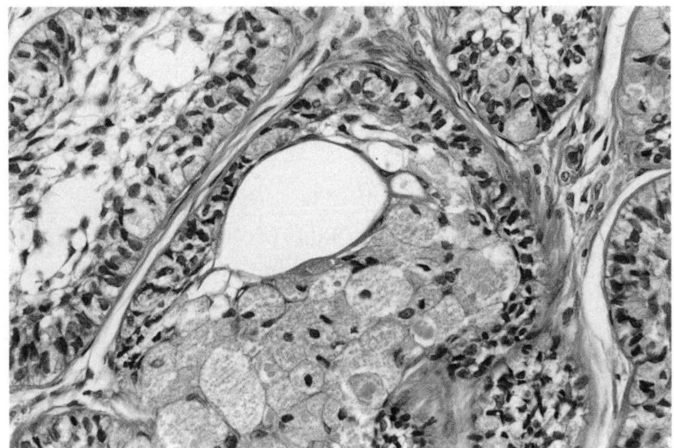

FIGURE 40. Ameloblastoma, granular cell pattern.

that the "dentinogenic ghost-cell tumor" should be considered a form of ameloblastoma because of its microscopic resemblance to that tumor and its aggressive, infiltrative behavior that is typical of ameloblastoma.

The desmoplastic ameloblastoma (45,46) is another recently described variant. It is peculiar because it tends to involve the anterior maxilla, an unusual site for an ameloblastoma, and to exhibit a radiographic appearance that is more suggestive of a benign fibroosseous lesion than of ameloblastoma. It has been suggested that the desmoplastic ameloblastoma is less aggressive than other ameloblastomas, but this seems doubtful. In a recent case that I reviewed on consultation, a desmoplastic ameloblastoma destroyed the maxilla from the second premolar on one side to the second premolar on the other. The typical location of the desmoplastic ameloblastoma in the anterior maxilla makes it less dangerous than ameloblastomas of the posterior maxilla because it is further from the base of the skull and consequently less likely to invade intracranially. Microscopically, the epithelial islands of desmoplastic ameloblastoma are surrounded by a dense, collagenous stroma, that is, by a desmoplastic reaction (Fig. 42). This connective tissue tends to condense the epithelial islands, which often do not exhibit as prominently columnar basal cells as do other variants of ameloblastoma. However, they are clearly not simply rests of odontogenic epithelium because their basal cells exhibit nuclear hyperchromatism and there is some evidence of stellate reticulum, which is not found in most odontogenic rests. Consequently, confusion of desmoplastic ameloblatoma with odontogenic fibroma should not be a problem.

There are several other odontogenic tumors that may be mistaken microscopically for ameloblastoma, including the ameloblastic fibroma, adenomatoid odontogenic tumor, calcifying odontogenic cyst (tumor), and squamous odontogenic tumor. The characteristic loose connective tissue component of the ameloblastic fibroma serves to distinguish that tumor from ameloblastoma, and the microscopic features of the adenomatoid odontogenic tumor are really quite different from those of ameloblastoma. Moreover, both the ameloblastic fibroma and the adenomatoid odontogenic tumor tend to occur in patients under the age of 20 years, whereas intraosseous ameloblastomas

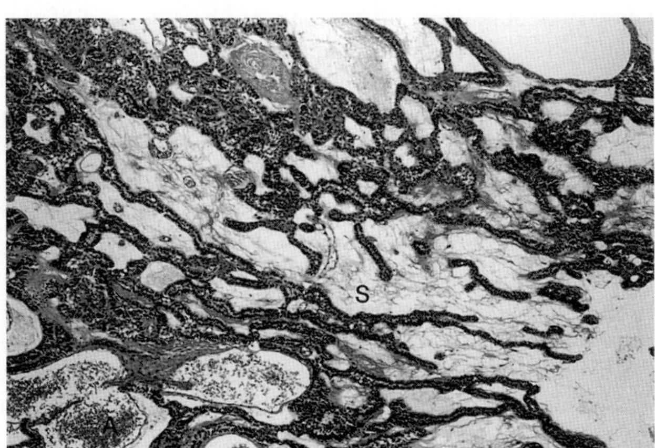

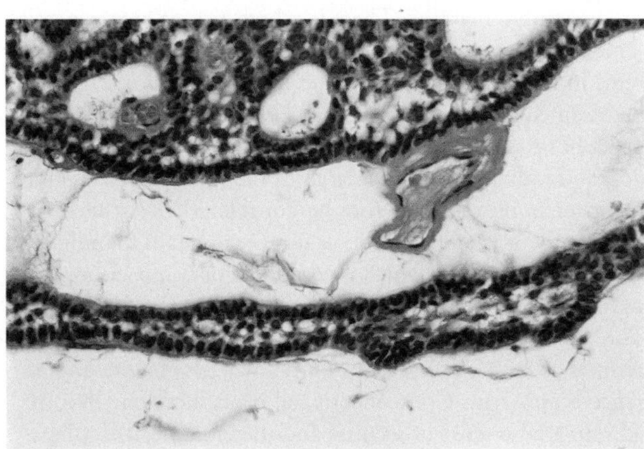

FIGURE 41. A: Solid or multicystic ameloblastoma (classical intraosseous ameloblastoma). Plexiform pattern exhibiting stromal degeneration and vascular areas. *S,* degenerate stroma. **B:** This pattern is composed of strands, rather than islands, of odontogenic epithelium; stellate reticulum is sparse.

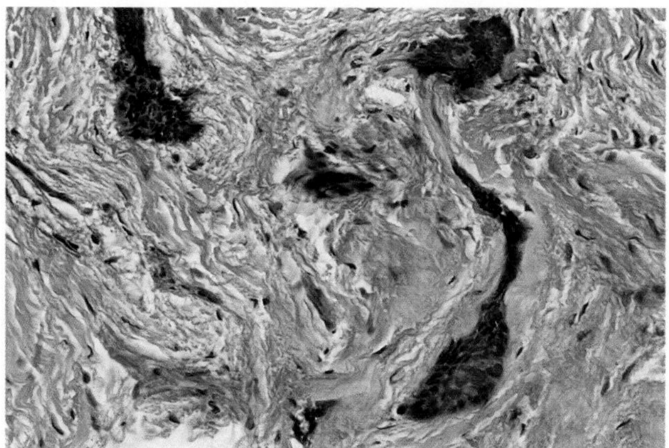

FIGURE 42. Desmoplastic ameloblastoma. The stroma in this histologic variant is very dense, and the epithelial islands are compressed.

seldom do so. The calcifying odontogenic cyst is a complicated lesion because several entities have been included under that designation and there are often microscopic similarities to ameloblastoma. However, the classical calcifying odontogenic cyst is usually readily diagnosable. The rare squamous odontogenic tumor resembles the acanthomatous pattern of ameloblastoma microscopically but does not exhibit the characteristic basal cells of ameloblastomas. Basal cell carcinomas have occasionally been diagnosed on the oral soft tissues, but probably all of them really represent the basaloid pattern of ameloblastoma or a salivary gland tumor, depending on their location. Although the histopathologic diagnosis of typical ameloblastomas is not difficult, it is advisable to seek expert consultation in questionable cases.

The biological behavior of the solid or multicystic ameloblastoma is that of a slow-growing, locally invasive tumor with a high rate of recurrence if not removed adequately. It very rarely metastasizes. The above points are important. The high rate of recurrence is caused by the ameloblastoma's marked tendency to infiltrate between the trabeculae of cancellous bone, leaving them intact for some time. Consequently, the actual margins of the tumor within cancellous bone are located well beyond its clinical and radiographic margins. There is a high risk of recurrence if the ameloblastoma is treated as if the clinical and radiographic margins in cancellous bone were the actual boundaries. In contrast, the ameloblastoma does not invade the haversian system of compact bone, although it will eventually erode that tissue. The clinical and radiographic boundaries of the tumor in the region of compact bone can therefore be considered the true ones. Consequently, it is often feasible at surgery to retain the inferior border of the mandible, which is composed of compact bone, if it has not been eroded.

The characteristic slow growth is important because years, sometimes as long as 10 years or more, may pass before any recurrence is apparent. Consequently, all concerned may become lulled into a false sense of security and therefore neglect follow-up examinations after the first few years. It is essential that the surgical site be examined, including radiographically, annually for at least 10 years. Very rarely, an ameloblastoma that exhibits no cytologic evidence of malignancy metastasizes. This phenomenon is so rare, however, that the possibility should not be considered when planning treatment.

The treatment of the solid or multicystic ameloblastoma is surgical and, depending on the size of the lesion, varies from marginal resection to segmental resection to resection of the affected jaw. To avoid recurrence it is necessary to excise beyond the radiographic margins of the lesion, but it is often possible to save the inferior border of the mandible. Curettage is generally followed eventually by recurrence but can be used in the body of the mandible, provided that the surgeon is sure that he or she will be able to follow the patient for at least 10 years. Curettage definitely should not be used in the posterior maxilla because recurrences in that site are difficult to control and there is a real danger of the tumor invading the cranium, possibly resulting in the death of the patient. Therapeutic irradiation should not be used in the treatment of ameloblastoma (47), although its use has been recommended by a major oncology hospital (48), except as a last resort in inoperable tumors of the pterygomaxillary fossa. It does not control the tumor and can lead to osteonecrosis. There is also at least the potential of inducing postradiation malignancies.

Unicystic Ameloblastoma

The unicystic ameloblastoma (38,49) is less common than the classical intraosseous ameloblastoma but is important because it has a much better prognosis. It occurs predominantly in the second and third decades, that is, in younger people than the classical intraosseous ameloblastoma. Almost all have occurred in the mandible, especially the posterior part.

This lesion generally appears radiographically as a dentigerous cyst and, if it is not too large, is enucleated on that basis. It is only when a pathologist examines such a lesion that it is apparent that it contains ameloblastoma. However, the larger ones are generally examined by incisional biopsy and present a real problem. In these cases the pathologist may suggest the diagnosis of unicystic ameloblastoma based on the patient's age, the radiographic appearance of the lesion, and its microscopic features, but he or she cannot be certain that the tumor has not breached the fibrous wall of the cyst in other parts of the specimen. One needs to examine the whole specimen to make that evaluation.

The existence of the unicystic ameloblastoma is the basis of statement that ameloblastomas may develop in preexisting dentigerous cysts. This point is moot because it is possible that these unicystic ameloblastomas are really neoplastic from inception. The important concept is that lesions that appear radiographically to be dentigerous cysts may in fact be unicystic ameloblastomas. A few unicystic ameloblastomas are not associated with the crown of a tooth and consequently may be diagnosed clinically as a residual cyst or as a possible odontogenic keratocyst.

On gross examination, this lesion appears to be a typical cyst

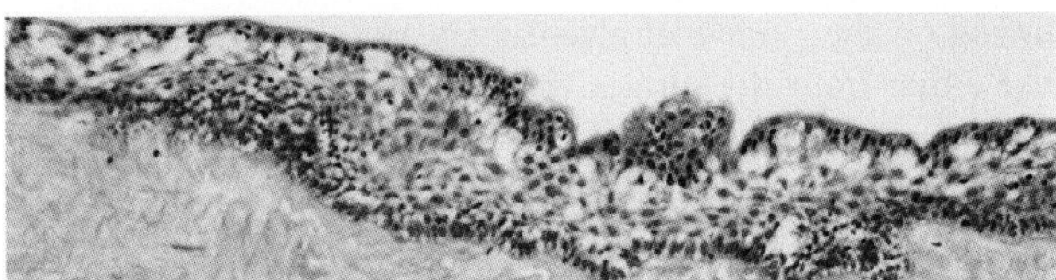

FIGURE 43. Unicystic ameloblastoma. The lining of this cystic lesion represents ameloblastoma because the basal cells are typical of that tumor and stellate reticulum is present.

if it has been enucleated cleanly. Some examples exhibit a focal growth into the lumen.

Histologically, one or more of the following features are present:

1. The lining epithelium is ameloblastomatous (Fig. 43).
2. One or more nodules of ameloblastoma project into the lumen (the so-called luminal ameloblastoma) (Fig. 44).
3. Islands of ameloblastoma have proliferated from the epithelial lining into the connective tissue capsule of the cyst (one form of so-called mural ameloblastoma) (Fig. 45).
4. Islands of ameloblastoma are present in the connective tissue capsule of the cyst, but the actual lining does not appear microscopically to be neoplastic (another form of mural ameloblastoma).

Many examples of unicystic ameloblastoma exhibit the typical basal cell features of ameloblastoma. This feature is very helpful in diagnosing situations 1 and 4 above. However, the intraluminal nodules often appear as an anastomosing network of epithelial strands, which resemble hyperplastic epithelium within a delicate vascular stroma. Although in many examples no classical ameloblastoma is present, this pattern (Fig. 46) has been shown to indeed represent that tumor (50,51). It has been referred to as plexiform unicystic ameloblastoma (50,51), but it is only a histologic variant.

There are several factors that should be taken into account when considering the histopathologic diagnosis of unicystic ameloblastoma.

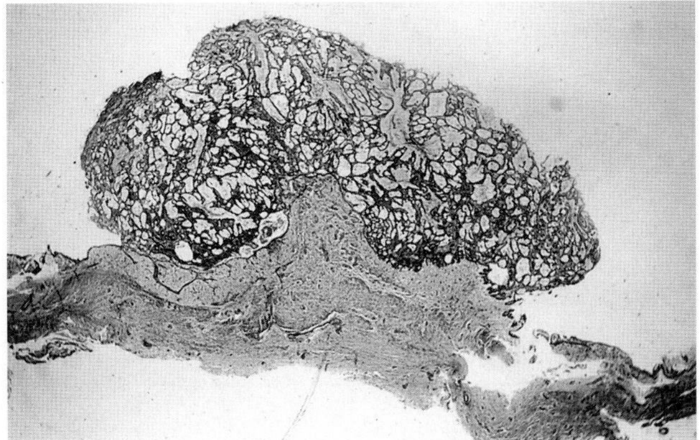

FIGURE 44. Unicystic ameloblastoma. In this example the nodule of ameloblastoma protrudes into the lumen (luminal ameloblastoma).

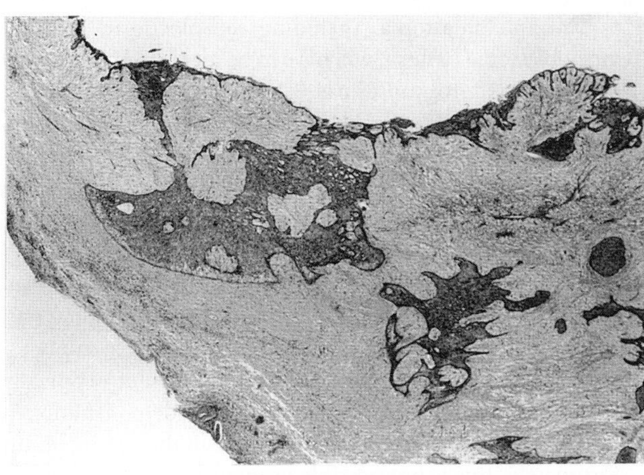

FIGURE 45. Unicystic ameloblastoma. The ameloblastoma has infiltrated into the connective tissue capsule of the cyst (mural ameloblastoma).

1. The diagnosis should be made only when the lesion in question is truly unicystic. In practice, this is generally when the lesion has already been enucleated on the basis of its being considered a dentigerous cyst, and the pathologist has the opportunity to examine the entire specimen. In less ideal situations the diagnosis of consistent with, or suggestive of, unicystic ameloblastoma is appropriate.
2. Not all unilocular ameloblastomas are examples of unicystic ameloblastoma. The classical intraosseous ameloblastoma may be unilocular, but it does not exhibit the fibrous capsule of the unicystic ameloblastoma; it does not appear to have arisen in a cyst.
3. Parts of the epithelial lining of a unicystic ameloblastoma may be flattened, consist simply of hyperchromatic basal cells, or otherwise not be typical of ameloblastoma. In suspicious cases,

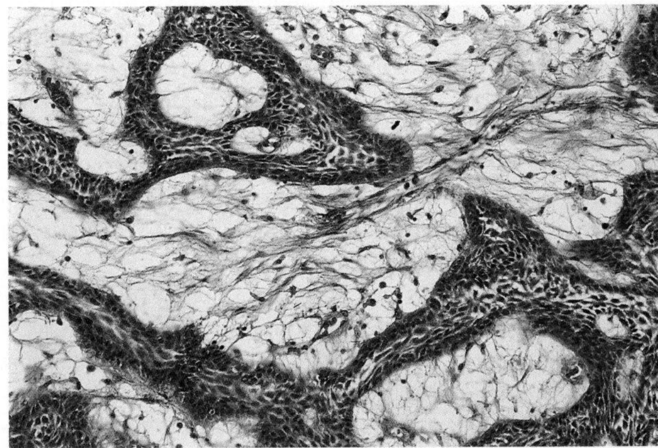

FIGURE 46. Unicystic ameloblastoma. This photomicrograph is from the luminal ameloblastoma in Fig. 44. It illustrates the pattern of anastomosing epithelial strands within a loose connective tissue stroma that is known as plexiform unicystic ameloblastoma. It is readily mistaken for hyperplastic epithelium.

typical ameloblastoma, including the plexiform unicystic ameloblastoma pattern, will have to be identified elsewhere in the specimen to substantiate the diagnosis of unicystic ameloblastoma. Features that should arouse the suspicion of the examining pathologist are when the lining of a putative dentigerous cyst appears atypical, the most important clue in the absence of frank ameloblastoma being hyperchromatic basal cells.

4. The plexiform unicystic ameloblastoma (50,51) (Figs. 44 and 46) pattern can be a real problem to the pathologist, but with experience it can generally be identified, even though it closely resembles hyperplastic epithelium microscopically. Obviously, the most useful feature is the demonstration of more classical ameloblastoma elsewhere in the specimen; unfortunately, this is not possible in many examples. There are other clues. First, there is the intraluminal location. Second, the very delicate, rather vascular connective tissue is typical. Third, hyperplastic epithelium is not a feature of uninflamed dentigerous cysts, although it occurs in those that have become infected. Even then, it does not typically appear as an intraluminal projection.
5. Another real problem is the differential diagnosis in the wall of a dentigerous cyst of rests of odontogenic epithelium from ameloblastoma. Some of these rests, which are an inconsistent feature, resemble closely islands of ameloblastoma, although this is rather uncommon. The issue is largely one of extent. One or two such foci do not warrant the diagnosis of ameloblastoma. In equivocal cases it is best to diagnose these islands as odontogenic rests but to note their resemblance to ameloblastoma and to recommend that the patient be followed closely.
6. The term *ameloblastomatous change* is sometimes encountered in the literature on the pathology of dentigerous cysts. It is best avoided because it has not been properly defined. It appears to have been used chiefly when pathologists were uncertain as to whether they were dealing with unicystic ameloblastomas.

Most unicystic ameloblastomas are diagnosed as such by a pathologist after they have been enucleated. No further treatment is indicated, other than radiographing the surgical site annually for 10 years if it can be demonstrated microscopically that the ameloblastoma is confined to the epithelial lining or is an intraluminal nodule. If, however, the ameloblastoma has invaded the cystic capsule, the surgeon may consider the option of further surgery, such as marginal resection, to ensure that the tumor has been completely removed. The overall recurrence rate for unicystic ameloblastomas after enucleation is 10% to 15%. The rare unicystic ameloblastomas of the posterior maxilla should be treated by marginal resection because recurrences in that location can involve the pterygomaxillary fossa and are therefore dangerous. Once a unicystic ameloblastoma has breached the fibrous connective tissue capsule of the cyst, it has become classical intraosseous ameloblastoma and has to be treated as such.

Peripheral Ameloblastoma

This rare entity (52) is defined as an odontogenic tumor having the histologic features of an intraosseous ameloblastoma but occurring on the gingiva or alveolar mucosa. Individual examples arise either from the surface epithelium of the gingiva or from rests of dental lamina within the gingiva. The peripheral ameloblastoma occurs as an epulis (gingival growth) of either jaw over a wide age range, with a peak in the fourth and fifth decades. It does not appear to occur before the age of 20. There is no sex predilection.

Grossly, peripheral ameloblastomas appear as focal enlargements of the gingiva or alveolar mucosa, sometimes with a papillary surface. Microscopically, they may exhibit all of the variants of the follicular pattern of intraosseous ameloblastoma, but they tend to be acanthomatous or basaloid. Occasionally, the basaloid pattern is interpreted as basal cell carcinoma and undoubtedly would be diagnosed as such were it to occur on the skin. However, basal cell carcinomas do not arise within the oral cavity. The few that have been reported there are almost certainly misdiagnoses of ameloblastomas, salivary gland tumors, or basaloid variants of squamous cell carcinomas.

The microscopic relationship of peripheral ameloblastoma to the surface epithelium varies. Some examples exhibit no continuity with the surface epithelium and presumably arise from rests of dental lamina within the gingiva. Others are joined to the surface epithelium at one site only (Fig. 47), and still others are joined at several separate sites. It is tempting to conclude that the ameloblastomas in these last two situations arose from the surface epithelium. They may have done so but they also could represent fusion of an underlying tumor with the surface epithelium.

These lesions should not be treated as aggressively as a solid or multicystic ameloblastoma because they lack that tumor's invasive characteristic. Peripheral ameloblastomas are usually excised without the diagnosis being suspected; it is made subsequently by the pathologist. If the tumor is excised with a margin of apparently normal tissue, no further treatment is necessary except for periodic examination of the surgical site. If not, a further operation to obtain a margin of normal tissue is indicated. The peripheral ameloblastoma should not recur if adequately excised. It should be noted that a solid or multicystic ameloblastoma may eventually break out of bone, but its extraosseous component should not be referred to as a peripheral ameloblastoma.

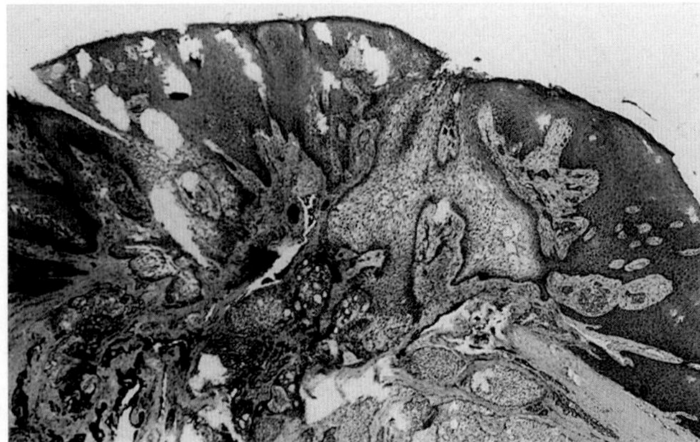

FIGURE 47. Peripheral ameloblastoma. In this example the tumor is continuous with the overlying epithelium.

The lesion most likely to be confused microscopically with the peripheral ameloblastoma is the peripheral complex odontogenic fibroma (also known as the WHO type) *(q.v.)*. In this tumor, the epithelium is in the form of odontogenic rests, unlike islands of ameloblastoma in which the basal cells should exhibit varying degrees of nuclear hyperchromatism, palisading and reverse polarity. Moreover, unlike the peripheral ameloblatoma, the peripheral odontogenic fibroma may also exhibit collagenous material that could be variously interpreted as osteoid, dentinoid, or cementum.

Squamous Odontogenic Tumor

This is a very rare tumor (53,54). Its importance lies in the possibility of its being misdiagnosed microscopically as squamous cell carcinoma or acanthomatous ameloblastoma. In both cases, the treatment would be more extensive than is required for the squamous odontogenic tumor (SOT). Moreover, proliferations of odontogenic epithelium, resembling SOT, occur occasionally in the linings of dentigerous and radicular cysts (55). Care should be taken not to diagnose them as the actual tumor.

The SOT occurs over a wide age range but chiefly in young adults of both sexes. It occurs in either jaw with a marked predilection for the alveolar processes. The tumor appears radiologically as a well-demarcated radiolucency that often resembles severe periodontal disease because of its association with the roots of adjacent teeth. Multiple lesions may occur. Most examples are small, up to 1.5 cm in diameter. There may be a painless or slightly tender swelling, but some examples have exhibited no symptoms and have been detected during a routine radiographic examination.

Microscopically, the SOT consists of islands of squamous epithelium, exhibiting no atypia, within a fibrous connective tissue stroma (Fig. 48A). The peripheral cells may be flattened and do not exhibit the morphologic features of preameloblasts, as ameloblastomas do *(q.v.)* (Fig. 48B). This feature is the major point in differentiating the SOT from ameloblastoma. The lack of dysplasia distinguishes it from squamous cell carcinoma. Moreover, the islands of that tumor are more irregularly shaped than in SOT. Microcysts, foci of keratinization, laminated calcifications, and eosinophilic globular structures all may occur within the epithelial islands but are not consistent features.

The treatment recommended for mandibular lesions is curettage with extraction of the adjacent teeth. A wider excision is advisable in the posterior maxilla, where there is the possibility of involvement of the maxillary sinus. There have been a few recurrences after curettage, but too few examples have been reported as yet to allow for firm statements concerning the long-term biological behavior of this tumor.

Adenomatoid Odontogenic Tumor

This lesion (AOT) (56) is rarer than the ameloblastoma, with which it has sometimes been confused. In fact, it was formerly known as the adenoameloblastoma, implying incorrectly that it is a variant of ameloblastoma. It is important that these two tumors be distinguished because the AOT has a much better prognosis than the classical intraosseous ameloblastoma and therefore requires less extensive treatment. The term *adenomatoid* refers to the tumor's resemblance microscopically to a benign glandular neoplasm. The AOT is considered to be a hamartoma rather than a neoplasm (1,56).

The AOT is generally asymptomatic, although it may cause a smooth swelling of the jaws. It has a predilection for the anterior maxilla but it also occurs elsewhere in the jaws. Many examples are first detected on radiologic examination. Occasional cases occur as extraosseous growths of the gingiva, that is, as peripheral tumors. This lesion is approximately twice as common in female as in male patients and occurs mainly in those between 5 and 30 years old; most examples occur before age 20, whereas the classical intraosseous ameloblastoma seldom occurs before the age of 20 years.

The radiologic features of the intraosseous examples illustrate an important characteristic of this lesion: it is often associated with the crown of an unerupted tooth and, being radiolucent and well circumscribed, resembles a dentigerous cyst. Frequently, small radiopaque foci are evident within the radiolucency, a feature not found in dentigerous cysts.

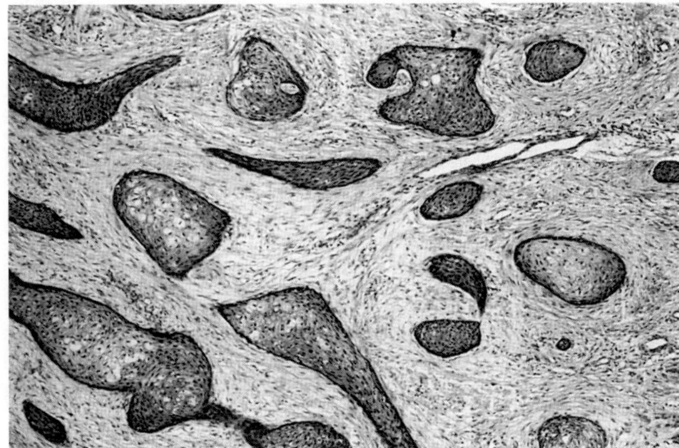

A

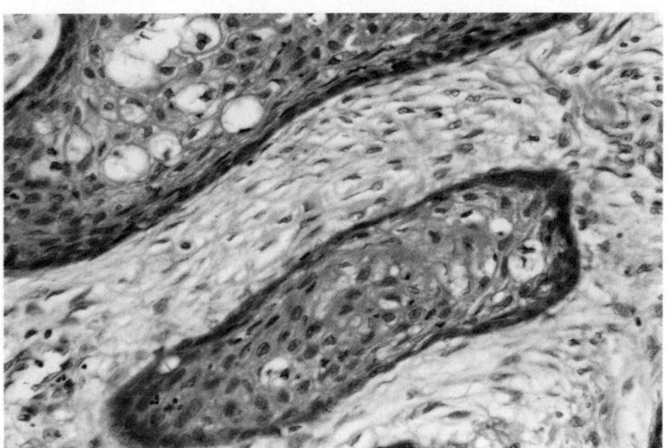

B

FIGURE 48. Squamous odontogenic tumor. **A:** Islands of squamous epithelium within a fibrous connective stroma. **B:** The basal cells do not exhibit the features of ameloblastoma.

The intraosseous AOT is seldom larger than 5 cm in diameter. If enucleated cleanly it often resembles a dentigerous cyst grossly and is usually well encapsulated. On being transected, the lesion may be found to be essentially cystic and attached to the crown of an associated tooth in a dentigerous relationship. These cystic examples exhibit intraluminal tumorous growths. Others are quite solid but may still surround the crown of a tooth, although not all examples of AOT contain a tooth. The peripheral lesions are gingival growths and are not associated with a tooth.

The microscopic features of the AOT are characteristic (Fig. 49). They consist of whorled masses of spindle-shaped epithelial cells that are intermingled with duct-like structures composed of columnar epithelial cells, the nuclei of which are located away from the lumina. Less characteristically, the epithelial cells in part of the tumor are arranged in sheets or plexiform strands. Apart from the fibrous capsule, the fibrous connective component is sparse, and the tumor may be solid or cystic. Eosinophilic deposits, which are probably an abortive form of enamel, may be present. Some may stain positively for amyloid. Calcifications are often present, but their number varies. An eosinophilic, collagenous matrix, which is usually interpreted as dysplastic dentin (dentinoid), occurs in some examples and is used in the 1992 WHO classification (1) as justification for considering the AOT to be other than a purely epithelial tumor.

Although the microscopic features of the AOT are characteristic, there are some important points to be noted. The duct-like structures may be sparse or even absent. However, the whorled epithelium is usually sufficiently characteristic without them to lead to the correct diagnosis. Some dentigerous cysts exhibit in their lining small foci that resemble AOT microscopically. Whether these foci should be considered incipient tumors or incidental findings is moot. Recently, there has been considerable interest in so-called hybrid tumors that exhibit features of both AOT and calcifying epithelial odontogenic tumor (CEOT) (56). Too much has been made of this finding. It is better to consider these tumors as AOTs that exhibit, as a microscopic variation, foci that resemble CEOT.

The intraosseous AOT enucleates readily and does not recur if removed adequately. The peripheral lesions have generally been removed completely without the correct diagnosis having been suspected. Recurrence is most unlikely, provided the margins are free of tumor.

Calcifying Epithelial Odontogenic Tumor

This neoplasm (CEOT) (57), which is often referred to as the Pindborg tumor, is considerably rarer than the ameloblastoma. Its importance lies, first, in that its epithelial cells may demonstrate sufficient pleomorphism to suggest malignancy, although it is benign (Fig. 50). Actually, its microscopic appearance is so characteristic that those pathologists who are familiar with odontogenic tumors will not fall into that trap. Second, it is a locally invasive tumor, much like the classical intraosseous ameloblastoma. However, taken collectively, CEOTs are not as aggressive as ameloblastomas. A few have been well circumscribed.

The CEOT occurs over a wide age range, commencing with the first decade, although it is most common in midlife, the mean age of diagnosis being 40. It affects men and women equally. There may be expansion of the jaw, or the lesion may be detected on routine radiographic examination. Occasional peripheral (extraosseous) lesions occur. The CEOT is twice as common in the mandible as in the maxilla and has a predilection for the posterior mandible. The radiographic appearance varies considerably. It is usually a relatively poorly demarcated radiolucency in which there may be focal or diffuse opacities; some cases are completely radiolucent. Trabeculae, breaking the lesion into apparent compartments, are a variable finding. The CEOT is often associated with an unerupted tooth.

The three characteristic histopathologic features of the CEOT are (a) sheets or widely dispersed islands of polyhedral epithelial cells, which may exhibit well-defined cell outlines and prominent intercellular bridges as well as considerable, albeit harmless, pleomorphism, (b) amyloid, and (c) calcifications (Fig. 50). The pleomorphism noted in many examples of CEOT consists of cells that exhibit nuclear hyperchromatism and/or giant nuclei, multinucleated cells, and some variation in the size of individual cells. Mitotic figures are not evident.

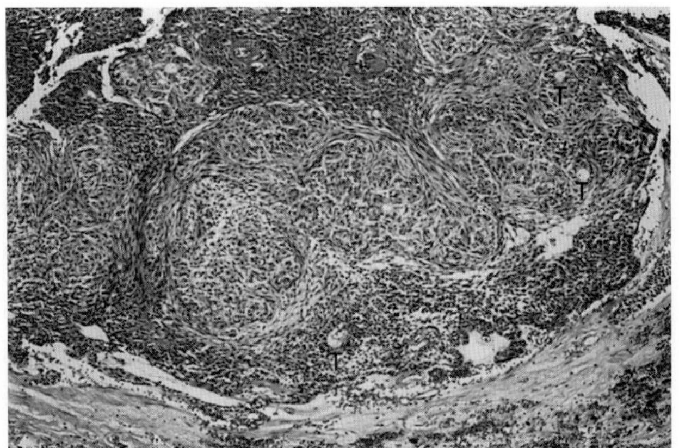

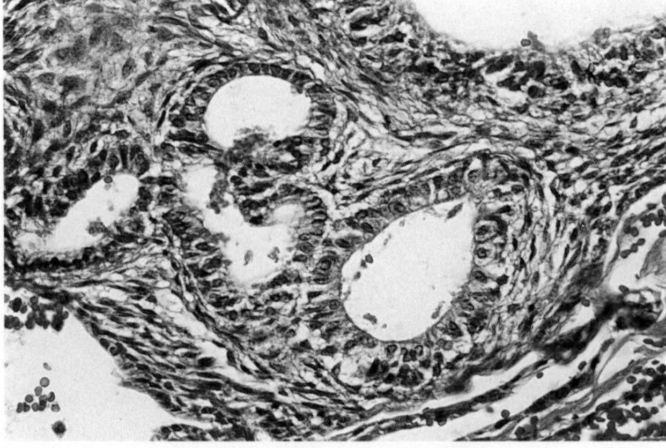

FIGURE 49. Adenomatoid odontogenic tumor. **A:** The tumor consists of whorled masses of spindle-shaped epithelial cells in which are interspersed duct-like structures *(T)*. **B:** Higher-power magnification illustrating the typical duct-like structures. The spindle-shaped epithelial cells are present in the upper left corner of the photomicrograph.

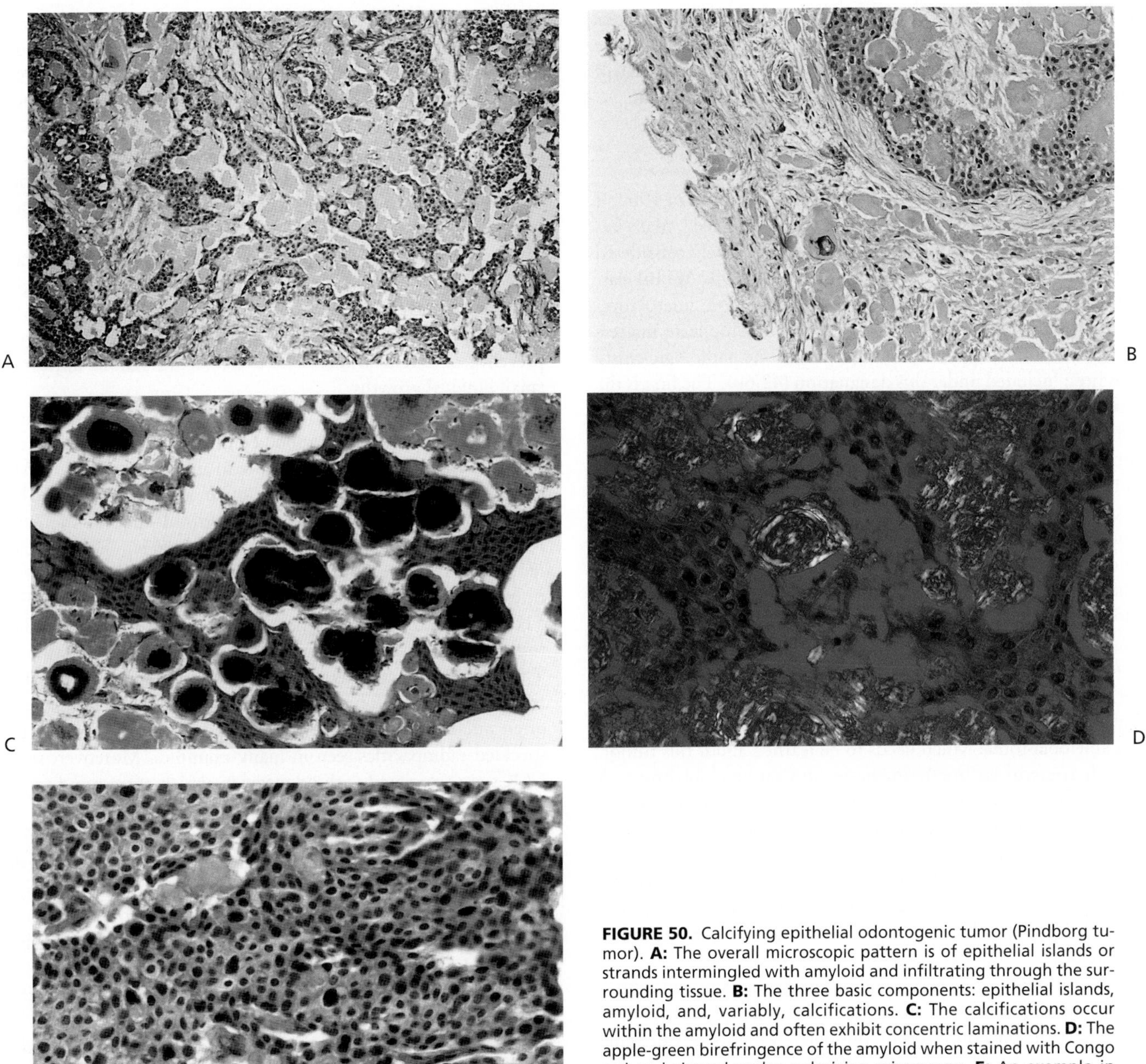

FIGURE 50. Calcifying epithelial odontogenic tumor (Pindborg tumor). **A:** The overall microscopic pattern is of epithelial islands or strands intermingled with amyloid and infiltrating through the surrounding tissue. **B:** The three basic components: epithelial islands, amyloid, and, variably, calcifications. **C:** The calcifications occur within the amyloid and often exhibit concentric laminations. **D:** The apple-green birefringence of the amyloid when stained with Congo red and viewed under polarizing microscopy. **E:** An example in which the epithelium exhibits considerable nuclear pleomorphism. The cell outlines and intercellular bridges are not as prominent as is sometimes the case.

The extent of calcification varies considerably (Fig. 50B,C) and is reflected in the radiographic appearance of the individual lesion. Some tumors exhibit none. It follows that the diagnosis of CEOT can be made in its absence, but the other two components are essential. The calcifications occur within the amyloid and often take the form of concentric laminations referred to as Liesegang rings. Of importance, in explaining the clinical behavior of this tumor, is that islands of tumor may be present in the intertrabecular spaces, illustrating that it has invaded adjacent tissue. Consequently, recurrence is probable if the lesion is not excised with a margin of apparently normal bone.

Although the microscopic features of the CEOT are characteristic, individual examples vary significantly because of the relative proportions of the three components. In addition, one variant exhibits clear cells, in which case demonstration of the other features of CEOT are necessary to substantiate the diagnosis. Some CEOTs exhibit foci that resemble adenomatoid odontogenic tumor microscopically. This feature should be considered a histologic variation, not a hybrid tumor.

The nature of the amyloid in CEOT and other odontogenic tumors is controversial. It stains positively with Thioflavine T, exhibits apple-green birefringence with Congo red (Fig. 50D)—properties it shares with traditional amyloid—and in practice can be referred to as odontogenic amyloid. In many accounts it continues to be referred to as amyloid-like material.

The CEOT is a slow-growing, locally invasive lesion. The

principles of treatment described for the classic intraosseous ameloblastoma are consequently equally applicable to the CEOT. The recurrence rate is, however, lower than that of ameloblastomas. Peripheral lesions respond well to excision.

Calcifying Odontogenic Cyst

When this rare lesion (COC) (58) was first described in 1962, it was considered to be a nonneoplastic cyst, and indeed, many examples are cystic. However, it is more appropriately considered a tumor (58,59), and it is listed as such in the 1992 WHO classification (1). It is certainly a more complex lesion, microscopically, than the other odontogenic cysts. To complicate matters further, it is now apparent that more than one pathologic entity has been included under this designation (42,60). The first is the "classical," unilocular, well-circumscribed lesion with characteristic microscopic features. It was referred to as type I COC by Praetorius et al. (42) and is described below as the classical COC. The second entity, which was included in type II COC by Praetorius et al. (42), is very rare and infiltrates adjacent tissue in the same way that an ameloblastoma does. It resembles that tumor microscopically but also exhibits features that are typical of the calcifying odontogenic cyst, namely ghost cells and dentinoid. Consequently, a number of terms have been used for this lesion, including *dentinogenic ghost cell tumor* (40), (epithelial) *odontogenic ghost cell tumor* (60), and *ghost cell ameloblastoma* (41). This last designation appears to be the most appropriate because the presence of dentinoid is variable and the lesion acts as an ameloblastoma. Much needs to be learned about this tumor, which is discussed briefly in the section on ameloblastoma. A third, very rare, entity that was also included as a type II COC (42) exhibits cytologic features of malignancy but also contains ghost cells, calcifications, and sometimes dentinoid. It should be considered a form of odontogenic carcinoma (61) and is consequently discussed briefly in that section. Again, our present knowledge of this lesion is incomplete, including its biological behavior.

To summarize this rather complicated subject in which concepts are still evolving, there appear to be three different entities that have all previously been considered variants of calcifying odontogenic cyst:

1. The "classical" calcifying odontogenic cyst (equivalent to type I COC).
2. Ghost cell ameloblastoma (also referred to as type II COC or dentinogenic ghost cell tumor).
3. Ghost cell odontogenic carcinoma (also previously included in type II COC).

Much confusion would be avoided in the future if the term calcifying odontogenic cyst were confined to the first of these three entities.

"Classical" Calcifying Odontogenic Cyst (Type I)

"Classical" calcifying odontogenic cysts (COC) occur principally in people under 40 years of age, with a peak in the second decade. Women are affected about twice as often as men, and 70% of the lesions occur in the maxilla. Most occur anterior to the first molars. A significant number occur as extraosseous growths of the gingiva. Clinically these peripheral lesions resemble irritation fibromas but on histologic examination are shown to contain small COCs.

Radiographically, the intraosseous lesions are well-defined radiolucencies that generally exhibit focal, speckled radiopacities. Some exhibit quite extensive radiopaque bodies, whereas others exhibit no radiopacities at all.

At gross examination, a cleanly enucleated COC is an encapsulated lesion, usually exhibiting a central lumen, although this feature may have become almost obliterated by epithelial proliferation. The tissue may feel gritty as it is being cut because of the presence of calcifications. The extraosseous lesions appear as small gingival growths.

Histologically, the "classical" COC, which may be obviously a cyst or in some examples a solid epithelial lesion, is lined by epithelium with a marked resemblance to ameloblastoma (Fig. 51). For instance, the basal cells are columnar, and their nuclei are hyperchromatic and are located at the distal ends of the cells. Moreover, these basal cells enclose epithelium similar to stellate reticulum. However, the stellate reticulum also exhibits two features—numerous "ghost cells" (Fig. 51B) and calcifications (Fig. 51C)—that are characteristic of COC but not of ameloblastoma, although both may occur occasionally in that tumor. These ghost cells are keratinized squamous cells that have lost their nuclear basophilia but still retain their original cellular and often nuclear outlines. They tend to calcify, accounting for the speckled radiopacities seen in many examples. Moreover, some COCs are associated with odontomas, which correspond to the larger radiopacities sometimes noted.

Another variable microscopic feature is the presence of foci of dentinoid (Fig. 51D) within the fibrous connective tissue directly adjacent to the epithelium. This eosinophilic, collagenous material is similar in appearance to osteoid. Sometimes the ghost cells are present in the surrounding connective tissue, where they induce a foreign body reaction.

The microscopic diagnosis of the classical COC is not difficult, although care should be taken not to diagnose it as an ameloblastoma. The more complicated examples may cause difficulty, even to the experienced oral and maxillofacial pathologist. Intraosseous COCs should be treated by enucleation; a few have recurred (62). There have been a few cases reported of malignant transformation of a previously benign COC, but this is extremely rare. The extraosseous COCs are usually excised before the definitive diagnosis is established by pathologic examination.

Odontogenic Myxoma

The odontogenic myxoma (63,64) is quite a rare lesion but, even then, is probably the second most frequent of the significant odontogenic tumors, after the ameloblastoma. It is important because its gelatinous nature allows it to infiltrate the intertrabecular spaces of bone, making it difficult to remove unless a marginal resection is performed. Consequently, it tends to recur if not treated properly. It is generally accepted that all myxomas of the jaw are of odontogenic origin because they resemble mi-

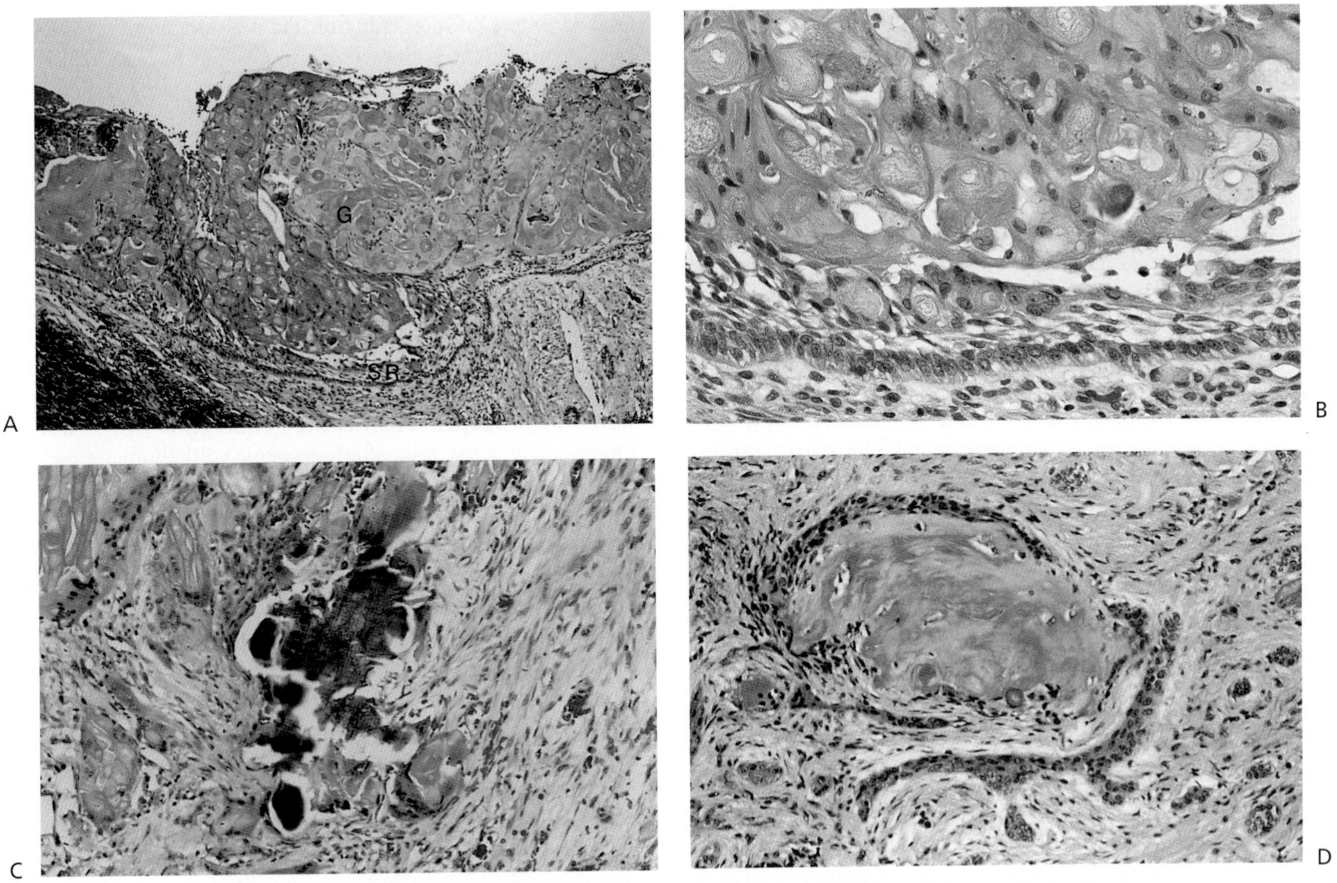

FIGURE 51. Calcifying odontogenic cyst. **A:** A typical field. *SR*, stellate reticulum; *G*, ghost cells. **B:** Higher magnification of part of **A** illustrating the typical basal cells, stellate reticulum, ghost cells, and one small calcification. **C:** Calcifications, ghost cells, and multinucleated giant cells within the adjacent connective tissue. **D:** Dentinoid within the connective tissue.

croscopically the dental papilla of the enamel organ, and, moreover, myxomas of bone apparently do not occur in extragnathic sites (63).

The odontogenic myxoma is usually a slow-growing lesion that may expand bone, although some examples have grown rapidly. It may also be detected on routine radiographic examination. It is generally symptomless, occurs equally in both sexes, over the age range of 10 to 50 years with a mean around 30, and throughout the jaws with no particular site of predilection. It is a radiolucent lesion with ill-defined borders and often exhibits trabeculae that give it a honeycomb appearance, much like the classical radiographic appearance of ameloblastoma. Adjacent teeth may be displaced.

On gross examination an odontogenic myxoma appears gelatinous, a so-called myxofibroma less so. It is not encapsulated, and in the case of a biopsy, the submitted specimen consists of gelatinous curettings.

The odontogenic myxoma (Fig. 52) is composed of abundant mucinous ground substance in which are interspersed relatively few stellate cells, which are fibroblasts that have not been compressed by the adjacent connective tissue, and sparse collagen fibrils. Rests of odontogenic epithelium occur only occasionally and are not necessary for the diagnosis. Mitoses are very rare, but some examples exhibit atypical nuclei. These lesions have sometimes been referred to as myxosarcomas, but, because none have metastasized, the significance of the atypical nuclei is questionable.

Some odontogenic myxomas contain more connective tissue than just described and consequently are sometimes termed myxofibromas or fibromyxomas. This variation does not warrant designation as a different tumor entity, but it is clinically signif-

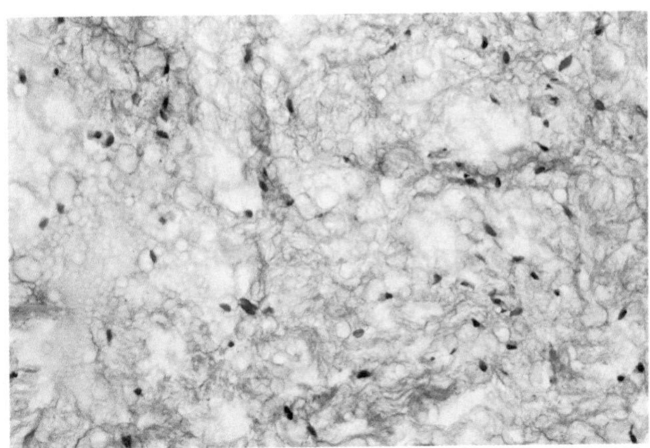

FIGURE 52. Odontogenic myxoma. Stellate cells and collagen fibrils within a mucinous ground substance.

icant. The more fibrous connective tissue present, the less infiltrative is the lesion and therefore the easier it is to remove.

The microscopic diagnosis of odontogenic myxoma is usually not difficult, but there are two possible pitfalls. Dental papillae that have been inadvertently curetted out of the jaw during surgery are sometimes mistaken microscopically for odontogenic myxomas. The history and clinical and radiographic findings are all important in reaching the correct diagnosis. Moreover, the characteristic well-defined shape and size of a dental papilla (it is the mesenchymal part of a tooth germ), together with the inconsistent finding of odontoblasts around its periphery, are useful in avoiding its misdiagnosis as an odontogenic myxoma. The dental follicle of an unerupted tooth may become slightly enlarged and exhibit considerable amounts of mucoid ground substance. Occasionally this hyperplastic dental follicle may be misdiagnosed as an odontogenic myxoma, myxofibroma, or, most commonly, as an odontogenic fibroma. That the tissue is from a fairly narrow band around the crown of an unerupted tooth is strong evidence that the lesion is an enlarged follicle, not an odontogenic myxoma.

A marginal resection, that is, removal of the tumor with, if possible, a 1- to 1½-cm margin of apparently normal tissue is the appropriate treatment for most odontogenic myxomas. Such treatment is essential for a lesion of the posterior maxilla because of the close proximity to the pterygomaxillary fossa and orbit. Small lesions in the mandible, or the anterior maxilla, may be curetted provided that the surgeon realizes that the chance of recurrence is high and, most important, is able to follow the patient closely for at least 5 years. Recurrence necessitates a second operation, but in the meantime the patient has been spared more extensive surgery.

Odontogenic Fibroma

This topic is somewhat confusing because several pathologic entities have been included under this term (8). One tumor, the simple odontogenic fibroma, is an uncomplicated intraosseous fibroma derived from the mesenchyme of the enamel organ. The second lesion is a more complex fibroblastic tumor that exhibits varying numbers of rests of odontogenic epithelium and, again variably, foci of collagenous matrix. Originally, this tumor was referred to as the WHO type of odontogenic fibroma because it was first illustrated in the 1971 WHO classification (36). *Complex odontogenic fibroma* would be a logical alternative designation. Finally, a third tumor exists that has been called a granular cell odontogenic fibroma, among other synonyms. It is discussed later as a separate tumor, the granular cell odontogenic tumor, because it is probably not a variant of odontogenic fibroma. All three are rare.

Simple Odontogenic Fibroma

Odontogenic fibromas have been reported over a wide age range and occur in either jaw. They may be asymptomatic, or they may cause swelling of the jaw with accompanying loosening of teeth. Radiographically, they may be either unilocular or multilocular radiolucencies that may or may not appear to be related to the adjacent teeth.

The simple odontogenic fibroma is an uncomplicated lesion microscopically; it is simply an intraosseous fibroma consisting of fibrous connective tissue that is usually fairly delicate, although denser examples occur, and may exhibit a considerable amount of ground substance. The designation *odontogenic myxofibroma* is sometimes used for those examples that exhibit this last feature. It is apparent that there is a microscopic spectrum ranging from a tumor consisting of chiefly fibrous connective tissue (the odontogenic fibroma) (Fig. 53) through a myxofibroma (Fig. 54), to the odontogenic myxoma (Fig. 52). However, the lesions at either end of this spectrum exhibit different biological behaviors and consequently should be considered separate pathologic entities. The odontogenic fibroma does not infiltrate surrounding tissues, whereas the odontogenic myxoma does. Occasionally, a few rests of odontogenic epithelium are present, but the diagnosis of odontogenic fibroma is routinely made without them. Foci of small calcifications sometimes occur.

One problem is the separation microscopically of the odontogenic fibroma from the desmoplastic fibroma of bone (intraosseous desmoid tumor). Doing so, in some cases, is virtually impossible, although it is not difficult if the tumor in question contains abundant ground substance and is therefore not desmoplastic, or if it exhibits odontogenic epithelium, in which case the diagnosis of odontogenic fibroma is appropriate. The problem lies with the tumors that consist of dense fibrous connective tissue with no epithelial component. Distinguishing between an odontogenic fibroma and a desmoplastic fibroma is theoretically an important distinction because the latter is an infiltrative lesion that requires more extensive surgery than the odontogenic fibroma, which does not infiltrate surrounding tissues. In practice, because of the difficulty in distinguishing microscopically between some examples of these two tumors, it may be necessary, in deciding on the appropriate treatment for an individual patient, to rely more on evaluating the clinical situation than on the exact histopathologic diagnosis.

A second diagnostic problem concerns the hyperplastic dental follicle. This lesion consists of a relatively narrow band of tissue around the crown of an unerupted tooth, although obviously it is wider than a normal dental follicle. Microscopically, it is identical to an odontogenic fibroma, a not surprising situation

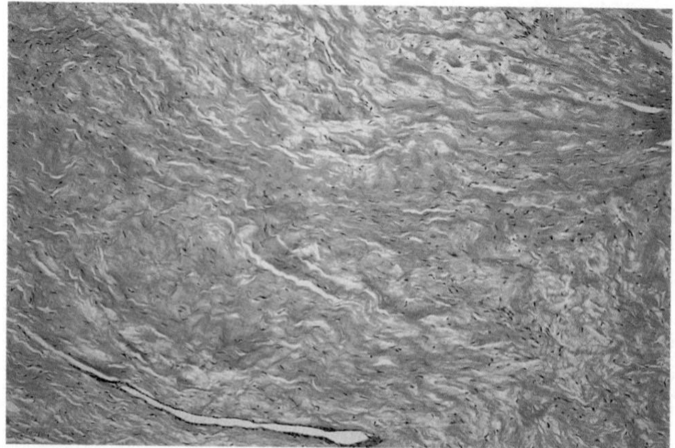

FIGURE 53. Simple odontogenic fibroma. Dense, relatively cellular, fibrous connective tissue, similar to that in some dental follicles.

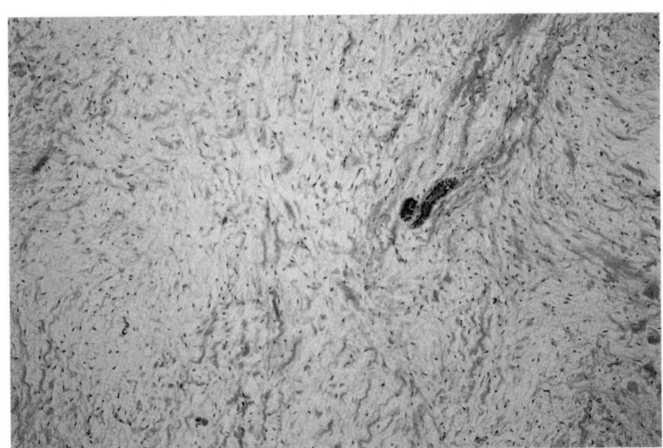

FIGURE 54. Myxofibroma. The connective tissue is less dense than that in Fig. 53, and abundant ground substance is present. Again, this appearance is similar to that of some dental follicles. Rests of odontogenic epithelium are a variable finding in both simple odontogenic fibromas and myxofibromas.

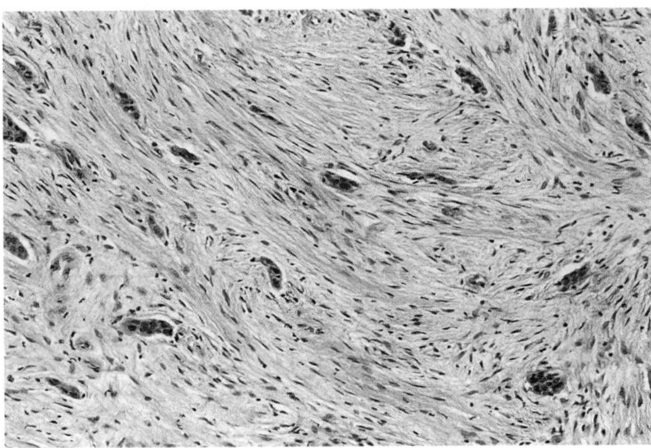

FIGURE 55. Complex odontogenic fibroma. The connective tissue is much more cellular than those in Figs. 53 and 54 and is arranged in interwoven bundles. Numerous odontogenic rests are evident. No dentinoid is present in this example.

because many odontogenic fibromas are presumably derived from dental follicles. The differential diagnosis is therefore based on the above clinical and radiologic findings. In the past, these hyperplastic dental follicles were often diagnosed as odontogenic fibromas, accounting for the impression that the odontogenic fibroma was a common lesion. This view is no longer held.

A third possible differential diagnosis is an intraosseous neurofibroma, which occurs occasionally within the jaws, especially within the mandible. In contrast to the odontogenic fibroma, the neurofibroma exhibits characteristic wavy nuclei and reacts positively to S-100 protein by immunohistochemistry.

The treatment recommended for the simple odontogenic fibroma is curettage or enucleation, although large examples may require more extensive surgery. There is little follow-up information available because of its rarity.

Complex Odontogenic Fibroma (Odontogenic Fibroma, WHO Type)

The clinical features of this lesion are similar to those of the simple odontogenic fibroma. There is one difference. The complex odontogenic fibroma may occur as a peripheral (extraosseous) lesion (65), that is, as an epulis, whereas the simple odontogenic fibroma does not.

There are several microscopic features (Fig. 55) that separate this lesion from the simple odontogenic fibroma. An important difference is that it is more cellular, and its cells tend to be plumper fibroblasts than those in the simple odontogenic fibroma. Moreover, the connective tissue may be arranged in interwoven bundles and exhibit quite prominent small blood vessels. Epithelial rests may be numerous, sometimes raising the question of an epithelial tumor rather than a fibroma. Third, foci of collagenous matrix that could be variously considered as osteoid, dentinoid, or cementum occur in many examples. This lesion appears to be a different tumor than the simple odontogenic fibroma, but its biological behavior is similar; the distinction is not, therefore, critical. The recommended treatment is also the same.

Recently, a few complex odontogenic fibromas have been reported as exhibiting a component that resembles central giant-cell granuloma (66). The production of giant cells may be an inductive effect of the tumor. However, one possibility that has to be considered is whether these lesions are really giant-cell granulomas that exhibit areas resembling odontogenic fibromas, that is, fibrous connective tissue containing rests of odontogenic epithelium. This question has yet to be resolved. In practice, this distinction is not going to affect treatment.

The peripheral complex odontogenic fibroma may be confused microscopically with the also rare *odontogenic gingival epithelial hamartoma* (67), which consists of strands and islands of epithelium within a dense fibrous connective tissue stroma. The basic difference is that the latter lesion is an epithelial, not a fibroblastic one. Because it is also readily curable by excision, the distinction is of no clinical importance.

Granular Cell Odontogenic Tumor (Granular Cell Ameloblastic Fibroma, Granular Cell Odontogenic Fibroma, Central Granular Cell Tumor of the Jaws)

This lesion (68–70) was originally reported as a granular cell ameloblastic fibroma, although it is clearly not a variant of ameloblastic fibroma because it does not exhibit that tumor's typical mesenchymal component. It has also been reported as a granular cell variant of odontogenic fibroma, a term that is also inappropriate because the tumor is composed of sheets of eosinophilic granular cells (Fig. 56) with some odontogenic epithelium, rather than consisting predominantly of fibrous connective tissue. *Granular cell odontogenic tumor* appears to be the most suitable designation because it emphasizes the tumor's putative odontogenic origin and avoids implying that it is related to granular cell tumor of soft tissues. The only known example that has been investigated for S-100 protein was negative, suggesting that the two tumors are not related.

Very few examples have been reported, and almost all have occurred in patients over 40 years of age. The lesion appears as a

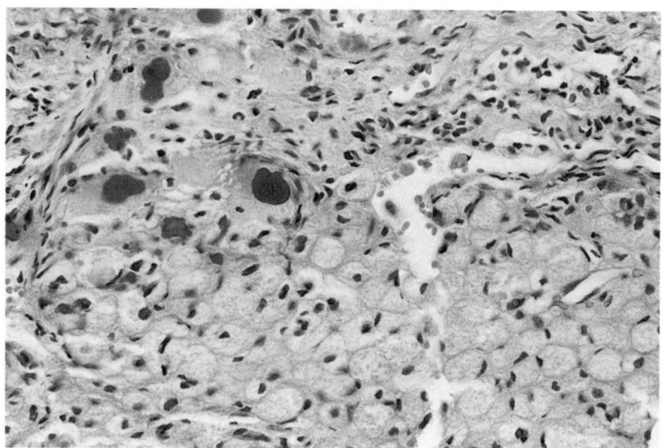

FIGURE 56. Granular cell odontogenic tumor. Eosinophilic granular cells with small calcifications, a variable feature. Rests of odontogenic epithelium are often present.

well-demarcated radiolucency in either jaw, predominantly in the posterior region. It is composed of sheets of eosinophilic granular cells, similar to those of the granular cell tumor of soft tissues. Islands or cords of odontogenic epithelium are interspersed among the granular cells, and some examples also exhibit small calcifications (Fig. 56). The granular cell odontogenic tumor responds well to curettage and does not recur.

The differential diagnosis of granular cell odontogenic tumor and the granular cell pattern of ameloblastoma *(q.v.)* should pose no problem because the latter is really a microscopic variation of the follicular pattern of ameloblastoma in which the central stellate reticulum cells have been replaced by granular cells; the peripheral cells are typical of ameloblastoma (Fig. 40). The granular cell odontogenic tumor does not exhibit this feature.

Cementum versus Bone

One longstanding problem in oral pathology has been the confusion generated by attempting to distinguish lesions considered to consist of bone from those thought to consist of cementum. However, there is no practical value in this distinction because the biological behavior of these lesions is identical.

The mineralized tissue that normally covers the roots of teeth is, by definition, cementum. However, elsewhere it is not really possible to distinguish microscopically between bone and cementum. Indeed, cementum is a form of bone. If this logic is followed, it is unnecessary to attempt to distinguish between ossifying fibromas and cementifying fibromas. Moreover, it is appropriate, as the WHO has done in its 1992 classification (1), to place three of the four lesions that were previously considered to be cementomas into the category "neoplasms and other lesions related to bone." The fourth one, the cementoblastoma, can be accepted as being of cemental origin because of its close association with the roots of teeth. It is discussed next. The other three "cementomas" from the 1971 WHO classification (36)—cementifying fibroma, periapical cemental dysplasia, and gigantiform cementoma (florid osseous dysplasia)—are discussed in Chapter 11.

Cementoblastoma (Benign Cementoblastoma, True Cementoma)

This lesion (71) is the most logical one to refer to as a cementoma because it consists of a relatively large mass of cementum attached to the root of a tooth—hence the term *true cementoma.* The adjective *benign* is not necessary, as there is no malignant counterpart other than osteosarcoma.

The cementoblastoma may be symptomless, being detected only on routine radiographic examination, or it may cause localized expansion of the jaw. It may or may not be painful but is never severely so. Usually involving the premolar–molar region of the mandible, it occurs with equal frequency in both sexes and is found in the age range of 8 to 30 years. Radiographically, the cementoblastoma occurs as a solitary 1- to 2-cm well-circumscribed radiopacity fused to the root of a tooth, usually a molar or premolar. There is generally a thin radiolucent zone around its periphery.

If a cementoma is removed intact, it appears grossly as an approximately spherical mass of hard tissue fused to the root of the affected tooth. If removed piecemeal, it will be received in the pathology laboratory as fragments of bone-like calcified material.

The microscopic appearance of an actively developing cementoblastoma is similar to that of the osteoblastoma. It consists of a mass of calcified material, which could be considered to be cementum, osteoid, or bone, associated with plump hyperchromatic cells that could, in turn, be considered to be either osteoblasts or cementoblasts (Fig. 57). Radiating trabeculae of this calcified material are often seen at its periphery (Fig. 57). Mature examples tend to exhibit more, relatively acellular, calcified material than do osteoblastomas, and reversal lines are often prominent. Osteoclasts may also be present. In some examples it is possible to demonstrate fusion of the tumor to the tooth's root. The root surface in that region exhibits irregular resorption.

The distinction between cementoblastoma and osteoblastoma is of academic interest only. A lesion is accepted as a cementoblastoma if it is fused to a tooth. Even then it could be argued that it represents an osteoblastoma that has become fused to an adjacent tooth. Osteoblastomas have been reported occasionally in the jaws.

It is more important that a cementoblastoma not be misinterpreted microscopically as a well-differentiated osteosarcoma; osteosarcomas of the jaws tend to be well differentiated. The problem arises if a small biopsy is examined of a cellular area composed of hyperchromatic plump cells resembling active osteoblasts. In such cases, the clinical and radiographic findings are all-important in determining the correct diagnosis. In addition, in cementoblastomas, the active hyperchromatic cells do not exhibit cytologic evidence of malignancy.

The usual treatment for cementoblastoma is extraction of the associated tooth and enucleation of the tumor. The tooth generally has to be divided surgically before either it or the tumor can be removed. An alternative treatment, used occasionally, consists of separating the tumor from the tooth before removing the cementoblastoma. The tooth is then treated endodontically.

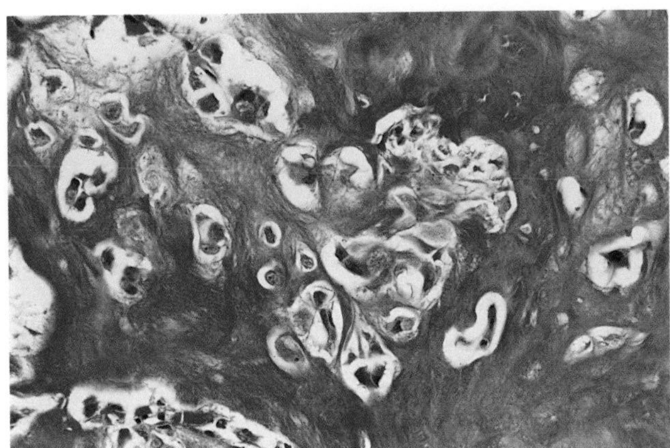
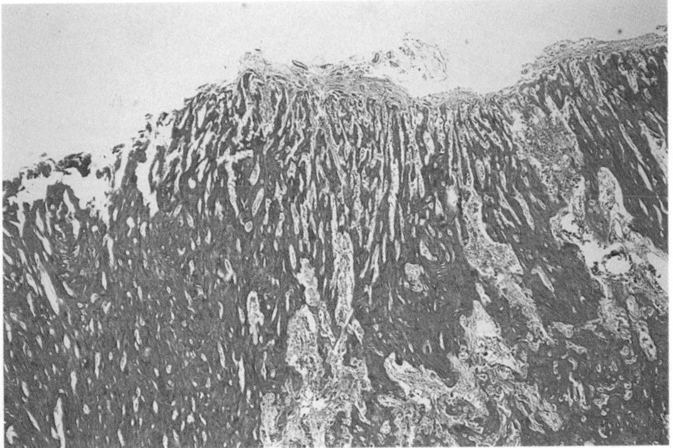

FIGURE 57. Cementoblastoma. **A:** Mineralized collagenous matrix with plump, hyperchromatic cells consistent with osteoblasts. **B:** Collagenous matrix arranged in radiating trabeculae at the lesion's periphery.

Odontoma

The most common odontogenic tumor, the odontoma (72), is a hamartoma and occurs in two forms. One, the *complex odontoma,* is an amorphous mass of dental hard tissues having no morphologic resemblance to a tooth. The complex odontoma may become quite large but is generally no more than 2 to 3 cm in diameter. The other, more common, type is the *compound odontoma,* which consists of tooth-like structures called denticles. These are generally smaller than normal teeth and are more conical; one compound odontoma may contain quite a number. This distinction between complex and compound odontomas is poorly defined; it is of no importance clinically.

Odontomas are generally discovered during the first three decades of life, especially the second, in keeping with their being developmental lesions. They occur equally in men and women and in all tooth-bearing parts of the jaws, although they are most common in the anterior region. Peripheral odontomas—those occurring on the gingiva rather than intraosseously—are extremely rare. In general, odontomas cause no symptoms. Their chief importance lies in that they cause disruption of the dentition, sometimes preventing the eruption of adjacent teeth or displacing them. When a tooth is impacted by an odontoma, the corresponding deciduous teeth may be retained. If sufficiently large, an odontoma may cause a smooth swelling of the alveolar process. On occasion, odontomas may be associated with dentigerous cysts or be a component of rarer odontogenic tumors such as the ameloblastic fibroodontoma, odontoameloblastoma, and calcifying odontogenic cyst. It is therefore important that all odontomas that are associated with more soft tissue than would normally be attributed to a dental follicle be examined by a pathologist.

It is often difficult to distinguish radiologically between compound and complex odontomas. The guideline is that a compound odontoma consists of a group of small tooth-like structures, whereas a complex odontoma appears as a well-circumscribed, amorphous radiodensity surrounded by a narrow radiolucent zone in the tooth-bearing part of the jaws. The radiolucent zone helps distinguish an odontoma from other radiodense lesions such as condensing osteitis. Developing odontomas exhibit various degrees of radiodensity, depending on the degree of calcification that has occurred. Compound odontomas can be diagnosed on gross examination and consequently need not be examined microscopically. Complex odontomas appear grossly as amorphous masses of hard tissue and are generally examined microscopically to confirm their nature. In both cases, parts of a dental follicle may be submitted along with the odontoma.

Compound odontomas exhibit the microscopic features of little teeth (Fig. 58), whereas complex odontomas are composed of a more disorganized mixture of enamel, dentin, cementum, dental pulp, and odontogenic epithelium. The morphology of teeth is not reproduced in complex odontomas; however, the interrelationship of the various tissues is normal. It is not strictly true, as is often stated, that the dental tissues in odontomas are completely normal. They commonly exhibit such aberrations as marked globular dentin, tubular dentin, and abnormal enamel matrix.

The histopathologic diagnosis of a fully developed odontoma is not difficult. However, the differential diagnosis between a developing odontoma and the much rarer ameloblastic fibroodontoma is a problem. This subject is discussed in the section on ameloblastic fibroodontoma (below).

Odontomas should be enucleated. They do not recur and are completely benign.

Ameloblastic Fibroma

The ameloblastic fibroma (73,74) is an important, although rather uncommon, tumor because it is readily confused microscopically with the classical intraosseous ameloblastoma, which exhibits a poorer prognosis.

This tumor, like the ameloblastoma, has a predilection for the posterior part of the mandible. It occurs predominantly in persons under 20 years of age, with the mean around 12 years. This age predilection is markedly different from that of the in-

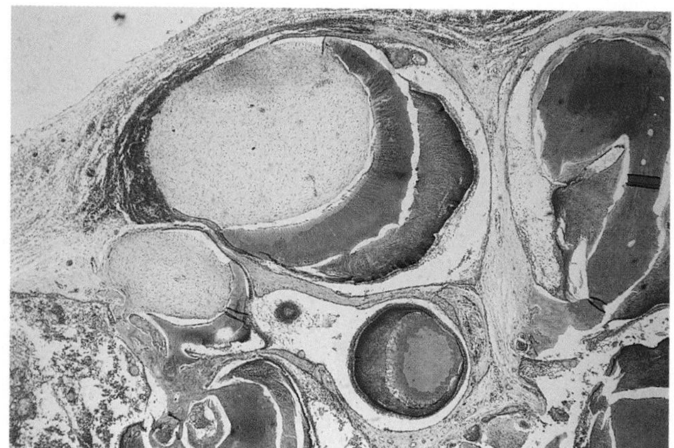

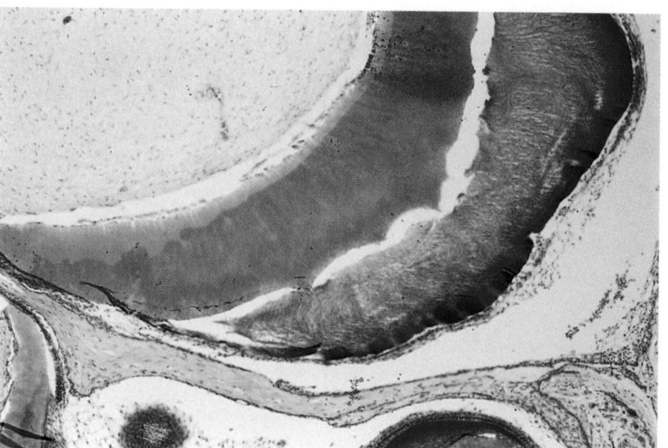

FIGURE 58. Odontoma. **A:** This example would be considered a compound odontoma because it exhibits several recognizable enamel organs. **B:** High magnification of one of the enamel organs in **A,** illustrating dental pulp, dentin, and enamel matrix in a normal anatomic relationship. Demineralized specimen.

traosseous ameloblastoma, which seldom occurs before 20 years of age. The ameloblastic fibroma occurs equally in both sexes. Clinically the patient may exhibit a swelling of the jaw, but many examples are detected radiographically. It is a well-defined radiolucent lesion that may be either multilocular or unilocular. It is often associated with the crown of an unerupted tooth and may therefore resemble a dentigerous cyst radiographically.

Grossly, the ameloblastic fibroma is a soft tissue mass that may be encapsulated. It consists of islands and strands of odontogenic epithelium that are dispersed throughout a cellular connective tissue component (Fig. 59). Both elements are neoplastic. The epithelial islands resemble the follicular pattern of ameloblastoma, although they seldom become cystic. Their basal cells exhibit the features of ameloblastoma, including palisading and reverse polarity, and surround stellate reticulum. The epithelial strands appear as slender anastomosing cords of cuboidal to columnar cells, usually two cells thick. Recognition of the characteristic connective tissue component is essential if the misdiagnosis of ameloblastoma is to be avoided. It resembles the dental papilla of the developing tooth and is richly cellular, delicate, and exhibits little collagen. The fibroblasts are plump and usually stellate. Quite commonly, there is a narrow zone of hyalinization of the connective tissue located immediately adjacent to the epithelial islands; more extensive hyalinization occurs occasionally. Ameloblastic fibromas do not form either dentin or enamel. Their presence in a tumor that otherwise resembles ameloblastic fibroma indicates a diagnosis of ameloblastic fibroodontoma *(q.v.)* or developing odontoma. Differentiating between ameloblastic fibroma and odontogenic fibroma is not difficult because of the former tumor's characteristic cellular connective tissue component. Moreover, the odontogenic epithelium in ameloblastic fibroma more closely resembles that of ameloblastoma than do the dormant epithelial rests of odontogenic fibroma, which in fact are absent in many examples.

The ameloblastic fibroma lacks the persistent infiltrative behavior that is characteristic of the intraosseous ameloblastoma and consequently has a better prognosis than that lesion. In the past, enucleation was considered to be the most appropriate

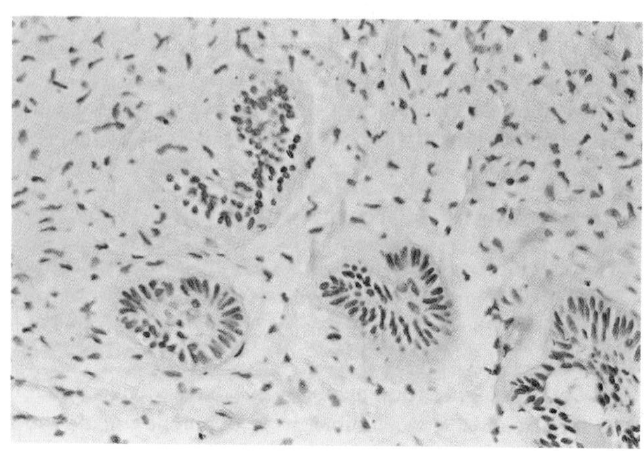

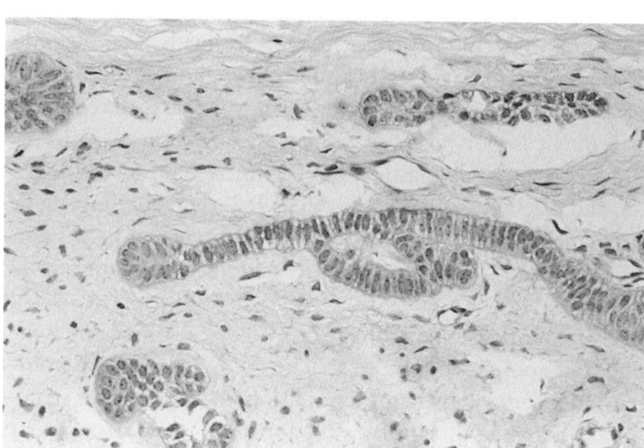

FIGURE 59. Ameloblastic fibroma. **A:** The islands of odontogenic epithelium resemble follicular ameloblastoma. The diagnostic connective tissue component is delicate and very cellular. **B:** In some examples the epithelium may consist of strands.

treatment, and recurrences have been rare. However, more recently it has become apparent that the recurrence rate after enucleation or curettage approaches 20% (74). Consequently, some surgeons are now advocating more extensive surgery for these tumors. There is also some evidence that the very rare ameloblastic fibrosarcomas may develop in recurrences of previously benign ameloblastic fibromas. A rare lesion that at one time was considered to be a variant of ameloblastic fibroma (the granular cell ameloblastic fibroma) is probably a different entity and is discussed elsewhere as the granular cell odontogenic tumor.

Ameloblastic Fibroodontoma

This is a rare tumor (75) that consists of an ameloblastic fibroma in which dentin and enamel have formed; that is, the process of odontogenesis has proceeded further in this tumor than in the ameloblastic fibroma. An intermediate tumor, the ameloblastic fibrodentinoma, in which dentin but not enamel has formed, is sometimes described.

A diagnostic problem is that odontomas, at one stage of their development, exhibit the same histologic features as the ameloblastic fibroodontoma. It follows that, because the differential diagnosis of these two lesions on microscopic findings is not possible, data concerning the clinical differences between the two lesions are unreliable.

The following is offered as a guide in the differential diagnosis of a lesion that exhibits the microscopic features that could equally be those of a developing odontoma or of an ameloblastic fibroodontoma. They are not definitive, and there is room for discussion when dealing with an individual lesion.

A small tumor that occurs during odontogenesis, especially if it is associated with an unerupted tooth or occurs instead of a tooth, is most likely a developing odontoma. This matter is complicated because odontogenesis commences *in utero* and occurs over the first two decades of life. Moreover, the timing varies with the teeth involved and, therefore, with the location in the jaws. For example, the second permanent molars should be completely formed by 14 years, as should the permanent canine teeth, whereas the third molars are not completely developed until 18 to 22 years of age. Large, expansile lesions, occurring in patients of any age, are more likely to be ameloblastic fibroodontomas. This is especially true of patients over 22 years of age.

The difficulty in distinguishing between these two lesions has undoubtedly led to the overdiagnosis of many developing odontomas as ameloblastic fibroodontomas. However, the distinction, other than resulting in an esoteric diagnosis that may alarm patients and clinicians alike, is not important because both lesions shell out readily and do not recur, unlike the ameloblastic fibroma, which sometimes recurs. This one point lends support to those who argue that the ameloblastic fibroodontoma is related more closely to the odontoma than it is to ameloblastic fibroma.

It has also been suggested that ameloblastic fibroodontomas are all developing odontomas. However, it is generally accepted that a true neoplasm, the ameloblastic fibroodontoma, exists. The evidence is that tumors exhibiting the microscopic features common to developing odontomas and ameloblastic fibroodontomas have occasionally occurred in patients of an age in whom odontogenesis is complete. Moreover, some have reached a size that suggest a neoplasm rather than an odontoma.

Tumors that are considered to be ameloblastic fibroodontomas occur as swellings in the jaw, either in the tooth-bearing region or sometimes in the ascending ramus of the mandible. Most have been reported in children. Their radiologic appearance varies depending on the amount of dental hard tissue that has formed. Those in which there is little dentin or enamel are radiolucent, whereas those examples in which these tissues are mineralized exhibit a mixed radiolucent–radiopaque appearance. Most examples are well circumscribed and unilocular. An ameloblastic fibroodontoma may be associated with an unerupted tooth.

There is nothing characteristic about the gross appearance of this tumor. An intact lesion will be encapsulated. Fragments of tissue may exhibit a gritty texture, depending on the degree of calcification present.

The ameloblastic fibroma component of the ameloblastic fibroodontoma is identical microscopically to that described for ameloblastic fibroma. In an ameloblastic fibroodontoma, enamel and dentin form to a varying extent within the ameloblastic fibroma component. In some examples rudimentary denticles are formed. These dental hard tissues are not formed adjacent to the ameloblastic fibroma, as in a collision tumor, but are an integral part of the tumor.

The treatment for ameloblastic fibroodontomas is enucleation. They do not recur.

Odontoameloblastoma

This is an even rarer tumor (75) than the ameloblastic fibroodontoma. It consists of an ameloblastoma associated with an odontoma and exhibits the biological behavior of the classical intraosseous ameloblastoma.

Ameloblastic odontoma is an obsolete term. It included lesions that are now known as ameloblastic fibroodontomas and odontoameloblastomas, respectively.

Odontogenic Carcinomas

These lesions (76) are very rare and consist of several types, some of which are better understood than others. It is not yet known whether separating them out as pathologic entities is justified by any significant difference in biological behavior. At present, they can all be considered simply as odontogenic carcinomas for clinical purposes. There is, however, academic justification in attempting to understand these various lesions better. Perhaps in the future doing so will be important clinically.

Malignant Ameloblastoma and Ameloblastic Carcinoma

There is some confusion associated with the term *malignant ameloblastoma* because it has been used in two different ways. It has been applied to those rare ameloblastomas that are cytologically benign but inexplicably metastasize. The metastatic lesions also appear as typical ameloblastomas.

On the other hand, the WHO classification (1) uses *malignant ameloblastoma* for a neoplasm in which the microscopic pattern of an ameloblastoma and cytologic features of malignancy are exhibited by the primary growth and/or any metastatic growth. This lesion has often been referred to as an ameloblastic carcinoma (77).

Making the diagnosis of ameloblastic carcinoma is not difficult if obvious dysplastic changes are present and the tumor otherwise has the features of an ameloblastoma (Fig. 60). There is a problem, however, in that the prognostic significance of mitotic figures in ameloblastomas is as yet unknown. Normally, ameloblastomas exhibit very few mitoses, but occasional examples possess obvious mitotic activity. As yet it is not known how extensive this feature should be to warrant the diagnosis of ameloblastic carcinoma.

There is a danger of misdiagnosing salivary gland tumors that have invaded bone as ameloblastic carcinomas. The adenoid cystic carcinoma, in particular, resembles the basaloid pattern of ameloblastoma and has occasionally been diagnosed as an ameloblastoma. One possible origin for the rare central mucoepidermoid carcinoma of the jaws are mucous cells in the lining of odontogenic cysts. However, this lesion is not generally considered an odontogenic carcinoma.

The best review of malignant ameloblastomas is that of Laughlin (78), who found the average age at which the primary tumor was treated to be 30.5 years (range 5 to 60 years). It is interesting that five of these patients were less than 10 years of age, which is an unusual age for ameloblastomas. Most metastases were to the lung. The median survival time after metastasis was detected was only 2 years. Laughlin concluded that surgery was the preferable treatment for solitary metastatic lesions and that disseminated ameloblastoma does not respond to chemotherapy.

The clinicopathologic features of ameloblastic carcinoma, which appears to be rarer than malignant ameloblastoma, have been well reviewed by Corio et al. (77). They found the mean age of their eight patients was 30 years. The clinical course was uniformly aggressive with extensive local destruction and frequent recurrences; one case metastasized to the neck nodes.

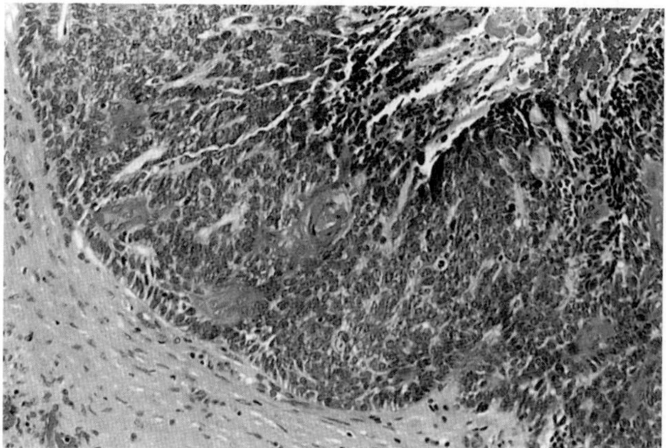

FIGURE 60. Ameloblastic carcinoma. The central epithelium is dysplastic, whereas the basal cells exhibit the typical morphology of preameloblasts.

Primary Intraosseous Carcinoma

This tumor (PIOC) (79) is a form of squamous cell carcinoma that occurs as a primary growth within the jaws. To justify this diagnosis there must be no connection with the overlying oral mucosa because otherwise it is impossible to determine whether the lesion arose intraosseously or extraosseously. These tumors presumably develop from rests of odontogenic epithelium within the jaws, but often they exhibit no microscopic evidence of odontogenic origin. In other examples the basal cells are palisaded and resemble those in ameloblastomas, occasionally to the point that their nuclei are located at the distal ends of the cells. It may be difficult in this situation to decide whether the tumor is a PIOC or an ameloblastic carcinoma, but this distinction is not important clinically. Adding to the diagnostic problem is that palisading of basal cells, such as occurs in ameloblastomas, is not necessarily indicative of odontogenic origin; it can be seen in some squamous cell carcinomas of mucosal origin.

The standard article on this condition is that of Elzay (76), who carefully reviewed 12 examples. He found that they occurred mainly after the third decade, with a mean age of 45 years, although one patient was only 4 years old. Men were affected three times as often as women. The tumors occurred predominantly in the mandible, especially in the posterior region. The basic treatment was surgery. Six of nine patients developed recurrences, and 6 of 10 died within 2 years of treatment. Almost all the patients developed cervical metastases.

Carcinomas Arising in Odontogenic Cysts

This is a rare event. However, squamous cell carcinomas (SCC) can arise from the linings of various odontogenic cysts (80,81). It has been suggested that they do so most commonly in residual radicular cysts, but radicular, dentigerous, and odontogenic keratocysts have also been involved. The first three of these cysts are not generally keratinized, and some workers believe that SCC tends to occur chiefly in those rare examples that have in fact become keratinized, usually with orthokeratin (1), as opposed to in OKCs in which parakeratin is a characteristic feature. This hypothesis has not been proved, as yet.

Although the diagnosis of SCC is normally straightforward, and in some cases the SCC is obviously arising from a cystic lining, in other putative examples the proof that the SCC arose in a preexisting cyst may be difficult. One alternative possibility is that the SCC has secondarily involved a preexisting cyst. Another is that the SCC could have undergone cystic degeneration.

Waldron and Mustoe (81) have reviewed the clinicopathologic features of squamous cell carcinomas arising in odontogenic cysts. Apparently, these carcinomas have a better prognosis, probably because they are well-differentiated keratinizing lesions, than the primary intraosseous carcinomas, which tend to be more poorly differentiated carcinomas. Local recurrence appears to be the major problem if the surgical excision is not sufficiently extensive, but metastasis to the regional lymph nodes has occurred in one of the recently reported cases. In 14 examples reported between 1974 and 1989, eight patients were alive and well between 2 and 6 years after their last treatment. The

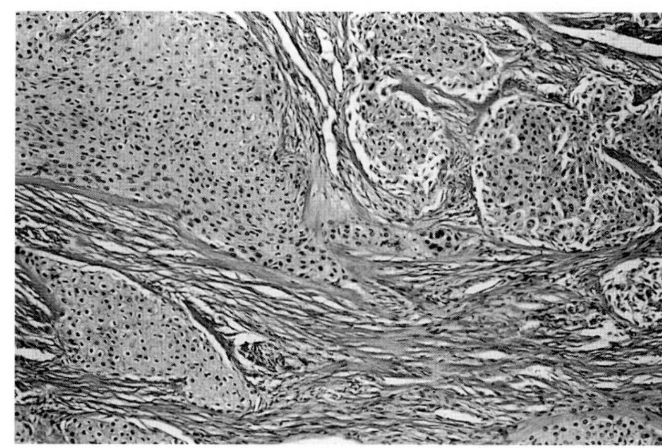

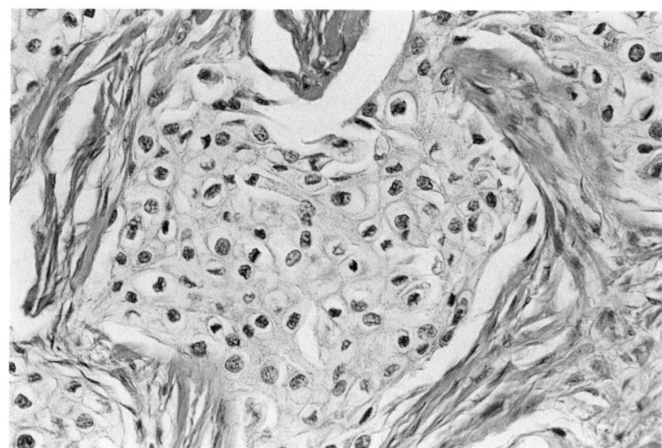

FIGURE 61. Clear-cell odontogenic carcinoma. **A:** Islands of epithelial cells with clear cytoplasm within a fibrous connective tissue stroma. **B:** The connective tissue around the epithelial islands tends to be dense and often hyalinized. The clear cells are actually faintly granular in some examples.

mean age of these 14 patients was 59 years, with a range of 22 to 85 years; 10 were male and 4 were female; and nine occurred in the mandible and five in the maxilla.

Other Odontogenic Carcinomas

Odontogenic Ghost Cell Carcinoma

This lesion (61) exhibits some of the microscopic features of the COC, including ghost cells, calcifications, and sometimes dysplastic dentin. Although our knowledge is sparse, some examples have apparently developed in preexisting COCs, and others have arisen *de novo.* Little is known about its biological behavior.

Clear-Cell Odontogenic Carcinoma

This tumor is included in the 1992 WHO classification of odontogenic tumors (1), under the designation *clear-cell odontogenic tumor,* as a benign but locally invasive tumor. It has now been confirmed, on the basis of proven metastases, to be a form of odontogenic carcinoma (82–84).

Microscopically, it consists of sheets, strands, or islands of clear cells, many of which exhibit abundant glycogen (Fig. 61). The epithelial islands are generally separated by dense hyalinized connective tissue bands. In some examples, the basal cells have resembled those of ameloblastoma; that is, they exhibit palisading, nuclear hyperchromatism, and cytoplasmic vacuolation. Some examples have exhibited quite numerous mitotic figures; others have not. The differential diagnosis includes metastatic clear-cell carcinomas, notably renal cell carcinoma, and mucoepidermoid carcinoma. The latter lesion may exhibit clear cells, but it will also demonstrate mucicarminophilia.

The relationship of the very rare ameloblastoma that exhibits clear cells (85) to the clear-cell odontogenic carcinoma remains unanswered. The one published example (85) of the former lesion responded well to marginal resection and showed no clinical or cytologic evidence of malignancy.

The calcifying epithelial odontogenic tumor (Pindborg tumor) may exhibit considerable cellular pleomorphism. However, it is a benign, generally infiltrative, lesion that should not be diagnosed as a malignancy.

Ameloblastic Fibrosarcoma

Ameloblastic fibrosarcoma is an extremely rare tumor, only 51 examples having been reported since 1960, according to a recent review (86). It is the malignant counterpart of the ameloblastic fibroma, and almost half of all reported cases have arisen in previously benign examples of that tumor. The mesenchymal component of the tumor is cytologically malignant, but the epithelium, which may be quite sparse and tends to become more so in recurrent lesions, is not. Related tumors have been designated as ameloblastic fibrodentinosarcoma and ameloblastic fibroodontosarcoma (the malignant counterparts of ameloblastic fibrodentinoma and ameloblastic fibroodontoma, respectively), but doing so seems excessive in view of their rarity. It is practical to consider these tumors, which exhibit the formation of dentin and/or enamel, as simply variants of ameloblastic fibrosarcoma. The microscopic diagnosis of malignancy is obvious in some examples, but it is unclear whether a small amount of pleomorphism such as the presence of a few mitotic figures in an otherwise benign-appearing ameloblastic fibroma is significant.

Most examples have occurred in the mandible in the third decade of life. However, it is interesting that those tumors that apparently arose in previously benign ameloblastic fibromas occur in older patients (mean 33 years) than those that apparently arose *de novo* (mean 22 years).

Ameloblastic fibrosarcomas are clinically aggressive and destroy bone. In some cases they have caused death by intracranial extension, but only one has been documented histologically (86,87) as having metastasized. About one fifth of patients have died of their disease. These tumors are best considered as low-grade sarcomas and should be treated by a sufficiently wide excision to include a substantial margin of apparently normal tissue if recurrence is to be avoided. Long-term follow-up is essential.

REFERENCES

1. Kramer IRH, Pindborg JJ, Shear M. *Histological typing of odontogenic tumours, 2nd ed.* Berlin: Springer-Verlag, 1992.

2. Gardner DG, Sapp JP, Wysocki GP. Epithelial cysts of the jaws. *Int Pathol* 1976;17:6–22.
3. Christ TF. The globulomaxillary cyst: an embryologic misconception. *Oral Surg Oral Med Oral Pathol* 1970;30:515–526.
4. Wysocki GP. The differential diagnosis of globulomaxillary radiolucencies. *Oral Surg Oral Med Oral Pathol* 1981;51:281–286.
5. Wysocki GP, Goldblatt LI. The so-called "globulomaxillary cyst" is extinct. *Oral Surg Oral Med Oral Pathol* 1993;76:185–186.
6. Gardner DG. An evaluation of reported cases of median mandibular cysts. *Oral Surg Oral Med Oral Pathol* 1988;65:208–213.
7. Stanley HR, Krogh H, Pannkuk E. Age changes in the epithelial components of follicles (dental sacs) associated with impacted third molars. *Oral Surg Oral Med Oral Pathol* 1965;19:128–139.
8. Gardner DG. The central odontogenic fibroma: an attempt at clarification. *Oral Surg Oral Med Oral Pathol* 1980;50:425–432.
9. Kim J, Ellis GL. Dental follicular tissue: misinterpretation as odontogenic tumors. *J Oral Maxillofac Surg* 1993;51:762–767.
10. Gardner DG, Sapp JP. Regional odontodysplasia. *Oral Surg Oral Med Oral Pathol* 1973;35:351–365.
11. Crawford PJM, Aldred MJ. Regional odontodysplasia: a bibliography. *J Oral Pathol Med* 1989;18:251–263.
12. Gardner DG, Radden B. Multiple calcifying hyperplastic dental follicles. *Oral Surg Oral Med Oral Pathol* 1995;79:603–606.
13. Sollecito TP, Greenberg MS. Plasma cell gingivitis. Report of two cases. *Oral Surg Oral Med Oral Pathol* 1992;3:690–693.
14. Anneroth G, Hall G, Stuge U. Nasopalatine duct cyst. *Int J Oral Maxillofac Surg* 1986;15:572–580.
15. Swanson KS, Kaugars GE, Gunsolley JC. Nasopalatine duct cyst: an analysis of 334 cases. *J Oral Maxillofac Surg* 1991;49:268–271.
16. Allard, RHB. Nasolabial cyst: review of the literature and report of 7 cases. *Int J Oral Surg* 1982;11:351–359.
17. Shear M. *Cysts of the oral regions, 3rd ed.* Bristol: John Wright & Sons, 1992.
18. Main DMG. Epithelial jaw cysts: 10 years of the WHO classification. *J Oral Pathol* 1985;14:1–7.
19. Shear M. Cysts of the jaws; recent advances. *J Oral Pathol* 1985;14: 43–59.
20. Craig GT. The paradental cyst: a specific inflammatory odontogenic cyst. *Br Dent J* 1976;141:9–14.
21. Ackermann G, Cohen MA, Altini M. The paradental cyst: a clinicopathologic study of 50 cases. *Oral Surg Oral Med Oral Pathol* 1987;64: 308–312.
22. Stoneman DW, Worth HM. The mandibular infected buccal cyst—molar area. *Dent Radiogr Photogr* 1983;56:1–14.
23. Browne RM. The odontogenic keratocyst—clinical aspects. *Br Dent J* 1970;128:225–231.
24. Browne RM. The odontogenic keratocyst—histological features and their correlation with clinical behaviour. *Br Dent J* 1971; 131:249–259.
25. Brannon RB. The odontogenic keratocyst—a clinicopathologic study of 312 cases. Part I. Clinical features. *Oral Surg Oral Med Oral Pathol* 1976;42:54–72.
26. Brannon RB. The odontogenic keratocyst—a clinicopathologic study of 312 cases. Part II. Histologic features. *Oral Surg Oral Med Oral Pathol* 1977;43:233–255.
27. Waldron CA. Odontogenic cysts and tumors. In: Neville BW, Damm DD, Allen CM, et al, eds. *Oral and maxillofacial pathology.* Philadelphia: WB Saunders, 1995:493–540.
28. Wright JM. The odontogenic keratocyst: orthokeratinized variant. *Oral Surg Oral Med Oral Pathol* 1981;51:609–618.
29. Gorlin RJ, Vickers RA, Kelln E, et al. The multiple basal cell nevi syndrome. *Cancer* 1965;18:89–103.
30. Fromm A. Epstein's pearls, Bohn's nodules and inclusion cysts of the oral cavity. *J Dent Child* 1967;34:275–287.
31. Wysocki GP, Brannon RB, Gardner DG, et al. Histogenesis of the lateral periodontal cyst and the gingival cyst of the adult. *Oral Surg Oral Med Oral Pathol* 1980;50:327–334.
32. Ramusson LG, Magnusson BC, Borman H. The lateral periodontal cyst. *Br J Oral Maxillofac Surg* 1991;29:54–57.
33. Greer RO, Johnson M. Botryoid odontogenic cyst: clinicopathologic analysis of ten cases with three recurrences. *J Oral Maxillofac Surg* 1988;46:574–579.
34. Gardner DG, Kessler HP, Morency R, et al. The glandular odontogenic cyst: an apparent entity. *J Oral Pathol Med* 1988;17:359–366.
35. Hussain K, Edmondson HD, Browne RM. Glandular odontogenic cysts. Diagnosis and treatment. *Oral Surg Oral Med Oral Pathol Oral Radiol Endo* 1995;79:593–602.
36. Pindborg JJ, Kramer IRH, Torloni H. *Histological typing of odontogenic tumours, jaw cysts, and allied lesions.* Geneva: World Health Organization, 1971.
37. Larson A, Almeren H. Ameloblastoma of the jaw. An analysis of a consecutive series of all cases reported to the Swedish Cancer Registry during 1958—1971. *Acta Pathol Microbiol Scand [A]* 1978;86:337–349.
38. Gardner DG, Peçak AMJ. The treatment of ameloblastoma based on pathologic and anatomic principles. *Cancer* 1980;46:2514–2519.
39. Ewing J. *Neoplastic diseases, 4th ed.* Philadelphia: WB Saunders, 1940:770–776.
40. Tajima Y, Ohno J, Ustumi N. The dentinogenic ghost cell tumor. *J Oral Pathol* 1986;15:359–362.
41. Scott J, Wood GD. Aggressive calcifying odontogenic cyst—a possible variant of ameloblastoma. *Br J Oral Maxillofac Surg* 1989;27:53–59.
42. Praetorius F, Hjøting-Hansen E, Gorlin RJ, et al. Calcifying odontogenic cyst. Range, variations and neoplastic potential. *Acta Odontol Scand* 1981;39:227–240.
43. Hirshberg A, Dayan D, Horowitz J. Dentinogenic ghost cell tumor. *Int J Oral Maxillofac Surg* 1987;16:620–625.
44. Shear M. Developmental odontogenic cysts. An update. *J Oral Pathol Med* 1994;24:1–11.
45. Eversole LR, Leider AS, Hansen LS. Ameloblastoma with pronounced desmoplasia. *J Oral Maxillofac Surg* 1984;42:735–740.
46. Waldron CA, El-Mofty S. A histopathologic study of 116 ameloblastomas with special reference to the desmoplastic variant. *Oral Surg Oral Med Oral Pathol* 1987;63:441–451.
47. Gardner DG. Radiotherapy in the treatment of ameloblastoma. *Int J Oral Maxillofac Surg* 1988;17:201–205.
48. Atkinson C, Harwood A, Cummings B. Ameloblastoma of the jaw: a reappraisal of the role of megavoltage irradiation. *Cancer* 1984;53: 869–873.
49. Ackermann GL, Altini M, Shear M. The unicystic ameloblastoma: a clinicopathological study of 57 cases. *J Oral Pathol* 1988;17:541–546.
50. Gardner DG, Corio RL. The relationship of plexiform unicystic ameloblastoma to conventional ameloblastoma. *Oral Surg Oral Med Oral Pathol* 1983;56:54–60.
51. Gardner DG, Corio RL. Plexiform unicystic ameloblastoma. *Cancer* 1984;53:1730–1735.
52. Gardner DG. Peripheral ameloblastoma: a study of 21 cases, including 5 reported as basal cell carcinomas of the gingiva. *Cancer* 1977;39: 1625–1633.
53. Pullon PA, Shafer WG, Elzay RP, et al. Squamous odontogenic tumor: report of six cases of a previously undescribed lesion. *Oral Surg Oral Med Oral Pathol* 1975;40:616–630.
54. Goldblatt LI, Brannon RB, Ellis GL. Squamous odontogenic tumor: report of five cases and review of the literature. *Oral Surg Oral Med Oral Pathol* 1982;54:187–196.
55. Wright JM. Squamous odontogenic tumor-like proliferations in odontogenic cysts. *Oral Surg Oral Med Oral Pathol* 1979;47:354–358.
56. Philipsen HP, Reichart PA, Zhang KH, et al. Adenomatoid odontogenic tumor: biologic profile on 499 cases. *J Oral Pathol Med* 1991; 20: 149–158.
57. Franklin CD, Pindborg JJ. Calcifying epithelial odontogenic tumor. A review and analysis of 113 cases. *Oral Surg Oral Med Oral Pathol* 1976; 42:753–765.
58. Freedman PD, Lumerman H, Gee JK. Calcifying odontogenic cyst. *Oral Surg Oral Med Oral Pathol* 1975;40:93–106.
59. Hong SP, Ellis GL, Hartman KS. Calcifying odontogenic cyst: a review of ninety-two cases with re-evaluation of their nature as cysts or neoplasms, the nature of the ghost cells and subclassification. *Oral Surg Oral Med Oral Pathol* 1991;72:56–64.
60. Ellis GL, Shmookler BM. Aggressive (malignant?) epithelial odonto-

genic ghost cell tumor. *Oral Surg Oral Med Oral Pathol* 1986;61: 471–478.

61. Grodjesk JE, Dolinsky HB, Schneider LC, et al. Odontogenic ghost cell carcinoma. *Oral Surg Oral Med Oral Pathol* 1987;63:576–581.
62. Wright BA, Bhardwaj AK, Murphy D. Recurrent calcifying odontogenic cyst. *Oral Surg Oral Med Oral Pathol* 1984;58:579–583.
63. Ghosh BC, Huvos AG, Gerold FP, et al. Myxoma of the jaw bones. *Cancer* 1973;31:237–240.
64. White DK, Chen S, Mohnac AM, et al. Odontogenic myxoma: a clinical and ultrastructural study. *Oral Surg Oral Med Oral Pathol* 1975; 39:901–917.
65. Gardner DG. The peripheral odontogenic fibroma; an attempt at clarification. *Oral Surg Oral Med Oral Pathol* 1982;54:40–48.
66. Allen CM, Hammond HL, Stimson PG. Central odontogenic fibroma, WHO type. A report of three cases with an unusual giant cell reaction. *Oral Surg Oral Med Oral Pathol* 1992;73:62–66.
67. Sciubba JJ, Zola MB. Odontogenic epithelial hamartomas. *Oral Surg Oral Med Oral Pathol* 1978;45:261–265.
68. White DK, Chen S-Y, Hartman KS, et al. Central granular-cell tumor of the jaws (the so-called granular-cell ameloblastic fibroma). *Oral Surg Oral Med Oral Pathol* 1978;45:396–405.
69. Vincent SD, Hammond HL, Ellis GL, et al. Central granular cell odontogenic fibroma. *Oral Surg Oral Med Oral Pathol* 1987;63: 715–721.
70. Shiro BC, Jacoway JR, Mirmiran SA, et al. Central odontogenic fibroma, granular cell variant. *Oral Surg Oral Med Oral Pathol* 1989;67: 725–730.
71. Ulmansky M, Hjørting-Hansen E, Praetorius F, et al. Benign cementoblastoma. A review and five new cases. *Oral Surg Oral Med Oral Pathol* 1994;77:48–55.
72. Kaugars GE, Miller ME, Abbey LM. Odontomas. *Oral Surg Oral Med Oral Pathol* 1989;67:172–176.
73. Trodahl JN. Ameloblastic fibroma: a survey of cases from the Armed Forces Institute of Pathology. *Oral Surg Oral Med Oral Pathol* 1972;33: 547–558.
74. Zallen RD, Preskar MH, McClary SA. Ameloblastic fibroma. *J Oral Maxillofac Surg* 1982;40:513–517.
75. Gardner DG. The mixed odontogenic tumors. *Oral Surg Oral Med Oral Pathol* 1984;58:166–168 (errata in 1984;58:574 only).
76. Elzay RP. Primary intraosseous carcinoma of the jaws. Review and update of odontogenic carcinomas. *Oral Surg Oral Med Oral Pathol* 1982; 54:299–303.
77. Corio RL, Goldblatt LI, Edwards PA, et al. Ameloblastic carcinoma: a clinicopathologic study and assessment of eight cases. *Oral Surg Oral Med Oral Pathol* 1987;64:570–576.
78. Laughlin EH. Metastasizing ameloblastoma. *Cancer* 1989;64:776–780.
79. Shear M. Primary intra-alveolar epidermoid carcinoma of the jaw. *J Pathol* 1969;97:645–651.
80. Van der Waal I, Rauhamaa R, van der Kwast WAM, et al. Squamous cell carcinoma arising in the lining of odontogenic cysts: report of 5 cases. *Int J Oral Surg* 1985;14:146–152.
81. Waldron CA, Mustoe TA. Primary intraosseous carcinoma of the mandible with probable origin in an odontogenic cyst. *Oral Surg Oral Med Oral Pathol* 1989;67:716–724.
82. Bang G, Loppang HS, Hansen LS, et al. Clear cell odontogenic carcinoma: report of three cases. *J Oral Pathol Med* 1989;18: 113–118.
83. Milles M, Doyle JL, Mesa M, et al. Clear cell odontogenic carcinoma with lymph node metastasis. *Oral Surg Oral Med Oral Pathol* 1993;76:82–89.
84. Eversole LR, Duffey DC, Powell NB. Clear cell odontogenic carcinoma. A clinicopathologic analysis. *Arch Otolaryngol Head Neck Surg* 1995;121:685–689.
85. Müller H, Slootweg P. Clear cell differentiation in an ameloblastoma. *J Maxillofac Surg* 1986;14:158–160.
86. Muller S, Parker DC, Kapadia SB, et al. Ameloblastic fibrosarcoma of the jaws. *Oral Surg Oral Med Oral Pathol* 1995;79:469–477.
87. Chomette G, Auriol M, Guilbert F, et al. Ameloblastic fibrosarcoma of the jaws—report of three cases. *Pathol Res Pract* 1983;178:40–47.

7

LARYNX AND HYPOPHARYNX

BEN Z. PILCH

ANATOMIC CONSIDERATIONS

The larynx and hypopharynx constitute the region of the upper aerodigestive tract where air on the one hand and food and water on the other part company, the former to travel to the lungs via the larynx, trachea, and bronchi, and the latter to the stomach via the hypopharynx and esophagus. In addition, the larynx is the seat of phonation. Thus, diseases of this region can affect respiration, deglutition, and speech.

The anatomy of the larynx is complex, and the reader is referred to standard texts for detailed description and discussion. Selected points relevant to laryngeal surgical pathology are mentioned here. The larynx is continuous superiorly with the oropharynx (anteriorly) and the hypopharynx (posteriorly) and inferiorly with the trachea at the inferior border of the cricoid cartilage. The larynx is divided into three portions, from superior to inferior, that have relevance for the staging, spread, and behavior of laryngeal cancer. The supraglottic larynx consists of the epiglottis, aryepiglottic folds, arytenoids, and the vestibular (ventricular) folds (or false vocal cords). The glottic larynx (or vocal cord region) consists of the anterior commissure, true vocal cords (vocal folds), and posterior commissure. The subglottic larynx lies inferior to the true cords and is continuous with the trachea at its upper border (1) (Fig. 1A).

The epiglottic cartilage is composed of elastic cartilage, is fan-shaped, wider superiorly and narrowing inferiorly, and is perforated by several spaces through which nerves, vessels, and glands pass. These perforations, as well as the epiglottis' narrow inferior portion, provide an avenue for the spread of tumors from the inner (or laryngeal) surface of the epiglottis to its outer (or lingual) surface and the preepiglottic space. The aryepiglottic folds, paired folds connecting the lateral borders of the epiglottis to the arytenoid cartilages, divide the supraglottic larynx medially from the pyriform sinuses laterally. The paired vestibular folds, or false vocal cords, are at the inferior portion of the supraglottis and are separated from the vocal folds or true vocal cords by a mucosa-lined space, the laryngeal ventricle (Fig. 1B). The ventricle provides a barrier (though an incomplete one, see below) to the spread of tumors between the supraglottic and glottic compartments. A narrow central finger-like prolongation of the ventricle, the appendix of the ventricle or saccule, extends superiorly at the midcord level (Fig. 1A). The saccule can become dilated, leading to a laryngocele if air-filled and unobstructed or to a saccular cyst if secretion-filled with an obstructed orifice (see below). The true cords meet in the midline anteriorly at the anterior commissure. The junction of the glottis and subglottis is somewhat controversial. It may be defined by an imaginary horizontal plane 1 cm inferior to the apex of the ventricle or, alternatively, 0.5 cm inferior to the free margin of the vocal cord (i.e., the area where the laryngeal mucosa changes from glottic squamous epithelium to subglottic respiratory epithelium) (2). A conceptually attractive separation because it consists of an anatomic structure is the conus elasticus, an elastic tissue–containing membrane that extends from the superior border of the cricoid cartilage to the vocal cord (Fig. 1A). Thus, the glottic compartment would be superolateral to the conus elasticus and include the vocalis muscle, and the subglottic compartment would be inferomedial to the conus elasticus.

The lingual surface of the epiglottis and the true vocal cords are lined by stratified squamous epithelium. The remainder of the larynx is lined by respiratory epithelium; however, the laryngeal surface of the epiglottis and false cords often develop patches of squamous metaplasia, especially in smokers and others likely to develop laryngeal lesions leading to biopsy. The ventricle and subglottis are virtually always lined by ciliated respiratory epithelium.

The hypopharynx, or laryngopharynx, lies posterior to the larynx and is continuous with it anteriorly. It is the most inferior of the three portions of the pharynx (nasopharynx, oropharynx, and hypopharynx) and extends from the level of the tip of the epiglottis superiorly, where it is continuous with the oropharynx, to the lower border of the cricoid cartilage, where it is continuous with the esophagus. The hypopharynx is divided into three regions: the pyriform sinuses, which lie between the aryepiglottic folds medially and the laminae of the thyroid cartilage laterally, constituting a pair of spaces the shape of upside-down pears, with the apex (or stem of the pear) inferiorly; the postcricoid region, which is the posterior surface of the cricoid lamina; and the posterior pharyngeal wall, which lies anterior to the cervical spine. The hypopharynx is lined by stratified squamous epithelium.

INFLAMMATORY LESIONS

Infectious

Most of the laryngeal infectious lesions the surgical pathologist can expect to encounter are chronic, mass-producing infections and may lead to biopsy.

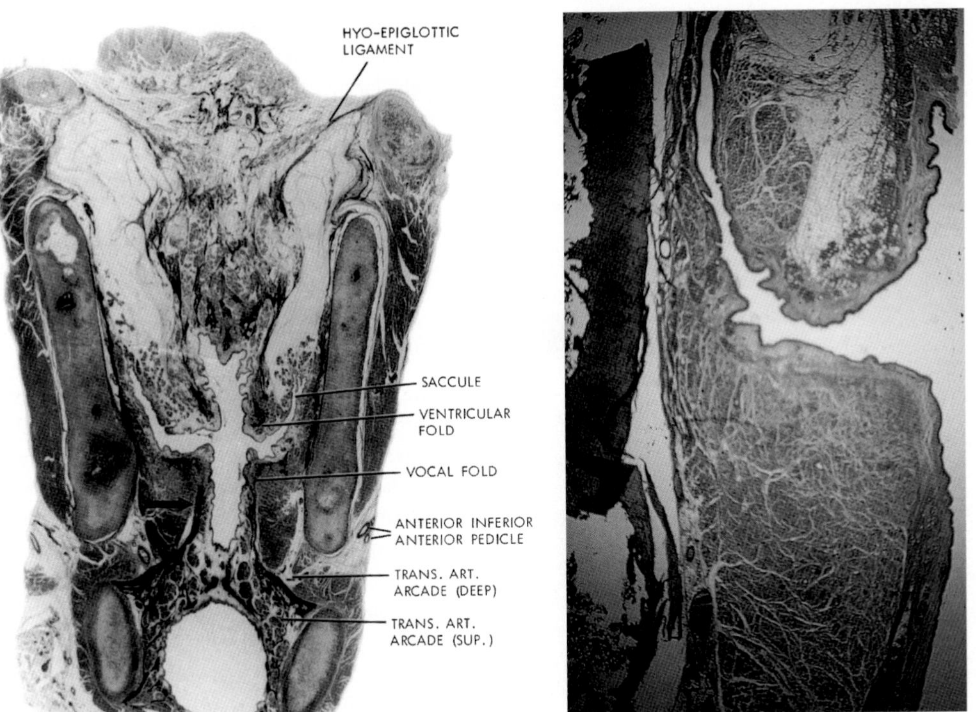

FIGURE 1. Normal larynx. **A:** Whole-organ coronal section of larynx at approximately midcord level. (From Tucker GF. Human larynx—coronal section atlas. Washington, DC: AFIP, 1971:12R, with permission.) The *arrow* points to the conus elasticus (see text). **B:** Histologic section at midcord level showing false vocal cord, ventricle and saccule, and true vocal cord. The thyroid cartilage is at the extreme left of the figure.

Tuberculosis

The incidence of tuberculosis (TB), especially in Western countries, had diminished markedly from the turn of the century to the 1970s and 1980s. There has been, however, a disturbing resurgence in the incidence of TB in recent years, such that in 1993 the World Health Organization (WHO) declared TB to be a global emergency (3). This increased incidence has coincided with the occurrence of the acquired immunodeficiency syndrome (AIDS) epidemic, and the problem is worsened by the emergence of drug-resistant strains of the tubercle bacillus. TB is common in human immunodeficiency virus (HIV)-infected individuals, and the disease is extrapulmonary in about half of these patients (3). Laryngeal TB, once considered the most common disease of the larynx (4–6) and the dreaded near-terminal sequela to advanced pulmonary disease, has become uncommon, less morbid, and associated with less advanced pulmonary TB, occurring in an older population and more likely to be confused with a neoplastic lesion (7). It is, however, as with other head and neck mycobacterial infections, of increased interest in this age of AIDS (3,8).

Most patients with laryngeal TB present with hoarseness, and some have dysphagia or odynophagia or both (5–7). The average age of patients is approximately the fifties, and most are men (6). Most patients have pulmonary disease, observable on x-ray (3), though generally of only mild to moderate severity (6). The vocal cords are most commonly affected, but supraglottic areas can be involved as well. Lesions can vary from hyperemic mucosal thickening to nodular masses (7). These mass lesions in patients with only mild chest disease can mimic laryngeal neoplasms, specifically carcinoma (9,10).

Histologically, one sees the classic picture of necrotizing epithelioid granulomas, with Langhans' giant cells and often with palisading histiocytes. Identification of beaded acid-fast rods confirms the diagnosis of mycobacterial disease (Fig. 2). Bacteriologic cultures or the use of newer molecular biological techniques is needed to determine the species.

Differential diagnosis includes other granulomatous diseases, specifically fungal infections, whose granulomas look essentially identical to those of TB, and sarcoidosis. Sarcoidal granulomas are characteristically nonnecrotizing, though some slight degree of necrosis may be seen, and organisms will generally not be found. The lesions of Wegener's granulomatosis do not form tight tubercles, and there is characteristically a fibrinoid, rheumatoid-like degeneration of collagen, often serpiginous or geographic in configuration. Vasculitis is often present.

Laryngeal TB responds quite well to treatment with antituberculous drugs to which the organism is sensitive. The degree of infectivity is somewhat controversial (6), and appropriate precautions should be taken.

Fungal Infections

Clinically significant mycotic lesions of the larynx are very uncommon, although, like many rare infections, they may possibly become more frequent in the HIV era. Laryngeal *histoplasmosis* (11) *coccidioidomycosis* (12,13), *cryptococcosis* (14), *blastomycosis*

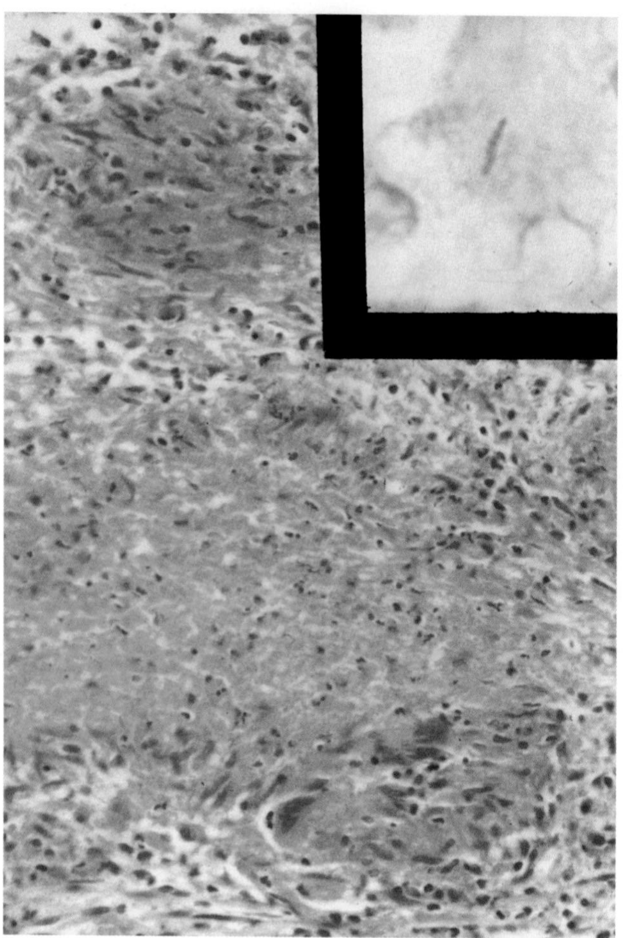

FIGURE 2. Laryngeal tuberculosis. A necrotizing granuloma (tubercle) contains epithelioid histiocytes and Langhans' giant cells. The **inset** shows a beaded acid-fast mycobacterial bacillus from this case.

(15,16), *aspergillosis* (17), *candidiasis* (18), and *actinomycosis* (19) (actually a bacterial infection) have been reported. Laryngeal lesions may present as ulcerations, mucosal thickenings, or masses and often mimic carcinoma (11,16–18). Histopathologic changes range from chronic granulomatous inflammation, reported with histoplasma, cryptococcus, and coccidioides, to abscess formation in blastomycosis and actinomycosis. Interestingly, laryngeal blastomycosis is characterized by prominent mucosal pseudoepitheliomatous hyperplasia, which must be distinguished from carcinoma histologically (11,15,16). This pseudocarcinomatous mucosal squamous epithelial hyperplasia has also been reported associated with *Candida* and *Aspergillus* infection of the larynx (17,18). Demonstration of the causative organisms in the lesions confirms the diagnosis.

Rarities (in the United States)

The larynx is involved in a significant number of cases of lepromatous (but not tuberculoid) *leprosy* (11,20,21). The disease is quite rare in Western countries and is rarely diagnosed by biopsy. The larynx was involved in cases of tertiary *syphilis,* with the formation of laryngeal gummas, many years ago; however, laryngeal syphilis is vanishingly rare in developed countries today (20). The larynx is not uncommonly involved in *rhinoscleroma* (11), rarely as an isolated site of involvement (22). The histomorphology of laryngeal disease is similar to that in the nose (see Chapter 4).

Encysted larvae of *Trichinella spiralis* are rarely encountered incidentally in laryngeal muscle (Fig. 3), primarily the vocalis muscle (20), and an exceptional case of laryngeal *schistosomiasis* has been reported (23).

Acute Infections

Biopsy of the larynx is rarely done in cases of acute laryngeal infections, most of which are viral in origin; however, a brief mention of *acute epiglottitis* seems in order. Epiglottitis, more accurately termed supraglottitis, is a bacterial infection of the larynx that results in marked erythema and swelling of supraglottic structures, including the epiglottis, aryepiglottic folds, and mucosa of the arytenoid region. It occurs in children, chiefly as a result of infection with *Haemophilus influenzae* type B (HIB), and in adults with a more varied bacteriologic etiology (24). In both children and adults the marked supraglottic swelling and pooling of secretions can lead to airway obstruction that may be of

A

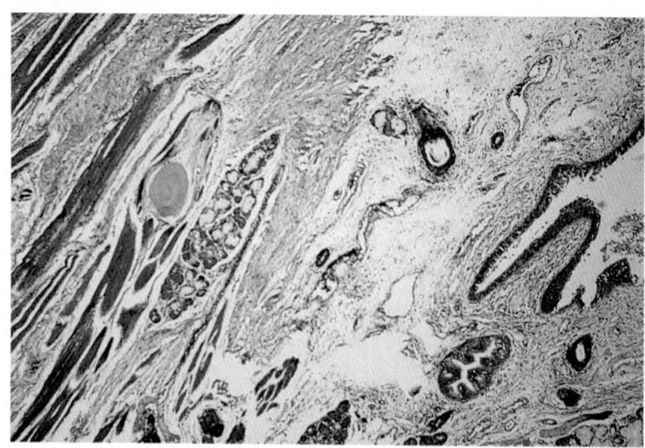

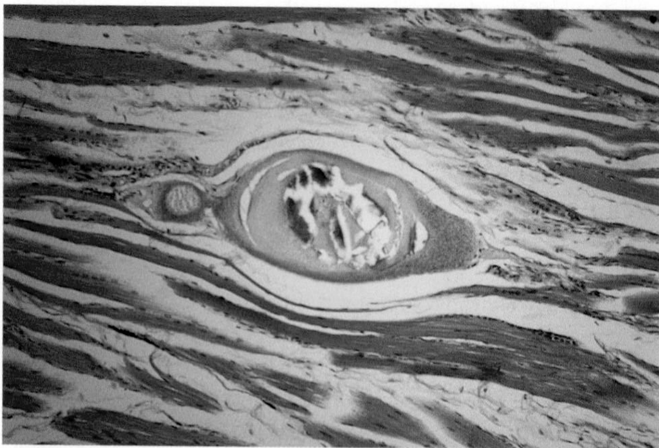

B

FIGURE 3. *Trichinella* infestation of larynx. **A:** A *Trichinella* cyst is present in skeletal muscle just to the left of a seromucinous gland. **B:** A high-power view of the encysted degenerated partially calcified larva of *Trichinella spiralis* in a laryngectomy specimen.

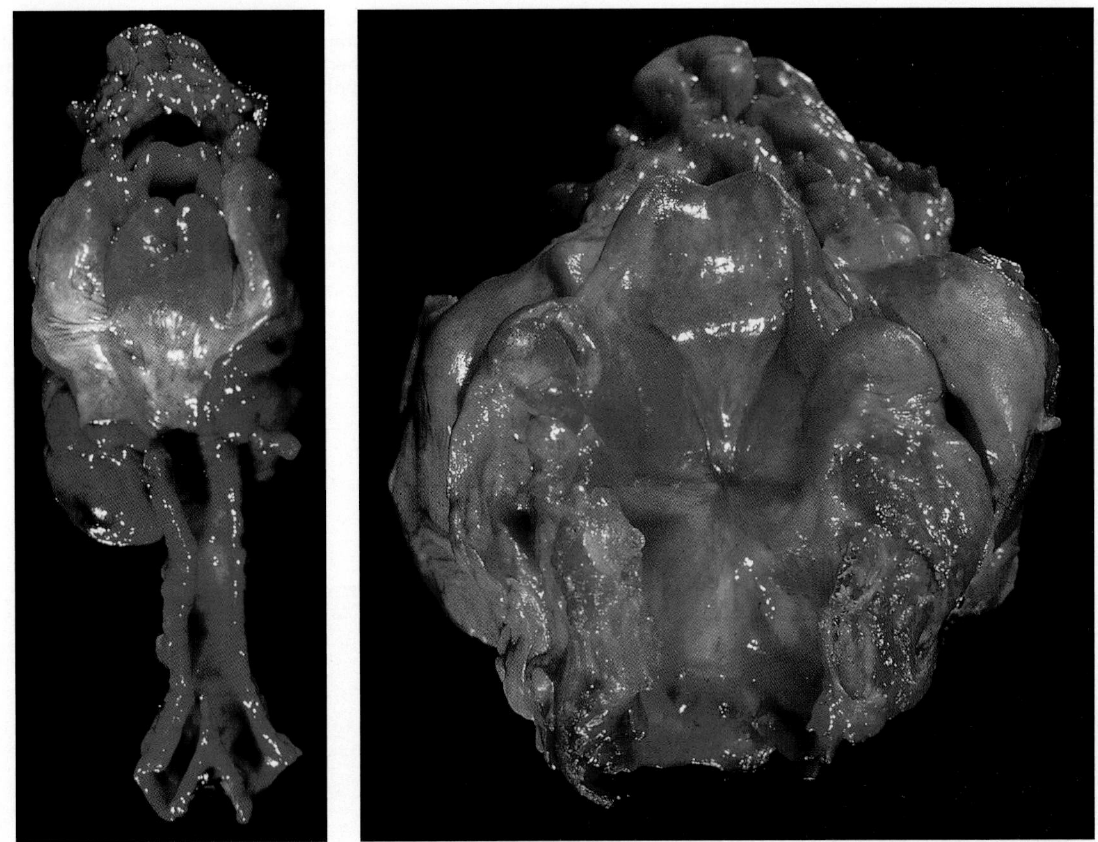

FIGURE 4. Acute supraglottitis (epiglottis). **A:** Posterior view of the larynx, showing congestion and swelling of the mucosa. Note the marked erythema and swelling of the epiglottis and arytenoids. (From Case Records of the Massachusetts General Hospital—Case 17-1967. *N Engl J Med* 1967;276:920–926. Copyright 1967 Massachusetts Medical Society. All rights reserved.) **B:** Erythema involves primarily the false cords, with an abrupt reduction in redness at the level of the ventricle.

alarmingly rapid onset and progression with a fatal outcome possible if not properly managed. Fortunately, following the availability of HIB vaccine in 1985, the incidence of epiglottitis (supraglottitis) has decreased markedly in children (25), and it is now mainly an uncommon disease of adults. Presenting symptoms in adults are primarily severe sore throat with dysphagia (26,27). Dyspnea does not typically occur in adults until relatively late in the course (27). A rapid pulse rate in the face of a normal respiratory rate in an adult with acute severe sore throat and dysphagia may be a diagnostic clue (27).

Pathologically, one sees reddened, markedly edematous supraglottic structures (Fig. 4). The swelling ends abruptly at the level of the vocal cords, possibly because of the lax supraglottic mucosa as opposed to the glottic mucosa, which is more adherent to underlying structures. Histologically, edema with a marked infiltrate of neutrophils, at times with microabscess formation, involving supraglottic structures is seen (24). Proper airway management, with intubation if necessary, is crucial in treating this disease.

Laryngeal *diphtheria* is currently very rarely seen, fortunately, although uncommon cases occasionally surface (28,29). The diphtheritic membrane is composed of abundant fibrin and a neutrophilic inflammatory infiltrate, overlying a mucosal surface whose epithelium becomes necrotic and disappears, leaving the membrane adherent to the subepithelial tissue, yielding a bleeding surface when peeled off, usually with some difficulty (Fig. 5).

Noninfectious

Sarcoidosis

Sarcoidosis is a granulomatous inflammatory disease of uncertain etiology and pathogenesis. It has a propensity to affect the lung and pulmonary hilar lymph nodes but can involve many other organs, including those of the head and neck and specifically the larynx (30,31). The disease generally does not cause severe problems, is characterized by remissions and exacerbations, and often eventually "burns out" (30). The larynx is rarely affected. When it is, symptoms may include hoarseness, dysphagia, and dyspnea (30), or the laryngeal involvement may be asymptomatic (31). At times, significant airway compromise may occur (32). The supraglottic larynx is most commonly affected with a characteristic laryngoscopic appearance of pale pink swollen and enlarged supraglottic structures (30).

Histologically, sarcoidosis is characterized by the presence of predominantly nonnecrotizing epithelioid granulomas (Fig. 6). At times some central necrosis in granulomas may be seen. The granulomas are discrete tubercles, with close apposition of the

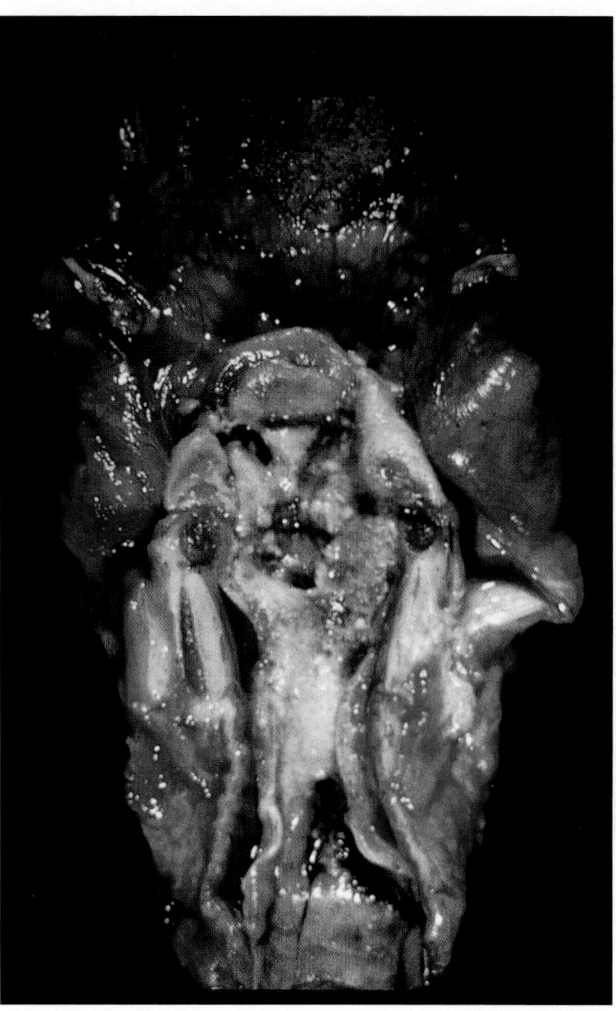

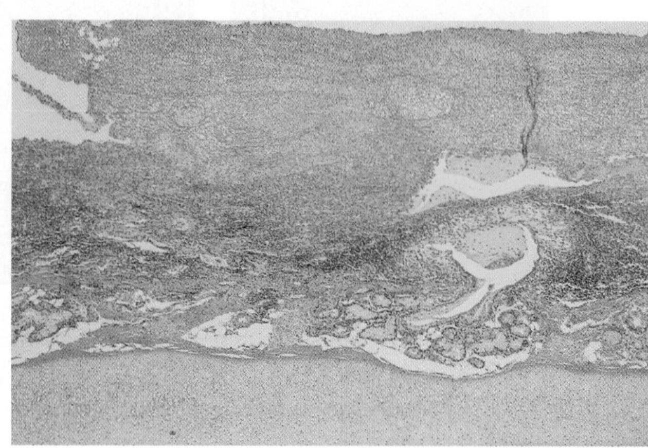

FIGURE 5. Larynx: diphtheria. **A:** Gross photo of the gray-white diphtheritic membrane lining the larynx and trachea. **B:** Microscopic view of the diphtheritic fibrinous true membrane (replacing a destroyed mucosal epithelium) overlying epiglottic cartilage.

epithelioid cells. When structures are floridly involved, as is often the case in hilar lymph nodes, the granulomas can become confluent. Multinucleated histiocytic giant cells of Langhans' type are often present, and the giant cells may contain stellate pink asteroid bodies or crystalline laminated Schaumann bodies (31), although these structures are not specific for sarcoidosis. In older lesions, fibrosis is often present in granulomatous areas (31).

The differential diagnosis of sarcoidosis includes other granulomatous diseases, especially infectious diseases. There is no specific pathognomonic histologic feature of sarcoidosis, and so the diagnosis, histopathologically, has traditionally been considered one of exclusion. Although microorganisms will generally not be found in sarcoidal granulomas, recent evidence suggests that mycobacteria, possibly cell wall–deficient forms, are present in cases of sarcoidosis (33–35), and exhaustive search may reveal the presence of acid-fast bacilli (36). In general, the granulomas of tuberculosis and histoplasmosis tend to be necrotizing or caseating, as opposed to those of sarcoidosis. Wegener's granulomatosis does not have tight discrete tubercles, and has features absent in sarcoidosis, such as fibrinoid degeneration of collagen and necrotizing vasculitis (see below).

Treatment may be expectant or involve administration of steroids for troublesome symptoms. In cases of marked airway compromise, tracheostomy may be indicated (30).

Others

Necrotizing sialometaplasia is a nonneoplastic condition of salivary glands that is characterized by infarct-type necrosis of salivary lobules with squamous metaplasia of adjacent salivary structures, set in an inflammatory background. It occurs spontaneously in the palate and following prior injury (e.g., surgery, trauma, irradiation, infection) in other sites and is thought probably to have an ischemic etiology and pathogenesis (see Chapter 8). This lesion can occur in the seromucinous glands of the sinonasal tract and in the corresponding glands of the larynx as well (31,37,38). The histomorphology in the larynx is identical to that in the salivary glands (see Chapter 8) and is of importance because it can mimic and must be distinguished from mucoepidermoid and/or squamous cell carcinoma. *Crohn's disease* can be associated with extraintestinal manifestations including oral ulceration (39). Very rarely,

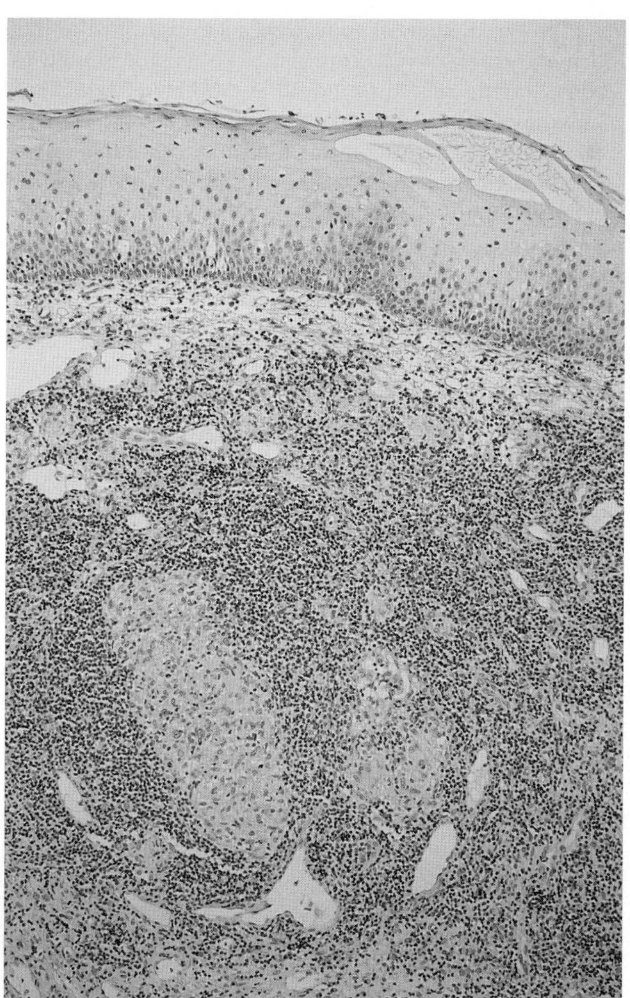

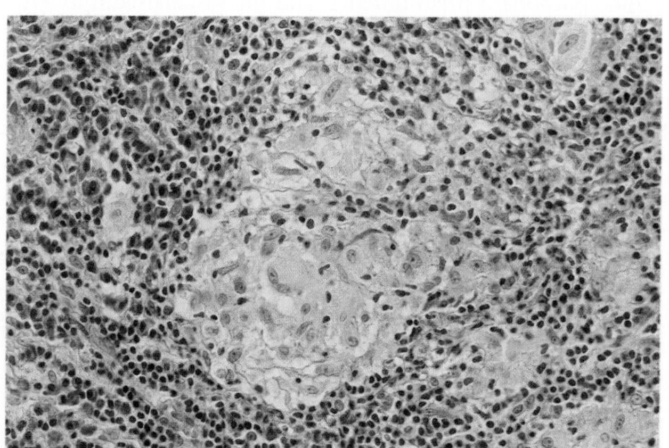

FIGURE 6. Larynx: nonnecrotizing granulomas consistent with sarcoid. **A:** Two granulomas, one very discrete and "tight," are present in inflamed tissue deep to mucosal epithelium. **B:** Higher-power view of a granuloma from the aryepiglottic fold composed of epithelioid histiocytes with a central giant cell.

laryngeal involvement in Crohn's disease can occur, with supraglottic edema and chronic inflammation and possibly granuloma formation seen histologically (39) (Fig. 7). An exceptional case of *Kimura's disease* of the epiglottis has been reported (40).

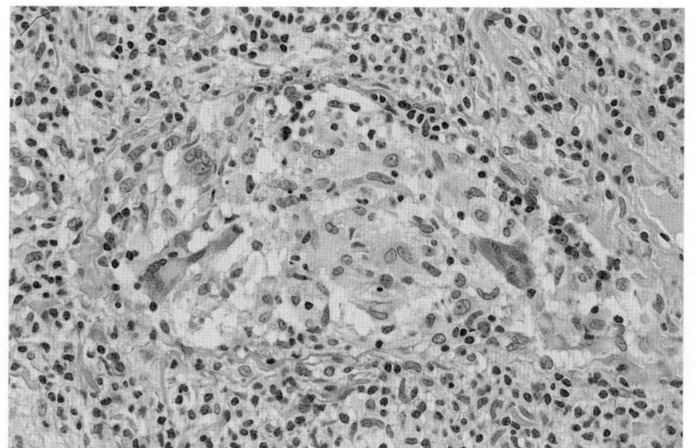

FIGURE 7. Larynx: granuloma in a patient with Crohn's disease. The granuloma, amid chronic inflammation, is composed of epithelioid histiocytes and giant cells. This patient has a history of intestinal Crohn's disease. Note the marked resemblance to a sarcoidal granuloma.

MECHANICAL AND CHEMICAL LESIONS

Vocal Cord Polyps

Vocal cord polyps are nonneoplastic swellings of subepithelial tissue on the vocal cords. They are characteristically related to vocal abuse or phonotrauma (41–43), and several colorful synonymous terms attest to this association, such as singer's nodule, teacher's nodule, preacher's nodule, and screamer's nodule. The lesions present in both sexes over a wide age range and may be unilateral or bilateral. Hoarseness is the main presenting symptom. Clinically, this type of lesion is divided into three major subtypes (43). Vocal cord *polyps* are unilateral or bilateral sessile or pedunculated localized swellings of varying sizes, generally in the midcord region. Polyps with a major vascular or fibrinous component (see below) can present as bluish nodules reminiscent of dilated vascular structures, and, hence, these types have been called "varix of the cord" in older terminology. *Reinke's edema* refers to a more diffuse myxoid swelling involving a larger portion of the vocal cord (Reinke's space is the area of the vocal cord between the mucosal epithelium and the vocal ligament). Vocal cord *nodules* are small bilateral and symmetric localized swellings in the anterior to midcord area.

There is significant histologic overlap among these three forms. Vocal cord polyps can be predominantly myxoid, predominantly vascular, or a mixture of these patterns. The myxoid type contains an accumulation of loose edematous, generally light bluish and mucinous tissue, often deep to a thickened mucosal basement membrane (Fig. 8A). There may be lakes of edematous fluid, especially in cases of clinical Reinke's edema. The vascular type contains dilated vascular structures with intravascular and extravascular deposits of fibrin (Fig. 8B). The fibrin not uncommonly undergoes organization, with an ingrowth and proliferation of endothelial cells resembling an organizing thrombus (42). This eosinophilic material had formerly been confused with amyloid but is now known to be fibrinous. Often, there is a mixture of the myxoid, edematous and vascular, fibrinous patterns in the same polyp (Fig. 8C). The polyp can undergo fibrosis and manifest a cellular, fibrotic pattern (Fig. 8D), but this type of polyp is rare in my experience. Reinke's edema and vocal nodules have similar pathologic features, although the myxoid component predominates, and the vascular component is quite limited in these clinical lesions (43). Inflammation is sparse in vocal cord polyps. The overlying squamous epithelium can be hyperplastic and often has a thin layer of overlying keratin (the vocal cord mucosa is normally nonkeratinizing).

The pathogenesis of vocal cord polyps is related to the mechanical trauma of vocal cord abuse (41–43) and possibly to airborne irritants related to industrial exposure or smoking (41). This causes increased vascular permeability (42,44), with transudation of proteinaceous edema fluid and, depending on the extent of the permeability or endothelial damage, the escape of blood and fibrinous products.

Treatment consists of voice therapy and, if necessary, surgical excision.

Contact Ulcers and "Granulomas"

Contact ulcers are laryngeal ulcerations that develop in response to mechanical or chemical (i.e., gastric acid) injury. They most frequently occur in the posterior third of the vocal cord, in the area of the vocal process of the arytenoid cartilage. The mucosa in this region is very thin (31,45), and the two vocal processes of the arytenoid cartilages, being situated posteriorly, are subjected to the greatest degree of excursion and, hence, impact during vocal cord vibration (31), as in phonation, cough, or throat clearing. For these reasons, the mucosa covering the vocal process is particularly susceptible to mechanical injury. Contact ulcers may be unilateral or bilateral. If the pathologic process continues, per-

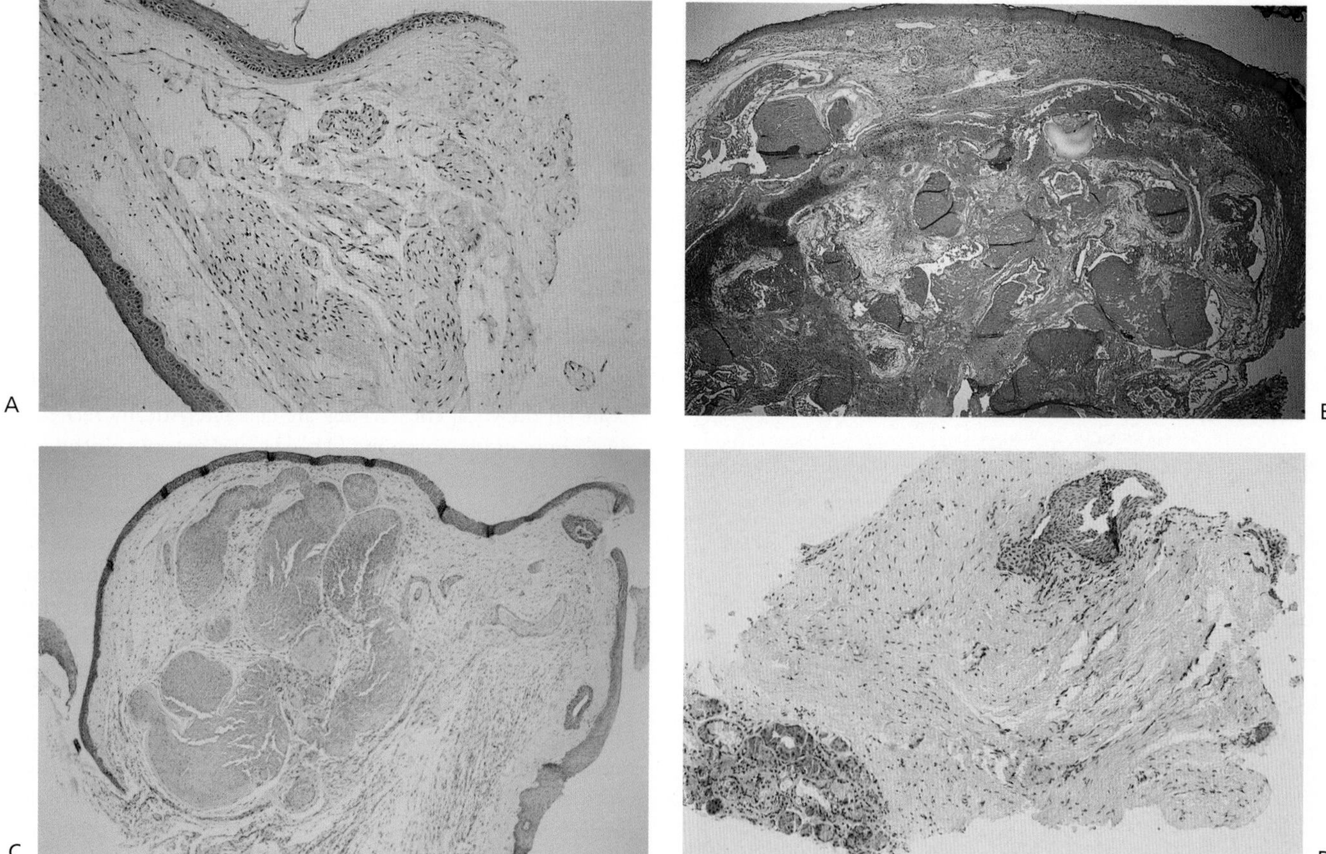

FIGURE 8. Vocal cord polyp. **A:** Myxoid polyp with loose myxomatous tissue deep to mucosal epithelium. **B:** Vascular polyp with marked intra- and extravascular fibrin deposition. **C:** Mixed polyp with loose myxoid tissue admixed with fibrinous material. **D:** Vocal cord "nodule" with fibrous tissue subepithelially.

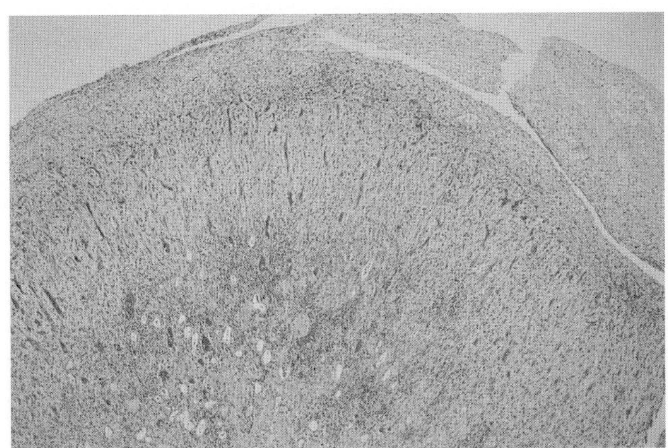

FIGURE 9. Vocal cord contact ulcer or "granuloma." An ulcerated fibrin-lined surface overlies polypoid granulation tissue, whose capillaries are oriented parallel to each other and perpendicular to the surface.

haps with an additional boost from supervening infection, reddish soft masses of granulation tissue (or "granulomas" in clinical parlance, although the lesions are not true epithelioid histiocytic granulomas) may develop as well, as contact "granulomas."

The pathogenesis of vocal cord contact ulcers or "granulomas" has been considered to be related to vocal abuse (e.g., excessive shouting, explosive glottic attack with initiating speech) or persistent habitual coughing or throat clearing (31,45,46). This lesion may also follow prolonged or traumatic laryngotracheal intubation (47), resulting from the tube's pressing or rubbing against the thin mucoperichondrium covering the arytenoid vocal process. Interestingly, more recent evidence suggests that reflux of gastric contents may contribute to the pathogenesis of vocal cord ulcers. The refluxed acid can irritate the thin mucosa covering the vocal processes and lead to direct injury or contribute to it by promoting repeated cough or throat clearing (46,48). This notion is supported by the dramatic therapeutic effect of antireflux measures (49).

Contact ulcers or "granulomas" occur in adults over a wide age range. Men are affected more often than women in cases not related to intubation injury (31). Symptoms include hoarseness (31) as well as possibly throat tickling, throat discomfort, pain, and a sensation of something in the throat with a desire to clear the throat or cough (46).

Laryngoscopic examination reveals ulceration or soft red masses of "proud flesh" involving the posterior vocal cord, either unilateral or bilateral. Masses can range in size from a few millimeters to several centimeters (31).

Histologically, one sees mucosal ulceration with a surface deposition of fibrin that may be thick at times. In cases of contact "granulomas" (more likely than simple ulcers to be excised surgically), there is a rounded polypoid mass of granulation tissue, usually with acute and chronic inflammatory cells (50). The capillaries of the granulation tissue are characteristically oriented radially, perpendicular to the surface of the ulcer (Fig. 9). This is in contrast to the case in pyogenic granulomas or lobular capillary hemangiomas, in which there is a lobular architectural arrangement of capillaries, often around central larger vessels (51,52). One may encounter fibrosis with hemosiderin deposition at the base of the contact "granulomas." In older lesions there may be partial or total reepithelialization of the ulcerated surface, with hyperplastic squamous epithelium, possibly exhibiting plump nuclei, prominent nucleoli, and mitotic figures—features of "regenerative" atypicality (31). Regenerating epithelium may even be fragmented in a background of fibrin (not solid tissue), thus simulating invasion. Obviously, it is important not to mistake such changes for carcinoma.

Most postintubation lesions heal spontaneously. Other contact ulcers may be treated by vocal therapy, antacids and antireflux measures, and, if necessary, surgical excision. Recurrence is common if treatment is ineffective.

Laryngocele and Saccular Cyst

The laryngeal saccule (or appendix of the ventricle) is a narrow prolongation of the ventricle at its superior extent, extending superiorly between the false vocal cord and the lamina of the thyroid cartilage. An abnormal dilation of the saccule that communicates with the laryngeal lumen via a patent saccular orifice is termed a laryngocele (53,54). Laryngoceles may be congenital or acquired (55,56). Practices that promote the repeated incidence of increased intralaryngeal pressure (or valsalva maneuvers with an open glottis against closed or partially closed lips), as in glass blowers or wind instrument players, may predispose to acquired laryngoceles (53). Laryngoceles may project medially, causing enlargement of the false cord or aryepiglottic fold. These are termed internal laryngoceles. They can extend through the opening in the thyrohyoid membrane for the superior laryngeal vessels and nerve to present as neck masses; these are called external laryngoceles. Combined laryngoceles represent saccular dilations that involve and cause masses in both locations (54). Laryngoceles are seen radiographically as air-filled saccular dilations (Fig. 10). They can expand or collapse because of their continuity with the laryngeal lumen. They can intermittently con-

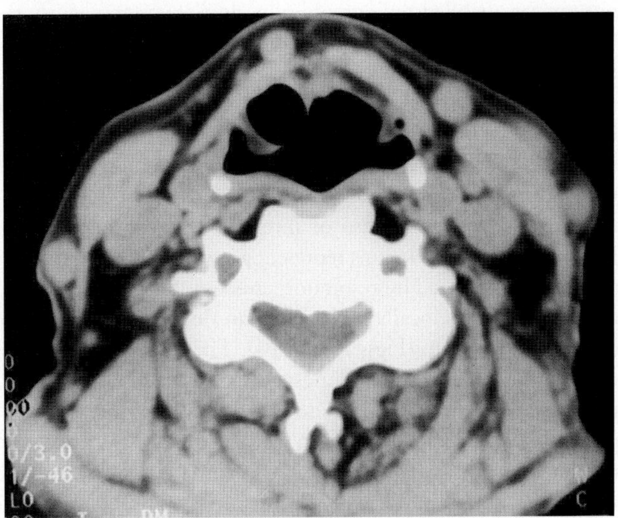

FIGURE 10. Laryngocele. This computed tomographic scan shows an air-filled laryngocele forming an outpouching abutting the inner surface of the thyroid cartilage in the supraglottic area.

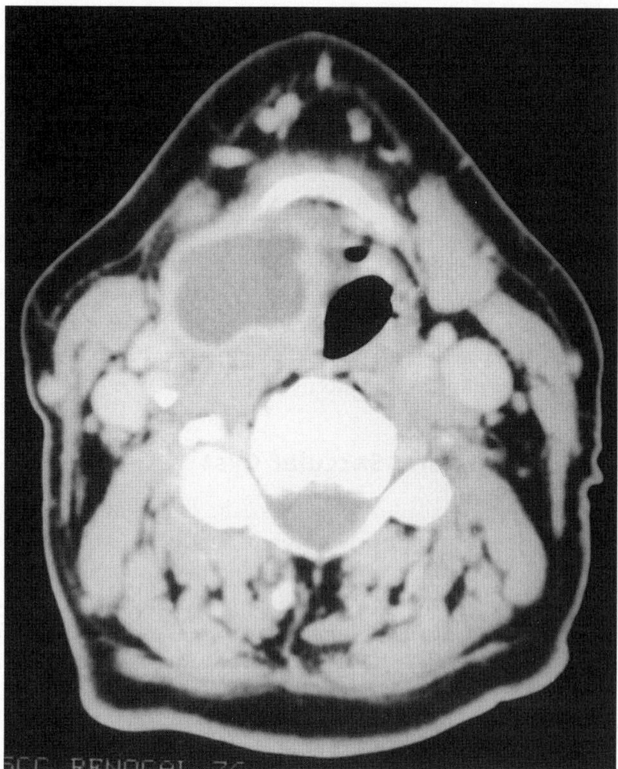

FIGURE 11. Saccular cyst. This computed tomographic scan shows a large fluid-filled saccular cyst at the level of the hyoid bone, narrowing the airway and protruding into the neck.

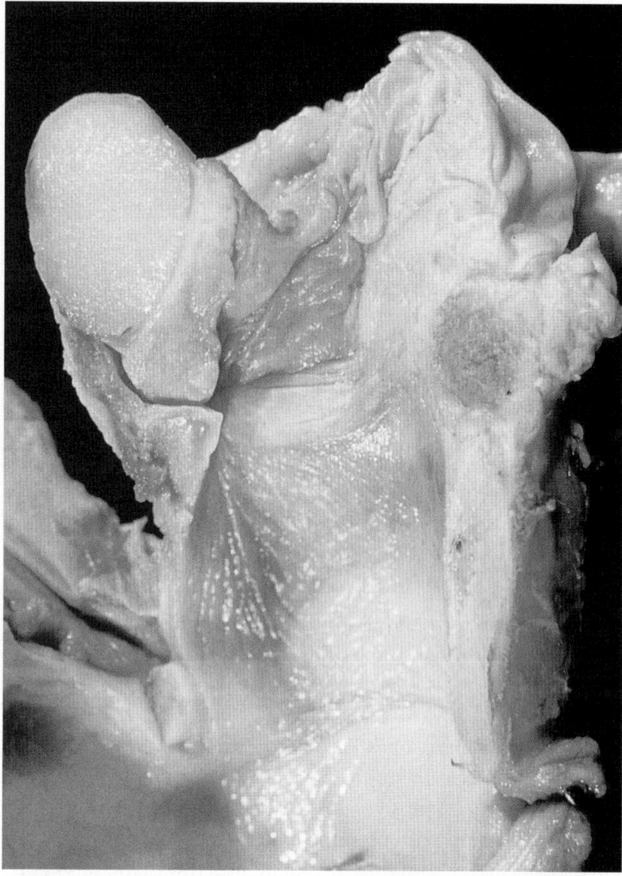

FIGURE 12. Larynx: saccular cyst. A mucus-filled cystic dilation is located at the tip of the laryngeal ventricle. (From Fig. 2-2 of Goodman ML, Pilch BZ. Airway pathology. In: Roberts JT, ed. *Clinical management of the airway.* Philadelphia: WB Saunders, 1994:28, with permission.)

tain fluid, as multiple seromucinous glands empty into the saccule. If they are infected, purulent laryngopyoceles may result (53,56). Saccular cysts are saccular dilations that are fluid-filled and do not communicate with the laryngeal lumen (Figs. 11 and 12). The saccular orifice in such cases is obstructed either congenitally, by fibrosis, such as after repeated inflammation, or by compression, for example by a neoplasm (54). Saccular cysts do not appear air-filled radiographically, do not spontaneously deflate, nor are they easily compressible, as are air-filled laryngoceles.

Patients are typically either infants or babies with congenital lesions or adults with acquired lesions. Symptoms may include hoarseness, muffled voice, dyspnea, or the appearance of a neck mass. Laryngoscopic examination usually reveals a bulge in the false cord area in the case of internal or combined lesions. Histologically, these lesions represent a cystic enlargement of the saccule and are lined by respiratory mucosa that is often attenuated and at times focally replaced by an oncocytic columnar or cuboidal epithelium (Figs. 13 and 14). The wall may be chronically inflamed. In large and longstanding cases, cholesterol clefts may be seen in the wall (57). The lumen may be empty (in laryngoceles) or filled with mucus (in saccular cysts). It is important to remember that laryngoceles may at times be associated with carcinoma, so any surgical specimens of laryngoceles should be examined for this eventuality (54–56).

Treatment involves aspiration, marsupialization, or excision in stubborn, multiply recurrent cases.

Teflon Granuloma

Teflon is the commercial name for polytetrafluoroethylene (58). It has been used, in paste form, for intralaryngeal injections in the treatment of unilateral vocal cord paralysis in abduction. Such paralysis can accompany tumors (e.g., laryngeal or pul-

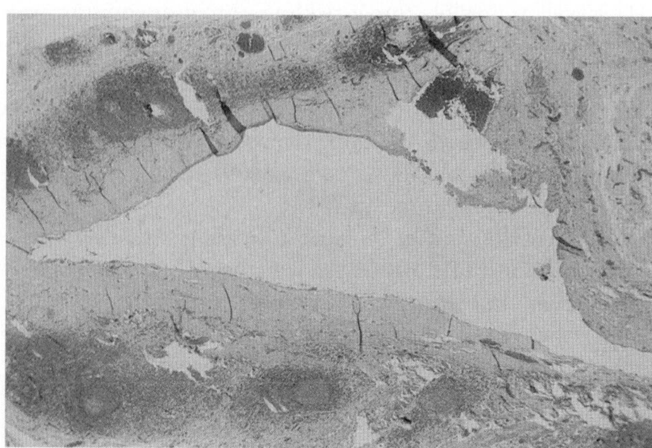

FIGURE 13. Larynx: laryngocele. A ventricular dilation is lined by attenuated mucosal epithelium and has a fibrotic wall with prominent chronic inflammation.

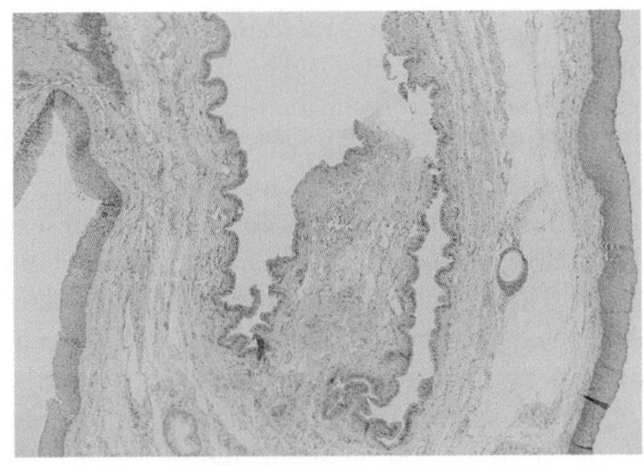
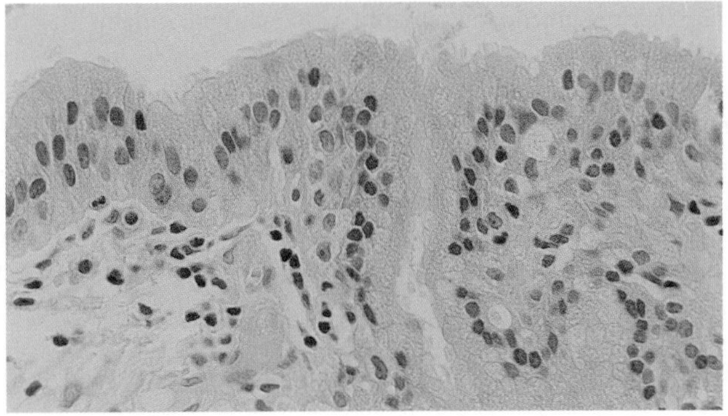

FIGURE 14. Larynx: saccular cyst. **A:** The cyst lies deep to mucosal epithelium. **B:** The cyst is lined by oncocytic focally ciliated epithelium.

monary) that involve the recurrent laryngeal nerve, can follow trauma to the nerve (e.g., as a complication of surgery), or can be idiopathic (59). Unilateral vocal cord paralysis in abduction (i.e., with the cord fixed laterally) may result in a breathy poor-quality voice and/or aspiration. Injection of Teflon into the paralyzed cord serves to increase the cord's bulk and bring its free edge medially to more closely approximate the opposite cord and thereby improve phonation and decrease aspiration (31,58). The Teflon usually stays localized and encased in fibrous tissue. Although this procedure often works well, complications may occur. These involve migration and extension of the Teflon such as through the cricothyroid space anterolaterally into the neck or by injection below the conus elasticus into the subglottic compartment (58) (see anatomic considerations). Alternatively, too large a bolus can enlarge the cord too much, compromising speech and breathing.

Symptoms of such complications of Teflon injections include the presence of a neck mass, hoarseness, or airway obstruction (31). Laryngoscopic examination reveals a submucosal mass caused by Teflon accumulation and the tissue reaction to it. Histologically, Teflon elicits a brisk foreign body giant-cell response, and the Teflon granuloma, on removal, has a characteristic appearance. The Teflon appears as numerous crystalline deposits in the tissue, with a florid associated multinucleated foreign body giant-cell response (59) (Fig. 15A). The crystals are markedly birefrigent when viewed under polarized light (Fig. 15B). A densely fibrotic response with few, if any, chronic inflammatory cells is usually present. Treatment is by surgical excision.

Recently, alternative methods of vocal cord medialization to Teflon injection have been developed. These include thyroplasty procedures, with plastic implants inserted through the thyroid cartilage to push the paralyzed cord medially (60).

Zenker's (Hypopharyngeal) Diverticulum

A hypopharyngeal, or Zenker's, diverticulum represents an outpouching of hypopharyngeal mucosa posterolaterally between the fibers of the cricothyroid and cricopharyngeus muscles, forming a diverticular sac. The condition occurs primarily in elderly individuals, men more often than women (61). The etiology is incompletely understood, but abnormalities of esophageal sphincters with increased hypopharyngeal pressure may be contributing factors (61). Symptoms most commonly include dysphagia or regurgitation of food. The diverticulum may easily be visualized radiographically with a barium swallow.

Histologically, the sac is composed of essentially unremarkable appearing squamous epithelial lined hypopharyngeal mu-

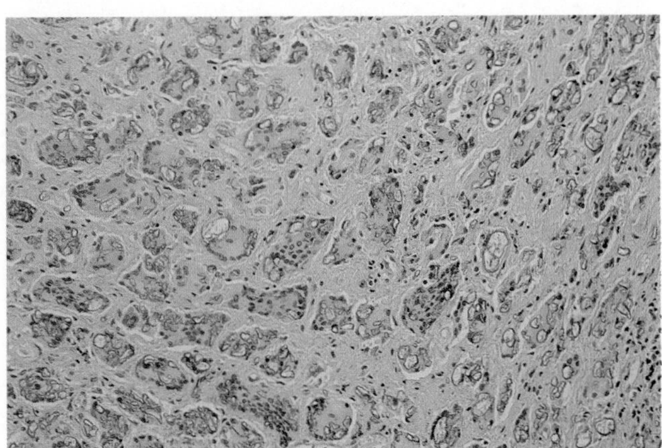
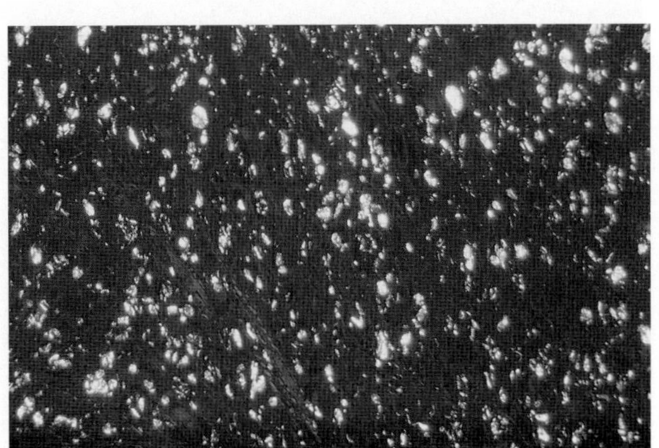

FIGURE 15. Larynx: Teflon granuloma. **A:** Teflon particles are being phagocytized by foreign body giant cells. **B:** The Teflon is brightly birefringent when viewed under polarized light.

cosa, perhaps a bit thinned, and possibly with a chronic inflammatory infiltrate.

Although the classic treatment in symptomatic cases has been surgical diverticulectomy, recently more conservative procedures (diverticulopexy or suspending the sac by suturing it to the prevertebral fascia, imbrication into the hypopharynx, or myotomy) have been employed with success (61).

DEGENERATIVE, AUTOIMMUNE, AND METABOLIC DISEASE

Wegener's Granulomatosis

Classic systemic Wegener's granulomatosis is characterized by involvement of the upper respiratory tract, lungs, and kidneys and occasionally other organs as well (62,63). Pathologically, degenerative granulomatous lesions somewhat akin to rheumatoid nodules involving the upper and lower respiratory tract, necrotizing and at times granulomatous vasculitis, and necrotizing glomerulonephritis are seen (64). The disease used to be frequently fatal, most patients expiring with renal failure, before the advent of successful treatment with cytotoxic immunosuppressive drugs such as cyclophosphamide (62). Limited forms of the disease occur, often with involvement of the respiratory tract without renal involvement (63).

Most patients with Wegener's granulomatosis, generalized or limited, present with symptoms and signs related to the upper respiratory tract. These are characteristically nonspecific, such as rhinorrhea, pain, and nasal mucosal ulceration (see Chapter 4). Recently, it has become apparent that a significant proportion of patients have laryngeal involvement, characteristically manifesting as a subglottic lesion, often with subglottic stenosis (65). Thus, 16% (25 of 158) of patients with Wegener's granulomatosis in the series of Lebovics et al. (66) had subglottic narrowing. Interestingly, this percentage is substantially higher in children and adolescents, 48% (11 of 23) in the Lebovics et al. series compared to 10% (14 of 135) of adults (66).

The histopathology of Wegener's granulomatosis (see Chapter 4) is varied, and it is important to remember that often not all of the characteristic features are seen on a biopsy in the head and neck area (67). The histopathologic features of Wegener's granulomatosis in the head and neck, including the larynx, include fibrinoid degeneration of collagen, often with palisading histiocytes, reminiscent of a palisading granuloma such as is seen in rheumatoid nodules. Such an area may be large and have a serpiginous appearance of "geographic necrosis" (67). These foci characteristically have a bluish or basophilic hue, a feature of diagnostic value. One may see microabscesses or small focal collections of neutrophils, at times with a component of epithelioid histiocytes, in extravascular tissue or centered on a small blood vessel (Fig. 16A). Multinucleated histiocytic giant cells may be few or numerous, scattered or clustered (Fig. 16B); however, frank tight discrete granulomas resembling tubercles or sarcoidal granulomas are not encountered. Necrotizing vasculitis with fibrinoid necrosis may involve arteries and/or veins, of small or large caliber. Vasculitis may also be granulomatous, with the presence of giant cells, and may have an infiltrate containing neutrophils and/or lymphocytes. These findings are usually seen in a background of dense chronic inflammation, often with fibrosis. Fibrosis may be extensive in older lesions. When all three major components (granulomatous changes, degeneration of collagen, and vasculitis) are present, in the absence of infectious agents such as acid-fast bacilli or fungi on special stains, one may be highly suspicious if not convinced of the diagnosis of Wegener's granulomatosis. All three components, however, were present in only 16% of head and neck biopsies in Wegner's patients in the Devaney et al. series (67). One may suspect the diagnosis if fewer of these pathologic features are present. Antineutrophil cytoplasmic antibodies (ANCA) are present in the serum in the great majority of patients with generalized Wegener's granulomatosis and in most patients (but not all) with limited forms, and this is a very helpful confirmatory diagnostic test (68–70).

Although therapy with cytotoxic agents such as cyclophosphamide is very effective in the treatment of Wegener's granulomatosis (62), many patients with symptomatic subglottic stenosis require surgical intervention (66).

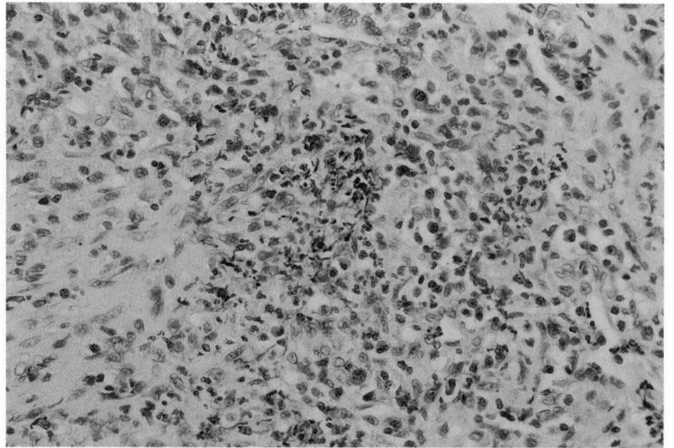
A

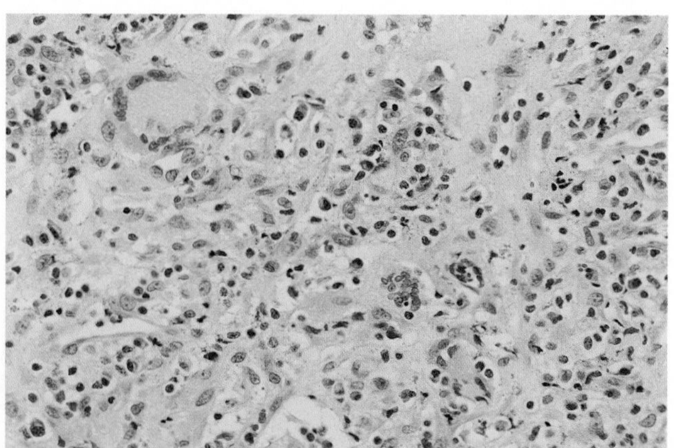
B

FIGURE 16. Subglottic larynx: Wegener's granulomatosis. **A:** A microabscess is present amid a mixed inflammatory background containing mononuclear cells, neutrophils, and eosinophils. **B:** Occasional multinucleated giant cells are present in the mixed inflammatory infiltrate.

Amyloid

Amyloid is the term applied to a group of fibrillar proteins deposited extracellularly that have certain physicochemical properties in common. Thus, they exhibit amorphous eosinophilic staining with hematoxylin and eosin, they exhibit an apple-green birefringence when stained with Congo red and viewed under polarized light, and they have a structural β pleated sheet conformation (71,72). Amyloidosis comprises a group of diseases in which extracellular deposits of amyloid accumulate. Several classification schemes for amyloidosis have been proposed over the years. Amyloidosis may be systemic or localized, primary or associated with chronic inflammatory conditions such as tuberculosis or rheumatoid arthritis, associated with multiple myeloma, familial or sporadic, present as deposits in the elderly in the brain or heart, or associated with renal dialysis (71,72). Several different proteins have been identified and are associated with various clinical forms of amyloidosis, and currently, amyloidosis is often classified according to its constituent protein (72,73).

Although the larynx may be involved in cases of systemic amyloidosis, significant symptomatic laryngeal amyloid deposition is almost always a manifestation of localized amyloidosis. In fact, the larynx is the most common site of localized amyloidosis of the respiratory tract. It has recently been shown that the protein of localized laryngeal amyloidosis is AL protein or immunoglobulin light chain, similar to cases of primary systemic amyloidosis and myeloma-associated amyloidosis (72,74).

Within the larynx, the false vocal cord area is most commonly affected, although glottic and subglottic foci may be involved as well. Multiple sites can be affected. Occasionally laryngeal amyloidosis (usually subglottic) is associated with tracheal or tracheobronchial amyloid deposits, and rarely, laryngeal amyloidosis (usually supraglottic) is associated with nasopharyngeal involvement. Symptoms of laryngeal disease include hoarseness, most commonly, as well as occasionally cough or the sensation of a lump in the throat; with more extensive involvement, stridor, dyspnea, or hemoptysis may occur (75). Laryngeal amyloid may manifest endoscopically as one or more discrete tumor-like masses or as a more diffuse submucosal thickening.

Histologically, amyloid appears as a homogeneous amorphous eosinophilic material deposited extracellularly (Fig. 17). It takes the form of sheets or large globules. A characteristic separation of masses of amyloid by thin linear spaces forming a "cracked" appearance is a useful diagnostic clue (Fig. 17A). Amyloid deposition may be accompanied by mutlinucleated giant cells in an attempt at phagocytosis (Fig. 17B). There may be a scattering of mononuclear inflammatory cells, characteristically rich in plasma cells in laryngeal cases. Focal dystrophic calcifica-

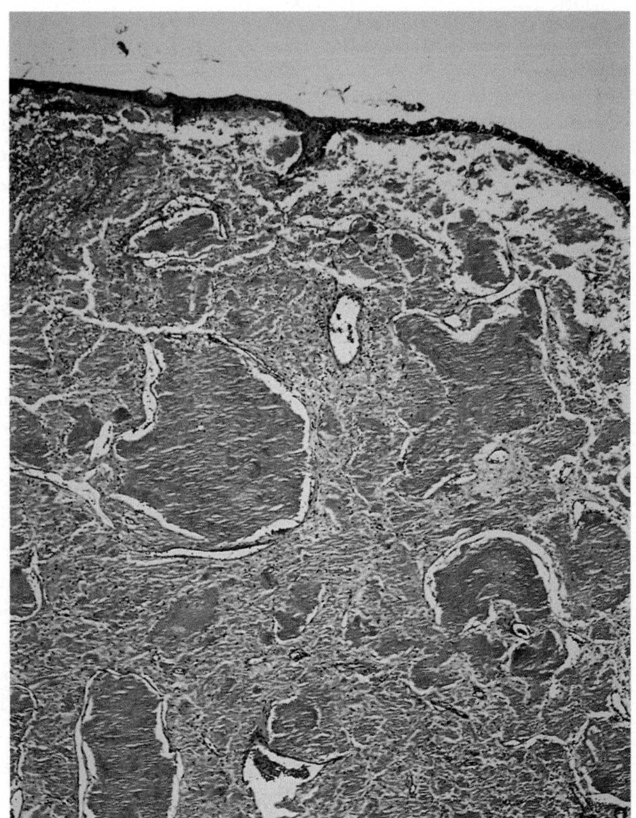
A

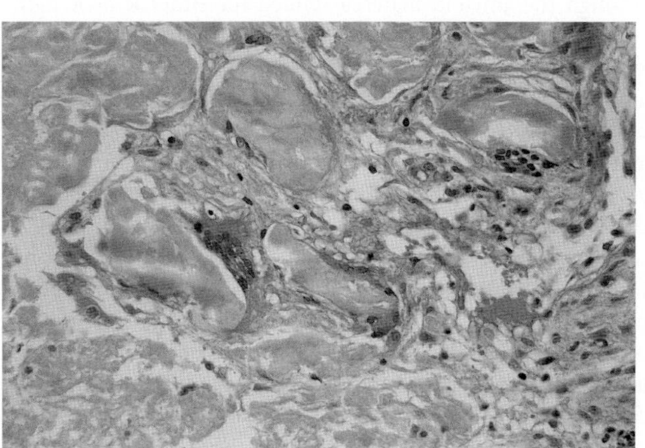
B

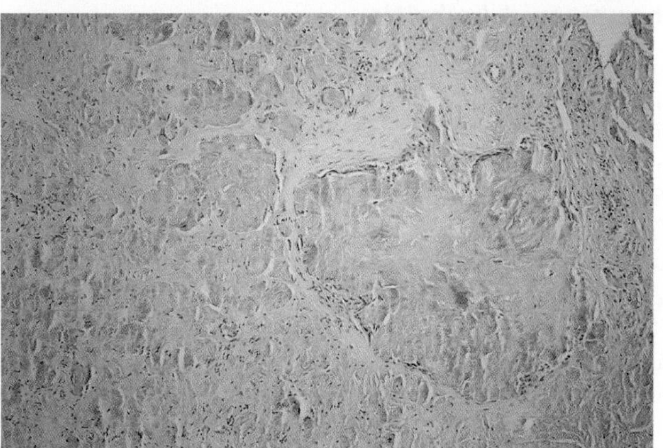
C

FIGURE 17. Larynx: amyloid deposition. **A:** Homogeneous eosinophilic amyloid is diffusely present deep to mucosal epithelium. Note the "cracked" appearance caused by artifactual spaces around masses of amyloid. **B:** The amyloid elicits a foreign body giant-cell reaction. **C:** The amyloid stains orange with Congo red. Under polarized light, apple-green birefringence would be expected.

tion or rarely even ossification may occasionally occur. The amyloid material may be deposited diffusely in soft tissue, and it has a propensity to be deposited in vascular walls, as rings around fat cells, and around laryngeal seromucinous glands, as though squeezing them into atrophy. The material stains metachromatically with crystal violet or Thioflavin T, but the most characteristic and pathognomonic staining pattern is with Congo red. This produces an intense orange staining microscopically (Fig. 17C), with a pathognomonic apple-green birefringence of the amyloid material when viewed under polarized light.

Differential diagnostic considerations include fibrosis, vocal cord polyps, and amyloid associated with plasmacytoma. Collagen appears more fibrillar under light microscopy than amyloid, which has a more homogeneous, amorphous character. Collagen does not polarize apple-green with Congo red. The fibrinous material in vocal cord polyps of vascular type (see above) can simulate amyloid, but this material has the granular staining characteristics of fibrin and also does not polarize apple-green with Congo red. Amyloid may be associated with plasmacytomas. This is more common in the nasopharynx but is rarely encountered in the larynx (75). Tumor-like sheets of plasma cells should be seen in plasmacytomas, as opposed to scattered collections in non-plasmacytoma–related amyloidosis, and the cytoplasm in the sheeted neoplastic plasma cells generally stains monotypically for either κ or λ immunoglobulin light chain. Although the amyloid material stained for either κ or λ light chain in 17 of 20 of Lewis et al's cases, associated plasma cells were polyclonal in their series (72). Interestingly, however, the amyloid-associated plasma cells in a case of laryngeal amyloidosis reported by Berg et al. (73) stained for κ light chain, as did the amyloid. This finding raises the intriguing possibility that, at least in some cases, localized amyloidosis may represent the product of a localized plasma cell dyscrasia (73).

Laryngeal amyloidosis is generally satisfactorily managed by surgical excision, although multiple procedures may be necessary, and recurrences may occur. The prognosis is generally good. Some extensive cases may be more problematic, and, rarely, extensive tracheobronchial involvement may eventuate in a fatal outcome.

Rheumatoid Arthritis

Both the cricoarytenoid and cricothyroid joints are synovial diarthrodial joints (76), and both may be affected by arthritis. The cricoarytenoid joint is the more clinically significant, and its involvement produces the more serious symptomatology. Different kinds of arthritis may involve the cricoarytenoid joint (77–79), but rheumatoid arthritis is probably the most significant, with as many as 26% of patients with rheumatoid arthritis having symptoms related to cricoarytenoid joint involvement (78,79). Symptoms and signs of acute arthritis include mainly pain and tenderness and at times hoarseness, and the arytenoid areas are swollen and red on examination. In chronic arthritis, pain is generally not prominent, and symptoms relate to dyspnea and airway compromise; arytenoids become stiff, less mobile, and, in severe cases, fixed (79).

Although larynges are rarely removed surgically for arthritis, the histopathology of cricoarytenoid rheumatoid arthritis mirrors that of other more commonly examined joints. Thus, in early involvement one sees a lymphoplasmacytic inflammatory infiltrate. With chronicity, a fibrous pannus covers the articular surface, and erosion and destruction of articular hyaline cartilage occur. Eventually, a fibrous ankylosis gradually obliterates the joint space, and bony ankylosis may rarely eventuate in end-stage disease (76).

Occasionally the surgical pathologist may encounter examples of rheumatoid nodules involving the vocal cord (80,81). These, like subcutaneous rheumatoid nodules, show fibrinoid degeneration of collagen with surrounding palisading histiocytes. Interestingly, methotrexate therapy, increasingly used in the treatment of rheumatoid arthritis, is associated with increased formation of rheumatoid nodules, and so perhaps one may encounter more cases of laryngeal rheumatoid nodules (81). Treatment for acute cricoarytenoid arthritis involves medical therapy with steroids and other antiinflammatory agents. For chronic disease with arytenoid immobility, surgical procedures aimed at restoring the airway are utilized (78).

Laryngeal involvement may also accompany other rheumatoid diseases. The larynx may be affected in cases of *systemic lupus erythematosus,* producing either cricoarytenoid arthritis (78,82), vocal cord nodules (83), including histologically typical rheumatoid nodules (84), or rarely, subglottic stenosis (82). *Sjogren's syndrome* may also involve the larynx, with pathologic findings of rheumatoid-like nodule formation in the vocal cord (85) and dense lymphoplasmacytic infiltration (86) being reported.

Others

Relapsing polychondritis is a disease characterized by inflammatory destruction of cartilage, most notably auricular, nasal, and laryngotracheobronchial cartilages. The etiology of the disease has not been entirely clarified, but it is considered to be related to the rheumatic and autoimmune diseases (87,88). Involvement of the eyes and inner ears is not uncommon as well (87). Painful recurrent swelling of the auricular pinnae is characteristic (see Chapter 3), polyarthralgias are common, and nasal involvement may eventuate in a saddle-nose deformity (88). Involvement of the cartilages of the respiratory tree is the most dangerous, with respiratory compromise resulting from chondromalacia and subsequent subglottic or tracheobronchial stenosis.

The histopathology is similar for all cartilages involved (87) (see Chapter 3). The initial change is a loss of the characteristic basophilia of the cartilaginous ground substance with transformation to an eosinophilic staining quality. Acute and chronic perichondritis and then chondritis ensue, with eventual chondronecrosis and fibrous replacement.

The larynx may rarely be involved in the bullous diseases *pemphigus vulgaris* and *cicatricial pemphigoid* (see Chapter 13). The first is the more serious of the two diseases and, before the use of steroid therapy, was almost always fatal (89). In pemphigus vulgaris, laryngeal involvement may present with hoarseness or odynophagia (89,90). Examination reveals mucosal blistering with frequent sloughing and denuded mucosal areas. Histologically, pemphigus vulgaris is characterized by acantholysis and bulla formation with suprabasal clefting, with intercellular IgG demonstrated by immunofluorescence. Cicatricial pemphigoid shows bullous change with subepithelial rather than suprabasal clefting and with IgG localized to the basement membrane on immunofluorescence (89). The larynx has very rarely been reported to be involved in the bullous disease *epidermolysis bullosa dystrophica* (91). For a more complete discussion, see Chapter 13.

The larynx may rarely be involved in cases of *gout.* Such patients generally have severe multifocal disease. Laryngeal pathology may include gouty cricoarytenoid arthritis (78,92) as well as the occurrence of gouty tophi of the vocal cord (93,94). Histopathologic changes typical of gouty tophi elsewhere are seen with foreign body granulomatous reaction to tissue deposits of amorphous material containing innumerable refractile needle-like urate crystals.

IDIOPATHIC CONDITIONS

Oncocytic Cyst

There is an interesting group of lesions involving seromucinous glands in the upper respiratory tract, predominantly the larynx but occasionally the nasopharynx (see Chapter 5), that are characterized by a proliferation of oncocytic cells, usually of a cystic character, with varying degrees of oncocytic cellular proliferation, often papillary. These lesions bear a striking resemblance to Warthin's tumors and to some oncocytomas of the salivary glands (see Chapter 8), though without the striking lymphoid component of the former tumor. These lesions have been called by various names, including oncocytic cyst, papillary cystadenoma, and oncocytic papillary cystadenoma, among others. Patients are usually middle-aged to elderly. Symptoms are usually hoarseness and rarely some degree of respiratory difficulty (95). Some are discovered incidentally and are asymptomatic. They occur predominantly in the area of the ventricle or false vocal cord, a region rich in seromucinous glands, and appear as cystic submucosal masses.

The histopathology of these lesions is characterized by the presence of typical oncocytic cells: large columnar to polygonal cells with ample granular eosinophilic cytoplasm representing a marked proliferation of mitochondria, which typically fill the cytoplasm on ultrastructural examination. These oncocytes often line cystic structures, with varying degrees of mural infolding or papillary proliferation (Fig. 18). Sometimes solid masses of oncocytes may be present. There may be a variety of oncocytic lesions in the same larynx (96), varying from oncocytic metaplasia of acinar cells to oncocytic hyperplasia and the formation of small to larger cystic structures. When large, these laryngeal lesions bear a marked resemblance to oncocytic tumors of major salivary glands. The cystic lesions, in fact, often have a double layer of lining cells, the luminal layer of which is columnar and oncocytic while the basal layer is composed of smaller cells, as in a Warthin's tumor (see Chapter 8). The link between these conditions is illustrated by a case of familial Warthin's tumor associated with a laryngeal oncocytic cystic lesion (97).

Although the larger more cellular examples resemble neoplasms, most current opinion is that these lesions represent non-neoplastic oncocytic metaplasia and hyperplasia with varying degrees of cyst formation (98). This concept is supported by the multiple lesions occasionally present, the finding of oncocytic metaplasia in seromucinous glands of older individuals, and the range and variety of oncocytic lesions encountered. Because most of these are cystic, we prefer the term oncocytic cyst of the larynx for this group of lesions.

These proliferations are benign, and simple excision is curative, although incomplete excision may be associated with recurrence. The lesions may rarely be extensive (95).

Tracheopathia Osteoplastica

Tracheopathia osteoplastica is a condition in which numerous generally small mucosa-covered cartilaginous and/or bony nodules protrude into the lumen from tracheal cartilage. Although at first considered primarily a lesion of the lower trachea, the disease has been reported in areas from the subglottic larynx to the bronchi (99). Thus, the cumbersome term laryngotracheobronchopathia chondroosteoplastica (100) may be more precise;

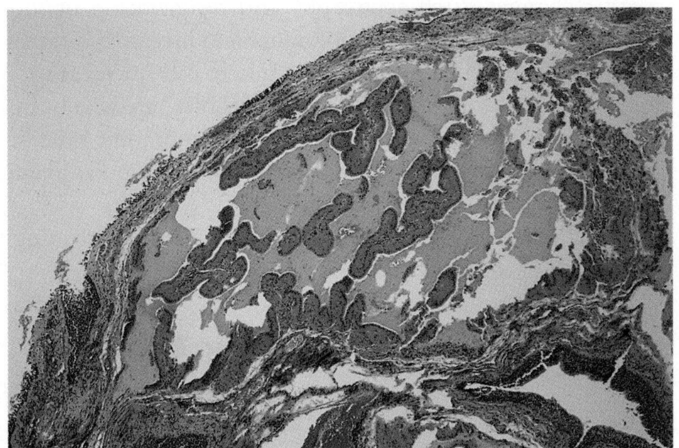
A

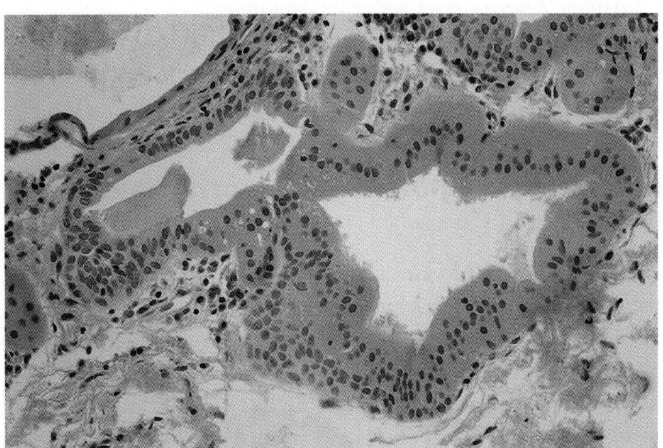
B

FIGURE 18. Larynx: oncocytic cyst. **A:** Cystic enlargement and papillary oncocytic metaplasia or hyperplasia in a laryngeal seromucinous gland. **B:** Focal oncocytic metaplasia and early dilation of the duct of a laryngeal gland.

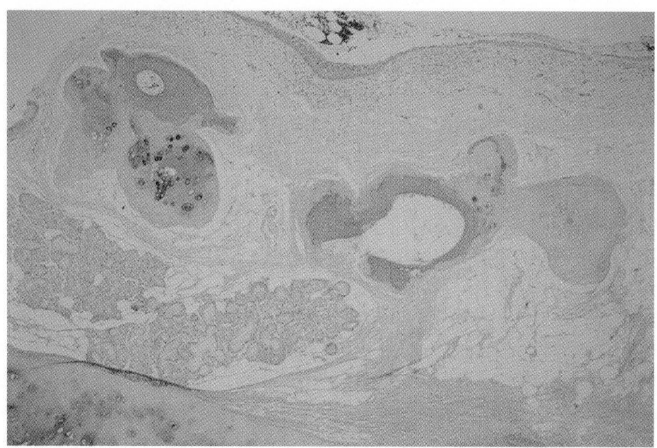

FIGURE 19. Tracheopathia osteoplastia. Osteocartilaginous nodules are present between the mucosal epithelium and cartilage wall.

however, the mercifully shorter term tracheopathia osteoplastica is generally used.

The lesion is often asymptomatic, and many early examples were discovered incidentally at autopsy (101). More recently, with increasing use of endoscopy and more sophisticated imaging techniques, more cases are being discovered during life. If extensive, the condition may evoke symptoms such as cough, hemoptysis, exertional dyspnea, or wheezing (99). The lesion may cause unanticipated difficulty in intubation (102). The classic radiologic appearance is a characteristic calcific radiopaque tracheal mucosal beading that protrudes into the lumen (99).

Histologically, one encounters foci of cartilage and/or bone, generally mature lamellar in type, below a usually intact mucosal epithelium (Fig. 19). These osteocartilaginous foci have been reported to be connected, either directly or via a fibrous band, to underlying tracheal cartilage, as in the manner of an osteocartilaginous ecchondrosis (101). One frequently encounters calcification and ossification of laryngeal and tracheal cartilage with advancing age, but such ossification occurs within the confines of preexisting laryngotracheal cartilage, and, in the case of tracheal rings, this ossification is primarily located in the antiluminal (peripheral) half of the cartilage. This is in contrast to the submucosal ossification seen outside the confines of the preexisting cartilage rings in tracheopathia osteoplastica.

The etiology of the condition has not been definitively elucidated. If significantly symptomatic, the condition may warrant surgical intervention, either excision or laser ablations (102).

Idiopathic (Subglottic) Laryngotracheal Stenosis

The great majority of cases of subglottic stenosis are of known cause, such as postintubation injury, congenital stenosis, infection, Wegener's granulomatosis, amyloid, sinus histiocytosis with massive lymphadenopathy (see below), and others. There remain, however, a few cases of subglottic or laryngotracheal stenosis for which no apparent cause is identified. Curiously, the vast majority of patients with this condition are female (103,104), with ages ranging from 15 to over 70, but with most patients ranging from the forties to the sixties (103,104). Symptoms include dyspnea, stridor, and occasionally voice change. Radiographically and on exam, one sees narrowing of the subglottic airway that is generally circumferential and symmetric. Most lesions begin in the subglottic larynx, occasionally just beneath the vocal cords, and extend into the upper trachea, the stenotic segment generally being 2 to 3 cm long (103).

Histologically, there is dense fibrosis in the lamina propria that has been described as keloidal in type (103). There is a generally scant chronic inflammatory infiltrate of lymphocytes and occasional histiocytes (Fig. 20). The fibrosis is generally paucicellular, but occasionally foci of greater cellularity of fibroblasts are seen. Granulomas, amyloid deposition, or fibrinoid degeneration of collagen are not part of the picture.

The etiology is unknown, although a subgroup of cases characterized by softer areas of stenosis with less dense collagen has been reported that may be related to gastroesophageal reflux and that seems to benefit from antireflux therapy (105). Although the morphology of the condition is reminiscent of fibrosclerotic entities such as retroperitoneal fibrosis, sclerosing mediastinitis, sclerosing orbital pseudotumor, and Riedel's struma, the occurrence of such conditions in association with idiopathic (subglottic) laryngotracheal stenosis has not been observed.

Therapy ranges from periodic dilation to surgical resection and reconstruction, with tracheostomy occasionally necessary.

Oculopharyngeal Muscular Dystrophy

Oculopharyngeal muscular dystrophy is an inherited autosomal dominant myopathy of late onset that primarily affects the eyelid elevator and pharyngeal constrictor muscles. The prime symptoms are ptosis and dysphagia, although facial and proximal limb weakness may also occur (106). The disease was given its current name by Victor et al. in 1962 (107), who described an affected American Jewish family of Eastern European origin (107). Most patients, however, are French Canadian; other affected communities are Spanish American as well as French and Spanish (106). More recently, the disease has been encountered among other groups, including Bukharan and Uzbekistan Jews (108).

Muscle biopsy, as well as hypopharyngeal muscle removed during cricopharyngeal myotomy, reveals degenerative myopathic changes, such as atrophy and regeneration of muscle fibers, with a disorganized appearance and increased internal (as opposed to peripherally located) muscle cell nuclei (Fig. 21). Characteristic cytoplasmic "rimmed vacuoles" are seen in frozen section specimens of muscle, and a pathognomonic type of intranuclear inclusion consisting of short straight tubular filaments can be identified ultrastructurally (109).

Cricopharyngeal myotomy has proved useful in treating the dysphagia of these patients (110).

Inflammatory Myofibroblastic Tumor

Inflammatory myofibroblastic tumor (IMT) is a rather controversial lesion, some examples of which are akin to so-called plasma cell granuloma and some histologically mimicking a spindle cell sarcoma (111). These lesions occur most commonly in the lung and abdomen and pelvis and tend to involve

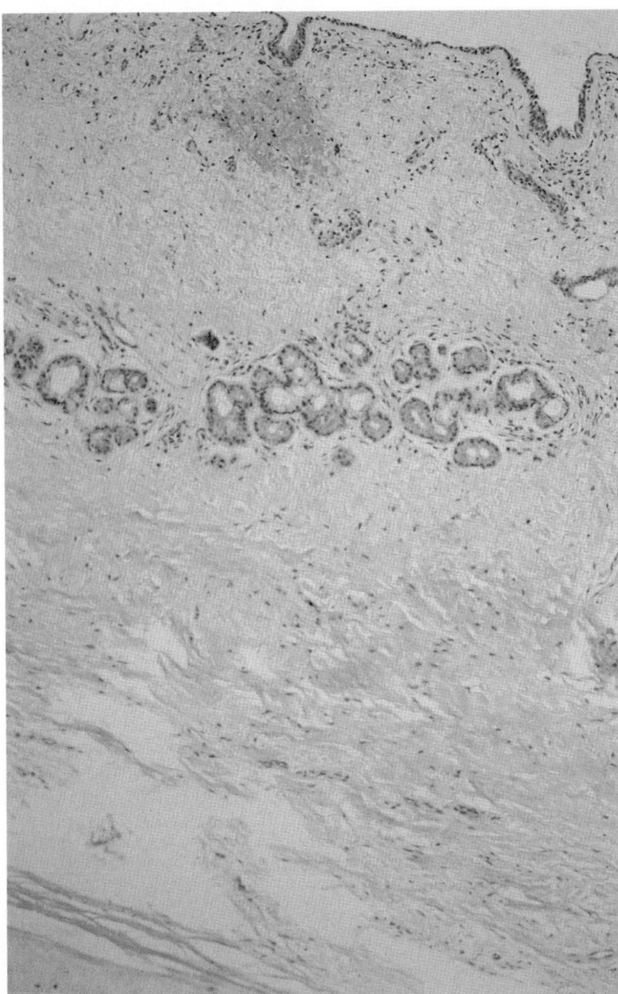

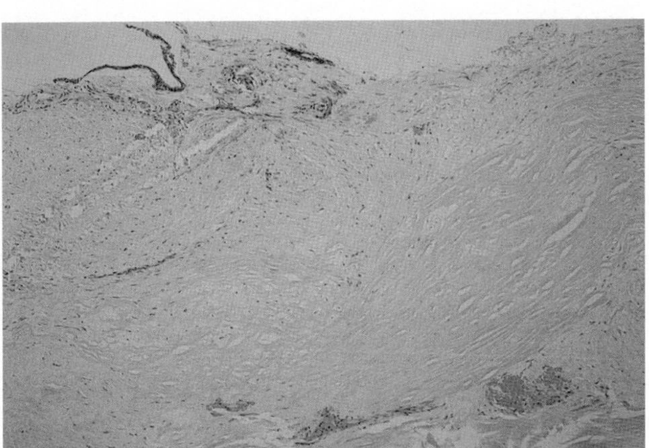

FIGURE 20. Idiopathic (subglottic) laryngotracheal stenosis. **A:** Fibrosis surrounds seromucinous glands. There is slight chronic inflammation deep to surface mucosal epithelium. **B:** In this area, fibrosis is dense, and inflammation is minimal.

children, but rare examples have been reported in the larynx in children (111) and adults (112–114). Laryngeal lesions need to be differentiated from spindle cell carcinoma (see below) or rarely occurring laryngeal sarcomas, as the reported adult laryngeal lesions of IMT have behaved in a benign fashion (113,114).

Patients with laryngeal IMT in the series of Wenig et al. (113) have been adults (age range 19–69 years, mean 59 years), although Coffin et al. (111) have reported a laryngeal IMT in a 7-year-old child. Symptoms include hoarseness, dysphonia, and stridor, and the lesions appear as polypoid or pedunculated masses, usually on the true vocal cord (113).

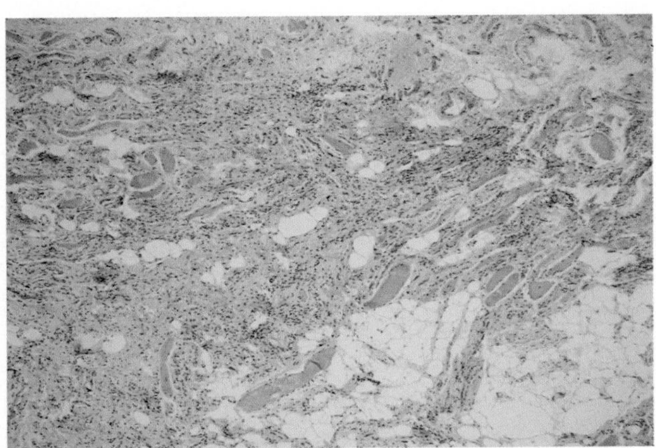

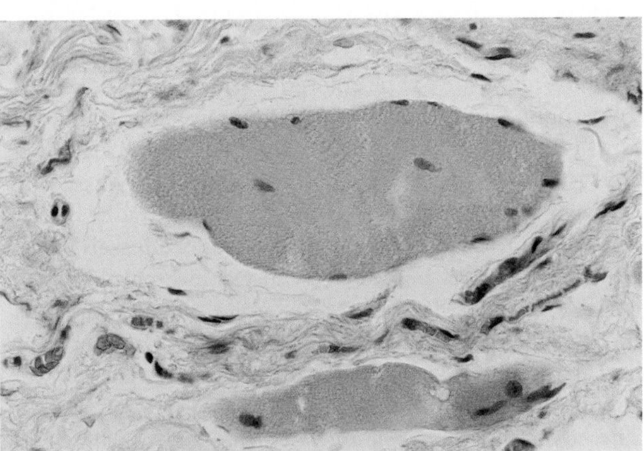

FIGURE 21. Hypopharynx, cricopharyngeus muscle: oculopharyngeal muscular dystrophy. **A:** Atrophic skeletal muscle with a reduced number of abnormally oriented fibers admixed with fibrous tissue and fat. **B:** A regenerative muscle fiber with abnormally placed central (rather than peripheral) nuclei.

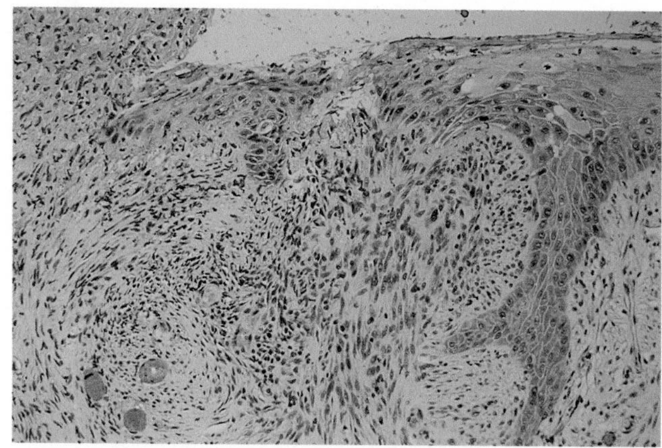

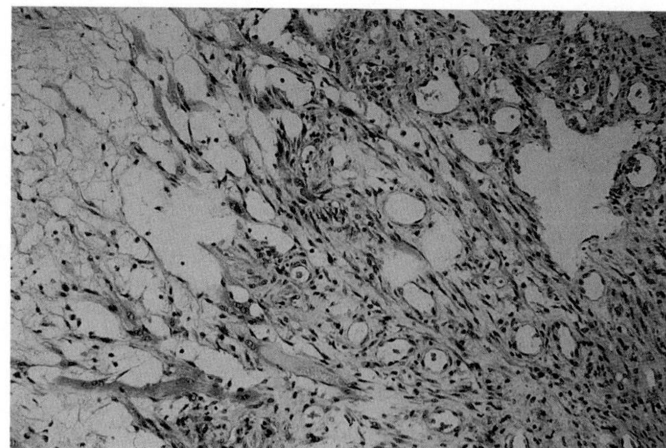

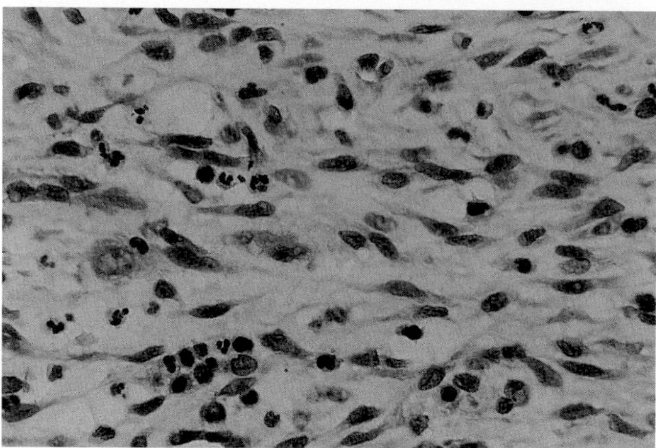

FIGURE 22. Larynx: inflammatory myofibroblastic tumor. **A:** A cellular proliferation of spindle cells underlies mucosal epithelium with regenerative atypia. **B:** There is focal marked edema and scattered inflammatory cells. **C:** A high-power view shows the spindled cells to have bland, nonpleomorphic nuclei.

Histologically one sees a proliferation of spindled cells of varying cellularity admixed with inflammatory cells, including lymphocytes, plasma cells, and neutrophils (Fig. 22). The spindled cells are cytologically bland, and neither significant pleomorphism nor atypical mitotic figures are observed (Fig. 22C). Immunohistochemical stains show the cells to stain with vimentin and actin, and the lesion is considered to be a myofibroblastic proliferation. We have seen one case that we consider to represent laryngeal IMT in an adult following irradiation for carcinoma.

Differential diagnosis from spindle cell carcinoma is important. There is an absence of an associated histologically characteristic squamous cell carcinoma or carcinoma *in situ* component in IMT, the nuclei are not pleomorphic, and the spindle cells in adult laryngeal cases neither stain immunohistochemically for keratin nor exhibit epithelial differentiation ultrastructurally (113,114). Weidner et al. (115) reported a hypopharyngeal case of a benign spindle cell proliferation following irradiation for carcinoma that they termed a bizarre (pseudosarcomatous) granulation-tissue reaction. In their cases, nuclear pleomorphism was appreciable, as opposed to cases of laryngeal IMT, and the atypia extended to endothelial cells as well (115). The lack of significant nuclear atypicality also serves to help differentiate laryngeal IMT from rare examples of laryngeal sarcoma.

The laryngeal lesion is nonmetastasizing and usually cured by conservative total surgical excision (113). No predisposing factors were found in five of seven cases reported by Wenig et al. (114).

The precise nature of IMT in general, especially in children, is still not entirely clear. It is generally thought to be a benign myofibroblastic proliferation, but recent results have shown clonality in some cases and raise the possibility that some lesions may be neoplastic (116).

Others

Sinus histiocytosis with massive lymphadenopathy (or Rosai-Dorfman disease) is a condition of obscure etiology generally pre-

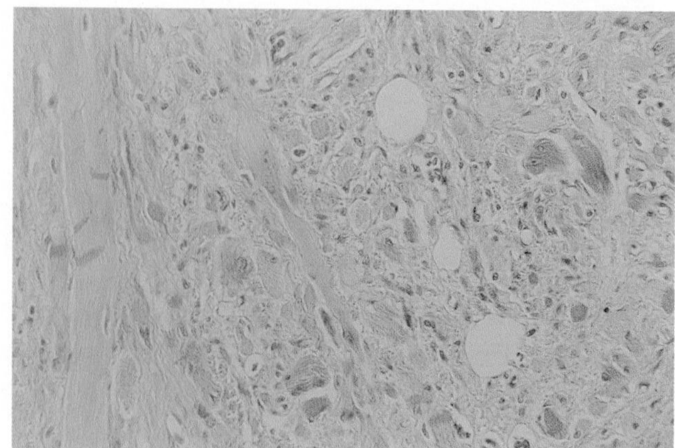

FIGURE 23. Hypopharynx: hamartoma. An abnormal proliferation of skeletal muscle with fibrous tissue and fat.

senting as cervical lymphadenopathy with marked nodal enlargement (see Chapter 12). The lesion can involve extranodal sites, including those in the head and neck. Rare examples have been reported in the larynx (117,118), with characteristic large histiocytes containing intracytoplasmic lymphocytes occupying sinus-like ("sinusal") spaces (see Chapter 12). *Hamartomas* of the larynx and hypopharynx are rarely encountered (119–122) (Fig. 23). Two cases of so-called *eosinophilic angiocentric fibrosis* have been reported involving the subglottic larynx (123,124) (see Chapter 4).

NEOPLASMS

Benign Neoplasms

Squamous Papilloma

Squamous papillomas are the most common laryngeal tumors in children (125–127). Their characteristics of multiplicity, unpredictability of behavior with frequent recurrences, often after long latent periods of quiescence, their frustrating recalcitrance to treatment, and their potential for airway compromise in children make these lesions a thorny clinical problem indeed. Laryngeal squamous papillomas in the past have traditionally been separated into juvenile and adult types; however, it is currently generally recognized that the multiple, nonkeratinizing, viral-associated type of papillomas, whether of childhood or adult onset, represent essentially the same disease, albeit with a few differences between them (127–129). The solitary and keratinizing papillary squamous lesion of adults, on the other hand, appears not to be viral-associated, may be associated with preneoplastic histologic dysplasia, may be a forerunner of squamous cell carcinoma, and is best considered as a different entity, a papillary type of leukoplakia or squamous epithelial hyperplasia or keratosis (128,129); the present discussion is not concerned with this latter type of papillomatous lesion.

It is now generally accepted that the multiple, often frequently recurring laryngeal squamous papillomas are associated with human papillomavirus (HPV) as an etiologic factor, specifically HPV types 6 and 11 (127,130–133). These are the same types of HPV associated with condylomas of the anogenital tract as well as squamous lesions of the uterine cervix. HPV types 16 and 18, associated with malignant lesions of the cervix, are almost never found in laryngeal papillomas (130,132–135). This identity of viral types in genital condylomas and laryngeal papillomas lends credence to the theory that many cases of juvenile-onset papillomas are acquired via infection during passage through a contaminated birth canal (136,137).

There are other possible means of prenatal infection (e.g., transplacental passage of virus), however, and many vaginally delivered children of mothers with genital condylomas do not develop laryngeal papillomas. Furthermore, cases of children with papillomas who had been delivered by cesarean section are reported (127). Thus, the role of cesarean section in the control of laryngeal papillomas is not clear-cut and appears to be, in fact, quite limited (138,139). Adult onset laryngeal papillomas, although also HPV-associated, may be related to post-natal infection with HPV, e.g., via sexual contact (127,137). Alternatively, cases of adult onset may reflect prolonged latency of congenitally acquired HPV (128).

Squamous papillomas have a bimodal age distribution of presentation. In children, most present during the first five years of life, and in adults, most cases appear to present in the 20's and 30's (126–128,140). The predominant presenting symptom is dysphonia or hoarseness, with rare childhood cases presenting with respiratory distress (140). Lesions most commonly involve the true cords, with involvement of false cords and subglottic areas also reported (127,129). Rarely, involvement of the epiglottis and palate, as well as trachea and bronchi may occur (129). Thus, the disease is often currently referred to as recurrent respiratory papillomatosis (RRP) (137,138,141). The incidence of RRP is estimated at 4.3 per 100,000 population in children and 1.8 per 100,000 in adults (138). Interestingly, in adults, a male prevalence is noted, whereas this is not the case in children (127,140). In most cases, multiple mulberry-like soft papillomatous growths are seen (129). Most are small, but when numerous, they can coalesce to form larger masses.

Histologically, squamous papillomas are characterized by thickened mucosal stratified squamous epithelium thrown up into papillary folds and fronds with thin fibrovascular cores (Fig. 24). Branching of papillae may occur. There is frequently a lesser degree of cellular maturation in papillomas as compared with normal squamous mucosal epithelium, with less surface flattening of cells. When papillomas involve areas of transition between squamous and respiratory epithelium, as they often do (142), the transitional-type epithelium often seen in these areas, with less surface cell flattening than is seen in pure squamous mucosa, adds to the appearance of a lack of traditional stratified squamous mucosal epithelial maturation. Mitotic figures may be prominent in basal layers, and mitoses may extend to the mid-epithelial level. Occasionally, a slight disturbance of cellular polarity may impart a disorganized or slightly jumbled appearance to the epithelium. These changes most likely represent a viral effect on the tissue rather than dysplastic or premalignant changes. The classic changes of koilocytosis, as seen in the uterine cervix, may often be observed, although the koilocytotic alterations are generally less pronounced than in the cervix (Fig. 24D). Thus, cytoplasmic clearing around wrinkled, often dark nuclei may be seen, as well as occasional multinucleated epithelial cells, with two or more nuclei present in a single cell. Additional histologic features of papillomas include occasional dyskeratotic cells and vacuoles of intercellular or intracellular edema. Very rare cases of histologically benign papillomatous lesions of the larynx (143) or trachea (144) that have invaded adjacent tissues but have not metastasized have been reported as invasive papillomatosis. Radical surgery may be required to deal with these unusual lesions (143,144). Abnormal mitotic figures, necrosis, and nuclear pleomorphism as seen in dysplastic or malignant epithelial lesions are generally not observed in papillomas.

Although the clinicopathologic features of laryngeal squamous papillomas are characteristic and generally cause little diagnostic difficulty, several entities enter into the differential diagnosis of these lesions, most notably papillary or exophytic squamous cell carcinoma and verrucous carcinoma. *Papillary and exophytic squamous cell carcinoma* of the larynx, especially the papillary variety, has an architecture similar to that of squamous

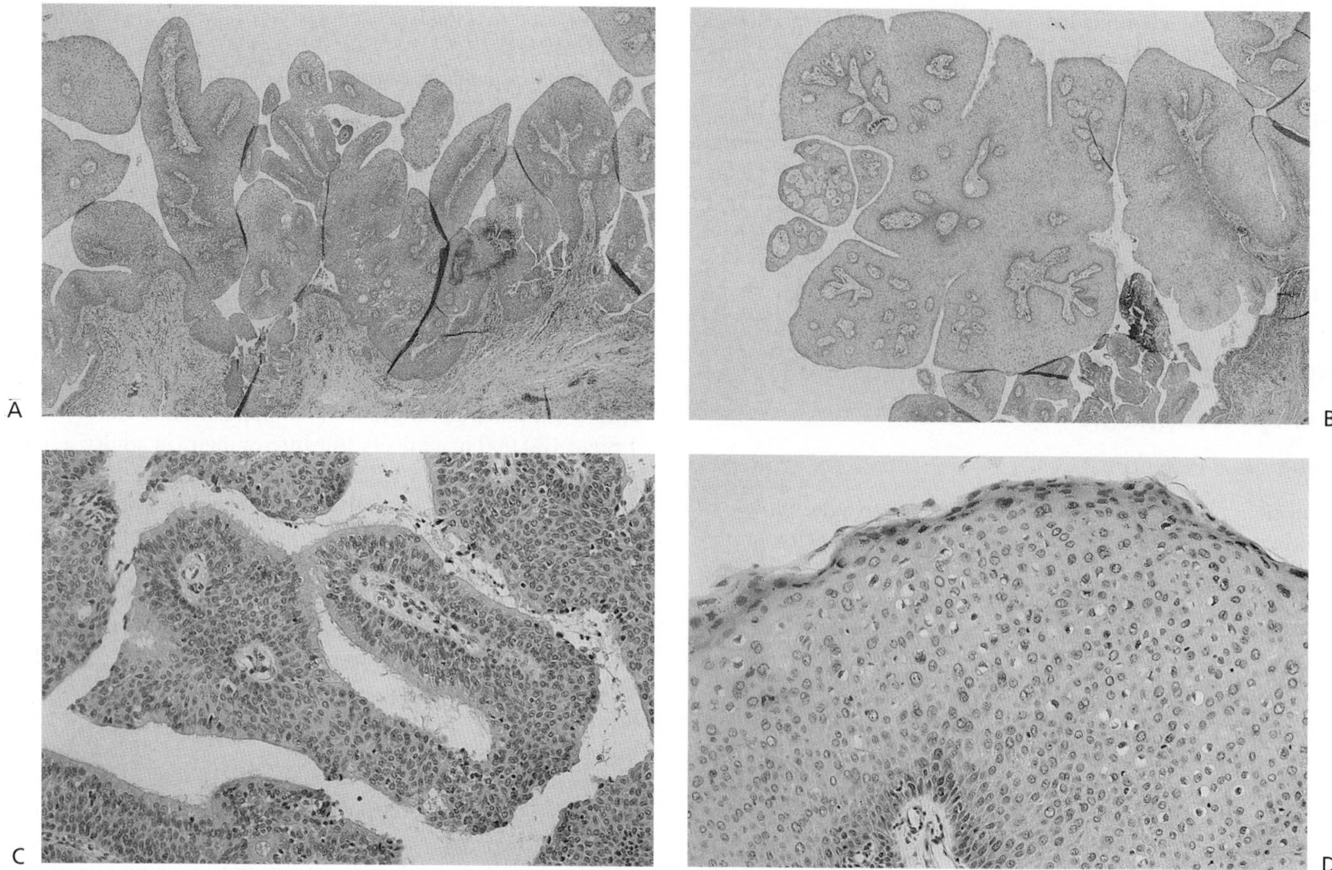

FIGURE 24. Larynx: squamous papilloma. **A:** The mucosal epithelium is thrown up into papillary fronds with thin fibrovascular cores. Keratosis is typically minimal to absent. **B:** There is focal branching of papillae. The epithelium is generally nonpleomorphic stratified squamous. **C:** The papillomatous process can extend to involve ciliated respiratory epithelium. **D:** Viral epithelial change may manifest as delay or arrest of squamous maturation, irregular polarity of nuclei, multinucleated epithelial cells, and classical koilocytosis with cells with dark wrinkled nuclei and perinuclear clearing.

papillomas. In addition, definite stromal invasion is often difficult to identify in these papillary carcinomas, and ragged single-cell infiltration is generally not seen. The cytologic features of papillary carcinoma, however, are those of a malignant neoplasm, and this tumor often has the histologic appearance of a papillary squamous cell carcinoma *in situ.* This is in contrast to the viral-associated though not malignant cytologic appearance of papillomas. *Verrucous carcinomas* are cytologically bland neoplasms that also do not invade stroma in an infiltrating finger-like fashion but in a blunted pushing fashion (see Chapter 2 and below). Verrucous carcinoma, however, is characterized by thicker squamous fronds and by keratinization that may at times be prominent. Koilocytosis is generally not a feature of verrucous carcinoma. Furthermore, verrucous carcinoma may extend into underlying tissues and cause resorption of cartilaginous and bony structures, a feature not shared with squamous papillomas (but see invasive papillomas, above). Exceptional cases diagnosed as verruca vulgaris of the larynx have been described (145,146). These lesions morphologically resemble cutaneous warts, with significant keratosis and a prominent granular layer with large keratohyaline granules, accentuated in interpapillary crevices. Interestingly, in the case reported by Barnes et al. (146), *in situ* hybridization studies of the lesion showed HPV types 6 and 11 to be present, as in typical laryngeal squamous papillomas, rather than types 2 and 4, the HPV types associated with cutaneous verrucae. Isolated usually solitary squamous papillomas are common incidental occurrences in the palate or tonsillar area. These tend not to recur and do not have koilocytic changes. The solitary so-called keratinizing squamous papilloma in larynges of adults has been referred to above.

Biological Behavior and Treatment

As mentioned previously, laryngeal squamous papillomas are notorious for their multiplicity and frequent and unpredictable recurrences. Recent findings of HPV DNA in clinically uninvolved mucosa in patients with RRP suggest that apparently "normal" mucosa may serve as a reservoir for HPV, helping to explain the repeated recurrence of papillomas (135,147). Papillomas may extend all along the respiratory tract, from the pharynx to the trachea, bronchi, and even alveoli. Fortunately, such occurrences are rare. Distal spread of papillomas into the lung is a serious manifestation of the disease, and it can cause obstruction to distal air spaces with obstructive pneumonia and abscesses possibly developing as a result. Such distal spread has traditionally been associated with previous tracheostomy (127,129), and thus tracheostomy is often avoided if possible (127). A recent study, however, reports that posttracheostomy distal spread of papillomas was usually limited to the tracheostomy site and that tracheostomy was not a catastrophic event in cases of papillomatosis (148). The concept of spontaneous regression of juvenile papillomatosis with the onset of puberty has not found support in current literature (127,149).

Malignant transformation of laryngeal papillomas is, fortunately, uncommon. When it occurs, it is usually associated with previous irradiation (129). Perhaps this in part related to the association of the "benign" HPV types 6 and 11 with the vast majority of laryngeal papillomas. HPV types 16 and 18, associated with carcinoma of the uterine cervix, are very rarely found in laryngeal papillomas. Interestingly, in a rare case of RRP progression to carcinoma, HPV types 6 and 11 were gradually replaced by HPV type 16 (150), and a recent report showed the presence of HPV-16 as well as HPV-11 in a case of laryngeal papilloma with severe dysplastic changes (151).

Therapy for RRP has been frustrating and problematic. Surgical removal is the mainstay of treatment, and use of the CO_2 laser is the generally preferred current surgical technique (138). Multiple recurrences, however, necessitate multiple surgical procedures. More recently, adjunctive therapy with interferon and methotrexate has shown potential promise in treating this condition (152).

Benign Salivary Gland–Type Tumors

Benign neoplasms of salivary gland type are quite uncommon in the larynx and trachea. About 30 cases of *pleomorphic adenoma* of the larynx have been reported (153–155). Patients have been adults, primarily in the fourth through seventh decades. Most lesions have been supraglottic, with the epiglottis being the single most common site. The subglottis is the next most common site, with very few lesions reported in the vocal cord (154). Symptoms are primarily dysphonia for supraglottic lesions and dyspnea for subglottic lesions. The histology is that of the much more common tumors in the salivary glands (see Chapter 8). Treatment is surgical, and the prognosis is excellent. Rare pleomorphic adenomas have been reported in the trachea, an even rarer site than the larynx (156,157). These tumors are often present for a long time before being diagnosed, and symptoms include wheezing as well as dyspnea.

Oncocytic tumors have been noted in the larynx. Almost all of these belong to the group of lesions described above under the heading of oncocytic cyst. A rare solid oncocytic proliferation analogous to a salivary gland oncocytoma (see Chapter 8) may occur in the larynx, but such solid tumors are much less frequent than the cystic or papillocystic oncocytic laryngeal proliferations (158).

Subglottic Hemangioma

Subglottic hemangiomas are vasoproliferative lesions of infancy that are considered to be congenital (159–161) and that may represent malformations or neoplasms (162). For convenience they are discussed here with the benign neoplasms. Although rare, their importance lies in their considerable potential to obstruct the narrow and vulnerable infant airway.

Patients generally present during the first 6 months of life, though rarely at birth (161). Girls are more commonly affected than boys in a ratio of about 2:1 (159,163). Symptoms most commonly include stridor, at first inspiratory and progressing to biphasic (164), and, at times, a croupy cough (165), resulting in a common initial diagnosis of croup (161). About half of the patients have cutaneous hemangiomas, an important diagnostic clue (159,163). Symptoms tend to wax and wane, being accentuated during periods of crying or agitation. This may be related to variations in pressure in the component vessels leading to their filling with blood or emptying (159). Significant airway compromise may occur, and if left untreated, the condition may be lethal.

On endoscopic examination, the lesions are subglottic in location, almost all beginning just below the vocal cords and most not extending below the inferior border of the cricoid cartilage. Rarely, extension to the level of the first few tracheal rings may occur. The lesions are most commonly predominantly one-sided and eccentric in location, usually posterolateral. Rarely, they may be multiple or circumferential. Considerable airway compromise, up to 90% or more, may be present. The endoscopic findings of a round submucosal subglottic mass, soft and compressible, bluish to red in color, are virtually pathognomonic, and biopsy is rarely necessary for diagnosis, although it can be performed safely.

Histologically, the lesions are capillary hemangiomas of juvenile type. They are not encapsulated or circumscribed, and the capillaries infiltrate and surround submucosal structures such as seromucinous glands (Fig. 25). The tumors are primarily submucosal in location, but extension to involve the perichondrium or the area between tracheal rings may occasionally occur (159). Endothelial cells are plump, and mitotic figures may be present. The vessels may be empty or blood-filled. The lesions are often cellular, at times so much so that individual vessels may be obscured and a more solid appearance may be imparted to parts of the lesion. The papillary endothelial proliferations, nuclear pleomorphism, and dissection of collagen by endothelial cells as seen in angiosarcomas are not encountered.

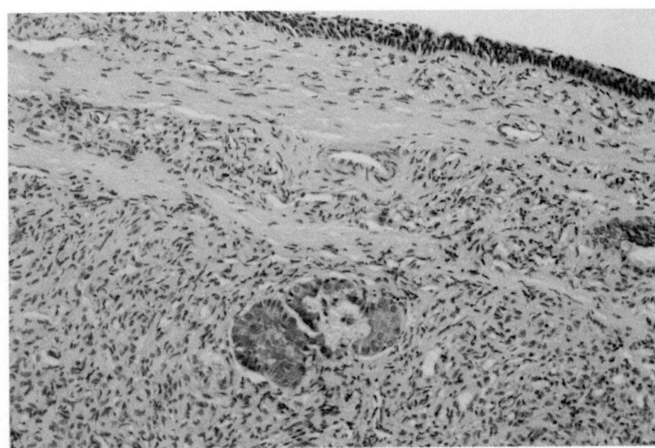

FIGURE 25. Larynx: subglottic hemangioma. A cellular proliferation of small capillaries occupies the subepithelial area and surrounds a seromucinous gland.

The natural history of these lesions is to regress spontaneously and involute after an initial period of proliferation, similarly to many cutaneous vascular lesions of infancy (161,164). Thus, the therapeutic goal is to stabilize the airway and hasten involution or to remove excess tissue until involution occurs, with the least possible morbidity. Numerous therapeutic modalities have been tried, including tracheostomy, steroids administered systemically or injected intralesionally (166), CO_2 laser ablation (164), and, more recently, surgical excision (161,167) or interferon administration. The currently most popular treatment in the United States appears to be CO_2 laser ablation and steroid administration, with tracheostomy if indicated, and with surgical ablation in selected cases, usually with large tumors.

Paraganglioma

Paraganglia are neuroendocrine structures of neuroectodermal neural crest derivation analogous to cells of the adrenal medulla (168). Most paraganglia of the head and neck region are intimately associated with nerves and blood vessels of branchiomeric distribution, that is, in close association with structures derived from mesoderm of the branchial arches (169), such as the carotid artery, aortic arch, and jugular vein. This group of paraganglia has been called the branchiomeric paraganglia by Glenner and Grimley (170). The carotid body is the best known and most studied of this group (169), and its tumor, the carotid body paraganglioma or carotid body tumor, is the most frequent and familiar of the branchiomeric paragangliomas (171). The carotid bodies have a chemoreceptor function, responding to changes in arterial Po_2 or pH, but the function of laryngeal paraganglia is unknown (168,169).

Laryngeal paraganglia are divided into superior and inferior groups. The superior laryngeal paraganglia are more constant in location and are located in the supraglottic larynx, mainly in the upper anterior false cord area near the superior border of the thyroid cartilage and in relation to the internal branch of the superior laryngeal nerve (172). The inferior laryngeal paraganglia may be found subglotically in the cricothyroid or cricotracheal area, at times associated with the capsule of the thyroid gland (172). Rare laryngeal paraganglia are sometimes found in other locations, and there are tracheal paraganglia present in the upper tracheal region (168,172).

Laryngeal paragangliomas are uncommon neoplasms, almost always benign, and significantly rarer than carotid body, vagal, or jugulotympanic paragangliomas. Most arise from the superior laryngeal paraganglia and present as supraglottic masses, often in the area of the aryepiglottic fold or false vocal cord. The rarer paragangliomas of the inferior laryngeal paraganglia are subglottic masses that may project intralaryngeally or, very rarely in a dumbbell fashion, a portion of the tumor intralaryngeal and a portion extralaryngeal, adjacent to the thyroid gland (173). One inferior laryngeal paraganglioma reported in the literature had most of its mass outside the larynx and presented originally as a thyroid tumor (174). The average age of patients is 47 years, and women outnumber men by more than 2:1 (168). Symptoms include hoarseness, dysphagia, and dyspnea (168). Pain, despite occasional assertions to the contrary (175), is generally considered not to be a common symptom of true laryngeal paragangliomas (176) but rather an indicator of moderately differentiated neuroendocrine carcinoma (see below). Tumors present as smooth rounded submucosal masses (177). The lesions are quite vascular, and biopsy may result in significant hemorrhage (177,178).

Grossly, the tumors are rounded firm rubbery and solid masses that may be smooth or granular on cut section (168). They are pink-tan to reddish-brown in color and may have fibrous streaks or areas of hemorrhage (168).

Histologically, paragangliomas are characterized by an arrangement of tumor cells in round nests and balls termed *Zellballen*. The tumor cells in the nests, or chief cells, are epithelioid cells with inconspicuous cell borders and a syncytial appearance (Fig. 26). Cytoplasm is ample, and nuclei are mainly round and dark. Nuclei can vary in size, however, and they may be large, irregular in size, and hyperchromatic. This nuclear irregularity is not associated with malignant behavior. Mitoses are few, and necrosis is usually absent. There may be a thick fibrous capsule with fibrous bands traversing the tumor, but this is variable. The characteristic *Zellballen* may be highlighted by a retic-

A 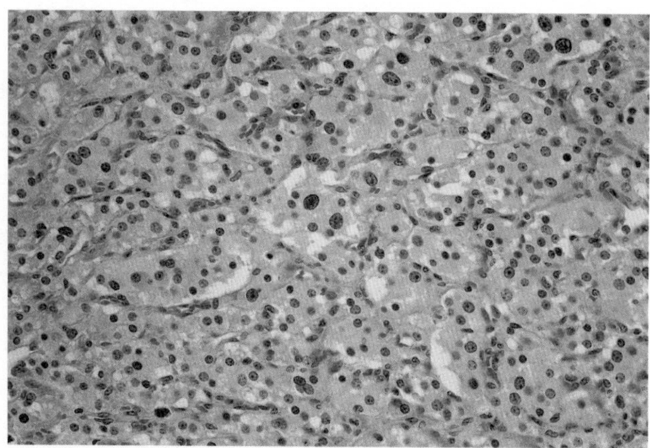

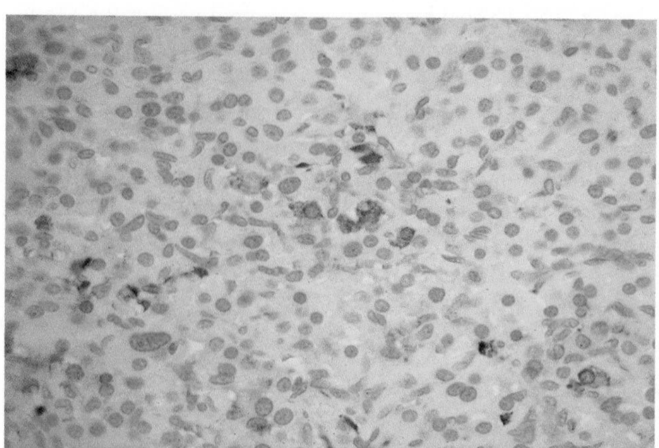 B

FIGURE 26. Larynx: paraganglioma. **A:** Characteristic *"Zellballen"* or balls of cells, surrounded by capillaries, composed of chief cells with occasionally large nuclei. **B:** Many chief cells are positive immunohistochemically for chromogranin.

ulin stain. Small elongated sustentacular cells are present at the periphery of the rounded cell nests, but they are inconspicuous on hematoxylin and eosin stain and are seen to best advantage with immunohistochemical staining for S-100 protein. The chief cells are argyrophilic and stain with Grimelius and Churukian-Schenk stains. They are argentaffin negative. The tumor is very vascular, as is usual for endocrine neoplasms, with an abundance of capillaries surrounding the *Zellballen.* The cell nests may be squeezed and not readily apparent on biopsy specimens, and the lesion may mimic granulation tissue or a primary vascular proliferation. Careful scrutiny of the entire specimen will usually reveal the characteristic *Zellballen.*

Immunohistochemistry is an extremely useful adjunct in the diagnosis of paragangliomas. The chief cells stain for neuroendocrine markers such as chromogranin, neuron-specific enolase (NSE), and synaptophysin but not for S-100 protein (179,180) (Fig. 26B). Paragangliomas do not stain for epithelial markers such as keratin proteins in the vast majority of cases, although rare exceptions may occur; but keratin-positive laryngeal paragangliomas have not as yet been reported (180). The elongated peripheral sustentacular cells stain for S-100 protein and for glial fibrillary acidic protein (GFAP) and are chromogranin negative. This pattern of chromogranin-positive chief cells and S-100 protein–positive sustentacular cells is quite characteristic for paragangliomas (179). Ultrastructurally, chief cells contain characteristic dense-core neuroendocrine granules and have cell junctions without tonofilaments, and the dendritic sustentacular cells are devoid of neurosecretory granules (173).

The most significant and troublesome differential diagnosis is with neuroendocrine carcinomas of the larynx, specifically the moderately differentiated neuroendocrine carcinoma (MDNC, atypical carcinoid, large-cell neuroendocrine carcinoma; see below). This differentiation is very important, as the malignant potential and prognosis of these two lesions differ significantly. MDNCs are also neuroendocrine neoplasms that may have an architectural pattern resembling *Zellballen.* There are a number of helpful differentiating features. MDNCs of the larynx frequently have glandular differentiation with mucin positivity. Pargangliomas are mucin negative. Perhaps the most useful differential features are the immunohistochemical staining patterns of the two lesions. MDNCs are characteristically keratin positive, and paragangliomas are, with rare exceptions, keratin negative (177,179–182). Interestingly, many laryngeal MDNCs stain for calcitonin, and paragangliomas do not. The characteristic chromogranin-positive chief cell and peripheral S-100 protein-positive sustentacular cell pattern of paragangliomas is also helpful. The neuroendocrine marker positivity also helps differentiate paragangliomas from nonneuroendocrine carcinomas and vascular tumors. Melanomas are S-100 protein positive but chromogranin negative, and most epithelioid melanomas stain immunohistochemically for HMB45 and MART-1.

The similar histologic appearance of laryngeal paragangliomas and laryngeal MDNC, combined with the only fairly recent use of immunohistochemical techniques to distinguish them, have led to some confusion and controversy regarding the biology and natural history of laryngeal paragangliomas. Hence, it was thought that a significant percentage of laryngeal paragangliomas were malignant and characterized by cutaneous metastases and considerable pain (175,179). Virtually all of these malignant cases, however, are currently thought to represent misdiagnosed MDNCs (168,177,179). True laryngeal paragangliomas are, in fact, almost invariably benign, with Barnes, Wenig, and Ferlito willing to accept only one case in the literature as a bona fide malignant laryngeal paraganglioma (168,179). No reliable histologic criteria (e.g., mitotic activity, vascular invasion, peripheral infiltration, necrosis) appear to be able to predict accurately malignant behavior in paragangliomas of the head and neck (168). Although multiple familial paragangliomas and functional paragangliomas are reported in other sites, such associations are extremely uncommon with laryngeal paragangliomas. Surgery, preferably involving local *en bloc* excision or partial laryngectomy if possible, is the recommended treatment.

Granular Cell Tumor

Granular cell tumor (GCT) refers to a group of lesions of soft tissues, almost all of which are benign, that are characterized by cells with a distinctive granular cytoplasm. These tumors can occur virtually anywhere in the body (183,184), most commonly in the skin and subcutaneous tissues (183). The head and neck is a common site for GCTs (185), and the tongue is the single noncutaneous organ most commonly involved (183). The larynx is an uncommon but well-recognized site of occurrence (185–188). The trachea is even more rarely involved (189).

Laryngeal GCTs occur with approximately equal frequency in men and women, most commonly in patients in the third to fifth decades (186,188), although ages of reported cases have ranged from 5 to 92 years (188,190). The patients typically present with hoarseness (186), but lesions can be asymptomatic (185,187). Rarely will respiratory obstruction be a problem (191,192). The posterior vocal cord is the most frequent location (187,188). Lesions are typically small, rounded, sessile, mucosal covered masses, often resembling vocal cord polyps (186,187).

Histologically, GCTs are characterized by nests and sheets of large rounded to polygonal cells with ample granular eosinophilic cytoplasm (Fig. 27). Cell borders are characteristically indistinct, imparting a syncytial appearance to the tumor cells. Tumor cells occasionally can assume a somewhat spindled appearance. Nuclei are generally small dark and rounded but can sometimes be larger, with moderately sized nucleoli. Nuclear pleomorphism suggestive of malignancy is rarely observed but has been noted in an unusual laryngeal GCT that exhibited locally aggressive behavior (191). The characteristic granules are usually small and fine but may occasionally be larger. They are PAS positive and diastase resistant. The tumor is not encapsulated or well circumscribed, and granular cells often infiltrate into surrounding tissue. The ample eosinophilic granular cytoplasm led early observers to note a resemblance to muscle cells, hence the old term granular cell "myoblastoma." It is currently realized that the tumors are not of muscle origin, however (see below).

A highly distinctive feature of GCTs arising deep to squamous mucosal surfaces, particularly in the tongue and larynx, is their frequent but not universal intimate association with a char-

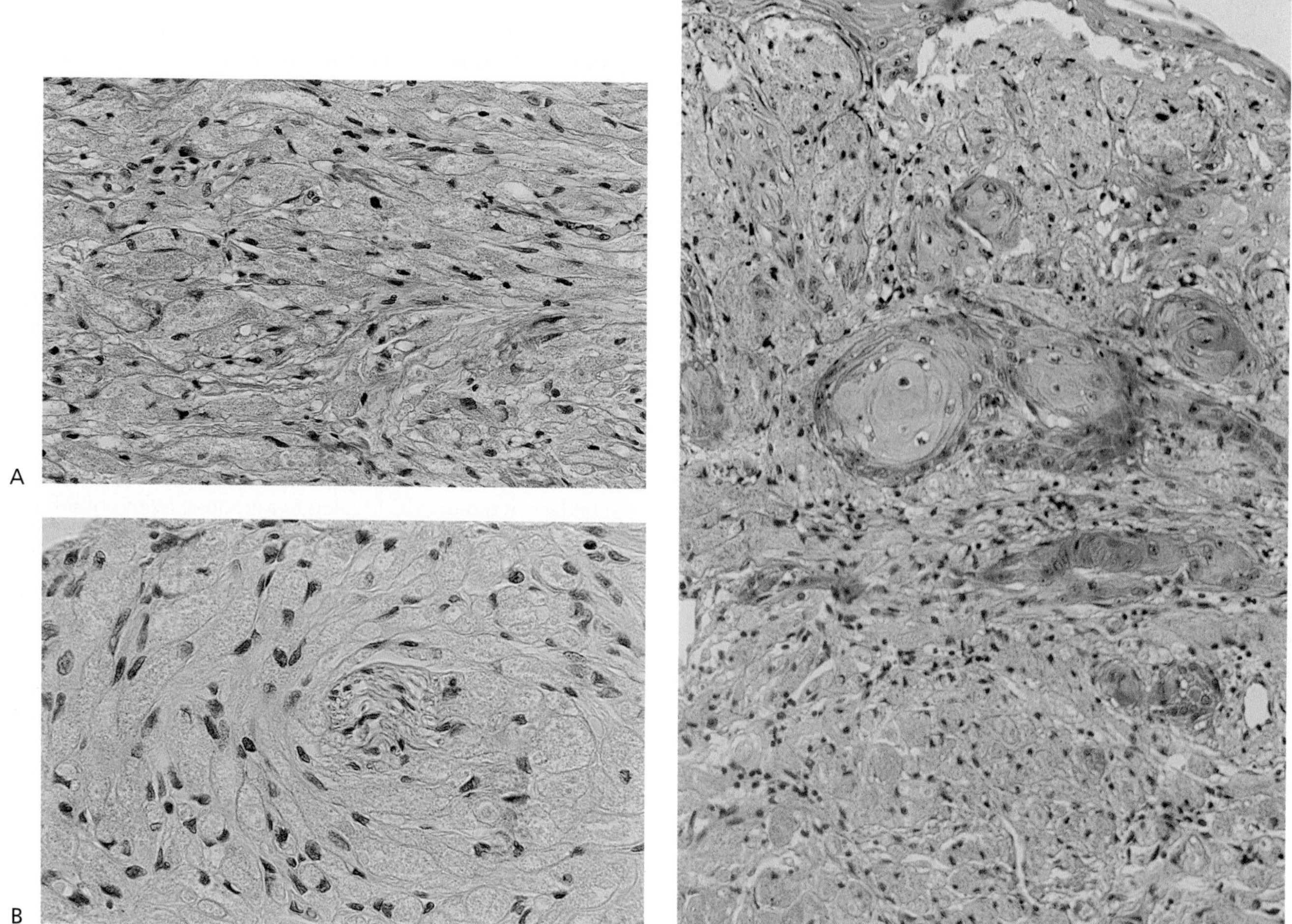

FIGURE 27. Larynx: granular cell tumor. **A:** Large cells with ample highly granular eosinophilic cytoplasm. The granules are less uniform in size, and cellular borders are less distinct than in oncocytic lesions. **B:** Granular cells in intimate association with a small nerve fiber (center of figure) consistent with the cells' derivation from schwann cells. **C:** Marked pseudoepitheliomatous hyperplasia overlying a granular cell tumor. This should not be misconstrued as invasive squamous cell carcinoma.

acteristic pseudoepitheliomatous hyperplasia of the overlying squamous mucosa (Fig. 27C). This irregular hyperplastic epithelium can appear to infiltrate the underlying granular cell lesion, simulating a malignant process, but such epithelial proliferations are virtually always benign, and the cytology of the hyperplastic mucosal epithelial cells is quite bland. Very rarely, a coexisting squamous cell carcinoma is present in the tongue or larynx (187,193), but these have been separate lesions, distinct from the GCT.

Immunohistochemical studies have found GCTs in the head and neck area to be S-100 positive, vimentin positive, frequently neuron-specific enolase (NSE)-positive, positive for CD68, but keratin negative (184,194,195), in keeping with the current generally held concept of schwann cell derivation for most GCTs (see below). Ultrastructural studies have shown the granules in the tumor cells to correspond to lysosomal autophagic vacuoles or autophagosomes as well as larger coated vesicles (183).

The histogenesis of GCTs has been much debated over the years. The predominant current opinion is that most GCTs are of schwann cell origin (Fig. 27B). This concept has been bolstered by histochemical studies that have shown that most GCTs mark for S-100 protein and NSE but not for keratin or for muscle markers (184,194–196). Further, studies have shown GCTs to stain immunohistochemically for myelin proteins (197,198). Not all GCTs mark with S-100 protein, however. Uncommon tumors containing granular cells that have the morphologic features of GCT have been found in the brain and neurohypophysis, and these as well as a tumor from the soft tissue near the clavicle have marked for the nonspecific histiocytic marker α_1-antichymotrypsin (AAC) but were negative or only weakly positive for S-100 protein (194,195). In addition, an interesting tumor found in the gingival area in newborns, usually girls, termed variously gingival granular cell tumor of the newborn (199), congenital granular cell tumor, or granular cell epulis, resembles other GCTs but uniformly stains for histiocytic but not schwannian markers (184,194). Interestingly, some odontogenic tumors, including some cells of occasional ameloblastomas, have granules histologically identical to those of GCTs, but these cells have been shown to be epithelial in origin (see Chapter 6). Thus, it would appear that GCTs or tumors with cells with the histologic appearance of typical cells of GCTs may be of heterogeneous origins, and that the granular appearance may be related to autophagic lysosomal vacuoles rather than to cell type. Nonetheless, virtually all GCTs in the head and neck, including the larynx, are considered most likely of schwannian origin.

The main differential diagnostic consideration regarding GCT relates to distinguishing its associated mucosal pseudoepitheliomatous hyperplasia from *squamous cell carcinoma.* This can best be accomplished by recognizing the underlying GCT as well as by noting the bland cytologic appearance of the epithelial cells. *Rhabdomyomas* also have cells with ample granular pink cytoplasm, but GCTs do not have cross striations, rhabdomyomas contain glycogen (PAS positive but diastase sensitive rather than resistant), and adult type rhabdomyomas often have partially clear cytoplasm or "spider cells"—cells with thin cytoplasmic strands extending from the nucleus to the cell border, as in a spider's web. Further, rhabdomyomas are well circumscribed rather than infiltrative, and adult rhabdomyomas have discrete cell borders and do not appear syncytial. Other tumors, such as *ameloblastomas* and some *neurofibromas,* may have occasional granular cells but are not composed virtually exclusively of such cells.

Most GCTs of all sites are benign tumors, and most laryngeal GCTs do not recur, even if excisional margins are microscopically positive. Exceptional malignant GCTs have been reported (191,196). Surgical excision is usually curative.

Others

Benign mesenchymal neoplasms of the larynx and hypopharynx are quite rare. Benign *nerve sheath tumors* can occur, either as solitary lesions or as part of neurofibromatosis (200–203). These lesions morphologically resemble their compatriots that occur in more common locations (Fig. 28). An exceptional case of a hypopharyngeal *cellular neurothekeoma* has recently been reported (204). Muscular neoplasms also are occasionally encountered, including *leiomyomas,* both conventional (205) and vascular (i.e., *angiomyoma*) (206), and *rhabdomyomas,* both adult (207) and fetal (208,209) (Fig. 29). *Fibromatosis* of the larynx rarely occurs in infants and children and may be a component of multicentric fibromatosis (210,211). Benign *lipomas* of the larynx are very rare and may be difficult to distinguish morphologically from liposarcoma, most cases of which in the larynx are low grade and rather indolent (212,213).

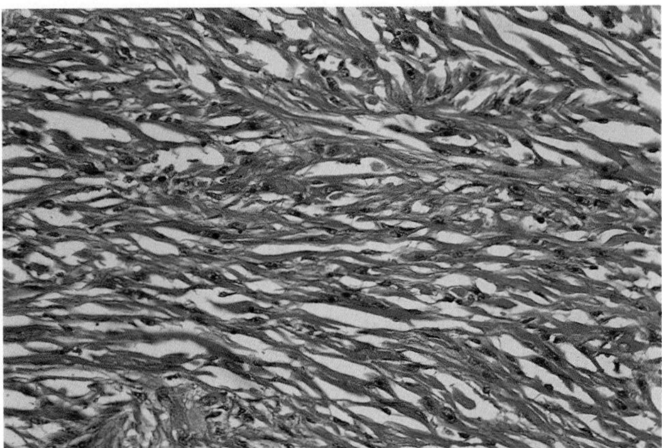

FIGURE 29. Larynx: fetal rhabdomyoma. There is a proliferation of cytologically bland spindled cells reminiscent of fetal skeletal muscle. Rare cross striations are appreciated.

Other rarities that have been reported in the larynx or hypopharynx include *hemangiopericytoma* (214), *fibrous histiocytoma* (215), *teratoma* (216), *chondroblastoma* (217), and *hamartoma* (120).

Malignant Neoplasms

Squamous Cell Carcinoma

Preinvasive Lesions

The preinvasive mucosal squamous epithelial lesions of the upper aerodigestive tract (UADT), including the larynx and hy-

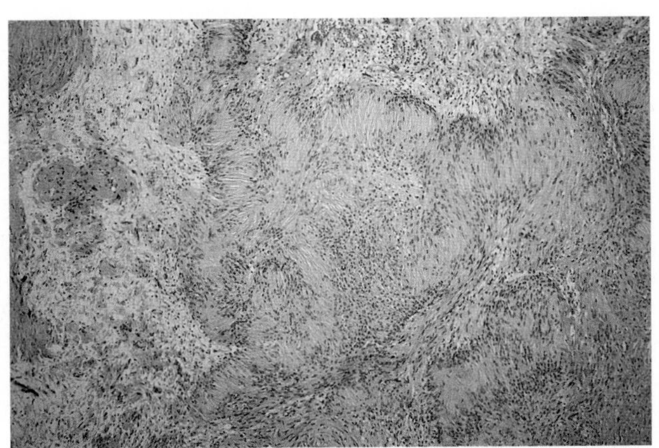

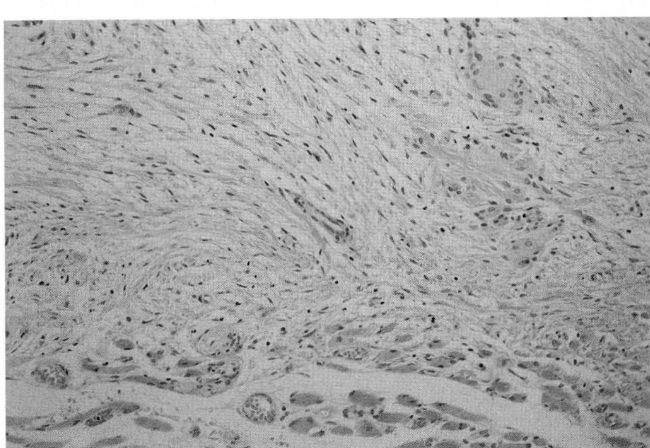

FIGURE 28. Larynx: schwannoma. **A:** Cellular Antoni A tissue occupies the right two thirds to three fourths of the figure, with nuclear palisading and Verocay body formation (see Chapter 10). Loose Antoni B tissue is at the left of the figure. **B:** In contrast to most soft tissue schwannomas, this laryngeal example does not have a discrete structural capsule but tends to blend in with the adjacent skeletal muscle. A similar lack of discrete encapsulation is seen in schwannomas of the nasal cavity.

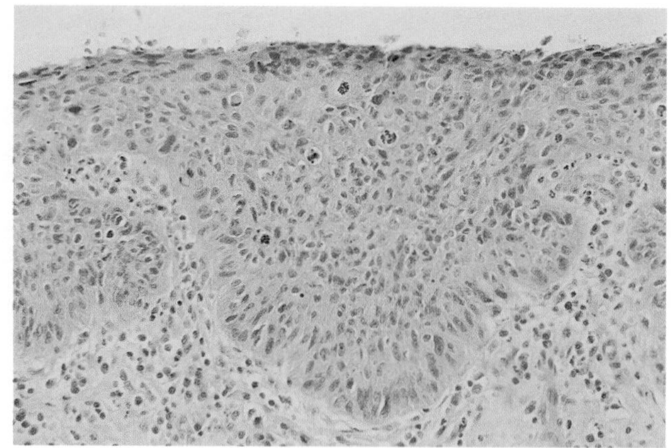

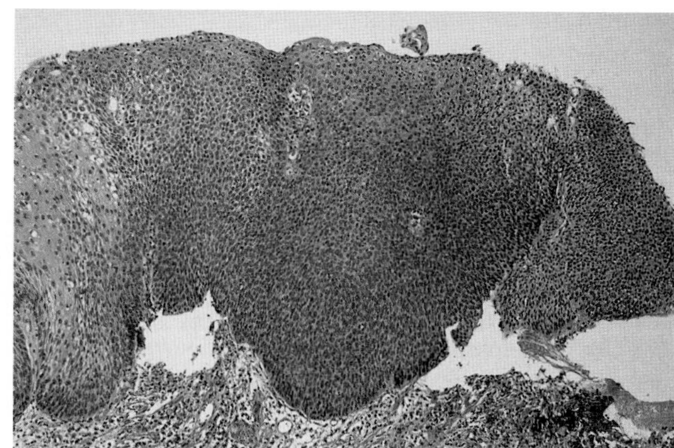

FIGURE 30. Larynx: squamous intraepithelial neoplasia (SIN) or high-grade carcinoma *in situ* (see Chapter 2). **A:** There is full-thickness atypicality of the mucosal epithelial layer with lack of maturation, disturbance of polarity, nuclear pleomorphism, and mitoses at different levels of the epithelium. **B:** This carcinoma *in situ* (CIS) with a basaloid pattern, reminiscent of classical CIS of the uterine cervix, is uncommonly encountered in the larynx.

popharynx, have been covered in Chapter 2, to which the reader is referred for a detailed discussion of squamous intraepithelial neoplasia (SIN) (Fig. 30). Briefly, the same carcinogenic agents that predispose to laryngeal cancer, including alcohol and tobacco products, also predispose to the precursor lesions of SIN. These lesions can manifest clinically as erythroplasia (a red mucosal patch) or leukoplakia (a white, often keratotic mucosal patch). Erythroplasia corresponds histologically to SIN without significant surface keratin and with atypical changes extending close to the surface and thus is generally a clinically serious lesion. Leukoplakia results from surface keratin deposition, which can reflect changes ranging from the low-risk lesions of hyperplasia and keratosis with minimal if any cytologic atypicality to the high-risk lesion of high-grade keratinizing SIN. Leukoplakia, therefore, can be associated with histologic lesions of varying clinical severity.

It is important to remember that reactive and regenerative epithelial changes that are not neoplastic or preinvasive may mimic lesions of bona fide SIN. Thus, lesions associated with trauma (e.g., tracheostomy, intubation, irradiation, previous surgery) and ulceration should be viewed with this differential diagnosis in mind. Reactive or regenerative lesions may exhibit features such as large nuclei, frequent mitoses, and some disordered polarity, especially in basal layers, but these changes generally do not extend to the surface of a mucosal epithelium of normal or increased thickness, or they involve an attenuated, not yet fully regenerated, mucosal epithelial layer. Severe changes, such as abnormal mitotic figures and prominent individual epithelial cell necrosis, generally do not occur in reactive or regenerative lesions.

Although it may be difficult to differentiate high-grade SIN from microinvasive squamous cell carcinoma (Fig. 31), studies suggest that the clinical significance of these two lesions is similar (218,219) and that the prognosis of glottic microinvasive carcinoma is excellent (219).

High-grade laryngeal or hypopharyngeal SIN is associated with a significant risk of development of subsequent invasive squamous cell carcinoma (see Chapter 2). Treatment for high-grade lesions, including those diagnosed as carcinoma *in situ,* generally consists of local excision of the gross lesion (e.g., "stripping" of the vocal cord) and subsequent frequent careful clinical follow-up. Radiation therapy is occasionally utilized in treatment (220).

Invasive Squamous Cell Carcinoma

Epidemiologic Considerations. Squamous cell carcinoma is by far the most common malignant neoplasm of the larynx and hypopharynx, accounting for about 96% of laryngeal cancers in the United States (221). Although laryngeal cancer is not one of the most prevalent cancers, it is not uncommon, and an incidence of 11,100 new cases was estimated for the United States in 1998 (222). In the United States, in fact, the larynx is the most common noncutaneous organ in which a primary cancer of the head and neck occurs (222,223). Men are affected significantly more

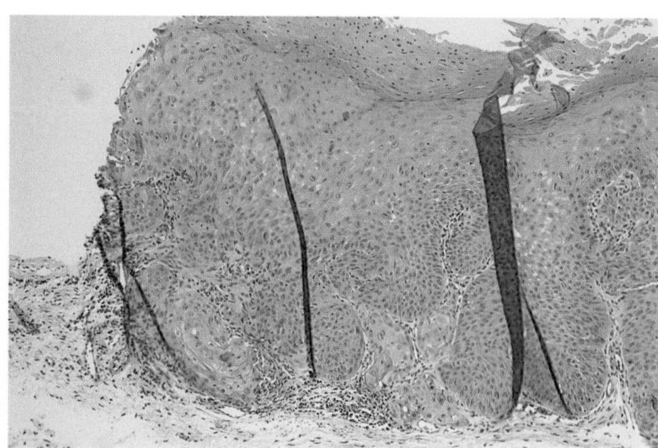

FIGURE 31. Larynx: squamous intraepithelial neoplasia, high grade with focal microinvasive carcinoma. Focal small tongues of tumor protrude into the stroma with loss of the palisading basal layer and apparent basement membrane in the lower middle of the figure. Note the prominent keratosis.

frequently than women, in a ratio of about 5:1 in one recent study (223); the male-to-female ratio in cases predicted to occur in the United States in 1998 was 4.3:1 (222). The male prevalence is even higher among black individuals (223). Men also outnumber women in cases of cancer of the hypopharynx, with about 75% of cases in the United States occurring in men (224). Most patients with laryngeal and hypopharyngeal cancer are in the 60s and 70s with a lower incidence among patients in the 50s; this cancer is uncommon in younger individuals (224,225).

Smoking and alcohol consumption are strongly etiologically related to laryngeal cancer (see Chapter 2), and more recently, additional possible etiologic factors such as human papilloma virus (HPV) infection and *ras* oncogene activation are being considered as well (226–228). Smoking and alcohol use are also associated with hypopharyngeal cancers (224,229).

Clinical Findings. Hoarseness or alteration of voice is the classic and most common symptom of laryngeal carcinoma, followed in frequency by throat pain and dysphagia (221). Hemoptysis, shortness of breath, and the presence of a neck mass can also occur. When tumors become large and bulky, significant airway compromise may ensue. Tumors involving the three different compartments of the larynx (supraglottic, glottic, and subglottic; see anatomic considerations) have somewhat different properties.

Glottic carcinomas are the most common laryngeal cancers (221,230) (Fig. 32A,B). Because of their strategic location, glottic tumors characteristically cause symptoms (usually hoarseness) early while still small and therefore curable. The carcinomas that are only superficially invasive and confined to Reinke's space—the area between the vocal ligament and the deep surface of the mucosal epithelium of the vocal cord (a region said to contain relatively few lymphatics) (226)—metastasize only infrequently to cervical lymph nodes. The incidence of nodal metastasis increases as the tumor invades more deelpy into the vocalis muscle but is still lower than that of supraglottic tumors, which inhabit an area richer in lymphatics.

Supraglottic cancers represent the next most frequent laryngeal malignancies, accounting for about a third of laryngeal cancers (221,230) (Fig. 32C). They tend to be associated with

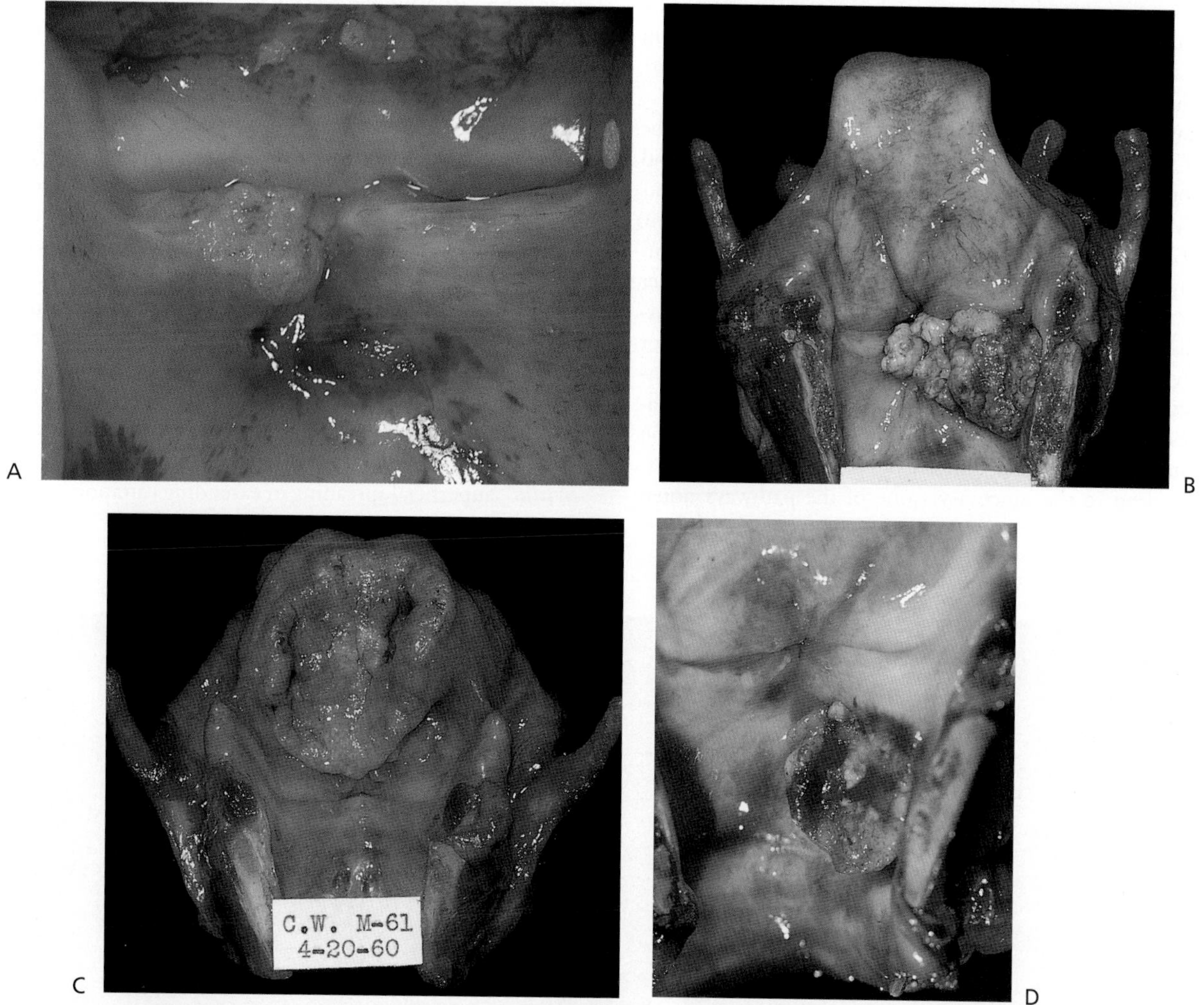

FIGURE 32. Larynx: squamous cell carcinoma, gross morphology. **A:** Exophytic tumor of left true vocal cord. **B:** Fungating exophytic tumor of right true cord with subglottic extension. **C:** Large fungating supraglottic tumor with focal ulceration. **D:** Subglottic laryngeal cancer, an uncommon location.

hoarseness later in their course than glottic tumors, and a muffled voice, foreign body sensation, pain, and hemoptysis may be initial symptoms. Supraglottic tumors, especially epiglottic lesions, are more prone to extend across the midline than glottic ones (226). They are also more likely to metastasize to lymph nodes (230), especially tumors located in the aryepiglottic fold region. Epiglottic and false cord tumors may infiltrate the preepiglottic space, abetted by the fenestrations present in the epiglottic cartilage as well as that cartilage's narrowing inferiorly. This may result in involvement of the vallecula or base-of-tongue area and a more serious clinical situation.

The anterior commissure, technically a part of the glottic larynx but immediately abutting the supraglottis, is the area of closest approximation of laryngeal mucosal epithelium to the thyroid cartilage, and in addition, there is no perichondrium at the site of the anterior commissure tendon (226); thus, the thyroid cartilage is particularly vulnerable to invasion by laryngeal carcinoma at this location.

Although glottic carcinomas not infrequently extend subglottically (Fig. 32B), primary subglottic carcinomas are quite rare, representing only between 1% and 2% of laryngeal cancers (221,230) (Fig. 32D). Because of the narrow and rigid nature of the subglottic laryngeal airway, the cricoid cartilage being the only circumferential cartilage in the respiratory tract, tumors in this location often present with stridor or some degree of airway obstruction (230).

The laryngeal ventricle has traditionally been considered to be a barrier to the spread of carcinoma between supraglottic and glottic compartments, and supraglottic laryngectomies have consequently been successfully performed for many supraglottic cancers (231). Recent studies indicate, however, that large tumors may spread between glottic and supraglottic areas, either posterior to and behind the ventricle to the arytenoid region, laterally adjacent to the thyroid cartilage in the paraglottic space, or anteriorly, through the region of the anterior commissure tendon or anterior thyroid cartilage (231–233). Thus, although relatively few laryngeal cancers appear transglottic on examination of the mucosal surface, a significant number may extend transglottically deep to the mucosa via one of the pathways noted above. Increasingly sensitive radiologic imaging techniques may be used productively in the pretreatment investigation of staging of laryngeal carcinomas.

Hypopharyngeal carcinomas often present late in their course, when tumors are large and therefore difficult to cure. Carcinomas of the pyriform sinus are by far the most common hypopharyngeal malignancies (Fig. 33A), followed in incidence by tumors of the posterior pharyngeal wall (Fig. 33B); and postcricoid carcinomas, involving the mucosa covering the posterior surface of the cricoid lamina, are the least common (224). Dysphagia is the most common symptom of hypopharyngeal cancer, and otalgia, a neck mass, sore throat, and general cachexia and inanition may also be present (224,229). Tumors of the pyriform sinus may extend anterosuperiorly to the base of tongue and oropharynx and posteriorly to the postcricoid region. Advanced tumors may involve the thyroid gland or extend around or through the thyroid cartilage to the lateral neck.

It is well recognized that patients with squamous cell carcinoma of the upper aerodigestive tract (UADT) develop one or more additional synchronous or metachronous cancers (see Chapter 2). This phenomenon has generally been related to the concept of "field cancerization" or a "field effect" of carcinogenic agents predisposing large areas to develop presumably different and independent cancers (see Chapter 2). This theory may need to be modified somewhat, as a study by Worshman et al. (234), utilizing cytogenetic and molecular biological techniques, has elegantly demonstrated that two topographically separate synchronous UADT cancers, one in the floor of the mouth and one in the pyriform sinus, were actually both monoclonal, or genetically identical, implying origin from a common progenitor cell. Such monoclonal origin of disparate tumors has also been described in the urinary bladder (235). This concept raises intriguing questions as to the significance of lateral or intramucosal extension of carcinoma cells in squamous cell carcinoma of the UADT (234), with implications for the clinical significance of histologically malignant intramucosal ("pagetoid") clusters of cells that do not occupy the full thickness of the mucosal epithelium and hence do not fulfill traditional criteria for "carcinoma *in situ*." Superficial spreading or extending carcinomas have been

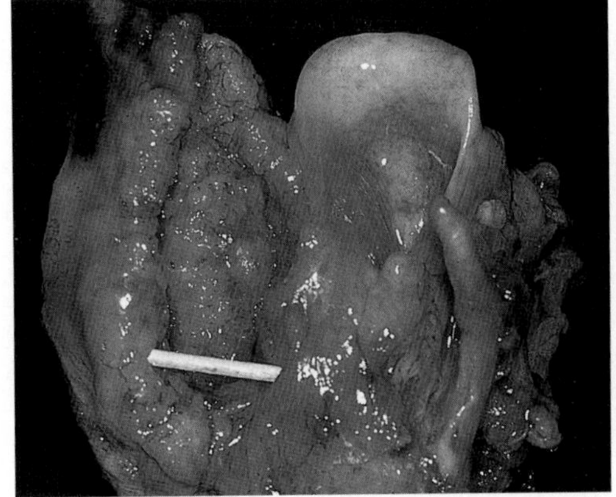
A

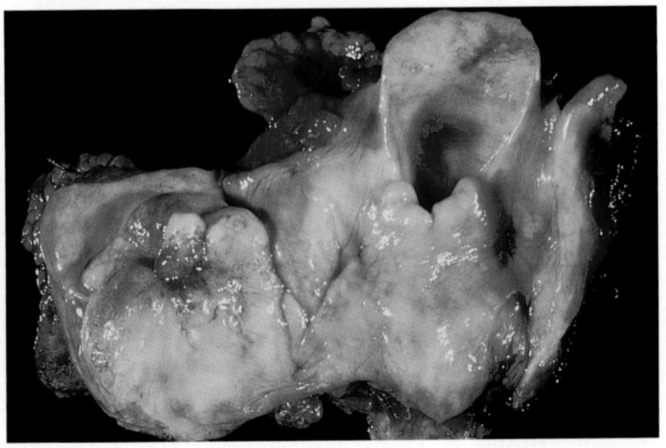
B

FIGURE 33. Hypopharynx: squamous cell carcinoma. **A:** A large centrally ulcerated tumor of the left pyriform sinus. **B:** An exophytic tumor of the posterior hypopharyngeal wall.

A 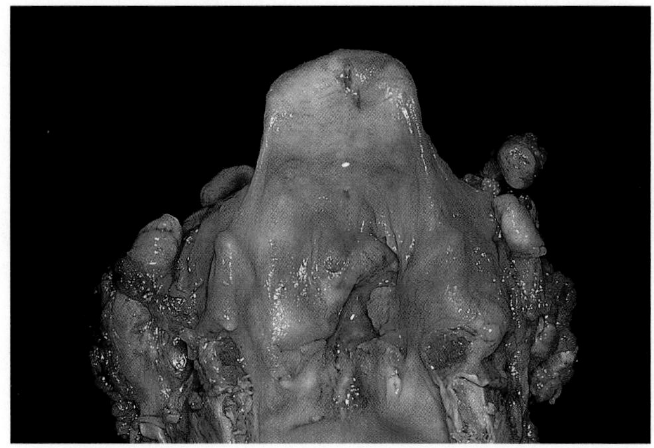

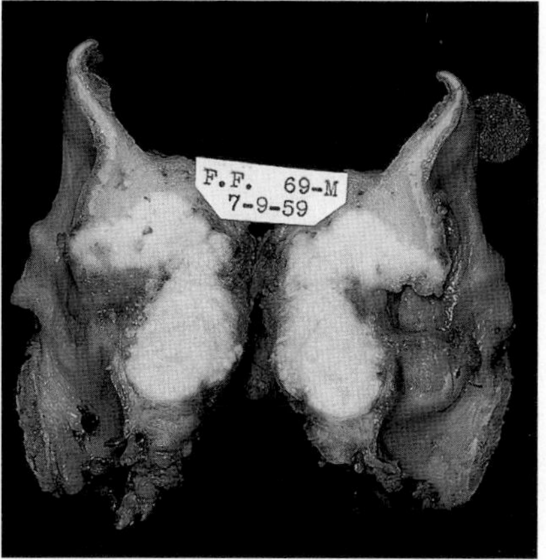 B

FIGURE 34. Larynx: squamous cell carcinoma, ulceroinfiltrating. **A:** Transglottic tumor involves the anterior commissure area. **B:** A cross section shows deeply infiltrative tumor.

reported in the stomach (236), esophagus (237,238), colon (239), and even the hypopharynx (240) and larynx (241). Interestingly, a recent study revealed most superficial depressed-type gastric carcinomas investigated to be monoclonal (242).

Pathologic Findings. Grossly, squamous cell carcinomas of the larynx and hypopharynx can manifest as exophytic, fungating masses, at times papillary and friable (Fig. 32). There may be central ulceration and necrosis (Fig. 33A). Alternatively, laryngeal cancers can be ulceroinfiltrative and appear as craters invading deeply, perhaps surrounded by an elevated rim of firm tissue (Fig. 34). On cut section, the tumors, especially keratinizing carcinomas, are usually white, firm, and somewhat gritty. At times focal necrosis, or soft keratin debris, possibly with a superimposed necroinflammatory component, may be present. Rarely, carcinomas may have a minimal surface or mucosal component, with most of the tumor lying deep to intact surface mucosa. Tumors centered around the ventricle or saccule (so-called ventriculosaccular carcinomas) (Fig. 35) (243) are often of this type and may exhibit minimal surface changes on examination.

Histologically, the tumors are characteristic of squamous cell carcinomas in general, in the head and neck and elsewhere. They can be well, moderately, or poorly differentiated (Fig. 36), with larger or lesser amounts of keratin, or they may be nonkeratinizing. SIN of varying degrees of severity often surrounds areas of frank invasive carcinoma and may also appear as distinct foci in the mucosa separate from invasive foci. The reader is referred to Chapter 2 for a more detailed discussion of the pathology of squamous cell carcinoma. Some points to mention here include the fact that squamous cell carcinoma may at times have a component of spindled cells that may occasionally be prominent, possibly resulting in confusion with a sarcoma. Areas of more conventional squamous cell carcinoma, however, can usually be found, and immunohistochemical stains for keratin proteins will generally be positive. When this spindle cell change is marked, a spindle cell or sarcomatous carcinoma may result. This particular subtype of squamous cell carcinoma is discussed in Chapter 2, and some comments are offered later in this chapter. Another pattern that may lead to confusion is the acantholytic pattern,

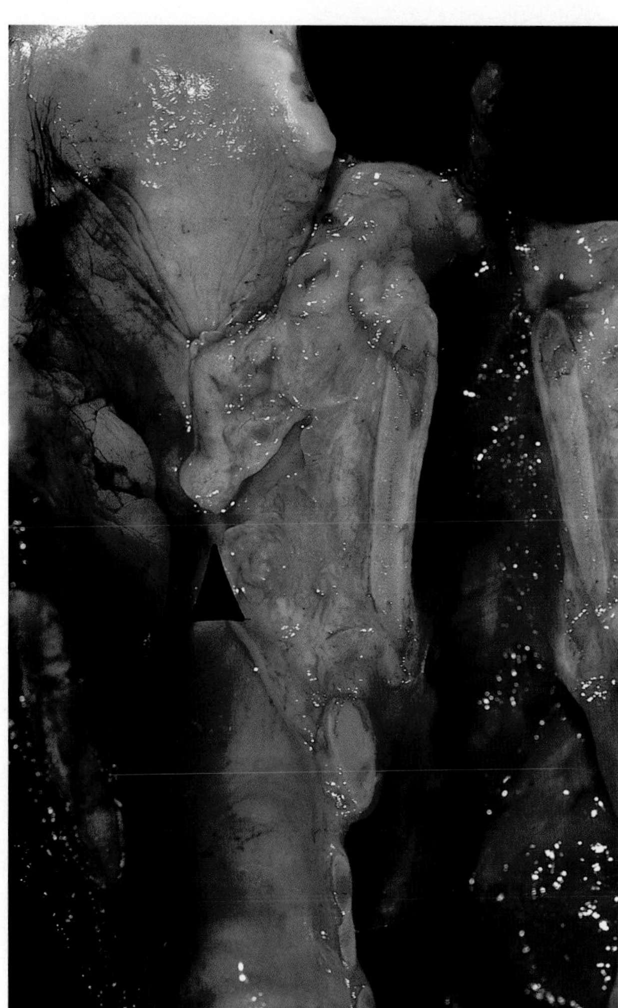

FIGURE 35. Larynx: squamous cell carcinoma, ventriculosaccular. The largely subepithelial tumor surrounds the laryngeal ventricle (*arrowhead* points to medial opening of ventricle).

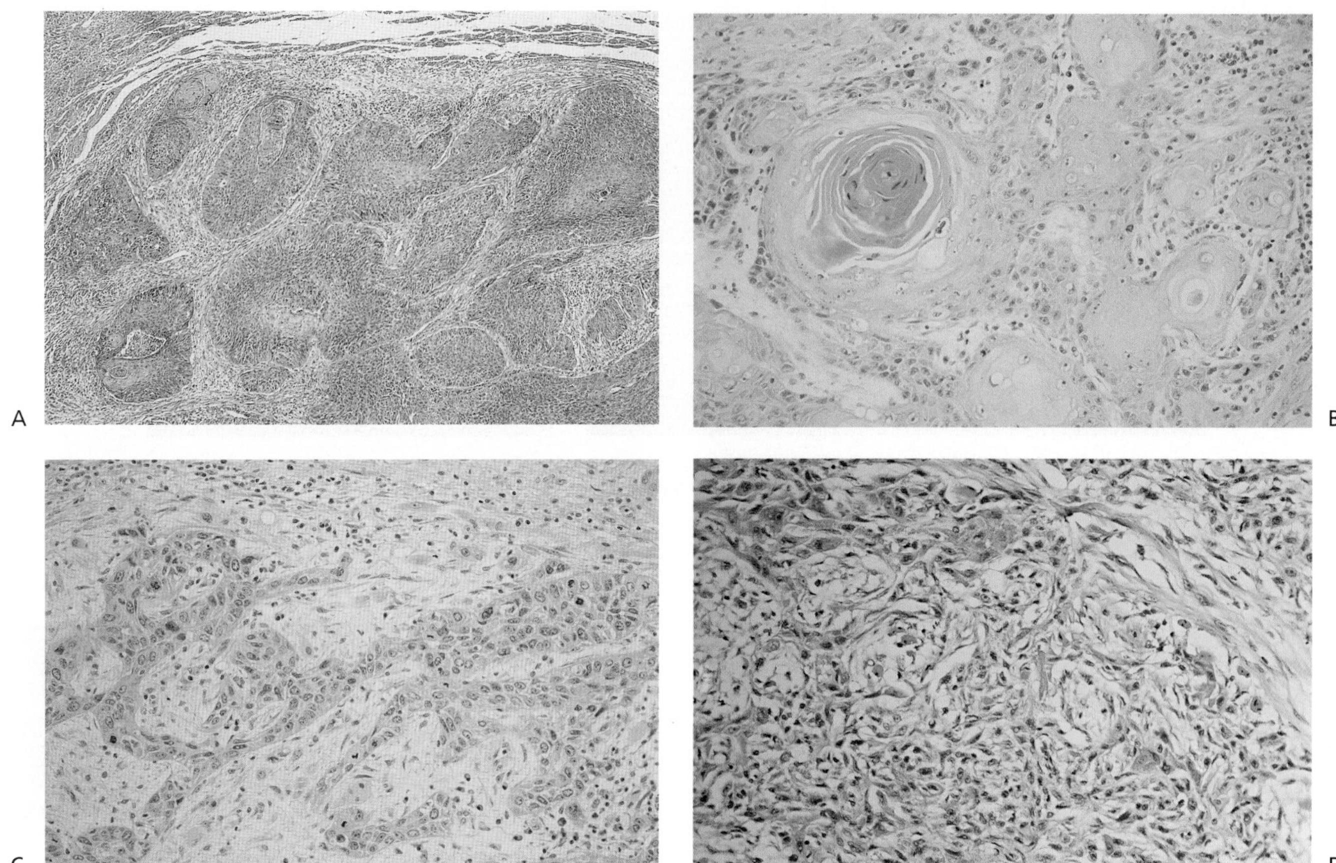

FIGURE 36. Larynx: squamous cell carcinoma. **A:** Nests of carcinoma with focal keratinization infiltrate soft tissue in a desmoplastic stroma. **B:** In this well-differentiated focus of carcinoma, there is prominent squamous differentiation with ample eosinophilic cytoplasm and keratin production. **C:** A moderately differentiated focus of squamous cell carcinoma. **D:** Poorly differentiated squamous cell carcinoma, with convincing squamous differentiation notable only at the top of the figure.

wherein acantholysis of cells in nests of tumor results in the appearance of pseudoglandular spaces, at times with rounded tumor cells that appear to be floating in the spaces. This so-called "adenoid squamous" pattern is well recognized in the skin, and it can also appear in the larynx and hypopharynx. At times, the peripheral squamous cells in these pseudoglandular spaces can be thin and flattened, resulting in a pseudovascular appearance that may mimic an angiosarcoma (so-called pseudovascular adenoid squamous cell carcinoma) (244) (Fig. 37).

Not uncommonly one is faced with the task of interpreting a biopsy of a patient who has undergone irradiation therapy or previous surgery for squamous cell carcinoma. Radiation can result in histologic changes such as mesenchymal cell nuclear atypia as well as atypical changes in epithelial cells. Especially noteworthy regarding diagnosis of posttherapy persistence or recurrence of carcinoma are radiation-induced changes in seromucinous glands. These glands are often atrophic following therapy, and small remaining ducts can exhibit significant atypical changes (e.g., nuclear enlargement and mitotic activity). A useful clue that helps differentiate benign irradiated ductal remnants from carcinoma is the recognition that the residual ducts, perhaps with some remnants of additional glandular epithelium, occupy the original site of the seromucinous glands and are not infiltrating or abnormally located. Enlarged prominent endothelial cells can also be a problem in evaluating postradiation biopsies. Regenerative mucosal epithelium, encountered for example during reepithelialization of an ulcerated surface, may look atypical, with enlarged nuclei and (normal) mitotic figures. If these epithelial cells are "floating" in surface fibrin, a misleading appearance of superficial invasion may result. Again, recognition of the underlying ulceration, reepithelialization, and fibrinous membrane may help to prevent serious interpretative errors.

Laryngeal squamous cell carcinoma can invade blood vessels and lymphatics. Lymphatic permeation can be difficult to identify, for an artifactual tissue space around a small clump of tumor cells must be distinguished from cells in the lumen of a lymphatic channel. A clue to recognizing cells lining a space containing tumor cells as endothelial cells is that the nuclei of endothelial cells often protrude into the lumen. Laryngeal carcinoma invades veins much more commonly than arteries. Use of an elastic tissue stain may help delineate the wall of a blood vessel of appreciable size, and the presence of tumor thrombi, or carcinoma cells enmeshed in a fibrin clot, can also help identify intravascular tumor.

Much work has been done regarding the correlation of histologic factors of laryngeal squamous cell carcinomas, such as tu-

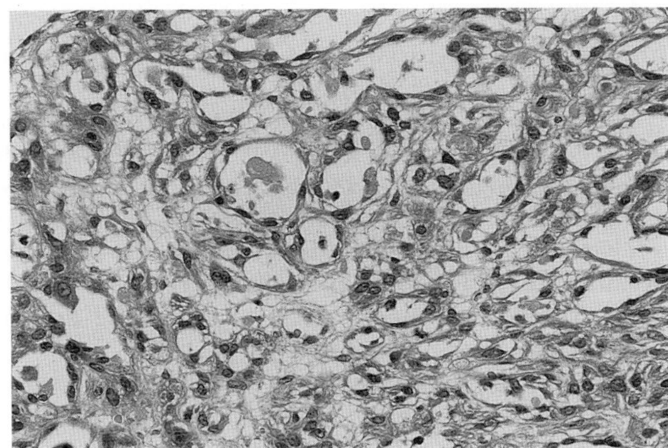

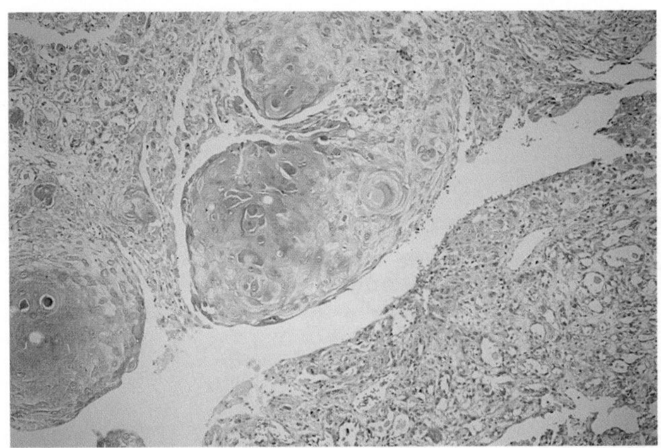

FIGURE 37. Larynx: acantholytic or "pseudovascular adenoid" squamous cell carcinoma. **A:** Marked acantholysis with central dropout of cells in tumor nests leaving flattened peripheral cells intact and creating a gland-like or vascular appearance. **B:** Another focus in the tumor shows recognizable squamous differentiation.

mor grade, with biological behavior and prognosis. These numerous attempts at correlation have met with varying degrees of success (245). It appears that the presence of lymph node metastases, and especially of extracapsular extension of metastatic nodal carcinoma, is indeed related to a poorer outcome (245). Histologic grading of the invasive tumor front (tumor–host tissue interface) is another promising method of correlating histology and prognosis (246,247). Recently, more sophisticated techniques such as DNA cytometry (247) assessment of proliferation markers such as Ki 67 (MIB I) (247), cyclin D1 protein expression (248), and p53 protein overexpression (249), have shown some promise in predicting the clinical outcome of laryngeal carcinomas.

Most of the differential diagnostic problems of squamous cell carcinoma relate to their variants, discussed in Chapter 2 and mentioned below. Identification of keratin or unequivocal intercellular bridges serves to establish squamous differentiation, and formation of a rounded squamous "pearl" and the enveloping or surrounding of a tumor cell or cells by the cytoplasm of another are also helpful features suggestive of squamous differentiation. Immunohistochemical stains for keratin may help differentiate carcinomas from sarcomas, melanomas (negative for keratin, positive for S-100 protein and possibly for HMB 45), and lymphoma (negative for keratin, positive for leukocytic common antigen or cytoplasmic immunoglobulins if plasmacytic). Ultrastructural demonstration of tonofilaments and desmosomes is indicative of squamous differentiation, and immunohistochemical [neuron-specific enolase (not entirely specific), synaptophysin, chromogranin] and ultrastructural methods (presence of dense-core membrane-bound neurosecretory granules) can help distinguish neuroendocrine neoplasms. Differentiation from mucoepidermoid and adenosquamous carcinoma is discussed below.

Therapy and Biological Behavior. Treatment for carcinoma of the larynx and hypopharynx includes surgery, radiation, and chemotherapy. For the larynx, the most common therapy has traditionally been surgery combined with radiation or radiation alone, followed in incidence by surgery alone (221). Organ-sparing therapy for advanced disease involving radiation and chemotherapy without surgery as primary therapy is receiving significant current attention (250). The 5-year disease-specific survival for cases of cancer of the larynx in the United States diagnosed from 1980 through 1985 was 74.5%; it was higher for glottic (85.4%) than for supraglottic tumors (61.4%) (221). This may be in part because patients with glottic tumors present with lower-stage lesions than those with supraglottic tumors (221). Patients with cervical nodal metastases fared significant worse than those without (221).

More patients with hypopharyngeal cancer received combined-modality therapy than single-modality treatment (224). The 5-year disease-specific survival for patients with hypopharyngeal cancer in the United States diagnosed from 1980 through 1985 is poorer than that for laryngeal cancer patients, being only 33.4% (224). Five-year survival rates were somewhat better for patients with postcricoid tumors (45.4%) than for those with pyriform sinus (33.6%) or posterior wall (36.9%) lesions (224).

Variants of Squamous Cell Carcinoma

The pathology of the variants of squamous cell carcinoma in the upper aerodigestive tract has been discussed in Chapter 2. A few comments relating to their laryngeal and hypopharyngeal manifestations are made here.

Verrucous Carcinoma. Verrucous carcinoma is a slow-growing, exophytic, warty, broad-based squamous epithelial neoplasm that invades deep tissue via a broad pushing front. It can be locally destructive but, in the pure form, virtually never metastasizes. It occurs most commonly in the oral cavity, particularly the buccal area, but also presents as a laryngeal tumor (251–254). It also occurs on the skin, most commonly on the extremities and genitalia.

In three large series, the incidence of laryngeal verrucous carcinomas was reported as 1.7% of laryngeal carcinomas (254,255) and 3.82% of laryngeal malignancies (253). There is a marked

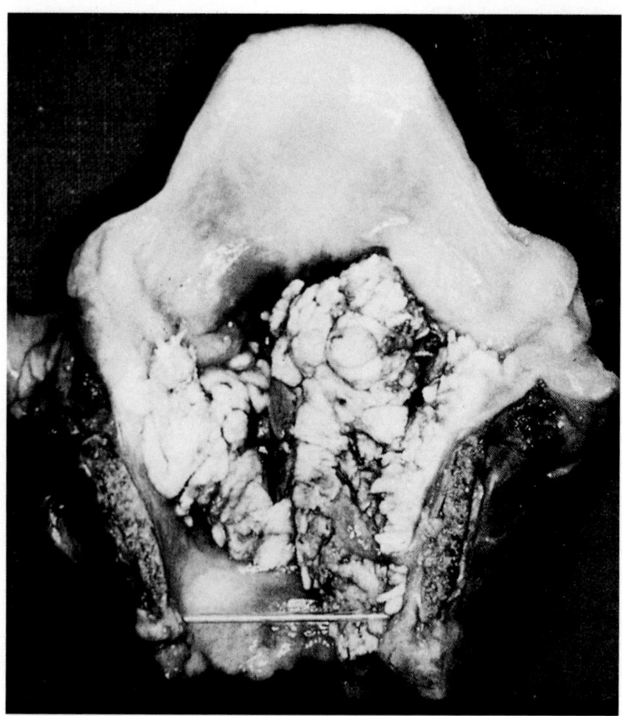

FIGURE 38. Larynx: verrucous carcinoma. A gross photo shows a large and extensive exophytic shaggy, warty neoplasm. (From Ferlito A. Diagnosis and treatment of verrucous squamous cell carcinoma of the larynx: a critical review. *Ann Otol Rhinol Laryngol* 1985;94:575–579, with permission.)

male predominance, most patients are or had been smokers, and the average age of patients at presentation was about 60 (252,254,255); most patients are in their 50's or 60's (252). Most tumors are glottic, and the presenting symptom is most often hoarseness (254).

The pathology is as described in Chapter 2. Briefly, a broad based, shaggy, exophytic, warty tumor is present grossly (Fig. 38). The histology of the tumor is characterized by well-differentiated squamous epithelial tongues and fronds with minimal cyto-architectural atypia that invade with a broad blunt pushing margin, often accompanied by a chronic inflammatory infiltrate at the base of the tumor (Fig. 39). Close collaboration between clinician and pathologist is generally necessary for an accurate biopsy diagnosis to be made because of the deceptively bland histologic appearance of the tumor; and recognition of the clinical manifestations of the lesion by the pathologist combined with the provision of a generous biopsy sample including the invasive portion of the tumor by the surgeon may help in this regard. Differentiation from verrucous hyperplasia is accomplished by recognizing that the hyperplastic lesion does not invade below the level of adjacent uninvolved mucosa, whereas verrucous carcinoma does (256). The lack of significant atypia distinguishes verrucous carcinoma from papillary squamous cell carcinoma.

A point worth emphasizing is that foci of conventional squamous cell carcinoma, at times small, with greater atypicality or a more jagged infiltrative pattern, may occur within lesions of otherwise classic verrucous carcinoma (254). Thus, verrucous tumors should be thoroughly sampled to exclude such foci of conventional squamous cell carcinoma, which can impart the more serious biological behavior and metastatic potential associated with the latter lesion (254).

Pure verrucous carcinomas do not metastasize and are generally considered best treated by surgical excision, although radiation therapy has its proponents (257). Anaplastic transformation of verrucous carcinoma following radiation therapy, previously prominently mentioned in the literature (258,259), is rarely encountered currently (254) any may perhaps have been related to unrecognized concurrent conventional squamous cell carcinoma in the original lesion.

It is worth noting the position of pure nonmetastasizing verrucous "carcinoma" in the spectrum of squamous proliferative lesions, situated between hyperplasia on the one hand and combined verrucous–squamous carcinomas and metastasizing squamous cell carcinomas on the other. In this context, some authors suggest recognizing this behavior by substituting the term verrucous acanthosis for verrucous carcinoma (260).

Spindle Cell Carcinoma (Sarcomatoid Carcinoma). Spindle cell carcinoma (SpCC) (sarcomatoid carcinoma) of the head and neck is an uncommon but fascinating neoplasm that has engendered much controversy in the past, but about which more consensus is currently being reached. The entity occurs most commonly in the larynx and oral cavity and also in the hypopharynx and esophagus (usually the upper esophagus) and more rarely in the sinonasal tract (261,262). SpCC is discussed in Chapter 2, but some comments related to the lesion in the larynx and hypopharynx are made here.

Men are significantly more commonly affected than women, with the ratio in one large study from 1975 and a review of the literature to 1980 being 12:1 and 10:1, respectively (263,264); a ratio of 4:1 was reported in a more recent series (265). The true vocal cord is most commonly affected, followed in incidence by the hypopharynx (usually the pyriform sinus) and the supraglottis (263–266). The mean age at diagnosis ranges from the mid- to late sixties (263–265). Hoarseness is the most common presenting symptom, with dysphagia, pain, and airway obstruction also reported (265,267). Interestingly, a significant number (about one fourth) of patients have a history of prior radiation to the site (266,268,269). The pedunculated nature of many of these tumors may explain the interesting observation that some patients cough up or expectorate a portion of their tumor (266,269).

As discussed in Chapter 2, these tumors are generally polypoid, often pedunculated, generally ulcerated masses. Most, though bulky, do not appear deeply invasive into underlying tissue (263). The spindle cell or sarcomatoid component of the neoplasm almost always predominates (Fig. 40A,B), with the squamous component often scant and difficult to find, at times necessitating examining multiple sections for its detection. The squamous component may be severe dysplasia or carcinoma *in situ* (or SIN), superficially invasive or frankly invasive squamous cell carcinoma (Fig. 40C). Often, the base of the polypoid lesion is a productive place in which to seek the carcinomatous component (266,269). The sarcomatous component usually resembles malignant fibrous histiocytoma or fibrosarcoma (266) (Fig. 40A,B). Occasionally, osseous or cartilaginous differentiation

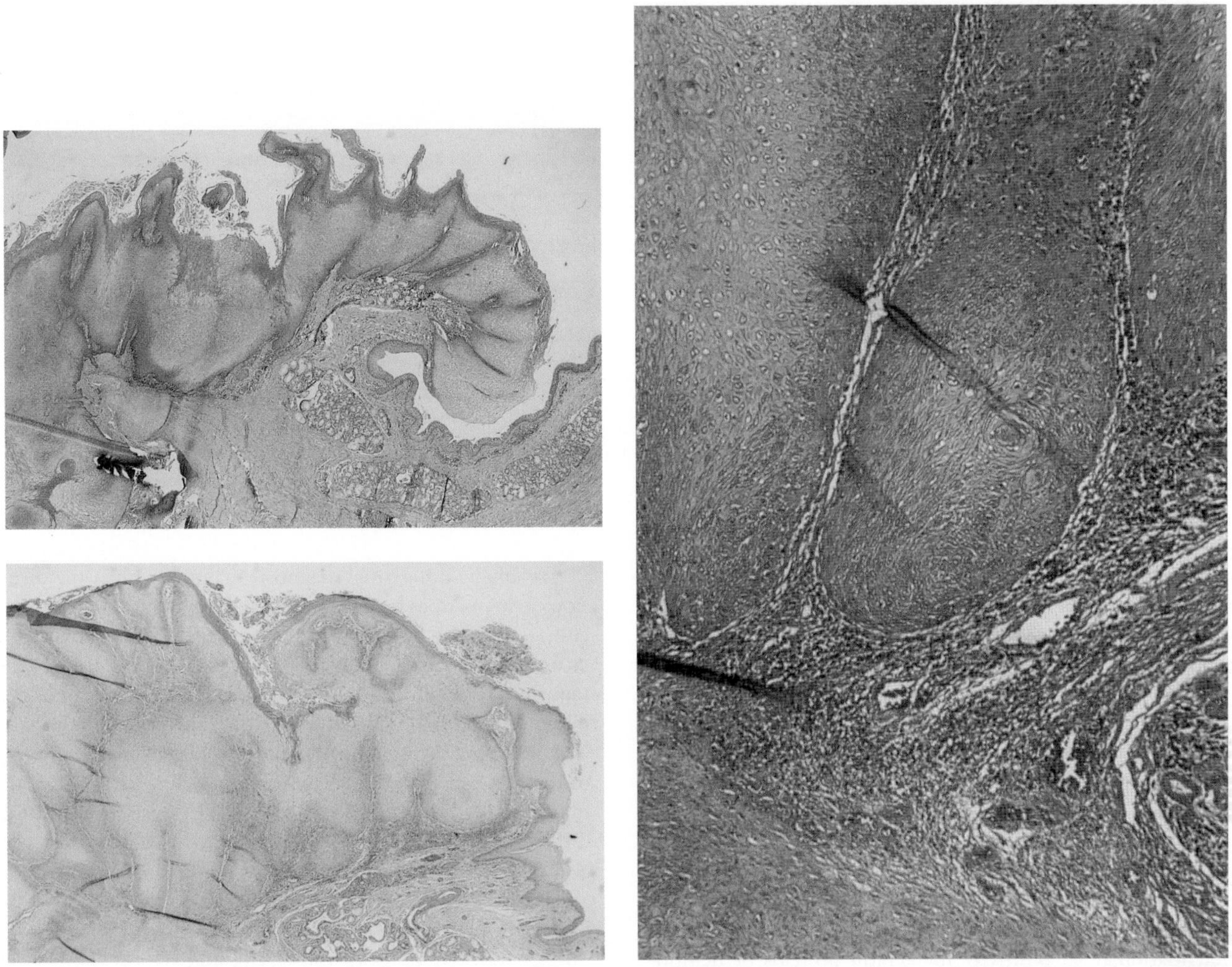

FIGURE 39. Larynx: verrucous carcinoma. **A:** A thick well-differentiated squamous epithelial proliferation has a warty papillary surface. **B:** Well-differentiated epithelial fronds infiltrating in a pushing, broad-based manner. **C:** A higher-power view of the pushing, smooth infiltrating edge of the very well-differentiated tumor. Note the chronic inflammatory infiltrate at the tumor's base.

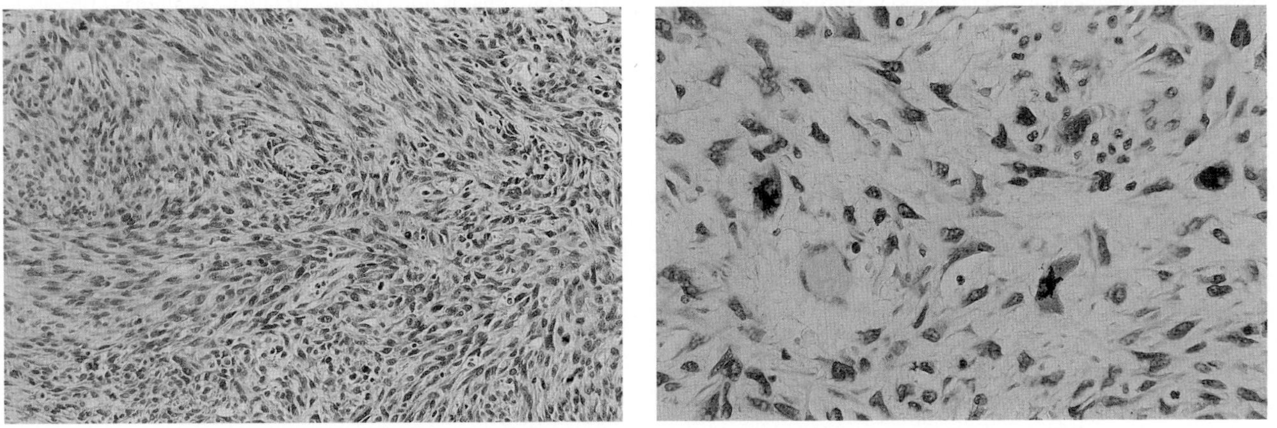

FIGURE 40. Larynx: spindle cell carcinoma. **A:** Fascicles of malignant spindle cells with a histomorphology reminiscent of fibrosarcoma. **B:** A high-power view of a looser area with stellate cells, some with atypical mitotic figures. This field is reminiscent of a malignant fibrous histiocytoma.

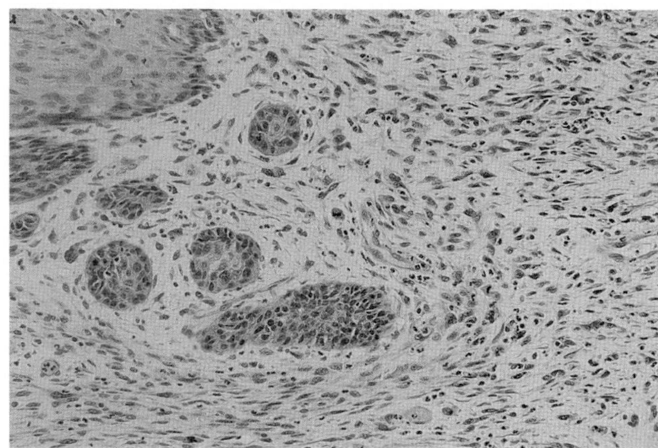

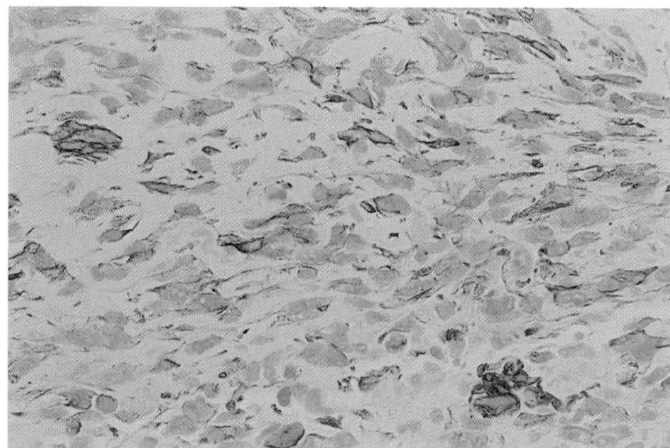

C D

FIGURE 40. ***(Continued)*** **C:** Nests of conventional squamous cell carcinoma are interspersed among the spindle cells. **D:** The spindle cells are immunohistochemically positive for keratin proteins (AE1,3/Cam 5.2).

may be seen. Interestingly, such matrix-producing differentiation often occurs in patients with a history of prior radiation (264,266). Metastases may have a squamous or spindle cell morphology.

Monophasic SpCCs have been reported in which only a sarcomatoid pattern is identified, without a histologic component of squamous cell carcinoma being recognized (266,270). Such cases present a diagnostic dilemma. In our laboratory, we take the position, as do Lewis et al. (266), that to make a definitive diagnosis of SpCC, one must identify either a definite histologic squamous as well as a sarcomatous component to the tumor or, in a histologically monophasic lesion, immunohistochemical or ultrastructural evidence of carcinomatous differentiation (e.g., positivity for keratin proteins or demonstration of tonofilaments or desmosomes). Keratin positivity in the sarcomatous foci may be capricious and focal, and utilization of a battery of keratin stains is suggested. Most lesions will show keratin positivity in spindled areas with at least one keratin marker (266) (Fig. 40D).

The histogenesis of this intriguing lesion has been the subject of considerable speculation and discussion. Suffice it to say here that most current opinion is that SpCC is a variant of squamous cell carcinoma of epithelial origin, in which metaplastic alteration has given rise to a sarcomatoid or mesenchymal morphology in a large portion of the tumor (261,263,266,268,271). Recent experimental evidence of epithelial–mesenchymal interconversion has provided a further argument in favor of this concept (272,273).

A recent study of ploidy and proliferative activity in esophageal SpCCs found that the sarcomatous component had a higher tumoral proliferative index as well as higher aneuploidy than the carcinomatous component in the series of cases examined (262). The authors surmise that these features may convey a growth advantage to the sarcomatous component, explaining at least in part its predominance over the carcinomatous component as is seen in SpCCs. Interestingly, in a study of laryngeal SpCCs, Lewis et al. found a greater degree of concordance in ploidy between the sarcomatous and carcinomatous components of tumors in their series (266).

Histologic differential diagnosis mainly involves the distinction of SpCC from benign spindle cell proliferations or from sarcomas. Atypical-appearing granulation tissue in the larynx simulating a malignant neoplasm following radiation has been reported by Weidner et al. (115). A frank carcinomatous component is not present in this lesion; the atypical spindle cells were keratin-negative; and capillary endothelial cells shared the atypia of the mesenchymal cells. The recently described inflammatory myofibroblastic tumor of the larynx (113) also enters into the differential diagnosis of SpCC (see above). The former lesion also does not have a carcinomatous component, its spindle cells are keratin-negative, and the spindle cells are generally more bland appearing and less cytologically atypical than those in SpCC. Rare sarcomas of the larynx and hypopharynx occur. They do not have a squamous carcinomatous component. Some sarcomas, notably synovial sarcoma, stain for keratin, but the epithelioid component in that sarcoma is glandular appearing rather than squamous, and the spindle cells of that lesion are usually more densely packed and smaller than those in SpCCs. Further, the hemangiopericytoma-like pattern often seen in synovial sarcomas is not a feature of SpCC. Malignant fibrous histiocytomas may rarely have a degree of keratin positivity, but they do not exhibit squamous differentiation either histologically or ultrastructurally.

Surgery is generally considered the mainstay of treatment for SpCC. The biological behavior of this lesion was found in the series of Olsen et al. to be about the same as for comparably staged conventional squamous cell carcinomas (265). The 5-year survival rate in their series was 68% (265). Adverse prognostic factors appear to be location in hypopharyngeal or extraglottic laryngeal sites, large size, presence of nodal metastases, and, interestingly, keratin positivity (264,265).

Basaloid–Squamous Carcinoma. Basaloid–squamous carcinoma (BSC) is an aggressive variant of squamous cell carcinoma of the UADT, originally described by Wain et al. in 1986 (274), with a predilection for the base of tongue, pyriform sinus, and supraglottic larynx (274–277). Patients are generally male (the male:female ratio is about 4:1), and the average age is in the

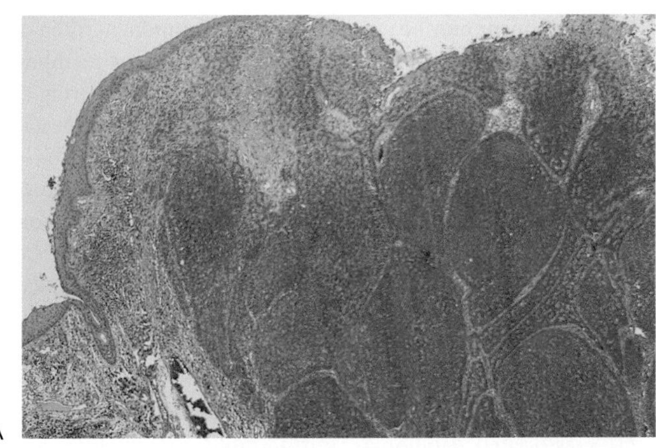

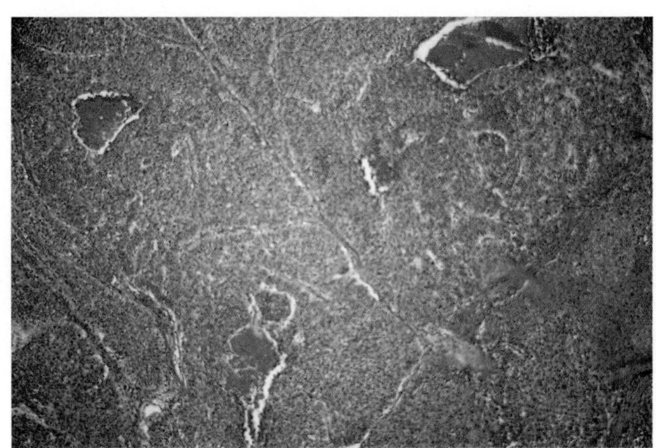

FIGURE 41. Larynx: basaloid–squamous carcinoma. **A:** Rounded nests of compact small basaloid cells infiltrate subepithelial tissue. **B:** The basaloid tumor nests show central comedo-type necrosis.

sixties (276). This tumor type has been recognized to occur in the esophagus (278,279), and similar tumors are described in the lung, anus, and uterine cervix (277). Presenting symptoms for UADT cases have included sore throat, hoarseness, the presence of a neck mass, and dysphagia (275,276). A significant number of patients have cervical metastatic disease at presentation.

The pathologic features of BSC are described in Chapter 2. In summary, the tumor is composed of rounded nests and strands of basaloid tumor cells, with a high nuclear:cytoplasmic ratio, often with central comedo-type necrosis (Fig. 41), peripheral palisading of tumor cells, and an intriguing pseudoglandular pattern with deposition of basement membrane material reminiscent of adenoid cystic carcinoma (Fig. 42A,B). There is always a squamous component to the lesion (SIN, distinct foci of squamous cell carcinoma, or squamous differentiation in basaloid nests) (Fig. 42B,C). Interestingly, foci of spindle cell carcinoma are rarely observed in cases of BSC (277,280) (Fig. 43). Differentiation from adenoid cystic carcinoma (ACC) is by the

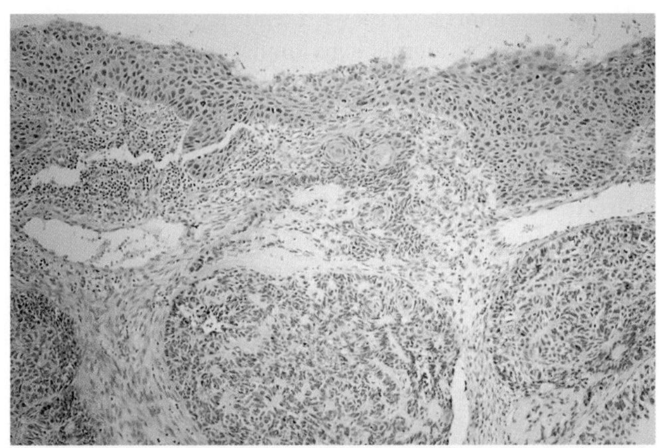

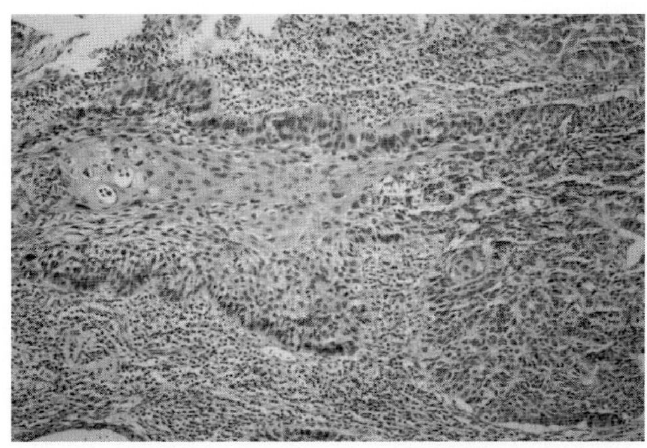

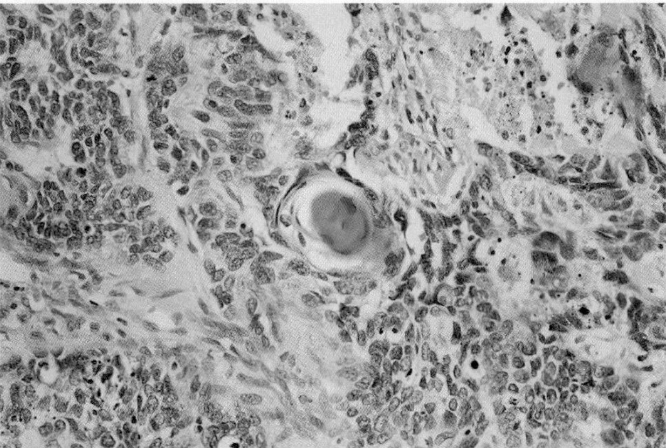

FIGURE 42. Hypopharynx: basaloid–squamous carcinoma. **A:** Nests of basaloid cells containing basement membrane-like hyaline material are reminiscent of adenoid cystic carcinoma and underlie a mucosa that shows squamous cell carcinoma *in situ*. **B:** A large basaloid tumor nest has prominent peripheral palisading, reminiscent of cutaneous basal cell carcinoma. Squamous differentiation can be seen at the left of the figure. **C:** A squamous pearl is present in the midst of small basaloid tumor cells.

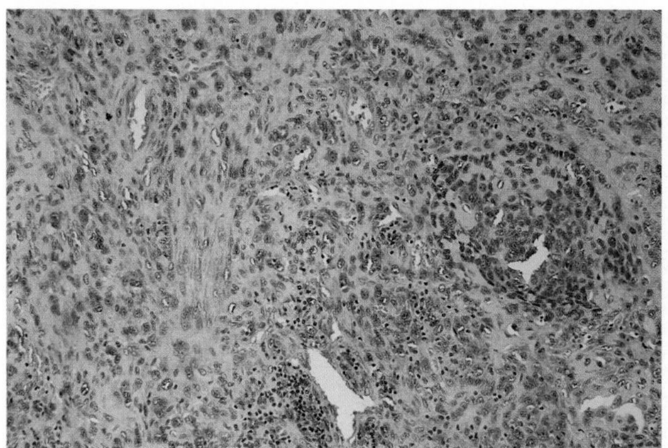

FIGURE 43. Pharynx: combined spindle cell and basaloid–squamous carcinoma. A basaloid tumor cell nest is at the right of the figure, on a background of malignant sarcoma-like tumor tissue.

absence of squamous differentiation and the presence of a myoepithelial component in most cases of the latter tumor. In addition, dendritic S-100 protein–positive cells have been found in tumor cell nests in cases of BSC and not in cases of ACC (275,281). The basaloid adenoid cystic-like pattern differentiates BSC from conventional squamous cell carcinomas, and the absence of neuroendocrine differentiation and of prominent nuclear smearing and the presence of a somewhat organoid pattern helps differentiate this lesion from small-cell (poorly differentiated neuroendocrine) carcinoma of pure or combined type (see below).

BSC is a biologically aggressive neoplasm with a high rate of cervical and distant metastases and a 38% mortality rate at 17 months median follow-up (276). Surgery is the usual mode of therapy.

Papillary Squamous Cell Carcinoma. Some squamous cell carcinomas have a prominent surface papillary component. These may be problematic on biopsy, for only the surface papillary component may be sampled, and this component often does not exhibit stromal invasion deep to the basement membrane. This possibility should be borne in mind on encountering a laryngeal or hypopharyngeal biopsy specimen with the appearance of a papillary high-grade SIN or carcinoma *in situ* (Figs. 44 and 45). The atypicality of this lesion differentiates it from verrucous carcinoma, which is characterized by bland cytology. The koilocytotic atypia of benign viral squamous papillomas may cause problems in differential diagnosis. The clinicopathologic picture of recurrent papillomatous lesions in a child or adolescent is characteristic of the HPV-associated papillomas, which rarely undergo malignant transformation (see above), and koilocytosis is rarely as prominent in papillary squamous cell carcinoma as in HPV-associated papillomas. Furthermore, the cytologic atypicality is characteristically greater in the former lesion than in the latter. Papillary laryngeal squamous cell carcinoma generally behaves less aggressively than conventional invasive squamous cell carcinoma (282–284).

Lymphoepitheliomatous (Nasopharyngeal-type) Carcinoma
Many nasopharyngeal carcinomas, especially in Southern Chinese patients, have a striking undifferentiated morphology associated with a prominent lymphoid infiltrate and association with Epstein-Barr virus (EBV) (nasopharyngeal carcinoma, nonkeratinizing, undifferentiated or "lymphoepithelioma," see Chapter 5). Carcinomas of similar, if not identical, morphology have very rarely been encountered in the larynx and hypopharynx (285–289). Interestingly, most of these tumors appropriately studied have also shown association with EBV (287–289). These rare tumors have shown a tendency to have a clinical behavior, as well as morphology, similar to their nasopharyngeal counterparts (287,289).

Neuroendocrine Carcinomas

Neuroendocrine neoplasms of the larynx have been receiving increasing attention in recent years. The use of adjunctive diagnostic modalities such as immunohistochemistry and electron

A

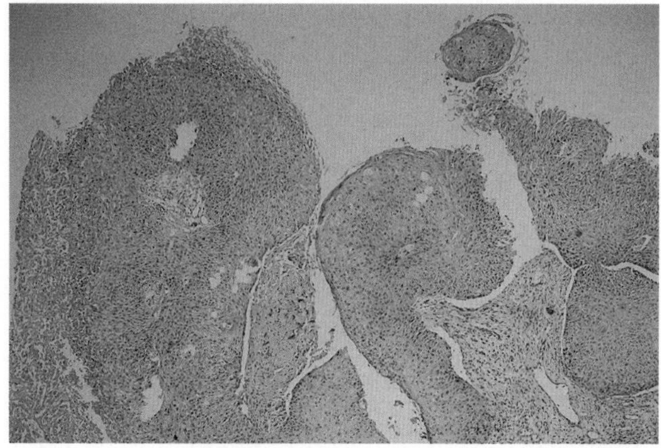

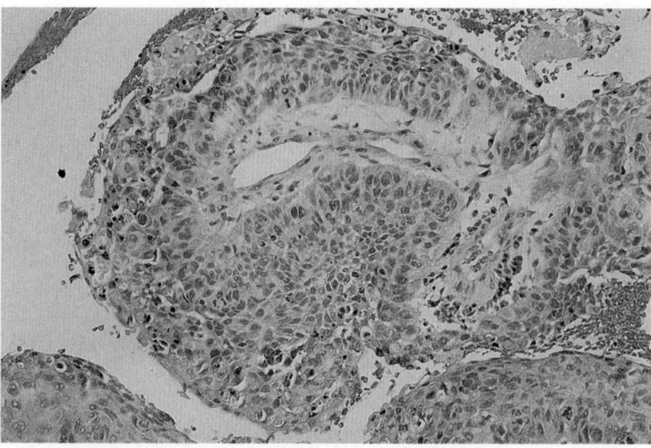

B

FIGURE 44. Larynx: papillary squamous cell carcinoma. **A:** Papillary squamous neoplasm with desmoplastic stroma and cellular atypia. **B:** High-power view of a neoplastic papilla in a papillary laryngeal squamous cell carcinoma showing marked cytologic atypia, suggestive of a "papillary carcinoma *in situ.*"

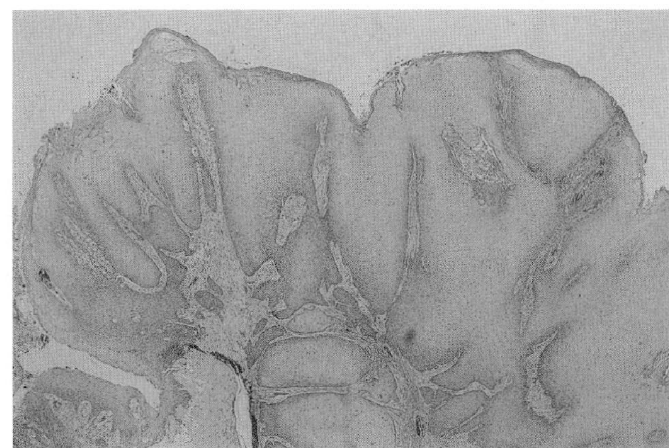
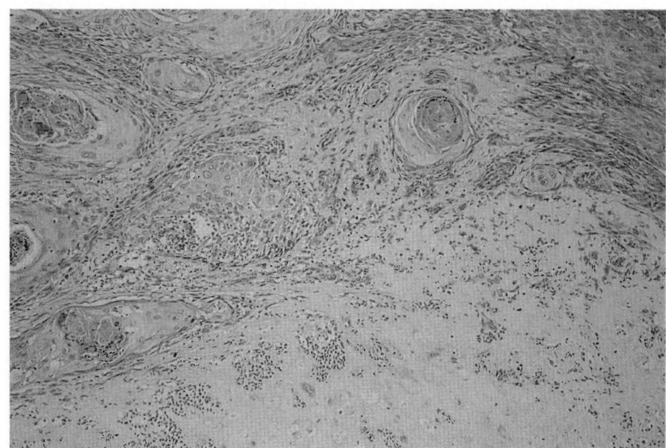

FIGURE 45. Larynx: exophytic squamous cell carcinoma. **A:** Low-power view of an exophytic well-differentiated squamous tumor. Parts of the bases of the tumor fronds are more pointed and angular than the smooth bases of verrucous carcinoma. **B:** Elsewhere the same tumor has areas of typical infiltrative squamous cell carcinoma.

microscopy has allowed greater precision in diagnosis, and the number of these lesions being diagnosed has been increasing. Concurrent with the increased awareness and diagnosis of these lesions is the realization that some cases previously reported as adenocarcinomas and malignant paragangliomas most probably represent examples of neuroendocrine carcinoma. In fact, several authors have stated that neuroendocrine carcinomas are the most common variety of nonepidermoid laryngeal carcinomas (290,291). Nonetheless, laryngeal neuroendocrine carcinomas are much less common that the comparable lesions of the lung and bronchi. Kulchitsky-type argyrophilic cells have been identified in human laryngeal respiratory mucosa, but these have been few, present in only a few of larynges examined, and difficult to find (292). These cells have been considered by some as a possible cell of origin for laryngeal neuroendocrine carcinomas, as have cells associated with seromucinous glands and a primitive pleuripotential cell.

Laryngeal paragangliomas are nonepithelial, generally benign neuroendocrine neoplasms and have been discussed earlier in this chapter. The neuroendocrine carcinomas constitute the remainder of the laryngeal neuroendocrine tumors. Numerous terms have been used for these lesions in the past, including carcinoid, atypical carcinoid, large-cell neuroendocrine carcinomas, well-differentiated neuroendocrine carcinoma, oncocytic or oncocytoid carcinoid tumor, oat cell carcinoma, small-cell carcinoma, undifferentiated small-cell carcinoma, etc. In 1988, Weing et al. (293) proposed a classification scheme for laryngeal neuroendocrine carcinomas using the terms well-differentiated, moderately differentiated, and poorly differentiated neuroendocrine carcinoma to designate the three well-recognized types of these lesions. I find this classification attractive because it recognizes that all of these lesions are carcinomas (i.e., epithelial neoplasms capable of metastatic behavior) and share features of neuroendocrine differentiation (i.e., production of neuropeptides and presence of dense-core membrane-bound "neurosecretory" granules on ultrastructural examination) but vary in their degree of histologic differentiation and biological aggressiveness. The WHO has proposed the terms carcinoid tumor (typical carcinoid tumor), atypical carcinoid tumor, and small-cell carcinoma (small-cell neuroendocrine carcinoma) for these three entities in its classification (294,295). Both classifications are used in this discussion.

Well-Differentiated Neuroendocrine Carcinoma (Carcinoid Tumor, Typical Carcinoid Tumor)

Well-differentiated neuroendocrine carcinoma (WDNEC) (carcinoid tumor, typical carcinoid tumor) is the rarest of the laryngeal neuroendocrine carcinomas. Only 12 or 13 recognized and accepted cases are reported in the literature (291,296). Most patients are men between 50 and 80 years of age (291,296). Lesions are predominantly supraglottic in location and present with dysphagia, hoarseness, a lump, or sore throat. Some are asymptomatic (296). Only one patient developed the carcinoid syndrome after developing hepatic metastases (291,296).

On gross examination, laryngeal WDNECs are submucosal round solid masses about 1 to 2 cm in diameter. Histologically, they resemble their much more common bronchopulmonary counterparts and are composed of organoid rounded nests, trabeculae, ribbons, and/or gland-like structures composed of relatively uniform, rounded cells with scant, clear, or occasionally eosinophilic or oncocytoid cytoplasm (Fig. 46). There is little, if any, nuclear pleomorphism, mitoses are scanty at best, and necrosis is negligible (Fig. 46B). The tumor cells are argyrophil but usually not argentaffin. Immunohistochemical stains show neuroendocrine differentiation with positivity for markers such as chromogranin and synaptophysin (173,291), and most tumors stain for epithelial markers such as keratin and epithelial membrane antigen (EMA). Ultrastructural examination reveals numerous dense-core neurosecretory granules (173,291,296) as well as intercellular junctional complexes (291,296).

Differential diagnosis primarily involves differentiation of laryngeal WDNEC from moderately differentiated neuroendocrine carcinoma (MDNEC) (atypical carcinoid), paraganglioma, and adenocarcinoma. Adenocarcinomas do not demonstrate neuroendocrine differentiation immunohistochemically or ultrastructurally. Paragangliomas usually are not

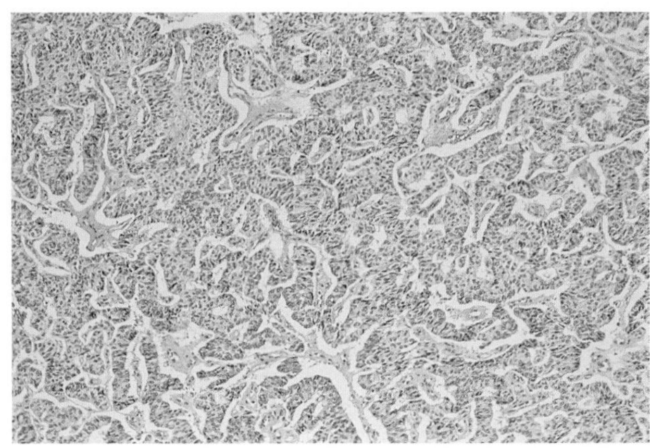

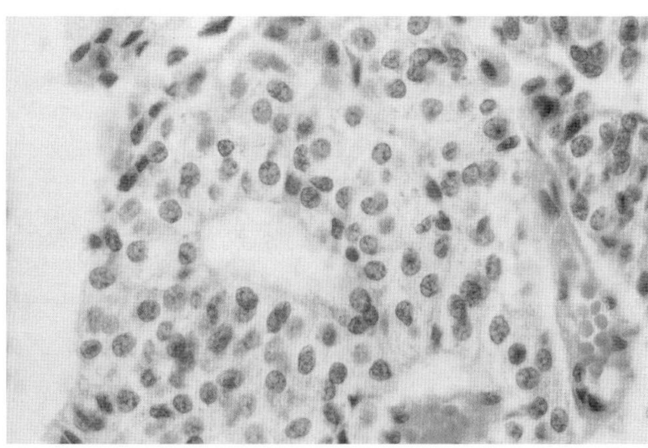

FIGURE 46. Larynx: well-differentiated neuroendocrine carcinoma (WDNEC, carcinoid). **A:** A trabecular architecture of organoid neuroendocrine pattern. **B:** High-power view of the tumor shows neuroendocrine-type nuclei that are round, regular, and have finely stippled chromatin with inconspicuous nucleoli. Pleomorphism is essentially absent.

keratin positive, and WDNECs usually are. In addition, the characteristic *"Zellballen"* architecture is generally more prominent in the former tumor (see above), as are S-100 protein–positive sustentacular cells. Both lesions display neuroendocrine differentiation. Perhaps the most difficult differential is between WDNECs and MDNECs. This distinction is clinically significant, for treatment as well as biological behavior and prognosis differ for these two entities. The distinction between WDNEC and MDNEC of the larynx is based on hematoxylin and eosin morphology, as both lesions show immunohistochemical and ultrastructural neuroendocrine and epithelial differentiation. MDNECs are less well differentiated then WDNECS, with nuclear pleomorphism, mitotic activity, and tumor necrosis significantly more prominent (see below). In addition, the distinctive painfulness of both primary MDNECs and their metastases, with a notable percentage of cutaneous metastases in the latter condition, may help differentiate the two lesions.

WDNEC of the larynx has an excellent prognosis, with most patients disease-free after appropriate therapy. Metastases occur but are rare (291,296,297). Conservative but complete surgical excision is the treatment of choice, and elective neck dissection is not indicated (291,297).

Moderately Differentiated Neuroendocrine Carcinoma (MDNEC) (Atypical Carcinoid Tumor)

MDNEC, the most common of the laryngeal neuroendocrine carcinomas, is a very interesting lesion that has probably been underdiagnosed in the past. Some tumors that were reported in the literature as malignant laryngeal paragangliomas, or possibly adenocarcinoma, most likely represent cases of MDNEC (298). As with WDNECs, most patients are men in their sixth or seventh decades, and most tumors are supraglottic. Common presenting symptoms are dysphagia and hoarseness. Interestingly, significant pain, described as glossopharyngeal neuralgia (177,291), throat pain, or sore throat (293,298), was present in a third of patients in the Milroy et al. series (177). Some patients have cervical metastases at presentation, and rare patients have been reported with the carcinoid syndrome or as asymptomatic. Another curious clinical feature of laryngeal MDNEC is that a substantial number of patients (22% in Woodruff and Senie's review) (298) develop cutaneous or subcutaneous metastases, and many are painful; a recently reported patient had scalp metastases as her initial complaint (299).

Grossly, laryngeal MDNECs appear as rounded exophytic or pedunculated masses, occasionally papillomatous, most often deep to an intact mucosa (293). Most lesions are supraglottic, with a mean size of about 1.5 cm in diameter (298), and are firm or solid.

Histologically, laryngeal MDNECs are characterized by organoid rounded nests, trabeculae, ribbons, and glandular structures of rounded cells with round nuclei and a moderate amount of slightly eosinophilic to oncocytoid cytoplasm (Fig. 47). Glandular differentiation is usually present. In contrast to WDNECs, nuclear pleomorphism is appreciable, mitotic figures are not uncommon, and necrosis is frequently seen (Fig. 47C). A *"Zellballen"* pattern, reminiscent of paragangliomas, may at times be present (182). Immunohistochemical studies typically show tumor cells to be positive for keratin and for neuroendocrine markers such as chromogranin, synaptophysin, bombesin, or neuron-specific enolase (Fig. 47D). Interestingly, the majority of laryngeal MDNECs are positive for calcitonin. This feature, and the occasional presence of amyloid material, may cause a remarkable similarity between laryngeal MDNECs and medullary thyroid carcinomas (290). Ultrastructural examination reveals many intracytoplasmic dense-core neurosecretory granules.

Differential diagnostic considerations involve paraganglioma, other laryngeal neuroendocrine carcinomas, adenocarcinoma, and medullary thyroid carcinoma. As with WDNEC, demonstration of neuroendocrine differentiation distinguishes MDNEC from adenocarcinoma. Distinction from WDNEC has been discussed above. Differentiation between MDNEC and poorly differentiated neuroendocrine carcinoma (PDNEC) or small-cell carcinoma is important, as treatment is very different for these two lesions. As with pulmonary lesions, laryngeal PDNECs are less organoid, more undifferentiated appearing, and generally composed of smaller cells than MDNEC. Glandular differentiation is only rarely apparent (in cases of combined small-cell carcinoma). The tumor cells in PDNEC are rarely argyrophil, but they usually are in MDNEC. Neuroendocrine differentiation is less pronounced in PDNEC; for example, immunohistochemical staining for chromogranin and synaptophysin is less strong and ultrastructural neurosecretory granules are fewer than in MDNEC. The cells in PDNEC are usually calcitonin-negative as well (177,300). Paragangliomas share neuroendocrine differentiation and at times a *"Zellballen"* architectural pattern with MDNECs, but the tumor cells of the former lesion are almost never keratin positive, and S-100–positive sustentacular cells are usually more prominent.

Differentiating MDNEC from medullary carcinoma of the thyroid can be a thorny problem, especially when one is dealing with a cervical nodal metastasis. Laryngeal MDNECs will have a laryngeal (usually supraglottic) primary site, whereas medullary carcinoma manifests as a thyroid tumor. Also, serum calcitonin level is elevated in thyroid rather than laryngeal tumors.

MDNEC of the larynx is an aggressive, metastasizing and potentially lethal neoplasm. In Woodruff and Senie's review (298), 49% of patients with follow-up died with tumor, and 5- and 10-year survival rates were 48% and 30%, respectively. Surgical therapy is the treatment of choice, with neck dissection indicated (in contrast to the situation with WDNECs) because of frequent cervical metastases.

Poorly Differentiated Neuroendocrine Carcinoma (PDNEC) (Small-Cell Carcinoma, Small-Cell Neuroendocrine Carcinoma)

PDNEC is the most aggressive and least differentiated of the neuroendocrine carcinomas of the larynx and hypopharynx. It is histologically virtually identical to, although much rarer than, its bronchopulmonary counterpart. As with the other laryngeal neuroendocrine carcinomas, patients are predominantly men in their sixth and seventh decades, and most lesions are supraglottic in location. Hoarseness is the most common presenting symptom, although many patients (about half) have cervical nodal metastases on initial presentation (301). Interestingly, as with pulmonary small-cell carcinomas, occasional paraneoplastic syndromes are reported associated with laryngeal PDNECs, including inappropriate antidiuretic hormone secretion, myasthenic or Eaton-Lambert syndrome, and ectopic adrenocorticotropic hormone production (302,303).

Most tumors are submucosal, and some have surface ulceration. Histologically, PDNECs of the larynx and hypopharynx

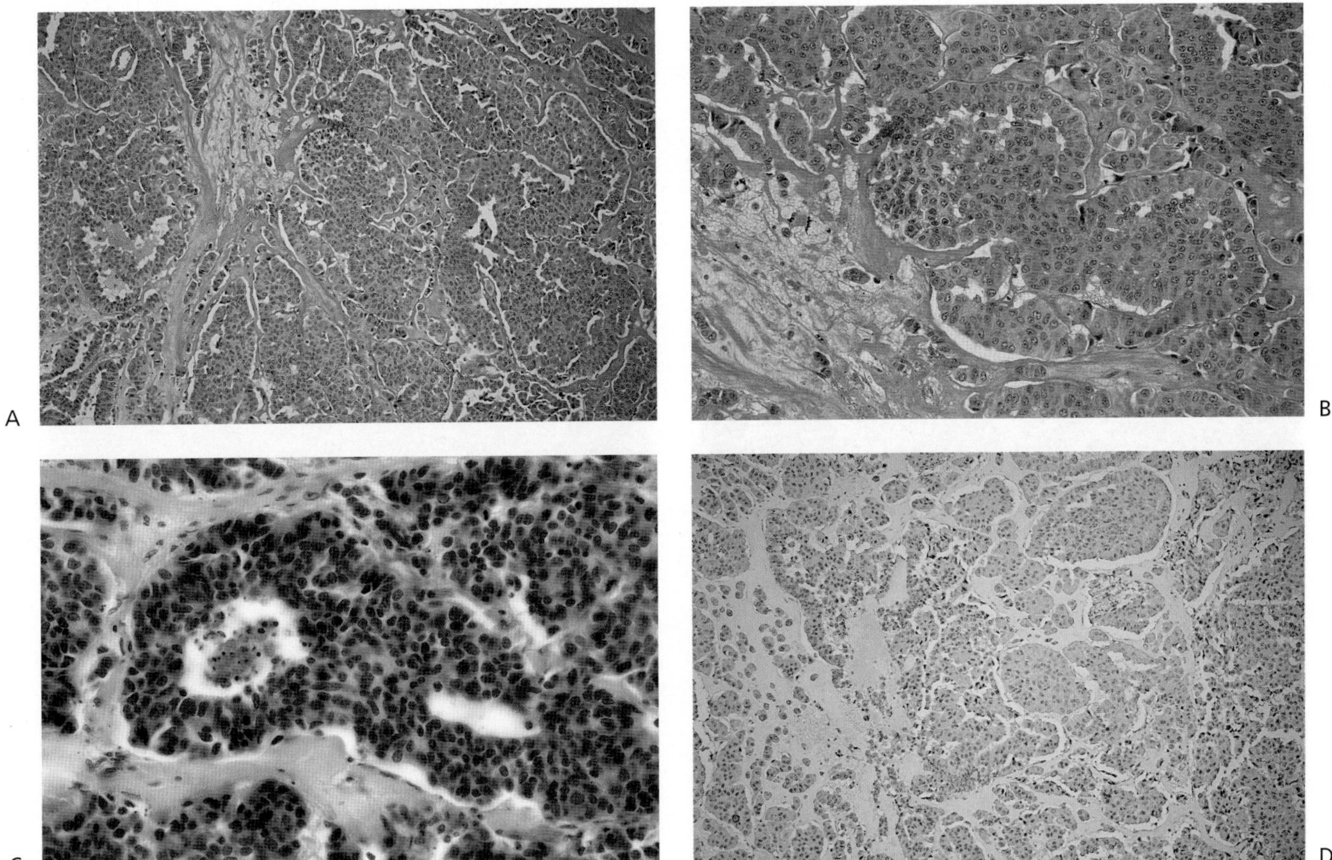

FIGURE 47. Larynx: moderately differentiated neuroendocrine carcinoma (MDNEC, atypical carcinoid). **A:** There is a vaguely trabecular architecture as well as formation of gland-like spaces. **B:** There is a mixture of gland-like and solid patterns in tumor cell nests. Nuclei are larger and more variable than in WDNEC. **C:** Focal necrosis is present in this tumor cell nest. **D:** An immunohistochemical stain for chromogranin is diffusely positive.

are essentially indistinguishable from the corresponding pulmonary lesions. The tumor is composed of sheets and nests and occasionally ribbons and trabeculae of small undifferentiated cells with nuclei containing finely stippled chromatin and generally inconspicuous nucleoli and with scant to almost absent cytoplasm (Fig. 48A,B). Mitoses are plentiful, as is tumor necrosis. Invasion of perineural and vascular spaces may be prominent. The tumor cells are fragile, and nuclear smearing is often seen (300). DNA encrustation on vascular walls (the so-called Azzopardi effect) has been described (301). Rare rosette-like structures may occasionally be noted; organoid architecture is subtle at best. Like pulmonary small-cell carcinomas, laryngeal PDNECs have been divided into oat-cell, intermediate-cell, and combined types (295,301,303). The oat-cell type consists of small round cells with minimal cytoplasm and generally hyperchromatic nuclei, whereas the intermediate cell type comprises slightly larger cells with a bit more cytoplasm and nuclei that are often less hyperchromatic than those of the oat-cell type (Fig. 48C). Nucleoli may be a bit more prominent in this histotype, and tumor cells may occasionally be fusiform or spindly. The combined type represents the oat-cell or intermediate-cell type (or both) admixed with a component of histologically recognizable squamous cell or adenocarcinoma (304,305) (Fig. 49). Although argyrophilia and immunohistochemical positivity for chromogranin is rare in laryngeal PDNECs, neuroendocrine differentiation may be seen in tumors, manifested as immunohistochemical positivity for neuroendocrine markers such as neuron-specific enolase (not a specific neuroendocrine marker, despite its name), synaptophysin, bombsein, protein gene product 9, calcitonin, and calcitonin gene-related peptide (182,306,307), or ultrastructural demonstration of dense-core neurosecretory-type granules. The granules are significantly more sparse, however, and immunohistochemical evidence of neuroendocrine differentiation is less striking than in the other laryngeal neuroendocrine carcinomas, reflecting the more poorly differentiated character of this neoplasm.

It is admittedly more difficult to demonstrate neuroendocrine differentiation in laryngeal PDNECs than in other neuroendocrine carcinomas. The question then arises as to whether some PDNECs can be so poorly differentiated that conventional techniques fail to demonstrate neuroendocrine differentiation or that such differentiation must be demonstrable to warrant a diagnosis of PDNEC. Gnepp (301) takes this latter position. Aguilar et al. (308), however, maintain that laryngeal small-cell carcinoma may or may not show neuroendocrine differentiation and that the biological behavior of laryngeal neoplasms manifesting the hematoxylin and eosin morphologic appearance of PDNEC is similar whether or not neuroendocrine differentiation is demonstrated. Furthermore, the WHO classification of upper respiratory neoplasms states under their heading of small-cell carcinoma (small-cell neuroendocrine carcinoma) that "there is variable neuroendocrine differentiation" and that ". . . dense-core granules are occasionally present . . ." (294). Perhaps

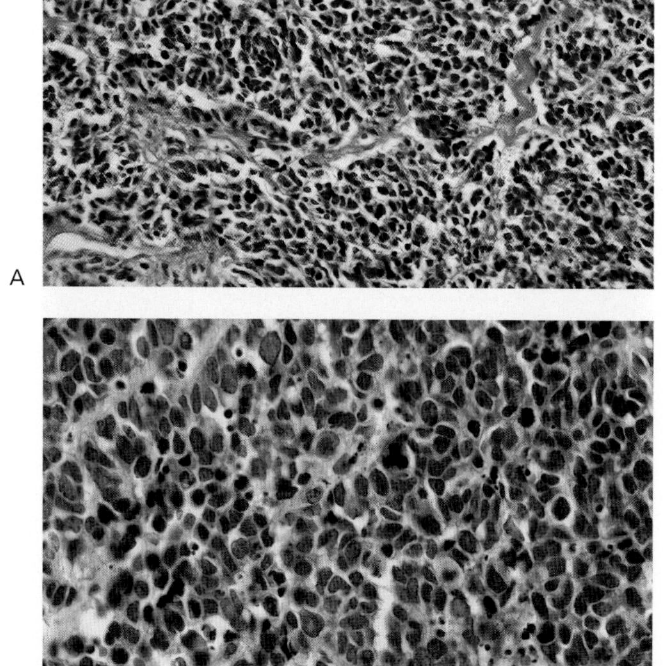

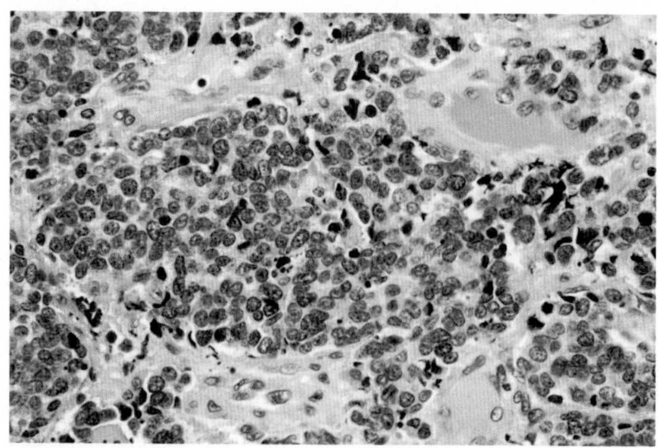

FIGURE 48. Larynx: poorly differentiated neuroendocrine carcinoma (PDNEC, small-cell carcinoma). **A:** Nests and sheets of small undifferentiated tumor cells with dark nuclei and scant cytoplasm. **B:** The small undifferentiated tumor cells almost look lymphocytic, but they cluster to form nests, more typical of epithelial tumors. **C:** In this intermediate cell variant of PDNEC, the nuclei are larger, cytoplasm is still scant, and nuclear pleomorphism, necrotic nuclear debris, and an atypical tripolar mitotic figure can be seen.

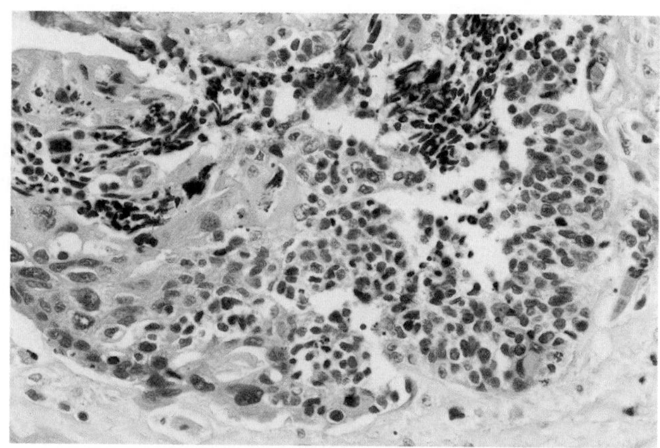

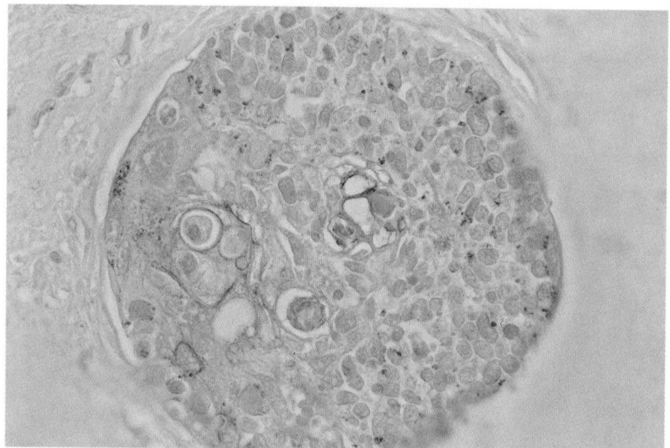

FIGURE 49. Larynx: poorly differentiated neuroendocrine carcinoma (PDNEC, combined small-cell carcinoma). **A:** The small-cell component is to the right of the figure, and neoplasm with squamous differentiation is present to the left. **B:** An immunohistochemical stain for keratin (AE1,3/CAM 5.2) shows more diffuse cytoplasmic staining in the squamous component and perinuclear dot-like staining (a pattern seen in neuroendocrine neoplasms) in the small-cell component.

a practical approach might be to investigate a potential laryngeal or hypopharyngeal PDNEC for neuroendocrine differentiation and, if such differentiation is found, to use that term, and if such differentiation is not identified, to use the term "small-cell carcinoma," recognizing that the tumor might be but is not unequivocally an example of a very poorly differentiated neuroendocrine carcinoma but is a neoplasm whose biological behavior is probably similar to that of PDNEC.

Differential diagnosis includes other poorly differentiated small-cell neoplasms such as lymphoma, the small-cell variant of malignant melanoma, the solid variant of adenoid cystic carcinoma (ACC), and basaloid–squamous carcinoma (BSC). Lymphomas can usually be differentiated by their reactivity to lymphoid markers such as leukocyte common antigen and B- or T-cell markers and by their lack of epithelial or neuroendocrine differentiation. Malignant melanomas lack keratin immunohistochemical positivity and stain for S-100 protein, MART-1, and often for HMB 45. ACC will not demonstrate neuroendocrine differentiation and often demonstrates myoepithelial differentiation as manifested by immunohistochemical actin or S-100 protein positivity. The cells of BSC are usually larger than those of PDNEC, lack neuroendocrine differentiation, and tend to stain immunohistochemically for high-molecular-weight keratin proteins such as with the marker 34βE12, whereas PDNEC cells do not (307). Differentiation from other neuroendocrine carcinomas is discussed above. Primitive neuroectodermal tumor (PNET) occurs in a significantly younger age group and is generally keratin-negative and CD99 (or MIC2)-positive.

PDNEC is a biologically highly aggressive malignancy with a propensity for metastatic spread and with a poor prognosis. In Gnepp's review (301), 73% of patients died of disease, and the 2- and 5-year survival rates were only 16% and 5%, respectively. A combined regimen of irradiation and chemotherapy is generally indicated as optimal therapy for this disease, and radical surgical procedures are advised against (291,297,300,301,308).

Adenocarcinoma

Adenocarcinomas of the larynx and hypopharynx are rare neoplasms. They comprise only about 1% of laryngeal malignancies (309,310). In recent years, most lesions originally subsumed under the general rubric of adenocarcinoma have been subcategorized, and most appear to be carcinomas of salivary gland type (311). Some tumors originally classified as adenocarcinomas are probably MDNECs (see above), and examples of more recently described types of salivary gland carcinomas have been reported in the larynx, including salivary duct carcinoma (312) and epithelial–myoepithelial carcinoma (313). Rare examples of laryngeal acinic cell carcinoma have been reported as well (314,315). The most common types of laryngeal adenocarcinomas are adenoid cystic and mucoepidermoid carcinoma.

Adenoid cystic carcinoma (ACC) is well known as a tracheobronchial neoplasm, but it also occurs in the larynx, most commonly in the subglottic larynx (158,309–311,316). Patients tend to be somewhat younger than those with other laryngeal adenocarcinomas, with the peak incidence in the fifth decade, although the age range is wide (316). Interestingly, in contrast to other laryngeal carcinomas, the male and female incidence is roughly equal (158,311). Symptoms are comparable to those of other laryngeal tumors, with patients experiencing hoarseness, dyspnea, and dysphagia. Pain is not infrequently a prominent symptom, possibly because of the tendency of ACC for perineural invasion (158,311,316). Tumors are often advanced at presentation and are generally submucosal masses. Laryngeal ACCs share with their salivary gland compatriots the clinical features of slow but relentless growth, long survival, frequent ultimate metastatic spread, low cure rate, and the morphologic features of the cribriform, tubular, and, least commonly, solid architectural patterns of small basaloid tumor cells in a mucinous or eosinophilic basement membrane–like matrix with a propensity to perineural spread (see Chapter 8) (Fig. 50). Interestingly, laryngeal ACCs do not characteristically metastasize to lymph nodes, although they may involve lymph nodes by direct exten-

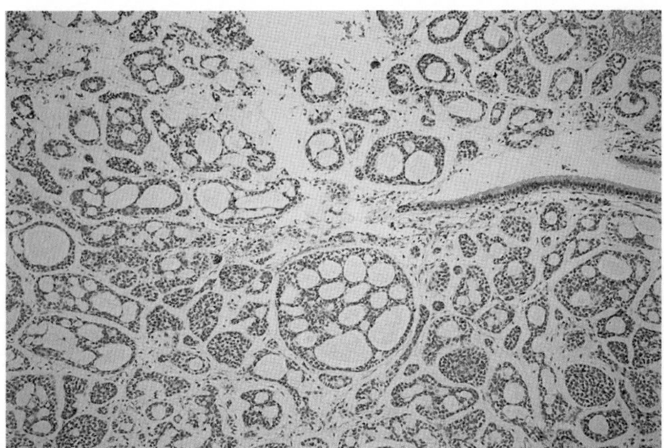

FIGURE 50. Larynx and trachea: adenoid cystic carcinoma. Cribriform nests of basaloid cells with the classic appearance of adenoid cystic carcinoma (see Chapter 8). Respiratory mucosal epithelium can be seen on the right of the figure.

sion, but tend to metastasize via the bloodstream in the manner of sarcomas (311). Surgery is the recommended therapeutic modality.

Mucoepidermoid carcinoma (MEC) is rare in the larynx and hypopharynx. About 100 laryngeal cases had been reported as MEC in the literature up to 1993 (311). Men are significantly more commonly affected than women, and the average age is reported as in the late fifties or 60 years of age (317–319). The supraglottic larynx is most commonly involved, but glottic and infraglottic cases are reported, as well as rare hypopharyngeal lesions (311,317). Symptoms, as with most laryngeal neoplasms, most commonly involve hoarseness, with dysphagia, foreign body sensation, and hemoptysis also reported (311,317).

Histologically, MECs of the larynx and hypopharynx resemble their counterparts in the salivary glands (see Chapter 8). Tumors are composed of mucus-containing, occasionally cuboidal to columnar cells, squamoid cells, and "intermediate" cells (Fig. 51). Architectural patterns vary from largely cystic in low-grade lesions to largely solid in high-grade lesions.

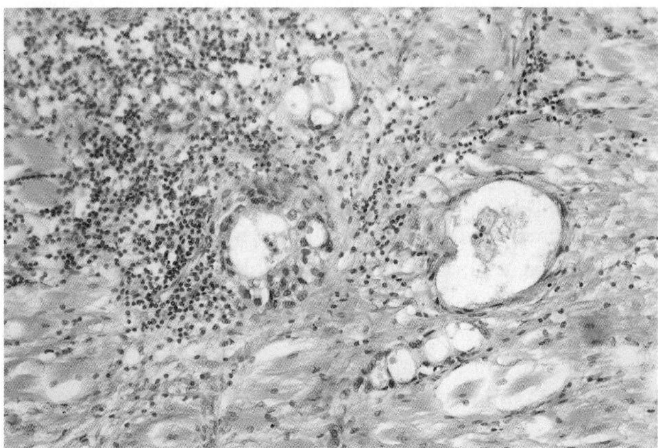

FIGURE 51. Larynx: mucoepidermoid carcinoma. Mucin-containing spaces are lined by intermediate cells in this focus of low-grade mucoepidermoid carcinoma (see Chapter 8).

Keratinization is usually sparse if present, and nuclear pleomorphism is absent to minimal in low-grade lesions and generally not more than moderate even in high-grade lesions (see Chapter 8).

A tumor type occurring in the upper aerodigestive tract including the larynx, closely related to MEC, was described and designated as adenosquamous carcinoma by Gerughty et al. (320). This is reported as a high-grade and biologically aggressive neoplasm and is distinguished by Gerughty et al. from MEC by the occurrence in the former tumor of separate and distinct areas of adenocarcinoma and squamous cell carcinoma as well as mixed foci (320). Although some authors maintain that this tumor should be distinguished from MEC (318), Damiani et al. include it with high-grade MECs in their series from the Armed Forces Institute of Pathology ("mucoepidermoid–adenosquamous" carcinoma) (317).

In recent years, the term adenosquamous carcinoma has been used to refer to a lesion with a prominent component of conventional-appearing squamous cell carcinoma, including definite surface mucosal involvement and with definite focal glandular differentiation, usually with intracellular mucin as well (321). I find this usage appealing and consider this type of adenosquamous carcinoma to be essentially or primarily a tumor of mucosal epithelial origin, as opposed to MEC, which I feel is best thought of as a glandular neoplasm. Squamous cell carcinomas of respiratory epithelial origin are rarely recognized as containing scant mucus-containing cells in the lung, and such a situation has been mentioned as likely occurring in the upper aerodigestive tract as well (318). A neoplasm probably corresponding to this latter, and I feel more useful, designation of adenosquamous carcinoma has been reported in the hypopharynx (322), and we have encountered such a neoplasm in the larynx (Fig. 52).

MECs of salivary gland type in the larynx are preferentially treated surgically. As with salivary gland tumors, low-grade laryngopharyngeal lesions have a better prognosis than high-grade lesions (318), with an overall 5-year survival rate for all MECs in the larynx and hypopharynx reported as 77% in the Damiani et al. series (318).

Cartilaginous Tumors

Laryngeal sarcomas are rare lesions, accounting for fewer than 1% of laryngeal malignancies (323–326). In recent years, chondrosarcoma has come to be recognized as the most common laryngeal sarcoma (325,327,328) and not fibrosarcoma as originally thought (329,330). About 250 cases of laryngeal chondrosarcomas have been reported in the literature (328). The precise classification of laryngeal cartilaginous tumors has been problematic because many such tumors are histologically low-grade chondrosarcomas, morphologically difficult to differentiate from chondromas (326,327,331) and biologically not very aggressive (331,332). It is currently generally considered that the vast majority of laryngeal cartilaginous tumors are chondrosarcomas and that true histologically benign chondromas are quite rare (326,330). Thus, in the largest single series of laryngeal cartilaginous tumors published to date, of 47 lesions studied, 44 were classified as chondrosarcoma, and only three as chondroma

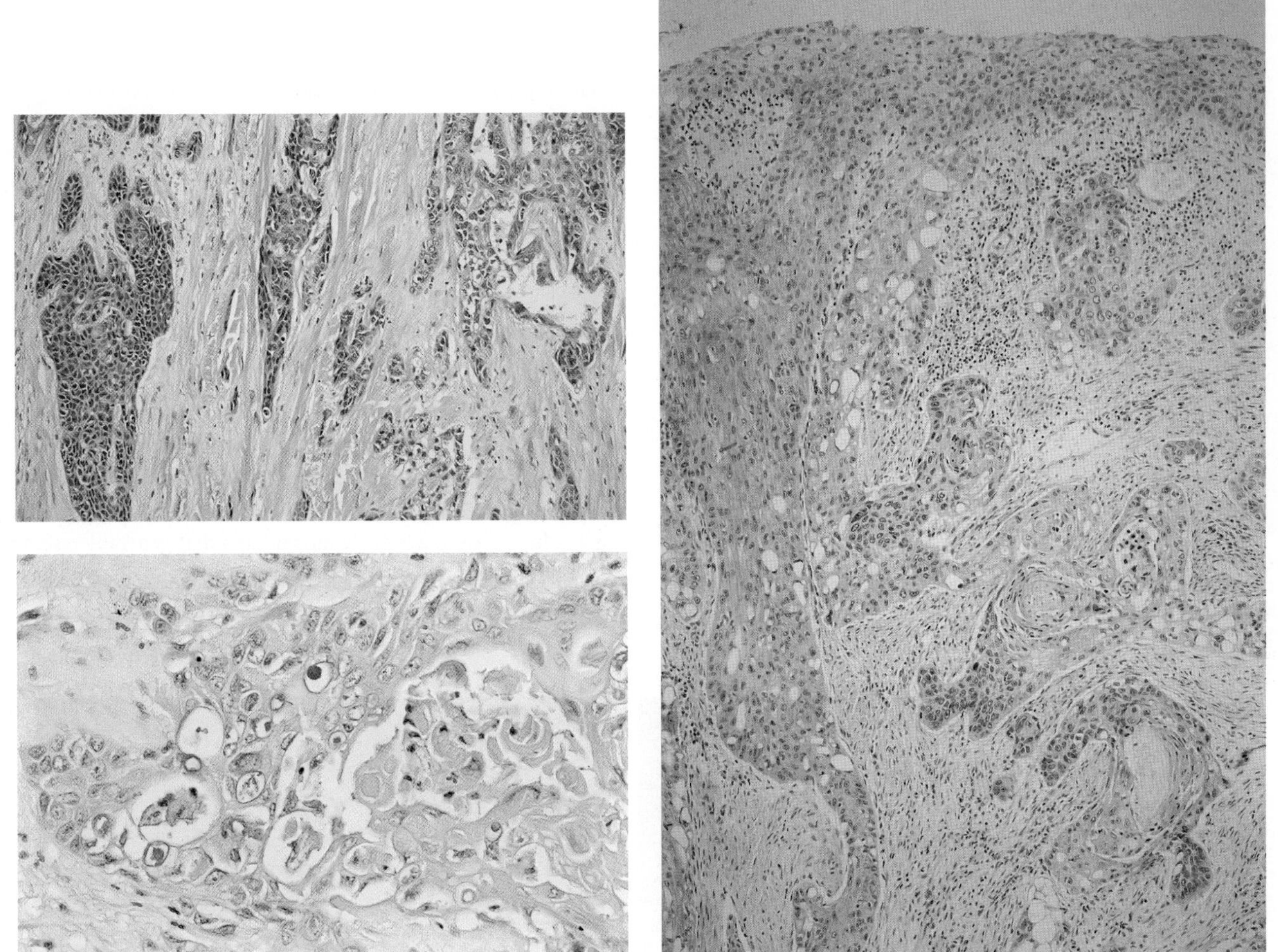

FIGURE 52. Larynx: adenosquamous carcinoma. **A:** To the left of the figure are nests of squamous cell carcinoma; to the right of the figure, the tumor is forming gland-like spaces. **B:** A mucicarmine stain shows red mucin in a tumor cell nest with squamous differentiation. Keratin is present to the right of the figure. **C:** Strands of squamous cell carcinoma connect to cytologically atypical mucosal squamous epithelium.

(333). True neoplastic chondromas are to be distinguished from the much more common metaplastic elastic cartilaginous nodules of the vocal cord (334), also referred to as chondrometaplasia (335). Thus, a group of nine "chondromas" composed of elastic cartilage of the vocal cord reported by Hyams and Rabuzzi (336) were considered metaplastic in origin.

Chondrosarcomas of the larynx occur most commonly in patients in the sixth or seventh decade (324,326). The mean age of patients in the Lewis et al. series (333) was 63. Men are more commonly affected than women, in a ratio of about 3:1 (330,333). The cricoid cartilage is the most frequent laryngeal cartilage involved (about 75%) (330,337), especially the posterior lamina or posterolateral area (328). The thyroid cartilage is the next most common site (about 15%) (328,337). Other laryngeal cartilages (arytenoid, epiglottic) are rarely involved. Symptoms include hoarseness (the most common) (327,328,333,337). Symptoms are largely related to the site and size of the tumor. Thus, cricoid lesions projecting anteriorly into the airway may cause dyspnea, whereas lesions projecting posteriorly into the hypopharynx may result in dysphagia. More anteriorly placed lesions of the thyroid cartilage may present as a neck mass. If the tumor significantly comprises the airway, wheezing may result (338,339), and the patient may mistakenly be thought to have asthma (333).

On endoscopic examination the tumor presents as a rounded submucosal hard mass. Adequate biopsy may be tricky, and the overlying mucosa usually should be incised and the slippery cartilaginous mass securely grasped and sampled.

Radiographic findings are characteristic. The tumor appears as a soft tissue mass, usually with coarse or stippled calcification (338,340) (Fig. 53). These calcifications in a laryngeal mass are highly suggestive, and some say pathognomonic, of a cartilaginous tumor (338,340). Computed tomography (CT) is the preferred imaging modality for these lesions.

Grossly, laryngeal chondrosarcomas are characteristically rounded, well-delineated, lobulated, bluish or gray masses that

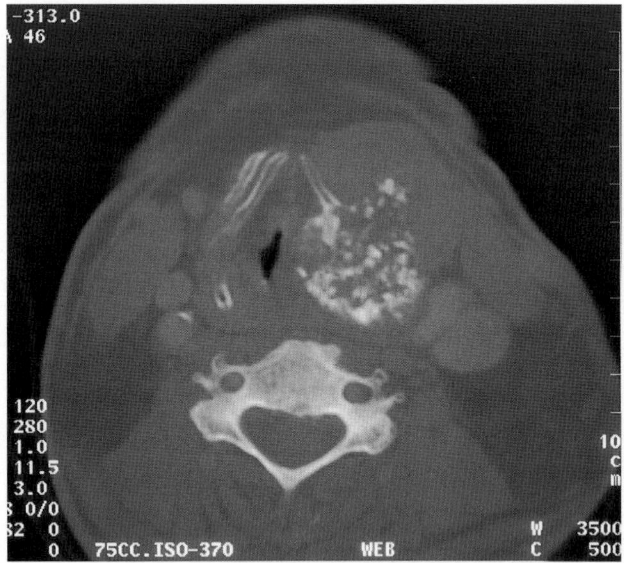

FIGURE 53. Larynx: chondrosarcoma. The radiograph (CT scan) shows a tumor of the right lamina of the thyroid cartilage with characteristic stippled calcification. The soft tissue mass lateral to the calcified area represents the dedifferentiated component of this dedifferentiated chondrosarcoma.

expand the cartilage of origin (Fig. 54). They are usually solid, but cystification and focal hemorrhage may occur.

Histologically, the lesions have an abundant cartilaginous matrix, mainly hyaline but occasionally myxoid, containing clusters of chondrocytes in lacunae (Fig. 55A,B). The cells are more clustered, and the cellularity is greater than in normal cartilage. Cellular pleomorphism is generally slight to moderate, with occasional to more frequently occurring multinucleated cells and enlarged nuclei with a discernible chromatin pattern. Thus, the findings are usually those of a low-grade chondrosarcoma, grade 1/3 or sometimes grade 2/3 (Fig. 55C,D). The histologic appearance may sometimes vary somewhat from area to area in a given tumor (Fig. 55C). Rarely, higher-grade chondrosarcomas, myxoid chondrosarcomas (324,326,341), or dedifferentiated chondrosarcomas (325,342) may be encountered. The latter type, also called chondrosarcoma with additional malignant mesenchymal component (CAMMC) (342,343), represents a tumor with a component of low-grade chondrosarcoma as well as a component of a high-grade sarcoma that generally resembles another type of sarcoma histologically (e.g., malignant fibrous histiocytoma) (Fig. 56).

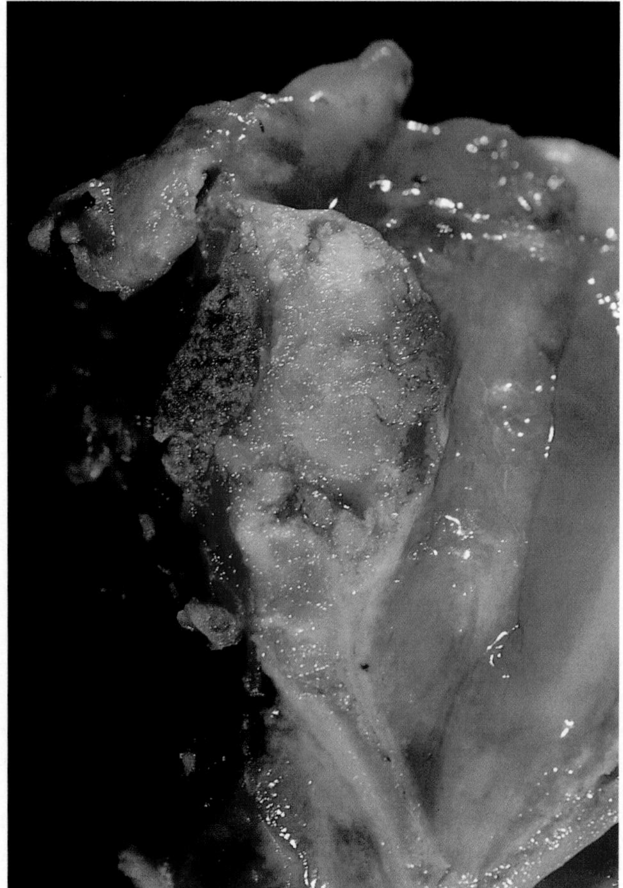

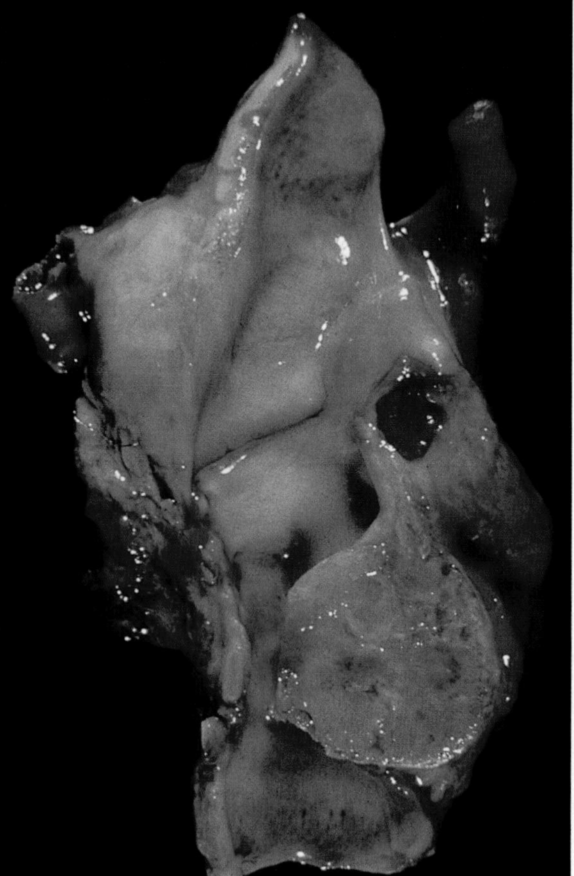

FIGURE 54. Larynx: chondrosarcoma. **A:** This gross photo shows the chondrosarcoma of the thyroid cartilage depicted in the previous figure. The perichondrum medially is largely intact. Most of the lateral dedifferentiated component has been removed at a previous operation. **B:** This cartilaginous neoplasm of the cricoid cartilage (the most common location) significantly comprises the airway. (From Shapshay SM, Aretz HT. *Benign lesions of the larynx.* Washington, DC: American Academy of Otolaryngology, Head and Neck Surgery Foundation, 1984:35, with permission.)

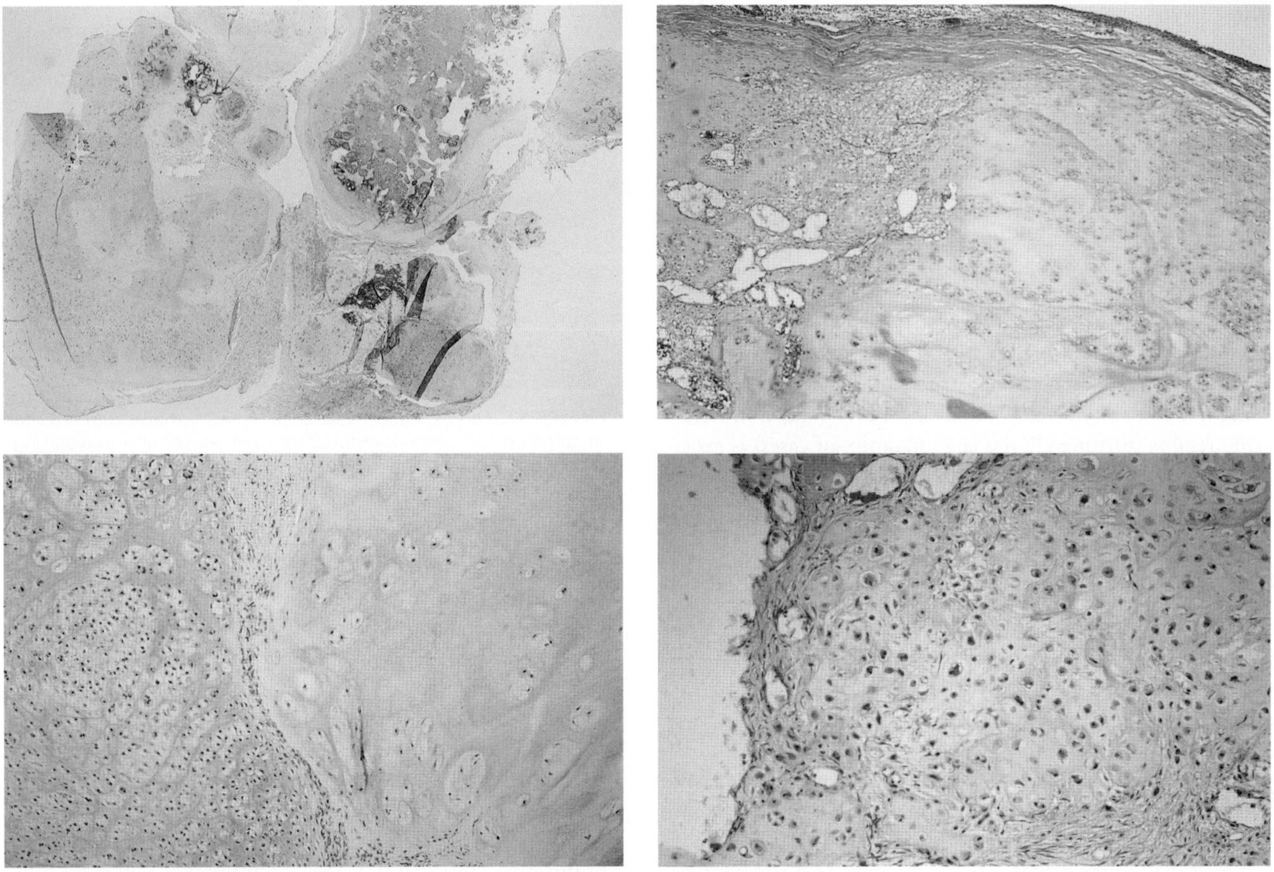

FIGURE 55. Larynx: chondrosarcoma. **A:** Multiple fairly well-delineated nodules of a low-grade laryngeal chondrosarcoma. **B:** Submucosal lobular chondrosarcoma. **C:** Varying degrees of cellularity in this laryngeal cartilaginous neoplasm. **D:** Cellular area with large atypical chondrocyte nuclei in the chondrosarcoma. This focus is grade 2/3.

Differential diagnosis primarily involves separating chondromas from chondrosarcomas. This may indeed be extremely difficult when dealing with very low-grade (grade 1) chondrosarcomatous lesions. In general, chondromas are rarer and smaller than chondrosarcomas and are histologically less cellular with less nuclear pleomorphism, following the criteria originally proposed for skeletal chondrosarcomas by Lichtenstein and Jaffe (344). Elastic cartilaginous metaplasia of the vocal cords occurs in extracartilaginous laryngeal tissue and is composed of a focal loose aggregate of myxoid and elastic tissue with occasional progression to recognizable elastic cartilage. Such a lesion is considered reactive rather than neoplastic.

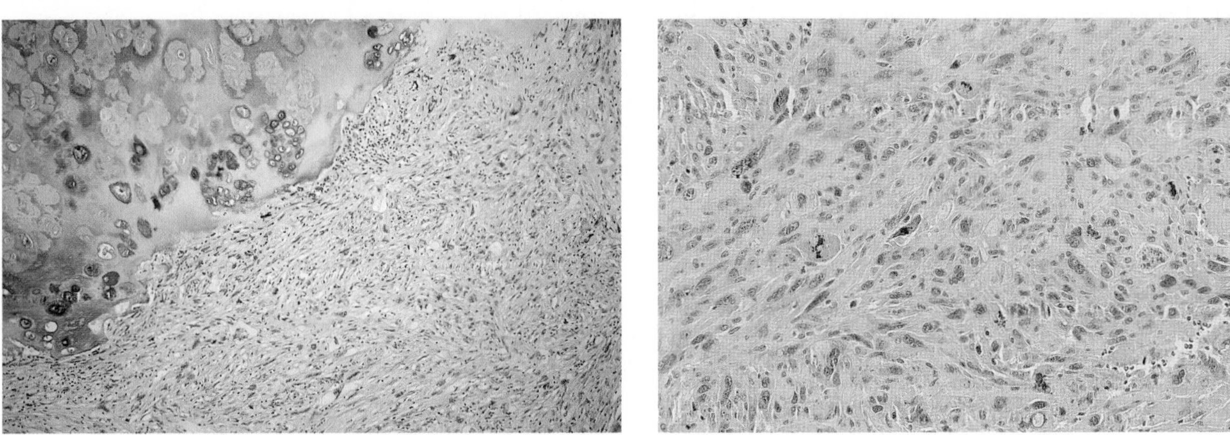

FIGURE 56. Larynx: dedifferentiated chondrosarcoma. **A:** Junction of the low-grade chondrosarcoma with the dedifferentiated component. **B:** The dedifferentiated component has the appearance of a high-grade non–matrix-producing sarcoma.

Most laryngeal cartilaginous tumors have a biological behavior of slow progressive growth with a tendency to recur if incompletely excised but with a low metastatic potential. In fact, the overall biological aggressiveness of laryngeal chondrosarcoma is considered less than that of chondrosarcomas in other sites by most observers (331,332) although not by all (345). Only rare metastatic laryngeal chondrosarcomas are reported, and these mainly involve the uncommon high-grade or dedifferentiated variants (325,326). Because of this predominantly nonaggressive behavior, conservative surgical excision, avoiding total laryngectomy if possible, is recommended, even for recurrences (327,333,337,339). Radiation therapy is generally considered ineffective, although an occasional case with a favorable response to radiation is reported (328). Survival for low-grade nonmetastasizing lesions (fortunately the large majority of cases) is excellent. It was 90.1% at 5 years and 80.9% at 10 years in the Lewis et al. series (333).

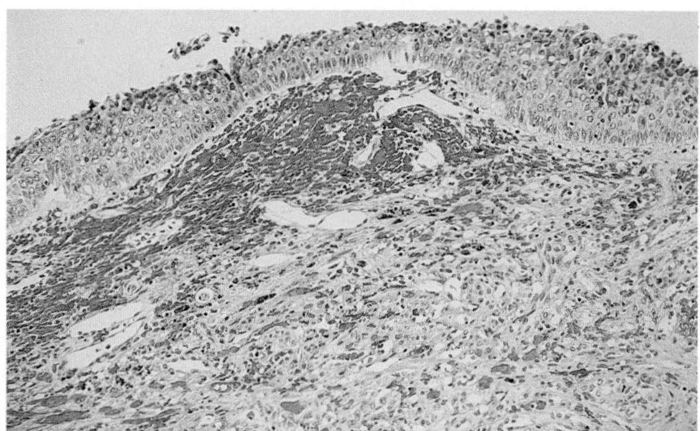

FIGURE 57. Larynx: Kaposi's sarcoma. A hemorrhagic tumor composed of spindled cells with ill-defined vascular spaces and percolating erythrocytes.

Other Sarcomas

Sarcomas of the larynx and hypopharynx other than chondrosarcomas are extremely uncommon. Laryngeal *rhabdomyosarcomas* have been reported in both children and adults (346–350). Interestingly, as opposed to most soft tissue rhabdomyosarcomas, most of which occur in children and adolescents, about half of laryngeal rhabdomyosarcomas occur in patients younger and half in patients older than 30 years (348). Embryonal, alveolar, botryoid, and pleomorphic variants have all been described, with embryonal rhabdomyosarcoma being the most frequent subtype (348). As might be expected, the embryonal, alveolar, and botryoid variants were found most commonly in patients younger than 31 years, and the pleomorphic variant occurred in older adults (33–72 years of age) (348,350). Survival among children with embryonal laryngeal rhabdomyosarcomas has improved dramatically since the institution of modern treatment protocols including combined therapy utilizing radiation and chemotherapy (347,350).

Synovial sarcomas are unusual in that, although very rare, they are much more frequent in the hypopharynx than in the endolarynx (351–355). Patients tend to be adolescents or young adults (354,355). The tumor can occasionally be pedunculated or attached to the hypopharynx by a stalk (351,354). Most tumors are classic biphasic synovial sarcomas histologically (see Chapter 10), although a monophasic spindle cell variant has been reported in the larynx (353).

Kaposi's sarcoma (KS) was, before the onset of the acquired immunodeficiency syndrome (AIDS) epidemic, an extremely rare laryngeal tumor (356). An occasional case of laryngeal involvement in cases of classic KS is reported, usually in elderly patients of Mediterranean descent, and usually (but not invariably) is associated with multiple cutaneous lesions (356,357). With the advent of the AIDS epidemic, an AIDS-associated variety of KS has developed that affects younger patients, is more aggressive, and has more extracutaneous involvement than in classical cases (358). KS is, in fact, the most frequent AIDS-associated malignancy (359,360). KS not uncommonly involves the mucosa of the head and neck in AIDS patients, and consequently more cases of laryngeal involvement are now being encountered among AIDS patients (359,360). These laryngeal AIDS-related cases usually involve the supraglottis and are seen in patients with numerous cutaneous lesions (357,360), thus making diagnosis of the laryngeal lesions usually straightforward. The histologic appearance of laryngeal KS, both classic and epidemic, is similar to that of the classically described cutaneous variety (see Chapter 13) (Fig. 57). Therapies such as irradiation, surgical dubulking, chemotherapy, and interferon have been utilized in the treatment of laryngeal KS (356,359,360).

Malignant fibrous histiocytoma (MFH) has also been reported in the larynx (361,362). Cases of laryngeal MFH have tended to behave aggressively (362). Of the various histologic subtypes of MFH, the storiform-pleomorphic, giant cell, and myxoid variants have been reported in the larynx (362) (see Chapter 10). Differentiation of laryngeal MFH from the spindle cell (sarcomatoid) component of spindle cell carcinoma is important (see above).

Liposarcomas are very rare in the larynx and hypopharynx (213,363,364). They tend to occur in the supraglottis and pyriform sinus, and men are much more frequently affected than women. Most lesions are described as pedunculated or exophytic (364). Almost all cases have been histologically well differentiated or low grade liposarcomas (Fig. 58) (361,364), but an exceptional case of laryngeal pleomorphic liposarcoma is encountered in the literature (365). Prognosis is generally favorable, with local recurrences not uncommon but distant metastases very rare (361,364). Because most laryngeal liposarcomas are well differentiated, distinction from the extremely rare laryngeal lipoma can be a problem. We have encountered a case in our laboratory that bore a resemblance to a spindle cell lipoma (Fig. 58A). Differentiation from lipomas can be aided by noting pleomorphic nuclei in spindled areas and the presence of lipoblasts (see Chapter 10).

Although considered in older literature to be one of the most common laryngeal sarcomas (162,323), true *fibrosarcomas* of the larynx are currently considered quite rare (329,366). Laryngeal tumors initially reported as fibrosarcomas have probably represented other benign as well as malignant spindle cell lesions (329). Differential diagnosis is now aided greatly by adjunctive immunohistochemical, ultrastructural, and even cytogenetic and

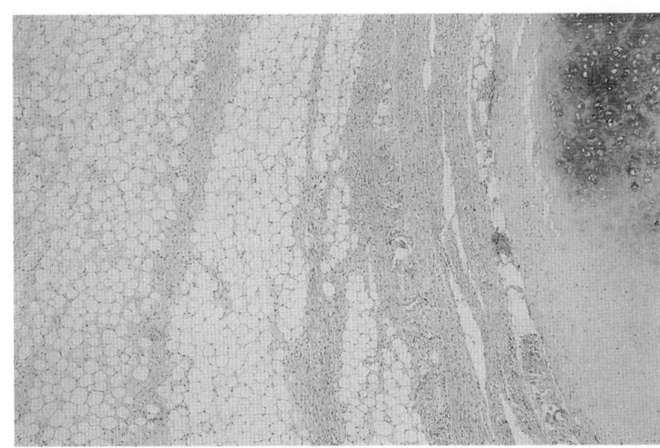
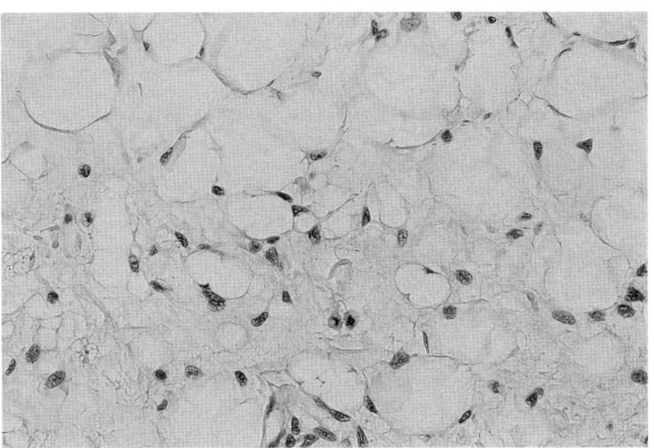

FIGURE 58. Larynx: liposarcoma. **A:** Fibrous bands with spindle cells are present in this well-differentiated fatty liposarcoma. Laryngeal cartilage is present on the right. **B:** A high-power view showing occasional enlarged nuclei and multivacuolar lipoblasts.

molecular genetic techniques, and the designation of fibrosarcoma is properly reserved for spindle cell sarcomas not evidencing any differentiation other than fibroblastic. With these restrictions, true fibrosarcomas of the larynx are extremely rare but are occasionally encountered (367).

Other extremely rare sarcomas reported in the larynx or hypopharynx include *leiomyosarcoma* (361,368), *malignant peripheral nerve sheath tumor* (369), *angiosarcoma* (370), *malignant hemangiopericytoma* (371), *Ewing's sarcoma* or *primitive neuroectodermal tumor* (372), *osteosarcoma* (373–375), and *malignant mesenchymoma* (376). A unique case of a laryngeal blastoma, analogous to pulmonary blastoma, was reported by Eble et al. in 1985 (377).

Other Malignant Neoplasms

Malignant lymphoma may rarely involve the larynx primarily, either with or without the involvement of regional lymph nodes (378,379) (Fig. 59). Most primary laryngeal lymphomas appear to be high-grade B-cell neoplasms, and most involve the supraglottic larynx (378). Since the recognition of marginal zone lymphoma or so-called lymphoma of MALT (mucosal associated lymphoid tissue) (see Chapter 12), an occasional rare case of laryngeal MALT lymphoma has been reported (380,381). Interestingly, *extramedullary plasmacytoma* appears to be the most common of the hematopoetic laryngeal malignancies, with about 90 cases reported in the literature (378). Symptomatic laryngeal involvement in cases of disseminated lymphoma or leukemia is reported rarely, although an autopsy study has shown that the marrow of ossified laryngeal cartilage as well as the laryngeal mucosa were frequently involved histologically in patients with disseminated lymphoma or with leukemia (378). *Granulocytic sarcoma* is extremely rarely encountered in the larynx (382), and a single case of laryngeal *mast cell sarcoma* has appeared in the literature (383). Laryngeal involvement in cases of advanced *mycosis fungoides* is extremely uncommon (384,385).

Primary *malignant melanoma* of the larynx is extremely rare (386–388), although melanoma is the most common metastatic

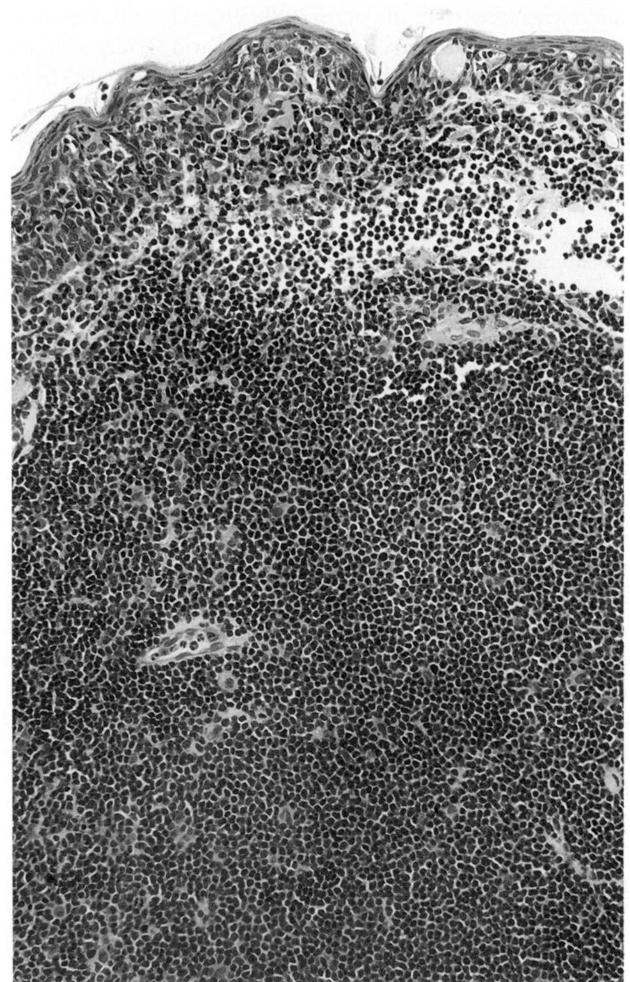

FIGURE 59. Hypopharynx (pyriform sinus): malignant lymphoma. A diffuse sheet of small lymphoid cells lies in the submucosa. Lymphoid cells infiltrate the mucosal epithelium. This proved to be a B cell-lymphoma, probably mantle cell type.

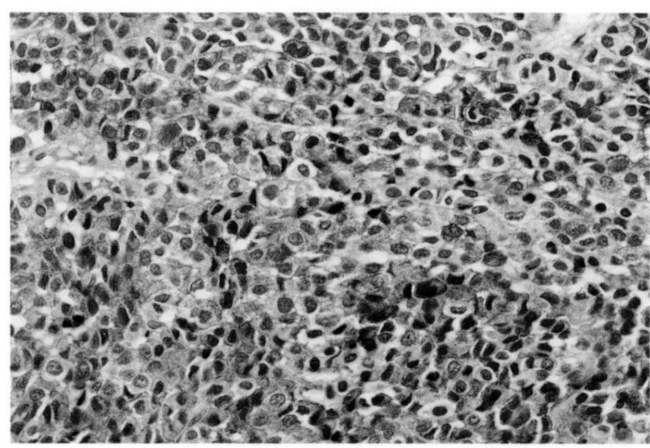

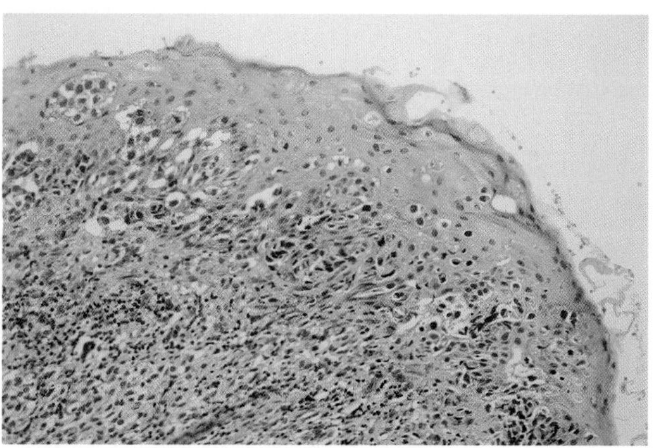

FIGURE 60. Larynx: metastatic malignant melanoma. **A:** A sheet of pigment-containing melanoma cells. **B:** There is junctional activity and pagetoid extension of melanoma cells into the mucosal epithelium. These findings may be present in metastatic as well as primary malignant melanoma.

tumor encountered in the larynx (389,390) (Fig. 60). Reports of laryngeal nevi, lentigines, and melanosis provide evidence of possible precursor lesions (391–393). Patients with primary laryngeal melanoma are generally men in their sixth and seventh decades, and most lesions are supraglottic in location (387,388). Pagetoid involvement of laryngeal mucosa is often seen (387,388). The morphologic features are those of the more common cutaneous melanomas (see Chapter 13) and mucosal melanomas of the nasal and oral cavities. Prognosis is poor, although local recurrences appear less common in the larynx than in other sites (387,388).

Although aggressive thyroid malignancies may invade the larynx secondarily by direct extension, hematogenous *metastases* to the larynx are distinctly uncommon (389,390,394). As noted above, cutaneous melanoma is the most frequent malignancy to metastasize to the larynx (389,390), followed by renal cell carcinoma (390). Other tumors with documented laryngeal metastases include carcinomas of the lung, breast, ovary, colon, stomach, and prostate, among others (390). Melanomas and renal cell carcinomas tend to metastasize to laryngeal soft tissue, with lung and breast cancers tending to metastasize to ossified laryngeal cartilage. Interestingly, the laryngeal metastasis has occasionally been the presenting feature of the patient's malignancy (390). Although generally associated with a poor prognosis, occasional reports exist of patients with prolonged survival following laryngeal metastasis (390).

REFERENCES

1. American Joint Committee on Cancer. *AJCC Cancer Staging Manual, 5th ed.* Philadelphia: Lippincott-Raven, 1997:41–46.
2. Snow GB, Gerritsen GF. TNM classification according to the UICC and AJCC. In: Ferlito A, ed. *Neoplasms of the larynx.* New York: Churchill Livingstone, 1993:425–434.
3. Williams RG, Douglas-Jones T. *Mycobacterium* marches back. *J Laryngol Otol* 1995;109:5–13.
4. Bull TR. Tuberculosis of the larynx. *Br Med J* 1966;2:991–992.
5. Hunter AM, Millar JW, Wightman AJ, et al. The changing pattern of laryngeal tuberculosis. *J Laryngol Otol* 1981;95:393–398.
6. Case records of the Massachusetts General Hospital. Weekly clinicopathological exercises. Case 51—1983. A 60-year-old man with progressive hoarseness. *N Engl J Med* 1983;309:1569–1574.
7. Thaller SR, Gross JR, Pilch BZ, et al. Laryngeal tuberculosis as manifested in the decades 1963–1983. *Laryngoscope* 1987;97:848–850.
8. Cleary KR, Batsakis JG. Mycobacterial disease of the head and neck: current perspective. *Ann Otol Rhinol Laryngol* 1995;104:830–833.
9. Yarnal JR, Golish JA, van der Kuyp F. Laryngeal tuberculosis presenting as carcinoma. *Arch Otolaryngol* 1981;107:503–505.
10. Lightfoot SA. Laryngeal tuberculosis masquerading as carcinoma. *J Am Board Fam Pract* 1997;10:374–376.
11. Pillsbury HCD, Sasaki CT. Granulomatous diseases of the larynx. *Otolaryngol Clin North Am* 1982;15:539–551.
12. Ward PH, Berci G, Morledge D, et al. Coccidioidomycosis of the larynx in infants and adults. *Ann Otol Rhinol Laryngol* 1977;86: 655–660.
13. Platt MA. Laryngeal coccidioidomycosis. *JAMA* 1977;237:1234–1235.
14. Kerschner JE, Ridley MB, Greene JN. Laryngeal cryptococcus. Treatment with oral fluconazole. *Arch Otolaryngol Head Neck Surg* 1995;121:1193–1195.
15. Blair PA, Gnepp DR, Riley RS, et al. Blastomycosis of the larynx. *South Med J* 1981;74:880–882.
16. Dumich PS, Neel HBD. Blastomycosis of the larynx. *Laryngoscope* 1983;93:1266–1270.
17. Kheir SM, Flint A, Moss JA. Primary aspergillosis of the larynx simulating carcinoma. *Hum Pathol* 1983;14:184–186.
18. Hicks JN, Peters GE. Pseudocarcinomatous hyperplasia of the larynx due to *Candida albicans. Laryngoscope* 1982;92:644–647.
19. Brandenburg JH, Finch WW, Kirkham WR. Actinomycosis of the larynx and pharynx. *Otolaryngology* 1978;86:ORL-739–ORL-742.
20. Michaels L. *Pathology of the larynx.* Berlin: Springer-Verlag, 1984.
21. Soni NK. Leprosy of the larynx. *J Laryngol Otol* 1992;106:518–520.
22. Jay J, Green RP, Lucente FE. Isolated laryngeal rhinoscleroma. *Otolaryngol Head Neck Surg* 1985;93:669–673.
23. Toppozada HH. Laryngeal bilharzia. *J Laryngol Otol* 1985;99: 1039–1041.
24. Case records of the Massachusetts General Hospital. Weekly clinicopathological exercises. Case 42—1977. *N Engl J Med* 1977;297: 878–883.
25. Senior BA, Radkowski D, MacArthur C, et al. Changing patterns in pediatric supraglottitis: a multi-institutional review, 1980 to 1992. *Laryngoscope* 1994;104:1314–1322.
26. Dort JC, Frohlich AM, Tate RB. Acute epiglottitis in adults: diagnosis and treatment in 43 patients. *J Otolaryngol* 1994;23:281–285.
27. Deeb ZE. Acute supraglottitis in adults: early indicators of airway obstruction. *Am J Otolaryngol* 1997;18:112–115.

28. Goutas N, Simopoulou S, Papazoglou K, et al. A fatal case of diphtheria. *Pediatr Pathol* 1994;14:391–395.
29. Garlicki A, Bociaga M, Krukowiecki J, et al. Laryngeal diphtheria in a young woman causes diagnostic difficulties—case report. *Przegl Lek* 1996;53:761–762.
30. Neel HBD, McDonald TJ. Laryngeal sarcoidosis: report of 13 patients. *Ann Otol Rhinol Laryngol* 1982;91:359–362.
31. Wenig BM, Devaney K, Wenig BL. Pseudoneoplastic lesions of the oropharynx and larynx simulating cancer. *Pathol Annu* 1995;30: 143–187.
32. Leahy F, Mina M, deSa D. Sarcoidosis of the larynx in a child. *J Otolaryngol* 1985;14:372–374.
33. Popper HH, Winter E, Hofler G. DNA of *Mycobacterium tuberculosis* in formalin-fixed, paraffin-embedded tissue in tuberculosis and sarcoidosis detected by polymerase chain reaction. *Am J Clin Pathol* 1994;101:738–741.
34. Almenoff PL, Johnson A, Lesser M, et al. Growth of acid fast L forms from the blood of patients with sarcoidosis. *Thorax* 1996;51: 530–533.
35. el-Zaatari FA, Naser SA, Markesich DC, et al. Identification of *Mycobacterium avium* complex in sarcoidosis. *J Clin Microbiol* 1996;34:2240–2245.
36. Vanek J, Schwarz J. Demonstration of acid-fast rods in sarcoidosis. *Am Rev Respir Dis* 1970;101:395–400.
37. Walker GK, Fechner RE, Johns ME, et al. Necrotizing sialometaplasia of the larynx secondary to atheromatous embolization. *Am J Clin Pathol* 1982;77:221–223.
38. Wenig BM. Necrotizing sialometaplasia of the larynx. A report of two cases and a review of the literature. *Am J Clin Pathol* 1995;103: 609–613.
39. Case records of the Massachusetts General Hospital. Weekly clinicopathological exercises. Case 35-1978. *N Engl J Med* 1978;299: 538–544.
40. Cho MS, Kim ES, Kim HJ, et al. Kimura's disease of the epiglottis. *Histopathology* 1997;30:592–594.
41. Kambic V, Radsel Z, Zargi M, et al. Vocal cord polyps: incidence, histology and pathogenesis. *J Laryngol Otol* 1981;95:609–618.
42. Kleinsasser O. Pathogenesis of vocal cord polyps. *Ann Otol Rhinol Laryngol* 1982;91:378–381.
43. Dikkers FG, Nikkels PG. Benign lesions of the vocal folds: histopathology and phonotrauma. *Ann Otol Rhinol Laryngol* 1995;104:698–703.
44. Frenzel H, Kleinsasser O, Hort W. [Light and electron microscopic observations on polyps of human vocal cords]. *Virchows Arch [Pathol Anat]* 1980;389:189–204.
45. Holinger PH, Johnston KC. Contact ulcer of the larynx. *JAMA* 1960;172:93–97.
46. Ward PH, Zwitman D, Hanson D, et al. Contact ulcers and granulomas of the larynx: new insights into their etiology as a basis for more rational treatment. *Otolaryngol Head Neck Surg* 1980;88: 262–269.
47. Barton RT. Observation of the pathogenesis of laryngeal granuloma due to endotracheal anesthesia. *N Engl J Med* 1953;248:1097–1099.
48. Miko TL. Peptic (contact ulcer) granuloma of the larynx. *J Clin Pathol* 1989;42:800–804.
49. Hanson DG, Kamel PL, Kahrilas PJ. Outcomes of antireflux therapy for the treatment of chronic laryngitis. *Ann Otol Rhinol Laryngol* 1995;104:550–555.
50. Wenig BM, Heffner DK. Contact ulcers of the larynx. A reacquaintance with the pathology of an often underdiagnosed entity. *Arch Pathol Lab Med* 1990;114:825–828.
51. Mills SE, Cooper PH, Fechner RE. Lobular capillary hemangioma: the underlying lesion of pyogenic granuloma. A study of 73 cases from the oral and nasal mucous membranes. *Am J Surg Pathol* 1980;4: 470–479.
52. Fechner RE, Cooper PH, Mills SE. Pyogenic granuloma of the larynx and trachea. A causal and pathologic misnomer for granulation tissue. *Arch Otolaryngol* 1981;107:30–32.
53. Canalis RF, Maxwell DS, Hemenway WG. Laryngocele—an updated review. *J Otolaryngol* 1977;6:191–199.
54. Holinger LD, Barnes DR, Smid LJ, et al. Laryngocele and saccular cysts. *Ann Otol Rhinol Laryngol* 1978;87:675–685.
55. Baker HL, Baker SR, McClatchey KD. Manifestations and management of laryngoceles. *Head Neck Surg* 1982;4:450–456.
56. Szwarc BJ, Kashima HK. Endoscopic management of a combined laryngocele. *Ann Otol Rhinol Laryngol* 1997;106:556–559.
57. Raveh E, Inbar E, Shvero J, et al. Huge saccular cyst of the larynx: a case report. *J Laryngol Otol* 1995;109:653–656.
58. Schmidt PJ, Wagenfeld D, Bridger MW, et al. Teflon injection of the vocal cord: a clinical and histopathologic study. *J Otolaryngol* 1980;9:297–302.
59. Varvares MA, Montgomery WW, Hillman RE. Teflon granuloma of the larynx: etiology, pathophysiology, and management. *Ann Otol Rhinol Laryngol* 1995;104:511–515.
60. Montgomery WW, Blaugrund SM, Varvares MA. Thyroplasty: a new approach. *Ann Otol Rhinol Laryngol* 1993;102:571–579.
61. Nguyen HC, Urquhart AC. Zenker's diverticulum. *Laryngoscope* 1997;107:1436–1440.
62. Wolff SM, Fauci AS, Horn RG, et al. Wegener's granulomatosis. *Ann Intern Med* 1974;81:513–525.
63. Batsakis JG. Wegener's granulomatosis and midline (nonhealing) "granuloma." *Head Neck Surg* 1979;1:213–222.
64. Godman GC, Churg J. Wegener's granulomatosis. *AMA Arch Pathology* 1954;58:533–553.
65. Case records of the Massachusetts General Hospital. Weekly clinicopathological exercises. Case 31-1986. A 39-year-old woman with stenosis of the subglottic area and pulmonary artery. *N Engl J Med* 1986;315:378–387.
66. Lebovics RS, Hoffman GS, Leavitt RY, et al. The management of subglottic stenosis in patients with Wegener's granulomatosis. *Laryngoscope* 1992;102:1341–1345.
67. Devaney KO, Travis WD, Hoffman G, et al. Interpretation of head and neck biopsies in Wegener's granulomatosis. A pathologic study of 126 biopsies in 70 patients. *Am J Surg Pathol* 1990;14: 555–564.
68. Hoare TJ, Jayne D, Rhys Evans P, et al. Wegener's granulomatosis, subglottic stenosis and antineutrophil cytoplasm antibodies. *J Laryngol Otol* 1989;103:1187–1191.
69. Yumoto E, Saeki K, Kadota Y. Subglottic stenosis in Wegener's granulomatosis limited to the head and neck region. *Ear Nose Throat J* 1997;76:571–574.
70. Merkel PA, Polisson RP, Chang Y, et al. Prevalence of antineutrophil cytoplasmic antibodies in a large inception cohort of patients with connective tissue disease. *Ann Intern Med* 1997;126:866–873.
71. Simpson GTD, Strong MS, Skinner M, et al. Localized amyloidosis of the head and neck and upper aerodigestive and lower respiratory tracts. *Ann Otol Rhinol Laryngol* 1984;93:374–379.
72. Lewis JE, Olsen KD, Kurtin PJ, et al. Laryngeal amyloidosis: a clinicopathologic and immunohistochemical review. *Otolaryngol Head Neck Surg* 1992;106:372–377.
73. Gertz MA, Kyle RA. Primary systemic amyloidosis—a diagnostic primer. *Mayo Clin Proc* 1989;64:1505–1519.
74. Berg AM, Troxler RF, Grillone G, et al. Localized amyloidosis of the larynx: evidence for light chain composition. *Ann Otol Rhinol Laryngol* 1993;102:884–889.
75. Michaels L, Hyams VJ. Amyloid in localised deposits and plasmacytomas of the respiratory tract. *J Pathol* 1979;128:29–38.
76. Bridger MW, Jahn AF, van Nostrand AW. Laryngeal rheumatoid arthritis. *Laryngoscope* 1980;90:296–303.
77. Montgomery WW. Pathology of cricoarytenoid arthritis. *N Engl J Med* 1959;260:66–69.
78. Montgomery WW. Cricoarytenoid arthritis. *Laryngoscope* 1963;73: 801–836.
79. Simpson GTD, Javaheri A, Janfaza P. Acute cricoarytenoid arthritis: local periarticular steroid injection. *Ann Otol Rhinol Laryngol* 1980;89:558–562.
80. Abadir WF, Forster PM. Rheumatoid vocal cord nodules. *J Laryngol Otol* 1974;88:473–478.
81. Sorensen WT, Moller-Andersen K, Behrendt N. Rheumatoid nodules of the larynx. *J Laryngol Otol* 1998;112:573–574.

82. Smith GA, Ward PH, Berci G. Laryngeal lupus erythematosus. *J Laryngol Otol* 1978;92:67–73.
83. Tsunoda K, Soda Y. Hoarseness as the initial manifestation of systemic lupus erythematosus. *J Laryngol Otol* 1996;110:478–479.
84. Schwartz IS, Grishman E. Rheumatoid nodules of the vocal cords as the initial manifestation of systemic lupus erythematosus. *JAMA* 1980;244:2751–2752.
85. Prytz S. Vocal nodules in Sjogren's syndrome. *J Laryngol Otol* 1980;94:197–203.
86. Barrs DM, McDonald TJ, Duffy J. Sjogren's syndrome involving the larynx: report of a case. *J Laryngol Otol* 1979;93:933–936.
87. Damiani JM, Levine HL. Relapsing polychondritis—report of ten cases. *Laryngoscope* 1979;89:929–946.
88. Batsakis JG, Manning JT. Relapsing polychondritis. *Ann Otol Rhinol Laryngol* 1989;98:83–84.
89. Block LJ, Caldarelli DD, Holinger PH, et al. Pemphigus of the air and food passages. *Ann Otol Rhinol Laryngol* 1977;86:584–587.
90. Frangogiannis NG, Gangopadhyay S, Cate T. Pemphigus of the larynx and esophagus [letter]. *Ann Intern Med* 1995;122:803–804.
91. Thompson JW, Ahmed AR, Dudley JP. Epidermolysis bullosa dystrophica of the larynx and trachea. Acute airway obstruction. *Ann Otol Rhinol Laryngol* 1980;89:428–429.
92. Goodman M, Montgomery W, Minette L. Pathologic findings in gouty cricoarytenoid arthritis. *Arch Otolaryngol* 1976;102:27–29.
93. Marion RB, Alperin JE, Maloney WH. Gouty tophus of the true vocal cord. *Arch Otolaryngol* 1972;96:161–162.
94. Guttenplan MD, Hendrix RA, Townsend MJ, et al. Laryngeal manifestations of gout. *Ann Otol Rhinol Laryngol* 1991;100:899–902.
95. Oliveira CA, Roth JA, Adams GL. Oncocytic lesions of the larynx. *Laryngoscope* 1977;87:1718–1725.
96. Yamase HT, Putman HCD. Oncocytic papillary cystadenomatosis of the larynx: a clinicopathologic entity. *Cancer* 1979;44: 2306–2311.
97. Noyek AM, Pritzker KP, Greyson ND, et al. Familial Warthin's tumor. 1. Its synchronous occurrence in mother and son. 2. Its association with cystic oncocytic metaplasia of the larynx. *J Otolaryngol* 1980;9:90–96.
98. Newman BH, Taxy JB, Laker HI. Laryngeal cysts in adults: a clinicopathologic study of 20 cases. *Am J Clin Pathol* 1984;81:715–720.
99. Nienhuis DM, Prakash UB, Edell ES. Tracheobronchopathia osteochondroplastica. *Ann Otol Rhinol Laryngol* 1990;99:689–694.
100. Smid L, Lavrencak B, Zargi M. Laryngo-tracheo-bronchopathia chondro-osteoplastica. *J Laryngol Otol* 1992;106:845–848.
101. Young RH, Sandstrom RE, Mark GJ. Tracheopathia osteoplastica: clinical, radiologic, and pathological correlations. *J Thorac Cardiovasc Surg* 1980;79:537–541.
102. Birzgalis AR, Farrington WT, O'Keefe L, et al. Localized tracheopathia osteoplastica of the subglottis. *J Laryngol Otol* 1993;107: 352–353.
103. Grillo HC, Mark EJ, Mathisen DJ, et al. Idiopathic laryngotracheal stenosis and its management. *Ann Thorac Surg* 1993;56:80–87.
104. Benjamin B, Jacobson I, Eckstein R. Idiopathic subglottic stenosis: diagnosis and endoscopic laser treatment. *Ann Otol Rhinol Laryngol* 1997;106:770–774.
105. Jindal JR, Milbrath MM, Shaker R, et al. Gastroesophageal reflux disease as a likely cause of "idiopathic" subglottic stenosis. *Ann Otol Rhinol Laryngol* 1994;103:186–191.
106. Tomé FMS, Fardeau M. Oculopharyngeal muscular dystrophy. In: Engel AG, Franzini-Armstrong C, eds. *Myology, 2nd ed, vol 2.* New York: McGraw-Hill, 1994:1233–1245.
107. Victor M, Hayes R, Adams RD. Oculopharyngeal muscular dystrophy. A familial disease of late life characterized by dysphagia and progressive ptosis of the eyelids. *N Engl J Med* 1962;267: 1267–1272.
108. Blumen SC, Sadeh M, Korczyn AD, et al. Intranuclear inclusions in oculopharyngeal muscular dystrophy among Bukhara Jews. *Neurology* 1996;46:1324–1328.
109. Tomé FMS, Chateau D, Helbling-Leclerc A, et al. Morphological changes in muscle fibers in oculopharyngeal muscular dystrophy. *Neuromusc Dis* 1997;7:S63–S69.
110. Montgomery WW, Lynch JP. Oculopharyngeal muscular dystrophy treated by inferior constrictor myotomy. *Trans Am Acad Ophthalmol Otolaryngol* 1971;75:986–993.
111. Coffin CM, Watterson J, Priest JR, et al. Extrapulmonary inflammatory myofibroblastic tumor (inflammatory pseudotumor). A clinicopathologic and immunohistochemical study of 84 cases. *Am J Surg Pathol* 1995;19:859–872.
112. Manni JJ, Mulder JJ, Schaafsma HE, et al. Inflammatory pseudotumor of the subglottis. *Eur Arch Otorhinolaryngol* 1992;249:16–19.
113. Wenig BM, Devaney K, Bisceglia M. Inflammatory myofibroblastic tumor of the larynx. A clinicopathologic study of eight cases simulating a malignant spindle cell neoplasm. *Cancer* 1995;76:2217–2229.
114. Wenig BM, Devaney K. Myofibroblastic pseudotumors of the larynx (MPL). *Mod Pathol* 1995;8:104A.
115. Weidner N, Askin FB, Berthrong M, et al. Bizarre (pseudomalignant) granulation-tissue reactions following ionizing-radiation exposure. A microscopic, immunohistochemical, and flow-cytometric study. *Cancer* 1987;59:1509–1514.
116. Su LD, Atayde-Perez A, Sheldon S, et al. Inflammatory myofibroblastic tumor: cytogenetic evidence supporting clonal origin. *Mod Pathol* 1998;11:364–368.
117. Case records of the Massachusetts General Hospital. Weekly clinicopathological exercises. Case 52-1981. A 51-year-old man with upper-airway obstruction and lymphadenopathy. *N Engl J Med* 1981;305: 1572–1580.
118. Asrar L, Facharzt EH, Haque I. Rosai-Dorfman disease: presenting as isolated extranodal involvement of larynx. *J Otolaryngol* 1998; 27:85–86.
119. Wey W, Torhorst J. [Hamartoma of the hypopharynx]. *HNO* 1974;22:217–219.
120. Patterson HC, Dickerson GR, Pilch BZ, et al. Hamartoma of the hypopharynx. *Arch Otolaryngol* 1981;107:767–772.
121. Zapf B, Lehmann WB, Snyder GGD. Hamartoma of the larynx: an unusual cause for stridor in an infant. *Otolaryngol Head Neck Surg* 1981;89:797–799.
122. Archer SM, Crockett DM, McGill TJ. Hamartoma of the larynx: report of two cases and review of the literature. *Int J Pediatr Otorhinolaryngol* 1988;16:237–243.
123. Roberts PF, McCann BG. Eosinophilic angiocentric fibrosis of the upper respiratory tract: a mucosal variant of granuloma faciale? A report of three cases. *Histopathology* 1985;9:1217–1225.
124. Fageeh NA, Mai KT, Odell PF. Eosinophilic angiocentric fibrosis of the subglottic region of the larynx and upper trachea. *J Otolaryngol* 1996;25:276–278.
125. Quick CA, Foucar E, Dehner LP. Frequency and significance of epithelial atypia in laryngeal papillomatosis. *Laryngoscope* 1979;89: 550–560.
126. Cohen SR, Geller KA, Seltzer S, et al. Papilloma of the larynx and tracheobronchial tree in children. A retrospective study. *Ann Otol Rhinol Laryngol* 1980;89:497–503.
127. Abramson AL, Steinberg BM, Winkler B. Laryngeal papillomatosis: clinical, histopathologic and molecular studies. *Laryngoscope* 1987; 97:678–685.
128. Kleinsasser O, Olieveira e Cruz G. ["Juvenile" and "adult" papillomas of the larynx]. *HNO* 1973;21:97–106.
129. Batsakis JG, Raymond AK, Rice DH. The pathology of head and neck tumors: papillomas of the upper aerodigestive tracts, Part 18. *Head Neck Surg* 1983;5:332–344.
130. Terry RM, Lewis FA, Griffiths S, et al. Demonstration of human papillomavirus types 6 and 11 in juvenile laryngeal papillomatosis by *in situ* DNA hybridization. *J Pathol* 1987;153:245–248.
131. Quiney RE, Wells M, Lewis FA, et al. Laryngeal papillomatosis: correlation between severity of disease and presence of HPV 6 and 11 detected by *in situ* DNA hybridisation. *J Clin Pathol* 1989;42:694–698.
132. Duggan MA, Lim M, Gill MJ, et al. HPV DNA typing of adult-onset respiratory papillomatosis. *Laryngoscope* 1990;100:639–642.
133. Gabbott M, Cossart YE, Kan A, et al. Human papillomavirus and host variables as predictors of clinical course in patients with juvenile-onset recurrent respiratory papillomatosis. *J Clin Microbiol* 1997;35: 3098–3103.

134. Pignatari S, Smith EM, Gray SD, et al. Detection of human papillomavirus infection in diseased and nondiseased sites of the respiratory tract in recurrent respiratory papillomatosis patients by DNA hybridization. *Ann Otol Rhinol Laryngol* 1992;101:408–412.
135. Rihkanen H, Aaltonen LM, Syrjanen SM. Human papillomavirus in laryngeal papillomas and in adjacent normal epithelium. *Clin Otolaryngol* 1993;18:470–474.
136. Quick CA, Watts SL, Krzyzek RA, et al. Relationship between condylomata and laryngeal papillomata. Clinical and molecular virological evidence. *Ann Otol Rhinol Laryngol* 1980;89:467–471.
137. Kashima HK, Mounts P, Shah K. Recurrent respiratory papillomatosis. *Obstet Gynecol Clin North Am* 1996;23:699–706.
138. Derkay CS. Task force on recurrent respiratory papillomas. A preliminary report. *Arch Otolaryngol Head Neck Surg* 1995;121:1386–1391.
139. Kosko JR, Derkay CS. Role of cesarean section in prevention of recurrent respiratory papillomatosis—is there one? *Int J Pediatr Otorhinolaryngol* 1996;35:31–38.
140. Lindeberg H, Elbrond O. Laryngeal papillomas: clinical aspects in a series of 231 patients. *Clin Otolaryngol* 1989;14:333–342.
141. Bauman NM, Smith RJ. Recurrent respiratory papillomatosis. *Pediatr Clin North Am* 1996;43:1385–1401.
142. Kashima H, Mounts P, Leventhal B, et al. Sites of predilection in recurrent respiratory papillomatosis. *Ann Otol Rhinol Laryngol* 1993;102:580–583.
143. Fechner RE, Goepfert H, Alford BR. Invasive laryngeal papillomatosis. *Arch Otolaryngol* 1974;99:147–151.
144. Fechner RE, Fitz-Hugh GS. Invasive tracheal papillomatosis. *Am J Surg Pathol* 1980;4:79–86.
145. Fechner RE, Mills SE. Verruca vulgaris of the larynx: a distinctive lesion of probable viral origin confused with verrucous carcinoma. *Am J Surg Pathol* 1982;6:357–362.
146. Barnes L, Yunis EJ, Krebs FJD, et al. Verruca vulgaris of the larynx. Demonstration of human papillomavirus types 6/11 by *in situ* hybridization. *Arch Pathol Lab Med* 1991;115:895–899.
147. Smith EM, Pignatari SS, Gray SD, et al. Human papillomavirus infection in papillomas and nondiseased respiratory sites of patients with recurrent respiratory papillomatosis using the polymerase chain reaction. *Arch Otolaryngol Head Neck Surg* 1993;119:554–557.
148. Shapiro AM, Rimell FL, Shoemaker D, et al. Tracheotomy in children with juvenile-onset recurrent respiratory papillomatosis: the Children's Hospital of Pittsburgh experience. *Ann Otol Rhinol Laryngol* 1996;105:1–5.
149. Doyle DJ, Gianoli GJ, Espinola T, et al. Recurrent respiratory papillomatosis: juvenile versus adult forms. *Laryngoscope* 1994;104:523–527.
150. Doyle DJ, Henderson LA, LeJeune FE Jr, et al. Changes in human papillomavirus typing of recurrent respiratory papillomatosis progressing to malignant neoplasm. *Arch Otolaryngol Head Neck Surg* 1994;120:1273–1276.
151. Lin KY, Westra WH, Kashima HK, et al. Coinfection of HPV-11 and HPV-16 in a case of laryngeal squamous papillomas with severe dysplasia. *Laryngoscope* 1997;107:942–947.
152. Avidano MA, Singleton GT. Adjuvant drug strategies in the treatment of recurrent respiratory papillomatosis. *Otolaryngol Head Neck Surg* 1995;112:197–202.
153. MacMillan RHD, Fechner RE. Pleomorphic adenoma of the larynx. *Arch Pathol Lab Med* 1986;110:245–247.
154. Dubey SP, Banerjee S, Ghosh LM, et al. Benign pleomorphic adenoma of the larynx: report of a case and review and analysis of 20 additional cases in the literature. *Ear Nose Throat J* 1997;76:548–550,552,554–557.
155. Sawatsubashi M, Tuda K, Tokunaga O, et al. Pleomorphic adenoma of the larynx: a case and review of the literature in Japan. *Otolaryngol Head Neck Surg* 1997;117:415–417.
156. Ma CK, Fine G, Lewis J, et al. Benign mixed tumor of the trachea. *Cancer* 1979;44:2260–2266.
157. Bizal JC, Righi PD, Kesler KA. Pleomorphic adenoma of the trachea. *Otolaryngol Head Neck Surg* 1997;116:139–140.
158. Heffner DK. Sinonasal and laryngeal salivary gland lesions. In: Ellis GL, Auclair PL, Gnepp DR, eds. *Major problems in pathology, vol 25.* Philadelphia: WB Saunders, 1991:544.
159. Brodsky L, Yoshpe N, Ruben RJ. Clinical–pathological correlates of congenital subglottic hemangiomas. *Ann Otol Rhinol Laryngol Suppl* 1983;105:4–18.
160. Cotton RT, Richardson MA. Congenital laryngeal anomalies. *Otolaryngol Clin North Am* 1981;14:203–218.
161. Phipps CD, Gibson WS, Wood WE. Infantile subglottic hemangioma: a review and presentation of two cases of surgical excision. *Int J Pediatr Otorhinolaryngol* 1997;41:71–79.
162. Batsakis JG, Fox JE. Supporting tissue neoplasms of the larynx. *Surg Gynecol Obstet* 1970;131:989–997.
163. Shikhani AH, Jones MM, Marsh BR, et al. Infantile subglottic hemangiomas. An update. *Ann Otol Rhinol Laryngol* 1986;95:336–347.
164. Sie KC, McGill T, Healy GB. Subglottic hemangioma: ten years' experience with the carbon dioxide laser. *Ann Otol Rhinol Laryngol* 1994;103:167–172.
165. Healy G, McGill T, Friedman EM. Carbon dioxide laser in subglottic hemangioma. An update. *Ann Otol Rhinol Laryngol* 1984;93:370–373.
166. Meeuwis J, Bos CE, Hoeve LJ, et al. Subglottic hemangiomas in infants: treatment with intralesional corticosteroid injection and intubation. *Int J Pediatr Otorhinolaryngol* 1990;19:145–150.
167. Wiatrak BJ, Reilly JS, Seid AB, et al. Open surgical excision of subglottic hemangioma in children. *Int J Pediatr Otorhinolaryngol* 1996;34:191–206.
168. Barnes L. Paraganglioma of the larynx. A critical review of the literature. *J Otorhinolaryngol Rel Spec* 1991;53:220–234.
169. Lack EE. *Atlas of tumor pathology, vol 19, Tumors of the adrenal gland and extra-adrenal paraganglia, 3rd ed.* Washington, DC: Armed Forces Institute of Pathology, 1997.
170. Glenner GG, Grimley PM, eds. *Atlas of tumor pathology, vol 9, Tumors of the extra-adrenal paraganglion system (including chemoreceptors), 2nd ed.* Washington, DC: Armed Forces Institute of Pathology, 1974.
171. Lack EE, Cubilla AL, Woodruff JM. Paragangliomas of the head and neck region. A pathologic study of tumors from 71 patients. *Hum Pathol* 1979;10:191–218.
172. Lawson W, Zak FG. The glomus bodies ("paraganglia") of the human larynx. *Laryngoscope* 1974;84:98–111.
173. Googe PB, Ferry JA, Bhan AK, et al. A comparison of paraganglioma, carcinoid tumor, and small-cell carcinoma of the larynx. *Arch Pathol Lab Med* 1988;112:809–815.
174. Olofsson J, Grontoft O, Sokjer H, et al. Paraganglioma involving the larynx. *J Otorhinolaryngol Rel Spec* 1984;46:57–65.
175. el-Silimy O, Harvy L. A clinico-pathological classification of laryngeal paraganglioma. *J Laryngol Otol* 1992;106:635–639.
176. Barnes L. Paragangliomas of the larynx [Letter]. *J Laryngol Otol* 1993;107:664–667.
177. Milroy CM, Rode J, Moss E. Laryngeal paragangliomas and neuroendocrine carcinomas. *Histopathology* 1991;18:201–209.
178. Konowitz PM, Lawson W, Som PM, et al. Laryngeal paraganglioma: update on diagnosis and treatment. *Laryngoscope* 1988;98:40–49.
179. Ferlito A, Barnes L, Wenig BM. Identification, classification, treatment, and prognosis of laryngeal paraganglioma. Review of the literature and eight new cases. *Ann Otol Rhinol Laryngol* 1994;103:525–536.
180. Ferlito A, Milroy CM, Wenig BM, et al. Laryngeal paraganglioma versus atypical carcinoid tumor. *Ann Otol Rhinol Laryngol* 1995;104:78–83.
181. Martinez-Madrigal F, Bosq J, Micheau C, et al. Paragangliomas of the head and neck. Immunohistochemical analysis of 16 cases in comparison with neuro-endocrine carcinomas. *Pathol Res Pract* 1991;187:814–823.
182. Milroy CM, Ferlito A. Immunohistochemical markers in the diagnosis of neuroendocrine neoplasms of the head and neck. *Ann Otol Rhinol Laryngol* 1995;104:413–418.
183. Lack EE, Worsham GF, Callihan MD, et al. Granular cell tumor: a clinicopathologic study of 110 patients. *J Surg Oncol* 1980;13:301–316.

184. Filie AC, Lage JM, Azumi N. Immunoreactivity of S100 protein, alpha-1-antitrypsin, and CD68 in adult and congenital granular cell tumors. *Mod Pathol* 1996;9:888–892.
185. Victoria LV, Hoffman HT, Robinson RA. Granular cell tumour of the larynx. *J Laryngol Otol* 1998;112:373–376.
186. Compagno J, Hyams VJ, Ste-Marie P. Benign granular cell tumors of the larynx: a review of 36 cases with clinicopathologic data. *Ann Otol Rhinol Laryngol* 1975;84:308–314.
187. Coates HL, Devine KD, McDonald TJ, et al. Granular cell tumors of the larynx. *Ann Otol Rhinol Laryngol* 1976;85:504–507.
188. Nolte E, Kleinsasser O. [Granular cell tumors of the larynx]. *HNO* 1982;30:333–339.
189. Burton DM, Heffner DK, Patow CA. Granular cell tumors of the trachea. *Laryngoscope* 1992;102:807–813.
190. Garud O, Bostad L, Elverland HH, et al. Granular cell tumor of the larynx in a 5-year-old child. *Ann Otol Rhinol Laryngol* 1984;93:45–47.
191. Brandwein M, LeBenger J, Strauchen J, et al. Atypical granular cell tumor of the larynx: an unusually aggressive tumor clinically and microscopically. *Head Neck* 1990;12:154–159.
192. Farmer RW, Scher RL. Granular cell tumor of the larynx presenting with airway obstruction. *Otolaryngol Head Neck Surg* 1998;118: 874–876.
193. Said-al-Naief N, Brandwein M, Lawson W, et al. Synchronous lingual granular cell tumor and squamous carcinoma. A case report and review of the literature. *Arch Otolaryngol Head Neck Surg* 1997;123: 543–547.
194. Nathrath WB, Remberger K. Immunohistochemical study of granular cell tumours. Demonstration of neurone specific enolase, S 100 protein, laminin and alpha-1-antichymotrypsin. *Virchows Arch [A] Pathol Anat Histopathol* 1986;408:421–434.
195. Ulrich J, Heitz PU, Fischer T, et al. Granular cell tumors: evidence for heterogeneous tumor cell differentiation. An immunocytochemical study. *Virchows Arch [B] Cell Pathol Mol Pathol* 1987;53:52–57.
196. Mazur MT, Shultz JJ, Myers JL. Granular cell tumor. Immunohistochemical analysis of 21 benign tumors and one malignant tumor. *Arch Pathol Lab Med* 1990;114:692–696.
197. Mukai M. Immunohistochemical localization of S-100 protein and peripheral nerve myelin proteins (P2 protein, P0 protein) in granular cell tumors. *Am J Pathol* 1983;112:139–146.
198. Penneys NS, Adachi K, Ziegels-Weissman J, et al. Granular cell tumors of the skin contain myelin basic protein. *Arch Pathol Lab Med* 1983;107:302–303.
199. Lack EE, Worsham GF, Callihan MD, et al. Gingival granular cell tumors of the newborn (congenital "epulis"): a clinical and pathologic study of 21 patients. *Am J Surg Pathol* 1981;5:37–46.
200. Cummings CW, Montgomery WW, Balogh K Jr. Neurogenic tumors of the larynx. *Ann Otol Rhinol Laryngol* 1969;78:76–95.
201. Schaeffer BT, Som PM, Biller HF, et al. Schwannomas of the larynx: review and computed tomographic scan analysis. *Head Neck Surg* 1986;8:469–472.
202. Cohen SR, Landing BH, Isaacs H. Neurofibroma of the larynx in a child. *Ann Otol Rhinol Laryngol Suppl* 1978;87:29–31.
203. al-Otieschan AT, Mahasin ZZ, Gangopadhyay K, et al. Schwannoma of the larynx: two case reports and review of the literature. *J Otolaryngol* 1996;25:412–415.
204. Chow LT, Ma TK, Chow WH. Cellular neurothekeoma of the hypopharynx. *Histopathology* 1997;30:192–194.
205. Karma P, Hyrynkangas K, Rasanen O. Laryngeal leiomyoma. *J Laryngol Otol* 1978;92:411–415.
206. Shibata K, Komune S. Laryngeal angiomyoma (vascular leiomyoma): clinicopathological findings. *Laryngoscope* 1980;90:1880–1886.
207. Boedts D, Mestdagh J. Adult rhabdomyoma of the larynx. *Arch Otorhinolaryngol* 1979;224:221–229.
208. Di Sant'Agnese PA, Knowles DMD. Extracardiac rhabdomyoma: a clinicopathologic study and review of the literature. *Cancer* 1980; 46:780–789.
209. Granich MS, Pilch BZ, Nadol JB, et al. Fetal rhabdomyoma of the larynx. *Arch Otolaryngol* 1983;109:821–826.
210. Rosenberg HS, Vogler C, Close LG, et al. Laryngeal fibromatosis in the neonate. *Arch Otolaryngol* 1981;107:513–517.
211. McIntosh WA, Kassner GW, Murray JF. Fibromatosis and fibrosarcoma of the larynx and pharynx in an infant. *Arch Otolaryngol* 1985;111:478–480.
212. Wenig BM. Lipomas of the larynx and hypopharynx: a review of the literature with the addition of three new cases. *J Laryngol Otol* 1995;109:353–357.
213. Wenig BM, Heffner DK. Liposarcomas of the larynx and hypopharynx: a clinicopathologic study of eight new cases and a review of the literature. *Laryngoscope* 1995;105:747–756.
214. Schwartz MR, Donovan DT. Hemangiopericytoma of the larynx: a case report and review of the literature. *Otolaryngol Head Neck Surg* 1987;96:369–372.
215. Van Laer C, Hamans E, Neetens I, et al. Benign fibrous histiocytoma of the larynx: presentation of a case and review of the literature. *J Laryngol Otol* 1996;110:474–477.
216. Cannon CR, Johns ME, Fechner RE. Immature teratoma of the larynx. *Otolaryngol Head Neck Surg* 1987;96:366–368.
217. Gates GA, Tucker JA. Sliding flap tracheoplasty. *Ann Otol Rhinol Laryngol* 1989;98:926–929.
218. Crissman JD, Zarbo RJ, Drozdowicz S, et al. Carcinoma *in situ* and microinvasive squamous carcinoma of the laryngeal glottis. *Arch Otolaryngol Head Neck Surg* 1988;114:299–307.
219. Nguyen C, Naghibzadeh B, Black MJ, et al. Glottic microinvasive carcinoma: is it different from carcinoma *in situ? J Otolaryngol* 1996; 25:223–226.
220. Fried MP, Gopal H. Carcinoma of the glottis. In: Fried MP, ed. *The larynx: a multidisciplinary approach, 2nd ed.* St Louis: CV Mosby, 1996:503–517.
221. Shah JP, Karnell LH, Hoffman HT, et al. Patterns of care for cancer of the larynx in the United States. *Arch Otolaryngol Head Neck Surg* 1997;123:475–483.
222. Landis SH, Murray T, Bolden S, et al. Cancer statistics, 1998. *CA Cancer J Clin* 1998;48:6–29. [Published errata appear in *CA Cancer J Clin* 1998;48:192, 329.]
223. Muir C, Weiland L. Upper aerodigestive tract cancers. *Cancer* 1995;75:147–153. [Published erratum appears in *Cancer* 1995; 75:2978.]
224. Hoffman HT, Karnell LH, Shah JP, et al. Hypopharyngeal cancer patient care evaluation. *Laryngoscope* 1997;107:1005–1017.
225. Cann CI, Rothman KJ, Fried MP. Epidemiology of laryngeal cancer. In: Fried MP, ed. *The larynx: a multidisciplinary approach, 2nd ed.* St Louis: CV Mosby, 1996:425–436.
226. Pilch BZ, Dorfman DM, Brodsky GL, et al. Pathology of laryngeal malignancies. In: Fried MP, ed. *The larynx: a multidisciplinary approach, 2nd ed.* St Louis: CV Mosby, 1996:425–436.
227. Koufman JA, Burke AJ. The etiology and pathogenesis of laryngeal carcinoma. *Otolaryngol Clin North Am* 1997;30:1–19.
228. McKaig RG, Baric RS, Olshan AF. Human papillomavirus and head and neck cancer: epidemiology and molecular biology. *Head Neck* 1998;20:250–265.
229. Fabian RL, Varvares MA. Carcinoma of the laryngopharynx and cervical esophagus. In: Fried MP, ed. *The larynx: a multidisciplinary approach, 2nd ed.* St Louis: CV Mosby, 1996:549–560.
230. Wang CC. *Radiation therapy for head and neck neoplasms, 3rd ed.* New York: Wiley-Liss, 1997.
231. Kirchner JA. Glottic–supraglottic barrier: fact or fantasy? *Ann Otol Rhinol Laryngol* 1997;106:700–704.
232. Ferlito A, Olofsson J, Rinaldo A. Barrier between the supraglottis and the glottis: myth or reality? *Ann Otol Rhinol Laryngol* 1997;106: 716–719.
233. Weinstein GS, Laccourreye O, Brasnu D, et al. Reconsidering a paradigm: the spread of supraglottic carcinoma to the glottis. *Laryngoscope* 1995;105:1129–1133.
234. Worsham MJ, Wolman SR, Carey TE, et al. Common clonal origin of synchronous primary head and neck squamous cell carcinomas: analysis by tumor karyotypes and fluorescence *in situ* hybridization. *Hum Pathol* 1995;26:251–261.
235. Sidransky D, Frost P, Von Eschenbach A, et al. Clonal origin of bladder cancer. *N Engl J Med* 1992;326:737–740.

236. Mori M, Adachi Y, Kakeji Y, et al. Superficial flat-type early carcinoma of the stomach. *Cancer* 1992;69:306–313.
237. Barge J, Molas G, Maillard JN, et al. Superficial oesophageal carcinoma: an oesophageal counterpart of early gastric cancer. *Histopathology* 1981;5:499–510.
238. Soga J, Tanaka O, Sasaki K, et al. Superficial spreading carcinoma of the esophagus. *Cancer* 1982;50:1641–1645.
239. Yasuda K, Ajioka Y, Watanabe H, et al. Morphogenesis and development of superficial spreading tumor of the colon and rectum. *Pathol Int* 1997;47:769–774.
240. Carbone A, Micheau C, Bosq J, et al. Superficial extending carcinoma of the hypopharynx: report of 26 cases of an underestimated carcinoma. *Laryngoscope* 1983;93:1600–1606.
241. Carbone A, Volpe R, Barzan L. Superficial extending carcinoma (SEC) of the larynx and hypopharynx. *Pathol Res Pract* 1992;188: 729–735.
242. Bamba M, Sugihara H, Okada K, et al. Clonal analysis of superficial depressed-type gastric carcinoma in humans. *Cancer* 1998;83: 867–875.
243. Michaels L, Hassmann E. Ventriculosaccular carcinoma of the larynx. *Clin Otolaryngol* 1982;7:165–173.
244. Nappi O, Wick MR, Pettinato G, et al. Pseudovascular adenoid squamous cell carcinoma of the skin. A neoplasm that may be mistaken for angiosarcoma. *Am J Surg Pathol* 1992;16:429–438.
245. Cappellari JO. Histopathology and pathologic prognostic indicators. *Otolaryngol Clin North Am* 1997;30:251–268.
246. Bryne M, Jenssen N, Boysen M. Histological grading in the deep invasive front of T1 and T2 glottic squamous cell carcinomas has high prognostic value. *Virchows Arch* 1995;427:277–281.
247. Welkoborsky HJ, Hinni M, Dienes HP, et al. Predicting recurrence and survival in patients with laryngeal cancer by means of DNA cytometry, tumor front grading, and proliferation markers. *Ann Otol Rhinol Laryngol* 1995;104:503–510.
248. Capaccio P, Pruneri G, Carboni N, et al. Cyclin D1 protein expression is related to clinical progression in laryngeal squamous cell carcinomas. *J Laryngol Otol* 1997;111:622–626.
249. Narayana A, Vaughan AT, Gunaratne S, et al. Is p53 an independent prognostic factor in patients with laryngeal carcinoma? *Cancer* 1998;82:286–291.
250. The Department of Veterans Affairs Laryngeal Cancer Study Group. Induction chemotherapy plus radiation compared with surgery plus radiation in patients with advanced laryngeal cancer. *N Engl J Med* 1991;324:1685–1690.
251. Batsakis JG, Hybels R, Crissman JD, et al. The pathology of head and neck tumors: verrucous carcinoma, Part 15. *Head Neck Surg* 1982;5:29–38.
252. Ferlito A, Recher G. Ackerman's tumor (verrucous carcinoma) of the larynx: a clinicopathologic study of 77 cases. *Cancer* 1980;46: 1617–1630.
253. Ferlito A. Diagnosis and treatment of verrucous squamous cell carcinoma of the larynx: a critical review. *Ann Otol Rhinol Laryngol* 1985;94:575–579.
254. Orvidas LJ, Olsen KD, Lewis JE, et al. Verrucous carcinoma of the larynx: a review of 53 patients. *Head Neck* 1998;20:197–203.
255. Lundgren JA, van Nostrand AW, Harwood AR, et al. Verrucous carcinoma (Ackerman's tumor) of the larynx: diagnostic and therapeutic considerations. *Head Neck Surg* 1986;9:19–26.
256. Shear M, Pindborg JJ. Verrucous hyperplasia of the oral mucosa. *Cancer* 1980;46:1855–1862.
257. Burns HP, van Nostrand AW, Bryce DP. Verrucous carcinoma of the larynx management by radiotherapy and surgery. *Ann Otol Rhinol Laryngol* 1976;85:538–543.
258. Kraus FT, Perezmesa C. Verrucous carcinoma. Clinical and pathologic study of 105 cases involving oral cavity, larynx and genitalia. *Cancer* 1966;19:26–38.
259. Van Nostrand AW, Olofsson J. Verrucous carcinoma of the larynx. A clinical and pathologic study of 10 cases. *Cancer* 1972;30: 691–702.
260. Glanz H, Kleinsasser O. Verrucous carcinoma of the larynx—a misnomer. *Arch Otorhinolaryngol* 1987;244:108–111.
261. Weidner N. Sarcomatoid carcinoma of the upper aerodigestive tract. *Semin Diagn Pathol* 1987;4:157–168.
262. Lauwers GY, Grant LD, Scott GV, et al. Spindle cell squamous carcinoma of the esophagus: analysis of ploidy and tumor proliferative activity in a series of 13 cases. *Hum Pathol* 1998;29:863–868.
263. Hyams VJ. Spindle cell carcinoma of the larynx. *Can J Otolaryngol* 1975;4:307–313.
264. Lambert PR, Ward PH, Berci G. Pseudosarcoma of the larynx: a comprehensive analysis. *Arch Otolaryngol* 1980;106:700–708.
265. Olsen KD, Lewis JE, Suman VJ. Spindle cell carcinoma of the larynx and hypopharynx. *Otolaryngol Head Neck Surg* 1997;116:47–52.
266. Lewis JE, Olsen KD, Sebo TJ. Spindle cell carcinoma of the larynx: review of 26 cases including DNA content and immunohistochemistry. *Hum Pathol* 1997;28:664–673.
267. Thompson LD. Diagnostically challenging lesions in head and neck pathology. *Eur Arch Otorhinolaryngol* 1997;254:357–366.
268. Leventon GS, Evans HL. Sarcomatoid squamous cell carcinoma of the mucous membranes of the head and neck: a clinicopathologic study of 20 cases. *Cancer* 1981;48:994–1003.
269. Batsakis JG, Rice DH, Howard DR. The pathology of head and neck tumors: spindle cell lesions (sarcomatoid carcinomas, nodular fasciitis, and fibrosarcoma) of the aerodigestive tracts, Part 14. *Head Neck Surg* 1982;4:499–513.
270. Zarbo RJ, Crissman JD, Venkat H, et al. Spindle-cell carcinoma of the upper aerodigestive tract mucosa. An immunohistologic and ultrastructural study of 18 biphasic tumors and comparison with seven monophasic spindle-cell tumors. *Am J Surg Pathol* 1986;10:741–753.
271. Ellis GL, Langloss JM, Heffner DK, et al. Spindle-cell carcinoma of the aerodigestive tract. An immunohistochemical analysis of 21 cases. *Am J Surg Pathol* 1987;11:335–342.
272. Guarino M. Epithelial-to-mesenchymal change of differentiation. From embryogenetic mechanism to pathological patterns. *Histol Histopathol* 1995;10:171–184.
273. Guarino M, Giordano F. Experimental induction of epithelial–mesenchymal interconversions. *Exp Toxicol Pathol* 1995;47:325–334.
274. Wain SL, Kier R, Vollmer RT, et al. Basaloid–squamous carcinoma of the tongue, hypopharynx, and larynx: report of 10 cases. *Hum Pathol* 1986;17:1158–1166.
275. Banks ER, Frierson HF Jr, Mills SE, et al. Basaloid squamous cell carcinoma of the head and neck. A clinicopathologic and immunohistochemical study of 40 cases. *Am J Surg Pathol* 1992;16:939–946.
276. Raslan WF, Barnes L, Krause JR, et al. Basaloid squamous cell carcinoma of the head and neck: a clinicopathologic and flow cytometric study of 10 new cases with review of the English literature. *Am J Otolaryngol* 1994;15:204–211.
277. Barnes L, Ferlito A, Altavilla G, et al. Basaloid squamous cell carcinoma of the head and neck: clinicopathological features and differential diagnosis. *Ann Otol Rhinol Laryngol* 1996;105:75–82.
278. Tsang WY, Chan JK, Lee KC, et al. Basaloid–squamous carcinoma of the upper aerodigestive tract and so-called adenoid cystic carcinoma of the oesophagus: the same tumour type? *Histopathology* 1991;19: 35–46.
279. Abe K, Sasano H, Itakura Y, et al. Basaloid–squamous carcinoma of the esophagus. A clinicopathologic, DNA ploidy, and immunohistochemical study of seven cases. *Am J Surg Pathol* 1996;20:453–461.
280. Muller S, Barnes L. Basaloid squamous cell carcinoma of the head and neck with a spindle cell component. An unusual histologic variant. *Arch Pathol Lab Med* 1995;119:181–182.
281. Klijanienko J, el-Naggar A, Ponzio-Prion A, et al. Basaloid squamous carcinoma of the head and neck. Immunohistochemical comparison with adenoid cystic carcinoma and squamous cell carcinoma. *Arch Otolaryngol Head Neck Surg* 1993;119:887–890.
282. Thompson LD, Wenig BM, Heffler DK, et al. Exophytic and papillary squamous cell carcinomas of the larynx: a clinicopathologic series of 105 cases. *Mod Pathol* 1997;10:117A.
283. Thompson LDR, Wenig BM, Heffner DK, et al. Exophytic and papillary squamous cell carcinomas of the larynx: a clinicopathologic series of 104 cases. *Otolaryngol Head Neck Surg* 1999;120:718–724.
284. Batsakis JG, Suarez P. Papillary squamous carcinoma: Will the real one please stand up? *Adv Anat Pathol* 2000;7:2–8.

285. Toker C, Peterson DW. Lymphoepithelioma of the vocal cord. *Arch Otolaryngol* 1978;104:161–162.
286. Micheau C, Luboinski B, Schwaab G, et al. Lymphoepitheliomas of the larynx (undifferentiated carcinomas of nasopharyngeal type). *Clin Otolaryngol* 1979;4:43–48.
287. Frank DK, Cheron F, Cho H, et al. Nonnasopharyngeal lymphoepitheliomas (undifferentiated carcinomas) of the upper aerodigestive tract. *Ann Otol Rhinol Laryngol* 1995;104:305–310.
288. Andryk J, Freije JE, Schultz CJ, et al. Lymphoepithelioma of the larynx. *Am J Otolaryngol* 1996;17:61–63.
289. Zbaren P, Borisch B, Lang H, et al. Undifferentiated carcinoma of nasopharyngeal type of the laryngopharyngeal region. *Otolaryngol Head Neck Surg* 1997;117:688–693.
290. Woodruff JM, Huvos AG, Erlandson RA, et al. Neuroendocrine carcinomas of the larynx. A study of two types, one of which mimics thyroid medullary carcinoma. *Am J Surg Pathol* 1985;9:771–790.
291. Ferlito A, Barnes L, Rinaldo A, et al. A review of neuroendocrine neoplasms of the larynx: update on diagnosis and treatment. *J Laryngol Otol* 1998;112:827–834.
292. Pesce C, Tobia-Gallelli F, Toncini C. APUD cells of the larynx. *Acta Otolaryngol (Stockh)* 1984;98:158–162.
293. Wenig BM, Hyams VJ, Heffner DK. Moderately differentiated neuroendocrine carcinoma of the larynx. A clinicopathologic study of 54 cases. *Cancer* 1988;62:2658–2676.
294. Shanmagurathnam K. *Histologic typing of tumours of the upper respiratory tract and ear, 2nd ed.* Berlin: Springer-Verlag, 1991.
295. Ferlito A, Rosai J. Terminology and classification of neuroendocrine neoplasms of the larynx. *ORL J Otorhinolaryngol Rel Spec* 1991; 53:185–187.
296. el-Naggar AK, Batsakis JG. Carcinoid tumor of the larynx. A critical review of the literature. *ORL J Otorhinolaryngol Rel Spec* 1991; 53:188–193.
297. Moisa II, Silver CE. Treatment of neuroendocrine neoplasms of the larynx. *ORL J Otorhinolaryngol Rel Spec* 1991;53:259–264.
298. Woodruff JM, Senie RT. Atypical carcinoid tumor of the larynx. A critical review of the literature. *ORL J Otorhinolaryngol Rel Spec* 1991;53:194–209.
299. Ereno C, Lopez JI, Sanchez JM. Atypical carcinoid of larynx: presentation with scalp metastases. *J Laryngol Otol* 1997;111:89–91.
300. Gripp FM, Risse EK, Leverstein H, et al. Neuroendocrine neoplasms of the larynx. Importance of the correct diagnosis and differences between atypical carcinoid tumors and small-cell neuroendocrine carcinoma. *Eur Arch Otorhinolaryngol* 1995;252:280–286.
301. Gnepp DR. Small cell neuroendocrine carcinoma of the larynx. A critical review of the literature. *ORL J Otorhinolaryngol Rel Spec* 1991;53:210–219.
302. Baugh RF, Wolf GT, McClatchey KD. Small cell carcinoma of the head and neck. *Head Neck Surg* 1986;8:343–354.
303. Ferlito A, Friedmann I. Review of neuroendocrine carcinomas of the larynx. *Ann Otol Rhinol Laryngol* 1989;98:780–790.
304. Ferlito A, Recher G, Caruso G. Primary combined small cell carcinoma of the larynx. *Am J Otolaryngol* 1985;6:302–308.
305. Chen DA, Mandell-Brown M, Moore SF, et al. "Composite" tumor—mixed squamous cell and small-cell anaplastic carcinoma of the larynx. *Otolaryngol Head Neck Surg* 1986;95:99–103.
306. Salim SA, Milroy C, Rode J, et al. Immunocytochemical characterization of neuroendocrine tumours of the larynx. *Histopathology* 1993;23:69–73.
307. Morice WG, Ferreiro JA. Distinction of basaloid squamous cell carcinoma from adenoid cystic and small cell undifferentiated carcinoma by immunohistochemistry. *Hum Pathol* 1998;29:609–612.
308. Aguilar EAd, Robbins KT, Stephens J, et al. Primary oat cell carcinoma of the larynx. *Am J Clin Oncol* 1987;10:26–32.
309. Whicker JH, Neel HBD, Weiland LH, et al. Adenocarcinoma of the larynx. *Ann Otol Rhinol Laryngol* 1974;83:487–490.
310. Fechner RE. Adenocarcinoma of the larynx. *Can J Otolaryngol* 1975;4:284–289.
311. El-Jabbour JN, Ferlito A, Friedmann I. Salivary gland neoplasms. In: Ferlito A, ed. *Neoplasms of the larynx.* New York: Churchill Livingstone, 1993:231–264.
312. Ferlito A, Gale N, Hvala H. Laryngeal salivary duct carcinoma: a light and electron microscopic study. *J Laryngol Otol* 1981;95:731–738.
313. Mikaelian DO, Contrucci RB, Batsakis JG. Epithelial–myoepithelial carcinoma of the subglottic region: a case presentation and review of the literature. *Otolaryngol Head Neck Surg* 1986;95:104–106.
314. Crissman JD, Rosenblatt A. Acinous cell carcinoma of the larynx. *Arch Pathol Lab Med* 1978;102:233–236.
315. Squires JE, Mills SE, Cooper PH, et al. Acinic cell carcinoma: its occurrence in the laryngotracheal junction after thyroid radiation. *Arch Pathol Lab Med* 1981;105:266–268.
316. Olofsson J, van Nostrand AW. Adenoid cystic carcinoma of the larynx: a report of four cases and a review of the literature. *Cancer* 1977;40:1307–1313.
317. Damiani JM, Damiani KK, Hauck K, et al. Mucoepidermoid–adenosquamous carcinoma of the larynx and hypopharynx: a report of 21 cases and a review of the literature. *Otolaryngol Head Neck Surg* 1981;89:235–243.
318. Ferlito A, Recher G, Bottin R. Mucoepidermoid carcinoma of the larynx. A clinicopathological study of 11 cases with review of the literature. *ORL J Otorhinolaryngol Rel Spec* 1981;43:280–299.
319. Ho KJ, Jones JM, Herrera GA. Mucoepidermoid carcinoma of the larynx: a light and electron microscopic study with emphasis on histogenesis. *South Med J* 1984;77:190–195.
320. Gerughty RM, Hennigar GR, Brown FM. Adenosquamous carcinoma of the nasal, oral and laryngeal cavities. A clinicopathologic survey of ten cases. *Cancer* 1968;22:1140–1155.
321. Ellis GL, Auclair PL, Gnepp DR, et al. Other malignant epithelial neoplasms. In: Ellis GL, Auclair PL, Gnepp DR, eds. *Surgical pathology of the salivary gland.* Philadelphia: WB Saunders, 1991: 455–488.
322. Sanderson RJ, Rivron RP, Wallace WA. Adenosquamous carcinoma of the hypopharynx. *J Laryngol Otol* 1991;105:678–680.
323. Gorenstein A, Neel HBD, Weiland LH, et al. Sarcomas of the larynx. *Arch Otolaryngol* 1980;106:8–12.
324. Moran CA, Suster S, Carter D. Laryngeal chondrosarcomas. *Arch Pathol Lab Med* 1993;117:914–917.
325. Nakayama M, Brandenburg JH, Hafez GR. Dedifferentiated chondrosarcoma of the larynx with regional and distant metastases. *Ann Otol Rhinol Laryngol* 1993;102:785–791.
326. Devaney KO, Ferlito A, Silver CE. Cartilaginous tumors of the larynx. *Ann Otol Rhinol Laryngol* 1995;104:251–255.
327. Bogdan CJ, Maniglia AJ, Eliachar I, et al. Chondrosarcoma of the larynx: challenges in diagnosis and management. *Head Neck* 1994;16:127–134.
328. Gripp S, Pape H, Schmitt G. Chondrosarcoma of the larynx: the role of radiotherapy revisited—a case report and review of the literature. *Cancer* 1998;82:108–115.
329. Ferlito A. Laryngeal fibrosarcoma: an over-diagnosed tumor. *ORL J Otorhinolaryngol Rel Spec* 1990;52:194–195.
330. Ferlito A. Cartilaginous and osteogenic neoplasms. In: Ferlito A, ed. *Neoplasms of the larynx.* New York: Churchill Livingstone, 1993: 305–326.
331. Ferlito A, Nicolai P, Montaguti A, et al. Chondrosarcoma of the larynx: review of the literature and report of three cases. *Am J Otolaryngol* 1984;5:350–359.
332. Sztern J, Sztern D, Fonseca R, et al. Chondrosarcoma of the larynx. *Eur Arch Otorhinolaryngol* 1993;250:173–176.
333. Lewis JE, Olsen KD, Inwards CY. Cartilaginous tumors of the larynx: clinicopathologic review of 47 cases. *Ann Otol Rhinol Laryngol* 1997;106:94–100.
334. Burtner D, Goodman M, Montgomery W. Elastic cartilaginous metaplasia of vocal cord nodules. *Ann Otol Rhinol Laryngol* 1972;81: 844–847.
335. Ferlito A, Recher G. Chondrometaplasia of the larynx. *ORL J Otorhinolaryngol Rel Spec* 1985;47:174–177.
336. Hyams VJ, Rabuzzi DD. Cartilaginous tumors of the larynx. *Laryngoscope* 1970;80:755–767.
337. Cantrell RW, Reibel JF, Jahrsdoerfer RA, et al. Conservative surgical treatment of chondrosarcoma of the larynx. *Ann Otol Rhinol Laryngol* 1980;89:567–571.

338. Weber AL, Shortsleeve M, Goodman M, et al. Cartilaginous tumors of the larynx and trachea. *Radiol Clin North Am* 1978;16:261–267.
339. Goethals PL, Dahlin DC, Devine KD. Cartilaginous tumors of the larynx. *Surg Gynecol Obstet* 1963;117:77–82.
340. Wippold FJD, Smirniotopoulos JG, Moran CJ, et al. Chondrosarcoma of the larynx: CT features. *Am J Neuroradiol* 1993; 14:453–459.
341. Wilkinson AHD, Beckford NS, Babin RW, et al. Extraskeletal myxoid chondrosarcoma of the epiglottis: case report and review of the literature. *Otolaryngol Head Neck Surg* 1991;104:257–260.
342. Brandwein M, Moore S, Som P, et al. Laryngeal chondrosarcomas: a clinicopathologic study of 11 cases, including two "dedifferentiated" chondrosarcomas. *Laryngoscope* 1992;102:858–867.
343. Bleiweiss IJ, Kaneko M. Chondrosarcoma of the larynx with additional malignant mesenchymal component (dedifferentiated chondrosarcoma). *Am J Surg Pathol* 1988;12:314–320.
344. Lichtenstein L, Jaffe HL. Chondrosarcoma of bone. *Am J Pathol* 1943;19:553–587.
345. Escher A, Escher F, Zimmermann A. [Clinical aspects and pathology of chondromatous tumors of the larynx.] *HNO* 1984;32:269–285.
346. Winther LK, Lorentzen M. Rhabdomyosarcoma of the larynx. Report of two cases and a review of the literature. *J Laryngol Otol* 1978;92:417–424.
347. DeGroot TR, Frazer JP, Wood BP. Combination therapy for laryngeal rhabdomyosarcoma. *Am J Otolaryngol* 1980;1:456–460.
348. Dodd-o JM, Wieneke KF, Rosman PM. Laryngeal rhabdomyosarcoma. Case report and literature review. *Cancer* 1987;59:1012–1018.
349. Balazs M, Egerszegi P. Laryngeal botryoid rhabdomyosarcoma in an adult. Report of a case with electron microscopic study. *Pathol Res Pract* 1989;184:643–649; discussion 649–651.
350. Da Mosto MC, Marchiori C, Rinaldo A, et al. Laryngeal pleomorphic rhabdomyosarcoma. A critical review of the literature. *Ann Otol Rhinol Laryngol* 1996;105:289–294.
351. Gapany-Gapanavicius B, Behar AJ, Chisin R. Synovial sarcoma of the hypopharynx. *Ann Otol Rhinol Laryngol* 1978;87:356–359.
352. Quinn HJ Jr. Synovial sarcoma of the larynx treated by partial laryngectomy. *Laryngoscope* 1984;94:1158–1161.
353. Pruszczynski M, Manni JJ, Smedts F. Endolaryngeal synovial sarcoma: case report with immunohistochemical studies. *Head Neck* 1989;11:76–80.
354. Chew KK, Sethi DS, Stanley RE, Sng I. View from beneath: pathology in focus. Synovial sarcoma of hypopharynx. *J Laryngol Otol* 1992;106:285–287.
355. Ramamurthy L, Nassar WY, Hasleton PS, et al. Synovial sarcoma of the pharynx. *J Laryngol Otol* 1995;109:1207–1210.
356. Gridelli C, Palmieri G, Airoma G, et al. Complete regression of laryngeal involvement by classic Kaposi's sarcoma with low-dose alpha-2b interferon. *Tumori* 1990;76:292–293.
357. Schiff NF, Annino DJ, Woo P, et al. Kaposi's sarcoma of the larynx. *Ann Otol Rhinol Laryngol* 1997;106:563–567.
358. Goldberg AN. Kaposi's sarcoma of the head and neck in acquired immunodeficiency syndrome. *Am J Otolaryngol* 1993;14:5–14.
359. Friedman M, Venkatesan TK, Caldarelli DD. Intralesional vinblastine for treating AIDS-associated Kaposi's sarcoma of the oropharynx and larynx. *Ann Otol Rhinol Laryngol* 1996;105:272–274.
360. Mochloulis G, Irving RM, Grant HR, et al. Laryngeal Kaposi's sarcoma in patients with AIDS. *J Laryngol Otol* 1996;110:1034–1037.
361. Barnes L, Ferlito A. Soft tissue neoplasms. In: Ferlito A, ed. *Neoplasms of the larynx.* New York: Churchill Livingstone, 1993:265–304.
362. Ferlito A, Nicolai P, Recher G, et al. Primary laryngeal malignant fibrous histiocytoma: review of the literature and report of seven cases. *Laryngoscope* 1983;93:1351–1358.
363. Allsbrook WC Jr, Harmon JD, Chongchitnant N, et al. Liposarcoma of the larynx. *Arch Pathol Lab Med* 1985;109:294–296.
364. Wenig BM, Weiss SW, Gnepp DR. Laryngeal and hypopharyngeal liposarcoma. A clinicopathologic study of 10 cases with a comparison to soft-tissue counterparts. *Am J Surg Pathol* 1990;14:134–141.
365. Ferlito A. Primary pleomorphic liposarcoma of the larynx. *J Otolaryngol* 1978;7:161–166.
366. Ferlito A, Nicolai P, Barion U. Critical comments on laryngeal fibrosarcoma. *Acta Otorhinolaryngol Belg* 1983;37:918–925.
367. Rohn GN, Close LG, Vuitch F, et al. Fibrous neoplasms of the adult larynx. *Head Neck* 1994;16:227–231.
368. McKiernan DC, Watters GW. Smooth muscle tumours of the larynx. *J Laryngol Otol* 1995;109:77–79.
369. DeLozier HL. Intrinsic malignant schwannoma of the larynx. A case report. *Ann Otol Rhinol Laryngol* 1982;91:336–338.
370. Ferlito A, Nicolai P, Caruso G. Angiosarcoma of the larynx. Case report. *Ann Otol Rhinol Laryngol* 1985;94:93–95.
371. Ferlito A. Primary malignant haemangiopericytoma of the larynx (a case report with autopsy). *J Laryngol Otol* 1978;92:511–519.
372. Abramowsky CR, Witt WJ. Sarcoma of the larynx in a newborn. *Cancer* 1983;51:1726–1730.
373. Dahm LJ, Schaefer SD, Carder HM, et al. Osteosarcoma of the soft tissue of the larynx: report of a case with light and electron microscopic studies. *Cancer* 1978;42:2343–2351.
374. Berge JK, Kapadia SB, Myers EN. Osteosarcoma of the larynx. *Arch Otolaryngol Head Neck Surg* 1998;124:207–210.
375. Myssiorek D, Patel M, Wasserman P, et al. Osteosarcoma of the larynx. *Ann Otol Rhinol Laryngol* 1998;107:70–74.
376. Kawashima O, Kamei T, Shimizu Y, et al. Malignant mesenchymoma of the larynx. *J Laryngol Otol* 1990;104:440–444.
377. Eble JN, Hull MT, Bojrab D. Laryngeal blastoma. A light and electron microscopic study of a novel entity analogous to pulmonary blastoma. *Am J Clin Pathol* 1985;84:378–385.
378. Horny HP, Kaiserling E. Involvement of the larynx by hemopoietic neoplasms. An investigation of autopsy cases and review of the literature. *Pathol Res Pract* 1995;191:130–138.
379. Ansell SM, Habermann TM, Hoyer JD, et al. Primary laryngeal lymphoma. *Laryngoscope* 1997;107:1502–1506.
380. Hisashi K, Komune S, Inoue H, et al. Coexistence of MALT-type lymphoma and squamous cell carcinoma of the larynx. *J Laryngol Otol* 1994;108:995–997.
381. Horny HP, Ferlito A, Carbone A. Laryngeal lymphoma derived from mucosa-associated lymphoid tissue. *Ann Otol Rhinol Laryngol* 1996; 105:577–583.
382. Ferguson JL, Maragos NE, Weiland LH. Granulocytic sarcoma (chloroma) of the epiglottis. *Otolaryngol Head Neck Surg* 1987; 97:588–590.
383. Horny HP, Parwaresch MR, Kaiserling E, et al. Mast cell sarcoma of the larynx. *J Clin Pathol* 1986;39:596–602.
384. Gordon LJ, Lee M, Conley JJ, et al. Mycosis fungoides of the larynx. *Otolaryngol Head Neck Surg* 1992;107:120–123.
385. Kuhn JJ, Wenig BM, Clark DA. Mycosis fungoides of the larynx. Report of two cases and review of the literature. *Arch Otolaryngol Head Neck Surg* 1992;118:853–858.
386. el-Barbary Ae-S, Fouad HA, el-Sayed AF. Malignant melanoma involving the larynx: report of two cases. *Ann Otol Rhinol Laryngol* 1968;77:338–343.
387. Reuter VE, Woodruff JM. Melanoma of the larynx. *Laryngoscope* 1986;96:389–393.
388. Wenig BM. Laryngeal mucosal malignant melanoma. A clinicopathologic, immunohistochemical, and ultrastructural study of four patients and a review of the literature. *Cancer* 1995;75:1568–1577.
389. Whicker JH, Carder GA, Devine KD. Metastasis to the larynx. Report of a case and review of the literature. *Arch Otolaryngol* 1972; 96:182–184.
390. Ferlito A. Secondary neoplasms. In: Ferlito A, ed. *Neoplasms of the larynx.* New York: Churchill Livingstone, 1993:349–360.
391. Wenig BM. Malignant melanoma. In: Ferlito A, ed. *Neoplasms of the larynx.* New York: Churchill Livingstone, 1993:207–230.
392. Pesce C, Toncini C. Melanin pigmentation of the larynx. *Acta Otolaryngol (Stockh)* 1983;96:189–192.
393. Travis LW, Sutherland C. Coexisting lentigo of the larynx and melanoma of the oral cavity: report of a case. *Otolaryngol Head Neck Surg* 1980;88:218–220.
394. Freeland AP, van Nostrand AW, Jahn AF. Metastases to the larynx. *J Otolaryngol* 1979;8:448–456.

8

SALIVARY GLANDS

MARIO A. LUNA

GENERAL CONSIDERATIONS

Embryogenesis

All of the major salivary glands are ectodermally derived, and they all arise in fundamentally the same manner, by the growth of oral epithelium into the underlying mesenchyme (1). The epithelial buds that form the parotid and submandibular glands appear in the sixth week of embryonic life, and those of the sublingual glands appear during the seventh to eighth week.

At the future site of the exit of the excretory ducts of the salivary glands, the oral epithelium thickens and forms a solid bud of epithelial cells that grow into the underlying mesenchyme. Cell proliferation and cleavage between terminal cell groups eventually result in the development of a multiply branched structure of epithelial strands. Each strand is completely surrounded by richly vascularized mesenchymal tissue. Terminal clusters of epithelial cells are found at the tips of the most distal branches. A tubuloalveolar pattern is formed when terminal cell clusters differentiate into round or oblate alveoli. After this tubuloalveolar character is established, the individual cells undergo further cytodifferentiation of ductal and secretory end pieces in preparation for their various functions (2). The secretory end pieces are connected to the developing ductal system by the terminal tubule complex. It is generally accepted that the reserve cells of the excretory duct and the intercalated duct act as stem cells for the most differentiated cells of the salivary gland unit. Excretory duct stem cells give rise to the columnar and squamous cells of those ducts, and intercalated duct stem cells give rise to the acinar cells, other intercalated duct cells, striated duct cells, and probably to the myoepithelial cells (3). The first salivary gland to appear is the parotid, when the crown–rump length of the embryo is about 10 mm. The submandibular and sublingual glands appear at 18 mm and 22 mm, respectively.

Histologic Appearance

Salivary glands in histologic sections appear as numerous lobules separated from each other by connective tissue septa. Each gland is entirely surrounded by a connective tissue capsule that may be substantial in some glands and rather insignificant in others.

The ducts of the salivary glands form a tree-like pattern. The finest branches are the intercalated ducts; the larger branches on the stem form the excretory ducts. Striated ducts usually are present between the intercalated and excretory ducts. The acini are terminally located at the tips of the intercalated ducts. Excretory and striated ducts are located in the connective tissue septa, and smaller striated ducts, intercalated ducts, and acini make up the bulk of the lobules.

The acini consist of a number of pyramidal cells arranged around a central lumen with myoepithelial cells interposed between the acinus and the basement membrane. The acinar cells may be serous, mucinous, or seromucinous. Serous cells are found predominantly in the parotid gland and in variable amounts in the submandibular gland (Fig. 1). Mucinous cells are found in the sublingual and submandibular glands, in many minor salivary glands, and in small amounts in the parotid glands of young individuals (Fig. 2). The sublingual gland generally contains a higher percentage of mucinous cells than the submandibular gland. Seromucinous cells are found in the sublingual glands and in many minor salivary glands. The intercalated ducts are formed by a single layer of cuboidal cells; myoepithelial cells may appear between these cells and the basal lamina (Fig. 3). The striated ducts are lined by a single layer of tall to low columnar eosinophilic cells, and fine striations are present at the basal portion of the cytoplasm (Fig. 2). The excretory ducts are located entirely within connective tissue septa; they are lined by usually two (but sometimes multiple) layers of epithelial cells that may vary in shape from cuboidal to squamous (Fig. 4).

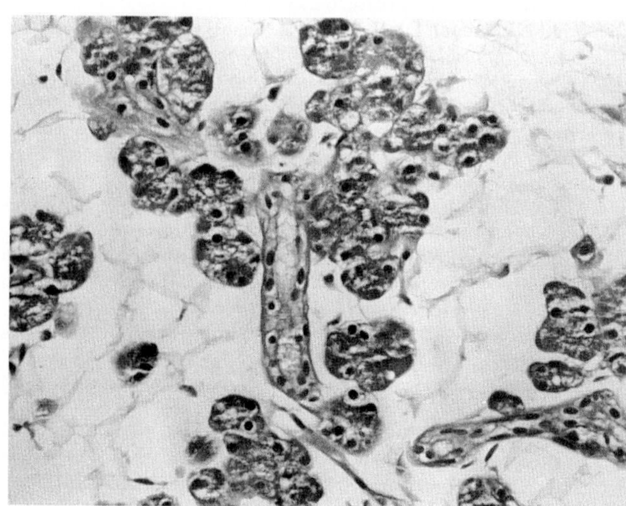

FIGURE 1. Parotid intercalated ducts lie in contact with the acinus. Note serous character of parotid acini.

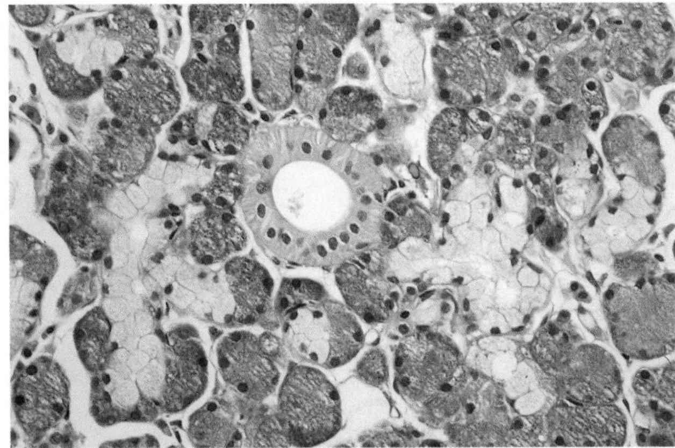

FIGURE 2. Transverse section of striated duct lined by columnar epithelium with a basal striated appearance. Note acini with mucous and serous cells of the submandibular gland.

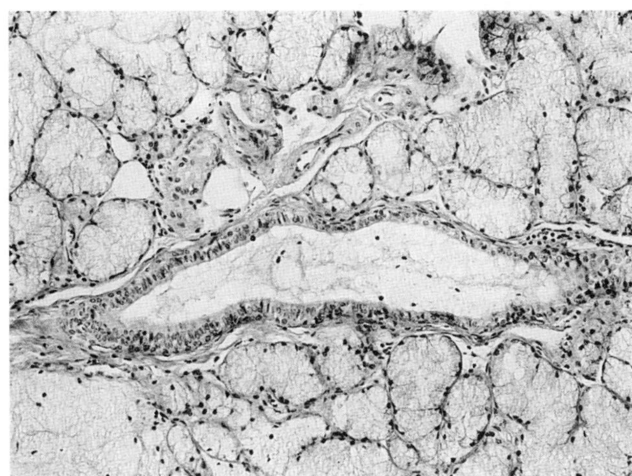

FIGURE 4. Excretory duct lined by columnar pseudostratified epithelium. Note mucous type of acini of minor salivary glands of palate.

The most active part of the salivary gland duct unit is at the junction of the intercalated ducts and the acini (Fig. 1). Intercalated ducts are probably the source of reserve cells. Under certain influences, the reserve cells may proliferate and differentiate into a number of cellular types, such as acinar cells, intercalated duct cells, and myoepithelial cells. It is also from this cellular zone of the salivary duct unit that most tumors of the salivary glands arise (3).

Under normal circumstances, sebaceous cells occur in the parotid gland. They arise from intercalated and striated ducts (Fig. 5). Oncocytic changes in salivary glands are not infrequent accompaniments of aging. The preexisting epithelial cells become enlarged and acquire a granular eosinophilic cytoplasm (Fig. 6).

The lymphoid tissue of the salivary glands is represented by lymph nodes located near or within the parotid gland and by scattered lymphoid cells located in the connective tissue around the acini and ducts. The latter are thought to be part of the mucosa-associated lymphoid tissue (MALT) (4). As early as the sixth week of intrauterine life in the 16-mm embryo, a complete anatomic relationship exists between the parotid anlage and the developing system of the upper cervical lymph nodes. Proximity and contact of these anlagen explain both the entrapment of salivary tissue within lymph nodes and the development of lymph nodes within the parotid gland.

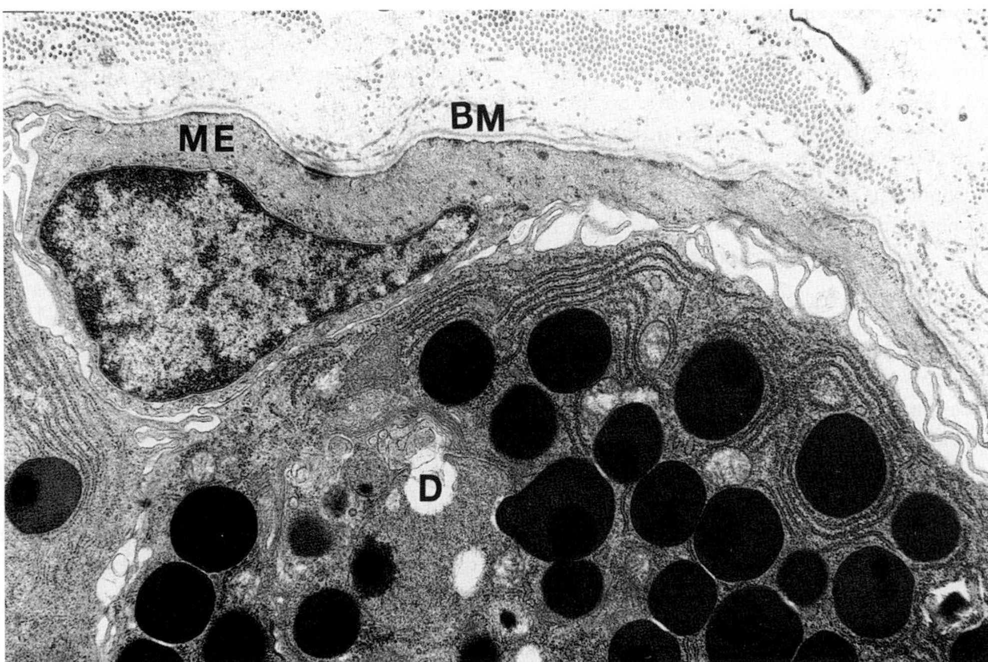

FIGURE 3. Electron microscopic appearance of intercalated duct with a myoepithelial cell (ME) situated between the ductal cell (D) and the basal membrane (BM).

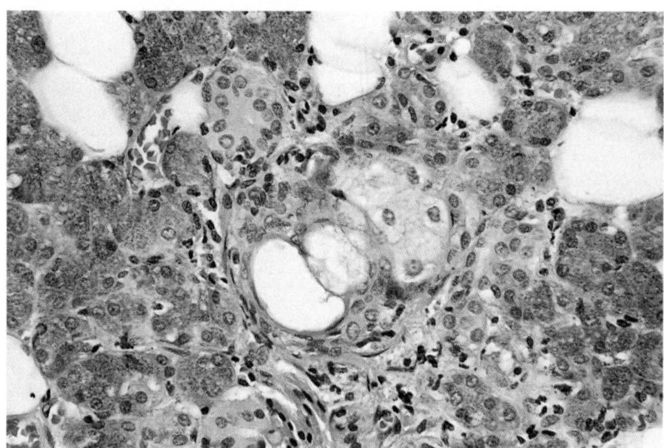

FIGURE 5. Sebaceous cells in parotid gland.

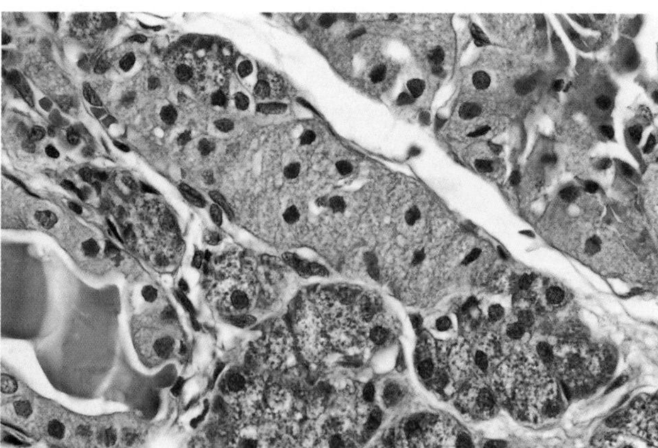

FIGURE 6. Oncocytic changes in parotid gland. Note the abundant and granulated eosinophilic cytoplasm.

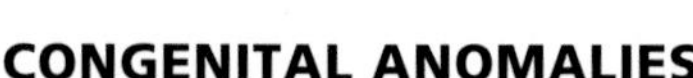

CONGENITAL ANOMALIES

Heterotopia

The presence of salivary gland tissue outside the major salivary glands and the upper aerodigestive tract is considered heterotopia. Such heterotopia may be intralymphatic or extralymphatic.

Intralymphatic heterotopia is more common, and it occurs more often in the lymph nodes near the parotid gland; it is much less frequent in the submandibular region and other upper cervical nodes (5). The glandular elements are either normal or atrophic; they consist mainly of intercalated and intralobular ducts, but acini are also found. They are localized in the medullary region and make up a variable proportion of lymphoid and salivary tissue.

Extralymphatic heterotopias are rare and often latent, but they may be symptomatic. Depending on their location, they are classified as high or low forms. High heterotopia is limited to the mandible, ear, mylohyoid muscle, pituitary gland, and cerebellopontine angle (6). Heterotopia in all of these sites except the last may be related to the embryonic migration of the salivary glands. The low type of heterotopia is localized in the base of the neck, particularly around the sternoclavicular joint and in the thyroid gland. Low heterotopia is related to the branchial apparatus and is found in association with cysts and sinuses in the lower neck (7).

Neoplastic transformation in heterotopic salivary tissue is very rare. Most instances reported are in the mandible (8) and in the upper cervical lymph nodes (9,10). Pleomorphic adenoma, mucoepidermoid carcinoma, adenoid cystic carcinoma, and acinic cell carcinoma are the most common neoplasms arising in heterotopic salivary tissue. In fact, heterotopia may be an explanation for many aberrant salivary neoplasms and some cervical lymph node metastases that are regarded as metastases of unknown primary origin (3).

Accessory Salivary Glands

Accessory parotid gland tissue is defined as salivary tissue adjacent to Stensen's duct and separate from the main body of the parotid gland (11). This serves to distinguish accessory parotid glands from an anterior facial process in which parotid tissue extends anteriorly from the main gland but remains in continuity with it. As judged by anatomic dissections, approximately 20% of human parotid glands manifest accessory tissue (11). The accessory parotid tissue is variable in size, position, and shape. They are, however, usually pea- to kidney-bean-sized and flat. The tissue most often lies on or above the parotid duct and between the buccal branch of the facial nerve and the duct. There is no histologic difference between the accessory tissue and the parotid gland proper. Accessory parotid tissue is heir to all diseases afflicting the parotid gland (11).

Other Congenital Anomalies

Aplasia, hypoplasia, and *duct atresia* of the salivary glands are fairly rare and usually of no functional significance. Duct anomalies include *diverticula,* especially of the submandibular gland, and *congenital sialectasia* of the parotid gland (11).

INFLAMMATORY AND NONNEOPLASTIC LESIONS

Cysts

Cysts of salivary gland origin belong to one of three types: dysgenetic cysts, secondary acquired cysts lined by epithelium (duct cysts, lymphoepithelial cysts, and retention mucoceles), and pseudocysts without epithelial lining (extravasation mucoceles) (11). The nonneoplastic cysts and pseudocysts form about 6% of all lesions of the salivary glands at the salivary gland register of the Pathological Institute of the University of Hamburg (Table 1) (12). Seventy-five percent of these lesions are mucoceles of the minor salivary glands, followed in decreasing order of frequency by parotid duct cysts (11%), lymphoepithelial cysts (7%), and ranulas (5%). Congenital sialectasia and dysgenetic cysts are vary rare (2%).

One should also keep in mind that some salivary gland neoplasms may undergo prominent cystic changes. This is particularly true of mucoepidermoid carcinoma, sebaceous lymphade-

TABLE 1. FREQUENCY OF SALIVARY GLAND DISEASES

Salivary Gland Diseases	Number of Cases	Percentage of Total
Salivary gland tumors	2,704	37.4
Sialadenitis	2,050	28.3
Neck dissection with salivary glands	709	9.8
Other lesions	605	8.4
Salivary gland cysts	499	6.9
Lymph node diseases of the salivary glands	372	5.1
Sialadenosis	297	4.1
Total	7,236	100.0

Modified from Seifert G, Michlke A, Hanubrich J, et al. *Diseases of the salivary glands: Pathology, diagnosis, treatment, facial nerve surgery*. Stuttgart: Georg Thieme, 1986.

noma, Warthin's tumor, cystic adenocarcinoma, and occasionally pleomorphic adenoma. Nonneoplastic cysts must also be distinguished from cystic changes in the ducts occurring in certain forms of chronic sialadenitis such as chronic sialectatic parotitis and the chronic myoepithelial parotitis of Sjögren's syndrome.

Polycystic (dysgenetic) disease of the parotid glands is the rarest of the nonneoplastic cystic lesions. Its clinical characteristics include the following:

1. It has been found almost exclusively in females.
2. Overt clinical signs are usually delayed, even in adulthood.
3. There is almost always bilateral parotid gland involvement.
4. A history of fluctuating nontender parotid gland swelling for several years is antecedent to surgical intervention.
5. Sialograms show cystic alterations with the main parotid duct uninvolved.
6. Surgical procedures are used for diagnosis or cosmesis (13).

Viewed microscopically, the cysts vary in size and are lined by different types of duct epithelium (Fig. 7). Their structure resembles that of the intercalated or striated ducts and also that of the primitive duct bulbs of the embryonal period. Secretory products within the cysts range from a watery fluid to inspissated, often laminated, microliths or spheroliths. These may be congophilic. Remnants of gland tissue with acini are recognized between the cysts, but inflammatory changes are absent.

The abnormality leading to polycystic parotid disease is likely developmental. Its pathogenesis has been related to disturbance in the ramification and canalization of the duct system during the second stage of the development of the salivary gland that extends to the end of the seventh embryonal month (14). Another unusual dysgenetic cyst is the Merkel cyst of the submandibular gland. It is caused by distortion and segmentation of the duct. The cysts are usually lined by flattened epithelium (11).

Salivary duct cysts occur mainly in the parotid gland and constitute about 10% of all nonneoplastic cysts of the salivary glands (11). The peak incidence is in the second decade, and 77% occur in male patients. The cysts are lined by several layers of ductal epithelium, but they may also be flat (Fig. 8). Oncocytic and squamous metaplasia can occur. The lumen is filled with secretions containing spheroliths and crystalline precipitate. Small granulomas formed by extravasated mucin can be seen in the interstitium. In the course of time, focal obstructive parotitis develops in the majority of patients (11). Duct obstruction plays an important role in the pathogenesis of these cysts (e.g., kinking of the duct, duct stenosis, microliths).

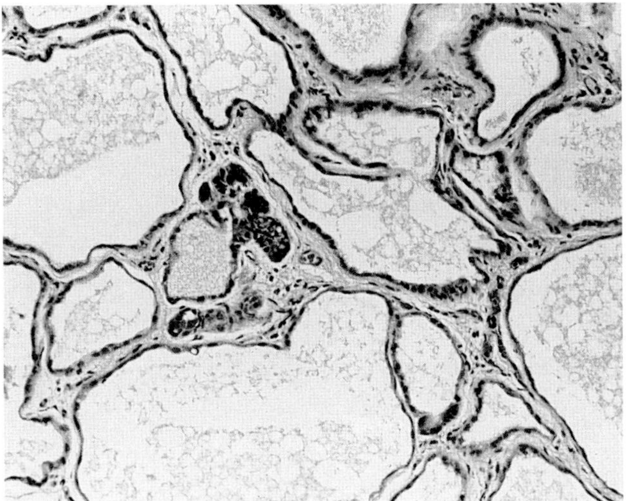

FIGURE 7. Polycystic (dysgenetic) disease of parotid gland showing multiple epithelial cysts of varying size.

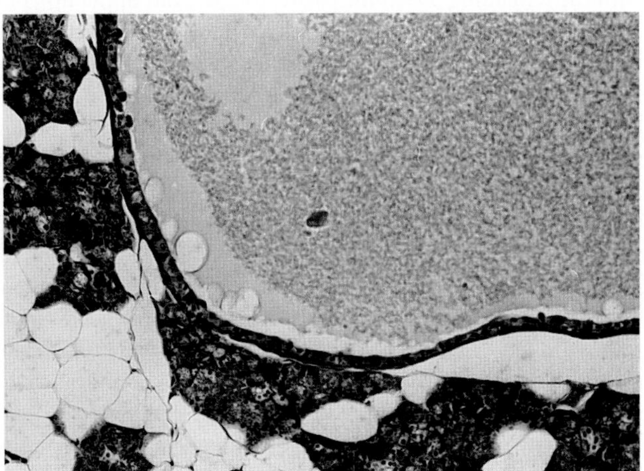

FIGURE 8. Salivary duct cyst with characteristic epithelial lining.

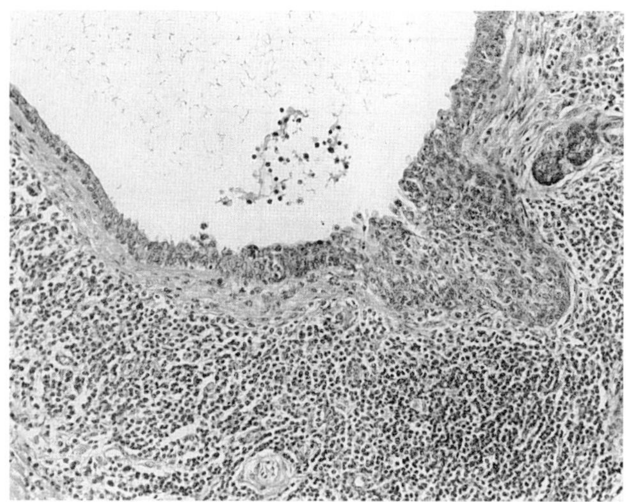

FIGURE 9. Lymphoepithelial cyst of the parotid gland lined by stratified epithelium.

Lymphoepithelial cysts are found in the parotid gland, parotid lymph nodes, and in the floor of the mouth (15,16). Histologically, the cysts are lined by flattened, multilayered epithelium that is always surrounded by lymphoid stroma with lymphoid follicles (Fig. 9) (15,17). Occasional sebaceous gland and goblet cells may be present within the epithelial lining. The formation of these cysts seems to be related to the displacement of epithelium into lymphoid stroma, analogous to that of salivary gland inclusions in the parotid lymph nodes (5). Proliferation of branchial pouch–derived epithelium induced by the lymphoid proliferation has been suggested by several authors as the cause (7). This cyst belongs to the group of lymphoepithelial salivary gland lesions including benign lymphoepithelial lesion, chronic myoepithelial sialadenitis, and HIV-related cystic lymphohyperplasia (11).

Mucoceles are mucosal swellings of varying sizes that contain mucus. Two types are recognized: extravasation and retention. *Extravasation mucoceles* are by far the most common; 85% of mucoceles are of this type. Their most common location is the lower lip (80%), followed by the cheek or floor of the mouth (15%), with the remaining 5% in the palate, tongue, and upper lip (11). Extravasation mucoceles are more common in boys and men (60%), and their peak incidence occurs in the second decade of life. Histologically, three stages of development of the lesion have been described. The initial stage is characterized by the formation of ill-defined lakes of mucin in the interstitium and parenchyma. In the resorption phase, mucous granulomas are formed. They contain histiocytes, macrophages, foamy cells, and giant cells in whose cytoplasm resorbed masses of mucus can be demonstrated. The end phase is marked by the formation of mucus-filled pseudocysts with a connective tissue capsule lacking epithelial lining (Fig. 10) (11). A *ranula* is a special form of extravasation mucocele from the sublingual gland or duct; the lesion extends into the soft tissue of the floor of the mouth above the mylohyoid muscle. There are two types of ranula: simple (intraoral) and deep (plunging). The latter are referred to also as cervical ranulas because they invade downward into the tissues of the neck (18).

Retention mucoceles are common in people older than 20 years, and they are distributed evenly among the minor salivary glands (lower lip, cheek, upper lip, palate, and floor of the mouth) (11). Microscopically, the cysts are lined by epithelium and contain mucous material; a thick connective tissue capsule surrounds the structure (11). The epithelial lining may be flat, cuboidal, or multilayered, resembling the various segments of the duct system. Microliths, an inspissated secretion, or bends in the duct system play the main role in the pathogenesis of the retention mucoceles (11).

Sialolithiasis

Lithiasis (the formation of calculi) in the head and neck occurs in two forms: sialolithiasis and angiolithiasis. The former is much more common and is exclusively salivary; the later is vascular-based, sometimes salivary, but more often found in oral or perioral soft tissues (19). Salivary calculi are usually diagnosed by clinical and radiographic findings. Angioliths may be asymptomatic. They are often incidental findings and can be mistaken clinically for sialoliths.

Sialoliths can originate in any salivary gland, but the submandibular gland is by far the preponderant gland. This may be related to the more tortuous course of the submanibular, as opposed to the parotid, duct and to the more mucinous nature of submandibular, as opposed to parotid, secretion. In a review of 1,200 cases of salivary calculi, 83% occurred in the submandibular gland, 10% in the parotid gland, and 7% in the sublingual gland (11). The frequency was minor in the salivary tissue of the upper lip and buccal mucosa (20).

The consequence of salivary calculi is that they cause ductal obstructions. Recurrent bouts of tender glandular swelling, especially during meals when secretions are stimulated, are typical. If the obstruction is not relieved, chronic obstructive sialadenitis follows. Because of the large size and location of the submandibular glands, sialoliths found therein may often be palpated. Radiographic examination is diagnostically effective for calculi at this duct's bending point, but it is less contributory for intraparenchymal sialoliths. Radiographic examination is more

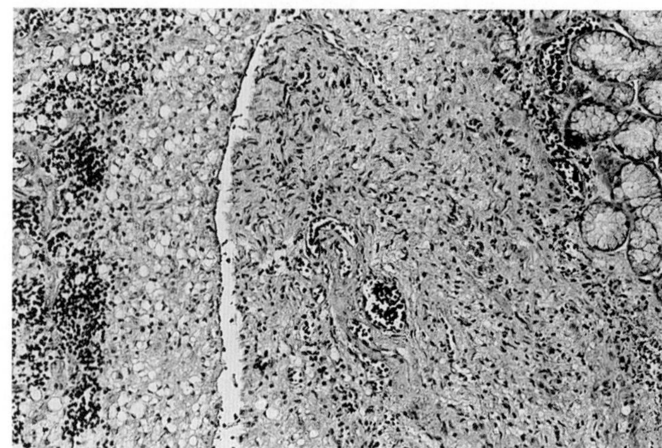

FIGURE 10. Extravasation mucocele. Extravasation of mucus into connective tissue, with abundant muciphages.

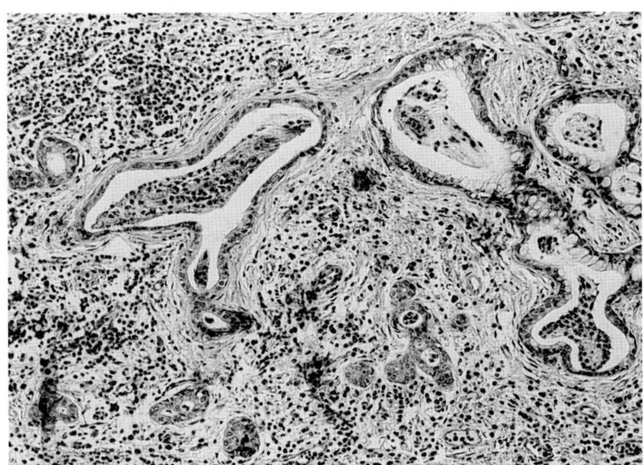

FIGURE 11. Ductal ectasia with periductal fibrosis and inflammation in a case of sialolithiasis.

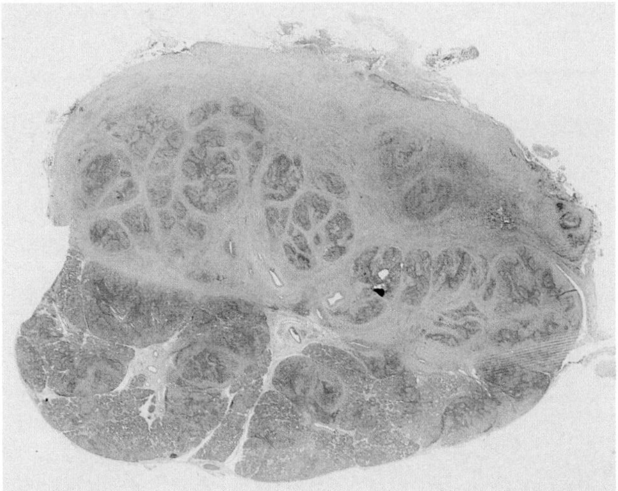

FIGURE 12. Whole organ section of chronic sclerosing sialadenitis of the submandibular gland, also known as "Kuttner's tumor."

more important in parotid gland sialoliths because they are less likely to be palpable (11).

Microscopic examination of tissue from glands that were affected by calculi shows dilation of ducts, often with squamous metaplasia, variable destruction of acinar tissue, modest or severe chronic inflammation, and varying degrees of fibrosis (Fig. 11) (21).

Surgical treatment for submandibular and parotid duct calculi depends on the accessibility of the calculi. If they are near the ostium of the duct, their removal may be feasible (11). Disintegration of the calculus may be achieved with techinques such as intracorporeal or extracorporeal shock wave lithotripsy (22).

Sialadenitis

The majority of specific acute and chronic inflammatory diseases that may affect the major salivary glands and their internal or nearby lymph nodes are primarily diagnosed by clinical symptomatology (11). Acute suppurative sialadenitis is caused by *Staphylococcus aureus, Streptococcus* spp., and gram-negative bacteria. Once an abscess has formed, surgical excision of the gland may be necessary. Viral sialadenitis can be caused by cytomegalovirus, paramyxovirus, Epstein-Barr virus, influenza and parainfluenza viruses, and coxsackievirus (23). The histologic patterns of these infectious diseases in salivary glands are similar to those in other sites.

Granulomatous inflammation in salivary tissue is most often a response to liberated ductal contents, particularly mucin, in various degrees of obstructive sialadenopathy (24). Far less often, granulomatous sialadenitis is the result of specific infective granulomas or a systemic granuloma-forming disease. In these instances, the involvement of the salivary gland parenchyma is usually secondary to disease localization in regional lymph nodes (24). The parotid parenchyma, however, may be involved by multiple granulomas in the variant of sarcoidosis known as *Heerfordt's disease,* or uveoparotid fever (11). In our experience, the granulomatous diseases that are often mistaken clinically for a neoplasm are tuberculosis, cat-scratch disease, and toxoplasmosis (25,26) (see Chapter 12).

Chronic sclerosing sialadenitis of the submandibular gland (Kuttner's tumor) is a unilateral disorder histologically characterized by a plasmacytic and lymphocytic periductal infiltrate that eventually leads to encasement of the ducts in thick fibrous tissue (Fig. 12) (27). Clinically, the lesion cannot be distinguished from a neoplasm. The diagnosis is made after the submandibular gland has been removed. Smith et al. (28) recently described a distinctive histopathologic sclerotic lesion, under the name of sclerosing polycystic adenosis, that is histologically reminiscent of fibrocystic disease of the breast.

Irradiation Effects

The parotid and submandibular glands are often included in the field of irradiation for tumors of the head and neck. These glands, particularly the submandibular, may become enlarged, firm, and clinically may simulate metastatic carcinoma following radiation treatment (29,30). Microscopic examination shows a decrease in acinar elements, the presence of chronic inflammatory cells, and interstitial fibrosis (Fig. 13).

Sialadenosis

Sialadenosis, characterized by uniform hypertrophy and hyperplasia of the acinar parenchyma of salivary glands, is associated with a variety of systemic diseases or functional disorders (31). Present evidence relates the clinical and morphologic changes in the salivary tissues to a neuropathic alteration of the autonomic innervation of the salivary acini. Sialadenosis has been classified into three major types: neurogenic, dystrophic-metabolic, and hormonal (32). In most instances, sialadenosis presents as a painless, recurrent bilateral swelling of the parotid glands.

Microscopic examination of tissue from experimental animals and from humans with parotid sialadenosis shows a characteristic increase in acinar diameter. Control tissue samples of parotid

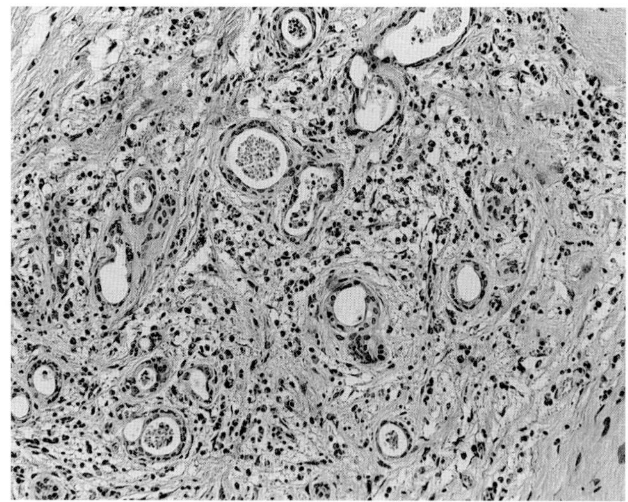

FIGURE 13. Irradiation changes in submandibular gland. Note absence of acini, persistence of ducts, and presence of chronic inflammatory cells.

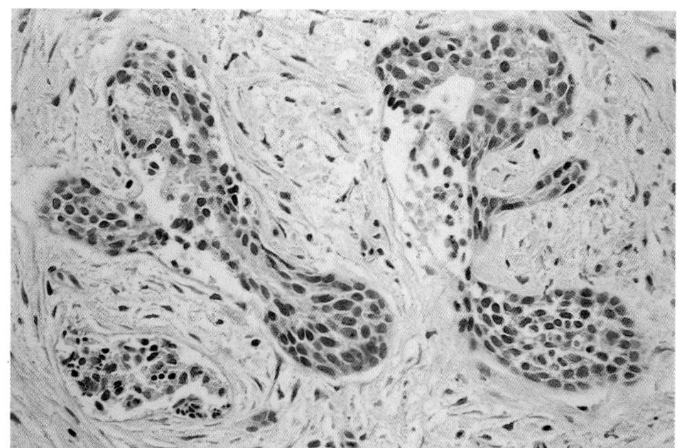

FIGURE 14. Necrotizing sialometaplasia showing squamous metaplasia of ducts and acini in affected lobule.

acini have a diameter of 30 μm. Sialadenotic acini have a mean diameter of up to 100 μm (32). There is uniform hypertrophy and hyperplasia of the functional acinar parenchyma. Inflammation is characteristically absent. Donath and Seifert (33) ultrastructurally distinguish three types of sialadenosis: a type with dark granules, one with light granules, and one with mixed granules. It should be noted, however, that there is no correlation between these electron optic forms and the clinical presentation of sialadenosis (31).

Necrotizing Sialometaplasia

Necrotizing sialometaplasia is a benign, self-healing, reactive, necroinflammatory process of salivary gland tissue that histologically and clinically simulates malignancy (34). Necrotizing sialometaplasia most commonly involves the intraoral minor salivary glands, particularly those of the palate (35–37). However, the major salivary glands and the minor salivary glands of the upper aerodigestive tract can be affected (36,38,39). Review of the literature shows that the most common site of occurrence of necrotizing sialometaplasia is the palate with 77% of cases identified at this location. Ten percent of the cases are found in other oral cavity sites, 9% in the major salivary glands, and 4% in miscellaneous sites of the upper aerodigestive tract (35).

Necrotizing sialometaplasia occurs primarily in patients between the ages of 40 and 60 and has been reported more frequently in men than in women (35). Pathogenesis remains the subject of some controversy. Most authors feel that the likely cause is vascular compromise to the affected salivary glands, which results in infarction and subsequent tissue necrosis (38,39). In mucosal sites, it often takes the form of a deep-seated ulcer, with or without an antecedent swelling or mass. A nonulcerated mass accounts for only about one third of the reported cases, including mucosal and nonmucosal parenchymal cases. Painful lesions are about twice as common as those without symptoms (35). Paresthesias or anesthesias may also be noted. The ulcers typically heal in 6 to 12 weeks.

Histologically, there is a zonal or lobular distribution of the changes (34,39). Centrally, the preexisting salivary duct system exhibits squamous metaplasia (Fig. 14). Peripheral to this are necrotic acini with acute and chronic inflammation. Surrounding this area of necrosis, uninvolved intact salivary gland tissue is present. The recognition of this zonal or lobular distribution is necessary for proper diagnois (39).

Histologic features that are helpful in diagnosing necrotizing sialometaplasia can be summarized as follows: (a) lobular infarction and necrosis of the affected salivary gland; (b) benign-appearing squamous cells; (c) metaplasia of ducts and acini producing rounded or smooth edges; (d) prominent granulation tissue reaction and inflammatory tissue components; and (e) maintenance of lobular architecture (Fig. 15). Identification of these features will help to differentiate necrotizing sialometaplasia from squamous cell carcinoma or mucoepidermoid carcinoma (36,39).

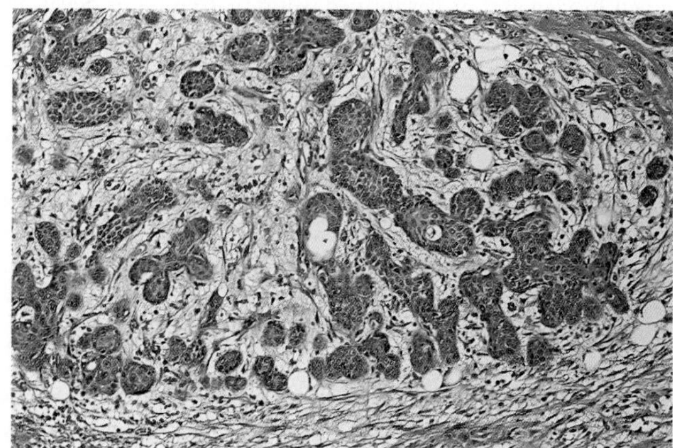

FIGURE 15. Necrotizing sialometaplasia. The preservation of lobular architecture is a hallmark of this lesion. Note that salivary lobules are in different stages of evolution of the disease process.

Lymphoepithelial Lesions and Sjögren's Syndrome

Benign lymphoepithelial lesions or myoepithelial sialadenitis of salivary glands begin with a focal periductal lymphoreticular proliferation and progress to partial or total replacement of the functioning acinar parenchyma. These lesions are associated with several clinical disorders (40). A lesion may signify a salivary gland disease without systemic manifestations, or it may be a tissue manifestation of autoimmune disease or primary or secondary Sjögren's syndrome (41,42). The incidence of similar lesions is markedly increased in human immunodeficiency virus (HIV)-infected patients (43) and in intravenous drug users at high risk for HIV infection (44) (See below).

Microscopically, the lesion is charaterized by a heavy lymphocytic infiltration of the salivary parenchyma and by the presence of epimyoepithelial islands (45) (Fig. 16). The lymphoid tissue contains well-formed germinal centers and is composed of a mixed population of B and T lymphocytes, plasma cells, histiocytes, and dendritic reticulum cells. The epithelial islands consist of two distinct cell types, basal epithelial cells and modified myoepithelial cells; there is very little involvement of the ductal cells (46). The hyaline material deposited between cells is shown by electron microscopy to represent basal lamina material (47). The changes are similar in minor salivary glands of the oral cavity, except for the fact that the epimyoepithelial islands are usually scant or absent (48).

Sjögren's syndrome is a clinical diagnosis that may be made if any two or all three of the following symptoms are present: keratoconjunctivitis sicca, xerostomia, and rheumatoid arthritis or any other connective tissue disease such as disseminated lupus erythematosus, progressive scleroderma, polymyositis, or polyarteritis nodosa (11).

The presence or absence of a coexisting autoimmune disease has led to classification of the syndrome as either primary or secondary (49). The primary form is a disease process resulting from lymphocyte-mediated destruction of exocrine glands that leads to decreased or absent glandular secretions and consequent mucosal dryness. Principal exocrine targets are the major salivary glands in the head and neck, but exocrine elements in the lungs, gastrointestinal tract, and elsewhere have also been affected (50). The secondary form of the syndrome is defined as the exocrinopathy associated with, or followed by, another autoimmune systemic disease (49).

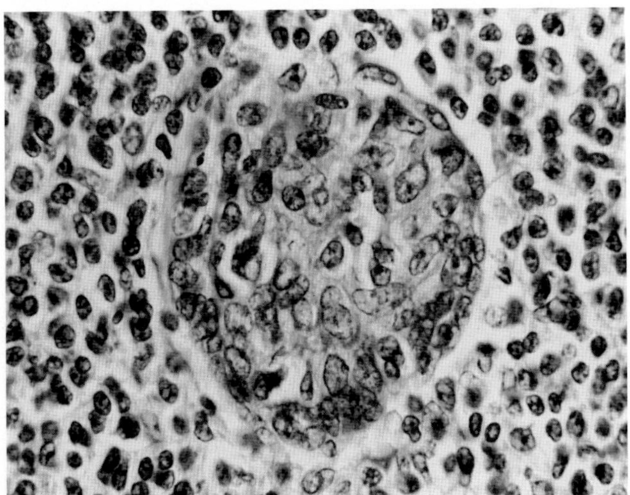

FIGURE 16. Lymphoepithelial lesion of parotid gland with lymphocytic infiltrate and epimyoepithelial island.

Clinicians often seek to confirm a diagnosis of either primary or secondary Sjögren's syndrome by the histologic demonstration of a salivary gland component (42). The labial glands are now established as the preferred site from which to take a biopsy specimen (48,51). The specimen should be taken only from normal-appearing lower labial mucosa between the midline and the commissure. The best biospy technique for procuring labial salival tissue is the one described by Daniels (52). A trephine or "punch biopsy" is not recommended because it usually does not provide enough glandular tissue for microscopic evaluation.

The routine histologic preparation of a labial biopsy specimen demonstrates a wide range in the degree to which salivary glands are affected by inflammation, acinar atrophy, and fibrosis. Periductal and perivascular hyaline deposits may also be noted (53). Further characterization of the focal sialadenitis may be achieved by a focus score. The focus score is defined as the number of foci of inflammatory cells per 4 mm^2 of gland in the tissue section (52,54). A focus is considered to represent a localized collection of at least 50 lymphoid cells. Correlative studies have consistently indicated that a salivary gland biospy score >1 focus per 4 mm^2 is an acceptable threshold for a diagnosis of the salivary component of Sjögren's syndrome. A focus score of 1 suggests the possiblilty of syndrome, but specimens with score <1 or nonfocal chronic inflammation should be considered as being either within normal limits or nondiagnostic (52,54).

The advent of lymphoma in patients with Sjögren's syndrome is significant, especially in women. The lymphomas are almost exclusively non-Hodgkin's in type and may be salivary or extrasalivary (55,56). Most of these neoplasms are of MALT type. Others have the appearance of small cleaved-cell or small lymphocytic lymphomas, with some of the latter exhibiting plasmacytoid features (56). The proposal has been made that these neoplasms belong to the group of lymphomas of mucosa-associated lymphoid tissue (MALT) of the parotid gland (56) (see Chapter 12). Occasionally, a unilaterial, poorly differentiated salivary carcinoma (lymphoepithelial carcinoma) may arise in patients with a benign lymphoepithelial lesion (57,58). This represents a poorly differentiated carcinoma with prominent lymphoid stroma and should not be confused with lymphoma.

The risk of the development of a malignant neoplasm in patients with benign lymphoepithelial lesion, with or without Sjögren's syndrome, has been analyzed carefully by Kassan et al. (59). The relative risk for nonlymphatic malignancy (malignant lymphoepithelial lesion) is increased only slightly to 1.2:1. For non-Hodgkin's lymphoma, the relative risk increases dramatically to 43.8:1.

Cystic Lymphoid Hyperplasia in HIV-Positive Patients

Cystic lymphoid hyperplasia or cystic lymphoepithelial lesion is a nodular or diffuse enlargement of salivary glands observed in

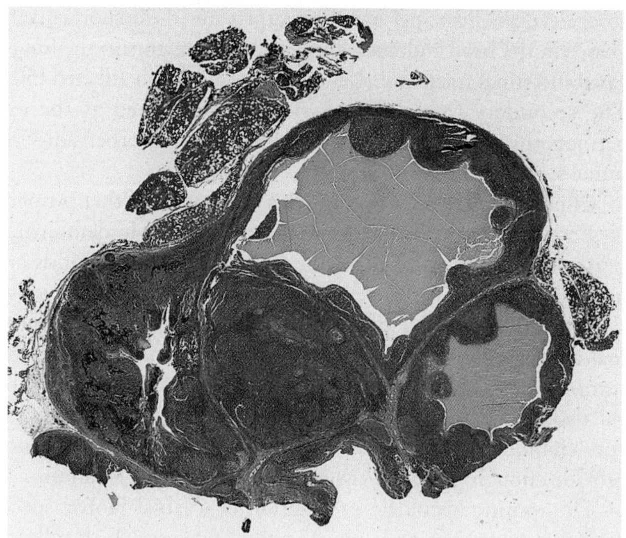

FIGURE 17. Whole organ section of cystic lymphoid hyperplasia in an HIV-positive patient. Note cystic spaces and prominent lymphoid hyperplasia.

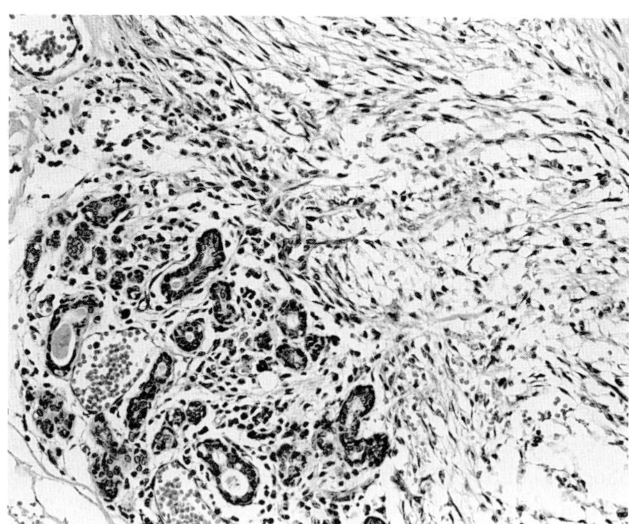

FIGURE 18. Haphazardly arranged fascicles of spindle cells in an inflammatory pseudotumor of the parotid gland.

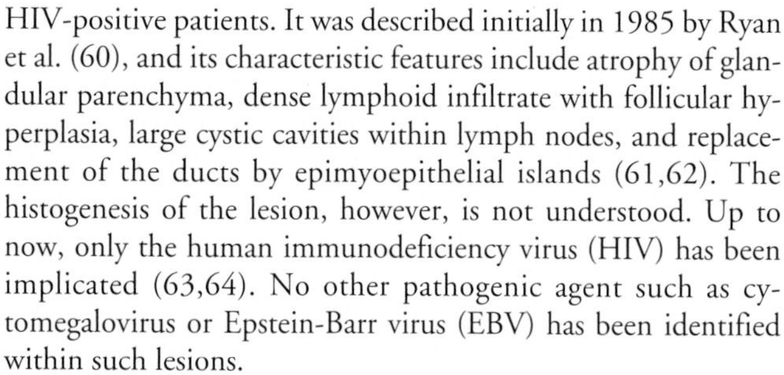

HIV-positive patients. It was described initially in 1985 by Ryan et al. (60), and its characteristic features include atrophy of glandular parenchyma, dense lymphoid infiltrate with follicular hyperplasia, large cystic cavities within lymph nodes, and replacement of the ducts by epimyoepithelial islands (61,62). The histogenesis of the lesion, however, is not understood. Up to now, only the human immunodeficiency virus (HIV) has been implicated (63,64). No other pathogenic agent such as cytomegalovirus or Epstein-Barr virus (EBV) has been identified within such lesions.

The pathologic features consist of hyperplastic lymphoid tissue analogous to that described in HIV-associated, persistent generalized lymphadenopathy in association with gross epithelial cysts within lymph nodes (Fig. 17). The cystic cavities are filled with a mucoid and gelatinous substance. The cystic spaces are lined by epithelium of variable thickness infiltrated by lymphocytes. The lining epithelium is derived from salivary duct inclusions within lymph nodes. The proliferative epithelial cystic component might represent an exuberant reaction to HIV infection (63,64).

Inflammatory Pseudotumors

Inflammatory pseudotumor is a pathologic term used to describe reactive pseudoneoplastic phenomena that can occur in many parts of the body. Among the salivary glands, all the cases described have occurred in the parotid gland. The lesions contain an admixture of four histologic elements: myofibroblasts, histiocytes, plasma cells, and lymphocytes (Fig. 18). Immunohistochemical studies by Williams et al. (65) have shown a biphasic spindle cell population of myofibroblasts and histiocytes with variable staining for smooth muscle actin (SMA), muscle specific actin (MSA), vimentin, and KP 1(CD3).

Histologic Changes Induced by Fine-Needle Aspiration

Fine-needle aspiration (FNA) is widely used to investigate salivary gland masses (see Chapter 14). Although FNA usually causes only minor histologic changes that do not interfere with subsequent histologic assessment, it may on occasion result in changes that obscure the underlying pathologic process or mislead the unwary to an erroneous diagnosis of malignancy (66). Particularly vulnerable to this are Warthin's tumor, oncocytoma, and pleomorphic adenoma with a myoepithelial preponderance (66). The histologic changes include necrosis, hemorrhage, acute and subacute inflammation, and epithelial or connective tissue cell proliferation in response to injury (Fig. 19). Squamous metaplasia is frequent, and cellular atypia can be seen. All of these are potential pitfalls in histologic interpretation (66,67).

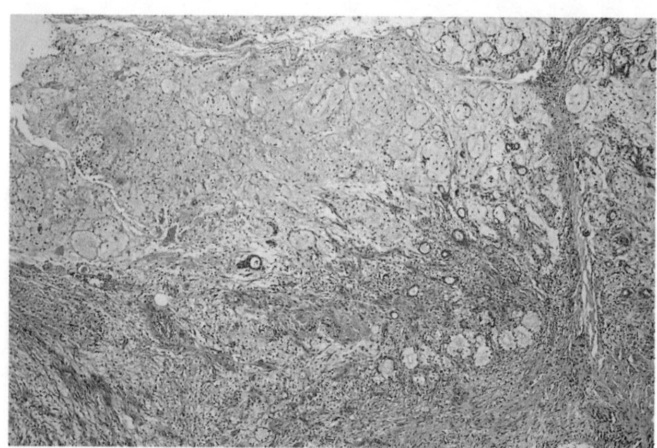

FIGURE 19. Spindle cell proliferation and mucous extravasation after fine-needle aspiration of a parotid tumor.

Other Nonneoplastic Conditions

Nodular fasciitis (68), amyloidosis (69,70), sinus histiocytosis with massive lymphadenopathy (or Rosai-Dorfman disease) (71), Wegener's granulomatosis (72), trichomoniasis (73), and lymphoid disorders of a reactive nature affecting the parotid lymph nodes all have been described in the salivary glands, especially in the parotid glands.

NEOPLASTIC DISEASES: GENERAL CONSIDERATIONS

Salivary gland neoplasms are uncommon, but they generate considerable interest and debate because of their remarkable variation in histologic appearance, clinical presentation, and behavior.

Histogenesis and Classification

Three types of tumors must be distinguished in the region of the salivary glands:

1. *Sialadenoma* or *sialoma* is a tumor of the salivary gland parenchyma.
2. *Synsialadenoma* or *synsialoma* is a tumor that arises within the salivary gland capsule and stroma from the supporting connective tissues such as fibrous tissue, blood vessels, and nerves.
3. *Parasialadenoma* or *parasialoma* is a neoplasma of the surrounding tissues that may simulate a salivary gland tumor.

Tumors of the salivary parenchyma, or sialomas, are the most common and by far the most important of all neoplasms involving these structures. Current classifications of tumors of the salivary gland parenchyma are based on their morphologic, cytologic, and biological features (74–78). Because observers do not universally agree on the cell of origin, for the present, histogenetic classifications are premature. The classification used in this chapter, presented in Table 2, is the one suggested by the World Health Organization (WHO) (75) with slight modifications. This classification has proved to be useful in daily practice and has been by and large adopted by the Armed Forces Institute of Pathology (AFIP) (74,76). It is also the basis of the tumor classifications used by the Salivary Gland Registry at the Pathology Institute of the University of Hamburg (11) and by the British Salivary Gland Panel (77,78).

At least two theories of tumorigenesis have been proposed for salivary gland neoplasms (79,80). In the bicellular theory, two basal cell or stem cell populations give rise to mature cells and also to neoplasms in the salivary glands. From one population, intercalated duct cells and myoepithelial cells arise, and from the other set, excretory duct cells arise. Hence, despite the seeming heterogeneity of these tumors, all of them are predicted to arise from one of two cell populations. In this model, gland-like tumors including pleomorphic adenoma, oncocytoma, acinic cell carcinoma, and adenoid cystic carcinoma are all derived from one set of basal cells, and epidermoid tumors such as mucoepidermoid carcinomas are derived from the second set.

TABLE 2. HISTOLOGIC CLASSIFICATION OF SALIVARY GLAND TUMORS

- Adenomas
  - Pleomorphic adenoma (mixed tumor)
  - Myoepithelioma (myoepithelial adenoma)
  - Basal cell adenoma
  - Warthin's tumor (adenolymphoma)
  - Oncocytoma (oncocytic adenoma)
  - Canalicular adenoma
  - Sebaceous adenoma
  - Ductal papilloma
    - Inverted ductal papilloma
    - Intraductal papilloma
    - Sialadenoma papilliferum
  - Cystadenoma
  - Papillary cystadenoma
  - Mucinous cystadenoma
- Carcinomas
  - Acinic cell carcinoma
  - Mucoepidermoid carcinoma
  - Adenoid cystic carcinoma
  - Terminal duct adenocarcinoma (polymorphous low-grade adenocarcinoma)
  - Epithelial–myoepithelial carcinoma
  - Basal cell adenocarcinoma
  - Sebaceous carcinoma
  - Papillary cystadenocarcinoma
  - Mucinous adenocarcinoma
  - Oncocytic carcinoma
  - Salivary duct carcinoma
  - Hyalinizing clear cell carcinoma
  - Adenocarcinoma NOS
  - Myoepithelial carcinoma (malignant myoepithelioma)
  - Malignant mixed tumor
    - Carcinoma *ex* pleomorphic adenoma
    - Carcinosarcoma (true malignant mixed tumor)
    - Metastasizing mixed tumor
  - Squamous cell carcinoma
  - Small-cell carcinoma
  - Undifferentiated carcinoma
  - Other carcinomas
- Nonepithelial tumors
- Malignant lymphomas
- Secondary tumors
- Unclassified tumors
- Tumor-like lesions

Modified from Seifert G. Histological typing of salivary gland tumors. In: *World Health Organization International Histological Classification of Tumours, 2nd ed.* Berlin: Springer-Verlag, 1991.

In the multicellular theory, each neoplasm is matched to a cell type within the salivary gland unit. Warthin's and oncocytic tumors are thought to arise from striated ductal cells, squamous and mucoepidermoid carcinomas from excretory duct cells, and pleomorphic adenomas from intercalated duct cells and myoepithelial cells. The experimental observation that all differentiated salivary cell types retain the ability to undergo mitosis and regenerate further supports this theory and suggests that no limitations exist for a potential neoplastic cell of origin (81). An important question associated with these two theories is whether the tumor cell population is formed by derangement of a differentiated cell (82) or whether it arises from one or more pluripotent stem cells (83).

Recent studies using molecular techniques appear to support the unicellular origin of the salivary gland tumors from a stem cell, and the results are not consistent with the bicellular or multicellular theory (84,85).

Incidence

The annual incidence of salivary gland tumors varies around the world from approximately 0.4 to 13.5 per 100,000 people (86). Auclair et al. (87) estimated that the annual incidence of both benign and malignant salivary gland neoplasms in the United States is between 2.2 and 2.5 cases in 100,000 people. Spiro and associates reported that at Memorial Sloan-Kettering Cancer Center, patients with salivary gland tumors accounted for about 1% of all admissions and for 6.5% of all the tumors seen in the Head and Neck Service of that center (88).

Clinical Findings

Epithelial tumors are the most common neoplasms of the major salivary glands. In most large series, benign tumors are three to four times more common than are malignant tumors. The percentage varies from 54.5% to 79.0% (11,74–79).

The age and sex of patients with salivary gland tumors varies so much that firm conclusions cannot be drawn, although the following general guidelines can be stated. Salivary gland tumors are encountered in people of all ages, but the peak incidence is the third decade of life. Women are affected more than men; the proportion reported varies from 9:1 to 2.1:1. Patients with malignant tumors are older. The median ages of patients with benign and malignant tumors are 46 and 55 years, respectively. In adults, the great majority of neoplasms are epithelial tumors, whereas the nonepithelial tumors, hemangiomas, and lymphangiomas occur mainly in children (11,74–79).

In the United States, salivary gland tumors are more common in white than in black patients (87). Warthin's tumors are notable for their rarity among blacks, but pleomorphic adenomas, carcinoma *ex* pleomorphic adenoma, and adenocarcinoma not otherwise specified (NOS) appear to be disproportionately more common in African-American patients than among white patients (87,88). According to Auclair et al., the greatest proportion of tumors among patients of Asian extraction (from the files of the AFIP) are pleomorphic adenomas and cystadenomas (87).

The most common neoplasm of salivary origin in all series is the pleomorphic adenoma, representing 70% of the benign neoplasms and 45% of all tumors. The most common malignant tumor in most series is the mucoepidermoid carcinoma, accounting for one third of all malignant neoplasms (11,87,88). Following in decreasing order of frequency are adenoid cystic carcinoma, acinic cell carcinoma, adenocarcinoma NOS, and carcinoma *ex* pleomorphic adenoma.

A salivary gland tumor may be localized or diffuse, mobile or fixed, painless or painful. It may affect only a specific part of the gland, or it may affect the entire body of the gland. The function of the facial nerve may be affected by a parotid tumor because of the close relationship between the gland and the nerve. Partial or complete paralysis of the facial nerve provides important information about the nature of the tumor. Facial paralysis is observed almost exclusively in malignant tumors (11).

Distribution

Although the distribution of salivary gland tumors appears to vary from series to series, an estimated 80% of tumors occur in the parotid gland, and 5% to 10% in the submandiabular, 1% in the sublingual, and 9% in the minor salivary glands (11,74–79,87,88). In addition, the proportion of malignant neoplasms varies by sites. In the parotid gland, about 20% of all tumors are malignant, whereas in the submandibular and minor salivary glands, 45% are malignant. In the sublingual gland, as many as 90% of all tumors are malignant (88,89).

Etiology

Little is known about the cause or causes of salivary gland tumors. An association between external radiotherapy to the head and neck and subsequent salivary tumors has been noted (90). A similar association has been noted in Japanese survivors of the atomic bomb (91), in children irradiated for tinea capitis (92), and in persons whose enlarged tonsils and adenoids were irradiated during childhood (93).

Elevated proportionate mortality ratios for salivary cancers have been demonstrated in the rubber industry in Ohio (94), in plumbers in Washington (95), and in woodworkers employed in the automobile industry (96). In all instances, the observed numbers were extremely small. Hormonal factors, severe malnutrition, and exposure to viruses have also been implicated in the cause of salivary gland tumors (97,98). The association of salivary gland carcinomas with breast and skin cancers is of interest; however, the conflicting conclusions among various studies diminsh their value and their clinical applications (99).

Unilateral or Bilateral Tumors

Multiple salivary tumors in the same patient are recorded repeatedly (100). The tumors may be unilateral or bilateral, with the same or a different histologic picture; and they may be synchronous or metachronous (101). The neoplasms that more often are bilateral, either synchronous or metachronous, are Warthin's tumor, pleomorphic adenoma, acinic cell carcinoma, and oncocytoma (101,102).

Biopsy

The results of a biopsy form the foundation on which the diagnosis and treatment plan of any neoplasm is based. Therefore, biospy becomes the *sine qua non* of oncologic surgery. The frozen section technique, the preoperative fine-needle aspiration cytologic examination, the core needle biopsy, and the incisional and excisional biopsy are discussed.

Incisional Biopsy

Except for tumors of the minor salivary glands and perhaps for neoplasms of the sublingual gland, an incisional biospy should not be performed (see below).

Excisional Biopsy

For tumors in the lateral lobe of the parotid gland, the minimal procedure is superficial or lateral parotidectomy (79). This procedure allows the surgeon to remove the tumor in question in its entirety, to identify the facial nerve and its branches, and to remove the parotid lymph nodes. In addition, it provides the pathologist with the best possible diagnostic material. For tumors in the submandibular gland, the gland should be removed completely along with the regional lymph nodes and periglandular soft tissues. This technique allows the surgeon to determine clearly the relationships among the gland, the neoplasm, and the lingual, hypoglossal, and mylohyoid nerves (79).

Frozen Section

The accuracy of frozen section diagnosis of salivary gland lesions (98%) compares favorably with the accuracy rate when this technique is used on tissue from other organs of the body (98.6%) (87,103). However, in 21 series reviewed by Auclair et al. (87), the overall average accuracy rate was slightly lower (96.2%). Furthermore, if salivary gland lesions are divided into benign and malignant groups, it is apparent that the accuracy rates for the benign group are excellent. In the malignant group the accuracy rates with and without deferred diagnoses are 77% and 85.7%, respectively (87). Most problems arise in recognition of cellular pleomorphic adenomas, in some oncocytomas, in mucoepidermoid carcinomas, and in lymphomas (87,103–105).

Unless a precise diagnosis modifies the surgical procedure, the indication for frozen section is to evaluate the surgical margins of excision (79,88). The plan for surgical treatment of parotid gland tumors and submandibular gland tumors is based primarily on their size, the anatomic structures involved by the tumor, and the clinical stage of disease (79,88). These variables cannot be assessed accurately until the tumor is surgically exposed.

Preoperative Fine-Needle Aspiration Cytology

The overall type-specific diagnostic accuracy of preoperative FNA for benign and malignant neoplasms of salivary glands is high (more than 80%). The accuracy rate is higher for benign tumors (96.5%) than it is for malignant tumors (74.3%). The sensitivity of the diagnosis is about 80%, and the specificity is higher than 98% (87,106). Difficulties arise, particularly in distingushing poorly differentiated mucoepidermoid carcinoma, poorly differentiated acinic cell carcinoma, and pleomorphic adenomas of variable histologic patterns (107). Cystic changes can also lead to difficulties in interpretation. Carcinoma arising in pleomorphic adenoma can be missed in limited samples, and a false-negative result may be generated.

For this reason, correct typing of the wide variety of salivary gland neoplasms on the basis of cytologic smears is difficult and requires a highly qualified cytologist and a well-trained procurer of the specimen to ensure a correct interpretation.

The pros and cons of this procedure have been extensively discussed by several authors (87,106–110). In my opinion and those of others, FNA is indicated in the following circumstances: when the surgeon is not sure if the lesion represents a nonneoplastic process or a neoplasm; when the patient is a poor surgical risk; when the neoplasm is not resectable; in patients with a history of a previous malignancy; in children (because of the high incidence of nonneoplastic lesions); and as triage in certain institutions so that patients with malignant neoplasms may receive early surgery (66). It is important to recall the statement of Johns and Kaplan (79): "The lack of a preoperative tissue diagnosis (of salivary gland neoplasms) does not alter the surgical approach." In the same vein, Spiro (88) states that treatment decisions were not significantly influenced by aspiration results even when a correct diagnosis was obtained.

Core Needle Biopsy

Core needle biopsy is helpful in differentiating neoplastic from nonneoplastic disorders, in diagnosing metastatic cancers, and in patients in whom surgical intervention is contraindicated. In other circumstances, this procedure is not reliable. In contrast to FNA, core needle biopsy has not achieved popularity in the diagnosis of salivary gland diseases. Furthermore, core needle biopsy has many disadvantages compared with aspiration cytology, and the risk of complications is considerably greater after core biospy (87).

Ancillary Histologic Diagnostic Methods

Hematoxylin and eosin (H&E) has long been the standard tissue stain used by pathologists; in the large majority of cases, this type of stain alone permits an accurate diagnosis. Histochemistry, immunohistochemistry, and electron microscopy studies are ancillary rather than primary diagnostic methods (11). Molecular techniques are so far used primarily for investigation, but they take third place behind histologic and ancillary methods. Histologic diagnosis is the only certain foundation for correct treatment.

Histochemistry

No specific battery of histochemistry studies is unique for the demonstration of diseases of the salivary glands (11). The histochemistry of mucins and enzymes in tumors of these glands has been extensively studied, though its value as a diagnostic measure has not been particularly impressive (111). Mucin stains (mucicarmine, alcian blue) (pH 2.5), and periodic acid–Schiff (PAS) (with and without diastase digestion) are the most useful special stains for establishing a diagnosis. Mucoepidermoid carcinomas are differentiated from squamous cell carcinoma by the presence of goblet or signet-ring cells with large mucicarmine- and alcian blue-positive droplets in their cytoplasm (11,112). The cytoplasm of at least some of the cells in acinic cell carcinomas contains PAS-positive, diastase-resistant secretory granules (112). Epithelial–myoepithelial carcinomas of salivary gland origin and metastatic renal cell carcinomas do not exibit PAS-positive, diastase-resistant granules in the cytoplasm, and they may or may not contain glycogen. In addition, these tumors do not have mucicarmine- or alcian blue-positive secretions (11,112).

Electron Microscopy

The extent to which electron microscopy can aid in identifying neoplasms of the salivary glands varies. It may provide a specific diagnosis not otherwise obtainable, or it may offer information that is as easily available on routine light microscopy (11). Despite its variable contribution, it is especially reliable in the identification of atypical acinic cell carcinomas, in questionable oncocytic tumors, in clear cell carcinomas and in distingushing undifferentiated carcinomas from lymphomas (113). However, electron microscopy does not distinguish benign from malignant tumors.

Immunohistochemistry

There are several reasons why it is important to determine the immunohistochemical profile of salivary gland tumors. A profile may be useful in the differential diagnosis of poorly differentiated neoplasms (i.e., carcinoma, lymphomas, melanoma), of certain primary tumors (myoepithelial tumors, acinic cell carcinoma, neuroendocrine carcinomas), and of metastatic lesions (i.e., thyroid carcinoma, melanoma) (11,75). The immunohistochemical profile of each type of tumor is discussed along with the pathology of each.

DNA Content

Assessment of DNA content by means of scanning cytophotometry or flow cytometry can be helpful in the evaluation of salivary gland neoplasms. DNA aneuploidy and S-phase fractions are potential prognostic indicators for malignant salivary tumors, and DNA analysis may assist in the characterization of such neoplasms (114,115). This technique is of value in the analysis of mucoepidermoid carcinomas, adenoid cystic carcinomas, and adenocarcinoma NOS. However, the tests do not provide additional information for acinic cell carcinomas, epithelial–myoepithelial carcinomas, and terminal duct adenocarcinomas, as virtually all of these tumors have diploid histograms (75).

Molecular Techniques and Cytogenetics

The study of oncogene alterations in salivary gland tumors remains an important tool in oncogenesis research (116–119). The utility of oncogenic biomarkers is not that they can furnish prognostic information but rather that they may predict recalcitrance of disease to specific therapies (120,121).

Cytogenetic studies of salivary gland neoplasms have been limited mainly to pleomorphic adenomas (122) and used less for terminal duct carcinomas and mucoepidermoid carcinomas (123,124).

Clinical Staging

A clinical staging system using the TNM classification scheme for salivary gland tumors has been designed. This system is based on five parameters: size of the primary tumor, local extension, palpability of the regional lymph nodes, degree of suspicion for positivity of the regional lymph nodes, and the presence or absence of distant metastases (75,125). The TNM classification provides a uniform system for recording, reporting, and comparing this data.

EPITHELIAL NEOPLASMS

Approximately 88% of salivary gland neoplasms are of epithelial origin (11,74–80), and there are two distinct groups of epithelial tumors. Benign adenomas account for 65.5% of salivary tumors, and malignant epithelial neoplasms account for 22.5% (11,74–79,88). In this chapter, when possible, the benign neoplasms are discussed together with their malignant counterparts.

Pleomorphic Adenoma and Malignant Mixed Tumor

Pleomorphic Adenoma (Mixed Tumor)

Definition

Pleomorphic adenoma is

> a tumor of variable capsulation characterized microscopically by architectural rather than cellular pleomorphism. Epithelial and modified myoepithelial elements intermingle with tissue of mucoid, myxoid, or chondroid appearance. The epithelial and myoepithelial components form ducts, strands, sheets, or structures resembling a swarm of bees. Squamous metaplasia is found in about 25% of pleomorphic adenomas. (75)

Clinical Data

Pleomorphic adenomas (mixed tumors) are the most common neoplasms of the salivary glands and account for 55% to 70% of all neoplasms of the major glands (11,74–79,88). They are most frequent in women in the fourth decade of life, but they are also found in children and elderly persons of either sex (126–129). The usual clinical manifestation is that of a painless, slowly growing, firm mass located in the parotid gland, the submandibular region, or the palate. Paralysis of the facial nerve by pleomorphic adenoma of the parotid gland is rare (130). Approximately 84% of these tumors are located in the parotid glands, 10% in the minor glands of the upper aerodigestive tract, 5% in the submandibular glands, and 0.1% in the sublingual glands (126,127). In the parotid gland, 90% arise within the superficial lobe, most from either the lower (50%) or the anterior portion (25%). The remaining 10% arise in the deep lobe and often present as an oropharyngeal submucosal mass without external evidence of tumor (131).

Radiologic Studies

Magnetic resonance imaging and computed tomography studies have been applied to the study of parotid tumors and may yield valuable information, especially for tumors situated in the deep lobe of the gland. Both techniques can show the tumor margins and whether the mass is multicentric or a single lobulated mass. Computed tomography is less effective in demonstrating tumor margins, but it shows the calcifications that are often present in pleomorphic adenomas (132,133).

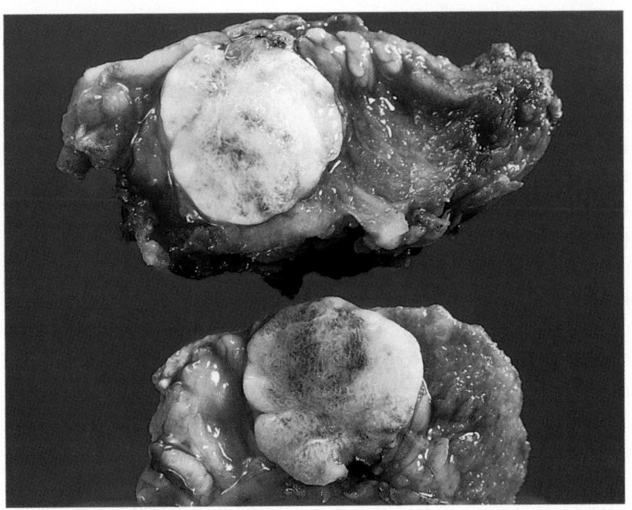

FIGURE 20. Gross appearance of pleomorphic adenoma.

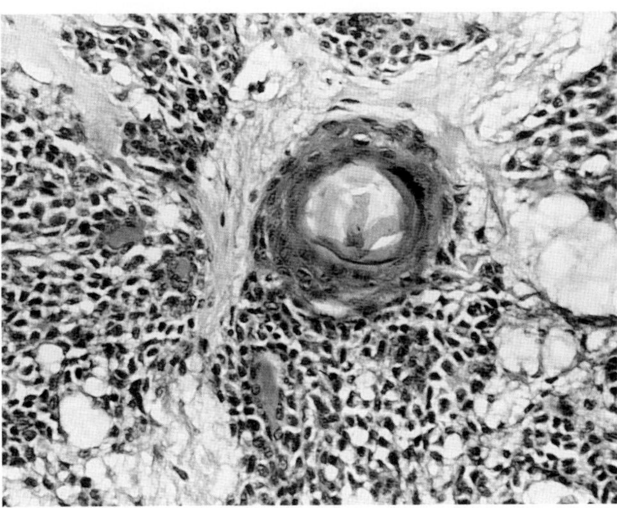

FIGURE 22. Squamous differentiation in pleomorphic adenoma.

Gross Appearance

Grossly, mixed tumors are often irregular, lobulated, and bosselated. The cut surface is gray or blue, depending on the amount of chondroid tissue present. The tumors are enclosed within an uneven connective tissue capsule that is well developed and thick in some areas and thin and incomplete in others (Fig. 20). Regardless of the completeness of the capsule or its absence, the tumor is clearly demarcated (134). Only 0.5% of mixed tumors are initially multicentric (128). Recurrent mixed tumors have a strong tendency to be multinodular.

Histologic Features

Microscopically, the tyical pleomorphic adenoma has a biphasic appearance resulting from the intimate admixture of ductal epithelium, myoepithelium, and stroma (Fig. 21). The ductal epithelial cells are arranged in numerous patterns, forming glands, tubules, solid nests, ribbons, or files. Squamous, sebaceous, or oncocytic metaplasia is often present in the epithelial elements (Fig. 22). The myoepithelial cells are mainly of two types: spindle and plasmacytoid. The spindle cells are usually arranged in fascicles simulating smooth muscle or neurogenic tumors, and the plasmacytoid cells are usually arranged in solid nests or cords (135). The stroma of the mixed tumor is also pleomorphic and consists of an admixture of mucoid, myxoid, chondroid, and hyaline tissues (Fig. 23) and, on rare occasions, of bone or fat (Fig. 24). Several types of crystal-like structures have been recognized in the extracellular component of pleomorphic adenomas, including tyrosine-rich crystalloids, calcium oxalate crystals, collagenous spherules, and amyloid (136). The proportion of ductal, myoepithelial, and stromal elements as well as the degree of stromal and epithelial metaplasia are responsible for the structural variation and diversity of the histologic appearance within and between tumors.

A subdivision of pleomorphic adenomas based on the stroma content and differentiation of the epithelial cells has been pro-

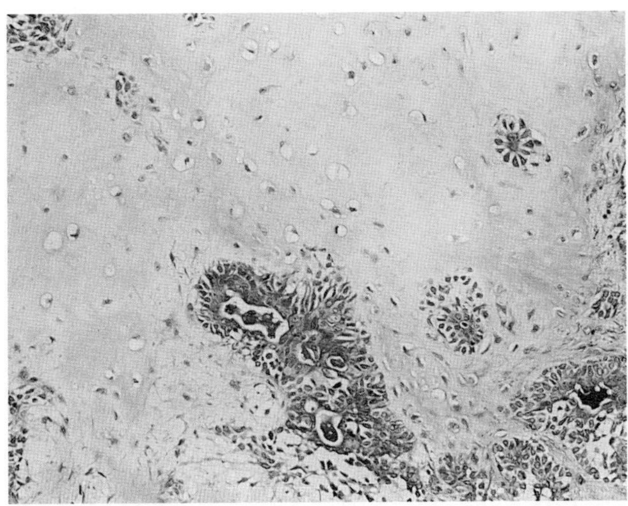

FIGURE 21. Pleomorphic adenoma. Note ductal and stromal components.

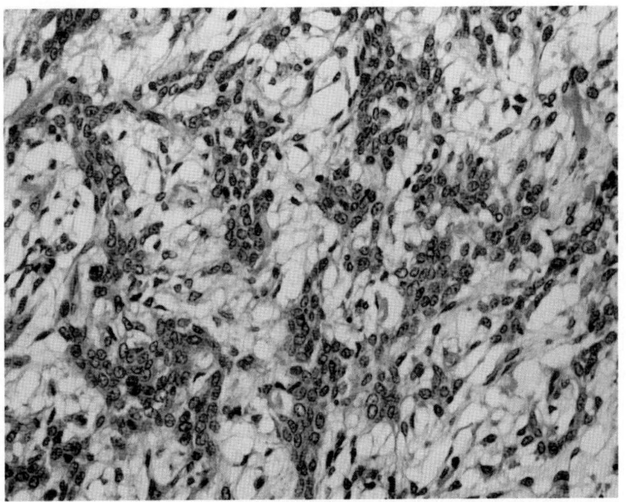

FIGURE 23. Spindled myoepithelial structures in myxoid stroma.

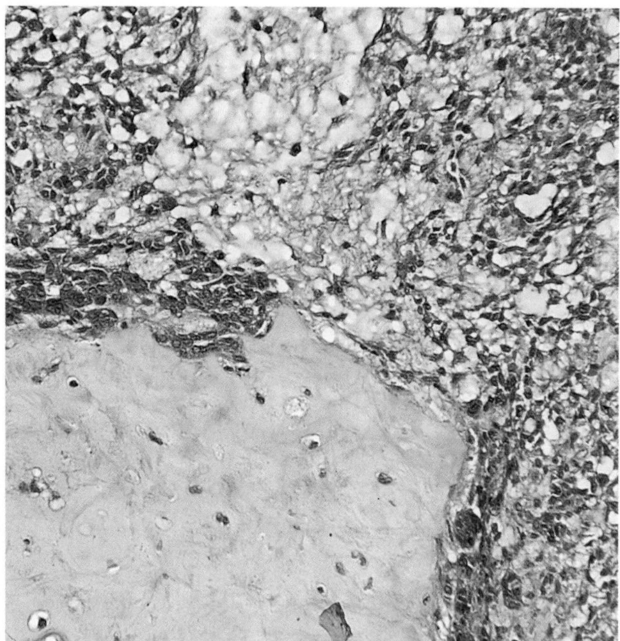

FIGURE 24. Chondroid tissue and myoepithelial cell in pleomorphic adenoma.

posed by Seifert et al. (11). Type 1 is the classic tumor type in which the stroma constitutes 30% to 50% of the tumor mass. In type 2, the stroma content is about 80% of the tumor mass. In types 3 and 4, the stroma content is low (<20%), but type 3 shows diverse epithelium akin to types 1 and 2, whereas type 4 has a uniformly differentiated epithelial component resembling a basal cell adenoma. In addition, type 4 is characterized by an absence of mucoid stroma. It has been suggested that cell-rich variants have a higher risk of malignant transformation and that the cell-poor tumors have a higher risk of recurrence. However, the range of histologic appearance within an individual tumor can be extremely variable, which makes subclassification difficult (11).

Some pleomorphic adenomas exhibit atypical features that are not seen in the majority of cases. These features are hypercellularity, hyalinization, focal spontaneous necrosis, cellular anaplasia, and capsular violation (Fig. 25). Follow-up studies have indicated that these tumors do not behave differently from the ordinary variety (137,138). However, if extensive hyalinization and increased mitotic activity are found, additional sections should be examined to exclude the presence of a carcinoma.

Special Studies

Ultrastructural studies have been widely employed in the study of pleomorphic adenomas. Ultrastructural identification of desmosomes, cytoplasmic actin microfilaments, and remnants of basal lamina may be used to help confirm the myoepithelial origin of both spindle and plasmacytoid cells present in mixed tumors. In addition, electron microscopic studies of these tumors have demonstrated cells with ductal characteristics such as precursor cells and transitional forms (139). A range of cytoplasmic features from epithelium to mesenchymal cells have also been found (139).

Immunohistochemical methods have been applied to the study of pleomorphic adenomas (139–141). Although immunohistochemical studies are not necessary or useful for routine diagnosis of mixed tumors, these analyses have provided considerable information regarding histogenesis of the tumors, especially the role of myoepithelial cells. The ductal epithelium of pleomorphic adenomas shows positive markers for keratin, carcinoembryonic antigen (CEA), lactoferrin, epithelial membrane antigen (EMA), and lectin receptors (141). Interestingly, about half of the cases of mixed tumors contain prostate-specific antigen (PSA)- and prostate-specific acid phosphatase (PSAP)-reactive cells (142). The myoepithelial component is immunoreactive for keratin, actin, myosin, S-100 protein, and vimentin. S-100 protein is also strongly positive in the chondroid areas and in a subtype of ductal epithelial cells (143). The demonstration of glial fibrillary acidic protein (GFAP) and astroprotein, two glial markers, is more difficult to explain (144). These findings combined with ultrastructural observations support the conclusion that the epithelial component is similar to that of the normal intercalated duct cells.

The intercellular matrix contains laminin, fibronectin, glycosaminoglycans, and type IV collagen. Type II collagen and tenascin are expressed in connection with the chondroid areas (145). The cell proliferation index is low, whether measured with flow cytometry, proliferating cell nuclear antigen (PCNA), or Ki-67 (146,147).

Pleomorphic adenomas have been cytogenetically investigated better than any other epithelial tumor in humans (122–124). The three major subgroups of these lesions are characterized by an apparent normal karyotype, rearrangement of 8q12, or rearrangement of 12q14–15 (122). These cytogenetic alterations have been correlated with some success with the histologic types described by Seifert et al. (11). Overexpression of p53 gene is rare in a mixed tumor but not in its malignant counterpart (148).

Differential Diagnosis

In a few cases, a mixed tumor might be confused with an adenoid cystic carcinoma. The most helpful feature in distinguishing be-

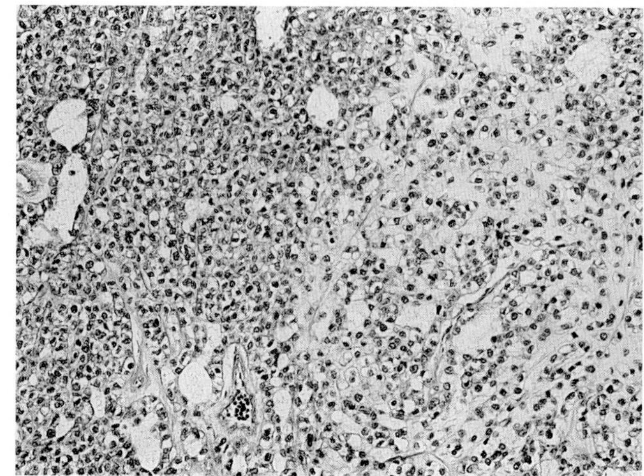

FIGURE 25. Cellular pleomorphic adenoma with atypia.

tween the two is the presence of myxoid or chondroid stroma in the mixed tumor, as opposed to the poorly cellular collagenous stroma of the adenoid cystic carcinoma. The mucoid change, however, which is so typical of the mixed tumor, sometimes is found in an adenoid cystic carcinoma. Here, the distinguishing feature is the clear demarcation between epithelial cells and mucoid intercellular material in adenoid cystic carcinoma. In contrast, the cells in mixed tumors often appear to blend with the mucin. Other features that confirm a diagnosis of adenoid cystic carcinoma are its highly invasive growth pattern and its tendency to involve nerves. Diagnostic problems usually can be resolved if a sufficient amount of tissue from the tumor is examined. Differential diagnosis from terminal duct carcinoma is discussed with that neoplasm.

Treatment and Clinical Behavior

The clinical course of a mixed tumor depends on the type of initial treatment more than on the microscopic appearance of the tumor (79,126). The rate of recurrence of parotid mixed tumors following lateral lobectomy or total parotidectomy, as indicated by the position of the tumor, varies from zero to 2%, in contrast to a much higher recurrence rate after enucleation of the tumor (149–151).

The proper therapy for pleomorphic adenoma is complete surgical removal along with a margin of normal tissue. In the parotid gland, parotidectomy with preservation of the facial nerve is the ideal treatment (79,152,153). Consideration should be given to postoperative radiotherapy for patients in whom there was tumor spillage, residual disease, or both (154).

Most disease recurrences will appear during the first 18 months after surgery, but others supervene over an exceedingly long period (151). Because of this, long-term follow-up is essential.

Recurrent Mixed Tumor

A recurrent mixed tumor is grossly characterized by the presence of multiple, round, well-circumscribed nodules growing in the salivary gland tissue, in the adipose tissue adjacent to the gland, or in scar tissue from a previous surgical procedure. Histologically, recurrent mixed tumors exhibit the same growth pattern observed in other benign mixed tumors, and the tumor cells have benign cytologic features (Fig. 26).

Carcinoma may arise in recurrent mixed tumors; therefore, when a resection has been performed for recurrence, each nodule should be examined microscopically because carcinoma may be found in any one of the nodules (155,156). The proper treatment for recurrent mixed tumor is complete surgical excision including margins of normal tissue, if possible. Postoperative radiotherapy may be considered (126,154).

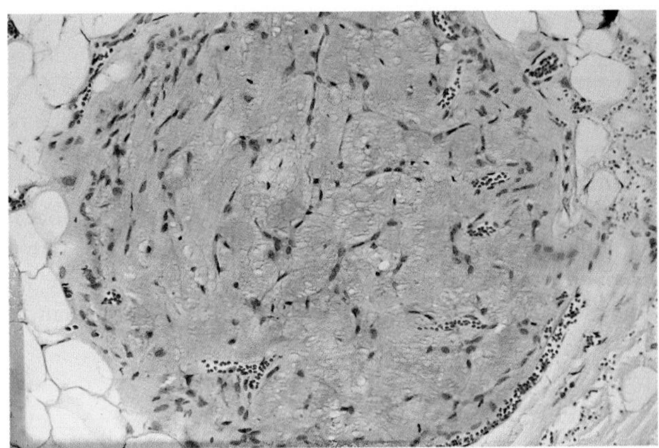

FIGURE 26. A largely myxoid recurrent pleomorphic adenoma.

Malignant Mixed Tumor

The incidence of malignant mixed tumors varies from series to series but usually falls within the more frequent types of salivary gland carcinomas: mucoepidermoid carcinoma, adenoid cystic carcinoma, and acinic cell carcinoma. Malignant mixed tumors account for between 3% and 12% of all cancers of the salivary glands and 2% of all tumors in these glands (11,74–80). Within the broad heading of "malignant mixed tumors" are incuded three different clinical and pathologic entities: carcinoma *ex* pleomorphic adenoma or carcinoma arising in mixed tumor, carcinosarcoma or true malignant mixed tumor, and metastasizing mixed tumor (75,157).

Carcinoma ex Pleomorphic Adenoma

Definition

These include "tumors showing definitive evidence of malignancy, such as cytological and histological characteristics of anaplasia, abnormal mitoses, progressive course, and infiltrative growth, and in which evidence of pleomorphic adenoma can still be found" (75).

Clinical Data

This is the most common form of malignant mixed tumor and can be viewed as a malignant transformation of a preexisting pleomorphic adenoma. This complication occurs in about 5% to 10% of these benign neplasms (158). The average incidence is 3.6% (range between 1% and 14%) of all salivary gland tumors and 11.6% of all malignant salivary tumors (range between 2.8% and 42.4%) (11,74–80).

Fifty-five percent of the cases occur in women. Most observers have recorded a peak incidence for this neoplasm in the sixth to eighth decades, and it is exceptional in patients under 20 (159–164). Only 4 of 326 carcinomas *ex* pleomorphic adenoma in a recent series occurred in patients younger than 20 years of age (161).

Approximately 82% of cases of carcinoma *ex* pleomorphic adenoma involve the major glands, and only 18% are found in the minor salivary glands. In the major glands, the parotid is involved in 81.7% of cases, the submandibular gland in 18%, and the sublingual gland in 0.3% (164). The palate is the most common site in the minor glands, followed by the sinonasal tract (159–164).

Carcinoma *ex* pleomorphic adenoma seems to arise in two different clinical situations: *de novo* or in recurrent mixed tumor. A history of a longstanding tumor with recent rapid growth is found in only 15% of the patients (164). The most frequent symptom in more than 80% of patients is a painless mass (164). Thirty-eight percent of the patients develop facial nerve palsy, and up to 65% of patients have fixation of the tumor to adjacent tissues (164). The incidence of malignant transformation of a preexisting pleomorphic adenoma increases progressively with the preoperative duration of the tumor. In the series studied by Eneroth and Zetterberg (165), the rate of malignant transformation was 1.6% in tumors present for less than 5 years and 9.4% in tumors present for more than 15 years.

Gross Appearance

Grossly, the majority of carcinomas *ex* pleomorphic adenoma are poorly circumscribed and infiltrative lesions with extensive areas of necrosis and hemorrhage. In general, the average size of such a neoplasm is more than twice as large as the ususal benign pleomorphic adenoma (166).

Histologic Features

Microscopically, foci of residual mixed tumor and of carcinoma are present in the same neoplasm (11,74) (Fig. 27). To find the preexisting benign tumor may require thorough sampling of the neoplasm. Sometimes the benign residual tumor is represented only by a totally hyalinized round nodule surrounded by carcinoma. In this latter case, the neoplasm can only be strongly presumed, rather than proven, to be a carcinoma *ex* pleomorphic adenoma. The most common types of carcinoma present are, in order of descending frequency, salivary duct carcinoma, undifferentiated carcinoma, terminal duct carcinoma, myoepithelial carcinoma, and adenocarcinoma not otherwise specified (NOS) (157) (Fig. 28). Epithelial–myoepithelial carcinoma has also been observed (167). A point of origin of adenoid cystic carcinoma, mucoepidermoid carcinoma, or acinic cell carcinoma in benign mixed tumor seldom can be demonstrated (168). LiVolsi and Perzin (160) introduced the term carcinoma *in situ* (or intracapsular carcinoma) *ex* pleomorphic adenoma to designate tumors without evidence of capsular invasion of adjacent tissues and that are therefore malignant neoplasms of no clinical or biological significance. If no invasion outside the main mass is identified, the carcinoma should not metastasize.

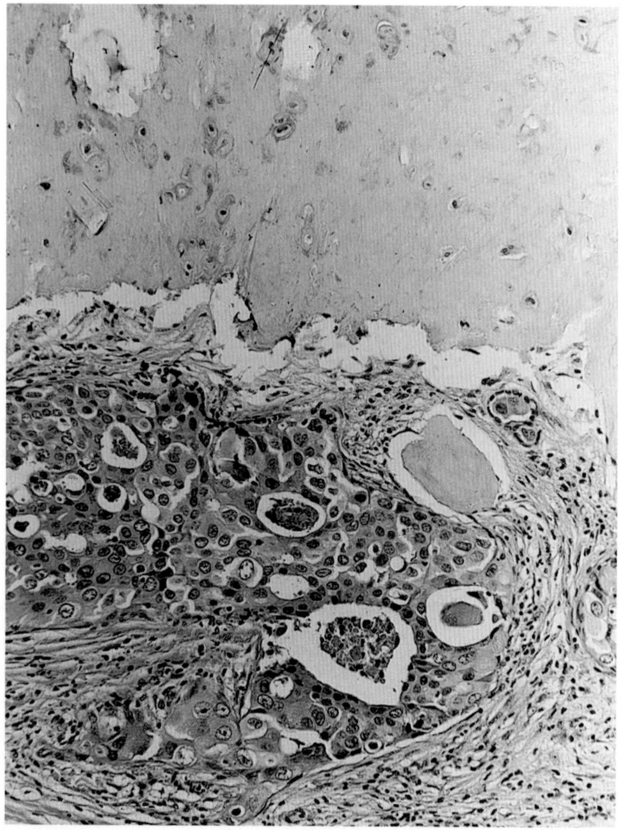

FIGURE 27. Carcinoma *ex* mixed tumor. Residual mixed tumor **(upper half)** with adenocarcinoma **(lower half).**

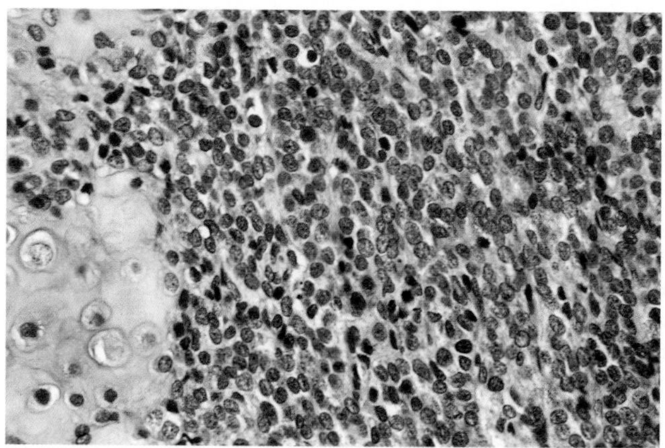

FIGURE 28. Carcinoma *ex* pleomorphic adenoma with small-cell carcinoma component.

The metastases contain only carcinoma. The most common sites of metastases are the cervical lymph nodes, lungs, bone (especially the vertebral column), and liver (164,169).

Special Studies

Immunohistochemically, carcinoma *ex* pleomorphic adenoma closely resembles pleomorphic adenoma, demonstrating antigen reactivity for epithelial and myoepithelial cells (170). Diffuse immunoreactivity for B72.3 is more common in carcinoma *ex* pleomorphic adenoma than in benign mixed tumors (171). The proliferative markers PCNA and Ki-67 exhibit diffuse reaction in these tumors (170) as well as overexpression of p53 (148). Cytogenetic analysis of pleomorphic adenomas and carcinomas *ex* pleomorphic adenoma has shown progression from diploid pleomorphic adenomas to tetraploid carcinoma *ex* pleomorphic adenoma (170).

Differential Diagnosis

Occasionally, it may be difficult to distinguish between benign and malignant mixed tumors. The malignant mixed tumor is a destructive, infiltrating lesion, in stark contrast to the benign tumor with its expanding, encapsulated margins. No single criterion unequivocally defines the malignancy of these tumors.

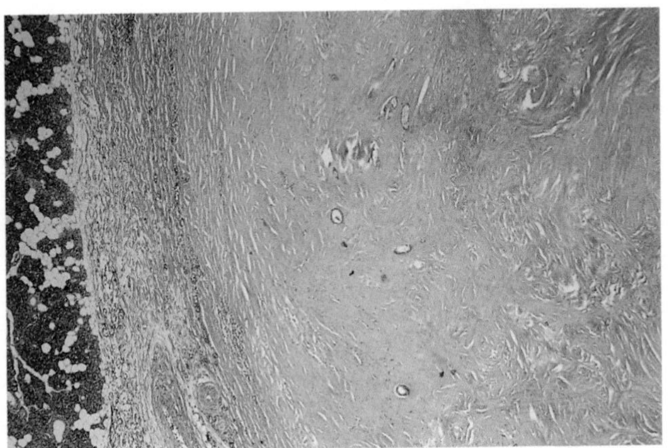

FIGURE 29. Intracapsular carcinoma (carcinoma *in situ ex* pleomorphic adenoma). Carcinoma in prominent hyalinized stroma.

Some useful diagnostic features of borderline tumors are as follows (172,173):

- Micronecrosis
- Dystrophic calcification
- Atypical mitosis
- Extensive hyalinization of the residual mixed tumor (Fig. 29)
- Solid areas resembling lobular carcinoma of the breast

When all of these features are observed in a mixed tumor, it qualifies as being malignant.

Clinical Behavior and Treatment

Carcinoma *ex* pleomorphic adenoma is an agressive neoplasm. Approximately 40% of patients develop one or more recurrences (157,164). The metastatic rate varies from series to series with up to 70% of patients developing regional or distant metastases (165). The prognosis of these neoplasms depends on the extension of the carcinoma outside the capsule and on the histologic type of carcinoma.

Tortoledo et al. (157) reviewed 37 patients and found that no patient with less than 8 mm of invasion measured from the capsule died of disease. However, all patients with invasive tumors extending more than 9 mm beyond the capsule died of disease. Tortoledo et al. also examined recurrence rates in the context of adjacent tissue invasion and found them to be 70.5% when invasion exceeded 6 mm and 16.6% when invasion was less than 6 mm. In addition, Tortoledo et al. (157) correlated the histologic type of carcinoma with prognosis and found 5-year survival rates of 30% for undifferentiated carcinomas, 50% for ductal carcinomas, 63% for myoepithelial carcinomas, and 92% for terminal duct carcinomas. They also examined the effect that surgical margins had on survival. Only 2 of 12 patients with histologically positive resection margins remained free of disease; however, negative margins were no assurance against recurrence. Nodal metastases or death occurred in 8 of 24 (33%) patients with negative surgical margins.

The best form of therapy seems to be wide surgical excision together with continuous lymph node dissection and adjuvant radiation therapy (161,164). The adjuvant role of chemotherapy needs further evaluation. However, because of the high rate of distant metastasis with these tumors, adjuvant chemotherapy would appear to offer the potential of increased survival as better protocols become available. Radiotherapy alone has not proven effective.

Carcinosarcoma

Definition

"Carcinosarcomas or true malignant mixed tumors are neoplasms of the salivary gland in which both the epithelial and the stromal components are malignant. When these tumors metastasize, both components are almost always present" (75,164).

Clinical Data

Carcinosarcomas are extremely rare neoplasms of the salivary glands. Only eight neoplasms were found in the files of the AFIP Salivary Gland Registry (164). They accounted for 0.06% of 13,749 benign and malignant salivary gland tumors and 0.16% of 5,053 malignant tumors (164). The clinical presentation, age, and gender of the patients are similar to the more common carcinoma *ex* pleomorphic adenoma. The anatomic location is also similar (174–182).

Histologic Features

Microscopically, the neoplasms are biphasic. Both the epithelial and the mesenchymal elements are malignant, the former often in the form of ductal carcinoma and the latter in the form of chondrosarcoma (Fig. 30). Tumors may, in addition, contain areas of osteosarcoma, malignant fibrous histiocytoma, and undifferentiated sarcoma (183).

Special Studies

Flow cytometry analysis has demonstrated diploidy and high S-phase in the carcinomatous component and aneuploidy in the sarcomatous areas (170). These tumors exhibit variable positivity for Ki-67, proliferative cell nuclear antigen (PCNA), and p53 (148). Immunohistochemical and ultrastructural studies have confirmed two separate populations of tumor cells corresponding to the histologic growth pattern (170,184).

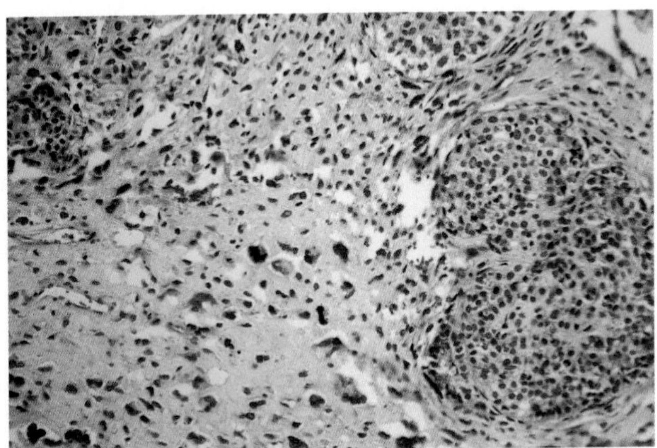

FIGURE 30. Carcinosarcoma. Islands of carcinoma surrounded by malignant stroma.

Differential Diagnosis

Differential diagnosis includes spindle cell carcinoma and other primary sarcomas, especially synovial sarcoma. The uniform stromal cells arranged in tight bundles and the simple gland-like structures, if present, will help differentiate synovial sarcoma from a true malignant mixed tumor. In addition, the stromal elements of true malignant mixed tumors are more pleomorphic than one would expect to find in synovial sarcoma. Spindle-cell carcinoma will exhibit spindle cells and keratinizing epithelium, and, as demonstrated with immunohistochemistry and electron microscopy studies, both components will exhibit squamous characteriestics.

Clinical Behavior and Treatment

Carcinosarcomas are aggressive, often rapidly lethal neoplasms. Only occasionally does a patient survive 3 years (164). Approximately 70% of the patients will develop lung metastases within 18 months after treatment (174–182). There are insufficient data available regarding treatment of these neoplasms. However, radical surgery with postoperative irradiation seems to be the most prudent approach.

Metastasizing Pleomorphic Adenoma

Definition

"Metastasizing pleomorphic adenoma is a salivary gland neoplasm that is histologically identical to a benign tumor. Nevertheless, for some unknown reason, the tumor metastasizes. The metastases of these tumors contain both epithelial and stromal components found in typical mixed tumors" (74,75,164). The existence of this neoplasm has been challenged by some authors who believe that the lesion most likely represents a peculiar form of myoepithelial carcinoma (185–187).

Clinical Data

The age and gender of the patients are similar to those of patients with benign pleomorphic adenoma. The location in the salivary glands is also identical. The main difference is that 75% of the patients had a history of one or more previous excisions of a benign pleomorphic adenoma. The length of time from excision of the original tumor to finding the first metastasis ranged from 1.5 to 51 years and averaged 16.3 years (185–195). El-Naggar et al. (186) postulated that repeated surgical manipulation possibly allows access to vascular spaces.

Histologic Features

Both primary and metastasizing pleomorphic adenomas are composed of cells typical of those seen in benign pleomorphic adenomas of salivary gland origin (Fig. 31). Several cases contain only or mostly myoepithelial cells (185–187).

Special Studies

Flow cytometry studies performed in six cases demonstrated a diploid cell population in all primary and metastatic lesions (186,191); however, in a recent case report an aneuploid population was revealed in one metastasizing mixed tumor (185).

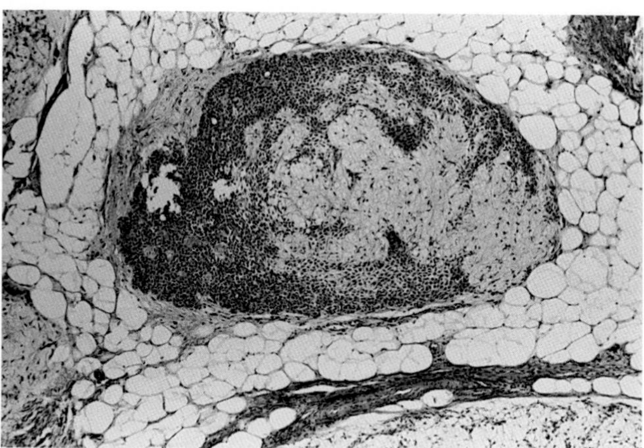

FIGURE 31. Metastasizing mixed tumor in mediastinal soft tissues.

Differential Diagnosis

The diagnosis of metastatic pleomorphic adenoma usually is not difficult because both epithelial and mesenchymal elements are present. However, when the metastases are in the lungs and vertebrae, this tumor must be distinguished from chondroid hamartoma and chondroid chordoma. The presence of ductal differentiation excludes chondroid chordoma. In pulmonary hamartoma, the cartilage nests are surrounded by a fibrous capsule. Also, the epithelial component is more complex, and it can be seen to arise from the alveoli or bronchioles (161). In addition, pulmonary hamartomas do not have a prominent myoepithelial component, as do pleomorphic adenomas.

Clinical Behavior and Treatment

The outcome of the patients depends on the location and extent of the metastases. In the cases collected by Gnepp (161,164), 37% of the patients died of distant metastases, 53% of the patients were alive and free of tumor, and 10% of the patients were alive with metastases. The best treatment appears to be wide excision of the primary tumor, metastatic tumors, or both. Irradiation and chemotherapy do not appear to have a role in disease management unless the neoplasm is unresectable.

Myoepithelioma and Myoepithelial Carcinoma

Myoepithelioma

Definition

"Myoepithelioma is a benign tumor composed of sheets and islands of various proportions of spindle, plasmacytoid, epithelioid, and clear cells that exhibit myoepithelial but not ductal differentiation" (74). A considerable number of these neoplasms may exhibit acellular, mucoid, or hyalinized stroma but lack chondroid or myxochondroid tissues (74,196–201). Some investigators have stipulated that no more than 10% of a microscopic section of myoepithelioma be composed of ductal elements (126,197). In the past, this neoplasm was considered to be one end of the spectrum of pleomorphic adenoma (199).

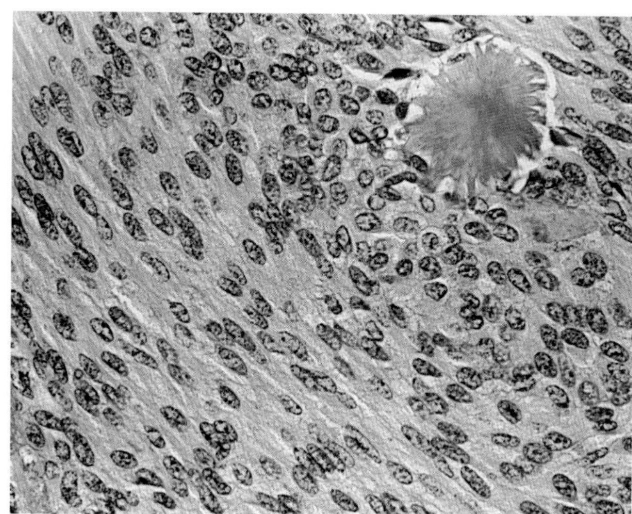

FIGURE 32. Myoepithelioma, spindle cell variant. Note the collagenous crystalloid in the upper right of the figure.

Clinical Data

Myoepitheliomas account for 1.5% of all salivary gland tumors of the major and minor salivary glands in the AFIP files (74,75,126). They represent 2.2% and 5.7% of all benign major and minor salivary gland tumors, respectively (74,127). Men and women are affected with equal frequency (74,126,196–201). The age of the patients with myoepithelioma ranges from 9 to 98 years, with an average of 44 years (74,126,196–201). The parotid gland and the palate are the most common sites, but all salivary glands can be affected as well as the larynx and sinonasal tract (196,201).

Gross Appearance

The tumors are solid and well circumscribed and seldom are larger than 6 cm.

Histologic Features

Four major morphologic types of myoepitheliomas have been identified: spindle, hyaline or plasmacytoid, epithelioid, and clear cell (135,196–201). However, it should be noted that combined forms exist. The *spindle cell tumors* have a stroma-like appearance. The cells are arranged in interlacing fascicles (Fig. 32) and can be confused with smooth muscle tumors, neurogenic tumors, and fibroblastic lesions. These tumors are hypercellular and have limited myxoid or mucoid stroma but often have scattered clusters of epithelioid and clear cells. The *hyaline or plasmacytoid myoepitheliomas* are composed of polygonal cells with eccentric nuclei and abundant nongranular or "hyaline" eosinophilic cytoplasm (Fig. 33). Collagenous crystalloids are often present in the stroma. The appearance of the hyaline cells may simulate that of neoplastic plasma cells, skeletal muscle, or "rhabdoid" cells. These cells occur more often in the palate than in the parotid gland. *Clear cell myoepitheliomas* are composed of sheets, cords, or tubules of cells with clear cytoplasm that contain glycogen but not fat or mucin (Fig. 34). Some myoepitheliomas are composed predominantly of *epithelioid cells* arranged in interconnected cords surrounded by abundant mucoid stroma. The spindle cells and plasmacytoid cells are scanty. Dardick et al. (198) have designated this as a *reticular* type of myoepithelioma (Fig. 35). Most of the reported cases of spindle cell and clear cell myoepitheliomas have occurred in the major glands, whereas most plasmacytoid and epithelioid myoepitheliomas have been

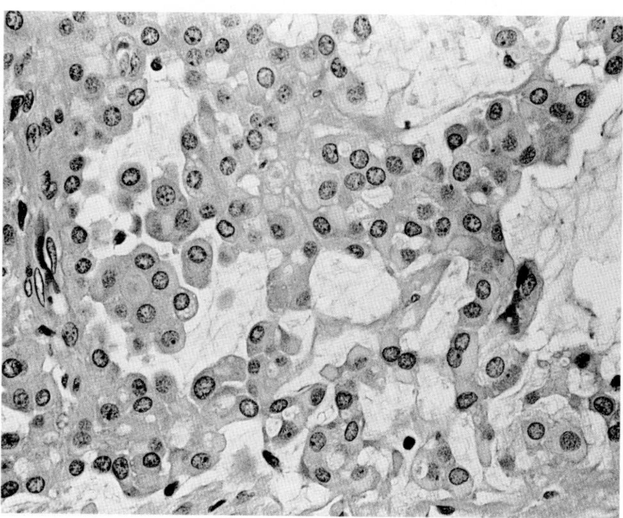

FIGURE 33. Myoepithelioma, plasmacytoid (hyaline) cell type.

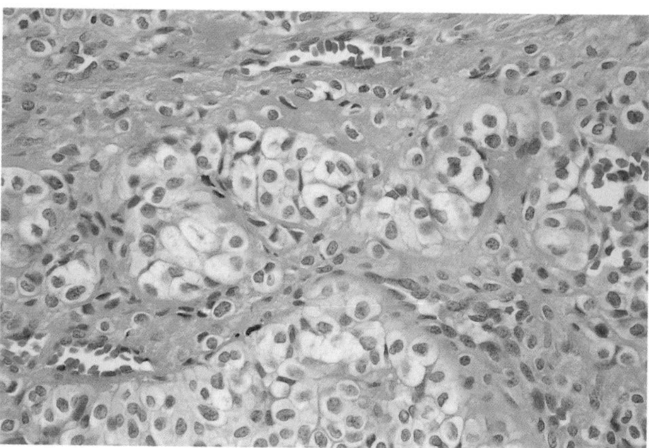

FIGURE 34. Myoepithelioma with prominent clear epithelioid cells.

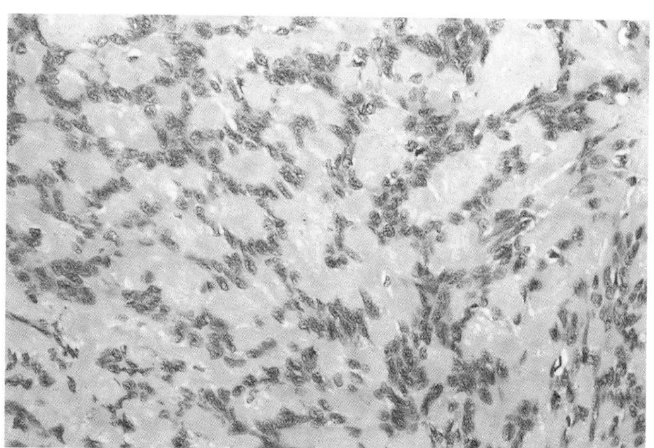

FIGURE 35. Reticular variant of myoepithelioma.

described in minor salivary glands of the palate, paranasal sinus, and larynx (196–201).

Special Studies

Each myoepithelioma subtype has a different immunohistochemical profile, but there is as well a great deal of heterogeneity within each category (196–202). The neoplastic cells of myoepithelioma consistently demonstrate keratin immunoreactivity, especially to keratin 14, although reactivity of the spindle cells is variable. There is considerable variation of tumor expression of muscle-specific actin (MSA). The spindle cells immunoreact strongly for MSA, the epithelioid cells react sporadically, and hyaline and clear cells are generally nonreactive (202). Immunoreactivity for S-100 protein is usually strong, whereas it is more variable for vimentin, GFAP, and EMA (202–205). The immunoreaction to desmin is generally negative (196).

Ultrastructurally, spindle cell myoepithelioma often contains microfilaments of both keratin and actin types in addition to pinocytotic vesicles, desmosomes, glycogen, and basal lamina formation (Fig. 36) (143,198). The main feature of hyaline cells is the presence of abundant, uniformly dispersed microfilaments measuring 50 to 100 Å in diameter (202). The epithelioid and clear cells often contain a limited number of filaments, many polyribosomes, and glycogen (143,196,198).

Flow cytometric analysis indicates that the majority of benign myoepitheliomas are diploid with a normal S fraction, whereas recurrent and malignant myoepitheliomas tend to be aneuploid with high proliferative indices (196,206). Nucleolar organizer regions (NORs) studied by an argyrophilic staining technique (AgNOR) did not correlate well with DNA cytometric indices or with the clinical outcome in patients with myoepitheliomas (207).

Differential Diagnosis

Spindle cell myoepitheliomas must be distinguished from leiomyomas, leiomyosarcomas, nerve sheath tumors, synovial sarcoma, and nodular fasciitis. The infiltrative growth pattern seen in leiomyosarcomas, synovial sarcomas, and malignant peripheral nerve sheath tumors and the demonstration of nuclear abnormalities in these tumors will exclude myoepithelioma. Strong diffuse staining for keratin would help to rule out other mesenchymal neoplasms and nodular fasciitis.

The perinuclear clearing, negative stain for keratin, and positive immunoreactivity for immunoglobulin separate plasmacytoma from plasmacytoid myoepithelioma. An organoid neoplasm with increased vascularity, hemorrhage, and nuclear atypia would favor metastatic renal cell carcinoma rather than clear cell myoepithelioma. The presence of chondroid tissue and ductal differentiation would support the diagnosis of pleomorphic adenoma in a neoplasm composed of spindle, plasmacytoid, and clear myoepithelial cells. The infiltrative growth pattern is characteristic of myoepithelial carcinoma in contrast to the well-circumscribed borders of the benign neoplasms (74,206).

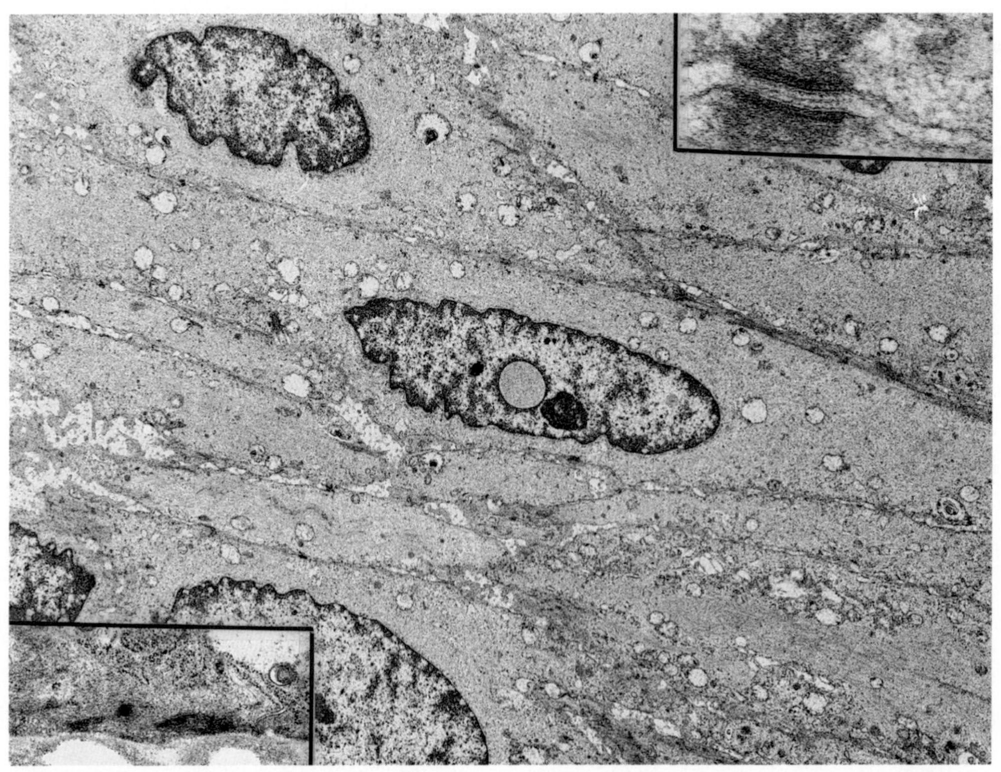

FIGURE 36. Ultrastructural appearance of myoepithelioma. Cell junctions **(insert right upper corner).** Dense bodies of actin-type microfilaments **(insert left lower corner).**

Clinical Behavior and Treatment

According to the AFIP experience, myoepitheliomas are less likely to recur than are mixed tumors (74). In a series of 16 cases published by Sciubba and Brannon (199), only one case recurred after 7 years. However, higher recurrence rates have been reported by El-Naggar et al. (206) and Alos et al. (196). Complete surgical excision with free surgical margins is the recommended treatment. Each of the recurrences was presaged by positive margins at the first excision in the series of patients studied by El-Naggar et al. (206).

Myoepithelial Carcinoma

Definition

"Myoepithelial carcinoma is a rare malignant epithelial tumor composed of atypical myoepithelial cells with increased mitotic activity and aggressive growth" (75). Two requirements must be met to establish a diagnosis of myoepithelial carcinoma: the neoplastic cells must be characterized as myoepithelial, and the tumor must be morphologically and biologically malignant (74). These carcinomas can arise *de novo* or as a malignant transformation of a pleomorphic adenoma (74,157,208,209).

Clinical Data

Myoepithelial carcinomas constitute only 0.2% of all epithelial salivary gland neoplasms accessioned in the AFIP files (74). The parotid gland is the most common location for this tumor, followed by the palate and the submandibular gland (208–213). Reported patients range in age from 14 to 86 years with a mean age of 62 years (208–213). Men and women are affected in equal numbers by these carcinomas.

Gross Appearance

These neoplasms are unencapsulated, and the cut surfaces show necrosis, hemorrhages, and cystic degeneration.

Histologic Features

The cellular composition of myoepithelial carcinoma is the same as that found in myoepitheliomas and includes spindle, plasmacytoid, clear cell, and epithelioid elements (208–213) (Fig. 37).

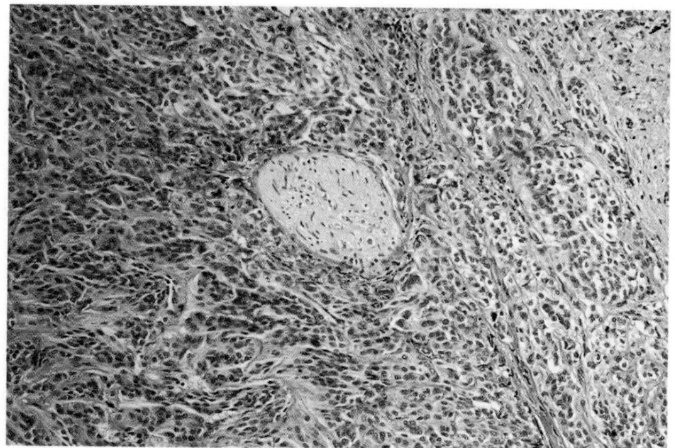

FIGURE 37. Myoepithelial carcinoma. Pleomorphic spindle cells with atypical nuclei surrounding a nerve.

Cellular and nuclear pleomorphisms vary from slight to severe. The highly cellular neoplasms have scanty stroma. Desmoplasia is often present at the infiltrative borders of the tumor. The mitosis rate is variable; one to five mitoses are usually seen per high-power field. Necrosis is a frequent feature of myoepithelial carcinomas. An important diagnostic feature is the invasive and destructive character of these carcinomas.

Special Studies

Tissue samples from each of the 10 cases of myoepithelial carcinomas in the series of Di Palma and Guzzo (213) and from the four in the series of Alos et al. (196) were immunoreactive for S-100 protein, high- or low-molecular-weight keratins, and vimentin. Other investigators reported a negative reaction for keratin but positive reactions with S-100, vimentin, and actin (208–212). At the ultrastructural level, filaments with focal dense bodies, pinocytic vesicles, desmosomes, and basal lamina have been described in several myoepithelial carcinomas (208,210). Flow cytometric studies performed by El Naggar et al. (206) and Alos and associates (196) showed that the majority of these carcinomas are aneuploid with a high proliferative phase. El Naggar et al. (206) found that a high S-phase fraction as determined by flow cytometry is a better indication of aggressiveness than DNA content analysis.

Differential Diagnosis

Leiomyosarcoma, malignant peripheral nerve sheath tumor, malignant fibrous histiocytoma, synovial sarcoma, and metastatic melanoma must be considered in the differential diagnosis. The immunohistochemical profile of each one of these mesenchymal neoplasms helps to separate them from myoepithelial carcinoma. In addition, ultrastructural differences set myoepithelial carcinoma apart.

Clinical Behavior and Treatment

Local invasion and destruction characterize all cases of myoepithelial carcinoma. However, metastases were documented in the lungs, liver, bones, and lymph nodes (74,196,209–213). In the AFIP series, 33% of the patients were alive and well, 33% were living with disease, and 33% had died as a result of their tumor (74). Complete excision of the neoplasm with clear surgical margins appears to be the best treatment. Total parotidectomy or wide excision of minor salivary gland tumors is recommended (74,196,209–213). Radiotherapy alone has been unsatisfactory (74,209–213).

Oncocytoma and Oncocytic Carcinoma

Oncocytoma

Definition

"Oncocytoma is a rare tumor composed of a well-demarcated mass of polyhedral eosinophilic cells with small, dark nuclei. It has a solid, trabecular or tubular pattern and frequently contains both light and dark cells" (75). Hamperl (214) considered oncocytes to differ from other epithelial cells by their excessive proliferation of mitochondria. Because of their size and characteristic abundant acidophilic cytoplasm and altered DNA, oncocytic cells may be classified as somatic mutants (214,215). Oncocytic transformation is not a degenerative process, as has often been professed, but rather a redifferentiation of the cells as they attempt to increase their output of high-energy phosphate (215–217). Oncocytes have the following properties: they appear after the gland in which they occur has reached histologic maturity; they manifest a high level of oxidative activity; they possess an unusually large number of mitochondria; and they have no special cytoarchitectural features such as basal infoldings or brush borders, although regression of these features may have occurred (215–219). Proliferations of oncocytic cells in salivary glands can be categorized as oncocytic metaplasia, nodular or diffuse hyperplasia (oncocytosis), oncocytoma, or oncocytic carcinoma.

Clinical Data

Oncocytomas arise in the parotid gland, the submandibular gland, and the minor salivary glands. They account for fewer than 1% of all salivary gland tumors (11,74–76,88). Patients with this type of tumor are usually older; the average age is 72 years. More women than men are affected, by a slight margin (220–226). Brandwein and Huvos (220) estimated that bilateral parotid gland or submandibular gland disease, synchronous or metachronous, occurs in at least 7% of patients. Swelling is the single complaint of patients in nearly all cases of oncocytoma; only rarely is pain associated with these tumors (220–226).

Gross Appearance

An oncocytoma has an average diameter of 3 to 4 cm, is encapsulated, and has a typical brown-red lobular cut surface (Fig. 38). The capsule varies in thickness, definition, and completeness. Oncocytomas are almost always solitary, although focal oncocytic hyperplasia may frequently be observed apart from the main tumor.

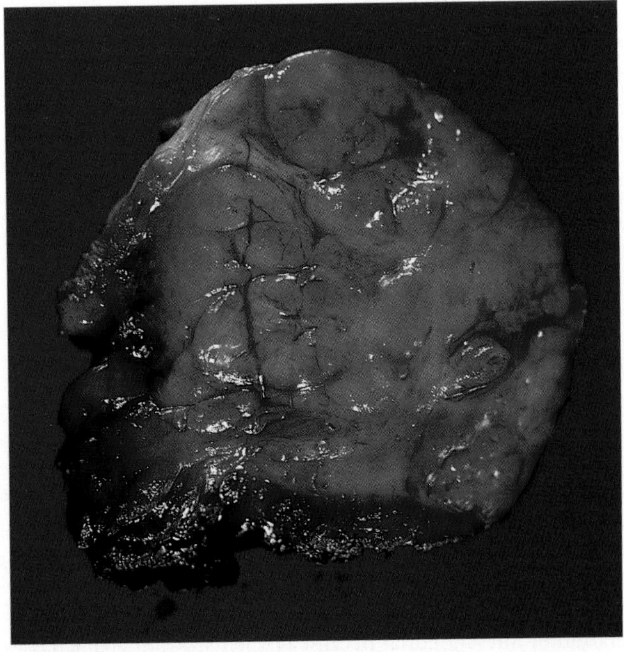

FIGURE 38. Oncocytoma. Homogeneous brown-red surface.

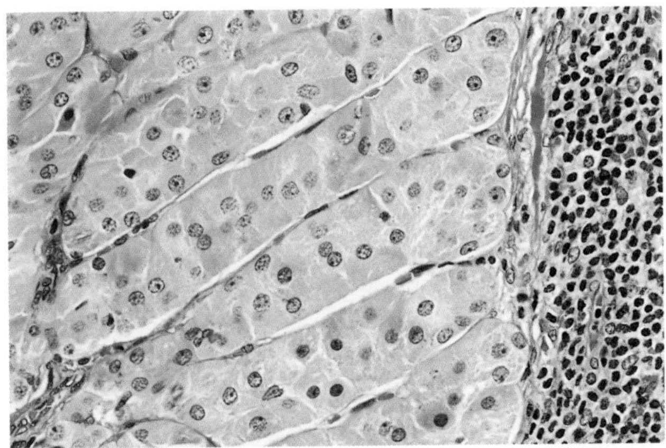

FIGURE 39. Oncocytoma composed of granular cells in organoid pattern.

Histologic Features

Microscopically, oncocytomas are composed of large cells with round nuclei and abundant granular acidophilic cytoplasm (Fig. 39). The cells are arranged in columns, solid cords, or in a few tumors, in tubular and acinar formations. Mitotic figures are virtually absent, and squamous or mucinous metaplasia can occur (225). Clear cells may dominate some lesions (Fig. 40). The clear cytoplasm results from an accumulation of cytoplasmic glycogen in the oncocytes. Clear cell oncocytomas have the same organoid arrangement as conventional oncocytomas (223). Focal oncocytic hyperplasia is often seen outside the capsule. Papillary oncocytoma is rare in the major salivary glands, but when seen, its appearance is that of an exaggerated Warthin's tumor without the lymphoid tissue.

Oncocytosis is the accumulation and proliferation of oncocytes in the salivary glands. It can be nodular or diffuse. The former consists of multiple nonencapsulated nodules of oncocytic cells in the parotid gland. The nodules have a lobular distribution, and normal acinar tissue may be included at the periphery. In the diffuse form nearly the entire gland is replaced by oncocytes.

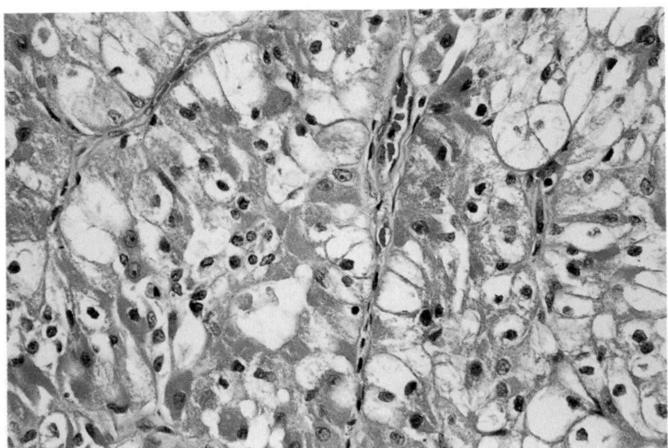

FIGURE 40. Clear cell oncocytoma. Clear and granular cells in organoid pattern.

Histopathologically, the distinction between an oncocytic hyperplasia and an oncocytoma can be difficult to define, especially in glands with multiple nodules clinically or surgically evident. It is largely a semantic distinction. One criterion has been the presence or absence of fibrous encapsulation, which is often incomplete: oncocytoma is encapsulated, whereas oncocytic hyperplasia is not (221,227). The process of oncocytic metaplasia transforms ductal and acinar epithelium to oncocytes (219). Oncocytic metaplasia occasionally occurs in tumor cells of salivary gland neoplasms other than oncocytoma. It is most frequently observed in mixed tumors and mucoepidermoid carcinomas but has been seen in nearly every type of salivary gland neoplasm (74).

Special Studies

Ultrastructurally, the cytoplasm is packed with mitochondria that have long cristae mitochondriales and a partially lamellar internal structure (Fig. 41). Some of the mitochondria contain large amounts of glycogen, and others are partitioned, suggesting division (218). Desmosomal cell attachments are usually evident. Enzyme histochemisty shows that the tumor cells contain oxidative and hydrolytic mitochondrial enzymes, in particular phosphatase and esterases (222). These tissues stain strongly with Luxol fast blue but display metachromasia with thionin and cresyl violet (222). In addition, Mallory's modified phosphotungstic acid hematoxylin (PTAH) demonstrates numerous mitochondrial clumps. Bradwein and Huvos (220) recommend a 48-hour incubation period rather than the routine overnight incubation for PTAH staining of mitochondria. Immunohistochemical studies conducted by Gustafsson et al. (228) indicate that the oncocyte is immunoreactive for keratin and negative for S-100 protein and muscle-specific actin. Felix et al. (229) studied the nuclear DNA content by image cytophotometry in nine oncocytic tumors; benign tumors had a DNA diploid pattern, and the oncocytic carcinomas displayed a DNA aneuploid pattern. These observations point to DNA nuclear assessment as an additional criterion with which to categorize neoplasms with divergent clinical behavior.

Differential Diagnosis

Pleomorphic adenoma, mucoepidermoid carcinoma, and acinic cell carcinoma are the salivary gland neoplasms that most often demonstrate oncocytic metaplasia. Oncocytomas lack the pleomorphic appearance, the myxochrondroid tissue, and proliferation of spindle and plasmacytoid myoepithelial cells that characterize pleomorphic adenoma. Positive PTAH staining for mitochondria and the absence of intracellular mucin demonstrated with the help of mucicarmine stain can be useful in differentiating oncocytoma from mucoepidermoid carcinoma. Unlike acinic cell carcinoma, oncocytoma lacks well-differentiated acinar cells and contains glycogen.

Clear cell oncocytoma must be distinguished from epithelial–myoepithelial carcinoma and metastatic carcinoma, mainly renal cell carcinoma. The characteristic biphasic pattern of ductal cells surrounded by clear cells in epithelial–myoepithelial carcinoma is not present in clear cell oncocytoma. The lack of invasion and the presence of hyperplastic nodules of oncocytes outside the capsule would favor oncocytoma over renal cell car-

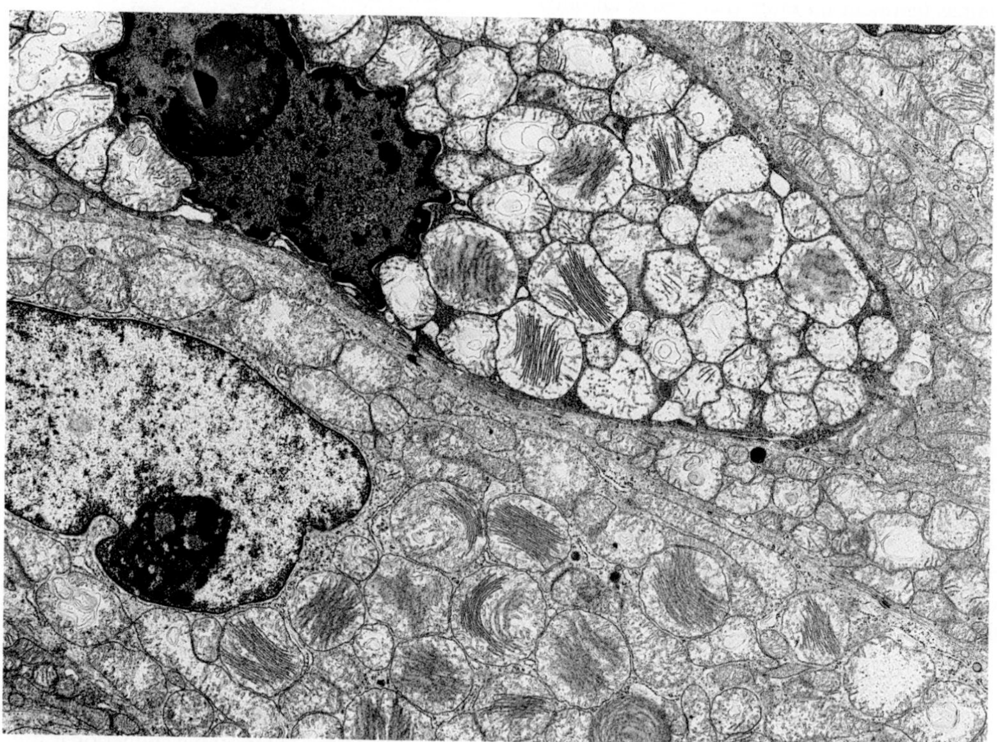

FIGURE 41. Electron micrograph of oncocytoma shows numerous enlarged mitochondria in cytoplasm.

cinoma. Clinical evaluation of the patient for primary renal cell carcinoma is worthy of consideration if any doubt persists.

Clinical Behavior and Treatment

The prognosis for patients with oncocytoma is excellent. Multifocal tumor growth and incomplete excision appear to be factors in the incidence of recurrence. Brandwein and Huvos (220) reported that 4 of 39 patients had recurrences and that three of these patients had multifocal primary tumors. Recurrences developed 0.5 to 13 years after initial treatment. Nasal oncocytomas have a tendency to be more aggressive, without being malignant, than do oncocytomas in any other location (222,226). Excision is the principal modality of treatment (219–226).

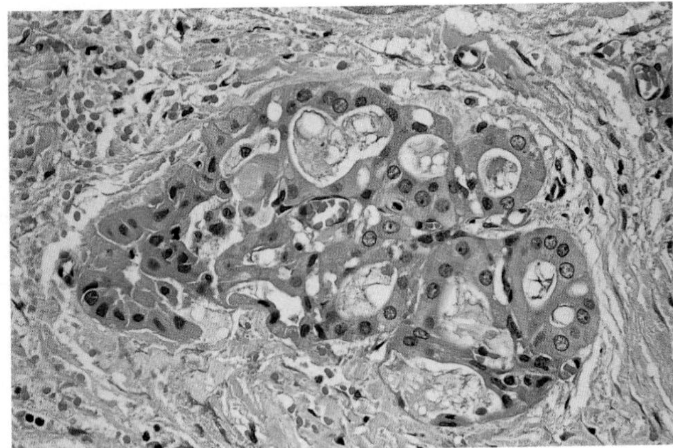

FIGURE 42. Oncocytic carcinoma. Pleomorphic cells with nuclear atypia.

Oncocytic Carcinoma

Definition

"A very rare tumor composed of malignant oncocytic cells" is Seifert's description of oncocytic carcinoma (75). The oncocytic nature of the tumor cells is confirmed with either histochemical or electron microscopic studies. Johns et al. (226) and later Goode and Corio (230) emphasized that the diagnosis of oncocytic carcinoma should rely principally on invasive features, for example, perineural invasion, intravascular and intralymphatic extension, and invasion into soft tissues including adjacent salivary gland parenchyma (74,222). Metastatic deposits in regional lymph nodes are irrefutable evidence that the tumor is malignant.

Clinical Data

Oncocytic carcinomas represent no more than 5% of all oncocytomas and, hence, only 0.005% of all epithelial neoplasms (74–76,88,230). These tumors arise most often in the major salivary glands, particularly the parotid glands, but oncocytic carcinomas have been reported in the intraoral and sinonasal minor glands also (230–233). As with oncocytoma, older women are affected by this tumor slightly more than any other patient group. Parotid masses that cause pain or paralysis typically develop in one third of the patients (231,232).

Gross Appearance

Oncocytic carcinoma appears as a single, firm, infiltrative, unencapsulated tumor with necrosis and hemorrhage.

Histologic Features

The tumor is composed of large round and polyhedral cells that are arranged in solid sheets, islands, and cords or scattered individually (Fig. 42). The cells have the appearance of oncocytes with cellular pleomorphism and polymorphism along with nuclear enlargement and mitoses. Invasion of nerves, vessels, soft tissue, or normal parenchyma is easily visible.

Special Studies

Histochemical, electron microscopic, and immunohistochemical studies reveal that these tumors appear identical to benign oncocytomas (231).

Differential Diagnosis

The main differential diagnoses are benign oncocytoma and salivary duct carcinoma. Compared to oncocytomas, oncocytic carcinomas usually show considerably greater mitotic activity, cellular pleomorphism, and unequivocal evidence of invasion into surrounding tissues. Salivary duct carcinoma has cells with an apocrine appearance that form duct-like spaces with cribriform and papillary areas, often with comedonecrosis. The cells of salivary duct carcinoma do not react with the PTAH stain for mitochondria.

Clinical Behavior and Treatment

The ability to predict the biological behavior of these carcinomas is hampered by their low frequency. A number of studies have reported multiple recurrences and distant metastases (214,220, 224,226,230–233). Good and Corio (230) indicated that carcinomas smaller than 2 cm seem to offer a better prognosis. In the series examined by Goode and Corio (230), three patients died less than 2 years after initial treatment, and the other died after 7 years. As with other carcinomas of the salivary glands, aggressive surgical intervention seems to be warranted. Radiotherapy and chemotherapy have been used in too few cases to afford any meaningful conclusions.

Warthin's Tumor and Carcinoma in Warthin's Tumor

Warthin's Tumor or Papillary Cystadenoma Lymphomatosum (Adenolymphoma)

Definition

"Warthin's tumor is composed of glandular and often cystic structures, sometimes with a papillary cystic arrangement, lined by characteristic eosinophilic epithelium. The stroma contains a variable amount of lymphoid tissue and follicles" (75). According to the most widely accepted theory concerning its histogenesis, Warthin's tumor originates in a heterotopic salivary gland duct in the lymph nodes of the parotid gland, both inside and outside the parenchyma. Functional immunologic studies, in conjunction with morphologic observations, support the concept that the lymphoid component of Warthin's tumor is derived from a preexisting lymph node (234–241).

Clinical Data

Warthin's tumor accounts for 2% to 15% of all parotid tumors and is the second most common benign neoplasm of the salivary glands (74). It almost always involves only the parotid gland, although it may arise in lymph nodes superficial or medial to this gland (239). A significant number of patients have bilateral or multiple growths or both (237). Warthin's tumor may develop in patients of any age, although it is usually observed in those over 40 years old. The incidence is eight times higher in men than it is in women (234–236).

Similar to other parotid salivary tumors, Warthin's tumor is usually nodular and enlarges and swells slowly. Located superficially, it may cause facial asymmetry. Typically, such tumors are found in the inferior pole of the parotid gland next to the angle of the mandible. When the tumors are located inferior to and outside the parotid gland, the clinical impression may be that a branchial cleft cyst, chronic lymphadenitis, or lymphoma is present (240,241).

Gross Appearance

Grossly, Warthin's tumor is well circumscribed, soft, and cystic. The lumen contains a creamy, often brownish, substance resembling pus or caseous material (Fig. 43).

Histologic Features

Microscopically, the tumor is composed of papillary elements lining cystic spaces in a lymphoid stroma (Fig. 44). The epithelium typically is arranged in two layers, the inner layer consisting of tall, cylindrical oncocytic cells and the outer layer consisting of cuboidal cells abutting the basement membrane. Other types of epithelial cells such as goblet, sebaceous, and squamous cells may also be found. The associated lymphoid tissue is benign, yet it may manifest varying degrees of reactivity. Germinal centers are virtually always present. The lymphoid stroma is composed predominantly of E-rosette–forming T lymphocytes and a smaller number of surface immunoglobulin–positive B lymphocytes. The relative distribution of the T and B lymphocytes is similar to that found in normal and reactive lymph nodes (242).

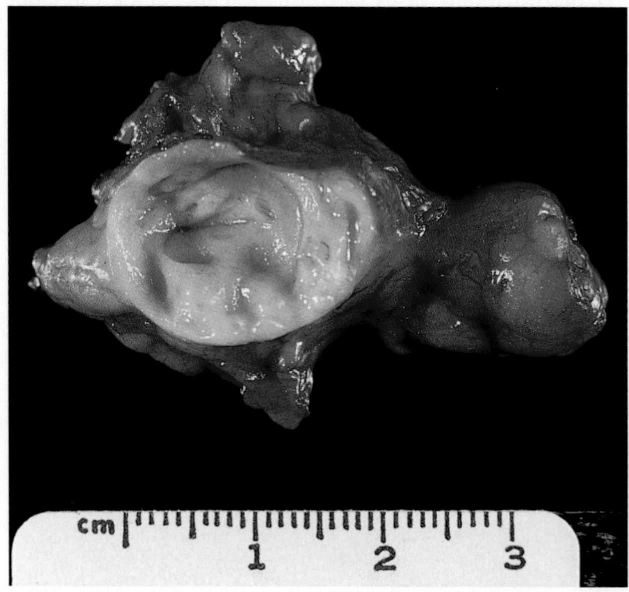

FIGURE 43. Warthin's tumor. Note cystic cavity with papillary projections.

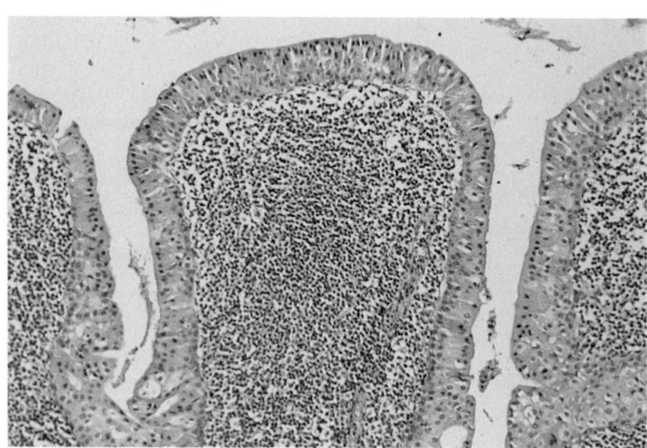

FIGURE 44. Warthin's tumor. Cystic spaces lined by a double layer of oncocytes bordered by lymphoid tissue.

On the basis of having examined 275 Warthin's tumors, Seifert et al. (240) histologically classified Warthin's tumors into four subtypes. The classification is based primarily on the ratio of epithelium to lymphoid stroma of the tumors. Subtype 1 or "typical" Warthin's tumor has an epithelial component of 50% of the tumor mass. Subtype 2 is stroma poor, with an epithelial component of 70% to 80%. Seventy-five percent of the Warthin's tumors seen by Seifert et al. were of subtype 1, and 90% of the tumors were of types 1 and 2. Stroma-rich Warthin's tumors are those with an epithelial component of 20% to 30%. These comprised 2% of the tumors in the study group. They occurred only in men. Subtype 4 (metaplastic) tumors accounted for 7.5% of the tumors. They were Warthin's tumors with large areas of squamous metaplasia and regressive secondary changes (Fig. 45). Of interest is the observation that 20% of the subtype 4 Warthin's tumors had been irradiated or had been sampled by fine needle aspiration (FNA) biopsy (243,244). No prognostic implications are associated with any of these subtypes.

Special Studies

Warthin's tumors show diffuse cytoplasmic staining for cytokeratin and apical cellular reactivity for EMA, and they are uniformly negative for S-100 protein and salivary amylase (245,246). Secretory component and secretory IgA have been identified in these lesions, and their lymphoid component consists of a mixture of B cells, T cells, and scattered histiocytes.

Electron microscopic studies reveal that apical oncocytic cells show structural characteristics similar to those of the neoplastic oncocytes in other oncocytic tumors. These features include permeation of the cytoplasm with mitochondria, which are characterized by long, densely layered cristae mitochondriales. Giant mitochondria and lyosomes are also seen (246). The pyramid-shaped basal cells occasionally contain crystalloids. Cytogenetic

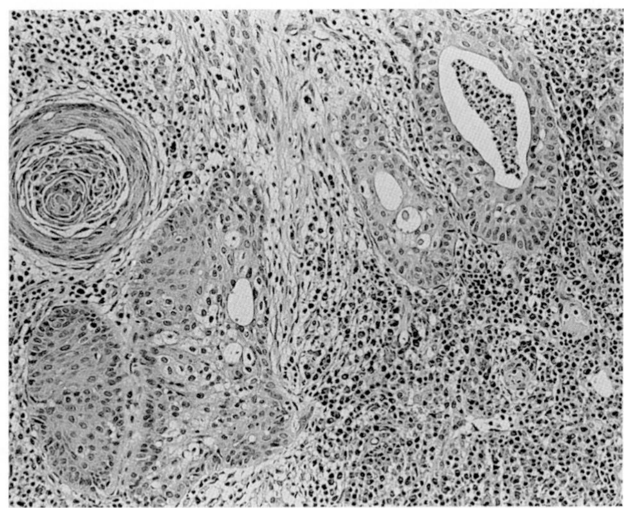

FIGURE 45. Metaplastic Warthin's tumor. Note squamous epithelium lining spaces.

studies revealed genetic aberrations in the epithelium of Warthin's tumors involving chromosome 7 (247), and in some tumors the Epstein-Barr viral genome was detected in the cytoplasm of ductal cells. This was seen most often in bilateral or multiple Warthin's tumor and only occasionally in cases of solitary Warthin's tumor (248).

Differential Diagnosis

Subtype 1 presents no difficulties in differential diagnosis. Subtype 2, which is poor in stroma, may be distinguished from an oncocytoma by the presence of the lymphoid stromal component of Warthin's tumor. The metaplastic subtype 4 must be distinguished from sebaceous adenoma, from mucoepidermoid carcinoma, from squamous cell carcinoma, and from necrotizing sialometaplasia. These may be confused with one another, especially if aspiration cytology specimens are examined.

Clinical Behavior and Treatment

Recurrence rates for Warthin's tumors are difficult to assess accurately because of the nature of the lesion. The largest series reporting recurrence rates were by Chaudhry and Gorlin (236) and Eveson (234); they found rates of 6.7% and 5.5%, respectively. Surgical management includes excisional biopsy, enucleation without removing a margin of normal parotid tissue, subtotal parotidectomy, and total parotidectomy with preservation of the facial nerve (241). Each method has its advocates, and perhaps each case should be approached individually.

Carcinoma in Warthin's Tumor

Definition

"Like carcinoma in pleomorphic adenoma, the development of carcinoma in a Warthin's tumor is observed rarely. Reported cases have been mostly squamous cell carcinomas, oncocytic carcinomas, and adenocarcinomas. Metastatic carcinoma in a Warthin's tumor must be excluded" (75). Excluding involvement by disseminated lymphomas, malignant lymphomas in Warthin's tumor are rare. Those seen were non-Hodgkin's lymphoma; nearly all were low grade (249). Equally rare is carcinoma in Warthin's tumors. If present, the carcinoma must have arisen from the epithelial elements of the Warthin's tumor; a transition zone between benign and malignant epithelium should be clearly visible (240). This definition may help exclude metastases to the lymphoid stroma and malignant neoplasms that coincide with the Warthin's tumor (241).

Clinical Data

Carcinoma in Warthin's tumor is extremely rare. The majority of these carcinomas are located in the parotid gland or the lymph nodes therein. More men than women are affected (a ratio of 4.5:1); the median age is 63.4 years and ranges from 49 to 79 years (240,241,250–255). Radiotherapy to the Warthin's tumor was antecedent in four of the eight cases reported by Seifert et al. (240).

Gross Appearance

These neoplasms have been described as solid and cystic with ill-defined margins.

Histologic Features

Microscopically, these tumors reveal residual Warthin's tumor with transition to carcinoma (Fig. 46). The most common type of carcinoma is oncocytic; squamous carcinoma, adenocarcinoma NOS, and undifferentiated carcinoma are seen less frequently (251).

Special Studies

Immunohistochemistry and electron microscopy studies demonstrate features of Warthin's tumor in addition to the type of carcinoma present in each case (251,254,255).

Differential Diagnosis

A visible area of transition between the benign residual tumor and the carcinoma helps to distinguish metastatic carcinoma and concomitant salivary gland tumors. The physician should

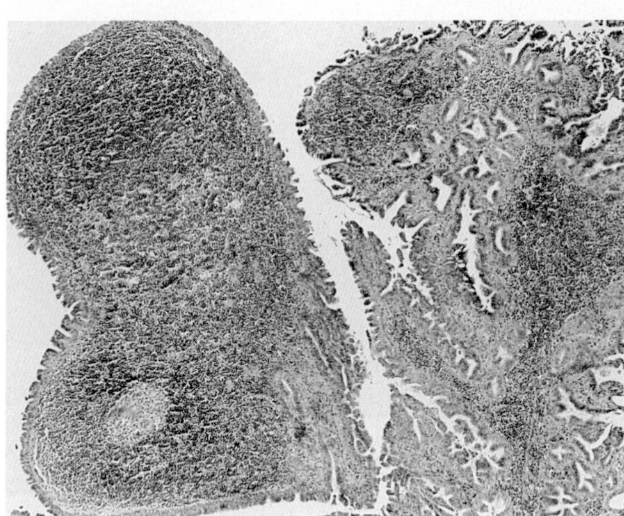

FIGURE 46. Malignant Warthin's tumor with marked cellular atypia.

know the clinical history of the patient before excluding metastatic carcinoma.

Clinical Behavior and Treatment

Because of the rarity of these carcinomas, an estimate of the biological behavior is not possible. In six of the 17 cases collected by Therkildsen and associates (251), disease metastasized to the regional lymph nodes, and one patient developed distant metastases. Similar experiences were reported by Seifert et al. (240) and Batsakis and El-Naggar (241). Complete surgical excision of the tumor with disease-free surgical margins appears to be the ideal treatment. Neck dissection depends on the presence of clinically positive lymph nodes (240,241,250–255).

Sebaceous Adenomas and Sebaceous Carcinomas

Sebaceous Cells

Sebaceous cells are commonly present within normal salivary gland tissue, yet neoplasms consisting partially or entirely of such cells within salivary glands are seldom observed. Sebaceous cells are also found in a variety of salivary gland tumors. They have been observed in Warthin's tumor, pleomorphic adenoma, mucoepidermoid carcinoma, and adenoid cystic carcinoma (256–262). Benign sebaceous cell neoplasms of the salivary glands exhibit two forms: sebaceous lymphadenoma and sebaceous adenoma.

Sebaceous Lymphadenoma

Definition

"Sebaceous lymphadenoma is a benign tumor that is composed of irregular proliferating nests and islands of epithelium, including solid and gland-like sebaceous elements, surrounded by lymphoid stroma" (75). The sebaceous lymphadenoma is so named because it originates, as does Warthin's tumor, from enclaved salivary tissue in parotid or periparotid lymph nodes (263–265). It requires both sebaceous and lymphoid components for histopathologic diagnosis.

Clinical Data

Sebaceous lymphadenomas represent about 0.1% of all adenomas in the AFIP file (75). The parotid gland is by far the most common site. Patients range in age from 25 to 89 years, with an average age of 62 years. Men and women are affected nearly equally. A painless mass is the most frequent complaint.

Gross Appearance

These tumors are usually encapsulated. Their gross appearance is similar to that of Warthin's tumor.

Histologic Features

Histologically, sebaceous lymphadenomas are characterized by islands of cells with sebaceous differentiation and metaplastic salivary ducts diffusely distributed in lymphoid tissue (Fig. 47). The islands may be solid but more often are cystic, with secretory products within the cysts. A localized foreign body reaction is provoked after escape of the cystic contents into the lymphoid tissue.

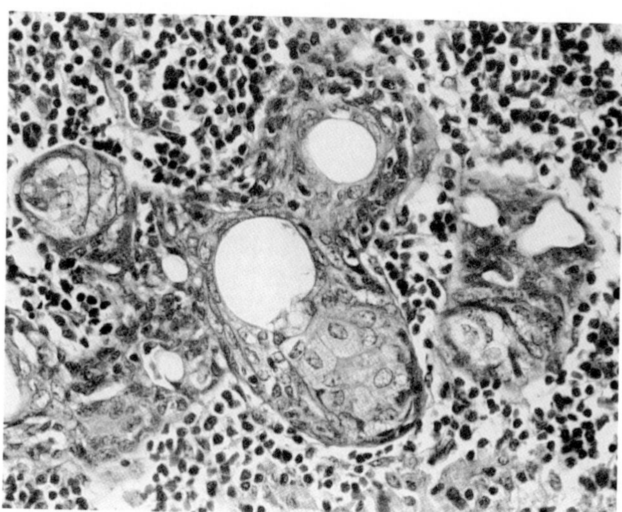

FIGURE 47. Sebaceous lymphadenoma. Nests of sebaceous cells in lymphoid stroma.

Clinical Behavior and Treatment

Sebaceous lymphadenoma seldom recurs. In the series studied by Auclair et al. (261), only one case recurred. Partial parotidectomy has often proven to be adequate treatment.

Sebaceous Adenoma

Definition

"Sebaceous adenoma is a benign tumor consisting of irregular nests of sebaceous cells without cellular atypia. The tumor is typically well circumscribed" (74).

Clinical Data

The sebaceous adenoma accounts for 0.1% of all salivary gland tumors (11,74). Seifert et al. found only three cases in 2,913 tumors in the Salivary Gland Registry of the University of Hamburg (11). The mean age at presentation is 58 years; the range is 22 to 90 years (74). Men are affected more than women by a slight margin. The adenomas have been reported to occur in the parotid gland, the submandibular gland, and the oral cavity (262).

Gross Appearance

The tumors have been described as encapsulated, varying in color from gray to pink.

Histologic Features

Sebaceous adenoma consists of numerous sebaceous glands and large cystic cavities lined by epithelium. They are supported by connective tissue stroma and are devoid of a lymphoid component (Fig. 48).

Clinical Behavior and Treatment

No recurrences of this adenoma have been reported (74,261). Complete excision or parotidectomy is the surgical procedure usually performed (261) with curative intent.

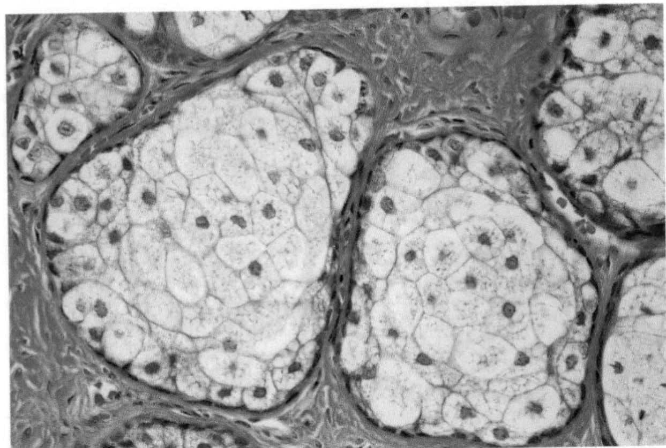

FIGURE 48. Sebaceous adenoma. Nests of sebaceous cells in connective tissue.

Sebaceous Carcinomas

Two forms of malignant sebaceous tumors of the salivary glands exist: the "pure" sebaceous carcinoma and the sebaceous lymphadenocarcinoma (74,258,262,266).

Sebaceous Carcinoma

Definition
Sebaceous carcinoma is classified as "a rare variety of carcinoma composed of sebaceous cells of varying degrees of maturity" (75).

Clinical Data
The parotid gland is the only gland affected by this extremely rare type of carcinoma. Sebaceous carcinoma of the parotid gland exhibits a bimodal age distribution with peak incidences in the third decade and also in the sixth to ninth decades of life (262). The incidence in men and women is the same. A painless mass is the most common presentation, but some patients do experience pain. Very few patients suffer facial paralysis.

Histologic Features
The carcinomas vary in their degree of cytodifferentiation. For an unequivocal diagnosis, there should be areas of recognizable sebaceous cells, with transition to less differentiated cells (Fig. 49). Intracellular mucin may be found. The carcinomas' high lipid content is helpful in the differential diagnosis. Some carcinomas may be circumscribed, but the majority show areas of necrosis, fibrosis, and invasion of nerves and other tissue.

Special Studies
Electron microscopic and immunohistochemical examinations have revealed coexistence of sebaceous and glandular differentiation. Tumor cells with lipid granules participate in the formation of glandular structures with intracytoplasmic lumina and immunohistochemical localization of lactoferrin and secretory components (267).

Differential Diagnosis
The presence of sebaceous cells and the absence of the histologic patterns seen in the most common types of salivary gland carcinomas characterize sebaceous carcinomas of the parotid gland. These tumors must always be clinically and pathologically distinguished from secondary involvement by a contiguous or more remote sebaceous carcinoma of the skin of the head and neck, especially the eyelid (262).

Clinical Behavior and Treatment
Treatment varies from local excision to parotidectomy with or without postoperative radiotherapy (266). The 5-year survival rate is 62% for patients with sebaceous carcinoma (262). The carcinomas have the ability to recur locally. Lymph node metastases and distant metastases may develop late in the clinical course of these carcinomas (266).

Sebaceous Lymphadenocarcinoma

Definition
"Sebaceous lymphadenocarcinoma is an extremely rare malignant tumor that represents carcinomatous transformation of a sebaceous lymphadenoma. The carcinomatous element may be sebaceous carcinoma or some other specific or nonspecific form of salivary gland carcinoma" (74). Sebaceous lymphadenocarcinomas are medical curiosities. The clinical data and clinical behavior are similar to those seen with the more common sebaceous carcinoma (262).

Basal Cell Adenomas and Basal Cell Adenocarcinoma

Basal Cell Adenomas

Definition
Basal cell adenoma is "a tumor of isomorphic basaloid cells with a prominent basal cell layer, a distinct basement-membrane-like structure, and no mucoid stromal component as in pleomorphic adenomas. Three cellular patterns occur: solid, trabecular–tubular, and membranous" (75).

Clinical Data
Basal cell adenoma represents 1% to 3% of the major salivary gland neoplasms (11,74,75). Although it is most often observed

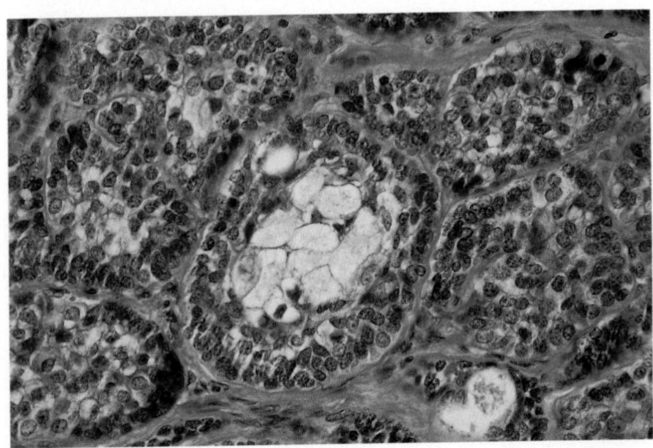

FIGURE 49. Sebaceous carcinoma. Atypical epithelial cell nests containing sebaceous cells.

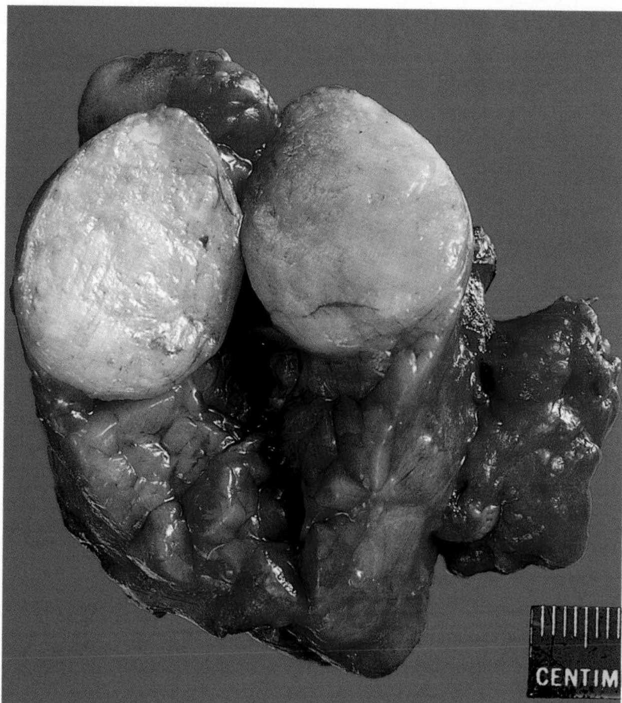

FIGURE 50. Basal cell adenoma. Well-circumscribed solid white-gray tumor.

in women over 60 years of age, the broad range of age distribution (32 to 87 years) indicates that basal cell adenoma should be considered in the differential diagnosis of salivary gland tumors, even in persons in the eighth and ninth decades of life (268–272). The parotid gland is the usual site of this type of tumor. A few adenomas have been found in the submandibular glands. Basal cell adenoma may also arise within cervical lymph nodes (273,274).

Gross Appearance

Grossly, basal cell adenomas are round or oval in shape and are encapsulated by fibrous connective tissue. The cut surface is grayish-white. In many cases, cystic formations containing mucinous fluid are present in the center of the tumor. In general, basal cell adenomas tend to be smaller than mixed tumors; their greatest diameter is less than 2 cm (Fig. 50).

Histologic Features

Three basic histologic patterns are found in basal cell adenomas: trabecular–tubular, solid, and membranous (268). The trabecular–tubular and solid types are often combined, demonstrating that there is no firm dividing line between these histologic subtypes. Microscopically, the tumors are composed of dark, round to oval nuclei set in a scant basophilic cytoplasm. The cells are arranged in solid nests, buds, and cords with palisading peripheral rows (Fig. 51); in the minor glands, the tumor cells are usually arranged in tubules rather than in solid nests. The parenchyma and stroma are well demarcated by a prominent basement membrane. Batsakis and Brannon (274) used the term dermal analogue tumors to describe basal cell

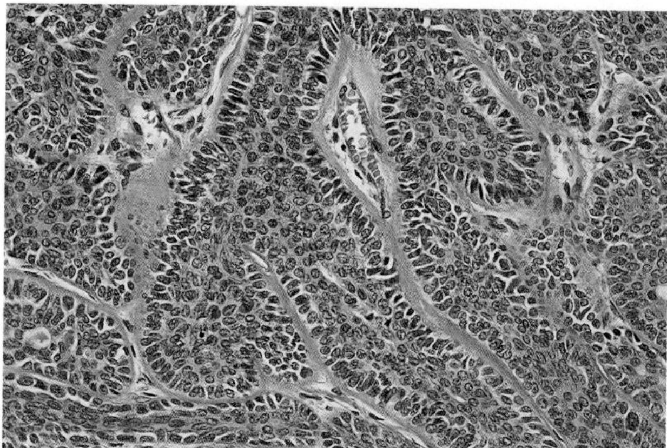

FIGURE 51. Basal cell adenoma, trabecular type.

adenomas with a prominent membranous component. The biological behavior of these adenomas appears to be somewhat different from that of other basal cell adenomas; in three of the eight cases observed, evidence of recurrence was apparent (274–276).

Membranous basal cell adenomas are often multicentric, multilobular, and nonencapsulated (Fig. 52); as a consequence, an invasive quality is imparted to this group. Microscopically, these adenomas are characterized by excessive production of an eosinophilic basal laminar material presenting the following features: hyaline cuffs around blood vessels within the tumor, small droplets surrounded by epithelial cells, and large coalescent masses entrapping pyknotic cells (Fig. 53). The parenchymal cells are similar to those found in solid basal cell adenomas and, like many of them, manifest epidermoid changes, formation of whorled morula-like structures, and keratinization. Sebaceous differentiation is seen less often.

Although the majority of these adenomas are located in the parotid gland, they have been observed in the submandibular gland and arising within periparotid or intraparotid lymph nodes (273). Synchronous or metachronous cutaneous adnexal tumors, including dermal cylindromas, trichoepitheliomas, and eccrine spiradenomas, have been reported in patients with salivary

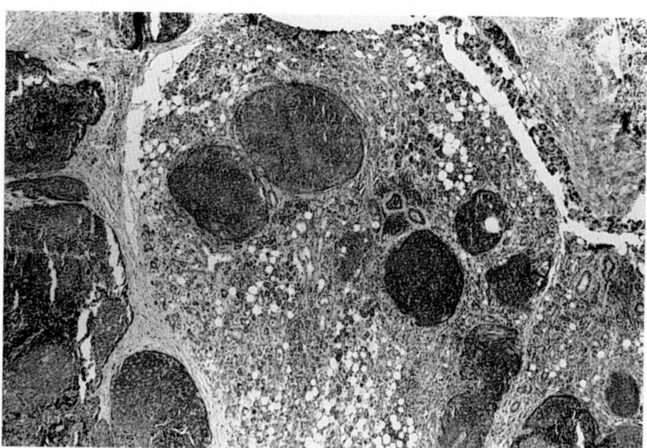

FIGURE 52. Membranous basal cell adenoma with multiple nodules.

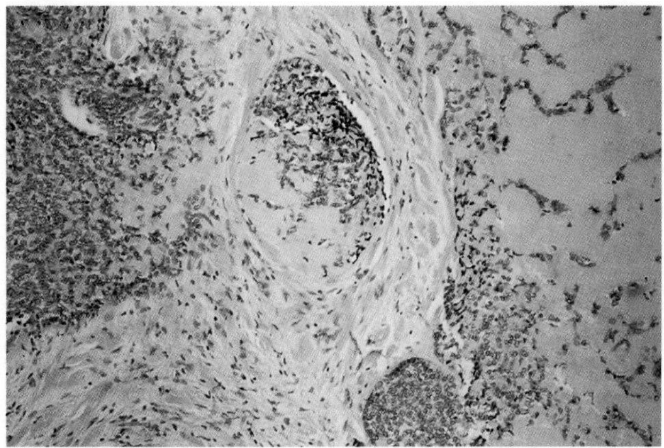

FIGURE 53. Hyaline intercellular deposits in membranous basal cell adenoma.

dermal analogue adenomas (274–276). No other type of basal cell adenoma exhibits such combinations (Table 3).

Special Studies

Most authors concur on the presence of cells that stain positively for S-100, vimentin, and SMA in most basal cell adenomas, but these cells are typically located at the periphery of the epithelial islands adjacent to the connective tissue stroma (277–280). Keratin is demonstrable in nearly all types of basal cell adenomas. CEA and EMA reactivity is mostly confined to luminal cells (278). Glial fibrillary acidic protein (GFAP) and myosin have been reported to be focally positive (279).

Ultrastructurally, basal cell adenoma may be predominately, but not exclusively, composed of an isocellular population. It may in addition contain a few progenitor cells, as well as some cells that achieve a more advanced stage of cytodifferentiation beyond the predominant cell (281–283). These studies have confirmed ductal, myoepithelial, and basal cell differentiation. One of the most distinctive electron microscopic characteristics of basal cell adenomas is the presence of reduplicated, multilayered basal lamina that surrounds the epithelial cell clusters (283).

Differential Diagnosis

The monomorphic appearance and the absence of chondroid tissue and myxoid stroma differentiate basal cell adenoma from mixed tumor. The basal cell adenoma has sometimes been mistaken for adenoid cystic carcinoma. There are two features that help to distinguish these lesions. One is the circumscription of the basal cell adenoma, which contrasts with the invasive pattern of adenoid cystic carcinoma. The other is the lack of vascularity in the microcystic areas of adenoid cystic carcinoma, which contrasts with the numerous endothelial-lined channels in basal cell adenoma. The vascular pattern should be interpreted with caution, however, especially in limited biopsy material. I have observed focal areas in adenoid cystic carcinoma of the same vascular pattern as that encountered in basal cell adenoma. Similarly, the vascular pattern of the basal cell adenoma can be obscured in the presence of fibrosis. In the experience of the author and oth-

TABLE 3. COMPARISON BETWEEN BASAL CELL ADENOMAS AND CANALICULAR ADENOMA

	Membranous Basal Cell Adenoma	Other Types of Basal Cell Adenoma	Canalicular Adenoma
Number of patients	25[a]	102	121
Sex of patients (M/F ratio)	10/1	1/1	1.7/1
Age at diagnosis (years)	34 to 74 (mean 58.1)	Neonate to 83 (mean 58.6)	34 to 88 (mean 65.1)
Number of patients with synchronous dermal appendage tumors	9 (37.7%)	0	0
Salivary gland site			
Parotid	25	92	2
Submandibular	2	5	0
Upper lip	0	5	89
Nasal cavity	1	0	0
Other minor glands	1	0	30
Multicentric salivary gland involvement	12 (48%)	1	29 (24%)
Size of adenoma (cm)	1.5 to 4.5 (mean 3.4)	1.5 to 4.0 (mean 2.6)	0.5 to 2.0 (mean 1.7)
Number of patients with recurrences	6 (24%)	0	0
Malignant "transformation"	7 (28%)	4 (3.9%)	0

[a] Twenty-five patients with dermal analogue basal cell adenomas had 29 tumors.

Sources: Batsakis JG, Luna MA, El-Naggar AK. Basaloid monomorphic adenomas. *Ann Otol Rhinol Laryngol* 1991;100:687–690. Kratochvil FJ. Canalicular adenoma and basal cell adenoma. In: Ellis GL, Auclair PL, Gnepp DR, eds. *Surgical pathology of the salivary glands.* Philadelphia: WB Saunders, 1991: 202–224.

ers, special stains are of no value in distinguishing between these tumors (277–280).

Basal cell adenocarcinoma is characterized by invasive destructive growth, in contrast to the noninvasive appearance of basal cell adenoma. Even in the multinodular forms of membranous basal cell adenoma, the individual tumor nodules are well circumscribed and non-infiltrative. In cases of basal cell adenocarcinoma, invasion of the salivary gland parenchyma and adjacent tissue is the rule.

Clinical Behavior and Treatment

The recurrence rate for the solid and trabecular-tubular variants is almost nonexistent (268). This contrasts with the high recurrence rate (24%) of the membranous type, which is perhaps a result of the multicentricity of this lesion (268). Malignant transformation is more common in the membranous type than in the other types (268). Local excision with disease-free surgical margins is adequate treatment for basal cell adenomas, whereas the membranous subtype requires parotidectomy with preservation of the facial nerve (268–272).

Basal Cell Adenocarcinoma

Definition

Basal cell adenocarcinoma is "an epithelial neoplasm that has the cytological characteristics of basal cell adenoma but morphological growth pattern indicative of malignancy" (75). Basal cell adenocarcinoma is the malignant counterpart of basal cell adenoma and it arises in two ways: *de novo* (284) or by evolution from a basal cell adenoma (285).

Clinical Data

Basal cell adenocarcinomas are rare, accounting for 2% of malignant epithelial salivary gland tumors and 1.6% of all salivary gland neoplasms (284,286,287). Most of these carcinomas are found in the parotid glands, and a few cases have involved the submandibular and the minor salivary glands (284–295). Recently, Fonseca and Soares (286) reported on 12 patients with basal cell adenocarcinomas involving the minor salivary glands and the seromucous glands of the upper aerodigestive tract. These carcinomas occur with approximately equal frequency among men and women. The average age at diagnosis is 60 years, with ages ranging from 27 to 92 years. A few cases have been reported in children (291). Swelling is the main symptom, but pain or tenderness is occasionally associated with this disease. In approximately 12% of the patients there is a diathesis of multiple dermal adenomas and parotid basal cell adenocarcinomas (284–292).

Gross Appearance

The tumors are well circumscribed but not encapsulated. Some are infiltrative. The cut surfaces are homogeneous with an occasional cystic area.

Histologic Features

Two distinct cell populations are recognized in every neoplasm in variable proportions (Fig. 54). The predominant cell type is a small, round to ovoid cell. The nuclei are dark and hyperchromatic with coarse chromatin, sometimes showing a small, inconspicuous nucleolus. The cytoplasm is sparse, usually with poorly defined borders. The other cell type is larger, and it has vast and clear or slightly eosinophilic cytoplasm as well as a nucleus similar to that of the smaller cell type. A palisade-like arrangement of the tumor cells is observed at the periphery of the neoplastic nodules (Fig. 55) along the epithelial–stromal interface and is formed mostly by neoplastic small cells. Nuclear atypia is usually inconspicuous. Focal squamous metaplasia is seen in about 25% of the cases. Counts of mitotic figures vary from less than 1 to as many as 10 per 10 high-power fields.

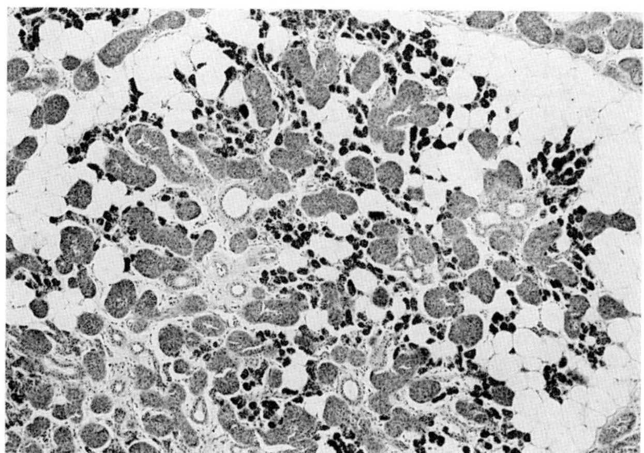

FIGURE 54. Basal cell adenocarcinoma infiltrating soft tissues.

The cells are arranged in four main patterns: solid, trabecular, tubular, and membranous (284,287). In many cases, areas of more than one microscopic pattern are seen. The solid type is characterized by contiguous tumor cells arranged in islands and masses with fibrous, connective-tissue stroma (Fig. 54). Anastomosing cords and bands of basaloid cells characterize the trabecular type (Fig. 56). Small lumina or pseudolumina are typical of the tubular variant (Fig. 57). These lumina appear to be more like tiny cystic spaces than true duct lumina. The membranous variant is distinguished by thick eosinophilic, periodic acid–Schiff-positive hyaline drops that surround and separate tumor nests and may create a jigsaw puzzle appearance (Fig. 58).

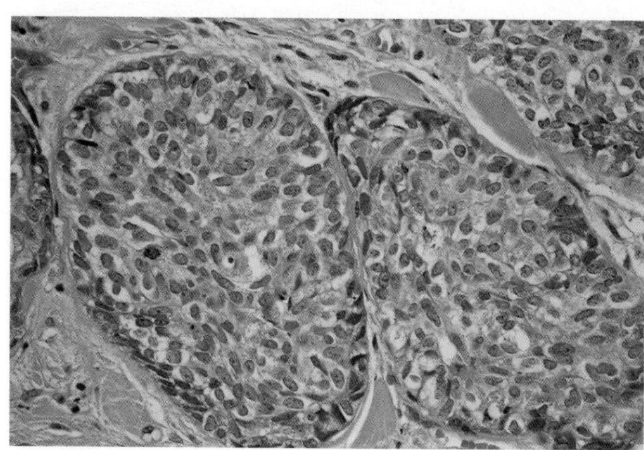

FIGURE 55. Basal cell adenocarcinoma. Islands of pale and dark cells.

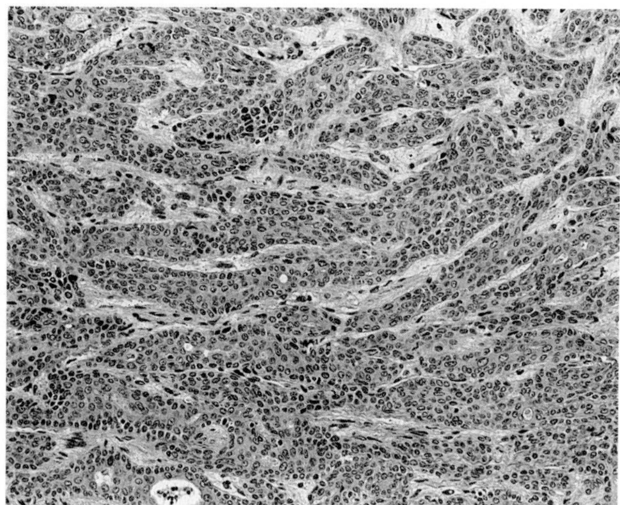

FIGURE 56. Basal cell adenocarcinoma, trabecular type.

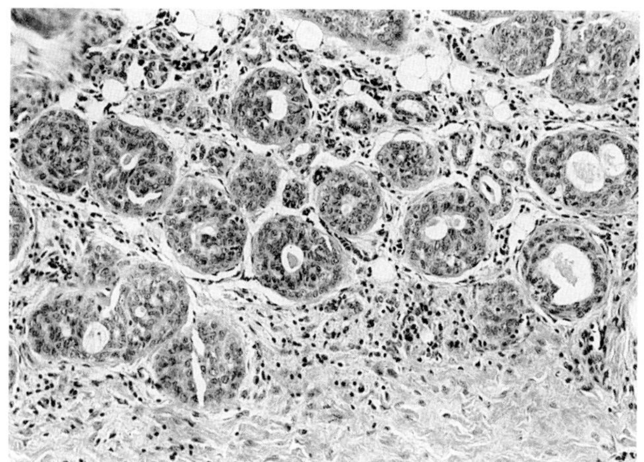

FIGURE 57. Basal cell adenocarcinoma, tubular type.

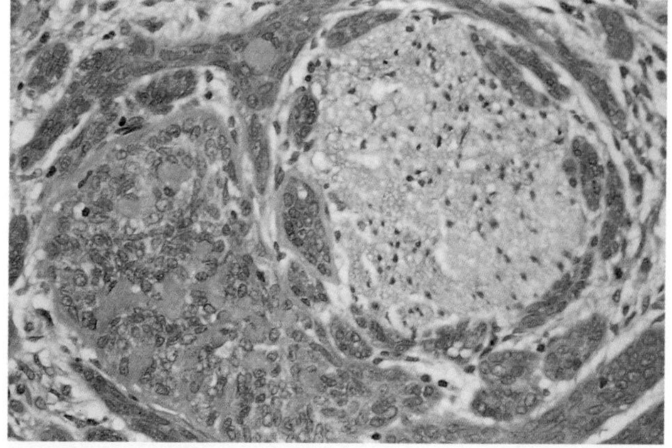

FIGURE 58. Basal cell adenocarcinoma, membranous type. Note hyaline deposits and perineural invasion.

A distinctive diagnostic feature of basal cell adenocarcinomas is this infiltrative growth pattern. Nests and strands of neoplastic cells insinuate themselves into the salivary gland lobules between the acini, into adjacent structures such as skeletal muscle, fat, and dermis, or into acini and adjacent structures. About 30% of the carcinomas show perineural infiltration, and 25% exhibit neoplastic intravascular invasion (271,284–286).

Special Studies

Immunohistochemical staining is variable from case to case, but these carcinomas express keratins in 100% of the cases. CEA, EMA, S-100 protein, actin, and vimentin are each positive about 75% of the time (271,286,292–295). In the series by Fonseca and Soares (286), all cases lacked evidence of neuroendocrine differentiation.

Ultrastructurally, the cells of basal cell adenocarcinoma are mostly oval to polygonal in shape; they are tightly apposed and interconnected by small desmosomes as well as by a few tight junctions. Well-developed desmosomes with related tonofilaments are seen occasionally, usually in relation to true or abortive basal laminae (286,292). All cells are equipped with rough endoplasmic reticulum that usually has large numbers of free ribosomes and some small mitochondria with a dense matrix. Neurosecretory granules are never present (286).

A continuous basal lamina delineates the solid tumor nodules. There is also deposition of basal lamina-like material within the tumor aggregates, frequently in the form of intercellular droplets. Elongated slender cells with a few pinocytotic vesicles and occasional smooth muscle-like filaments can be seen at the periphery of the tumor nests; these represent myoepithelial differentiation.

There are only three studies reporting the results of flow cytometry of basal cell adenocarcinoma. Atula et al. (292) reported a parotid gland carcinoma that was diploid. The submandibular neoplasm reported by McCluggage and associates (295) was aneuploid. In the largest series (286), DNA aneuploidy was documented in six tumors, and two others were diploid. A relationship between ploidy and tumor prognosis was not demonstrated.

Proliferating cell nuclear antigen (PCNA) studies performed by Fonseca and Soares (286) were positive 32% to 95.7% of the time with a mean value of 48.2 ± 23.6%. This rather high expression of proliferative markers might be related to the fact that the neoplasms are formed by basal cells, undifferentiated cells, or both, with few elements of mature epithelial or ductal phenotype.

Differential Diagnosis

The differential diagnosis of basal cell adenocarcinoma of salivary glands includes basal cell adenoma, basal cell carcinoma of the skin, solid adenoid cystic carcinoma, undifferentiated small-cell carcinoma, and basaloid squamous carcinoma.

Basal cell adenomas have cytologic and architectural characteristics similar to those of basal cell adenocarcinoma, but they lack invasive growth features (271,284). The presence of basal cell carcinoma of the skin on the face, especially if it is a recurrent lesion of the cheek, should indicate caution in the diagnosis of basal cell adenocarcinoma, although both tumors have similar histologic patterns. Clinical information and the absence of myoepithelial markers in the tumor cells are both helpful in the differential diagnosis (271).

Adenoid cystic carcinoma of the solid type is another neoplasm with histologic features like those of basal cell adenocarcinoma. However, there are distinctive histologic features that favor the diagnosis of basal cell adenocarcinoma: the palisading appearance of the peripheral cells of the neoplastic islands, the foci of squamous metaplasia, and less frequent epithelial–ductal differentiation. The pattern of deposition of basement membrane-like material can also be helpful in distinguishing the two entities. In adenoid cystic carcinoma, basal lamina is observed at the periphery of the tumor islands, especially within the pseudolumina, whereas in basal cell adenocarcinoma, hyaline basal lamina-like material is frequently irregularly distributed inside the tumor islands, dissecting between the neoplastic cells (11,271).

Previous studies of series of undifferentiated small-cell carcinoma of the salivary glands include cases that are not neuroendocrine in derivation and cases that exhibit an unequivocal bicellular composition of dark elements and clear larger cells with some characteristics of basal cell adenocarcinoma (294). Immunohistochemical characterization of the tumor cells using both neuroendocrine and myoepithelial markers usually supports a diagnosis of undifferentiated small-cell carcinoma.

The basaloid squamous carcinoma is a specific clinicopathologic entity of mucosal-lined structures that must be differentiated from basal cell adenocarcinoma of minor salivary gland origin because its clinically aggressive behavior justifies a multimodal therapeutic approach. Similarly to basal cell adenocarcinoma, basaloid squamous carcinoma presents a lobular pattern with peripheral nuclear palisading and marginal stromal fibrosis. Comedo-type necrosis is common in basaloid squamous carcinomas. Basaloid squamous carcinomas show multiple attachments to the overlying mucosal epithelium, which must be searched for. Features of squamous cell carcinoma are also present. Definitive differential diagnosis is achieved by the demonstration of either high-grade dysplasia or invasive squamous cell carcinoma arising at the overlying epithelium. Moreover, immunohistochemical and ultrastructural features do not provide evidence of dual differentiation in this neoplasm; this is in contrast to what is seen with basal cell adenocarcinoma (296).

Clinical Behavior and Treatment

Basal cell adenocarcinomas are low-grade malignancies. They have a strong tendency to recur locally but have a low rate of distant metastases. The recurrence rate varies from 28% to 76% with a mean rate of 35% (284–292). Metastasis occurs in only about 12% of cases. In the minor salivary glands, the recurrence is 72.7%, with a rate for metastases to cervical lymph nodes of 18.2% (286). Complete surgical excision with disease-free margins of resection appears to be the appropriate treatment (284–292).

Canalicular Adenoma

Definition

Canalicular adenoma is not a variant of basal cell adenoma but a separate entity with distinct clinical and pathologic features (75,270,297). It is defined as "a tumor of columnar epithelial cells which are arranged in anastomosing bilayered strands that form a beading pattern. The stroma is loose, highly vascular and not fibrous" (75).

Clinical Data

Canalicular adenoma constitutes about 1% of all salivary gland neoplasms and 4% of all minor salivary gland tumors (74,270). The neoplasm is localized to the upper lip in 73% of cases; the second most common location is the buccal mucosa, followed by the palate (270,297–301). Batsakis et al. (302) found four canalicular adenomas in the parotid gland in a study of 96 monomorphic adenomas of the major salivary glands. The average age of patients with canalicular adenoma is 65 years, with a range of 34 to 88 years. The tumor definitely affects women more commonly than men in a ratio of 1.7 to 1.0 (270, 297–301). The most common symptom is a painless nonulcerated nodule that exhibits gradual enlargement. Canalicular adenomas are not found in patients with the salivary basal cell adenoma dermal appendage tumor syndrome (268).

Gross Appearance

These tumors range in size from 0.5 to 2.0 cm with a mean of 1.7 cm (270). They are circumscribed but nonencapsulated nodules; it is not uncommon for canalicular adenoma to be multinodular or multifocal (303). Daley et al. (297) reported that 22.4% of the canalicular adenomas in their series were multifocal.

Histologic Features

Canalicular adenomas are composed largely of bilayered strands of columnar cells (Fig. 59). The characteristic columnar cells exhibit a moderate to abundant amount of eosinophilic or amphophilic cytoplasm. The stroma is loose and highly vascular with a few fibroblasts and little collagen. A characteristic peri-

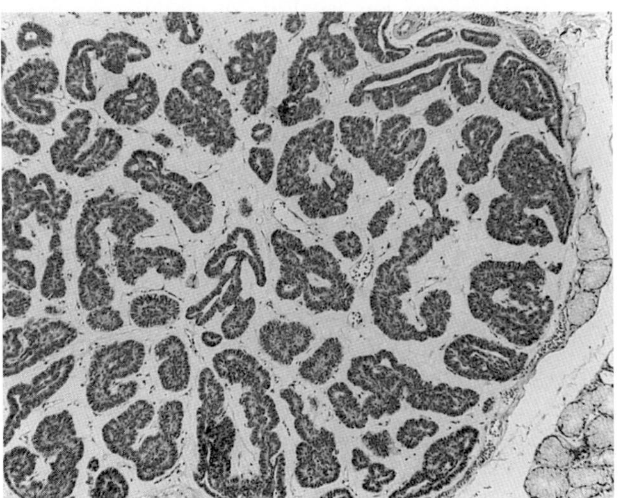

FIGURE 59. Canalicular adenoma. Note loose myxoid stroma.

odic separation of the bilayered epithelial strands, referred to as "beading," is present in most canalicular adenomas (Fig. 59). Sometimes large cystic spaces are present with papillary projections into the lumina. These projections also are lined by columnar or cuboidal cells, and psammoma bodies may be present in these areas. For the most part, the lesions are well circumscribed and appear to be surrounded by a thin fibrous capsule. However, many tumors are unencapsulated and multifocal (297,303).

Special Studies

Histochemical studies have demonstrated that alcian blue staining is greatly decreased after hyaluronidase digestion in the loose stroma of canalicular adenomas. This result indicates the presence of large quantities of hyaluronic acid, chondroitin sulfate, or both. Immunohistochemical studies by Zarbo et al. (304) revealed that the epithelium in canalicular adenomas shows immunoreactivity for S-100 protein, but the stromal cells do not. Of the canalicular adenoma tissue samples studied at the AFIP by immunohistochemistry, nearly all of the tumor cells were immunoreactive for keratin and S-100 protein. Generally, none of the tumor cells were reactive with SMA, and focal staining for GFAP occurred in one case (74). The implication is that there is little or no myoepithelial involvement in these adenomas.

Electron microscopic analysis by Daley et al. (297) and Guccion and Redman (301) revealed a uniform single layer of low columnar cells with a few short desmosomes joining them. The cytoplasm contained abundant free polysomes, scattered tubules of granular endoplasmic reticulum, and a moderate number of mitochondria. The basement membrane was a single thick sheet without intervening myoepithelial cells between it and the columnar cells.

Differential Diagnosis

The principal differential diagnoses for canalicular adenomas are basal cell adenoma and adenoid cystic carcinoma. Distinguishing canalicular adenoma from basal cell adenoma is of academic interest but has little therapeutic significance (268,297,300). Canalicular adenoma is frequently mistaken for the tubulotrabecular variant of basal cell adenoma. However, basal cell adenoma lacks the peripheral row and branching canaliculi of columnar cells that are characteristic of canalicular adenoma. Table 3 displays the clinicopathologic differences among membranous basal cell adenoma, other types of basal cell adenoma, and canalicular adenoma.

Making the distinction between canalicular adenoma and adenoid cystic carcinoma may sometimes be difficult. Both are composed of morphologically bland basaloid cells that form numerous duct-like structures. Daley (300) pointed out two important distinguishing features: circumscription of canalicular adenoma contrasted with the invasive pattern of adenoid cystic carcinoma, and the lack of vascularity in the cribriform areas of adenoid cystic carcinoma in contrast to the numerous endothelial-lined channels in the adenomas. These criteria are generally true, although not absolute.

Clinical Behavior and Treatment

The prognosis for patients with canalicular adenoma is excellent. Recurrences are extremely rare after surgical treatment, even though many canalicular adenomas have been treated with lumpectomy (74,268,270,297–301). Local excision is the appropriate therapy.

Other Benign Epithelial Neoplasms

Sialadenoma papilliferum, inverted ductal papilloma, and intraductal papillomas are rare variants of ductal papillomas of the minor glands and occasionally of the parotid and submandibular glands (305). Other unusual benign epithelial neoplasms are papillary cystadenoma, which resembles a Warthin's tumor without the lymphoid stroma, mucinous cystadenoma lined by mucus-producing cells, and a squamous papillary tumor (305–307).

Acinic Cell Carcinoma

Definition

Acinic cell carcinoma is characterized as "a malignant epithelial neoplasm that demonstrates some cytological differentiation toward acinar cells" (75). In the past, this neoplasm was considered biologically benign with only an occasional unpredictable malignancy. The term "acinic cell tumor" was often used to indicate the ambiguity in biological behavior (11). At present, most investigators recognize these neoplasms as adenocarcinomas with low-grade malignant potential (308–314). They can recur and metastasize to regional lymph nodes or to distant viscera. Thus, the term carcinoma should be used (74,75).

Clinical Data

These tumors chiefly affect middle-aged and elderly patients, although they may be encountered in patients of any age. They are more prevalent in women than in men and frequently arise in the salivary glands of children (308–315). A few cases have been reported in ectopic salivary gland tissue in the middle and low cervical lymph nodes (316). In 99% of the cases, the parotid gland is the primary site; rarely, acinic cell carcinomas originate in the submandibular gland and the oral cavity (310,315).

Acinic cell carcinomas account for between 2% and 4% of all parotid gland tumors and between 12% and 17% of all cancers of this gland. They rank second only to Warthin's tumor in bilaterality; the incidence of bilateral occurrence in the parotid glands is approximately 3% (11,14,76,88).

Gross Appearance

Upon gross examination, acinic cell carcinomas are frequently fairly well circumscribed by a large layer of dense fibrous tissue. They are much the same consistency and color as the normal salivary gland.

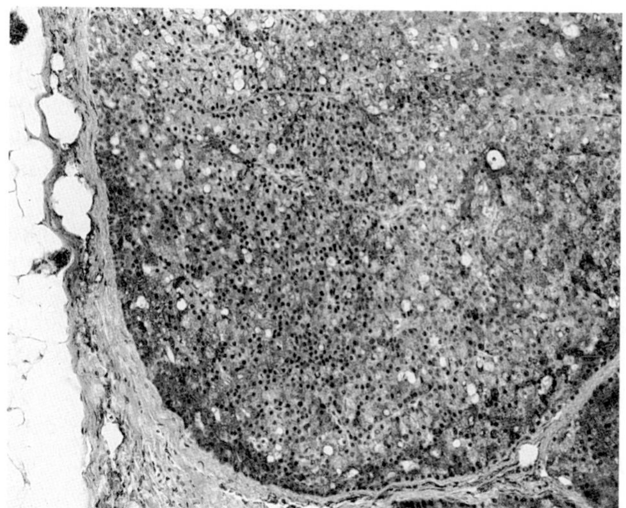

FIGURE 60. Acinic cell carcinoma, solid pattern.

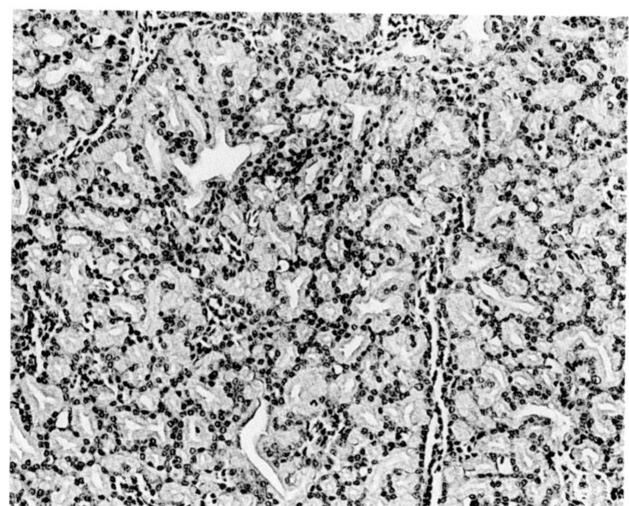

FIGURE 62. Acinic cell carcinoma, microcystic pattern.

Histologic Features

On low-power microscopic examination, many cancer cells can be seen growing in large, fairly well circumscribed nests of cells with basophilic cytoplasm. The individual cells can be categorized as acinar, intercalated duct-like, vacuolated, clear, or nonspecific glandular. The stroma is sparse and consists of fibrovascular septa. A lymphoid infiltrate may be prominent, at times containing germinal centers. The margins of the tumors are usually of the pushing type, though the more aggressive tumors may have destructive infiltrating margins with vascular or lymphatic invasion.

The cytoplasm of at least some of the cells in acinic cell carcinoma contains PAS-positive, diastase-resistant secretory granules. The number of granules varies from field to field and from tumor to tumor.

The neoplastic cells are arranged in a wide variety of architectural patterns: solid (Fig. 60), papillary and/or papillocystic (Fig. 61), microcystic (Fig. 62), and follicular. None of the four histologic patterns nor predominance of any of the cell types has been found to reliably predict aggressive or favorable disease behavior. Batsakis et al. (317) proposed a grading system for acinic cell carcinomas. Stanley and associates (318) described six cases of dedifferentiated forms of acinic cell carcinoma. Three of the cases were associated with an undifferentiated carcinoma, and the other three with poorly differentiated adenocarcinoma (Fig. 63).

Special Studies

Electron microscopic examination reveals three types of cells: ductal cells with few cytoplasmic organelles and microvilli oriented toward irregular lumina; serous cells with abundant cytoplasmic organelles in the form of rough endoplasmic reticulum and large secretory granules with a variably electron-dense content; and undifferentiated cells with sparse cytoplasm and no se-

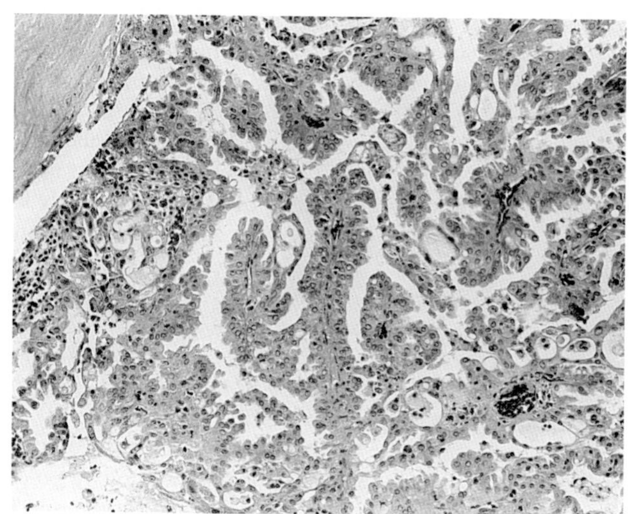

FIGURE 61. Acinic cell carcinoma, papillary pattern.

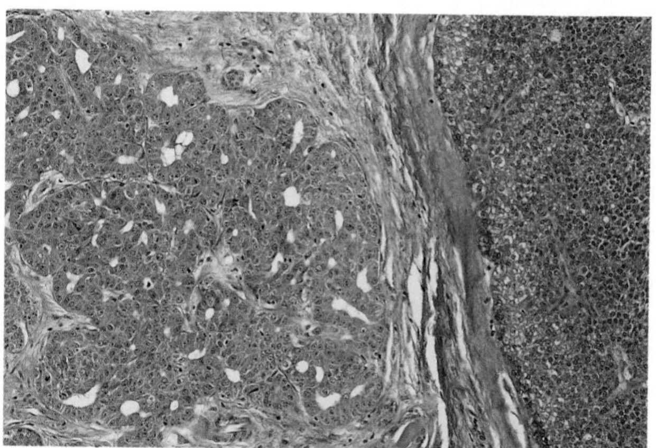

FIGURE 63. Acinic cell carcinoma with dedifferentiated component. Classic acinic cell carcinoma is on the right of the figure, with a more pleomorphic adenocarcinoma on the left.

cretory granules. These epithelial cells are situated between the ductular and the serous cells (319,320).

Immunohistochemical studies show acinic cell carcinomas to react to keratin, transferrin, lactoferrin, carcinoembryonic antigen (CEA), Leu M1 antigen, and amylase (321,322). In formalin-fixed, paraffin-embedded tumor tissue samples, however, amylase stain has not been useful (74,322).

DNA analysis by flow cytometry has not been useful in predicting clinical behavior of these carcinomas because the majority are diploid (323,324). Argyrophilic nucleolar organizer region (AgNOR) studies have produced disparate results. Chomette et al. (325) found a correlation between number of AgNORs and biological behavior in a study of 17 acinic cell carcinomas, whereas Timon and associates (326) found no significant correlation in 45 cases.

Differential Diagnosis

Solid tumors composed of well-differentiated acinar cells pose few problems in diagnosis. However, when these cells are inconspicous and the tumor is made up predominantly of clear cells or when the carcinoma has a papillary pattern, the neoplasm may be difficult to recognize as acinic cell carcinoma. Acinic cell carcinomas with a preponderance of clear cells must be differentiated from the clear cell variant of mucoepidermoid carcinoma, from metastatic renal cell carcinoma, and from epithelial–myoepithelial carcinoma. In the vast majority of acinic cell carcinomas, the histologic pattern, the focal cytoplasmic granularity with basophilia, and the postdiastase PAS-positive reaction are the most distinct features. Mucoepidermoid carcinoma, renal cell carcinoma, and epithelial–myoepithelial carcinoma are recognized by the fact that they contain cells rich in glycogen. Electron microscopic examination is valuable in the differential diagnosis of atypical acinic cell carcinomas (319,320).

Papillocystic acinic cell carcinoma should be differentiated in the major glands from cystadenocarcinoma of salivary glands and from metastatic papillary carcinoma of thyroid; in the minor salivary glands, from terminal duct carcinoma. The presence of vacuolated areas, microcystic formations, and cells with granular cytoplasm would favor papillary acinic cell carcinoma. The clear nuclei and immunostaining for thyroglobulin should readily identify papillary thyroid carcinoma. The demonstration of moderate to strongly positive mucin-positive cells argues strongly against acinic cell carcinoma and would favor cystadenocarcinoma.

There are many similarities between terminal duct carcinoma and acinic cell carcinoma. Both have cytologic uniformity and manifest various histologic patterns. Terminal duct carcinoma predominates in the minor salivary glands, whereas acinic cell carcinoma is by far more common in the parotid gland. Furthermore, terminal duct carcinoma has a more homogeneous cell population, tendency to form single cell or single file cell formations, and a greater affinity for perineural invasion than acinic cell carcinoma.

Clinical Behavior and Treatment

As a group, acinic cell carcinomas behave as low-grade malignant tumors in that they have a strong tendency to recur locally, yet they seldom metastasize. Thus, patients with this tumor should be followed up for long periods of time. In Spiro's series (312) the "determinate cure" rates were 76%, 63%, and 55% at 5, 10, and 15 years, respectively. Perzin and LiVolsi (314) reported the determinate 5-, 10-, and 15-year survival rates at 76%, 63%, and 44%, respectively. Similar results have been reported by Ellis and Corio (310) and more recently by Lewis et al. (311).

Complete surgical excision of the carcinoma in the form of parotidectomy or submandibular triangle dissection offers the best opportunity for cure (88,312,327,328). Radiotherapy should be given if the tumor was incompletely excised or for tumors with extensive vascular, lymphatic, or perineural invasion (74,88).

Adenoid Cystic Carcinoma

Definition

Seifert describes adenoid cystic carcinoma as

> an infiltrative malignant tumor having various histological features with three growth patterns: glandular (cribriform), tubular, or solid. The tumor cells are of two types: duct-lining cells and cells of myoepithelial type. Perineural or perivascular spread without stromal reaction is very characteristic. All structural types of adenoid cystic carcinoma can be associated in the same tumor (75).

Of all salivary gland tumors, the adenoid cystic carcinoma is one of the most biologically deceptive and difficult to manage. Its rather bland histologic appearance and favorable short-term therapeutic results mask its ultimate biological aggressiveness (329,330). Adenoid cystic carcinoma is thought to arise from cells in the intercalated or terminal ducts that can differentiate into epithelial and myoepithelial cell forms (331). Ultrastructural and immunohistochemical studies have demonstrated that the state of cellular differentiation parallels that of developing intercalated duct cells (331–334).

Clinical Data

In a review of 2,807 epithelial salivary gland neoplasms, 281 (10%) were adenoid cystic carcinomas (88). This frequency is very close to that provided by an analysis of the Salivary Gland Register at the Pathology Institute of the University of Hamburg, where 6.5% of epithelial salivary gland tumors were of the adenoid cystic type (11). The tumor constitutes between 2% and 4% of parotid tumors, approximately 15% of submandibular gland neoplasms, and 30% of minor salivary gland tumors (74,76,88,335). In the minor glands, the tumors are mainly located in the palate (18%), the nasal cavity and sinuses (17%), the tongue (6.9%), the buccal mucosa and lip (5.8%), and the floor of the mouth (2.5%) (335). Adenoid cystic carcinoma may occur at any age, although most patients are middle-aged or older. It is seen more frequently in women when it occurs in the submandibular gland but occurs equally in men and women when found in minor salivary glands (329,330,335–341).

The overall growth rate is rather slow, and the most common initial symptom is the presence of a firm, unilobular mass generally measuring 2 to 4 cm in diameter at the time of diagnosis. It has a strong tendency to invade the perineural spaces. This behavior probably accounts for the unusual neurologic symptoms and signs observed in patients with adenoid cystic carcinomas. Facial nerve paralysis has been noted in 4% of the cases as an initial finding. Furthermore, 18% of the patients reported pain as a symptom when first seen by their physicians (329,330).

Gross Appearance

The average carcinoma measures from 1.5 to 4 cm before the patient seeks treatment and comes to surgery. When resected, the tumor is a firm monolobular growth whose cut surface is moist and solid. Some carcinomas appear to be grossly circumscribed, but there is a lack of true encapsulation. In many cases, the infiltrative character of the tumor is quite apparent.

Histologic Features

Microscopically, adenoid cystic carcinoma is distinguished by its stroma and by the morphology of the cells comprising the tumor. The cells are small, round, and isomorphic with large, dark-staining nuclei with scant cytoplasm and ill-defined borders. Little or no nuclear atypism or mitotic activity is present. The cells can be arranged in four basic patterns: tubular, cribriform, cylindromatous, and solid or basaloid.

The *tubular* pattern consists of well-formed ducts or tubules with central lumina lined by two or three layers of cells. An inner ductal cell layer and outer, generally more fusiform and/or clear, myoepithelial cell layer are apparent in this architectural pattern. When cut longitudinally, these structures appear as long, fairly thin tubules. In cross section, they have a round glandular configuration (Fig. 64).

The *cribriform* pattern is the most important and classical feature of adenoid cystic carcinoma. In this pattern, nests of tumor cells have a "sieve-like" or "Swiss cheese" configuration. The cribriform appearance results from the presence of numerous microcystic pseudoglandular spaces (Fig. 65). Hyaline cylinders surrounded by tumor cells are the signs of the *cylindromatous* variant.

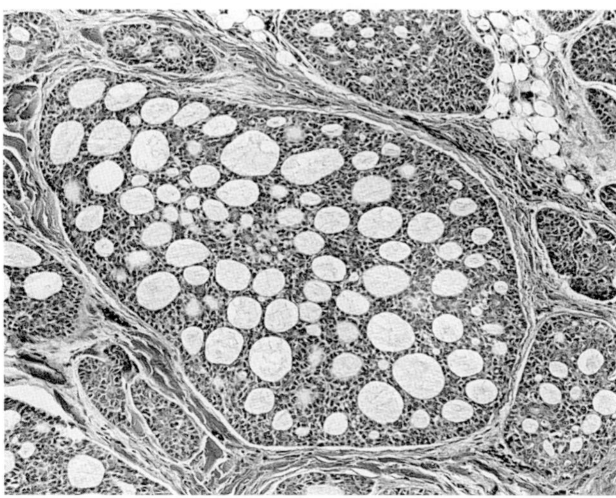

FIGURE 65. Adenoid cystic carcinoma, cribriform (glandular) type.

The *solid* or *basaloid* form is composed of solid epithelial islands completely filled with cells; only a few lumina may be seen. Small foci of necrosis in the centers of the cell masses are often present. The solid pattern can form small nests as well as larger units (Fig. 66).

In most cases, all four patterns can be observed, although their distribution varies greatly between different tumors. The pattern may also vary in different areas of the same tumor.

In most adenoid cystic carcinomas, the stroma is hyalinized and often takes the form of cylindrical cores surrounded by epithelial cells. Sometimes the stroma acquires a mucinous or myxoid appearance, but in contrast to the myxoid component of pleomorphic adenoma, the stroma of adenoid cystic carcinoma contains no epithelial cells scattered throughout the mucinous or myxoid substance, and there is a clear demarcation between the epithelial component and the myxoid stroma.

Eneroth and Zajicek (342) describe the cytologic features of this carcinoma seen in samples taken by fine-needle aspiration. The tumor cells have round or oval nuclei surrounded by a barely

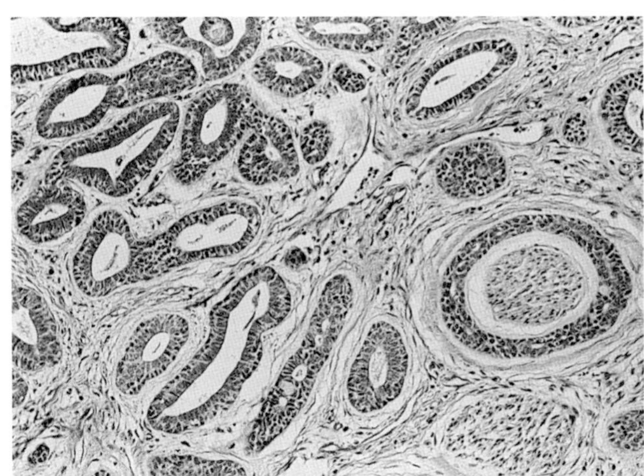

FIGURE 64. Adenoid cystic carcinoma, tubular type. Note perineural invasion.

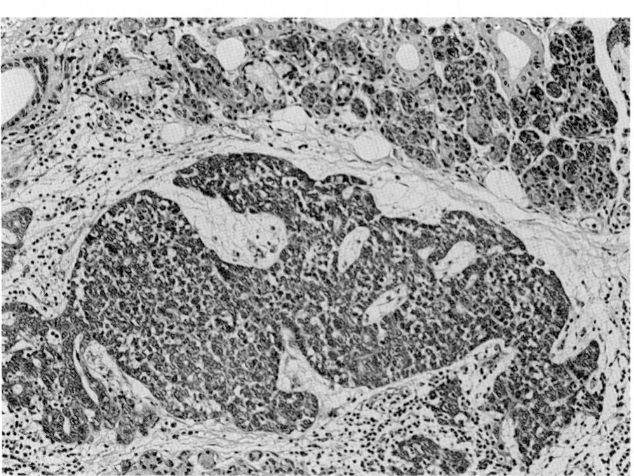

FIGURE 66. Adenoid cystic carcinoma, solid type.

noticeable rim of cytoplasm, vary little in size, and are usually tightly packed in clusters. The majority of the cases also show globules of mucus or mucoid structures, which are colorless when stained with Papanicolaou's stain and appear pink when stained with the May-Grünwald-Giemsa method.

Special Studies

Ultrastructural studies demonstrate that the neoplasm is composed of both undifferentiated cells and cells with ductal and myoepithelial differentiation (331). The cellular composition of adenoid cystic carcinoma varies between different tumors and within the same tumor. Cells with ductal differentiation are seen in the tubular and cribriform structures and, to a lesser extent, in the solid basaloid areas of the tumor. In these structures, small true lumina lined by cells with microvilli and junctional complexes are identified. Most of the undifferentiated cells are observed in the cribriform and solid basaloid areas. Chaudhry et al. (331) used light microscopy to demonstrate that the cyst-like formations in areas of acellular hyaline represent extracellular circular compartments containing replicated multilayered basal lamina substance without junctional complexes and microvilli.

Cells with myoepithelial differentiation are observed mainly in the peripheries of the tubular and ductal structures and around the acellular hyaline pseudocysts, but they are not associated with the solid basaloid areas of the tumor (331).

Immunohistochemical staining confirms the presence of at least two cell types: ductal cells that express carcinoembryonic antigen (CEA) and epithelial membrane antigen (EMA) and nonductal cells that express muscle-specific actin characteristic of myoepithelium (332–334). The immunophenotypes depend on the histologic patterns of the tumor. Cells in morphologically recognizable ductal formation express CEA, EMA, keratin, low-molecular-weight keratin (54 kDa), and S-100. This group of cells consists of true luminal cells in the cribriform, solid, and tubular growth patterns.

Cells with myoepithelial differentiation are seen in the layers around the pseudocysts in the cribriform and cylindromatous areas and in cells facing the stroma in the tubular structures. These cells express muscle-specific actin and low-molecular-weight keratin (54 kDa); occasionally these cells also express S-100 or keratin (332–334). In pseudocysts, replicated basal lamina reacts with antisera to laminin and to type IV collagen (343).

Studies of nuclear DNA content analysis are available regarding the prognostic value of cytometric DNA assessment of adenoid cystic carcinomas. Franzen and associates (344) and Eibling et al. (345) found, using flow cytometric analysis, a potentially important role for flow cytometry in evaluation of adenoid cystic carcinoma. Tytor et al. (346) observed that in some tumors both diploid and aneuploid stem lines can coexist. They emphasized, however, that two samples from different tumor areas are needed for consistency.

Greiner et al. (347) reviewed 37 paraffin-embedded adenoid cystic carcinoma tissue samples by flow cytometry and reported that 35 (95%) of the tumors were diploid. The authors found that diploid tumors with high S-phase fraction were more frequently associated with death from tumor and that S-phase appeared to be a more useful marker than was ploidy. In the series, 58% of 19 patients with tumors with high S-phase died of their tumor in contrast to 37% of 16 patients with low–S-phase tumors.

In our experience with 26 adenoid cystic carcinomas of the submandibular gland retrospectively studied by flow cytometry, 10 (38.4%) tumors were aneuploid, and 16 were diploid (348). Six of 10 patients with aneuploid tumor died of their disease, and only one of 16 patients with diploid tumor died. Aneuploidy correlated with above-median S-phase, clinical stage, histologic pattern, and invasion of large nerves and blood vessels.

There are significantly increased numbers of AgNORs in adenoid cystic carcinoma compared with normal salivary gland tissue (349,350). Higashi et al. (351) reported anomalies of the terminal part of chromosomes 6q and 9p in adenoid cystic carcinoma of the respiratory tract.

Differential Diagnosis

If the surgical specimen is large, the diagnosis of adenoid cystic carcinoma can be made without difficulty. In small biopsy specimens, however, distinguishing this tumor from mixed tumor, basal cell adenoma, and poorly differentiated mucoepidermoid carcinoma may be a problem. Mucoepidermoid carcinoma can be determined by the presence of glandular structures composed of mucinous, transitional, and squamous cells. The histologic differences between adenoid cystic carcinoma, basal cell adenoma, and benign mixed tumor have already been discussed.

The presence of squamous cell differentiation separates basaloid squamous carcinoma and basal cell adenocarcinoma from adenoid cystic carcinoma. The biphasic pattern is usually more prominent in epithelial–myoepithelial carcinoma than in adenoid cystic carcinoma. Furthermore, the periductal cells in epithelial–myoepithelial carcinoma are larger and polygonal with rounded nuclei rather than smaller and angular as in adenoid cystic carcinoma. The difference between polymorphous low-grade adenocarcinoma and adenoid cystic carcinoma is discussed in the adenocarcinoma section.

Clinical Behavior and Treatment

Adenoid cystic carcinomas have a slow but relentlessly malignant natural course, which is marked by a high incidence of local recurrence and distant metastases. The success of treatment and ultimate prognosis cannot be evaluated in a 5-year term but rather must be considered in terms of 15 to 20 years. In 40 large studies, only 31% to 35% of patients died of disease after only 5 years, and 80% to 90% of the patients succumbed to the tumor after 15 years. It appears, however, that for prognostic purposes the most critical period lies between 5 and 10 years (330,331,342).

Recurrence of an adenoid cystic carcinoma is common and often occurs within 3 years after therapy. The local recurrence rates reported vary widely, from 16% to 67% (329,330, 335–341). Perzin et al. (336) examined 130 cases of recurrence in 49 patients; 97 (75%) occurred less than 3 years after treatment. However, late local recurrences were not uncommon, especially for the tubular and cribriform types of adenoid cystic carcinoma. In the series reported by Spiro and associates (329), the disease-free interval varied from a few months to as long as 15 years; the median time was less than 1 year for lesions of the sinonasal tract and about 2 years for all others. A recurrence usually indicates incurability; only 5 of 54 patients in this category in Szanto's series (352) and 5 of 56 in Conley's series (330) were free of disease over a 10-year interval.

Reports on metastases to cervical lymph nodes have shown great variation. The reported rate ranges from 4% to 25%, with the pooled incidence of regional metastases being 15% (329,330,335–341). More metastases originate from primary tumors of the submandibular gland than from those of the parotid and minor salivary glands (330). According to Conley (330), when lymph node involvement occurs, it is commonly a result of direct or contiguous invasion rather than embolic metastases. Lymph node involvement is an ominous sign; in Spiro's material (331) only 1 of 33 patients having involvement of lymph nodes was alive and well 10 years after therapy.

The incidence of distant metastases varies from 25% to 54% in various studies and increases as time since initial treatment lengthens. Metastatic disease is more likely to occur as the result of vascular or hematogenous spread; the lung is the common site. The largest series is that of Spiro et al. (331). They recorded remote spread of the disease in 93 (43%) of 218 cases of adenoid cystic carcinoma of the major and minor salivary glands. Sixty-six of these subjects demonstrated lung metastases. According to Koka et al. (339), lung metastases outnumber those to lymph nodes by a 3:1 margin. Bone, brain, and liver metastases occur less often.

Distant metastasis often occurs late in the course of the disease. As a rule, patients with distant metastases usually have uncontrolled disease in the primary site or in the neck. Spiro's data (329) showed that 20% of the patients survived for more than 5 years after the appearance of pulmonary metastases, and one third of the patients died within 1 year of the appearance of distant metastases. In Matsuba's series, the median survival time was 40 months after metastases developed (338).

Several investigators have attempted to correlate the different architectural patterns of adenoid cystic carcinoma with biological behavior and survival, but they have not achieved uniform results (336,337,352–354). Perzin et al. (336) in 1978 studied the tubular form separately and suggested that this was the most differentiated form of adenoid cystic carcinoma and had the best prognosis. This observation was corroborated by Chomette (353) and Szanto et al. (352). Nascimento et al. (337) were unable to corroborate this finding and, in fact, found that the tubular form had a worse prognosis than did the cribriform tumors. There are, however, indications that the solid pattern entails a worse prognosis than cribriform carcinomas, often with death occurring in the first 3 years after diagnosis (11,74,75,352,353). A uniform grading system has been developed by Batsakis and associates to avoid differences among various histologic grading criteria (354).

Some factors that affect survival time are more important than histologic grade; these include the size of the tumor, its location, the clinical disease stage, perineural and bone invasion, and the presence or absence of tumor at the surgical margins (355–359).

Although details of treatment vary among institutions, surgery is the primary choice. Casler et al. (360) and Stell et al. (361) found that patients who survived for extended periods without residual tumors had been treated surgically. Recurrent resectable lesions are better managed by surgery followed by radiotherapy (362), whereas unresectable tumors can be treated with irradiation alone (363).

The increasing use of planned postoperative fast-neutron irradiation has resulted in notable improvement in local disease control but apparently has not altered survival time (362,363). Sophisticated modifications of this technique are necessary if it is to be used on tumors close to the brain and intracranial structures.

The use of systemic chemotherapy for adenoid cystic carcinoma has not yet been clarified. Occasional regression of a tumor or its metastasis after chemotherapy has been reported in the literature (364).

Mucoepidermoid Carcinoma

Definition

"A tumor characterized by the presence of squamous, mucus-producing cells and cells of intermediate type" is how Seifert describes mucoepidermoid carcinoma (75). Electron microscopic studies indicate that both mucous and squamous cells may differentiate from intermediate cells and that these cells are also a feature of the tumors (365). Myoepithelial cells are not found. All salivary gland mucoepidermoid neoplasms must be considered to have a malignant potential, and thus the previously used, noncommittal term "mucoepidermoid tumor" is no longer considered appropriate. They can recur or metastasize to regional lymph nodes or to distant viscera. They should be classified as carcinomas (366–376).

Clinical Data

Mucoepidermoid carcinoma is the most common malignant neoplasm of the salivary glands. It represents 15.5% of all salivary gland tumors and 22% and 41% of the malignant tumors of the major and minor glands, respectively (366–376). The prevalence of mucoepidermoid carcinoma is highest among people in the fifth decade of life, although it is the most common malignant salivary gland tumor in children (375). In the majority of reported series, its predominance in women is striking, ranging from two to four times more common than it is in men (371). Approximately 60% to 70% of the tumors are located in the parotid gland, 15% to 20% in the oral cavity, and 6% to 10% in the submandibular glands (366–376). Occasionally, this tumor is centrally located in the mandible (377) or in the paraparotid lymph nodes (378).

Tumors of low-grade malignancy manifest themselves clinically in a manner similar to that of benign mixed tumor and generally undergo a prolonged period of painless enlargement. Highly malignant tumors grow rapidly and are often accompanied by pain and ulceration. The mean time interval between the initial swelling and histologic verification of low-grade tumors is quite long, an average of 6.8 years, whereas that of high-grade lesions is approximately 1.5 years (369,371).

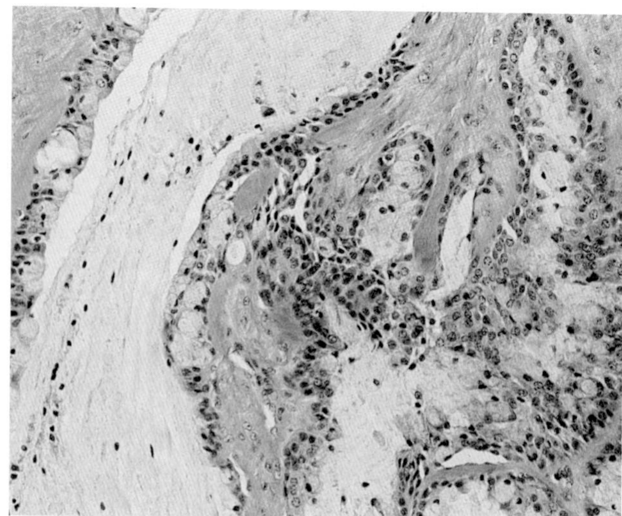

FIGURE 67. Mucoepidermoid carcinoma, low grade.

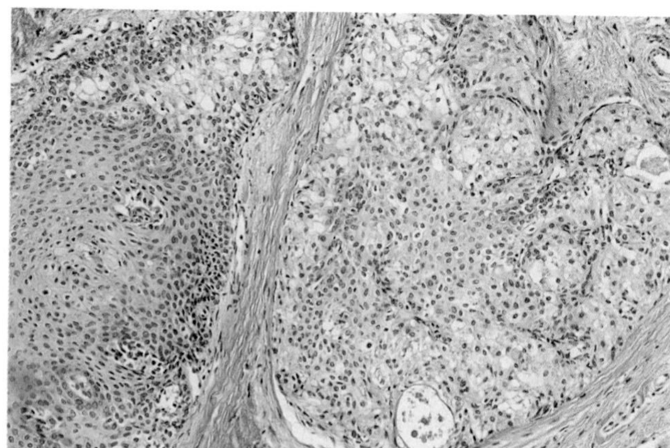

FIGURE 68. Mucoepidermoid carcinoma, intermediate grade, composed predominantly of intermediate cells.

Gross Appearance

Grossly, tumors of low-grade malignancy resemble mixed tumors. They are usually well circumscribed, and the cut surfaces often show dilated cystic structures containing mucous material. Although low-grade tumors vary in size, they rarely measure more than 3 cm in diameter. Intermediate and high-grade carcinomas are poorly circumscribed, and infiltration of adjacent tissues is a prominent feature. The cut surfaces lack the cystic formation usually observed in the low-grade tumors.

Histologic Features

Our practice is to divide mucoepidermoid carcinomas into low-, intermediate-, and high-grade types (see below). Microscopically, most low-grade mucoepidermoid carcinomas consist of multiple well-developed cystic or microcystic structures lined by mucin-producing, intermediate, or epidermoid cells (Fig. 67). Solid cellular areas are not prominent. Keratinization s seldom found. Microcystic formations coalescing into larger cysts are often prominent. A prominent fibrous stroma is often present. If the mucinous material present in the cysts escapes into the stroma, an intense inflammatory reaction may obscure the true neoplastic character of the lesion. The growth pattern of low-grade carcinomas is generally a broad advancing front, and they are not highly invasive.

As mucoepidermoid carcinomas become less differentiated and higher grade, the nests of tumor cells become larger, more irregular, and more solid, and fewer cystic spaces containing mucous secretions are apparent. In intermediate-grade carcinomas, the nests are composed of epidermoid or even squamous cells or intermediate basaloid elements; if the latter cells predominate, fewer goblet cells are present (Fig. 68).

High-grade mucoepidermoid carcinomas exhibit more extensive local invasion and are likely to have infiltrated beyond a point grossly visible. Microscopically, the high-grade carcinomas tend to form solid nests or cords composed of intermediate and epidermoid cells, with a few mucin-producing cells (Fig. 69). Anaplasia, atypical mitoses, nuclear pleomorphism, and invasion of normal structures are obvious. Perineural invasion and lymph node metastases are frequently associated. In the metastases, all these cell types are present, though not necessarily in the same proportions as they are in the primary tumor. A focal component of sebaceous cells is occasionally present, and varying degrees of oncocytic changes have been reported rarely (379).

Grades of Mucoepidermoid Carcinoma

The first attempt to grade mucoepidermoid carcinomas divided these tumors into two groups: benign (somewhat favorable) and malignant (highly unfavorable) (366). The authors of this system, Foote and Frazell (367), noting the arbitrary nature of this type of grading and also that some of their "benign lesions" had metastasized, concluded that all mucoepidermoid tumors were malignant, albeit in degrees: low, intermediate, and high grades. This three-level grading system found general acceptance among pathologists, and differences in biological behavior could be demonstrated even though clinical stage became a better prognosticator (369–372). However, lack of universal agreement regarding which histologic grading criteria are most useful and

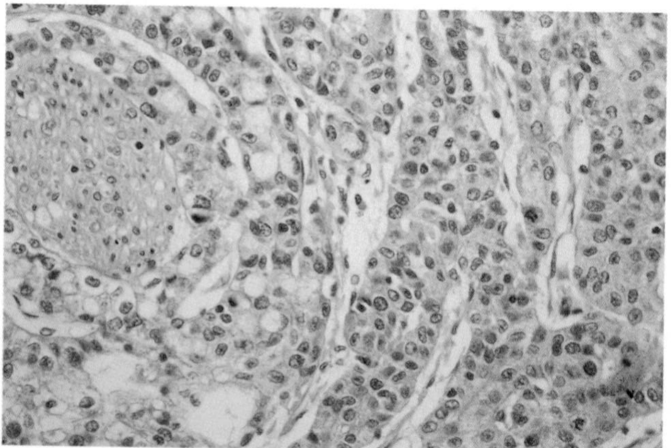

FIGURE 69. Mucoepidermoid carcinoma, high grade. Note isolated mucous cells, anaplasia, and neural invasion.

whether two or three grades should be applied led to the investigation of other systems (368,373,380).

Jakobsson et al. and later Evans championed two-tiered grading systems using low and high grades. Jakobsson et al. (368) based their version solely on the presence or absence of "invasive growth." Evans (373) ignored cell type and differentiation and defined high-grade carcinomas as those that had more than 90% solid architecture; all others were considered low grade.

Batsakis and Luna (381) designed a three-level grading system modified after the one proposed by Healy et al. (369). It incorporates cytodifferentiation as well as growth patterns, emphasizes the intermediate-cell population as an integral histogenetic and histologic component, and recognizes poorly differentiated types of the carcinoma. This three-level grading system was clinically tested by Hicks et al. (382) with success. In their series, the mortality rates were 0%, 30%, and 78% at 5 years for grades 1, 2, and 3, respectively (383).

A quantitative grading system was devised by Auclair et al. (376) in 1992. They analyzed the histologic features most useful in predicting high-grade aggressive behavior: a cystic component of less than 20%, 4 or more mitotic figures per 10 HPFs, neural invasion, necrosis, and anaplasia. Each one of these histologic features was given a fixed score. A total score of 0 to 4 was considered low grade; 5 to 6, intermediate grade; and 7 or more, high grade. Using this point system, the mortality rates were 3.3%, 9.7% and 46.3% for low, intermediate, and high grade, respectively (74).

Special Studies

Three cell types may be distinguished by electron microscopic examination: typical epidermoid prickle cells with tonofilaments and desmosomes, mucus-forming cells with mucous vacuoles, and intermediate, poorly differentiated cells with glycogen granules in the cytoplasm. Small, hollow spaces are bounded by microvilli and contain secretory particles. Other features include clear cells with glycogen and oncocytic areas rich in mitochondria (365,384).

Immunohistochemical studies of mucoepidermoid carcinoma have shown three cell types to be reactive to keratin, but the well-developed mucous cells generally do not react. Most tumor cells are immunoreactive to vimentin, S-100 protein, muscle-specific actin, α-fetoprotein, and carcinoembryonic antigen (385–387). The immunohistochemical staining pattern does not correlate with histologic grade of differentiation.

Nuclear DNA content of mucoepidermoid carcinomas assessed by cytophotometric analysis and by flow cytometry have demonstrated that diploid tumors have a favorable course whereas aneuploid tumors have an unfavorable course (383,388–390). Frankenthaler et al. (383) found a high correlation of proliferating cell nuclear antigen (PCNA) with survival. Patients with high PCNA have a poor prognosis. This allows for further stratification of patients with mucoepidermoid carcinoma, especially for patients with grade 2 tumors, a group that historically follows a variable and unpredictable course. Expression of p53 protein was seen in only 3 of 12 mucoepidermoid carcinomas (118). The proliferative capacity of mucoepidermoid carcinomas has been evaluated by quantitation of the AgNORs and by the expression of PCNA. By both techniques, the intermediate cells have shown more activity than the mucous and epidermoid cells (391).

Differential Diagnosis

Many benign mixed tumors contain prominent areas of squamous metaplasia and thus may pose a diagnostic problem. Mucoepidermoid carcinomas of any grade of malignancy, however, exhibit no evidence of myoepithelial cells or of chondroid or myxochondroid stroma, all of which are so characteristic of mixed tumor.

High-grade mucoepidermoid carcinoma is differentiated from squamous cell carcinoma by the presence of intracellular mucin. If mucin-producing cells are entirely absent, the lesion is classified as squamous cell carcinoma. The confinement of cytologically benign squamous epithelium to the preexisting lobular pattern of the salivary gland distinguishes necrotizing sialometaplasia from mucoepidermoid carcinoma.

Clinical Behavior and Treatment

The prognosis of mucoepidermoid carcinoma depends on adequacy of treatment, clinical stage, tumor grade, and tumor location (11,74,369–372). Patients are more likely to have recurrences if the margins of resection are positive, regardless of grade. Healey et al. (369) reported that 0 of 33 low- and intermediate-grade lesions recurred when the margins were free of carcinoma, but 6 of 12 of the same grade recurred when the margins were positive. Similarly, 13 of 16 high-grade lesions recurred when margins were involved by tumor. Most of the tumors that recur do so within 1 year of therapy (74). However, delayed recurrences may occur (366–371).

Spiro et al. (371) have observed that metastases to regional lymph nodes are more frequent with submandibular tumors than with tumors of any other major or minor glands. Distant metastases of mucoepidermoid carcinoma imply a poor prognosis. Patients with distant metastasis survive an average of 2.3 years and 2.6 years with minor and major gland tumors, respectively (74,370).

Survival is closely related to the clinical stage and histologic grade. Although staging and grading are interrelated, they appear to work independently of each other. Low-grade lesions behave less aggressively than do high-grade lesions regardless of stage, and conversely, a lower-stage tumor has a better prognosis than do stage III or IV lesions, regardless of grade (371). Spiro and associates (371) reported 5-year, 10-year, and 15-year cure rates of 49%, 42%, and 33%, respectively, for intermediate- and high-grade carcinomas. In a more recent series, Hicks et al. (382) reported a mortality rate at 5 years of 0%, 30%, and 78% for low-, intermediate-, and high-grade tumors, respectively. Fonseca and co-workers (390) reported a 5-year survival rate of 100% for low-grade and 40.7% for high-grade carcinomas. In the series by Ellis and Auclair (74) the mortality rates were 3.3%, 9.7%, and 46.3% for low-, intermediate-, and high-grade carcinomas, respectively.

Parotid tumors should be treated by parotidectomy with preservation of the facial nerve; however, if the cervical lymph nodes are involved, neck dissection is indicated. For tumors of the submandibular gland, dissection of the triangle is recommended, and if cervical nodes are involved, then a neck dissection is indicated (369,371). For carcinomas of the minor glands, complete excision with normal tissue margins is the ideal treatment. Radiotherapy is indicated for high-grade carcinomas, for tumors with extensive perineural or vascular invasion, and for incompletely excised tumors (392–394).

Salivary Duct Carcinoma

Definition

Salivary duct carcinoma is defined as

> an epithelial tumor of high malignancy with formation of relatively large cell aggregates resembling distended salivary ducts. The neoplastic epithelium presents a combination of cribriform, looping (Roman bridging), and solid growth patterns, often with central necrosis both in the primary lesions and the lymph node metastases. (75)

Several names have been suggested for this neoplasm: cribriform salivary duct carcinoma (395), infiltrating salivary duct carcinoma (396), and intraductal carcinoma (397). However, salivary duct carcinoma has become the established term (398–408, 411–413). The term "intraductal carcinoma" is inappropriate because it implies a noninvasive tumor with little metastatic potential. Quite the contrary, most salivary duct carcinomas are very aggressive neoplasms with a poor prognosis (395,396, 398–405). The carcinoma exists in two clinicopathologic forms: as the malignant component in some carcinomas *ex* pleomorphic adenoma and as a *de novo* malignancy (411).

Clinical Data

The parotid gland was the site of occurrence in nearly 85% of the cases, approximately 7% of the reported carcinomas occurred in the submandibular gland, and fewer than 5% were found in the minor glands (74,408,411). Other sites of occurrence are the sublingual gland and extraparotid Stensen's duct (74). The incidence of salivary duct carcinoma is difficult to determine. In a review of 4,068 salivary gland tumors, Seifert and Caselitz (409) reported 37 cases of salivary duct carcinoma (0.9%). In the AFIP files, the carcinomas represent only 0.2%, 0.5% and 1.1% of all epithelial salivary gland neoplasms, salivary gland carcinomas, and parotid gland carcinomas, respectively (74). Kane et al. (410) identified 12 cases in 194 parotid malignancies seen at the Mayo Clinic from 1970 to 1987, an incidence of 6%.

Seventy-six percent of the patients are men. The peak incidence is in the sixth and seventh decades of life, but patients' ages range from 22 to 91 years (74,407,408). Parotid swelling is the most frequent sign. Facial nerve dysfunction or paralysis occurs in more than one fourth of the patients. Cervical lymphadenopathy is evident in more than one third of the patients.

Gross Appearance

The tumors are generally poorly demarcated and infiltrative. Sometimes they are evenly and diffusely distributed within and beyond the parotid or submandibular gland. They range in size from less than 1 cm to greater than 6 cm in diameter.

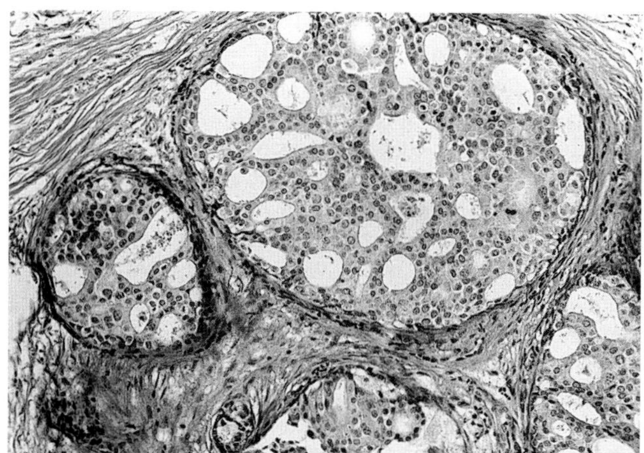

FIGURE 70. Salivary duct carcinoma, cribriform pattern.

Histologic Features

Histopathologically, it is important to be cognizant of the fact that the most currently accepted appellation for this tumor was derived from its resemblance to ductal carcinoma (especially comedocarcinoma) of the breast. Intraductal and infiltrative ductal elements are both commonly observed. The most frequently encountered patterns are comedonecrotic, papillary, and cribriform (Figs. 70–72). Solid areas are also seen. A desmoplastic reaction with variable hyalinization is common. Individual tumor cells are cuboidal to polygonal and have a moderate amount of eosinophilic or amphophilic cytoplasm that may appear powdery or finely granular. Luminal cells may have an apocrine appearance in some tumors, with prominent apical eosinophilic cytoplasm. There is variable cellular and nuclear pleomorphism, and mitotic figures are usually evident. Neither epidermoid nor myoepithelial differentiation is apparent. Mucin

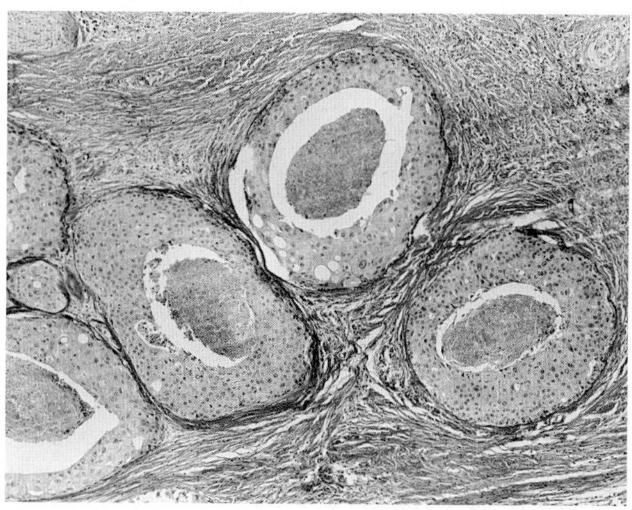

FIGURE 71. Salivary duct carcinoma, solid nests with comedonecrosis.

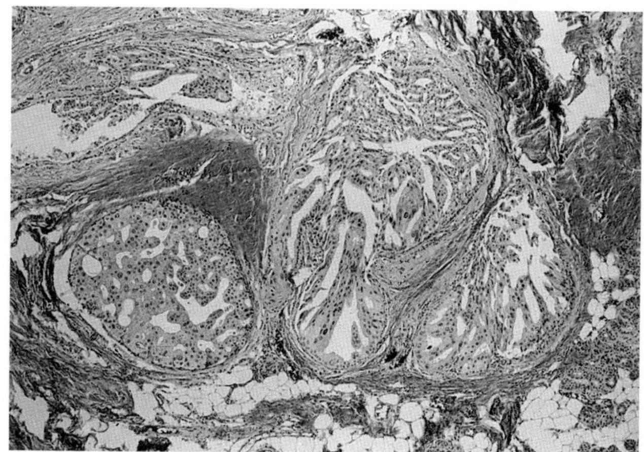

FIGURE 72. Salivary duct carcinoma, papillary and cribriform patterns.

is generally not prominent. Infiltration of salivary gland lobules and surrounding tissue is frequently seen, as is vascular and neural invasion. Duct changes adjacent to the neoplasm may include goblet cell metaplasia with occasional atypical goblet cells and basal cell hyperplasia, frequently with atypical cells.

Special Studies

Ultrastructural studies (400,404) have revealed cuboidal tumor cells forming a duct-like arrangement with projection of microvilli and rare cilia into the lumina. Irregular sheets of cells with scattered small acini and islands of stroma are also seen. Small desmosomes forming tight cell junctions are observed at the margins of lumina. A basal lamina is frequently observed surrounding many tumor cell groups. Scattered cells contain small lakes of glycogen, and small numbers of lipid droplets are also present. Myoepithelial cells are not observed.

Special stains for mucin (alcian blue and mucicarmine) are generally negative with the exception of some luminal positivity. Immunohistochemical studies show a positive reaction for epithelial membrane antigen (100%), keratin (95%), α-lactoalbumin (88%), gross cystic disease fluid protein-15 (GCDFP-15) (76%), and CEA (72%). S-100 protein has rarely been detected (395,406,407,411). Lewis Y and B72.3 antigens are also markers that have been demonstrated to be present in these carcinomas (395). Stains for estrogen receptors are generally negative. An occasional tumor stains positive for progesterone receptors (406,407,411). Salivary duct carcinomas have shown constant overexpression of *c-erbB-2* as detected by membrane accentuation and p53 protein nuclear immunostaining (407,412).

Flow cytometry studies have shown that most of the tumors are aneuploid (58% to 79%) with a highly proliferative S-phase (401,411,412). Similarly, high proliferative activity as detected by Ki-67 and PCNA studies has been demonstrated in the majority of the neoplasms (407,412). DNA aneuploidy, p53 immunopositivity, high growth, and proliferative fractions as measured by PCNA, Ki-67, and flow cytometry studies did not correlate with the clinical behavior of the carcinomas (401,412).

Differential Diagnosis

Microscopic differential diagnosis for salivary duct carcinoma should include entities with ductal and papillary components and cells with eosinophilic cytoplasm. Any of the following may be considered: mucoepidermoid carcinoma, mucus-producing adenopapillary adenocarcinoma (MPAPC), acinic cell carcinoma, oncocytic carcinoma, terminal duct carcinoma, and metastatic (particularly from the breast) adenocarcinoma. Although solid areas of salivary duct carcinoma may resemble mucoepidermoid carcinoma, intermediate or goblet cells are not seen with the former. High-grade mucoepidermoid carcinoma also does not display cribriform or papillary growth patterns.

Although MPAPC displays cysts and ducts with cribriform tumor elements, it is composed of cells that are columnar, goblet-shaped, or signet ring-shaped, whereas salivary duct carcinoma has larger cuboidal cells. An MPAPC does not produce the comedonecrosis seen in salivary duct carcinoma. Acinic cell carcinoma displays less cellular pleomorphism and eosinophilia, a greater variety of cell types, and no intraductal component. Although large eosinophilic cells are seen in oncocytic carcinoma, this tumor's cells are usually more granular, more eosinophilic, and larger than are those of salivary duct carcinoma. Oncocytic carcinoma has neither papillary nor cribriform growth patterns and no comedonecrosis. Terminal duct adenocarcinoma, in contrast to salivary duct carcinoma, is preponderantly associated with the minor salivary glands, displays no comedonecrosis, and is cytologically bland, with few mitoses. Metastatic adenocarcinoma, especially metastatic breast carcinoma, may be the most difficult malignancy to distinguish from salivary duct carcinoma because the microscopic features can be essentially identical. Salivary duct carcinoma is found four times as often in men as in women. As mentioned earlier, Brandwein et al. (395) suggested, where the exclusion of metastatic adenocarcinoma is difficult, the use of anti-B72.3 to identify "*in situ* premalignant change."

Clinical Behavior and Treatment

Barnes et al. (408) presented a summary report concerning the prognosis for 104 cases of salivary duct carcinoma reported with follow-up in the world literature. Thirty-three percent of the carcinomas showed local recurrence or persistence, 60% had lymphatic involvement, and 46% had distant metastases. Sixty-five percent of patients from all series were dead of disease within a mean period of 48 months. According to Hui et al. (404), in addition to the size and glandular locations previously mentioned, the features that correlate with a poorer prognosis are local recurrence, infiltrative margins, and local and distant metastases. Delgado et al. (413) believe that a low-grade variant of this carcinoma may exist.

Aggressive clinical management appears to offer the only hope for long-term survival (411). Complete local excision with radical neck dissection and adjuvant radiotherapy and chemotherapy are advocated. Because of the paucity of cases, however, statistics relevant to the efficacy of adjuvant therapy are inconclusive.

Epithelial–Myoepithelial Carcinoma

Definition

Epithelial–myoepithelial carcinoma (EMC) is "a tumor composed of variable proportions of two cell types that typically form duct-like structures. There is an inner layer of duct-lining cells and an outer layer of clear cells," according to Seifert (75). The neoplasm represents clearly definable participation of myoepithelial cells in a salivary neoplasm helping to lift the veil from the mysterious myoepithelial cell (196).

Clinical Data

This rare carcinoma represents 1% of all salivary gland tumors (74). It is predominantly a tumor of the major salivary glands, especially the parotid, as 75% of the tumors arise in this gland. The remaining 25% arise from the submandibular and minor salivary glands in equal parts (414–422). Patient age ranges from 31 to 89 years with a mean of 62 years. The tumor is twice as common in women as it is in men (414–422). The most common symptom is a painless mass in the parotid region, present over a period of several months to years. Pain, facial paralysis, or both occur only occasionally.

Gross Appearance

Most of the untreated neoplasms are solitary, well-circumscribed, firm, lobulated white masses measuring between 2 and 8 cm in greatest dimension. Recurrent carcinomas are multilobulated or multicentric with areas of necrosis and irregular roughened margins.

Histologic Features

The histologic appearance of EMC varies not only from carcinoma to carcinoma but also within the same neoplasm. In its classic form, this carcinoma demonstrates a multinodular growth pattern composed of well-defined tubules of varying size lined by two layers of cells (Fig. 73). The inner layer is composed of cuboidal to low columnar ductal cells with an eosinophilic cytoplasm. The outer layer consists of ovoid cells with pale abundant optically clear cytoplasm overlying an external well-developed basement membrane (Fig. 73).

The cuboidal cells have a finely granular dense eosinophilic cytoplasm and a central or basal round nucleus. The clear cells are polyhedral with well-defined cell borders and eccentric vesicular nuclei. They contain abundant diastase-digestible periodic acid–Schiff (PAS)-positive cytoplasmic granules. The lumina of the tubules contain PAS-positive diastase-resistant material. Mucicarmine stain is negative. There is minimal nuclear pleomorphism, and necrosis or mitoses are noted only infrequently. On occasion, the neoplastic cells may be found in perivascular and perineural spaces.

In some of the carcinomas, the biphasic pattern is less apparent, and the appearance is dominated by solid groups of clear cells separated by fibroconnective tissue or trabeculae of clear cells separated by thick, hyaline, PAS-positive basement membrane material. In others, there are areas of pronounced hypertrophy of the ductal component with minimal clear cell proliferation or areas composed almost exclusively of clear spindle cells.

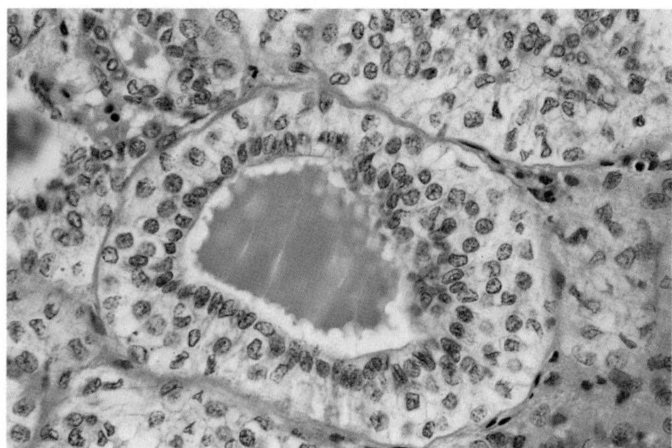

FIGURE 73. Epithelial–myoepithelial carcinoma. Ductal cells surrounded by clear cells.

In most instances, transition between these areas and the classic biphasic pattern can be found.

Special Studies

Immunocytochemical techniques using antibodies against keratin, S-100 protein antigen, smooth muscle actin, and amylase have enabled pathologists to characterize the different cell components in epithelial–myoepithelial carcinoma (415,416,423). Immunocytochemical staining for smooth muscle actin and S-100 protein produces intense staining of the outer clear cells; the inner ductal cells remain unstained (Fig. 74). Immunostaining for keratin shows a strong reaction in the inner ductal cells, whereas the peripheral clear cells have a weak and focal reaction. Some neoplasms may also show focal areas of immunoreactivity for amylase. This staining occurs only in the ductal cells and tends to be stronger toward the apex of the cells.

There is a correlation between the ultrastructural and immunocytochemical findings in epithelial–myoepithelial carcinoma (415,417). The cells forming the biphasic ductal structures display two distinct lines of differentiation. The inner cells have luminal microvilli, tonofilaments, desmosomes, and zymogen

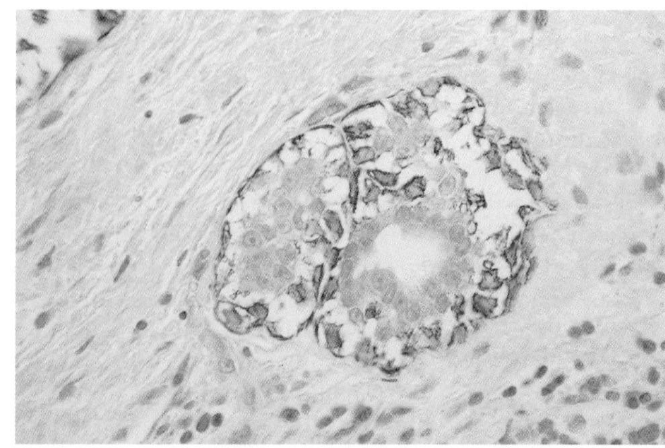

FIGURE 74. Epithelial–myoepithelial carcinoma. Clear cells immunoreactive to smooth muscle actin. Ductal cells are nonreactive.

granules (415). The outer cells form a single layer immediately within the basal lamina, typical of myoepithelial cells, and contain abundant glycogen and a peripheral band of smooth muscle myofilaments (417). Transitional forms of cells can be found.

A few studies are attempting to investigate the influence of DNA ploidy on the behavior of epithelial–myoepithelial carcinoma (421,424,425). Hamper et al. (424) studied 21 epithelial–myoepithelial carcinomas by cytophotometry and concluded that all 21 tumors were diploid and that ploidy, therefore, was of no value in predicting disease behavior. Using the same technique, Fonseca and Soares (421) found 3 of 18 epithelial–myoepithelial carcinomas to be aneuploid; in all three cases, the carcinoma recurred, and the patients died of disease. Cho and associates (425) used flow cytometry studies to find that 5 of 26 epithelial–myoepithelial carcinomas were aneuploid; all aneuploid carcinomas were near diploid (hyperdiploid) and showed low proliferative activity. In their series, there was no difference in the behavior of diploid and aneuploid tumors; all aneuploid tumors and 60% of diploid tumors recurred, metastasized, or both.

Immunohistochemical analysis of Ki-67 proliferation markers also showed low overall growth fractions. Interestingly, Ki-67 immunoreactivity was largely restricted to myoepithelial cells, suggesting a central role for this cell in the development of these tumors (425). In the same study by Cho et al. (425), *HER-2/neu* oncogene analysis failed to demonstrate overexpression in any of the 31 tumors examined.

Differential Diagnosis

The differential diagnosis of epithelial–myoepithelial carcinoma includes mucoepidermoid carcinoma, acinic cell carcinoma, mixed tumor, sebaceous carcinoma, and metastatic renal cell carcinoma. Mucoepidermoid carcinoma differs from epithelial–myoepithelial carcinoma in that the cells form acid mucopolysaccharides, and the tumors lack a myoepithelial component. The clear cells, which may be seen in some acinic cell carcinomas, are usually PAS-positive after diastase digestion, and if multiple sections are examined, the characteristic secretory granule–containing cells are eventually identified. Sebaceous carcinoma does not contain glycogen, stains positively for fat, and may have keratin pearls. Epithelial–myoepithelial carcinoma lacks the complex growth pattern and the stromal complexity of the mixed tumor.

Histologic distinction between epithelial–myoepithelial carcinoma and metastatic renal cell carcinoma may at times be difficult, especially if the classic biphasic pattern of epithelial–myoepithelial carcinoma is absent. The presence of necrosis and hypervascularity with hemorrhage favors a diagnosis of metastatic renal cell carcinoma. On occasion, the differential diagnosis rests only on the clinical exclusion of carcinoma in the kidneys (414,415,417).

Clinical Behavior and Treatment

From a review of the literature and our experience with epithelial–myoepithelial carcinoma, it is apparent that this tumor is biologically a malignant neoplasm despite its innocuous cytologic features (415,417,421). Of the 89 patients reported in the literature (Table 4), local recurrence occurred in 31.3%. The time interval between initial treatment and recurrence has varied from 9 months to 28 years. Cervical lymph node metastases were documented in 17.9%, and 13 patients died as a result of epithelial–myoepithelial carcinoma with distant metastases (417,421). Surgical excision with disease-free margins is the treatment of choice.

Terminal Duct Adenocarcinoma (Polymorphous Low-Grade Adenocarcinoma)

Definition

"A malignant epithelial tumor characterized by cytological uniformity, morphological diversity, and a low metastatic potential" is Seifert's description of terminal duct adenocarcinoma (TDC)

TABLE 4. SALIVARY GLAND ADENOCARCINOMAS

	TDC[a]	EMC	BCA	SDC
Number of patients	206	89	29	130
Male-to-female patient ratio	2:1	2:1	1.3:1	5:1
Site				
Major glands (%)	1	87	99	96
Minor glands (%)	99	13	1	4
Local recurrence (%)	21.3	31.3	28	35
Metastases to regional lymph nodes (%)	6.5	17.9	12	59
Distant metastases (%)	1.8	7.5	4	56
Mortality (%)	0.9	7.5	4	65

[a] TDC, terminal duct adenocarcinoma; EMC, epithelial–myoepithelial carcinoma; BCA, basal cell adenocarcinoma; SDC, salivary duct carcinoma, high grade.

Modified from the following sources:

(a) Ellis GL, Wiscovitch JG. Basal cell adenocarcinomas of the major salivary glands. *Oral Surg Oral Med Oral Pathol Oral Radiol Endod* 1990;69:461–469. (b) Luna MA, Batsakis JG, Tortoledo MF, et al. Carcinomas ex monomorphic adenoma of salivary glands. *J Laryngol Otol* 1989;103:756–759. (c) Barnes L, Rao U, Krause J, et al. Salivary duct carcinoma. Part I. A clinicopathologic evaluation and DNA image analysis of 13 cases with review of the literature. *Oral Surg Oral Med Oral Pathol Oral Radiol Endod* 1994;78:64–73. (d) Lewis JE, McKinney BC, Weiland LH, et al. Salivary duct carcinoma. Clinicopathologic and immunohistochemical review of 26 cases. *Cancer* 1996;77:223–230. (e) Batsakis JG, El-Naggar AK, Luna MA. Epithelial–myoepithelial carcinoma of salivary glands. *Ann Otol Rhinol Laryngol* 1992;101:540—542. (f) Kemp BL, Batsakis JG, El-Naggar AK, et al. Terminal duct adenocarcinoma of the parotid gland. *J Laryngol Otol* 1995;109:466–468.

(75). This neoplasm was first identified as a specific salivary gland carcinoma in 1983 by two independent groups of investigators. Batsakis et al. (426) reported 12 cases as TDC. Freedman and Lumerman (427) reported the neoplasm under the term "lobular carcinoma" because its histologic appearance focally reminded them of infiltrating lobular carcinoma of the breast. The following year, the term polymorphous low-grade adenocarcinoma was suggested as a clinically and morphologically descriptive term by Evans and Batsakis (428).

Clinical Data

The hard palate is the most frequent site of this tumor (426–432), although it may arise from any minor salivary gland and also, rarely, as a primary neoplasm in major salivary glands (433–436). In our experience, TDC may also occur in the major glands as a malignant component of carcinoma *ex* pleomorphic adenoma (157). Other locations in the oral cavity are the buccal mucosa, retromolar region, upper lip, and the base of the tongue (429). The most frequent clinical sign is a painless mass of variable duration. The age of the patient has ranged from 23 years old to 79 years old, and more women than men are affected (Table 4). TDC comprises 7.4% of minor salivary gland tumors and 19.6% of those that are malignant (74). Thus, it is the most common of the more recently delineated subgroups of salivary gland adenocarcinoma (i.e., TDC, EMC, and salivary duct carcinoma).

Gross Appearance

Grossly, the tumors are described as firm, circumscribed, yellow-tan lobulated nodules from 1 cm to several centimeters in greatest dimension.

Histologic Features

Microscopically, TDC is characterized by cytologic uniformity and histologic diversity. The cells are cuboidal or columnar, small to medium in size, and with ovoid to spindle nuclei with fine chromatin and inconspicuous nucleoli. The cytoplasm is scanty and usually eosinophilic. In some carcinomas, the cell's cytoplasm is optically clear; less often it is mucoid or granular. Nuclear atypia is absent. The mitotic rate is low, and necrosis is not a typical feature.

In contrast to cytologic uniformity, histologically, TDC displays a variety of growth patterns, many of which may be found within the same carcinoma. The spectrum of growth patterns includes tubular (Fig. 75), cribriform, papillary (Fig. 76), solid, and fascicular (Fig. 77). Combinations of and transition among these patterns are frequent. The stroma may be mucoid, hyaline, or mucohyaline.

Despite its innocuous cytologic appearance, the carcinoma always invades adjacent soft tissues and is unencapsulated. Infiltration is either by single ducts or by groups of neoplastic ducts and elongated cords of cells forming a single-file pattern. Neurotropism is particularly prominent and is manifested by perineural and intraneural invasion. Invasion of adjacent bone may be seen in tumors of the palate or those near the mandible.

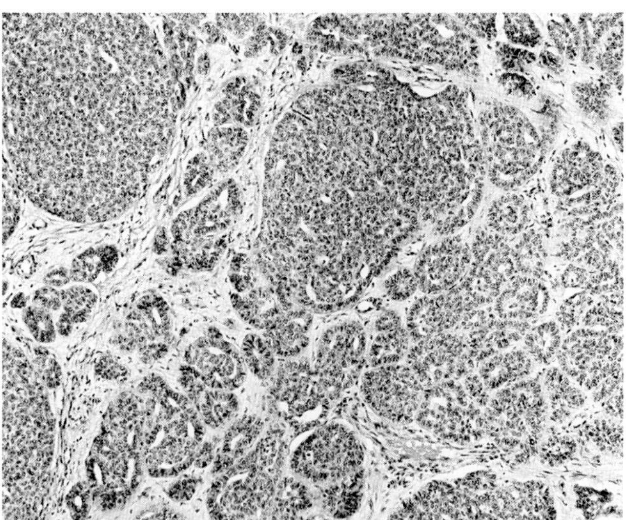

FIGURE 75. Terminal duct adenocarcinoma, tubular pattern.

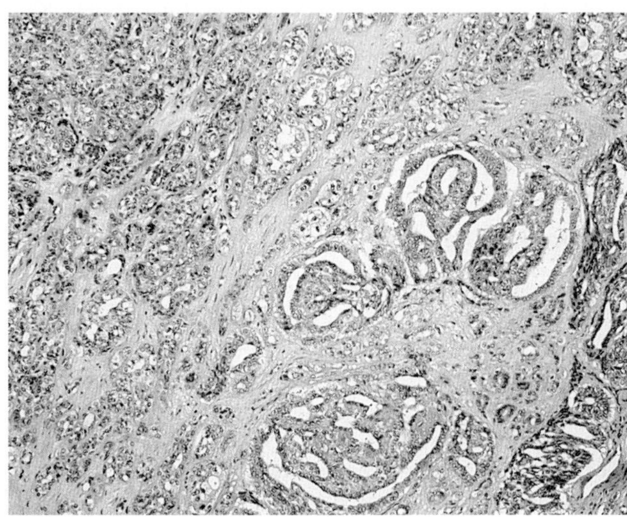

FIGURE 76. Terminal duct adenocarcinoma. Papillary and glandular formations.

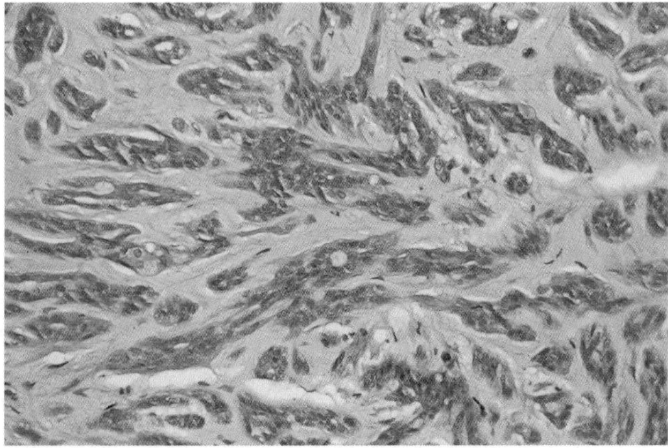

FIGURE 77. Terminal duct adenocarcinoma. Streaming row of cells with microlumen formations, reminiscent of lobular or tubulolobular carcinoma of the breast.

Special Studies

Ultrastructurally, the neoplastic ducts contain cuboidal cells containing a central round to oval nucleus. The nuclear membrane is usually smooth or may have a few indentations. The chromatin is fine and evenly distributed through the nucleus. Nucleoli are small, eccentric, and often located in direct contact with the nuclear membrane. In many cells, the cytoplasm contains abundant intermediate filaments that often appear to form bundles around the nucleus (430,437,438). Cells are joined by well-formed junctional complexes and surrounded by a continuous thin basal lamina. Short microvilli project into luminal spaces, which often contain amorphous material or cellular debris. Some carcinomas have tubules or solid areas with clear cells that contain abundant glycogen (438).

The neoplastic cells of TDC are immunoreactive to keratin, vimentin, muscle-specific actin, epithelial membrane antigen, and carcinoembryonic antigen (430,439,440). All TDCs studied by Regezi et al. (440) stain for S-100 protein antigen. Our findings confirm this observation; S-100 protein antigen was present in all of the carcinomas we studied and was strongly positive in the spindle and clear cells as opposed to the ductal cells (441). This finding is consistent with the light microscopic appearance of myoepithelial cells.

Differential Diagnosis

TDC should be distinguished from other salivary neoplasms such as pleomorphic adenoma, basal cell adenoma, and adenoid cystic carcinoma (ACC). Unlike TDC, pleomorphic adenoma is nearly always well circumscribed and is composed of a proliferation of stromal and epithelial cells. It lacks the infiltrative nonencapsulated character of TDC. The key distinguishing feature of TDC, a locally infiltrative nonencapsulated pattern, separates it from the different types of basal cell and canalicular adenomas (tubular, solid–trabecular, canalicular, and basaloid). Many clinical and pathologic similarities exist between TDC and ACC. The distinction of TDC from ACC is primarily based on cytologic features. Cells of TDC are cuboidal or columnar. They have vesicular nuclei and an often conspicuous eosinophilic cytoplasm without the basaloid features characteristic of ACC. Furthermore, papillary and fascicular growth patterns are extremely unusual in ACC and common in TDC. Clinically, ACC exhibits a more aggressive behavior and a worse prognosis.

Clinical Behavior and Treatment

A recent review of 204 published cases revealed a 17% recurrence rate and a regional metastasis rate of 9% (431). Some patients have multiple recurrences, and recurrences develop from months to many years after initial treatment, which indicates a need for long-term follow-up. In large series with follow-up data, metastasis to regional lymph nodes occurred in just under 10% of the patients, and there were no metastases to distant sites (426–431).

Eight of nine TDCs *ex* pleomorphic adenoma reported by Tortoledo et al. (157) had a protracted course. One patient died of distant metastases. It is unclear whether TDC in association with a pleomorphic adenoma has the same biological potential as TDC alone. Data from Slootweg and Muller (432) indicate that the papillary variant of terminal duct carcinoma is more aggressive in clinical behavior than is the nonpapillary type. A comparison between parotid gland TDC and more than 200 minor salivary gland TDCs indicated that there is little difference in biological behavior and confirmed the low-grade quality of the carcinomas, regardless of site of origin (435).

Other Types of Adenocarcinomas

Other well-defined types of adenocarcinomas are mucus-producing adenopapillary carcinoma (442,443), cystadenocarcinoma (444,445), hyalinizing clear cell adenocarcinoma (446), and adenosquamous carcinoma (447). Finally, a group of adenocarcinomas not otherwise specified has been retained for the occasional tumors that defy classification. They are the least common of salivary gland carcinomas and manifest a cytoarchitecture ranging from a well-differentiated, low-grade appearance to high-grade, invasive lesions (448,449). Table 4 compares the clinical behavior of the four most common types of adenocarcinoma.

Primary Squamous Cell Carcinoma

Definition

Primary squamous cell carcinoma is "a malignant epithelial tumor with cells forming keratin or having intercellular bridges. Mucus secretion is not present" (75).

Clinical Data

The reported frequency of primary squamous carcinoma among all major salivary gland tumors varies from 0.9% to 4.7% (11,74,88). In the parotid gland, the frequency varies from 0.3% to 1.5% (450–455), and in the submandibular gland from 2.4% to 7.0% (456–461). The average age of patients with primary squamous cell carcinoma is between 61 and 68 years, with an age range of 20 to 89 years old (74). This carcinoma afflicts three times as many men as women (450–461). The most common complaint refers to a salivary gland mass (50% of patients so report). Some patients complain of pain associated with the tumor (33%), and fewer than 17% of the patients notice facial nerve paralysis (74,456).

Gross Appearance

The tumors are infiltrative with ill-defined borders and firm consistency.

Histologic Features

Microscopically, these tumors are identical to the squamous cell carcinomas of any other site. They vary from well to poorly differentiated. However, most of the carcinomas are well to moderately differentiated with different degrees of keratinization. The cells are arranged in strands, islands, or files. The borders of the carcinoma infiltrate and replace the normal salivary parenchyma

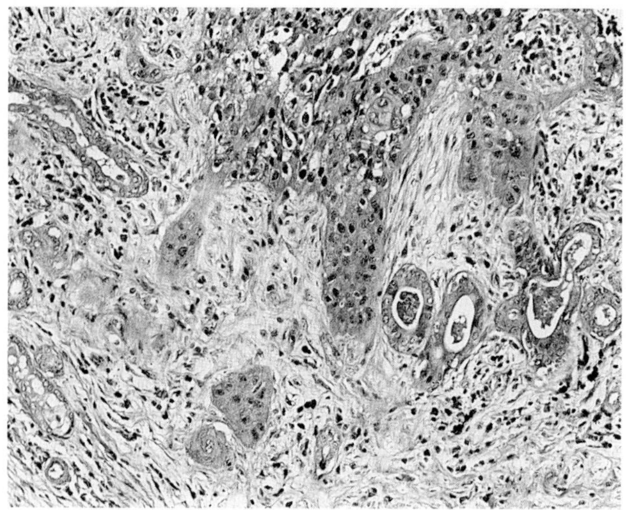

FIGURE 78. Primary squamous cell carcinoma.

(Fig. 78). Occasionally, sections reveal origin from dysplastic ductal epithelium.

Differential Diagnosis

The most difficult diagnosis is between primary and metastatic squamous cell carcinoma. If the tumor is found only within the parotid or submandibular lymph nodes, most likely the carcinoma is metastatic. In other circumstances, the clinical history is of paramount importance unless the tumor is fortuitously found to originate from the salivary duct. The absence of mucin-producing and transitional cells distinguishes squamous cell carcinoma from mucoepidermoid carcinoma. The invasive character of the neoplasia and the absence of lobular preservation favors squamous cell carcinoma over necrotizing sialometaplasia.

Clinical Behavior and Treatment

Local disease recurrence and regional lymph node metastases are the usual outcome for patients with primary squamous carcinoma of the parotid gland (450–455). Distant metastases are not common. The overall survival rate at 5 years is 50% (455). With submandibular carcinomas, the regional recurrence rate is 66%, and metastasis to cervical lymph nodes is 48% at the time of initial treatment (74). Surgery with postoperative radiation therapy is the treatment of choice for primary squamous cell carcinoma (453,455). Concurrent neck dissection is performed for tumors in either major salivary gland if cervical metastases are detected or clinically suspected (450–461).

Undifferentiated Carcinomas

An undifferentiated carcinoma of salivary glands is defined as one without enough distinguishing light-optic features to allow placement in another classification of salivary gland carcinoma (462). That this seemingly exclusive definition has not been uniformly applied is evidenced by the reported incidence of undifferentiated carcinomas ranging from 1% to 30% of all malignant salivary gland tumors (463). Hui et al. (463) have suggested at least three reasons for the wide spread in estimated frequency: failure to exclude metastases, notably those of Merkel cell carcinomas and metatypical basal cell carcinomas, to salivary glands; inclusion of otherwise classifiable primary carcinomas, e.g., high-grade adenoid cystic carcinomas and carcinomas *ex* pleomorphic adenoma; and inappropriate use of the term undifferentiated as the qualifying diagnostic adjective for nonmalignant salivary tumors such as basal cell adenomas and the rarely occurring embryomas. Undifferentiated carcinomas are classified as small-cell, large-cell, or undifferentiated carcinoma with lymphoid stroma or lymphoepithelial carcinoma (with an ethnic, geographic, and Epstein-Barr virus relationship akin to the analogous nasopharyngeal neoplasm) (74) (see Chapter 5).

Small-Cell Carcinoma

Definition

"A malignant tumor similar in histology, behavior, and histochemistry to the small cell carcinoma of the lungs" is how Seifert describes this undifferentiated tumor (75).

Clinical Data

It is estimated that 4% of all small-cell carcinomas arise in extrapulmonary tissues (464). In the head and neck, besides originating from the major salivary glands (usually the parotid gland), the carcinomas have been reported as having origin in the larynx, sinonasal tract, oral cavity, and cervical esophagus. Of the cases in the AFIP files, small-cell carcinoma represents 1.7% of primary malignant epithelial parotid tumors, 2.2% of submandibular gland malignancies, and 1.8% of all major salivary gland malignancies (74). The mean age of the patient is 56 years, ranging from 5 years to 86 years old (463–469). The ratio of male to female patients is 6:1 (74).

Histologic Features

Microscopically, the tumors are composed of solid sheets, nests, or trabeculae. The cells are larger than lymphocytes and have dense, round to oval nuclei with diffuse chromatin (Fig. 79).

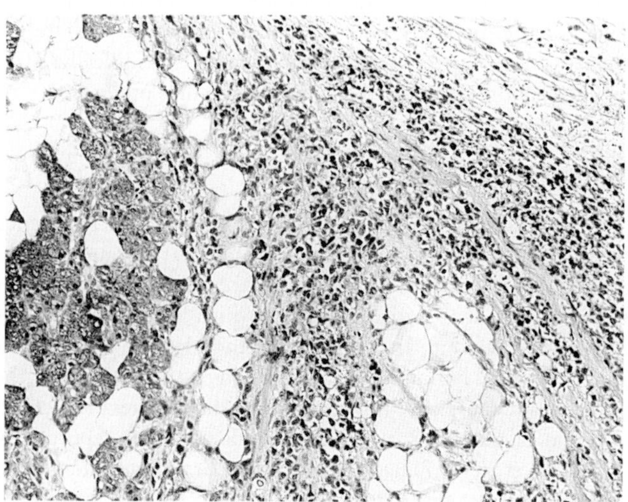

FIGURE 79. Small-cell undifferentiated carcinoma.

Ductal differentiation occasionally is evident. Limited squamous differentiation is evident only rarely (468).

Special Studies

Ultrastructural examination of small-cell carcinomas of the major salivary glands revealed that some will be so undifferentiated that they exhibit no distinguishing electron-optic features other than epithelial findings. A ductal or epidermoid appearance will be present in others, and a good number of tumors will also manifest neuroendocrine differentiation (463,470).

Immunohistochemical studies revealed that most of the cells are immunoreactive for keratin, although focal areas are nonreactive (464,465,467). Immunoreactivity to synaptophysin, chromogranin, and neuron-specific enolase is present in cells in some cases, indicating neuroendocrine differentiation (464, 465).

Differential Diagnosis

The differential diagnosis includes lymphoma, the solid variant of adenoid cystic carcinoma, and metastatic small-cell carcinoma from the skin (Merkel cell), the lung, or elsewhere. Negative immunoreactivity to keratin together with immunoreactivity for leukocyte common antigen (LCA) will indicate lymphoma. The presence of a focal cribriform pattern, tubules, or both favors a diagnosis of solid adenoid cystic carcinoma. In addition, adenoid cystic carcinoma lacks immunoreactivity for neuroendocrine markers. Distinguishing primary small-cell carcinoma from metastatic small-cell carcinomas may be difficult. Sometimes only the relevant clinical information is of help.

Clinical Behavior and Treatment

This is a high-grade malignancy. Gnepp and associates (464) found that the 2-year and 5-year survival rates for major salivary gland tumors were 70% and 46%, respectively. Hui et al. (463) found that the most important prognostic factor was the tumor size. All patients with tumors measuring more than 4 cm died of their tumor. Most patients were treated with surgery and postoperative irradiation (463–470). Chemotherapy has been used to treat systemic disease (463).

Large-Cell Carcinoma

Clinical Data

The majority of large-cell carcinomas occur in the parotid gland; they occur occasionally in the submandibular and minor salivary glands (463,471). Patients have ranged in age from 40 to 96 years, with a peak incidence in the seventh and eighth decades of life (471–473). Other clinical features are similar to those seen in the small-cell carcinomas.

Histologic Features

Most cells are two or more times the size of those of small-cell carcinoma. They are polygonal with abundant amphophilic to eosinophilic cytoplasm. The cells are arranged in nests, cords, and trabeculae (Fig. 80). Mitotic figures are common.

Special Studies

Large-cell carcinomas are seen well in electron microscopy studies. Ductal, epidermoid, and neuroendocrine features can be found among undifferentiated tumor cells (463,471).

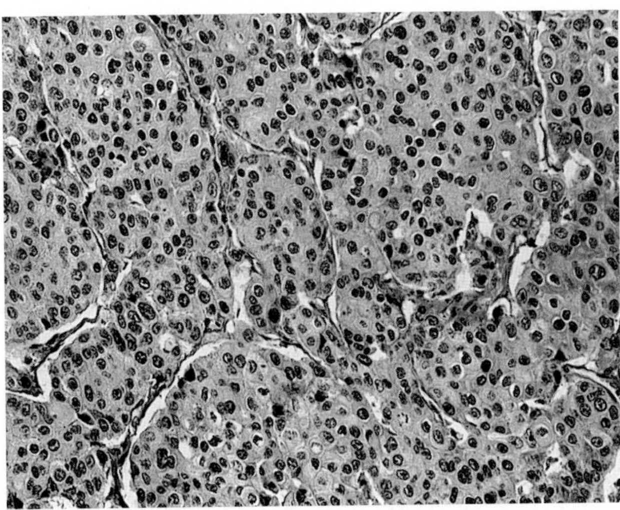

FIGURE 80. Large-cell undifferentiated carcinoma.

Differential Diagnosis

The differential diagnosis includes large-cell lymphoma and metastatic melanoma. Immunohistochemical studies are useful in identifying these tumors. LCA is positive in large-cell lymphoma. Melanoma cells are immunoreactive for S-100 protein and sometimes for HMB 45 antigen and are negative for keratin. Large-cell carcinomas are immunoreactive for keratin (471–473).

Clinical Behavior and Treatment

Large-cell undifferentiated carcinomas are very aggressive neoplasms. North et al. (472) found that none of five patients with this type of carcinoma survived 10 years. Treatment is identical to that for small-cell carcinoma.

Lymphoepithelial Carcinoma

Definition

Seifert defines lymphoepithelial carcinoma as "a tumor characterized by syncytial clumps of large cells with vesicular nuclei and prominent nucleoli, admixed with abundant small lymphocytes and plasma cells" (75). Other terms for this carcinoma are carcinoma *ex* lymphoepithelial lesion (474), undifferentiated carcinoma with lymphoid stroma (475), and malignant lymphoepithelial lesion (476). We prefer the term "lymphoepithelial carcinoma" for brevity and clarity.

Clinical Data

Lymphoepithelial carcinoma comprises only about 0.4% of the salivary gland neoplasms accessioned at the files of the AFIP (74). This carcinoma has a striking prevalence among native Greenlanders and the North American Inuit (Eskimo) people. The incidence of salivary gland cancer in the Eskimo population is the highest in the world, 10 times the expected rate, and most of these cancers are lymphoepithelial carcinomas (477–481). Mongolian ethnicity is certainly a risk factor for this salivary gland carcinoma. Greenlanders, North American Inuit, and Southern Chinese people living in Hong Kong make up nearly three-fourths of the reported cases (479). Of patients with this disease, the ratio of women to men is 1.5 to 1. Patients range in age from 10 years to 86 years, with a median age of about 40 years (477–481). The major salivary glands appear to be the exclusive site of origin for lymphoepithelial carcinoma, with the parotid gland affected seven times more often than the submandibular gland. Familial clustering of affected patients has been reported (482). These patients showed enhanced antigenic stimulation by Epstein-Barr virus (EBV) as evidenced by EBV-specific serum antibody titers. EBV genome equivalents were demonstrated in the salivary gland carcinomas of these patients (483–484).

Histopathologic Features

Supposedly indistinguishable from its nasopharyngeal analogue by either light- or electron-optic studies, the lymphoepithelial carcinoma of salivary glands can assume different architectural growth patterns. These may be epithelial islands, anastomosing or syncytial masses or cords, and isolated cells usually set in a lymphoid stroma (Fig. 81). In some areas, the lymphoid component is minimal or replaced by fibrous connective tissue. Usually, the carcinoma is demarcated from nonepithelial elements and can appear to be a malignant caricature of the epimyoepithelial islands seen in lymphoepithelial lesions of the salivary glands. Foci of squamous differentiation may be found, but the overall histopathologic appearance is that of an undifferentiated carcinoma whose phenotypic expression ranges from rather large cells with vesicular nuclei and prominent nucleoli to spindle-shaped cells. The degree of anaplasia also varies, from severe, with pleomorphic nuclei and numerous mitoses, to a uniform cell population and rare mitoses.

Differential Diagnosis

Regardless of patient ethnicity, the pathologist must exclude a metastasis from the nasopharynx or Waldeyer's ring epithelium when presented with a case of undifferentiated carcinoma with lymphoid stroma of the parotid or submandibular gland. As noted, EBV antibody titers may not be of use in the differential diagnosis. The catchment areas of the parotid lymph nodes include the nasopharynx and oropharynx, but unilateral parotid swelling as a presenting sign of a nasopharyngeal carcinoma is very unusual, and parotid node involvement in cases of known nasopharyngeal carcinoma is uncommon (485).

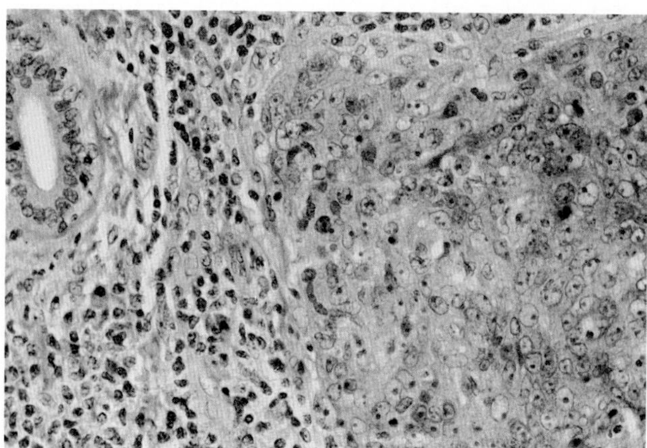

FIGURE 81. Nasopharyngeal-like lymphoepithelial carcinoma of salivary gland. A syncytial-appearing nest of large epithelial cells with vesicular nuclei and prominent nucleoli sits in a lymphoid-rich stroma.

Clinical Behavior and Treatment

Early metastasis to regional lymph nodes is a feature of the undifferentiated carcinoma with lymphoid stroma. At least 40% of patients are said to have histologically proven nodal metastases at their first presentation to a physician. Local recurrence and systemic spread of disease have been recorded in 20% to 50% of patients (474–481).

Most of the patients with this carcinoma have been treated with a combination of surgical removal of the salivary gland (with or without neck dissection) and irradiation. Each of these treatments has also been used alone (472,476).

NONEPITHELIAL TUMORS

Nonepithelial tumors, both benign and malignant, constitute fewer than 5% of all neoplasms in the salivary glands of adults (74). Collectively, they are termed synsialomas or synsialadenomas. They arise in the supporting tissues of the salivary glands such as blood vessels, lymphatic vessels, nerves, and surrounding connective tissue. Angiomas, lipomas, neurofibromas, and hemangiopericytomas are the most frequently observed benign synsialomas (486–491). With the exception of neurofibromas, these tumors have been reported only in the parotid gland. Benign mesodermal tumors often arise in the parotid glands of children; the majority of these are hemangiomas, which are discussed subsequently in the section on salivary gland tumors in children.

Grossly, many mesenchymal tumors are poorly demarcated, and the infiltrating margins suggest malignancy. The microscopic patterns and histologic criteria are identical to those of tumors in other tissues. Lipoma and neurofibroma may penetrate deeply into the intraglandular septa, and such tumors may recur. Sarcomas arising primarily in the major salivary glands or growing into them make up an interesting group of neoplasms. They affect all age groups, although they are more prevalent in patients less than 40 years of age. They cover almost the entire gamut of mesenchymal tumors: rhabdomyosarcomas, malignant fibrous histiocytomas, fibrosarcomas, malignant peripheral nerve sheath tumors, and synovial sarcomas (Fig. 82). Although they are unusual, these are the types of sarcomas involving the major salivary glands that are most often reported (492–496).

Primary Malignant Lymphomas

Primary malignant lymphomas of the salivary glands are rarely encountered; Batsakis and Regezi (497) found two among 589 tumors of the parotid gland. Freeman and associates (498), reviewing 1,467 cases of extranodal lymphomas, discovered 69 in the major salivary glands. The parotid glands are involved much more often than are the submandibular glands, the ratio of involvement being 5 to 1. Most patients with salivary gland lymphomas are in the sixth or seventh decade of life (497–504).

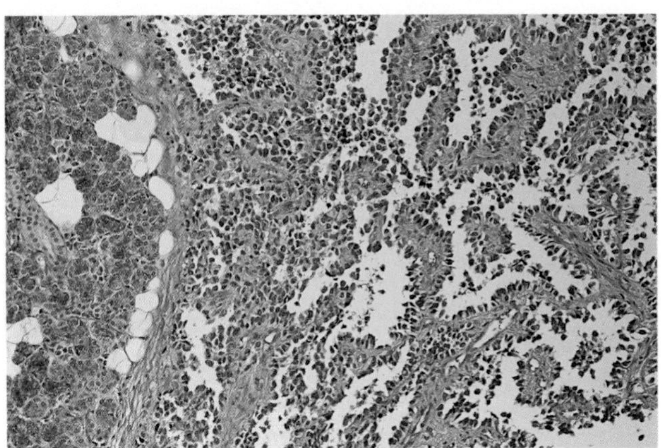

FIGURE 82. Salivary gland alveolar rhabdomyosarcoma.

Malignant lymphomas in the parotid region may arise from an intraglandular lymph node or in the parotid gland itself (499). In the former instance, the patient requires the same type of staging as would a patient with a lesion in the cervical lymph nodes (499). Involvement of salivary gland tissue may represent the expression of disseminated involvement or, more commonly, a primary disease of this organ.

The majority of lymphomas of the salivary glands are of follicular center cell origin (499–504). Nearly all are of B-cell derivation; a few cases of T-cell lymphoma of the salivary glands have been reported (505). Sclerosis is a common feature among the large-cell types (504).

The lymphomas composed of small lymphoid cells often arise against a background of a benign lymphoepithelial lesion (497–505). As in other epithelial organs, it has been proposed that most, if not all, of these lymphomas are of MALT type (506). See Chapter 12 for further discussion.

It is noteworthy that many types of malignant reticuloendothelial neoplasms are encountered in the salivary glands, although Hodgkin's disease appears to be extremely unusual (499). Plasmacytomas have been reported; some later develop into multiple myeloma (507). Cases of malignant lymphoma have also been observed in association with Warthin's tumor (508).

The end result of therapy in patients with large-cell lymphoma of the salivary glands is discouraging; approximately 30% are free of disease after a 5-year follow-up period (499–505). Lymphomas composed of small lymphocytes are characterized by a very slow evolution and an excellent long-term prognosis (499,504).

METASTASIS TO SALIVARY GLANDS

Metastasis to the major salivary glands may take place by lymphatic spread, hematogenous dissemination, or contiguous extension. The last is especially likely with sarcomas arising from facial bones or soft tissues as well as of cancers of the skin (509–511). The majority of lymphatic and hematogenous metastases to the major salivary glands are found in the parotid glands (509–512). The submandibular glands are seldom invaded. The absence of intraglandular lymph nodes is the apparent reason for the rarity of lymphatic metastatic lesions to the submandibular glands. Hematogenous dissemination of carcinoma of lung, breast, or kidney to the submandibular glands occasionally has been reported (513,514).

Secondary neoplastic involvement of the parotid gland is probably less rare than the literature would lead one to believe. Yarington (515), in a series of 250 consecutive parotidectomies performed for clinically primary parotid tumors, found 10 (4%) metastatic neoplasms from an unsuspected primary source. Similar experiences were described by Gnepp (516) and by Nichols and associates (517).

As noted by Conley and Arena (518) and by McKean et al. (519), the parotid gland contains as many as 20 to 30 lymph nodes and a rich network of intercommunicating lymph vessels. Paraparotid lymph nodes are present around the external surface of the gland, being particularly numerous in the pretragal and supratragal areas. Intraglandular and paraglandular lymph nodes communicate freely with each other and drain into the cervical chains. Because the lymphatic drainage of the scalp, face, external ear, eyelids, and nose is to both intraglandular and periglandular parotid lymph nodes, it is not surprising that cutaneous squamous cell carcinoma and melanoma arising in these areas are the metastatic malignant tumors most often found in the parotid lymph nodes (520).

In a review of 81 cases of secondary parotid lesions, Conley and Arena (518) found that 40% were squamous cell carcinomas and 42% were melanomas. Other authors have observed the propensity of cutaneous tumors of the head and neck to metastasize to the parotid lymph nodes. Occasionally, the palate, tonsil, and nasopharynx are sites of origin of metastases to the intra- or paraparotid lymph nodes (521).

Blood-borne metastatic carcinomas from infraclavicular organs to the parotid gland region arise most often from a primary tumor in the lung, and less often, from one in the breast, kidney, or the gastrointestinal tract (512,514,522). When it becomes difficult to assign a given salivary gland neoplasm to a particular category, the pathologist must remember that it may possibly be a secondary tumor.

Malignant secondary neoplasms of the parotid gland carry a grave prognosis: the overall 5-year survival rate is estimated at 12.5% (509–517). Survival of the patient is influenced by the cell type, regional spread of the disease, site of origin of metastases, and prevention of local recurrence. Jackson and Ballantyne (523) and Rees and associates (524) have reported a 67% 5-year survival rate for cutaneous metastatic squamous carcinoma. The 5-year survival rate for metastatic melanoma to the parotid lymph nodes varies from 10% to 30%. Metastatic parotid tumors that arise from noncutaneous sites also have a poor prognosis: the 5-year survival rate is less than 5%, indicating the aggressive nature of systemically metastatic carcinomas of the lungs, breasts, kidneys, and tonsillar and nasopharyngeal regions (512,514,522).

SALIVARY GLAND TUMORS IN CHILDREN

No more than 5% of all salivary gland neoplasms occur in children (525–532). Several features distinguish the neoplasms of children as compared with those of adults. In children, there is a much greater frequency of nonepithelial tumors. There is a higher proportion (50%) of malignant neoplasms when nonepithelial tumors are excluded. Finally, there is a preponderance of cases with parotid gland involvement; these occur seven times more often than those with submandibular gland involvement.

Vasoformative, nonepithelial tumors are the most common tumors in neonates and infants. The rarely occurring embryoma is almost confined to the perinatal–neonatal period. Pleomorphic adenoma, mucoepidermoid carcinoma, and acinic cell carcinoma occur later in childhood, with nearly 80% occurring in children between the ages of 10 years and 16 years (530).

Hemangioma

Parotid gland hemangiomas are by far the most common supportive tissue tumors (527,532–534). They are the most frequent salivary gland tumor of any type in the first year of life; they occur most often in girls and most often on the left side of the body. Spontaneous involution over a few years is the usual course. Indications for surgical intervention include persistence, sustained growth, extensive hemorrhage, and an uncertainty of the clinical diagnosis.

Clinical Data

Hemangiomas are located at the angle of the mandible. They may be well defined, although they are more often diffuse, with margins extending below the ramus of the mandible and into the neck itself. The masses seem to increase in size when the patient cries or strains. Another important clinical observation is the bluish discoloration of the overlying skin; it is transmitted from the cavernous component of the hemangioma. Much has been made of associated regional and cutaneous hemangiomas as a preoperative diagnostic aid. Such a relationship varies greatly and in the opinion of several authors is more uncommon than usual (532,534). Arteriography and sialography are of diagnostic value in complicated cases (527,534).

Gross Appearance

Grossly, the involved gland is enlarged, apparently incident to an increase in the size of individual lobules; the latter are purple-red, spongy, and distinctly congested.

Histologic features

Microscopically, numerous capillary blood vessels ramify in the parenchyma of the gland (Fig. 83). Occasionally, endothelial cells with mitoses are present in the capillary lumina. Nuclear pleomorphism and atypism are lacking.

Clinical Behavior

Approximately 50% of hemangiomas will undergo spontaneous involution, particularly during the second and third years of life (527,532–534). After excision of the tumor, recurrence is unusual, although it is more likely if the patient is less than 4 months old (527,532–534).

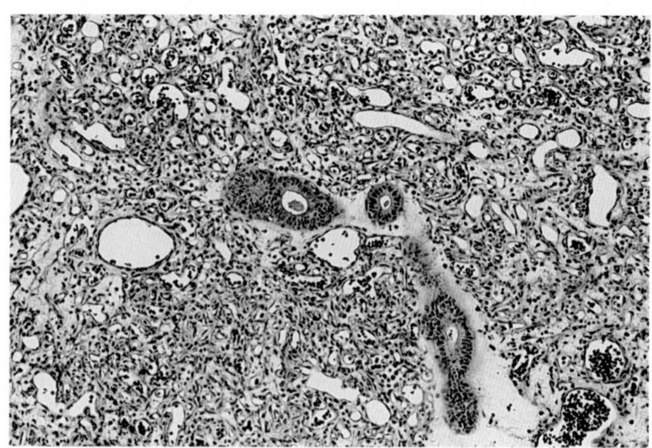

FIGURE 83. Hemangioma separating parotid ducts.

Embryoma or Sialoblastoma

Definition

Embryomas and sialoblastomas are rare, congenital or perinatal, aggressive, potentially low-grade malignant basaloid salivary gland neoplasms that occur in the major salivary glands (74). Batsakis and Frankenthaler (535) suggested separating these tumors into benign and malignant types. Their criteria for malignancy include invasion of nerves or vessels, necrosis, and cytologic atypia beyond that expected for embryonic epithelium. These criteria are valid based on their correlation with behavior in a number of cases reported thus far.

Clinical Data

Most embryomas are recognized in newborns or during the first year of life. The majority are described as being in the parotid gland. They range in size from 1.5 cm to 15 cm. There is no gender predilection. In nearly all cases, the tumor is asymptomatic, but one infant had facial paralysis at birth (535–540).

Gross Appearance

Grossly, the tumor appears partially encapsulated, well circumscribed, and lobulated. The cut surfaces are yellowish-tan, firm, and usually solid. Central necrosis may be present.

Histologic Features

Morphologically, embryomas are similar to the tissue that develops into the embryonic epithelial cells of the major salivary glands in its various stages of differentiation. Thus, embryoma tissue cannot be identified with that of any of the other types of salivary gland tumors described in adults. Embryomas are composed of primitive basaloid cells separated by fibrous or fibromyxomatous stroma (Fig. 84). Many areas resemble the primitive epithelium seen in sebaceous adenomas; focal sebaceous differentiation may occur. The peripheral layer cells demonstrate palisaded nuclei. Small ducts lined by cuboidal cells may be seen in the epithelial islands. Cribriform spaces are evident in some tumors. The malignant tumors show necrosis, perineural or vascular invasion, or both, or destructive invasion of surrounding tissues.

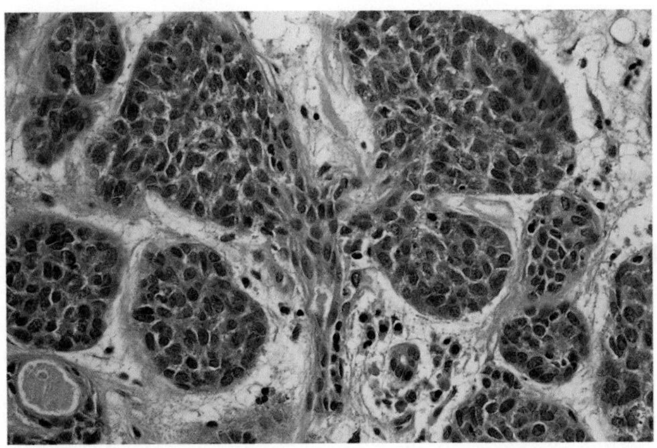

FIGURE 84. Embryoma (sialoblastoma). Basaloid epithelium in primitive stroma. Note the resemblance to the budding off of embryologically developing acini.

Special Studies

The immunoreactivity of sialoblastomas with antibodies to cytokeratin, smooth muscle actin, and S-100 protein is similar to that of basal cell adenocarcinoma (293). Ultrastructurally, embryomas indicate their embryonic quality by containing primitive cells having numerous free ribosomes and limited development of endoplasmic reticulum in the nonductal cells. The cells with ductal character are connected to the surrounding cells by junctions (537,538). Spindle cells with myoepithelial differentiation can be observed at the periphery of the epithelial islands (538).

Differential Diagnosis

In contrast to basal cell adenoma, embryomas are composed of more primitive cells that have less prominent peripheral palisading of nuclei, often with greater mitotic activity and primitive stroma. Adenoid cystic carcinoma or basal cell adenocarcinoma is extremely rare in the first decade of life.

Clinical Behavior and Treatment

The majority of embryomas follow a benign course. Fewer than 25% of the tumors manifested histologically and biologically malignant characteristics (535). Until additional experience is accumulated with these unusual tumors, embryomas should be treated by complete surgical excision; enucleation is inadequate even for tumors that appear well circumscribed (535–540).

Benign Epithelial Tumors

Pleomorphic adenomas are by far the most commonly observed epithelial salivary tumor in children, despite the fact that they are rare in this age group. Only 1.4% of a total of 3,875 pleomorphic adenomas accessioned at the AFIP were found in the pediatric population (528). Other types of benign salivary gland tumors are rare in patients under 16 years of age. Warthin's tumor, cystadenomas, myoepitheliomas, and basal cell adenomas are seldom seen in children. Recently, Dehner et al. (541) described a nasopharyngeal tumor that morphologically resembled pleomorphic adenoma. The authors named this neoplasm "salivary gland anlage tumor" (see Chapter 5).

Malignant Epithelial Tumors

Three characteristics of malignant salivary gland neoplasms in children deserve emphasis. The tumor may have epithelial or mesenchymal origin. The biological activity of malignant salivary epithelial neoplasms in children does not differ from that of their counterpart in adults. Well-differentiated mucoepidermoid carcinoma is the malignant neoplasm usually observed in the salivary glands of children.

Mucoepidermoid carcinoma and acinic cell carcinoma together account for almost 60% of the malignant salivary gland tumors in children (525–532,542). Adenoid cystic carcinoma, adenocarcinoma, and undifferentiated carcinoma are found in lower percentages (543). Carcinoma *ex* pleomorphic adenoma and squamous cell carcinomas are extremely rare.

Lymphomas and Sarcomas

Malignant lymphoma and sarcomas are seldom observed in children, although they should be considered in the differential diagnosis of an enlargement of any of the salivary glands. Of the 59 patients with lymphomas in the salivary glands reported by Colby and Dorfman (499), only four patients were under 16 years of age. All of these patients had lymphoblastic lymphoma. Rhabdomyosarcoma accounted for 16 of 74 specimens of sarcoma of the salivary glands collected by Luna et al. (493).

REFERENCES

Embyrogenesis and Histology

1. Arey LB. *Developmental anatomy.* Phildelphia: WB Saunders, 1974.
2. Lee S, Lim CY, Chi J, et al. Prenatal development of human salivary glands and immunohistochemical detection of keratins, using monoclonal antibodies. *Acta Histochem* 1990;89:213–235.
3. Martinez-Madrigal F, Micheau C. Histology of the major salivary glands. *Am J Surg Pathol* 1989;13:879–899.
4. Seifert G. The pathology of the salivary gland immune system. Diseases and correlations with other organ systems. *Surg Pathol* 1993;5:161–180.

Congenital Anomalies

5. Shinohara M, Harada T, Nakamura S, et al. Heterotopic salivary gland tissue in lymph nodes of the cervical region. *Int J Oral Maxillofac Surg* 1992;21:166–171.
6. Curry B, Yaylor CW, Fisher AWF. Salivary gland heterotopia: an unique cerebellopontine angle tumor. *Arch Pathol Lab Med* 1982; 106:35–38.
7. Young LA, Scofield HH. Heterotopic salivary gland tissue in the lower neck. *Arch Pathol Lab Med* 1967;83:550–556.
8. Bruner JM, Batsakis JG. Salivary neoplasms of the jaw bones with particular reference to central mucoepidermoid carcinomas. *Ann Otol Rhinol Laryngol* 1991;100:954–955.
9. Zajtchuk ST, Paton CA, Hyams VJ. Cervical heterotopic salivary gland neoplasms: a diagnostic dilemma. *Otolaryngol Head Neck Surg* 1982;80:178–181.
10. Luna MA, Monheit J. Salivary gland neoplasms arising in lymph nodes. A clinicopathologic analysis of 13 cases. *Lab Invest* 1988;58: 58A.

11. Seifert G, Michlke A, Hanubrich J, et al. *Diseases of the salivary glands: pathology, diagnosis, treatment, facial nerve surgery.* Stuttgart: George Thieme, 1986.

Cysts

12. Seifert G, Donath K. Classfication of the pathology of diseases of the salivary glands: review of 2,600 cases in the Salivary Gland Register. *Beitr Pathol* 1976;159:1–32.
13. Batsakis JG, Bruner JM, Luna MA. Polycystic (dysgenetic) disease of the parotid gland. *Arch Otolaryngol Head Neck Surg* 1988;114 1146–1148.
14. Smyth AG, Ward-Booth RP, High AS. Polycystic disease of the parotid glands. Two familial cases. *Br J Oral Maxillofac Surg* 1993; 31:38–40.
15. Elliot JN, Ortel YC. Lymphoepithelial cysts of the salivary glands. Histological and cytological features. *Am J Clin Pathol* 1990;93: 39–43.
16. Buchner A, Hansen LS. Lymphoepithelial cysts of oral cavity. A clinicopathologic study of thirty-eight cases. *Oral Surg Oral Med Oral Pathol* 1980;50:441–449.
17. Weidner N, Geisinger KR, Sterling RT, et al. Benign lymphoepithelial cysts of the parotid gland. A histologic, cytologic, and ultrastructural study. *Am J Clin Pathol* 1986;85:395–401.
18. Batsakis JG, McClatchey KD. Cervical ranula. *Ann Otol Rhinol Laryngol* 1988;97:561–562.

Sialolithiasis

19. Raymond RK, Batsakis JG. Angiolithiasis and sialolithiasis in the head and neck. *Ann Otol Rhinol Laryngol* 1992;101:445–457.
20. Ho V, Currie WJ, Walker A. Sialolithiasis of minor salivary glands. *Br J Oral Maxillofac Surg* 1992;30:273–275.
21. Shinohara M, Oka M, Yamada K, et al. Immunohistochemical and electronmicroscopic studies of obstructive lesions in submandibular glands. *J Oral Pathol Med* 1992;21:370–375.
22. Konigsberg R, Feyh J, Goetz A, et al. Endoscopically controlled electrohydraulic intracorporeal shock wave lithotripsy (EISL) of salivary stones. *J Otolaryngol* 1993;22:12–13.

Sialadenitis

23. Brook I. Diagnosis and managment of parotitis. *Arch Otolaryngol Head Neck Surg* 1992;118:469–471.
24. Batsakis JG. Granulomatous sialadenitis. *Ann Otol Rhinol Laryngol* 1991;101:166–169.
25. Singh B, Maharaj TJ. Tuberculosis of the parotid gland. Clinically indistinguishable from a neoplasm. *J Laryngol Otol* 1992;106:929–931.
26. Akiner MN, Saatci MR, Yilmaz O, et al. Intraglandular toxoplasmosis lymphadenitis of the parotid gland. *J Laryngol Otol* 1991; 105: 860–862.
27. Seifert G, Donath K. Zur pathogenese des kuttner-tumorous der submandibularis analysis von 349 fallen mit. *HNO* 1981;25:81–93.
28. Smith BC, Ellis GL, Slater LJ, et al. Sclerosing polycystic adenosis of major salivary glands. A clinicopathologic analysis of nine cases. *Am J Surg Pathol* 1996;20:161–170.

Irradiation Effects

29. Evans JC, Ackerman LV. Irradiation and obstructed submandibular salivary glands simulating cervical lymph node metastasis. *Radiology* 1954;62;550–555.
30. Leslie MD, Dische S. Changes in serum and salivary amylase during radiotherapy for head and neck cancer. A comparison of conventionally fractionated radiotherapy with CHART. *Radiother Oncol* 1992; 24:27–31.

Sialadenosis

31. Batsakis JG. Sialadenosis. *Ann Otol Rhinol Laryngol* 1988;97:94–95.
32. Chilla R. Sialadenosis of the salivary glands of the head and neck. *Adv Otorhinolaryngol* 1981;26:1–38.
33. Donath K, Seifert G. Ultrastructural studies of the parotid glands in sialadenosis. *Virchows Arch* 1975;365:119–135.

Necrotizing Sialometaplasia

34. Abrams AM, Melrose RJ, Howell FV. Necrotizing sialometaplasia: a disease simulating malignancy. *Cancer* 1973;32:130–135.
35. Brannon RB, Fowler CB, Hartman KS. Necrotizing sialometaplasia. A clinicopathologic study of sixty-nine cases and review of the literature. *Oral Surg Oral Med Oral Pathol Oral Radiol Endod* 1991;72: 317–325.
36. Sniege N, Batsakis JG. Necrotizing sialometaplasia. *Ann Otol Rhinol Laryngol* 1992;101:282–284.
37. Grillon GL, Lally ET. Necrotizing sialometaplasia: literature review and presentation of five cases. *J Oral Maxillofac Surg* 1981;39: 747–753.
38. Walker GK, Lally ET. Necrotizing sialometaplasia of the larynx, secondary to atheromatous embolization. *Am J Clin Pathol* 1982; 77:221–223.
39. Wenig BN. Necrotizing sialometaplasia of the larynx. A report of two cases and a review of the literature. *Am J Clin Pathol* 1995;103: 609–613.

Lymphoepithelial Lesion and Sjögren's Syndrome

40. Batsakis JG. The pathology of the head and neck: the lymphoepithelial lesion and Sjögren's syndrome. *Head Neck* 1982;5:150–165.
41. Shaha AR, Di Maio T, Webber C, et al. Benign lymphoepithelial lesions of the parotid. *Am J Surg* 1993;166:403–406.
42. Batsakis JG. Lymphoepithelial lesion and Sjögren's syndrome. *Ann Otol Rhinol Laryngol* 1987;96:354–355.
43. Terry JH, Loree TR, Thomas MD, et al. Major salivary gland lymphoepithelial lesions and the acquired immunodeficiency syndrome. *Am J Surg* 1991;162:324–329.
44. Smith FB, Rajdeo N, Bhuta K, et al. Benign lymphoepithelial lesion of the parotid gland in intravenous drug users. *Arch Pathol Lab Med* 1981;111:554–556.
45. Morgan WS, Castleman BA. Clinicopathologic study of "Mikulicz's disease." *Am J Pathol* 1953;29:471–503.
46. Caselitz J, Osborn M, Wustrow J, et al. Immunohistochemical investigations on the epimyoepithelial islands in lymphoepithelial lesions. Use of monoclonal keratin antibodies. *Lab Invest* 1986;55:427–432.
47. Chaudhry AP, Cutler LS, Yamane GM, et al. Light and ultrastructural features of lymphoepithelial lesions of the salivary glands in Mikulicz's disease. *J Pathol* 1986;146:239–250.
48. Bodeutsch C, de Wilde PC, Kater L, et al. Quantitative immunohistochemical criteria are superior to the lymphocytic focus score criterion for the diagnosis of Sjögren's syndrome. *Arthritis Rheum* 1992;35:1075–1087.
49. Moutsopoulos HM. Sjögren's syndrome (sicca syndrome): current issues. *Ann Intern Med* 1980;92:212–226.
50. Molina R, Provost TT, Arnett FC, et al. Primary Sjögren's syndrome in men: clinical, serologic, and immunogenetic features. *Am J Med* 1986;80:23–31.
51. Cleary KR, Batsakis JG. Biopsy of the lip and Sjögren's syndrome. *Ann Otol Rhinol Laryngol* 1990;90:323–325.
52. Daniels TE. Labial salivary biopsy in Sjögren's syndrome: assessment as a diagnostic criterion in 362 suspected cases. *Arthritis Rheum* 1984;27:147–156.
53. Greenspan JS, Daniels TE, Talal N, et al. The histopathology of Sjögren's syndrome in labial biopsies. *Oral Surg Oral Med Oral Pathol* 1974;37:217–229.

54. Daniels TE. Salivary histopathology in diagnosis of Sjögren's syndrome. *Scand J Rheumatol [Suppl]* 1986;61:36–43.
55. Hsi ED, Zukerberg LR, Schnitzer B, et al. Development of extrasalivary lymphoma in myoepithelial sialadenitis. *Mod Pathol* 1995;8: 817–824.
56. Diss TC, Wotherspoon AC, Speight P, et al. B-cell monoclonality, Epstein Barr virus, and *t*(14;18) in myopithelial sialadenitis and low grade B-cell MALT lymphoma of the parotid gland. *Am J Surg Pathol* 1995;19:531–536.
57. Redondo C, Garcia A, Vazquez F. Malignant lymphoepithelial lesion of the parotid gland. *Cancer* 1981;48:289–292.
58. Batsakis JG. Carcinoma *ex* lymphoepithelial lesion. *Ann Otol Rhinol Laryngol* 1983;92:657–758.
59. Kassan SS, Thomas HM, Moutsopoulos R, et al. Increased risk of lymphoma in sicca syndrome. *Ann Intern Med* 1978;89:888–892.

Cystic Lymphoid Hyperplasia in HIV-Postive Patients

60. Ryan JR, Ioachim HL, Marmer J, et al. Acquired immune deficiency syndrome-related lymphadenopathies presenting in the salivary gland lymph nodes. *Arch Otolaryngol Head Neck Surg* 1985;11:554–556.
61. Cleary KR, Batsakis JG. Lymphoepithelial cysts of the parotid region: a "new face" of an old lesion. *Ann Otol Rhinol Laryngol* 1990;99: 162–164.
62. D'Agay MF, de Roguancourt A, Peuchmaur M, et al. Cystic benign lymphoepithilial lesion of the salivary glands in HIV-positive patients. Reports of two cases with immunohistochemical study. *Virchows Arch* 1990;417:353–356.
63. Bruner JM, Cleary KR, Smith FB, et al. Immunohistochemical identification of HIV(p 24) antigen in parotid lymphoid lesions. *J Laryngol Otol* 1989;103:1063–1066.
64. Labouyrie E, Merlio JP, Beylot-Barry M, et al. Human immunodeficiency virus type I. Replication within cystic lymphoepithelial lesion of the salivary glands. *Am J Clin Pathol* 1993;100:41–46.
65. Williams SB, Foss RD, Ellis GL. Inflammatory pseudotumors of the major salivary glands. *Am J Surg Pathol* 1992;16:896–902.
66. Batsakis JG, Sneige N, El-Naggar AK. Fine-needle aspiration of salivary glands: its utility and tissue effects. *Ann Otol Rhinol Laryngol* 1992;101:185–188.
67. Chan JK, Tang SK, Tsang WYW, et al. Histologic changes induced by fine-needle aspiration. *Adv Anat Pathol* 1996;3:71–90.

Other Nonneoplastic Lesions

68. Fischer JR, Abdul-Karim FW, Robinson RA. Intraparotid fasciitis. *Arch Pathol Lab Med* 1989;113:1276–1278.
69. Stimson PG, Tortoledo ME, Luna M. Localized primary amyloid tumor of the parotid gland. *Oral Surg Oral Med Oral Pathol Oral Radiol Endod* 1988;66:466–469.
70. Myssiorek D, Alvi A, Bhuiya T. Primary salivary gland amyloidosis causing sicca syndrome. *Ann Otol Rhinol Laryngol* 1992;101: 487–490.
71. Foucar E, Rosai J, Dorfman RD. Sinus histiocytosis with massive lymphoadenopathy (Rosai-Dorfman disease). Review of the entity. *Semin Diagn Pathol* 1990;7:19–73.
72. Specks U, Coldy TV, Olsen KD, et al. Salivary glands involvement in Wegener's granulomatosis. *Arch Pathol Lab Med* 1991;117:218–223.
73. Duboucher C, Mogenet M, Perie G. Salivary trichomoniasis. A case report of infestation of a submaxillary gland by trichomonas tenax. *Arch Pathol Lab Med* 1995;119:277–279.

Classification of Tumors

74. Ellis GL, Auclair PL. *Tumors of the salivary glands. Atlas of tumor pathology, 3rd ser, Fasc 17.* Washington, DC: Armed Forces Institute of Pathology, 1996.
75. Seifert G. *Histological typing of salivary gland tumors. World Health Organization International Histological Classification of Tumours, 2nd ed.* Berlin: Springer-Verlag, 1991.
76. Ellis GL, Auclair PL. Classification of salivary gland neoplasms. In: Ellis GL, Auclair PL, Gnepp DR, eds. *Surgical pathology of salivary glands.* Philadelphia: WB Saunders, 1991:129.
77. Eveson JW, Cawson RA. Salivary gland tumors. A review of 2410 cases with particular reference to histological types, site, age and sex distribution. *J Pathol* 1985;146:51–58.
78. Simpson RHW. Classification of tumours of the salivary glands. *Histopathology* 1994;24:187–191.
79. Johns M, Goldsmith M. Incidence, diagnosis, and classification of salivary gland tumors, 1. *Oncology* 1989;3:47–56.

Histogenesis of Tumors

80. Yoshida H, Azuma M, Yanagawa TM, et al. Effect of dibutyl cyclic AMP on morphologic features and biologic markers of a human salivary gland adenocarcinoma cell line in culture. *Cancer* 1986;57: 1011–1018.
81. Dardick I, Byard R, Carnegie J. A review of the proliferative capacity of major salivary glands and the relationship to current concepts of neoplasia in salivary glands. *Oral Surg Oral Med Oral Pathol Oral Radiol Endod* 1990;69:53–67.
82. Burford-Mason A, Byard RW, Dardick I, et al. The pathobiology of the salivary gland, I: growth and development of rat submandibular gland organoids cultured in a collagen gel matrix. *Virchows Arch* 1991;418:387–400.
83. Batsakis J, Regezi J, Luna M, et al. Histogenesis of salivary gland neoplsms: a postulate with prognostic implications. *J Laryngol Otol* 1989;103:939–944.
84. Levin RJ, Bradley MK. Neuroectodermal antigens persist in benign and malignant salivary gland tumor cultures. *Arch Otolaryngol Head Neck Surg* 1996;122:551–558.
85. Noguchi S, Aihara T, Yoshino K, et al. Demonstration of monoclonal origin of human parotid pleomorphic adenoma. *Cancer* 1996;77: 431–435.

Incidence

86. Waterhouse J, Muir C, Correa P. Cancer incidence in five continents, Vol III. Lyon: International Agency for Research on Cancer, 1976:16–25.
87. Auclair PL, Ellis GL, Gnepp DR, et al. Salivary gland neoplasms: general considerations. In: Ellis GL, Auclair PL, Gnepp DR, eds. *Surgical pathology of salivary glands.* Philadelphia: WB Saunders, 1991:135.
88. Spiro RH. Salivary neoplasms: overview of a 35-year experience with 2,807 patients. *Head Neck* 1986;8:177–184.
89. Batsakis JG. Sublingual gland. *Ann Otol Rhinol Laryngol* 1991;100: 521–522.

Etiology

90. Spitz MR, Sider JG, Newell GR, et al. Incidence of salivary gland cancer in the United States relative to radiation exposure. *Head Neck* 1988;10:305–308.
91. Belsky JL, Takeichi N, Yamamoto T, et al. Salivary gland neoplasms following atomic radiation: additional cases and reanalysis of combined data in a fixed population. 1957–1970. *Cancer* 1975;35: 555–559.
92. Modan B, Baidatz D, Mart H, et al. Radiation-induced head and neck tumors. *Lancet* 1974;1:277–279.
93. Shore-Freedman E, Abrahams C, Recant W. Neurilemmomas and salivary gland tumors of the head and neck following childhood irradiation. *Cancer* 1983;51:2159–2163.
94. Mancuso TF, Breannan MJ. Epidemiological considerations of cancer of the gallbladder, bile ducts and salivary glands in rubber industry. *J Occup Environ Med* 1970;12:333–341.

95. Milham S Jr. Cancer mortality patterns associated with exposure to metals. *Ann NY Acad Sci* 1976;271:243–259.
96. Sawanson GW, Belle SH. Cancer morbidity among woodworkers in the US automotive industry. *J Occup Environ Med* 1982;24: 313–319.
97. Spitz M, Tilley BC, Batsakis JG, et al. Risk factors for major salivary gland carcinoma. A case comparison study. *Cancer* 1984;54: 1854–1859.
98. Lamey PJ, Waterhouse JP, Ferguson MM. Pleomorphic salivary adenoma. Virally induced pleomorphic salivary adenoma in the CFLP mouse. *Am J Pathol* 1982;14:129–132.
99. Abbey LM, Schwab BH, Landau GC. Incidence of second primary breast cancer among patients with a first primary salivary gland tumor. *Cancer* 1984;54:1439–1442.

Multiple Tumors

100. Gnepp DR, Schroeder W, Heffner D. Synchronous tumors arising in a single major salivary gland. *Cancer* 1989;63:1219–1224.
101. Seifert G, Donath K. Multiple tumours of the salivary glands. Terminology and nomenclature. *Eur J Cancer B Oral Oncol* 1996; 32:3–7.
102. Johns ME, Shikhani AH, Kashima HK, et al. Multiple primary neoplasms in patients with salivary and thyroid gland tumors. *Laryngoscope* 1986;96:718–721.

Biopsy

103. Dandour-Edwards RF, Donald PJ, Wise DA. Accuracy of intraoperative frozen section diagnosis in head and neck surgery: experience at a university medical center. *Head Neck* 1993;15:33–38.
104. Miller RH, Calcaterra TC, Paglia DE. Accuracy of frozen section diagnosis of salivary gland disorders in the community hospital setting. *Ann Otol Rhinol Laryngol* 1979;88:573–576.
105. Hillel AD, Fee WE. Evaluation of frozen section in parotid gland surgery. *Arch Otolaryngol Head Neck Surg* 1983;109:230–232.
106. Pitts DB, Hilsenger RL, Karandy E, et al. Fine needle aspiration in the diagnosis of salivary gland disorders in the community hospital setting. *Arch Otolaryngol Head Neck Surg* 1992;118:479–482.
107. Frable MAS, Frable WJ. Fine-needle aspiration biopsy of salivary glands. *Laryngoscope* 1991;101:245–249.
108. Layfield LJ, Glasgow BJ. Diagnosis of salivary gland tumors by fine needle aspiration cytology: a review of clinical utility and pitfalls. *Diagn Cytopathol* 1991;7:267–272.
109. Layfield LF, Tan P, Glasgow BJ. Fine-needle aspiration of salivary gland lesions. Comparision with frozen sections and histologic findings. *Arch Pathol Lab Med* 1987;111:346–353.
110. Cross DL, Gansler TS, Morris RC. Fine-needle aspiration and frozen section of salivary gland lesions. *South Med J* 1990;83:283–286.
111. Batsakis JG. *Tumors of the head and neck, 2nd ed.* Baltimore: Willams & Willams, 1979.
112. Perzin KH. Systematic approach to the pathologic diagnosis of salivary gland tumors. *Prog Surg Pathol* 1982;4:137–179.

Ancillary Methods

113. Donath K. Ultrastrukturelle marker bei speicheldrusentumoren. *Dtsch Zeitschr Mund Kiefer Ges Chir* 1983;7:119–127.
114. Bang G, Donath K, Thorsesen S. DNA flow cytometry of reclassified subtypes of malignant salivary gland tumors. *J Oral Pathol Med* 1994;7:628–631.
115. Carrillo R, Batsakis JG, Weber R. Salivary neoplasms. *J Laryngol Otol* 1993;107:858–861.
116. Muller S, Vignesawran N, Gansler T. c-erbB-2 oncoprotein expression and amplification in pleomorphic adenoma and carcinoma *ex* pleomorphic adenoma: relationship to prognosis. *Mod Pathol* 1994; 7:628–931.
117. Soini Y, Kamel D, Nourva K. Low p53 protein expression in salivary gland tumours compared with lung carcinomas. *Virchows Arch* 1992;421:415–420.
118. Stenman G, Sahlin P, Mark J. Structural alterations of the *c-mos* locus in benign pleomorphic adenomas with chromosome abnormalities of 8q12. *Oncogene* 1991;6:1105–1108.
119. van Halteren HK, Top B, Mooi WJ. Association of *H-ras* mutations with adenocarcinomas of the parotid gland. *Int J Cancer* 1994;57: 362–364.
120. Batsakis JG. Staging of salivary gland neoplasms: role of histopathologic and molecular factors. *Am J Surg* 1994;168:386–390.
121. Schantz SP. Head and neck oncology research. *Curr Opin Oncol* 1994;168:386–390.
122. Bullerdiek-Wobst G, Meyer-Bolte K, Chilla R. Cytogentic subtyping of 220 salivary gland pleomorphic adenomas: correlation to occurrence, histologic subtype, and *in vitro* cellular behavior. *Cancer Genet Cytogenet* 1993;65:27–31.
123. Mark J, Wedell B, Dahlenfors R, et al. Karyotypic variability and evolutionary charateristics of polymorphous low grade adenocarcinomas of the parotid gland. *Cancer Genet Cytogenet* 1991;55:19–29.
124. Bullerdick J, Vollrath M, Witteking C, et al. Mucoepidermoid tumor of the parotid gland showing a translation (3;8) (p21;q12) and a deletion (5) (q22) as sole chromosome abnormalities. *Cancer Genet Cytogenet* 1990;50:161–164.
125. Levitt SH, McHugh RB, Gomez-Marin O, et al. Clinical staging system for cancer of the salivary gland: a retrospective study. *Cancer* 1981;47:2712–2724.

Plemorphic Adenoma and Malignant Mixed Tumors

126. Waldron CA. Mixed tumor (pleomorphic adenoma) and myoepithelioma. In: Ellis GL, Auclair PL, Gnepp DR, eds. *Surgical pathology of the salivary glands.* Philadelphia: WB Saunders, 1991:165–186.
127. Chau MN, Radden BG. A clinical-pathological study of 53 intra-oral pleomorphic adenomas. *Int J Oral Maxillofac Surg* 1989;18:158–162.
128. Krolls SO, Boyers RC. Mixed tumors of salivary glands: long-term follow-up. *Cancer* 1972;30:176–281.
129. Lack EE, Upton MP. Histopathologic review of salivary gland tumors in childhood. *Arch Otolaryngol Head Neck Surg* 1988;114:898–906.
130. Koide C, Imai A, Nagaba A, et al. Pathological findings in the facial nerve palsy associated with benign parotid tumor. *Arch Otolaryngol Head Neck Surg* 1994;120:410–412.
131. Fliss DM, Rival R, Gullane P, et al. Pleomorphic adenoma: preliminary histopathologic comparison between tumors occurring in the deep and superficial lobes of the parotid gland. *Ear Nose Throat J* 1992;71:254–257.
132. Som PM, Shugar JMA, Sacher M, et al. Benign and malignant pleomorphic adenoma: CT and MR studies. *J Comput Assist Tomogr* 1988;12:65–69.
133. Mirich DR, McArdle CB, Kulkarni MV. Benign pleomorphic adenoma of the salivary glands: surface coil MR imaging versus CT. *J Comput Assist Tomogr* 1987;11:620–623.
134. Lam KH, Wei WI, Ho HC, et al. Whole organ sectioning of mixed parotid tumors. *Am J Surg* 1990;160:377–381.
135. Lomax-Smith JD, Azzopardi JJ. The hyaline cell: a distinctive feature of mixed salivary tumors. *Histopathology* 1978;2:77–92.
136. Humphrey PA, Ingram P, Tucker A, et al. Crystalloids in salivary gland pleomorphic adenomas. *Arch Pathol Lab Med* 1989;113: 390–393.
137. Ryan RE Jr, DeSanto LW, Weiland LH, et al. Cellular mixed tumors of the salivary glands. *Arch Otolaryngol Head Neck Surg* 1978;104:451–453.
138. Auclair PL, Ellis GL. Atypical features in salivary gland mixed tumors: their relationship to malignant transformation. *Mod Pathol* 1996;9: 652–657.
139. Erlandson RA, Cardon-Cardo C, Higgins PJ. Histogenesis of benign pleomorphic adenoma (mixed tumor) of the major salivary glands. An

ultrastructural and immunohistochemical study. *Am J Surg Pathol* 1984;8:803–820.

140. Gandour-Edwards R, Kapadia SB, Gumerlock PH, et al. Immunolocalization of interleukin-6 in salivary gland tumors. *Hum Pathol* 1995;26:501–503.
141. Takahashi M, Tsuda N, Tezuka F, et al. Immunohistochemical localization of carcinoembryonic antigen in carcinoma in pleomorphic adenoma of salivary gland: use in the diagnosis of benign and malignant lesions. *Tohoku J Exp Med* 1986;149:329–340.
142. van Krieken JH. Prostate marker immunoreactivity in salivary gland neoplasms. A rare pitfall in immunohistochemistry. *Am J Surg Pathol* 1993;17:410–414.
143. Dardick I, Cavell S, Boivin M. Salivary gland myoepithelioma variants. Histological, ultrastructural and immunocytological features. *Virchows Arch* 1989;416:25–42.
144. Anderson C, Knibbs DR, Abbott SJ, et al. Glial fibrillary acidic protein expression in pleomorphic adenoma of salivary gland. An immunoelectron microscopic study. *Ultrastruct Pathol* 1990;14:263–271.
145. Landini G. Immunohistochemical demonstration of type II collagen in the chondroid tissue of pleomorphic adenomas of the salivary glands. *Acta Pathol Jpn* 1991;41:270–276.
146. Murakami M, Ohtani I, Hojo H, et al. Immunohistochemical evaluation with Ki-67. An application to salivary gland tumours. *J Laryngol Otol* 1992;106:35–38.
147. Martin AR, Mantravadi J, Kotylo PK, et al. Proliferative activity and aneuploidy in pleomorphic adenomas of the salivary glands. *Arch Pathol Lab Med* 1994;118:252–259.
148. Deguchi H, Hamano H, Hayashi Y. *c-myc, ras* p21 and p53 expression in pleomorphic adenoma and its malignant form of the human salivary glands. *Acta Pathol Jpn* 1993;43:413–422.
149. Donovan DT, Conley JJ. Capsular significance in parotid tumor surgery: reality and myths of lateral lobectomy. *Laryngoscope* 1984; 94:324–329.
150. Touquet R, Mackenzie IJ, Carruth JA. Management of the parotid pleomorphic adenoma, the problem of exposing tumour tissue at operation. The logical pursuit of treatment policies. *Br J Oral Maxillofac Surg* 1990;28:404–408.
151. Myssiorek D, Ruah CB, Hybels RL. Recurrent pleomorphic adenomas of the parotid gland. *Head Neck* 1990;12:332–336.
152. Hancock BD. Pleomorphic adenomas of the parotid: removal without rupture. *Ann R Coll Surg Engl* 1987;69:293–295.
153. Yamashita T, Tomoda K, Kumazawa T. The usefulness of partial parotidectomy for benign parotid gland tumors. A retrospective study of 306 cases. *Acta Otolaryngol Suppl (Stockh)* 1993;500:113–116.
154. Liu FF, Rotstein L, Davison AJ, et al. Benign parotid adenomas: a review of the Princess Margaret Hospital experience. *Head Neck* 1995;17:177–183.
155. Naeim R, Forsberg MI, Waisman J, et al. Mixed tumor of the salivary gland. Growth pattern and recurrence. *Arch Pathol Lab Med* 1976; 100:271–275.
156. Eneroth CM. Mixed tumors of major salivary glands: prognostic role of capsular structure. *Ann Otol Rhinol Laryngol* 1965;74:944–954.
157. Tortoledo ME, Luna MA, Batsakis JG. Carcinomas *ex* pleomorphic adenoma and malignant mixed tumors: histomorphologic indexes. *Arch Otolaryngol Head Neck Surg* 1984;110:172–176.
158. Duck SW, McConnel FM. Malignant degeneration of pleomorphic adenoma—clinical implications. *Am J Otolaryngol* 1993:14:175–178.
159. Spiro RH, Huvos AG, Strong EW. Malignant mixed tumor of salivary gland origin. A clinicopathologic study of 146 cases. *Cancer* 1977; 39:388–396.
160. LiVolsi C, Perzin KH. Malignant mixed tumor arising in salivary glands. *Cancer* 1977;39:2209–2230.
161. Gnepp DR, Wenig BM. Malignant mixed tumors. In: Ellis GL, Auclair PL, Gnepp DR, eds. *Pathology of salivary gland.* Philadelphia: WB Saunders, 1991:350–368.
162. Eneroth CM, Blanck C, Jakobsson PA. Carcinoma in pleomorphic adenoma of the parotid gland. *Acta Otolaryngol (Stockh)* 1968;66: 477–492.
163. Gerughty RM, Scofield HH, Brown FM, et al. Malignant mixed tumors of salivary gland origin. *Cancer* 1969;24:471–486.
164. Gnepp DR. Malignant mixed tumors of the salivary glands: a review. *Pathol Annu* 1993;28(Pt 1):279–328.
165. Eneroth CM, Zetterberg A. Microspectrophotometric DNA analysis of malignant salivary gland tumours. *Acta Otolaryngol (Stockh)* 1974;77:289–294.
166. Eneroth CM, Zetterberg A. Malignancy in pleomorphic adenoma. A clinical and microspectrophotometric study. *Acta Otolaryngol (Stockh)* 1974;77:426–432.
167. Littman CD, Alguacil-Garcia A. Clear cell carcinoma arising in pleomorphic adenoma of the salivary gland. *Am J Clin Pathol* 1987;88: 239–243.
168. Jacobs JC. Low grade mucoepidermoid carcinoma *ex* pleomorphic adenoma. A diagnostic problem in fine needle aspiration biopsy. *Acta Cytol* 1994;38:93–97.
169. Moberger JG, Eneroth CM. Malignant mixed tumors of the major salivary glands. Special reference to the histologic structure in metastases. *Cancer* 1968;21:1198–1211.
170. Bocklage T, Feddersen R. Unusual mesenchymal and mixed tumors of the salivary gland. An immunohistochemical and flow cytometric analysis of three cases. *Arch Pathol Lab Med* 1995;119:69–74.
171. Brandwein MS, Huvos AG, Patil J, et al. Tumor associated glycoprotein distribution detected by monoclonal antibody B72.3 in salivary neoplasias. *Cancer* 1992;69:2623–2630.
172. Batsakis JG, Regezi JA, Bock D. The pathology of the head and neck tumors. Part 3. *Head Neck* 1979;1:260–276.
173. Dardick I, Hardie J, Thomas MJ, et al. Ultrastructural contributions to the study of morphological differentiation in malignant mixed (pleomorphic) tumors of salivary gland. *Head Neck* 1989;11:5–21.
174. Stephen J, Batsakis JG, Luna MA, et al. True malignant mixed tumors (carcinosarcoma) of salivary glands. *Oral Surg Oral Med Oral Pathol* 1986;61:597–602.
175. Suzuki J, Takagi M, Okada N, et al. Carcinosarcoma of the submandibular gland. An autopsy case. *Acta Pathol Jpn* 1990;40: 827–831.
176. Toynton SC, Wilkins MJ, Cook HT, et al. True malignant mixed tumour of a minor salivary gland. *J Laryngol Otol* 1994;108:76–79.
177. Yamashita T, Kameda N, Katayama K, et al. True malignant mixed tumor of the submandibular gland. *Acta Pathol Jpn* 1990;40: 137–142.
178. Bleiweiss IJ, Huvos AG, Lara J, et al. Carcinosarcoma of the submandibular salivary gland. Immunohistochemical findings. *Cancer* 1992;69:2031–2035.
179. Chen KT, Weinberg RA, Moseley D. Carcinosarcoma of the salivary gland. *Am J Otolaryngol* 1984;5:415–417.
180. Garner SL, Robinson RA, Maves MD, et al. Salivary gland carcinosarcoma: true malignant mixed tumor. *Ann Otol Rhinol Laryngol* 1989;98:611–614.
181. Granger JK, Houn HY. Malignant mixed tumor (carcinosarcoma) of parotid gland diagnosed by fine-needle aspiration biopsy. *Diagn Cytopathol* 1991;7:427–432.
182. Hellquist H, Michaels L. Malignant mixed tumour. A salivary gland tumour showing both carcinomatous and sarcomatous features. *Virchows Arch* 1986;409:93–103.
183. Rumnong V, Banerjee AK, Joshi K, et al. Carcinosarcoma of parotid gland having osteosarcoma as sarcomatous component: a case report. *Indian J Pathol Microbiol* 1993;36:492–494.
184. Huntington HW, Dardick I. Intracranial metastasis from a malignant mixed tumor of parotid salivary gland. *Ultrastruct Pathol* 1985;9:169–173.
185. Cresson DH, Godsmith M, Askin FB, et al. Metastasizing pleomorphic adenoma with myoepithelial cell predominance [Discussion]. *Pathol Res Pract* 1990;186:795–800.
186. El-Naggar A, Batsakis JG, Kessler S. Benign metastatic mixed tumours or unrecognized salivary carcinomas? *J Laryngol Otol* 1988;102: 810–812.
187. Freeman SB, Kennedy KS, Parker GS, et al. Metastasizing pleomorphic adenoma of the nasal septum. *Arch Otolaryngol Head Neck Surg* 1990;116:1331–1333.
188. Morrison PD, McMullin JP. A case of metastasizing benign pleomorphic adenoma of the parotid. *Clin Oncol* 1984;10:173–176.

189. Pitman MB, Thor AD, Goodman ML, et al. Benign metastasizing pleomorphic adenoma of salivary gland: diagnosis of bone lesions by fine-needle aspiration biopsy. *Diagn Cytopathol* 1992;8:384–387.
190. Sim DW, Maran AG, Harris D. Metastatic salivary pleomorphic adenoma. *J Laryngol Otol* 1990;104:45–47.
191. Wenig BM, Hitchcock CL, Ellis GL, et al. Metastasizing mixed tumor of salivary glands. A clincopathologic and flow cytometric analysis. *Am J Surg Pathol* 1992;16:845–858.
192. Wermuth DJ, Mann CH, Odere F. Metastasizing pleomorphic adenoma arising in the soft palate. *Otolaryngol Head Neck Surg* 1988;99: 505–508.
193. Youngs GR, Scheuer PJ. Histologically benign mixed parotid tumour with hepatic metastasis. *J Pathol* 1973;109:171–172.
194. Chen KT. Metastasizing pleomorphic adenoma of the salivary gland. *Cancer* 1978;42:2407–2411.
195. Collina G, Eusebi V, Carasoli PT. Pleomorphic adenoma with lymph-node metastases: report of two cases. *Pathol Res Pract* 1989;184: 188–193.

Myoepithelioma and Myoepithelial Carcinoma

196. Alos L, Cardesa A, Bombi JA, et al. Myoepithelial tumors of salivary glands: a clinicopathologic, immunohistochemical, ultrastructural and flow cytometric study. *Semin Diagn Pathol* 1996;13: 138–147.
197. Barnes L, Appel BN, Perez H, et al. Myoepithelioma of the head and neck: case report and review. *J Surg Oncol* 1985;28:21–28.
198. Dardick I, Thomas MJ, van Nostrand AW. Myoepithelioma—new concepts of histology and classification: a light and electron microscopic study. *Ultrastruct Pathol* 1989;13:187–224.
199. Sciubba JJ, Brannon RB. Myoepithelioma of salivary glands: report of 23 cases. *Cancer* 1982;49:562–572.
200. Redman RS. Myoepithelium of salivary glands. *Microsc Res Tech* 1994;27:25–45.
201. Martinez-Madrigal F, Santiago Payan H, Meneses A, et al. Plasmacytoid myoepithelioma of the laryngeal region: a case report. *Hum Pathol* 1995;26:802–804.
202. Franquemont DW, Mills SE. Plasmacytoid monomorphic adenoma of salivary glands. Absence of myogenous differentiation and comparison to spindle cell myoepithelioma. *Am J Surg Pathol* 1993;17: 146–153.
203. Batsakis JG, Ordóñez NG, Ro J, et al. S-100 protein and myoepithelial neoplasms. *J Laryngol Otol* 1986;100:687–698.
204. de Araújo VC, de Araújo NS. Vimentin as a marker of myoepithelial cells in salivary gland tumors. *Eur Arch Otorhinolaryngol* 1990;247: 252–255.
205. Jones H, Moshtael F, Simpson RH. Immunoreactivity of alpha smooth muscle actin in salivary gland tumours: a comparison with S-100 protein. *J Clin Pathol* 1992;45:938–940.
206. El-Naggar A, Batsakis JG, Luna MA, et al. DNA content and proliferative activity of myoepitheliomas. *J Laryngol Otol* 1989;103: 1192–1197.
207. Carrillo R, El-Naggar AK, Luna MA, et al. Nucleolar organizer regions (NORs) and myoepitheliomas: a comparison with DNA content and clinical course. *J Laryngol Otol* 1992;106:616–620.
208. Singh R, Cawson RA. Malignant myoepithelial carcinoma (myoepithelioma) arising in a pleomorphic adenoma of the parotid gland. An immunohistochemical study and review of the literature. *Oral Surg Oral Med Oral Pathol Oral Radiol Endod* 1988;66:65–70.
209. Di Palma S, Pilotti S, Rilke F. Malignant myoepithelioma of the parotid gland arising in a pleomorphic adenoma. *Histopathology* 1991;19:273–275.
210. Crissman JD, Wirman JA, Harris A. Malignant myoepithelioma of the parotid gland. *Cancer* 1977;40:3042–3049.
211. Dardick I. Malignant myoepithelioma of parotid salivary gland. *Ultrastruct Pathol* 1985;9:163–168.
212. Takeda Y. Malignant myoepithelioma of minor salivary gland origin. *Acta Pathol Jpn* 1992;42:518–522.
213. Di Palma S, Guzzo M. Malignant myoepithelioma of salivary glands: clinicopathological features of ten cases. *Virchows Arch* 1993;423: 389–396.

Oncocytoma and Oncocytic Carcinoma

214. Hemperl H. Benign and malignant oncocytoma. *Cancer* 1962;15: 1019–1027.
215. Green DE. Mitochondria—structure, function, and replication. *N Engl J Med* 1983;309:182–183.
216. Ernster L, Schatz G. Mitochondria: a historical review. *J Cell Biol* 1981;91:227–255.
217. Smith RA, Ord MJ. Mitochondrial form and function relationships *in vivo:* their potential in toxicology and pathology. *Int Rev Cytol* 1983;83:63–134.
218. Carlsöö B, Domeij S, Helander HF. A quantitative ultrastructural study of a parotid oncocytoma. *Arch Pathol Lab Med* 1979;103: 471–474.
219. Chang A, Harawi SJ. Oncocytes, oncocytosis, and oncocytic tumors. *Pathol Annu* 1992;27(Pt 1):263–304.
220. Brandwein MS, Huvos AG. Oncocytic tumors of major salivary glands. A study of 68 cases with follow-up of 44 patients. *Am J Surg Pathol* 1991;15:514–528.
221. Palmer TJ, Gleeson MJ, Eveson JW, et al. Oncocytic adenomas and oncocytic hyperplasia of salivary glands: a clinicopathological study of 26 cases. *Histopathology* 1990;16:487–493.
222. Hartwick RW, Batsakis JG. Non-Warthin's tumor oncocytic lesions. *Ann Otol Rhinol Laryngol* 1990;99:674–677.
223. Ellis GL. "Clear cell" oncocytoma of salivary gland. *Hum Pathol* 1988;19:862–867.
224. Gray SR, Cornog JL, Seo IS. Oncocytic neoplasms of salivary glands. A report of fifteen cases including two malignant oncocytomas. *Cancer* 1976;38:1306–1317.
225. Taxy J. Necrotizing squamous/mucinous metaplasia in oncocytic salivary gland tumors. *Am J Clin Pathol* 1992;97:40–45.
226. Johns ME, Batsakis JG, Short CD. Oncocytic and oncocytoid tumors of the salivary glands. *Laryngoscope* 1973;83:1940–1952.
227. Lidang Jensen M. Multifocal adenomatous oncocytic hyperplasia in parotid glands with metastatic deposits or primary malignant transformation? Pathol Res Pract 1989;185:514–521.
228. Gustafsson H, Kjörell U, Carlsöö B. Cytoskeletal proteins in oncocytic tumors of the parotid gland. *Arch Otolaryngol Head Neck Surg* 1985;111:99–105.
229. Felix A, Fonseca I, Soares J. Oncocytic tumors of salivary gland type: a study with emphasis on nuclear DNA ploidy. *J Surg Oncol* 1993;52:217–222.
230. Goode RK, Corio RL. Oncocytic adenocarcinoma of salivary glands. *Oral Surg Oral Med Oral Pathol Oral Radiol Endod* 1988;65: 61–66.
231. Sugimoto T, Wakizono S, Uemura T, et al. Malignant oncocytoma of the parotid gland: a case report with an immunohistochemical and ultrastructural study. *J Laryngol Otol* 1993;107:69–74.
232. Ramakrishna B, Perakath B, Chandi SM. Malignant multinodular oncocytoma of parotid gland—a case report and literature review. *Indian J Cancer* 1992;29:230–233.
233. DiMaio S, DiMaio VJM, DiMaio TM, et al. Oncocytic carcinoma of the nasal cavity. *South Med J* 1980;73:803–806.

Warthin's Tumor and Malignant Warthin's Tumor

234. Eveson JW, Cawson RA. Warthin's tumor cystadenolymphomas of salivary glands. A clinicopathologic investigation of 278 cases. *Oral Surg Oral Med Oral Pathol Oral Radiol Endod* 1986;61: 256–262.
235. Fantasia JE, Miller AS. Papillary cystadenoma lymphomatosum arising in minor salivary gland. *Oral Surg Oral Med Oral Pathol Oral Radiol Endod* 1981;52:411–416.

236. Chaudhry AP, Gorlin R. Papillary cystadenoma lymphomatosum (adenolymphoma): a review of the literature. *Am J Surg* 1958;95: 923–931.
237. Lefor AT, Ord RA. Multiple synchronous bilateral Warthin's tumors of the parotid glands with pleomorphic adenoma. Case report and review of the literature. *Oral Surg Oral Med Oral Pathol Oral Radiol Endod* 1993;76:319–324.
238. Warnock GR. Papillary cystadenoma lymphomatosum (Warthin's tumor) In: Ellis GL, Auclair PL, Gnepp DR, eds. *Surgical pathology of the salivary glands.* Philadelphia: WB Saunders, 1991: 187–201.
239. Snyderman C, Johnson JT, Barnes EL. Extraparotid Warthin's tumor. *Otolaryngol Head Neck Surg* 1986;94:169–175.
240. Seifert G, Bull HG, Donath K. Histologic subclassification of the cystadenolymphoma of the parotid gland. Analysis of 275 cases. *Virchows Arch* 1980;388:13–38.
241. Batsakis JG, El-Naggar AK. Warthin's tumor. *Ann Otol Rhinol Laryngol* 1990;99:588–591.
242. Chin KW, Billings KR, Ishiyama A, et al. Characterization of lymphocyte subpopulations in Warthin's tumor. *Laryngoscope* 1995; 105:928–933.
243. Kern SB. Necrosis of a Warthin's tumor following fine needle aspiration. *Acta Cytol* 1988;32:207–208.
244. Newman L, Loukota RA, Bradley PF. An infarcted Warthin's tumour presenting with facial weakness. *Br J Oral Maxillofac Surg* 1993;31: 311–312.
245. Foulsham CK II, Johnson GS, Snyder GG III, et al. Immunohistopathology of papillary cystadenoma lymphomatosum (Warthin's tumor). *Ann Clin Lab Sci* 1984;14:47–63.
246. Dardick I, Claude A, Parks WR, et al. Warthin's tumor: an ultrastructural and immunohistochemical study of basilar epithelium. *Ultrastruct Pathol* 1988;12:19–32.
247. Mark J, Dahlenfors R, Stenman G, et al. Chromosomal patterns in Warthin's tumor. A second type of human benign salivary gland neoplasm. *Cancer Genet Cytogenet* 1990;46:35–39.
248. Santucci M, Gallo O, Calzolari A, et al. Detection of Epstein-Barr viral genome in tumor cells of Warthin's tumor of parotid gland. *Am J Clin Pathol* 1993;100:662–665.
249. Madeiros LJ, Rizzi R, Lardelli P, et al. Malignant lymphoma involving a Warthin's tumor: a case with immunophenotypic and gene rearrangement analysis. *Hum Pathol* 1990;21:974–977.
250. Podlesak T, Doleckovo V, Sibl O. Malignancy of a cystadenolymphoma of the parotid gland. *Eur Arch Otorhinolaryngol* 1992;249: 233–235.
251. Therkildsen MH, Christensen N, Andersen IJ, et al. Malignant Warthin's tumour: a case study. *Histopathology* 1992;21:167–171.
252. Bengoechea O, Sanchez F, Larrnaga B, et al. Oncocytic adenocarcinoma arising in Warthin's tumor. *Pathol Res Pract* 1989;185: 907–911.
253. Batsakis JG. Carcinoma *ex* papillary cystadenoma lymphomatosum. Malignant Warthin's tumor. *Ann Otol Rhinol Laryngol* 1987;96: 234–235.
254. Damjanov I, Sneff EM, Delerme AN. Squamous cell carcinoma arising in Warthin's tumor of the parotid gland. A light, electron microscopic and immunohistochemical study. *Oral Surg Oral Med Oral Pathol Oral Radiol Endod* 1983;55:286–290.
255. Brown L, Aparicio SP. Malignant Warthin's tumor: an ultrastructural study. *J Clin Pathol* 1984;37:170–175.

Sebaceous Adenomas and Carcinomas

256. Linhartova A. Sebaceous glands in salivary gland tissue. *Arch Pathol Lab Med* 1974;98:320–324.
257. Lipani C, Woytash JJ, Greene GW Jr. Sebaceous adenoma of the oral cavity. *J Oral Maxillofac Surg* 1983;41:56–60.
258. Gnepp DR. Sebaceous neoplasms of salivary gland origin. A review. *Pathol Annu* 1983;18:71–102.
259. Rulon DB, Helwig EB. Cutaneous sebaceous neoplasms. *Cancer* 1974;33:82–102.
260. Batsakis JG, Littler ER, Leahy MS. Sebaceous cell lesions of the head and neck. *Arch Otolaryngol Head Neck Surg* 1972;95:151–157.
261. Auclair PL, Ellis GL, Gnepp DR. Other benign epithelial neoplasms. In: Ellis GL, Auclair PL, Gnepp DR, eds. *Surgical pathology of the salivary glands.* Philadelphia: WB Saunders, 1991:252–268.
262. Batsakis JG, El-Naggar AK. Sebaceous lesions of salivary glands and oral cavity. *Ann Otol Rhinol Laryngol* 1990;99:416–418.
263. McGavran MH, Bauer WC, Ackerman LV. Sebaceous lymphadenoma of the parotid gland. *Cancer* 1960;13:1185–1187.
264. Tschen JA, McGavran MG. Sebaceous lymphadenoma. Ultrastructural observations and lipid analysis. *Cancer* 1979;44: 1388– 1392.
265. Baratz M, Loewenthal M, Rozin M. Sebaceous lymphadenoma of the parotid gland. *Arch Pathol Lab Med* 1976;100:269–270.
266. Ellis GL, Auclair PL, Gnepp DR, et al. Other malignant epithelial neoplasms. In: Ellis GL, Auclair PL, Gnepp DR, eds. *Surgical pathology of the salivary glands.* Philadelphia: WB Saunders, 1991:455–488.
267. Takata T, Ogawa I, Nikai H. Sebaceous carcinoma of the parotid gland. An immunohistochemical and ultrastructural study. *Virchows Arch* 1989;414:459–464.

Basal Cell Adenomas and Basal Cell Adenocarcinoma

268. Batsakis JG, Luna MA, El-Naggar AK. Basaloid monomorphic adenomas. *Ann Otol Rhinol Laryngol* 1991;100:687–690.
269. Maurizi M, Salvinelli F, Capelli A, et al. Monomorphic adenomas of the major salivary glands: clinicopathological study of 44 cases. *J Laryngol Otol* 1990;104:790–796.
270. Kratochvil FJ. Canalicular adenoma and basal cell adenoma. In: Ellis GL, Auclair PL, Gnepp DR, eds. *Surgical pathology of the salivary glands.* Philadelphia: WB Saunders, 1991:202–224.
271. Seifert G. Classification and differential diagnosis of clear and basal cell tumors of the salivary glands. *Semin Diagn Pathol* 1996;13: 95–103.
272. Fantasia JE, Neville BW. Basal cell adenomas of the minor salivary glands. A clinicopathologic study of seventeen new cases and a review of the literature. *Oral Surg Oral Med Oral Pathol Oral Radiol Endod* 1980;50:433–440.
273. Luna MA, Tortoledo ME, Allen M. Salivary dermal analogue tumors arising in lymph nodes. *Cancer* 1987;59:1165–1169.
274. Batsakis JG, Brannon RB. Dermal analogue tumours of major salivary glands. *J Laryngol Otol* 1981;95:155–164.
275. Headington JT, Batsakis JG, Beals TF, et al. Membranous basal cell adenoma of parotid gland, dermal cylindromas, and trichoepitheliomas. Comparative histochemistry and ultrastructure. *Cancer* 1977;39:2460–2469.
276. Schmidt KT, Ma A, Goldberg R, et al. Multiple adnexal tumors and a parotid basal cell adenoma. *J Am Acad Dermatol* 1991;25:960–964.
277. Ogawa I, Nikai H, Takata T, et al. The cellular composition of basal cell adenoma of the parotid gland: an immunohistochemical analysis. *Oral Surg Oral Med Oral Pathol Oral Radiol Endod* 1990;70:619–626.
278. Takahashi H, Fujita S, Okabe H, et al. Immunohistochemical characterization of basal cell adenomas of the salivary gland. *Pathol Res Pract* 1991;187:145–156.
279. Gupta RK, Naran S, Dowle C, et al. Coexpression of vimentin, cytokeratin and S-100 in monomorphic adenoma of salivary gland; value of marker studies in the differential diagnosis of salivary gland tumours. *Cytopathology* 1992;3:303–309.
280. Hamano H, Abiko Y, Hashimoto S. Immunohistochemical study of basal cell adenoma in the parotid gland. *Bull Tokyo Dent Coll* 1990;31:23–31.
281. Abiko Y, Shimono M, Hashimoto S. Ultrastructure of basal cell adenoma in the parotid gland. *Bull Tokyo Dent Coll* 1989;30:145–153.
282. Jao W, Keh PC, Swerdlow MA. Ultrastructure of the basal cell adenoma of parotid gland. *Cancer* 1976;37:1322–1333.
283. Dardick I, Lytwyn A, Bourne AJ, et al. Trabecular and solid–cribriform types of basal cell adenoma. A morphologic study of two cases of

an unusual variant of monomorphic adenoma. *Oral Surg Oral Med Oral Pathol Oral Radiol Endod* 1992;73:75–83.
284. Ellis GL, Wiscovitch JG. Basal cell adenocarcinomas of the major salivary glands. *Oral Surg Oral Med Oral Pathol Oral Radiol Endod* 1990;69:461–469.
285. Luna MA, Batsakis JG, Tortoledo MF, et al. Carcinomas *ex* monomorphic adenoma of salivary glands. *J Laryngol Otol* 1989; 103:756–759.
286. Fonseca I, Soares J. Basal cell adenocarcinoma of minor salivary and seromucous glands of the head and neck. *Semin Diagn Pathol* 1996; 13:128–137.
287. Ellis GL, Auclair PL. Basal cell adenocarcinoma. In: Ellis GL, Auclair PL, Gnepp DR, eds: *Surgical pathology of the salivary glands.* Philadelphia: WB Saunders, 1991:441–454.
288. Batsakis JG, Luna MA. Basaloid salivary carcinoma. *Ann Otol Rhinol Laryngol* 1991;100:785–787.
289. Murty GE, Welch AR, Soames JV. Basal cell adenocarcinoma of the parotid gland. *J Laryngol Otol* 1990;104:150–151.
290. Chen KT. Carcinoma arising in monomorphic adenoma of the salivary gland. *Am J Otolaryngol* 1985;6:39–41.
291. Adkins GF. Low grade basaloid adenocarcinoma of salivary gland in childhood–the so-called hybrid basal cell adenoma—adenoid cystic carcinoma. *Pathology* 1990;22:187–190.
292. Atula T, Klemi PJ, Donath K, et al. Basal cell adenocarcinoma of the parotid gland: a case report and review of the literature. *J Laryngol Otol* 1993;107:862–864.
293. Williams SB, Ellis GL, Auclair PL. Immunohistochemical analysis of basal cell adenocarcinoma. *Oral Surg Oral Med Oral Pathol Oral Radiol Endod* 1993;75:64–69.
294. Gallimore A, Spraggs P, Allen J. Basaloid carcinoma of salivary glands, a clinicopathologic and immunohistochemical study. *Histopathology* 1994;24:139–144.
295. McCluggage G, Sloan J, Cameron S, et al. Basal cell adenocarcinoma of the submandibular gland. *Oral Surg Oral Med Oral Pathol Oral Radiol Endod* 1995;79:342–350.
296. Luna MA, El-Naggar A, Parichatikanond P, et al. Basaloid squamous carcinoma of the upper aerodigestive tract. Clinicopathologic and DNA flow cytometric analysis. *Cancer* 1990;66:537–542.

Canalicular Adenoma and Other Benign Epithelial Tumors

297. Daley TD, Gardner DG, Smout MS. Canalicular adenoma: not a basal cell adenoma. *Oral Surg Oral Med Oral Pathol Oral Radiol Endod* 1984;57:181–188.
298. Nelson JF, Jacoway JR. Monomorphic adenoma (canalicular type). Report of 29 cases. *Cancer* 1973;31:1511–1513.
299. Chen SY, Miller AS. Canalicular adenoma of the upper lip: an electron microscopic study. *Cancer* 1980;46:552–556.
300. Daley TD. The canalicular adenoma: considerations on differential diagnosis and treatment. *J Oral Maxillofac Surg* 1984;42: 728–730.
301. Guccion JG, Redman RS. Canalicular adenoma of the buccal mucosa. An ultrastructural and histochemical study. *Oral Surg Oral Med Oral Pathol Oral Radiol Endod* 1986;61:173–178.
302. Batsakis JG, Brannon RB, Sciubba JJ. Monomorphic adenomas of major salivary glands: a histologic study of 96 tumours. *Clin Otolaryngol* 1981;6:129–143.
303. Khullar SM, Best PV. Adenomatosis of minor salivary glands. Report of a case. *Oral Surg Oral Med Oral Pathol Oral Radiol Endod* 1992;74:783–787.
304. Zarbo RJ, Regezi JA, Batsakis JG. S-100 protein in salivary gland tumors: an immunohistochemical study of 129 cases. *Head Neck* 1986;8:268–275.
305. Ellis GL, Auclair PL. Ductal papillomas. In: Ellis GL, Auclair PL, Gnepp DR, eds. *Surgical pathology of the salivary glands.* Philadelphia: WB Saunders, 1991:238–251.
306. Ellis GL, Gnepp DR. Unusual salivary gland tumors. In: Gnepp DR, ed. *Pathology of the head and neck.* New York: Churchill Livingston, 1988:585–661.
307. Sher L. The papillary cystadenoma of salivary gland origin. *Diastema* 1982;10:37–41.

Acinic Cell Carcinoma

308. Abrams AM, Cornyn J, Scofield HH, et al. Acinic cell adenocarcinoma of the major salivary glands: a clinicopathologic study of 77 cases. *Cancer* 1965;18:1145–1162.
309. Colmenero C, Patron M, Sierra I. Acinic cell carcinoma of the salivary glands. A review of 20 new cases. *J Craniomaxillofac Surg* 1991;19: 260–266.
310. Ellis GL, Corio RL. Acinic cell adenocarcinoma. A clinicopathologic analysis of 294 cases. *Cancer* 1983;52:542–549.
311. Lewis JE, Olsen KD, Weiland LH. Acinic cell carcinoma. Clinicopathologic review. *Cancer* 1991;67:172–179.
312. Spiro RH, Huvos AG, Strong EW. Acinic cell carcinoma of salivary origin. A clinicopathologic study of 67 cases. *Cancer* 1978;41: 924–935.
313. Oliveira P, Fonseca I, Soares J. Acinic cell carcinoma of the salivary glands. A long-term follow-up study of 15 cases. *Eur J Surg Oncol* 1992;18:7–15.
314. Perzin KH, LiVolsi VA. Acinic cell carcinomas arising in salivary glands: a clinicopathologic study. *Cancer* 1979;44: 1434–1457.
315. Zbaeren P, Lehmann W, Widgren S. Acinic cell carcinoma of minor salivary gland origin. *J Laryngol Otol* 1991;105:782–785.
316. Lidang-Jensen M, Kiaer H. Acinic cell carcinoma with primary presentation in an intraparotid lymph node [Discussion]. *Pathol Res Pract* 1992;188:226–231.
317. Batsakis JG, Luna MA, El-Naggar AK. Histopathologic grading of salivary gland neoplasms: II. Acinic cell carcinomas. *Ann Otol Rhinol Laryngol* 1990;99:929–933.
318. Stanley RJ, Weiland LH, Olsen KD, et al. Dedifferentiated acinic cell (acinous) carcinoma of the parotid gland. *Otolaryngol Head Neck Surg* 1988;98:155–161.
319. Chaudhry AP, Cutler LS, Leifer C, et al. Histogenesis of acinic cell carcinoma of the major and minor salivary glands. An ultrastructural study. *J Pathol* 1986;148:307–320.
320. Dardick I, George D, Jeans MT, et al. Ultrastructural morphology and cellular differentiation in acinic cell carcinoma. *Oral Surg Oral Med Oral Pathol Oral Radiol Endod* 1987;63:325–334.
321. Caselitz J, Seifert G, Grenner G, et al. Amylase as an additional marker of salivary gland neoplasms. An immunoperoxidase study. *Pathol Res Pract* 1983;176:276–283.
322. Takahashi H, Fujita S, Okabe H, et al. Distribution of tissue markers in acinic cell carcinomas of salivary gland. *Pathol Res Pract* 1992;188:692–700.
323. Hamper K, Mausch HE, Caselitz J, et al. Acinic cell carcinoma of the salivary glands: the prognostic relevance of DNA cytophotometry in a retrospective study of long duration (1965–1987). *Oral Surg Oral Med Oral Pathol Oral Radiol Endod* 1990;69:68–75.
324. El-Naggar AK, Batsakis JG, Luna MA, et al. DNA flow cytometry of acinic cell carcinomas of major salivary glands. *J Laryngol Otol* 1990;104:410–416.
325. Chomette G, Auriol M, Wann A, et al. Acinic cell carcinomas of salivary glands histoprognosis. Value of NORs stained with AgNOR technique and examined with semi-automatic image analysis. *J Biol Bucc* 1991;19:205–210.
326. Timon CI, Dardick I, Panzarella T, et al. Acinic cell carcinoma of salivary glands: prognostic relevance of DNA flow cytometry and nucleolar organizer regions. *Arch Otolaryngol Head Neck Surg* 1994; 120:727–733.
327. Chong GC, Beahrs OH, Woolner LB. Surgical management of acinic cell carcinoma of the parotid gland. *Surg Gynecol Obstet* 1974;138: 65–68.

328. Spafford PD, Mintz DR, Hay J. Acinic cell carcinoma of the parotid gland: review and management. *J Otolaryngol* 1991;20:262–266.

Adenoid Cystic Carcinoma

329. Spiro RH, Huvos AG, Strong EW. Adenoid cystic carcinoma of salivary origin. A clinicopathologic study of 242 cases. *Am J Surg* 1974;128:512–520.
330. Conley J, Dingman DL. Adenoid cystic carcinoma in the head and neck (cylindroma). *Arch Otolaryngol Head Neck Surg* 1974;100: 81–90.
331. Chaudhry AP, Leifer C, Cutler LS, et al. Histogenesis of adenoid cystic carcinoma of the salivary glands. Light and electron microscopic study. *Cancer* 1986;58:72–82.
332. Azumi N, Battifora H. The cellular composition of adenoid cystic carcinoma. An immunohistochemical study. *Cancer* 1987;60:1589–1598.
333. Caselitz J, Schulze I, Seifert G. Adenoid cystic carcinoma of the salivary glands: an immunohistochemical study. *J Oral Pathol Med* 1986;15:308–318.
334. Chen JC, Gnepp DR, Bedrossian CW. Adenoid cystic carcinoma of the salivary glands: an immunohistochemical analysis. *Oral Surg Oral Med Oral Pathol Oral Radiol Endod* 1988;65:316–326.
335. Tomich CE. Adenoid cystic carcinoma. In: Ellis GL, Auclair PL, Gnepp DR, eds. *Surgical pathology of salivary glands.* Philadelphia: WB Saunders, 1991:333–349.
336. Perzin KH, Gullane P, Clairmont AC. Adenoid cystic carcinoma arising in salivary glands: a correlation of histologic features and clinical course. *Cancer* 1978;42:265–282.
337. Nascimento AG, Amaral AL, Prado LA, et al. Adenoid cystic carcinoma of salivary glands. A study of 61 cases with clinicopathologic correlation. *Cancer* 1986;57:312–319.
338. Matsuba HM, Spector GJ, Thawley SE, et al. Adenoid cystic salivary gland carcinoma. A histopathologic review of treatment failure patterns. *Cancer* 1986;57:519–524.
339. Koka VN, Tiwari RM, van der Waal I, et al. Adenoid cystic carcinoma of the salivary glands: clinicopathological survey of 51 patients. *J Laryngol Otol* 1989;103;675–679.
340. Cowie VJ, Pointon RC. Adenoid cystic carcinoma of the salivary glands. *Clin Radiol* 1984;35:331–333.
341. Hickman RE, Cawson RA, Duffy SW. The prognosis for specific types of salivary gland tumors. *Cancer* 1984;54:1620–1624.
342. Eneroth CM, Zajicek J. Aspiration biopsy of salivary gland tumors. IV. Morphologic studies on smears and histologic sections from 45 cases of adenoid cystic carcinoma. *Acta Cytol* 1969; 13:59–63.
343. d'Ardenne AJ, Kirkpatrick P, Wells CA, et al. Laminin and fibronectin in adenoid cystic carcinoma. *J Clin Pathol* 1986;39: 138–144.
344. Franzen G, Klausen OG, Grenko RT, et al. Adenoid cystic carcinoma: DNA as a prognostic indicator. *Laryngoscope* 1991;101:669–673.
345. Eibling DE, Johnson JT, McCoy JP Jr, et al. Flow cytometric evaluation of adenoid cystic carcinoma: correlation with histologic subtype and survival. *Am J Surg* 1991;162:367–372.
346. Tytor M, Gemryd P, Grenko R, et al. Adenoid cystic carcinoma: significance of DNA ploidy. *Head Neck* 1995;17:319–327.
347. Greiner TC, Robinson RA, Maves MD. Adenoid cystic carcinoma. A clinicopathologic study with flow cytometric analysis. *Am J Clin Pathol* 1989;92:711–720.
348. Luna MA, El-Naggar A, Batsakis JG, et al. Flow cytometric DNA content of adenoid cystic carcinoma of submandibular gland. Correlation of histologic features and prognosis. *Arch Otolaryngol Head Neck Surg* 1990;116:1291–1296.
349. Fonseca I, Soares J. Adenoid cystic carcinoma: a study of nucleolar organizer regions (AgNOR) counts and their relation to prognosis. *J Pathol* 1993;169:255–258.
350. Fujita S, Takahashi H, Okabe H. Nucleolar organizer regions in malignant salivary gland tumors. *Acta Pathol Jpn* 1992;42:727–733.
351. Higashi K, Jin Y, Johansson M, et al. Rearrangement of 9p13 as the primary chromosomal aberration in adenoid cystic carcinoma of the respiratory tract. *Genes Chromosomes Cancer* 1991;3:21–23.
352. Szanto PA, Luna MA, Tortoledo ME, et al. Histologic grading of adenoid cystic carcinoma of the salivary glands. *Cancer* 1984;54: 1062–1069.
353. Chomette AP, Auriol M, Tranbaloc P, et al. Adenoid cystic carcinoma of salivary glands. Analysis of 86 cases. Clinico-pathological, histoenzymological and ultrastructural studies. *Virchows Arch A Pathol Anat Histol* 1982;395:289–307.
354. Batsakis JG, Luna MA, El-Naggar A. Histopathologic grading of salivary gland neoplasms: III. Adenoid cystic carcinomas. *Ann Otol Rhinol Laryngol* 1990;99:1007–1009.
355. Spiro RH, Huvos AG. Stage means more than grade in adenoid cystic carcinoma. *Am J Surg* 1992;164:623–628.
356. Ampil FL, Misra RP. Factors influencing survival of patients with adenoid cystic carcinoma of the salivary glands. *J Oral Maxillofac Surg* 1987;45:1005–1010.
357. Hamper K, Lazar F, Dietel M, et al. Prognostic factors for adenoid cystic carcinoma of the head and neck: a retrospective evaluation of 96 cases. *J Oral Pathol Med* 1990;19:101–107.
358. Vrielinck LJ, Ostyn F, van Damme B, et al. The significance of perineural spread in adenoid cystic carcinoma of the major and minor salivary glands. *Int J Oral Maxillofac Surg* 1988;17:190–193.
359. van der Wal JE, Snow GB, van der Waal I. Intraoral adenoid cystic carcinoma. The presence of perineural spread in relation to site, size, local extension, and metastatic spread in 22 cases. *Cancer* 1990;66: 2031–2033.
360. Casler JD, Conley JJ. Surgical management of adenoid cystic carcinoma in the parotid gland. *Otolaryngol Head Neck Surg* 1992;106: 332–338.
361. Stell PM, Cruikshank AH, Stoney PJ, et al. Adenoid cystic carcinoma: the results of radical surgery. *Clin Otolaryngol* 1985;10:205–208.
362. van der Wal JE, Snow GB, Karim AB, et al. Intraoral adenoid cystic carcinoma: the role of postoperative radiotherapy in local control. *Head Neck* 1989;11:497–499.
363. Hosokawa Y, Ohmori K, Kaneko M, et al. Analysis of adenoid cystic carcinoma treated by radiotherapy. *Oral Surg Oral Med Oral Pathol Oral Radiol Endod* 1992;74:251–255.
364. Slichenmyer WJ, LeMaistre CF, Von Hoff DD. Response of metastatic adenoid cystic carcinoma and Merkel cell tumor to high-dose melphalan with autologous bone marrow transplantation. *Invest New Drugs* 1992;10:45–48.

Mucoepidermoid Carcinoma

365. Chen S-Y. Ultrastructure of mucoepidermoid carcinoma in minor salivary glands. *Oral Surg Oral Med Oral Pathol Oral Radiol Endod* 1979;47:247–255.
366. Stewart FW, Foote FW, Becker WF. Mucoepidermoid tumors of salivary glands. *Ann Surg* 1945;122:820–844.
367. Foote FW, Frazell EL. Tumors of major salivary glands. *Cancer* 1953;6:1065–1133.
368. Jakobsson PA, Blanck C, Eneroth CM. Mucoepidermoid carcinoma of the parotid gland. *Cancer* 1968;22:111–124.
369. Healey WV, Perzin KH, Smith L. Mucoepidermoid carcinoma of salivary gland origin. *Cancer* 1970;26:368–388.
370. Thorvaldsson SE, Beahrs OH, Woolner LB, et al. Mucoepidermoid tumors of the major salivary glands. *Am J Surg* 1970;120:432–438.
371. Spiro RH, Huvos AG, Berk R, et al. Mucoepidermoid carcinoma of salivary gland origin. A clinicopathologic study of 367 cases. *Am J Surg* 1978;136:461–468.
372. Nascimento AG, Amaral ALP, Prado LAF, et al. Mucoepidermoid carcinoma of salivary glands: a clinicopathologic study of 46 cases. *Head Neck* 1986;8:409–417.
373. Evans HL. Mucoepidermoid carcinoma of salivary glands: a study of 69 cases with special attention to histologic grading. *Am J Clin Pathol* 1984;81:696–701.

374. Jensen OJ, Poulsen T, Schiodt T. Mucoepidermoid tumors of salivary glands. A long-term follow-up study. *APMIS* 1988;96:421–427.
375. Auclair PL, Ellis GL. Mucoepidermoid carcinoma. In: Ellis GL, Auclair PL, Gnepp DR, eds. *Surgical pathology of the salivary glands.* Philadelphia: WB Saunders, 1991:269–298.
376. Auclair PL, Goode RK, Ellis GL. Mucoepidermoid carcinoma of intraoral salivary glands. Evaluation and application of grading criteria in 143 cases. *Cancer* 1992;69:2021–2030.
377. Brookstone MS, Huvos AG. Central salivary gland tumors of the maxilla and mandible: a clinicopathologic study of 11 cases with an analysis of the literature. *J Oral Maxillofac Surg* 1992;50:229–236.
378. Adkins GF, Hinckley DM. Primary muco-epidermoid carcinoma arising in a parotid lymph node. *Aust NZ J Surg* 1989;59:433–435.
379. Hamed G, Shmookler BM, Ellis GL, et al. Oncocytic mucoepidermoid carcinoma of the parotid. *Arch Pathol Lab Med* 1994;118: 313–314.
380. Laudadio P, Caliceti U, Cerasoli PT, et al. Mucoepidermoid tumour of the parotid gland: a very difficult prognostic evaluation. *Clin Otolaryngol* 1987;12:177–182.
381. Batsakis JG, Luna MA. Histopathologic grading of salivary gland neoplasms: I. Mucoepidermoid carcinoma. *Ann Otol Rhinol Laryngol* 1990;99:835–838.
382. Hicks MJ, El-Naggar AE, Byers R, et al. Prognostic factors in mucoepidermoid carcinoma of major salivary glands: a clinicopathologic and flow cytometric study. *Eur J Cancer B Oral Oncol* 1994;30: 329–334.
383. Frankenthaler RA, El-Naggar AE, Ordóñez NG, et al. High correlation with survival of proliferating cell nuclear antigen expression in mucoepidermoid carcinoma of the parotid gland. *Otolaryngol Head Neck Surg* 1994;111:460–466.
384. Dardick I, Gliniecki MR, Heathcote JG, et al. Comparative histogenesis and morphogenesis of mucoepidermoid carcinoma and pleomorphic adenoma. An ultrastructural study. *Virchows Arch* 1990;417: 405–417.
385. Kumasa S, Yuba R, Sagara S, et al. Mucoepidermoid carcinomas: immunohistochemical studies on keratin, S-100 protein, lactoferrin, lysozyme and amylase. *Basic Appl Histochem* 1988;32:429–441.
386. Huang JW, Mori M, Yamada K, et al. Mucoepidermoid carcinoma of the salivary glands: immunohistochemical distribution of intermediate filament proteins, involucrin and secretory proteins. *Anticancer Res* 1992;12:811–820.
387. Regezi JA, Zarbo RJ, Batsakis JG. Immunoprofile of mucoepidermoid carcinomas of minor salivary glands. *Oral Surg Oral Med Oral Pathol Oral Radiol Endod* 1991;71:189–192.
388. Schimmelpenning H, Hamper K, Flakmer UG, et al. Methodologic aspects of DNA assessment by means of image cytometry in tumors of the salivary glands. *Acta Cytol* 1989;11:379–383.
389. Hamper K, Schimmelpenning, Caselitz J, et al. Mucoepidermoid tumors of the salivary glands. Correlation of cytophotometrical data and prognosis. *Cancer* 1989;63:708–717.
390. Fonseca I, Clode AL, Soares J. Mucoepidermoid carcinoma of the major and minor salivary glands. A survey of 43 cases with study of prognostic indicators. *Int J Surg Pathol* 1993;1:3–12.
391. Fujita S, Takahashi H, Okabe H. Nucleolar organizer regions in malignant salivary gland tumors. *Acta Pathol Jpn* 1992;42:727–733.
392. McNaney D, McNeese MD, Guillamondegui OM, et al. Postoperative irradiation in malignant epithelial tumors of the parotid. *Int J Radiat Oncol Biol Phys* 1983;9:1289–1295.
393. Armstrong JG, Harrison LB, Spiro RH, et al. Malignant tumors of major salivary gland origin. A matched-pair analysis of the role of combined surgery and postoperative radiotherapy. *Arch Otolaryngol Head Neck Surg* 1990;116:290–293.
394. Kaplan MJ, Johns ME, Cantrell RW. Chemotherapy for salivary gland cancer. *Otolaryngol Head Neck Surg* 1986;95:165–170.

Salivary Duct Carcinoma

395. Brandwein MS, Jagirdar J, Patil J, et al. Salivary duct carcinoma (cribriform salivary carcinoma of excretory ducts). A clinicopathologic and immunohistochemical study of 12 cases. *Cancer* 1990; 65:2307–2314.
396. Chen KT, Hafez GR. Infiltrating salivary duct carcinoma. A clinicopathologic study of five cases. *Arch Otolaryngol* 1981;107:37–39.
397. Anderson C, Muller R, Piorkowski R, et al. Intraductal carcinoma of major salivary gland. *Cancer* 1992;69:609–614.
398. Butterworth DM, Jones AW, Kotecha B. Salivary duct carcinoma: report of a case and review of the literature. *Virchows Arch* 1992;420: 371–374.
399. Colmenero Ruiz C, Patrön Romero M, Martin P. Salivary duct carcinoma: a report of nine cases. *J Oral Maxillofac Surg* 1993; 51:641–646.
400. de Araújo VC, de Souza SO, Sesso A, et al. Salivary duct carcinoma: ultrastructural and histogenetic considerations. *Oral Surg Oral Med Oral Pathol Oral Radiol Endod* 1987;63:592–596.
401. Dee S, Masood S, Issacs JH Jr, et al. Cytomorphologic features of salivary duct carcinoma on fine needle aspiration biopsy. A case report. *Acta Cytol* 1993;37:539–542.
402. Delgado R, Vuitch F, Albores-Saavedra J. Salivary duct carcinoma. *Cancer* 1993;72:1503–1512.
403. Garland TA, Innes DJ Jr, Fechner RE. Salivary duct carcinoma: an analysis of four cases with review of literature. *Am J Clin Pathol* 1984;81:436–441.
404. Hui KK, Batsakis JG, Luna MA, et al. Salivary duct adenocarcinoma: a high grade malignancy. *J Laryngol Otol* 1986;100:105–114.
405. Simpson RH, Clarke TJ, Sarsfield PT, et al. Salivary duct adenocarcinoma. *Histopathology* 1991;18:229–235.
406. Barnes L, Rao U, Contis L, et al. Salivary duct carcinoma. Part II. Immunohistochemical evaluation of 13 cases for estrogen and progesterone receptors, cathepsin D, and c-erbB-2 protein. *Oral Surg Oral Med Oral Pathol Oral Radiol Endod* 1994;78:74–80.
407. Hellquist HB, Karlsson MG, Nilsson C. Salivary duct carcinoma—a highly aggressive salivary gland tumour with over-expression of c-erbB-2. *J Pathol* 1994;172:35–44.
408. Barnes L, Rao U, Krause J, et al. Salivary duct carcinoma. Part I. A clinicopathologic evaluation and DNA image analysis of 13 cases with review of the literature. *Oral Surg Oral Med Oral Pathol Oral Radiol Endod* 1994;78:64–73.
409. Seifert G, Caselitz J. Epithelial salivary gland tumors: tumor markers. *Prog Surg Pathol* 1989;9:157–187.
410. Kane WJ, McCaffrey TV, Olsen KD, et al. Primary parotid malignancies. A clinical and pathologic review. *Arch Otolaryngol Head Neck Surg* 1991;117:307–315.
411. Lewis JE, McKinney BC, Weiland LH, et al. Salivary duct carcinoma. Clinicopathologic and immunohistochemical review of 26 cases. *Cancer* 1996;77:223–230.
412. Felix A, El-Naggar AK, Press MF, et al. Prognostic significance of biomarkers (c-erbB-2, p53, proliferating cell nuclear antigen, and DNA content) in salivary duct carcinoma. *Hum Pathol* 1996;27: 561–566.
413. Delgado R, Klimstra D, Albores-Saavedra J. Low grade salivary duct carcinoma. *Cancer* 1996;78:958–967.

Epithelial–Myoepithelial Carcinoma

414. Corio RL, Sciubba JJ, Brannon RB, et al. Epithelial–myoepithelial carcinoma of intercalated duct origin. A clinicopathologic and ultrastructural assessment of sixteen cases. *Oral Surg Oral Med Oral Pathol Oral Radiol Endod* 1982;53:280–287.
415. Luna MA, Ordóñez NG, Mackay B, et al. Salivary epithelial–myoepithelial carcinomas of intercalated ducts: a clinical, electron microscopic, and immunocytochemical study. *Oral Surg Oral Med Oral Pathol Oral Radiol Endod* 1985;59:482–490.
416. Collina G, Gale N, Visona A, et al. Epithelial–myoepithelial carcinoma of the parotid gland: a clinico-pathologic and immunohistochemical study of seven cases. *Tumori* 1991;77:257–263.
417. Batsakis JG, El-Naggar AK, Luna MA. Epithelial–myoepithelial carcinoma of salivary glands. *Ann Otol Rhinol Laryngol* 1992;101: 540–542.

418. Morinaga S, Hashimoto S, Tezuka F. Epithelial–myoepithelial carcinoma of the parotid gland in a child. *Acta Pathol Jpn* 1992;42: 358–363.
419. Simpson RH, Clarke TJ, Sarsfield PT, et al. Epithelial–myoepithelial carcinoma of salivary glands. *J Clin Pathol* 1991;44:419–423.
420. Simpson RH, Sarsfield PT, Clarke T, et al. Clear cell carcinoma of minor salivary glands. *Histopathology* 1990;17:433–438.
421. Fonseca I, Soares J. Epithelial–myoepithelial carcinoma of the salivary glands. A study of 22 cases. *Virchows Arch* 1993;422:389–396.
422. Noel S, Brozna JP. Epithelial–myoepithelial carcinoma of salivary gland with metastasis to lung: report of a case and review of the literature. *Head Neck* 1992;14:401–406.
423. Palmer RM. Epithelial–myoepithelial carcinoma: an immunocytochemical study. *Oral Surg Oral Med Oral Pathol Oral Radiol Endod* 1985;59:511–515.
424. Hamper K, Brugmann M, Koppermann R, et al. Epithelial–myoepithelial duct carcinoma of salivary glands: a follow-up and cytophotometric study of 21 cases. *J Oral Pathol Med* 1989;18:299–304.
425. Cho KJ, El-Naggar AK, Ordóñez NG, et al. Epithelial myoepithelial carcinoma of salivary glands. A clinicopathologic, DNA flow cytometric, and immunohistochemical study of Ki-67 and HER-2/neu oncogen. *Am J Clin Pathol* 1995;103:432–437.

Terminal Duct Adenocarcinoma

426. Batsakis JG, Pinkston GR, Luna MA, et al. Adenocarcinomas of the oral cavity: a clinicopathologic study of terminal duct carcinomas. *J Laryngol Otol* 1983;97:825–835.
427. Freedman PD, Lumerman H. Lobular carcinoma of intraoral minor salivary gland origin. Report of twelve cases. *Oral Surg Oral Med Oral Pathol Oral Radiol Endod* 1983;56:157–165.
428. Evans HL, Batsakis JG. Polymorphous low-grade adenocarcinoma of minor salivary glands. A study of 14 cases of a distinctive neoplasm. *Cancer* 1984;53:935–942.
429. Wenig BM, Gnepp DR. Polymorphous low-grade adenocarcinoma of minor salivary glands. In: Ellis GL, Auclair PL, Gnepp DR, eds. *Surgical pathology of the salivary glands.* Philadelphia: WB Saunders, 1991:390–411.
430. Anderson C, Krutchkoff D, Pedersen C, et al. Polymorphous low-grade adenocarcinoma of minor salivary gland: a clinicopathologic and comparative immunohistochemical study. *Mod Pathol* 1990;3:76–82.
431. Vincent SD, Hammond HL, Finkelstein MW. Clinical and therapeutic features of polymorphous low-grade adenocarcinoma. *Oral Surg Oral Med Oral Pathol Oral Radiol Endod* 1994;77:41–47.
432. Slootweg PJ, Muller H. Low-grade adenocarcinoma of the oral cavity. A comparison between the terminal duct and the papillary type. *J Craniomaxillofac Surg* 1987;15:359–364.
433. Haba R, Kobayashi S, Miki H, et al. Polymorphous low-grade adenocarcinoma of submandibular gland origin. *Acta Pathol Jpn* 1993;43: 774–778.
434. Wenig BM, Harpaz N, DelBridge C. Polymorphous low-grade adenocarcinoma of seromucous glands of the nasopharynx. A report of a case and a discussion of the morphologic and immunohistochemical features. *Am J Clin Pathol* 1989;92:104–109.
435. Kemp BL, Batsakis JG, El-Naggar AK, et al. Terminal duct adenocarcinoma of the parotid gland. *J Laryngol Otol* 1995;109:466–468.
436. Ritland F, Lubensky I, LiVolsi VA. Polymorphous low grade adenocarcinoma of the parotid gland. *Arch Pathol Lab Med* 1993;117: 1261–1263.
437. Nicolatou O, Kakarantza-Angelopoulou E, Angelopoulos AP, et al. Polymorphous low-grade adenocarcinoma of the palate: report of a case with electron microscopy. *J Oral Maxillofac Surg* 1988;46: 1008–1013.
438. Dardick I, van Nostrand AW. Polymorphous low-grade adenocarcinoma: a case report with ultrastructural findings. *Oral Surg Oral Med Oral Pathol Oral Radiol Endod* 1988;66:459–465.
439. Gnepp DR, Chen JC, Warren C. Polymorphous low-grade adenocarcinoma of minor salivary gland. An immunohistochemical and clinicopathologic study. *Am J Surg Pathol* 1988;12:461–468.
440. Regezi JA, Zarbo RJ, Stewart JE, et al. Polymorphous low-grade adenocarcinoma of minor salivary gland. A comparative histologic and immunohistochemical study. *Oral Surg Oral Med Oral Pathol Oral Radiol Endod* 1991;71:469–475.
441. Luna MA, Batsakis JG, Ordóñez NG, et al. Salivary gland adenocarcinomas: a clinicopathologic analysis of three distinctive types. *Semin Diagn Pathol* 1987;4:117–135.
442. Blanck C, Eneroth CM, Jakobsson PA. Mucus-producing adenopapillary (non-epidermoid) carcinoma of the parotid gland. *Cancer* 1971;28:676–685.
443. de Araujo VC, de Souza SO, Lopes EA, et al. Mucus-producing adenopapillary carcinoma of the minor salivary gland origin with signet ring cells and intracytoplasmic lumina. A light and electron microscopic study. *Arch Oto-Rhino-Laryngol* 1988;245:145–150.
444. Foss RD, Ellis GL, Auclair PL. Salivary gland cystadenocarcinoma: a clinicopathologic analysis of 57 cases. *Am J Surg Pathol* 1996;20; 1440–1447.
445. Mostofi R, Wood RS, Christison W, et al. Low grade papillary adenocarcinoma of minor salivary glands. Case report and literature review. *Oral Surg Oral Med Oral Pathol Oral Radiol Endod* 1992;73: 591–595.
446. Milchgrub S, Gnepp DR, Vuitch F, et al. Hyalinizing clear cell carcinoma of salivary gland. *Am J Surg Pathol* 1994;18:74–82.
447. Martinez Madrigal F, Baden E, Casiraghi O, et al. Oral and pharyngeal adenosquamous carcinoma. A report of four cases with immunohistochemical studies. *Eur Arch Otorhinolaryngol* 1991;248:255–258.
448. Batsakis JG, El-Naggar AK, Luna MA. "Adenocarcinoma not otherwise specified": a diminished group of salivary carcinomas. *Ann Otol Rhinol Laryngol* 1992;101:102–104.
449. Spiro RH, Huvos AG, Strong EW. Adenocarcinoma of salivary origin. Clinicopathologic study of 204 patients. *Am J Surg* 1982;144: 423–431.

Primary Squamous Cell Carcinoma

450. Batsakis JG, McClathey KD, Johns ME, et al. Primary squamous cell carcinoma of the parotid gland. *Arch Otolaryngol Head Neck Surg* 1976;102:355–357.
451. Eneroth CM. Salivary gland tumors in the parotid gland, submandibular gland, and the palate region. *Cancer* 1971;27:1415–1418.
452. Woods JE, Chong GC, Beahrs OH. Experience with 1,360 primary parotid tumors. *Am J Surg* 1975;130:460–462.
453. Spiro RH, Huvos AG, Strong EW. Cancer of the parotid gland: a clinicopathologic study of 288 primary cases. *Am J Surg* 1975;130: 452–459.
454. Sterman BM, Kraus DH, Sebek BA, et al. Primary squamous cell carcinoma of the parotid gland. *Laryngoscope* 1990;100:146–148.
455. Gaughan RK, Olsen KD, Lewis JE. Primary squamous cell carcinoma of the parotid gland. *Arch Otolaryngol Head Neck Surg* 1992;118: 798–801.
456. Spiro RH, Hajdu SI, Strong EW. Tumors of the submaxillary gland. *Am J Surg* 1976;132:463–468.
457. Eneroth CM, Hjertman L, Moberger G. Malignant tumors of the submandibular gland. *Acta Otolaryngol (Stockh)* 1967;64:514–536.
458. Simons JN, Beahrs OH, Woolner LB. Tumors of the submaxillary gland. *Am J Surg* 1964;108:485–494.
459. Conley J, Meyers E, Cole R. Analysis of 115 patients with tumors of the submandibular gland. *Ann Otol Rhinol Laryngol* 1972;81: 323–330.
460. Trail ML, Lubritz J. Tumors of the submandibular gland. *Laryngoscope* 1974;84:1225–1232.
461. Rafla S. Submaxillary gland tumors. *Cancer* 1970;26:821–826.

Small- and Large-Cell Undifferentiated Carcinoma

462. Patey DH, Sobin LH. *Histological typing of salivary gland tumors. International histological classification of tumors, no. 7.* Geneva: World Health Organization, 1972.

463. Hui KK, Luna MA, Batsakis JG, et al. Undifferentiated carcinomas of the major salivary glands. *Oral Surg Oral Med Oral Pathol Oral Radiol Endod* 1990;69:76–83.
464. Gnepp DR, Corio RL, Brannon RB. Small cell carcinoma of the major salivary glands. *Cancer* 1986;58:705–714.
465. Hayashi Y, Nagamine S, Yanagawa T, et al. Small cell undifferentiated carcinoma of the minor salivary gland containing exocrine, neuroendocrine, and squamous cells. *Cancer* 1987;60:1583–1588.
466. Nagao K, Matsuzaki O, Saiga H, et al. Histopathologic studies of undifferentiated carcinoma of the parotid gland. *Cancer* 1982;50: 1572–1579.
467. Kraemer BB, Mackay B, Batsakis JG. Small cell carcinoma of the parotid gland. A clinicopathologic study of three cases. *Cancer* 1983;52:2115–2121.
468. Rollins CE, Yost BA, Costa MJ, et al. Squamous differentiation in small cell carcinoma of the parotid gland. *Arch Pathol Lab Med* 1995;119:183–185.
469. Koss LG, Spiro RH, Hajdu S. Small cell (oat cell) carcinoma of minor salivary gland origin. *Cancer* 1972;30:737–741.
470. Yaku Y, Kanda T, Yoshihara T, et al. Undifferentiated carcinoma of the parotid gland. Case report with electron microscopic findings. *Virchows Arch* 1983;401:89–97.
471. Hayashi Y, Aoki N. Undifferentiated carcinoma of the parotid gland with bizarre giant cells. Clinicopathologic report with ultrastructural study. *Acta Pathol Jpn* 1983;33:169–176.
472. North CA, Lee DJ, Piantadosi S, et al. Carcinoma of the major salivary glands treated by surgery or surgery plus postoperative radiotherapy. *Int J Radiat Oncol Biol Phys* 1990;18:1319–1326.
473. Takata T, Caselitz J, Seifert G. Undifferentiated tumours of salivary glands. Immunocytochemical investigations and differential diagnosis of 22 cases. *Pathol Res Pract* 1987;182:161–168.

Lymphoepithelial Carcinoma

474. Batsakis JG. Pathology consultation. Carcinoma *ex* lymphoepithelial lesion. *Ann Otol Rhinol Laryngol* 1983;92:657–658.
475. Cleary KR, Batsakis JG. Undifferentiated carcinoma with lymphoid stroma of the major salivary glands. *Ann Otol Rhinol Laryngol* 1990; 99:236–238.
476. Kott ET, Goepfert H, Ayala AG, et al. Lymphoepithelial carcinoma (malignant lymphoepithelial lesion) of the salivary glands. *Arch Otolaryngol* 1984;110:50–53.
477. Nielsen NH, Mikkelsen F, Hansen JPH. Incidence of salivary gland neoplasms in Greenland with special reference to an anaplastic carcinoma. *Acta Pathol Microbiol Scand* 1978;86:185–193.
478. Imperato PJ. Health and disease in Greenland (Kalaallit Nunaat). *NY State J Med* 1988;88:300–317.
479. Saw D, Lau WH, Ho JHC, et al. Malignant lymphoepithelial lesion of the salivary gland. *Hum Pathol* 1986;17:914–923.
480. Povah WB, Beecroft W, Hodson I, et al. Malignant lymphoepithelial lesion—the Manitoba experience. *J Otolaryngol* 1984;13:153–158.
481. Wallace AG, McDougall JT, Hildes JA, et al. Salivary gland tumors in Canadian Eskimos. *Cancer* 1963;16:1338–1353.
482. Merrick Y, Albeck H, Nielsen NH, et al. Familial clustering of salivary gland carcinoma in Greenland. *Cancer* 1986;57:2097–2102.
483. Saemundsen AK, Albeck H, Hansen JPH, et al. Epstein-Barr virus in nasopharyngeal and salivary gland carcinomas of Greenland Eskimos. *Br J Cancer* 1982;46:721–728.
484. Sehested M, Hainau B, Albeck H, et al. Ultrastructural investigation of anaplastic salivary gland carcinomas in Eskimos. *Cancer* 1985;55: 2732–2736.
485. Saw D, Ho JHC, Lau WH, et al. Parotid swelling as the first manifestation of nasopharyngeal carcinoma: a report of two cases. *Eur J Surg Oncol* 1986;12:71–75.

Mesenchymal Tumors

486. McDaniel RK. Benign mesenchymal neoplasms. In: Ellis GL, Auclair PL, Gnepp DR, eds. *Surgical pathology of the salivary glands.* Philadelphia: WB Saunders, 1991:489–513.
487. Seifert G, Oehne H. Die mesenchymalen (nichtepithelialen) speicheldrusentumorens. Analyse von 167 tumorfallen des speicheldrusenregisters. *Laryngorhinootologie* 1986;65:485–491.
488. Baker SE, Jensen JL, Correll RW. Lipomas of the parotid gland. *Oral Surg Oral Med Oral Pathol Oral Radiol Endod* 1981;52: 167–171.
489. Layfield LJ, Glasgow BJ, Goldstein N, et al. Lipomatous lesions of the parotid gland. Potential pitfalls in fine needle aspiration biopsy diagnosis. *Acta Cytol* 1991;35:553–556.
490. Wiley EL, Stewart D, Brown M, et al. Fibrous histiocytoma of the parotid gland. *Am J Clin Pathol* 1992;97:512–516.
491. Sullivan MJ, Babyak JW, Kartush JM. Intraparotid facial nerve neurofibroma. *Laryngoscope* 1987;97:219–223.
492. Auclair PL, Langloss JM, Weiss SW, et al. Sarcomas and sarcomatoid neoplasms of the major salivary gland regions. A clinicopathologic and immunohistochemical study of 67 cases and review of the literature. *Cancer* 1986;58:1305–1315.
493. Luna MA, Tortoledo ME, Ordóñez NG, et al. Primary sarcomas of the major salivary glands. *Arch Otolaryngol Head Neck Surg* 1991; 117:302–306.
494. Stimson PG, Valenzuela-Espinoza A, Tortoledo ME, et al. Primary osteosarcoma of the parotid gland. *Oral Surg Oral Med Oral Pathol Oral Radiol Endod* 1989;68:80–86.
495. Bonzanini M, Togni R, Barabareschi M, et al. Primary Kaposi's sarcoma of intraparotid lymph node. *Histopathology* 1992;21: 489–491.
496. Whittam DE, Hellier W. Haemangiopericytoma of the parotid salivary gland: report of a case with literature review. *J Laryngol Otol* 1993;107:1159–1162.

Malignant Lymphoma

497. Batsakis JG, Regezi JA. Selected controversial lesions of salivary tissue. *Otolaryngol Clin North Am* 1977;10:309–328.
498. Freeman C, Berg JW, Culter SJ. Occurrence and prognosis of extranodal lymphomas. *Cancer* 1972;29:252–257.
499. Colby TV, Dorfman RF. Malignant lymphomas involving the salivary gland. *Pathol Annu* 1979;14:307–324.
500. Gleeson MJ, Bennett MH, Cawson RA. Lymphomas of salivary glands. *Cancer* 1986;58:699–704.
501. Hyman GA, Wolff M. Malignant lymphomas of the salivary glands. Review of the literature and report of 33 new cases, including four cases associated with the lymphoepithelial lesion. *Am J Clin Pathol* 1976;65:421–438.
502. Mehle ME, Kraus DH, Wood BG, et al. Lymphoma of the parotid gland. *Laryngoscope* 1993;103:17–21.
503. Nime FA, Cooper HS, Eggleston JC. Primary malignant lymphomas of the salivary glands. *Cancer* 1976;37:906–912.
504. Schmid U, Helbron D, Lennert K. Primary malignant lymphomas localized in salivary glands. *Histopathology* 1982;6:673–687.
505. James M, Norton AJ, Akosa AB. Primary T-cell lymphoma of submandibular salivary gland. *Histopathology* 1993;22:83–85.
506. Takahashi H, Cheng J, Fujita S, et al. Primary malignant lymphoma of the salivary gland. A tumor of mucosa-associated lymphoid tissue. *J Oral Pathol Med* 1992;21:318–325.
507. Kerr PD, Dort JC. Primary extramedullary plasmacytoma of the salivary glands. *J Laryngol Otol* 1991;105:687–692.
508. Banik S, Howell JS, Wright DH. Non-Hodgkin's lymphoma arising in adenolymphoma. A report of two cases. *J Pathol* 1985;146: 167–177.

Metastatic Tumors to Salivary Glands

509. Batsakis JG. Pathology consultation. Parotid gland and its lymph nodes as metastatic sites. *Ann Otol Rhinol Laryngol* 1983;92:209–210.
510. Seifert G, Hennings K, Caselitz J. Metastatic tumors to the parotid and submandibular glands—analysis and differential diagnosis of 108 cases. *Pathol Res Pract* 1986;181:684–692.

511. Batsakis JG, Bautina E. Metastases to major salivary glands. *Ann Otol Rhinol Laryngol* 1990;99:501–503.
512. Bissett D, Bossell EM, Bradley PJ, et al. Parotid metastases from carcinoma of the breast. *Clin Radiol* 1989;40:309–310.
513. Bedrosian SA, Goldman RL, Dekelboum AM. Renal carcinoma presenting as a primary submandibular gland tumor. *Oral Surg Oral Med Oral Pathol Oral Radiol Endod* 1984;58:699–701.
514. Brodsky G, Rabson AB. Metastasis to the submandibular gland as the initial presentation of small cell (oat cell) lung carcinoma. *Oral Surg Oral Med Oral Pathol Oral Radiol Endod* 1984;58:76–80.
515. Yarington CT. Metastatic malignant disease to the parotid gland. *Laryngoscope* 1981;91:517–519.
516. Gnepp DR. Metastatic disease to the major salivary glands. In: Ellis GL, Auclair PL, Gnepp DR, eds. *Surgical pathology of the salivary glands.* Philadelphia: WB Saunders, 1991:560–569.
517. Nichols RD, Pinnock LA, Szymanowski RI. Metastasis to parotid nodes. *Laryngoscope* 1980;90:1324–1328.
518. Conley J, Arena S. Parotid gland as a focus of metastasis. *Arch Surg* 1963;87:757–764.
519. McKean ME, Lee K, McGregor IA. The distribution of lymph nodes in and around the parotid gland: an anatomical study. *Br J Plast Surg* 1985;38:1–5.
520. Shah JP, Kraus DH, Dubner S, et al. Patterns of regional lymph node metastases from cutaneous melanomas of the head and neck. *Am J Surg* 1991;162:320–323.
521. Ord RA, Ward-Booth RP, Avery BS. Parotid lymph node metastases from primary intra-oral squamous carcinomas. *Int J Oral Maxillofac Surg* 1989;18:104–106.
522. Ravi R, Tongaonkar HB, Kulkarni JN, et al. Synchronous bilateral parotid metastases from renal cell carcinoma. A case report. *Indian J Cancer* 1992;29:40–42.
523. Jackson GL, Ballantyne AJ. Role of parotidectomy for skin cancer of the head and neck. *Am J Surg* 1981;142:464–469.
524. Rees R, Maples M, Lynch JB, et al. Malignant secondary parotid tumors. *South Med J* 1981;74:1050–1052.

Salivary Gland Tumors in Children

525. Castro EB, Huvos AG, Strong EW, et al. Tumors of the major salivary glands in children. *Cancer* 1972;29:312–317.
526. Catania VC, Bozzetti F, Santangelo A, et al. Parotid gland tumors in infants and children. *Tumori* 1977;63:195–198.
527. Chong GC, Beahrs OH, Chen MLC, et al. Management of parotid gland tumors in infants and children. *Mayo Clin Proc* 1975;50: 279–283.
528. Krolls SG, Trodahl NJ, Boyers RC. Salivary gland lesions in children: a survey of 430 cases. *Cancer* 1972;30:459–469.
529. Schuller DE, McCabe BF. Salivary gland neoplasms in children. *Otolaryngol Clin North Am* 1977;10:399–412.
530. Seifert G, Okabe H, Caselitz J. Epithelial salivary gland tumors in children and adolescents: analysis of 80 cases. *J Otorhinolaryngol Rel Spec* 1986;48:137–149.
531. Callender DL, Frankenthaler RA, Luna MA, et al. Salivary gland neoplasms in children. *Arch Otolaryngol Head Neck Surg* 1992;118: 472–476.
532. Lack EE, Upton MP. Histopathologic review of salivary gland tumors in childhood. *Arch Otolaryngol Head Neck Surg* 1988;113:898–906.
533. Kauffman SL, Stout AP. Tumors of the major salivary glands in children. *Cancer* 1963;16:1317–1331.
534. Batsakis JG. Vascular tumors of the salivary glands. *Ann Otol Rhinol Laryngol* 1986;95:649–650.
535. Batsakis JG, Frankenthaler R. Embryomas (sialoblastoma) of salivary glands. *Ann Otol Rhinol Laryngol* 1992;101:958–960.
536. Batsakis JG, Mackay B, Ryka AF, et al. Perinatal salivary gland tumours (embryomas). *J Laryngol Otol* 1988;102:1007–1011.
537. Harris MD, McKeever P, Robertson JM. Congenital tumours of the salivary gland: a case report and review. *Histopathology* 1990;17: 155–157.
538. Hsueh C, Gonzalez-Crussi F. Sialoblastoma: a case report and review of the literature on congenital epithelial tumors of salivary gland origin. *Pediatr Pathol Lab Med* 1992;12:205–214.
539. Taylor GP. Congenital epithelial tumor of the parotid—sialoblastoma. *Pediatr Pathol Lab Med* 1988;8:447–452.
540. Roth A, Micheau C. Embryoma (or embryonal tumour) of the parotid gland: report of two cases. *Pediatr Pathol Lab Med* 1986;5:9–10.
541. Dehner L, Valbuena L, Perez-Atayde A, et al. Salivary gland anlage tumor (congenital pleomorphic adenoma). A clinicopathologic, immunohistochemical and ultrastructural study of nine cases. *Am J Surg Pathol* 1994;18:25–36.
542. Gustafsson H, Dahlqvist A, Anniko M, et al. Mucoepidermoid carcinoma in minor salivary glands in childhood. *J Laryngol Otol* 1987;101:1320–1323.
543. Jones DC, Bainton R. Adenoid cystic carcinoma of the palate in a 9-year-old boy. *Oral Surg Oral Med Oral Pathol Oral Radiol Endod* 1990;69:483–486.

9A

PATHOLOGY OF THE THYROID

MARIA J. MERINO
LAVINIA P. MIDDLETON

ANATOMIC CONSIDERATIONS

The thyroid gland is one of the largest organs in the endocrine system. It ranges in weight from 1.5 to 3 g in the newborn, and 25 to 40 g in the adult. The gland, located on the anterior, upper portion of the trachea, is composed of two lateral lobes joined by a medial isthmus. Occasionally an extra lobe, the pyramidal lobe, can be found, extending superiorly from the isthmus or from either of the lateral lobes.

Embryologically, the thyroid gland forms during the first few weeks of fetal life and is recognized as early as 24 days. It forms from a diverticulum at the floor of the tongue, the foramen caecum, and remains connected to the base of the tongue through the thyroglossal duct. Normally, during the 7th week of life the duct becomes obliterated. Aberrant thyroid tissue can sometimes be found along the duct's tract from the base of the tongue to the trachea, producing a lingual or aberrant subhyoid thyroid.

In its early stages of development, the gland is composed of cords of cells that eventually give origin to the follicles or acini that constitute the functional unit of the thyroid gland. These follicles are lined by a single row of cuboidal cells surrounded by a delicate basement membrane. The follicles eventually become filled with an eosinophilic colloid material (1). Approximately 20 to 40 follicles, supplied by a lobular artery and sustained by a diffuse meshwork of fibrous stroma, lymphatics, and connective tissue, comprise a thyroid lobule.

In the upper, lateral aspects of both thyroid lobes, intimately associated with the follicles, the C cells can be found. These calcitonin-secreting cells are derived from the ultimobranchial bodies and have features of neuroendocrine cells by ultrastructural and immunohistochemical studies (1). They are associated with other cells of ultimobranchial derivation (with which they migrate) that form solid cell nests, found in many thyroid glands (1) (Fig. 1).

The main function of the thyroid gland is the production of thyroid hormone (thyroxine), essential in controlling metabolic rate, growth, and development.

CONGENITAL ABNORMALITIES

Athyrosis

Complete absence of thyroid tissue or athyrosis is a rare congenital abnormality, usually not discovered until several weeks after birth due to the passage of maternal thyroid hormone through the placenta (1).

Ectopic Thyroid

As a result of congenital abnormalities or abnormal migration, thyroid tissue can be found outside the thyroid gland in a variety of places. Studies with radioactive iodine can confirm the presence of thyroid tissue in ectopic locations (2–5).

Lingual Thyroid

The term *lingual thyroid* refers to the presence of thyroid tissue at the base of or beneath the tongue. The amount of thyroid tissue present is variable; in some cases the total thyroid gland persists in this location. It occurs more frequently in females and usually is discovered secondary to difficulties in swallowing, phonation, or breathing. Enlargement of the ectopic thyroid can occur under certain physiologic conditions such as puberty or pregnancy (1,6–9).

Grossly, the ectopic tissues have a polypoid or pedunculated appearance and are red—brown, similar to the normal thyroid. Histologically, the tissues also resemble normal thyroid, but extension of thyroid tissue into adjacent muscle can mimic carcinoma. Primary malignant tumors, albeit rare, have occasionally been reported to arise from ectopic thyroidal tissue.

Treatment is directed toward removal of the tissues. However, proper radioactive scanning should be done prior to surgical therapy to search for the presence of additional thyroid tissue, as complete removal of a lingual thyroid that represents the patient's only thyroid tissue results in hypothyroidism and myxedema.

Substernal or Intrathoracic Thyroid

The thyroid is located close to the heart during early fetal life. As the heart relocates, fragments of thyroid tissue can be carried down with it into the thoracic cavity and even into the myocardium. These portions of thyroid can not only be functionally active, but also can give rise to disease (1,5–9).

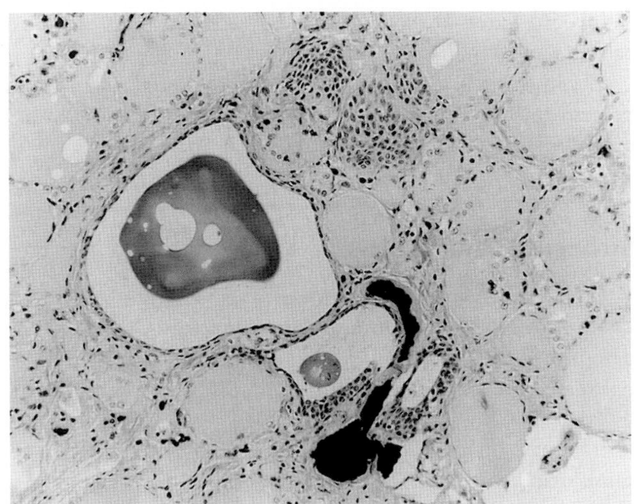

FIGURE 1. Normal histology of the thyroid. The follicles are lined by cuboidal cells and are distended by eosinophilic material. These are located at the periphery of the photomicrograph. Several solid cell nests, derived from the ultimobranchial body, with which C cells migrate to the thyroid, are present in the upper central portion of the figure. In addition, three central follicular structures, two with dense luminal secretion, are likely at least partially composed of these ultimobranchial-derived cells (hematoxylin and eosin stain, original magnification ×150).

Thyroglossal Duct Cysts

Persistence of the thyroglossal duct is frequently linked with cysts, sinuses, and fistulas, usually found near the mid-anterior portion of the neck, passing behind or through the hyoid bone (see also Chapter 1).

The clinical presentation is that of cystic masses of variable sizes (1–4 cm) often in the mid-portion of the neck and attached to the hyoid bone or soft tissues, although the overlying skin is easily movable. These cysts can present at any age and affect both sexes equally (10). Not infrequently, sinuses or fistulas can develop that drain the contents of the cyst into the adjacent soft tissues. The cysts are filled with clear mucoid material that becomes purulent if infected.

Histologically, the duct can be lined by stratified squamous or columnar epithelium, or a transitional type of epithelium intermediate between the two. Infection and ulceration of the lining epithelium occurs frequently. Healing causes subsequent fibrosis, which can be extensive and can contain chronic inflammatory cells (10–15).

Because islands of thyroid tissue can be found anywhere along the duct from the base of the tongue to the thyroid, a carcinoma can arise wherever this displaced thyroidal tissue is found. The majority of such malignancies reported are papillary thyroid carcinomas (classic or follicular variants) (11–15). In approximately 25% to 30% of these cases, cancers of the same histologic type have been found in the thyroid gland (10). The question as to whether these are actually metastases from a clonal lesion or represent two independent clonal growths remains to be answered.

Lateral Aberrant Thyroid

This term is used to describe the presence of thyroid tissue in a location lateral to the jugular veins (16). This abnormally located thyroid tissue is frequently found contained within cervical lymph nodes, which often raises the question as to whether or not it represents metastatic spread from a primary thyroid cancer. It is generally accepted that if thyroid tissue is present within the nodal parenchyma and has a papillary configuration, with characteristic nuclear clearing, nuclear grooves, and psammoma bodies, then the lesion should be considered a metastasis (1,9,16–18).

Some clinicians recognize the existence of few benign-appearing thyroid follicles contained within the capsule of a lymph node and call such lesions benign ectopic thyroid tissue (17). However, the presence of thyroid tissue in intranodal locations is difficult to explain embryologically. Therefore, it is generally recommended for therapeutic purposes, that if thyroid tissue is found in a cervical lymph node, including those in the lateral neck, consideration of an ipsilateral thyroid lobectomy is warranted, as is a careful search for a primary malignancy (1,9).

INFLAMMATION AND INFECTION

Acute Thyroiditis

Acute thyroiditis is an inflammation of the thyroid gland usually caused by bacterial or fungal infections. The disease usually develops in the course of systemic infections that reach the thyroid by hematogeneous spread. Patients of all ages can be affected, but acute thyroiditis appears to predominate at the two extremes of life, childhood and old age (19–21). Female predominance has been reported by some researchers (21).

Clinically, patients may present with fever, chills, malaise, and a painful, swollen neck. The pain can radiate to the ear or skull and is exacerbated by movement. Ipsilateral lymphadenopathy can be present; however, thyroiditis also can occur in immunocompromised patients without any of the above associated symptoms. The infection can be localized to one lobe or involve the entire gland. After acute symptoms subside, the gland may remain enlarged. The most common causes of acute thyroiditis are the gram-positive bacteria *Streptococcus haemolyticus, Staphylococcus aureus,* and *Diplococcus pneumoniae.* Other causative bacterial organisms include *Escherichia coli* and *Pseudomonas* species (19–24).

Histologically, there is diffuse infiltration of the gland by neutrophils and lymphocytes with focal microabscess formation. There is also destruction of thyroid follicles and colloid depletion. The causative organisms often can be demonstrated by special stains.

Immunocompromised patients may have extensive infiltration of the gland by infectious organisms without a significant host response due to their immunosuppressed status and reduced number of inflammatory cells. Fungal organisms such as *Aspergillus* can cause extensive infarction of the gland due to their avidity for vascular invasion, causing thrombosis and associated hemorrhage (25). Infections by organisms such as *Pneumocystis carinii* are not unusual in these types of patients who have sys-

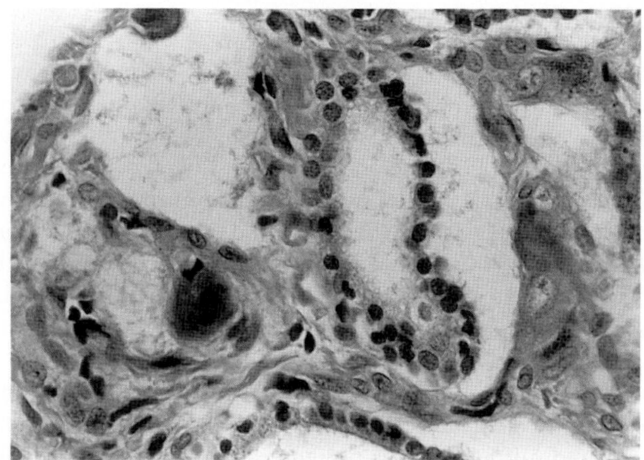

FIGURE 2. Cytomegalovirus inclusion in the thyroid of an immunocompromised patient (hematoxylin and eosin stain, original magnification ×200).

temic infections. Immunocompromised patients also can exhibit a variety of viral infections such as with cytomegalovirus. In these instances, the viral inclusions are found predominantly in the follicular epithelium (26) (Fig. 2).

The treatment of acute thyroiditis is directed toward the eradication of the causative organism. Prognosis is excellent, with total recovery when the infection is recognized and promptly treated. Rarely, complications can occur with extension of the infection into the trachea, mediastinum, and esophagus. In cases of recurrent, suppurative thyroiditis, the pyriform sinuses should be evaluated to rule out the possibility of a pyriform sinus fistula (27–29).

Tuberculosis

Tuberculous (TB) thyroiditis is a rare occurrence, and is frequently secondary to a TB infection elsewhere in the body, although sometimes the primary focus of the disease cannot be clearly eludicated. Clinically, the thyroid gland may be fixed to the adjacent cervical soft tissues and will be swollen and firm, with multiple or single nodules on examination (30–32).

Grossly, the red—brown parenchyma can show several or isolated white—yellow foci of caseous necrosis, which histologically show the characteristic necrotizing granulomata of TB. Variable degrees of fibrosis with calcifications also can be present. Demonstration of the causative organisms by acid-fast stains confirms the diagnosis.

Sarcoidosis

Involvement of the thyroid by Boeck's sarcoid has been reported but is extremely rare. Autopsy studies have demonstrated an incidence of involvement of approximately 4% (33). Grossly, small white to gray nodules can be found scattered throughout the dark red parenchyma.

Histologically, the characteristic noncaseating granulomas of sarcoidosis are identified surrounding vascular structures and in fibrous septa. Generally, the disease is interstitial and does not cause destruction of the follicles, but variable degrees of fibrosis can be seen (34–36).

Because this is a diagnosis of exclusion, special stains should be performed to rule out an infectious process. A clinical history of sarcoidosis is almost always obtained in these patients.

Subacute Thyroiditis

Subacute thyroiditis, also known as granulomatous, de Quervain's disease, or nonsuppurative thyroiditis, was originally described by de Quervain in 1904 (37). But it was Jaffe who later postulated a nontuberculous or noninfectious etiology for this disease (38).

The true incidence of subacute thyroiditis is unknown because many infectious types of thyroiditis have been reported under this name. The disease is reportedly rare, although it is possible that many cases are not correctly diagnosed or spontaneously resolve. It affects patients at all ages, but most commonly in the third to sixth decade of life, and has a 3:1 female to male ratio (39). Subacute thyroiditis has been found to be strongly associated with HLA-B35 haplotype (40).

Clinically, the presentation of subacute thyroiditis may vary; it can present as an acute event with fever, malaise, fatigue, and pain localized to the neck or radiating to the jaw. Other patients follow a mild course with only minimal symptoms. Painless thyroiditis is not uncommon in young females (39). Postmenopausal women may present with weight loss, heart palpitations, and depression and have biochemical and clinical features of hyperthyroidism due to painless subacute thyroiditis. Fluctuations of thyroid hormone levels can be detected in the serum according to the phase of the disease. The disease is usually self-limited and patients usually recover after several weeks.

The cause of subacute thyroiditis remains controversial, but a viral etiology is favored (41,42). Epidemiologic studies support this theory, because many cases present in clusters or as an epidemic and are frequently associated with viral infections such as mumps, measles, adenovirus infection, mononucleosis, influenza, and others. A viral etiology is also supported by the fact that an increase in T cells has been found in the serum of patients with this disease. The disease does not respond to antibiotics; however, patients usually recover completely with supportive therapy.

Grossly, the thyroid is enlarged and sometimes shows an asymmetrical involvement with one lobe larger than the other. The surface of the gland has scattered, yellow or white, ill-defined nodules surrounded by normal uninvolved red—brown tissue. These nodules can be firm in advanced stages of disease. The capsule is preserved because the process does not extend into the adjacent soft tissue; consequently, the gland is not attached to the neck and is easily movable.

Histologically, there is destruction of the follicular epithelium by foreign body giant cell granulomas, as well as a mixture of inflammatory cells, including lymphocytes, plasma cells, polymorphonuclear leukocytes, and epithelioid histocytes. The giant cells are of variable size and are frequently found surrounding colloid or colloid remnants. Residual outlines of preexisting follicles can be detected in early stages, destroyed predominantly by chronic inflammatory cells. As the process advances, fibrosis occurs in both the interfollicular and lobular areas, and inflammatory cells can be identified in the fibrous tissue. Colloid material, highlighted by periodic acid-Schiff stain, is frequently found in the cytoplasm of the giant cells.

Microabscess formation occasionally can be found in subacute thyroiditis. In contradistinction to TB thyroiditis or fungal infections, this process lacks caseating necrosis.

Eventually, there is healing and follicle regeneration, although mild fibrosis may persist. Normal thyroid function returns both clinically and biochemically after several weeks. Hypothyroidism is a rare complication of the disease (42,43).

Palpation Thyroiditis

This entity, reported by Carney et al. in 1975, describes the presence of small granulomas involving usually one to three follicles that are surrounded by chronic inflammatory cells, histiocytes, lymphocytes, and occasional giant cells (44).

These small granulomas can be found in an otherwise normal parenchyma. It is believed that such changes are the result of trauma to the gland, because these histologic findings are not generally seen in nonmanipulated thyroids. Palpation granulomas do not have clinical significance, nor do they cause alterations in thyroid function.

AUTOIMMUNE PROCESSES

Hashimoto's Thyroiditis

In his original report (45), Hashimoto described four patients with what he called *struma lymphomatosa.* The patients had an enlarged thyroid, but he recognized the lesion that bears his name as a different process than Riedel's or de Quervain's thyroiditis.

Hashimoto's thyroiditis is a relatively common form of thyroiditis that predominantly affects women 30 to 50 years of age. No age group is spared, however, and the incidence increases with age. Patients present with diffuse thyroid enlargement accompanied by either mild hyperthyroidism or hypothyroidism. The disease can affect several members of the same family who often also suffer from a variety of autoimmune conditions such as systemic lupus erythematosus, Graves' disease, arteritis, and scleroderma. Preliminary studies by Dorman et al. and others have shown an increased prevalence of Hashimoto's thyroiditis in women with insulin-dependent diabetes mellitus (46). Hashimoto's thyroiditis is the most common cause of goitrous hypothyroidism in the United States.

The disease is apparently caused by a defect in suppressor T-lymphocytes, a defect that can occur randomly in genetically predisposed individuals. With suppressor T-lymphocytes lacking, killer lymphocytes attack the thyroid cells, and plasma cells are induced to produce antithyroid antibodies. Patients have high titers of circulating antibodies, including antimicrosomal antibody (detected in 95% of patients), antithyroglobulin, and cell membrane antibodies. Laboratory data for such patients show low T4 and elevated serum thyrotropin and thyroxine index, consistent with hypothyroidism. Serum thyroid-stimulating hormone (TSH) also can be elevated (47–51).

The affected gland is enlarged, with diffuse involvement that does not spare even the pyramidal lobe. Weights of up to 300 g have been reported. The capsule is preserved and there is no involvement of perithyroidal soft tissues, differentiating this lesion from malignant lymphoma and Riedel's thyroiditis. The cut surface shows lobules of various sizes separated by fibrous tissue and with a characteristic tan to pale yellow appearance.

Histologically, two major variants of Hashimoto's thyroiditis are recognized: the classic and the fibrosing variants (1,47,49).

Classic Variant

The classic type is characterized by a diffuse lymphocytic and plasmacytic cellular infiltrate accompanied by the formation of well-developed germinal centers (Fig. 3). Immunoblasts and macrophages are also present. The thyroid follicles are small and can contain small amounts of colloid. The epithelial cells are enlarged and contain abundant dense eosinophilic or orangiophilic cytoplasm and a hyperchromatic large nucleus. This so-called Hürthle cell change or metaplasia can be extensive, forming cell clusters or nests, and these cells are frequently found adjacent to or admixed with lymphoid aggregates. This cellular change is characterized ultrastructurally by a large amount of cytoplasmic mitochondria. Müller-Hocker et al. recently demonstrated that this cell change is associated with functional and molecular genetic defects in cytochrome-c oxidase of the respiratory chain (52). The epithelial cells also can show changes to a paler, more cuboidal type of cell with clear-appearing nuclei reminiscent of the nuclear changes observed in papillary carcinoma. Not infrequently, both types of cells can be seen in areas of thyroid follicular proliferation. Fibrosis begins as the epithelium starts to regenerate and is apparent first in the interlobular areas, but eventually can replace areas of normal follicles. Immunophenotypic studies highlight the lymphoid aggregates and demonstrate a mixture of B and T cells (51).

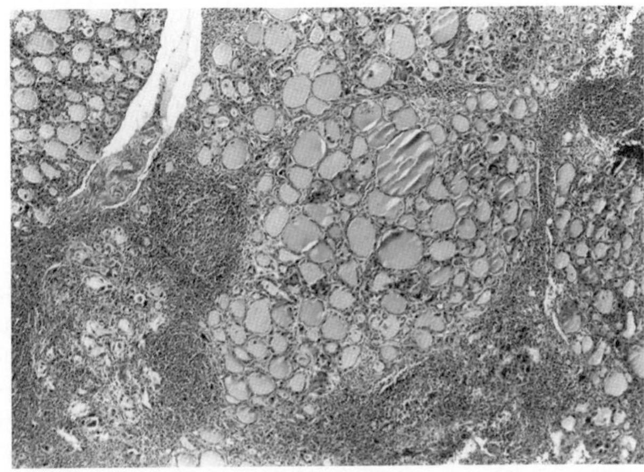

FIGURE 3. Low-power view of Hashimoto's thyroiditis. Follicular cells are surrounded by lymphoid aggregates with germinal centers (hematoxylin and eosin stain, original magnification ×100).

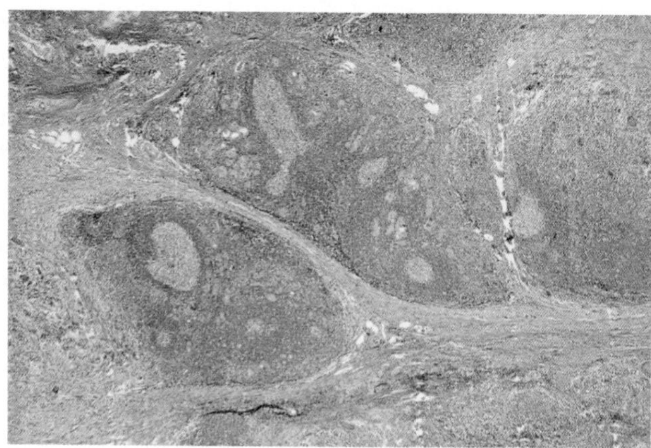

A

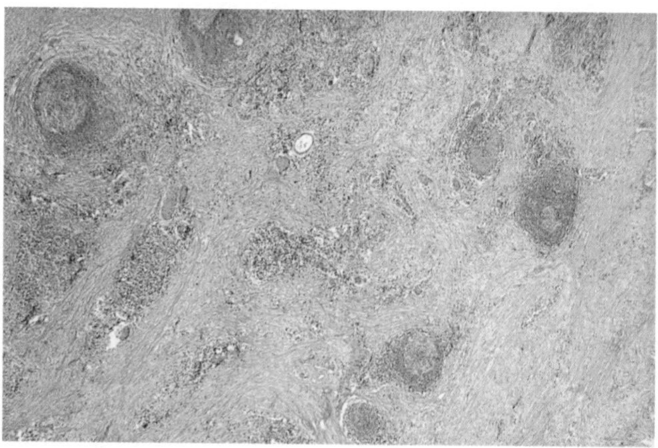

B

FIGURE 4. Fibrosing variant of Hashimoto's thyroiditis. **A:** Focally broad fibrous bands are present. **B:** A severe case in which the normal parenchyma is extensively replaced by fibrous tissue containing abundant lymphocytes (hematoxylin and eosin stain, original magnification ×200).

Fibrosing Variant

This type accounts for about 10% of all cases of Hashimoto's thyroiditis. Elderly patients present with large goitrous glands, severe hypothyroidism, and pressure symptoms in the neck. Grossly, the large, well-encapsulated gland has preservation of the lobular architecture. The histologic changes of typical Hashimoto's thyroiditis are altered by diffuse broad bands of fibrous tissue containing lymphocytes and plasma cells that extensively replace the thyroid parenchyma (Fig. 4). Follicular atrophy and squamous metaplasia are common. It is possible that this variant represents a "burned-out" progression from earlier stages of Hashimoto's thyroiditis (49).

Because the fibrosing variant of Hashimoto's thyroiditis does not extend beyond the thyroid capsule, it can be distinguished from Riedel's disease. The latter involves the thyroid as well as contiguous neck structures.

Hashimoto's thyroiditis frequently coexists with other thyroid diseases, including both hematologic malignancies and epithelial neoplasias. Malignant lymphoma is the most common neoplasm associated with Hashimoto's thyroiditis (53,54). Coexisting papillary carcinoma is usually occult and often difficult to appreciate. Areas that show cellular crowding with distinct nuclear clearing and grooves should alert the pathologist to this possibility. When occult or micropapillary carcinoma is identified in a thyroid that had been removed for Hashimoto's thyroiditis, no additional treatment is usually necessary.

Diffuse Thyroid Hyperplasia

Diffuse hyperplasia of the thyroid, Graves' disease, or diffuse toxic goiter is a systemic disorder of autoimmune etiology that affects predominantly young women with a female:male ratio of 9:1. Graves' disease is the predominant cause of pediatric hyperthyroidism, and a female preponderance persists (55). The most common signs and symptoms include exophthalmus, tachycardia, muscle weakness, and tibial myxedema. Clinically there is either an elevated T4 (either bound or free) or elevated T3 with an increased radioactive iodine uptake and decreased TSH level. Graves' disease is thought to be caused by the production of immunoglobulin G (IgG) autoantibodies against specific domains of the thyrotropin receptor (56,57).

Grossly, the gland usually shows modest symmetrical enlargement, with weights ranging from 40 to 100 g. The capsule is intact and the parenchyma is firm. The cut surface is red to brown, perhaps due to increased vascularity. If there has been preoperative radioactive iodine administration, there is colloid production by the gland, making the cut surface shiny, like that of nodular goiter.

The histologic appearance also varies according to whether the patient has received therapy prior to surgery, and depending on the type of therapy administered. In untreated cases, there is marked follicular hyperplasia. The follicles are round to oval in shape and are lined by tall columnar cells with pale, granular, or vacuolated cytoplasm. The nuclei of these cells are also large and can show a degree of clearing, but marked atypicality is absent. The follicles can be devoid of colloid or contain variable amounts of pale eosinophilic colloid with a scalloped appearance at the periphery. Formation of papillary structures is common, and sometimes very prominent, mimicking papillary cancer (58,59) (Fig. 5).

Lymphocytes and well-developed germinal centers can be found scattered throughout the stroma. These lymphocytes usually persist after treatment and involution of the gland, and immunophenotypically they are both cytotoxic and T-helper cell in type (60). Immunologic remissions can occur in patients with a less severe or only partial organ-specific defect of their suppressor T lymphocytes.

With preoperative radioiodine therapy there is a decrease in hyperplastic papillary proliferations, with follicular involution, decreased vascularity, and some fibrosis. Medications such as propylthiouracil, on the other hand, exaggerate the hyperplastic pattern (58,59).

Malignant tumors are known to develop in association with Graves' disease; however, controversies remain as to the frequency and clinical significance of such tumors. Some researchers support the point of view that when these tumors develop they are predominantly papillary in type, but with worse

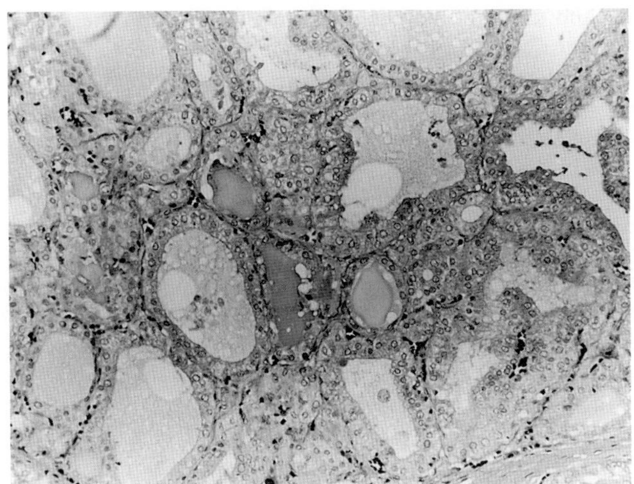

FIGURE 5. Hyperplastic follicles with focally clear nuclei and incipient papillary formation in a patient with Graves' disease (hematoxylin and eosin stain, original magnification ×150).

prognosis because of the continued stimulation of the tumor and normal thyroid tissue by antithyroid antibodies. Further studies with larger series of patients are needed before any definite conclusions can be drawn.

Riedel's Disease

Also known as Riedel's struma or fibrous or ligneous thyroiditis, the disease bears the name of Riedel, who in 1896 described the clinical features of three patients, each of whom presented with a rapidly growing thyroid mass and dyspnea (61). During surgery, the thyroid gland was noted to be extremely hard, and tissue infiltrated extensively into the neck, trachea, and adjacent structures. Later this lesion was considered to be a variant of Hashimoto's thyroiditis, and eventually it was reclassified as an invasive type of fibrous thyroiditis.

Despite the careful description of Hashimoto's thyroiditis by Hashimoto, including his recognition of the fibrosing variant and its distinction from Riedel's disease, these two entities were regarded as the same disease by many pathologists. For example, in 1922, Ewing (62) stated that "the two lesions are different manifestations of the same process." With few exceptions, this confusion remained until 1974, when Katz and Vickery "rediscovered" (49) and more fully described the fibrosing variant of Hashimoto's thyroiditis. It is now accepted that the fibrosing variant of Hashimoto's thyroiditis and Riedel's thyroiditis represent distinct entities (63,64). Recently, however, Taubenberger et al. (65) reported the case of a patient with a thyroid lesion showing histologic features of both Riedel's and fibrosing Hashimoto's thyroiditis.

Riedel's fibrous thyroiditis is rare. Patients with this disorder present with a thyroid mass and also may have fibrosing lesions in other sites, including the retroperitoneum, mediastinum, and retroorbital tissues (66). The clinical impression of the thyroid lesion is frequently carcinoma. Grossly, the process infiltrates extensively into the thyroid gland and adjacent tissues of the neck, including skeletal muscle and nerves, and may surround and infiltrate lymph nodes and the parathyroid glands. Histologically, there is abundant keloid-like fibrocollagenous tissue with a variable amount of inflammatory cells, including lymphocytes, plasma cells, and eosinophils. The entrapped thyroidal vessels often show a lymphocytic vasculitis (67). Immunophenotypic studies demonstrate that there is a predominance of T cells with few infiltrating B cells. Although not considered as an autoimmune disease, a study by Schwaegerle et al. demonstrated low serum titers of antithyroid antibodies in the majority of patients studied. It was hypothesized that these antibodies may occur secondarily to destruction of thyroid parenchyma by the fibrosing process (68,69).

The evolution of this disease is slow, and spontaneous recurrences can occur. If pressure symptoms are troublesome, surgical therapy may be indicated.

BENIGN TUMORS

Nodular (Adenomatous) Goiter

Nodular hyperplasia or nodular goiter is a common process involving the thyroid gland, which then appears enlarged and multinodular on palpation. Patients are usually euthyroid, but may present with tracheal obstruction or respiratory distress in extreme cases when thyroid enlargement is marked. Occasionally, a prominent single nodule is palpated, which requires further investigation to rule out the presence of a malignancy. Rapid enlargement with pain can be indicative of hemorrhage into the nodule. Nodular goiter is associated with a state of hyperfunction, which can be secondary to low iodine in the diet, or increased clearance of iodide, which stimulates the production and secretion of thyroid hormone (1).

Grossly, the thyroid is enlarged, often diffusely, and can attain weights of over 1,000 g. The capsule is intact, and upon sectioning, diffuse parenchymal nodularity is noted. The characteristic red–brown color of the normal parenchyma is preserved; however, areas of hemorrhage, fibrosis, cystic degeneration, and calcifications can be identified (Fig. 6).

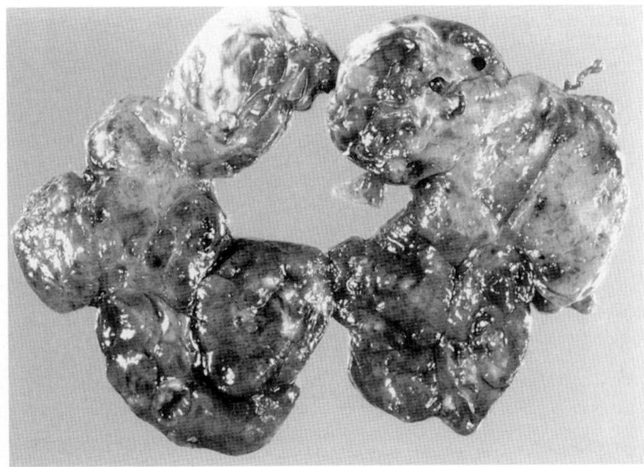

FIGURE 6. Cross-section of a retrosternal goiter in a patient complaining of difficulties in breathing. The large mass was homogeneously red and showed benign thyroid follicles.

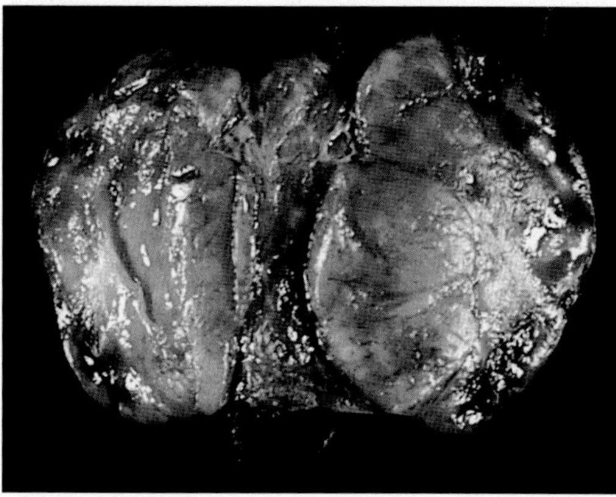

FIGURE 7. Gross photograph of a follicular adenoma compressing the normal thyroid parenchyma.

By light microscopy there is a spectrum of changes. Frequently in cases where a dominant nodule is clinically suspected, several different-sized nodules may be observed histologically. Some follicles appear normal, some hyperplastic with scant amounts of colloid, and some markedly dilated and filled with dense eosinophilic colloid. Hemorrhage, fibrosis, and chronic inflammatory cells are frequently found. Adjacent to these areas, it is not unusual to find cells with clear nuclei, which should not be mistaken for occult papillary cancer. Focal areas of papillary hyperplasia with the formation of small abortive papillae lined by a row of follicular cells, called Sanderson's polsters, can be seen. Occasionally, clusters of small hyperplastic follicles can be seen protruding into the lumen of larger follicles. These areas probably represent the result of episodes of hyperactivity and involution.

The follicles are of variable size, but are usually large. If there is a predominant nodule found, it should be differentiated from a follicular adenoma. The latter usually shows predominantly uniform small follicles surrounded by a more developed capsule, with the adjacent thyroid tissue having a compressed or normal appearance.

Mild cases of nodular hyperplasia need no treatment. Administration of exogenous thyroid hormone to suppress nodular hyperplasia is not efficacious. Subtotal thyroidectomy is reserved for patients with pressure symptoms or prominent unsightly glands (70).

Follicular Adenomas

Follicular adenoma is a common thyroid neoplasm. It occurs predominantly in the lateral lobes, rarely in the isthmus, and characteristically as a single lesion. When more than one adenoma is identified within the gland, LiVolsi (1) suggests that the term *multinodular goiter with adenomatous change* is more appropriate.

Follicular adenomas have been shown to be independent clonal growths (71–73). They can occur in both sexes at all ages, but predominate in middle-aged women. Similar to nodular goiter, rapid growth of the mass can be caused by intralesional hemorrhage. At presentation, patients are usually euthyroid, with a painless lump.

Grossly, adenomas are well circumscribed and encapsulated, oval to round solitary masses, and clearly demarcated from the surrounding normal parenchyma. The capsule is usually thin and delicate. The size of these nodules is variable, but most are 1 to 4 cm in diameter. They have a homogeneous, pink, tan to brown appearance on cut surfaces, although cystic changes as well as hemorrhage and necrosis can be seen in larger lesions (Fig. 7).

Microscopically, a variety of patterns have been reported: trabecular (embryonal), microfollicular (fetal), macrofollicular, and solid (Fig. 8). These histologic types have no clinical significance. The capsule is complete and often thin, and may contain blood vessels. Degenerative changes such as hemorrhage, fibrosis, calcifications, inflammatory cells, and hyalinization of the stroma can be seen in some long-standing tumors (1,9).

Benign adenomas do not often show marked nuclear pleomorphism, although occasional enlarged or hyperchromatic nuclei may be seen, and mitoses are rare. The follicular pattern of

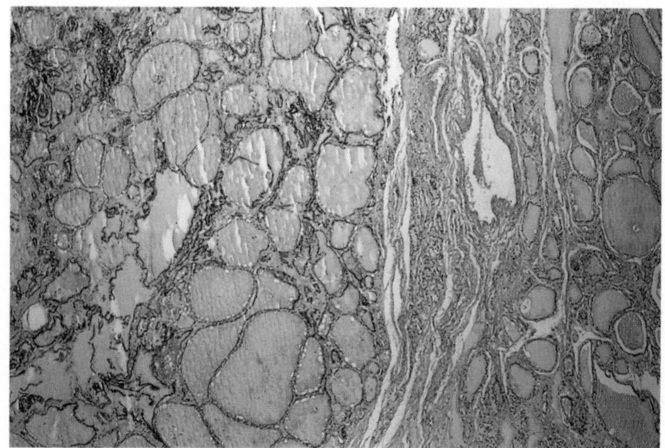

A

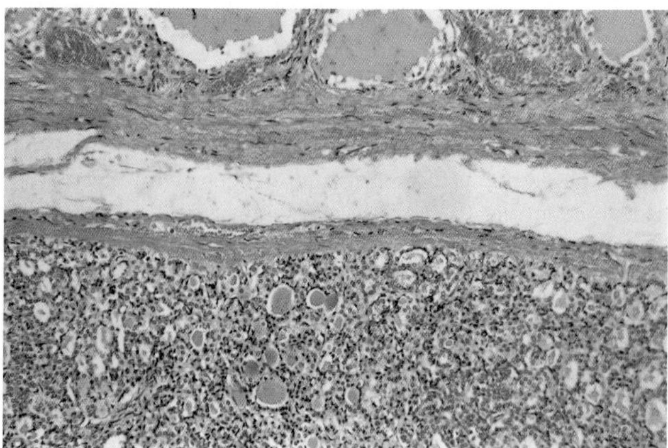

B

FIGURE 8. Follicular adenomas. **A:** Follicular adenoma, focally macrofollicular. **B:** Microfollicular or fetal adenoma. In both of these examples, the tumors are sharply demarcated from adjacent thyroid parenchyma.

growth of adenomas generally contrasts sharply with the normal or compressed adjacent thyroid tissue.

These benign lesions are treated with lobectomy and should be differentiated from well-differentiated follicular carcinomas. The latter usually exhibit a thicker capsule. Careful evaluation of the capsule for evidence of capsular or vascular invasions is mandatory. If no invasion is seen, the lesion is considered to be benign (see later section on Follicular Carcinoma); however, it is important to know that malignancies can develop in association with or within benign nodules.

Atypical Follicular Adenoma

This diagnosis encompasses a group of follicular neoplasms that show worrisome histologic features such as increased cellularity, mitotic figures, necrosis, or marked nuclear pleomorphism. In addition there are areas suggestive of but not definite for capsular or vascular invasion. Again, careful evaluation of the capsule is mandatory. These lesions usually behave in a benign fashion, although careful follow-up of the patient is still recommended (1,9).

Hyalinizing Trabecular Adenoma

This neoplasm recently was redefined by Carney et al. (74). Similar lesions have been described in the literature as "paraganglioma" and "paraganglioma-like" tumors (9). The significance of recognizing this subtype of adenoma is that it is frequently misdiagnosed as papillary or medullary carcinoma, both in surgical specimens and fine-needle aspirates.

The gross appearance of hyalinizing trabecular adenoma (HTA) is similar to that of the other types of adenomas. Histologically, the follicular cells have a predominantly trabecular arrangement. Follicle formation is minimal or absent. The cells are large and have an oval, spindled, or fusiform configuration with abundant eosinophilic or clear cytoplasm.

The nuclear shape is also variable, and the nucleus may focally contain either grooves or cytoplasmic nuclear pseudoinclusions. Prominent nesting of the cells is frequently identified, giving the tumor an organoid or paraganglioma-like appearance (Fig. 9). The stroma can have marked fibrosis and eosinophilic degeneration and can contain calcifications as well as well-formed psammoma body-like structures (75).

Although the biology of these lesions is generally benign, Rosai et al. (9) and others (76) report having seen cases of HTA associated with papillary carcinomas. At this point, careful evaluation and ample histologic sampling of these lesions is recommended to avoid missing a true malignant lesion.

Immunohistochemically, HTA cells react positively for thyroglobulin and negatively for calcitonin, which helps to differentiate them from medullary carcinomas. High molecular weight cytokeratin, CK 19, laminin, and collagen IV also have been reported to be immunoreactive in HTA (76). Occasional focal immunoreactivity for neuroendocrine markers has been observed (75).

Hyalinizing trabecular adenoma is different from the true, rare, intrathyroidal paraganglioma, which shows tumor cells

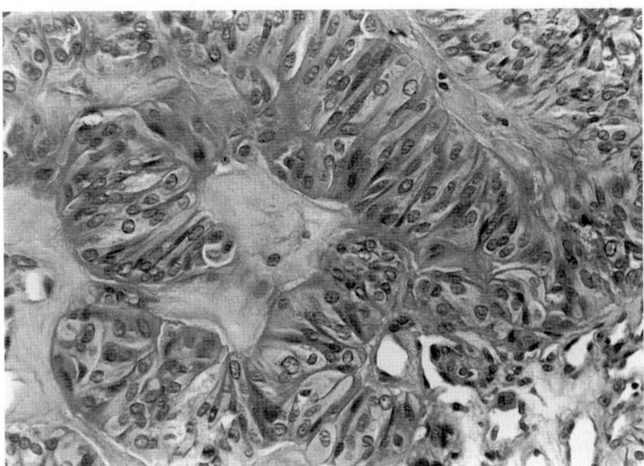

FIGURE 9. High-power view of a hyalinizing trabecular adenoma. The cells are spindled and fusiform, and there are prominent nuclei, some with grooves (hematoxylin and eosin stain, original magnification ×200).

with granular cytoplasm in a *Zellballen* configuration being bathed by a prominent vascular network. Paragangliomas can contain two cell populations (chief cells and sustentacular cells), exhibit prominent cytoplasmic vacuolization, contain large bizarre nuclei, and have dense hyalinized stroma. Importantly, there is an absence of follicles or a true trabecular pattern in paragangliomas, and the nuclear features of HTA are not appreciated. Immunohistochemistical stains show immunoreactivity with neuroendocrine markers, neuron-specific enolase (NSE), chromogranin, and synaptophysin. Epithelial markers and thyroglobulin are negative (77).

Papillary Hyperplastic Nodule

These are solitary lesions that occur predominantly in children and young females. Histologically, these nodules are well circumscribed and encapsulated, and they are composed of papillae of different sizes in which the stalk may contain small follicles. These papillae are lined by cuboidal cells with characteristic follicular nuclei (i.e., dense and dispersed chromatin). Usually there is one nucleus per cell, arranged in a linear fashion along the papillae. The center of the nodule is frequently cystic and can contain colloid-like material (1).

These benign nodules must be distinguished from the encapsulated variant of papillary cancer, which has follicles lined by cells with clear ground-glass nuclei. Psammoma bodies are also not observed in the hyperplastic nodules. Staining for cytokeratins is focal in these benign lesions; papillary cancer stains diffusely and intensely.

MALIGNANT TUMORS

Malignant neoplasms of the thyroid are the most common type of endocrine cancers. Approximately 12,000 to 14,000 new cases are diagnosed each year, accounting for 0.4% of all cancer deaths in the United States (78–83).

Although the exact cause of thyroid cancer is not known, epidemiologic studies have shown that many factors may play important roles in the development of these tumors. For example, it is well known that exposure to radiation during childhood increases the incidence of papillary carcinoma (1,9,78–81). These tumors are also more frequently found in patients living in areas where there is an excess of iodine in the diet. Conversely, diets poor in iodine are associated with the development of follicular carcinoma, and these tumors are common in countries known for endemic goiters (82,83). Medullary carcinoma can occur in a genetic form and frequently occurs as a part of the multiple endocrine neoplasia syndrome (MEN) (1,9).

The age distribution of patients with thyroid cancer is variable, and it can occur even in children, but it is more frequently a disease of young adults. Thyroid cancer is more frequent in women than in men, with a ratio of 2.5:1.

The usual clinical presentation is nodular enlargement of the gland, sometimes (in cases of papillary carcinoma) with enlarged ipsilateral lymph nodes. Less commonly, the initial manifestation may be enlarged cervical nodes in the absence of a palpable thyroid mass. The appearance of a single thyroid nodule in children or adult males should be always vigorously investigated to rule out malignancy. A single nodule has a probability of up to 12% of being malignant, whereas the probability of malignancy decreases significantly (3%) if multiple nodules are palpated. In patients exposed to significant amounts of radiation, up to 30% of nodules can be malignant (1,9).

Radioscintigraphy of the gland is helpful in differential diagnosis because hyperfunctioning ("hot") nodules are usually benign. "Cold" or nonfunctioning nodules, on the other hand, although more occasionally malignant, also can be benign. Thus, histologic examination of some sort is often needed.

TABLE 1. THYROID CANCER CLASSIFICATION

- Papillary carcinoma
  - Prognosis as good or better than classical papillary carcinoma
    - Classical papillary
    - Microcarcinoma
    - Encapsulated
    - Follicular variant
    - Solid
  - Prognosis poorer than classical papillary carcinoma
    - Diffuse sclerosing
    - Tall cell
    - Columnar cell
- Follicular carcinoma
  - Minimally invasive
  - Invasive
- Hürthle cell carcinoma
- Medullary carcinoma
  - Small cell
  - Giant cell
  - Papillary
  - Glandular
  - Other types
- Insular carcinoma
- Anaplastic carcinoma
- Squamous cell carcinoma
- Sclerosing mucoepidermoid carcinoma with eosinophilia
- Small cell carcinoma
- Thymic-like Malignancies ("SETTLE" and "CASTLE")
- Malignant lymphoma
- Sarcomas: angiosarcoma
- Metastases

Classification

Some researchers classify thyroid cancer into only two groups: (a) differentiated (papillary, follicular) carcinomas (tumors characterized by indolent biological behavior and good prognosis) and (b) undifferentiated or anaplastic carcinomas (associated with aggressive behavior, metastases, and eventual death of the patient).

Carcangiu et al. (84) reported a special type of thyroid cancer, the poorly differentiated or "insular" carcinoma, that seems to fit between these two categories, and could, therefore, be recognized as an intermediate type of tumor (Table 1).

Papillary Carcinoma

Papillary carcinoma is the most common form of thyroid cancer, accounting for up to 80% of all thyroid malignancies in the United States. This slow-growing tumor can occur at any age, but the peak incidence at the time of diagnosis is 30 to 40 years. It is also the most common thyroid tumor type in the prepubertal or young adolescent group. Women are affected more commonly than men, and elderly men appear to have a worse prognosis when afflicted with this type of thyroid cancer (1,9,81,85).

The etiology of papillary thyroid cancer is not well known; however, it has been well documented that children who were exposed to ionizing radiation for medical treatment of thymic masses, acne, tonsillitis, lymphadenitis, and hemangiomas have a higher predisposition to develop papillary carcinoma. The incidence of thyroid cancers in these patients varies, but it is proportional to the amount of radiation exposure and the age of the patient at exposure and has been reported to be as high as 10% (86). Recent studies from the Chernobyl region indicate that the incidence of thyroid carcinoma increased from 4 to 6 cases per year before the accident to 29 to 55 cases per year in the 4 years directly following the nuclear power plant explosion (87). However compelling these data are, it is important to recognize that the majority of patients who develop papillary carcinoma have no history of radiation exposure.

There is controversy as to whether an increased incidence of papillary carcinoma exists in patients with Hashimoto's thyroiditis (88). The surgical literature indicates that there is a strong relationship. The suggested mechanism is that of increased levels of TSH related to the thyroiditis. It is thought that uninterrupted and long stimulation of thyroid cells with TSH can cause thyroid cancer. Other studies, however, have found no association between the two diseases and point out that some of the reported studies lack serologic proof of preexisting thyroiditis in these patients (1,9).

Papillary carcinoma can develop in the setting of preexisting adenomas; however, as LiVolsi (1) pointed out, there is no evidence that these host nodules or adenomas are premalignant.

Clinically, papillary cancer is usually found by palpation of a nodule or mass of variable size in the thyroid. Occasionally papillary carcinomas can present with ipsilateral lymph node involvement or distant metastases. In a series of cases studied by Carcangiu et al. (85), 67% of the patients presented only with a thyroid tumor, 19% had a mass in the neck and 13% had thyroid and cervical lymph node involvement. These tumors are frequently multicentric (up to 75% of cases).

Scintigraphy with radionuclides is the most useful imaging procedure for the detection of papillary cancer. Approximately 15% to 25% of cold nodules are thyroid cancers. Calcification is the sole significant radiographic feature associated with papillary cancer, but it is only found in 10% of patients with this malignancy.

Grossly, papillary cancer may be located anywhere in the gland, including the isthmus. These tumors are firm, solid, and white to yellow, with irregular and infiltrative borders. The center of the lesion may show fibrosis and sclerosis. The tumors can be encapsulated and sometimes calcified, and in about 10% of the cases cystic changes are noted (Fig. 10). Occasionally, small papillary fronds lining the cyst wall can be seen grossly. Hemorrhage and necrosis as well as extension into adjacent perithyroidal tissues can be seen in large tumors and aggressive variants.

Histologically, the hallmark of classic papillary cancer is the presence of true papillae composed of stalks of fibroconnective tissue containing blood vessels and lined by cuboidal cells with characteristic clear nuclei (Fig. 11). Nuclear characteristics of the tumor cells are more crucial for diagnosis than papillary architecture, however, and the follicular variant of papillary cancer maintains the characteristic nuclear features without the papillary architecture. The nuclear features consist of "Orphan Annie," empty-appearing, clear, or ground-glass nuclei that are larger than normal follicular nuclei with a round nuclear membrane encasing condensed chromatin in the periphery, giving the nuclei an empty or washed-out appearance (89) (Fig. 12). The reason for this nuclear appearance is unclear, but it is probably an artifact of fixation because it is almost never seen in frozen sections or fine-needle aspiration (FNA) preparations. Overlapping of the nuclei is also frequently found at the top of papillae. The papillae can be edematous and hyalinized, and show myxomatous changes or contain clusters of chronic inflammatory cells.

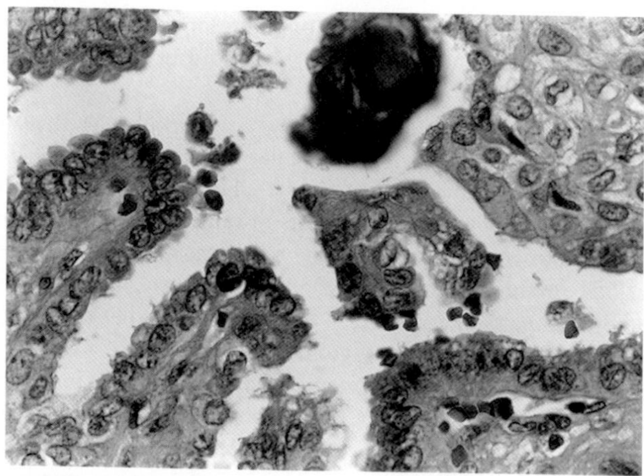

FIGURE 11. High-power view of well-formed papillary structures characteristic of papillary carcinoma. A psammoma body is also present (hematoxylin and eosin stain, original magnification ×200).

Other nuclear features include nuclear grooves or infoldings of the nuclear membrane, as well as cytoplasmic intranuclear pseudoinclusions or invaginations of the cytoplasm into the nucleus (90). The reliability of nuclear grooves as an important diagnostic feature in papillary cancers has been questioned by some researchers (91).

Another characteristic feature of papillary cancer is the presence of psammoma bodies. These laminated basophilic concretions probably represent tumor papillae that have undergone necrosis and calcification. Although psammoma bodies are reliable markers of papillary cancer, they are only present in 40% to 50% of cases. The presence of psammoma bodies either in lymph nodes or thyroid tissue should make one highly suspicious of the presence of papillary cancer (92). These calcified bodies must be distinguished from the dystrophic calcifications frequently found in other thyroid lesions such as goiters or as the

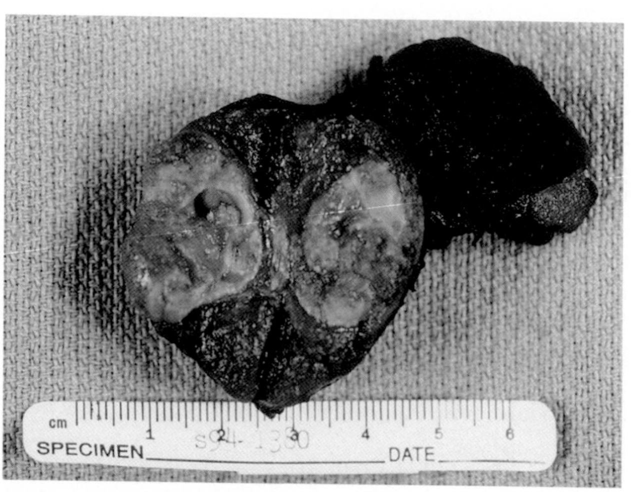

FIGURE 10. Papillary carcinoma in a 22-year-old woman. Areas of necrosis as well as papillary formation are noted.

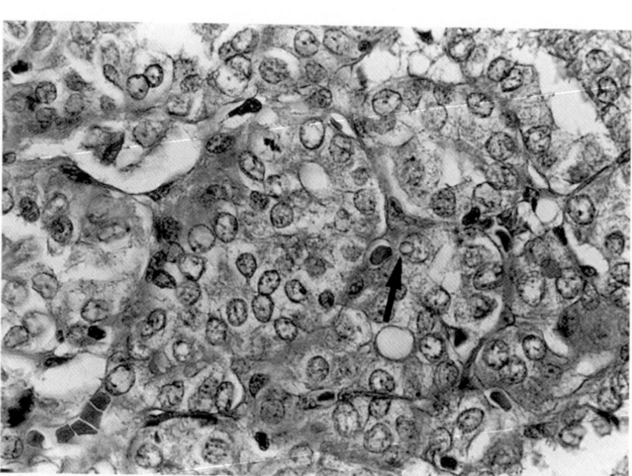

FIGURE 12. Clear cell nuclei are the hallmark of papillary carcinoma. Intranuclear pseudoinclusion (*arrow*) and grooves are identified as well (hematoxylin and eosin stain, original magnification ×200).

result of FNA. An example of a nonpsammomatous calcification is the intrafollicular calcification of colloid not uncommonly present in sections of thyroid.

Immunohistochemically, papillary carcinoma reacts positively for thyroglobulin, low molecular weight cytokeratins, and epithelial membrane antigen (EMA). High molecular weight keratins have shown positive results in some studies, but not in others. Estrogen and progesterone receptors also have been described in these tumors (1,9,93,94). Recently, the putative mesothelioma marker HBME-1 has been shown to be reactive in papillary carcinoma of the thyroid (95).

Molecular genetic rearrangements of the tyrosine kinase domain of the *RET* oncogene are found in 3% to 33% of papillary carcinomas not associated with radiation and in up to 80% of patients with papillary carcinoma from the region north of Chernobyl or who have a history of therapeutic radiation (96–102). The histology of these papillary carcinomas is well differentiated. Rearrangements of the *TRK* gene is a less common finding in papillary thyroid carcinomas occurring in a young population (97).

Variants of Papillary Carcinoma with Generally Favorable Prognosis

Microcarcinoma (Occult-Type Papillary Carcinoma)

Historically, these are tumors that measure less than 1.0 cm in diameter, although recently this definition has been expanded to include lesions up to 1.5 cm. Most of the lesions, however, fall in the range of 3 to 7 mm. The tumors can be nonencapsulated, have marked fibrosis and sclerosis, or be surrounded by a dense fibrous capsule. The clear nuclei are frequently present and the tumors may have either a follicular or papillary architectural pattern (Fig. 13).

These tumors, although small, can give rise to cervical lymph node metastases. The incidence of these metastases is variable according to different researchers, varying from 23% (103) to 71% (85). Sampson and collaborators reported an incidence of only 16% in a series of 128 cases of microcarcinomas found at autopsy (104). However, distant metastases from these tumors are infrequent (104–110).

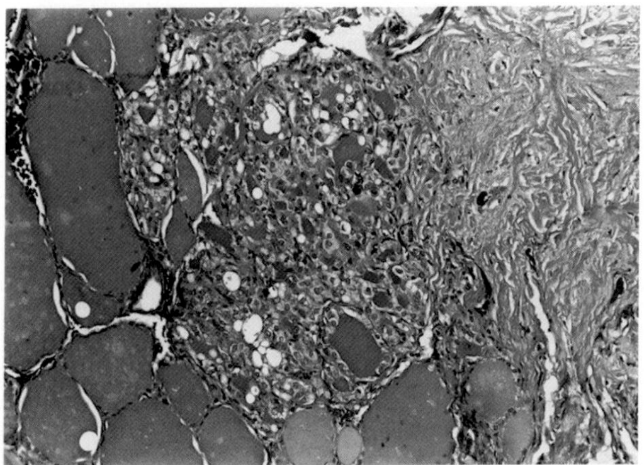

FIGURE 13. Microcarcinoma. This variant of papillary carcinoma is usually about 0.7 mm in size (hematoxylin and eosin stain, original magnification ×150).

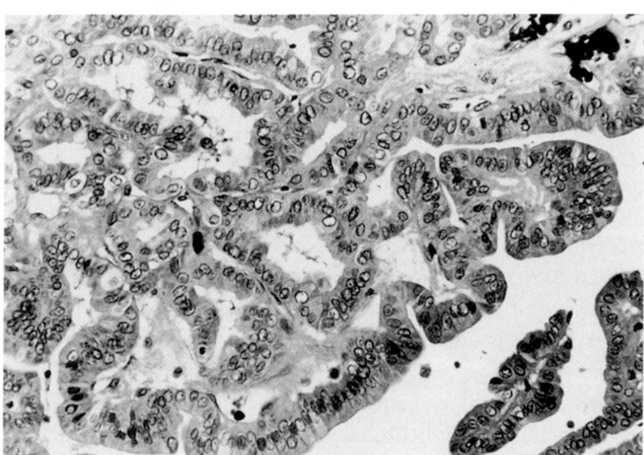

FIGURE 14. Follicular variant of papillary carcinoma. The follicles are lined by cells in which the characteristic clear nuclei are present (hematoxylin and eosin stain, original magnification ×150).

Microcarcinomas must be differentiated from benign clusters of solid squamoid or basaloid solid cell nests of ultimobranchial body origin. These nests are interfollicular or involve a portion of a follicle, are quite small (usually less than 1.0 mm), and may contain central mucin, and their cells do not have clear nuclei. When closely associated with follicular cells, staining for thyroglobulin can appear to be positive (111).

Follicular Variant

For many years tumors composed of both follicles and papillae were classified as mixed carcinomas, implying that these neoplasms may behave somewhat differently from pure follicular or pure papillary carcinomas.

In 1960, Lindsay first described this variant of papillary cancer as a tumor characterized by a follicular pattern of growth in which the follicles are lined by the clear or papillary-type nuclei, and that clinically and biologically resembled papillary cancer (112).

These tumors may or may not be encapsulated on gross or histologic examination. The follicles often contain dense eosinophilic colloid with a scalloped border. Other histologic characteristics of this tumor include the presence of occasional psammoma bodies, formation of rudimentary or abortive papillae, and a desmoplastic reaction. These tumors frequently are composed entirely of follicles (Fig. 14). This tumor is difficult to diagnosis at the time of operation because the clear nuclei may or may not be appreciated on frozen section (9,113). Albores-Saavedra and collaborators described a macrofollicular type of papillary cancer in which the tumor showed large follicular spaces filled with colloid, architecturally and histologically similar to nodular goiter, but which had the typical papillary nuclei (114).

The incidence of the follicular variant of papillary thyroid carcinoma (PTC) is variable; Carcangiu reported it to be 14%, whereas other researchers believe it to be as high as 25% (9,85).

Metastases to regional lymph nodes are frequent and can be present at the time of diagnosis. These metastases can have either a follicular or papillary pattern of growth.

Evidence that these tumors might be papillary in origin include, in addition to the nuclear features, multifocal involvement of the gland in some cases, rarity of vascular permeation and dissemination, frequency of lymph nodal involvement, and an immunophenotype similar to PTC.

The biologic behavior of this variant of PTC remains to be better defined, because there are cases in which this variant had an aggressive behavior characterized by extensive capsular and vascular invasion, diffuse involvement of the gland with extension into the adjacent soft tissues, and even distant metastases. These cases are definitely composed of follicles in which the PTC can be recognized cytologically, but they also exhibit increased mitosis and cellular pleomorphism. Further study of this aggressive follicular variant with a larger number of cases is needed.

Encapsulated

This variant of papillary cancer is recognized grossly by its thick capsule and gross appearance similar to that of follicular adenomas. They account for 10% to 15% of all papillary cancers, and are associated with an excellent prognosis, although metastases to regional lymph nodes can occur in up to 25% of the cases despite encapsulation (115).

Histologically, both papillary and follicular structures can be present, always lined by clear papillary carcinoma type nuclei. The amount of each component is variable, and in the experience of some pathologists, these tumors are frequently of a predominant follicular pattern. Psammoma bodies, as well as areas of hemorrhage, inflammation, and cystic degeneration of the nodules, can be present. Invasion of the capsule is not uncommon (1,9,85,103) (Fig. 15).

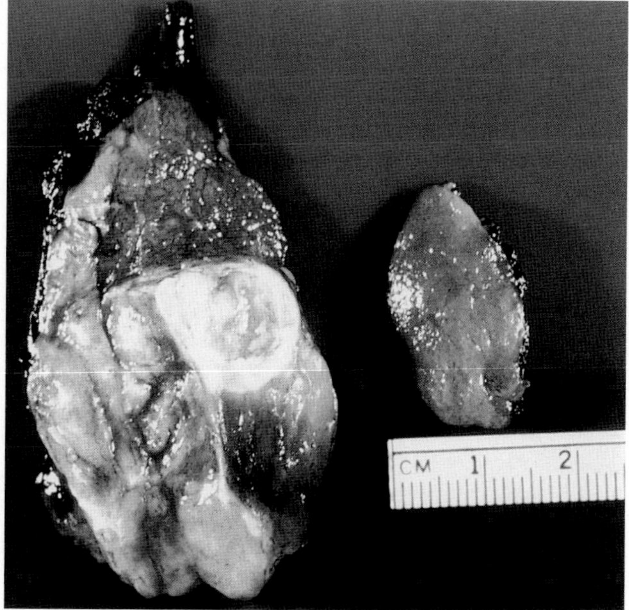

FIGURE 15. Gross photograph of an encapsulated variant of papillary carcinoma. Note the thick fibrous capsule.

Solid Variant

Carcangiu and collaborators recognized a rare type of papillary cancer with a solid or trabecular pattern of growth involving all or almost all of the neoplasm. The presence of clear or papillary cell nuclei is necessary, however, in order to make this diagnosis. Psammoma bodies also may be present (9,85).

Solid patterns of growth can be seen as part of other papillary and follicular neoplasms and are often associated with squamous metaplasia. This finding does not seem to affect prognosis.

Tumors with these morphologic features should be distinguished from poorly differentiated malignant thyroid neoplasms, which often have biologic behavior worse than that of most papillary carcinomas.

Variants of Papillary Cancer Associated with Aggressive Behavior

Diffuse Sclerosing

This unusual form of papillary cancer was originally described by Vickery and collaborators, who noticed that it developed more frequently in children and was associated with a grave prognosis (105). In our experience, it has been associated with total body irradiation. It accounts for 2% to 4% of all thyroid cancers. The tumors are characterized by diffuse involvement of one or both thyroid lobes; however, a dominant nodule can be detected in more than half of the cases. Grossly, the diffuse fibrosis and marked calcifications give the tumor a gritty cut surface.

Histologically, the tumor extensively infiltrates the gland with diffuse spread into the gland's lymphatic system. Small papillary structures are found scattered throughout the lobe in close association with numerous psammoma bodies and accompanied by dense sclerosis (Fig. 16). Marked squamous metaplasia that resembles squamous morulas and dense lymphocytic infiltration are also a common finding (Fig. 17).

Patients with this type of cancer have a higher incidence of lymph node and lung metastases, as well as an overall less favor-

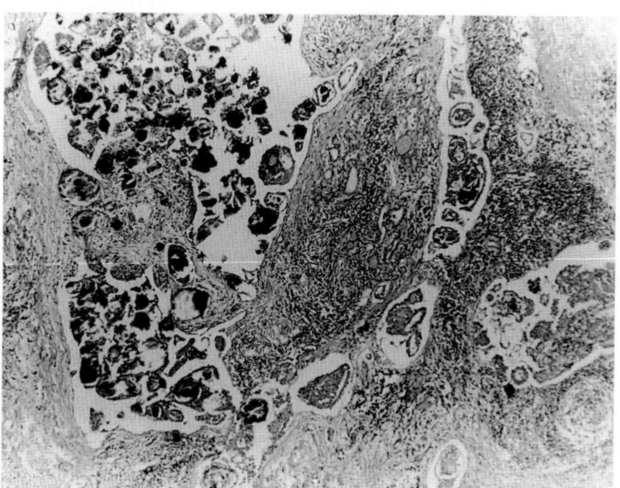

FIGURE 16. Low-power view of diffuse sclerosing variant of papillary carcinoma. Prominent lymphatic invasion and psammoma bodies are present (hematoxylin and eosin stain, original magnification ×100).

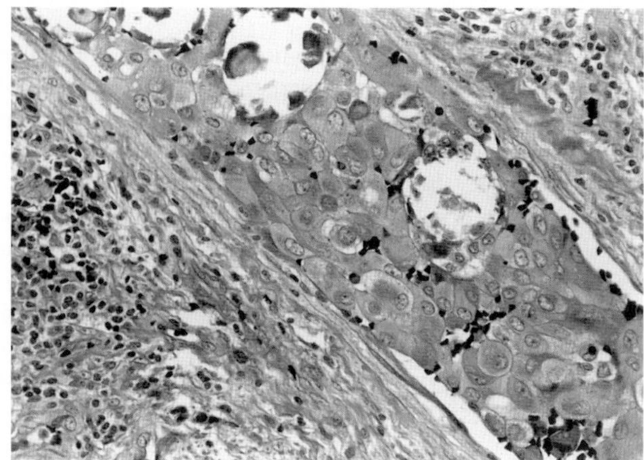

FIGURE 17. Diffuse sclerosing variant of papillary carcinoma. At high power, squamous metaplasia can be appreciated (hematoxylin and eosin stain, original magnification ×200).

able outcome when compared with traditional papillary cancer. However, other investigators have reported a prognosis similar to that of common variants, reflecting perhaps differences in the populations studied. The tumor biology of this unusual variant needs better definition (1,9,85,106).

Tall Cell Variant

In 1968, Hazard (116) described a rare type of papillary cancer whose main histologic features were tall columnar cells with heights that were twice the widths and with an eosinophilic cytoplasm. The tall cell features should be present in more than 30% of the tumor cells to warrant this diagnosis. The tumors are often quite large (>5cm) and extend beyond the thyroid, involving the adjacent soft tissues, a fact that is frequently noted at the time of surgery. Although the tumors more frequently affect elderly patients, all ages have been reported to have this variant.

Tall cell cancers comprise about 10% of all papillary carcinomas. They have a predominant papillary pattern of growth, but they also may form follicles devoid of colloid. Ground-glass nuclei are rarely present, but nuclear grooves and intranuclear invaginations are common (Fig. 18). Marked dense fibrous desmoplasia accompanies the tumor as it infiltrates the thyroid parenchyma and soft tissues. Heavy lymphocytic infiltration can be observed within the well-formed papillary structures as well as the stroma, which suggests that some of these neoplasms can arise in association with chronic thyroiditis (116,117).

This aggressive variant of papillary cancer may show associated squamous or anaplastic changes, suggesting the possibility of dedifferentiation and tumor progression. Another interesting feature of these tumors is the fact that once they metastasize, they may lose their ability to concentrate iodine, making follow-up and treatment of the patients difficult.

Tall cell cancers follow a more aggressive course than the usual papillary cancer, and recurrences are common in the neck, with tracheal invasion. Metastases to distant sites such as lung, bone, liver, pleura, and brain have been documented (117). Johnson and collaborators (118) compared 12 patients with tall cell carcinomas to an equal number of age- and sex-matched patients with classic papillary tumors. They found statistically significant differences in distant metastases, recurrences, and disease-specific mortality.

Tall cell papillary tumors are frequently misdiagnosed as Hürthle cell carcinomas because of their eosinophilic cytoplasm. Hürthle cell tumors, however, have a more intensely stained and dense cytoplasm, and the nucleus is smaller and hyperchromatic. Electron microscopy has shown abundant intracytoplasmic mitochondria filling the cells in both tumors; however, tall cell cancers lack all of the structural findings that are seen in Hürthle cells.

Columnar Cell

In 1986, Evans reported two cases of aggressive papillary cancer occurring in middle-aged men. The tumors were large and unencapsulated, with formations of papillary and follicular structures, but morphologically looked like secretory endometrium with marked subnuclear cytoplasmic clearing. The tumors lacked the typical nuclear features of papillary cancer and had areas of spindle, microfollicular, and tall cell differentiation (119). Pseudostratification of tumor cells was a prominent feature.

Both patients died of this disease within 2 years of diagnosis. Sobrinho-Simoes et al. have reported another case of columnar cell cancer and emphasized the poor prognosis associated with this type of cancer (120). It is possible that these tumors are part of the spectrum of tall cell carcinomas; two cases reported in the literature show overlap with tall cell histology (121,122).

Prognosis of Papillary Cancer

The prognosis of papillary cancer depends on the histologic tumor type, sex of the patient (male patients seem to follow a more aggressive course), age of the patient (age over 50 is associated with worse prognosis), and size (larger tumors have a tendency to infiltrate and metastasize more frequently) (123).

The role of hormone receptors, flow cytometry, and oncogene determination in the prognosis and treatment of these tumors remains to be determined (1,9,85,117,118).

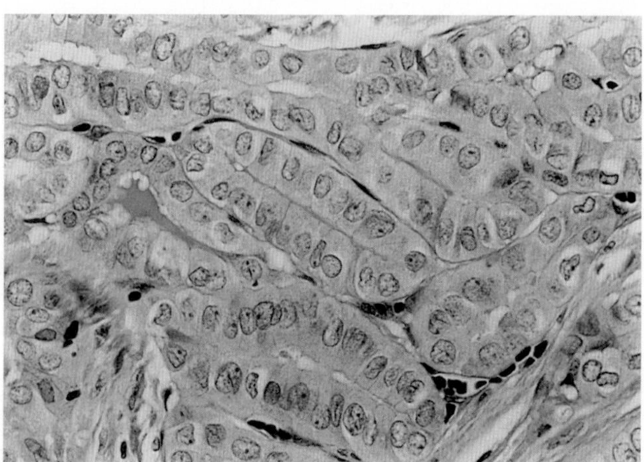

FIGURE 18. The tall cell variant of papillary carcinoma is composed of tall cells, at least twice as tall as they are wide (hematoxylin and eosin stain, original magnification ×200).

Treatment

The treatment of papillary cancer is still controversial, in part due to the multicentric nature of these tumors. Forms of therapy include lobectomy, total thyroidectomy with or without neck dissection, or radiation therapy via administration of iodine 131. In a study of 241 patients, Carcangiu et al. (85) compared all modalities of treatment and concluded that conservative surgery (lobectomy) was adequate therapy in the majority of cases. They recommended that total thyroidectomy and adjuvant therapy be reserved for older patients and patients with extrathyroidal extension or metastases. Total thyroidectomy, however, is the most common current form of treatment in the United States, not only because of possible multicentric involvement of the gland, but also because of the difficulties that arise when trying to treat and follow these patients with radioiodine when normal thyroid tissue is left behind.

Follicular Carcinoma

Follicular cancers are rare, accounting for 5% to 10% of all thyroid malignancies. The incidence, however, can be as high as 40% in endemic iodine-deficient regions, suggesting that iodine deficiency with subsequent high levels of TSH stimulation and goiter formation play a role in carcinogenesis. The incidence of follicular carcinoma may be artificially elevated, because many of the tumors previously classified as follicular cancers may currently be best classified as follicular variants of papillary cancer.

The disease affects middle-aged women more frequently than men, and rarely occurs in children. The incidence of well-differentiated follicular carcinoma in blacks is over twice the incidence in whites (80). This cancer has the strongest propensity of all thyroid tumors to concentrate radioiodine. Patients usually present with a single palpable cold nodule. On rare occasions, the initial manifestation is that of distant metastases, frequently in bone, lung, or brain (1,9,124,125).

Grossly, follicular cancer varies in size, has a yellow–tan cut surface, and often shows a thick white fibrous capsule. Areas of hemorrhage and necrosis are sometimes observed, as are foci of cystic degeneration. Unlike papillary carcinomas, these lesions are usually solitary. The gross differential diagnosis between adenomas and carcinomas sometimes may be difficult or impossible; a useful feature, when present, is a thick fibrous capsule seen around carcinomas.

Histologically, two main types are recognized, and they are described below.

Minimally Invasive

These tumors grossly and histologically resemble follicular adenomas. However, they are generally more cellular and may exhibit solid patterns of growth as well as marked trabecular configuration, with cellular pleomorphism and an increased number of mitoses. The diagnosis of cancer, however, is made when definite capsular or vascular invasion is found. Capsular invasion is defined as penetration of the entire thickness of the capsule by tumor cells (9) (Fig. 19). The presence of small clusters of follicular cells within the capsule is not definite evidence of invasion, because trapping of follicular epithelium can frequently occur. Frequently, this finding is seen as a sequela of FNA. Vascular dilatation, small hemorrhagic areas, inflammatory cells, and hemosiderin are also frequently identified after this procedure (126). In suspicious and worrisome cases, additional sectioning or levels deeper in the block may help to further clarify the diagnosis.

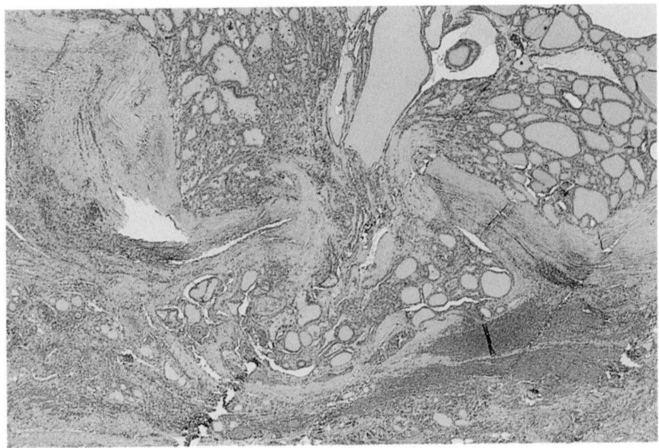

FIGURE 19. Follicular carcinoma showing capsular invasion with a mushroom or volcanic eruption-like pattern.

The other important histologic finding is vascular invasion. This parameter is defined as the presence of tumor thrombi in vascular structures or tumor invading vascular structures within the capsule or in vessels outside the capsule (Fig. 20). It is well recognized that thyroid neoplasms are rich in vessels, creating their own vascular framework as they grow. Consequently, clusters of tumor cells found in vessels within the main tumor mass have no prognostic significance.

The intravascular tumor may or may not be covered by endothelial cells. Immunohistochemical stains for Factor VIII–related antigens, CD34 or CD31, can be used. One should remember, however, that endothelial cells may not always be present in the sections examined, and in these cases the stains will be negative.

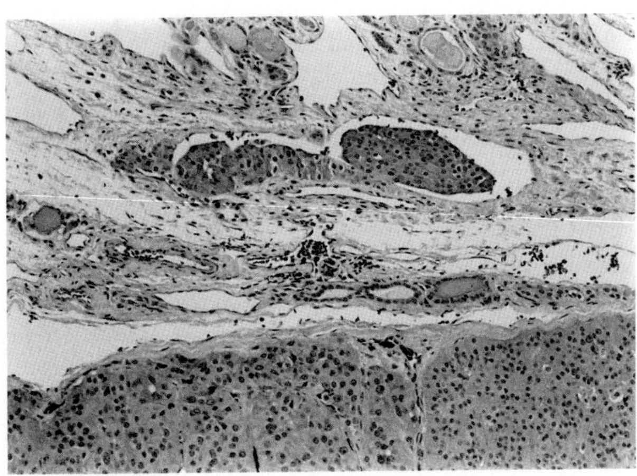

FIGURE 20. Follicular carcinoma showing vascular invasion (hematoxylin and eosin stain, original magnification ×200).

Controversies exist as to how to diagnose and treat cases in which only focal capsular invasion is noted, in the absence of vascular invasion. Some pathologists prefer to use the diagnosis of atypical follicular adenoma for such lesions and avoid altogether the diagnosis of cancer. However, these patients rarely may present many years later with bone, lung, or brain metastasis, and upon re-review of the original thyroid tumor, only minimal capsular invasion is noted. Some of these cases may represent improper evaluation of the capsule secondary to insufficient sampling or histologic misinterpretation. Another possible explanation is that the biologic behavior of these tumors is not uniform, and perhaps some tumors have a higher propensity to invade and eventually metastasize more often than others. In the future, molecular biologic studies may assist us in recognizing this group of aggressive tumors.

What is clear is that many of these lesions represent a diagnostic dilemma. For the present, the general consensus is that the presence of definitive, unequivocal complete transcapsule invasion merits a diagnosis of follicular carcinoma, to assure close follow-up of the patients, keeping in mind those cases that have had late recurrences. Further studies with large series of cases may help to elucidate further the true biology of these neoplasms.

Kahn and Perzin (127) evaluated histologic criteria in 68 cases of follicular carcinoma and concluded that the most important parameter to make the diagnosis of cancer was unequivocal invasion—capsular, vascular, or into adjacent thyroid tissue. Their definition of capsular invasion is similar to that previously described. They also found an increased incidence of metastatic disease when there was vascular invasion, invasion into extrathyroidal tissues, a microfollicular pattern, increased size of the primary lesion, and local recurrences.

Minimally invasive carcinoma is treated with unilateral lobectomy. These tumors disseminate via blood vessels, and metastases may occur to the lung, bone, and brain. Metastases can be treated with radioiodine. However, when tumors lose their ability to concentrate iodine, treatment of extracervical metastases is difficult. Administration of the radioisotope as a conjugate of monoclonal antibodies is being studied as an alternative modality of therapy.

The prognosis of minimally invasive thyroid cancer is excellent. However, factors associated with worse outcome have included lesions that have a solid pattern of growth, are aneuploid by flow cytometry studies, and occur in elderly males. The differential diagnosis of minimally invasive follicular cancer includes follicular variants of papillary carcinoma and the follicular variant of medullary carcinoma.

Widely Invasive

These tumors, as their name implies, infiltrate extensively through the capsule into the thyroid parenchyma, have prominent vascular invasion, nuclear pleomorphism, mitotic activity, and necrosis (1). There is frequent extension into the adjacent soft tissues of the neck, and patients carry a poor prognosis.

RAS and GSP point mutations have been identified by polymerase chain reaction (PCR) in both follicular adenomas and carcinomas, suggesting that these mutations occur early in thyroid tumorigenesis (128,129). Activating mutations of the genes for the thyrotropin receptor and the alpha subunit of the stimulatory G protein also have been reported in follicular carcinomas (129,130).

Hürthle Cell Tumors (Benign and Malignant)

Hürthle cell tumors, also known as oncocytic or oxyphilic tumors, are neoplasms of follicular origin that LiVolsi defined as having more than 75% of the lesion composed of Hürthle cells or oncocytes (1). Hürthle cell tumors occur most commonly in adult women and present as a hypofunctioning nodule.

Thyroid oncocytes are follicular cells characterized by their granular eosinophilic or orangiophilic cytoplasm, large, dark hyperchromatic nucleus with prominent nucleolus, and well-demarcated cellular borders. Electron microscopic studies have shown that these cells contain abundant abnormal mitochondria and few other residual cytoplasmic organelles. The mitochondria may be irregularly shaped and dilated with few other cristae, and may have pleomorphic bodies. It is not known why these cells are so rich in mitochondria. These changes were originally felt to be part of a degenerative process. However, it has been demonstrated that these cells are rich in oxidative enzymes and are biochemically active, with the capacity to produce and contain thyroglobulin (131). Oncocytic cells can occur in a variety of benign and malignant neoplasms throughout the body, and therefore are not specific to thyroid disease.

The prognosis of Hürthle cell tumors in the thyroid has been controversial for many years. Some researchers have considered all oncocytic tumors as malignant, suggesting total thyroidectomy as the best modality of treatment. However, as the biology of these tumors has come to be better understood (131–139), it appears that not all Hürthle cell neoplasms are malignant; rather, the majority can be classified as Hürthle cell (oncocytic) adenomas and the remainder as carcinomas. In essence, the same criteria for malignancy are applied to Hürthle cell tumors as to non–Hürthle cell tumors of the thyroid. An oncocytic variant of papillary cancer also has been recognized.

Hürthle Cell Adenomas

These are well circumscribed and encapsulated lesions that are homogeneous and brown on cut section (Fig. 21). Areas of hemorrhage may be present in large lesions or as the result of recent FNA (126).

Histologic evaluation of the specimen is performed to distinguish benign from malignant lesions following established criteria for follicular tumors (i.e., identifying the presence or absence of capsular and vascular invasion) (1,9).

Oncocytic adenomas have an intact capsule and no evidence of vascular invasion. The cells can grow in a solid, trabecular, or follicular pattern. Papillary structures can be present, but usually they do not have well-formed fibrous stalks. Rare nuclear pseudoinclusions and occasional nuclear grooves can be seen. Hürthle cell tumors can undergo spontaneous hemorrhage and infarction, which does not imply malignancy. These changes are frequently found following FNA. Lobectomy is the modality of treatment, and patients follow a benign clinical course.

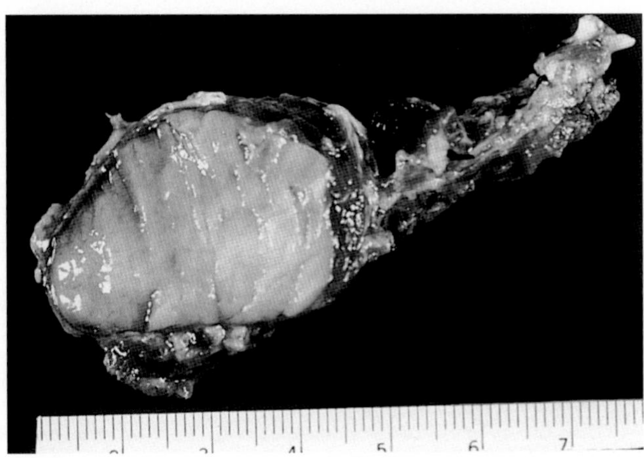

FIGURE 21. Follicular adenoma, Hürthle cell type. A homogeneous appearance is evident.

Hürthle Cell Carcinoma

Oncocytic carcinomas represent about 3% of all thyroid cancers and account for about 20% of all follicular lesions (9). The clinical presentation is similar to that of follicular cancers. Unfortunately, Hürthle cell tumors frequently do not take up radioiodine and appear as hypofunctioning nodules, making metastases difficult to identify and treat (133–139).

Grossly, these are large tumor masses with a characteristic brown cut surface. Areas of hemorrhage and necrosis are common. Histologically, there is evidence of capsular and vascular invasion. Carcinomas also may have an increased number of mitoses, nuclear hyperchromasia, cellular pleomorphism, and necrosis. It has been suggested that within the spectrum of Hürthle cell carcinomas, patients harboring tumors with solid or trabecular architectural patterns fare worse (140). In some cases, these patterns mixed with common forms of follicular cancer also can be seen. Rosai classifies these lesions as minimally invasive and widely invasive, following previously described criteria for follicular carcimomas.

Total thyroidectomy is recommended for cases of Hürthle cell carcinoma. These carcinomas have a capacity to metastasize to regional lymph nodes as well as to spread hematogenously to lung, bone, and liver. The 5-year survival rate varies between 50% and 60%, but late metastases can occur (133–139, 141,142).

In a recent review comparing Hürthle cell and classic follicular carcinomas of the thyroid, Evans and Vassilopoulou-Sellin concluded that when cases were stratified according to extent of invasion, the behavorial differences of these two tumors were not statistically significant (143).

Flow cytometry has not proven useful to distinguish between benign and malignant Hürthle cell tumors, because more than 50% of adenomas can show aneuploidy. However, aneuploidy may characterize a subset of patients with oncocytic carcinomas that may follow a more aggressive course (144).

Rare Hürthle cell tumors that are histologically similar to Warthin's tumors have been described. These tumors are composed of oncocytic cells with a papillary architecture arising in glands with chronic lymphocytic thyroiditis. The majority of these cases affect women and appear to behave similarly to typical papillary cancer (145).

Takiyama et al. have found that Hürthle cell carcinomas have more genetic alterations on chromosome 1q and 2p than Hürthle cell adenomas and that all Hürthle cell neoplasms have a significantly higher frequency of alterations in chromosome 1p as compared with the normal thyroid (146).

Poorly Differentiated (Insular) Carcinoma

Carcangiu et al. (84) reported 25 cases of a special variant of thyroid cancer that appears to have distinct morphologic features and biologic behavior. These tumors occur in an older population and frequently metastasize to lymph nodes, lung, and bone, ultimately leading to death. The researchers suggested that this aggressive behavior places insular carcinoma in an intermediate position between differentiated papillary and follicular cancers and the highly malignant anaplastic carcinoma.

Histologically, these tumors are recognized by the formation of solid cellular clusters containing a variable number of follicles filled with uniform small round cells with scant cytoplasm. These cells are characteristically arranged in a trabecular pattern with spaces, often containing thin-walled blood vessels, between them, creating trabecular islands or insulae (Fig. 22). Capsular and vascular invasion, necrosis, and high mitotic rates are also often present.

Unlike anaplastic carcinomas, these tumors usually concentrate radioiodine (147,148). By immunohistochemistry, there is reactivity for thyroglobulin. Calcitonin is negative, differentiating this neoplasm from medullary thyroid carcinoma (MTC). Most of the cases of insular carcinoma have been reported in European patients (149).

Anaplastic Carcinoma (Undifferentiated Carcinoma)

Anaplastic carcinoma accounts for only 4% to 10% of all thyroid tumors; however, it is one of the most rapidly growing and lethal of all malignancies. The tumors occur predominantly in elderly women, with a female:male ratio of 3:1. Very few cases have been reported in patients under 40 years of age (1,9,150–152).

Clinically, anaplastic tumors present as rapidly enlarging neck masses associated with symptoms such as dysphagia, hoarseness, dyspnea, and enlargement of cervical lymph nodes (150). Commonly, symptoms are of rapid onset. Distant metastases are found at presentation in a small percentage of patients. Not infrequently, the patients have a prior history of nodular goiter. The etiology of this highly aggressive neoplasm is not known; however, some researchers have associated its development with previous external neck irradiation for treatment of more indolent forms of thyroid cancer (153).

Grossly, the tumors appear as large bulky masses extending into adjacent soft tissues, trachea, and lymph nodes. Cut surfaces show replacement of normal thyroid tissues by solid or focally necrotic, hemorrhagic and yellow tumor.

Microscopically, three basic patterns are recognized: spindle cell, giant cell, and squamoid. The spindle cell type may be

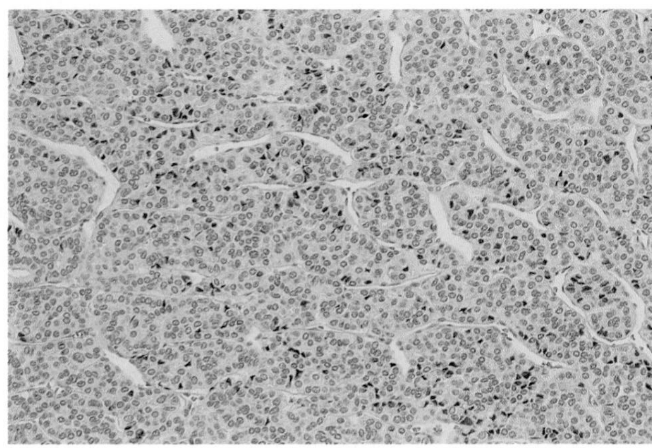

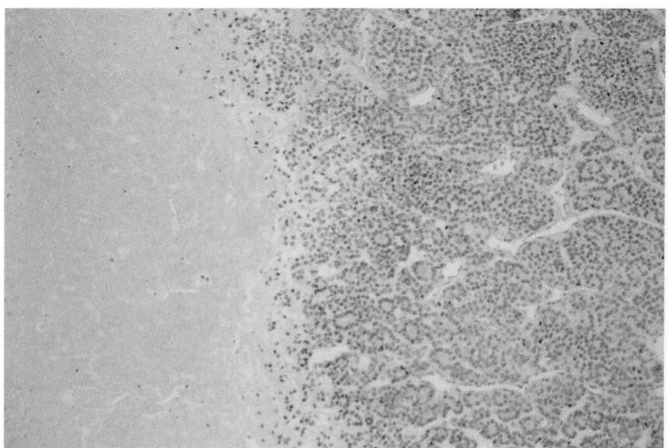

FIGURE 22. Insular carcinoma. **A:**. Trabecular nests (insulae) of tumor cells are separated by spaces containing thin-walled blood vessels. **B:** The tumor is focally necrotic.

arranged in a storiform or fascicular pattern of growth and may resemble sarcomas such as fibrosarcoma, rhabdomyosarcoma, hemangiopericytoma, or malignant fibrous histiocytoma. The cells have varying degrees of nuclear pleomorphism and mitotic activity (Fig. 23). Occasionally, these sarcoma-like areas also may contain inflammatory cells, giant cells, and epithelioid cells. Necrosis is common and may be extensive, perhaps due to the high propensity these tumors have to invade blood vessels. This pattern can be found singly or in combination with the other two types (150).

The giant cell type is predominantly composed of multinucleated giant cells with multiple, large, hyperchromatic (and sometimes bizarre) nuclei and abundant eosinophilic cytoplasm. These giant cells may be the sole or predominant component, or they may be mixed with a smaller more histiocyte-like cell. Occasional tumors contain a component of more bland-appearing osteoclast-like giant cells. These cells have ultrastructural features suggestive of histiocytic derivation. These osteoclast-like cells stain positively with KP-1, a macrophage-associated antigen highly specific for histiocytes. Tumor cells also stain for acid phosphatase. These tumors are similar to the giant cell tumors reported in the breast, uterus, and pancreas (154,155).

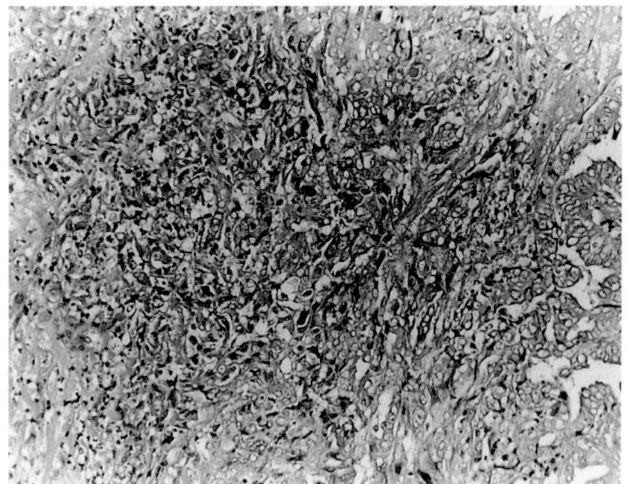

FIGURE 23. Anaplastic carcinoma of thyroid. Poorly differentiated malignant fusiform cells (hematoxylin and eosin stain, original magnification ×150).

The squamous pattern is similar to nonkeratinizing, poorly differentiated squamous cell carcinoma. Mucin production occasionally can be demonstrated in the cytoplasm of the cells. Immunohistochemical stains for carcinoembryonic antigen (CEA) can be positive.

Residual areas of well-differentiated carcinoma, usually papillary and infrequently follicular, are often found in cases of anaplastic thyroid carcinoma, suggesting that anaplastic carcinoma may represent the dedifferentiated expression of these well-differentiated tumors (156,157).

The differential diagnosis for undifferentiated or anaplastic carcinoma includes the rare true thyroid sarcoma, medullary carcinoma, insular carcinoma, and metastasis. Electron microscopy of anaplastic carcinoma reveals epithelial differentiation in about 50% of cases, with the presence of intercellular junctions, microvilli, and filaments. Immunohistochemical staining for cytokeratin and EMA may be helpful in the differential diagnosis (150,158,159). Anaplastic thyroid carcinoma also can stain positively for CEA and vimentin. Immunoreactivity with thyroglobulin is an unreliable marker because some researchers (150,160) did not find positivity in any of their cases, whereas focal reactivity was found in a very low percentage of cases by others (151,156–160).

Mutations in the p53 gene have been identified in anaplastic carcinomas and anaplastic carcinoma cell lines (161–163).

The prognosis of patients with anaplastic carcinoma is dismal, with the majority of patients dying within 1 year as a result of involvement of contiguous neck structures by tumor. Metastases can occur to the lungs, or to the brain, adrenal tissues, or other distant sites. Radiation and chemotherapy have been used in combination therapy, but without much success (1,9,150–153,164).

Squamous Cell Carcinoma

Primary squamous cell carcinoma of the thyroid is rare, accounting for less than 1% of all thyroid tumors (Fig. 24). The

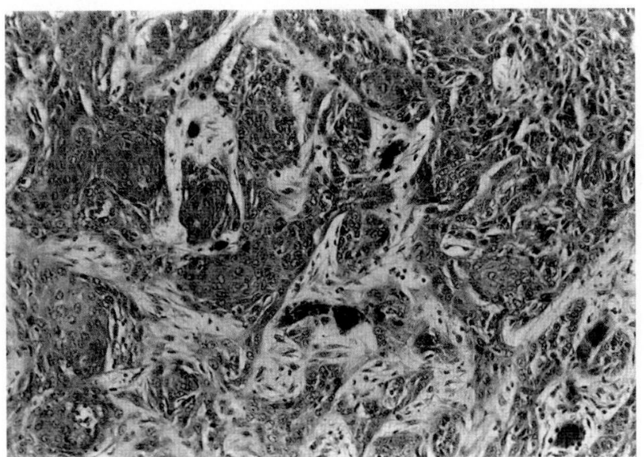

FIGURE 24. High-power view of a squamous cell carcinoma (hematoxylin and eosin stain, original magnification ×150).

histogenesis of this malignancy is not entirely understood, but nests of squamous epithelium have been found in the ultimobranchial bodies of some mammals and as the result of metaplastic changes of the follicular cells in certain chronic thyroid diseases (165).

Cases of squamous and adenosquamous carcinomas of the thyroid have been reported in patients who have received local radiation therapy for malignant lymphoma. Patients with this type of tumor carry a poor prognosis (166).

Tumors with Clear Cells

Follicular cells with abundant clear cytoplasm have long been recognized to be present in a variety of thyroid neoplasms that include otherwise typical follicular, papillary, Hürthle cell, and even anaplastic carcinoma. Most primary clear cell carcinomas of the thyroid display features of follicular carcinoma (Fig. 25).

The reason for the clear appearance of the cytoplasm in these cells is not completely understood. Civantos et al. (167) have postulated that this change may be the result of chronic TSH overstimulation. Studies by Carcangiu et al. (168) reported glycogen, mucin, and distended mitochondria as potential causes of the clear appearance of the cytoplasm. The presence or amount of clear cells does not affect the biology of the tumors; rather, the significance of recognizing a primary thyroid tumor with clear cells rests in its differentiation from metastases of other tumors with similar features, such as parathyroid cancer and renal cell carcinoma.

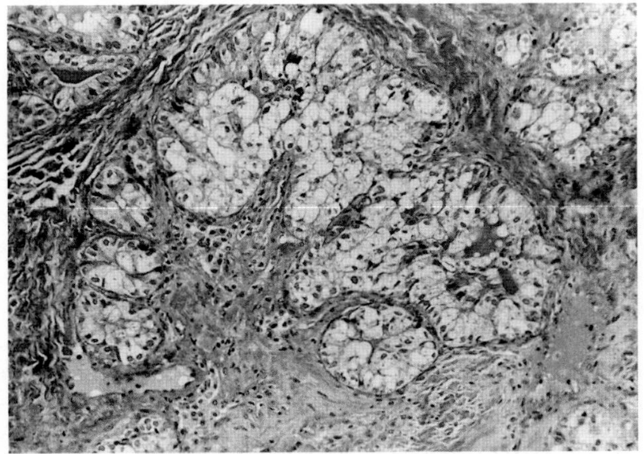

FIGURE 25. Clear cell changes in the cytoplasm are present in this follicular carcinoma (hematoxylin and eosin stain, original magnification ×100).

Clear cell change also can occur in a variety of benign conditions, including Hashimoto's thyroiditis and dyshormonogenetic goiter (168); however, the presence of clear cells in a follicular neoplasm should be regarded with suspicion, because these findings are more often associated with cancer.

Medullary Carcinoma

Medullary thyroid carcinoma (MTC), first described by Horn (169), was recognized as a specific clinicopathologic entity by Hazard (170), who believed it was a variant of poorly differentiated carcinoma based on its solid pattern of growth.

It was later demonstrated that these tumors derived from the C cells that originate from the cells of the branchial pouches and differentiate to have neuroendocrine features. These cells are the source of the hormone calcitonin and, infrequently, other peptides, including serotonin, adrenocorticotrophic hormone, and somatostatin (171).

There are two major types of MTC: the sporadic, which is the most common form, accounting for 70% to 80% of all tumors, and the familial or genetically determined form, which is inherited as an autosomal dominant trait and accounts for the remaining 20% to 30% of cases. Mutations of the *RET* protooncogene have been identified in both familial and sporadic medullary carcinoma. Patients in affected families may have other syndromes such as Sipple's syndrome (MEN type 2 or 2a), in which coexistence of thyroid, adrenal gland, and parathyroid tumors may be found. In MEN type 2b, patients also have endocrine tumors, marfanoid phenotype, mucosal neuromas, and ganglioneuromas. Studies indicate that MTC is frequently preceded by C-cell hyperplasia in these patients (172–176).

Medullary carcinoma accounts for 3% to 10% of all thyroid tumors and affects both sexes nearly equally. It can occur at any age, with most patients diagnosed with the sporadic form being 40 to 50 years of age. These patients usually present with a solitary thyroid mass, cervical adenopathy, and rarely diarrhea, flushing, and Cushing's syndrome. In the familial form, the tumors are frequently multiple and bilateral and affect a younger age group. Because these tumors are common among children in affected families, it is recommended that thyroid screening begin by age 3 in this population (1,9,175).

The tumors are located in the lateral aspects of the middle and upper segments of the thyroid, areas that have the highest concentration of C cells. Grossly, MTC can be circumscribed or infiltrative. The cut surface of the tumors is white to yellow. Areas of hemorrhage and necrosis can be seen in larger lesions. Frequently, only small tumors or C-cell hyperplasia is

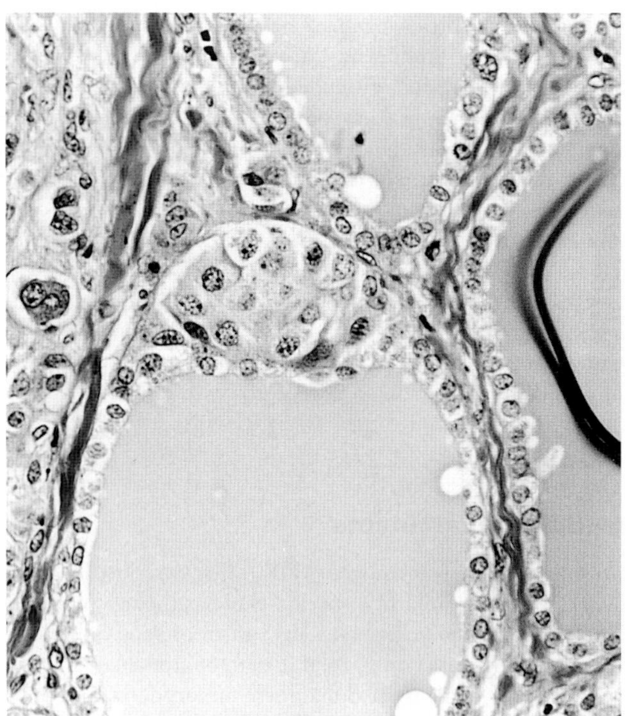

FIGURE 26. C-cell hyperplasia, typically seen in patients with MEN syndrome (hematoxylin and eosin stain, original magnification ×150).

found when screening members of a MEN syndrome family (Fig. 26).

Histology

The classic medullary cancer is composed of nests, cords, and trabeculae of tumor cells, which are of medium size and have abundant, sometimes eosinophilic cytoplasm. The cells can take on a spindled or epithelioid appearance (Fig. 27). The nuclei are round, quite uniform, and regular with minimal pleomorphism. Intranuclear inclusions and mitoses are frequent findings. The nests of cells are surrounded by a delicate vascular network and fibrous tissue. Necrosis and hemorrhage are rare. A helpful feature, identified in about 75% of tumors, is the presence of masses of dense eosinophilic amyloid material that stain positively with Congo red and crystal violet (177) (Fig. 28). Several variations from the classic pattern are recognized.

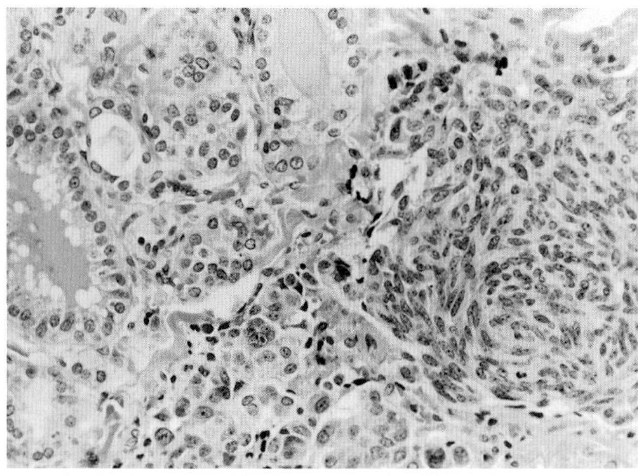

FIGURE 27. Medullary carcinoma, spindle cell type (at right) (hematoxylin and eosin stain, original magnification ×150).

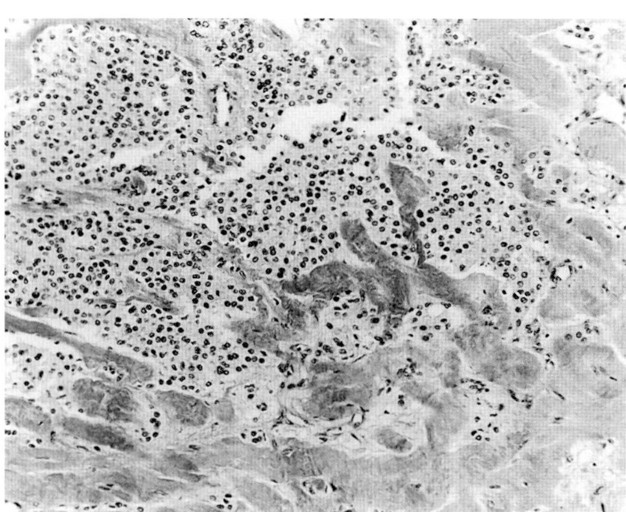

FIGURE 28. Medullary carcinoma. The abundant amyloid that is present associated with nests of tumor cells (hematoxylin and eosin stain, original magnification ×150).

Papillary structures may occur in these lesions, with scant stroma. The papillary fronds have fibrovascular stalks containing amyloid-rich material. These tumors have to be distinguished from true papillary carcinomas. The presence of amyloid and immunohistochemical reactivity for calcitonin assist in making the correct diagnosis. However, a true papillary pattern is rare.

Tubular or glandular formation is frequently found in medullary cancer; the lumina of the glands may contain eosinophilic proteinaceous material.

Rarely MTC is composed of uniform small cells with hyperchromatic nuclei and scant cytoplasm similar to the intermediate variant of small cell cancer of the lung and other sites. Again, amyloid deposits are usually appreciated.

Medullary thyroid carcinoma with prominent clear cells has been described and should be distinguished from metastases to the thyroid. Mucin has been demonstrated in the clear or pale cytoplasm.

Giant cell formation may coexist with other types of medullary cancer. It is important to distinguish this variant from anaplastic carcinoma. Anaplastic carcinomas usually extend beyond the thyroid gland, have bizarre cells with increased nuclear to cytoplasmic ratios and frequent mitoses, and are associated with extensive necrosis (1,9,172,173,176–184).

In addition to amyloid, medullary carcinoma may contain mucin (185), melanin (186,187), and, as mentioned before, other polypeptide hormones demonstrable by immunohistochemical stains (173). MTC also shows positive staining for CEA, chromogranin, synaptophysin, and NSE (188–191). Thyroglobulin is rarely positive (192,193). The characteristic feature of MTCs is the production of calcitonin, a peptide that is present in the great majority of cases, and can be demonstrated in the cytoplasm of the cells by immunohistochemial staining with anticalcitonin antibodies. *In situ* hybridization using probes for calcitonin messenger RNA (mRNA) and other gene-related peptide mRNAs shows positive signals in the tumor cells (194). By electron microscopy, the tumor cells usually contain moderate numbers of dense-core neurosecretory-type granules, granular endoplasmic reticulum, and polyribosomes (173).

Cases of calcitonin-free medullary carcinoma exist in familial settings or in association with C-cell hyperplasia. However, these are extremely rare and usually stain for CEA, synaptophysin, and chromogranin. Absence of amyloid also has been reported up to 25% of the time (195).

Medullary thyroid carcinoma has a tendency to metastasize to regional lymph nodes, lung, liver, and bone. Lymph nodal dissection of the central compartment yields metastases over 50% of the time in both sporadic and familial MTC (196–198). The prognosis depends on age, sex (younger patients and women have a better prognosis), size of the tumor, and stage. Reportedly, patients with MEN type 2B have the most clinically aggressive tumors, with early metastases and death from disease (175). Other established prognostic parameters include histologic type, mitotic count, necrosis, and amount of calcitonin and amyloid present. The 5-year survival rate is 60% to 70%. Total thyroidectomy is the modality of treatment for both sporadic and familial patients. Follow-up of MTC is based on monitoring basal and stimulated plasma calcitonin levels (1,9,176,196–199).

Mixed Medullary and Follicular Carcinoma

Hales and collaborators described a thyroid cancer with a predominant medullary pattern but in which areas of follicular differentiation were also present. The tumor stained positive for calcitonin and thyroglobulin. Histologically, these tumors usually have a combination of both trabecular and follicular patterns. These patterns can be present in the metastases as well (200).

Mixed tumors may behave aggressively. Special stains for CEA, chromogranin, somatostatin, and other markers of medullary carcinoma should be performed (200,201).

Sclerosing Mucepidermoid Carcinoma with Eosinophilia

First described by Chan et al. in 1991, sclerosing mucoepidermoid carcinoma with eosinophilia is a rare primary malignancy of the thyroid usually seen in association with Hashimoto's thyroiditis (202). The majority of the cases described in the literature have occurred in females. Histologically the tumors are infiltrative with dense sclerotic stroma. Characteristically there are abundant eosinophilia and nests and islands of pleomorphic squamous cells and scattered mucous cells. The adjacent gland is usually involved by Hashimoto's thyroiditis. Peripherial eosinophilia has not been described (202,203).

Immunohistochemical studies show the tumor cells to be cytokeratin and CEA positive, but negative for thyroglobulin and calcitonin. Although many of the tumors have pursued a less aggressive course, in some of the reported cases, tumor extended locally to involve other structures in the neck. Metastases to regional lymph nodes and bone have been reported (202–204).

Small Cell Carcinoma

Small cell carcinomas of the thyroid are unusual and controversial lesions, difficult to differentiate from lymphomas by light microscopy. Meissner (205) described two types of small cell carcinoma: the compact and the diffuse type.

The compact type is composed of nests of small uniform epithelial cells with prominent nuclei, eosinophilic cytoplasm, frequent mitoses, and hyalinized stroma. This type probably represents a variant of medullary carcinoma.

The diffuse type histologically resembles malignant lymphoma and is rare. Probably most cases of small cell carcinoma reported in the literature would be best classified as malignant lymphoma. In all suspected cases, lymphoma should be ruled out by either immunohistochemistry or electron microscopy. Thus, the existence of this tumor type is open to some question.

In addition to malignant lymphoma, a putative small cell carcinoma also must be distinguished from medullary and poorly differentiated or insular carcinomas. The tumor cell uniformity and occasional follicle formation in the latter lesion may be helpful clues to assist in the diagnosis. Additionally, insular carcinomas contain abundant necrosis in the absence of amyloid. Studies with immmunohistochemistry are essential to make this differential diagnosis (1,9,54).

Thyroid Tumors of Probable Thymic/Branchial Origin

Spindle Epithelial Tumor with Thymus-like Differentiation (SETTLE)

SETTLE is the term given by Chan and Rosai in 1991 to a rare group of thyroid neoplasms of presumed thymic or related branchial derivation (9,206). The tumors occur in children and young adults, the mean age of 14 patients reported in the literature being 16.9 years (206–211). The tumors usually present as a mass in the region of the thyroid gland. Grossly, the tumor may be circumscribed or occasionally infiltrative, mainly firm and solid but with occasional small cysts present. Histologically, the tumor is composed of masses of bland, uniform-appearing spindled cells with scant cytoplasm and with few mitotic figures that merge with more epithelial-appearing structures. These latter structures may be duct-like or tubular, papillary, or solid and squamoid (Fig. 29). The abrupt occurrence of cystic spaces lined by mucus-containing epithelial cells or respiratory epithelium is noted at times, although the frankly epithelial structures may not be prominent and the tumor may appear predominantly monophasic (spindled) (210). The tumors have a fibrotic stroma with fibrous bands traversing the lesion. The spindled cells are epithelial, as shown by strong immunohistochemical staining for keratin as well as ultrastruc-

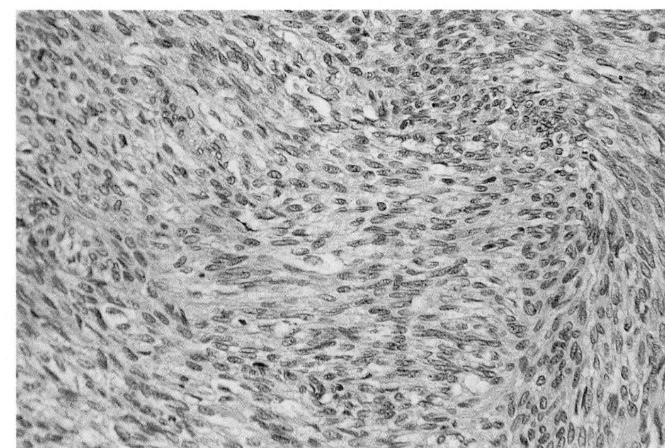

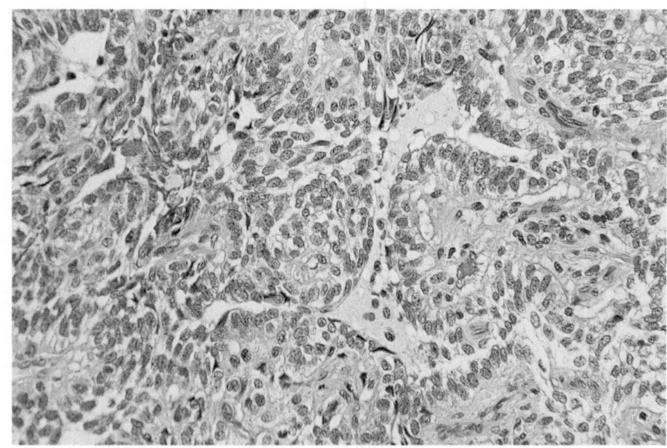

FIGURE 29. Spindle epithelial tumor with thymus-like differentiation (SETTLE). **A:** Cellular array of cytologically bland spindle cells. **B:** The spindled cells merge with epithelial-lined tubular structures.

tural evidence of tonofilaments and desmosomes (209). The spindled epithelial cells and tubular structures are reminiscent of thymic differentiation, and the immunonegativity of the tumor for thyroglobulin reinforces the notion that the tumor is not derived from follicular epithelium. Interestingly, an area of prominent solid cell nests adjacent to the tumor in the case illustrated lends further support to a relationship to branchial (or ultimobranchial) structures (Fig. 30). The biologic behavior of SETTLE is generally favorable, although occasional late metastases have been reported (9,206). Thus, the tumor should probably be considered as a low-grade malignancy.

Differential diagnosis is from the rare intrathyroidal thymoma and from the more aggressive synovial cell sarcoma. A thymoma generally has a more conspicuous lymphoid component without mucus-containing or respiratory epithelium, whereas synovial cell sarcoma is generally more atypical appearing, more mitotically active, and has less prominent keratin staining in its spindle cell component than SETTLE, and often has a focally prominent hemangiopericytomatous vascular pattern, not seen in SETTLE.

Carcinoma Showing Thymus-like Differentiation (CASTLE)

CASTLE, like SETTLE, is a rare tumor, usually involving the thyroid gland, that is thought to arise from thymic or related branchial tissue (9,206,212–214). It occurs in an older patient population than SETTLE, the average age of patients with CASTLE being about 48 years (9,206). The usual clinical presentation is as a thyroid mass. The tumor was originally called an intrathyroid thymoma, but it actually most closely resembles a lymphoepitheliomatous type of thymic carcinoma. Thus, it is composed of large epithelial tumor cells with ill-defined cell borders and with large vesicular nuclei with prominent nucleoli admixed with lymphocytes, reminiscent of nasopharyngeal lymphoepitheliomatous carcinoma (Fig. 31). Frank squamous differentiation is occasionally seen. CASTLE is immunohistochemically positive for keratin and negative for thyroglobulin and calcitonin. Ultrastructural studies show the tumor cells to have tonofilaments and desmosomes (9). As opposed to nasopharyngeal carcinoma, mitotic figures are infrequent, and the

FIGURE 30. Spindle epithelial tumor with thymus-like differentiation (SETTLE). A proliferation of solid cell nests is present near the tumor.

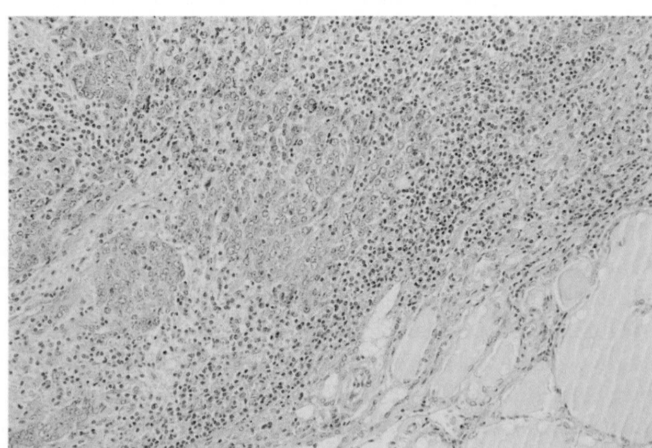

FIGURE 31. Carcinoma showing thymus-like differentiation (CASTLE). A poorly differentiated carcinoma in lymphoid stroma, reminiscent of the lymphoepitheliomatous type of thymic carcinoma, is present in the thyroid gland. (Case courtesy of Dr. David Dorfman.)

one case of CASTLE so investigated in a Chinese patient did not show *in situ* hybridization for Epstein-Barr virus nucleic acid (215). In addition, the biologic behavior of CASTLE is significantly less aggressive than nasopharyngeal carcinomas, and although lymph node metastases occur, the clinical course is usually indolent, with local recurrence generally occurring late (206).

Malignant Lymphoma

For years the existence of primary malignant lymphoma of the thyroid as an entity was debated, and the majority of the lesions were classified as epithelial small cell cancers. The development of diagnostic immunohistochemical and molecular techniques has allowed the confirmation of the existence of this entity, and it is now believed that non-Hodgkin's lymphoma of the thyroid, albeit rare, accounts for 1.6% to 8% of malignant thyroid disease (216–220).

Lymphoma is commonly found in the setting of Hashimoto's thyroiditis. These tumors generally occur in patients over the age of 50 with a peak incidence around 65 (although cases have been reported in younger individuals). It is more common in women than men (ratio of 3:1) and in whites. Patients usually complain of either a rapidly enlarging neck mass, hoarseness, dysphasia, stridor, or dyspnea; some have vocal cord paralysis. The symptoms can last from days to months. Thyroid function tests show that most patients are euthyroid or hypothyroid, but occasional cases of hyperthyroidism have been reported. Thyroid scans show either single or multiple cold nodules (54,221,222).

Grossly, the gland may be markedly enlarged and bulky, weighing up to 500 g or more. The tumors are usually white or tan with a fish-flesh appearance, similar to nodal lymphomas (Fig. 32). Extension beyond the capsule into adjacent tissues is quite frequent.

Histologically, most tumors are diffuse B-cell lymphomas, although all types of malignant lymphoma, including Hodgkin's disease, have been reported. Pedersen and Pedersen evaluated 50 cases of primary non-Hodgkin's lymphoma of the thyroid. In 83% of their cases, they found tumor morphology exhibiting the histologic spectrum of disease from Hashimoto's thyroiditis to low-grade lymphoma of mucosa-associated lymphoid tissue (MALT) to a transformation to high-grade non-Hodgkin's lymphoma (222). Pledge et al. (223) and Hyjek and Isaacson (54) found similar findings in a series of 43 patients.

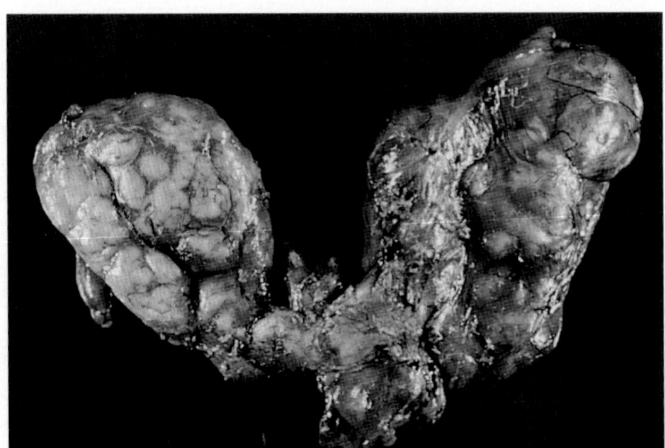

FIGURE 32. Gross appearance of malignant lymphoma involving the entire thyroid.

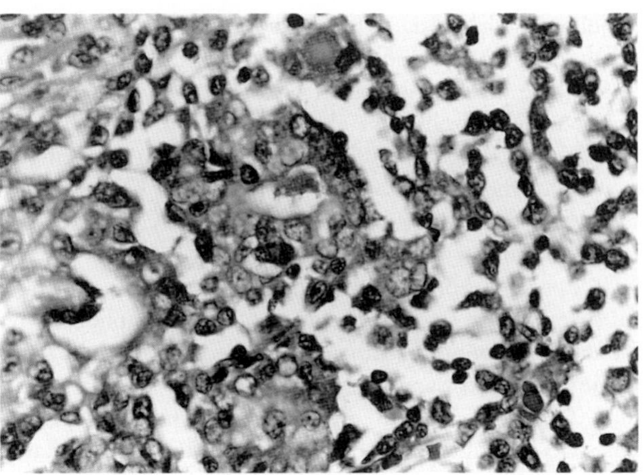

FIGURE 33. Remnants of thyroid follicular epithelium destroyed by malignant lymphoid cells (hematoxylin and eosin stain, original magnification ×100).

The histology of MALT lymphoma of the thyroid consists of the triad of centrocyte-like cells, lymphoepithelial lesions, and large lymphoid follicles (see Chapter 12). The centrocyte-like cells sheet out and replace the thyroid parenchyma and infiltrate follicles. Immunohistochemical expression of monoclonal immune globulin is necessary for the diagnosis. Stains for cytokeratin help delineate the lymphoepithelial lesions.

Immunoblastic sarcoma of the B-cell type is the second most common type of lymphoma (224). These tumors can occur in both the diffuse or follicular form. In general, the normal thyroid architecture is replaced by a diffuse homogeneous infiltrate of immature lymphocytes that have vesicular nuclei and moderate amounts of cytoplasm. The malignant cells have plasmacytoid features with prominent nucleoli and abundant eosinophilic cytoplasm. Mitoses, as well as necrosis and extension into perithyroidal fat, are common. Multinucleated and Reed-Sternberg–like cells are present. Occasionally, atrophic follicles or single epithelial cells with oncocytic features are found intermixed with the tumor cells (Fig. 33). Evidence of Hashimoto's thyroiditis has been found histologically in 30% to 95% of these patients as well, but a preexisting disease may be difficult to demonstrate in cases in which the tumor replaces the entire gland.

Although the majority of the cases of malignant lymphoma of the thyroid are immunoreactive for leukocyte common antigen and B-cell markers, immunohistochemical stains for surface immunoglobulins can show variable results (225–227).

A monomorphic proliferation of cells replacing the thyroid parenchyma, formation of lymphoepithelial lesions, and the presence of lymphoid cells within the follicular lumina of the thyroid are important diagnostic clues that support the diagnosis of lymphoma over chronic lymphocytic thyroiditis. The differential diagnosis of malignant lymphoma also includes insular carcinoma, anaplastic carcinoma, and metastatic disease.

Following diagnosis and appropriate subtyping of malignant lymphoma of the thyroid, appropriate staging techniques are required. The primary treatment of thyroid lymphoma includes surgery with removal of the gland for decompression of the trachea or other neck organs followed by radiation or chemotherapy; use of the latter modalities is predicated on subtype and stage of the tumor. Lesions localized to the thyroid have an excellent response to radiation therapy.

The prognosis of thyroid lymphomas depends mainly on the cell type and the stage of the disease. Small lymphocytic lymphomas commonly present in an advanced stage with bone marrow involvement; therefore, some researchers feel that involvement of the thyroid by this type of lymphoma probably represents systemic spread of the disease. These tumors have an excellent prognosis despite the advanced stage of the disease.

Patients with large cell, noncleaved tumors confined to the thyroid have a 30% to 40% 5-year survival rate. Those patients that have involvement of cervical nodes at the time of diagnosis usually have a course similar to that of primary nodal disease (220,224,228–232).

Plasma cell proliferations involving the thyroid gland are rare. Sporadic cases of solitary plasmacytoma involving only the gland or as a systemic part of multiple myeloma have been reported in the literature (233). Differentiating this disease from benign plasma cell granuloma or inflammatory pseudotumor can be achieved with the help of immunohistochemical studies. Histologically, plasma cell granuloma has a more polymorphous infiltrate with admixed histiocytes, multinucleated giant cells, and lymphocytes (234).

Angiosarcoma

For many years there was controversy between European and American pathologists regarding the existence of angiosarcoma as a true thyroid tumor. In the Alpine areas of Europe and Switzerland, angiosarcoma was reported to constitute 10% to 20% of all thyroid malignancies, whereas in the United States these tumors were found extremely rarely and probably were being classified as variants of anaplastic carcinoma until recently (235,236). The utilization of techniques such as electron microscopy and immunohistochemical markers for endothelial cells, especially Factor VIII–related antigen, CD34, and CD31, have confirmed the vascular nature of these neoplasms. Ruchti et al. (237) demonstrated the presence of Factor VIII–related antigen in 13 of 20 tumors that had been classified as angiosarcoma, and found Weibel-Palade bodies in one case in which tissue was obtained for electron microscopic studies. These researchers hypothesized that angiosarcomas probably develop (although not always) as a complication of long-standing nodular goiter.

The tumors affect predominantly elderly patients who present with a history of goiter and a rapidly enlarging neck mass. Grossly, the gland is markedly enlarged and with extensive areas of hemorrhage and necrosis. However, similar gross findings have been reported by Axiotis et al. (238) as an exuberant reaction after FNA. Without the appropriate history, post-FNA artifact can easily be mistaken grossly for poorly differentiated malignancies.

Histologically, these vascular neoplasms are identical to angiosarcomas in other locations and are composed of anastomosing channels of endothelial cells frequently showing atypia (see Chapter 10). However, some tumors may have a prominent epithelioid pattern with tumor cells that are cytokeratin positive (239). The tumors are usually invasive, causing destruction of the normal follicular architecture, involving blood vessel walls, and extending into the adjacent soft tissues. Areas of fresh and old hemorrhage are frequently found (239,240).

Angiosarcomas are frequently misdiagnosed as anaplastic carcinomas because these tumors may share coexpression of epithelial and vascular markers by immunohistochemistry (241). In contrast to angiosarcoma, ultrastructural studies often demonstrate the presence of desmososomes and microvilli in anaplastic carcinoma cells (242).

The prognosis of angiosarcomas is poor, with frequent distant hemorrhagic metastases to the lung, pleura, and lymph nodes. Treatment has not proven to be successful in this aggressive type of neoplasm.

Teratomas

Teratomas of the thyroid are quite unusual lesions, with fewer than 200 cases recorded in the literature. These tumors affect predominantly the pediatric population, and although many have a benign histologic appearance, some cases have proven fatal because of respiratory compromise (243). Histologically, the tumors can be cystic or solid and show an admixture of mature tissues with elements of the endoderm, ectoderm, and mesoderm in either an organized or disorganized pattern (see Chapter 1).

These lesions usually follow an indolent course. The presence of an immature neural component supports the diagnosis of teratoma and differentiates the lesion from carcinosarcomas.

In the adult, teratomas are malignant with rare exceptions. The origin of these tumors is not clear, but they are believed to arise from totipotential cells. The prognosis of the patients is poor due to the high propensity of these tumors to locally recur and metastasize (244,245).

Use of Frozen Sectioning in Thyroid Surgery

The role of frozen sectioning in diagnosing nodular lesions of the thyroid has recently been questioned because of the difficulty in rendering a final diagnosis. Bronner et al. (246) reviewed 103 patients with follicular nodules and concluded that frozen sectioning was not particularly helpful if the preoperative FNA diagnosis was that of follicular or Hürthle cell tumor, but it could be helpful in cases of the follicular variant of papillary cancer.

Several other diagnoses, however, can be rendered by proper interpretation of frozen section: benign lesions such as thyroiditis, goiter, and some tumors (lymphoma, papillary, anaplastic, and poorly differentiated and medullary carcinoma). However, the follicular variant of papillary carcinoma of the thyroid is a more difficult diagnosis to render on frozen sections because the characteristic optically clear nuclei of these lesions may not be appreciated. Cytologic evaluation of a touch preparation of the lesion may be helpful (247). If a definite diagnosis is not possible, the diagnosis of "follicular lesion, defer to permanent sections" is warranted.

Hamburger and Hamburger reviewed 359 patients who underwent preoperative FNA and intraoperative frozen sectioning of thyroid nodules. They concluded that frozen section results influenced surgery in only 3 of the 359 cases (248).

Metastases to the Thyroid

Metastases to the thyroid gland are unusual. Autopsy studies indicate that the frequency with which the thyroid is involved in patients with disseminated carcinomatosis is variable, ranging from 4% to 24% depending on the extent of gland sampling at autopsy.

Thyroid involvement by nonthyroid malignancies can occur by direct extension from adjacent tumors, retrograde lymphatic spread, and hematogeneous metastases.

Laryngeal, pharyngeal, and upper esophageal carcinomas may extend directly into the thyroid gland. In these cases, the tumor histology is usually squamous cell carcinoma, and clinical and pathologic distinction from primary thyroid tumors usually does not present a problem. Retrograde lymphatic spread occurs most often with breast carcinoma, but any tumor involving cervical lymph nodes could extend via lymphatics into the thyroid.

Clinically, a metastasis to the thyroid may present as a solitary thyroid nodule, which, by palpation appears suspicious for carcinoma. Unless the histology is obviously incompatible with a thyroid primary, the pathologic diagnosis of a metastasis may be missed. Some patients give a history of a previously diagnosed malignancy; in these instances, the clinician's and pathologist's awareness of the past history aids in reaching the correct diagnosis of a metastasis to the thyroid (249–252).

In a recent autopsy study of 79 Chinese patients, the mean latency period for developing thyroid metastases was 9 months and the mean survival after diagnosis was just 3 months (253).

The most common sites of origin of the metastasis include the kidney, lung, breast, stomach, and primary cutaneous melanoma (Fig. 34); however, virtually any carcinoma may secondarily involve the thyroid gland (249–253). Metastatic renal cell carcinoma can be extremely difficult to differentiate from a primary thyroid tumor with clear cell features, especially in the absence of the appropriate history. Features favoring a metastasis include multiple discreet nodules, prominent tumor vascularity, and intracytoplasmic glycogen and fat. Mucicarmine stains and immunohistochemical analysis for thyroglobulin and calcitonin are helpful in difficult cases. Only rarely have disturbances in thyroid function been described with metastases to the thyroid (167,168,254).

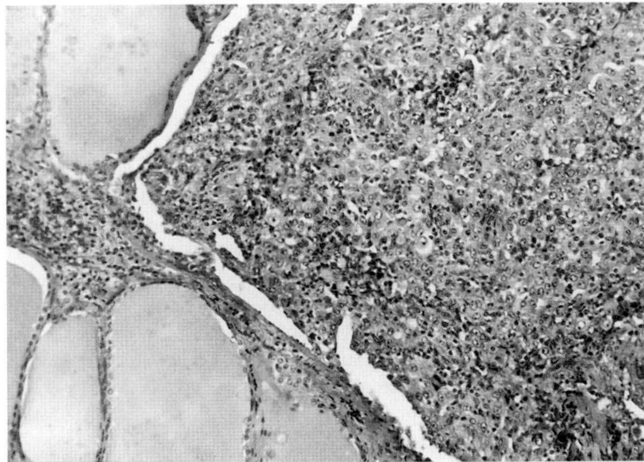

FIGURE 34. Metastatic malignant melanoma in thyroid (hematoxylin and eosin stain, original magnification ×150).

REFERENCES

1. LiVolsi VA. *Surgical pathology of the thyroid.* Philadelphia: WB Saunders, 1990.
2. Fish J, Moore RM. Ectopic thyroid tissue and ectopic thyroid carcinoma. *Ann Surg* 1963;157:212–222.
3. Pollice L, Caruso G. Stroma cordis. Ectopic thyroid goiter in the right ventricle. *Arch Pathol Lab Med* 1986;110:452–453.
4. Taylor MA, Bray M, Roberts WC. Aberrant thyroid gland attached to ascending aorta. *Am J Cardiol* 1986;57:708.
5. De Andrade MA. A review of 128 cases of posterior mediastinal goiter. *World J Surg* 1977;1:789–797.
6. Baughman RA. Lingual thyroid and lingual thyroglossal tract remnants. *Oral Surg* 1972;34:871–879.
7. Neinas FW, Gorman CA, Devine KD, et al. Lingual thyroid: clinical characteristics of 15 cases. *Ann Intern Med* 1973;79:205–210.
8. Kansal P, Sakati N, Rifai A, Woodhouse N. Lingual thyroid-diagnosis and treatment. *Arch Intern Med* 1987;147:2046–2048.
9. Rosai J, Carcangiu ML, DeLellis D. *Tumors of the thyroid gland.* Series 3. Washington, DC: Armed Forces Institute of Pathology, 1992.
10. LiVolsi VA, Perzin KH, Savetsky L. Carcinoma arising in median ectopic thyroid (including thyroglossal duct tissue). *Cancer* 1974; 34: 1303.
11. Page CP, Memmerer WT, Haff RC, et al. Thyroid carcinomas arising in thyroglossal ducts. *Ann Surg* 1974;74:799.
12. Shepard GH, Rosenfeld L. Carcinoma of thyroglossal duct remnants. *Am J Surg* 1968;116:125.
13. Roses DF, Snively SL, Phelps RG, et al. Carcinoma of the thyroglossal duct. *Am J Surg* 1983;145:266–269.
14. Silverman PM, Degesys GE, et al. Papillary carcinoma in a thyroglossal duct cyst. *J Comput Assist Tomogr* 1985;9:806–808.
15. Tori F, Fliss DM, Inbar-Yania I. Hürthle cell adenoma of the thyroglossal duct. *Head Neck Surg* 1988;10:346–349.
16. Frantz VK, Forsythe R, Hanford JM, et al. Lateral aberrant thyroid. *Ann Surg* 1942;115:161–183.
17. Meyer JS, Steinberg LS. Microscopically benign thyroid follicles in cervical lymph nodes. *Cancer* 1969;24:302–331.
18. Roth LM. Inclusions of non-neoplastic thyroid tissue within cervical lymph nodes. *Cancer* 1965;18:105–111.
19. Volpe R. Acute suppurative thyroiditis. In: Werner SC, Ingbar SH, eds. *The thyroid.* New York: Harper & Row 1971:849.
20. Volpe R. The pathology of thyroiditis. *Hum Pathol* 1987;9:429.
21. Robertson WS. Acute inflammation of the thyroid gland. *Lancet* 1911;1:930.
22. Berger SA, Zonszein J, et al. Infectious diseases of the thyroid gland. *Rev Infect Dis* 1983;5:108–122.
23. Elias AN, Kyaw T, et al. Acute suppurative thyroiditis. *J Otolaryngol* 1985;14:17–19.
24. Walter RM, McMonagle JR. Salmonella thyroiditis, apathetic thyrotoxicosis and follicular carcinoma in a Laotian woman. *Cancer* 1982;50:2493–2495.
25. Meyer RD, Young LS, et al. Aspergillosis complicating neoplastic disease. *Am J Med* 1973;54:6–15.
26. Frank TS, LiVolsi VA, Connor AM. Cytomegalovirus infection of the thyroid in immunocompromised adults. *Yale J Biol Med* 1987;60:1–8.

27. Miyauchi A, Matsuzuka F, Kuma K, Takai S. Pyriform sinus fistula: an underlying abnormality common in patients with acute suppurative thyroiditis. *World J Surg* 1990;14:400–405.
28. Rossiter JL, Topf P. Acute suppurative thyroiditis with bilateral pyriform sinus fistulae. *Otolaryngol Head Neck Surg* 1991;105;625–628.
29. Skuza K, Rapaport R, Fieldman R, et al. Recurrent acute suppurative thyroiditis. *J Otolaryngol* 1994;20:126–129.
30. Goldfar H, Schifrin D, Graig FA. Thyroiditis caused by tuberculous abscess of the thyroid gland. *Am J Med* 1965;38:825–828.
31. Klassen KP, Curtis GM. Tuberculous abscess of the thyroid gland. *Surgery* 1945;17:552–559.
32. Laohapand T, Ratanarapee S, Chantarakul N, et al. Tuberculous thyroiditis: a case report. *J Med Assoc Thai* 1981;64:256–260.
33. Birchall G. Sarcoidosis and thyroiditis. *Br J Clin Pract* 1966;20: 586–587.
34. Hughes JN, Modigliani E, Baltest JP, et al. Thyroid disorders during sarcoidosis. *Ann Med Intern* 1981;132:367–371.
35. Hemmings IL, McLean DC. Thyroid involvement in systemic sarcoidosis. *J Pediatr* 1971;87:131–134.
36. Cilley RE, Thompson NW, Lloyd RV, et al. Sarcoidosis of the thyroid presenting as a painful nodule. *Thyroidology* 1988;1:61–62.
37. de Quervain F, Giordanengo G. Die akute und subakute thyreoditis. *Mitt Grenzgeb Med Chir* 1935;44:538.
38. Jaffe RH. Tubercle-like structures in human goiters. *Arch Surg Chicago* 1930;21:717.
39. Volpe R. Subacute (nonsuppurative) thyroiditis. In: Werner SC, Ingbar SH, eds. *The thyroid.* New York: Harper & Row, 1987:986.
40. Nyulassy S, Hnilica P, Buc M, et al. Subacute (de Quervain) thyroiditis associated with HLA b 35 antigen and abnormalities of the complement system, immunoglobulins and other serum proteins. *J Clin Endocrinol Metab* 1977;45:270–274.
41. Werner J, Gelderblom H. Isolation of foamy virus from patients with de Quervain thyroiditis. *Lancet* 1979;2:258–259.
42. Eylan E, Zmucky R, Sheba C. Mumps virus and subacute thyroiditis—evidence of a causal association. *Lancet* 1957;1:1062–1063.
43. Totterman TH, Gordin A, Hayry P, et al. Accumulation of thyroid antigen-reactive T-lymphocytes in the gland of patients with subacute thyroiditis. *Clin Exp Immunol* 1978;32:153–158.
44. Carney JA, Moore SB, Northcutt RC, et al. Palpation thyroiditis (multifocal granulomatous thyroiditis). *Am J Clin Pathol* 1975; 64: 639–647.
45. Hashimoto H. Zur Kenntniss der lymphomatosen Veranderung der Schilddruse (Struma lymphomatosa). *Arch Klin Chir* 1912;97: 219–248.
46. Dorman J, Kramer MK, O'Lear LA, et al. Molecular epidemiology of autoimmune thyroid disease. *Gac Med Mex* 1997;133(suppl 1): 97–103.
47. Woolf PD. Thyroiditis. *Med Clin North Am* 1985;69:1035–1048.
48. Masi AT. Hashimoto's disease. An epidemiological study based on community-wide hospital survey. *J Chronic Dis* 1965;18:35–37.
49. Katz SM, Vickery AL. The fibrous variant of Hashimoto's thyroiditis. *Hum Pathol* 1974;5:161–170.
50. Grubeck-Loebenstein B, Derfler K, Kassal H, et al. Immunological features of nonimmunogenic hyperthyroidism. *J Clin Endocrinol Metabol* 1985;60:150–155.
51. Feldt-Rasmussen U, Bech K, Bliddal H, et al. Autoantibodies, immune complexes and HLA-D in thyrogastric autoimmunity. *Tissue Antigens* 1983;22:342–347.
52. Müller-Hocker J, Jacob U, Seibel P. Hashimoto's thyroiditis is associated with defects of dytochrome-c oxidase in oxyphil Askanazy cells and with the common deletion (4,977) of mitochondrial DNA. *Ultrastruct Pathol* 1998;22:91–100.
53. Holm LE, Blomgren H, Lowhagen T. Cancer risks in patients with chronic lymphocytic thyroiditis. *N Engl J Med* 1985;312:60–64.
54. Hyjek E, Isaacson PG. Primary B cell lymphoma of the thyroid and its relationship to Hashimoto's thyroiditis. *Hum Pathol* 1988;19: 1315–1326.
55. Zimmerman D, Lteif AN. Thyrotoxicosis in children. *Endocrinol Metab Clin North Am* 1998;27:109–126.
56. McIver B, Morris JC. The pathogenesis of Graves' disease. *Endocrinol Metab Clin North Am* 1998;27:73–79.
57. Wilkin TJ. Receptor autoimmunity in endocrine disorders. *N Engl J Med* 1990;323:1318–1324.
58. Kennedy JS, Thomson JA. The changes in the thyroid gland after irradiation with I131 or partial thryoidectomy for thyrotoxicosis. *J Pathol* 1974;112:65–82.
59. Valdeseri RO, Borochovitz D. Histologic changes in previously irradiated glands. *Arch Pathol Lab Med* 1980;104:150–152.
60. Margolick JB, Hsu S, Volkman DJ, Burman KD, Fauchi AS. Immunohistochemical characterization of intrathyroidal lymphocytes in Graves' disease. *Am J Med* 1984;76:815–821.
61. Riedel BMKL. Die cronische, zur Bildung eisenharter Tumoren fuhrende Entzundung der Schilddruse. *Verh Dtsch Ges Chir* 1896; 25: 101–105.
62. Ewing J. *Neoplastic diseases,* 2nd ed. Philadelphia: WB Saunders, 1922:908
63. Graham A. Riedel's struma in contrast to struma lymphomatosa (Hashimoto). *West J Surg* 1931;39:681–689.
64. Woolner LB, McConahel WM, Beahrs OH. Invasive fibrous thyroiditis (Riedel's struma). *J Endocrinol Metab* 1957;17:201–220.
65. Taubenberger JK, Merino MJ, Medeiros J. A thyroid biopsy with histologic features of both Riedel's thryoiditis and the fibrosing variant of Hashimoto's thyroiditis. *Hum Pathol* 1991;23:1072–1075.
66. Turner-Warwick R, Nabarro JDN, Doniach D. Riedel's thyroiditis and retroperitoneal fibrosis. *Proc R Soc Med* 1966;59:596–598.
67. Harach HR, Williams ED. Fibrous thyroiditis, an immunohistochemical study. *Histopathology* 1983;7:739–751.
68. McClintock JC, Wright AW. Riedel's struma and struma lymphomatosa (Hashimoto). *Ann Surg* 1937;106:11–32.
69. Schwaegerle SM, Bauer TW, Esselstyn CB. Riedel's thyroiditis. *Am J Clin Pathol* 1988;90:715–722.
70. Surgnova A, Masuda H, Komatsu M, et al. Adenomatous goitre. Therapeutic strategy, post-operative outcome, and study of epidermal growth factor receptor. *Br J Surg* 1992;79:404–406.
71. Hicks DG, LiVolsi VA, Neidich JA, et al. Clonal analysis of solitary follicular nodules in the thyroid. *Am J Pathol* 1990;137:553–562.
72. Thomas GA, Williams D, Williams ED. The clonal origin of thyroid nodules and adenomas. *Am J Pathol* 1989;134:141–147.
73. Namba H, Matsuo K, Fagin JA. Clonal composition of benign and malignant human thyroid tumors. *J Clin Invest* 1990;86:120–125.
74. Carney JA, Ryan J, Goellner JR. Hyalinizing trabecular adenoma of the thyroid gland. *Am J Surg Pathol* 1987;11:583–591.
75. Katoh R, Jansan B, Williams ED. Hyalinizing trabecular adenoma of the thyroid. A report of three cases with immunohistochemical and ultrastructural studies. *Histopathology* 1989;15:211–224.
76. Papotti M, Riella P, Montemurro F, et al. Immunophenotypic heterogeneity of hyalinizing trabecular tumor of the thyroid. *Histopathology* 1997;31:525–533.
77. LaGuette J, Matias-Guiu, Rosai J. Thyroid paraganglioma: a clinicopathologic and immunohistochemical study of three cases. *Am J Surg Pathol* 1997;21:748–753.
78. Williams ED. Pathology and natural history. In: Duncan W, ed. *Thyroid cancer.* Berlin: Springer-Verlag, 1980.
79. Woolner LW. Thyroid carcinoma: pathologic classification with data on prognosis. *Semin Nucl Med* 1971;1:481–502.
80. Correa P, Chen VW. Endocrine gland cancer. *Cancer* 1995;75:338.
81. Woolner LB, Beahrs OL, Black BM, et al. Classification and prognosis of thyroid carcinoma. A study of 885 cases observed in a thirty year period. *Am J Surg* 1961;102:354–387.
82. Harach HR, Escalante DA, Onativia A, et al. Thyroid carcinoma and thyroiditis in an endemic goiter region before and after iodine prophylaxis. *Acta Endocrinol* 1985;108:55–60.
83. Williams ED, Doniach I, Bjarnason O, et al. Thyroid cancer in an iodide rich area. A histopathologic study. *Cancer* 1977;39:215–222.
84. Carcangiu ML, Zampi G, Rosai J. Poorly differentiated ("insular") thyroid carcinoma. *Am J Surg Pathol* 1984;8:655–668.
85. Carcangiu ML, Zampi G, Pupi A, et al. Papillary carcinoma of the thyroid. A clinicopathologic study of 241 cases treated at the University of Florence, Italy. *Cancer* 1985;55:805–828.

86. Schneider AB, Recant W, Pickny SM, et al. Radiation induced thyroid carcinoma. Clinical course and results of therapy in 296 patients. *Ann Intern Med* 1986;105:405.
87. Kazakov VS, Demidchik EP, Asakhova LN. Thyroid cancer after Chernobyl. *Nature* 1992;359:21–22.
88. Carcangiu ML, Zampi G, Pupi A, et al. The incidence of thyroid carcinoma in Hashimoto's thyroiditis. *Am Surgeon* 1987;53:442–445.
89. Hapke MR, Dehner LP. The optically clear nucleus. A reliable sign of papillary carcinoma of thyroid. *Am J Surg Pathol* 1979;3:31–38.
90. Chan JK, Saw D. The grooved nucleus. A useful diagnostic criterion of papillary carcinoma of thyroid. *Am J Surg Pathol* 1986;10:672–679.
91. Scopa CD, Melachrinou M, Saradopoulou C, et al. The significance of the grooved nucleus in thyroidal lesions. *Mod Pathol* 1993;6: 691–694.
92. Johannessen JV, Sobrinho-Simoes M. Origin and significance of thyroid psammoma bodies. *Lab Invest* 1980;43:287–296.
93. Inoue H, Oshimo K, Miki H, et al. Immunohistochemical study of estrogen receptors and the responsiveness to estrogen in papillary thyroid carcinoma. *Cancer* 1993;72:1364–1368.
94. Miki H, Oshimo K, Inoue H. Sex hormone receptors in human thyroid tissues. *Cancer* 1990;66:1759–1862.
95. van Hoeven KH, Kovatich AJ, Miettinen M. Immunohistochemical evaluation of HBME, Ca-19-9 and CD 15 (Leu M1) in fine needle aspiration of thyroid nodules. *Diagn Cytopathol* 1997;18:9397.
96. Santoro M, Carlomango F, Hay ID, et al. Ret oncogene activation in human thyroid neoplasms is restricted to papillary cancer subtype. *J Clin Invest* 1992;89:1517–1522.
97. Bongarzone I, Fugazzola L, Vingeri P, et al. Age related activation of the tyrosine kinase receptor protooncogenes RET and NTRK1 in papillary thyroid cancer. *J Clin Endocrinol Metab* 1996;81: 2006–2009.
98. Zou M, Shi Y, Farid NY. Low rate of ret proto-oncogene activation (PTC/RET TPC) in papillary thyroid cancer from Saudia Arabia. *Cancer* 1994;73:176–180.
99. Fugazzola L, Pilotti S, Pinchera A, et al. Oncogenic rearrangements of the RET protooncogene in papillary thyroid cancers in children exposed to the Chernobyl nuclear accident. *Cancer Res* 1995;55: 5617–5620.
100. Klugbauer S, Lengfelder E, Demidchik EP, et al. High prevalence of RET rearrangement in thyroid tumors of children from Belarus after the Chernobyl reactor accident. *Oncogene* 1995;11:2459–2467.
101. Nikiforov YE, Rowland JM, Bove KE, et al. Distinct pattern of RET oncogene rearrangements in morphological variants of radiation-induced and sporadic thyroid papillary cancer in children. *Cancer Res* 1997;57:1690–1694.
102. Bounacer A, Wicker R, Calillou B, et al. High prevalence of activating RET protooncogene rearrangements in thyroid tumors from patients who have received external radiation. *Oncogene* 1997;15:1263–1273.
103. Hazard JB. Small papillary carcinoma of the thyroid. *Lab Invest* 1960;9:86–97.
104. Sampson RJ, Woolner LB, Bahn RC, et al. Occult thyroid carcinoma in Olmsted County, Minnesota: prevalence at autopsy compared with that in Hiroshima and Nagasaki, Japan. *Cancer* 1974;34:2072–2076.
105. Vickery AL. Thyroid papillary carcinoma. Pathological and philosophical controversies. *Am J Surg Pathol* 1983;7:777–807.
106. LiVolsi VA. Papillary neoplasms of the thyroid. Pathologic and prognostic features. *Am J Clin Pathol* 1992;97:426–437.
107. Lloyd RV, Beierwaltes WH. Occult sclerosing carcinoma of the thyroid: potential for aggressive biologic behavior. *South Med J* 1983;76: 437–439.
108. Kasai N, Sakamoto A. New subgrouping of small thyroid carcinoma. *Cancer* 1987;60:1767–1770.
109. Naruse T, Koike A, Kanemitsu T, et al. Minimal thyroid carcinoma: a report of nine cases discovered by cervical lymph node metastases. *Jpn J Surg* 1984;14:118–121.
110. Strate SM, Lee EL, Childers JH. Occult papillary carcinoma of the thyroid with distant metastases. *Cancer* 1984;54:1093–1100.
111. Mizukami Y, Nonomura A, Takatoshi M, et al. Solid cell nests of the thyroid: a histological and immunohistochemistry study. *Am J Clin Pathol* 1994;101:186–191.
112. Lindsay S. *Carcinoma of the thyroid gland.* Springfield: Charles C Thomas, 1960.
113. Chen KTK, Rosai J. Follicular variant of thyroid papillary carcinoma: a clinicopathologic study of six cases. *Am J Surg Pathol* 1977;1: 123–131.
114. Albores-Saavedra J, Gould E, Vardaman C, Vuitch F. The macrofollicular variant of papillary thyroid carcinoma: a study of 17 cases [Abstract]. *Lab Invest* 1991;63:31.
115. Evans HL. Encapsulated papillary neoplasms of the thyroid: a study of 14 cases followed for a minimum of 10 years. *Am J Surg Pathol* 1987; 11:592–597.
116. Hazard JB. Nomenclature of thyroid tumors. In: Inman DR, Young S, eds. *Thyroid neoplasia.* London: Academic, 1968:2–22.
117. Merino MJ, Kennedy S, Norton J, et al. Pleural involvement by metastatic thyroid carcinoma "tall cell variant." *Surg Pathol* 1990;3: 59–64.
118. Johnson TL, Lloyd RV, Thompson NW, et al. Prognostic implications of the tall cell variant of papillary thyroid carcinoma. *Am J Surg Pathol* 1988;12:22–27.
119. Evans HL. Columnar cell carcinoma of the thyroid. A report of two cases of an aggressive variant of thyroid carcinoma. *Am J Clin Pathol* 1986;88:77–80.
120. Sobrinho-Simoes M, Nesland JM, Johannessen JV. Columnar cell carcinoma: another variant of poorly differentiated carcinoma of the thyroid. *Am J Clin Pathol* 1988;89:264–267.
121. Asklen LA, Varhaug JE. Thyroid carcinoma with mixed tall cell and columnar features. *Am J Clin Pathol* 1990;94;422–445.
122. Berends D, Mouthaan RJ. Columnar cell cancer of the thyroid. *Histopathology* 1992;20:360–362.
123. Franssila KO. Prognosis in thyroid carcinoma. *Cancer* 1975;36: 1138–1146.
124. Evans HL. Follicular neoplasms of the thyroid. A study of 44 cases followed for a minimum of 10 years, with emphasis on differential diagnosis. *Cancer* 1984;54:535–540.
125. Hazard JB, Kenyon R. Encapsulated angioinvasive carcinoma (angioinvasive adenoma) of thyroid gland. *Am J Clin Pathol* 1954;24: 755–766.
126. LiVolsi VA, Merino MJ. Worrisome alterations following fine needle aspiration of thyroid. *Pathol Annu* 1994;29(part 2):99–120.
127. Kahn NF, Perzin KH. Follicular carcinoma of the thyroid. An evaluation of the histologic criteria used for diagnosis. *Pathol Annu* 1983;18(part 1):221–253.
128. Fagin JA. Molecular pathogenesis. In: Braverman LE, Utiger RD, eds. *Werner and Ingbar's the thyroid: a fundamental and clinical text,* 7th ed. Philadelphia: Lippincott-Raven, 1996:909–916.
129. Challeton C, Bounacer A, DuVillard JA, et al. Pattern of ras and gsp oncogene mutations in radiation associated human thyroid tumors. *Oncogene* 1995;11:601–603.
130. Russo D, Arturi F, Schlumber M, et al. Activating mutations of the TSH receptor in differentiated thyroid cancers. *Oncogene* 1995; 11:1907–1911.
131. Valenta LJ, Michel-Bechet M, Warshaw JB, et al. Human thyroid tumors composed of mitochondria-rich cells: electron microscopic and biochemical findings. *J Clin Endocrinol Metab* 1974;39:719–733.
132. Gosain AK, Clark OH. Hürthle cell neoplasms: malignant potential. *Arch Surg* 1984;119:515–519.
133. Gundry SR, Burney RE, Thompson NW, Lloyd R. Total thyroidectomy for Hürthle cell neoplasm of the thyroid. *Arch Surg* 1983; 118:529–532.
134. Bondeson L, Bondeson AG, Ljungberg O, et al. Oxyphil tumors of the thyroid. Follow-up of 42 surgical cases. *Ann Surg* 1981;194: 677–680.
135. Caplan RH, Abellera M, Kisken WA. Hürthle cell tumors of the thyroid gland: a clinicopathologic review and long-term follow-up. *JAMA* 1984;251:3114–3117.
136. Bondeson L, Bondeson AG, Ljungberg O. Treatment of Hürthle cell neoplasms of the thyroid. *Arch Surg* 1983;118:1453.
137. Bronner MP, LiVolsi VA. Oxyphilic (Askanazy/Hürthle cell) tumors of the thyroid: microscopic features predict biologic behavior. *Surg Pathol* 1988;1:137–150.

138. Hill JH, Werkhaven JA, DeMay RM. Hürthle cell variant of papillary carcinoma of the thyroid gland. *Otolaryngol Head Neck Surg* 1988;98:338–341.
139. Flint A, Lloyd RV. Hürthle cell neoplasms of the thyroid. *Pathol Annu* 1990;25:37–52.
140. Papotti M, Torchio B, Grassi L, et al. Poorly differentiated oxyphilic (Hürthle cell) carcinomas of the thyroid. *Am J Surg Pathol* 1996; 20:686–694.
141. Azadian A, Rosen IB, Walfish PG, Asa SL. Management considerations in Hürthle cell carcinoma. *Surgery* 1995;118:711–715.
142. McDonald MP, Sanders LE, Silverman ML, et al. Hürthle cell carcinoma of the thyroid gland: prognostic factors and results of surgical treatment. *Surgery* 1996;120:1000–1005.
143. Evans HL, Vassilopoulou-Sellin R. Follicular and Hürthle cell carcinomas of the thyroid: a comparative study. *Am J Surg Pathol* 1998; 22:1512–1520.
144. Bronner MP, Clevenger CV, Edmonds PR, et al. Flow cytometric analysis of DNA content in Hürthle cell adenomas and carcinomas of the thyroid. *Am J Clin Pathol* 1988;89:764–769.
145. Apel RL, Asa SL, LiVolsi VA. Papillary Hürthle cell carcinoma with lymphocytic stroma "Warthin-like tumor" of the thyroid. *Am J Surg Pathol* 1995;19:810–814.
146. Takiyama Y, Saji M, Clark DP, et al. Polymerase chain reaction-based microsatellite analysis of fine needle aspirations from Hürthle cell neoplasms. *Thyroid* 1997;7:853–857.
147. Justin EP, Seabold JE, Robinson RA, et al. Insular carcinoma. A distinct thyroid carcinoma associated with iodine-131 localization. *J Nucl Med* 1991;32:1358–1363.
148. Papotti M, Botto F, Favero A, et al. Poorly differentiated thyroid carcinoma with primordial cell component. *Am J Surg Pathol* 1994;18: 1054–1064.
149. Sakamoto A, Kasai N, Sugano H. Poorly differentiated carcinoma of the thyroid. A clinicopathologic entity for a high-risk group of papillary and follicular carcinomas. *Cancer* 1983;52:1849–1855.
150. Carcangiu ML, Steeper T, Zampi G, et al. Anaplastic thyroid carcinoma: a study of 70 cases. *Am J Clin Pathol* 1985;83:135–158.
151. LiVolsi VA, Brooks JJ, Arendash-Durand B. Anaplastic thyroid tumors: immunohistology. *Am J Clin Pathol* 1987;87:434–442.
152. Venkatesh Y, Ordonez N, Schultz P, et al. Anaplastic carcinoma of the thyroid. *Cancer* 1990;66:321–330.
153. Becker HW. Anaplastic thyroid carcinoma 12 years after radioiodine therapy. *Cancer* 1969;23:885–890.
154. Hashimoto H, Koga S, Watanabe H, et al. Undifferentiated carcinoma of the thyroid gland with osteoclast like giant cells. *Acta Pathol Japan* 1980;30:323–334.
155. Silverberg SG, DeGiorfi LS. Osteoclastoma-like giant cell tumor of the thyroid gland. *Cancer* 1973;31:621–625.
156. Ordonez NO, El-Naggar AK, Hickey RC, et al. Anaplastic thyroid carcinoma. Immunocytochemical study of 32 cases. *Am J Clin Pathol* 1991;96:15–24.
157. Bocker W, Dralle H, Husselmann H, et al. Immunohistochemical analysis of thyroglobulin synthesis in thyroid carcinomas. *Virchows Arch* 1980;385:187–200.
158. Hurlimann J, Gardiol D, Scazziga B. Immunohistology of anaplastic thyroid carcinoma: a study of 43 cases. *Histopathology* 1987;11: 567–580.
159. Albores-Saavedra J, Nadji M, Civantos F, et al. Thyroglobulin in carcinoma of the thyroid: an immunohistochemical study. *Hum Pathol* 1983;14:62–66.
160. Ryff-de Leche A, Staub JJ, Kholer-Faden R, et al. Thyroglobulin production by malignant thyroid tumors. An immunohistochemistry and radioimmunoassay study. *Cancer* 1986;57:1145–1153.
161. Fagin JA, Matsuo K, Karmaker A, et al. High prevalence of mutations of the p53 gene in poorly differentiated human thyroid cancer. *J Clin Invest* 1993;91:179–184.
162. Ito T, Seyama T, Mizuno T, et al. Unique association of p53 mutation with undifferentiated but not differentiated cancer of the thyroid gland. *Can Res* 1992;52:1369–1371.
163. Nakamura T, Yana I, Kobayashi T, et al. p53 gene mutation associated with anaplastic transformation of human thyroid cancer. *Jpn J Can Res* 1992;83:1293–1298.
164. Tallroth E, Walling-Lundell G. Multinodality treatment in anaplastic giant cell thyroid carcinoma. *Cancer* 1987;7:1428–1431.
165. LiVolsi VA, Merino MJ. Squamous cells in the human thyroid gland. *Am J Surg Pathol* 1978;2:133–139.
166. Huang T, Assor D. Primary squamous cell carcinoma of the thyroid gland: a report of four cases. *Am J Clin Pathol* 1971;55:93–98.
167. Civantos F, Albores-Saavedra J, Nadji M, et al. Clear cell variant of thyroid cancer. *Am J Surg Pathol* 1984;8:187–192.
168. Carcangiu ML, Sibley RK, Rosai J. Clear cell change in primary thyroid tumors: a study of 38 cases. *Am J Surg Pathol* 1985;9:705–722.
169. Horn RC. Carcinoma of the thyroid. Description of a distinctive morphological variant and report of seven cases. *Cancer* 1951;4:697–707.
170. Hazard JB, Hawk WA, Crile G. Medullary (solid) a clinicopathologic entity. *J Clin Endocrinol Metab* 1959;19:152–161.
171. Sundler F, Alumets J, Hakanson R, et al. Somastostatin-immunoreactive C-cells in medullary carcinoma of the thyroid. *Am J Pathol* 1977;88:381–386.
172. Albores-Saavedra J, LiVolsi VA, Williams ED. Medullary carcinoma. *Semin Diagn Pathol* 1985;2:137–146.
173. Capella C, Bordi C, Monga G, et al. Multiple endocrine cell types in thyroid medullary carcinoma: evidence of calcitonin, somatostatin, ACTH, 5HT, and small granule cells. *Virchows Arch* 1978; 377: 111–128.
174. Hofstra RM, Landsvater RM, Ceccherini I, et al. A mutation in the RET protooncogene associated with multiple endocrine neoplasia type 2B and sporadic medullary thyroid cancer. *Nature* 1994;367: 375–376.
175. Heshmati HM, Gharib H, van Heerden JA, et al. Advances and controversies in the diagnosis and management of medullary thyroid cancer. *Am J Med* 1997;103:60–69.
176. Uribe M, Grimes M, Fenoglio-Preiser CM, et al. Medullary carcinoma of the thyroid gland. *Am J Surg Pathol* 1985;9:577–894.
177. Albores-Saavedra J, Rose GG, Ibanez ML, et al. The amyloid in solid carcinoma of the thyroid gland: staining characteristics, tissue culture and electron microscopic observations. *Lab Invest* 1964;13:77–93.
178. Landon G, Ordonez NG. Clear cell variant of medullary carcinoma of the thyroid. *Hum Pathol* 1985;16:844–847.
179. Fernandes BJ, Bedard VC, Rosen I. Mucous producing medullary cell carcinoma of the thyroid gland. *Am J Clin Pathol* 1982;78:536–540.
180. Mendelsohn G, Bigner SH, Eggleston JC, et al. Anaplastic variants of medullary thyroid carcinoma. *Am J Surg Pathol* 1980;4:333–341.
181. Harach HR, Williams ED. Glandular (tubular and follicular) variants of medullary carcinoma of the thyroid. *Histopathology* 1983;7:83–89.
182. Hazard JB, Hawk WA, Crile G. Medullary (solid) carcinoma of the thyroid: a clinicopathologic entity. *J Clin Endocrinol Metab* 1959; 19:152–161.
183. Huss LJ, Mendelsohn G. Medullary carcinoma of the thyroid gland: an encapsulated variant resembling hyalinizing trabecular (paraganglioma-like) adenoma of thyroid. *Mod Pathol* 1990;3:581–585.
184. Kakudo K, Miyauchi A, Ogihara T, et al. Medullary carcinoma of the thyroid: giant cell type. *Arch Pathol Lab Med* 1987;102:445–447.
185. Zaatari GS, Saigo PE, Huvos AG. Mucin production in medullary carcinoma of the thyroid. *Arch Pathol Lab Med* 1983;107:70–74.
186. Burman H, Rigaud C, Bogemolitz WV, et al. Melanin production in medullary thyroid carcinoma. *Histopathology* 1990;16:227–233.
187. Marcus JN, Dise CA, LiVolsi VA. Melanin production in a medullary thyroid carcinoma. *Cancer* 1982;49:2518–2526.
188. DeLellis RA, Rue AH, Spiler L, et al. Calcitonin and CEA as tumor markers in medullary thyroid cancer. *Am J Clin Pathol* 1978;70: 578–594.
189. Lloyd RV, Sisson JC, Marangos PJ. Calcitonin, CEA and NSE in medullary thyroid cancer: an immunohistochemical study. *Cancer* 1983;51:2234–2239.
190. Schroder S, Kloppel G. CEA and non-specific cross reactive antigen in thyroid cancer. *Am J Surg Pathol* 1987;11:100–108.

191. Dasovic-Knezevic M, Bormer U, Holm R, et al. CEA in medullary thyroid cancer. An immunohistochemical study applying six novel monoclonal antibodies. *Mod Pathol* 1989;2:610–617.
192. De Micco C, Chapel F, Dor A, et al. Thyroglobulin in medullary thyroid cancer. Immunohistochemical study with polyclonal and monoclonal antibodies. *Hum Pathol* 1993;24:256–262.
193. Holm R, Sobrinho-Simoes M, Nesland JM, et al. Medullary thyroid carcinoma with thyroglobulin immunoreactivity: a special entity. *Lab Invest* 1987;57:258–267.
194. Boultwood J, Wynford-Thomas D, Richards GP, et al. In-situ analysis of calcitonin and CGRP expression in medullary thyroid cancer. *Clin Endocrinol* 1990;33:381–390.
195. Eusebi V, Damiani S, Riva C, et al. Calcitonin free oat-cell cancer of the thyroid gland. *Virchows Arch* 1990;417:267–271.
196. Russell CF, van Heevden HA, Sizemore GW, et al. The surgical management of medullary thyroid cancer. *Ann Surg* 1983;197:42–48.
197. Block MA. Surgery treatment for medullary carcinoma of the thyroid. *Otolaryngol Clin North Am* 1990;23:453–473.
198. Dralle H, Scheumann GFW, Proye C, et al. The value of lymph node dissection in medullary thyroid cancer; a retrospective, European, multicentre study. *J Intern Med* 1995;238:357–361.
199. Schroder S, Bocker W, Baiseh H, et al. Prognostic factors in medullary thyroid carcinoma: survival in relation to age, sex, histology, immunohistochemistry and DNA content. *Cancer* 1988;61:806–816.
200. Hales M, Rosenau W, Okerland M, et al. Carcinoma of the thyroid with a mixed medullary and follicular pattern. *Cancer* 1982;50: 1352–1359.
201. Ljungberg O, Bondeson L, Bondeson AG. Differentiated thyroid carcinomas, intermediate type. A new tumor entity with features of follicular and parafollicular cell carcinoma. *Hum Pathol* 1984;15: 218–228.
202. Chan JKC, Albores-Saavedra J, Batifora H, et al. Sclerosing mucoepidermoid thyroid carcinoma with eosinophilia: a distinctive low-grade malignancy arising from the metaplastic follicles of Hashimoto's thyroiditis. *Am J Surg Pathol* 1991;15:438–448.
203. Geisinger KR, Steffee CH, McGee RS, et al. The cytomorphic features of sclerosing mucoepidermoid carcinoma of the thyroid gland with eosinophilia. *Am J Clin Pathol* 1998;109:294–301.
204. Sim SJ, Ro JY, Ordonez NG, Cleary KR, Ayala AG. Sclerosing mucoepidermoid carcinoma with eosinophilia of the thyroid: report of two patients, one with distant metastases, and review of the literature. *Hum Pathol* 1997;28:1091–1096.
205. Miessner WA, Warren S. *Tumors of the thyroid gland.* Series 2, fascicle 4. Washington, DC: Armed Forces Institute of Pathology, 1969.
206. Chan JKC, Rosai J. Tumors of the neck showing thymic or related branchial pouch differentiation: a unifying concept. *Hum Pathol* 1991;22:349–367.
207. Hofman P, Mainguené C, Michiels JF, et al. Thyroid spindle epithelial tumor with thymus-like differentiation (the "SETTLE" tumor). An immunohistochemical and electron microscopic study. *Eur Arch Otorhinolaryngol* 1995;252:316–320.
208. Saw D, Wu D, Chess Q, Shemen L. Spindle epithelial tumor with thymus-like element (SETTLE), a primary thyroid tumor. *Int J Surg Pathol* 1997;4:169–174.
209. Su L, Beals T, Bernacki EG, Giordano TJ. Spindle epithelial tumor with thymus-like differentiation: a case report with cytologic, histologic, immunohistologic, and ultrastructural findings. *Mod Pathol* 1997;10:510–514.
210. Chetty R, Goetsch S, Nayler S, et al. Spindle epithelial tumour with thymus-like element (SETTLE): the predominantly monophasic variant. *Histopathology* 1998;33:71–74.
211. Bradford CR, Devaney KO, Lee JI. Spindle epithelial tumor with thymus-like differentiation: a case report and review of the literature. *Otolaryngol Head Neck Surg* 1999;120:603–606.
212. Dorfman DM, Shahsafaei A, Miyauchi A. Immunohistochemical staining for bcl-2 and mcl-1 in intrathyroidal epithelial thymoma (ITET)/carcinoma showing thymus-like differentiation (CASTLE) and cervical thymic carcinoma. *Mod Pathol* 1998;11:989–994.
213. Dorfman DM, Shahsafaei A, Miyauchi A. Intrathyroidal epithelial thymoma (ITET)/carcinoma showing thymus-like differentiation (CASTLE) exhibits CD5 immunoreactivity: new evidence for thymic differentiation. *Histopathology* 1998;32:104–109.
214. Berezowski K, Grimes MM, Gal A, Kornstein MJ. CD5 immunoreactivity of epithelial cells in thymic carcinoma and CASTLE using paraffin-embedded tissue. *Am J Clin Pathol* 1996;106:483–486.
215. Shek TW, Luk IS, Ng IO, et al. Lymphoepithelioma-like carcinoma of the thyroid gland: lack of evidence of association with Epstein-Barr virus. *Hum Pathol* 1996;27:851–853.
216. Logue JP, Hale RJ, Stewart AL, et al. Primary malignant lymphoma of the thyroid: a clinicopathological analysis. *Int J Radiat Oncol Biol Phys* 1992;22:929–933.
217. Goudie RB, Angouridakis LE. Autoimmune thyroiditis associated with malignant lymphoma of the thyroid. *Am J Clin Pathol* 1970; 23:377.
218. Selzer G, Kahn L, Albertyn L. Primary malignant tumors of the thyroid gland. *Cancer* 1977;40:1501–1510.
219. Souhamini L, Simpson W, Carruthers J. Malignant lymphoma of the thyroid gland. *Int J Radiat Oncol Biol Phys* 1980;6:1143–1147.
220. Heimann R, Vannineuse A, DeSloover C, et al. Malignant lymphoma and undifferentiated small cell carcinoma of the thyroid gland: a clinicopathological review in light of the Kiel classification for malignant lymphoma. *Histopathology* 1987;2:201–213.
221. Isaacson PG. Malignant lymphoma of mucosal associated lymphoid tissue. *Histopathology* 1987;11:445–462.
222. Pedersen RK, Pedersen NT. Primary non-Hodgkin's lymphoma of the thyroid gland: a population based study. *Histopathology* 1996; 28:25–32.
223. Pledge S, Bessell EM, Leach IH, et al. Non-Hodgkin's lymphoma of the thyroid: a retrospective review of all patients diagnosed in Nottinghamshire from 1973 to 1992. *Clin Oncol (R Coll Radiol)* 1996;8:371–375.
224. Aosasa K, Inoue A, Tajima K, et al. Malignant lymphoma of the thyroid gland. Analysis of 79 cases with emphasis on histological prognostic factors. *Cancer* 1986;58:100–104.
225. Maurer R, Taylor CR, Tery R. Non Hodgkin lymphomas of the thyroid. A clinicopathological review of 29 cases applying the Lukes-Collins classification and immunoperoxidase. *Virchows Arch* 1979;383:293–317.
226. Faure P, Chittal S, Woodman-Memeteau W, et al. Diagnostic features of primary malignant lymphoma of the thyroid with monoclonal antibodies. *Cancer* 1988:61:1852–1861.
227. Mizukami Y, Michigishi T, Nonomura A, et al. Primary lymphoma of the thyroid. A clinical, histological and immunohistochemical study of 20 cases. *Histopathology* 1990;17:201–209.
228. Woolner LB, McConahey WM, Beahrs OH, et al. Primary malignant lymphoma of the thyroid. *Am J Surg* 1966;111:501.
229. Cadman EC, Capizzi RL, Bertino JR. Acute non-lymphocytic leukemia, a delayed complication of Hodgkin's disease therapy: analysis of 109 cases. *Cancer* 1977;40:1280.
230. Burke JS, Butler JJ, Fuller LM. Malignant lymphoma of the thyroid. *Cancer* 1977;39:1587.
231. Compagno J, Oertel JE. Malignant lymphomas and other lymphoproliferative disorders of the thyroid gland: a clinicopathologic study of 245 cases. *Am J Clin Pathol* 1980;74:1.
232. Aozasa K, Ueda T, Katagiri S, et al. Immunologic and immunohistologic analysis of 27 cases with thyroid lymphoma. *Cancer* 1987;60:969–973.
233. Shimaoka K, Gailani S, Tsukada Y, et al. Plasma cell neoplasm involving the thyroid. *Cancer* 1978;14:1140–1146.
234. Holck S. Plasma cell granuloma of the thyroid. *Cancer* 1981;48: 830–832.
235. Hedinger C. Geographic pathology of thyroid diseases. *Pathol Res Pract* 1981;171:285–292.
236. Krisch K, Holzner JH, Kokoschka R, et al. Hemangioendothelioma of the thyroid gland: true endothelioma or anaplastic carcinoma. *Pathol Res Pract* 1980;170:230–242.
237. Ruchti C, Gerber HA, Schaffner T. Factor VII-related antigen in malignant hemangioendothelioma of thyroid. *Am J Clin Pathol* 1984; 82:474–480.

238. Axiotis C, Merino MJ, Aim K, et al. Papillary endothelial hyperplasia of the thyroid following fine needle aspiration. *Arch Pathol Lab Invest* 1991;115:240–242.
239. Eusebi V, Carcangiu ML, Dina R, et al. Keratin positive epithelioid angiosarcoma of the thyroid. A report of four cases. *Am J Surg Pathol* 1990;14:737–747.
240. Lamovec J, Zidar A, Zidanik B. Epithelioid angiosarcoma of the thyroid gland. *Arch Pathol Lab Med* 1994;118:642–646.
241. Mills SE, Stallings RG, Austin MB. Angiomatoid carcinoma of the thyroid gland: anaplastic carcinoma with follicular and medullary features mimicking angiosarcoma. *Am J Clin Pathol* 1986;86:674–687.
242. Tanda F, Massarelli G, Bosinar L. Angiosarcoma of the thyroid: a light, electorn microscopic and histoimmunological study. *Hum Pathol* 1988;19:742–745.
243. Fisher JE, Cooney DR, Voorhees ML, et al. Teratoma of thyroid gland in infancy: review of the literature and two case reports. *J Surg Oncol* 1992;21:135–140.
244. Kimler SC, Muth WF. Primary malignant teratoma of the thyroid: case report and literature review of cervical teratomas in adults. *Cancer* 1987;42:311–317.
245. Buckley NJ, Burch WM, Leight GS. Malignant teratoma of the thyroid gland in an adult: a case report and review of the literature. *Surgery* 1986;100:932–937.
246. Bronner MP, Hamilton R, LiVolsi VA. Utility of frozen section analysis on follicular lesions of the thyroid. *Endocrin Pathol* 1994;5: 154–161.
247. Basolo F, Baloch ZW, Baldanzi A, et al. Usefulness of ultra fast Papanicolaou-stained scrape preparations in intraoperative management of thyroid lesions. *Mod Pathol* 1999;12:653–657.
248. Hamburger JI, Hamburger SN. Declining role of frozen section in surgical planning for thyroid nodules. *Surgery* 1985;98:307–312.
249. Elliot RHE, Frantz VK. Metastatic carcinoma masquerading as primary thyroid cancer. *Ann Surg* 1960;151:551.
250. Silverberg SG, Vidone RA. Metastatic tumors in the thyroid. *Pacif Med Surg* 1966;74:175.
251. Harcourt-Webster JN. Secondary neoplasm of the thyroid presenting as a goiter. *J Clin Pathol* 1965;18:282.
252. Ivy HK. Cancer metastatic to the thyroid: a diagnostic problem. *Mayo Clin Proc* 1984;59:856.
253. Lam KY, Lo CY. Metastatic tumors of the thyroid gland. A study of 79 cases in Chinese patients. *Arch Pathol Lab Med* 1998;22:37–41.
254. Gault EW, Leung TH, Thomas DP. Clear cell renal carcinoma masquerading as thyroid enlargement. *J Pathol* 1974;113:21.

9B

THE PARATHYROID GLANDS

LAVINIA P. MIDDLETON
MARIA J. MERINO

ANATOMIC AND FUNCTIONAL CONSIDERATIONS

The parathyroid glands are derived from the third and fourth pharyngeal pouches. They are first recognized as such at 5 to 6 weeks' gestation, when they can be identified as thickenings of the branchial pouch epithelium (1). The superior parathyroids, derived from the dorsal edge of the fourth branchial pouch and the fourth and fifth branchial complex, are collectively known as parathyroid (IV). The position of these glands creates an important anatomic landmark, because they are usually within 1 mm of where the inferior thyroid artery crosses the recurrent laryngeal nerve at the cricothyroid articulation (1,2). Both the inferior bilateral parathyroid glands (III) and the lobes of the thymus gland arise as diverticula of the third branchial pouch. The thymic lobes and inferior parathyroids descend together, and continued migration of an inferior parathyroid into the anterior mediastinum can result in an intrathymic parathyroid (Fig. 1).

The normal combined weight for the encapsulated ovoid to reniform parathyroid glands are 117 mg for men and 131 mg for women (3). Akerström et al., in reviewing a series of 368 autopsies, observed a mean glandular weight of 22 mg, with a maximum normal weight of 39 mg (4). The majority of adults (84%–97%) have two paired parathyroid glands, but as many as 11 glands and as few as 1 have been recorded (5). Supernumerary glands are usually rudimentary and have been reported in up to 13% of patients.

The color of the parathyroids ranges from red to brown to tan depending on the degree of vascular congestion and fat content of the gland. The percentage of stromal fat increases with age and the amount of body fat (Fig. 2) (6). In addition to being located aberrantly in the thymus, on rare occasions parathyroid glands (III) can be intrathyroidal (1) (Fig. 3), and exceptionally can be found in the carotid sheath and vagus nerve (7,8). Parathyroids (IV) can be identified aberrantly in the neck, tracheoesophageal groove, and posterior superior mediastinum (2,5,7). The blood flow to the paired parathyroids is usually supplied by the inferior thyroid arteries.

The parathyroid glands regulate serum calcium and phosphate levels via the secretion of parathyroid hormone (parathormone). Parathormone is an 84–amino acid peptide that is encoded by a gene mapped on chromosome 11p15 (9), and is secreted by parathyroid chief cells. Parathormone mediates direct action on bone by increasing the rate of osteoclastic resorption and promoting the breakdown of bone matrix (10). Parathormone's direct action on the kidney increases renal tubular resorption of calcium ions with concomitant phosphate tubular secretion, causing phosphaturia (11). Combined with 1,25 dihydroxy vitamin D, parathormone promotes the absorption of calcium in the small intestines. Calcitonin, secreted by the C cells of the thyroid gland, has a lesser effect on serum calcium. It functions as a moderate calciuric agent with a rapid, but short-lived effect on serum calcium.

HYPOPARATHYROIDISM

Hypoparathyroidism can be divided into congenital and idiopathic origins. Hypoparathyroidism associated with DiGeorge's syndrome is an example of selective T-cell deficiency, derived from inadequate development of the facial neural crest tissues and resulting in defective organogenesis of the third and fourth pharyngeal pouches. This disorder creates hypoplasia or absence of the thymus, parathyroids, and C cells of the thyroid. Patients are susceptible to recurrent viral and fungal infections, as well as tetany resulting from absence of the parathyroids. Facial, skeletal, and cardiovascular abnormalities are common. DiGeorge's syndrome is part of a group of disorders that share a common chromosome 22q11 deletion (12–15).

Idiopathic hypoparathyroidism is an autoimmune disorder primarily affecting females. The disease is characterized by the presence of antibodies against endocrine organs, including the parathyroids, thyroid gland, ovaries, and adrenals. The underlying abnormality is a defect in suppressor T-cell function. Circulating autoantibodies may or may not be identified within the blood. Patients can present with mucocutaneous candidiasis, pernicious anemia, adrenal insufficiency, autoimmune insulin-dependent diabetes mellitus, premature ovarian failure, autoimmune thyroid disease, and, in children, hypoparathyroidism (16). Microscopic evaluation of the parathyroid glands reveals atrophy and fatty replacement with diffuse infiltration by lymphocytes and plasma cells. Familial examples of idiopathic hypoparathyroidism and seizures have been described. These patients usually present in early childhood and do not have an associated autoimmune disorder (17–19).

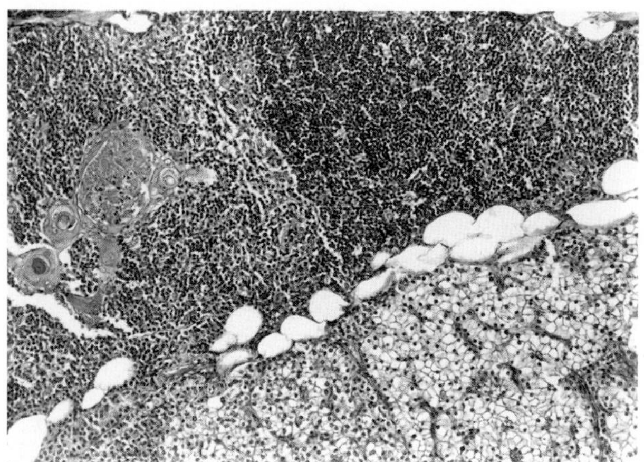

FIGURE 1. An ectopic parathyroid gland (at lower right) present in the thymus.

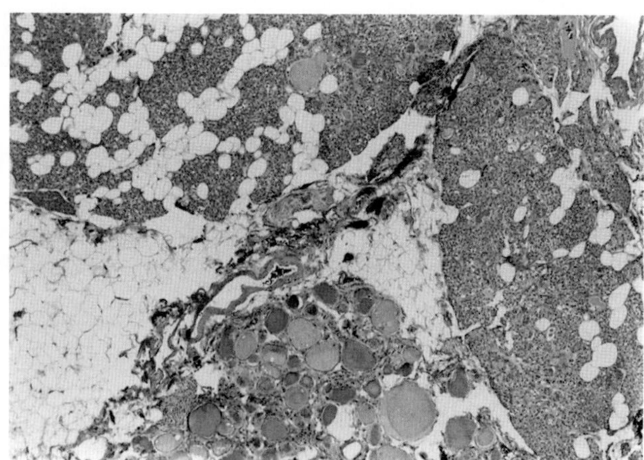

FIGURE 3. Inferior parathyroid glands can be intrathyroidal on rare occasions.

PARATHYROID ADENOMA

Primary hyperparathyroidism occurs in 0.1% to 0.3% of the general population, and up to 100,000 cases of primary hyperparathyroidism are diagnosed annually (20). The most common cause of primary hyperparathyroidism is the presence of a parathyroid adenoma, accounting for about 80% of cases (1). Parathyroid adenomas represent true monoclonal proliferations (21–23), affecting women more commonly than men at a ratio of 3:1 (1). Approximately half of the patients are asymptomatic, with hypercalcemia being picked up as part of a routine screening test. The mean age of incidence is 56 years. Similar to thyroid neoplasms, radiation to the head and neck has been causally related to the development of parathyroid adenomas (1,24–29).

The majority of parathyroid adenomas are solitary, and the average weight ranges from 200 to 1,000 mg (30). Examples of double and triple adenomas may exist, but they are much less common (31). Adenomas can arise in any location; however, the lower glands, parathyroid (III), are most frequently involved. The hypothesis that parathyroid adenomas are derived from clonal growth of preexisting single gland hyperplasia has been raised by several investigators (27,31–34).

Large adenomas can cause shadows or deformities of the neck structures on plain radiographs (35,36). Computerized tomographic (CT) scanning, ultrasonography, magnetic resonance imaging (MRI), venography with selective sampling of parathormone levels, nuclear imaging with thallium scanning, and thermography are several techniques that can be used alone or in combination to identify adenomas (37). Localization studies have about 80% accuracy in identifying lesional tissue (38).

Grossly, parathyroid adenomas are thinly encapsulated neoplasms (Fig. 4). The cut surface is a homogeneous red to tan. Cystic degeneration occurs occasionally. A correlation between the weight of the glands and the amount of hypercalcemia has been identified, with the average patient presenting with severe symptoms harboring an adenoma that weighs 10 g (1), although most parathyroid adenomas weight less than that.

Microscopically, the presence of an uninvolved rim of parathyroid tissue adjacent to the adenomatous proliferation, although helpful, is found only about half the time (Fig. 5). These cells, which can be compressed against the adenoma, are compact and admixed with stromal fat. The adenomas are circumscribed and sometimes thinly encapsulated, and contain proliferations of predominantly chief cells. Although the majority of the cells are monomorphic, marked nuclear irregularity is

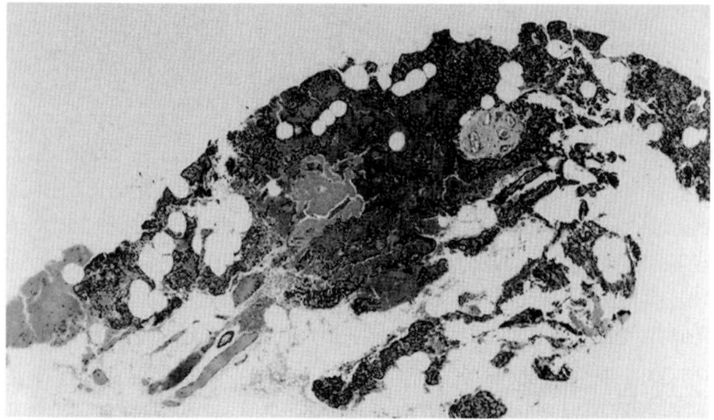

FIGURE 2. The normal accumulation of adipose tissue within the parathyroid gland during aging.

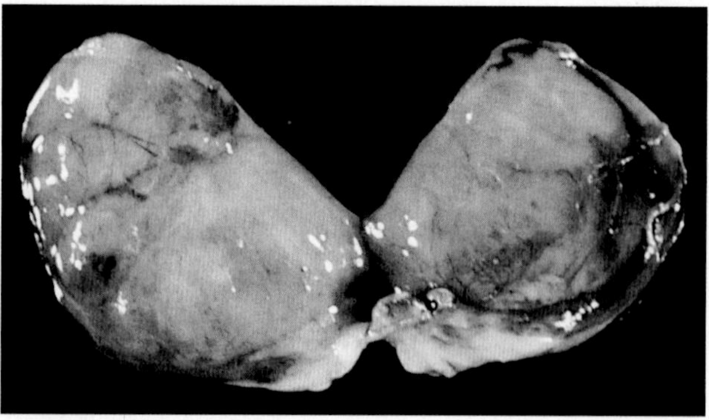

FIGURE 4. A gross photo of a parathyroid adenoma showing a thin capsule and homogeneous tan cut surface.

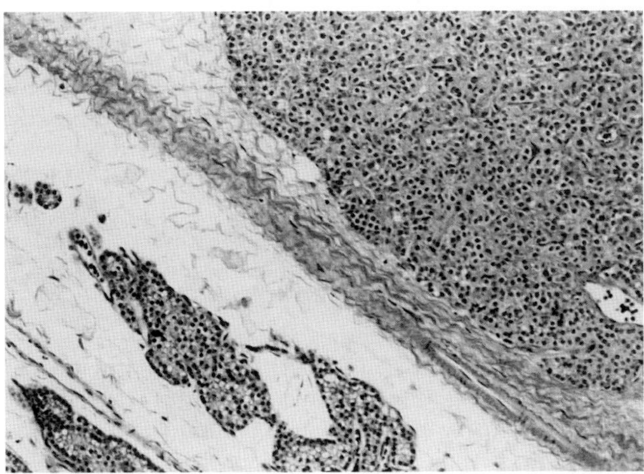

FIGURE 5. The edge of a parathyroid adenoma, with an adjacent rim of normal parathyroid tissue.

not uncommon and by itself is not a criterion of malignancy. The cells may grow in cords, nests, or sheets, or in a follicular arrangement. The follicles may contain periodic acid-Schiff (PAS)-positive colloid-like material, and they may be confused with thyroid follicles. Adenoma cells are polygonal and contain scant amounts of clear to amphophilic cytoplasm. The fact that these cells have regular, round nuclei and a more dense chromatin pattern aids in the differential diagnosis with thyroid follicular cells (Fig. 6).

The presence of mitoses in parathyroid adenomas is a well-recognized phenomenon. Mitotic figures by themselves have been reported in 80% of hyperplasias and 71% of adenomas (39). However, mitoses are not atypical, nor do they number more than five per 10 high-power fields (HPFs). Rare cases of reactive lymphocytic infiltration with destruction of parathyroid adenomas have been reported (40). In one of the two cases reported in the literature, there was considerable secondary fibrosis and atrophy in the adenoma. The diagnosis of atypical parathyroid adenoma is reserved for those infrequent cases that have some but not all of the features of malignancy (41). Patients given the diagnosis of atypical parathyroid adenoma should be followed carefully to identify recurrence or metastases.

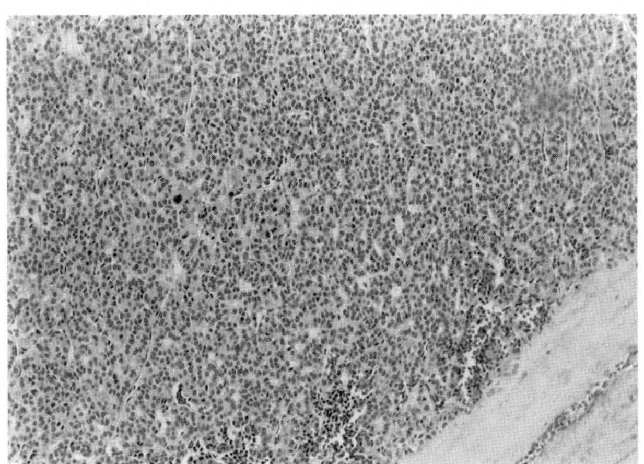

FIGURE 6. A parathyroid adenoma with the cells growing in a follicular fashion. The histology is similar to follicular cells of the thyroid, but the chromatin has a more dense pattern.

It is important to obtain a proper clinical history, because parathyroid specimens obtained from repeat operations for hyperparathyroidism can have histologic features that suggest malignancy. In addition to increased cellularity, broad intraglandular bands of fibrous tissue can contain entrapped cells mimicking invasive carcinoma. The surgeon may report experiencing difficulty in removing the parathyroid due to previous fibrosis and scarring.

At the time of frozen section or intraoperative consultation, the diagnosis of parathyroid adenoma should be made only after accounting for and evaluating at least one of the remaining glands. Small atrophic or normal-sized glands usually accompany a parathyroid adenoma. The presence of a double adenoma of the parathyroid is exceedingly rare, accounting for 1% to 3% of primary hyperparathyroidism (29,42–44). This diagnosis should be made with caution and in the absence of a familial endocrinopathy (44). After evaluation of the abnormal gland, at least one of the remaining glands should be examined via biopsy and histologically evaluated. If one gland is enlarged and hypercellular with decreased fat and the others are normal or atrophic, the diagnosis of adenoma is supported. If more than one gland is abnormally enlarged and hypercellular, the diagnosis of hyperplasia is favored.

The *PRAD1* oncogene is rearranged with the parathyroid hormone gene in a small subset of sporadic parathyroid adenomas (23). Hsi et al. studied cyclin D1/PRAD1 protein expression in 65 parathyroid adenomas and found diffuse nuclear immunoreactivity in 18% (45).

The treatment for patients with parathyroid adenomas ranges from removal of the diseased gland and biopsy of at least one remaining (usually ipsilateral) parathyroid to total four-gland parathyroidectomy. After conservative removal of just one gland, Rudberg et al. found recurrent hypercalcemia in only 3% of patients with adenomas (46). Reoperation in two of these 10 patients with persistent hypercalcemia revealed new single adenoma formation, suggesting that the stimuli for adenoma formation persisted. In this group, recurrent hypercalcemia developed 9 to 17 years after the initial surgery.

PARATHYROMATOSIS

Parathyromatosis is defined by finding multiple nodules of parathyroid tissue throughout the lower neck and anterior mediastinum (47–50). Parathyromatosis can be found as a result of autoimplantation of tissue after surgery, or even during an initial neck exploration. Nests of parathyroid tissue outside the normal anatomic location of the patient's glands have been described in patients during their primary surgery, essentially ruling out spillage as a mode of dissemination (47). A proposed mechanism is that these nests are present from early development and have become clinically significant after hyperplasia or adenoma formation. Patients may have symptoms of recurrent hypercalcemia. Histologically, foci of parathyroid tissue insinuate in soft tissue without desmoplasia (47–50). Stehman-Breen and colleagues reported a series of five patients with parathyromatosis secondary to chronic renal failure. Forty percent were unresponsive to combined surgical and medical treatment and ultimately died from their disease (48).

ONCOCYTIC CELL ADENOMA

Oncocytic or oxyphil cell adenomas of the parathyroid gland are unusual in their pure form, accounting for 3% of all parathyroid adenomas in a series by Wolpert et al. (51). As their name suggests, these adenomas are composed of large oncocytic cells with abundant granular eosinophilic cytoplasm and basophilic nuclei. Electron microscopic evaluation reveals abundant mitochondria and membrane-associated secretory granules, accounting for this tumor's characteristic histologic appearance (52). These adenomas may or may not be functional, with patients occasionally presenting with hypercalcemia. Immunohistochemical and *in situ* hybridization analysis show parathormone protein expression (53).

LIPADENOMA

Lipadenomas are hamartomatous proliferations of parathyroid cells and adipose tissue. Most patents present with hypercalcemia. The lesion can be circumscribed but is rarely encapsulated. Microscopically, islands of chief cells, oxyphilic cells, and mature fat can be identified, separated by myxoid stroma. The chief cells can form trabeculae and ribbons and be arranged in a canalicular pattern (54–58).

HYPERPARATHYROIDISM—JAW TUMOR SYNDROME

In 1958, Jackson reported a single family with hereditary hyperparathyroidism and jaw tumors (59). In 1987, Mallette et al. reported a similar kindred with cystic hyperparathyroidism and fibrous maxillary and mandibular tumors (60). Other families have since been identified, kidney tumors have been added to the spectrum of disease, and an autosomal dominant pattern of disease inheritance has been established (61–67). A gene has been identified (*HRPT 2*) and mapped to chromosome 1q21-31 (67). The histology of the parathyroids in hyperparathyroidism–jaw tumor syndrome is that of single and multiple parathyroid adenomas, some of which are cystic. Rarely, carcinoma of the parathyroid gland has been identified (61,62).

PARATHYROID CYSTS

Parathyroid cysts are uncommon, occurring more frequently in women and involving the lower parathyroid glands (parathyroid III) (68–73). Rarely, parathyroid cysts can be located in the upper glands or in ectopic locations such as the mediastinum, where they can mimic thymic cysts. The cysts range in size from 1 to 6 cm and are unilocular. Fine-needle aspiration of these cysts can be diagnostic, because the clear aspirated fluid contains high levels of assayable parathormone (71). It is important to sample the thickest portion of the cyst wall to evaluate for the presence of adenomatous tissue or hyperplasia. It has been postulated that the cyst formation can develop secondarily to cystic degeneration of an adenoma (68–73).

PARATHYROID CARCINOMA

Parathyroid carcinoma is rare, accounting for 0.5% to 5% of primary hyperparathyroidism (1,74–78). Serum calcium is usually greater than 14 mg/dL. Uncommonly, parathyroid carcinomas are nonfunctional, without hormonal production (79–80). This latter group is reportedly more clinically aggressive (80). The male:female ratio is almost equal, and the mean age of presentation is 45 years, about 10 years younger than for benign parathyroid disease (1,77,81). Patients can present with a palpable neck mass, polydipsia, polyuria, renal colic secondary to stones, pancreatitis, generalized weakness, anorexia, and gastrointestinal complaints. Rarely is the diagnosis of parathyroid carcinoma rendered preoperatively. Rather, it is not uncommon for patients initially to be given the diagnosis of parathyroid adenoma, with the development of metastases occurring many years later. In several retrospective studies there has been histologic evidence of carcinoma arising from both adenomatous and hyperplastic glands (82–85). Frequently this association is seen in a familial setting (79).

Grossly, the parathyroid carcinomas are usually larger than adenomas, with the average tumor measuring 3 cm in diameter and weighing 12 g (77,78,81). The surgeon often entertains the diagnosis of parathyroid carcinoma when he encounters a firm gland stuck to contiguous structures in a patient who has not had a previous neck exploration. Frequently the tumor will have a thick capsule. On cut surface, firm gray to tan tissue with necrosis, calcification, or cystic degeneration can be observed (1).

Microscopically, the presence of a thick capsule, thick intralesional fibrous bands, capsular or vascular invasion, a trabecular growth pattern, spindle cells, large nuclei, necrosis, and frequent mitoses have been described as discerning features distinguishing carcinoma from benign lesions (1,85–89). In a recent histologic study by Evans (85), 27 parathyroid tumors, including hyperplasias, adenomas, and carcinomas with a minimum 9-year follow-up were reviewed. He concluded that the majority of the carcinomas had eight or more mitoses per 10 HPFs, whereas the maximum number of mitoses in the benign lesions was five per 10 HPFs. He identified thick intralesional fibrous bands, spindle cells, and areas of trabecular growth in near equal frequency in both benign and malignant neoplasms. His findings reinforce the concept that these latter histologic features, taken by themselves, are not sufficient for the diagnosis of carcinoma. Vascular invasion, although virtually diagnostic of malignancy in parathyroid carcinoma, should be evaluated using the same criteria as for follicular neoplasms of the thyroid (90). True capsular invasion (i.e., penetration of tumor outside the capsule) should be distinguished from entrapped tumor cells resulting from long-standing disease and fibrosis (Fig. 7).

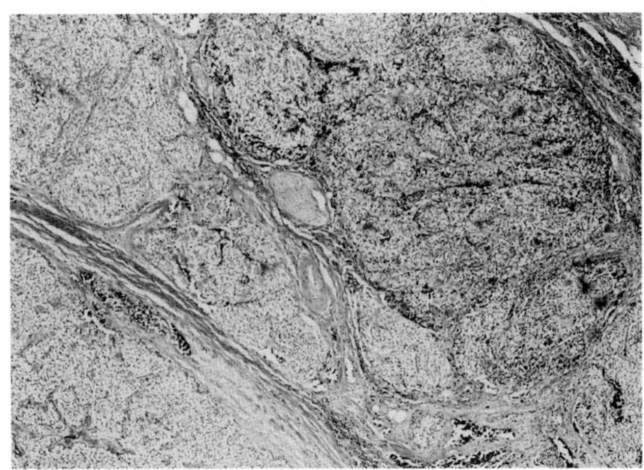

FIGURE 7. A parathyroid carcinoma showing extension beyond the capsule and entrapment of adjacent nerves and blood vessels.

Rarely, carcinomas will not exhibit any histologic features diagnostic of malignancy, their true nature only being revealed after long-term follow-up and the development of recurrences and metastases. Several investigators have looked at immunohistochemical studies and molecular techniques to try to separate adenomas from carcinoma. The retinoblastoma (RB) tumor suppressor gene was found to be inactive in all informative parathyroid carcinomas and only 1 of 19 parathyroid adenomas (91). Additionally, 88% of patients with cancer had abnormal immunohistochemical expression for RB protein, whereas none of the adenomas had abnormal staining.

Hakim et al., using the polymerase chain reaction (PCR) technique, found that p53 point mutations were absent in three parathyroid carcinomas and 26 adenomas (92). Vargas et al. identified one atypical adenoma and 2 of 11 parathyroid carcinomas that were immunoreactive for p53 (93). In a similarly designed study by Naccarato et al., 0 of 3 parathyroid carcinomas were immunoreactive for p53 (94).

Studies evaluating DNA ploidy in carcinomas and adenomas have shown statistically significant differences between the two, with aneuploidy being identified in 100% of metastases from parathyroid carcinoma, 60% of primary cancers, and 9% of adenomas in a study by Obara et al. (95). However, Joensuu and Klemi found aneuploidy in 35% of their adenomas and concluded that ploidy should not be used as a criterion for malignancy (96). Reportedly, aneuploidy, when seen in association with parathyroid carcinoma, is a valuable predictor of recurrence and metastases (95).

The primary treatment for parathyroid carcinoma is surgery, with an en bloc resection recommended for tumors that present with disease outside the gland (87,97,98). About 30% of patients are cured with surgery, and approximately 33% develop metastases in regional lymph nodes of the neck and mediastinum within 3 years of initial diagnosis (81). In a recent study of 16 patients with parathyroid carcinoma, Favia et al. reported that the sequelae of surgery included prolonged hypocalcemia (38%) and recurrence (63%), with a median disease-free period of 24 months postsurgery (78). Distant metastases to the lung, liver, pancreas, and bone are less common (77). Although recurrences usually develop within three years of initial diagnosis, multiple recurrences spanning a 15- to 20-year period are not uncommon (77,96). Recent studies advocate aggressively resecting foci of metastatic disease to achieve longer patient survival (99,100).

Most deaths result from complications of persistent hypercalcemia, with a 5-year survival rate of around 50%. Nonfunctioning carcinomas have been reported to behave more aggressively than their functioning counterparts (79,97,98). Historically, parathyroid carcinomas have been reported as not being radiosensitive (79,97,98). However, a recent communication by Chow et al. (101) reported success with adjuvant radiation therapy for microscopic residual disease in seven patients followed for a mean of 62 months.

PRIMARY PARATHYROID HYPERPLASIA

Primary parathyroid hyperplasia may occur sporadically or in the setting of multiple endocrine neoplasia (MEN). One to 18% of patients with primary hyperparathyroidism has familial hyperparathyroidism or MEN (102). The histology of these lesions is usually diffuse or nodular chief cell hyperplasia (Fig. 8). In an autopsy study of 422 patients, Akerström et al. found primary parathyroid hyperplasia in 7% of routinely examined parathyroid glands (103). The clinical presentation of patients with sporadic primary chief cell hyperplasia is not significantly different from patients with parathyroid adenoma. Most patients with MEN type 1 present with hyperparathyroidism before developing symptoms of other endocrinopathies (104). In the familial setting, males and females are affected equally, and the onset of hyperparathyroidism usually begins before age 40. Elevated serum levels of calcium can be detected much earlier in younger, asymptomatic patients.

Grossly there is generally four-gland enlargement, which may be asymmetrical. The lower glands (parathyroid III) are usually larger in asymmetrical cases (1). The cut surface is lobular and red to brown. The combined weight of all glands usually ranges from 1 to 3 g (1). Microscopically the hyperplasia may be diffuse

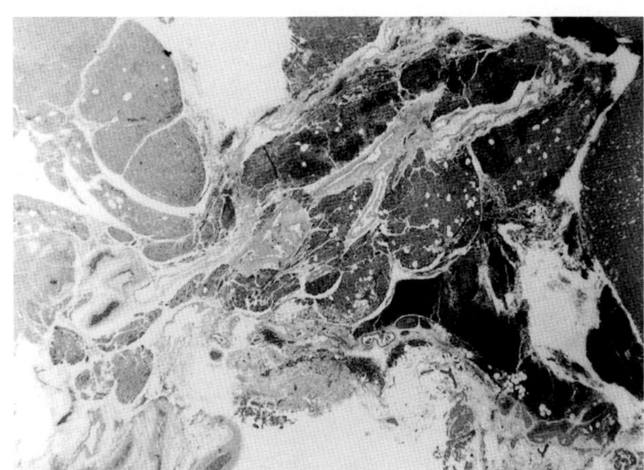

FIGURE 8. Primary parathyroid hyperplasia showing a multinodular growth pattern.

or nodular, as is frequently the case in MEN (Fig. 8). Histologic evaluation also may show asymmetrical involvement. Primary hyperparathyroidism may be divided into chief cell and water clear cell hyperplasia. Chief cell hyperplasia represents the majority of hyperplasias. As the name suggests, the predominant cell population is that of chief cells, but nodular proliferations of water clear cells and aggregates of oxyphilic cells are frequently interspersed. A delicate fibrovascular framework insinuates between proliferating cells. Architectural patterns include nests, follicular and acinar formation, and solid sheets of cells. Individual cells are generally uniform, with the bizarre cells and binucleate forms seen in parathyroid adenoma rarely identified. Intracellular and stromal fat is decreased, and mitoses are rare. Mature fat cells often can be found in the stroma, interspersed between proliferating cells. Unlike the case of parathyroid adenoma, a rim of residual compressed parathyroid tissue is generally not observed (1).

FROZEN SECTIONING OF THE PARATHYROID

The primary role of the pathologist at the time of frozen sectioning is to identify the lesional tissue as parathyroid. Lymph nodes, thymus, thyroid, and fibroconnective tissue must be ruled out. The weight and size of the glands should be recorded as well as whether the gland is histologically hypercellular. Nodularity and the presence of acini, fat, and water clear cells are helpful to note in assisting in the diagnosis of hyperplasia (105). The surgical pathologist should refrain from trying to be heroic when evaluating just one gland. Conveying to the surgeon the diagnosis of hypercellular parathyroid and reviewing subsequent parathyroids will help to determine whether the gland is considered hyperplastic or adenomatous. Uneven involvement of the glands by hyperplasia also can make the diagnosis difficult. Occasionally one gland is much larger than the others, suggesting a diagnosis of adenoma. It is imperative to choose the darkest, most solid and firm areas of the parathyroid to section and evaluate, because microscopic evaluation of the glands may show uneven areas of proliferating cells. Estimation of the amount of cellular and stromal fat by use of intraoperative Sudan IV or oil red O can be used with caution as an adjunctive technique in the differential diagnosis of adenoma and hyperplasia (44,105,106). However, both adenoma and hyperplasia will have a decreased amount of stromal and intracellular fat.

Surgical identification of more than one and optimally of all four glands is necessary in the evaluation of hyperparathyroidism. If all four glands appear normal in a patient with hypercalcemia, the possibility of supernumerary parathyroid glands should be entertained with evaluation of the mediastinum (107). Kraimps et al. reported that 135 patients with MEN had supernumerary parathyroids (108). Primary hyperparathyroidism is treated by subtotal parathyroidectomy, with total removal of three glands and subtotal excision of the fourth, leaving behind 50 to 80 mg of viable tissue (109–111). The thymic tongue also should be removed.

Several series report a higher recurrence rate of hyperparathyroidism in patients with familial disease (108,112). Thus, the current recommendation for patients with hyperparathyroidism and familial disease is total parathyroidectomy with autotransplantation of a small amount of parathyroid tissue in the patient's nondominant forearm (113–115). Patients also may have parathyroid tissue cryopreserved in case hypoparathyroidism develops from autograft failure (37). Conversely, the autotransplanted tissue may proliferate, with resultant hyperparathyroidism. Caution must be observed when reviewing the surgically removed autograft, because regrowth of the tissue between skeletal muscle fibers may simulate invasion by cancer (116,117).

The cure rate is about 90% in sporadic cases of primary hyperparathyroidism (1). As previously stated, familial hyperparathyroidism is more difficult to treat. The incidence of recurrent hyperparathyroidism in these patients postsurgery ranges from 9% to 67%, depending on the expertise of the surgeon (108,112,118,119).

WATER CLEAR CELL HYPERPLASIA

Water clear cell hyperplasia is extremely rare (1). The aggregate weight of the glands is usually greater than that seen in primary chief cell hyperplasia. In a series of water clear cell hyperplasias from the Massachusetts General Hospital, 50% of cases had total weights ranging from 10 to 60 g (120,121). Similar to primary chief cell hyperplasia, there can be asymmetrical enlargement. In contrast to primary chief cell hyperplasia, however, cases of water clear cell hyperplasia have affected the upper glands (parathyroid IV) to a greater extent than the lower glands. On gross inspection, the glands are red to brown and lobular. Microscopically, the glands show diffuse sheets of clear cells without a mixture of other cell types. The cells are polyhedral with enlarged hyperchromatic nuclei and small basophilic nucleoli. The cytoplasm is filled with multiple fine vacuoles. Important in the differential diagnosis of water clear cell hyperplasia is metastatic renal cell carcinoma (1,122,123).

MULTIPLE ENDOCRINE NEOPLASIA

In 1954, Wermer described a family in which several members, spanning two generations, had hyperparathyroidism and tumors of the pituitary and pancreas (124). It was not the first time that this relationship had been observed either sporadically (125,126) or in the familial setting (127). MEN type 1 or Wermer's syndrome is an autosomal dominant disorder defined by involvement of at least two of the following organs: parathyroid (80%–98%), pituitary (30%–60%), pancreas and duodenum (40%–85%). Adrenal cortical involvement, thyroid tumors, and multiple lipomatous tumors are much less common (128,129). Parathyroid involvement is in the form of chief cell hyperplasia. Parathyroid adenomas and carcinomas have been rarely described in patients with MEN type 1 (84,130).

In 1988, the gene for MEN type 1 was mapped on chromosome 11q13 (131). This study and others established the monoclonality of the parathyroid proliferations in MEN type 1 (131,132). Loss of heterozygosity in this region is a frequent finding in parathyroid tumors (132,133), supporting the hypothesis that the gene responsible for MEN type 1 is a tumor suppressor gene.

Some parathyroid tumors occurring on a sporadic basis also show loss of heterozygosity on 11q13, suggesting indirectly that the MEN type 1 gene also contributes to sporadic tumor formation (134).

First described by Sipple in 1961, MEN type 2 is also an autosomal dominant disorder with a high degree of penetrance and variable expression. Three clinical types of MEN type 2 are currently recognized (MEN type 2A, MEN type 2B, and familial medullary thyroid cancer). If left untreated, virtually all patients with MEN type 2 will develop medullary thyroid cancer (135–137). Parathyroid hyperplasia and adenoma formation occur in 0 to 53% of patients with MEN type 2, with a mean incidence of 35% (138,139). Parathyroid involvement is usually asymptomatic, with the symptoms of medullary thyroid cancer overshadowing hyperparathyroidism. Serum calcium is lower and hyperparathyroidism less severe than in patients with MEN type 1. However, treatment recommendations of total parathyroidectomy and heterotopic autotransplantation are the same (119).

Patients with MEN type 2B develop C-cell hyperplasia and medullary thyroid carcinoma. Approximately 40% develop pheochromocytoma. Additionally, mucosal neuromas, marfanoid body habitus, and ganglioneuromatosis characterize this disease. Parathyroid involvement is extremely rare with MEN type 2B (140).

As discussed earlier in the description of medullary thyroid cancer, genetic studies of families with MEN type 2A and 2B have identified germline mutations in the *RET* protooncogene, located on chromosome 10q11.2 (141,142). No *RET* protooncogene somatic mutations have been identified in sporadic parathyroid adenomas (143,144). Other familial endocrinopathies associated with hyperparathyroidism include mixed MEN syndrome and familial hyperparathyroidism with MEN.

FAMILIAL HYPOCALCIURIC HYPERCALCEMIA

Familial hypocalciuric hypercalcemia (FHH) is an autosomal dominant form of hypercalcemia, which, in its heterozygous form, is characterized by life-long nonprogressive hypercalcemia. These patients are asymptomatic; serum parathormone and urine calcium are normal. Patients are diagnosed with FHH when their ratio of calcium clearance over creatinine clearance is below 0.01, whereas patients with primary hyperparathyroidism have a ratio greater than 0.1. The homozygous form of FHH results in severe neonatal hyperparathyroidism with patients presenting by 3 weeks of age with severe hypercalcemia, lethargy, hypotonia, and mental retardation (119,145,146). In 1993, Pollak et al. reported mutations in the calcium-sensing receptor gene located on the long arm of chromosome 3 in patients with FHH (147).

The heterozygous form of FHH does not require surgery. However, when examined, the parathyroids show a mild degree of primary chief cell hyperplasia (148–150). Total parathyroidectomy and thymectomy with heterotopic autotransplantation of a small amount of parathyroid tissue in the arm of infants is recommended for patients with the homozygous form of FHH (119).

SECONDARY HYPERPARATHYROIDISM

Secondary hyperparathyroidism occurs as a sequela of chronic renal disease or intestinal malabsorption refractory to medical treatment. Persistent hypercalcemia with detection of enlarged parathyroid glands and bone disease are indications for surgical removal of the parathyroid glands. The histologic features of primary and secondary chief cell hyperplasia are similar (150). Initially the proliferations are diffuse and consist of chief cell hyperplasia with interspersed nodules of oxyphil cells.

Arnold et al. reported that 64% of their patients with secondary hyperparathyroidism had at least one monoclonal parathyroid mass (151). Interestingly, in parathyroid hyperplasia secondary to uremia, the nodular aggregates in nodular hyperplasia are monoclonal, and glands that are diffusely hyperplastic are polyclonal (152). Parathyroid hyperplasia secondary to uremia also can show allelic loss on chromosome 11q13 (153). These results show that not only can parathyroid adenoma be monoclonal, but primary and secondary hyperplasia with multigland involvement also can have clonal growth. The presence of both monoclonal and polyclonal proliferation zones within a single gland lends molecular support to the histologic impression of a monotypic expansion arising in the background of a polymorphous population.

REFERENCES

1. Delellis RA. Tumors of the parathyroid gland. In: Rosai J, Sobin LH, eds. *Atlas of tumors pathology.* Series 3, fascicle 6. Washington, DC: Armed Forces Institute of Pathology, 1993.
2. Wang C. The anatomic basis of parathyroid surgery. *Ann Surg* 1976;183:271–275.
3. Gilmore JR, Martin WJ. The weight of the parathyroid glands. *J Pathol* 1937;44:431–462.
4. Akerström G, Grimelius L, Johansson H, et al. The parenchymal cell mass in normal parathyroid glands. *Acta Pathol Microbiol Scand* 1981;89:367–375.
5. Akerström G. Malmaeus J, Bergström R. Surgical anatomy of human parathyroid glands. *Surgery* 1984;95:14–21.
6. Carney JA. Pathology of hyperparathyroidism: a practical approach. *Monogr Pathol* 1993;35:34–62.
7. Gilmore JR. Some developmental abnormalities of the thymus and parathyroids. *J Pathol Bacteriol* 1941;52:213–218.
8. Lack EE, Delay S, Linnoila I. Ectopic parathyroid tissue within the vagus nerve. Incidence and possible clinical significance. *Arch Pathol Lab Med* 1988;112:304–306.
9. Parisien M, Silverberg SJ, Shane E, et al. Bone disease in primary hyperparathyroidism. *Endocrinol Metab Clin North Am* 1990;19:19–34.
10. Raisz LG, Kream BE. Regulation of bone formation. *N Engl J Med* 1983;309:83–89.
11. Knox FG, Haramati A. Renal regulation of phosphate secretion. In: Seldin DW, Giebisch G, eds. *The kidney: physiology and pathophysiology.* New York: Raven, 1985.
12. Burke BA, Johnson D, Gilbert EF, et al. Thyrocalcitonin containing cells in the DiGeorge anomaly. *Hum Pathol* 1987;18:355–360.
13. Huber J, Zegers PJ, Schourman HJ. Pathology of congenital immunodeficiencies. *Semin Diagn Pathol* 1992;9:31–62.

14. Hong R. The DiGeorge anomaly (Catch 22, DiGeorge velocardiofacial syndrome). *Semin Hematol* 1998;35:282–290.
15. Leanna-Cox J, Pangkanon S, Eanet KR, et al. Familial DiGeorge velocardiofacial syndrome with deletion of chromosome area 22q11.2. Report of 5 families with review of literature. *Am J Med Genet* 1996;65:309–316.
16. Vazquez AM, Kenney FM. Ovarian failure and anti-ovarian antibodies in association with hypoparathyroidism, moniliasis, and Addison's and Hashimoto's diseases. *Obstet Gynecol* 1973;41:414–418.
17. Bronsky D, Kiamko RT, Waldstein SS. Familial idiopathic hypoparathyroidism. *J Clin Endocrinol Metab* 1968;28:61–65.
18. Peden VH. True idiopathic hypoparathyroidism as a sex-lined recessive trait. *Am J Hum Genet* 1960;12:323–335.
19. Whyte MP, Weldon VW. Idiopathic hypoparathyroidism presenting with seizures during infancy. X-linked recessive inheritance in a large Missouri kindred. *J Pediatr* 1981;99:608–611.
20. NIH Conference: Diagnosis and management of asymptomatic primary hyperparathyroidism: consensus development conference statement. *Ann Intern Med* 1991;114:593–597.
21. Arnold A, Kin HG. Clonal loss of one chomosome 11 in a parathyroid adenoma. *J Clin Endocrinol Metab* 1989;69:496–499.
22. Arnold A, Kim HG, Gaz RD, et al. Molecular cloning and chromosomal mapping of DNA rearranged with the parathyroid hormone gene in parathyroid adenoma. *J Clin Invest* 1989;83:2034–2040.
23. Arnold A, Staunton LE, Kim HG, et al. Monoclonality and abnormal parathyroid hormone genes in parathyroid adenomas. *N Engl J Med* 1988;318:658–662.
24. Tisell LE, Carlson S, Lingberg S, et al. Autonomous hyperparathyroidsm: a possible late complication of neck radiotherapy. *Acta Chir Scand* 1976;142:367–373.
25. Russ JE, Scanlon EF, Sener SF. Parathyroid adenomas following irradiation. *Cancer* 1979;43:1078–1083.
26. Fiorica V, Males JL. Hyperparathyroidism after radiation of head and neck: a case report and review of the literature. *Am J Med Sci* 1979; 278:223–228.
27. Prinz RA, Barabato AZ, Braithwaite SS, et al. Prior irradiation and the development of co-existent differentiated thyroid cancer and hyperparathyroidism. *Cancer* 1982;49:874–877.
28. Gillis D, Hirsch HJ, Landau H, et al. Parathyroid adenoma after radiation in an 8 year old boy. *J Pediatr* 1998;132:892–893.
29. Grimelius L, Johansson H. Pathology of parathyroid tumors. *Semin Surg Oncol* 1997;13:142–154.
30. Harness JK, Hiyama RH, Thompson NW. Multiple adenomas of the parathyroids: do they exist? *Arch Surg* 1979;114:468–474.
31. Golden, A, Canary JJ, Kerwin DM. Concurrence of hyperplasia and neoplasia of the parathyroid glands. *Am J Med* 1965;38:562–578.
32. Kramer WM. Parathyroid hyperplasia with neoplasia. *Am J Clin Pathol* 1970;53:275–283.
33. Akerström G, Rudberg C, Grimelius L, et al. Histologic parathyroid abnormalities in an autopsy series. *Hum Pathol* 1986;17:520–527.
34. Ghandur-Mnaymeh L, Kimura N. The parathyroid adenoma. A histopathologic definition with a study of 172 cases of primary hyperparathyroidism. *Am J Pathol* 1984;115:70–83.
35. Wyman SM, Robbins, LL. Roentgen recognition of parathyroid adenoma. *Am J Roentgenol Radium Ther Nucl Med* 1954;71:777–784.
36. Kebebew E, Clark OH. Parathyroid adenoma, hyperplasia and cancer localization, technical details of primary neck exploration and treatment of hypercalcemic crisis. *Surg Oncol Clin North Am* 1998;7: 721–748.
37. Miller DL. Preoperative localization and interventional treatment of parathyroid tumors: when and how? *World Surg* 1991:15:6.
38. Mitchell BK, Merrell RC, Kinder BK. Localization studies in patients with hyperparathyroidism. *Surg Clin North Am* 1995;75:483–498.
39. Snover DC, Foucar K. Mitotic activity in benign parathyroid disease. *Am J Clin Pathol* 1981;5:345–347.
40. Veress B, Nordenstrom J. Lymphocytic infiltration and destruction of parathyroid adenomas: a possible tumor-specific autoimmune reaction in two cases of primary hyperparathyroidism. *Histopathology* 1994;25:373–377.
41. Levin KE, Chew KL, Ljung BM, et al. Deoxyribonucleic acid cytometry helps identify parathyroid cancer. *J Clin Endocrinol Metab* 1988; 67:779–784.
42. Attie JN, Auguste LJ. Multiple parathyroid adenomas. Report of 33 cases. *Surgery* 1990;108:1014–1019.
43. Verdonk CA, Edis AJ. Parathyroid "double adenomas": fact or fiction? *Surgery* 1981;90:523–526.
44. Livolsi VA, Hamilton R. Intraoperative assessment of parathyroid gland pathology. A common view from the surgeon and the pathologist. *Am J Clin Pathol* 1994:102:365–373.
45. Hsi ED, Zukerberg, LR, Yang WI, et al. Cyclin D/PRAD1 expression in parathyroid adenoma. *J Clin Endocrinol Metab* 1996;81: 1736–1739.
46. Rudberg C. Akerström G, Palmer M, et al. Late results of operation for primary hyperparathyroidism in 441 patients. *Surgery* 1986;99: 643–650.
47. Reddick RL, Costa JC, Marx SJ. Parathyroid hyperplasia and parathyromatosis. *Lancet* 1977;1:549.
48. Stehman-Breen C, Muirhead N, Thorning D, et al. Secondary hyperparathyroidism complicated by parathyromatosis. *Am J Kidney Dis* 1996;28:502–507.
49. Kollmorgen CF, Aust MR, Ferreiro JA, et al. Parathyromatosis: an important cause of persistent or recurrent hyperparathyroidism. *Surgery* 1994;116:111–115.
50. Fitko R, Roth SI, Hines JR, et al. Parathyromatosis in hyperparathyroidism. *Hum Pathol* 1990;21:234–237.
51. Wolpert HR, Vickery AL Jr, Wang CA. Functioning oxyphil cell adenomas of the parathyroid gland. A study of 15 cases. *Am J Surg Pathol* 1989;13:500–504.
52. Selman HM, Fechner RE. Oxyphil adenoma and primary hyperparathyroidism: clinical and ultrastructural observations. *JAMA* 1967;199:359–361.
53. Stork PJ, Herteux C, Frazier R, et al. Expression and distribution of parathyroid hormone and parathyroid messenger RNA in pathological conditions of the parathyroid [Abstract]. *Lab Invest* 1989;60:92.
54. Abul-Haj SK, Conklin H, Hewitt WC. Functioning lipadenoma of the parathyroid gland: report of an unique case. *N Engl J Med* 1962;266:121–123.
55. Geelhoed GW. Parathyroid adenolipoma: clinical and morphological features. *Surgery* 1982;92:806–810.
56. LeGoluan DP, More BP, Nishiyama RH. Parathyroid hamartoma. Report of two cases and review of the Literature. *Am J Clin Pathol* 1997;67:31–35.
57. Weiland LH, Garrison RC, Remine WH, et al. Lipadenoma of the parathyroid gland. *Am J Surg Pathol* 1978;2:3–7.
58. Ober WB, Kaiser GA. Hamartoma of the parathyroid. *Cancer* 1958;11:601–606.
59. Jackson CE. Hereditary hyperparathyroidism associated with recurrent pancreatitis. *Ann Intern Med* 1958;49:829–836.
60. Mallette LE, Malini S, Rappaport MP, et al. Familial cystic parathyroid adenomatosis. *Ann Intern Med* 1987:107:54–60.
61. Dinnen JS, Greenwood RH, Jones JH, et al. Parathyroid cancer in familial hyperparathyroidism. *J Clin Pathol* 1977;30:966–975.
62. Rosen LB, Palmer JA. Fibro-osseous tumors of the facial skeleton in association with primary hyperparathyroidism. *Am J Surg* 1981;142: 494–498.
63. Inoue H, Miki H, Oshimi K, et al. Familial hyperparathyroidism associated with jaw fibroma. Case report and literature review. *Clin Endocrinol* 1995;43:225–229.
64. Teh BT, Farnebo F, Kristiffersson U, et al. Autosomal dominant primary hyperparathyroidism and jaw tumor syndrome associated with renal hamartomas and cystic kidney disease: linkage to lq21-32 and loss of the wild type allele in renal hamartomas. *J Clin Endocrinol Metab* 1996;81:4204–4211.
65. Jackson CE, Norum RA, Boyd SB, et al. Hereditary hyperparathyroidism and multiple jaw ossifying fibromas: a clinically and genetically distinct syndrome. *Surgery* 1990;108:1006–1012.
66. Hobbs MR, Pole AR, Pidwirny GN, et al. Hyperparathyroidism—jaw tumor syndrome: the HRPT2 locus is within an 0.7-cM region on chromosome 1q. *Am J Hum Genet* 1999:64:518–525.

67. Szabo J, Heath B, Hill VM, et al. Hereditary hyperparathyroidism—jaw tumor syndrome: the endocrine tumor gene HRPT2 maps to chromosome lq 21-31. *Am J Hum Genet* 1995;56:994–950.
68. Gordon A, Harcourt-Webster JN. Parathyroid cysts. A report of 2 cases. *J Pathol Bacteriol* 1965;89:374–377.
69. Simkin EP. Hyperparathyroidism associated with a parathyroid cyst: an unusual presentation. *Br J Surg* 1976;63:927–928.
70. Miyauchi A, Kakudo K, Fujimoto T, et al. Parathyroid cyst: analysis of the cyst fluid and ultrastructural observance. *Arch Pathol Lab Med* 1981;105:497–499.
71. Alva A, Myssiorek D, Wasserman P. Parathyroid cyst. Current diagnostic and management principles. *Head Neck* 1996;18:370–373.
72. Gurbuz AT, Peetz ME. Giant mediastinal parathyroid cyst. An unusual cause of hypercalcemic crisis—case report and review of literature. *Surgery* 1996;120:795–800.
73. Van Fossen VL, Edis AJ. Clear parathyroid cysts and hyperparathyroidism. *Am Surg* 1998;64:1226–1228.
74. Barnes BA, Cope O. Cancer of the parathyroid glands. Report of 10 cases with endocrine function. *JAMA* 1961;178:556–559.
75. Black BK. Cancer of the parathyroid. *Ann Surg* 1954;139:355–363.
76. McKeown PP, McGarity WC, Sewell CW. Cancer of the parathyroid gland: is it over diagnosed? A report of 3 cases. *Am J Surg* 1984;147: 292–298.
77. Wang C, Gaz RD. Natural history of parathyroid cancer: diagnosis, treatment and results. *Am J Surg* 1985;149:522–527.
78. Favia G, Lumachi F, Polistina F, et al. Parathyroid cancer: sixteen new cases and suggestion for correct management. *World J Surg* 1998:22:1225–1230.
79. Holmes EC, Morton DL, Ketcham AS. Parathyroid cancer, a collective review. *Ann Surg* 1969;169:631–640.
80. Aldinger KA, Hickey RC, Ibanez ML, et al. Parathyroid cancer, a clinical study of 7 cases of functioning and 2 of non-functioning parathyroid cancer. *Cancer* 1982;49:388–397.
81. Schanz A, Castleman B. Parathyroid cancer: a study of 70 cases. *Cancer* 1972;31:600–605.
82. Dinne JS, Greenwood RH, Jones JH, et al. Parathyroid cancer in familial hyperparathyroidism. *J Clin Pathol* 1977;30:966–975.
83. Haghighi P, Astarita RW, Wepsic HT, et al. Concurrent primary parathyroid hyperplasia and parathyroid cancer. *Arch Pathol Lab Med* 1983;107:349–350.
84. Mallette LE, Bilezikian JP, Ketcham AS, et al. Parathyroid cancer in familial hyperparathyroidism. *Am J Med* 1974;57:642–648.
85. Evans HL. Criteria for diagnosis of parathyroid cancer: a critical study. *Surg Pathol* 1991;4:244–265.
86. Streeten EA, Weinstein LS, Norton JA, et al. Studies in a kindred with parathyroid cancer. *J Clin Endocrinol Metab* 1992;75:362–366.
87. Cohn K, Silverman M, Conado J, et al. Parathyroid cancer, the Lahey Clinic experiences. *Surgery* 1985;98:1095–1100.
88. Levin KE, Galante M, Clark OH. Parathyroid cancer vs. parathyroid adenoma in patients with profound hypercalcemia. *Surgery* 1987;101: 649–660.
89. Smith JF, Coombs RRH. Histologic diagnosis of cancer of the parathyroid gland. *J Clin Pathol* 1984;37:1370–1378.
90. Altenahr E, Saeger V. Light and electron microscopy of parathyroid cancer. Report of three cases. *Virchows Arch* 1973;360:107–122.
91. Cryns VL, Thor A, Xu H, et al. Loss of retinoblastoma tumor suppressor gene in parathyroid cancer. *N Engl J Med* 1994;330:757–761.
92. Hakim JP, Levin MA. Absence of p53 point mutation in parathyroid adenoma and cancer. *J Clin Endocrinol Metab* 1994;78:103–106.
93. Vargas MP, Vargas HI, Kleiner DE, et al. The role of prognostic markers (M1B1, RB, and BCL-2) in the diagnosis of parathyroid tumors. *Mod Pathol* 1997;10:12–17.
94. Naccarato AG, Marococci C, Miccoli P, et al. BCL-2, p53, and MIB1 expression in normal and neoplastic parathyroid tissues. *J Endocrinol Invest* 1998;21:136–141.
95. Obara T, Fujimoto Y, Kanaji Y, et al. Flow cytometric DNA analysis of parathyroid tumors. Implications of aneuploidy for pathologic and biologic classification. *Cancer* 1990;66:1555–1562.
96. Joensuu H, Klemi P. DNA aneuploidy in adenomas of endocrine organs. *Am J Pathol* 1988;132:145–151.
97. Shane E, Bilezikian JP. Parathyroid cancer: review of 62 patients. *Endocrinol Rev* 1982;3:218–226.
98. Fujimoto Y, Obara T, Ho Y, et al. Surgical treatment of 10 cases of parathyroid cancer: importance of en bloc tumor resection. *World J Surg* 1984;8:392–400.
99. Vainas IG, Tsilikas C, Grecu A, et al. Metastatic parathyroid cancer; natural history and treatment of a case. *J Exp Clin Cancer Res* 1997; 16:429–432.
100. Obara T, Okamoto T, Kanbe M, et al. Functioning parathyroid cancer: clinicopathologic features and rationale for treatment. *Semin Surg Oncol* 1997;13:134–141.
101. Chow E, Tsang RW, Brierley JD, et al. Parathyroid cancer—the Princess Margaret Hospital experience. *Int J Radiat Oncol Biol Phys* 1998;41:569–572.
102. Brandi ML, Marx SJ, Aurbach GD, et al. Familial multiple endocrine neoplasia type 1: a new look at pathophysiology. *Endocr Rev* 1987;8:391–405.
103. Akerström G, Rudberg C, Grimelius L, et al. Histologic parathyroid abnormalities in an autopsy series. *Hum Pathol* 1986;17:520–527.
104. Benson L, Ljunghall S, Akerström G, et al. Hyperparathyroidism presenting as the first lesion in multiple endocrine neoplasia type 1 and 2. *Surgery* 1993;114:1031–1039.
105. Dekker A, Watson CG, Barnes EL Jr. The pathologic assessment of primary hyperparathyroidism and its impact on therapy. A prospective evaluation of 50 cases with oil red O stain. *Ann Surg* 1979; 190:671–675.
106. Monchik JM, Farrugia R, Teplitz C, et al. Parathyroid surgery. The role of chief cell intracellular fat staining with osmium carmine in the intraoperative management of patients with primary hyperparathyroidism. *Surgery* 1983;94:877–886.
107. Russell CF, Grant CS, van Heerden JA. Hyperfunctioning supernumerary parathyroid glands. An occasional cause of hyperparathyroidism. *Mayo Clin Proc* 1982;57:121–124.
108. Kraimps JL, Duh QY, Demure M, et al. Hyperparathyroidism in multiple endocrine neoplasia syndrome. *Surgery* 1992;112:1080–1088.
109. Palmer JA, Brown WA, Kerr WH, et al. The surgical aspects of hyperparathyroidism. *Arch Surg* 1975;110:1004–1007.
110. Wang C, Castleman B, Cope O. Surgical management of hyperparathyroidism due to primary hyperplasia. A clinical and pathological study of 104 cases. *Ann Surg* 1982;195:384–392.
111. Malmaeus J, Benson L, Johansson H, et al. Parathyroid surgery in the multiple endocrine neoplasia type 1 syndrome: choice of surgical procedure. *World J Surg* 1986;10:668–672.
112. Rizzoli R, Green H, Marx SJ. Primary hyperparathyroidism in familial multiple endocrine neoplasia type 1. *Am J Med* 1985;78:468–473.
113. Herrera M, Grant C, van Heerden JA, et al. Parathyroid autotransplantation. *Arch Surg* 1992;127:825–829.
114. Saxe A. Parathyroid transplantation. A review. *Surgery* 1984;95: 507–526.
115. Wells SA, Ellis GJ, Gunnells JC, et al. Parathyroid autotransplantation in primary hyperplasia. *N Engl J Med* 1976;295:57–62.
116. Ellis HA. Fate of long term parathyroid autografts in patients with chronic renal failure treated by parathyroidectomy. A histopathological study of autografts, parathyroid glands and bone. *Histopathology* 1988;13:289–310.
117. Tanaka Y, Seo H, Tominaga Y, et al. Factors related to the recurrent hyperfunctioning of autografts after total parathyroidectomy in patients with severe secondary hyperparathyroidism. *Surg Today* 1993; 23:220–227.
118. Mallette LE, Blevins T, Jordan PH, et al. Autogenous parathyroid grafts for generalized primary hyperparathyroidism: contrasting outcome in sporadic hyperplasia vs. multiple endocrine neoplasia type 1. *Surgery* 1987;101:738–745.
119. Herfarth KK, Wells SA. Parathyroid glands and the multiple endocrine neoplasia syndromes and familial hypocalciuric hypercalcemia. *Semin Surg Oncol* 1997;13:114–124.
120. Albright F, Bloomberg E, Castleman B, et al. Hyperparathyroidism due to diffuse hyperplasia of all parathyroid glands rather than adenoma of one. Clinical studies of three such cases. *Arch Intern Med* 1934;54:315–329.

121. Castleman R, Roth SI. Tumors of the parathyroid glands. In: *Atlas of tumor pathology*. Series 2, fascicle 14. Washington, DC: Armed Forces Institute of Pathology, 1978:1–94.
122. Dorado AE, Hensley G, Castleman B. Water clear cell hyperplasia of the parathyroid. Autopsy report of a case with supernumerary glands. *Cancer* 1976;38:1676–1683.
123. Tominaga Y, Grimelius L, Johansson H, et al. Histological and clinical features of non-familial primary parathyroid hyperplasia. *Pathol Res Pract* 1992;188:115–122.
124. Wermer P. Genetic aspects of adenomatosis of endocrine glands. *Am J Med* 1954;16:363.
125. Erdheim J. Zur normalen und pathologischen histologie der glansula thyroidea, parathyrodea und hypophysis. *Beitr Z Pathol Anat* 1903;33:158.
126. Moldawer MP. Case record of the Massachusetts General Hospital. Case 39501. *N Engl J Med* 1953;249:990.
127. Moldawer MP, Nardi GL, Raker JW. Concomitance of multiple adenomas of the parathyroids and pancreatic islet cells with tumor of the pituitary. A syndrome with familial incidence. *Am J Med Sci* 1954; 228:190.
128. Ballard HS, Frame B, Hartsock RJ. Familial multiple endocrine adenoma-peptic ulcer complex. *Am J Med* 1964;43:481.
129. Darling TN, Skarulis MC, Steinberg SM, et al. Multiple facial angiofibromas and collagenomas in patients with multiple endocrine neoplasia type 1. *Arch Dermatol* 1997;133:853.
130. Allo MD, Thompson NW. Familial hyperpararthyroidism caused by solitary adenomas. *Surgery* 1982;92:486–490.
131. Larsson C, Skogseid B, Oberg K, et al. Multiple endocrine neoplasia type 1 gene maps to chromosome 11 and is lost in insulinoma. *Nature* 1988;332:85–87.
132. Thakker RV, Poulox P, Wooding C, et al. Association of parathyroid tumors in multiple endocrine neoplasia type 1 with loss of alleles on chromosome 11. *N Engl J Med* 1989;321:218–224.
133. Lubensky IA, Gnarra JR, Bertheau P, et al. Allelic deletions in chromosome 11q13 in multiple tumors from individual MEN patients. *Cancer Res* 1996;56:5272–5278.
134. Farnebo F, Teh B, Dotzenrath C, et al. Differential loss of heterozygosity in familial, sporadic, and uremic hyperparathyroidism. *Hum Genet* 1997;99:342–349.
135. Schimke KN, Hartmann WH, Prout TE, et al. Syndrome of bilateral pheochromocytoma, medullary thyroid cancer and multiple neuromas. *N Engl J Med* 1968;279:1–7.
136. Khairi MRA, Dexter RN, Burzynoki NJ, et al. Mucosal neuroma, pheochromocytoma and medullary thyroid cancer. Multiple endocrine neoplasia type 3. *Medicine (Baltimore)* 1975;54:89–112.
137. Farndon JR, Leight GS, Dilley WG, et al. Familial medullary thyroid cancer without associated endocrinopathies: a distinct clinical entity. *Br J Surg* 1986;73:278–281.
138. Van Herdeen JA, Kent RB, Sizemore GW, et al. Primary hyperparathyroidism in patients with multiple endocrine neoplasia syndromes. *Arch Surg* 1993;118:533–536.
139. Howe JR, Norton JA, Wells SA. Prevalence of pheochromocytoma and hyperparathyroidism in multiple endocrine neoplasia type 2A: results of long term follow-up. *Surgery* 1993;114:1070–1077.
140. Dralle H, Schurmeyer TH, Kotzerke TH, et al. Surgical aspects of familial phaeochromocytoma. *Horm Metab Res Suppl* 1989;21:34.
141. Mulligan LM, Kwok JBJ, Healey CS, et al. Germ-line mutations of the RET proto-oncogene in multiple endocrine neoplasia type 2A. *Nature* 1993;363:458–460.
142. Carlson KM, Dou S, Chi D, et al. Single missense mutation in the tyrosine kinase catalytic domain of the RET protooncogene is associated with multiple endocrine neoplasia tye 2B. *Proc Natl Acad Sci U S A* 1994;91:1579–1583.
143. Padberg BC, Schroder S, Jochum W, et al. Absence of RET protooncogene point mutations in sporadic hyperplastic and neoplastic lesions of the parathyroid. *Am J Pathol* 1995;147:1600–1607.
144. Williams GH, Rooney S, Carss A, et al. Analysis of the RET protooncogene in sporadic parathyroid adenomas. *J Pathol* 1996;180: 138–141.
145. Marx SJ, Spiegel AM, Levine MA, et al. Familial hypocalciuric hypercalcemia: the relationship to primary parathyroid hyperplasia. *N Engl J Med* 1982;307:416–426.
146. Pollak MR, Chou YH, Marx SJ, et al. Familial hypocalciuric hypercalcemia and neonatal severe hyperparathyroidism. Effects of mutant gene dosage on phenotype. *J Clin Invest* 1994;93:1108–1112.
147. Pollak MR, Brown EM, Chou YH, et al. Mutations in the human calcium sensing receptor gene cause familial hypocalciuric hypocalcemia and neonatal severe hyperparathyroidism. *Cell* 1993;75:1297–1303.
148. Law WM Jr, Carney JA, Heath H III. Parathyroid glands in familial benign hypercalcemia (familial hypocalciuric hypercalcemia). *Am J Med* 1984;76:1021–1026.
149. Thorgeirsson U, Costa J. The parathyroid glands in familial hypocalciuric hypercalcemia. *Hum Pathol* 1981;12:229–237.
150. Roth SI. Pathology of the parathyroids in hyperparathyroidism. *Arch Pathol* 1962;73:495–510.
151. Arnold A, Brown MF, Urena P, et al. Monoclonality of parathyroid tumors in chronic renal failure and primary parathyroid hyperplasia. *J Clin Invest* 1995;95:2047–2053.
152. Tominaga Y, Kohara S, Namii Y. Clonal analysis of nodular parathyroid hyperplasia in renal hyperparathyroidism. *World J Surg* 1996;20: 744–752.
153. Falchetti A, Bale AE, Amorosi A, et al. Progression of uremic hyperparathyroidism involves allelic loss on chromosome 11. *J Clin Endocrinol Metab* 1993;76:139–144.

10

SOFT TISSUE PATHOLOGY OF THE HEAD AND NECK

SUZANNE B. KEEL
ANDREW E. ROSENBERG

A variety of abnormalities occur in the soft tissues of the head and neck. Although most entities are more common at other anatomic sites, some entities, such as rhabdomyosarcoma (RMS), occur frequently in the head and neck. This chapter is not meant to be a comprehensive reference of soft tissue lesions, but a guide to what may be encountered in this anatomic region.

NON-NEOPLASTIC LESIONS

Vascular Proliferations

Bacillary Angiomatosis

Bacillary angiomatosis (BA), initially described in 1983, was considered to be an unusual type of subcutaneous infection (1). Within the past decade, BA has been proven to be a reactive endothelial proliferation in response to infection by *Bartonella henselae* and *B. quintana* (2,3). It usually affects immunocompromised hosts of all ages, especially adults, and is highly associated with human immunodeficiency virus (HIV) infection. Epidemiologic studies have shown that infection by *B. henselae* is related to exposure to flea-infested cats, whereas *B. quintana* is transmitted by the human body louse (4,5).

Bacillary angiomatosis may affect the skin, mucosal surfaces, skeleton, or viscera. Skin lesions, which may number in the hundreds, are common in the head and neck area. In comparison, mucosal lesions are rare but have been reported in the nasal and oral cavities, as well as the larynx. Individual cutaneous or mucosal lesions are usually less than 1 cm in greatest dimension and appear as ulcerated polyps, subcutaneous nodules, or hyperpigmented plaques. The vascular proliferation in BA produces a spectrum of microscopic findings. The vessels are frequently arranged in a lobular configuration and range from small, well-formed capillaries lined by flattened to plump endothelial cells, to interanastomosing cords or solid sheets of epithelioid endothelial cells (Fig. 1). The endothelial cells may have prominent nucleoli and cytoplasmic vacuoles, and they can be mitotically active and show regions of necrosis. Present in all cases are interstitial edema and perivascular collections of neutrophils with karyorrhectic and fine basophilic debris. The diagnosis of BA is confirmed by the identification of clumps of pleomorphic gram-negative bacilli, which are located in the basophilic debris. They are best demonstrated by the Warthin-Starry silver stain (Fig. 2), are 1 to 3 μm in length, and have trilaminar walls by electron microscopy (2).

The differential diagnosis of BA most often includes other vasoformative lesions such as pyogenic granuloma, epithelioid hemangioma (EH), Kaposi's sarcoma and epithelioid angiosarcoma. Pyogenic granuloma also has a lobular architecture and is composed of capillaries that may be lined by plump endothelial cells; however, pyogenic granuloma lacks the prominent deep neutrophilic infiltrate and the granular basophilic material, which corresponds to the bacilli in BA. The presence of neutrophils and granular debris is also helpful in separating BA from EH. In Kaposi's sarcoma, the endothelial cells are spindled and arranged in fascicles forming slit-like vascular spaces. These findings are not present in BA, and Kaposi's sarcoma often has a lymphoplasmacytic infiltrate rather than one rich in neutrophils. Epithelioid angiosarcoma lacks a lobular architecture, shows a greater degree of cytologic atypia, demonstrates atypical mitoses, lacks a significant inflammatory cell infiltrate, and does not contain microorganisms. BA is effectively treated with erythromycin but may prove to be a fatal infection without prompt therapy (6).

Pyogenic Granuloma

Pyogenic granuloma (PG) is a benign hemangioma-like proliferation of capillaries that occurs on the skin or mucosal surfaces. PG affects all age groups, with most patients under 18 years of age being male, those 18 to 39 predominantly female, and older patients having an equal gender distribution. The most common site on the head and neck is the nasal mucosa, followed by the maxillary gingiva, mandibular gingiva, lip, skin of the face, and tongue (7,8). The majority of lesions are painless, polypoid, purple–red, and a few millimeters to centimeters in diameter, and bleed easily. The lesion develops over a relatively short time span, and approximately one third occur after trauma.

Histologically, the overlying epithelium is thinned or ulcerated, and the pedunculated mass is surrounded by a collarette of hyperplastic squamous epithelium (Fig. 3). PG is characteristically arranged in lobules, with each lobule composed of a larger vessel that may have a thick, muscular wall surrounded by con-

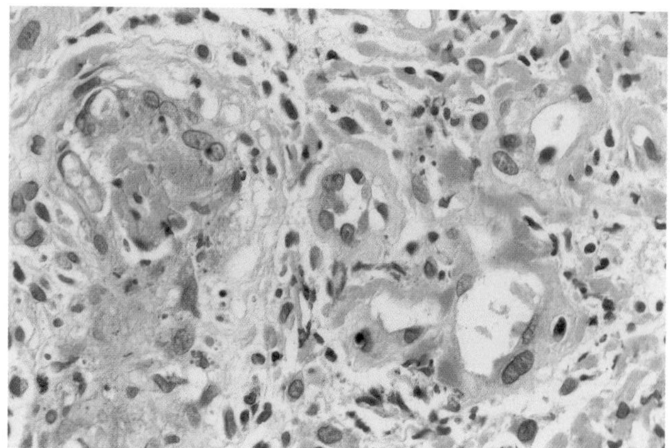

FIGURE 1. Bacillary angiomatosis with plump endothelial cells surrounded by basophilic finely particulate material and karyorrhectic debris.

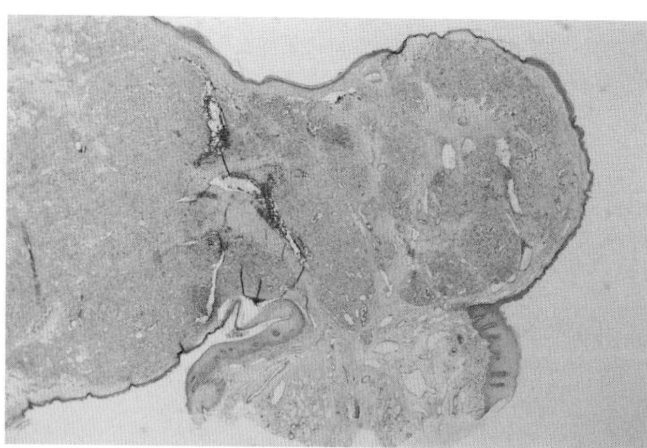

FIGURE 3. Pedunculated pyogenic granuloma surrounded by a collarette of hyperplastic squamous mucosa. A lobular pattern can be appreciated.

geries of smaller caliber capillaries (Fig. 4). The vessels are lined by banal flat or plump endothelial cells that may be mitotically active. Secondary inflammation due to ulceration is limited to the surface and is usually composed of neutrophils. The intervening stroma is edematous and composed of loose connective tissue. Because PG is not caused by infection, special stains for organisms are negative unless the surface ulceration is complicated by the growth of bacteria or fungi.

The differential diagnosis of PG is similar to BA. Importantly, PG can be distinguished from Kaposi's sarcoma and angiosarcoma by its lobular growth pattern, well-formed vessels, and cytologically bland endothelial cells. Treatment consists of surgery for troublesome lesions; however, up to 16% of lesions may recur, and some recurrences manifest as multiple deep satellite nodules that surround the site of the original lesion (Warner-Wilson Jones syndrome) (9).

Intravenous PG frequently affects the neck veins of patients who range in age from the second to the seventh decades of life (10). It is usually noted for only several months prior to diagnosis and manifests as a dark brown–red intravascular mass that may be mistaken for a thrombus. A typical lesion is polypoid, attached to the luminal surface of the vessel wall by a stalk, and covered by a layer of endothelium. Histologically, intravenous PG resembles PG occurring elsewhere, except that the stroma may contain smooth muscle. The treatment is excision. Recurrences have not been reported.

Granuloma gravidarum is a hormonally responsive PG that occurs on the gingiva between the teeth of women who are usually in their first trimester of pregnancy (11). Less than 1% of pregnant women develop these lesions, which are histologically indistinguishable from PG arising at other sites. Most spontaneously regress after delivery, but a small percentage persist in a diminished state, only to reappear during the next pregnancy.

Papillary Endothelial Hyperplasia

Initially described in 1923 by Masson as "hemangio-endotheliome vegetant intravasculaire" and thought to be a malignancy, papillary endothelial hyperplasia (PEH) is now considered to be an aberrant form of organization and recanalization of thrombi (12). PEH occurs in two settings. The primary type arises in an ectatic vessel, usually a vein, and the secondary type arises within

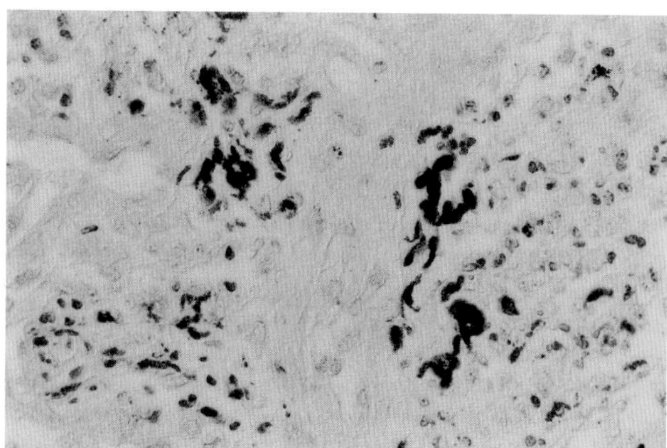

FIGURE 2. Clumps of *Bartonella henselae* in bacillary angiomatosis demonstrated by the Warthin-Starry silver stain.

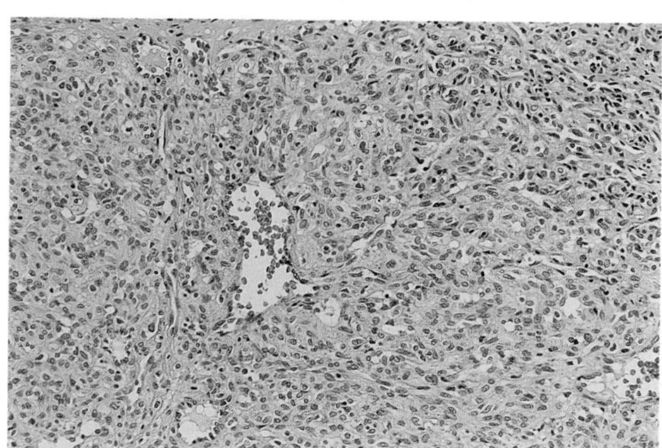

FIGURE 4. Central larger vessel surrounded by small capillaries in a pyogenic granuloma.

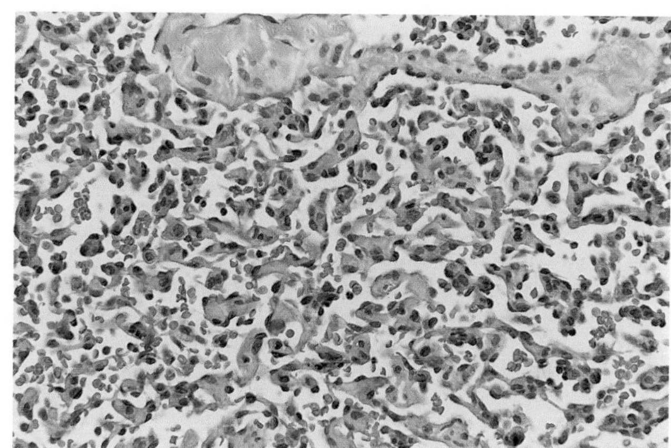

FIGURE 5. Tufts of fibrin lined by bland endothelial cells in papillary endothelial hyperplasia.

a preexisting vascular tumor or hematoma (13,14). The clinical features vary according to the type. The primary form presents as a slow-growing, sometimes painful, firm, small mass (<2 cm) that produces a red–blue discoloration. It has been described in virtually all organs and tissues, especially the superficial veins of the head and neck, where it affects all ages and has a predilection for women. The manifestations and epidemiology of the secondary form are variable and are determined by the underlying process within which it arises.

Macroscopically, PEH presents as a dark red–purple, focally microcystic mass of clotted blood. This correlates with the microscopic findings of dilated vascular channels containing round tufts or papillae of fibrin or fibrous tissue lined by endothelial cells (Fig. 5). The endothelial cells commonly cover the papillae in a single layer, but in foci they may grow as small solid fronds that protrude into the lumen. The endothelial cells are larger than their normal counterparts and have moderate amounts of eosinophilic cytoplasm. The nuclei are slightly enlarged and irregular, and nucleoli are generally small. Mitotic figures can be identified; however, they are not numerous and are not abnormal. In the early stages the cores of the papillary fronds are composed of fibrin, only to be eventually replaced by fibrous tissue. Over time, the fronds anneal to one another, forming a network of interanastomosing, irregularly shaped vascular channels lined by plump endothelial cells. This cellular process is usually confined by the wall of the affected vessel, except in the rare instance in which the vessel ruptures and the organization continues into the immediately adjacent tissue.

The most important tumor from which PEH should be differentiated is angiosarcoma. Angiosarcoma frequently arises in sun-exposed skin, especially on the head and neck. It has an infiltrative growth pattern and is rarely intravascular in location or associated with an underlying benign vascular tumor. The malignant endothelial cells use preexisting structures such as dermal collagen as scaffolding, and they demonstrate malignant cytologic features as well as numerous mitoses (including atypical forms) and necrosis.

Treatment of PEH consists of excision of the underlying lesion, if one exists, or removal of the ectatic vein and its intravascular growth. Recurrences of the primary form have not been reported; however, when PEH occurs within another lesion, recurrence of the underlying lesion is a possibility.

Fibroblastic Proliferations

Posttraumatic Spindle Cell Nodule

Lesions resembling postoperative or posttraumatic spindle cell nodule (PSCN) of the genitourinary tract have been reported to arise rarely in the buccal mucosa after trauma, at the site of a tooth extraction, or in the skin of the head and neck and elsewhere (15–17). PSCN is composed of a hypercellular proliferation of uniform spindled fibroblasts and myofibroblasts arranged in intersecting fascicles (Fig. 6). The cells have vesicular nuclei, finely distributed chromatin, and one or two small nucleoli. The cytoplasm is eosinophilic with indistinct cell borders. Mitotic activity is readily identifiable within PSCN, but no atypical mitoses are present. A network of small capillaries is present throughout the lesion, and edema and small foci of hemorrhage and lymphocytes are common findings. Infiltration into the surrounding tissue and ulceration of adjacent mucosa also may be present. The lesion bears some resemblance and may be related to nodular fasciitis (NF) (17).

Immunohistochemical studies reveal that the proliferating spindle cells stain with antibodies to vimentin, muscle-specific actin, and smooth muscle actin, but not with desmin or cytokeratin (16). This profile is consistent with a proliferation of fibroblasts and myofibroblasts.

The important differential diagnoses include spindle cell sarcoma and spindle cell carcinoma. Leiomyosarcoma (LMS), fibrosarcoma, and malignant fibrous histiocytoma (MFH) are the sarcomas most likely to be confused with PSCN. These tumors have different architectural arrangements of the fascicles of tumor cells (intersecting at right angles, herringbone, and storiform, respectively) than PSCN, and the tumor cells generally show a greater degree of cytologic atypia and atypical mitoses. Also, sarcomas do not rapidly develop after trauma or surgery. PSCN can be distinguished from spindle cell carcinoma because spindle cell carcinoma may be associated with overlying squamous cell carcinoma *in situ* if the mucosa is intact. Spindle

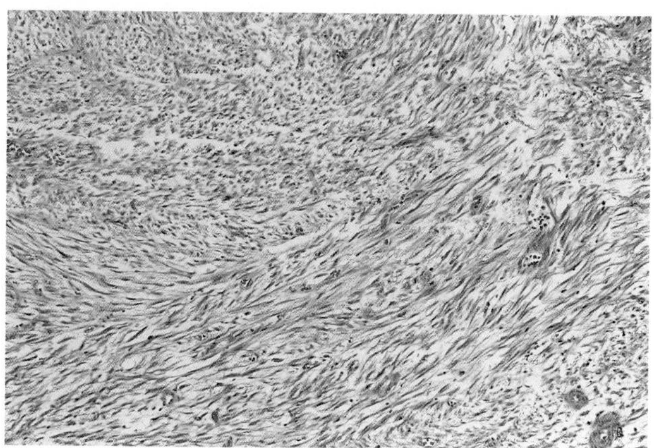

FIGURE 6. Posttraumatic spindle cell nodule composed of intersecting fascicles of bland spindle cells.

cell carcinoma also demonstrates a greater degree of pleomorphism and hyperchromasia than is seen in PSCN. Immunohistochemistry may be useful because spindle cell carcinoma is frequently focally cytokeratin positive. Electron microscopy also may be helpful if intercellular junctions or tonofibrils are identified; however, ultrastructural analysis of some spindle cell carcinomas may lack conventional features of epithelial differentiation (18). Treatment of PSCN consists of simple excision. Follow-up of a patient with a lesion in the buccal mucosa showed that 1 month after biopsy, the remainder of the lesion had regressed.

Nodular Fasciitis and Variants

Nodular fasciitis is a pseudosarcomatous, reactive proliferation of fibroblasts and myofibroblasts described initially by Konwaler et al. in 1955 (19). NF affects individuals of any age, including children, but is most common in the third through fifth decades of life (20). The frequency in males is slightly higher than in females. The upper extremity, especially the volar aspect of the forearm, is the most common site for NF; approximately 13% develop within the head and neck region (21). In the head and neck, NF most frequently affects the soft tissues of the face and neck, but also may arise in the superficial layers of the conjunctiva, buccal area, tongue, gingiva, and hypopharynx (21–24). The lesions are solitary and grow rapidly. The majority measure 1 to 4 cm in greatest dimension, but lesions of up to 6.5 cm have been reported.

Nodular fasciitis originates within the submucosa, subcutis, deep fascia, or skeletal muscle. Grossly it is circumscribed but not encapsulated and may have a stellate configuration. The cut surface is gray–white in color and frequently is myxoid or mucoid. Irrespective of its location, NF is richly cellular and consists of plump, immature-appearing fibroblasts arranged haphazardly or in intersecting short fascicles (Fig. 7). The cells vary in size and shape (spindle to stellate) and have discrete nucleoli and abundant mitotic figures of normal configuration. In early lesions the cells are embedded in a matrix rich in mucopolysaccharides with a paucity of collagen. This microscopic picture simulates fibroblasts grown in tissue culture or those present in granulation tissue. Extravasated red blood cells and inflammatory cells are common. In time, the fascicles of cells become broader and are frequently arranged in a storiform pattern with decreasing amounts of mucopolysaccharides and increasing amounts of collagen. The collagen may become glassy in appearance similar to that present in keloids. Ultrastructurally, the cells in NF have features of fibroblasts and myofibroblasts; immunohistochemically, greater than 90% of cases stain positively with antibodies to vimentin, smooth muscle actin, muscle-specific actin, and KP-1 (25). The cells do not stain for keratin or S-100 protein (21).

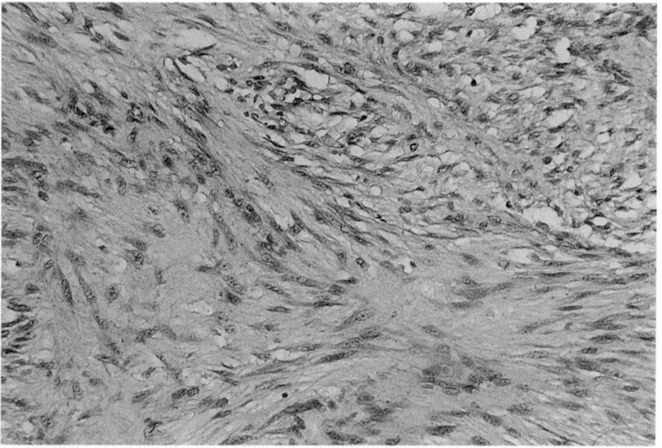

FIGURE 7. Nodular fasciitis characterized by plump fibroblasts arranged in short fascicles within myxoid stroma containing extravasated red blood cells.

Flow cytometry of NF reveals a high proliferative index and diploidy. Clonal chromosomal aberrations have been reported in several cases (26). Although the cytogenetic aberrations are not homogeneous, their presence suggests that reactive processes are not always composed of a polyclonal expansion of cells.

The differential diagnosis of NF is extensive; however, two important lesions that must be considered are fibromatosis and spindle cell sarcomas. Fibromatosis is usually situated in the deep soft tissue and is a large and infiltrative lesion. Unlike NF, it is composed of broad, sweeping fascicles of uniform bland spindle cells. The stroma is more collagenous and mitoses are less frequent. In a large series of NF, over 20% of cases were erroneously classified as sarcoma (21). Most malignant misdiagnoses are rendered because of the hypercellularity and high mitotic rate of NF. However, spindle cell sarcomas can be distinguished because they generally show a greater degree of cyologic atypia and contain atypical mitoses and areas of necrosis. The clinical history is also useful in the distinction in that sarcomas are slow growing and do not evolve as rapidly as NF. NF is a benign process, and local excision is curative in most cases. A very low recurrence rate has been reported, and the recurrences are believed to result from inadequate excision.

Cranial fasciitis (CF) is a subtype of NF that occurs on the scalp of children between birth and 6 years of age; the majority develop before 2 years of age (27). Lesions average 2.5 cm in diameter but may be as small as 1.5 cm and as large as 9 cm. Boys are affected twice as frequently as girls. The lesions grow rapidly, and the preoperative duration ranges from 2 weeks to 4 months. Usually there is no history of local trauma. CF originates in the deep layers of the scalp or periosteum and arises over the frontal, temporal, parietal, and occipital regions as well as on the petrous portion of the temporal bone, where it may present as a mass in the auditory canal (28). The calvarium may be eroded radiographically or demonstrate an adjacent rim of reactive sclerosis (29).

At surgery, CF may breach the inner table of the calvarium and even become adherent to the underlying dura. The lesion is typically gray–white and well circumscribed, and histologically it resembles NF; however, reactive woven bone may be present. Local excision is curative, and recurrence has not been reported.

Parosteal fasciitis or *ossifying fasciitis* is indistinguishable histologically from NF, except for the presence of reactive bone formation (30). The bone is located randomly within the lesion and does not have the zonation pattern that is typical of myositis ossificans (MO).

Proliferative Fasciitis and Proliferative Myositis

Proliferative fasciitis and proliferative myositis are similar clinicopathologic entities that involve the fascia and skeletal muscle, respectively. They are benign reparative processes that manifest as rapidly growing, tender masses that usually arise in an extremity, especially the forearm and thigh in fasciitis, and the shoulder girdle in myositis (31–33). Cases have been reported in the tongue, as well as the masseter, buccinator, and sternocleidomastoid muscles of the head and neck (34,35). The affected patient population tends to be older than in NF, with an average age of 50 years (32). Proliferative fasciitis and myositis uncommonly occur in children (36). Males predominate in proliferative myositis, whereas in proliferative fasciitis the sexes are equally affected.

The lesions are solitary and mobile, and range from 1.0 to 6.9 cm in diameter. Their macroscopic features are nonspecific; they are poorly demarcated, stellate, and consist of gray—tan firm tissue that extends along preexisting fibrous septae or fascial planes and may replace portions of skeletal muscle.

Microscopically, proliferative fasciitis and proliferative myositis are composed of a mixture of spindle and stellate fibroblasts similar in appearance to those in NF, along with larger more polygonal cells that morphologically mimic ganglion cells (Fig. 8). These latter cells have abundant basophilic cytoplasm, one or two nuclei, and large prominent nucleoli. Ultrastructurally, the ganglion-like cells have features of modified fibroblasts, and immunohistochemically they stain with antibodies to vimentin, actin, and KP-1 (34). The intervening stroma varies with respect to the quantity of the myxoid and collagenous components. In proliferative fasciitis the lesional cells extend along the fibrous septae that compartmentalize the subcutaneous fat. In proliferative myositis the cells expand the epimysium, perimysium, and endomysium and cause the separation and isolation of atrophic muscle fibers that usually do not show evidence of regeneration. Similar appearing reactive fibroblasts have infrequently been seen in other settings such as ulcerated polypoid lesions of the gastrointestinal tract.

Flow cytometry has shown that these lesions have a diploid pattern. Cytogenetic analysis has identified trisomy 2 in a case of proliferative fasciitis and proliferative myositis (37,38). As with NF, this finding indicates that reactive processes may result from a clonal proliferation of cells.

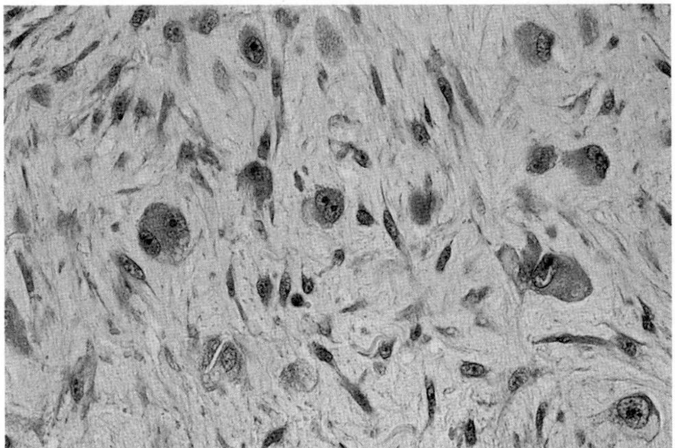

FIGURE 8. Ganglion-like cells in proliferative myositis surrounded by haphazardly arranged fibroblasts.

The large ganglion-like cells in proliferative fasciitis and myositis are often interpreted as ganglioneuroblasts or rhabdomyoblasts. However, ganglioneuroblastomas and RMS rarely occur in adults, and they tend to be large tumors that usually do not arise in the subcutis. In addition, the tumor cells demonstrate obvious malignant cytologic features, and a component of the tumor usually consists of primitive appearing hyperchromatic small round cells. As in NF, marginal excision is generally curative.

Head-bangers Tumor

In 1982 two cases of soft tissue swelling of the mid-forehead related to habitual head banging were reported (39). The lesions occurred in West Indian youths 12 and 16 years of age, both of whom banged their hand upon the forehead each night before going to bed. The skin overlying the swellings was deeply pigmented, and histologic examination revealed dense reactive fibrous tissue resembling scar tissue occupying the dermis and extending into the subcutis. This lesion is extremely rare, and clinical history should be sought before rendering such a diagnosis.

Nuchal Fibrocartilaginous Pseudotumor

A single case of a fibrocartilagenous nodule with calcification located in the ligamentum nuchae at the posterior cervical spine was reported in 1978 (40). Reports from 1997 and 1999 describe additional patients who developed histologically identical masses at the posterior base of the neck following trauma to the neck, and the researchers coined the term *nuchal fibrocartilagenous pseudotumor* (NFP) (41,42). The time interval between the injury and presentation of the mass may be as long as 25 years. The lesions are slow growing and sometimes painful. The masses arise at the junction of the nuchal ligament and deep cervical fascia, and cross-sectional imaging studies reveal thickening of the ligamentum nuchae between the C4 and C7 levels.

The nodules of NFP range in size from 1.0 to 3.0 cm. They are poorly defined, moderately cellular fibrocartilagenous masses within fascia and ligamentous tissue. No atypia, binucleate cells, mitotic activity or necrosis is present. The chondrocytes are embedded in a matrix of polarizable collagen and small amounts of mucopolysaccharides (Fig. 9). The ligamentous tissue at the periphery of the mass demonstrates degeneration, with fragmentation of the elastic fibers.

The histologic differential diagnosis of NFP includes nuchal fibroma, soft tissue chondroma, calcifying aponeurotic fibroma, and MO. Nuchal fibroma differs from NFP in that it may be found superficial to the fascia anywhere in the neck. Also, it is not related to trauma, does not have an association with ligaments, and cartilaginous differentiation is not a recognized component. Soft tissue chondroma is rarely observed in sites other than the distal extremities; however, in the head and neck it has been reported in the tongue. Although soft tissue chondromas may arise from a tendon sheath, histologically they are composed

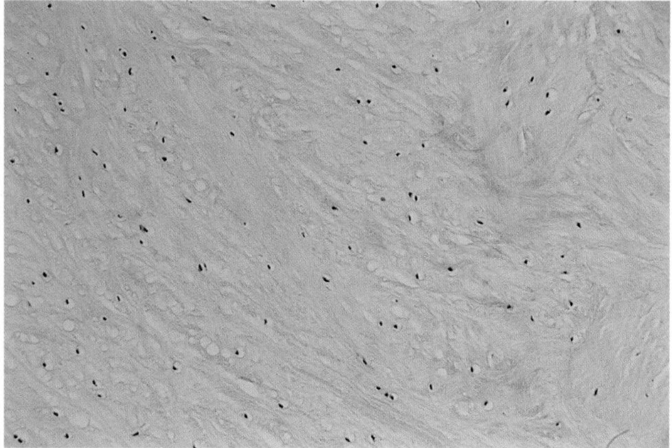

FIGURE 9. Fibrocartilagenous matrix in a nuchal fibrocartilagenous pseudotumor.

of well-defined lobules of hyaline cartilage and not fibrocartilage. Interestingly, however, fibrocartilaginous metaplasia of the lingual aponeurosis may occur, although quite rarely, and we have recently encountered such a case (43). Calcifying aponeurotic fibroma is also in the histologic differential diagnosis but is generally a lesion of the distal extremities although one case in the face has been reported, and it is composed predominantly of a cellular fibroblastic proliferation, with only small foci of chondroid differentiation, which are frequently calcified (44). MO is related to trauma and situated within muscle. It is much more cellular than NFP and is composed of a central zone of proliferating fibroblasts that merge peripherally with bone-forming osteoblasts. Bone is usually abundant and is most mature at the periphery. Fibrocartilage is not a component of MO.

Peripheral Ossifying Fibroma

Also known as fibrous epulis, calcifying fibroblastic granuloma, and peripheral fibroma with calcifications, peripheral ossifying fibroma (POF) is a reactive lesion that most commonly occurs in the maxillary gingiva (45). It is more common in women, and has a predilection for the second and third decades of life. POF presents as a pink or red, sessile or pedunculated, well-defined growth on the gingiva and ranges in size from 0.2 to 3.0 cm, but most are smaller than 1.0 cm. The majority of cases are of short duration and are present for less than 6 months prior to diagnosis.

Approximately 60% of POFs are ulcerated. Underlying the ulcer is a zone of cytologically banal proliferating fibroblasts arranged in a haphazard pattern. Dystrophic calcification in the form of small granules and larger globules are frequently prominent. Hyalinized collagen may or may not be present within the area of fibroblastic proliferation, and is most noticeable around blood vessels. Lymphocytic infiltration may be pronounced. Deep to the fibroblastic proliferation is a zone of matrix formation that contains trabeculae of unmineralized or mineralized woven bone, mature lamellar bone, or round deposits of cementum-like tissue (Figs. 10 and 11). Osteoblasts line the bony trabeculae, and loose connective tissue fills the intertrabecular

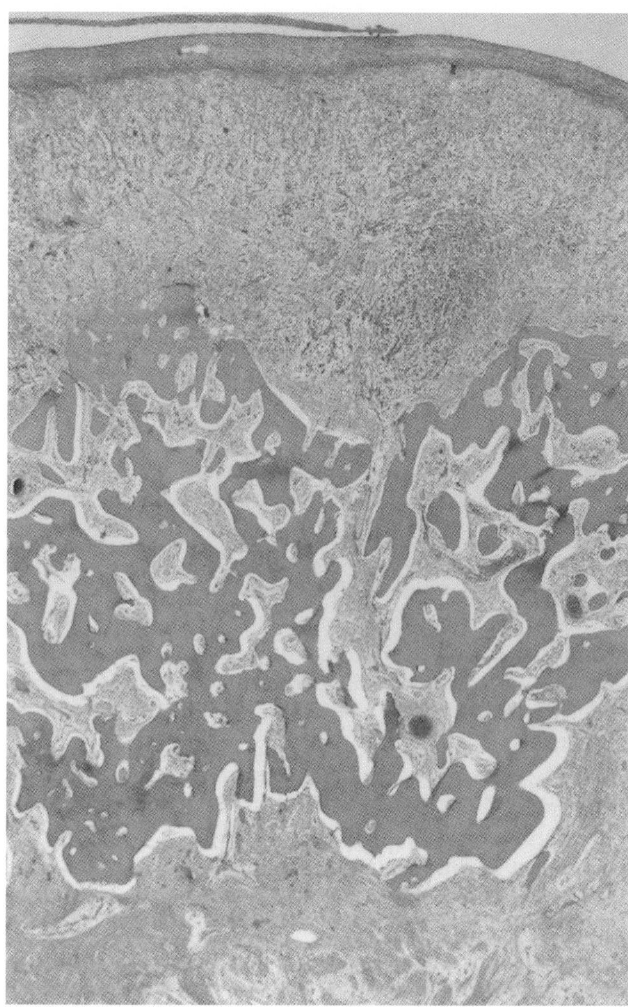

FIGURE 10. Peripheral ossifying fibroma bulging into the overlying squamous mucosa.

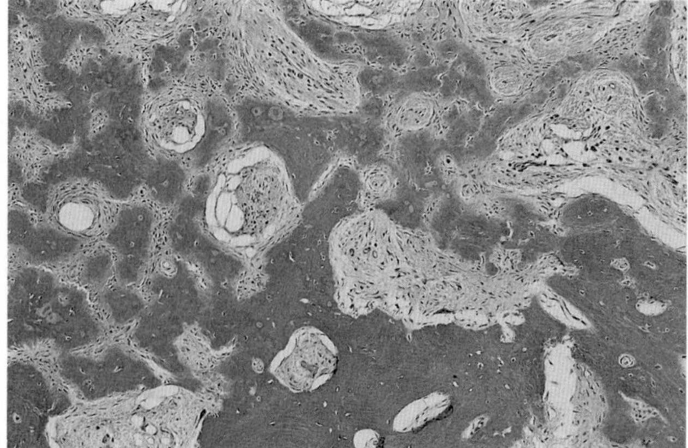

FIGURE 11. Peripheral ossifying fibroma demonstrating woven bone and intervening fibroblastic stroma.

spaces. Excision is the preferred treatment; however, the recurrence rate is approximately 15% (45).

The main differential diagnosis is with peripheral odontogenic fibroma and osteosarcoma. Peripheral odontogenic fibroma often contains prominent islands of odontogenic epithelium and may contain dentinoid tissue but does not have the wide spectrum of bone and cementum formation present in POF (see Chapter 6) (46). Osteosarcoma usually presents as a large mass and demonstrates considerably more cytologic atypia and mitotic activity, including atypical forms, all of which are absent in POF.

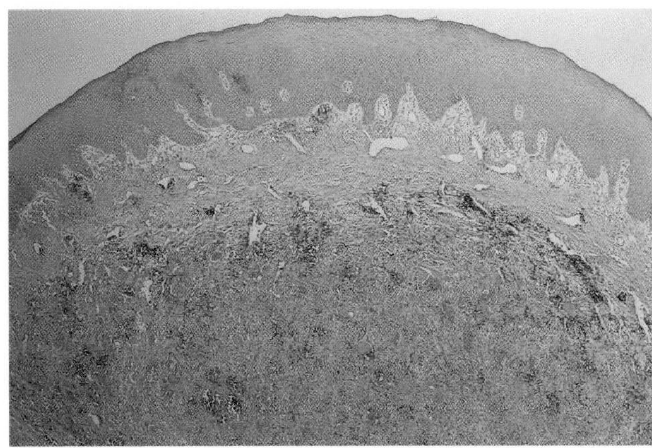

FIGURE 13. Submucosal location of a peripheral giant cell granuloma.

Others

Peripheral Giant Cell Granuloma

Peripheral giant cell granuloma (PGG), previously known as peripheral giant cell reparative granuloma, is probably not a neoplasm but a reactive lesion, and occurs on the alveolus and gingiva. It presents most often on the mandibular mucosa, affecting women slightly more often than men. The incidence peaks between the sixth and seventh decades of life. The lesion presents as a red to blue nodule that may be polypoid or sessile and is usually less than 2 cm in diameter (Fig. 12). Large lesions may erode the underlying bone or ulcerate the mucosa (Fig. 13). Histologically they resemble intraosseous giant cell reparative granulomas (see Chapter 11) and are composed of multinucleate osteoclast-like giant cells in a cellular stroma of fibroblasts and hemorrhage (Fig. 14). The multinucleated cells tend to congregate near the blood, and hemosiderin may be present. Mitotic activity can be pronounced in the background mononuclear cells (47). Treatment is simple excision.

Myositis Ossificans

Myositis ossificans is a painful, non-neoplastic, reparative process composed of a proliferation of fibroblasts and osteoblasts that deposit bone in various stages of maturation. It has been recognized since the early part of the 20th century, and because of its dense cellularity and abundant mitotic activity has been frequently mistaken for sarcoma (48). The process usually develops after trauma and arises within skeletal muscle, but it also may originate within the subcutis. MO rarely develops in the head and neck, but it has been reported to arise within the masseter, buccinator, digastric, medial pterygoid, and sternocleidomastoid muscles, as well as in the intrinsic muscles of the subglottic portion of the larynx (49–52). MO also has been known to develop after radical neck dissection and may be mistaken clinically for positive neck nodes in a patient with a history of carcinoma in the head and neck region (53). MO of the head and neck usually affects adults. The lesion is more common in males than females. The clinical findings are related to its stage of development; in the early phase the involved area is swollen and painful, and within 6 weeks of onset it becomes more circumscribed and firm. Eventually it evolves into a painless, hard, well-demarcated mass averaging 3 to 6 cm in greatest diameter.

Most surgically removed specimens demonstrate a well-delineated tan mass that has a soft glistening center and a firm, gray, bony periphery. The microscopic findings vary according to the age of the lesion. In the earliest phase the lesion is the most cel-

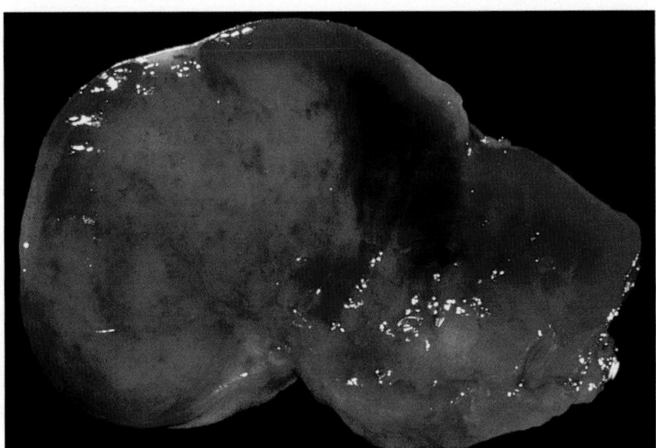

FIGURE 12. Polypoid peripheral giant cell granuloma with a tan-brown cut surface.

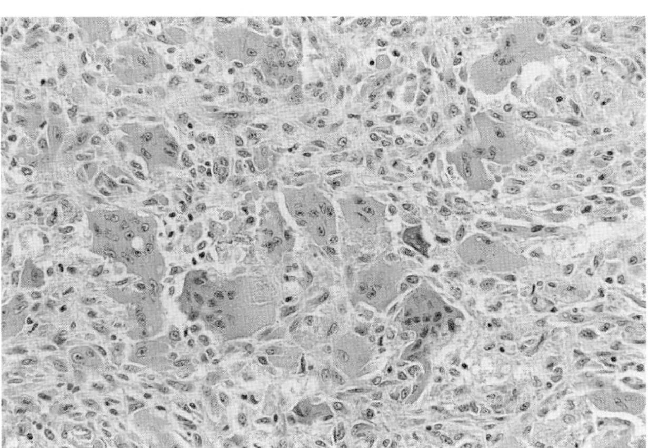

FIGURE 14. Peripheral giant cell granuloma composed of multinucleated giant cells and spindled stroma.

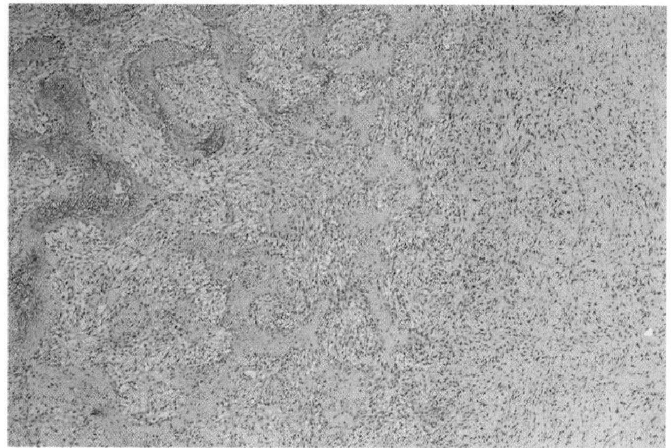

FIGURE 15. Myositis ossificans showing interanastomosing trabeculae of osteoid with prominent osteoblastic rimming adjacent to densely cellular stroma.

lular and consists of fibroblastic tissue similar to that in NF. After approximately 3 weeks morphologic zonation becomes apparent; the center retains its mixture of fibroblasts, abundant mucopolysaccharides, and delicate collagen fibers; however it merges with an adjacent intermediate zone that contains osteoblasts that form ill-defined trabeculae of woven bone (Figs. 15 and 16). In a minority of cases small islands of hyaline cartilage also may be present. In the most peripheral zone the bony trabeculae undergo remodeling and mineralization and more closely resemble cancellous bone. The proliferative process is demarcated from the surrounding soft tissues by a thin layer of loose fibrous tissue that may contain a sparse inflammatory infiltrate.

The radiographic changes parallel those noted on gross and microscopic study. Early in its development, a soft tissue fullness is appreciated that may show a blush on angiography. At about 3 weeks, peripheral calcification becomes apparent, usually as patchy irregular flocculent densities that, within another 3 weeks, mature into a prominent mineralized bony periphery that fades into a radiolucent center.

The differential diagnosis is chiefly with osteosarcoma. MO is a rapidly growing, painful lesion of adulthood and is nearly always associated with recent trauma or surgery. Extraskeletal osteosarcoma is a disease of late adulthood, is not as rapidly progressive, and the association with trauma is remote and likely to be coincidental. Histologically, osteosarcoma demonstrates a haphazard growth pattern that has been called the reverse zoning effect because the central portion of the mass may demonstrate the most mature bone. The cells of osteosarcoma demonstrate cytologic atypia and atypical mitotic figures, and the osteoid production is delicate and lace-like in comparison with the trabeculae in MO. Osteosarcoma generally infiltrates surrounding normal tissue, in contrast to the well-circumscribed nature of MO.

Treatment of MO consists of either local resection if the lesion remains painful, or watchful waiting. Reports of recurrence after local excision are uncommon and have been associated with incomplete excision of immature lesions. If surgery is not performed because of classic clinical and radiographic features or a diagnostic biopsy, careful follow-up to ensure the lesion matures and does not pursue a destructive course is indicated.

Traumatic Neuroma

Traumatic neuroma (TN) was first described by Odier in 1811 as a nerve tumor that arises from the distal end of the proximal segment of a sectioned peripheral nerve. It was not until the early 20th century that TNs of the oral cavity were first recognized (54). The most common intraoral sites are the lip, tongue, gingiva, and mandible, and they frequently develop after a tooth extraction (55). Pharyngeal TNs are also recognized, and they are heralded by hoarseness or dysphagia, and are hypothesized to form from the minor trauma of daily life, because small nerve twigs in this area reach up to the basal layer of epithelium (56). Up to 25% of TNs cause pain, and superficial TNs are more likely to be painful than those that are deep-seated.

Histologically, TNs form in the area of a severed nerve and are composed of haphazardly arranged nerve twigs of different sizes containing axons, Schwann cells, and endoneurial and perineurial connective tissue that are embedded in a fibrous scar (Fig. 17). TNs of the pharynx may contain ganglion cells from a

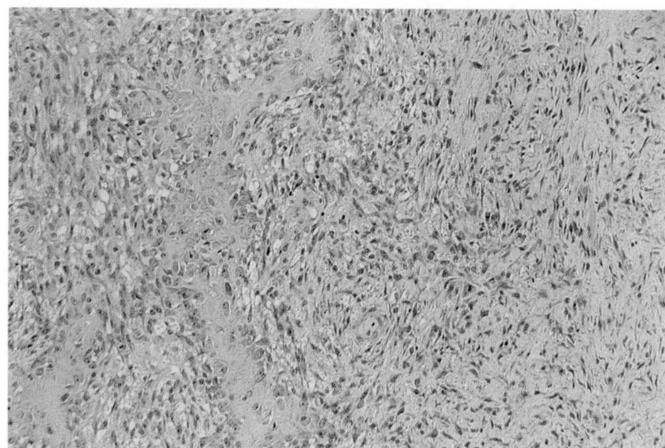

FIGURE 16. Woven bone formation adjacent to primitive fibroblastic stroma in myositis ossificans.

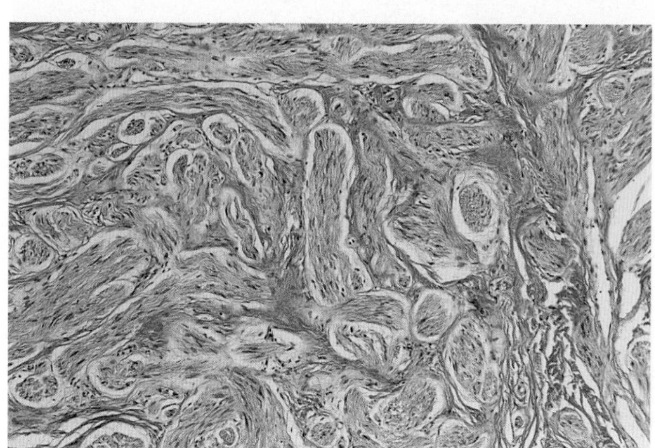

FIGURE 17. Disorganized nerve twigs in a traumatic neuroma.

neighboring ganglion, and this may cause confusion with ganglioneuroma on biopsy (56). The disorganized pattern of the well-formed nerve twigs is helpful in distinguishing TN from ganglioneuroma and other neural tumors. The treatment is excision; however, TN may recur or the pain may persist even after removal of the lesion.

NEOPLASMS

Adipocytic Tumors

Lipoma and Variants

Lipomas, benign neoplasms exhibiting adipocyte differentiation, are the most common mesenchymal neoplasms of adulthood. Approximately 13% of all lipomas arise in the head and neck region, usually the posterior neck, and they most commonly affect men in the seventh decade of life (57). The majority of lipomas are subcutaneous and superficial in location, which may cause cosmetic problems; however, lipomas of the parotid, oral cavity, tongue, pharynx, larynx, and nasopharynx may produce more serious complications, such as difficulty in speech, mastication, and respiration (57–59).

Subcutaneous lipomas are typically encapsulated, whereas the intramuscular variant tends to be ill-defined (60). Lipomas consist of yellow to white or light tan fatty tissue and are composed of lobules of mature-appearing white adipocytes. Cytogenetic analysis of conventional lipomas reveals that over 70% of cases have a cytogenetic abnormality in the region 12q13-q15 (61–64). Definitive diagnosis can be made reliably by computed tomography or magnetic resonance imaging techniques; therefore, excision may be necessary only if the mass is symptomatic.

Angiolipoma characteristically arises in young adults and is frequently multifocal. Although they infrequently affect the head and neck region, they have been reported to occur adjacent to the mandible, in the cheek, palate, and parotid gland, as well as in the soft tissue of the neck (65). Grossly, angiolipomas are usually well encapsulated, although infiltrating types have been described. The latter probably represent intramuscular lipomas with a prominent vasculature. Angiolipomas appear yellow to reddish yellow, depending on the amount of vascular tissue within the mass.

Microscopically, they are composed of mature adipose tissue with congeries of small capillaries that tend to predominate peripherally beneath the capsule. The endothelial cells within the vessels are inconspicuous, and fibrin thrombi are frequently found within the vessels (Fig. 18). Cellular angiolipomas in which the vascular component predominates may be confused with vascular malignancies such as Kaposi's sarcoma; however, the encapsulation of the mass and lack of cytologic atypia help exclude Kaposi's sarcoma. Angiolipoma is effectively treated by complete excision.

Spindle cell lipoma accounts for approximately 1.5% of adipocytic neoplasms. They classically occur on the upper shoulders, back, and neck of middle aged to elderly men, but also may involve the face. Characteristically the lesions measure 2 to 5 cm in diameter and are solitary, but a recent report suggests that in rare cases there may be a familial tendency toward multiple lesions (66). Microscopically, spindle cell lipomas are composed of varying proportions of mature white adipocytes, spindle cells admixed with wire-like collagen fibers, and myxoid stroma (Fig. 19). Mast cells are frequently numerous. Immunohistochemically the spindle cells express CD34 and, unlike adipocytes, are negative for S-100 protein. Rearrangements of chromosomes 13q or 16q are characteristic of this type of lipoma (61,67,68). The differential diagnosis is most often with diffuse neurofibroma that has infiltrated fat. Architecturally, spindle cell lipomas are well circumscribed and encapsulated, whereas diffuse neurofibroma has an infiltrative margin. Both tumors contain bland spindle cells with myxoid change, and mast cells may be plentiful; however, the spindle cells in neurofibroma are more randomly arranged, Wagner-Meissner bodies are frequently present, and the collagen bundles are less pronounced than in spindle cell lipoma. Both tumors stain with S-100 protein and CD34; however, the spindle cell component of a spindle cell lipoma stains strongly with CD34 and the fat cells with S-100 protein, whereas the spindle cells in a neurofibroma stain with S-100 protein, and only a minority of smaller, dendritic type cells with CD34 (69). The cytologic banality and architectural cir-

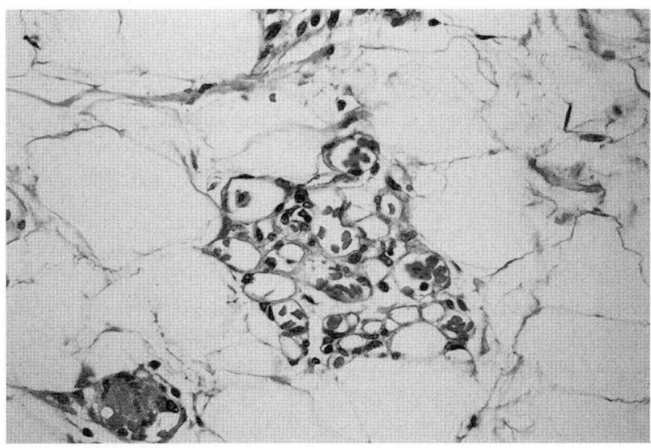

FIGURE 18. Aggregates of capillaries with fibrin thrombi within an angiolipoma.

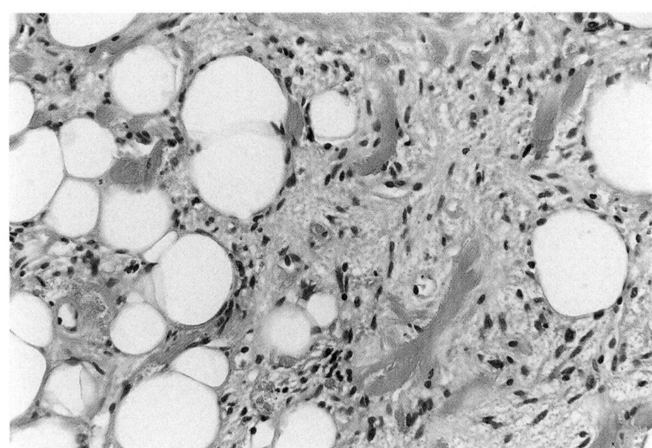

FIGURE 19. Spindle cell lipoma composed of mature adipocytes, wire-like collagen bundles, and bland spindle cells.

cumscription help to distinguish spindle cell lipoma from a sarcoma. Simple excision is the treatment of choice, and recurrence is rare.

Pleomorphic lipoma is a benign tumor related to spindle cell lipoma, and, like spindle cell lipoma, it has a predilection for the back, upper shoulder and neck of elderly men, with a small percentage of cases occurring on the head (70). They range in size from 1 to 12 cm, with an average of 4.5 cm, and grossly they are well encapsulated with a yellow–white cut surface. Pleomorphic mono- and multinucleated cells embedded in a myxoid stroma admixed with mature white adipocytes and thick collagen bundles typify this type of tumor. Floret-type giant cells that have peripherally arranged nuclei and abundant eosinophilic cytoplasm are commonly present (Fig. 20). The large atypical cells have dark, smudgy chromatin that is degenerative in appearance. Multivacuolated cells resembling lipoblasts also may be present. Approximately half of the tumors show a histologic transition to conventional spindle cell lipoma, and cytogenetic studies have shown that both spindle cell and pleomorphic lipomas have the same chromosomal abnormalities involving 13q or 16q (61,63,68,70). Differentiating pleomorphic lipoma from sclerosing liposarcoma may be difficult, because pleomorphic lipoma may contain lipoblasts. Clinical history of a long-standing, circumscribed, superficial mass on the back or neck of an elderly man is strongly suggestive of pleomorphic lipoma, whereas sclerosing liposarcoma usually presents as a large deep-seated mass. Histologically, sclerosing liposarcoma has more lipoblasts, fewer floret-like giant cells, and large areas of sclerosis that are not present in pleomorphic lipoma. Complete excision is curative.

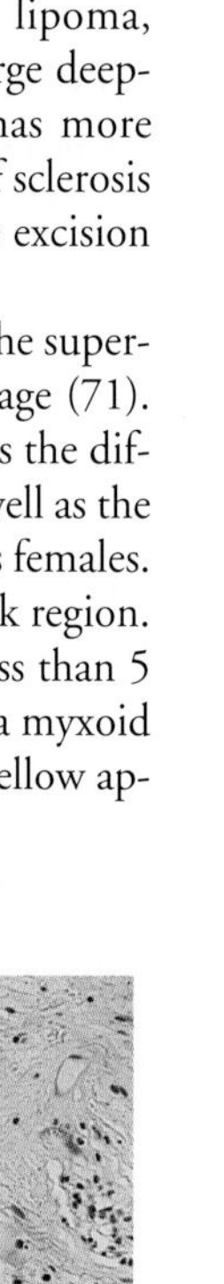

Lipoblastoma is a benign fatty tumor that occurs in the superficial soft tissues of children, usually under 3 years of age (71). The conventional variant is well circumscribed, whereas the diffuse variant is ill defined and infiltrates the subcutis as well as the skeletal muscle. Males are affected twice as frequently as females. Approximately 20% of cases occur in the head and neck region. They measure 1 to 21 cm in diameter, but most are less than 5 cm in greatest dimension. Grossly, lipoblastomas have a myxoid or mucinous, pale cut surface in comparison with the yellow appearance of conventional lipoma. Microscopically, they are composed of lobules of lipoblasts in varying stages of development, including spindle-shaped preadipocytes, multivacuolated lipoblasts, and univacuolated or signet ring cell adipocytes (Figs. 21 and 22). Maturation of the adipocytes has been observed with sequential biopsies. Areas of brown fat differentiation are infrequently present. The stroma is commonly myxoid and contains numerous delicate, branching, thin-walled vessels arranged in a plexiform pattern. Fibrous septa are prominent and characteristically compartmentalize the tumor into many lobules. Cytogenetic rearrangement of chromosome 8q has been identified in some of these tumors (61). The main differential diagnosis is with myxoid liposarcoma, which is rare in young children and lacks the lobulation seen in lipoblastoma. Excision is the treatment of choice for lipoblastoma. Recurrence rates of 9% to 22% have been reported, but they are generally associated with the diffuse type (71).

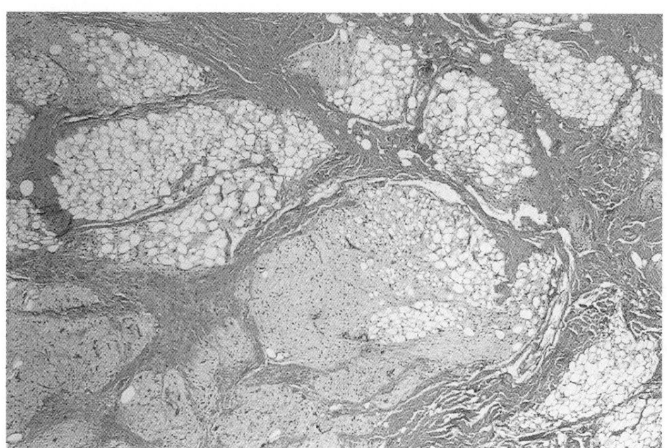

FIGURE 21. Lipoblastoma has a striking lobular architecture.

Hibernoma is a benign tumor of brown fat. Approximately 10% of cases arise in the neck, and it has been described to involve the parotid gland (72,73). On average the patients are in their third decade of life, with a range of 18 to 52 years.

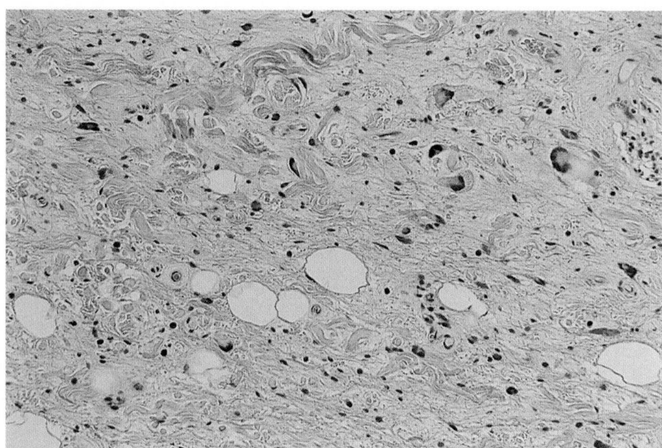

FIGURE 20. Floret-type giant cells with hyperchromatic nuclei typical of a pleomorphic lipoma.

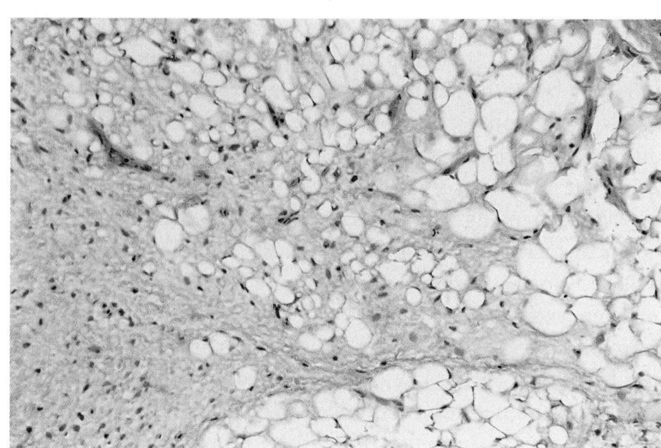

FIGURE 22. Lipoblastoma contains lipoblasts in varying stages of development.

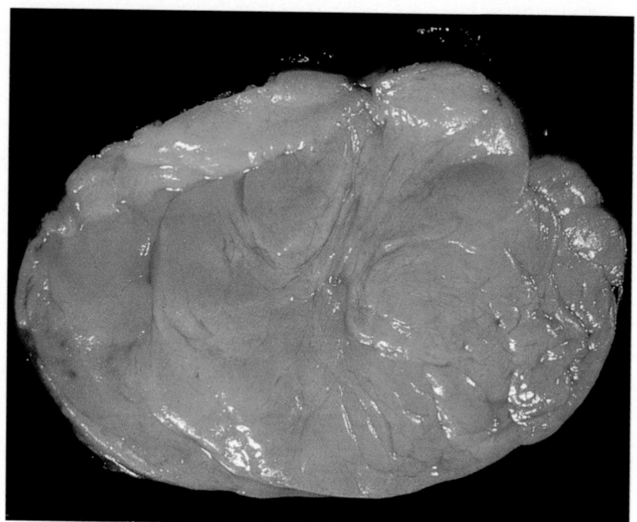

FIGURE 23. The tan–brown cut surface of a hibernoma.

Hibernomas are slowly growing, painless, well-circumscribed, subcutaneous masses that range from 5 to 18 cm in greatest diameter and have a tan to mahogany brown cut surface (Fig. 23). Hibernomas are composed of large, polyhedral cells with abundant granular eosinophilic cytoplasm that also contain multiple small round clear vacuoles that scallop the centrally located nuclei (Fig. 24). White fat cells are also present in variable numbers. Ultrastructural studies of the brown fat cells have revealed an abundance of mitochondria, which produces the granularity of their cytoplasm (72). Cytogenetic aberrations in chromosome 11q have been identified in a small number of these tumors (61). Simple excision is associated with a very low rate of recurrence.

Chondroid lipoma (CL) is an unusual benign tumor initially described in 1986 under the name extraskeletal chondroma with lipoblast-like cells (74). In 1993 Meis and Enzinger published a series of 20 cases and suggested the term *chondroid lipoma* (75). CL occurs more commonly in females, with a female:male ratio of 4:1. The tumors usually arise in the extremities and infrequently involve the head and neck region. Grossly they are well circumscribed, lobulated, and tan–yellow. By light microscopy they are composed of mature white adipocytes, vacuolated lipoblast-like cells, and polyhedral cells with eosinophilic cytoplasm that grow in cords, sheets, and clusters, as well as individually (Fig. 25). The stroma is myxohyaline and has a chondroid appearance (75–78). Immunohistochemical studies reveal that the tumor cells stain with vimentin, S-100 protein, and focally with cytokeratin and CD68. Ultrastructurally the tumor cells contain glycogen and lipid, and demonstrate features of white adipocytes (76,77). The unusual histomorphology and hypercellularity of this tumor may cause confusion with myxoid liposarcoma and extraskeletal myxoid chondrosarcoma. However, unlike myxoid liposarcoma, CL does not contain spindle and stellate cells and does not demonstrate a delicate plexiform vascular pattern. Extraskeletal myxoid chondrosarcoma does not contain adipocytes or lipoblast-like cells. CL is benign, and simple excision has been shown to be curative.

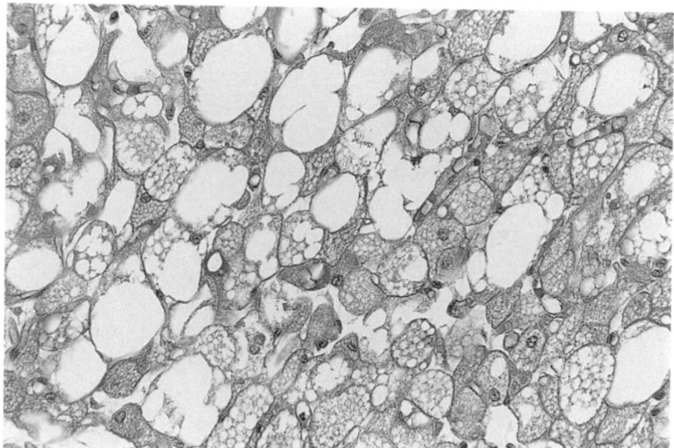

FIGURE 24. Granular eosinophilic cytoplasm and multiple small lipid vacuoles typical of hibernoma cells.

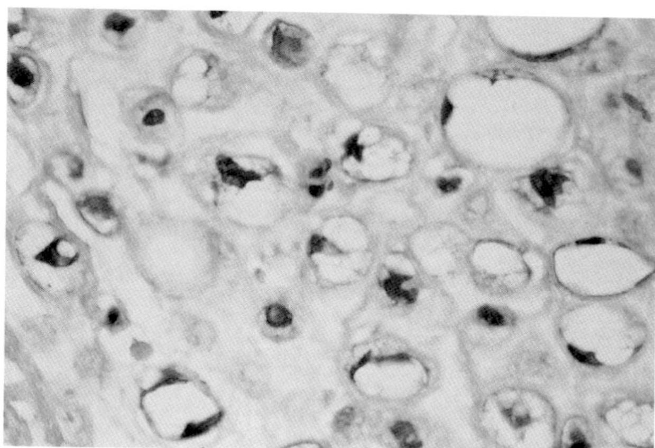

FIGURE 25. Vacuolated lipoblasts in myxohyaline stroma characteristic of chondroid lipoma.

Liposarcoma

Liposarcoma, originally described in 1857 by Virchow, is a malignant tumor demonstrating adipocytic differentiation (79). Although liposarcoma is one of the most common sarcomas of adulthood, only 4% of liposarcomas arise in the head and neck, where they account for only 1% of all sarcomas in this anatomic region (80–84). The mean age at the time of diagnosis is 46 years, with a range of 3 to 86 years. Males outnumber females by a ratio of nearly 2:1. The most common sites in the head and neck region are the neck, scalp, and face, followed by the larynx, pharynx, and oral cavity (80,81,83–88). Depending on the site, liposarcoma may be asymptomatic or may cause hoarseness, airway obstruction, or dysphagia (81,82,84).

The histologic classification of liposarcoma includes well-differentiated, myxoid, round cell, pleomorphic, and dedifferentiated types (86). Grossly, liposarcoma may be either infiltrative or well defined, and even encapsulated. The tumors range in size from 1 to 15 cm, and the cut surface depends on the subtype and ranges from yellow to gray–tan, glistening to fish-flesh–like in appearance (80).

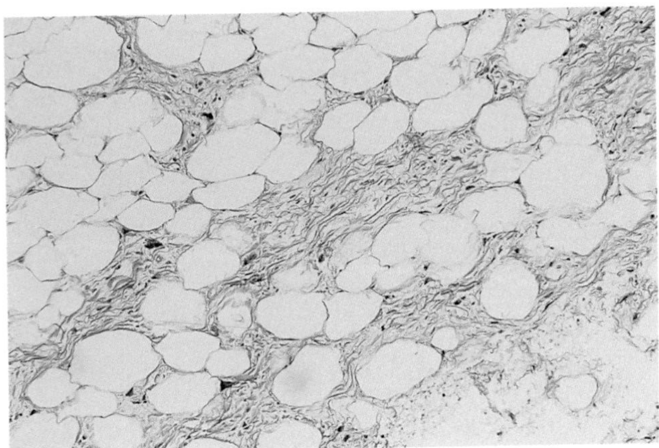

FIGURE 26. Large, hyperchromatic nuclei within fibrous septa of a well-differentiated lipoma-like liposarcoma.

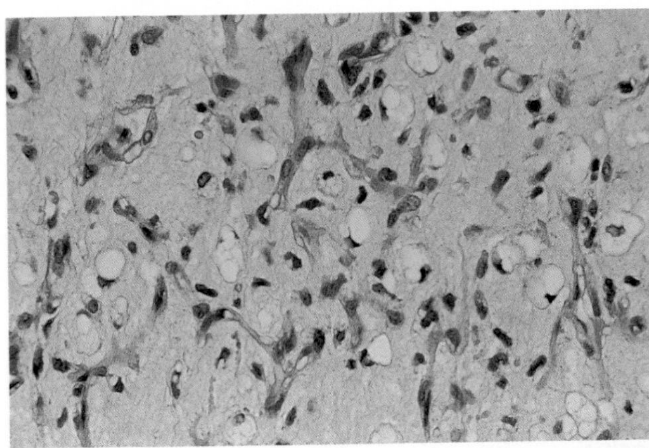

FIGURE 27. Myxoid liposarcoma consisting of multivacuolated lipoblasts within a myxoid stroma that has a delicate, branching capillary network.

Well-differentiated liposarcoma accounts for approximately 30% of head and neck liposarcomas, and is subclassified into lipoma-like, sclerosing, and inflammatory variants (86,87). Lipoma-like liposarcoma is composed of lobules of mature white adipocytes intermixed with occasional lipoblasts that have large, hyperchromatic nuclei that are scalloped by round, clear, lipid vacuoles which fill the cytoplasm of the cell. Fibrous septa divide the tumor into lobules and contain spindle cells with enlarged, hyperchromatic nuclei (Fig. 26). Scattered floret-type giant cells are also present. Ring chromosomes have been described in 78% of these tumors (61,89,90). A lesion that is important to distinguish from lipoma-like liposarcoma is fat necrosis with a histiocytic infiltrate. Fat necrosis lacks the atypical cells, including lipoblasts, and consists of histiocytes with foamy cytoplasm adjacent to necrotic adipocytes. The sclerosing subtype of well-differentiated liposarcoma contains areas of dense sclerotic collagen admixed with occasional lipoblasts and enlarged, hyperchromatic spindle cells. Inflammatory liposarcoma is the least common subtype of well-differentiated liposarcoma, but it has been reported to develop in the head and neck (91). In this variant of liposarcoma the lipoblasts are obscured by a densely cellular infiltrate containing lymphocytes that may be arranged in follicles with germinal centers and plasma cells, all in a sclerotic stroma. Many of these cases also contain areas of lipoma-like well-differentiated liposarcoma (91).

Myxoid liposarcoma comprises about 30% of all head and neck liposarcoma (80,87). Histologically it is composed of spindle and stellate cells and uni- and multivacuolated lipoblasts enmeshed within a myxoid stroma that contains a prominent network of delicate branching capillaries that are arranged in a plexiform pattern (Fig. 27). The differential diagnosis includes other neoplasms with myxoid stroma, such as myxofibrosarcoma, spindle cell lipoma, neurofibroma, and myxoma. However, none of these tumors display the delicate, branching vascular pattern characteristic of myxoid liposarcoma, nor do they contain true lipoblasts. Additionally, spindle cell lipoma and neurofibroma contain thick, wire-like collagen bundles that are not present in myxoid liposarcoma. Myxoid liposarcoma has a unique t(12;16) translocation that is present in 96% of cases, and its identification is useful in distinguishing it from other lesions in the differential diagnosis (61).

Round cell liposarcoma is closely related to myxoid liposarcoma because both types are frequently seen in the same neoplasm and both have the t(12;16) translocation (61,92,93). Round cell liposarcoma accounts for about 10% of head and neck liposarcomas (80,87). It is composed of sheets of uniform, small round cells with vesicular or hyperchromatic nuclei and a small amount of clear to pale pink cytoplasm (Fig. 28). Scattered uni- and multivacuolated lipoblasts are invariably present. The myxoid stroma and vascular pattern characteristic of myxoid liposarcoma are often difficult to appreciate because they are obscured by the dense cellularity of the tumor. Morphologically, round call liposarcoma may resemble other small round cell tumors. Immunohistochemistry and electron microscopy are helpful in distinguishing it from lymphoma, RMS, and extraskeletal Ewing's sarcoma. Round cell liposarcoma is positive for S-100 protein and negative for leukocyte common antigen (LCA), desmin, and mic-2, and electron microscopy detects the lipid within the cytoplasm of the tumor

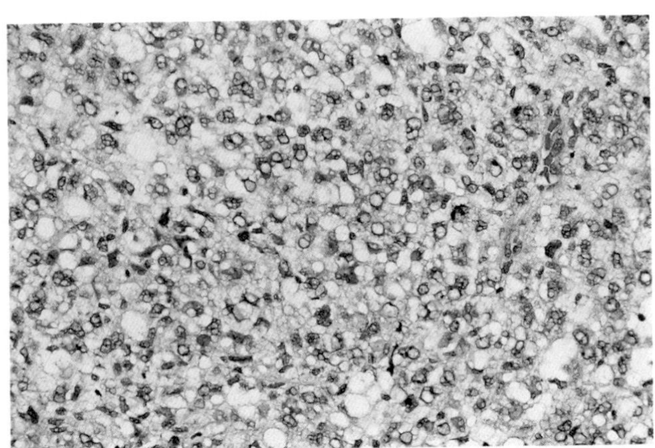

FIGURE 28. Round cell liposarcoma composed of sheets of small round cells with vesicular nuclei.

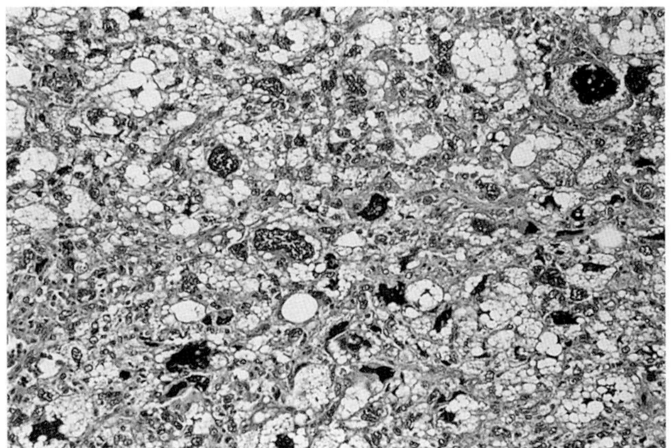

FIGURE 29. Large, bizarre tumor cells admixed with classic lipoblasts in pleomorphic liposarcoma.

cells. The identification of the unique t(12;16) translocation is another diagnostic aid.

Pleomorphic liposarcoma (PLS) was thought to account for about 30% of head and neck liposarcomas; however, this is likely to be a significant overestimate because many of the tumors previously diagnosed as PLS would be considered variants of MFH according to current morphologic criteria (80,87). PLS is characterized histologically by sheets of pleomorphic spindle or polyhedral cells with scattered lipoblasts (Fig. 29). Lipoblasts may be few in number or abundant, and when they are difficult to find, distinction from other high-grade sarcomas such as MFH can be very difficult. The problem is further exacerbated by the presence of degenerated cells within a high-grade sarcoma that may resemble lipoblasts (pseudolipoblasts). These can be distinguished from true lipoblasts by other evidence of degeneration such as nuclear vacuolization. True lipoblasts are S-100 positive, whereas most pleomorphic sarcomas, except malignant peripheral nerve sheath tumor (MPNST), are negative for this antibody.

Dedifferentiated liposarcoma was defined in 1979 as a high-grade sarcoma arising in association with a well-differentiated liposarcoma (94). The high-grade component most often resembles MFH; however, LMS, fibrosarcoma, and RMS components have been described. Dedifferentiated liposarcoma is extremely uncommon in the head and neck region.

The treatment for liposarcoma is wide excision with or without adjuvant radiation or chemotherapy, depending on the grade, size, and resectability of the tumor (81–83). Liposarcoma has the propensity to recur locally, and metastases may develop in the dedifferentiated, pleomorphic, and round cell subtypes (84,87). The overall 5-year survival rate for liposarcoma of the head and neck region is 67%. The 5-year survival rate for well-differentiated liposarcoma is approximately 100%, for pure myxoid liposarcoma it is 75%, and for PLS it is 40%; the few patients with round cell liposarcoma in this region died of disease (81,82,87). Patients with liposarcoma located in the larynx, face, and scalp have 5-year survival rates in the 80% to 90% range, possibly due to early detection. Patients with oral cavity tumors fare worse (80,87).

Fibroblastic and Myofibroblastic Tumors

Fibromatosis and Variants

Fibromatosis, also known as aggressive fibromatosis or extraabdominal desmoid tumor, is a benign but locally aggressive tumor. Approximately 10% of cases occur in the head and neck region, where the most common site is the supraclavicular fossa, but fibromatosis also may affect the orbital region, nose, paranasal sinuses, parotid, and oral and perioral regions (95–98). Females outnumber males by a ratio of 3:2. Approximately 25% of patients are younger than 15 years of age at presentation; however, all age groups may be affected. Fibromatosis has been associated with trauma, hormonal stimulation, as in the case of pregnancy, and genetic syndromes, such as Gardner's syndrome.

Patients present with a painless, slowly growing mass that may arise within the tendons, aponeuroses, subcutaneous soft tissues, or muscles. The tumor has ill-defined, infiltrative margins, and because of its invasive growth pattern, fibromatosis may encase vital structures in the head and neck such as the brachial plexus, trachea, and large arteries (95). Grossly fibromatosis is tan and firm. Microscopically, it is composed of broad, sweeping cellular fascicles of uniform spindle fibroblasts in a collagenous and sometimes focally myxoid background (Fig. 30). The nuclei have finely distributed chromatin and contain indistinct nucleoli. Up to one mitosis per high-power field may be seen, but atypical forms are not present. Ultrastructurally, the proliferating cells are fibroblasts and myofibroblasts, and immunohistochemically they express vimentin, muscle and smooth muscle actin, and sometimes desmin (99). Cytogenetic abnormalities of 5q and trisomy 8 have been identified in some nonsyndromic cases (see Gardner's syndrome) (100). The differential diagnosis with NF and fibrosarcoma is covered in the discussions of these latter entities.

Biologically, fibromatosis is locally aggressive, and in the head and neck region approximately 70% recur because of the difficulty in achieving complete excision (101). Deaths due to local disease in the head and neck are uncommon, but well documented (98). Treatment is wide local excision with adjuvant radiation therapy when necessary (102,103). Patients with fibro-

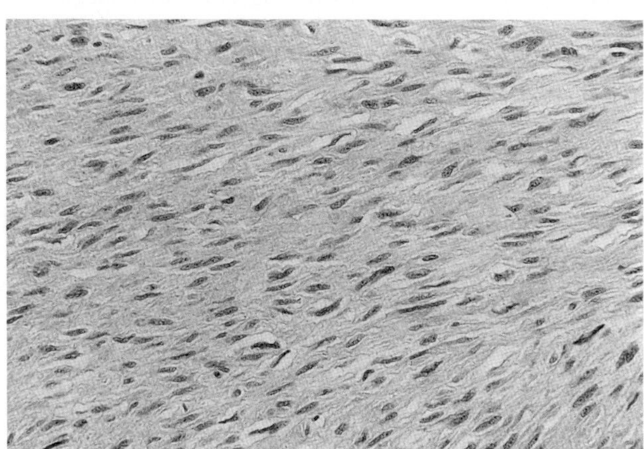

FIGURE 30. A broad fascicle of uniform spindled fibroblasts in fibromatosis.

matosis of the head and neck who receive surgery alone have a recurrence rate of up to 40%, compared with 30% for surgery plus radiation and 5% to 10% for radiation therapy alone (101–103).

Gardner's syndrome is the association of familial adenomatous polyposis and ectodermal or mesodermal tumors. It is a dominant trait determined by the heterozygous mutant *APC* gene that is located on the long arm of chromosome 5. Patients with familial adenomatous polyposis have an 850-fold increased risk of developing fibromatosis compared with the general population. The average age at presentation is 28 years, and most of the tumors develop in surgical wounds, especially in the abdomen of those patients who have had a colectomy. Only one case of fibromatosis of the head has been reported in Gardner's syndrome, and the tumor had a somatic mutation of both APC genes (100). This loss of heterozygosity has been demonstrated in eight additional desmoid tumors in patients with Gardner's syndrome, all of which were located in the abdominal wall (104). These results support the conclusion that fibromatosis in Gardner's syndrome is secondary to inactivation of the tumor suppressor *APC* gene in the uninvolved chromosome.

Infantile fibromatosis (IF) develops in the first 8 years of life. Approximately 35% of cases affect the head or neck (105), and it is slightly more common in boys. IF arises within the deep soft tissues or periosteum, is ill defined, and may cause bowing of the underlying bone. A single case has been reported to have developed in the deep lobe of the parotid (106). Histologically, IF may resemble the adult type of fibromatosis; however, it also may be more cellular and primitive in appearance, causing confusion with infantile fibrosarcoma. Variation in cellularity, the lack of a herringbone pattern and only occasional mitotic figures are features that help distinguish IF from infantile fibrosarcoma. When IF invades bone, its distinction from desmoplastic fibroma is difficult (107). Radiographic determination of the epicenter of the mass is helpful in this situation. The treatment of IF is surgical excision. Cases of spontaneous regression after incomplete surgery have been documented, but are rare (105).

Fibromatosis colli (FC) is a unique type of fibromatosis, which develops in the sternocleidomastoid muscle of newborn infants (108). When it causes a contracture that results in turning of the head, the term *congenital torticollis* is applied. Although birth trauma may play a role in its pathogenesis, well-documented cases involving infants delivered by uncomplicated vaginal and cesarean routes are present in the literature. FC presents as a 1- to 2-cm fusiform mass that is usually detected at 10 to 14 days of age. Approximately 75% occur on the right side. Grossly, FC has an infiltrative appearance and a gray–white glistening cut surface. Histologically it is composed of uniform spindle fibroblasts without pleomorphism in a collagenous background, infiltrating through the skeletal muscle (Fig. 31). Early lesions are cellular, with less collagen, but the amount of collagen increases with the age of the patient. In most cases, the mass regresses spontaneously by 8 months of age. The clinical differential diagnosis includes soft tissue tumors of infancy, which are easily distinguished from fibromatosis histologically, such as neuroblastoma, lymphoma, RMS, congenital cysts, and fibrosarcoma. Fine-needle aspiration in this clinical setting is an effective diagnostic technique (109,110).

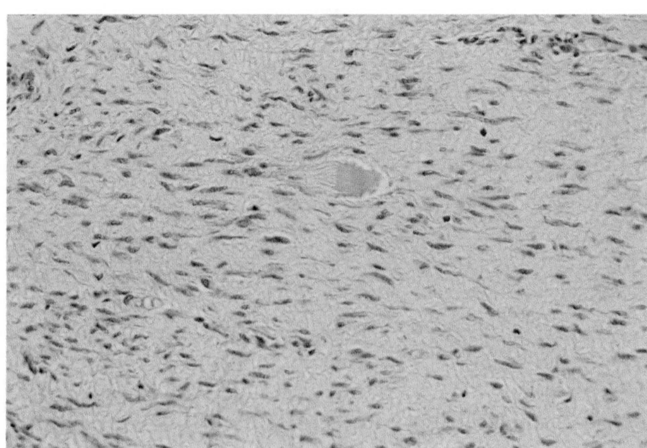

FIGURE 31. Bland appearing fibroblasts infiltrating through skeletal muscle in fibromatosis colli.

Juvenile Hyalin Fibromatosis

Juvenile hyalin fibromatosis (JHF), also known as fibromatosis hyalinica multiplex, is a rare disorder characterized by multiple soft tissue tumors, hypertrophic gingiva (Fig. 32), flexion contractures of the joints, and radiolucent bone abnormalities (111,112). Fewer than 50 cases have been reported in the world literature. Investigation of familial cases reveals that the pattern of inheritance is likely to be autosomal recessive. Patients present between 2 and 5 years of age with soft tissue nodules affecting multiple sites, most commonly the head and neck, as well as pearly gingival hypertrophy, joint swelling, and contractures. Osteopenia and osteolytic bone abnormalities may be present early or late in the course of the disease.

Regardless of site, the lesions are histologically similar. Spindle or round fibroblasts with contracted pink cytoplasm are embedded in an amorphous, hyalinized, eosinophilic stroma, where they form cords and loose fascicles (Fig. 33). The deposits may be surrounded by scattered inflammatory cells and dilated blood vessels. The stroma frequently contains abundant noncollagenous glycoproteins (113). Over time, the stroma predomi-

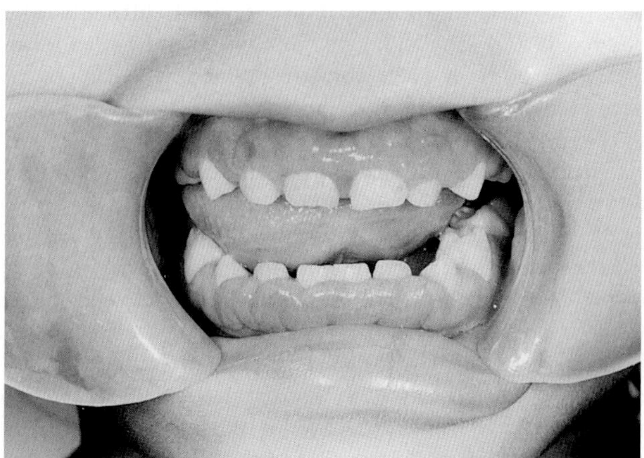

FIGURE 32. Gingival hyperplasia in a patient with juvenile hyalin fibromatosis. (Courtesy of Iyoko Miyake, M.D. Reprinted from Miyaki I, Tokumaru H, Sugino H, et al. Juvenile hyaline fibromatosis. Case report with five years' follow-up. *Am J Dermatopathol* 1995;15:584–590; with permission.)

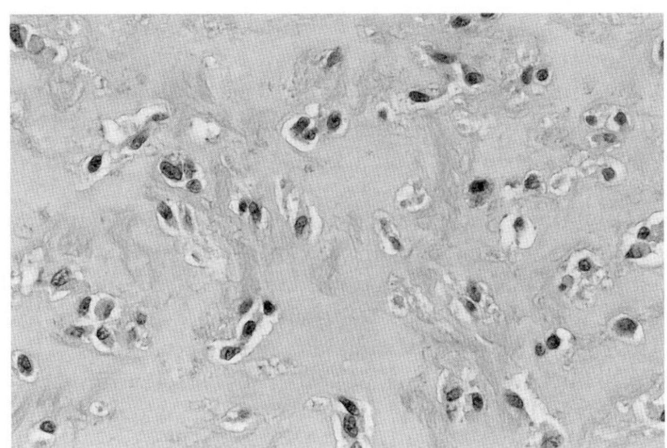

FIGURE 33. Juvenile hyalin fibromatosis composed of round fibroblasts embedded in hyalinized stroma. (Courtesy of Iyoke Miyake, M.D.)

nates as the tumor matures and becomes less cellular. Ultrastructural analysis shows that the cytoplasm of the fibroblasts contains cystic rough endoplasmic reticulum and Golgi filled with filamentous and granular material, which is eventually deposited into the surrounding matrix (111).

The cause of JHF is a defect in the synthesis of collagen (114). JHF is progressive, with no known treatment. Patients die by the third or fourth decade and are usually severely deformed. The clinical differential diagnosis includes other multicentric diseases that present in childhood, such as mucopolysaccharidosis, infantile myofibromatosis, and neurofibromatosis. Tissue biopsy is often necessary to make the distinction early in the disease course. Infantile systemic hyalinosis is a similar disease, but has an onset in early infancy and has a more severe clinical course (112).

Hereditary Gingival Fibromatosis

Hereditary gingival fibromatosis (GF) is not a true fibromatosis, but a rare autosomal-dominant fibrous hyperplasia of the gingiva (115). Sporadic cases and cases inherited in an autosomal-recessive fashion have been observed. GF may be associated with cognitive deficits, epilepsy, and hypertrichosis, and may be a component of a broader syndrome. The gingival proliferation causes delayed eruption of teeth and difficulty with proper hygiene and mastication. Histologic examination of the gingiva reveals elongation of the mucosal rete ridges and an underlying accumulation of dense collagen fibers intermixed with spindle and stellate fibroblasts. Although the cause of GF is unknown, *in vitro* studies have shown that the fibroblasts in GF produce greater amounts of fibronectin and type I collagen, and have increased proliferation rates when compared with normal fibroblasts (116). Primary hereditary GF may be mimicked by dilantin-induced gingival hyperplasia, which also demonstrates increased collagen synthesis *in vitro* when compared with normal (117).

Nuchal Fibroma

An uncommon benign tumor occurring in the cervical paraspinal and interscapular areas, nuchal fibroma occurs in patients between 19 and 60 years of age (118,119). It arises in the subcutis, and is well circumscribed but unencapsulated. It consists of large, hypocellular bundles of collagen that may extend for short distances into the subcutis and entrap nerves and small amounts of adipose tissue (Fig. 34). The differential diagnosis is with elastofibroma, fibrolipoma, and collagenous fibroma. Although nuchal fibroma may contain very small amounts of elastic fibers, the fibers are not beaded as in the classic elastofibroma. Fibrolipoma is a well-encapsulated tumor composed of adipose tissue and prominent bundles of collagen; however, the collagenous component is not as abundant as in nuchal fibroma, and entrapped normal structures, such as nerves, are generally absent. The distinction between nuchal fibroma and NFP is discussed in the earlier section on the latter lesion. The treatment of nuchal fibroma is excision.

Collagenous Fibroma

Originally termed *desmoplastic fibroblastoma* by Evans in 1995, collagenous fibroma is a benign fibrous tumor that is located on the neck or upper back in 6% of cases (120–123). Fewer than 80 cases have been reported. The age range is between 15 and 83 years, with a predilection for men in the sixth decade of life. Collagenous fibroma usually presents as a slowly growing, painless mass. The tumors range in size from 1 to 20 (mean 3) cm and the majority are subcutaneous, although those that are intramuscular account for 25% of cases. Grossly they are well circumscribed, and have a firm, tan cut surface. Collagenous fibroma is hypocellular and composed of widely spaced, haphazardly arranged, cytologically bland, medium to large stellate and spindle fibroblasts in a fibrous to fibromyxoid background containing wavy collagen fibers (Fig. 35). Occasionally the borders are focally infiltrative. Immunohistochemically collagenous fibroma may express actin, suggesting a myofibroblastic origin, and positive staining for S-100 protein has been reported in a minority of cases (122,123). Ultrastructural analysis reveals that the tumor cells have the features of fibroblasts and myofibroblasts (123). Treatment is conservative excision. To date none of the reported series have documented a local recurrence.

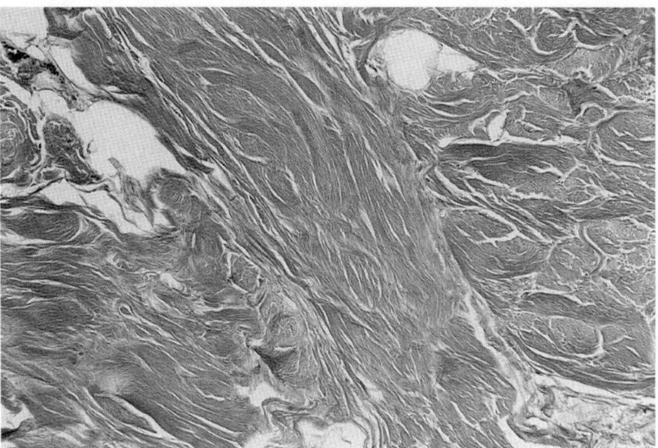

FIGURE 34. Large, hypocellular bundles of collagen in a nuchal fibroma.

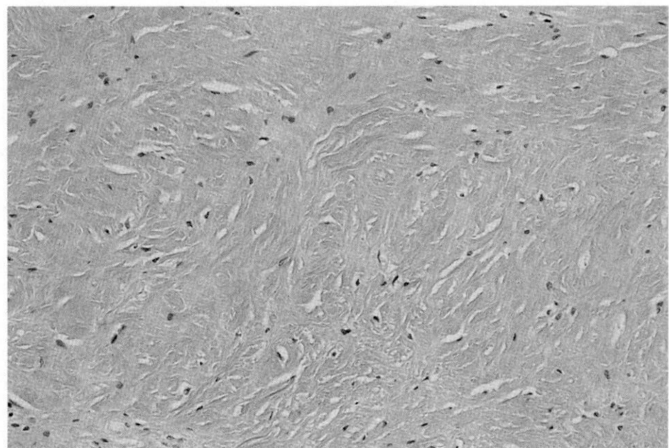

FIGURE 35. Haphazardly arranged banal-appearing stellate fibroblasts in a collagenous fibroma.

The differential diagnosis of collagenous fibroma includes fibromatosis, nuchal fibroma, neurofibroma, and low-grade fibromyxoid sarcoma. Fibromatosis is more cellular, its fascicular growth pattern better organized, and is more infiltrative than collagenous fibroma. Nodular fasciitis is also more cellular and less collagenous than collagenous fibroma, and the fibroblasts have a tissue culture appearance. Microcysts, appreciable mitotic activity, and extravasated erythrocytes are present in nodular fasciitis but are not features of collagenous fibroma. Neurofibroma also may be more cellular than collagenous fibroma, and the nuclei of the spindle cells are wavy and associated with bundles of wire-like collagen. Neurofibromas diffusely express S-100 protein, whereas collagenous fibroma shows only focal expression in a minority of cases. Low-grade fibromyxoid sarcoma contains focal areas that are more cellular than collagenous fibroma which have a characteristic whorled growth pattern, admixed with fewer cellular areas that contain myxoid stroma, and these features are not present in collagenous fibroma.

Myofibromatosis and Solitary Myofibroma

Myofibroma is a benign tumor of myofibroblasts first fully elucidated by Chung and Enzinger in 1981 (124). As long ago as 1954 similar cases were described under a variety of terms including *congenital generalized fibromatosis* and *multiple mesenchymal hamartomas* (125,126). Myofibroma is considered to be the most common fibrous tumor of infancy (127). The current understanding of the disease spectrum of myofibromatosis includes three forms: the multifocal form, a frequently congenital condition in which infants may have many lesions involving the soft tissues and bone; the rare but often fatal congenital generalized form, in which innumerable lesions involve the skin, soft tissue, bone, and viscera of infants; and the solitary form, in which a single lesions affects the skin and soft tissues of children and adults (128). Overall, males are affected more often than females. Evidence has been cited to support both autosomal dominant and recessive patterns of inheritance (129,130). The soft tissues of the head and neck and the oral cavity are the most common areas of involvement in the solitary form (131–134). The generalized and multicentric forms may develop at any site.

The gross and microscopic appearance of all forms of myofibromatosis is similar. Individual tumors are well circumscribed, up to 3 cm in diameter, and may be freely mobile or attached to the underlying fascia or bone. Myofibromas have a rubbery texture and a lobulated appearance. Histologically the classic myofibroma has a biphasic or zonated appearance. The central portion of the mass is composed of compact small round to oval cells with scant eosinophilic cytoplasm and vesicular nuclei arranged around hemangiopericytoma (HP)-like, branching vessels (Fig. 36). The cells are mitotically active and may show foci of necrosis. This zone blends into a peripheral, leiomyoma-like zone where the cells are larger and more spindle shaped, with abundant pale, eosinophilic cytoplasm and cigar-shaped nuclei. The cells in this zone are arranged in fascicles, may focally infiltrate into the surrounding tissue, and may even invade blood vessels. A small percentage of myofibromas are monomorphic and composed solely of the cellular component or the leiomyoma-like areas (135). Immunohistochemical studies reveal the cells within both zones of the myofibroma stain with antibodies to vimentin, smooth muscle actin, and muscle-specific actin (132). The spindle cells also can express desmin. Ultrastructural analysis confirms that the cells have characteristics of myofibroblasts and fibroblasts.

The clinical differential diagnosis of the multicentric and generalized forms includes entities that are ruled out by biopsy, such as metastatic neuroblastoma, lymphoma/leukemia, and neurofibromatosis. The histologic differential diagnosis of all forms includes nodular fasciitis, leiomyoma, HP, and sarcoma (136). Nodular fasciitis is also a myofibroblastic lesion but it does not contain the characteristic zonated pattern found in myofibroma. The tissue culture-like growth pattern of myofibroblasts in nodular fasciitis does not resemble either of the two zones of myofibroma. Although the peripheral zone of a myofibroma bears histologic similarity to leiomyoma, the cytoplasm of the smooth muscle cells of leiomyoma is more eosinophilic, and the cells are arranged in tight, well-formed fascicles that

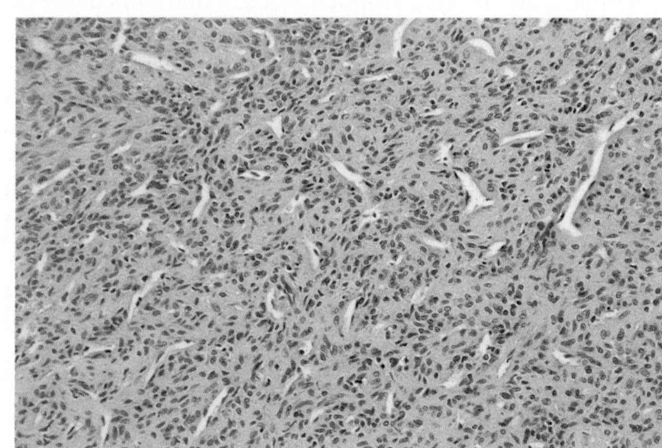

FIGURE 36. The central portion of a myofibroma composed of small round cells with vesicular nuclei and scant eosinophilic cytoplasm.

classically intersect at right angles. Clinical information regarding multicentricity and young age will help distinguish HP from myofibroma. HPs usually vary in cellularity and do not have areas in which the tumor cells resemble myofibroblasts or smooth muscle cells. HP stains for CD34, whereas myofibroma is negative for this antibody. Distinction from a sarcoma is usually not difficult if the biphasic pattern is evident on the biopsy. If only the cellular central portion is present in the specimen, the uniformity of the cells and lack of atypia make a malignant diagnosis unlikely.

The generalized form of infantile myofibromatosis has the worst prognosis. Many cases are fatal because of complications related to visceral disease (128). Chemotherapy is used in these cases, and some lesions respond, but the disease ultimately progresses. Patients with the multicentric and solitary forms usually do not have visceral involvement, and the disease has a benign course. Spontaneous tumor regression has been reported (127).

Intranodal Myofibroblastoma

In 1989 a benign tumor restricted to groin lymph nodes was described simultaneously by two groups of investigators as "palisaded myofibroblastoma of lymph node" and "intranodal hemorrhagic spindle cell tumor with amianthoid fibers" (137,138). Subsequently it has become known as intranodal myofibroblastoma (IMF) and has been shown to have a wider anatomic distribution, including submandibular lymph nodes (139,140). Affected patients are adults, ranging in age from 19 to 67 years, and men outnumber women by a ratio of 2:1. The lesion presents as a mobile, firm mass that may be present for years or grow rapidly over a short period of time. IMF is usually between 1 and 5 cm in greatest dimension and well circumscribed, and has a tan cut surface. Microscopically the lymph node is replaced by proliferating spindle cells but the capsule remains intact and a periphery of nodal tissue is usually present. The spindle cells are short and have a small amount of eosinophilic cytoplasm and slender, tapered nuclei. The cells are arranged in short, intersecting fascicles, and in areas the nuclei are arranged in pallisades adjacent to serpiginous areas of deeply eosinophilic, homogeneous collagen with peripheral hair-like fibrils rimmed by less eosinophilic, granular collagen. These latter areas are known as amianthoid fibers. Mitotic activity is minimal and nuclear atypia is absent. Immunohistochemical studies reveal that the spindle cells are positive for actin and not for desmin, S-100 protein, or Leu-7 (137,138). Ultrastructurally the spindle cell nuclei have indentations similar to myofibroblasts, and the cytoplasm contains abundant thin filaments with subplasmalemmal densities, pinocytotic vesicles, small amounts of mitochondria, and rough endoplasmic reticulum. Rare intercellular junctions are present (138).

The differential diagnosis should include metastatic sarcoma and schwannoma. Aside from epithelioid sarcoma (ES) and clear cell sarcoma, which do not morphologically resemble IMF, sarcomas infrequently metastasize to lymph nodes. When they do, they are generally high grade and demonstrate cytologic features of malignancy such as severe cytologic atypia, abnormal mitoses, and necrosis. An exception is Kaposi's sarcoma, which can extensively involve lymph nodes. Kaposi's sarcoma has a fascicular growth pattern like IMF, but it has slit-like vascular spaces containing erythrocytes that are not present in IMF, and Kaposi's sarcoma lacks amianthoid fibers. Immunohistochemical stains confirm the endothelial nature of Kaposi's sarcoma; it is positive for Factor VIII, CD31, CD34, and *Ulex europaeus,* whereas IMF is negative for these markers. A schwannoma can be distinguished from IMF because it contains hyalinized vessels and alternating areas of hyper- and hypocellularity. Immunohistochemistry is also helpful, because IMF is positive for actin and not for S-100 protein and schwannoma is positive for S-100 protein and negative for actin. All cases of IMF thus far have behaved in a benign fashion, and excision has been curative.

Solitary Fibrous Tumor

Solitary fibrous tumor (SFT) is a spindle cell neoplasm that most commonly develops in the pleura. Although a mesothelial origin had been postulated, immunohistochemical and ultrastructural studies indicate that SFT is of mesenchymal origin (141). In recent years SFT has been documented to arise in numerous areas unrelated to serosal membranes. In the head and neck SFT has been reported to originate in the soft tissues of the neck, face, orbit (Fig. 37), parapharyngeal space, epiglottis, nasopharynx, nasal cavity, thyroid, and major salivary glands (141–148). Affected patients have a broad age range (13–85 years), although most are adults at the time of diagnosis.

The tumors range in size from 2 to 25 cm. They are well demarcated and have a firm, gray–tan, whorled cut surface. Microscopically, SFT is usually well circumscribed and composed of an admixture of hypo- and hypercellular spindle cell areas. The spindle cells are haphazardly arranged, but in areas may

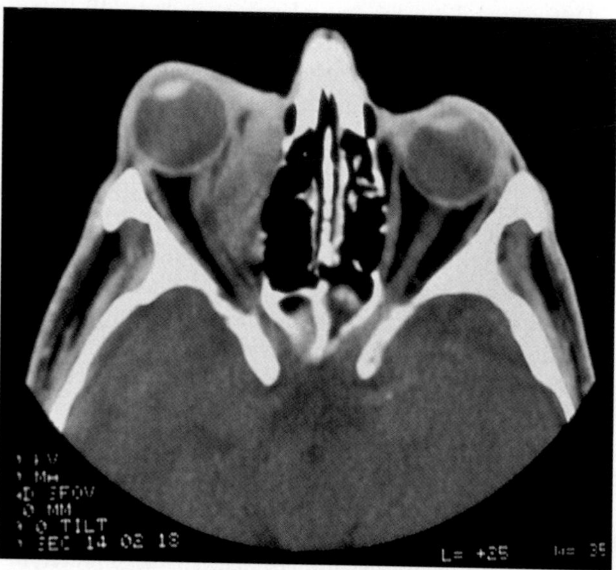

FIGURE 37. A solitary fibrous tumor occupies the soft tissues of the medial orbit.

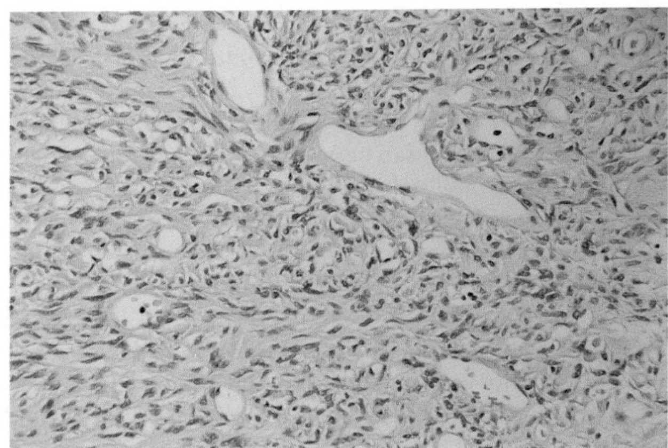

FIGURE 38. Haphazardly arranged spindle cells associated with dense collagen and branching vessels in a solitary fibrous tumor.

be oriented in a vague storiform pattern (Fig. 38). The cells have elongated, tapered nuclei and finely stippled chromatin and are intimately associated with wavy, dense, wire-like collagen that also may resemble amianthoid fibers. Mitotic activity is frequently present but is usually not more than one per 10 high-power fields. SFTs display a prominent vascularity that has an HP-like "staghorn" pattern. The vessels may be thick-walled and hyalinized. A minority of cases of SFT contain foci of adipocytes that may be entrapped (147–149).

Immunohistochemically, SFTs generally stain for vimentin and CD34. Some staining also has been demonstrated with actin, Leu-7, desmin, and CD99 (141,147,148). The tumors have not been shown to express cytokeratin, or S-100 protein. Ultrastructural analysis indicates that the tumor cells are fibroblastic in nature, arranged individually and in small groups within a matrix of banded collagen and amianthoid fibers (141). Focal myofibroblastic differentiation is present in a minority of cases.

Differential diagnostic considerations include HP, spindle cell lipoma, fibrous histiocytoma, and, especially in the nasal cavity, schwannoma. HP lacks the variability in cellularity and the collagenous, hyalinized stroma present in SFT. Ultrastructurally, HPs have features of pericyte differentiation and not of fibroblasts. An SFT that contains fat raises the histologic diagnosis of spindle cell lipoma with abundant collagen formation. Both stain positively with CD34; however, spindle cell lipomas usually have a myxoid stroma that is uncommonly seen in SFT, and they lack the hemangiopericytomatous vascular pattern. Deep-seated fibrous histiocytoma has a more uniform storiform growth pattern than SFT and is CD34 negative. Schwannomas may superficially resemble SFT because of the Antoni A and B areas; however, nuclear palisading and S-100 protein positivity make the distinction possible.

Most SFTs behave in a benign fashion. Malignant variants are uncommon but have been documented (141). Malignant SFTs are grossly indistinguishable from benign variants; however, histologically they are more uniformly cellular, have larger, more pleomorphic nuclei with more prominent nucleoli, contain 2 to 10 mitoses per 10 high-power fields, and may have areas of necrosis. Immunohistochemical and ultrastructural features of malignant SFT are similar to its benign counterpart. The treatment of benign SFT is simple excision, which is curative in most instances. Malignant SFTs should be widely excised with consideration of adjuvant therapy in appropriate instances because they can recur locally (150).

Giant Cell Angiofibroma

Giant cell angiofibroma (GCA) is a recently described, uncommon, benign but locally recurring soft tissue tumor that arises predominantly in the orbit, and rarely in the cheek (151). The tumor mainly affects adults with a mean age of 59 years. These tumors are slow growing and have been noted to be present for 6 months to 6 years prior to diagnosis.

Giant cell angiofibromas range from 1 to 3 cm in greatest dimension and are grayish in color, with focal glistening or myxoid areas. They are unencapsulated and may be well defined or infiltrative. GCAs are moderately cellular and are composed of haphazardly arranged spindle and stellate fibroblasts within a collagenous or myxoid stroma. Mulinucleate and uninucleate giant cells are a characteristic feature of the tumor. The multinucleate type has peripherally placed nuclei, which assume a floret appearance. Although the nuclei of the giant cells may be hyperchromatic, cytologic atypia is otherwise absent. Mitotic figures may be present but do not number more than two per 10 high-power fields. The stroma usually contains a prominent network of blood vessels that may be hyalinized, as well as irregular sinusoidal pseudovascular spaces that may harbor eosinophilic granular material (Fig. 39). The giant cells frequently line these pseudovascular spaces. Scattered inflammatory cells are common. Immunohistochemical stains are positive for vimentin and CD34 and negative for muscle and smooth muscle actins, desmin, S-100 protein, epithelial membrane antigen (EMA), and CD31. Electron microscopy reveals that the stromal cells have the characteristics of fibroblasts (151).

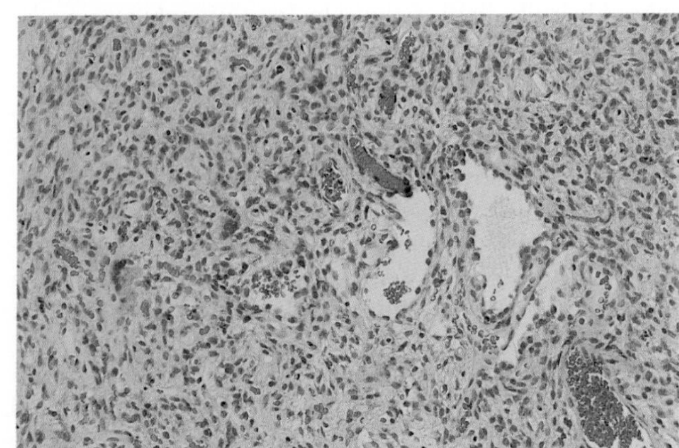

FIGURE 39. Giant cell angiofibroma with pseudovascular spaces lined by large, hyperchromatic cells and containing eosinophilic material and red blood cells.

The differential diagnosis of GCA includes SFT and giant cell fibroblastoma (GCF). SFT differs in that the cellularity is more variable and that giant cells are not a feature. In addition, most SFTs have an HP-like vascular tree, which is not a characteristic feature of GCA. However, we have seen orbital tumors that have features of both SFT and GCA, which raises the possibility that these tumors are closely related to one another. GCF is a lesion of childhood and rarely has been reported in the neck (152). It, too, contains multinucleate giant cells that line sinusoidal-like spaces, but it has a focally storiform pattern and sclerotic stroma, which are not present in GCA.

The treatment of GCA is excision. Only a small number of cases of GCA have been described in the literature, and their follow-up time is short, but GCA appears to have a benign course; only a small percentage of cases have recurred locally.

Giant Cell Fibroblastoma

Giant cell fibroblastoma, a fibroblastic tumor of childhood, may occur anywhere but infrequently arises in the head and neck. First described in 1982 by Schmookler et al., GCF bears resemblance to dermatofibrosarcoma protuberans (DFSP) and may be its childhood counterpart (153–155). Over 60% of patients are male, and greater than 80% occur in children under 12 years of age (152,156,157).

Giant cell fibroblastoma is a slowly enlarging, nontender subcutaneous mass that may be fixed to the overlying skin. Its size varies from less than a centimeter to 8 cm in diameter. It is ill defined, and has infiltrative borders and a rubbery consistency with foci of myxoid change. Although GCF is centered in the subcutis, it usually extends into the dermis, surrounds adenexal structures, and a small percentage of cases infiltrate the underlying skeletal muscle. By light microscopy GCF has a variety of histologic patterns. Solid areas predominate and are composed of slender stellate and spindled cells with normochromic nuclei and pale cytoplasm arranged in loose fascicles. Mitoses are infrequent. The stroma is somewhat myxoid and contains wavy collagen fibers and areas of hyalinization. Distributed throughout the solid areas are large mononucleate and multinucleate cells, the latter having nuclei arranged in a floret-type pattern. Large, irregularly shaped dilated spaces, known as angiectoid areas, are found throughout the tumors and contain granular pink material and occasional erythrocytes and are lined by the enlarged multi- and uninucleate cells as well as smaller bland spindle cells (Figs. 40 and 41). Cases of GCF arising adjacent to a DFSP and DFSP recurring as a GCF or GCF recurring as a DFSP are evidence that a relationship exists between these two neoplasms (154,155,158,159). This is further confirmed by the fact that GCF and DFSP both demonstrate the same t(17;22) translocation (160,161).

Immunohistochemical studies show that both the bland spindle component and the giant cells are positive for vimentin and CD34 and focally for muscle actin. No staining is present with S-100 protein, or endothelial markers, even in the cells lining the sinusoidal spaces (162). Ultrastructurally the cells resemble fibroblasts and myofibroblasts (163).

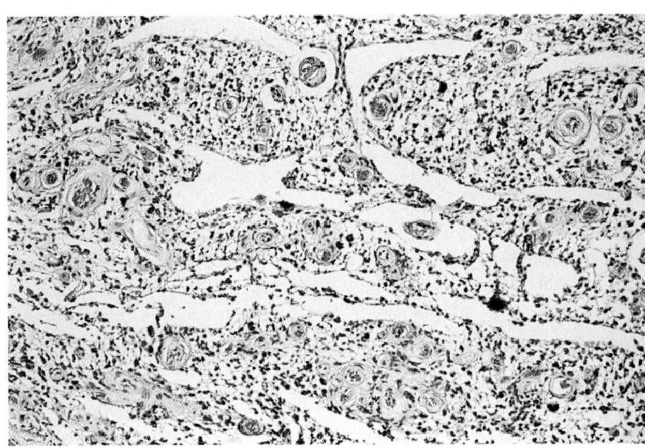

FIGURE 40. Giant cell fibroblastoma with prominent angiectoid areas.

The differential diagnosis includes GCA, lymphangioma, and high-grade sarcoma. GCA has a prominent vascular tree that is lacking in GCF. GCF also has infiltrative margins that are not characteristic of GCA. The dilated spaces of GCF may resemble a lymphangioma; however, lymphangioma can be ruled out by the presence of a solid spindle cell component as well as the presence of giant cells. Although the presence of giant cells may raise the differential diagnosis of a high-grade sarcoma, the uniformity of the cells and the lack of hyperchromasia and mitotic activity do not support the diagnosis of high-grade malignancy. Treatment of GCF is local excision. Although approximately 50% of GCF recur, none have been reported to metastasize.

Fibrosarcoma and Variants

Fibrosarcoma is one of the most common sarcomas of the head and neck, and approximately 5% to 10% of fibrosarcomas are located in this region (164,165). The neck and paranasal sinuses are the most prevalent primary sites, but fibrosarcoma may arise anywhere. Most tumors are deep seated and originate from fascia, aponeuroses, tendons, or intramuscular fibrous tissue. Fibrosarcomas affect all ages, but the average age at presentation

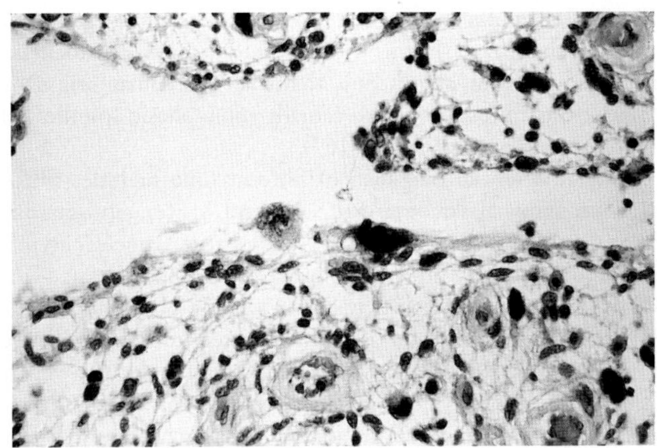

FIGURE 41. Multinucleate giant cells line the sinusoidal-like spaces in a giant cell fibroblastoma.

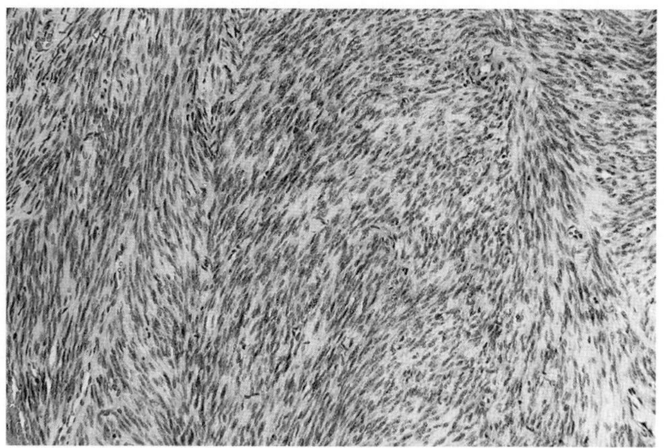

FIGURE 42. Hypercellular fascicles of spindle cells arranged in a herringbone pattern characteristic of fibrosarcoma.

is between 35 and 45 years. As many as 25% of patients have a history of prior radiation or thermal injury to the area (165,166).

Fibrosarcoma presents as a painless, enlarging mass that has a tan, firm cut surface. It may have well-delineated or infiltrative borders. Histologically the classic fibrosarcoma is composed of fascicles of uniform spindled fibroblasts arranged in a herringbone pattern in a background of collagen fibers (Fig. 42). The cytoplasm of the neoplastic cells is generally scant, eosinophilic, and ill defined. The degree of nuclear atypia, anaplasia, mitotic activity, and necrosis varies with the grade of the tumor. Myxoid change of the stroma is occasionally present, and areas of stromal hyalinization or sclerosis also may dominate, but mainly in the uncommon epithelioid variant of fibrosarcoma.

Immunohistochemically, fibrosarcoma uniformly stains with vimentin, and those with varying degrees of myofibroblastic differentiation also express actin and desmin. By electron microscopy the cells may be closely associated with or separated by intercellular collagen. The main cytoplasmic organelle is rough endoplasmic reticulum, with scattered mitochondria present as well. The cells lack external laminae and cytoplasmic junctions. Before immunohistochemistry and electron microscopy became routine in the diagnosis and subclassification of soft tissue tumors, fibrosarcoma was considered the most common sarcoma of the head and neck in adults. More recent published reviews of large series of head and neck fibrosarcomas have shown, with the aid of immunohistochemistry and electron microscopy, that many sarcomas originally classified as fibrosarcoma are actually monophasic spindle cell synovial sarcoma and MFH (167).

The differential diagnosis of fibrosarcoma includes fibromatosis, synovial sarcoma, MPNST, and MFH. Fibromatosis lacks the cellularity, herringbone growth pattern, nuclear atypia, and mitotic activity present in fibrosarcoma. Monophasic spindle cell synovial sarcoma may bear a striking histologic resemblance to fibrosarcoma but is easily separated from it by positive immunohistochemical stains for low and high molecular weight keratins and EMA. Electron microscopy reveals poorly developed intercellular junctions in synovial sarcoma, and these should not be present in fibrosarcoma. Lastly, fibrosarcoma lacks the t(X;18) translocation characteristic of synovial sarcoma. MFH may be confused with high grade fibrosarcoma. MFH generally occurs in an older population, and histologically is distinguished by a storiform growth pattern and presence of large, bizarre, multinucleated tumor cells.

The treatment for fibrosarcoma is primarily surgical, with chemotherapy reserved for patients with large high-grade tumors. Prognosis is based on tumor size, grade, and margin status. Adjuvant radiation therapy has been shown to improve local control, especially in the case of a positive margin (164). The overall 5-year survival rate for fibrosarcoma is 55% to 70% (164–166).

Congenital fibrosarcoma (CFS), also known as fibrosarcoma of infancy, is a locally aggressive fibroblastic tumor that occurs in children who are usually less than 2 years of age. Cytogenetic analysis of CFS has identified deletions on the long arm of chromosome 17 or a t(12;15)(p13;q25) rearrangement (168). The tumors are large in comparison to the size of the child and tend to grow rapidly, frequently eroding underlying bone (Fig. 43). CFS is composed of uniform sheets of small spindle to round cells that are arranged in a fascicular growth pattern (Fig. 44). The stroma usually contains only a small amount of collagen. Mitoses and necrosis are common, and a lymphocytic infiltrate is often present. Like most fibroblastic tumors, CFS does not have a specific immunohistochemical profile; however, these tumors express vimentin. A variety of markers, such as neuron-specific enolase (NSE), actins, estrogen receptors, desmin, CD34, Leu-7, and S-100 protein, have been positive in a small number of cases (169). The differential diagnosis of CFS is infantile

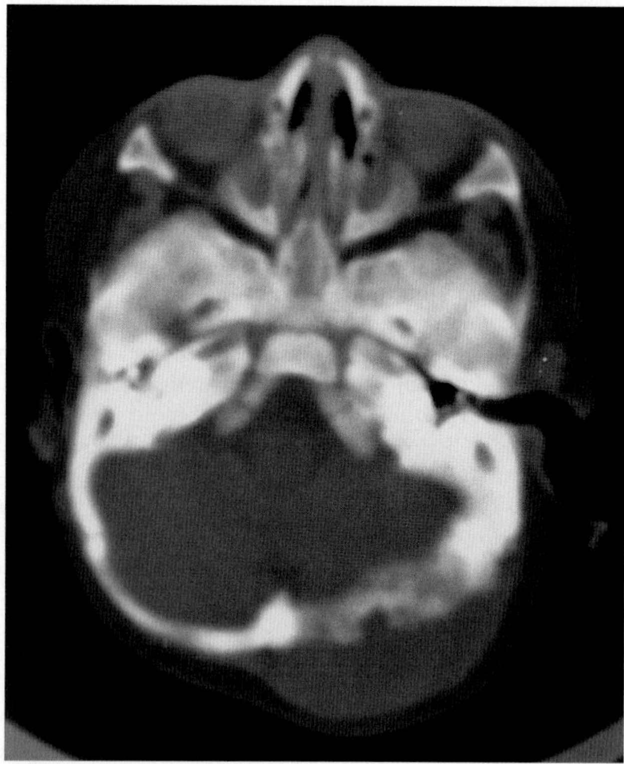

FIGURE 43. A large congenital fibrosarcoma present in the posterior neck soft tissue and invading the cranium.

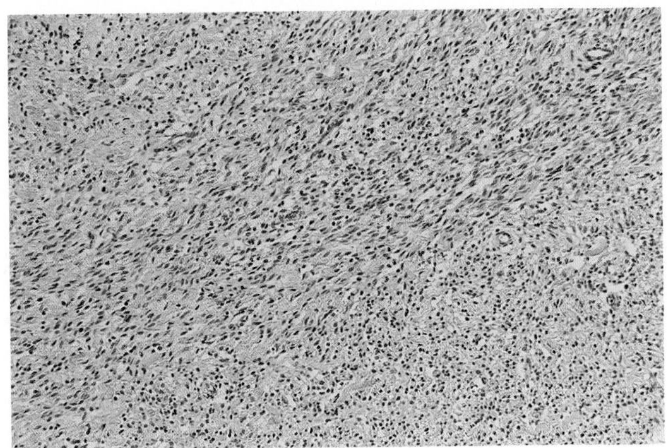

FIGURE 44. Congenital fibrosarcoma composed of fascicles of small fibroblasts admixed with lymphocytes.

fibromatosis (IF), which can be distinguished because it is less cellular and less atypical than CFS. Also, IF lacks the genetic derangements seen in CFS.

The treatment of choice for CFS is complete resection. Radiation and chemotherapy have been used successfully in patients in whom local control cannot be achieved by surgery alone (170). Although CFS may be histologically identical to the adult type of fibrosarcoma, its prognosis is more favorable (171). The 5-year survival rate for CFS is over 80%. A small percentage of tumors metastasize, and histologic features such as cellularity and atypia are not helpful in predicting this subset. Tumors of the head and neck have a poor prognosis due to their proximity to vital structures, such as the airway and large vessels.

Sclerosing epithelioid fibrosarcoma is a rare variant of fibrosarcoma in which the cells are smaller than the spindle cells of classic fibrosarcoma, have an epithelioid shape, and are surrounded by hyalinized stroma (172). The cells are frequently arranged in cords and nests. Rare cases are located in the head and neck region (172,173). Interestingly, this subtype of fibrosarcoma may express the epithelial-associated antigens keratin and EMA. Biologically, sclerosing epithelioid fibrosarcoma recurs locally and produces systemic metastases, resulting in death in 25% of patients (172).

Myofibrosarcoma has rarely been described in the head and neck (174). It is composed of spindled cells that may have a storiform or herringbone growth pattern. The cytoplasm is eosinophilic and fibrillar but lacks the cross-striations diagnostic of RMS. Antibodies for vimentin and actins are positive, and some cases also have stained with desmin. The cells have the ultrastructural features of myofibroblasts. Patients are treated with surgery, adjuvant chemotherapy, and radiation. In a small series of patients, two thirds died of either local or metastatic disease within 2 years of diagnosis (174).

Malignant Fibrous Histiocytoma

Malignant fibrous histiocytoma is a pleomorphic fibroblastic sarcoma first described by O'Brien and Stout in 1964 (175). Although it is the most common soft tissue sarcoma in adulthood, less than 3% arise in the head and neck region (176). MFH generally arises during the sixth to seventh decades of life. In the head and neck the most common sites are the sinonasal tract, larynx, and soft tissues of the neck (177). Tumors of the sinonasal tract present with symptoms of nasal obstruction and epistaxis, whereas tumors of the larynx cause hoarseness and dysphagia. MFH has four histologic subtypes: storiform–pleomorphic, myxoid, giant cell, and inflammatory; however, only the first two variants have been reported to arise in the head and neck.

Storiform–pleomorphic is the most prevalent histologic subtype. Grossly it is lobulated, tan–white, and well defined but not encapsulated. It is composed of atypical spindle cells oriented in fascicles that are arranged in a storiform pattern (Fig. 45). The cells demonstrate severe hyperchromasia and pleomorphism, and malignant giant cells are common. Some of the more anaplastic cells are epithelioid in shape and contain abundant eosinophilic cytoplasm, resembling malignant histiocytes. Mitotic activity is usually abundant with numerous atypical forms, and necrosis is common.

Myxoid MFH or *myxofibrosarcoma* is a variant of MFH that most commonly occurs in the extremities of elderly individuals, but also may arise in the head and neck region (178). The mean age at diagnosis is 60 years. These tumors may be superficial or deep, and gross inspection reveals a gelatinous mass with well-defined or infiltrative boarders. Microscopically, hypo- to moderately cellular nodules of spindle- and stellate-shaped cells in a myxoid background are separated by fibrous septae. The cell cytoplasm is wispy and ill defined, and the nuclei irregularly shaped and hyperchromatic (Fig. 46). Some cells may contain cytoplasmic vacuoles that scallop the nuclei, causing these cells to resemble lipoblasts. The vacuoles, however, contain nonsecreted myxoid matrix and are not optically clear as in true lipoblasts. Tumor cells tend to condense around elongated capillaries that course throughout the stroma. High-grade lesions contain more cellular areas that resemble standard fibrosarcoma or MFH with a fascicular growth pattern, abundant mitoses, and necrosis.

Immunohistochemical stains performed on MFH show positivity for vimentin, and many specimens may stain with the histiocyte-associated markers KP-1 (CD68), α_1-antichymotrypsin,

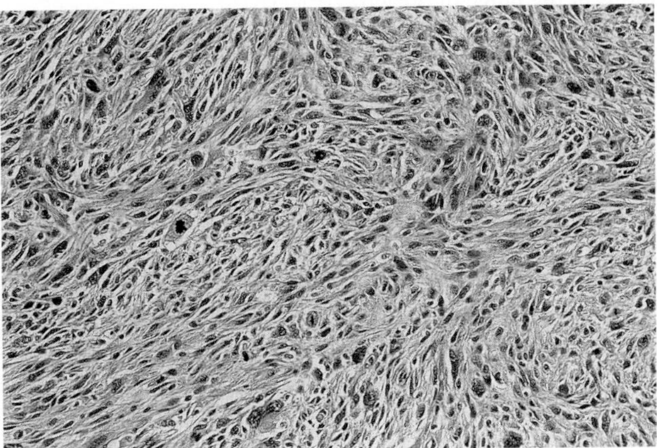

FIGURE 45. Cytologically malignant spindle cells arranged in a storiform pattern in a malignant fibrous histiocytoma.

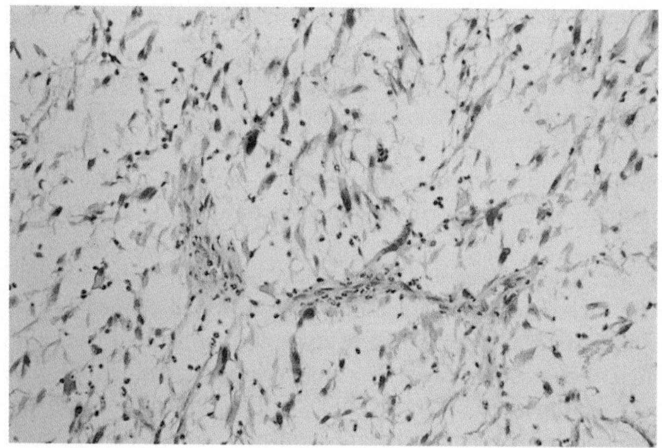

FIGURE 46. Atypical spindle cells in a myxoid stroma with prominent branching capillaries typical of myxoid malignant fibrous histiocytoma.

and α_1-antitrypsin. Myofibroblastic differentiation also may be demonstrated by staining with actin and desmin, and keratin staining has been described in 25% of cases (179). Ultrastructural analysis reveals that MFH is a tumor having fibroblastic and myofibroblastic differentiation, with a minority of cells containing prominent Golgi and lysosomes, features that are seen in histiocytes (180). Many chromosome abnormalities have been reported in MFH, but none of them are pathognomonic (181). The differential diagnosis is the same as with other pleomorphic sarcomas, principally liposarcoma, MPNST, and LMS. Although cells within an MFH may be vacuolated, true lipoblasts are not present. MPNSTs generally lack the pleomorphism and storiform growth pattern present in MFH, and immunohistochemical positivity for S-100 protein or Leu-7 favors the diagnosis of MPNST over MFH. Ultrastructurally, the presence of cytoplasmic processes containing microtubules surrounded by basal lamina, and the presence of junctional complexes is also evidence of schwannian differentiation, and these features are not seen in MFH.

Malignant fibrous histiocytoma of the head and neck is treated with surgery; when necessary, adjuvant chemotherapy and radiation therapy are used. The long-term survival rate for MFH of the head and neck is similar to that for fibrosarcoma and is in the range of 60% to 70% (182).

Pericytic and Vascular Tumors

Hemangiopericytoma

In 1942 Stout published the initial description of HP, a benign tumor of pericytes (183). Approximately 15% of these tumors arise in the head and neck area. The orbit, floor of the mouth, and nasal passage are the more common sites in this region. Typically, HP occurs in adulthood. Rarely, large pelvic tumors have been reported to cause hypoglycemia; however, head and neck tumors have not been associated with this endocrine abnormality (184–189).

Hemangiopericytoma is usually 1 to 8 cm in dimension, well circumscribed, and has a gray–white or brownish cut surface. It is composed of sheets of tightly packed oval to elongate and sometimes spindle-shaped cells with nuclei that are generally uniform and bland appearing cytologically. These cells are disposed amidst a network of thin-walled, branching vessels that form a staghorn configuration (Fig. 47). The cells are external to the vessels and are not endothelial cells. Although this vascular pattern is characteristic of HP, it is not specific and may be present in other tumors, such as mesenchymal chondrosarcoma, synovial sarcoma, myofibroma, and SFT, to name a few. HPs arising in the nasal cavity and paranasal sinuses tend to have more cytoplasm, a more prominent spindled pattern, and less striking vascularity than HPs in other anatomic locations (187).

The tumor that most closely resembles HP is SFT (see earlier section on Solitary Fibrous Tumor). Immunohistochemical studies are not helpful in distinguishing between them because the cells of HP stain with vimentin and CD34, similar to SFT. Electron microscopy is more helpful, because the cells in HP contain long cytoplasmic processes that are in intimate association with adjacent vascular channels and are surrounded by basal lamina that separates them from the endothelial cells. Their cytoplasm contains pinocytotic vesicles, rough endoplasmic reticulum, mitochondria, and some bundles of microfilaments. A few of the cells may appear more like smooth muscle cells with microfilaments containing focal condensations (190). In SFT the cells have the ultrastructural features of fibroblasts. HP does not have a specific chromosomal translocation; however, several different genetic abnormalities have been reported, including t(12;19) and t(13;22) (191).

Hemangiopericytomas are usually benign, but tumors with greater than four mitoses per 10 high-power fields, increased cellularity, and foci of necrosis should be considered malignant (192). Complete surgical excision is usually curative for benign tumors. Malignant HP should be treated like other sarcomas, with surgery and chemotherapy or radiation therapy as needed.

Infantile hemangiopericytoma (IHP) occurs in children and is often located in the mouth (193–196). The main difference between adult HP and IHP is the multilobulated growth pattern of IHP, which also may have satellite nodules, as well as the presence of necrosis and increased mitotic activity. In IHP these features do not indicate more aggressive behavior. Lipomatous HP,

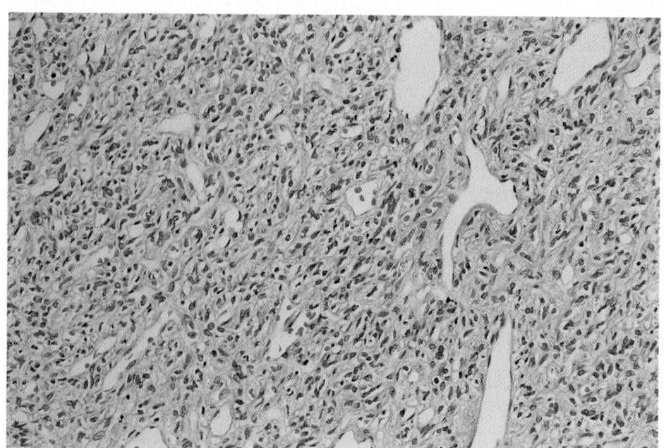

FIGURE 47. Hemangiopericytoma with staghorn pattern of branching vessels surrounded by bland spindle cells.

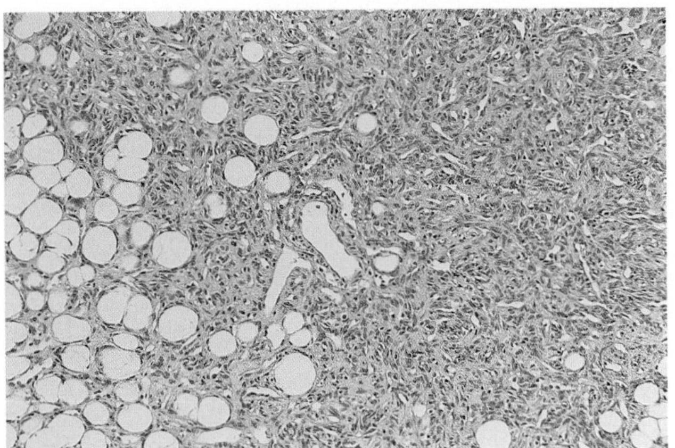

FIGURE 48. Lipomatous hemangiopericytoma with mature adipose tissue as an inherent component.

described in 1995, is a variant of HP with intermixed adipocytes (Fig. 48) (197). It should not be confused with a sarcoma infiltrating fat.

Glomus Tumor

In 1924 Masson described a group of tumors derived from the modified smooth muscle cells of the glomus body, an anastomosis between an arteriole and venule in the dermis that regulates blood flow (198). The most common site for a glomus tumor (GT) is the distal upper extremity, and only about 5% occur in the head and neck area (199,200). GTs are small, often painful, and are composed of nests of polyhedral cells with distinct cell borders and round nuclei that surround capillary-sized vessels (Fig. 49). Usually they are well circumscribed, but occasionally they may grow in an infiltrative fashion. Glomangioma is a specific subtype that contains similar cells; however the cells surround congeries of dilated vessels and therefore resemble a hemangioma. The least frequent subtype is glomangiomyoma which contains smooth muscle cells that merge with proliferating glomus cells.

Immunohistochemically, GTs stain for vimentin and actin. Desmin is positive in a number of cases as well (201). Ultrastructural studies reveal that the glomus cell contains shorter cell processes than the pericyte, and has more smooth muscle differentiation (202).

Most GTs are benign and are treated with simple excision. However, glomangiosarcoma is a rare tumor in which a component of the neoplasm has the features of a benign GT and in other areas the cells are malignant and may show smooth muscle or myofibroblastic differentiation (200,203). Glomangiosarcoma is treated like other sarcomas, with wide excision and possibly adjuvant chemotherapy or radiation therapy.

Lymphangioma

Whether lymphangiomas represent true neoplasms or developmental anomalies is controversial. They most commonly involve the soft tissues of the head, neck, and axilla, and the majority are present at birth or develop before the second birthday (204). Lymphangiomas may cause significant problems with the airway, feeding, and speech development (205,206). About 10% of neck lymphangiomas are extensive enough to involve the mediastinum. In addition to soft tissue involvement, lymphangiomas may involve solid organs of the head and neck, such as the parotid gland (207).

Lymphangiomas are divided into three categories: capillary, cavernous, and cystic. The capillary type consists of small thin walled spaces lined by attenuated endothelium, surrounded by adventitia. Small valves protrude into the lumina. There is histologic overlap between cavernous and cystic lymphangiomas. They both consist of larger spaces lined by endothelial cells surrounded by an adventitia and some smooth muscle cells. In the cavernous type, however, the vascular spaces are smaller than those in the cystic type (Fig. 50), in which the lumina are massively dilated. Lymphangiomas contain proteinaceous fluid within the vascular spaces and are invested by collagenous stroma that may contain lymphocytes. Cystic lymphangiomas, also called cystic hygromas, can be associated with fetal hydrops and Turner's syndrome (208).

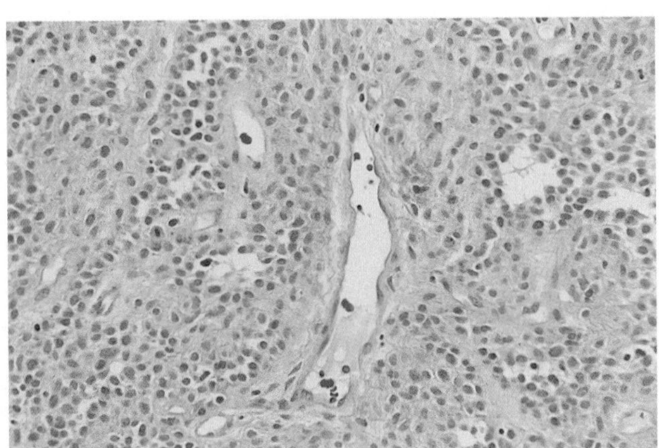

FIGURE 49. Polyhedral glomus cells surround a small vessel in a glomus tumor.

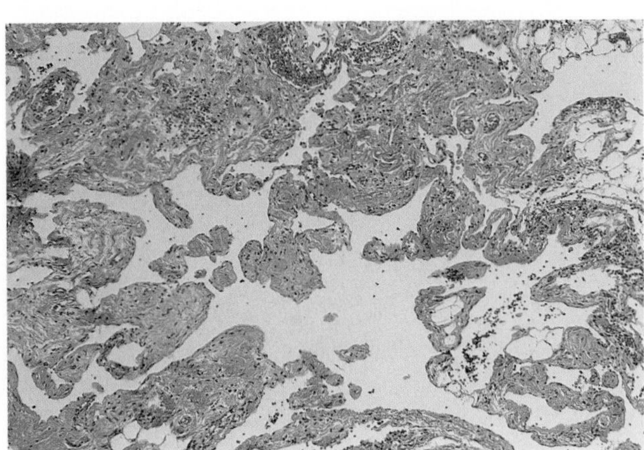

FIGURE 50. Large, irregular cystic spaces are lined by flattened endothelial cells in lymphangioma.

The main differential diagnosis of lymphangioma of the head and neck is with cavernous hemangioma. Lymphangiomas contain proteinaceous fluid and thin valves and the surrounding tissue is usually infiltrated by lymphocytes, whereas cavernous hemangiomas are filled with red blood cells and lack valve structures. Treatment of lymphangioma consists of surgery, which may require staged procedures for larger lesions. Recurrence rates range from 15% to 80% (206).

Hemangioma

Hemangiomas are a heterogeneous group of vascular lesions commonly located in the head and neck. Most hemangiomas in this region are superficial; however, they may arise within skeletal muscle and involve parenchymal tissue such as salivary gland and thyroid. Hemangiomas are classified by morphology into capillary, cavernous, arteriovenous, venous, and epithelioid types (209).

Capillary hemangioma is the most common type of hemangioma, and the most common benign tumor of infancy. About 2.5% of newborns are born with a hemangioma, and by 1 year of age they are present in about 12% of children (210). They arise in the skin, subcutaneous tissue, or mucosal surfaces and appear as raised red or blue papules. Capillary hemangiomas consist of lobules of small capillary-type vessels arranged around a larger "feeder" vessel. The cellular or juvenile hemangioma, also known as strawberry hemangioma, is an immature type of capillary hemangioma that is common in the head and neck and usually follows the distribution of cutaneous nerves and arteries. Early cellular hemangiomas are composed of plump endothelial cells lining inconspicuous lumina in a lobular pattern (Fig. 51). As the hemangioma matures, the endothelial cells flatten and the lumen of the capillary becomes visible. The maturation process begins at the periphery of the hemangioma and progresses toward the center. After a period of rapid enlargement, capillary hemangiomas may regress altogether, so surgery is not usually indicated.

Cavernous hemangiomas are also commonly located in the head and neck region. They are larger, more poorly circumscribed, and deeper than the capillary subtype. Cavernous hemangiomas are composed of round, dilated thin-walled vessels, larger than capillaries, that are filled with red blood cells, lined by flattened endothelium, and surrounded by a collagenous stroma. Focal calcifications may be present. *Arteriovenous hemangiomas* (or *arteriovenous malformations*) of the head and neck are poorly circumscribed, superficial lesions of adulthood (Fig. 52). They are composed of closely associated, structurally abnormal arteries, veins, and capillaries, with vessels present that cannot be readily categorized as arteries or veins (Fig. 53). *Venous hemangiomas* present in adulthood and are uncommon in the head and neck area. They are composed of dilated venous spaces with muscular walls that are lined by flattened endothelial cells. For the most part, cavernous, venous, and arteriovenous hemangiomas do not regress, and surgery is the treatment of choice (211,212).

Epithelioid hemangioma (EH), or angiolymphoid hyperplasia with eosinophilia, is a tumor of mid-adulthood first recognized in 1969 (213). It frequently occurs on the face or scalp and is classically located in the subcutis or dermis near the ear, although intravascular examples are well recognized (214,215). Grossly they present as single or multiple crusted plaques or nodules that

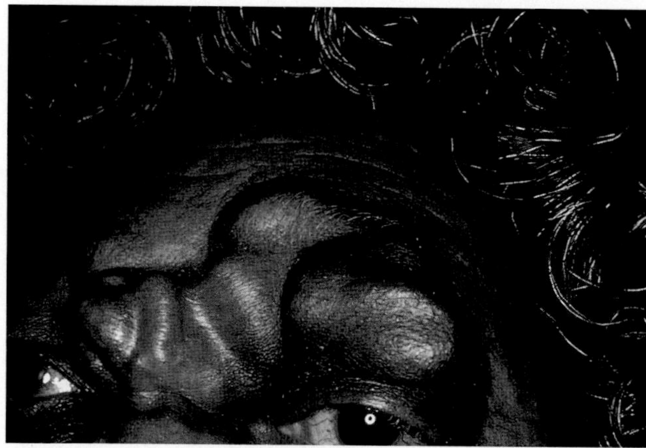

FIGURE 52. Longstanding arteriovenous hemangioma or malformation protruding from the forehead.

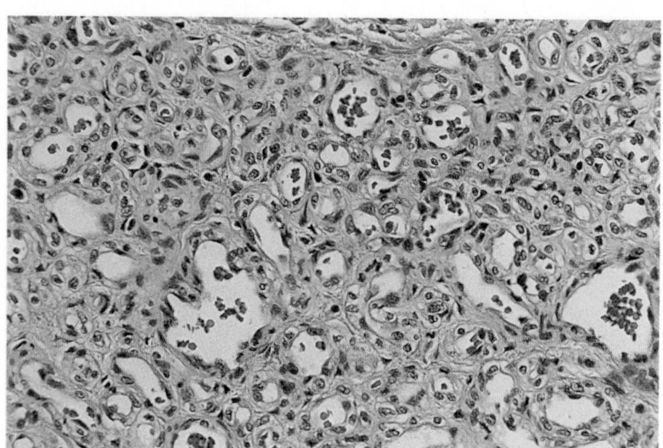

FIGURE 51. Cellular hemangioma composed of small capillaries lined by plump endothelial cells.

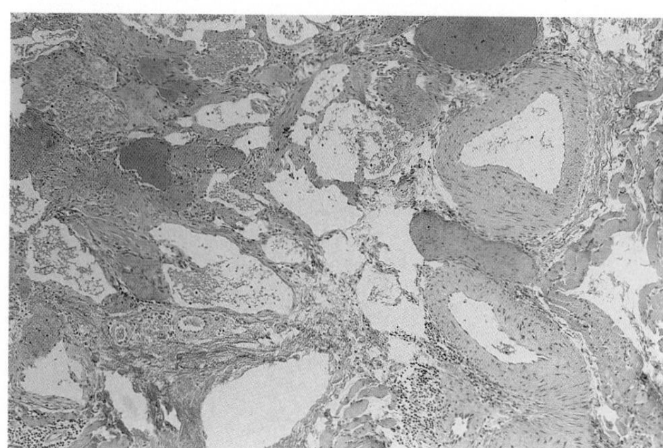

FIGURE 53. Abnormal vessels resembling veins, arteries, and capillaries in an arteriovenous hemangioma.

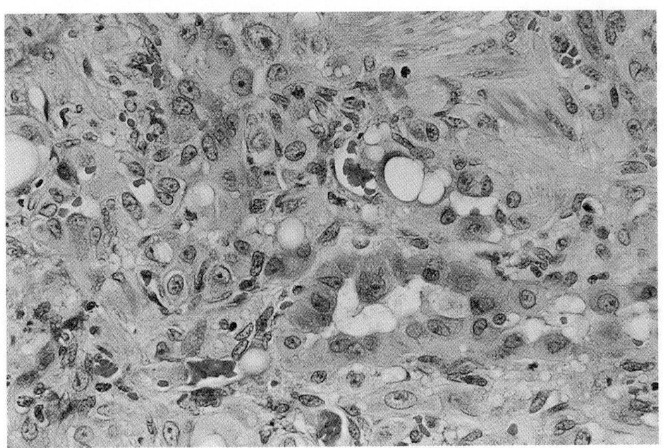

FIGURE 54. Epithelioid hemangioma composed of vessels lined by epithelioid endothelial cells with abundant eosinophilic cytoplasm and protruding into the lumen.

may itch. They are well circumscribed and composed of capillary-sized vessels clustered around a larger caliber vessel. The vessels are lined by large, epithelioid endothelial cells, with vesicular nuclei and abundant eosinophilic or amphophilic cytoplasm that may protrude into the lumen in a "tombstone" or "hobnail" fashion (Fig. 54). Intracytoplasmic vacuoles with or without fragmented or intact red blood cells, a feature of early vascular lumen differentiation, may be present. The vacuoles of neighboring cells may fuse, forming true lumina. In unusual cases the tumor cells may grow in solid sheets, with only occasional well-defined vascular spaces. The tumor cells demonstrate minimal cytologic atypia, and mitotic activity is limited. An inflammatory infiltrate composed of eosinophils, plasma cells, mast cells and lymphoid follicles is commonplace, but not always found throughout the tumor (216).

Immunohistochemistry shows that the epithelioid endothelial cells express the endothelial markers Factor VIII, CD31, CD34, and *Ulex europaeus.* In almost 50% of cases they may stain with the epithelial marker cytokeratin and less frequently with EMA (217). Ultrastructurally, the epithelioid cells have features indicative of endothelial differentiation, including Weibel-Palade bodies, but they also have increased numbers of cytoplasmic organelles such as mitochondria, endoplasmic reticulum, and thin filaments (214). This tumor also may occur in the bone (see Chapter 11).

The differential diagnosis of EH should include other epithelioid vascular tumors and Kimura's disease, and sometimes, because of the epithelioid morphology of the cells, carcinoma. Epithelioid hemangioendothelioma (EHE; see later section on Hemangioendothelioma) is composed of cords and clusters of epithelioid cells that demonstrate more cytologic atypia than those in EH. True vascular structures are less prominent in EHE, and characteristically the stroma is chondromyxoid or myxohyaline, a finding that is absent in EH. Also, inflammatory cells are usually not a feature of EHE. Angiosarcoma is commonly located on the face or scalp; however in epithelioid angiosarcoma the tumor cells show severe cytologic atypia and numerous mitoses, and grow in a highly infiltrative pattern using preexisting collagen as scaffolding. Kimura's disease has been confused with EH both clinically and histologically, but the lesions are distinct clinicopathologic entities (213,218,219). Kimura's disease lacks the arrangement of capillary-sized vessels oriented around a larger vessel, and although the endothelial cells in Kimura's disease may be enlarged, they are not epithelioid. In addition, Kimura's disease tends to have a denser lymphocytic inflammatory infiltrate than EH with abundant germinal center formation and interstitial fibrosis (see Chapter 12) (215). Carcinoma occurring in the superficial tissues of the head and neck does not characteristically have the distinct lobular pattern present in EH, and the tumor cells in carcinoma demonstrate a greater degree of cytologic atypia. Immunohistochemistry may be helpful, although both types of tumors may stain with cytokeratin. Carcinomas are usually negative for Factor VIII, CD31, and CD34.

Hemangioendothelioma

Hemangioendothelioma is a vascular tumor of intermediate malignant behavior that has the capacity to be locally aggressive and a somewhat limited potential to metastasize. EHE is the most common histologic type of hemangioendothelioma, and it does not commonly arise in the soft tissue of the head and neck (220). EHE usually develops during middle to late adulthood and infrequently affects children. These tumors are poorly defined and composed of cords and clusters of epithelioid and spindle cells arranged in a myxohyaline stroma (Fig. 55). The tumor cells have prominent eosinophilic cytoplasm that may have intracytoplasmic lumina that contain intact or fragmented erythrocytes (216). The nuclei generally do not show severe degrees of hyperchromasia or pleomorphism. Mitoses may be present, but they are usually not numerous. The tumor cells tend to form poorly defined vascular spaces composed of fused intracytoplasmic vacuoles of neighboring cells.

Immunohistochemical studies show that the tumor cells are positive for Factor VIII, *Ulex europaeus,* and CD31 and CD34. Cytokeratin also may be positive (217). The differential diagnosis is with carcinoma and angiosarcoma. Carcinoma generally lacks the myxohyaline stroma of EHE, and although carci-

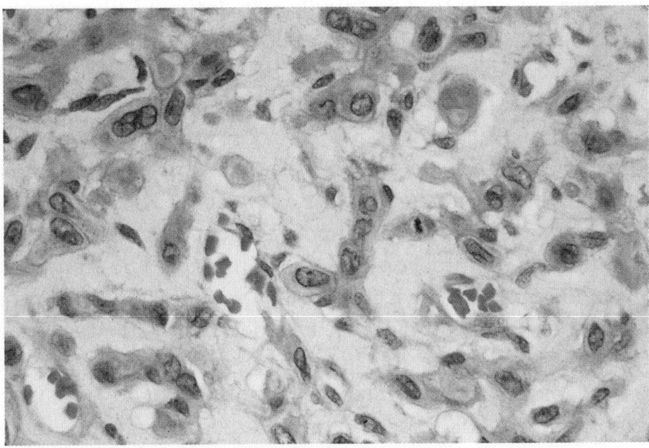

FIGURE 55. Epithelioid hemangioendothelioma composed of cords and clusters of epithelioid tumor cells with intracytoplasmic vacuoles embedded in a myxohyaline stroma.

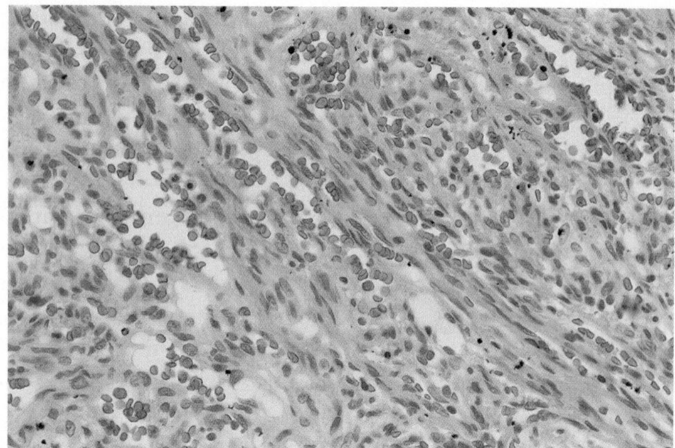

FIGURE 56. Cavernous spaces containing erythrocytes intermixed with fascicles of bland spindle cells in a spindle cell hemangioendothelioma.

noma is positive for keratin, it does not stain for endothelial markers. Angiosarcoma is more cytologically atypical than EHE and lacks the myxohyaline stroma, and the malignant cells dissect through the tissue using preexisting collagen as scaffolding, a feature not seen in EHE. Approximately 15% of patients with EHE will have a local recurrence and up to a third will develop metastases to regional lymph nodes, bones, or lung. Treatment of nonmetastatic cases is wide local excision. Chemotherapy or radiation therapy is used in addition to surgery for metastatic cases and cases in which the tumor appears cytologically high grade.

Spindle cell hemangioendothelioma (SCH) is an uncommon subtype of hemangioendothelioma that may be multifocal in anatomic location. Although initially thought to be a low-grade malignancy, large series have documented that SCH behaves in a benign fashion, and therefore spindle cell hemangioma may be a more appropriate term (221). Patients are usually 20 to 50 years of age at the time of diagnosis. SCH usually arises in the distal extremity and infrequently develops in the head and neck region. SCH is composed of small hemorrhagic nodules up to 2 cm in size which contain patulous, cavernous, flattened endothelial-lined, blood filled spaces resembling cavernous hemangiomas, admixed with fascicles of cytologically bland spindle cells (Fig. 56) (222). The spindle cells form slit-like vascular spaces that may contain red blood cells. Cords of epithelioid cells with intracytoplasmic vacuoles can be found coursing through the fascicles of spindle cells. Immunohistochemical studies reveal that the endothelial cells in the cavernous spaces and some of the epithelioid cells stain with endothelial markers, but the spindle cell component is negative for these antigens (223). The spindle cell component has the immunohistochemical and ultrastructural features of fibroblasts and myofibroblasts. These findings, in conjunction with the fact that SCH may arise in vessels or be associated with syndromes that include vascular abnormalities, lead some investigators to believe that it is a reactive lesion and not neoplastic. The primary differential diagnosis is with Kaposi's sarcoma. Kaposi's sarcoma does not contain cavernous spaces or epithelioid tumor cells. Furthermore, the spindle cell component of Kaposi's sarcoma shows more cytologic atypia than that of SCH, and the spindle cells express endothelial markers. The treatment of SCH is conservative excision, but up to 50% of cases recur locally. The recurrences can be successfully treated by reexcision.

Kaposi's Sarcoma

Kaposi's sarcoma is a malignant vascular tumor that affects the skin and mucosal surfaces. In Western nonendemic areas, primarily in patients infected with HIV, the head and neck is commonly affected. Approximately 40% of HIV-infected patients develop Kaposi's sarcoma, but for unknown reasons it is much more common in homosexual males than intravenous drug abusers or patients infected via contaminated blood products. Kaposi's sarcoma of the head and neck is often the presenting symptom of acquired immmunodeficiency syndrome (AIDS), possibly because lesions on the skin and mucosal surfaces are more easily detected in this area than elsewhere (224). Human herpes virus 8 has been implicated in the formation of AIDS-related Kaposi's sarcoma as well as the endemic form, which is commonly located on the lower extremities of elderly men (225,226).

Kaposi's sarcoma lesions begin as reddish brown macular discolorations and progress to plaques and nodules. Multifocality is the rule. Histologically the lesions progress from a proliferation of small banal-appearing vessels surrounded by a vague collar of spindle cells to a cellular plaque composed of fascicles of atypical spindle cells delineating slit-like vascular spaces, which contain erythrocytes (Fig. 57). Inflammatory cells, especially plasma cells, and hemosiderin deposits may be found within and at the periphery of the lesion. The spindle cells in well-developed tumors contain characteristic intracellular and extracellular periodic acid-Schiff (PAS)-positive, diastase-resistant hyaline globules. Immunohistochemical studies show that the spindle cells are positive for endothelial markers (225). The differential diagnosis with other vascular lesions is discussed in sections devoted to these other lesions. Radiation therapy, chemotherapy, and α-interferon are the main modalities of therapy. It has been suggested that anti–herpes virus therapy may have a role in controlling disease (224,227).

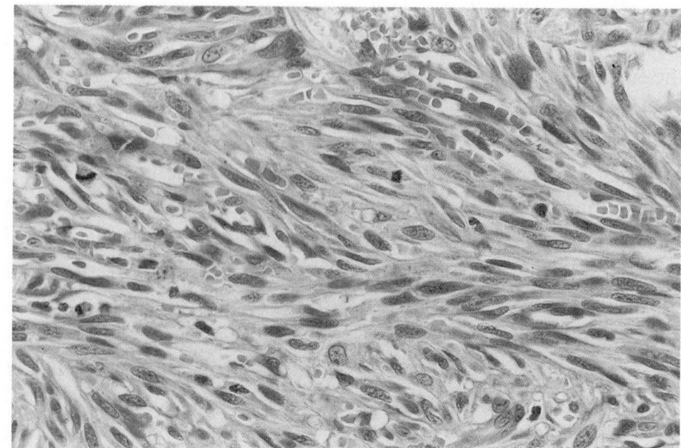

FIGURE 57. Kaposi's sarcoma composed of mitotically active mildly atypical spindle cells that delineate slit-like vascular spaces containing erythrocytes.

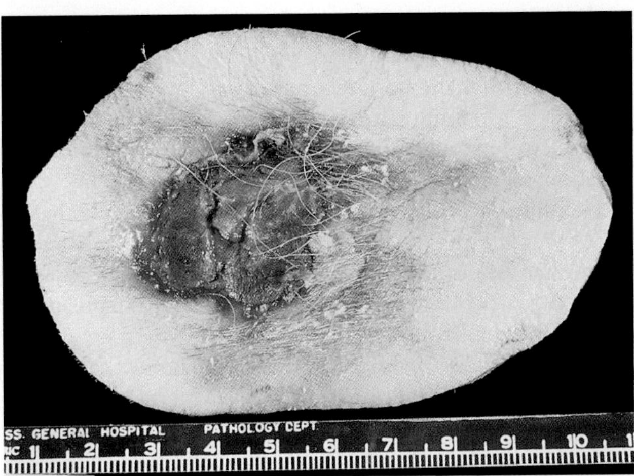

FIGURE 58. Ulcerated angiosarcoma of the scalp has poorly demarcated borders.

Angiosarcoma

Angiosarcoma is a malignant vascular tumor that most commonly arises in the skin and superficial soft tissue of the head and neck in the elderly (Fig. 58) (see Chapter 13). Fifty percent of cases are initially misdiagnosed as infection, hematoma, or hemangioma (228). Tumors present as plaques or nodules from 3 mm to over 20 cm in greatest diameter. They are composed of atypical cells with hyperchromatic nuclei and scant to ample eosinophilic cytoplasm. Mitotic activity is easily discernible, and necrosis may be present. The tumor grows in an infiltrative fashion, and the cells line interanastomosing vascular channels and sinusoids that may contain red blood cells (Fig. 59). Preexisting collagen and fat are used as scaffolding for the malignant cells. Less differentiated tumors may contain solid sheets of spindle or polyhedral tumor cells (Fig. 60). Well-formed vascular spaces are typically not present in angiosarcoma. Immunohistochemical stains for endothelial cells markers are positive in angiosarcoma, and cytokeratin may be positive in cells with an epithelioid phenotype (217). Treatment is surgery or radiation therapy. The 2-year survival rate is a dismal 20% (229).

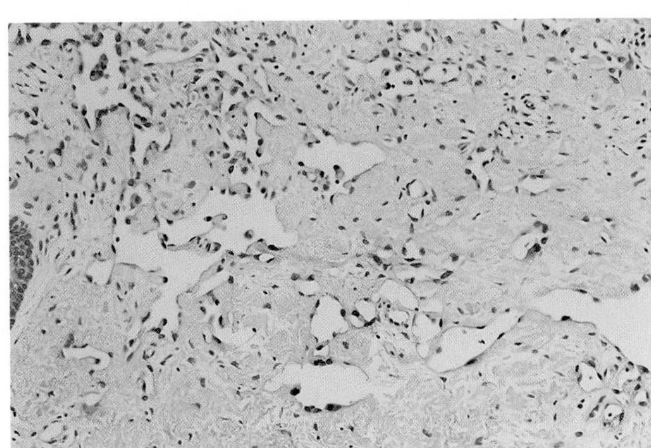

FIGURE 59. Hyperchromatic endothelial cell line dissecting vascular channels in a low-grade angiosarcoma.

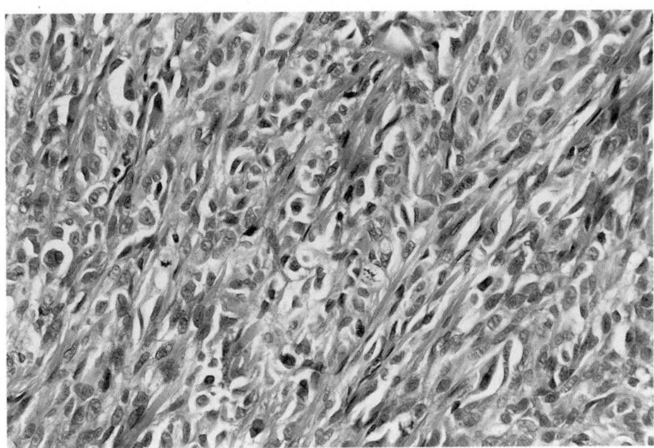

FIGURE 60. High-grade angiosarcoma containing large, atypical cells that line ill-defined vascular spaces.

Nerve Sheath Tumors

Granular Cell Tumor

Described initially by Weber in 1854 and later by Abrikossoff in 1926 as tumors of muscle lineage, granular cell tumors (GCTs) have been proven to have a Schwann cell phenotype (230–232). They occur in the superficial soft tissue, the mucosa, especially the tongue, and the minor and major salivary glands in patients of any age, but most are in the fourth to sixth decades of life (233,234). The larynx is also a characteristic location in the head and neck (see Chapter 7). For unknown reasons they occur more often in blacks than whites (233,235). GCT presents as a painless nodule, and most are solitary; however, 15% to 25% of patients have multiple nodules (232–234). The tumors are generally not associated with neurofibromatosis.

Granular cell tumors are usually less than 3 cm in diameter, are ill defined and infiltrative, and have a pale yellow or tan cut surface. They consist of uniform, plump or angulated, polygonal to fusiform cells with granular eosinophilic cytoplasm and central nuclei with vesicular chromatin (Fig. 61). The cells are arranged in nests, trabeculae, and sheets that are surrounded by a

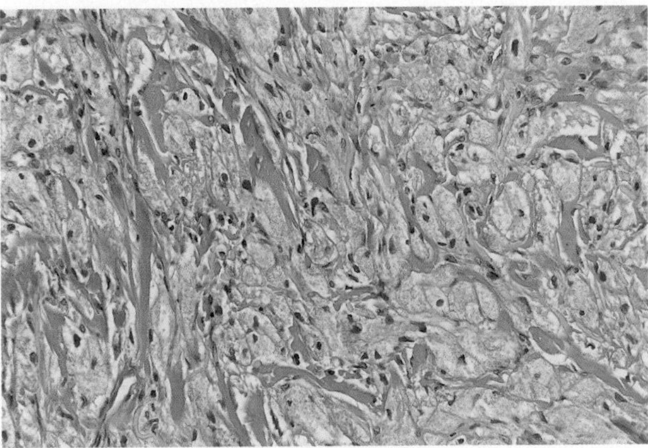

FIGURE 61. Granular cell tumor composed of large cells with granular eosinophilic cytoplasm and small round nuclei that are enmeshed in a hyalinized stroma.

desmoplastic stroma. Histochemical staining for Luxol fast blue demonstrates positive staining of the prominent and characteristic cytoplasmic granules, suggesting that they are of myelin origin (236). Granular cells stain positive with PAS with and without diastase predigestion. GCTs are positive with immunohistochemical stains for vimentin, S-100 protein, NK1/C3 (a melanocyte-associated antigen), and NSE, and also may express Leu-7 (CD57) and CD68 (237,238). Axons are not present with silver stains (239). Ultrastructural analysis reveals that cells of a GCT have numerous cell processes, basal lamina, and multiple secondary lysosomes that produce the cytoplasmic granularity. These lysosomal structures contain cellular debris and lipid-rich lamellar structures (232,240,241). Mitotic figures are rare in conventional GCTs. The tumors grow with an infiltrative pattern and may be closely associated with peripheral nerves, and even extend into them. Importantly, the overlying skin or mucosa of superficial lesions frequently demonstrates pseudoepitheliomatous hyperplasia that can be mistaken for invasive carcinoma (Fig. 62).

Simple excision is usually curative; however, the infiltrative nature of the GCT accounts for a low rate of recurrence (235).

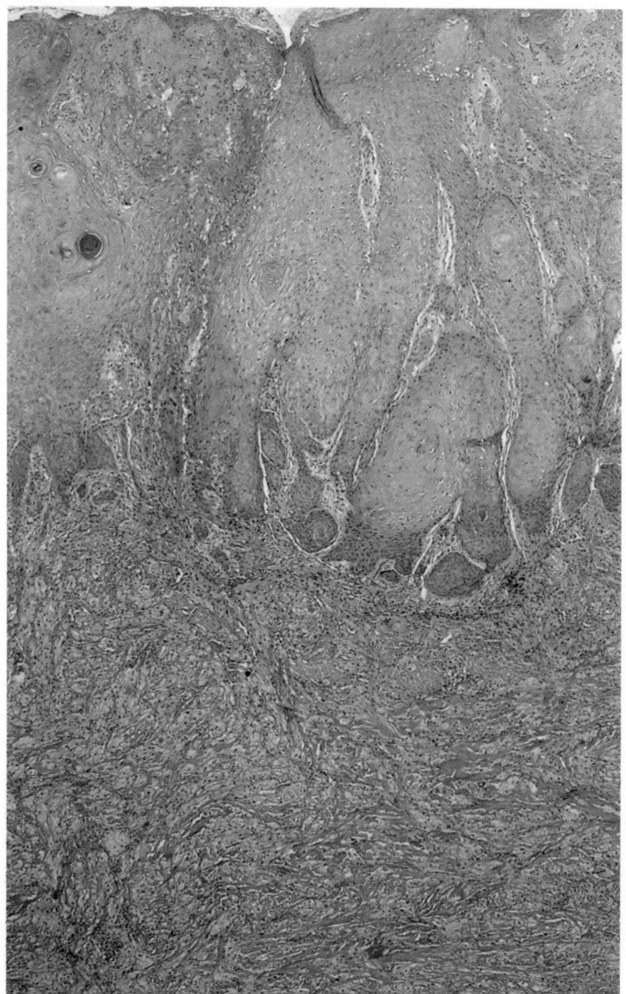

FIGURE 62. Hyperplastic squamous mucosa overlying a granular cell tumor.

Malignant GCTs are rare but well recognized, and although it may be difficult prospectively to predict which tumors will behave in a malignant fashion in all cases, tumors containing greater than two mitoses per 10 high-power fields, increased cellularity, cytologic atypia, necrosis, and spindling of tumor cells have been associated with malignant behavior (242,243).

The differential diagnosis of GCT should include other tumors containing granular or vacuolated cytoplasm. Rhabdomyoma can be distinguished by the presence of cross-striations and glycogen-rich cytoplasm, and hibernoma by the presence of lipid-laden cytoplasm.

Gingival GCT of infants (*congenital epulis*) is most common in newborn girls and usually occurs on the lateral ridge of the maxilla. About 10% of cases are multifocal. Histologically they are similar to adult-type GCTs (243).

Perineurioma

Perineurioma of soft tissue is a neoplastic proliferation of perineurites, the cells that surround the individual fascicles of normal nerves. Also termed *storiform perineurial fibroma,* the perineurioma is a rare benign tumor first described in 1978 (244,245). It usually arises in the deep soft tissues and occasionally in the neck, but one case of perineurioma of the maxillary sinus has been reported (246). The majority of patients are females who range in age from 14 to 66 years. Perineuriomas, unlike neurofibromas, are not associated with any syndromes.

The tumors are usually small, ranging in size from 1.5 to 6.5 cm, and may be fusiform in shape. They are well circumscribed but not encapsulated and are sometimes attached to a nerve. The cut surface is firm, tan–white, and gritty. Perineuriomas are composed of wavy elongate spindle cells that have small banal nuclei and long slender cytoplasmic processes that are enmeshed in a collagenous or myxoid background. The cells are arranged in short fascicles, usually in a storiform pattern (Fig. 63). Mast cells may be present. Electron microscopic examination of perineuriomas reveals that the tumor cells are similar to the perineurial cells of a normal nerve; they are long and thin with elongate polar processes, numerous surface vesicles, frequent

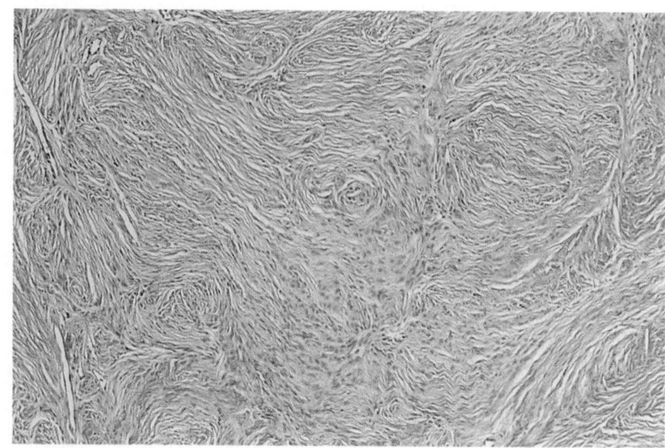

FIGURE 63. Spindle cells arranged in a storiform and whorled pattern typical of a perineurioma.

junctional complexes, and a variable basal lamina (247). A deletion or complete loss of chromosome 22 has been described in soft tissue perineuriomas (246).

Epithelial membrane antigen, which stains normal perineurial cells, also stains the spindle cells in perineurioma. Unlike nerve sheath tumors composed of Schwann cells, there is no staining for S-100 protein or Leu-7, and this profile distinguishes the perineurioma from the other tumors in the differential diagnosis, namely neurofibroma and solitary circumscribed neuroma (SCN). Also, neurofibroma may be infiltrative, it lacks the storiform growth pattern of a perineurioma, and the stroma is not as collagenous. The spindle cells in SCN are arranged in nerve twig–like fascicles and are S-100 protein positive, and only the spindle cells of the peripheral capsule are EMA positive. Soft tissue perineurioma also should be distinguished from localized hypertrophic neuropathy or intraneural perineurioma, in which an affected segment of nerve shows circumferential fibrosis around centrally placed axons with fibrosis and hyalinization of the perineurium. Intraneural perineurioma has distinct clinical findings related to nerve dysfunction and was thought to be a reactive process; however, the presence of chromosome 22 abnormalities similar to those found in soft tissue perineurioma is more supportive of a neoplastic process (245,248). Treatment of soft tissue perineurioma is simple excision. Malignant variants are exceedingly rare (249,250).

Solitary Circumscribed Neuroma (Palisaded Encapsulated Neuroma)

First described as palisaded encapsulated neuroma by Reed in 1972, the SCN commonly arises on the skin of the face near mucocutaneous junctions (251–255). Middle-aged individuals are usually affected, and some lesions may be present for decades prior to diagnosis (252). The flesh-colored, dome-shaped papules are usually less than 5 mm in diameter, do not ulcerate, and clinically mimic dermal nevi and cysts. They are not associated with neurofibromatosis or the multiple mucosal neuromas present in multiple endocrine neoplasia type II. SCNs are thought to be neoplastic, but some investigators argue that they are traumatic in origin (256,257). SCNs account for approximately 25% of dermal nerve sheath tumors (252,255).

Histologically SCN is a well-circumscribed, partially encapsulated dermal nodule that may be multilobular and extend into the fat. A small percentage of cases have a plexiform growth pattern or may be focally infiltrative. SCN is composed of small fascicles of Schwann cells that are spindle shaped with basophilic nuclei and indistinct, wavy eosinophilic cytoplasm. Their arrangement mimics small nerve twigs. Nuclear pallisading is uncommon (255). A single case of SCN that contains some epithelioid tumor cells has been described (258). Generally, mitoses are uncommon, and necrosis, ulceration, and hemorrhage are not seen. The fascicles are separated by artifactual clefts, and the capsule contains perineurial cells and collagen fibers. Axons are present within the fascicles of Schwann cells, and occasionally a peripheral nerve is identified adjacent to the tumor (255).

Immunohistochemical stains for S-100 protein are diffusely positive in the fascicles of spindle cells, but not the capsule. Neurofilament highlights the axons, which are dispersed between the spindle cells of the tumor, and the capsular cells are positive for EMA (257,259).

The differential diagnosis is with other superficial peripheral nerve sheath tumors. Neurofibromas are not encapsulated and do not contain well-formed fascicles. The cells in neurofibroma are admixed with wire-like collagen bundles, and the background is often myxoid. Axons are focally present in neurofibromas, but not to the extent they are found within SCN. Schwannomas are not common in the dermis, but occasionally occur there. They are encapsulated, not associated with axons and usually have prominent areas of nuclear pallisading and Verocay bodies. Antoni A and B areas, also a feature of schwannomas, are not present in SCN. SCNs are treated by simple excision that is usually curative; however, SCNs rarely may recur (255).

Neurofibroma

Solitary neurofibroma by definition affects patients that do not have neurofibromatosis. The solitary variety encompasses approximately 90% of neurofibromas and is usually a superficial lesion that may arise anywhere on the body (260,261). These lesions affect men and women equally, and usually appear in the third and fourth decades of life. Neurofibromas are usually painless, grow slowly, and present as a nodule. They arise within a nerve, producing a fusiform mass, and may remain encapsulated by the epineurium, or they may break out of the confines of the nerve and grow into the adjacent tissues.

Grossly, solitary neurofibroma has a gray–white cut surface. All neurofibromas are composed of a combination of Schwann cells, perineurial cells, and fibroblasts, but the microscopic appearance is variable. Wavy, spindled Schwann cells with small dark nuclei and delicate tapering cytoplasm are set in a variably myxoid background with wire-like bundles of collagen (Fig. 64). The spindle cells may be arranged in cellular fascicles. Occasional enlarged, hyperchromatic nuclei may be seen. Small neurites and mast cells are distributed throughout the tumor. Degenerative cytologic atypia, with enlarged, dark, "smudgy" nuclei, is com-

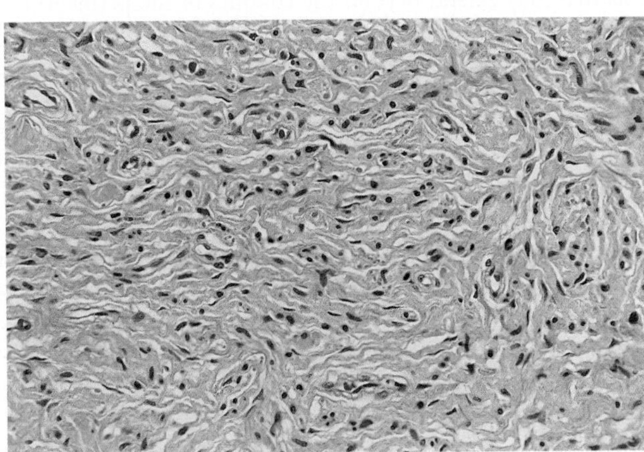

FIGURE 64. Solitary neurofibroma composed of Schwann cells with wavy cytoplasm and collagen bundles.

mon in benign neurofibroma and is termed *ancient change.*

Immunohistochemically, many but not all of the spindle cells are S-100 protein positive, and scattered neurofilament-positive axons are also present (262).

Neurofibromas with a prominent myxoid matrix may be confused histologically with myxomas. The spindle cells in a neurofibroma are usually more organized than in a myxoma, the vascular pattern in neurofibroma is more prominent, and myxomas do not stain with S-100 protein. A cellular neurofibroma may be confused with a schwannoma (see later section on Schwannoma); however, most schwannomas have hyper- and hypocellular Antoni A and B areas, and some degree of nuclear pallisading with Verocay bodies. Because schwannomas are composed primarily of Schwann cells, an S-100 protein stain is more diffusely positive than in neurofibroma. Solitary neurofibromas are treated conservatively with simple excision. Malignant potential is based on a combination of greater than four mitoses per 10 high-power fields, hypercellularity, and cytologic atypia. The chance of malignant progression of a solitary neurofibroma is unknown but is thought to be extremely low (263).

Neurofibromatosis is a disorder described in part by von Recklinghausen, which is now classified into two distinct disease entities that are distinguished by specific clinical and genetic findings. Neurofibromatosis type 1 is an autosomal dominant disease in which the affected gene has been localized to chromosome 17 (264). The diagnostic criteria include two or more neurofibromas of any type or one plexiform neurofibroma, six or more cutaneous café au lait spots, axillary or inguinal freckling, optic glioma, or two or more Lisch nodules. Neurofibromatosis type 2 is rarer than neurofibromatosis type 1. It is also an autosomal dominant disease, and the affected gene is on chromosome 22. Diagnostic criteria include bilateral acoustic schwannomas or neuromas, or unilateral acoustic neuroma and two of the following: neurofibroma, schwannoma, meningioma, or glioma.

Localized neurofibroma is histologically identical to solitary neurofibroma, but is found in patients with neurofibromatosis. The *plexiform neurofibroma* expands an existing nerve into a tortuous "bag of worms." This variant is usually the first type of neurofibroma to develop in a patient with neurofibromatosis type 1, and it may be extensive. The nerve is massively expanded by a combination of endoneurial ground substance and Schwann cells that may extend beyond the confines of the perineurium. Cross-section reveals multiple branches of the nerve in the same plane because of the serpiginous course of the affected nerve (Figs. 65 and 66). This type of neurofibroma may undergo malignant transformation. *Diffuse neurofibroma* commonly occurs on the skin of the head and neck as a plaque-like lesion. Affected individuals are children or young adults, and the majority are probably associated with neurofibromatosis type 1; however, because of the young age of the patients, most do not yet have an established clinical diagnosis of neurofibromatosis. In these lesions spindle cells with a wavy configuration surrounded by myxocollagenous stroma fill the dermis and subcutis, surrounding normal structures and extending along fibrous septa (Fig. 67). They may even extend into adjacent skeletal muscle. Mitotic activity is usually not appreciable. Foci containing Wagner-Meissner bodies (oval aggregates of eosinophilic, S-100 protein–positive material bordered by nuclei) are often present,

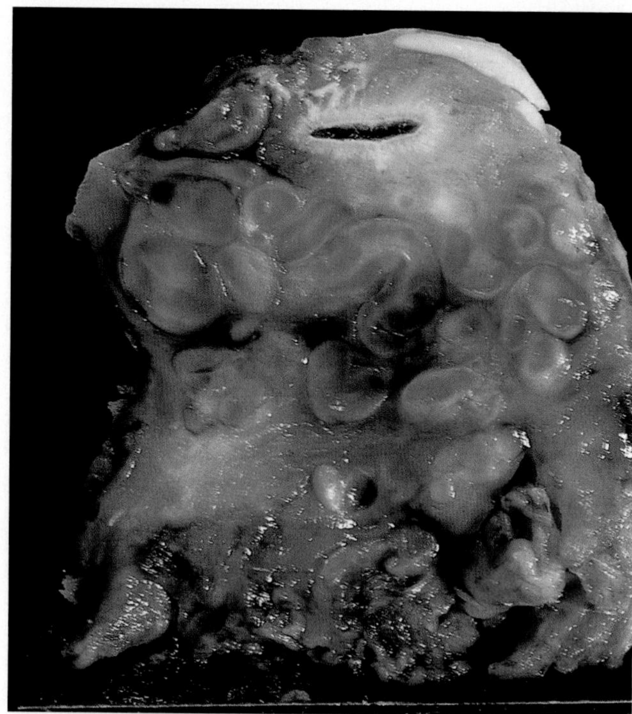

FIGURE 65. Plexiform neurofibroma encasing the auditory canal.

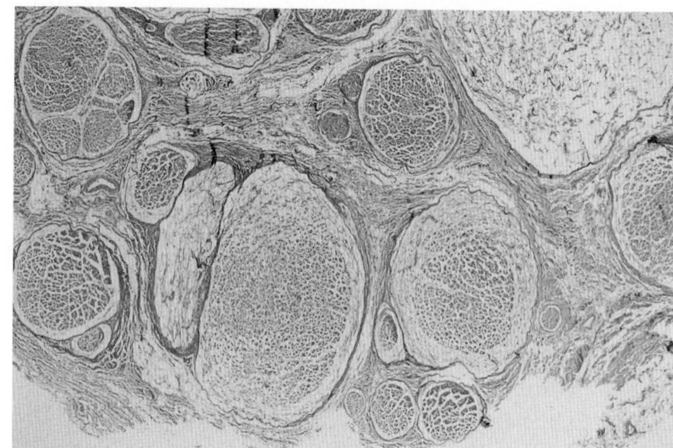

FIGURE 66. Neurofibroma expanding nerve twigs in a plexiform pattern.

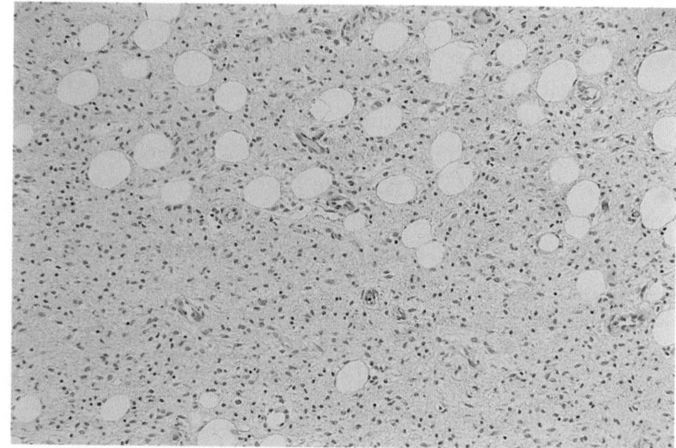

FIGURE 67. Diffuse neurofibroma invading adipose tissue.

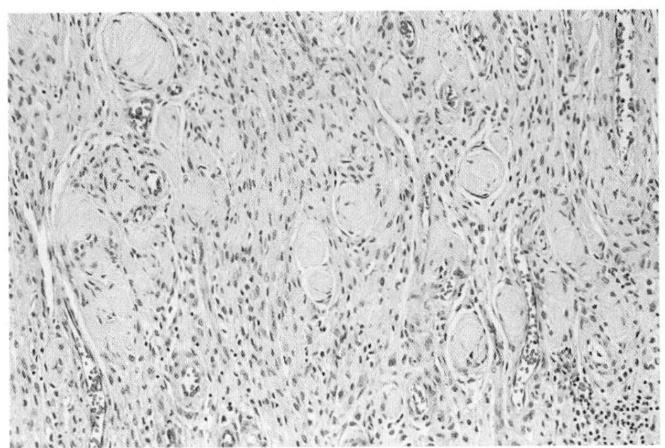

FIGURE 68. Wagner-Meissner bodies in a diffuse neurofibroma.

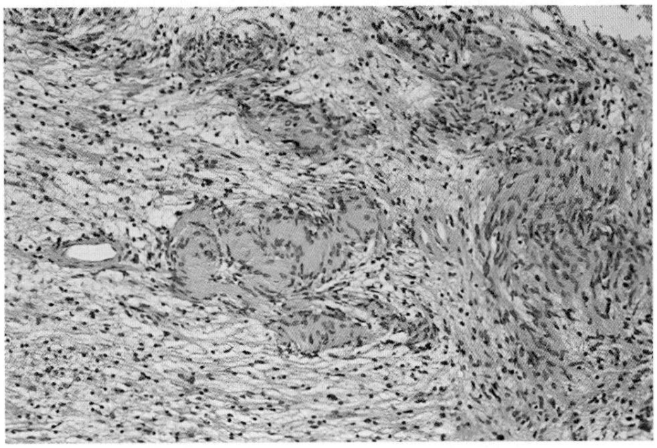

FIGURE 69. Schwannoma with Verocay bodies.

which help distinguish a diffuse neurofibroma from other lesions that infiltrate the dermis, such as DFSP (Fig. 68). Diffuse neurofibroma rarely undergoes malignant change (263).

Because patients with neurofibromatosis usually have multiple lesions, surgery is reserved for large or painful lesions (265). Studies have shown that approximately 5% of patients with neurofibromatosis will develop an MPNST (263,266). Rapid growth has been associated with malignant transformation, so close clinical follow-up is indicated.

Schwannoma

A schwannoma is a benign tumor of Schwann cells first described by Verocay in 1910 (267). Approximately 40% of schwannomas occur in the head and neck region. Cutaneous nerves may be affected, as well as the sympathetic chain and nerves in the orbit, nose, mouth, and parapharyngeal space (268–271). Aside from vestibular schwannoma (or acoustic neuroma), which may be associated with neurofibromatosis type 2, there is no well-defined link between schwannomas and neurofibromatosis. Patients are usually 20 to 50 years of age at presentation and frequently present with a slowly enlarging mass, which may be painful. Nerve function is generally not noticeably affected. In most cases schwannomas arise eccentrically within the nerve, causing fusiform expansion. In general, schwannomas are circumscribed and encapsulated; however, in the nasal cavity some may have ill-defined margins (268).

The cut surface of a schwannoma has a glistening, tan–gray and yellow appearance and may have areas of cystification. Histologically, schwannomas are composed of hypercellular and hypocellular regions, termed Antoni A and Antoni B areas, respectively. Cells in the Antoni A areas are spindle shaped with fibrillar eosinophilic cytoplasm and form short fascicles that may be arranged in a storiform or whorled pattern. Areas of nuclear palisading and Verocay bodies, two columns of aligned nuclei separated by fibrillar cytoplasm, are often present (Fig. 69). Antoni B areas are less cellular and are composed of spindle-shaped cells or short, plump cells that are arranged in a haphazard pattern and are enmeshed in an edematous myxoid stroma. Areas of cystic degeneration are common. Perivascular hyalinization is often predominant in the Antoni B regions. Ancient change of the nuclei manifesting as nuclear enlargement and hyperchromasia is often present and is not indicative of malignancy (Fig. 70).

Immunohistochemistry is helpful in separating schwannomas from other spindle cell lesions. Schwannoma stains diffusely positive with S-100 protein in 98% of cases. EMA highlights the surrounding perineurium. Ultrastructurally the proliferating cells have basal lamina, intertwining cell processes, and Luse bodies that are composed of collagen fibrils with a periodicity of 120 to 130 nm.

Cellular schwannoma is an uncommon lesion originally described as a large pelvic tumor in which the cellular Antoni A regions predominate and Verocay bodies are scarce or absent (Fig. 71) (272). Because of the cellularity, it may be confused with a sarcoma (Fig. 72). Cellular schwannomas are mitotically active, but the mitotic figures are not atypical. Hyalinized vessels, groups of foamy macrophages, and scattered lymphocytes are commonplace. Cellular schwannomas stain diffusely for S-100 protein, in contrast to MPNSTs, which generally contain more than four mitoses per 10 high-power fields, have atypical mitoses, and stain only focally for S-100 protein.

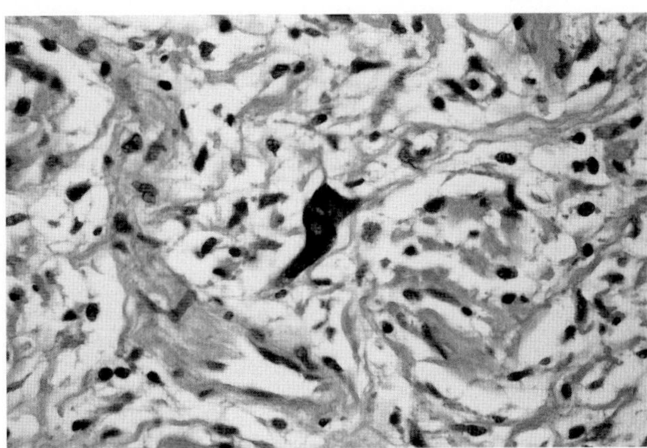

FIGURE 70. Enlarged nucleus with smudgy chromatin in an ancient schwannoma.

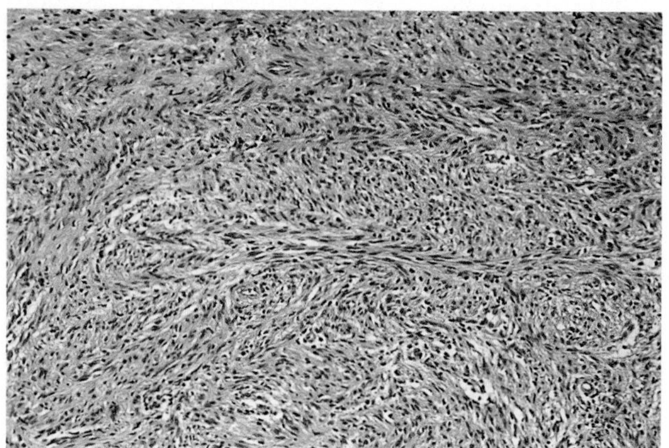

FIGURE 71. Short fascicles of spindle cells in a cellular schwannoma.

Approximately 5% of schwannomas grow in a multinodular or plexiform pattern and are termed *plexiform schwannomas.* Only a small fraction of these are associated with neurofibromatosis. They often lack significant Antoni B areas, and, because of the growth pattern and cellularity, may be confused with an MPNST (273).

Schwannomas are benign peripheral nerve sheath tumors with virtually no malignant potential. Only a handful of reports of an MPNST arising in association with a schwannoma have appeared in the literature (274,275). Complete excision of schwannomas is curative. Tumors that are not entirely excised may recur; this is especially true for those in the parapharyngeal area, where the local recurrence rate is high owing to surgical inaccessibility.

Malignant Peripheral Nerve Sheath Tumor

Malignant peripheral nerve sheath tumors, also known as neurofibrosarcoma, neurogenic sarcoma, and malignant schwannoma, account for about 5% to 10% of soft tissue sarcomas (276). Approximately 14% occur in the head and neck region, which follows the deep soft tissues of the extremities in frequency of occurrence (277). Fewer than 50% of cases arise in a preexisting neurofibroma in a patient with neurofibromatosis, and the remainder develop *de novo* in otherwise healthy patients (277). Rarely have they been documented to originate in a schwannoma (274). Approximately 10% of cases are associated with prior radiation therapy. Patients may be any age at the time of diagnosis, but the mean age for MPNST arising in a patient with neurofibromatosis is 29 to 36 years, which is 10 years younger than the mean age of patients without this disorder. MPNSTs have been described in a wide variety of head and neck locations, including the parotid, lip, cheek, mandible, sinus, and pharynx, and their symptomatology is related to their site of origin (276,278).

The gross appearance of an MPNST is nonspecific; however, it has a tan cut surface that may have foci of hemorrhage and necrosis. Occasionally a nerve may be associated with the tumor. Microscopic examination reveals spindle cells arranged in sheets and fascicles in a storiform, herringbone, or whorled pattern. The nuclei are enlarged, hyperchromatic, sometimes wavy, and have tapered ends (Fig. 73). Nuclear palisades are uncommon. The cytoplasm is pale and eosinophilic. A minority of tumors have an epithelioid morphology, and in these instances the stroma is frequently myxoid (279,280). Mitoses usually number greater than four per 10 high-power fields, and abnormal mitoses and necrosis may be present, especially in high-grade tumors. An immunohistochemical stain for S-100 protein is focally positive in up to 75% of cases (280–282). Ultrastructural studies reveal that malignant cells have some features of schwannian differentiation, including intertwining cell processes and a continuous basement membrane (276,283).

Recommended treatment is wide excision, with or without adjuvant chemotherapy and radiation therapy, depending on the size and grade of the tumor. Approximately 50% of head and neck MPNSTs recur (276). Neurofibromatosis patients who develop an MPNST fare worse than others; their 5-year survival rate is 30% compared with 65% for patients with sporadic tumors (277).

The differential diagnosis of MPNST is cellular schwannoma and a variety of spindle cell sarcomas. Cellular schwannomas generally have less cytologic atypia, fewer than four mitoses per 10 high-power fields, and do not have abnormal mitoses. In ad-

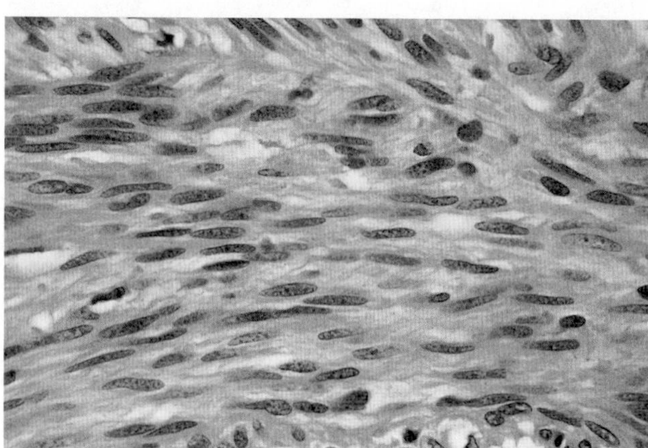

FIGURE 72. Spindle cells with tapered ends in a cellular schwannoma.

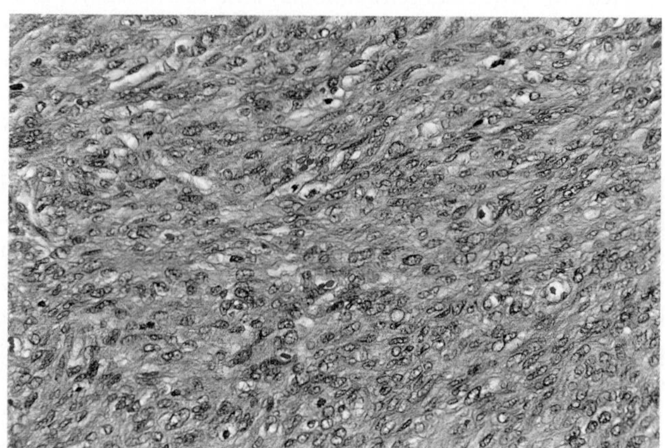

FIGURE 73. Hyperchromasia and mitotic activity are present in this malignant peripheral nerve sheath tumor.

dition, as previously stated, cellular schwannomas are diffusely S-100 protein positive, whereas S-100 protein staining is focal in MPNSTs. High grade MPNSTs may be morphologically similar to other sarcomas, and ancillary studies are frequently necessary to distinguish between them. LMS is composed of spindle cells with blunt-ended nuclei and abundant eosinophilic cytoplasm. The spindle cells are arranged in fascicles that intersect each other at right angles. Immunohistochemically, LMS stains for smooth muscle actin and desmin, antigens that are not typically expressed in MPNSTs. Electron microscopy is also helpful, because LMS demonstrates smooth muscle features, including actin filaments, dense bodies, mitochondria, and pinocytosis, features that are not present in MPNSTs. MFH and fibrosarcoma can be distinguished from MPNST because they are S-100 protein negative and manifest the ultrastructural features of fibroblasts and myofibroblasts.

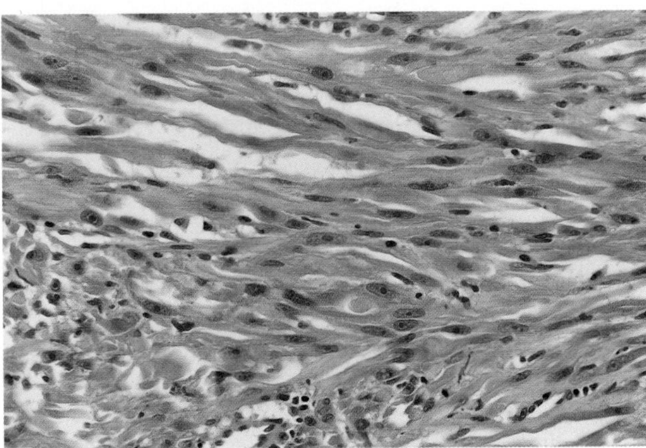

FIGURE 74. Elongate eosinophilic cytoplasm is characteristic of the spindle rhabdomyocytes of fetal rhabdomyoma.

Myogenetic Tumors

Rhabdomyoma

It is of interest that skeletal muscle comprises so much of the human body mass, and yet tumors of skeletal muscle differentiation are uncommon. Skeletal muscle neoplasms represent the only category of soft tissue tumors in which the malignant tumors outnumber their benign counterparts. Extracardiac rhabdomyomas are well described but exceedingly rare benign neoplasms of striated muscle. Those that affect the head and neck are classified into the fetal and adult types (284). Fetal rhabdomyomas are rarer than the adult type, with only a handful of case reports and small series having been reported in the literature. Nevertheless, fetal rhabdomyomas are further divided into the myxoid and intermediate or cellular subtypes.

The myxoid subtype of fetal rhabdomyoma occurs primarily in children under 3 years of age. It affects boys more often than girls and has a predilection for the postauricular region of the head. The tumors are tan–gray and soft and may be up to 4 cm in diameter. Myxoid fetal rhabdomyoma recapitulates the myotubule stage of normal muscle development and microscopically is composed of small round to oval, immature-appearing cells with little cytoplasm and that are intermixed with haphazardly arranged larger elongate, strap-like cells with abundant eosinophilic cytoplasm, all of which are surrounded by a prominent myxoid matrix. Mitotic activity is not appreciable. Cross-striations may be apparent in the larger strap cells, but are difficult to find and often are located in cells at the periphery of the tumor (285). The cellular type affects older children and adults more often than infants (286). It may arise in the orbit, tongue, palate, larynx, and pharynx, or in the subcutaneous soft tissue. The cellular fetal rhabdomyoma is grossly well defined and composed of oval cells with scant cytoplasm intermixed with haphazardly arranged fascicles of well-developed muscle cells containing a central nucleus and abundant eosinophilic cytoplasm with cross-striations. There is very scant stroma and virtually no pleomorphism, and mitotic figures are very few in number (Fig. 74).

The better differentiated cells in all types of fetal rhabdomyoma stain with antibodies to skeletal muscle: muscle-specific actin, desmin, and myoglobin. The less differentiated cells are desmin positive but may not stain with myoglobin. Ultrastructurally rhabdomyomas exhibit the features of developing striated muscle with organized bundles of thick and thin filaments and occasional banding in better differentiated cells (284). Glycogen is also present, but not in the same amount as in the adult type of rhabdomyoma. The more primitive cells of both the myxoid and cellular types of fetal rhabdomyoma do not contain ultrastructural evidence of skeletal muscle differentiation (287).

The main differential diagnosis for all fetal rhabdomyomas is RMS. The distinction is important because the therapy for RMS is aggressive and the prognosis significantly worse. Rhabdomyomas are well circumscribed and uniform in cytology, whereas RMS is infiltrative and shows cytologic atypia in the form of anaplasia, hyperchromasia, and increased mitotic activity.

Adult rhabdomyoma is more common than the fetal type. The mean age at diagnosis is 50 years, and the male:female ratio is 4:1 (288). Rhabdomyomas occur in all anatomic locations of the head, including the larynx, pharynx, palate, tongue, and cheek, as well as in the skeletal muscles of the neck. Mucosal rhabdomyomas may be polypoid or pedunculated. Most are solitary, but multifocal cases of adult rhabdomyoma are well documented (289). They range in size from 0.5 to 10 cm (median 3 cm), have a tan–red to brown cut surface, and are well circumscribed or encapsulated. Microscopically they are composed of large polygonal tumor cells with abundant granular, vacuolated cytoplasm and one or more peripherally placed nuclei that may contain prominent nucleoli (Fig. 75). The presence of abundant cytoplasmic glycogen imparts a distinct vacuolated appearance to the cytoplasm, causing a spider-like appearance. A minority of cells contain dense, eosinophilic crystalline structures termed jackstraw inclusions (Fig. 76). Strap cells and cross-striations are sometimes present, and they are accentuated by phosphotungstic acid hematoxylin (PTAH) and trichrome stains. Ultrastructurally the cells are surrounded by a continuous basal lamina and contain abundant mitochondria and glycogen as well as thin and thick myofilaments arranged in parallel or in a

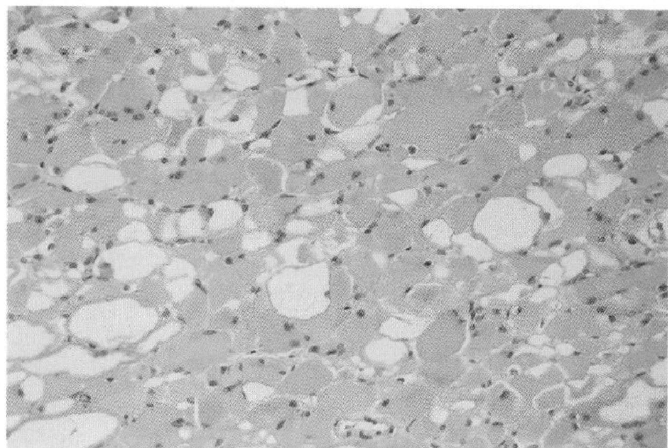

FIGURE 75. Adult rhabdomyoma of the tongue has granular eosinophilic cytoplasm and peripherally placed nuclei. (Courtesy of Robin Kirby, M.D.)

haphazard fashion (290). Focal electron densities resembling Z-band material are present, and the jackstraw inclusions have been shown to represent hypertrophied Z-band material (285). The immunohistochemical stains for vimentin, actins, desmin, and myoglobin are usually positive, whereas S-100 protein and Leu-7 are positive only in a minority of cases. A single case report of a reciprocal translocation of chromosomes 15 and 17 and an abnormality of the long arm of chromosome 10 may lend support to the hypothesis that extracardiac rhabdomyomas are neoplasms rather than hamartomas (291).

The differential diagnosis of adult rhabdomyoma includes GCT and hibernoma because of the abundant eosinophilic cytoplasm, which may be vacuolated as well as granular. GCT is usually infiltrative and associated with collagen production, and the cells do not contain vacuolated cytoplasm, crystalline inclusions, or cross-striations. GCTs are S-100 protein positive and negative for muscle markers (285). Ultrastructurally their cytoplasm contains abundant lysosomes and lacks the filaments present in rhabdomyomas. Although the cells of a hibernoma also are vacuolated, their cytoplasm is filled with lipid, not glycogen. Mature white adipocytes are frequently a component of hibernoma, and they are not present in rhabdomyoma. The vacuoles in a hibernoma are usually much smaller than the large vacuoles, which produce the spider-like change in the cytoplasm of rhabdomyoma cells. Hibernomas express S-100 protein and are negative for muscle markers. Treatment for all rhabdomyomas is excision. They rarely recur and do not metastasize.

Rhabdomyosarcoma

Rhabdomyosarcoma accounts for 19% of all soft tissue sarcomas, and it is the most common soft tissue sarcoma in children (288). Greater than 50% of patients are younger than 6 years of age at diagnosis, and tumors occurring in patients over 45 years of age are rare. Approximately 40% of pediatric cases occur in the head and neck area, including the orbit, nasopharynx, sinus, ear, mouth, and neck, whereas RMS in adults arises in the head and neck less frequently (292,293). RMS grows quickly and patient presentation varies according to the tumor site; proptosis, dysphagia, hoarseness, and nasal fullness may be present.

Grossly, RMS is firm, tan, and infiltrates the surrounding tissues. Areas of hemorrhage and necrosis are common. Three histologic subtypes of RMS exist and correlate with clinical and cytogenetic findings as well as outcome: embryonal, alveolar, and pleomorphic.

The embryonal type accounts for approximately 70% of RMS and is the most common histologic subtype to occur in the head and neck area (288). Patients are generally young children, but adolescents and adults also may be affected. Embryonal RMS is morphologically heterogeneous and may be composed of primitive small round cells with darkly staining nuclei that mimic lymphocytes or larger, oval to spindle-shaped strap cells with eccentric eosinophilic cytoplasm. Cross-striations are visible in these cells in 50% to 60% of cases (288). The tumor cells may be packed together tightly with little or no intervening matrix, or there may be abundant myxoid stroma (Figs. 77 and 78). Mitotic figures are easily appreciated, and nuclear pleomorphism is variable. The botryoid variant produces a polypoid mass in a submucosal location and has a cambium or densely cellular layer

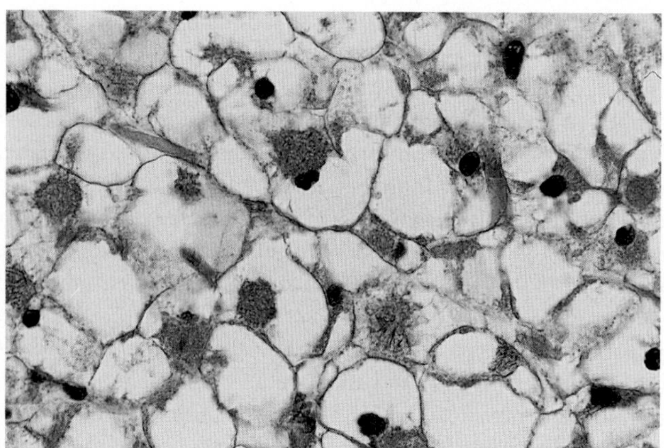

FIGURE 76. Adult rhabdomyoma containing jackstraw crystalline inclusions.

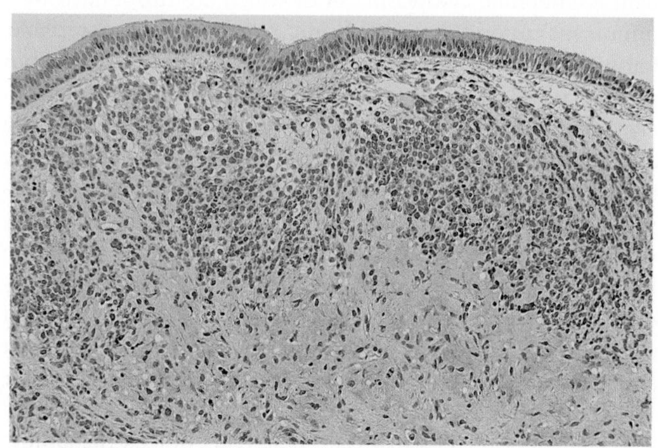

FIGURE 77. Polypoid rhabdomyosarcoma of the nasopharynx.

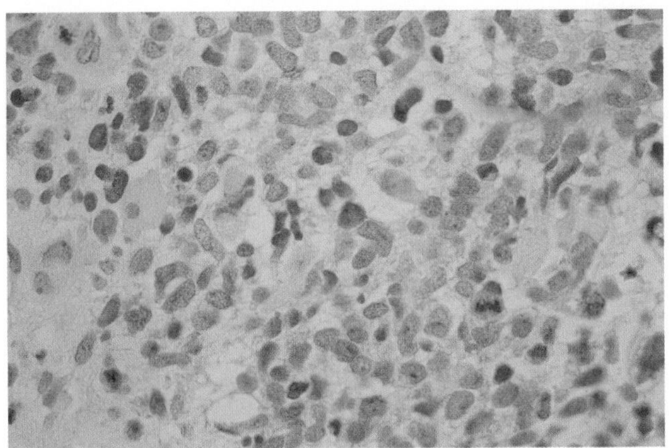

FIGURE 78. Eccentric eosinophilic cytoplasm is apparent in some rhabdomyoblasts in this rhabdomyosarcoma.

of cells, similar to the botryoid variant of RMS in the genital tract. It is otherwise histologically similar to conventional embryonal RMS. The spindle cell variant of RMS frequently occurs in the head and neck area and is composed of fascicles of spindle cells that have cross-striations and mimic the late stage of myotubule differentiation (294).

Alveolar RMS accounts for approximately 20% of RMS. It is more common in adolescents and young adults and occurs less often in the head and neck region than embryonal RMS. Microscopically the cells are small to medium sized and monomorphous with scant cytoplasm and irregular hyperchromatic nuclei. The cells are arranged in discohesive nests separated by fibrous septa, causing it to resemble somewhat pulmonary alveolar spaces (Fig. 79). In the solid variant there is no discohesion and the cells grow in solid sheets separated by the fibrous septa. Areas of classic alveolar morphology are generally present at least focally. Rhabdomyoblasts, tumor cells with eccentric eosinophilic cytoplasm, are present in 30% of cases and strap cells are infrequently present (288). Tumor cells with multiple peripherally placed nuclei are a characteristic finding of alveolar RMS, and spindled tumor cells also may be present.

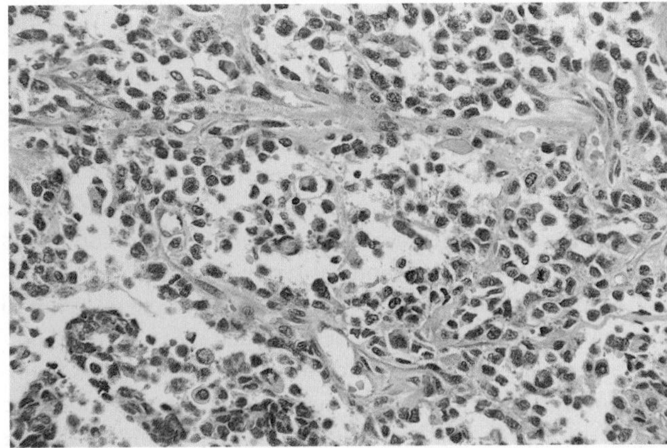

FIGURE 79. Rhabdomyoblasts arranged in discohesive nests in alveolar rhabdomyosarcoma.

Mitotic figures, including atypical mitoses, are numerous, and necrosis is often present.

Pleomorphic RMS, a variant most common in adulthood, occurs frequently in the extremities and does not involve the head and neck region.

Masson trichrome and PTAH stains may help in identifying cross-striations in better differentiated rhabdomyoblasts. Immunohistochemical studies show that the tumor cells express vimentin, muscle actin, desmin, myoglobin, and myo-D1. The level of desmin expression, as well as the degree of expression of striated muscle markers, is dependent on the degree of muscle differentiation; the better differentiated cells stain more intensely for desmin, as well as for muscle-specific actin, myoglobin, and myo-D1. Some RMS stain positively for keratin and S-100 protein, which may be misleading (295). Ultrastructural analysis reveals a wide range of differentiation within tumors, from undifferentiated cells containing mainly ribosomes, to cells with abundant rough endoplasmic reticulum similar to fibroblasts, to cells with numerous thick and thin filaments, Z bands, rough endoplasmic reticulum, and ribosomes. Pinocytotic vesicles, external basal lamina, and small intercellular junctions are also present. The degree of ultrastructural differentiation correlates with the light microscopic and immunohistochemical findings. Flow cytometry shows that nearly all RMS are aneuploid (296). The majority of alveolar RMS contain a characteristic t(2;13) (q37;q14) translocation not present in the other types of RMS (288,297). Embryonal RMS has been shown to have a hyperdiploid karyotype, but no specific chromosomal changes (298).

The differential diagnosis of RMS includes other small round cell tumors and, occasionally, fetal rhabdomyoma. Ewing's sarcoma/primitive neuroectodermal tumor (PNET) also may present as a soft tissue mass in the head of a child, but the cells have less cytoplasm than rhabdomyoblasts, and multinucleate and strap cells are not present. Ewing's sarcoma/PNET is negative for muscle markers and has a characteristic t(11;22) translocation. Small cell carcinoma may present as a soft tissue mass, but the average age at diagnosis is much older than that for patients with RMS. Small cell carcinoma displays nuclear molding and is cytokeratin positive and negative for muscle markers. Lymphoma grows in discohesive sheets of cells and is generally positive for LCA and negative for muscle markers. Malignant melanoma may mimic RMS, but may have prominent nucleoli and intracytoplasmic pigment that is absent in RMS. Melanoma is positive for S-100 protein, HMB-45, and Mart-1 and negative for muscle markers. Benign fetal rhabdomyoma often contains well-developed strap cells with obvious cross-striations. The cells in this tumor, however, lack the atypical nuclear features and mitotic activity characteristic of RMS.

Rhabdomyosarcoma of the head and neck is treated primarily with chemotherapy and often with adjuvant radiation therapy, depending on the location, size, and stage. The survival has improved with the use of multidrug chemotherapy and radiation therapy (293,299). The overall 5-year survival rate is 75%. Patient survival strongly correlates with stage of disease. Those with nonmetastatic disease have a 5-year survival rate of 90% (299,300). Patients under 16 years of age at diagnosis have a better prognosis, as do patients with the embryonal subtype, but the spindle cell variant of embryonal RMS has the best prognosis (294,300,301).

Leiomyoma and Leiomyosarcoma

Leiomyoma is a benign smooth muscle tumor that may occur in the cutaneous and subcutaneous tissues of the head and neck and oral cavity, but is uncommon in the deep soft tissue (302,303). Superficial leiomyomas may be painful and often arise from the pilar arrector muscles or vascular smooth muscle (see Chapter 13). The tumors are small, usually less than 3 cm in diameter, generally well circumscribed, and composed of broad fascicles of eosinophilic spindle cells with ample cytoplasm, bland, blunt-ended nuclei, and virtually no mitotic activity or atypia. The fascicles intersect one another at right angles (Fig. 80). Immunohistochemical studies are positive for actin, desmin, and sometimes keratin, and electron microscopy reveals nuclear membrane contractions, abundant mitochondria, collections of intermediate filaments with dense bodies, and pinocytotic vesicles.

Leiomyoma is treated by complete excision. Recurrence is uncommon. The differential diagnosis should include LMS, which is more cellular, cytologically atypical, and mitotically active, and may have necrosis. Leiomyoma may resemble the peripheral portion of a myofibroma, but the cells in myofibroma have a smaller amount of eosinophilic cytoplasm, and their nuclei do not have blunted ends. Importantly, the central area in myofibroma consists of sheets of primitive mesenchymal cells and has a hemangiopericytomatous vascular pattern.

Leiomyosarcoma is most common in the uterus and deep soft tissues of the extremities and retroperitoneum, but may occur in the head and neck region, where the scalp and superficial soft tissues and the oral cavity are most commonly involved (304,305). With regard to LMS in the head and neck region, males outnumber females by a ratio of at least 3:2. Although the age range at presentation is broad (1–88 years), most patients are adults at the time of diagnosis. LMS presents as a slowly growing soft tissue or polypoid submucosal mass that rarely may ulcerate. Depending on the location, stridor, hoarseness, and dysphagia may occur. Tumor size averages 3 cm, but ranges from 1 to 6 cm.

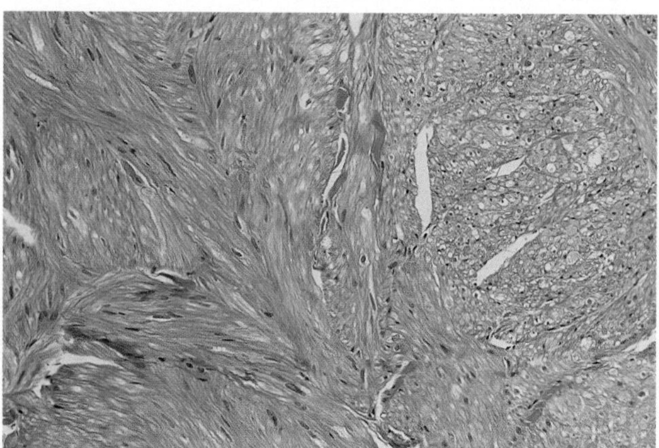

FIGURE 80. Fascicles of smooth muscle cells intersect at right angles in a leiomyoma.

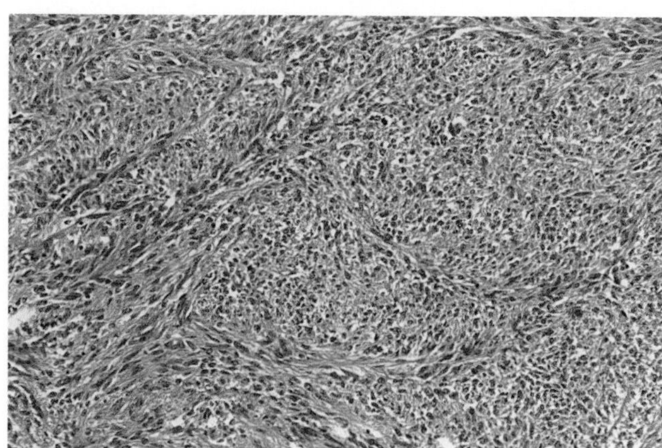

FIGURE 81. Increased cellularity and cytologic atypia in a leiomyosarcoma.

LMS is firm, has a whorled cut surface, and may have areas of hemorrhage or necrosis. LMS is more cellular than leiomyoma, with a greater degree of cytologic atypia, generally more than one or two mitoses per 10 high-power fields, atypical mitoses, and necrosis (Fig. 81). Immunohistochemistry and electron microscopy show findings similar to leiomyoma.

The differential diagnosis includes other spindle cell sarcomas. In MFH the cytoplasm of the cells is not as eosinophilic as in LMS and the fascicles are arranged in a storiform growth pattern, as compared with LMS, in which they are oriented at right angles to one another. Immunohistochemical studies for desmin are negative in most cases of MFH. MPNSTs lack the cytoplasmic eosinophilia of LMS, and the nuclei have tapered ends, compared with the blunted nuclei of LMS. Peripheral nerve sheath tumors may be S-100 protein positive and are usually desmin negative. Treatment of LMS is complete excision, with radiation therapy for incomplete resections. Chemotherapy is usually not effective. Patients generally do well because the tumors are small; however, large tumors may recur or metastasize (304).

Other Tumors

Synovial Sarcoma

Initially described as synovioma by Smith in 1927, synovial sarcoma accounts for approximately 10% of soft tissue sarcomas (306). It usually occurs in paraarticular areas of the extremities but rarely arises in the joint proper. It is estimated that 3% to 10% of synovial sarcomas occur in the head and neck region. In the head and neck the most common site of origin is the hypopharynx (see Chapter 7), but other sites include the tongue (Fig. 82), parapharyngeal area, paravertebral area, and soft tissues of the neck (307,308). Sinonasal synovial sarcoma is uncommon. Although the name implies synovial histogenesis, synovial sarcoma arises from primitive mesenchymal cells, not the modified mesothelial cells of the synovium. There is a male predominance of 1.4:1 (308,309). The age range at presentation is the second through the sixth decades of life. Depending on the site of the tumor, patients present with a mass, shortness of breath, hoarseness, or dysphagia, and the duration of symptoms prior to

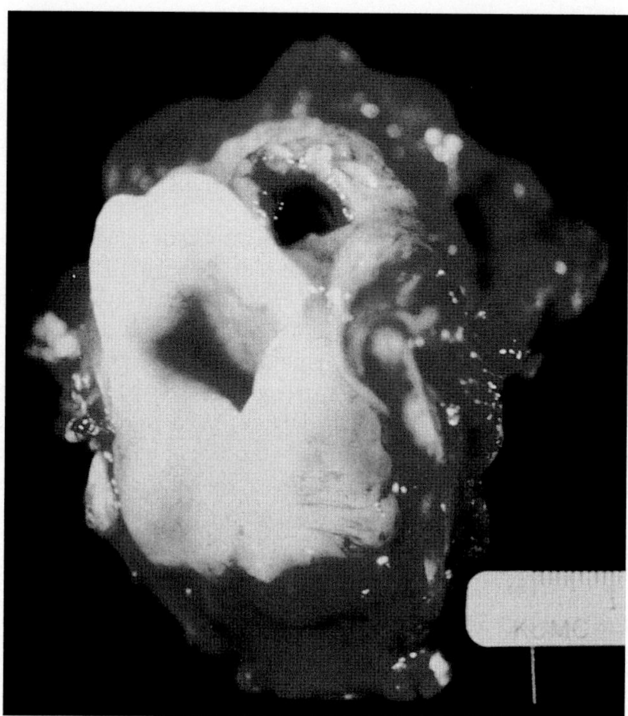

FIGURE 82. Large, ulcerating synovial sarcoma at the base of the tongue. (Courtesy of Julia A. Bridge, M.D.)

diagnosis ranges from 1 month to 1 or more years (309,310). Radiographic studies reveal calcifications or ossification, sometimes massive, within almost one third of cases (307).

Synovial sarcoma is well defined, lobulated, and often surrounded by a thin pseudocapsule. The cut surface is light tan–yellow and fleshy, with variable areas of necrosis, cystification, or hemorrhage. Calcifications may be grossly visible or manifest as grittiness within the tissue. Microscopically, synovial sarcoma is divided into the classic biphasic, monophasic spindle cell, the rare monophasic epithelial, and poorly differentiated subtypes.

The classic and most common biphasic subtype is composed of two cell populations: epithelial cells and spindle cells (Fig. 83).

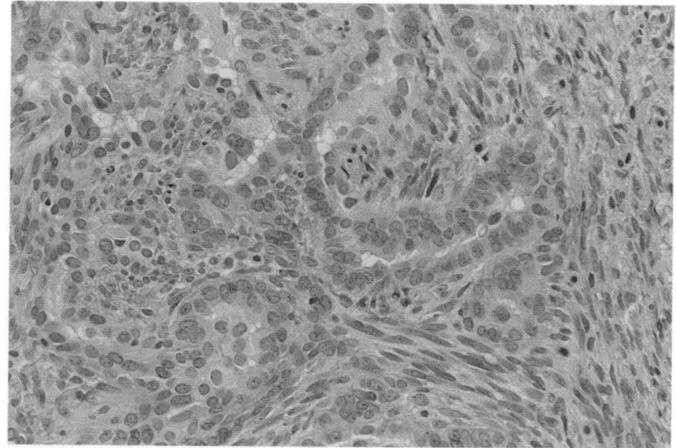

FIGURE 83. A biphasic pattern of glands and spindle cells in synovial sarcoma.

The epithelial cells demonstrate limited cytologic atypia and form nests and glands, line slit-like spaces or papillary projections, and have abundant eosinophilic cytoplasm, distinct cell borders, and vesicular nuclei. The glands contain eosinophilic, PAS-positive secretions. They are surrounded by sheets and fascicles of plump spindle cells that may have a storiform, herringbone, or random arrangement. The spindle cells have a uniform, monotonous appearance and contain scant pale cytoplasm and oval to spindle-shaped, hyperchromatic nuclei. Mitoses are the most numerous in the spindle cell component. The monophasic spindle or fibrous synovial sarcoma is composed exclusively of the spindle cells arranged in fascicles having a storiform or herringbone growth pattern. The monophasic epithelial pattern is the rarest subtype and is composed of plump epithelial cells with abundant eosinophilic cytoplasm and only focal areas of spindle cell differentiation. The poorly differentiated subtype of synovial sarcoma consists of round cells that are larger and plumper than the spindle cells, but not as large as the epithelial cells, and have less cytoplasm. The poorly differentiated cells are arranged in sheets and whorls with occasional foci of epithelial differentiation. The nuclei are more hyperchromatic than in the other subtypes, and mitoses are more readily identifiable.

Collagen deposition with hyalinization and calcification may be present in all subtypes of synovial sarcoma. In a minority of cases the stroma may have a prominent myxoid component. An HP-like vascular pattern is often quite striking. Immunohistochemical studies show that the epithelial cells stain positively with EMA and high and low molecular weight cytokeratin, as do a minority of the spindle cells. Synovial sarcoma also may be positive for S-100 protein and Leu-7. Electron microscopic study of the epithelial cells demonstrates smooth and rough endoplasmic reticulum, mitochondria, a prominent Golgi apparatus, intermediate filaments, and occasional tonofilaments within the cytoplasm. The cells contain microvilli on the luminal aspect, and they are connected by junctional complexes and surrounded by basal lamina. The spindle cells also contain smooth and rough endoplasmic reticulum, mitochondria, and a prominent Golgi, and early epithelial differentiation is manifested by slit-like spaces with poorly formed intercellular junctions and microvilli (311). A characteristic balanced t(X;18)(p11;q11) translocation is present in the majority of all synovial sarcoma subtypes and may be detected in paraffin-embedded tissue (312–314).

Treatment is radical surgery, with adjuvant radiation therapy or chemotherapy in the appropriate situation. The recurrence rate is high, about 60%, and recurrences may develop decades after the initial resection (307,310). Almost 50% of cases eventually metastasize to the lungs. The 5-year survival rate of patients with head and neck synovial sarcoma is 55%, similar to that for synovial sarcoma at other sites, and the 10-year survival rate decreases to 38% due to deaths related to late recurrences and metastases (307,309). Positive prognostic predictors include an age of less than 15 years at presentation, tumor size less than 5 cm, and massive calcifications (315,316). The poorly differentiated subtype behaves most aggressively.

Aside from the classic biphasic subtype, synovial sarcoma may be difficult to diagnose accurately. Cytogenetics is the most reliable means of distinction in most cases. The monophasic epithelioid subtype can be easily confused with carcinoma histologically; therefore, a thorough search for the spindle cell component should be undertaken to help make the correct diagnosis. Metastatic carcinoma is uncommon in the patient population usually affected by synovial sarcoma. The monophasic spindle cell variant resembles fibrosarcoma; however, a prominent HP-like vascular pattern is not a feature of fibrosarcoma. Immunohistochemical stains for keratin and EMA are positive in synovial sarcoma and not in fibrosarcoma, and the primitive epithelial differentiation present ultrastructurally in synovial sarcoma is not a feature of fibrosarcoma. Cellular schwannoma may have a monotonous spindle cell appearance similar to monophasic synovial sarcoma, but the cells lack the cytologic atypia of synovial sarcoma as well as the HP-like vascular pattern. MPNSTs are generally less monotonous than synovial sarcoma and show a greater degree of anaplasia. Both schwannoma and MPNST are frequently S-100 protein positive and negative for keratin and EMA.

Alveolar Soft Part Sarcoma

Alveolar soft part sarcoma (ASPS) was identified as a distinct but uncommon entity of unknown phenotype by Christopherson in 1952 (317). It accounts for less than 1% of soft tissue sarcomas, and about 25% of cases occur in the head and neck region, where the orbit and tongue are the most common sites (318–322). Adolescents and young adults are most commonly affected, and there is a female predominance (323). Most of the head and neck cases occur in younger individuals.

Alveolar soft part sarcoma presents as a slowly growing, painless mass. Grossly the tumors are frequently well circumscribed but unencapsulated. They have a soft consistency and are gray–red due to their vascularity. ASPS is characterized by organoid groups of large round tumor cells with abundant granular pink cytoplasm and prominent vesicular nuclei with conspicuous nucleoli. The aggregates of cells are surrounded by a thin layer of basal lamina and separated from neighboring cells by capillaries lined by flattened endothelial cells. The tumor cells in the center of the groups are discohesive, resulting in the characteristic alveolar pattern. Thick fibrous bands course through the tumor, further accentuating the alveolar pattern. Vascular invasion is frequently present.

A PAS stain highlights the abundant intracytoplasmic glycogen as well as the diagnostic rod-shaped crystals (Shipkey's crystals) that are present within the cytoplasm of some tumor cells (324). Ultrastructurally, the crystals have a regular lattice pattern, and the cytoplasm contains mitochondria, glycogen, smooth endoplasmic reticulum, and Golgi. Tumor cells may have desmosomes or hemidesmosomes (324). Immunohistochemical stains for vimentin, muscle-specific actin, desmin, and occasionally myoglobin, S-100 protein, and NSE are positive. ASPS usually does not stain for keratin, EMA, neurofilament, glial fibrillary acidic protein (GFAP), or synaptophysin. This staining pattern is confusing and has led some investigators to argue that ASPS is a myogenic neoplasm. To date the phenotype of ASPS remains unknown. Cytogenetic studies reveal abnormalities of 17q25 as well as less frequent abnormalities in chromosomes 1, 9, and 15 (325).

Treatment is radical surgery with adjuvant radiation and possibly chemotherapy (322,326). Metastases occur early and may be the presenting finding. The prognosis is guarded, with a 50% to 77% 5-year survival rate in patients without metastases, which decreases to a dismal 38% at 10 years (327–329). Pediatric patients tend to fare better, with survival reports of up to 82% at 10 years (330).

The differential diagnosis includes metastatic renal cell carcinoma, which generally occurs in an older population. Renal cell carcinoma does not contain the crystals present in ASPS and usually expresses cytokeratin and EMA, which is not seen in ASPS. Malignant GCT also resembles ASPS but lacks the vascular stroma and crystals and is strongly S-100 protein positive. Paraganglioma is distinguished from ASPS by the cohesive growth of the groups of tumor cells, the lack of intracytoplasmic crystals, the positivity of the tumor cells with neural markers such as chromogranin and the peripheral S-100 protein positive supporting sustentacular cells.

Epithelioid Sarcoma

Less than 1% of cases of ES occur in the head and neck region (331–334). ES usually affects individuals 10 to 35 years of age, and most commonly arises in the upper extremity (335). Males are affected twice as often as females. Tumors may arise superficially or in the deep soft tissue, and it is common for them to present as small firm nodules that may ulcerate. Because ES is often small and superficial, it is sometimes confused with a benign process such as a wart, resulting in a delay in diagnosis. ES has a propensity to grow along tendons, fascia, and aponeuroses and may grow for extensive distances.

Epithelioid sarcoma may measure up to 15 cm, but is usually only a few centimeters in diameter at the time of diagnosis. Grossly the cut surface is grayish and may show foci of necrosis and hemorrhage. Histologically, ES has a nodular growth pattern and is composed of polyhedral and spindle cells with abundant pale eosinophilic cytoplasm (Fig. 84). The nuclei are round or oval, may contain a small nucleolus, and are deceptively banal in appearance. Mitoses are usually easily identifiable. The stroma is collagenous and frequently hyalinized. As the tumor nodules

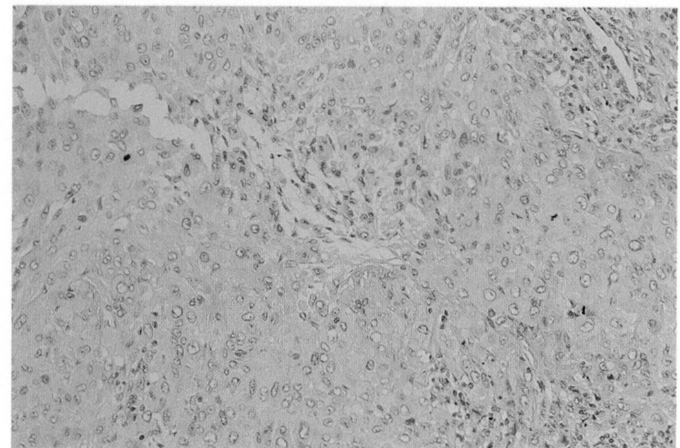

FIGURE 84. Granuloma-like cluster of malignant cells in epithelioid sarcoma.

enlarge, the area of central necrosis expands and the periphery of the nodule may contain inflammatory cells, mimicking a granuloma (336). Calcification is present in a minority of tumors, especially in areas of necrosis.

Immunohistochemically, the tumor cells are positive with low and high molecular weight keratin, EMA, and CD34 in the majority of cases (337,338). Electron microscopy demonstrates that the cells are full of whorls of intermediate filaments, rough endoplasmic reticulum, free ribosomes, and Golgi, and have small numbers of lysosomes, mitochondria, and droplets of osmiophilic material (339).

Epithelioid sarcoma is most often confused with a benign, granulomatous process such as granuloma annulare. The subtle atypia of the tumor cells and the mitotic activity should prevent one from rendering a benign diagnosis. If doubt exists, immunohistochemistry can help make the distinction. ES also may resemble squamous cell carcinoma, a common lesion of the skin of the face. Carcinoma, however, presents at a later age than ES and is usually accompanied by surface squamous epithelial atypia that is not present in ES. The treatment of head and neck ES is wide excision with radiation therapy. The recurrence rate is over 70%, and approximately 45% metastasize to regional lymph nodes; therefore, the draining lymph nodes should be clinically examined and even possibly sampled. The 5-year survival rate is approximately 50% to 70% (333,340).

Paraganglioma

Paraganglioma, often referred to as chemodectoma or GT, is a tumor derived from paraganglia, structures of neuroectodermal crest derivation that are found throughout the body. Paragangliomas are intimately associated with vascular and neural structures in the neck region and are most commonly classified according to their location; jugulotympanic, vagal, carotid body, and others, including laryngeal, nasal, and occular (341–343). Of these, carotid body and vagal paragangliomas are the most likely types to present as a soft tissue mass in the head and neck (see Chapters 3 and 7 for details on jugulotympanic and laryngeal paragangliomas).

The carotid body is the best understood of the paraganglia. Each is a tiny structure, 3 mm in greatest diameter, located on the medial aspect of the carotid bifurcation, which functions as a chemoreceptor, detecting and responding to changes in arterial Po_2 and pH (343). Neoplastic growth of the carotid body affects both sexes equally and peaks in the fifth decade of life. Tumors occurring in individuals living at high altitudes, however, preferentially affect females (344). Patients present with a slowly growing, painless mass near the angle of the mandible, which may have been noted for years. Imaging studies reveal lateral displacement of the carotid artery bifurcation and its branches, with characteristic widening of the bifurcation. Tumors average 3 to 4 cm in diameter, appear well delineated, and have a light tan cut surface which may show foci of vascular congestion.

The vagal region is the third most frequent site of involvement after the carotid body and jugulotympanic areas. Unlike the circumscribed carotid body, the vagal paraganglion represents a collection of microscopic nests placed along the vagus nerve distal to the ganglion nodosum. Because of the variability in location of the normal vagal paraganglia, paragangliomas arising from these structures also vary in location. At the time of diagnosis, patients are usually in the fourth to fifth decade of life, and there is a female predominance (341,345). Patients generally complain of a slowly growing neck mass, and, because of the intimate relationship with the vagus nerve, cranial nerve palsies also may be present (345). Vagal paragangliomas displace the carotid vessels anteriorly, are grossly rounded or fusiform, and abut the base of the skull.

Familial paragangliomas often follow an autosomal dominant mode of inheritance and occur at a slightly younger age. They affect the carotid bodies in 78% of cases and are bilateral in approximately 30% of cases. These patients may develop paragangliomas at other sites as well (341,343,346,347).

Paragangliomas have a tan, soft cut surface (Fig. 85). Paragangliomas from all regions of the head and neck are histologically similar. They are well circumscribed and composed of chief cells arranged in nests known as *Zellballen* (Fig. 86). The tumor cells have granular eosinophilic cytoplasm and round to oval nuclei with prominent nucleoli. Nuclear anaplasia may be present, but mitoses are rare, and necrosis is usually present only if the patient underwent preoperative embolization or if the nests of cells are very large. Compressed sustentacular cells and a rich capillary network surround each cell nest. Malignant varieties are difficult to distinguish on histologic grounds, but generally they

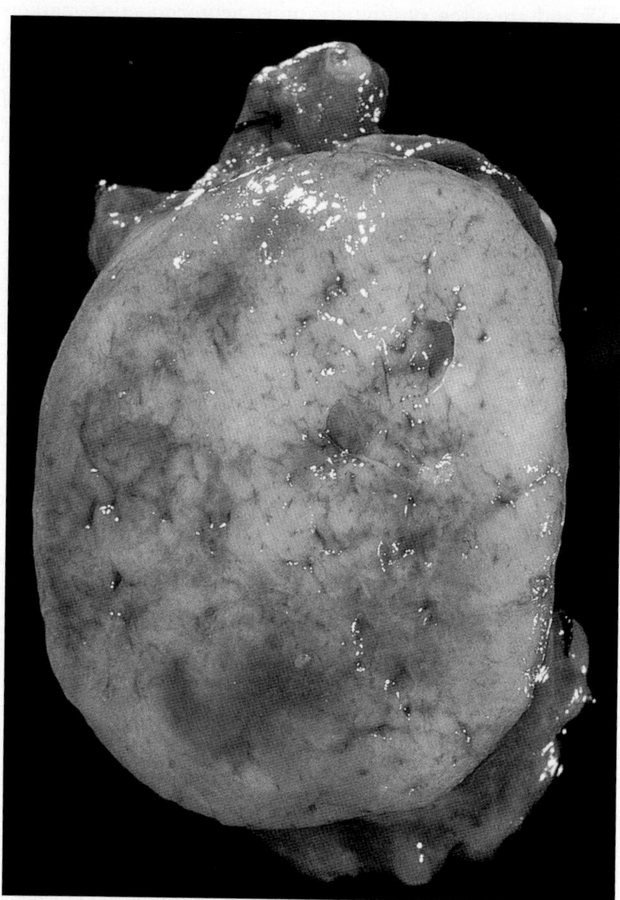

FIGURE 85. Paraganglioma with a tan, soft cut surface.

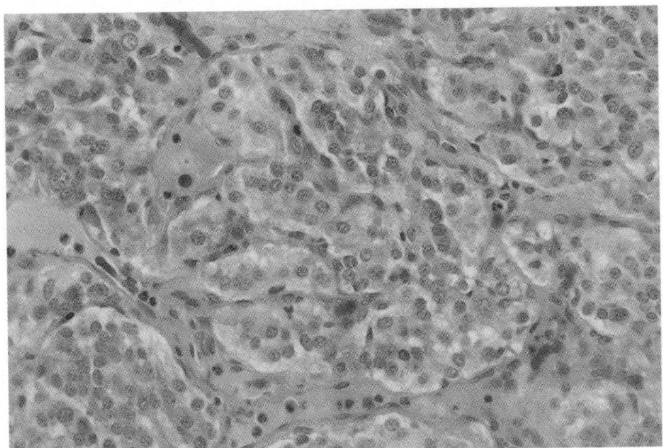

FIGURE 86. *Zellballen* are surrounded by sustentacular cells in a paraganglioma.

have a higher mitotic rate and more necrosis when compared with benign tumors. Vascular invasion may be present in both benign and malignant tumors. The absence of sustentacular cells has been associated with malignant behavior, but this is not a reliable method of distinction (348).

A reticulin stain highlights the nested arrangement of the cells, and an argyrophil stain demonstrates small cytoplasmic granules within the chief cells. The chief cells are positive for NSE and are often positive for other neuroendocrine markers such as chromogranin. Positivity for cytokeratin is rare, but has been reported (349). The sustentacular cells stain with S-100 protein (350). Ultrastructural studies demonstrate that the chief cells have cytoplasmic processes that surround neighboring cells, and the cytoplasm contains abundant large mitochondria, inconspicuous Golgi, smooth and rough endoplasmic reticulum, and membrane-bound, dense-core, neurosecretory granules (351,352).

Most paragangliomas behave in a benign fashion. About 15% recur, and 5% prove their malignant nature by metastasizing (341,345). Surgery is generally the treatment of choice, but radiation therapy alone, or in combination with surgery, is advocated by some, especially when tumors are difficult to remove, or in cases of multifocal tumors when resecting all lesions would leave the patient functionally impaired (353,354). Chemotherapy is effective in pain control for metastatic tumors, but seems to have no effect on the evolution of disease (355).

The differential diagnosis of paraganglioma is mainly with carcinoma, especially metastatic renal cell carcinoma. Although renal cell carcinoma often is a vascular tumor and arranged in nests, distinct sustentacular cells are not present in renal cell carcinoma. If in doubt, immunohistochemistry should be performed. Paragangliomas will be positive for NSE and chromogranin and rarely for keratin, and the peripheral sustentacular cells are highlighted with S-100 protein. Renal cell carcinoma, unlike paraganglioma, is frequently composed of clear cells, contains areas of hemorrhage and necrosis, and is usually positive for keratin and EMA. Renal cell carcinoma may express S-100 protein; however, the sustentacular cells surrounding the epithelial nests in paraganglioma are not present in renal cell carcinoma. Electron microscopy demonstrates neurosecretory granules in paraganglioma.

Extraskeletal Ewing's Sarcoma and Primitive Neuroectodermal Tumor

Although uncommon in the head and neck region, extraskeletal Ewing's sarcoma and PNET do occasionally arise in this area and may involve the scalp, nasal fossa and parotid gland (356–360). It is thought that Ewing's sarcoma and PNET are closely related small round cell tumors that demonstrate varying degrees of neuronal differentiation, with Ewing's sarcoma showing the least, and PNET with rosette formation the most. Both tumors occur over a wide age range but most commonly develop in patients under 30 years of age.

Ewing's sarcoma/PNET are rapidly growing multilobated, soft tumors that are usually tan–gray and may be friable. Their size varies from several centimeters to 10 cm or more, but in the head and neck region they are generally small. Microscopically, Ewing's sarcoma is composed of sheets and large nests of uniform small round cells (Fig. 87). The nuclei are round and have fine chromatin and a small nucleolus, and the cytoplasm is scant and may be clear or faintly eosinophilic. Necrosis and mitoses are easily found. The cells of PNET may be arranged in rosettes with thin eosinophilic cytoplasmic processes extending into the centers. PAS stain with and without diastase digestion demonstrates abundant glycogen within the cytoplasm of Ewing's sarcoma/PNET. Immunohistochemical stains for vimentin may be positive or negative, and over 95% of cases express the antibody to the *mic-2* gene–encoded protein (CD99) (361). A minority of cases of Ewing's sarcoma/PNET stain with keratin. Expression of one or more antibodies such as NSE, Leu-7, S-100 protein, synaptophysin, neurofilament, and chromogranin indicates neural differentiation, and these tumors are better classified as PNETs rather than Ewing's sarcoma. Ewing's sarcoma/PNET do not express LCA or desmin, which are helpful diagnostic features. Ultrastructurally Ewing's sarcoma is composed of primitive cells with few cytoplasmic organelles, but abundant glycogen. They are closely apposed, and primitive cell junctions may

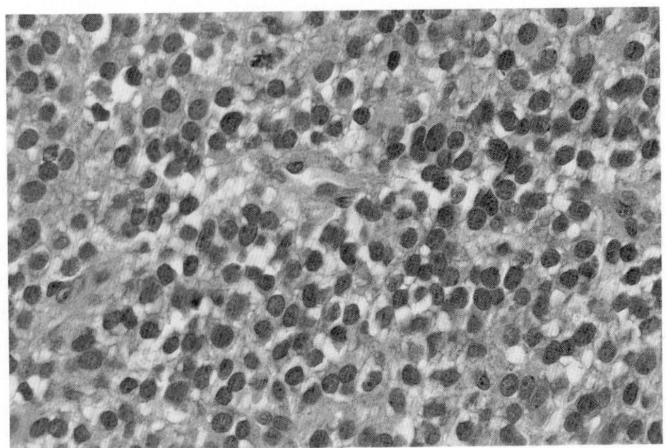

FIGURE 87. Extraskeletal Ewing's sarcoma composed of sheets of uniform small blue cells.

be present. PNET demonstrates interdigitating cell processes, cytoplasmic microtubules, and dense core granules. Both Ewing's sarcoma and PNET have a characteristic t(11;22) translocation.

The differential diagnosis of Ewing's sarcoma/PNET includes other small round cell tumors such as lymphoma, small cell carcinoma, RMS, and neuroblastoma. Lymphoma usually has an infiltrate of mature appearing lymphocytes within the tumor, and this is not a feature of Ewing's sarcoma/PNET. Most lymphomas are positive for LCA and negative for mic-2; however, lymphoblastic lymphoma is mic-2 positive. Small cell carcinoma occurs in an older patient population, is keratin positive, and is usually mic-2 negative, unlike Ewing's sarcoma. RMS may show histologic evidence of myoid differentiation in the form of eccentric eosinophilic cytoplasm and strap cells with cross-striations. RMS is strongly desmin positive and may be positive for muscle actin, myoglobin, and myo-D1. These antibodies are negative in Ewing's sarcoma/PNET. Neuroblastoma frequently has a fibrillar stroma typical of neuropils and evidence of ganglion cell differentiation which is usually not seen in Ewing's sarcoma/PNET. Unlike Ewing's sarcoma/PNET, neuroblastoma does not stain with the antibody to the mic-2 protein.

Chemotherapy is the first course of therapy and is usually combined with radiation therapy, with or without complete surgical resection, depending on the size and location of the tumor. The overall 5-year survival rate is 61%, and the disease free survival rate is 54% (362).

Chondroma/Osteoma

Soft tissue chondromas uncommonly develop in the head and neck, but when they do, they most frequently arise in the tongue, where they occur on the lateral surface and the dorsum (363–368). They are composed of lobulated nodules of mature-appearing hyaline cartilage. Focal myxoid degeneration may be present as well as mild hypercellularity and slight atypia. The cartilage may undergo enchondral ossification, and when the entire nodule is bone, it is referred to as an osteoma (Fig. 88) (366,369). These lesions may represent a non-neoplastic process, and therefore some favor the term *choristoma,* especially in reference to the tongue lesions. The true histogenesis of these benign mesenchymal nodules is uncertain (370,371). The differential diagnosis of a chondroma includes the rare cartilaginous metaplasia of the human aponeurosis linguae, a benign condition in which metaplastic fibrocartilage is present in a linear or multinodular configuration along the lingual aponeurosis (43). Simple excision of chondroma and osteoma is curative.

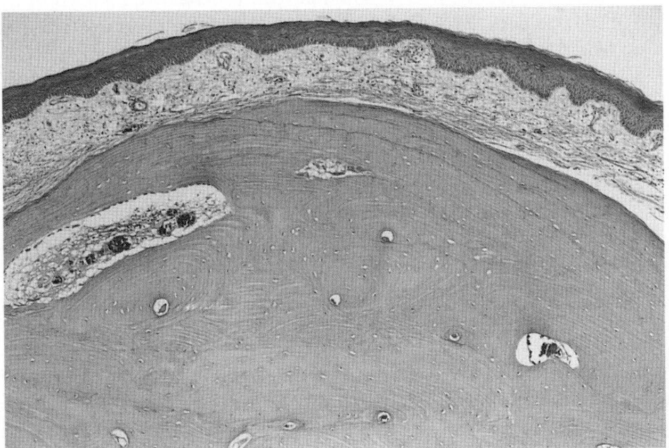

FIGURE 88. Submucosal osteoma composed of dense woven and lamellar bone.

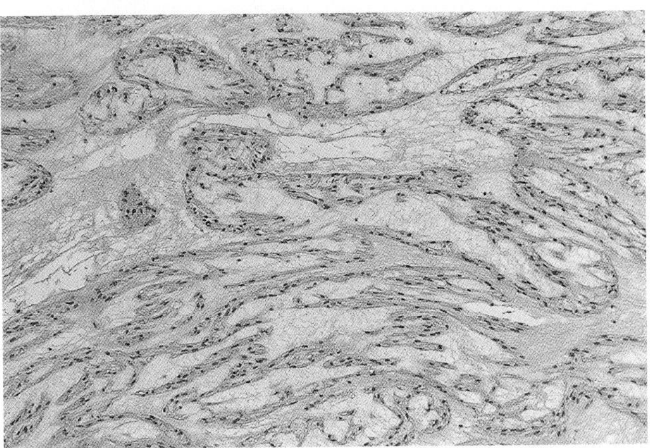

FIGURE 89. Nests and cords of epithelioid cells in a delicate myxoid background of an ectomesenchymal chondromyxoid tumor.

Ectomesenchymal Chondromyxoid Tumor

Ectomesenchymal chondromyxoid tumor (ECT) is an unusual tumor of uncertain histogenesis located in the tongue that was first described in 1995 (372). This type of tumor is rare, and just over 20 cases have been reported (373,374). ECTs occur in patients 9 to 78 years of age and do not seem to have a sex predilection. The tumors are slow growing and measure 0.5 to 2.0 cm upon presentation. They occur primarily on the dorsum of the tongue and are composed of well-defined, submucosal gray, tan, or yellow rubbery nodules that have a gelatinous cut surface. Histologically ECT grows in a lobular pattern, with the lobules separated by thin bands of fibroconnective tissue. Although the nodules are well defined, they are not encapsulated and may entrap normal structures. The tumor cells are round, fusiform, or spindle-shaped with uniform small dark nuclei, occasional nucleoli, or nuclear pseudoinclusions, and ample basophilic cytoplasm (Fig. 89). The cells have indistinct cell borders and are arranged in whorls, net-like sheets, and cords within a vacuolated myxoid and chondroid matrix that demonstrates foci of hyalinization (372). Mild cytologic atypia in the form of hyperchromasia, nuclear enlargement, and multinucleation may be present. Mitoses are not usually identified.

Ectomesenchymal chondromyxoid tumor is aldehyde fuchsin and Alcian blue positive, and PAS negative. Immunohistochemical stains are positive for GFAP, cytokeratin, smooth muscle actin, Leu-7, and S-100 protein at least focally in the majority of cases (372,374). Faint desmin staining also may be present, but none of the tumors have been positive for EMA. Ultrastructural analyses performed on a small number of cases have demonstrated concave nuclei with small nucleoli, and basal lamina. Tight junctions, pinocytotic vesicles, and well-developed rough endoplasmic reticulum are present, but thin filaments are absent.

Theories regarding histogenesis include an origin from undifferentiated mesenchymal cells within the tongue and salivary gland epithelial cells. ECT is thought to be a benign tumor, and simple excision should be curative; however, long-term follow-up is necessary to be certain. The differential diagnosis of ECT includes other chondroid tongue lesions. Chondroma or cartilaginous choristomas are composed of hyaline cartilage with foci of myxoid degeneration. They are not as cellular as ECT and are S-100 protein positive, but GFAP, keratin, and Leu-7 negative. Nerve sheath myxoma or neurothekeoma is a cutaneous tumor that also has a lobular growth pattern and myxoid stroma and has been reported in the oral cavity (see Chapter 13). Neurothekeoma may be S-100 protein and GFAP positive, but does not stain for cytokeratin or actin. ECT also may be confused with myoepithelial cell tumors, but these do not occur in the anterior dorsum of the tongue because this area is devoid of salivary glands. Histologically, myoepithelial cell tumors are at least focally composed of ductal structures and may have plasmacytoid cells, structures that are not present in ECT. Complete excision is recommended.

REFERENCES

1. Stoler MH, Bonfiglio TA, Steigbigel RT, et al. An atypical subcutaneous infection associated with acquired immune deficiency syndrome. *Am J Clin Pathol* 1983;80:714–718.
2. Batsakis JG, Ro JY, Frauenhoffer EE. Bacillary angiomatosis. *Ann Otol Rhinol Laryngol* 1995;104:668–672.
3. Hnatuk LA, Brown DH, Snell GE. Bacillary angiomatosis: a new entity in acquired immunodeficiency syndrome. *J Otolaryngol* 1994; 23:216–220.
4. Koehler JE, Sanchez MA, Garrido CS, et al. Molecular epidemiology of *Bartonella* infections in patients with bacillary angiomatosis-peliosis [Comment]. *N Engl J Med* 1997;337:1876–1883.
5. Tompkins LS. Of cats, humans, and *Bartonella* [Editorial, Comment]. *N Engl J Med* 1997;337:1916–1917.
6. Schwartzman W. *Bartonella* (*Rochalimaea*) infections: beyond cat scratch. *Annu Rev Med* 1996;47:355–364.
7. Bhaskar SN, Jacoway JR. Pyogenic granuloma—clinical features, incidence, histology, and result of treatment: report of 242 cases. *J Oral Surg* 1966;24:391–398.
8. Mills SE, Cooper PH, Fechner RE. Lobular capillary hemangioma: the underlying lesion of pyogenic granuloma. A study of 73 cases from the oral and nasal mucous membranes. *Am J Surg Pathol* 1980; 4:470–479.
9. Taira JW, Hill TL, Everett MA. Lobular capillary hemangioma (pyogenic granuloma) with satellitosis. *J Am Acad Dermatol* 1992; 27: 297–300.
10. Cooper PH, McAllister HA, Helwig EB. Intravenous pyogenic granuloma. A study of 18 cases. *Am J Surg Pathol* 1979;3:221–228.
11. McDonald RH. Granuloma gravidarum. Pregnancy tumor of the gingiva. *Am J Obstet Gynecol* 1956;75:1132–1136.
12. Masson P. Hemangioendotheliome vegetant intravasculaire. *Bull Soc Anat* 1923;93:517–523.
13. Kuo T, Sayers CP, Rosai J. Masson's "vegetant intravascular hemangioendothelioma": a lesion often mistaken for angiosarcoma: study of seventeen cases located in the skin and soft tissues. *Cancer* 1976; 38: 1227–1236.
14. Pins MR, Rosenthal DI, Springfield DS, et al. Florid extravascular papillary endothelial hyperplasia (Masson's pseudoangiosarcoma) presenting as a soft-tissue sarcoma. *Arch Pathol Lab Med* 1993;117: 259–263.
15. Proppe KH, Scully RE, Rosai J. Postoperative spindle cell nodules of genitourinary tract resembling sarcomas. A report of eight cases. *Am J Surg Pathol* 1984;8:101–108.
16. Zellers RA, Bicket WJ, Parker MG. Posttraumatic spindle cell nodule of the buccal mucosa. Report of a case. *Oral Surg Oral Med Oral Pathol* 1992;74:212–215.
17. Wick MR, Mills SE, Ritter JH, et al. Postoperative/posttraumatic spindle cell nodule of the skin: the dermal analogue of nodular fasciitis. *Am J Dermatopathol* 1999;21:220–224.
18. Balercia G, Bhan AK, Dickersin GR. Sarcomatoid carcinoma: an ultrastructural study with light microscopic and immunohistochemical correlation of 10 cases from various anatomic sites. *Ultrastruct Pathol* 1995;19:249–263.
19. Konwaler BE, Keasbey L, Kaplan L. Subcutaneous pseudosarcomatous fibromatosis (fasciitis). *Am J Clin Pathol* 1955;25:241–252.
20. Hutter RV, Stewart FW, Foote JW Jr. Fasciitis. A report of 70 cases with follow-up proving the benignity of the lesion. *Cancer* 1961; 15:992–1003.
21. Montgomery EA, Meis JM. Nodular fasciitis. Its morphologic spectrum and immunohistochemical profile. *Am J Surg Pathol* 1991;15: 942–948.
22. Davies HT, Bradley N, Bowerman JE. Oral nodular fasciitis. *Br J Oral Maxillofac Surg* 1989;27:147–151.
23. DiNardo LJ, Wetmore RF, Potsic WP. Nodular fasciitis of the head and neck in children. A deceptive lesion. *Arch Otolaryngol Head Neck Surg* 1991;117:1001–1002.
24. Werning JT. Nodular fasciitis of the orofacial region. *Oral Surg Oral Med Oral Pathol* 1979;48:441–446.
25. Wirman JA. Nodular fasciitis, a lesion of myofibroblasts: an ultrastructural study. *Cancer* 1976;38:2378–2389.
26. Sawyer JR, Sammartino G, Baker GF, Bell JM. Clonal chromosome aberrations in a case of nodular fasciitis. *Cancer Genet Cytogenet* 1994;76:154–156.
27. Barohn RJ, Kasdon DL. Cranial fasciitis: nodular fasciitis of the head. *Surg Neurol* 1980;13:283–285.
28. Clapp CG, Dodson EE, Pickett BP, et al. Cranial fasciitis presenting as an external auditory canal mass. *Arch Otolaryngol Head Neck Surg* 1997;123:223–225.
29. Lauer DH, Enzinger FM. Cranial fasciitis of childhood. *Cancer* 1980;45:401–406.
30. Daroca PJ Jr, Pulitzer DR, LoCicero JD. Ossifying fasciitis. *Arch Pathol Lab Med* 1982;106:682–685.
31. Batsakis JG, el-Naggar AK. Pseudosarcomatous proliferative lesions of soft tissues. *Ann Otol Rhinol Laryngol* 1994;103:578–582.
32. Enzinger FM, Dulcey F. Proliferative myositis. Report of thirty-three cases. *Cancer* 1967;20:2213–2223.
33. Kern WH. Proliferative myositis: a pseudosarcomatous reaction to injury. A report of seven cases. *AMA Arch Pathol* 1960;69:209–216.
34. Dent CD, DeBoom GW, Hamlin ML. Proliferative myositis of the head and neck. Report of a case and review of the literature. *Oral Surg Oral Med Oral Pathol* 1994;78:354–358.
35. Scher N, Dobleman TJ, Poe DS, et al. Proliferative myositis of the masseter muscle. *Laryngoscope* 1987;97:591–593.
36. Meis JM, Enzinger FM. Proliferative fasciitis and myositis of childhood. *Am J Surg Pathol* 1992;16:364–372.
37. Dembinski A, Bridge JA, Neff JR, et al. Trisomy 2 in proliferative fasciitis. *Cancer Genet Cytogenet* 1992;60:27–30.
38. McComb EN, Neff JR, Johansson SL, et al. Chromosomal anomalies in a case of proliferative myositis. *Cancer Genet Cytogenet* 1997;98: 142–144.
39. Sormann GW. The headbangers tumour. *Br J Plast Surg* 1982;35: 72–74.
40. Lewinnek GE, Peterson SE. A calcified fibrocartilagenous nodule in the ligamentum nuchae presenting as a tumor. *Clin Orthop* 1978: 163–165.
41. O'Connell JX, Janzen DL, Hughes TR. Nuchal fibrocartilaginous pseudotumor: a distinctive soft-tissue lesion associated with prior neck injury [Comments]. *Am J Surg Pathol* 1997;21:836–840.

42. Laskin WB, Fetsch JF, Miettinen M. Nuchal fibrocartilaginous pseudotumor: a clinicopathologic study of five cases and review of the literature. *Mod Pathol* 1999;12:663–668.
43. Takeda Y. Cartilaginous metaplasia of the human aponeurosis linguae: histologic and ultrastructural study. *J Oral Med* 1987;42: 35–37,66.
44. Corio RL, Goldblatt LI, Edwards PA. Paraoral cartilage analogue of fibromatosis. *Oral Surg Oral Med Oral Pathol* 1981;52:56–60.
45. Buchner A, Hansen LS. The histomorphologic spectrum of peripheral ossifying fibroma. *Oral Surg Oral Med Oral Pathol* 1987;63:452–461.
46. Kenney JN, Kaugars GE, Abbey LM. Comparison between the peripheral ossifying fibroma and peripheral odontogenic fibroma. *J Oral Maxillofac Surg* 1989;47:378–382.
47. Katsikeris N, Kakarantza-Angelopoulou E, Angelopoulos AP. Peripheral giant cell granuloma. Clinicopathologic study of 224 new cases and review of 956 reported cases. *Int J Oral Maxillofac Surg* 1988;17:94–99.
48. Ackerman LV. Extra-osseous localized non-neoplastic bone and cartilage formation (so-called myositis ossificans). *J Bone Joint Surg Am* 1958;40:279–298.
49. Ferlito A, Barion U, Nicolai P. Myositis ossificans of the head and neck. Review of the literature and report of a case. *Arch Otorhinolaryngol* 1983;237:103–113.
50. Pappas DG, Johnson LA. Laryngeal myositis ossificans. A case report. *Arch Otolaryngol* 1965;81:227–231.
51. Plezia RA, Mintz SM, Calligaro P. Myositis ossificans traumatica of the masseter muscle. Report of a case. *Oral Surg Oral Med Oral Pathol* 1977;44:351–357.
52. Shugar MA, Weber AL, Mulvaney TJ. Myositis ossificans following radical neck dissection. *Ann Otol Rhinol Laryngol* 1981;90:169–171.
53. Woolgar JA, Beirne JC, Triantafyllou A. Myositis ossificans traumatica of sternocleidomastoid muscle presenting as cervical lymph-node metastasis. *Int J Oral Maxillofac Surg* 1995;24:170–173.
54. Odier L. *Manual de medecine pratique.* Geneva: JJ Paschoud, 1811.
55. Peszkowski MJ, Larsson A. Extraosseous and intraosseous oral traumatic neuromas and their association with tooth extraction. *J Oral Maxillofac Surg* 1990;48:963–967.
56. Daneshvar A. Pharyngeal traumatic neuromas and traumatic neuromas with mature ganglion cells (pseudoganglioneuromas). *Am J Surg Pathol* 1990;14:565–570.
57. Som PM, Scherl MP, Rao VM, et al. Rare presentations of ordinary lipomas of the head and neck: a review. *AJNR* 1986;7:657–664.
58. Tsunoda A. Lipoma in the peri-tonsillar space. *J Laryngol Otol* 1994; 108:693–695.
59. Murty KD, Murty PS, George S, et al. Lipoma of the larynx. *Am J Otolaryngol* 1994;15:149–151.
60. Pelissier A, Sawaf MH, Shabana AH. Infiltrating (intramuscular) benign lipoma of the head and neck. *J Oral Maxillofac Surg* 1991; 49: 1231–1236.
61. Fletcher CD, Akerman M, Dal Cin P, et al. Correlation between clinicopathological features and karyotype in lipomatous tumors. A report of 178 cases from the chromosomes and morphology (CHAMP) collaborative study group. *Am J Pathol* 1996;148:623–630.
62. Sreekantaiah C, Leong SP, Chu D, et al. Translocation (X;12)(q27;q14) in a lipoma. *Cancer Genet Cytogenet* 1990;49: 235–239.
63. Mandahl N, Heim S, Johansson B, et al. Lipomas have characteristic structural chromosomal rearrangements of 12q13-q14. *Int J Cancer* 1987;39:685–688.
64. Mandahl N, Heim S, Arheden K, et al. Three major cytogenetic subgroups can be identified among chromosomally abnormal solitary lipomas. *Hum Genet* 1988;79:203–208.
65. Reilly JS, Kelly DR, Royal SA. Angiolipoma of the parotid: case report and review. *Laryngoscope* 1988;98:818–821.
66. Fanburg-Smith JC, Devaney KO, Miettinen M, et al. Multiple spindle cell lipomas: a report of 7 familial and 11 nonfamilial cases. *Am J Surg Pathol* 1998;22:40–48.
67. Mandahl N, Mertens F, Willen H, et al. A new cytogenetic subgroup in lipomas: loss of chromosome 16 material in spindle cell and pleomorphic lipomas. *J Cancer Res Clin Oncol* 1994;120:707–711.
68. Dal Cin P, Sciot R, Polito P, et al. Lesions of 13q may occur independently of deletion of 16q in spindle cell/pleomorphic lipomas. *Histopathology* 1997;31:222–225.
69. Weiss SW, Nickoloff BJ. CD-34 is expressed by a distinctive cell population in peripheral nerve, nerve sheath tumors, and related lesions [Comments]. *Am J Surg Pathol* 1993;17:1039–1045.
70. Shmookler BM, Enzinger FM. Pleomorphic lipoma: a benign tumor simulating liposarcoma. A clinicopathologic analysis of 48 cases. *Cancer* 1981;47:126–133.
71. Collins MH, Chatten J. Lipoblastoma/lipoblastomatosis: a clinicopathologic study of 25 tumors. *Am J Surg Pathol* 1997;21:1131–1137.
72. Worsey J, McGuirt W, Carrau RL, et al. Hibernoma of the neck: a rare cause of neck mass. *Am J Otolaryngol* 1994;15:152–154.
73. Vinayak BC, Reddy KT. Hibernoma in the parotid region. *J Laryngol Otol* 1993;107:257–258.
74. Chan JK, Lee KC, Saw D. Extraskeletal chondroma with lipoblast-like cells. *Hum Pathol* 1986;17:1285–1287.
75. Meis JM, Enzinger FM. Chondroid lipoma. A unique tumor simulating liposarcoma and myxoid chondrosarcoma. *Am J Surg Pathol* 1993;17:1103–1112.
76. Kindblom LG, Meis-Kindblom JM. Chondroid lipoma: an ultrastructural and immunohistochemical analysis with further observations regarding its differentiation [Comments]. *Hum Pathol* 1995; 26:706–715.
77. Nielsen GP, O'Connell JX, Dickersin GR, et al. Chondroid lipoma, a tumor of white fat cells. A brief report of two cases with ultrastructural analysis. *Am J Surg Pathol* 1995;19:1272–1276.
78. Gomez-Ortega JM, Rodilla IG, Basco Lopez de Lerma JM. Chondroid lipoma. A newly described lesion that may be mistaken for malignancy. *Oral Surg Oral Med Oral Pathol Oral Radiol Endod* 1996; 81:586–589.
79. Virchow R. Ein fau von Bo Sartigen Zum Theil in der form des neurons auftretenden fettgeshwulsten. *Virchows Arch* 1857;11:281.
80. Golledge J, Fisher C, Rhys-Evans PH. Head and neck liposarcoma. *Cancer* 1995;76:1051–1058.
81. Wenig BM, Weiss SW, Gnepp DR. Laryngeal and hypopharyngeal liposarcoma. A clinicopathologic study of 10 cases with a comparison to soft-tissue counterparts. *Am J Surg Pathol* 1990;14:134–141.
82. Wenig BM, Heffner DK. Liposarcomas of the larynx and hypopharynx: a clinicopathologic study of eight new cases and a review of the literature. *Laryngoscope* 1995;105:747–756.
83. Stewart MG, Schwartz MR, Alford BR. Atypical and malignant lipomatous lesions of the head and neck. *Arch Otolaryngol Head Neck Surg* 1994;120:1151–1155.
84. Mandell DL, Brandwein MS, Woo P, et al. Upper aerodigestive tract liposarcoma: report on four cases and literature review. *Laryngoscope* 1999;109:1245–1252.
85. Saddik M, Oldring DJ, Mourad WA. Liposarcoma of the base of tongue and tonsillar fossa: a possibly underdiagnosed neoplasm. *Arch Pathol Lab Med* 1996;120:292–295.
86. Yueh B, Bassewitz HL, Eisele DW. Retropharyngeal liposarcoma. *Am J Otolaryngol* 1995;16:331–340.
87. McCulloch TM, Makielski KH, McNutt MA. Head and neck liposarcoma. A histopathologic reevaluation of reported cases. *Arch Otolaryngol Head Neck Surg* 1992;118:1045–1049.
88. Miller D, Goodman M, Weber A, et al. Primary liposarcoma of the larynx. *Trans Am Acad Ophthalmol Otolaryngol* 1975;80:444–447.
89. Dal Cin P, Kools P, Sciot R, et al. Cytogenetic and fluorescence *in situ* hybridization investigation of ring chromosomes characterizing a specific pathologic subgroup of adipose tissue tumors. *Cancer Genet Cytogenet* 1993;68:85–90.
90. Rosai J, Akerman M, Dal Cin P, et al. Combined morphologic and karyotypic study of 59 atypical lipomatous tumors. Evaluation of their relationship and differential diagnosis with other adipose tissue tumors (a report of the CHAMP Study Group). *Am J Surg Pathol* 1996; 20:1182–1189.
91. Kraus MD, Guillou L, Fletcher CD. Well-differentiated inflammatory liposarcoma: an uncommon and easily overlooked variant of a common sarcoma. *Am J Surg Pathol* 1997;21:518–527.

92. Gibas Z, Miettinen M, Limon J, et al. Cytogenetic and immunohistochemical profile of myxoid liposarcoma. *Am J Clin Pathol* 1995; 103:20–26.
93. Smith TA, Easley KA, Goldblum JR. Myxoid/round cell liposarcoma of the extremities. A clinicopathologic study of 29 cases with particular attention to extent of round cell liposarcoma. *Am J Surg Pathol* 1996;20:171–180.
94. Evans HL. Liposarcoma: a study of 55 cases with a reassessment of its classification. *Am J Surg Pathol* 1979;3:507–523.
95. West CB Jr, Shagets FW, Mansfield MJ. Nonsurgical treatment of aggressive fibromatosis in the head and neck [Comments]. *Otolaryngol Head Neck Surg* 1989;101:338–343.
96. el-Sayed Y. Fibromatosis of the head and neck. *J Laryngol Otol* 1992; 106:459–462.
97. Maillard AA, Kountakis SE. Pediatric sino-orbital desmoid fibromatosis. *Ann Otol Rhinol Laryngol* 1996;105:463–466.
98. Masson JK, Soule EH. Desmoid tumors of the head and neck. *Am J Surg* 1966;112:615–622.
99. Gabbiani G, Majno G. Dupuytren's contracture: fibroblast contraction? An ultrastructural study. *Am J Pathol* 1972;66:131–146.
100. de Silva DC, Wright MF, Stevenson DA, et al. Cranial desmoid tumor associated with homozygous inactivation of the adenomatous polyposis coli gene in a 2-year-old girl with familial adenomatous polyposis. *Cancer* 1996;77:972–976.
101. Plaat BE, Balm AJ, Loftus BM, et al. Fibromatosis of the head and neck. *Clin Otolaryngol* 1995;20:103–108.
102. Spear MA, Jennings LC, Mankin HJ, et al. Individualizing management of aggressive fibromatoses. *Int J Radiat Oncol Biol Phys* 1998; 40:637–645.
103. Kamath SS, Parsons JT, Marcus RB, et al. Radiotherapy for local control of aggressive fibromatosis. *Int J Radiat Oncol Biol Phys* 1996;36:325–328.
104. Miyaki M, Konishi M, Kikuchi-Yanoshita R, et al. Coexistence of somatic and germ-line mutations of APC gene in desmoid tumors from patients with familial adenomatous polyposis. *Cancer Res* 1993; 53: 5079–5082.
105. Hoffman CD, Levant BA, Hall RK. Aggressive infantile fibromatosis: report of a case undergoing spontaneous regression. *J Oral Maxillofac Surg* 1993;51:1043–1047.
106. Ramanathan RC, Thomas JM. Infantile (desmoid-type) fibromatosis of the parotid gland. *J Laryngol Otol* 1997;111:669–670.
107. Carr RJ, Zaki GA, Leader MB, et al. Infantile fibromatosis with involvement of the mandible. *Br J Oral Maxillofac Surg* 1992;30: 257–262.
108. McQueen WJ, Johnson JT, Edwards PA. Fibromatosis colli: a case report. *Otolaryngol Head Neck Surg* 1980;88:49–51.
109. Gonzales J, Ljung BM, Guerry T, et al. Congenital torticollis: evaluation by fine-needle aspiration biopsy. *Laryngoscope* 1989;99:651–654.
110. Schwartz RA, Powers CN, Wakely PE Jr, et al. Fibromatosis colli. The utility of fine-needle aspiration in diagnosis. *Arch Otolaryngol Head Neck Surg* 1997;123:301–304.
111. Miyake I, Tokumaru H, Sugino H, et al. Juvenile hyaline fibromatosis. Case report with five years' follow-up. *Am J Dermatopathol* 1995;17:584–590.
112. Shehab ZP, Raafat F, Proops DW. Juvenile hyaline fibromatosis. *Int J Pediatr Otorhinolaryngol* 1995;33:179–186.
113. Remberger K, Krieg T, Kunze D, et al. Fibromatosis hyalinica multiplex (juvenile hyalin fibromatosis). Light microscopic, electron microscopic, immunohistochemical, and biochemical findings. *Cancer* 1985;56:614–624.
114. Iwata S, Horiuchi R, Maeda H, et al. Systemic hyalinosis or juvenile hyaline fibromatosis. Ultrastructural and biochemical study of cultured skin fibroblasts. *Arch Dermatol Res* 1980;267:115–121.
115. Ramer M, Marrone J, Stahl B, et al. Hereditary gingival fibromatosis: identification, treatment, control. *J Am Dent Assoc* 1996;127: 493–495.
116. Tipton DA, Howell KJ, Dabbous MK. Increased proliferation, collagen, and fibronectin production by hereditary gingival fibromatosis fibroblasts. *J Periodontol* 1997;68:524–530.
117. Huang JS, Ho KY, Chen CC, et al. Collagen synthesis in idiopathic and dilantin-induced gingival fibromatosis. *Kao Hsiung I Hsueh Ko Hsueh Tsa Chih* 1997;13:141–148.
118. Enzinger FM, Weiss SW. Benign fibrous tissue tumors. In: *Bone and soft tissue,* 3rd ed. St. Louis: CV Mosby, 1995:186–187.
119. Balachandran K, Allen PW, MacCormac LB. Nuchal fibroma. A clinicopathological study of nine cases [Comments]. *Am J Surg Pathol* 1995;19:313–317.
120. Evans HL. Desmoplastic fibroblastoma. A report of seven cases. *Am J Surg Pathol* 1995;19:1077–1081.
121. Hasegawa T, Shimoda T, Hirohashi S, et al. Collagenous fibroma (desmoplastic fibroblastoma): report of four cases and review of the literature. *Arch Pathol Lab Med* 1998;122:455–460.
122. Miettien JF, Fletch JF. Collagenous fibroma (desmoplastic fibroblastoma) a clinicopathologic study of 63 cases of a distinctive soft tissue lesion with stellate-shaped fibroblasts [Abstract]. *Mod Pathol* 1998; 11:12.
123. Nielsen GP, O'Connell JX, Dickersin GR, et al. Collagenous fibroma (desmoplastic fibroblastoma): a report of seven cases. *Mod Pathol* 1996;9:781–785.
124. Chung EB, Enzinger FM. Infantile myofibromatosis. *Cancer* 1981; 48:1807–1818.
125. Benjamin SP, Mercer RD, Hawk WA. Myofibroblastic contraction in spontaneous regression of multiple congenital mesenchymal hamartomas. *Cancer* 1977;40:2343–2352.
126. Stout AP. Juvenile fibromatoses. *Cancer* 1954;7:953–978.
127. Wiswell TE, Davis J, Cunningham BE, et al. Infantile myofibromatosis: the most common fibrous tumor of infancy. *J Pediatr Surg* 1988;23:315–318.
128. Coffin CM, Neilson KA, Ingels S, et al. Congenital generalized myofibromatosis: a disseminated angiocentric myofibromatosis. *Pediatr Pathol Lab Med* 1995;15:571–587.
129. Jennings TA, Duray PH, Collins FS, et al. Infantile myofibromatosis. Evidence for an autosomal-dominant disorder. *Am J Surg Pathol* 1984;8:529–538.
130. Baird PA, Worth AJ. Congenital generalized fibromatosis: an autosomal recessive condition? *Clin Genet* 1976;9:488–494.
131. Lingen MW, Mostofi RS, Solt DB. Myofibromas of the oral cavity. *Oral Surg Oral Med Oral Pathol Oral Radiol Endod* 1995;80:297–302.
132. Beham A, Badve S, Suster S, et al. Solitary myofibroma in adults: clinicopathological analysis of a series. *Histopathology* 1993;22:335–341.
133. Walsh RM, Leen EJ, Gleeson MJ. Solitary infantile and adult myofibromatosis of the nasal cavity: a report of two cases. *J Laryngol Otol* 1996;110:574–577.
134. Requena L, Kutzner H, Hugel H, et al. Cutaneous adult myofibroma: a vascular neoplasm. *J Cutan Pathol* 1996;23:445–457.
135. Zelger BW, Calonje E, Sepp N, et al. Monophasic cellular variant of infantile myofibromatosis. An unusual histopathologic pattern in two siblings. *Am J Dermatopathol* 1995;17:131–138.
136. Hartig G, Koopmann C Jr, Esclamado R. Infantile myofibromatosis: a commonly misdiagnosed entity. *Otolaryngol Head Neck Surg* 1993; 109:753–757.
137. Weiss SW, Gnepp DR, Bratthauer GL. Palisaded myofibroblastoma. A benign mesenchymal tumor of lymph node. *Am J Surg Pathol* 1989; 13:341–346.
138. Suster S, Rosai J. Intranodal hemorrhagic spindle-cell tumor with "amianthoid" fibers. Report of six cases of a distinctive mesenchymal neoplasm of the inguinal region that simulates Kaposi's sarcoma. *Am J Surg Pathol* 1989;13:347–357.
139. Alguacil-Garcia A. Intranodal myofibroblastoma in a submandibular lymph node. A case report. *Am J Clin Pathol* 1992;97:69–72.
140. Fletcher CD, Stirling RW. Intranodal myofibroblastoma presenting in the submandibular region: evidence of a broader clinical and histological spectrum. *Histopathology* 1990;16:287–293.
141. Nielsen GP, O'Connell JX, Dickersin GR, et al. Solitary fibrous tumor of soft tissue: a report of 15 cases, including 5 malignant examples with light microscopic, immunohistochemical, and ultrastructural data. *Mod Pathol* 1997;10:1028–1037.
142. Dorfman DM, To K, Dickersin GR, et al. Solitary fibrous tumor of the orbit. *Am J Surg Pathol* 1994;18:281–287.

143. Zukerberg LR, Rosenberg AE, Randolph G, et al. Solitary fibrous tumor of the nasal cavity and paranasal sinuses. *Am J Surg Pathol* 1991;15:126–130.
144. Safneck JR, Alguacil-Garcia A, Dort JC, et al. Solitary fibrous tumour: report of two new locations in the upper respiratory tract. *J Laryngol Otol* 1993;107:252–256.
145. Witkin GB, Rosai J. Solitary fibrous tumor of the upper respiratory tract. A report of six cases. *Am J Surg Pathol* 1991;15:842–848.
146. Ferreiro JA, Nascimento AG. Solitary fibrous tumour of the major salivary glands. *Histopathology* 1996;28:261–264.
147. Mentzel T, Bainbridge TC, Katenkamp D. Solitary fibrous tumour: clinicopathological, immunohistochemical, and ultrastructural analysis of 12 cases arising in soft tissues, nasal cavity and nasopharynx, urinary bladder and prostate. *Virchows Arch* 1997;430:445–453.
148. Brunnemann RB, Ro JY, Ordonez NG, et al. Extrapleural solitary fibrous tumor: a clinicopathologic study of 24 cases. *Mod Pathol* 1999; 12:1034–1042.
149. Taccagni G, Sambade C, Nesland J, et al. Solitary fibrous tumour of the thyroid: clinicopathological, immunohistochemical and ultrastructural study of three cases. *Virchows Arch* 1993;422:491–497.
150. Hanau CA, Miettinen M. Solitary fibrous tumor: histological and immunohistochemical spectrum of benign and malignant variants presenting at different sites. *Hum Pathol* 1995;26:440–449.
151. Dei Tos AP, Seregard S, Calonje E, et al. Giant cell angiofibroma. A distinctive orbital tumor in adults. *Am J Surg Pathol* 1995;19: 1286–1293.
152. Shmookler BM, Enzinger FM, Weiss SW. Giant cell fibroblastoma. A juvenile form of dermatofibrosarcoma protuberans. *Cancer* 1989;64:2154–2161.
153. Shmookler BM, Enzinger FM. Giant cell fibroblastoma: a peculiar childhood tumor [Abstract]. *Lab Invest* 1982;46:76.
154. Beham A, Fletcher CD. Dermatofibrosarcoma protuberans with areas resembling giant cell fibroblastoma: report of two cases. *Histopathology* 1990;17:165–167.
155. Michal M, Zamecnik M. Giant cell fibroblastoma with a dermatofibrosarcoma protuberans component. *Am J Dermatopathol* 1992; 14:549–552.
156. Fletcher CD. Giant cell fibroblastoma of soft tissue: a clinicopathological and immunohistochemical study. *Histopathology* 1988;13: 499–508.
157. Dymock RB, Allen PW, Stirling JW, et al. Giant cell fibroblastoma. A distinctive, recurrent tumor of childhood. *Am J Surg Pathol* 1987; 11:263–271.
158. Coyne J, Kaftan SM, Craig RD. Dermatofibrosarcoma protuberans recurring as a giant cell fibroblastoma [Comments]. *Histopathology* 1992;21:184–187.
159. Alguacil-Garcia A. Giant cell fibroblastoma recurring as dermatofibrosarcoma protuberans. *Am J Surg Pathol* 1991;15:798–801.
160. Craver RD, Correa H, Kao YS, et al. Aggressive giant cell fibroblastoma with a balanced 17;22 translocation. *Cancer Genet Cytogenet* 1995;80:20–22.
161. Dal Cin P, Polito P, Van Eyken P, et al. Anomalies of chromosomes 17 and 22 in giant cell fibroblastoma [Letter]. *Cancer Genet Cytogenet* 1997;97:165–166.
162. Bianchi PM, Tucci FM, Bosman C, et al. Paranasal giant cell fibroblastoma: case report and immunohistochemical findings. *Int J Pediatr Otorhinolaryngol* 1994;30:57–61.
163. Kanai Y, Mukai M, Sugiura H, et al. Giant cell fibroblastoma. A case report and immunohistochemical comparison with ten cases of dermatofibrosarcoma protuberans. *Acta Pathol Jpn* 1991;41:552–560.
164. Tran LM, Mark R, Meier R, et al. Sarcomas of the head and neck. Prognostic factors and treatment strategies. *Cancer* 1992;70:169–177.
165. Mark RJ, Sercarz JA, Tran L, et al. Fibrosarcoma of the head and neck. The UCLA experience. *Arch Otolaryngol Head Neck Surg* 1991; 117: 396–401.
166. Greager JA, Reichard K, Campana JP, et al. Fibrosarcoma of the head and neck. *Am J Surg* 1994;167:437–439.
167. Frankenthaler R, Ayala AG, Hartwick RW, et al. Fibrosarcoma of the head and neck. *Laryngoscope* 1990;100:799–802.
168. Knezevich SR, McFadden DE, Tao W, et al. A novel ETV6-NTRK3 gene fusion in congenital fibrosarcoma. *Nat Genet* 1998;18:184–187.
169. Coffin CM, Jaszcz W, O'Shea PA, et al. So-called congenital-infantile fibrosarcoma: does it exist and what is it? *Pediatr Pathol* 1994;14: 133–150.
170. Schofield DE, Fletcher JA, Grier HE, et al. Fibrosarcoma in infants and children. Application of new techniques. *Am J Surg Pathol* 1994;18:14–24.
171. Fisher C. Fibromatosis and fibrosarcoma in infancy and childhood. *Eur J Cancer* 1996;32A:2094–2100.
172. Meis-Kindblom JM, Kindblom LG, Enzinger FM. Sclerosing epithelioid fibrosarcoma. A variant of fibrosarcoma simulating carcinoma. *Am J Surg Pathol* 1995;19:979–993.
173. Eyden BP, Manson C, Banerjee SS, et al. Sclerosing epithelioid fibrosarcoma: a study of five cases emphasizing diagnostic criteria. *Histopathology* 1998;33:354–360.
174. Smith DM, Mahmoud HH, Jenkins JJ 3rd, et al. Myofibrosarcoma of the head and neck in children. *Pediatr Pathol Lab Med* 1995;15: 403–418.
175. O'Brien JE, Stout AP. Malignant fibrous xanthomas. *Cancer* 1964;17:1445–1455.
176. Enzinger FM, Weiss SW. Malignant fibrohistiocytic tumors. In: *Soft tissue tumors,* 3rd ed. St. Louis: CV Mosby, 1995:355–377.
177. Singh B, Shaha A, Har-El G. Malignant fibrous histiocytoma of the head and neck. *J Craniomaxillofac Surg* 1993;21:262–265.
178. Mentzel T, Calonje E, Wadden C, et al. Myxofibrosarcoma. Clinicopathologic analysis of 75 cases with emphasis on the low-grade variant. *Am J Surg Pathol* 1996;20:391–405.
179. Rosenberg AE, O'Connell JX, Dickersin GR, et al. Expression of epithelial markers in malignant fibrous histiocytoma of the musculoskeletal system: an immunohistochemical and electron microscopic study. *Hum Pathol* 1993;24:284–293.
180. Fu YS, Gabbiani G, Kaye GI, et al. Malignant soft tissue tumors of probable histiocytic origin (malignant fibrous histiocytomas): general considerations and electron microscopic and tissue culture studies. *Cancer* 1975;35:176–198.
181. Mairal A, Terrier P, Chibon F, et al. Loss of chromosome 13 is the most frequent genomic imbalance in malignant fibrous histiocytomas. A comparative genomic hybridization analysis of a series of 30 cases. *Cancer Genet Cytogenet* 1999;111:134–138.
182. Wanebo HJ, Koness RJ, MacFarlane JK, et al. Head and neck sarcoma: report of the Head and Neck Sarcoma Registry. Society of Head and Neck Surgeons Committee on Research. *Head Neck* 1992; 14:1–7.
183. Stout AP, Murray MR. Hemangiopericytoma. A vascular tumor featuring Zimmermann's pericytes. *Ann Surg* 1942;116:26–33.
184. Benn JJ, Firth RG, Sonksen PH. Metabolic effects of an insulin-like factor causing hypoglycaemia in a patient with a haemangiopericytoma. *Clin Endocrinol (Oxf)* 1990;32:769–780.
185. Croxatto JO, Font RL. Hemangiopericytoma of the orbit: a clinicopathologic study of 30 cases. *Hum Pathol* 1982;13:210–218.
186. Batsakis JG, Jacobs JB, Templeton AC. Hemangiopericytoma of the nasal cavity: electron-optic study and clinical correlations. *J Laryngol Otol* 1983;97:361–368.
187. Eichhorn JH, Dickersin GR, Bhan AK, et al. Sinonasal hemangiopericytoma. A reassessment with electron microscopy, immunohistochemistry, and long-term follow-up. *Am J Surg Pathol* 1990;14: 856–866.
188. Compagno J, Hyams VJ. Hemangiopericytoma-like intranasal tumors. A clinicopathologic study of 23 cases. *Am J Clin Pathol* 1976; 66:672–683.
189. Enzinger FM, Smith BH. Hemangiopericytoma. An analysis of 106 cases. *Hum Pathol* 1976;7:61–82.
190. Battifora H. Hemangiopericytoma: ultrastructural study of five cases. *Cancer* 1973;31:1418–1432.
191. Sreekantaiah C, Bridge JA, Rao UN, et al. Clonal chromosomal abnormalities in hemangiopericytoma. *Cancer Genet Cytogenet* 1991; 54:173–181.
192. Enzinger FM, Weiss SW. Perivascular tumors. In: *Soft tissue tumors,* 3rd ed. St. Louis: CV Mosby, 1995:713–729.

193. Alpers CE, Rosenau W, Finkbeiner WE, et al. Congenital (infantile) hemangiopericytoma of the tongue and sublingual region. *Am J Clin Pathol* 1984;81:377–382.
194. Seibert JJ, Seibert RW, Weisenburger DS, et al. Multiple congenital hemangiopericytomas of the head and neck. *Laryngoscope* 1978;88: 1006–1012.
195. Ordonez NG, Mackay B, el-Naggar AK, et al. Congenital hemangiopericytoma. An ultrastructural, immunocytochemical, and flow cytometric study. *Arch Pathol Lab Med* 1993;117:934–937.
196. Kauffman SL, Stout AP. Hemangiopericytoma in children. *Cancer* 1960;13:695–710.
197. Nielsen GP, Dickersin GR, Provenzal JM, et al. Lipomatous hemangiopericytoma. A histologic, ultrastructural and immunohistochemical study of a unique variant of hemangiopericytoma. *Am J Surg Pathol* 1995;19:748–756.
198. Masson P. Le glomus neuromyoarterial des regions tactilis et ses toumers. *Lyon Chir* 1924;21:257.
199. Enzinger FM, Weiss SW. Perivascular tumors. In: *Soft tissue tumors,* 3rd ed. St. Louis: CV Mosby, 1995:701–713.
200. Gould EW, Manivel JC, Albores-Saavedra J, et al. Locally infiltrative glomus tumors and glomangiosarcomas. A clinical, ultrastructural, and immunohistochemical study. *Cancer* 1990;65:310–318.
201. Dervan PA, Tobbia IN, Casey M, et al. Glomus tumours: an immunohistochemical profile of 11 cases. *Histopathology* 1989;14: 483–491.
202. Tsuneyoshi M, Enjoji M. Glomus tumor: a clinicopathologic and electron microscopic study. *Cancer* 1982;50:1601–1607.
203. Aiba M, Hirayama A, Kuramochi S. Glomangiosarcoma in a glomus tumor. An immunohistochemical and ultrastructural study. *Cancer* 1988;61:1467–1471.
204. Bill AH, Sumner DS. A unified concept of lymphangioma and cystic hygroma. *Surg Gynecol Obstet* 1965:79–86.
205. Emery PJ, Bailey CM, Evans JN. Cystic hygroma of the head and neck. A review of 37 cases. *J Laryngol Otol* 1984;98:613–619.
206. Ricciardelli EJ, Richardson MA. Cervicofacial cystic hygroma. Patterns of recurrence and management of the difficult case. *Arch Otolaryngol Head Neck Surg* 1991;117:546–553.
207. Work WP. Hemangiomas of the head and neck. *Ann Otol Rhinol Laryngol* 1978;87:633–635.
208. Chervenak FA, Isaacson G, Blakemore KJ, et al. Fetal cystic hygroma. Cause and natural history. *N Engl J Med* 1983;309:822–825.
209. Jackson IT, Carreno R, Potparic Z, et al. Hemangiomas, vascular malformations, and lymphovenous malformations: classification and methods of treatment. *Plast Reconstr Surg* 1993;91:1216–1230.
210. Stal S, Hamilton S, Spira M. Hemangiomas, lymphangiomas, and vascular malformations of the head and neck. *Otolaryngol Clin North Am* 1986;19:769–796.
211. Rossiter JL, Hendrix RA, Tom LW, et al. Intramuscular hemangioma of the head and neck. *Otolaryngol Head Neck Surg* 1993;108: 18–26.
212. Kohout MP, Hansen M, Pribaz JJ, et al. Arteriovenous malformations of the head and neck: natural history and management. *Plast Reconstr Surg* 1998;102:643–654.
213. Wells GC, Whimster IW. Subcutaneous angiolymphoid hyperplasia with eosinophilia. *Br J Dermatol* 1969;81:1–14.
214. Castro C, Winkelmann RK. Angiolymphoid hyperplasia with eosinophilia in the skin. *Cancer* 1974;34:1696–1705.
215. Urabe A, Tsuneyoshi M, Enjoji M. Epithelioid hemangioma versus Kimura's disease. A comparative clinicopathologic study. *Am J Surg Pathol* 1987;11:758–766.
216. Tsang WY, Chan JK. The family of epithelioid vascular tumors. *Histol Histopathol* 1993;8:187–212.
217. Gray MH, Rosenberg AE, Dickersin GR, et al. Cytokeratin expression in epithelioid vascular neoplasms. *Hum Pathol* 1990;21:212–217.
218. Don DM, Ishiyama A, Johnstone AK, et al. Angiolymphoid hyperplasia with eosinophilia and vascular tumors of the head and neck. *Am J Otolaryngol* 1996;17:240–245.
219. Googe PB, Harris NL, Mihm MC Jr. Kimura's disease and angiolymphoid hyperplasia with eosinophilia: two distinct histopathological entities. *J Cutan Pathol* 1987;14:263–271.
220. Ellis GL, Kratochvil FJD. Epithelioid hemangioendothelioma of the head and neck: a clinicopathologic report of twelve cases. *Oral Surg Oral Med Oral Pathol* 1986;61:61–68.
221. Perkins P, Weiss SW. Spindle cell hemangioendothelioma. An analysis of 78 cases with reassessment of its pathogenesis and biologic behavior. *Am J Surg Pathol* 1996;20:1196–1204.
222. Weiss SW, Enzinger FM. Spindle cell hemangioendothelioma. A low-grade angiosarcoma resembling a cavernous hemangioma and Kaposi's sarcoma. *Am J Surg Pathol* 1986;10:521–530.
223. Fletcher CD, Beham A, Schmid C. Spindle cell haemangioendothelioma: a clinicopathological and immunohistochemical study indicative of a non-neoplastic lesion [Comments]. *Histopathology* 1991;18: 291–301.
224. Goldberg AN. Kaposi's sarcoma of the head and neck in acquired immunodeficiency syndrome. *Am J Otolaryngol* 1993;14:5–14.
225. Li JJ, Huang YQ, Cockerell CJ, et al. Localization of human herpes-like virus type 8 in vascular endothelial cells and perivascular spindle-shaped cells of Kaposi's sarcoma lesions by in situ hybridization. *Am J Pathol* 1996;148:1741–1748.
226. O'Neill E, Henson TH, Ghorbani AJ, et al. Herpes virus–like sequences are specifically found in Kaposi sarcoma lesions. *J Clin Pathol* 1996;49:306–308.
227. Porter SR, Di Alberti L, Kumar N. Human herpes virus 8 (Kaposi's sarcoma herpesvirus). *Oral Oncol* 1998;34:5–14.
228. Aust MR, Olsen KD, Lewis JE, et al. Angiosarcomas of the head and neck: clinical and pathologic characteristics. *Ann Otol Rhinol Laryngol* 1997;106:943–951.
229. Naka N, Ohsawa M, Tomita Y, et al. Prognostic factors in angiosarcoma: a multivariate analysis of 55 cases. *J Surg Oncol* 1996;61: 170–176.
230. Weber CO. Anatonische untersuchung einer hypertrophischen zunge nebst bemerkungen uber dil neubildung quergestreifter muskelfasern. *Virchows Arch* 1854;7:115–125.
231. Abrikossoff A. Ubermyome, ausgehenot von der quergestreifter villkurlicher musculatur. *Virchows Arch* 1926;160:260–215.
232. Buley ID, Gatter KC, Kelly PM, et al. Granular cell tumours revisited. An immunohistological and ultrastructural study. *Histopathology* 1988;12:263–274.
233. Apisarnthanarax P. Granular cell tumor. An analysis of 16 cases and review of the literature. *J Am Acad Dermatol* 1981;5:171–182.
234. Said-Al-Naief N, Ivanov K, Jones M, et al. Granular cell tumor of the parotid. *Ann Diagn Pathol* 1999;3:35–38.
235. Kershisnik M, Batsakis JG, Mackay B. Granular cell tumors. *Ann Otol Rhinol Laryngol* 1994;103:416–419.
236. Mittal KR, True LD. Origin of granules in granular cell tumor. Intracellular myelin formation with autodigestion. *Arch Pathol Lab Med* 1988;112:302–303.
237. Billeret-Lebranchu V, Martin de la Salle E, Vandenhaute B, et al. Granular cell tumor and congenital epulis. Histochemical and immunohistochemical of 58 cases. *Arch Anat Cytol Pathol* 1999; 47: 31–37.
238. Mackie RM, Campbell I, Turbitt ML. Use of NK1 C3 monoclonal antibody in the assessment of benign and malignant melanocytic lesions. *J Clin Pathol* 1984;37:367–372.
239. Chrysomali E, Papanicolaou SI, Dekker NP, et al. Benign neural tumors of the oral cavity: a comparative immunohistochemical study. *Oral Surg Oral Med Oral Pathol Oral Radiol Endod* 1997;84:381–390.
240. Bedetti CD, Martinez AJ, Beckford NS, et al. Granular cell tumor arising in myelinated peripheral nerves. Light and electron microscopy and immunoperoxidase study. *Virchows Arch* 1983;402:175–183.
241. Fisher ER, Wechsler H. Granular cell myoblastoma—a misnomer: EM and histochemical evidence concerning its Schwann cell derivation and nature (granular cell schwannoma). *Cancer* 1962;936.
242. Fanburg-Smith JC, Meis-Kindblom JM, Fante R, et al. Malignant granular cell tumor of soft tissue: diagnostic criteria and clinicopathologic correlation. *Am J Surg Pathol* 1998;22:779–794 [erratum in *Am J Surg Pathol* 1999;23:136].
243. Khansur T, Balducci L, Tavassoli M. Granular cell tumor. Clinical spectrum of the benign and malignant entity. *Cancer* 1987;60: 220–222.

244. Scheithauer BW, Woodruff JM, Erlandson RA. Miscellaneous benign neurogenic tumors. In: *Tumors of the peripheral nervous system.* Washington, DC: Armed Forces Institute of Pathology, 1999: 219–236.
245. Tsang WY, Chan JK, Chow LT, et al. Perineurioma: an uncommon soft tissue neoplasm distinct from localized hypertrophic neuropathy and neurofibroma. *Am J Surg Pathol* 1992;16:756–763.
246. Giannini C, Scheithauer BW, Jenkins RB, et al. Soft-tissue perineurioma. Evidence for an abnormality of chromosome 22, criteria for diagnosis, and review of the literature. *Am J Surg Pathol* 1997;21: 164–173.
247. Lazarus SS, Trombetta LD. Ultrastructural identification of a benign perineurial cell tumor. *Cancer* 1978;41:1823–1829.
248. Stanton C, Perentes E, Phillips L, VandenBerg SR. The immunohistochemical demonstration of early perineurial change in the development of localized hypertrophic neuropathy. *Hum Pathol* 1988;19: 1455–1457.
249. Hirose T, Sumitomo M, Kudo E, et al. Malignant peripheral nerve sheath tumor (MPNST) showing perineurial cell differentiation [Comments]. *Am J Surg Pathol* 1989;13:613–620.
250. Hirose T, Scheithauer BW, Sano T. Malignant perineurioma: a study of 8 cases [Abstract]. *Mod Pathol* 1997;10:1075–1081.
251. Reed RJ, Fine RM, Meltzer HD. Palisaded, encapsulated neuromas of the skin. *Arch Dermatol* 1972;106:865–870.
252. Fletcher CD. Solitary circumscribed neuroma of the skin (so-called palisaded, encapsulated neuroma). A clinicopathologic and immunohistochemical study. *Am J Surg Pathol* 1989;13:574–580.
253. Megahed M. Palisaded encapsulated neuroma (solitary circumscribed neuroma). A clinicopathologic and immunohistochemical study [Comments]. *Am J Dermatopathol* 1994;16:120–125.
254. Magnusson B. Palisaded encapsulated neuroma (solitary circumscribed neuroma) of the oral mucosa. *Oral Surg Oral Med Oral Pathol Oral Radiol Endod* 1996;82:302–304.
255. Dakin MC, Leppard B, Theaker JM. The palisaded, encapsulated neuroma (solitary circumscribed neuroma). *Histopathology* 1992;20: 405–410.
256. Dover JS, From L, Lewis A. Palisaded encapsulated neuromas. A clinicopathologic study. *Arch Dermatol* 1989;125:386–389.
257. Argenyi ZB, Santa Cruz D, Bromley C. Comparative light-microscopic and immunohistochemical study of traumatic and palisaded encapsulated neuromas of the skin. *Am J Dermatopathol* 1992;14: 504–510.
258. Tsang WY, Chan JK. Epithelioid variant of solitary circumscribed neuroma of the skin. *Histopathology* 1992;20:439–441.
259. Albrecht S, Kahn HJ, From L. Palisaded encapsulated neuroma: an immunohistochemical study. *Mod Pathol* 1989;2:403–406.
260. Geschickter CF. Tumors of the peripheral nerves. *Am J Cancer* 1935;25:377.
261. Griffith BH, Lewis VL Jr, McKinney P. Neurofibromas of the head and neck. *Surg Gynecol Obstet* 1985;160:534–538.
262. Weiss SW, Langloss JM, Enzinger FM. Value of S-100 protein in the diagnosis of soft tissue tumors with particular reference to benign and malignant Schwann cell tumors. *Lab Invest* 1983;49:299–308.
263. Enzinger FM, Weiss SW. Benign tumors of peripheral nerves. In: *Soft tissue tumors,* 3rd ed. St. Louis: CV Mosby, 1995:843–863.
264. Barker D, Wright E, Nguyen K, et al. Gene for von Recklinghausen neurofibromatosis is in the pericentromeric region of chromosome 17. *Science* 1987;236:1100–1102.
265. Adkins JC, Ravitch MM. The operative management of von Recklinghausen's neurofibromatosis in children, with special reference to lesions of the head and neck. *Surgery* 1977;82:342–348.
266. Guccion JG, Enzinger FM. Malignant schwannoma associated with von Recklinghausen's neurofibromatosis. *Virchows Arch* 1979; 383:43–57.
267. Verocay J. Zur kenntinis der "neurofibrome." *Beitr Pathol Anat* 1910; 48:1–68.
268. Hasegawa SL, Mentzel T, Fletcher CD. Schwannomas of the sinonasal tract and nasopharynx. *Mod Pathol* 1997;10:777–784.
269. al-Ghamdi S, Black MJ, Lafond G. Extracranial head and neck schwannomas. *J Otolaryngol* 1992;21:186–188.
270. Jamal MN. Schwannoma of the larynx: case report, and review of the literature. *J Laryngol Otol* 1994;108:788–790.
271. Bruner JM. Peripheral nerve sheath tumors of the head and neck. *Semin Diagn Pathol* 1987;4:136–149.
272. White W, Shiu MH, Rosenblum MK, et al. Cellular schwannoma. A clinicopathologic study of 57 patients and 58 tumors. *Cancer* 1990;66:1266–1275.
273. Iwashita T, Enjoji M. Plexiform neurilemmoma: a clinicopathological and immunohistochemical analysis of 23 tumours from 20 patients. *Virchows Arch* 1987;411:305–309.
274. Rasbridge SA, Browse NL, Tighe JR, et al. Malignant nerve sheath tumour arising in a benign ancient schwannoma. *Histopathology* 1989;14:525–528.
275. Greager JA, Reichard KW, Campana JP, et al. Malignant schwannoma of the head and neck. *Am J Surg* 1992;163:440–442.
276. Bailet JW, Abemayor E, Andrews JC, et al. Malignant nerve sheath tumors of the head and neck: a combined experience from two university hospitals. *Laryngoscope* 1991;101:1044–1049.
277. Ghosh BC, Ghosh L, Huvos AG, et al. Malignant schwannoma. A clinicopathologic study. *Cancer* 1973;31:184–190.
278. Colmenero C, Rivers T, Patron M, et al. Maxillofacial malignant peripheral nerve sheath tumours. *J Craniomaxillofac Surg* 1991;19: 40–46.
279. Fernandez PL, Cardesa A, Bombi JA, et al. Malignant sinonasal epithelioid schwannoma. *Virchows Arch* 1993;423:401–405.
280. DiCarlo EF, Woodruff JM, Bansal M, et al. The purely epithelioid malignant peripheral nerve sheath tumor. *Am J Surg Pathol* 1986; 10:478–490.
281. Daimaru Y, Hashimoto H, Enjoji M. Malignant peripheral nerve-sheath tumors (malignant schwannomas). An immunohistochemical study of 29 cases. *Am J Surg Pathol* 1985;9:434–444.
282. Matsunou H, Shimoda T, Kakimoto S, et al. Histopathologic and immunohistochemical study of malignant tumors of peripheral nerve sheath (malignant schwannoma). *Cancer* 1985;56:2269–2279.
283. Taxy JB, Battifora H, Trujillo Y, et al. Electron microscopy in the diagnosis of malignant schwannoma. *Cancer* 1981;48:1381–1391.
284. Konrad EA, Meister P, Hubner G. Extracardiac rhabdomyoma: report of different types with light microscopic and ultrastructural studies. *Cancer* 1982;49:898–907.
285. Helliwell TR, Sissons MC, Stoney PJ, et al. Immunochemistry and electron microscopy of head and neck rhabdomyoma. *J Clin Pathol* 1988;41:1058–1063.
286. Di Sant'Agnese PA, Knowles DM 2d. Extracardiac rhabdomyoma: a clinicopathologic study and review of the literature. *Cancer* 1980; 46:780–789.
287. Dehner LP, Enzinger FM, Font RL. Fetal rhabdomyoma. An analysis of nine cases. *Cancer* 1972;30:160–166.
288. Agamanolis DP, Dasu S, Krill CE Jr. Tumors of skeletal muscle. *Hum Pathol* 1986;17:778–795.
289. Gardner DG, Corio RL. Multifocal adult rhabdomyoma. *Oral Surg Oral Med Oral Pathol* 1983;56:76–78.
290. Willis J, Abdul-Karim FW, di Sant'Agnese PA. Extracardiac rhabdomyomas. *Semin Diagn Pathol* 1994;11:15–25.
291. Gibas Z, Miettinen M. Recurrent parapharyngeal rhabdomyoma. Evidence of neoplastic nature of the tumor from cytogenetic study. *Am J Surg Pathol* 1992;16:721–728.
292. Nakhleh RE, Swanson PE, Dehner LP. Juvenile (embryonal and alveolar) rhabdomyosarcoma of the head and neck in adults. A clinical, pathologic, and immunohistochemical study of 12 cases. *Cancer* 1991;67:1019–1024.
293. Anderson GJ, Tom LW, Womer RB, et al. Rhabdomyosarcoma of the head and neck in children. *Arch Otolaryngol Head Neck Surg* 1990; 116:428–431.
294. Cavazzana AO, Schmidt D, Ninfo V, et al. Spindle cell rhabdomyosarcoma. A prognostically favorable variant of rhabdomyosarcoma. *Am J Surg Pathol* 1992;16:229–235.
295. Miettinen M, Rapola J. Immunohistochemical spectrum of rhabdomyosarcoma and rhabdomyosarcoma-like tumors. Expression of cytokeratin and the 68-kD neurofilament protein. *Am J Surg Pathol* 1989;13:120–132.

296. el-Naggar AK, Batsakis JG, Ordonez NG, et al. Rhabdomyosarcoma of the adult head and neck: a clinicopathological and DNA ploidy study. *J Laryngol Otol* 1993;107:716–720.
297. Dal Cin P, Brock P, Aly MS, et al. A variant (2;13) translocation in rhabdomyosarcoma. *Cancer Genet Cytogenet* 1991;55:191–195.
298. Polito P, Dal Cin P, Sciot R, et al. Embryonal rhabdomyosarcoma with only numerical chromosome changes. Case report and review of the literature. *Cancer Genet Cytogenet* 1999;109:161–165.
299. Kraus DH, Saenz NC, Gollamudi S, et al. Pediatric rhabdomyosarcoma of the head and neck. *Am J Surg* 1997;174:556–560.
300. La Quaglia MP, Heller G, Ghavimi F, et al. The effect of age at diagnosis on outcome in rhabdomyosarcoma. *Cancer* 1994;73:109–117.
301. Wharam MD, Beltangady MS, Heyn RM, et al. Pediatric orofacial and laryngopharyngeal rhabdomyosarcoma. An Intergroup Rhabdomyosarcoma Study report. *Arch Otolaryngol Head Neck Surg* 1987;113:1225–1227.
302. Natiella JR, Neiders ME, Greene GW. Oral leiomyoma. Report of six cases and a review of the literature. *J Oral Pathol* 1982;11:353–365.
303. Dharnidharka VR, Bahl NK, Kandoth PW, et al. Retropharyngeal leiomyoma: case report and review of the literature. *Head Neck* 1993;15:161–163.
304. Izumi K, Maeda T, Cheng J, et al. Primary leiomyosarcoma of the maxilla with regional lymph node metastasis. Report of a case and review of the literature. *Oral Surg Oral Med Oral Pathol Oral Radiol Endod* 1995;80:310–319.
305. Mindell RS, Calcaterra TC, Ward PH. Leiomyosarcoma of the head and neck: a review of the literature and report of two cases. *Laryngoscope* 1975;85:904–910.
306. Smith LW. Synoviomata. *Am J Pathol* 1927;3:355.
307. Carrillo R, Rodriguez-Peralto JL, Batsakis JG. Synovial sarcomas of the head and neck. *Ann Otol Rhinol Laryngol* 1992;101:367–370.
308. Pai S, Chinoy RF, Pradhan SA, et al. Head and neck synovial sarcomas. *J Surg Oncol* 1993;54:82–86.
309. Roth JA, Enzinger FM, Tannenbaum M. Synovial sarcoma of the neck: a followup study of 24 cases. *Cancer* 1975;35:1243–1253.
310. Amble FR, Olsen KD, Nascimento AG, et al. Head and neck synovial cell sarcoma. *Otolaryngol Head Neck Surg* 1992;107:631–637.
311. Dickersin GR. Synovial sarcoma: a review and update, with emphasis on the ultrastructural characterization of the nonglandular component. *Ultrastruct Pathol* 1991;15:379–402.
312. Argani P, Zakowski MF, Klimstra DS, et al. Detection of the SYT-SSX chimeric RNA of synovial sarcoma in paraffin-embedded tissue and its application in problematic cases. *Mod Pathol* 1998;11:65–71 [erratum in *Mod Pathol* 1998;11:592].
313. Cihak RA, Lydiatt WM, Lydiatt DD, et al. Synovial sarcoma of the head and neck: chromosomal translation (X;18) as a diagnostic aid. *Head Neck* 1997;19:549–553.
314. Kawai A, Woodruff J, Healey JH, et al. SYT-SSX gene fusion as a determinant of morphology and prognosis in synovial sarcoma [Comments]. *N Engl J Med* 1998;338:153–160.
315. Mullen JR, Zagars GK. Synovial sarcoma outcome following conservation surgery and radiotherapy. *Radiother Oncol* 1994;33:23–30.
316. Bergh P, Meis-Kindblom JM, Gherlinzoni F, et al. Synovial sarcoma: identification of low and high risk groups [Comments]. *Cancer* 1999;85:2596–2607.
317. Christopherson WM, Foot FW. Alveolar soft-part sarcomas. *Cancer* 1952;5:100–111.
318. Batsakis JG. Alveolar soft-part sarcoma. *Ann Otol Rhinol Laryngol* 1988;97:328–329.
319. Welsh RA, Bray DMD, Shipkey FH, et al. Histogenesis of alveolar soft part sarcoma. *Cancer* 1972;29:191–204.
320. De Sautel M, Gandour-Edwards R, Donald P, et al. Alveolar soft part sarcoma: report of a case occurring in the larynx. *Otolaryngol Head Neck Surg* 1997;117(suppl):95–97.
321. Marker P, Jensen ML, Siemssen SJ. Alveolar soft-part sarcoma of the oral cavity: report of a case and review of the literature. *J Oral Maxillofac Surg* 1995;53:1203–1208.
322. Hunter BC, Devaney KO, Ferlito A, et al. Alveolar soft part sarcoma of the head and neck region. *Ann Otol Rhinol Laryngol* 1998;107:810–814.
323. Simmons WB, Haggerty HS, Ngan B, et al. Alveolar soft part sarcoma of the head and neck. A disease of children and young adults. *Int J Pediatr Otorhinolaryngol* 1989;17:139–153.
324. Shipkey FH, Lieberman PH, Foote FW. Ultrastructure of alveolar soft part sarcoma. *Cancer* 1964;17:821.
325. van Echten J, van den Berg E, van Baarlen J, et al. An important role for chromosome 17, band q25, in the histogenesis of alveolar soft part sarcoma. *Cancer Genet Cytogenet* 1995;82:57–61.
326. Sherman N, Vavilala M, Pollock R, et al. Radiation therapy for alveolar soft-part sarcoma. *Med Pediatr Oncol* 1994;22:380–383.
327. Lieberman PH, Brennan MF, Kimmel M, et al. Alveolar soft-part sarcoma. A clinico-pathologic study of half a century. *Cancer* 1989;63:1–13.
328. Nakashima Y, Kotoura Y, Kasakura K, et al. Alveolar soft-part sarcoma. A report of ten cases. *Clin Orthop* 1993:259–266.
329. Jong R, Kandel R, Fornasier V, et al. Alveolar soft part sarcoma: review of nine cases including two cases with unusual histology. *Histopathology* 1998;32:63–68.
330. Pappo AS, Parham DM, Cain A, et al. Alveolar soft part sarcoma in children and adolescents: clinical features and outcome of 11 patients. *Med Pediatr Oncol* 1996;26:81–84.
331. Enzinger FM, Weiss SW. Malignant soft tissue tumors of uncertain type. In: *Soft tissue tumors,* 3rd ed. St. Louis: CV Mosby, 1995:1074–1083.
332. Vadmal M, Hajdu SI, Arlen M. Epithelioid sarcoma of the temporomandibular region: a case report. *J Oral Maxillofac Surg* 1997;55:754–758.
333. Batsakis JG. Epithelioid sarcoma. *Ann Otol Rhinol Laryngol* 1989;98:659–660.
334. White VA, Heathcote JG, Hurwitz JJ, et al. Epithelioid sarcoma of the orbit. *Ophthalmology* 1994;101:1680–1687.
335. Chase DR, Enzinger FM. Epithelioid sarcoma. Diagnosis, prognostic indicators, and treatment. *Am J Surg Pathol* 1985;9:241–263.
336. Enzinger FM. Epithelioid sarcoma. A sarcoma simulating a granuloma or a carcinoma. *Cancer* 1970;26:1029–1041.
337. Chase DR, Enzinger FM, Weiss SW, et al. Keratin in epithelioid sarcoma. An immunohistochemical study. *Am J Surg Pathol* 1984;8:435–441.
338. Miettinen M, Fanburg-Smith JC, Virolainen M, et al. Epithelioid sarcoma: an immunohistochemical analysis of 112 classical and variant cases and a discussion of the differential diagnosis. *Hum Pathol* 1999;30:934–942.
339. Fisher C. Epithelioid sarcoma: the spectrum of ultrastructural differentiation in seven immunohistochemically defined cases. *Hum Pathol* 1988;19:265–275.
340. Kraus DH, Dubner S, Harrison LB, et al. Prognostic factors for recurrence and survival in head and neck soft tissue sarcomas. *Cancer* 1994;74:697–702.
341. Lack EE, Cubilla AL, Woodruff JM. Paragangliomas of the head and neck region. A pathologic study of tumors from 71 patients. *Hum Pathol* 1979;10:191–218.
342. Paulus W, Jellinger K, Brenner H. Melanotic paraganglioma of the orbit: a case report. *Acta Neuropathol* 1989;79:340–346.
343. Lack EE. *Tumors of the adrenal gland and extra-adrenal paraganglia.* Washington, DC: Armed Forces Institute of Pathology, 1997.
344. Saldana MJ, Salem LE, Travezan R. High altitude hypoxia and chemodectomas. *Hum Pathol* 1973;4:251–263.
345. Lack EE, Cubilla AL, Woodruff JM, et al. Paragangliomas of the head and neck region: a clinical study of 69 patients. *Cancer* 1977;39:397–409.
346. Kahn LB. Vagal body tumor (nonchromaffin paraganglioma, chemodectoma, and carotid body-like tumor) with cervical node metastasis and familial association: ultrastructural study and review. *Cancer* 1976;38:2367–2377.
347. Parry DM, Li FP, Strong LC, et al. Carotid body tumors in humans: genetics and epidemiology. *J Natl Cancer Inst* 1982;68:573–578.
348. Linnoila RI, Becker RL Jr., Steinberg SM, et al. The role of S100 protein containing cells in the prognosis of symathoadrenal paragangliomas [abstract]. *Mod Pathol* 1993;6:39A.

349. Johnson TL, Zarbo RJ, Lloyd RV, et al. Paragangliomas of the head and neck: immunohistochemical neuroendocrine and intermediate filament typing. *Mod Pathol* 1988;1:216–223.
350. Schroder HD, Johannsen L. Demonstration of S-100 protein in sustentacular cells of phaeochromocytomas and paragangliomas. *Histopathology* 1986;10:1023–1033.
351. Grimley PM, Glenner GG. Histology and ultrastructure of carotid body paragangliomas. Comparison with the normal gland. *Cancer* 1967;20:1473–1488.
352. Toker C. Ultrastructure of a chemodectoma. *Cancer* 1967;20: 271–280.
353. Verniers DA, Keus RB, Schouwenburg PF, et al. Radiation therapy, an important mode of treatment for head and neck chemodectomas. *Eur J Cancer* 1992;28A:1028–1033.
354. Powell S, Peters N, Harmer C. Chemodectoma of the head and neck: results of treatment in 84 patients. *Int J Radiat Oncol Biol Phys* 1992;22:919–924.
355. Massey V, Wallner K. Treatment of metastatic chemodectoma. *Cancer* 1992;69:790–792.
356. Pontius KI, Sebek BA. Extraskeletal Ewing's sarcoma arising in the nasal fossa. Light- and electron-microscopic observations. *Am J Clin Pathol* 1981;75:410–415.
357. Suster S, Ronnen M, Huszar M. Extraskeletal Ewing's sarcoma of the scalp. *Pediatr Dermatol* 1988;5:123–126.
358. Lane S, Ironside JW. Extra-skeletal Ewing's sarcoma of the nasal fossa. *J Laryngol Otol* 1990;104:570–573.
359. Lim TC, Tan WT, Lee YS. Congenital extraskeletal Ewing's sarcoma of the face: a case report. *Head Neck* 1994;16:75–78.
360. Zachariades N, Koumoura F, Liapi-Avgeri G, et al. Extraskeletal Ewing's sarcoma of the parotid region: a case report with the detection of the tumour's immunophenotypical characteristics. *Br J Oral Maxillofac Surg* 1994;32:328–331.
361. Ambros IM, Ambros PF, Strehl S, et al. MIC2 is a specific marker for Ewing's sarcoma and peripheral primitive neuroectodermal tumors. Evidence for a common histogenesis of Ewing's sarcoma and peripheral primitive neuroectodermal tumors from MIC2 expression and specific chromosome aberration. *Cancer* 1991;67:1886–1893.
362. Ahmad R, Mayol BR, Davis M, et al. Extraskeletal Ewing's sarcoma. *Cancer* 1999;85:725–731.
363. Chung EB, Enzinger FM. Chondroma of soft parts. *Cancer* 1978; 41:1414–1424.
364. Blum MR, Danford M, Speight PM. Soft tissue chondroma of the cheek. *J Oral Pathol Med* 1993;22:334–336.
365. Kamysz JW, Zawin JK, Gonzalez-Crussi F. Soft tissue chondroma of the neck: a case report and review of the literature. *Pediatr Radiol* 1996;26:145–147.
366. Reiman HM, Dahlin DC. Cartilage- and bone-forming tumors of the soft tissues. *Semin Diagn Pathol* 1986;3:288–305.
367. Ramachandran K, Viswanathan R. Chondroma of the tongue. Report of a case. *Oral Surg Oral Med Oral Pathol* 1968;25:487–490.
368. Hankey GT, Waterhouse JP. A calcifying chondroma in the cheek. *Br J Oral Surg* 1968;5:239–244.
369. Schweitzer ME, Greenway G, Resnick D, et al. Osteoma of soft parts. *Skel Radiol* 1992;21:177–180.
370. Munro JM, Singh MP. Chondroma of the tongue. Report of a case and a consideration of the histogenesis of such lesions. *Arch Pathol Lab Med* 1990;114:541–542.
371. Segal K, Sidi J, Katzav Y, et al. Chondroma of the tongue. Report of two cases. *Ann Otol Rhinol Laryngol* 1984;93:271–272.
372. Smith BC, Ellis GL, Meis-Kindblom JM, et al. Ectomesenchymal chondromyxoid tumor of the anterior tongue. Nineteen cases of a new clinicopathologic entity [Comments]. *Am J Surg Pathol* 1995;19: 519–530.
373. van der Wal JE, van der Waal I. Ectomesenchymal chondromyxoid tumor of the anterior tongue. Report of a case. *J Oral Pathol Med* 1996;25:456–458.
374. Kannan R, Damm DD, White DK, et al. Ectomesenchymal chondromyxoid tumor of the anterior tongue: a report of three cases. *Oral Surg Oral Med Oral Pathol Oral Radiol Endod* 1996;82:417–422.

11

PATHOLOGY OF SELECTED DISEASES AFFECTING THE BONES AND JOINTS OF THE HEAD AND NECK

G. PETUR NIELSEN
JOHN X. O'CONNELL
ANDREW E. ROSENBERG

Almost every disease that affects the appendicular musculoskeletal system also can involve the bones and joints of the head and neck region. This chapter discusses the pathology of selected important examples of ischemic conditions, infection, metabolic processes, and benign and malignant neoplasms of the craniofacial skeleton. The majority of the chapter focuses on neoplasms, which pose the greatest diagnostic challenges to surgical pathologists. The head and neck region is a repository for all types of primary bone neoplasms; however, tumors such as osteomas, fibroosseous lesions, hemangiomas, giant cell reparative granulomas (GCRGs), and Langerhans' cell histiocytosis are more common in this area than elsewhere in the skeleton, whereas osteochondromas, enchondromas, osteoblastomas, and Ewing's sarcoma/primitive neuroectodermal tumor (PNET) are considerably less frequent. The basis of this relationship between anatomic site and tumor type is unknown except for cartilage neoplasms, because they do not arise in bones that do not form from the process of enchondral ossification during embryologic development. Although relatively uncommon, diseases of the craniofacial skeleton are important because of the clinical and pathologic heterogeneity and because they have significant impact on the well-being of the patient.

NON-NEOPLASTIC LESIONS

Inflammatory and Ischemic Lesions

Osteomyelitis

The term *osteomyelitis* is traditionally used to describe acute or chronic inflammation involving cortical and cancellous bone secondary to bacterial, mycobacterial, fungal, or viral infection. The inflammatory process usually is associated with bone necrosis and resorption, marrow fibrosis, and reactive bone formation. Although the pattern of inflammation provides a clue as to the causative organism, microbiologic culture is usually required to establish a definitive diagnosis. Two additional distinct clinical syndromes, namely osteoradionecrosis and so-called diffuse sclerosing osteomyelitis, are occasionally included within the general term *osteomyelitis* when it is applied to the craniofacial bones. These three conditions are discussed separately.

Infectious Osteomyelitis

Craniofacial osteomyelitis is relatively uncommon in developed countries. Most cases occur in men, and the mandible is the most common site (1–3). Maxillary osteomyelitis is more common in children (1). The most common predisposing condition to mandibular osteomyelitis is dental infection (1–3). Other conditions include trauma, postsurgical states, and infection of abnormal bone following radiation therapy for oral cancer (see later section on Osteoradionecrosis) (1–3). Patients typically present with pain and swelling overlying the affected portion of bone (1–3). Sinus formation, with draining pus, commonly supervenes. Many patients have a history of alcohol or tobacco abuse (particularly in the setting of osteoradionecrosis).

Radiographically, the most common finding is patchy regions of radiolucency (1). Necrosis of the mandible may lead to massive sequestrum formation, and in this setting marked periosteal new bone formation (involucrum) may develop.

In the acute phase the marrow cavity is filled with fibrin and an acute neutrophilic exudate. Bone necrosis involving cortical and cancellous bone is typically seen (Fig. 1). In chronic osteomyelitis various degrees of fibrosis with numerous plasma cells, lymphocytes, and macrophages are present. Usually chronic osteomyelitis of the facial bones coexists with foci of acute inflammation demonstrating attendant bone necrosis. Most types of bacterial osteomyelitis are caused by mixed bacterial infections, including *Streptococcus* species, *Peptostreptococcus,* diphtheroids, and various other anaerobic organisms (2,3).

Treatment involves surgical debridement, including the removal of carious teeth or necrotic bone, in addition to the administration of appropriate antibiotics (1–3). Most cases are cured with this approach.

It is important to note that in the non–marrow-containing bones of the ethmoid labyrinth, inflammatory cells within bone, usually in the setting of acute or chronic sinusitis, cannot by def-

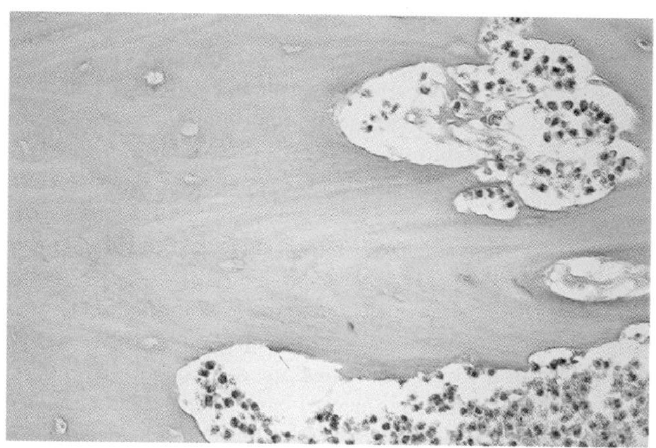

FIGURE 1. Acute suppurative osteomyelitis. Fibrinopurulent exudate surrounding fragments of necrotic bone that show evidence of previous osteoclastic resorption.

inition be osteomyelitis (*myelo* from the Greek for marrow). Thus, the proper term for bony inflammation in such areas is *osteitis.*

The differential diagnosis of infectious osteomyelitis includes osteoradionecrosis, sclerosing osteomyelitis, and Langerhans' cell histiocytosis, which are all discussed in detail in the relevant sections.

Osteoradionecrosis

Osteoradionecrosis is the term applied to the constellation of changes within bone secondary to the administration of therapeutic irradiation (4,5). The most common predisposing condition is squamous cell carcinoma of the oral cavity (4–9). Osteoradionecrosis is relatively common and develops in approximately 10% of patients irradiated for oral carcinoma; however, the incidence has decreased in recent years with the development of newer radiation therapy modalities (8). Therapeutic irradiation directly damages osteoblasts, osteoclasts, and osteoprogenitor cells, but it is the chronic effects on the vascular supply of bone (which results in chronic ischemia and necrosis) that accounts for most of the findings (4). The superficial epithelium overlying the affected bone is commonly ulcerated; therefore, patients frequently complain of pain and ulceration of the alveolar or gingival mucosa. A purulent discharge and secondary bacterial infection of the underlying bone are common findings (see preceding section on Osteomyelitis) (4–9).

Radiographically, the affected bone demonstrates osteopenia with mixed regions of medullary sclerosis.

Microscopically, the cortical bone demonstrates widened haversian canals with evidence of osteoclastic activity. The cancellous bone is thinned with Howship's lacunae and the adjacent fatty marrow is replaced by fine fibrillary fibrosis (4). Cytologically atypical radiation fibroblasts are uncommon (4). Hyalinization of blood vessel walls is frequently present, and irregular deposits of basophilic coarse woven bone in apposition to preexisting cancellous bone is a common finding (Fig. 2). This type of bone formation is characteristic of osseous ischemia. Necrosis of cortical and cancellous bone usually occcurs when secondary bacterial infection has supervened or in the presence of pathologic fracture. In the former setting, fibrinopurulent exudate will be seen as with conventional bacterial osteomyelitis, whereas callus may be present in the latter circumstance.

When bacterial infection is present, treatment involves surgical debridement and suitable antibiotic therapy. In addition, hyperbaric oxygen has been shown to help the mucosal ulcers to heal (6,8).

Diffuse Sclerosing Osteomyelitis (Sclerosing Osteomyelitis of Garré)

Diffuse sclerosing osteomyelitis is a disease of unknown etiology that typically affects the mandible in adult patients, although there is a wide age distribution of affected individuals (10). Men are affected more commonly than women. Patients complain of localized pain and swelling of the mandible, often in an asymmetrical distribution (10–14). Low-grade fever and trismus also may be present, but ulceration of oral mucosa or sinus tract formation are invariably absent.

Radiographically, the affected portion of the mandible is enlarged and sclerotic (10–14). Discrete lucencies of the type seen in bacterial osteomyelitis are not seen. Radionucleotide bone scanning exhibits intense uptake (10,11,14).

Microscopically, subperiosteal formation of lamellar and woven trabecular bone is prominent. Cortical thickening with sclerosis of preexisting cancellous bone is also present. Although there may be mild fibrosis of the marrow with occasional lymphocytes, plasma cells, and granulocytes, the degree of inflammation is never as marked as that seen in bacterial osteomyelitis (10,11,13). Overall, the pattern is that of minimally inflamed sclerotic cortical and cancellous bone (Fig. 3). Bacterial cultures are characteristically negative.

The treatment of diffuse sclerosing osteomyelitis is principally surgical debridement of the affected part of the mandible. Antibiotics are ineffective. Recurrences of the process are common; however, these diminish following additional surgery. Diffuse sclerosing osteomyelitis appears to exhibit a relationship with the so-called SAPHO syndrome (synovitis, acne, pustulosis, hyperostosis, and osteitis), in which patients exhibit a variety

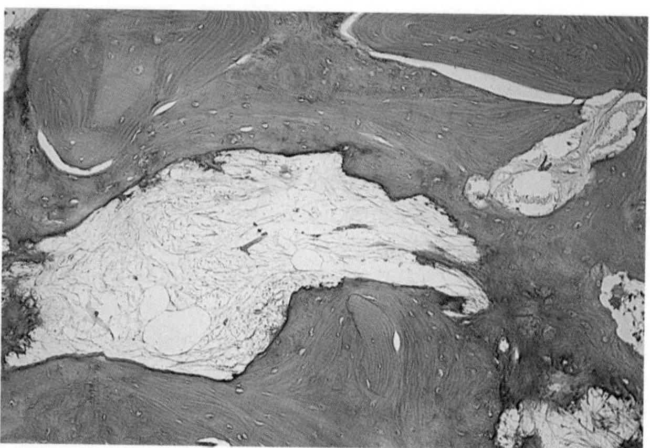

FIGURE 2. Osteoradionecrosis demonstrating medullary fibrosis and coarse woven bone adjacent to the preexisting cancellous bone.

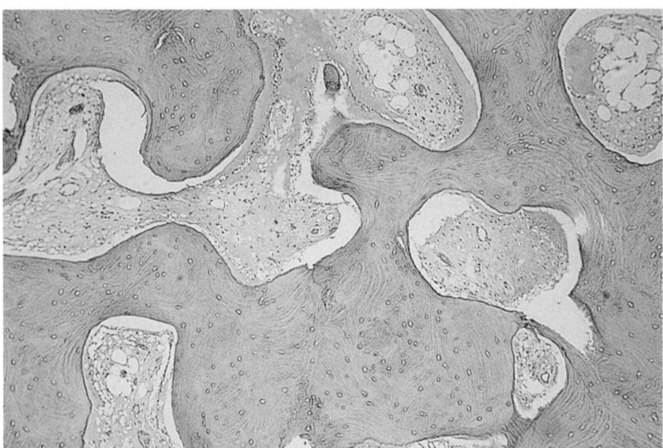

FIGURE 3. Sclerosing osteomyelitis. The bone is markedly thickened and the marrow is replaced by a fibrous stroma that contains scant chronic inflammatory cells.

of cutaneous abnormalities, skeletal and joint pains, and radiographic abnormalities throughout the skeleton (12,14).

The principal differential diagnosis of sclerosing osteomyelitis is infectious bacterial osteomyelitis. As outlined above, there are distinct clinical differences between these two entities. Additionally sclerosing osteomyelitis does not demonstrate the degree of acute inflammation, fibrinous exudate, or bone necrosis that is characteristic of acute bacterial osteomyelitis.

Metabolic

Paget's Disease of Bone

Paget's disease of bone is a disorder of remodeling that is probably caused by a slow virus infection such as a paramyxovirus (15–19). Ultrastructurally, viral particles may be found in osteoblasts, osteocytes, and osteoclasts (15,20,21). The infection causes uncoupling of bone resorption and bone formation that occurs normally during skeletal remodeling. Unlike most other metabolic bone diseases in which the skeleton is globally affected, in Paget's disease a single or multiple bones may be affected, but portions of the skeleton are invariably normal (21,22).

Paget's disease can be subclassified into three phases. The first is characterized by excessive osteoclastic activity and bone resorption. This is followed by the mixed osteoclastic and osteoblastic phase, which evolves into the final osteoblastic stage that is represented by abundant osteoblastic activity (21–23). Because the bone formed in Paget's disease is architecturally abnormal and unrelated to physiologic requirements, there is a tendency for the affected bones to be enlarged, misshapen, and functionally weak (21–23). Paget's disease of bone affects up to 10% of the population over 80 years of age and is more frequent in men than in women. It is common in Northern Europeans but rare in Asians and blacks. Most affected patients are asymptomatic; however, the incidence of symptoms increases steadily with age, and the vast majority of symptomatic patients are 50 years or older (21–23). The craniofacial skeleton is commonly affected in Paget's disease, and enlargement of the cranium is one of the cardinal signs of the disease (21–23). Additionally, craniofacial Paget's disease commonly causes hearing deficits, visual disturbances, an altered sense of smell, and various dental problems, including pain, swelling, and poor oral health (24–28).

Radiographs demonstrate focal radiolucency in the early stages of the disease (21–23). As the osteoblastic stage develops, the affected bones become enlarged and sclerotic, and exhibit cortical thickening and a coarse trabecular pattern (21–24) (Fig. 4).

Grossly, the bone is thickened and sclerotic (Fig. 5). The histomorphology of Paget's disease varies depending on the stage of the disease. In the lytic phase the bone demonstrates prominent osteoclastic resorption. Numerous large osteoclasts that have in excess of 12 nuclei are present within the bone. The external surfaces of cortical and cancellous bone show many large Howship's lacunae that represent recent osteoclastic resorption sites (Fig. 6). Because bone formation is coupled to bone resorption, new bone deposition always occurs in Paget's disease and may be in the form of woven bone or rebuttressing of preexisting cancellous bone. In the active cellular phase of Pagets's disease the marrow space is replaced by loose fibrovascular tissue. Visible cement lines within lamellar cortical and cancellous bone produce the typical jigsaw puzzle or mosaic appearance that is characteristic of Paget's disease. As the disease progresses to the quiescent stage, the osteoclasts and osteoblasts are few in number and the fibrotic

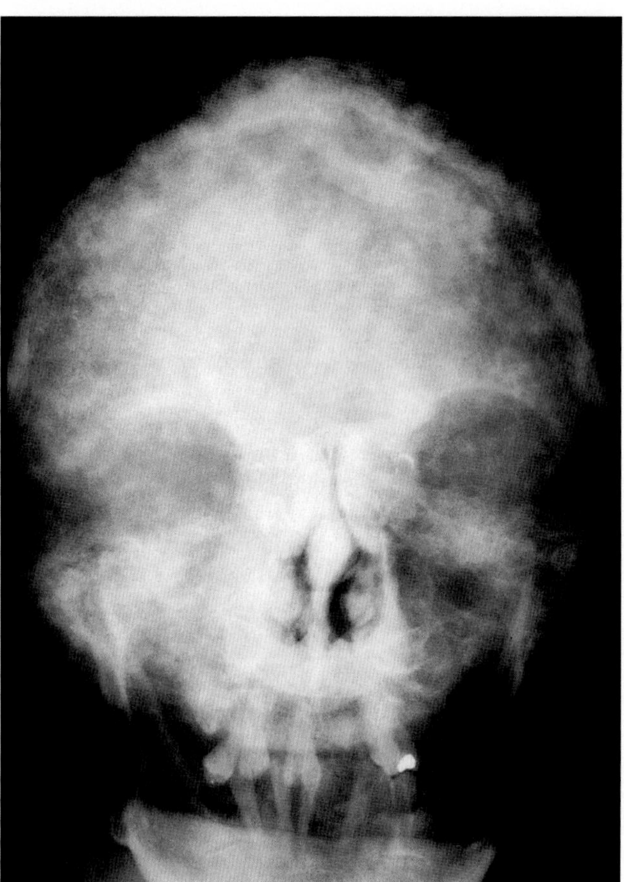

FIGURE 4. A radiograph of advanced Paget's disease showing the characteristic cotton wool–like opacities.

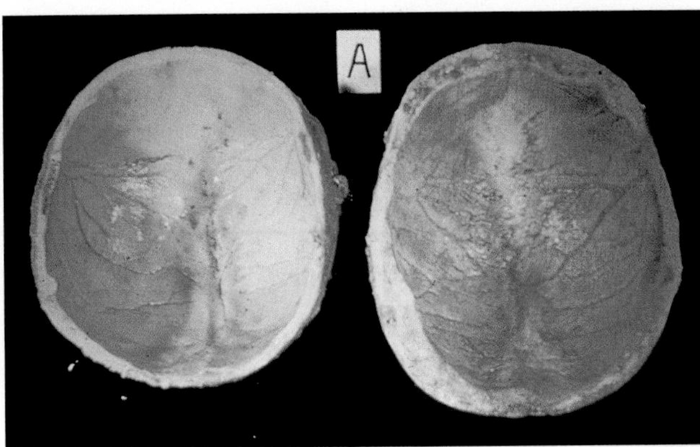

FIGURE 5. Abnormal thickened skull in Paget's disease **(right)** in comparison with a normal skull **(left)**.

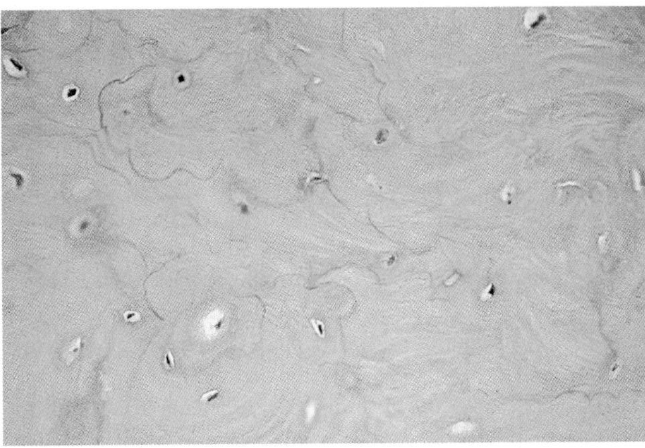

FIGURE 7. Sclerotic bone in late-stage Paget's disease demonstrating prominent cement lines (mosaic or jigsaw pattern).

marrow reverts to a fatty marrow. At this stage the bone demonstrates intense sclerosis and a prominent mosaic pattern (Fig. 7).

One of the most serious consequences of craniofacial Paget's disease is the development of a sarcoma, especially osteosarcoma (29–31). Rarely, giant cell tumors (GCTs) of bone arise within the craniofacial skeleton in the setting of Paget's disease (32–34). The morphology of these tumors is histologically similar to those tumors that arise *de novo* (29–34).

The treatment of Paget's disease involves physiotherapy and pain management for symptomatic relief (35). Biphosphonate drugs also may have a role in limiting the severity of the disease (35).

The differential diagnosis of Paget's disease includes hyperparathyroidism and hemangioma in the active phase and radiation osteitis in the burnt-out quiescent phase. In hyperparathyroidism, excessive osteoclastic activity is present, along with woven bone formation with osteoblastic rimming and paratrabecular fibrosis. Hyperparathyroidism lacks the prominent cement lines, which are always evident in Paget's disease. Clinical information, including serum calcium and phosphorus levels, also aids in the distinction. During the active phase of Paget's disease there is often vascular ectasia, particularly in those regions that exhibit the greatest degrees of bone resorption. Although some degree of bone remodeling occurs in osseous hemangioma, the extent of the changes are never as great as in Paget's disease. Also, prominent cement lines are not a feature of osseous hemangioma. Radiation osteitis, particularly in the later stages, may be associated with thickened bone trabeculae and marrow fibrosis and thus superfically resembles Paget's disease. The distinction is based on clinical information and careful evaluation of the bone trabeculae. In radiation osteitis the bone trabeculae demonstrate a coarse woven pattern similar to the type of bone formed adjacent to an infarct. Although the cement lines in affected bone may be disorganized, they do not exhibit the mosaic architecture of late-stage Paget's disease. Additionally, the vessels within the fibrotic marrow in radiation osteitis may show hyalinization and thickening, which are not present in Paget's disease.

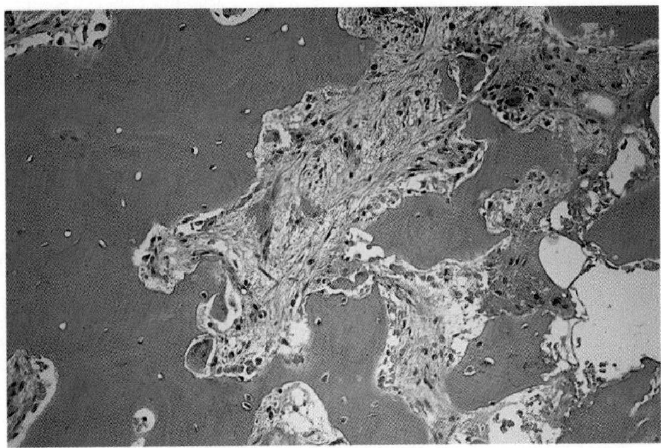

FIGURE 6. Active Paget's disease demonstrating prominent osteoclastic activity, marrow fibrosis, woven bone formation with osteoblastic rimming, and focally prominent cement lines.

Crystal-Induced Synovial and Joint Diseases

Deposition of crystals within synovium, articular cartilage, and periarticular soft tissue is associated with a spectrum of clinical conditions ranging from asymptomatic soft tissue aggregates through severe chronic destructive arthropathies (36,37). The two crystals that most commonly produce disease in humans are monosodium urate and calcium pyrophosphate dihydrate. The pathogenesis of joint destruction and synovial inflammation in these disorders is related to the ingestion of the crystals by phagocytic cells. These cells release chemotactic agents that support and propogate the inflammatory reaction (36). Ultimately, the bone, cartilage, and soft tissue injury that characterizes all of the crystal deposition diseases is produced by enzymatic degradation of the extracellular matrix (36).

Monosodium Urate Crystal Deposition Disease (Gout)

Gout is a systemic disease characterized by elevated serum uric acid levels, tissue deposits of monosodium urate (tophi), recurrent acute arthritis precipitated by urate deposits, and renal disease including uric acid lithiasis (36). Gout is relatively common, with an overall prevalence of 2 per 1,000 population; however, the prevalence increases dramatically with age, achieving a rate of 15 per 1,000 in men in their fourth and fifth decades of life (36). About 30% of patients have primary hyperuricemia. The remaining 70% exhibit hyperuricemia secondary to another disease, usually renal failure, or as a side effect of drug therapy (36).

Tophi may occur in any site of connective tissue; however, certain locations, including the first metatarsophalangeal joint, and the soft tissues around the pinna of the ear, are preferentially affected (37) (see Chapter 3). Involvement of the temporomandibular joint is uncommon (38,39). Acute attacks of gout may be precipitated by sudden changes in serum uric acid levels, trauma, and a variety of other causes. Clinically, acute gouty arthritis closely mimics acute septic arthritis and presents as a painful, swollen, red joint (36). Following resolution of the first attack, patients may remain asymptomatic or develop chronic gouty arthritis (36). Monosodium urate crystal deposits within synovium result in a papillary thickening and opacification of the membrane (37,40). The tophi are chalky white and usually soft. Larger tophi may be firmer and tan because of the presence of abundant admixed fibrous tissue, and these may present clinically as hard nodules. Because monosodium urate is dissolved by aqueous solutions, formalin fixation and conventional tissue processing usually dissolves in the crystals, so they are not seen on tissue sections (37,40). If white deposits are recognized on fresh or even partially fixed gross specimens, then cutting into the deposit and smearing the material on a slide is an effective way to identify the crystals. Microscopically, these smear preparations demonstrate elongate, needle-shaped crystals that are refractile and exhibit intense negative birefringence when viewed with red compensated polarized light. The crystals can usually be readily recognized based on their shape and intense birefringence alone. Because they are dissolved by water, the most efficient way to recognize them in tissue sections is either to perform a frozen section of the affected region or process tissue that has been fixed in absolute alcohol using a processing cycle that eliminates extended exposure to formalin or diluted alcohol (37,40) (Fig. 8).

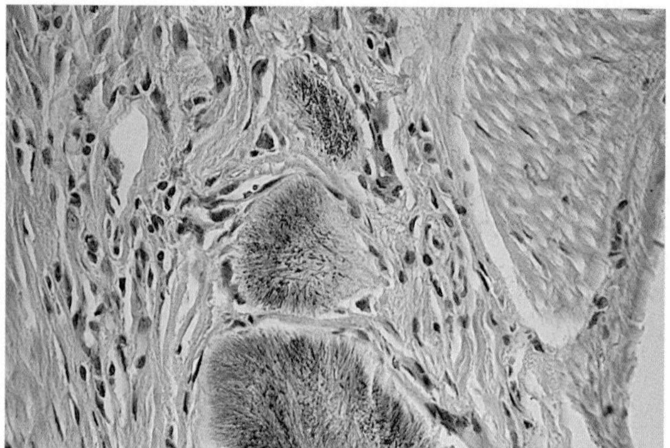

FIGURE 8. Frozen section preparation of a synovial deposit of monosodium urate crystals demonstrating the characteristic "dirty," brown, needle-like crystals.

Minor degrees of crystal loss occur during staining; however, usually enough crystals survive to be visible in hematoxylin and eosin–stained sections. The monosodium urate appears as amorphous granular aggregates of yellow–brown material embedded within thickened fibrotic synovium (37,40). Usually the deposits are associated with a prominent histiocytic and foreign body giant cell reaction. By light microscopy, pools of pale blue to eosinophilic amorphous material remain at the site of prior crystal deposition. This represents the proteinaceous matrix that surrounds the crystals. Frequently this matrix bears the imprint of the crystals, which are arranged as linear clusters, and hence a fibrillary or feathery pattern of lines may be seen within this substance (37,40) (Fig. 8). Larger tophi may exhibit ossification at their periphery, and, similarly, intraosseous deposits commonly show ossification. In acute attacks of gouty arthritis, the synovial membrane contains a dense neutrophilic infiltrate in addition to the crystal deposits. Joint aspiration is an equally effective way of identifying the needle-like crystals of monosodium urate during an acute attack.

The differential diagnosis of intraarticular monosodium urate crystals is principally calcium pyrophosphate crystal deposition disease, which is discussed in detail below.

Calcium Pyrophosphate Dihydrate Crystal Deposition Disease (Pseudogout)

Pseudogout is so named because it is a clinical syndrome characterized by recurrent paroxysmal attacks of severe arthritis that may proceed to a chronic destructive arthropathy (36,37,41). Like gout, the acute and chronic joint injury is a manifestation of intraarticular crystal deposition, in this case calcium pyrophosphate dihydrate ($Ca_2P_2O_7.2H_2O$). In addition to crystal deposits within the synovial membrane and periarticular tissues, in pseudogout, crystals are also found within hyaline articular cartilage, fibrocartilaginous menisci, and intervertebral discs (chondrocalcinosis) (42–45). Chondrocalcinosis affects up to 15% of adults over 65 years of age, and radiographically detectable deposits are present within the hyaline and fibrocartilage of the knees, symphysis pubis, and wrist (36,41). Tophaceous pseudogout, in which macroscopically detectable nodules of calcium pyrophosphate crystals occur within synovial joints, has a distinct predilection for the temporomandibular joint, which is affected in approximately 30% of cases (46). Chondrocalcinosis and pseudogout occur as a primary idiopathic abnormality in about 90% of affected individuals. Pseudogout also has an association with a number of other metabolic disorders, including hyperparathyroidism, gout, hemochromatosis, and hypophosphatasia (36).

Grossly, the synovial and meniscal deposits of calcium pyrophosphate dihydrate appear as flecks of chalky white material on the surface of the membrane and fibrocartilage. These only rarely achieve the large size of gouty deposits. Microscopically, pyrophosphate deposits appear dark blue to purple in undecalcified hematoxylin and eosin–stained slides (44,45) (Fig. 9). Examination with polarized light usually identifies short rhomboidal-shaped crystals (42,43). Within the articular and fibrocartilage the crystal deposits characteristically are not associated with a histiocytic or foreign body giant cell reaction; however,

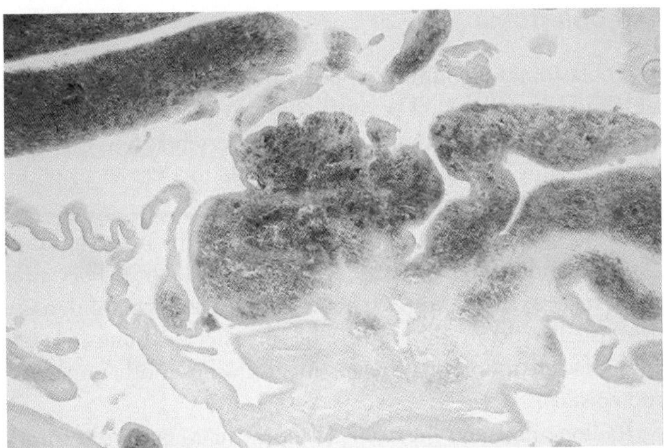

FIGURE 9. Calcium pyrophosphate deposit within degenerated fibrillar fibrocartilage.

the chondrocytes in the vicinity of the deposits may exhibit "degenerative" features, including swelling and a basophilic alteration of the adjacent cartilage matrix (44). It is these cells that are thought to represent the source of the pyrophosphate that forms the crystalline deposits (44). The synovial deposits may be associated with small foci of metaplastic cartilage, and these more commonly elicit a histiocytic reaction (44). If such cartilaginous deposits are extensive, the lesion may mimic synovial chondromatosis or even chondrosarcoma. Decalcification of tissue often results in complete removal of the crystals and in their place are oval to rounded pools of basophilic material. These often lack a cellular reaction and may be easily overlooked. Like the gouty deposits that have been dissolved in aqueous solution, the regions of decalcified pyrophosphate demonstrate a fibrillar or feathery appearance; however, the striations are shorter than those in gouty tophi.

The differential diagnosis of calcium pyrophosphate crystal deposition disease is principally gout, which is discussed in detail in the preceding section.

TUMORS AND TUMOR-LIKE LESIONS OF BONE

Bone-Forming Lesions

Osteoma

Osteoma is a benign, slow-growing bone-forming tumor that consists primarily of well-differentiated mature, compact, or cancellous bone. It is not clear whether osteomas are neoplasms or a manifestation of a reaction to an inflammatory process.

Osteomas usually arise on the surfaces of the cranial vault—either from the outer table (exostotic) or inner table (enostotic) (47)—or from the bones of the jaw (48,49), paranasal sinuses, or orbit. In the paranasal sinuses, osteomas most frequently involve the frontal sinus, followed in descending order by the ethmoid sinus, the maxillary antrum and the sphenoid sinus (50–53). Cranial osteomas are named according to the bone from which they arise, whereas osteomas of the paranasal sinuses are named according to which sinus they invade (54).

Although rare in children, they can affect all age groups but are most commonly diagnosed in the fourth or fifth decades of life (51,53).

Osteomas are often asymptomatic and found incidentally on radiographs taken for other reasons. Larger osteomas, however, can cause a variety of signs and symptoms such as painless swelling, facial asymmetry, and symptoms secondary to nasal or paranasal sinus obstruction, including sinusitis, nasal discharge, and mucocele formation (51,55–57). Orbital osteomas and paranasal sinus osteomas that protrude into the orbit can cause a variety of ocular abnormalities such as exophthalmos, proptosis, ptosis, diplopia, lid edema or swelling, and amaurosis fugax (56,58) (Fig. 10). In extraordinary cases the tumor may grow intracranially and cause neurologic complications (59).

Classically, osteomas manifest radiographically as well-circumscribed homogeneous radiodensities (Fig. 10); however, several different matrix patterns can be seen (52).

Grossly, osteomas are bosselated and well circumscribed and attach to the underlying bone by a broad base or occasionally by a small stalk. They can be dense or sclerotic, with narrow intertrabecular spaces (compact type) or spongiotic (osteoma spongiosum) (60).

Histologically, they arise subperiosteally and often blend imperceptibly with the underlying normal cortical bone. Compact osteomas are composed of sheets of predominantly lamellar bone with haversian-like systems of variable size and shape (cortical-type bone) (Fig. 11) and can be admixed with small amounts of woven bone and fibrous tissue, at times reminiscent of a fibroosseous lesion. Spongy osteomas are composed of cancellous

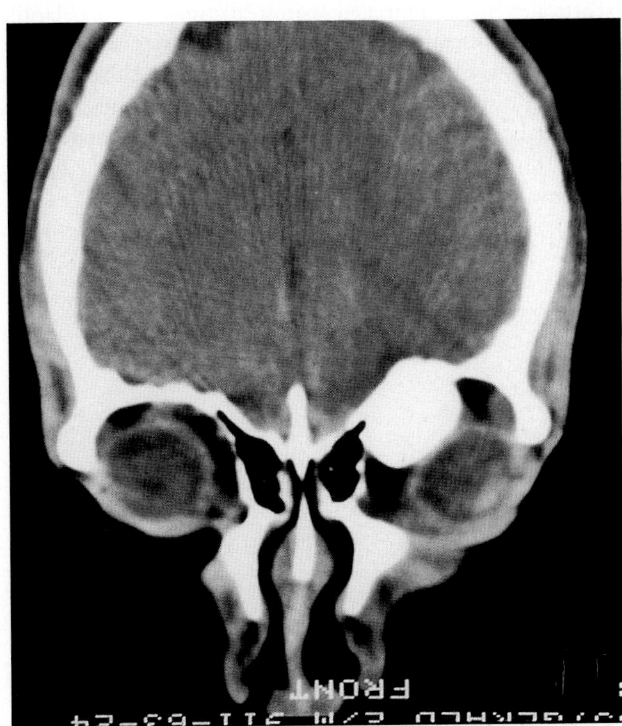

FIGURE 10. A well-circumscribed radiodense osteoma protruding into the orbit and causing exophthalmos.

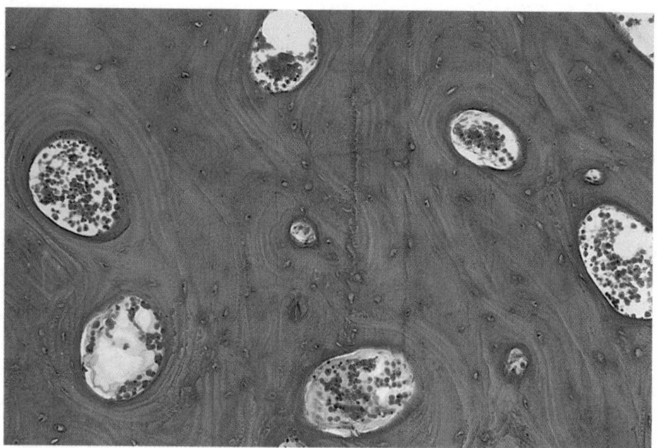

FIGURE 11. A compact osteoma composed of dense cortical-type bone with haversian systems of variable size.

bone with intertrabecular hemopoietic bone marrow or fat (Fig. 12). A thin layer of fibrous tissue (attenuated periosteum) often covers the external surface. There is little osteoblastic or osteoclastic activity.

Patients with Gardner's syndrome, an autosomal dominant disorder characterized by colonic polyps and soft tissue tumors, may have multiple osteomas. Osteomas of the skull are not infrequently the initial finding in these patients (53).

Only patients with symptomatic osteomas should be treated (53), generally by simple excision. Recurrences are rare, even in incompletely excised lesions. Malignant transformation has not been reported.

The most important entity in the differential diagnosis is juxtacortical well-differentiated (parosteal) osteosarcoma. Unlike osteomas that frequently arise in the skull bones, parosteal osteosarcomas are extremely rare in this location. Although bone formation can be extensive in parosteal osteosarcoma, the neoplastic trabeculae of woven or lamellar bone are separated by a cellular fibrous stroma that contains occasional mitotic figures, and these features are not seen in osteoma.

Osteoblastoma

Osteoblastomas account for approximately 1% of primary skeletal neoplasms (61,62). The most common location for these tumors is within the posterior elements of vertebrae and the metaphyses of long bones. Approximately 10% to 15% occur within the bones of the craniofacial skeleton (61–64).

Clinically, these tumors occur predominantly in young adults in the second through fourth decades of life (61–65). They affect males twice as frequently as females and present as painful masses that usually distort the outline of the affected bone (61–65). Craniofacial tumors may result in headache, tooth impaction, and epistaxis (61).

Radiographically, they typically present as expansile tumors with well-defined margins and peripheral reactive sclerosis, but poorly defined interfaces between the tumor and host bone occur in a minority of cases (61–63). Osteoblastomas commonly demonstrate intralesional mineralization, which may be minimal or extensive (61–63).

Grossly, most osteoblastomas measure between 1.0 and 5.0 cm and are solid dark red gritty nodules (61–65). Secondary aneurysmal bone cyst (ABC) formation develops in approximately 10% of tumors and produces blood-filled cysts within the solid components of the mass (61,63). Microscopically, osteoblastomas are characterized by haphazardly arranged trabeculae of neoplastic woven bone that are prominently rimmed by osteoblasts (Fig. 13). This trabecular architecture is usually not the exclusive pattern in any one tumor, and sheets of matrix with entrapped osteocytes also may be seen. Cellular aggregates of osteoblasts with scant lace-like osteoid are present in a minority of tumors (61,63). The bone is supported by a highly vascular stroma that frequently demonstrates vascular ectasia and interstitial hemorrhage. Between 5% and 10% of osteoblastomas may demonstrate foci of hyaline or fibrocartilaginous matrix (61,63,66). The osteoblasts that comprise the neoplastic cellular component of the tumor are oval to rounded in outline and have eosinophilic cytoplasm and eccentrically located uniform dark-staining nuclei. Mitoses are inconspicuous, and necrosis is usually not present unless there has been a prior pathologic fracture.

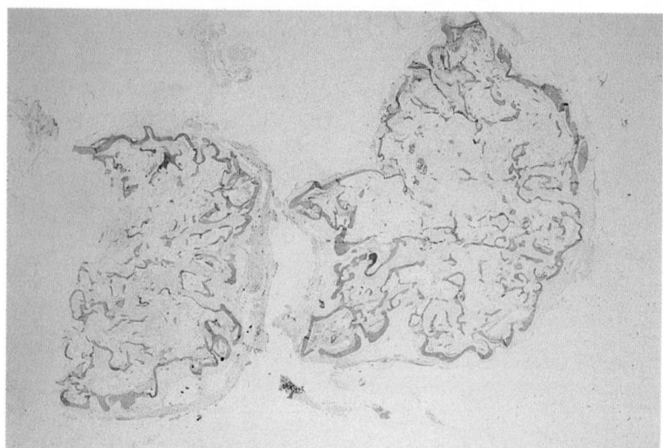

FIGURE 12. Spongy osteoma composed of thin interconnecting trabeculae of bone separated by fat.

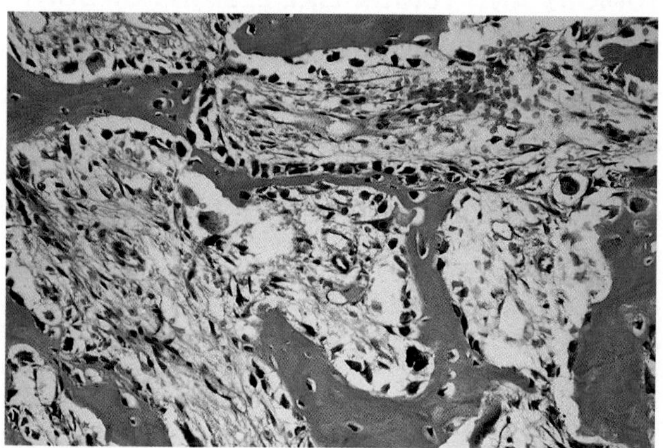

FIGURE 13. Intersecting trabeculae of woven bone in an osteoblastoma. The trabeculae demonstrate prominent osteoblastic rimming and are supported by a vascular fibrous stroma.

In approximately 10% to 15% of tumors epithelioid osteoblasts may comprise the majority of the neoplastic cells (61,63). These cells exhibit abundant eosinophilic cytoplasm and nuclei with vesicular chromatin and prominent nucleoli. A paranuclear region of pallor that corresponds ultrastructurally to a well-developed Golgi apparatus is frequently present. These epithelioid osteoblasts measure up to three times the size of conventional osteoblasts and in some cases appear to be a marker of more aggressive clinical behavior (61,63,65). Although osteoblastomas produce bone remodeling and expansion of the host bone, they do not demonstrate permeative growth. This latter feature is crucial in the distinction of these tumors from osteosarcoma. The preexisting cortical and cancellous bone surrounding the neoplasm frequently demonstrates reactive changes, including paratrabecular fibrosis, osteoclast activity, and woven bone formation; however, permeative growth with entrapment of existing cancellous or cortical bone by tumor cells and matrix does not occur. In approximately 15% of osteoblastomas, multiple separate foci of tumor cells may be seen within adjacent regions of cancellous bone (61,63). This phenomenon has been termed *multifocal nidi* and may simulate a permeative pattern of growth. The term *pseudomalignant osteoblastoma* has been applied to tumors that architecturally resemble conventional osteoblastoma but exhibit marked cytologic atypism of some of the osteoblasts (67,68). This atypia manifests as nuclear enlargement and intense hyperchromasia. It is not accompanied by increased mitotic activity or abnormal matrix production. The nuclear atypia is considered to be a degenerative type of change analogous to that which occurs in ancient schwannoma (67,68).

The treatment of osteoblastoma is principally surgical excision. En bloc resection is usually curative; however, curettage results in a local recurrence rate of approximately 20% (61,63,65). Malignant transformation of osteoblastoma to osteosarcoma is exceptionally rare. In a review of 306 osteoblastomas from the Mayo Clinic, malignant degeneration occurred in only 2 cases (61).

The differential diagnosis of osteoblastoma includes osteoid osteoma, osteosarcoma, and fibroosseous lesions of the craniofacial skeleton. Osteosarcomas demonstrate greater cytologic atypia, atypical mitoses, and a permeative growth pattern. The fibroosseous lesions contains a more uniform collagenous stroma that lacks the conspicuous dilated capillaries and hemorrhage typical of osteoblastoma, and although focal osteoblastic rimming may be seen in these lesions [especially in ossifying fibroma (OF)], it is rarely as well developed as in osteoblastoma. Clinical and radiographic findings also aid in distinguishing between these entities.

Osteoid Osteoma

Osteoid osteomas account for approximately 12% of benign bone tumors (56). These tumors share many morphologic similarities with osteoblastoma and, like the latter, predominantly affect children and young adults, particularly men (56,64,69–71). Most osteoid osteomas of the head and neck affect the posterior elements of the cervical vertebrae (70,72,73) (Fig. 14). Osteoid osteomas of the craniofacial and jaw bones are exceptionally uncommon (56,70). Between 5% and 10% of osteoid osteomas arise within the vertebral column, and approximately 25% of these affect the cervical vertebrae (69,70,73). Patients typically complain of severe localized pain that is often worse at night and relieved by aspirin (56,64,69–71). Additionally, the majority of patients with cervical osteoid osteoma exhibit torticollis and often scoliosis (72,73).

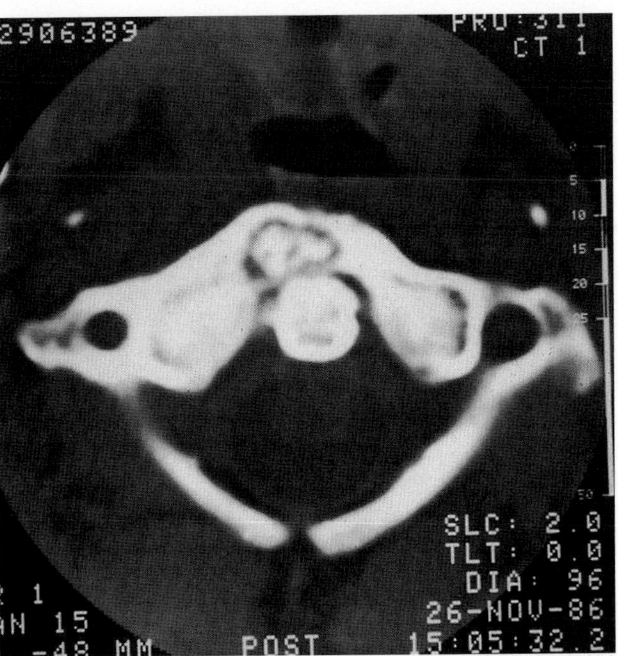

FIGURE 14. A cervical osteoid osteoma showing a central opacity (sclerotic nidus) surrounded by a lucent halo.

Radiographically, osteoid osteomas exhibit a central lucency (the nidus) surrounded by a zone of intense sclerosis (the reactive zone) (Fig. 14) (56,71). By definition, the nidus of the osteoid osteoma always measures less than 2.0 cm in maximum size.

Grossly, the nidus is usually gritty and dark red, representing the partially mineralized woven bone and rich capillary vascular supply, respectively. Microscopically, the nidus of the osteoid osteoma is composed of haphazardly intersecting trabeculae of woven bone that are rimmed prominently by osteoblasts (Fig. 15). The bone matrix is supported by a richly vascularized connective tissue that contains fibroblasts and fine fibers of collagen. All of the various patterns of bone matrix production, including solid sheets and focal lace-like arrangements, that may be seen in osteoblastoma also may be present within osteoid osteoma. In effect, the microscopic appearance of the nidus of an osteoid osteoma and osteoblastoma are indistinguishable (70,74). However, they differ in that the periphery of osteoid has a greater degree of reactive sclerotic bone (75) (Fig. 16). Additionally immunohistochemical stains for neurofilament and S-100 protein readily identify nerve fibers within the reactive zone and nidus of osteoid osteomas, whereas osteoblastomas lack these structures (75) (Fig. 17).

Osteoid osteomas are typically treated by surgical excision. The rate of persistent symptoms related to residual or recurrent tumor following such surgery is on the order of 5% to 10%

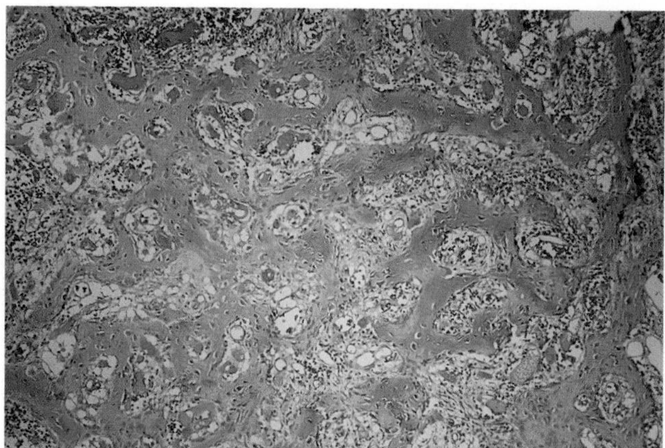

FIGURE 15. The nidus of an osteoid osteoma that appears histologically identical to an osteoblastoma.

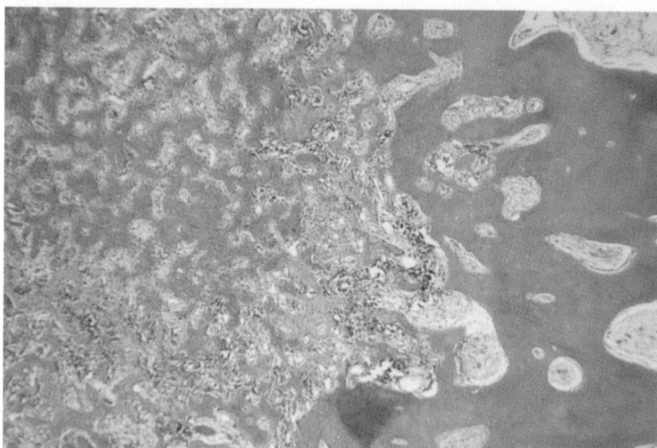

FIGURE 16. Low-power view of the nidus of an osteoid osteoma and the markedly sclerotic bone at the periphery. Note the circumscribed margin of the nidus.

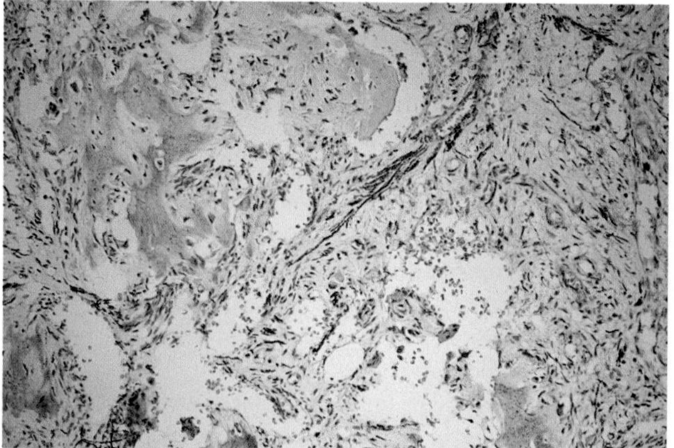

FIGURE 17. Immunohistochemical stain for neurofilament highlighting the nerve fibers at the edge of the nidus of the osteoid osteoma.

(70,76). More recently, percutaneous radiofrequency ablation has been used to treat osteoid osteomas (76). This less invasive procedure appears to be as successful in treating these patients as the traditional operative approach (76).

The differential diagnosis of osteoid osteoma includes osteoblastoma, osteosarcoma, and osteomyelitis. Osteoblastoma, although microscopically indistinguishable from osteoid osteoma, differs by virtue of its larger size, lack of marked reactive sclerosis, and absence of detectable nerve fibers. Additionally patients with osteoblastomas usually do not exhibit the characteristic pattern of nocturnal localized pain that is relieved by aspirin. Osteosarcoma is larger than osteoid osteoma, exhibits a poorly defined margin radiographically, and microscopically demonstrates greater cytologic atypia and mitoses. Localized chronic osteomyelitis (Brodie's abscess) may clinically and radiographically simulate osteoid osteoma; however, microscopically it is associated with acute and chronic inflammation, granulation tissue, and bone necrosis. The peripheral sclerotic rim surrounding a Brodie's abscess may be indistinguishable from the reactive zone of an osteoid osteoma. Microscopic evaluation of the central lucency (the nidus) is required to definitely separate these two lesions.

Osteosarcoma

Osteosarcoma is the most common primary malignant tumor of bone. It classically involves the long bones of the appendicular skeleton. In the craniofacial area osteosarcoma most frequently affects the jawbones, with approximately 6% of osteosarcomas (or 0.07 cases per 100,000 population per year) arising in the mandible or maxilla (77).

Although gnathic osteosarcomas can affect all age groups, they tend to occur approximately a decade later than osteosarcomas of the long bones, with the majority of patients being over 30 years of age (77,78). Men are affected more frequently than women (78,79). Some studies have shown a higher incidence of osteosarcoma in the mandible than in the maxilla (77,78), whereas other studies have shown the reverse (80). The most common sites of involvement are the body of the mandible and the alveolar ridge or the antral area of the maxilla (79). The majority of tumors arise within the medullary cavity of the affected bone, with rare examples developing on the bony surfaces (81,82).

Clinical signs and symptoms depend on the location of the tumor, its size, and rate of growth (83). Patients most frequently present with swelling and pain. Other symptoms include paresthesia, displacement or loosening of teeth, toothache, bleeding, and nasal obstruction (77,79).

Radiographic studies show a poorly defined destructive lesion that can be sclerotic, lytic, or mixed sclerotic and lytic, with or without soft tissue extension (78). Early tumors may show a symmetrical widening of the periodontal membrane space about one or more teeth (77).

Grossly, the tumors are gritty, tan–white, and sometimes myxoid (Fig. 18). They destroy the underlying bone with or without soft tissue extension. All subtypes of osteosarcomas can occur in the jaw bones; however, up to half of them show chondroid differentiation (chondroblastic osteosarcoma) (80). In

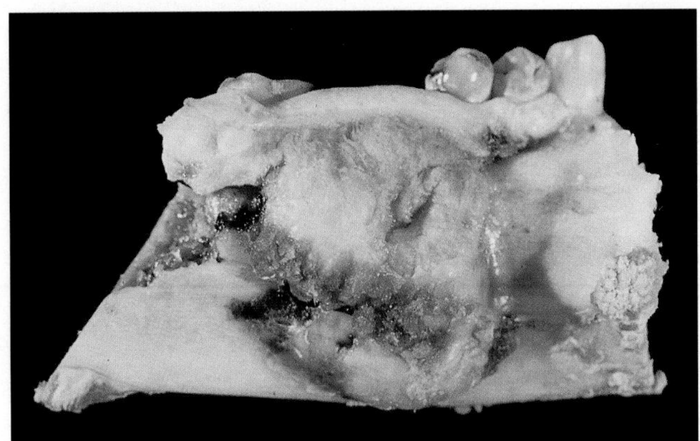

FIGURE 18. Osteosarcoma of the mandible showing a destructive tan–brown tumor with focal areas of hemorrhage.

chondroblastic osteosarcoma, the tumor has a lobular architecture with central cartilaginous areas that are surrounded by hypercellular regions, in which spindle or polygonal cells that demonstrate nuclear atypia and mitotic activity deposit neoplastic bone (Fig. 19). All types of osteosarcomas contain connective tissue cells, generally spindled or fusiform, with at least the focal production of neoplastic bone directly by tumor cells. Serum alkaline phosphatase is often elevated in primary osteosarcomas, although high levels generally suggest an osteosarcoma arising in Paget's disease (83).

The treatment of choice is radical surgery with or without adjuvant chemotherapy or radiation therapy. In our institution all high-grade osteosarcomas, regardless of location, are treated with adjuvant chemotherapy. The reported prognosis for osteosarcoma of the jawbones has been variable, and in some studies has been shown to be better than for those arising in the appendicular skeleton (79). Other studies have not shown biologic advantage for osteosarcomas of the jaw bones (78). The prognosis seems to be more favorable for mandibular osteosarcomas in comparison with those that arise in the maxilla. The site of origin within these bones also seems to affect prognosis, with maxillary antral tumors having the worst prognosis and tumors of the mandibular symphysis having the best prognosis (77). This may be related to the length of time the tumor has been present and its resectability. Lastly, in some studies the chondroblastic variant also has been associated with a better prognosis than other histologic types of osteosarcoma (79).

Gnathic osteosarcomas should be separated from osteosarcomas involving extragnathic craniofacial bones, because the latter are generally high grade and clinically extensive and have a much worse prognosis than jawbone osteosarcomas. In the study by Nora et al. of extragnathic craniofacial osteosarcoma (84), only 2 of 21 patients survived for 5 years, and only 1 patient was a long-term survivor. A high percentage of these patients also had a history of a predisposing condition such as Paget's disease of bone or prior radiation therapy.

Cartilage-Forming Lesions

Enchondroma and Osteochondroma

Although we have seen examples of enchondromas arising in the skull base, benign cartilaginous tumors of the skull and jawbones are uncommon, and any tumor that contains a significant amount of cartilage most likely represents a chondrosarcoma or a chondroblastic osteosarcoma. Ostechondromas rarely involve the bones of the head and neck (85–90), where (in our experience) they most frequently involve the cervical vertebrae. Osteochondromas can either arise from the outer surface of the vertebra, causing a mass effect, or it can protrude into the spinal canal and produce neurologic symptoms (91–93). Lesions of the head and neck have the same morphology as ostechondromas of the appendicular skeleton.

Soft tissue chondromas rarely arise in the palate and gingiva (94,95).

Chondroblastoma

Chondroblastoma of bone is a rare tumor accounting for approximately 1% of primary bone tumors (96,97). It most frequently arises in the epiphyses of long bones in skeletally immature individuals, and rarely involves the bones of the skull and

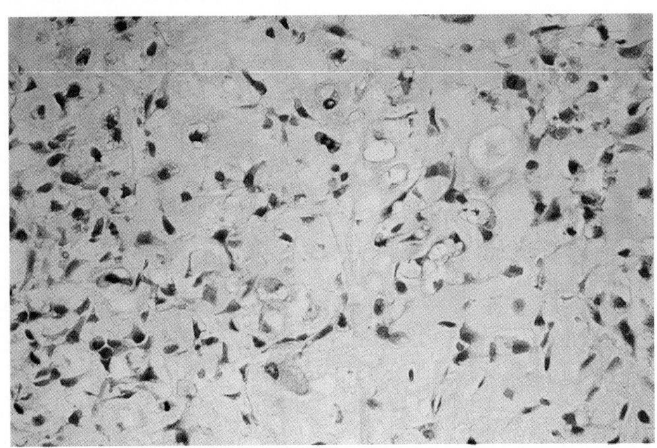

A

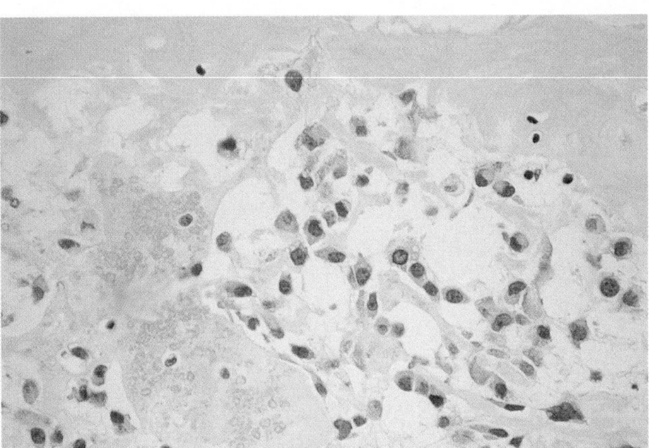

B

FIGURE 19. Chondroblastic osteosarcoma. Most of the tumor is composed of malignant cells separated by an extracellular chondroid matrix **(A)** with only focal neoplastic bone formation **(B)**.

cervical vertebrae. In a series of 495 cases of chondroblastomas, 34 (6.8%) arose in the skull and facial bones, and none involved the cervical vertebrae (although one tumor arose in a vertebral body at a different anatomic level) (98). In another study, less than 2% of chondroblastomas involved the bones of the skull and face (99). Exceptional cases of chondroblastoma develop within the cartilaginous components of the larynx or trachea.

All age groups are affected; however, patients with chondroblastoma of the skull bones have a median age of 44 (100), which is considerably older than patients with chondroblastomas of the appendicular skeleton. Men are affected more commonly than women.

In a series on 30 chondroblastomas of the skull and facial bones (101), 21 (70%) arose in the temporal bone, 6 (20%) in the mandible (3 in the condyles, 1 in the coronoid process, 1 in the angle, and 1 in the body), 1 in the parietal bone, and 2 in the region of the temporal bone and mandible. Chondroblastoma also has been reported to arise from the articular region of the temporomandibular joint (102).

The symptoms caused by the tumor are related to its site of origin. Patients with tumors arising in the temporal bone often complain of hearing loss, otalgia, plugged sensation, pain, tinnitus, vertigo, and headache. Mandible tumors can cause pain and swelling of the temporomandibular joint (100,101).

Radiographically, chondroblastomas have the appearance of a benign but locally aggressive lesion. They are generally well-marginated radiolucent lesions and may have foci of calcification. The bone may be expanded, and extension into soft tissues can be present.

Histologically, the tumor is composed of characteristic mononuclear, epithelioid cells with round, grooved nuclei and abundant eosinophilic cytoplasm with well-defined cell membranes (chondroblasts) (Fig. 20). The chondroblasts may be mitotically active and undergo necrosis. A frequent finding in craniofacial chondroblastomas is the presence of intracytoplasmic hemosiderin in the chondroblasts (Fig. 21). The matrix is usually sparse and cartilaginous (Fig. 20) and may calcify, entrapping individual cells, thereby producing a chicken wire-like pattern of mineralization. Osteoclast-type giant cells may be scattered throughout the tumor but are most numerous in areas of matrix production and hemorrhage (Figs. 20 and 21). Cystic changes, mimicking an ABC, and giant cell granuloma-like areas are commonly seen. The treatment of choice is total excision, if possible. Although curettage can lead to long periods of disease-free survival, there is a high rate of recurrence (100). Malignant transformation or metastases from a "benign" chondroblastoma, as seen in the appendicular skeleton, has not been reported in the skull.

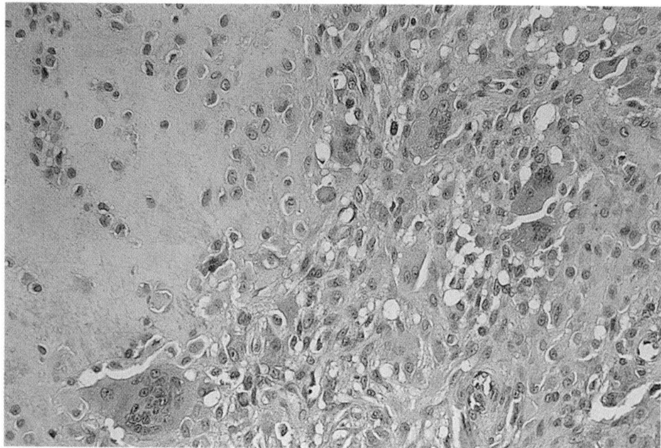

FIGURE 20. Chondroblastoma composed of an admixture of mononuclear epithelioid chondroblasts and osteoclast-type giant cells **(right)** and a chondroid matrix with individual cells residing in lacunae **(left)**.

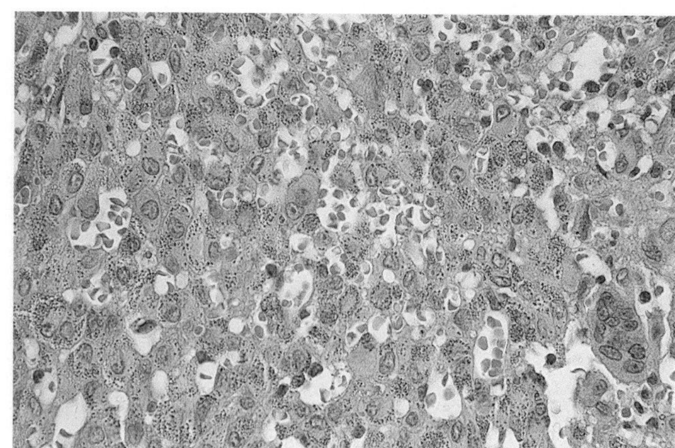

FIGURE 21. Chondroblastoma, showing the chondroblasts with eosinophilic cytoplasm and grooved nuclei. Many cells contain intracytoplasmic hemosiderin. A giant cell is also present (at lower right).

The histologic differential diagnosis includes clear cell chondrosarcoma and GCT of bone or GCRG. Clear cell chondrosarcoma has rarely been reported to involve the skull (103). Although chondroblastoma-like changes can be seen in clear cell chondrosarcoma, the latter is predominantly composed of sheets of large clear cells that contain abundant intracytoplasmic glycogen. Like chondroblastoma, GCT of bone is composed of an admixture of mononucleated and multinucleated giant cells. The giant cells in GCT of bone are evenly distributed throughout and contain a much higher number of nuclei than the giant cells seen in chondroblastoma. Also, the nuclear features of the stromal and multinucleated cells in GCT of bone are identical, whereas in chondroblastomas they are different. Lastly, GCTs do not contain neoplastic cartilage, and neither they nor giant cell granuloma contain the chicken wire mineralization of chondroblastomas.

Chondromyxoid Fibroma

Chondromyxoid fibroma (CMF) is a rare primary neoplasm of bone that accounts for less than 1% of all primary bone tumors. It was originally recognized as a distinct entity by Jaffe and Lichtenstein in 1948 in their review of previously diagnosed chondrosarcomas (104). CMF classically involves the metaphyses of long bones, most commonly presenting in the second and third decades of life (105).

Chondromyxoid fibroma of the cranial and facial bones is extremely rare. In a series of 278 CMFs, 15 (5.4%) arose in the bones of the skull and face (105), and 2 (0.7%) involved the cervical vertebrae. In another series of 36 CMFs, only 1 arose in the

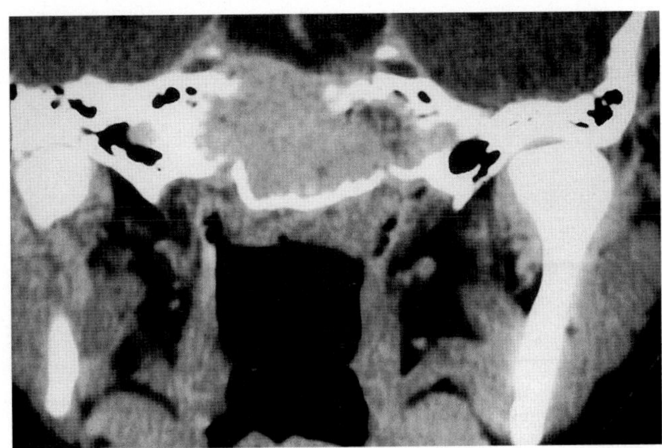

FIGURE 22. Base of skull chondromyxoid fibroma demonstrating an expansile mass within the clivus.

craniofacial bones and 1 in the body and the neural arch of the seventh cervical vertebra (106). In the cranial skeleton CMFs frequently arise in the mandible, but the tumor also has been reported in the maxilla, pterygopalatine space, zygoma, occipital bone, parietal bone, ethmoid labyrinth, frontal bone, and nasal bone (107–114). We have also seen a case arising in the temporal bone extending into the temporomandibular joint and presenting as a swelling of that joint. CMF also can involve the skull base, where it is often misdiagnosed as chordoma or chondrosarcoma (115,116).

Clinically, CMF frequently causes pain and swelling, but it also may be detected as an incidental finding on x-ray. Based on its size and location, CMF also may produce headaches, visual disturbances, nasal obstruction, hearing loss, and vertigo.

Radiographically, CMF is well defined, predominantly radiolucent, and locally destructive, especially when it arises in the skull base (Fig. 22) (115).

Chondromyxoid fibroma has a lobulated appearance and grows in a noninfiltrative fashion. It is composed of nodules of hypocellular chondroid or myxochondroid tissue that have peripheral hypercellular regions consisting of spindle or stellate cells with scattered multinucleated osteoclast-type giant cells (Fig. 23). Usually there is minimal cytologic atypia, and mitoses are infrequent. Rare cases, however, may contain enlarged hyperchromatic nuclei similar to those seen in ancient schwannoma. In our experience CMF of the head and neck has little if any well-formed hyaline cartilage.

Immunohistochemically, in our experience, the cartilaginous areas stain for S-100 protein, whereas the peripheral cellular areas stain for smooth muscle actin and muscle actin but not for S-100 protein. Ultrastructurally, the cells in the central areas have the features of chondrocytes but the cells in the peripheral regions show myofibroblastic and myochondroblastic differentiation (117).

Chondromyxoid fibroma has the potential to locally recur, and although complete resection is the treatment of choice, this is generally difficult in the craniofacial region. Therefore, the tumor should be thoroughly curetted and the patient carefully followed (107,108). In selected cases, especially those that involve the skull base, postoperative radiation therapy or proton beam therapy may be indicated (115).

The main differential diagnosis is chondrosarcoma. Chondrosarcoma, unlike CMF, has an infiltrative growth pattern, encasing trabecular bone. Chondrosarcoma is composed of hyaline type or myxoid type cartilage and does not have the lobular arrangement with central areas of cartilage surrounded by spindle shaped cells as seen in CMF.

Chondrosarcoma

Chondrosarcoma arising in the cranium is an uncommon tumor, and its exact incidence is unknown. In two large studies only 27 and 37 tumors among 16,557 and 24,197 proven intracranial tumors arising either within the cranium or brain, or its covering and supportive tissues, respectively, were cartilaginous tumors (118,119). In the head and neck region, chondrosarcoma most commonly affects the skull base, with rare tumors occurring in other bones, such as the maxilla and the mandible (120). Chondrosarcoma also can involve the cartilage of the larynx (see Chapter 7). In our experience and that of others, the conventional type of chondrosarcoma is the most common variant to develop in the skull base (121,122). A recent review of the literature identified almost 200 cases of skull base chondrosarcoma; however, the pathologic type was reported in only slightly more than half of the cases, and nearly 30% of them were mesenchymal chondrosarcomas rather than the conventional variant (121). In our experience with over 200 patients with skull base chondrosarcomas, the patients have ranged in age from 10 to 79 (mean 39) years, and women are affected slightly more frequently than men (122). The patients commonly present with symptoms related to the nervous system, including headache, cranial nerve palsies, hearing deficits, and disturbances in gait.

Radiographically, the tumors are destructive lobulated masses that show a variable degree of calcification (Fig. 24). Approximately two thirds of cases in the skull base arise in the temporooccipital skull base, 28% from the sphenoocciput

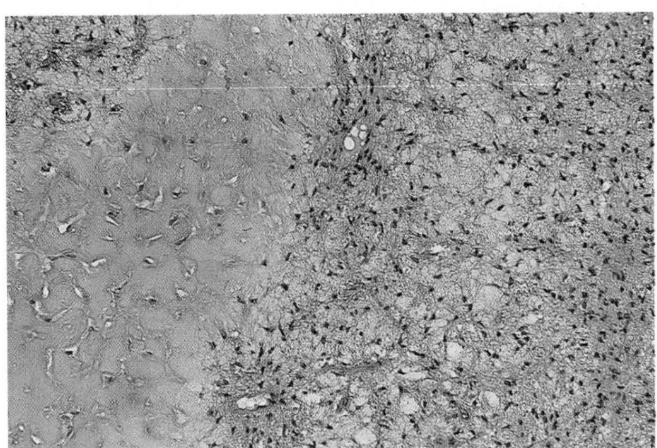

FIGURE 23. Nasal chondromyxoid fibroma showing a chondroid matrix **(left)** and spindle or stellate mesenchymal cells embedded in a myxoid stroma **(right)**.

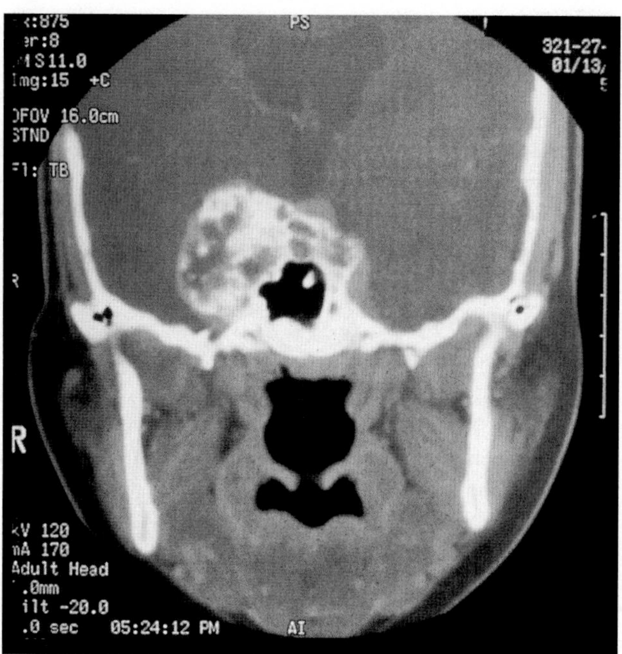

FIGURE 24. Base of skull chondrosarcoma showing a mixed sclerotic and lytic lesion.

(clivus), with the remaining tumors arising in the sphenoethmoid complex.

The vast majority of these tumors are conventional chondrosarcomas and are composed of either hyaline cartilage, myxoid cartilage, or an admixture of these matrices. Hyaline chondrosarcomas are characterized by hypercellular hyaline cartilage containing cytologically atypical chondrocytes residing within lacunae (Fig. 25). In contrast, the atypical chondrocytes of myxoid chondrosarcoma do not reside in lacunae but are enmeshed in a flocculent myxoid matrix (Fig. 26). Although they can have cords of cells, no nests or cohesive clusters, as in chordomas, are present.

Ultrastructurally, chondrosarcoma cells have an escalloped or villous surface and are surrounded by a clear zone between the cell and the surrounding extracellular matrix. The cytoplasm has abundant dilated rough endoplasmic reticulum. No junctions are present.

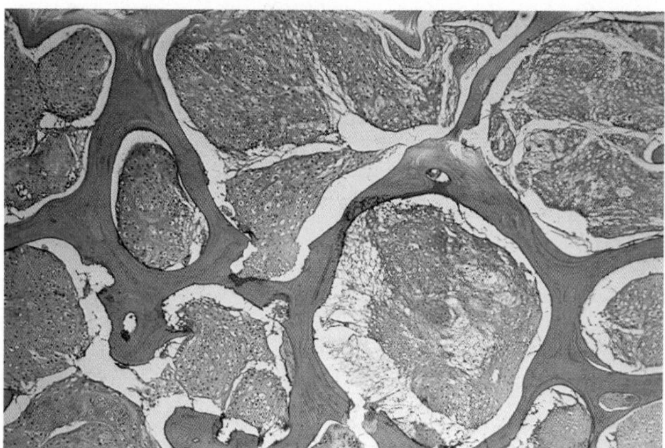

FIGURE 25. Conventional chondrosarcoma composed of nodules of hyaline cartilage infiltrating preexisting cancellous bone.

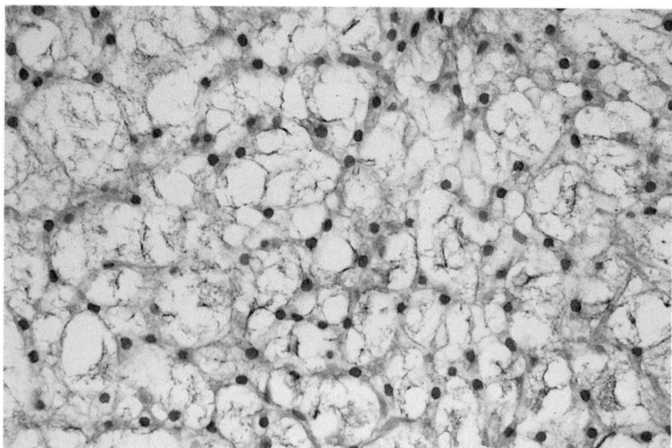

FIGURE 26. Myxoid chondrosarcoma composed of cords of cells embedded in a flocculent myxoid matrix.

Immunohistochemically, conventional chondrosarcomas express vimentin and S-100 protein but typically do not express epithelial markers such as keratin or epithelial membrane antigen (EMA) (122). Rare base of skull chondrosarcomas can, however, focally express EMA, but we have never encountered a keratin-positive skull base chondrosarcoma.

The natural history of conventional chondrosarcoma of the skull base is that of slow progressive growth, which can be fatal secondary to compression and invasion of adjacent vital structures (123,124). These tumors infrequently metastasize; therefore, local control is the goal of therapy. Traditionally this has been accomplished by piecemeal surgical resection; however, this mode of therapy has been associated with a local recurrence rate of up to 53% (121). More recently, radiation therapy has become an important adjuvant, and the combination of surgery and radiotherapy, particularly proton beam radiation therapy, has resulted in a reported 5-year progression-free survival rate of 99% (125).

The diagnosis of conventional chondrosarcoma is established by identifying its characteristic morphology and immunophenotype. It is well recognized, however, that the myxoid variant of chondrosarcoma has the potential to be confused with chordoma. Differentiating myxoid chondrosarcoma from chordoma on morphologic grounds alone can be difficult (125–127), and in our experience up to 37% of chondrosarcomas have been misclassified as conventional or chondroid chordomas. This distinction is extremely important because the prognosis for chordomas is significantly worse than for chondrosarcoma when treated with surgery and proton beam irradiation. Myxoid chondrosarcoma can be distinguished from chordoma on morphologic grounds because the neoplastic chondrocytes are relatively small, contain diminished amounts of cytoplasm, and do not grow in cohesive groups, nests, or sheets. In contrast, chordoma cells are large and have abundant eosinophilic cytoplasm. The numerous desmosome-type intercellular junctions cause the cells to be tightly apposed to one another, producing a cohesive nesting or sheet-like architectural pattern. In contrast, except for small contact points between the cytoplasmic processes of neighboring cells, in the myxoid variant of chondrosarcoma the matrix completely surrounds the neoplastic cells. Another distinctive feature of chordoma that is not present in chondrosarcoma is the wrapping of one cell around another. The physaliphorous cells also have been reported to be of diagnostic importance in chordoma; however, we have not found the presence of cytoplasmic vacuoles to be particularly helpful because they also may be found in chondrosarcoma. Immunohistochemistry is a useful diagnostic adjunct. Unlike chordomas, which stain strongly with vimentin, S-100 protein, keratin, and EMA, chondrosarcomas express vimentin and S-100 protein, very rarely stain for EMA, and, importantly, do not stain with keratin.

Mesenchymal Chondrosarcoma

Mesenchymal chondrosarcoma is the rarest subtype of chondrosarcoma (128,129) and may arise in bone or soft tissue (128,129). Unlike conventional chondrosarcoma that usually arises in patients over 50 years of age, mesenchymal chondrosarcoma typically occurs in younger patients in their second through fourth decades of life (128,129). Men and women are affected equally. Although this tumor is relatively rare, approximately 10% to 30% of skeletal tumors arise in the craniofacial bones (128–130). Most of the patients present complaining of pain and a mass, and depending on the exact location of the tumor, there may be site-specific symptoms such as loosened teeth or sinusitis (130).

Radiographically, mesenchymal CSA causes permeative destruction of bone (128–130); therefore, it has ill-defined margins. Intralesional dense irregular calcification is a frequent finding (128–130).

Grossly, mesenchymal chondrosarcoma is a gray, fleshy tumor that may exhibit recognizable foci of calcification. Microscopically, it is characterized by sheets of undifferentiated small blue cells resembling those of Ewing's sarcoma/PNET or small elongate spindle cells. Often there is a prominent branching supporting a capillary network that has a hemangiopericytoma-like pattern (Fig. 27). The mitotic rate is variable, and many microscopic fields may demonstrate few mitotic figures. The other diagnostic hallmark of mesenchymal chondrosarcoma is the presence of islands of mildly to moderately cellular hyaline and fibrocartilage (Fig. 28). These nodules of cartilage vary in size; however, they are often very small, measuring less than 1.0 mm in diameter, and as such may be absent on small biopsy fragments. Calcification and endochondral ossification occur within the cartilaginous foci, accounting for the radiodensities seen on radiographs. Individually, the cartilaginous nodules appear bland or demonstrate minimal chondrocyte atypia of the type seen in low-grade chondrosarcoma. High-grade nuclear atypia is not present within the cartilaginous components. The undifferentiated small blue cell components of the tumor express vimentin and CD99 (131). Because the latter antibody strongly labels Ewing's sarcoma/PNET, the possibility for misdiagnosis is considerable unless cartilaginous foci are present in the sample. This is particularly relevant for small biopsy samples. The chondrocytes in the cartilaginous foci stain positively for vimentin and S-100 protein (131).

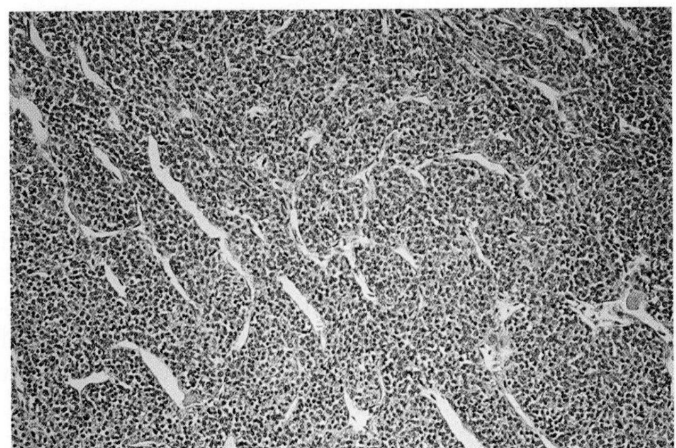

FIGURE 27. The cellular areas are composed of sheets of small blue cells supported by a branching hemangiopericytoma-like vascular pattern.

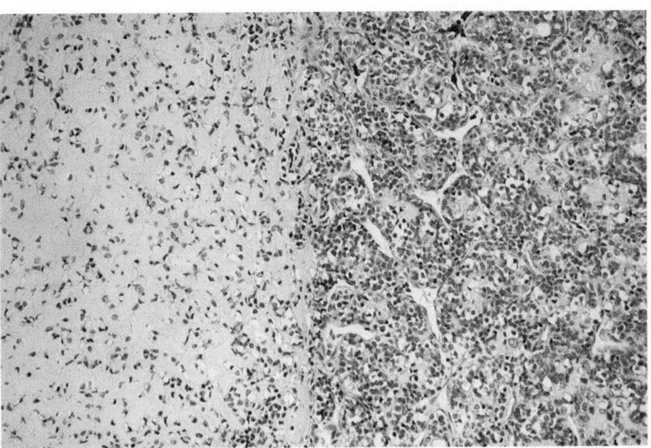

FIGURE 28. Mesenchymal chondrosarcoma showing the juxtaposition of the chondroid component (at left) with cells in lacunae and the cellular component with a prominent hemangiopericytoma-like vascular pattern.

Mesenchymal chondrosarcoma is treated by radical surgery with adjuvant radiation or chemotherapy. The overall 5- and 10-year survival rates for patients with this disease are poor and are 55% and 27%, respectively (129); however, the prognosis for tumors arising within the jaw bones appears to be better (82% and 56%, respectively) (130).

The differential diagnosis of mesenchymal chondrosarcoma is principally other small blue cell tumors of bone, which are discussed in detail in the section on Ewing's sarcoma/PNET.

Chordoma

Chordoma is a slow-growing malignant neoplasm that accounts for less than 5% of primary bone tumors. It is thought to arise from ectodermally derived notochordal remnants. This hypothesis is supported by the fact that chordomas have similar histologic, immunohistochemical, and ultrastructural characteristics to those of the notochord (132–140).

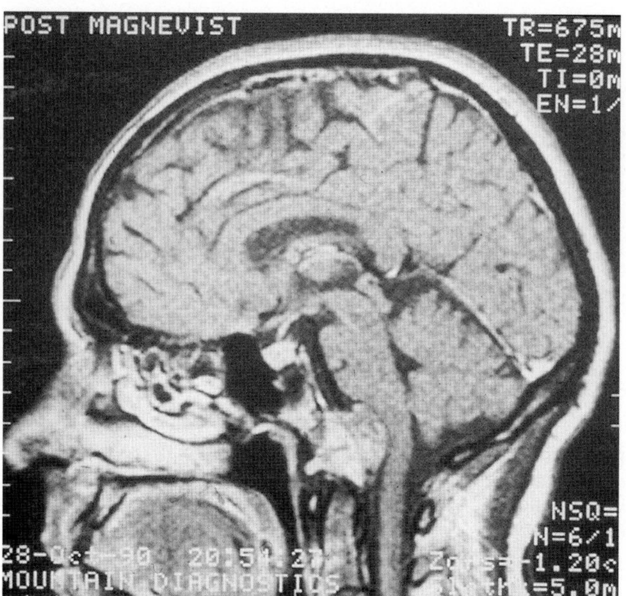

FIGURE 29. Clival chordoma impinging on the brainstem.

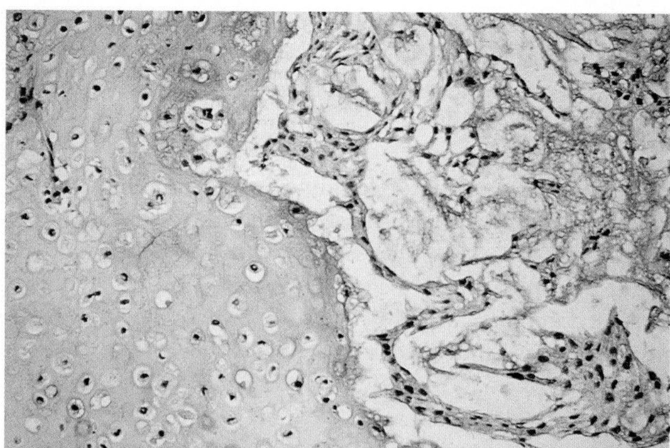

FIGURE 31. The chondroid component of chondroid chordoma has cells residing in lacunae in a chondroid matrix (at left) and more classic areas of chordoma with cohesive cells embedded in a myxoid matrix.

Chordomas arise in the axial skeleton, most commonly the sacrum, followed by the base of the skull in the area of the sella turcica, where cranial notochordal remnants are most plentiful (Fig. 29), and then the spine. Most patients are 30 to 70 years of age at the time of diagnosis, and men are affected more frequently than women. Chordomas in children and adolescents are uncommon: less than 5% are detected before the age of 20 (141,142).

Histologically, chordoma is subclassified into three different variants: conventional chordoma, chondroid chordoma, and dedifferentiated chordoma (143).

Conventional chordoma has a lobular growth pattern with the tumor cells arranged in cohesive nests or cords that are enmeshed in a frothy myxoid matrix. The neoplastic cells are large and epithelioid and have abundant eosinophilic cytoplasm that is occasionally vacuolated (Fig. 30). The vacuolated cells are known as physaliphorous cells. Chordoma cell nuclei vary slightly in size and shape, but occasionally they can demonstrate prominent nuclear pleomorphism that has no clinical significance. Another distinctive feature of chordoma is the wrapping of one cell around another, as if one cell is hugging the other.

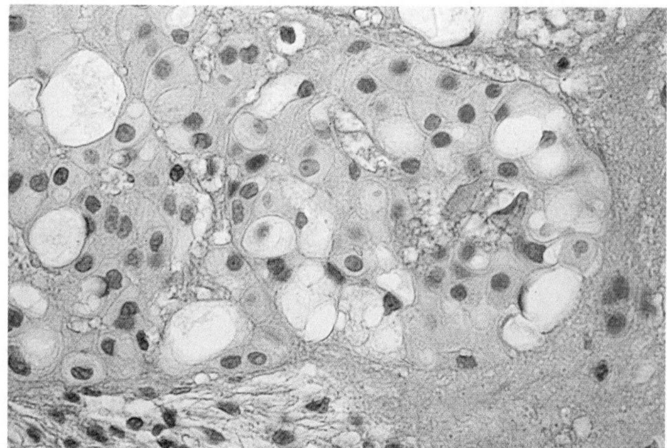

FIGURE 30. Chordoma composed of cohesive cells with abundant eosinophilic cytoplasm. Many cells have intracytoplasmic vacuoles (physaliferous cells).

Chondroid chordoma is composed of variable amounts of conventional chordoma and areas mimicking hyaline chondrosarcoma in which single tumor cells reside in lacunae surrounded by a hyaline-appearing stroma (Fig. 31). This entity has evoked a lot of controversy, and its existence has even been questioned (138,144–150). This stems from the fact that the tumors in many reported cases and series of chondroid chordomas are actually myxoid chondrosarcomas that were misinterpreted as chondroid chordoma. We believe that chondroid chordoma does indeed exist.

Dedifferentiated chordoma, by far the rarest variant of chordoma, is composed of areas of classic chordoma juxtaposed to a high-grade sarcoma that frequently has the appearance of malignant fibrous histiocytoma (MFH). This type of dedifferentiation can occur both as a primary event and secondary to radiation therapy.

The characteristic ultrastructural features of chordoma include villus-like projections, basal lamina, prominent desmosomes, intracytoplasmic glycogen and intermediate filaments, and mitochondria–rough endoplasmic reticulum complexes.

Immunohistochemically, the tumor cells in both the conventional variant and in the chondroid areas in chondroid chordomas express vimentin, S-100 protein, and epithelial markers such as keratin and EMA.

Base of skull chordomas are locally aggressive tumors, and surgery in conjunction with postoperative radiation is the standard form of therapy. Although chondroid chordoma was initially believed to have a better prognosis than the conventional variant (151), more recent studies have documented that their prognoses are not significantly different from one another (152). The dedifferentiated variant, however, has a much worse prognosis than the conventional or the chondroid type.

In our experience with almost 300 patients with skull base chordomas, the 5- and 10-year progression-free survival rates have been 70% and 45%, respectively, using combined surgery and proton beam radiation therapy (148).

Fibroosseous Lesions

Fibroosseous lesions are composed of an admixture of fibrous tissue and bone. These lesions are common in the craniofacial bones and are often difficult to subclassify. At one end of the spectrum is fibrous dysplasia (FD), which is composed of irregularly shaped trabeculae of woven bone devoid of osteoblastic rimming. At the other end is ossifying (or cementoossifying) fibroma, composed of trabeculae of woven or lamellar bone that have prominent osteoblastic rimming. Another variant of OF is juvenile (psammomatoid) OF, characterized by numerous psammomatoid-calcified structures. Many lesions, however, do not fall neatly into any category, and it is not uncommon for these fibroosseous lesions to show overlapping features. The radiographic findings can sometimes be very helpful in these instances, and, as in any bone tumor, the radiographic findings should be reviewed before a final diagnosis is rendered.

Fibrous Dysplasia (Fibroosseous Dysplasia)

Fibrous dysplasia is a benign process that was previously thought to be a developmental defect in the formation of lamellar bone such that bone formation is arrested at the stage of woven bone. Recently, monostotic and polyostotic FD has been shown to contain a mutation in the Gsα gene with resultant increased activity of the Gs protein and increased formation of cyclic adenosine monophosphate. It has been hypothesized that this results in overproduction of disorganized fibrous matrix and woven bone formation (153,154).

Fibrous dysplasia was first described by Lichtenstein and Jaffe as a distinct fibroosseous tumor of bone (155,156). It can involve a single bone (monostotic) or multiple bones (polyostotic). Albright's syndrome is the combination of polyostotic FD, cutaneous pigmentation (café au lait spots), and endocrine abnormalities, especially precocious puberty in girls, as well as hyperthyroidism (157,158). Mazabraud's syndrome is the combination of polyostotic FD and intramuscular myxomas (159). FD frequently involves the craniofacial bones, most commonly the maxilla followed by the mandible (80). FD of the craniofacial bones is slightly more common in women, and most patients are in their second or third decades of life at the time of diagnosis.

Clinically, FD can be asymptomatic and may be an incidental finding at radiography, or it can cause expansion of the affected bone and result in severe cosmetic deformities, especially in patients with polyostotic FD.

Radiographically, FD has a classic ground-glass appearance, but depending on the amount of bone present and its state of mineralization, it can be markedly radiodense, especially when it involves the jawbones and skull base. It has ill-defined margins that blend imperceptibly with the surrounding bone (Fig. 32) (160).

Grossly, FD has a gritty, leather-like consistency (Fig. 33). Histologically, it is composed of cellular fibrous tissue that surrounds irregular, curvilinear bony trabeculae. The fibrous tissue is composed of plump spindle cells, without cytologic atypia or mitotic figures, that are frequently arranged in a storiform pattern. The trabeculae are discontinuous (they do not interconnect), are composed predominantly of woven bone, and are formed directly by the spindle-shaped cells without osteoblastic rimming (fibroosseous metaplasia) (Fig. 34). The trabeculae of bone fuse with the surrounding host cancellous bone, which explains the lack of demarcation radiographically. Collagen fibers

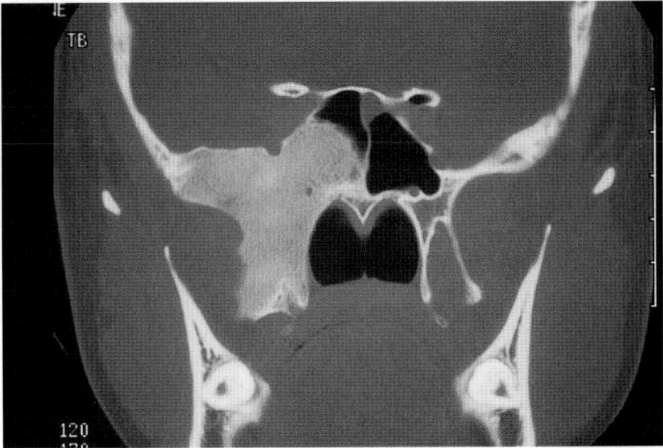

FIGURE 32. Radiograph of fibrous dysplasia. A ground-glass lesion involving the sphenoid region of the skull.

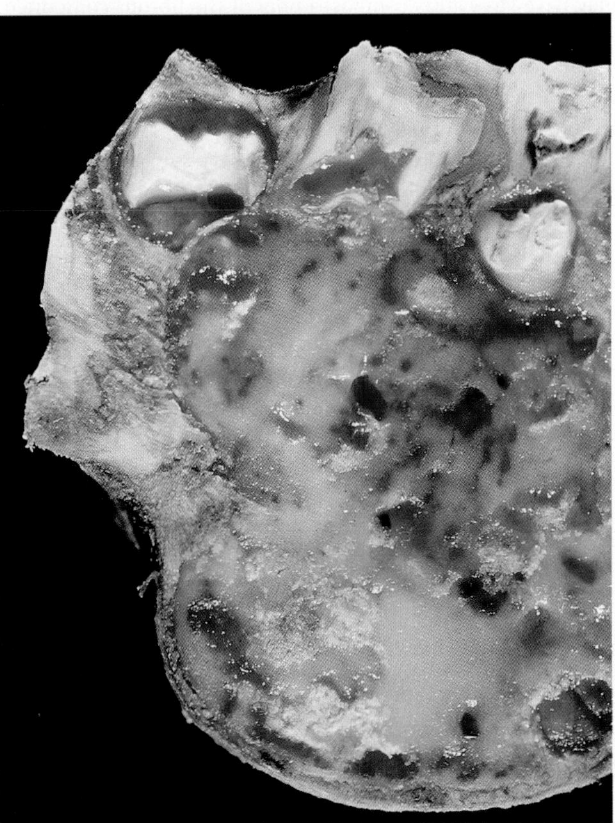

FIGURE 33. Fibrous dysplasia with a grayish tan cut surface, focally gritty bony areas, and small areas of hemorrhage.

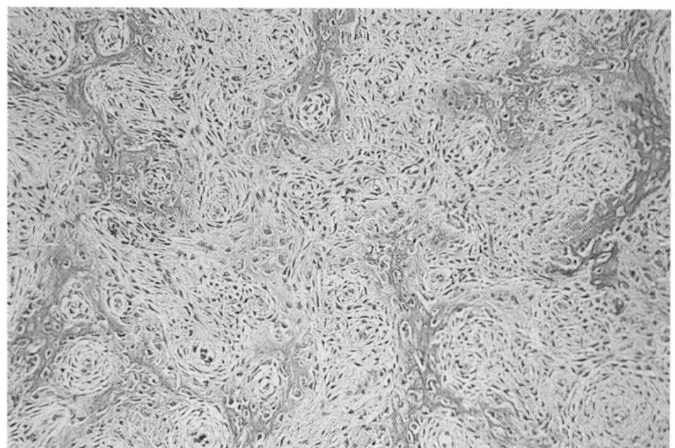

FIGURE 34. Fibrous dysplasia composed of discontinuous trabeculae of woven bone that lack osteoblastic rimming. The intertwining fibrous tissue is composed of plump spindle cells without cytologic atypia.

(Sharpey's-like fibers) are frequently seen extending from the bone and into the surrounding fibrous tissue. In the craniofacial bones, lamellar bone formation with osteoblastic rimming can be seen focally (161), and its presence should not argue against the diagnosis of FD as long as the clinical and radiographic features are consistent with that diagnosis (160). Cortical-type bone is not found in FD (160). Round ossicular or psammomatoid bodies also may be present in varying amounts. In some cases of FD, bone formation can be prominent, especially in those arising in the jawbones and skull base (80). Alternatively, other cases may have large areas composed only of the fibrous component. Cystic changes mimicking ABC are not uncommon. Although hyaline cartilage may be found in up to 20% of cases of FD of the appendicular skeleton, we have never seen cartilaginous differentiation in FD of the craniofacial bones. The treatment of choice for FD of the craniofacial bones is observation or conservative therapy when the lesion causes disfigurement.

Malignant transformation in FD (both monostotic and polyostotic) is rare, and only approximately 0.4% of cases undergo this process. Patients with Albright's syndrome have a higher incidence (~4%) (162). Although FD and sarcoma can be diagnosed simultaneously, sarcomas generally arise years after the initial diagnosis of FD (163). Many patients have a history of previous radiation therapy, so the possibility of radiation-induced sarcoma rather than malignant transformation of FD cannot be entirely excluded in these patients (162,163). The malignant tumors that develop in FD are sarcomas of various subtypes, including osteosarcoma, fibrosarcoma, chondrosarcoma, and MFH. They most frequently arise in the maxilla and mandible (162). In patients with FD, any change in the clinical course, especially in older individuals, such as increased pain and swelling, should raise the possibility of a malignant degeneration (162).

Ossifying Fibroma (Cementoossifying Fibroma, Cementifying Fibroma)

Ossifying fibroma is a well-demarcated fibroosseous lesion that consists of an admixture of fibrous tissue, interconnecting bony trabeculae lined by osteoblasts, and variable amounts of cementum-like material. Depending on the amount of bone and cementum-like tissue, these lesions have been called ossifying fibroma when bone predominates, cementifying fibroma when cementum-like material is in abundance, and cementoossifying fibroma when there is an admixture of both of these matrices. This subdivision has little if any clinical or prognostic significance (164).

Although OF has a wide age range, most patients are in the third and fourth decades of life at the time of diagnosis. Women are affected more frequently than men, with a female:male ratio as high as 5:1 (164,165). OF arises in tooth-bearing regions, and the vast majority (up to 90%) develop in the mandible. Within the mandible, the molar region is the most common site, followed by the premolar area, incisor area, and the cuspid region (165). Most lesions are detected incidentally; some patients complain of pain, numbness, asymmetry, or swelling (164).

Radiographically, OF is a unilocular, variably mineralized, well-demarcated lesion that does not blend with the surrounding bone as seen in FD (Fig. 35).

Grossly, the tumor is well demarcated with a gritty, nodular cut surface (Fig. 36). Histologically, it is well demarcated and easily separated from the surrounding bone. It is composed of fibrous tissue that classically contains an admixture of interconnecting trabeculae of woven (and sometimes lamellar) bone lined by osteoblasts and ovoid, basophilic cementum-like deposits (Fig. 37). ABC-like changes can be seen (165).

Due to the well-circumscribed nature of the lesion, it separates easily from the surrounding bone when shelled out. Local recurrence has been observed in up to 30% of cases; no specific clinical, radiographic, or microscopic features can predict which lesion will recur (165). Surgical curettage should be the initial treatment of choice, and en bloc resection should be considered for recurrent lesions. Malignant transformation has not been reported.

Psammomatoid (Juvenile) Ossifying Fibroma

Psammomatoid ossifying fibroma (POF) is a fibroosseous lesion that has a predilection for the supraorbital frontal and ethmoid

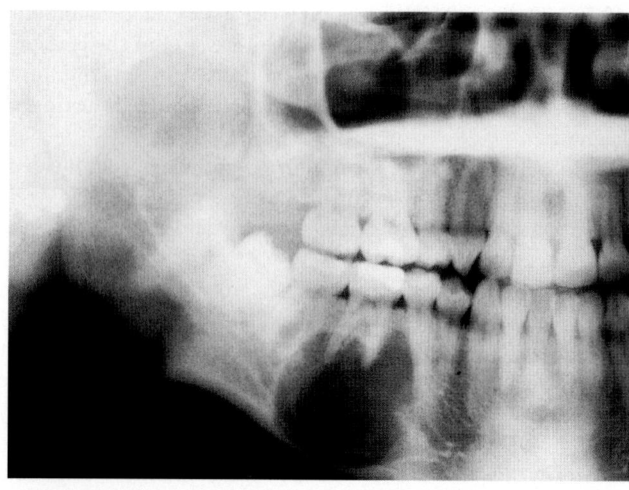

FIGURE 35. Cementoossifying fibroma. A unilocular, well-demarcated lesion arising in the mandible.

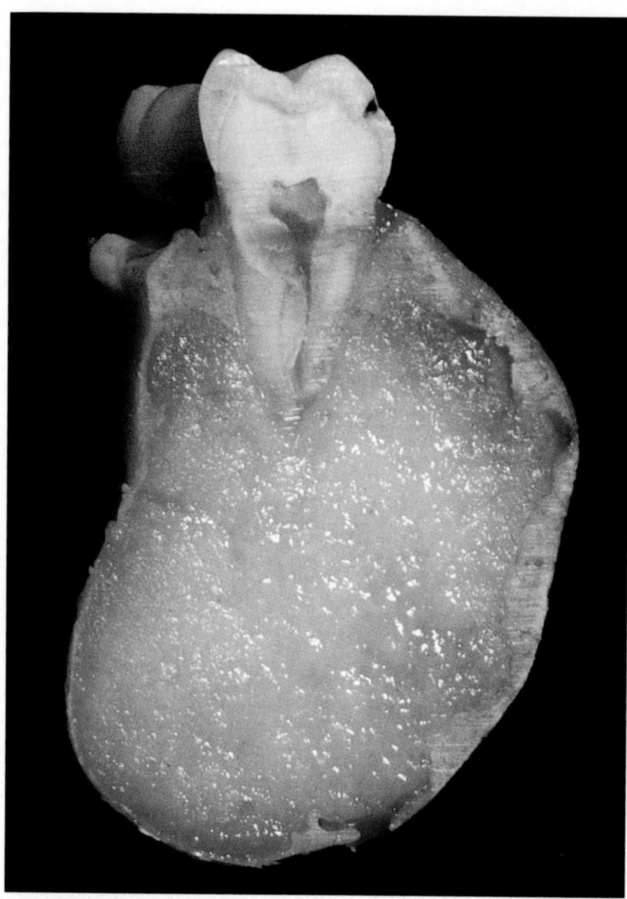

FIGURE 36. Cementoossifying fibroma is well circumscribed and has a gritty and nodular cut surface.

bones, and the ethmoid and the maxillary sinuses (166). In the literature it also has been known as ossifying fibroma, juvenile or young ossifying fibroma, juvenile active ossifying fibroma, cementifying fibroma, and cementoossifying fibroma (166). These terms reflect the uncertain histogenesis of this tumor and the presence of numerous "cementicle"-like structures.

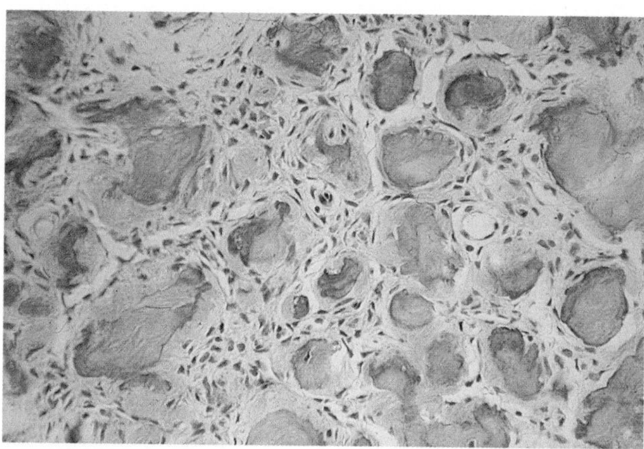

FIGURE 38. Psammomatoid ossifying fibroma with prominent cementicle-like deposits.

Psammomatoid ossifying fibroma arises primarily in young individuals: most patients are in their second decade of life. However, POF has been reported in patients as old as 54 years (166,167). The male:female ratio is approximately equal.

Clinical symptoms depend on the exact site of origin of the tumor, with the most common clinical manifestation being proptosis. Other signs and symptoms include visual disturbances, nasal obstruction, papilledema, strabismus, headaches, ptosis, and recurrent sinusitis (166,167).

Radiographically, POF shows an aggressive growth pattern, sometimes with invasion into adjacent anatomic structures; however, occasionally it can be well demarcated and expansile (166).

Grossly, the tumor is firm to hard and tan–white (166). Histologically, it is composed of a cellular fibrous component consisting of bland stellate or spindle cells, woven bone spicules, and small ossicular or cementicle-like structures having a concentric layering (psammomatoid) pattern (Fig. 38). The ossicles contain ostecytes and some are rimmed by osteoblasts. Large specimens often reveal a zoning pattern, with the hypercellular area having psammomatoid ossicles or cementicles in the center

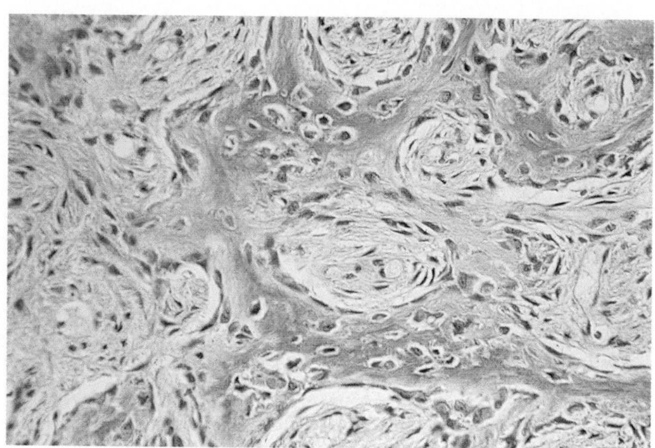

A

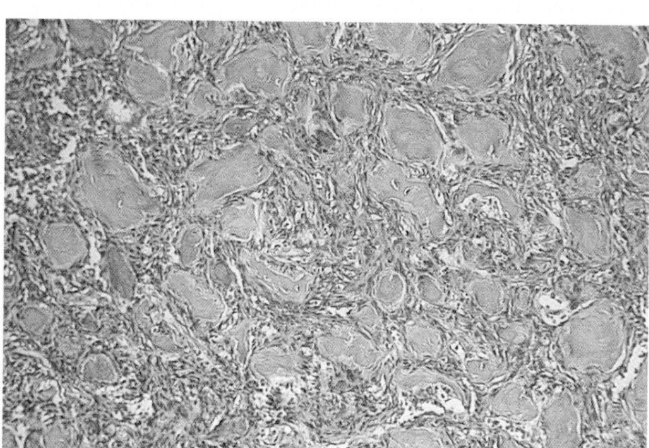

B

FIGURE 37. Cementoossifying fibroma is composed of fibrous tissue that contains an admixture of woven bone with osteoblastic rimming **(A)** and cementum-like deposits **(B)**.

merging with peripheral FD-like/OF-like areas that in turn merge with lamellar bone or bone with a pagetoid pattern (167). Cystic change and areas of hemorrhage with clustering of multinucleated osteoclast-type giant cells can be seen. Ultrastructural examination reveals an admixture of fibroblasts, osteoblasts, and osteoclasts, as well as calcium hydroxyapatite deposits either in areas occupied by collagen fibers or as amorphous dense aggregates, the latter corresponding to the psammoma bodies (168). The clinical behavior of POF is that of repeated local recurrences (169,170), and because of this aggressive behavior the term *aggressive POF* has been proposed (166). It is unclear why this fibroosseous lesion behaves more aggressively than other fibroosseous lesions of the head and neck, but it might be related to the "limited confines of the sinonasal tract," so that an expansile lesion ultimately causes bone erosion (166). Surgery is the treatment of choice and should be as complete as possible.

The main differential diagnosis of this tumor includes meningioma with numerous psammoma bodies invading bone. Knowledge of the patient's age, anatomic location, and radiographic findings is important. Also, meningioma involving bone shows a very infiltrative growth pattern, extending in between bony trabeculae in contrast to the relatively noninfiltrative growth pattern seen in POF. Also, the psammoma bodies in meningiomas are not associated with ostecytes or osteoblasts (166).

Giant Cell–Rich Lesions

Giant Cell Tumor

Giant cell tumor of bone rarely affects the craniofacial skeleton. It is difficult to evaluate its true incidence, because many reports of GCT of the craniofacial skeleton, when critically reviewed, actually represent examples of GCRG (171). Bona fide GCTs of the craniofacial bones do occur, however, and represent up to 2% of GCTs of bone (50,60).

Clinical signs and symptoms depend on the location of the tumor but include pain, swelling, headache, visual disturbance, dysphasia, memory loss, 5th or 7th cranial nerve dysfunction, olfactory hallucinations, and endocrine disorders (172,173).

Giant cell tumor of the craniofacial skeleton affects all age groups but tends to arise in patients who are older than those with GCT of long bones, with one third of patients being over 50 years of age at the time of diagnosis (172). There is a female predominance. The sphenoid bone is the most frequent site, followed by the temporal bone. Although GCTs also have been reported in the jawbones, some researchers believe that GCT does not arise in the mandible or maxilla except in association with Paget's disease (80). However, we have seen giant cell–rich tumors of the jawbones that we consider to be GCTs. Because approximately 50% of GCTs occurring in the setting of Paget's disease of bone arise in the skull and jaw (50), the possibility of Paget's disease should always be considered in a patient with a GCT in this location.

Radiologically, GCTs are locally destructive, radiolucent, and poorly defined and often have an associated soft tissue mass (Fig. 39) (172). These features are not unique for GCT, and in tumors arising in the sphenoid bone the radiographic differential diagnosis includes chordoma, pituitary tumor, and nasopharyngeal carcinoma (172).

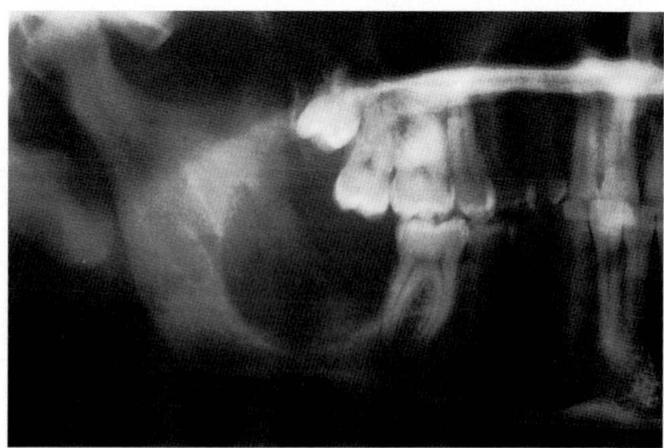

FIGURE 39. Giant cell tumor of mandible showing a well-demarcated radiolucent lesion.

Grossly, GCTs are red–brown and hemorrhagic. Microscopically, they are composed of evenly distributed osteoclast-type giant cells and oval mononuclear stromal cells that have nuclei identical to those in giant cells (Fig. 40). Other features include spindling of the mononuclear cells, sclerosis, hemosiderin deposition, peripheral reactive woven bone formation, and vascular invasion (172), all features that can be seen in conventional GCT of long bones. GCT of the skull can be very aggressive, resulting in local recurrence and even death. Subtotal excision with postoperative radiation therapy is the treatment of choice in many cases (172–174), and in some situations chemotherapy has been used as well (175).

The main differential diagnoses are GCRG and brown tumor, which are discussed below.

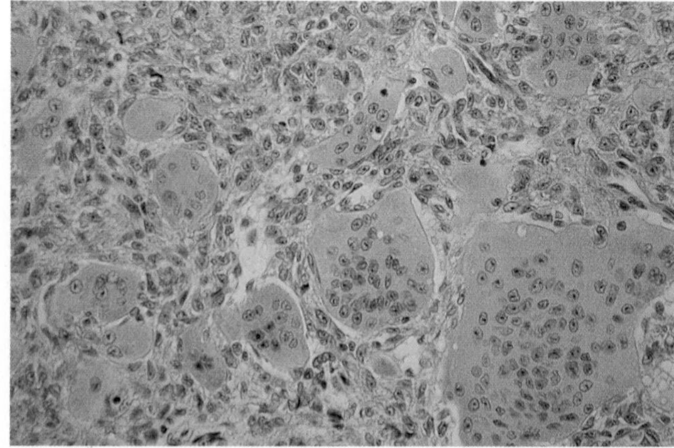

FIGURE 40. Giant cell tumor composed of giant cells with innumerable nuclei (more than is seen in giant cells in giant cell reparative granuloma) separated by mononucleated cells that have similar nuclear features.

Giant Cell Reparative Granuloma (Giant Cell Granuloma)

The term *giant cell reparative granuloma* was initially coined by Jaffe in 1953 (176) to describe a particular lesion of the jaw bones that had previously been diagnosed as GCT of bone (177). As the name implies, and as Jaffe believed, GCRG is considered to be a reparative or a reactive, non-neoplastic process. This term, however, is somewhat misleading, because this lesion can be destructive and does not contain true epithelioid histiocytic granulomas. Therefore, the noncommittal term *giant cell lesion* has been recommended by some investigators (177). GCRG characteristically arises in the mandible and less commonly in the maxilla, where it has a tendency to involve the anterior portions (incisor-cuspid-bicuspid region) of these bones and usually does not extend posterior to the first permanent molar area. It rarely affects other bones of the skull (171,178).

The term *central GCRG* is used to distinguish this intraosseous lesion from the peripheral or soft tissue GCRG, which is also known as giant cell epulis. Peripheral GCRG involves the soft tissues of the gingiva or alveolar mucosa and may arise from the periosteal surface of the bone (179,180).

The majority of central GCRGs occur in the first and second decades of life and are approximately twice as common in females as in males (171,181). Clinically, the patients complain of pain, swelling, or displacement of teeth. Some lesions are also incidentally discovered on x-rays that are taken for other reasons.

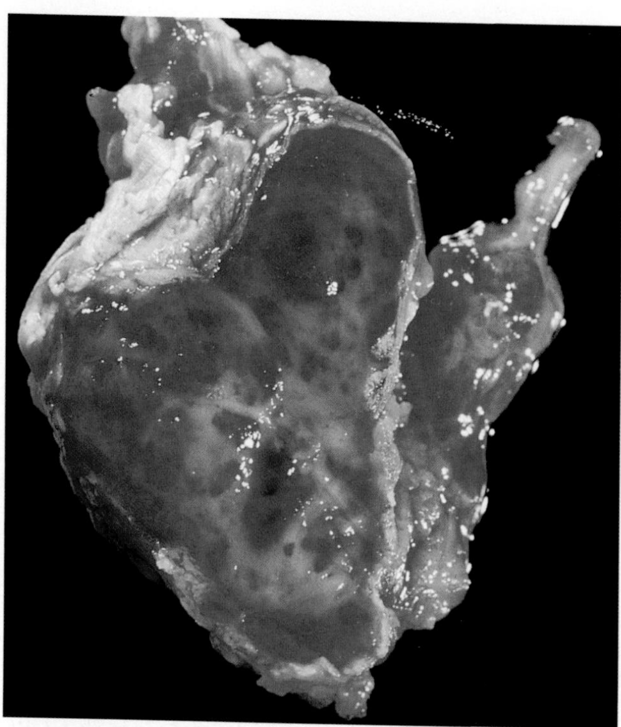

FIGURE 42. Giant cell reparative granuloma demonstrating a red–brown and focally tan sectioned surface. A thin shell of reactive bone surrounds the periphery of the tumor.

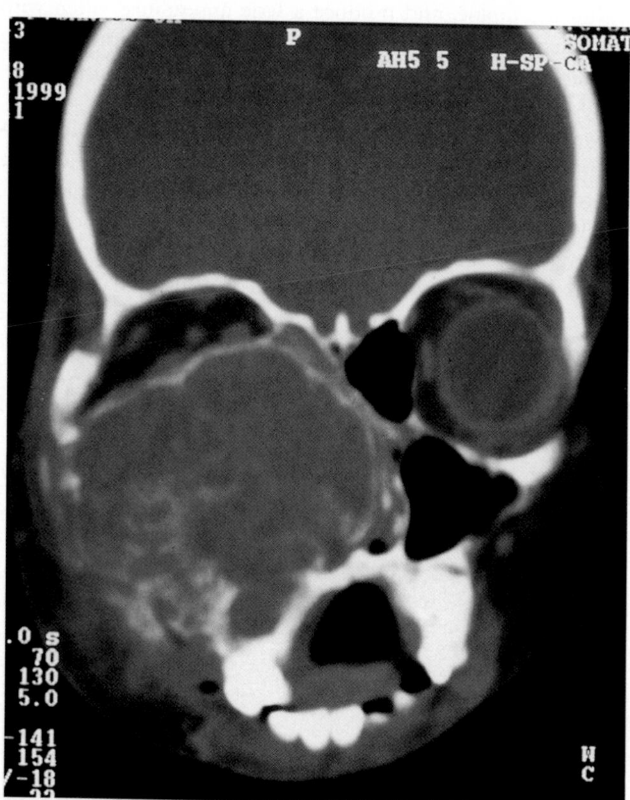

FIGURE 41. Large maxillary giant cell reparative granuloma demonstrating a radiolucent, trabeculated, and well-circumscribed expansile mass.

The rare case of GCRG arising in the body of a vertebra or the skull base produces other symptoms related to the site of origin.

Radiographically, central GCRG forms a well-demarcated, radiolucent, and often trabeculated or multiloculated ("soap bubble") lesion that may expand the bone (176,182) (Fig. 41). The multiloculated appearance is more common in larger tumors. Adjacent teeth are more frequently displaced than resorbed (181). The cortex is usually intact, and there is no periosteal reaction (143).

Grossly, the tumor is red–brown and hemorrhagic (Fig. 42), and, microscopically, it consists of lobules of spindled fibroblasts that are admixed with extracellular collagen, areas of hemorrhage, and numerous multinucleated osteoclast-like giant cells (Figs. 43 and 44). These giant cells tend to be arranged in small aggregates, contain fewer nuclei than seen in conventional GCT of bone, and are almost always associated with areas of hemorrhage (Fig. 44). Additionally, scattered lymphocytes, hemosiderin deposits, and reactive woven bone rimmed by osteoblasts (171) and small blood-filled spaces (ABC-like areas) are frequently present. Mitotic figures are usually few in number.

Although GCRG is believed to be a reactive/reparative process, a history of trauma is often not elicited. However, previous trauma may be forgotten or the traumatic episode can precede the appearance of GCRG by many years (171). It has been hypothesized that the giant cell–rich areas represent a reaction to recent hemorrhage and that the fibroblastic component represents the older or the healing part of the lesion (171).

The treatment for GCRG is curettage, after which the lesion usually heals and becomes ossified (180,183). The rate of recur-

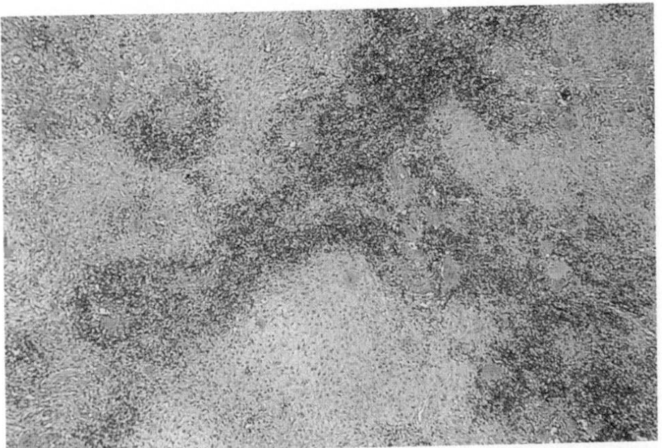

FIGURE 43. Giant cell reparative granuloma showing pale areas (containing predominantly the spindle cells) and large areas of hemorrhage (where the giant cells reside).

rence is less than 20% (180,184–186). In surgically inaccessible lesions such as the skull base, partial removal of the lesion, combined with radiation therapy, may be indicated (171,184,186)

The histologic differential diagnosis includes a variety of lesions. Morphologically, it is impossible to distinguish GCRG from brown tumor of hyperparathyroidism, and Jaffe in his original description actually believed that brown tumor of hyperparathyroidism "also represents a giant-cell reparative granuloma" (176). Therefore, every patient with GCRG should have the appropriate tests to rule out hyperparathyroidism. The jaw lesion present in patients with Jaffe-Companacci syndrome (multiple nonossifying fibromas, café au lait skin lesions, and other extraskeletal anomalies) is also histologically similar if not identical to GCRG (50), and the possibility of Jaffe-Companacci syndrome should always be raised in a patient with multiple jaw lesions. Some bone pathologists even believe that GCRG is identical to nonossifying fibroma of the long bones. Another tumor in the differential diagnosis is GCT of bone. Unlike GCRG, the giant cells in GCT of bone contain more nuclei than the giant cells in GCRG, and the nuclei in the giant cells are morphologically identical to those of the stromal cells. Another feature facilitating their distinction from one another is the distribution of the giant cells. In GCRG the giant cells tend to cluster around areas of hemorrhage, whereas in GCT of bone they are evenly distributed throughout the tumor.

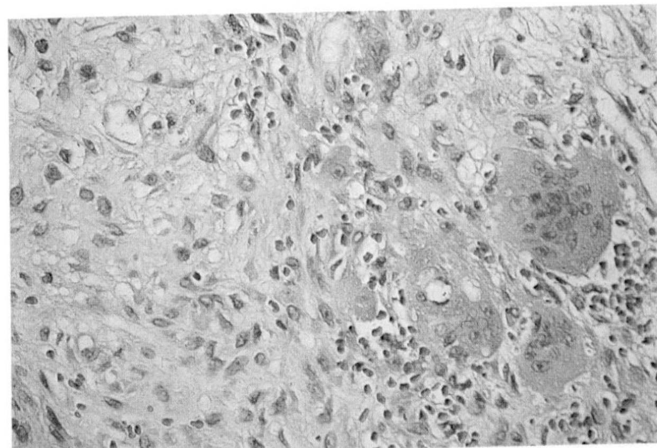

FIGURE 44. Giant cell reparative granuloma consisting of bland spindle cells **(left)** and osteoclast-type giant cells surrounded by red blood cells **(right)**.

Cherubism is characterized by multiple lesions closely resembling or identical to GCRG that predominantly involve the mandible and less commonly the maxilla. It is an autosomal dominant disorder with variable penetrance in females. The patients present with bilateral painless swelling of one or both jaws around the age of 1 to 7 years. The swelling continues for some years, but generally regresses at the time of puberty. It is usually a self-limited disorder; however, disfiguring lesions may be treated with curettage (187,188).

Vascular Tumors

Benign Vascular Tumors: Hemangioma

Although intraosseous hemangiomas may be found within vertebral bodies in up to 10% of autopsy specimens, clinically detectable hemangiomas of bone are uncommon (189). These tumors frequently develop in the vertebral bodies; however, the second most frequent site of occurrence is the craniofacial skeleton, where they involve the calvarium and present as painless or minimally painful lumps (189–193). Skeletal hemangiomas predominantly affect adults and are more common in women than men (189,190).

Radiographically, the cranial tumors are usually centered within the diploë, and produce a lytic appearance, often with prominent radiating intralesional spicules of bone producing a so-called sunburst appearance (189,190) (Fig. 45). The craniofacial skeletal hemangiomas are usually isolated lesions. However, they may be a component of multifocal bone involvement. Gorham's syndrome (disappearing bone disease) is a rare disorder characterized by osseous hemangiomas that produce extensive osteolysis and can extend from one bone to a neighboring one. The skull is commonly affected in this setting (194).

Grossly, an osseous hemangioma is a gritty dark red intraosseous mass that may have a distinct sponge-like appearance if resected intact (Fig. 46). Most are composed of dilated cavernous vascular spaces that may or may not be filled with red blood cells. The thin-walled vessels are lined by a single layer of uniform, cytologically bland, flattened endothelial cells. The vessels are surrounded by loose connective tissue, and they typically

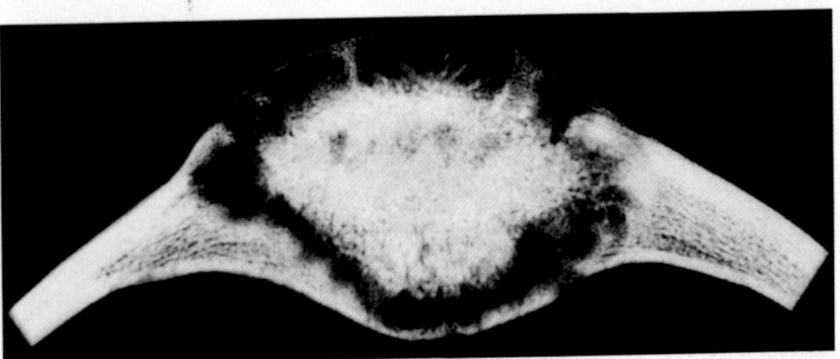

FIGURE 45. A specimen radiograph of a skull hemangioma demonstrating intralesional spicules of reactive bone.

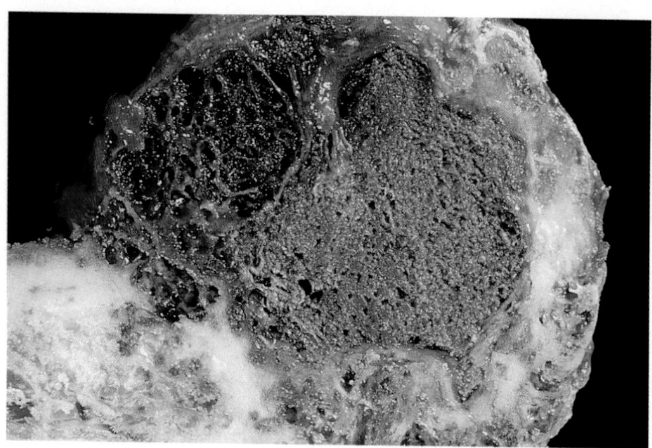

FIGURE 46. Hemangioma having a sponge-like cut surface.

infiltrate preexisting cancellous bone (Fig. 47). Entrapped thickened bony trabeculae produce the radiographically detectable intralesional spicules. Intraosseous epithelioid hemangioma is a variant of osseous hemangioma that may pose diagnostic difficulty because of the plump histiocyte-like or epithelioid appearance of the endothelial cells and the tendency for these cells to be arranged in solid cords and even sheets (195–198). A minority of endothelial cells typically contain one or more intracytoplasmic vacuoles that are believed to represent primitive vascular lumen formation at the single cell level. The stroma that surrounds epithelioid hemangiomas commonly contains numerous inflammatory cells, including plasma cells and eosinophils. Although these tumors almost always contain conventional-appearing vessels that are an inherent component of the tumor, they may be few in number, resulting in diagnostic difficulty.

Immunohistochemically, the endothelial cells in osseous hemangioma exhibit positive staining for the vascular markers Factor VIII–related antigen, *Ulex europaeus* lectin, CD34, and CD31 (195). Approximately 50% of epithelioid hemangiomas additionally stain for keratin and EMA (195).

Local excision is usually curative, because recurrences are uncommon (189,190). The differential diagnosis of conventional skeletal hemangioma is limited. On occasion the bone within osseous hemangiomas is well formed and the vascular spaces may not be recognized as part of a tumor. Under these circumstances, the pathologic material may be incorrectly considered to be nonspecific or within normal limits. Clinical and radiographic correlation to ensure that the sample represents the abnormality allows correct interpretation.

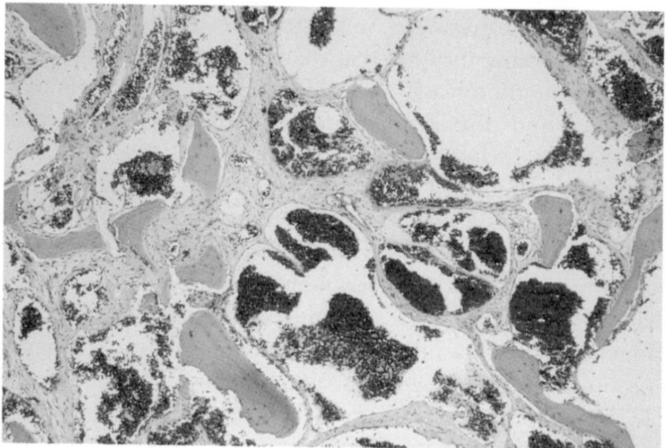

FIGURE 47. Hemangioma containing ectatic blood vessels and vascular channels that infiltrate between bone trabeculae.

The differential diagnosis of epithelioid hemangioma includes epithelioid hemangioendothelioma (EHE) and epithelioid angiosarcoma which are both discussed in detail below.

Malignant Vascular Tumors

Epithelioid Hemangioendothelioma

Epithelioid hemangioendothelioma is an uncommon endothelial tumor of borderline malignancy that was originally described in the soft tissues, liver, and lung; however, in recent years primary tumors of the skeleton have been recognized (199,200). Like other skeletal vascular tumors, multifocal osseous involvement occasionally occurs (185,199). The tumor is rarely reported in craniofacial bones. The literature that addresses skeletal EHE is confusing because many tumors reported as osseous EHE likely represent examples of epithelioid hemangioma or other vascular neoplasms (190,201–203). Osseous EHE presents as a punched-out lytic defect, typically without intralesional mineralization (184,199,200)

Grossly, osseous EHE appears pale tan in color, which belies its vascular nature. Microscopically, EHE is composed of lobules of epithelioid cells arranged in cords and nests, as well as scattered spindle cells, that are embedded within a myxoid to hyalinized ground substance (184,199,200). The latter often results in the tumor resembling a cartilaginous neoplasm. The neoplastic cells have eosinophilic cytoplasm and central round to oval nuclei that often exhibit readily visible nucleoli. Intracytoplasmic vacuoles which may contain red blood cell fragments represent primitive vascular differentiation. In fact, well-formed blood vessels lined by epithelioid endothelial cells are not prominent in most EHEs. This feature, in addition to the relative paucity of intralumenal or extravasated red blood cells, results in these tumors having a distinctly nonvascular appearance.

Immunohistochemically, the tumor cells demonstrate the full spectrum of endothelial markers and, like the cells in epithelioid hemangioma, also may exhibit positive staining for keratin antibodies.

Epithelioid hemangioendothelioma is treated by complete surgical excision if feasible. Predicting the prognosis for patients with osseous EHE is problematic, and the literature that refers to this subject is difficult to interpret because of the confusion in nomenclature applied to vascular tumors of the skeleton composed of epithelioid endothelial cells. Skeletal EHE may behave in a locally aggressive manner, and may often present with concurrent visceral disease, especially the lung and liver (184,199,200). The differential diagnosis of EHE is principally the other epithelioid vascular neoplasms discussed in detail in this section.

The epithelioid features of the tumor cells, their cohesive nature and intracytoplasmic vacuoles also can mimic metastatic carcinoma, especially metastatic adenocarcinoma. This distinction can be further complicated by the occasional staining of

EHE for epithelial markers. Most metastatic carcinomas, however, do not stain for endothelial markers. The myxoid or hyalinized stroma also can suggest a cartilaginous neoplasm. However, the cells in cartilaginous tumors do not form cohesive nests. Additionally, they stain immunohistochemically for S-100 protein and are negative for endothelial markers.

Angiosarcoma

Skeletal angiosarcomas are extremely rare tumors. The majority occur in adults and affect the axial and appendicular skeleton (189,190,204–207). Whereas most of these tumors affect a single bone, up to one third present with involvement of multiple bones (204).

Radiographically, angiosarcoma of bone appears as ill-defined lytic masses with prominent destruction of the underlying osseous matrix (189,190,204–207) with or without a soft tissue mass.

Grossly, skeletal angiosarcomas are hemorrhagic tumors that may exhibit necrosis and prominent bone destruction. Vessel formation is often rudimentary, and much of the tumor resembles an undifferentiated spindle and epithelioid cell malignant tumor. As with the other epithelioid vascular tumors, the cells may contain cytoplasmic vacuoles. Mitoses are numerous, and atypical mitotic figures are usually readily identified. Many of the tumors that historically were classified as low-grade hemangioendothelial sarcomas of bone likely represent examples of epithelioid hemangioma (195).

When the tumors that were formally classified as low-grade hemangioendothelial skeletal sarcomas are excluded, the prognosis for angiosarcoma is extremely poor (189,190,204–207).

The differential diagnosis of osseous angiosarcoma includes epithelioid hemangioma and EHE. In the case of epithelioid angiosarcoma, metastatic poorly differentiated carcinoma and metastatic malignant melanoma also enter into the differential diagnosis. Immunohistochemistry is very useful in distinguishing between these three possibilities, but it should be noted that angiosarcomas frequently demonstrate positive staining for cytokeratin in addition to endothelial cell markers. In this differential diagnosis, it is important to note that most carcinoma and melanoma cells are negative for Factor VIII–related antigen, CD31, and CD34.

Fibrous Lesions

Desmoplastic Fibroma

Desmoplastic fibroma is an extremely rare primary bone tumor that is considered the intraosseous counterpart of soft tissue fibromatosis. Like the latter lesion, it is locally aggressive but never metastasizes. In the craniofacial region, the mandible, particularly the ramus/angle region, is most commonly affected (208–211). Interestingly, the left side of the mandible is involved more frequently than the right side (211). Rarely the tumor arises in the maxilla, temporal bone, frontal bone, or parietal and sphenoid bone (211–217).

Desmoplastic fibroma affects a wide age range, including children, but generally develops in the second or third decade of life, similar to desmoplastic fibromas of the appendicular skeleton (218). The tumor is slow growing, and the most common presenting symptom is gradual swelling of the bone. Other symptoms include headache, recurrent otitis, and hearing loss; rarely it results in a pathologic fracture.

Radiographically, desmoplastic fibroma forms a unilocular or multilocular radiolucent lesion, often with a honeycomb or trabeculated appearance. Rarely it has a permeative or more aggressive appearance (208,213).

Histologically, desmoplastic fibroma is similar to soft tissue fibromatosis. The tumor is composed of spindle-shaped cells arranged in broad, sweeping fascicles, and the cells are surrounded by extracellular collagenous matrix. Cellular atypia or pleomorphism is not present, and mitoses are infrequent. Prominent vessels are found throughout the tumor. In areas, the tumor may be very hypocellular and show abundant collagen production. At the periphery of the tumor, there may be focal infiltration of the cancellous bone; however, extensive infiltration should raise concern for fibrosarcoma or low-grade osteosarcoma. Desmoplastic fibroma can break through the bone and infiltrate adjacent soft tissue in the same manner as soft tissue fibromatosis.

Desmoplastic fibroma is a locally aggressive tumor with a high rate of local recurrence. The treatment of choice is complete local excision (208,213). Desmoplastic fibroma does not metastasize, and we are aware of only one case of sarcomatous transformation in a recurrent desmoplastic fibroma (site not specified) (80).

The differential diagnosis of desmoplastic fibroma is a well-differentiated fibrosarcoma and intramedullary low-grade osteosarcoma. Well-differentiated fibrosarcoma is more cellular than desmoplastic fibroma and contains more nuclear atypicality and readily identified mitotic figures. It also has a more infiltrative growth pattern. Low-grade intramedullary osteosarcoma rarely arises in the bones of the skull and jaws. It is composed of a bland fibroblastic proliferation, similar to what is seen in desmoplastic fibroma. Unlike desmoplastic fibroma, well-differentiated osteosarcoma demonstrates neoplastic bone formation and extensively infiltrates the native bone.

Myofibroma/Myofibromatosis

Myofibromatosis was first recognized by Stout in 1954 as "congenital generalized fibromatosis" when he reported two infants with multiple fibrous nodules (219). Prior to his description, many of these tumors had been called *fibrosarcomas.* The term *infantile myofibromatosis* was later coined by Chung and Enzinger because they felt that the tumor cells were myofibroblasts and not fibroblasts (220). Myofibromas may be solitary or multifocal and arise in the dermis, soft tissues, internal organs, and skeleton, including the skull (220,221).

Unlike generalized myofibromatosis with visceral involvement, which has a poor prognosis, the solitary forms or those cases with multiple lesions without visceral involvement behave in a benign fashion. However, multifocal visceral disease, especially when it affects the gastrointestinal tract, may be fatal. When myofibroma involves the skeleton, it most frequently arises in the craniofacial bones, either the skull or the mandible (222).

Radiographically, myofibroma of bone manifests as a purely lytic lesion with a sclerotic rim of variable thickness (222–224).

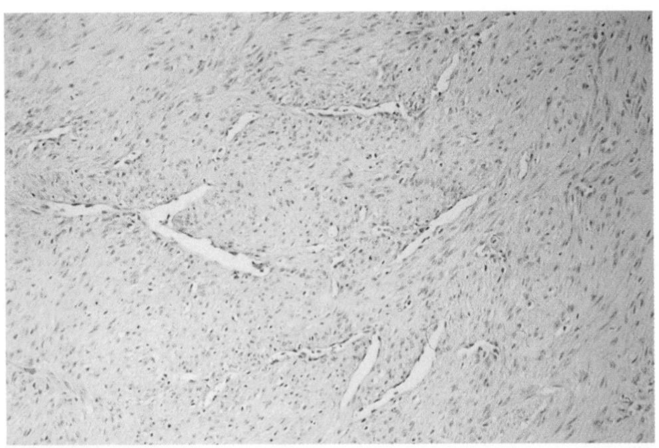

FIGURE 48. Myofibroma composed of pale spindle cells and a prominent hemangiopericytoma-like supportive vascular pattern.

Histologically, myofibroma of bone is similar to its soft tissue counterpart (see Chapter 10). In the center it is composed of sheets of small round or elongate cells that are associated with a supportive vascular network with a prominent hemangiopericytoma-like pattern. Peripherally the lesion consists of pale nodular areas composed of bland spindle cells with eosinophilic cytoplasm (Figs. 48 and 49). Ultrastructurally, the cells have the features of myofibroblasts, and immunohistochemically they stain for vimentin and smooth muscle actin and rarely for desmin, further supporting their myofibroblastic differentiation (223,225). Within bone, myofibroma has a pushing border, although focal infiltration can be seen at the periphery. Rare tumors show focal necrosis and calcification. Mitotic figures are generally rare, but in our experience can sometimes be numerous.

The differential diagnosis includes leiomyosarcoma. Leiomyosarcoma of the craniofacial skeleton is extremely rare. Unlike myofibroma, it has an infiltrative growth pattern and demonstrates significant cytologic atypia.

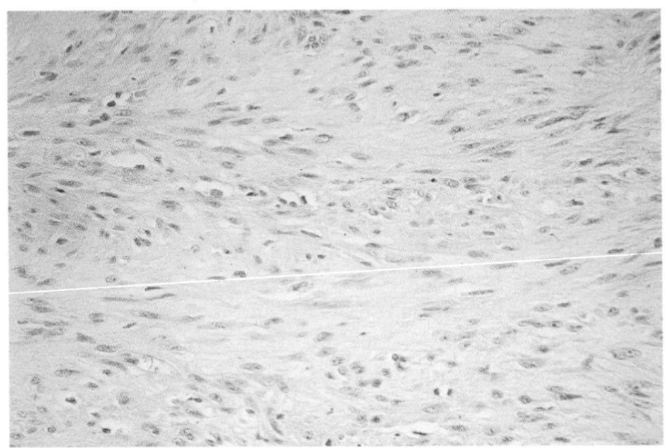

FIGURE 49. Myofibroma demonstrating bland spindle cells with elongated nuclei and pale eosinophilic cytoplasm.

Cystic Lesions of Bone

Simple Bone Cyst

Simple bone cyst (SBC), also known as unicameral bone cyst, is a fluid-filled, fibrous-walled cyst of unknown etiology. It most frequently affects the long bones, especially the proximal humerus and femur (80). In the craniofacial skeleton, most SBCs arise in the body or the symphysis of the mandible, and rarely do they involve other areas of the mandible or the maxilla (226–228). They are generally asymptomatic and are found incidentally on radiographs taken for other reasons. SBCs infrequently produce bone expansion or cause pain (229). They are usually diagnosed in children and adolescents and are rarely seen in adults (227). Their pathogenesis is unknown, but in the head and neck region, some investigators believe they are secondary to a traumatic event (hence the alternative terms *traumatic bone cyst, extravasation cyst,* and *hemorrhagic bone cyst*) and reflect the end stage of an organizing hematoma.

Radiographically, SBC is well demarcated and radiolucent. Grossly, it is filled with straw-colored or blood-stained fluid.

Histologically, the cyst is frequently unilocular and lined by a thin layer of fibrous tissue. Extravasated erythrocytes, osteoclast-type giant cells, and hemosiderin deposition may be present in traumatized cases (229). Matsumura and co-workers subdivided SBCs into two categories (228). The wall of type A cysts was composed only of a thin layer of connective tissue, whereas the wall of type B cysts also contained dysplastic bone formation. The latter may actually represent cystic degeneration of an underlying fibroosseous lesion. Most SBCs appear to undergo spontaneous resolution, because they are seldom seen in adults. In symptomatic cases the treatment is simple curettage, which is associated with a low rate of local recurrence. In the study by Matsumura and co-workers, type B cysts had a higher incidence of local recurrence (228).

The differential diagnosis of SBC includes ABC. An ABC generally demonstrates marked eccentric expansion of the affected bone. Histologically, an ABC is hemorrhagic and multilocular with thick walls containing plumb fibroblasts, histiocytes, and osteoclast-type giant cells.

Epidermoid Cyst

An epidermoid cyst forms when squamous epithelium becomes embedded in bone and proliferates, forming a mass and expanding the bone (80). Most epidermoid cysts occur in the skull bones, especially the frontal and parietal bones, and rarely do they arise in the maxilla or mandible. Radiographically, they present as a lytic, sharply defined lesion with sclerotic borders. Grossly, the cysts are filled with soft, white cheesy tissue (Fig. 50). The cyst lining is smooth and is easily detached from the adjacent bone. Histologically, the cyst wall is composed of squamous epithelium and the contents of the cyst consists of keratinous debris (Fig. 51). Epidermoid cysts behave in a benign fashion, although rare cases of squamous cell carcinoma have been reported to arise in the background of a preexisting epidermoid cyst (230).

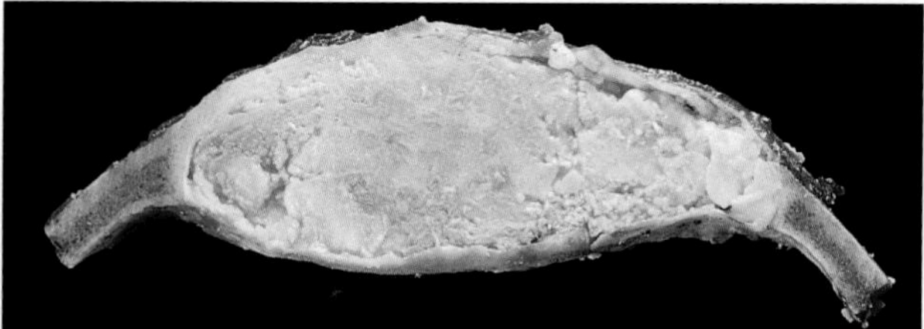

FIGURE 50. A large, well-demarcated epidermoid cyst filled with soft, keratinous white material.

Aneurysmal Bone Cyst

Aneurysmal bone cyst is the term applied to a benign, destructive, expansile, predominantly blood-filled cystic mass occurring in the skeleton (231–234). Although these lesions demonstrate many pathologic and radiographic features of an aggressive neoplasm, they behave in a benign fashion and there is controversy regarding whether they represent a neoplastic proliferation or a reactive process (231–234). Two distinct subtypes of ABC are recognized. Those that arise *de novo* are termed primary, whereas those that occur on the background of a preexisting neoplasm or other skeletal abnormality are termed secondary (231,232). Primary ABCs account for approximately 70% of cases (233). The majority of secondary ABCs complicate neoplasms such as GCT or osteoblastoma (231–233).

Primary ABC most commonly arises within the metaphyses of long bones and the axial skeleton (231,232). However, 2% to 5% occur within the craniofacial skeleton (232,235). Males and females are equally affected, and patients are usually under 30 years of age at the time of diagnosis (232–234,236). Patients typically present with a painful mass. Specific symptoms related to a craniofacial location include loosening of teeth, nasal stuffiness, diplopia, and raised intracranial pressure (235,237–239).

Radiographically, primary ABCs demonstrate expansion of the affected bone. The tumor is frequently well circumscribed and often contains a shell of reactive subperiosteal bone (231,232,234). Intralesional radiodensities are uncommon. Cross-sectional imaging with computed tomography and magnetic resonance imaging demonstrates the expanded nature of the bone, a relatively smooth interface with adjacent soft tissue structures, and, most characteristically, fluid–fluid levels within the multiloculated center of the lesion (231,232).

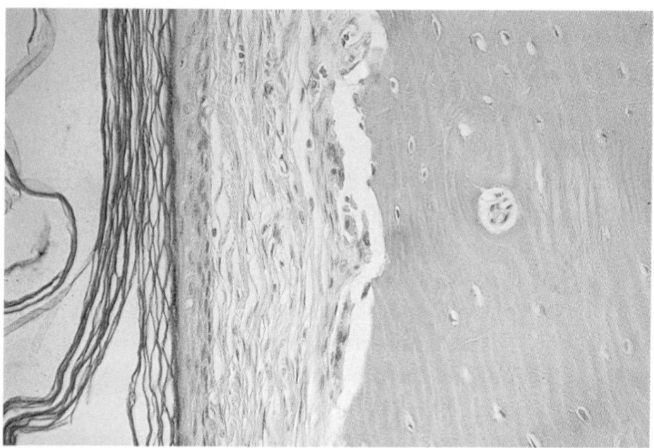

FIGURE 51. The epidermoid cyst is lined by keratinizing squamous epithelium.

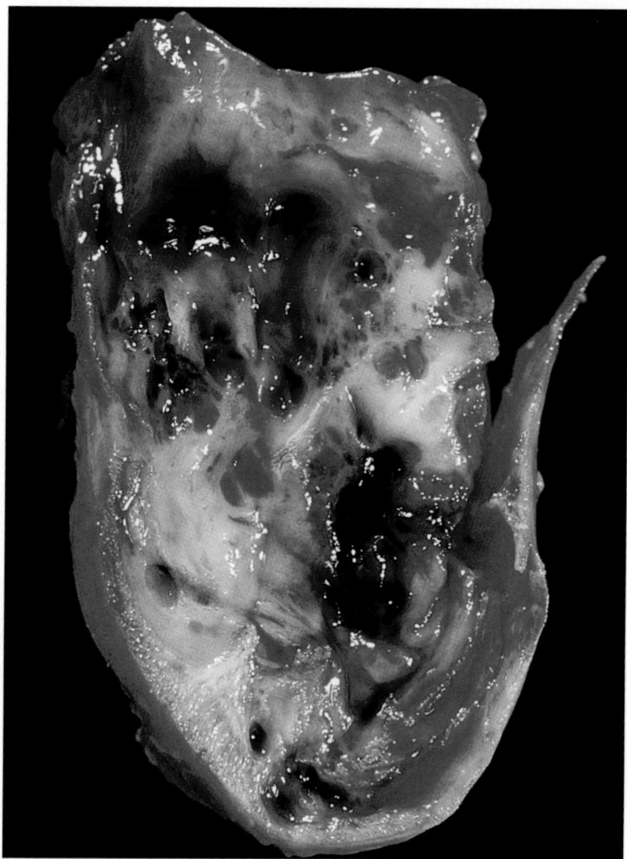

FIGURE 52. Aneurysmal bone cyst containing characteristic blood-filled cystic spaces that are separated by fibrous tissue.

Grossly, ABCs consist of blood-filled cystic spaces separated by thin strands of soft tissue resulting in a multilocular appearance (Fig. 52). The strands that traverse the blood-filled spaces are usually nonmineralized and easily cut with a knife. Solid tan, red, or gray nodules of tissue may be present adjacent to the cystic component of the mass, particularly in the setting of a secondary ABC. Microscopically, the blood-filled cystic spaces are not lined by endothelial cells but are covered by plump spindled or oval reactive fibroblasts or histiocytes. These cells along with osteoclast-type giant cells and reactive woven bone comprise the substance of the cyst wall and any solid component of the lesion (Fig. 53). Sometimes the osteoclast type giant cells may be so numerous that it can be difficult to distinguish the lesion from a GCT of bone. The reactive woven bone is usually trabecular in architecture and lined by osteoblasts and is deposited so that it follows the contours of the cyst lumen (232–234). Approximately one third of ABCs contain a partially calcified cartilage-like matrix adjacent to the cystic spaces (232). This material has been termed *lacy chondroid* and is considered by some to be virtually pathognomonic of ABC (50). Mitotic figures may be in the cyst walls, and necrosis is uncommon unless there has

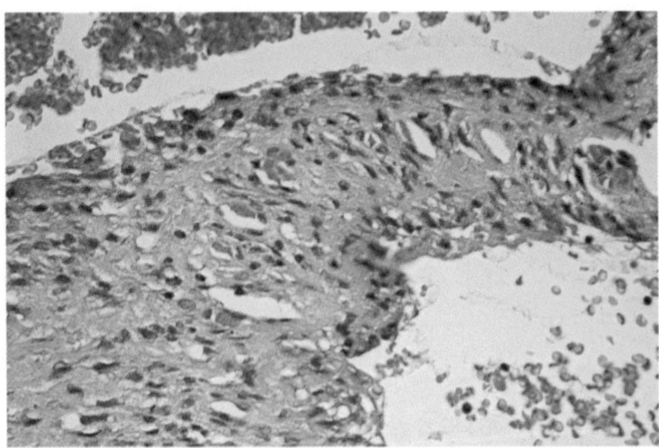

FIGURE 53. Septum from an aneurysmal bone cyst lined by plump fibroblasts. The septum is composed of highly vascular loose connective tissue.

been a previous fracture. The cortical and cancellous bone at the expanding edge of an ABC exhibits prominent osteoclastic resorption and reactive woven bone formation. The bone marrow adjacent to the mass typically shows mild fibrosis and edema. Marked nuclear pleomorphism, atypical mitotic figures, and permeative growth within cortical or cancellous bone are not seen in ABC and should raise the possibility of osteosarcoma. A minority of ABCs demonstrate a predominantly solid growth pattern with relatively few blood-filled cystic spaces (240,241). The tissue that comprises these tumors is essentially identical to the walls of conventional ABC. This variant of ABC has been given the paradoxical designation of solid ABC. Such lesions may be difficult to differentiate from GCRG, and some researchers believe that they are identical lesions.

Aneurysmal bone cysts are managed by surgical excision, usually in the form of curettage or partial resection. The overall recurrence rate is on the order of 10% to 44% (231,238). Maxillary ABCs demonstrate a rate of recurrence in the lower end of this range (235).

The differential diagnosis of ABCs includes all of the entities that may undergo secondary ABC-like change; however the most important tumor from which it must be distinguished is telangiectatic osteosarcoma. Grossly, telangiectatic osteosarcoma may closely simulate ABC, being composed of blood-filled cystic spaces separated by strands of predominantly nonmineralized soft tissue. However, high-power examination of the constituent cells in telangiectatic osteosarcoma always reveals marked pleomorphism, hyperchromatic nuclei, and a brisk mitotic rate including atypical forms. Necrosis is also commonly present in telangiectatic osteosarcoma, but it is uncommon in ABC unless preceded by pathologic fracture.

Miscellaneous

Melanotic Neuroectodermal Tumor of Infancy

Melanotic neuroectodermal tumor of infancy (MNTI) was originally described by Krompecher in 1918 when he reported a congenital melanoma (melanocarcinoma) arising in the maxilla in a 2 month-old infant (242). A variety of terms have been used for this tumor in the literature, such as melanotic ameloblastoma, pigmented ameloblastoma, melanoameloblastoma, melanotic progonoma, retinal anlage tumor, congenital melanocarcinoma, melanotic ameloblastic odontoma, and retinoblastic teratoma (51), reflecting its history of uncertain and controversial histogenesis. Currently it is believed to be a neoplasm of neural crest derivation (242,243).

Over 90% of MNTIs arise in the head and neck region, mainly in the anterior portion of the maxilla (approximately 70% of cases), followed by the skull and the mandible; the tumor also can arise in the brain and intracranial dura (244–247). A case arising in the temporal bone and soft tissues of the cheek also has been reported (248,249). Rarely, MNTI occurs outside the head and neck, for example, in the testis (250). Although MNTI has been reported in adults, the vast majority develop within the first year of life (245). Males and females are affected approximately equally.

Clinically, it presents as a rapidly growing, painless, expansile, pigmented mass that causes anterior protrusion of the upper lip and can interfere with feeding (244,246). Occasional cases have produced increased levels of vanillylmandelic acid that have returned to normal after removal of the tumor, similar to other tumors of neural crest origin such as neuroblastoma, ganglioneuroblastoma, and pheochromocytoma (242,243)

Radiographic studies show a destructive, osteolytic lesion displacing adjacent teeth and tooth buds (246,248).

Grossly, the tumor has a black or a gray cut surface (Fig. 54). Histologically, the tumor is composed of two populations of cells—namely, large and small cells—that are embedded in a dense fibrous stroma (Fig. 55). The larger, epithelioid, cells have a pseudoalveolar, glandular, or tubular arrangement and contain abundant eosinophilic cytoplasm, and many cells have large amounts of intracytoplasmic dark brown melanin pigment (Fig. 55A). The smaller cells form solid nests that are often sur-

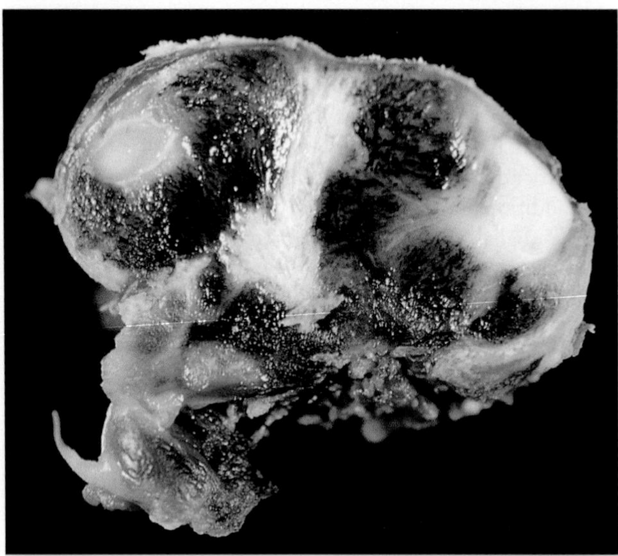

FIGURE 54. Melanotic neuroectodermal tumor of infancy has a characteristic black or gray cut surface. Two teeth are present.

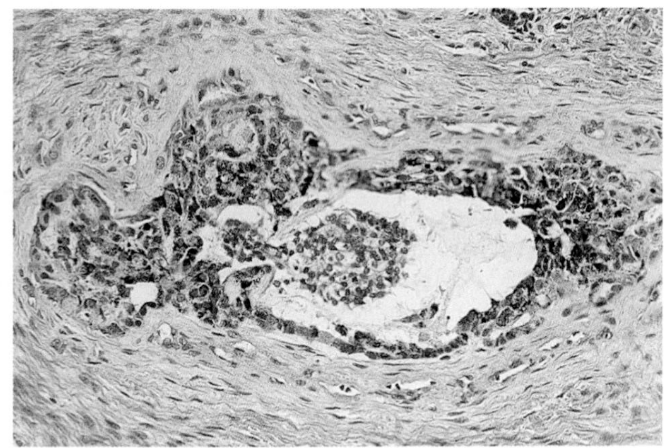
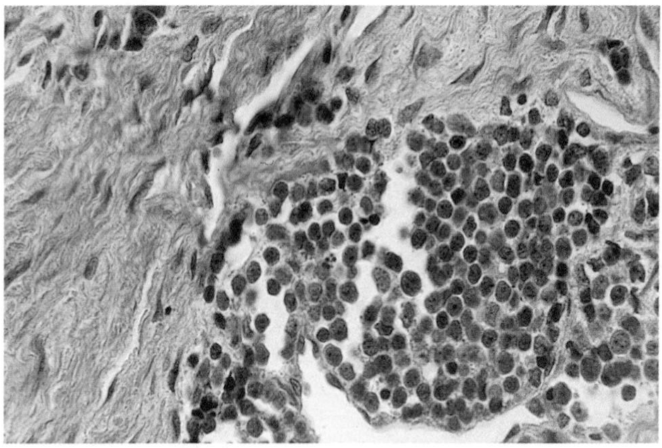

FIGURE 55. Melanotic neuroectodermal tumor of infancy showing two populations of cells. Large epithelioid cells with prominent intracytoplasmic melanin pigment surround a solid nest of small, round, nonpigmented cells **(A)**. The smaller cells are round, have dark nuclei, scant cytoplasm, and lack melanin pigment **(B)**.

rounded by the larger pigmented cells. These cells have scant cytoplasm and mimic small lymphocytes (Fig. 55B). They also can have more tapering, eosinophilic cytoplasmic processes, suggestive of neuroblastic differentiation. The smaller cells are generally nonpigmented, although pigment occasionally can be present within them. Mitotic figures are rare.

Ultrastructurally, the neoplastic cells form nests that are surrounded by an external basal lamina. As by light microscopy, two cell types can be identified ultrastructurally. The larger cells contain abundant intracytoplasmic melanosomes in different stages of maturation. Additionally these cells have numerous mitochondria and free ribosomes and are connected by numerous intercellular junctions, including desmosomes. The smaller cells are more primitive, they have nuclei that are slightly irregular in size and shape with clumped chromatin, and the cytoplasm contains predominantly mitochondria and free ribosomes. Melanosomes are not identified in these cells.

Immunohistochemical studies have shown different results with respect to the staining pattern of the large epithelioid cells and the smaller cells. The former cells generally show epithelial and melanocytic differentiation, with positive staining for keratin and HMB-45, whereas the smaller cells show predominantly neural differentiation with positive staining for a variety of neuroendocrine markers (248). Interestingly, rare tumors have additionally shown positive staining for desmin, muscle actin, and glial fibrillary acidic protein. Both cell types are generally negative for S-100 protein. This immunohistochemical profile suggests MNTI as being a PNET whose phenotypic expression includes the presence of epithelial markers, neural markers, melanin production, and occasional muscle and glial differentiation. These findings have suggested that this tumor might represent a dysembryogenetic neoplasm that recapitulates the retina at 5 weeks of gestation (248).

The treatment of choice is surgical excision. Although some studies have shown up to a 60% local recurrence rate (248), the overall local recurrence rate is generally about 10% to 15% (244,245). Metastases occur in less than 5% of cases (246). It is not possible to predict clinically or pathologically which cases will behave in a malignant fashion. Rare malignant cases also have been reported where the malignant component has acquired the features of a neuroblastoma (242,249,251).

Melanotic neuroectodermal tumor of infancy has classic light microscopic features that should not cause diagnostic difficulties on a large biopsy specimen. However, a small biopsy could be problematic in its accurate interpretation. The tumors that are in the histologic differential diagnosis include retinoblastoma, metastatic neuroblastoma, metastatic melanoma, and PNET. The presence of cytokeratin expression and HMB-45 distinguishes MNTI from retinoblastoma and neuroblastoma. Keratin expression is extremely rare in melanomas, and melanomas stain for HMB-45 in addition to S-100 protein. PNET can show positive staining for cytokeratin but does not stain for HMB-45.

Langerhans' Cell Histiocytosis (Eosinophilic Granuloma) of Bone

Langerhans' cell histiocytosis is characterized by infiltrates of Langerhans' cells, which are specialized antigen-presenting dendritic cells that normally occur in various body sites. Whether Langerhans' cell histiocytosis represents a reactive inflammatory process similar to sarcoidosis or a unifocal/multifocal neoplasm is not entirely clear (252). Recent evidence suggesting that Langerhans' cells in individual lesions are a clonal population supports the theory that the lesions are neoplastic in origin (253).

The clinical symptoms associated with this disease vary depending on the number, site, and size of the tumor(s). Traditionally, single or multiple skeletal lesions have been termed *eosinophilic granuloma* whereas multifocal disease associated with specific clinical symptoms has been included under the eponymic designations Hand-Schuller-Christian disease (exophthalmos, multifocal skeletal lesions, diabetes insipidus) and Letterer-Siwe disease (aggressive multifocal skeletal disease in infancy) (252,254–256). The skeleton is the most commonly affected organ in Langerhans' cell histiocytosis (252,254,255), and other body sites that may be affected include the skin, lung, and lymph nodes, although virtually any site may be involved. In general, monostotic skeletal lesions occur twice as frequently as polyostotic disease, and the most frequent presenting symptom is localized pain (252,254,255). The skull and facial bones, including the mandible, are involved in approximately one fourth to one third of cases (252,254,255). Mandibular lesions may cause toothache, tooth impaction, and oral ulcers, whereas mastoid involvement can produce hearing loss and otitis media. Headaches are associated with cranial involvement (252,254,255). Langerhans' cell histiocytosis manifests most commonly in the first three decades of life, and males are affected approximately twice as often as females (252,254,255).

Radiographically, the bone lesions, whether as part of monostotic or polyostotic disease, typically present as well-defined lytic masses (252,254,255). A minority of cases demonstrate ill-defined margins with a permeative pattern. Periosteal reaction may be present if the lesion involves the cortex of the affected bone (252,254,255). Most craniofacial lesions measure less than 3.0 cm in diameter. Complete resolution of radiographic abnormalities may follow treatment or occasionally occurs spontaneously.

Grossly, the lesional tissue has a nonspecific gritty tan appearance. Microscopically, it is characterized by an infiltrate of mononuclear oval to rounded histiocyte-like cells. These cells may be arranged in sheets or individually dispersed within a loosely fibrous stroma distributed among cortical and cancellous bone. The cells measure 10.0 to 15.0 μ in diameter and have eosinophilic cytoplasm (Fig. 56). Nuclei are central, oval in outline, and characteristically demonstrate deeply indented clefted nuclear membranes that result in readily visible nuclear grooves (Fig. 57). These are often prominent in the long axis of the nucleus, resulting in a coffee bean appearance. The chromatin is pale staining, and nucleoli are not prominent. Mitotic figures are variable in number; however, atypical mitotic figures are not seen. The mononuclear cells are admixed with scattered multinucleated osteoclast-like and Langhans' giant cells. Typically eosinophils are admixed with the Langerhans' cells and multinucleated cells, and these may be distributed evenly but commonly are arranged in clusters resulting in so-called eosinophilic abscesses (255) (Fig. 57). Additionally, mature lymphocytes and

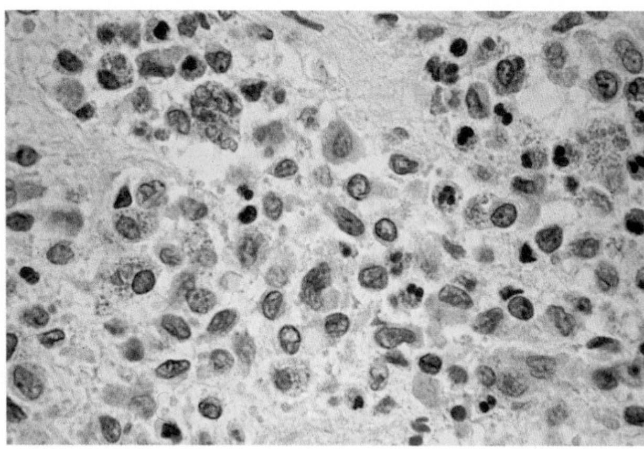

FIGURE 57. Langerhans' cells with characteristic clefted nuclei and eosinophilic cytoplasm. Note the scattered eosinophils in the background.

neutrophils are commonly present within the lesions (255). Necrosis is present in a minority of cases and may be prominent if pathologic fracture has occurred. The diagnosis of Langerhans' cell histiocytosis is principally based on the light microscopic appearance of the Langerhans' cells and the appropriate cellular background; however, adjuvant diagnostic techniques including electron microscopy and immunohistochemistry allow specific identification of Langerhans' cells (252,257). CD1a recognizes a cell membrane antigen that is specific for Langerhans' cells (252,257). Similarly, anti–S-100 protein antibodies strongly label Langerhans' cells, and although this latter staining reaction is not specific, it is characteristic for Langerhans' cells. Ultrastructurally, Langerhans cells' contain tubular, pentalaminar, membrane-bound cytoplasmic bodies, with central electron-dense granular material, that frequently demonstrate terminal oval protrusions, resulting in an appearance that has been likened to a tennis racket or lollypop (Fig. 58). They are thought to arise from an invagination and fusion of the plasma mem-

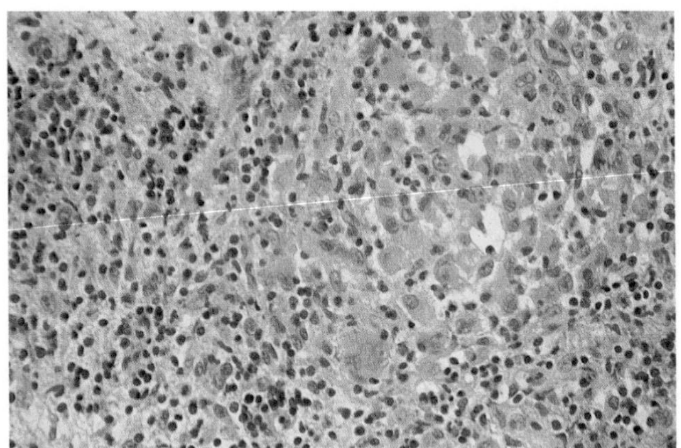

FIGURE 56. Eosinophilic granuloma, showing a mixed inflammatory infiltrate of Langerhans' cells, chronic inflammatory cells, and eosinophils.

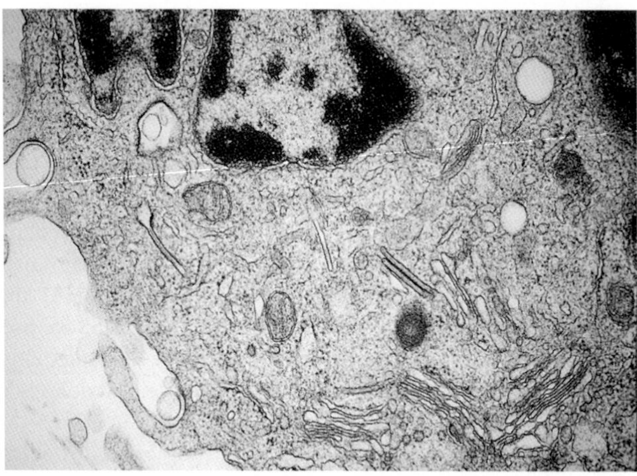

FIGURE 58. Ultrastructurally, the Langerhans' cells contain pentalaminar intracytoplasmic bodies, some with bulbous ends (Birbeck granules).

branes and are known as Birbeck granules and are a specific marker of Langerhans' cells (252).

The treatment and prognosis of Langerhans' cell histiocytosis depends on the site and size of the lesion, the age of the patient, and the presence or absence of multifocal disease. In general, monostotic disease is managed by curettage with or without low-dose radiation therapy, depending on the site of involvement (252,254,255). Single or multiagent chemotherapy may be administered when disseminated disease is present. Ultimately, there is a greater than 95% disease-free survival for patients with monostotic skeletal involvement (254).

The differential diagnosis of Langerhans' cell histiocytosis includes osteomyelitis (discussed earlier) and malignant lymphoma. Acute osteomyelitis typically demonstrates a prominent neutrophilic inflammation and fibrinous exudate in addition to bone necrosis. Chronic osteomyelitis exhibits a mixed inflammatory infiltrate similar to Langerhans' cell histiocytosis; however, it lacks the characteristic mononuclear Langerhans' cells and usually contains only a few eosinophils. Chronic osteomyelitis may contain numerous histiocytes. Primary skeletal malignant lymphomas or secondary bone involvement by generalized disease typically occurs with large cell non-Hodgkin's lymphoma. In these cases the mononuclear cells manifest a greater degree of nuclear atypia and mitotic activity. Immunohistochemistry for CD-1a, S-100 protein, and lymphoid markers will aid in establishing the correct diagnosis.

Schwannoma

Intraosseous peripheral nerve sheath tumors are uncommon and account for less than 1% of all primary bone tumors (258). Schwannomas account for the majority of these, although there have been rare reports of neurofibromas and malignant peripheral nerve sheath tumors arising in bone (258,259). The most common location for intraosseous schwannoma is the mandible (258,260–262), and rarely have they been described within other craniofacial bones (263,264).

Typically intraosseous schwannoma presents with the nonspecific symptoms of pain and swelling. Depending on the location of the tumor, patients may develop malaligned or loosened teeth.

Radiographically, the tumors are lucent and usually have a well-defined sclerotic border (258,260). Some bone expansion may be present, but there is usually no extraosseous soft tissue extension.

Intraosseous schwannomas grossly resemble their much more commonly occurring soft tissue counterparts (see Chapter 10) (258–264). They are usually well defined and tan–yellow on cut section. Focal regions of hemorrhage and cystic change also may be present. Microscopically, the hypercellular (Antoni A) and hypocellular (Antoni B) regions typical of schwannoma are present. The proliferating spindle cells have elongate, serpiginous, dark-staining nuclei with pointed ends. The cell cytoplasm is eosinophilic with ill-defined cell membranes. In some cases the nuclei are arranged in palisaded arrays forming Verocay bodies. Mitotic figures are uncommon. Foamy macrophages, mast cells, and mature lymphocytes commonly occur in the background. A helpful diagnostic feature of schwannoma in any site is the presence of scattered clusters of irregular medium-sized blood vessels whose walls demonstrate intense hyalinization. These vessels commonly exhibit lumenal thrombosis.

Immunohistochemically, schwannomas stain intensely for S-100 protein and vimentin.

Schwannomas are treated by conservative excision, which may include en bloc resection or curettage depending on the location of the tumor. Following resection the prognosis is excellent. Recurrence is extremely uncommon (258–264).

The differential diagnosis of osseous schwannoma includes other non–matrix-producing spindle cell tumors of bone, including desmoplastic fibroma and sarcomas such as MFH and leiomyosarcoma. Desmoplastic fibroma is more architecturally uniform than schwannoma, which characteristically exhibits regions of variable cellularity. Additionally the uniform spindle cells that compose desmoplastic fibroma are associated with abundant extracellular collagen in contrast to the collagen in schwannoma, which is patchy in its distribution. High-grade sarcomas such as MFH and leiomyosarcoma usually exhibit greater nuclear pleomorphism and readily detectable mitotic figures in contrast to schwannoma.

Leiomyosarcoma

Primary leiomyosarcomas of bone are extremely rare tumors (265). Although all age groups are affected, these tumors most commonly occur during middle age and late adulthood (265). Approximately one half of the leiomyosarcomas of the craniofacial skeleton that have been described have been associated with prior therapeutic irradiation (265). Patients typically complain of pain or swelling in the region of the tumor.

Radiographic images demonstrate a poorly defined lytic tumor, typically without intralesional mineralization (265).

The histologic features of osseous leiomyosarcoma are essentially similar to those of the much more commonly encountered primary soft tissue tumors (see Chapter 10). As such, the tumors are composed of sheets and fascicles of plump spindle cells with eosinophilic fibrillar cytoplasm. The nuclear atypia varies with the grade of the tumor. Low-grade tumors exhibit elongate spindle cells with classical blunt-ended nuclei, whereas high-grade tumors exhibit greater degrees of nuclear atypia (265). Necrosis is commonly present.

Immunohistochemically, the tumor cells exhibit positive staining for muscle actin, smooth muscle actin, and desmin. Focal cytokeratin staining also may be present (265).

Osseous leiomyosarcomas are managed by surgical resection with or without adjuvant radiation and chemotherapy. In the largest reported series of osseous leiomyosarcoma, the 5-year survival rate was 68% and the 5-year metastatic rate was 46% (265). In general, high-grade tumors behave in a more aggressive manner than low-grade tumors.

The differential diagnosis of osseous leiomyosarcoma is principally MFH. In fact, poorly differentiated regions of osseous leiomyosarcoma may be histologically indistinguishable from MFH. The distinction between these tumors is based on the presence of smooth muscle differentiation in the tumor cells. This usually means spindle-shaped cells with linear cytoplasmic fibrils or ultrastructural or immunohistochemical evidence of smooth muscle differentiation. Electron microscopy is the most definitive way to distinguish between these tumors because there is significant overlap between the immunohistochemical profile of myofibroblasts (the predominant cell type in MFH) and true smooth muscle cells.

Malignant Fibrous Histiocytoma

Malignant fibrous histiocytoma of bone is a non–matrix-producing sarcoma that formerly was included in the designation fibrosarcoma of bone (266). Similar to its much more common soft tissue counterpart (see Chapter 10), osseous MFH typically affects middle-aged and elderly adults (266). Although these tumors are distinctly uncommon, approximately 12% of osseous MFHs arise in the craniofacial skeleton (266). Typically, affected patients present complaining of pain or a mass (267–270). Radiographically, the tumors appear as a poorly circumscribed, nonmineralized lytic mass (266–270).

Most skeletal MFHs are high grade and are composed of fascicles of pleomorphic spindle cells arranged in a storiform pattern (266–270). Multinucleated tumor giant cells are frequently present. Necrosis and a high mitotic rate, including the presence of atypical mitotic figures, are commonplace. By definition these tumors do not produce neoplastic bone or cartilage matrix, but the neoplastic cells are often embedded within a collagen-rich stroma that may be hyalinized. Myxoid change, which is a common feature of soft tissue MFH, is less frequently encountered in the skeletal tumors.

Osseous MFH is usually managed in a manner similar to osteosarcoma. The 5-year survival rate for osseous MFHs from a variety of different sites, including the craniofacial skeleton, is approximately 50% (266). The lung is the most common site for distant metastases.

As discussed above, the principal differential diagnosis for osseous MFH is leiomyosarcoma.

Ewing's Sarcoma/Primitive Neuroectodermal Tumor

Ewing's sarcoma/PNET is a distinctive small round cell tumor that most frequently arises in the bones of the appendicular skeleton. Rarely does Ewing's sarcoma/PNET involve the bones of the craniofacial skeleton. In two large series, 7 of 512 (1.4%) (80) and 2 of 871 (0.23%) tumors (50) arose in the craniofacial skeleton. In a series of pediatric Ewing's sarcoma, 5 of 70 tumors (7.1%) arose in the head and neck region (271). In the intergroup Ewing's sarcoma study, only 4% of Ewing's sarcoma involved the bones of the head and neck (272). The clinical symptoms are those of pain or swelling of the affected bone.

Radiographically, Ewing's sarcoma/PNET produces a destructive and poorly defined tumor that often extends into the adjacent soft tissue.

Histologically, Ewing's sarcoma/PNET is composed of uniform small, round cells. The nuclei have finely dispersed chromatin and may contain small nucleoli. The cytoplasm is scant and in classic Ewing's sarcoma contains abundant intracytoplasmic glycogen (Fig. 59). Immunohistochemically, the tumor cells stain for vimentin and the vast majority are also positive for Mic-2 (CD99). PNET shows additional staining for one or more neural markers, such as neuron-specific enolase, Leu-7, S-100 protein, synaptophysin, neurofilament, or chromogranin. Ultrastructurally, classic Ewing's sarcoma is composed of small cells that have a high nuclear to cytoplasmic ratio. The nuclei are round and euchromatic. The cytoplasm contains glycogen, scattered free ribosomes, and occasional mitochondria. Small intercellular junctions may be present. In addition to these findings, PNET may have, in addition to the preceding findings, interdigitating cell processes and microtubules, but neuroendocrine granules are rare. Cytogenetically, the vast majority of these tumors have a t(11,22) translocation. The treatment is a combination of surgery, chemotherapy, and radiation therapy in selected cases. The differential diagnosis includes a variety of other small round cell tumors such as lymphoma, metastatic small cell carcinoma, rhabdomyosarcoma, and metastatic neuroblastoma (see Chapter 10).

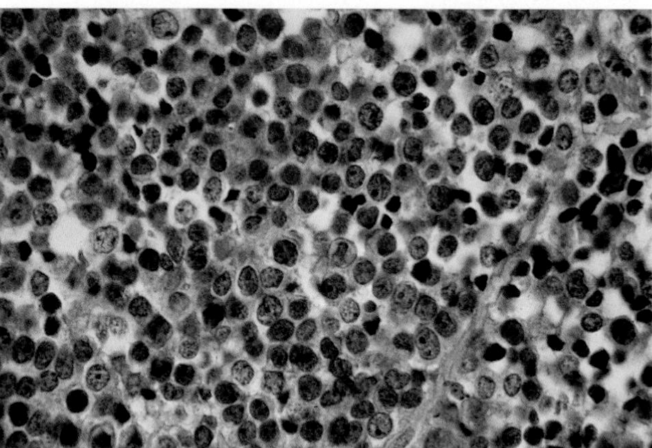

FIGURE 59. Ewing's sarcoma, composed of uniform, small, round cells with scant cytoplasm.

TUMORS AND TUMOR-LIKE LESIONS OF JOINTS

Primary Synovial Chondromatosis

In primary synovial chondromatosis, multiple nodules of hyaline cartilage expand the subsynovial connective tissue (273–275). At present, it is unclear whether the proliferating cartilage is metaplastic or neoplastic, but recent cytogenetic abnormalities found in synovial chondromatosis support a neoplastic process (276). This disorder affects patients of all ages and has no gender predilection (273–275). Any joint may be affected (277,278), and fewer than 100 examples of synovial chondromatosis involving the temporomandibular joint have been reported (279). There is no association between synovial chondromatosis and antecedent trauma, although on occasion an injury draws attention to an involved joint. Patients complain of pain and swelling related to the involved joint (273–275). Synovial chondromatosis appears as numerous glistening blue–gray nodules within the synovial membrane (273–275,277,278). Nodules range in size from 2.0 mm to over 1.0 cm and are firm on cut sectioning. They often demon-

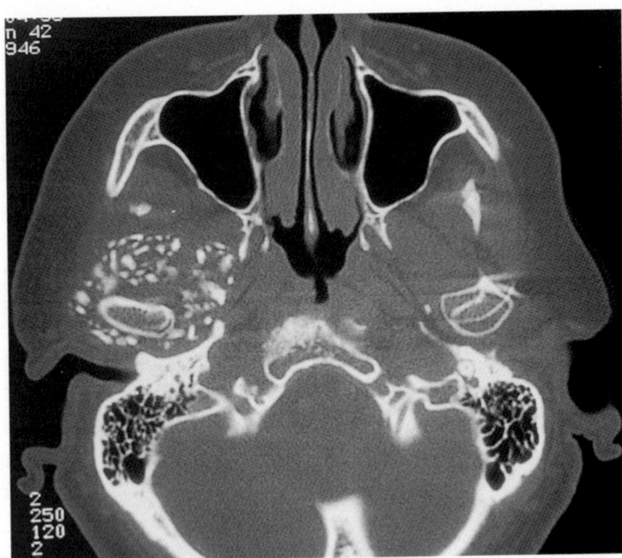

FIGURE 60. Computed tomography scan of synovial chondromatosis involving the temporomandibular joint. Many of the discrete nodules of hyaline cartilage exhibit endochondral ossification.

strate chalky yellow regions that represent calcification or foci of endochondral ossification (Fig. 60). Endochondral ossification proceeds from the periphery toward the center of the lobules. Microscopically, nodules of hypercellular hyaline cartilage are embedded within the synovial connective tissue (273–275,277,278) (Fig. 61). Individual nodules are circumscribed and round and demonstrate greater cellularity than hyaline articular cartilage. The chondrocytes are typically clustered rather than evenly distributed throughout the matrix (273–275,277,278). The individual cells exhibit a considerable range in size and nuclear chromaticity. Most have pyknotic dark-staining nuclei, but many cells exhibit atypical features, including large nuclei, dispersed chromatin, and visible nucleoli. Occasional mitoses may be found. The degree of cellularity and nuclear atypia found in synovial chondromatosis in most cases equals or exceeds that seen in low-grade intraosseous

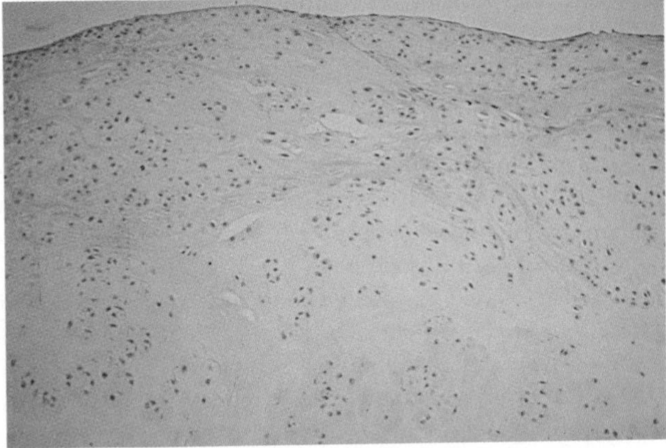

FIGURE 61. Cellular nodules of hyaline cartilage in synovial chondromatosis expand the subsynovial connective tissue.

chondrosarcoma (273–275,277,278). Hence, care must be taken not to overdiagnose malignancy in this setting. Knowledge of the radiographic and clinical features is therefore essential. Synovial chondromatosis is managed by synovectomy of the involved joint. Recurrence develops in up to 15% of cases, but the recurrence rate with the temporomandibular joint is lower (279). Bona fide chondrosarcomas of synovium are extremely rare neoplasms (280,281). These may arise *de novo* or secondary to preexisting primary synovial chondromatosis (280,281). The exact incidence of the latter event is unknown; however, it is generally considered to be rare. A single case of a synovial chondosarcoma of the temporomandibular joint has been described (282).

The differential diagnosis of synovial chondromatosis includes synovial chondrosarcoma and intraarticular loose bodies. Fragments of articular cartilage, bone, or fibrocartilaginous meniscus that come to lie free within a synovial joint are usually rapidly incorporated within the synovial membrane of the joint. At this site these loose bodies frequently act as a nidus for the formation of nodules of reactive fibrocartilage. These may be multiple and thus simulate primary synovial chondromatosis. Loose bodies, and the fibrocartilaginous reaction to them, typically are fewer in number than the nodules of synovial chondromatosis. Additionally, they are composed centrally of the inciting fragment and peripherally by layers of sheet-like fibrocartilage in contrast to the pure multinodular hyaline cartilage of synovial chondromatosis. Synovial chondrosarcomas are characterized by dense cellularity, spindling of the tumor cells, and a high mitotic rate. Bona fide chondrosarcomas, which are extremely rare, also demonstrate permeative destructive growth in contrast to the expansile, noninfiltrative growth of synovial chondromatosis.

Pigmented Villonodular Synovitis

Pigmented villonodular synovitis (PVNS) is a proliferative disorder of the synovial lining of joints that produces localized or diffuse nodular thickening of the synovial membrane (283–287). Any synovial-lined joint may be affected (283–287). PVNS of the temporomandibular joint is uncommon, with fewer than 50 cases having been reported (288,289). It typically presents with pain and difficulty opening the mouth. A minority produce erosions of the adjacent bones (283,288,289). PVNS affects men and women with equal frequency, and its greatest incidence is in the second to fourth decades of life (283–287). Whether PVNS represents a neoplasm or an exuberant reactive proliferation is still controversial. Recently cytogenetic abnormalities, including trisomy 7, have been identified in short-term cell cultures of PVNS. In a more recent study, the most common chromosomal abnormality was rearrangement of the short arm of chromosome 1 (1p11-13) (290). These results indicate the neoplastic nature of this lesion (291,292).

Pigmented villonodular synovitis produces a villous and nodular thickening of the synovial membrane. Diffuse involvement of the synovium results in thin, finger-like excrescences admixed with 0.5- to 2.0-cm rounded nodules that cover the normally smooth synovial membrane. Microscopically, surface synovial cells overlie a lobular and sheet-like arrangement of

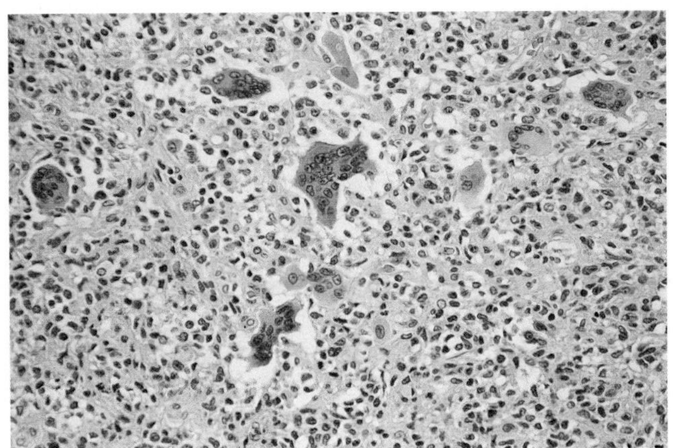

FIGURE 62. A nodule of pigmented villonodular synovitis exhibiting the sheet-like arrangement of mononuclear cells and scattered multinucleated giant cells.

mononuclear epithelioid cells, multinucleated osteoclast-like giant cells, and foamy macrophages (283–287) (Fig. 62). The mononuclear cells frequently contain large hemosiderin granules and have central round nuclei. Mild nuclear pleomorphism and prominent nucleoli are often present. Mitotic counts rarely exceed five per 10 high-power fields. Necrosis is rare. The sheets and nodules of mononuclear cells, which likely represent proliferating synovial cells, are embedded in a collagenous stroma. In some examples the nodular growth pattern is accentuated by broad bands of collagen. Immunohistochemically, PVNS exhibits a similar staining reaction to normal and reactive synovium (i.e., the mononuclear cells and multinucleated osteoclast-like giant cells react positively with antibodies to CD68 and vimentin) (293).

Pigmented villonodular synovitis is treated by surgical excision. Localized disease responds well to this approach; however, those examples that diffusely affect the synovium and that are incompletely excised have a high rate of local recurrence (>50%) (286,287).

The differential diagnosis of PVNS is principally with hemosiderotic synovitis. Hemorrhage into a synovial joint typically results in hemosiderin accumulation within synovial cells, which are actively phagocytic. Additionally, minor degrees of synovial hyperplasia often occur in the acute phase. This combination of findings is termed *hemosiderotic synovitis* and may simulate PVNS. Hemosiderotic synovitis lacks the nodule formation and sheet-like proliferation of synovial-like cells that are characteristic of PVNS.

REFERENCES

1. Adekeye EO, Cornah J. Osteomyelitis of the jaws: a review of 141 cases. *Br J Oral Maxillofac Surg* 1985;23:24–35.
2. Calhoun KH, Shapiro RD, Stiernberg CM, et al. Osteomyelitis of the mandible. *Arch Otolaryngol Head Neck Surg* 1988;114:1157–1162.
3. Koorbusch GF, Fotos P, Goll KT. Retrospective assessment of osteomyelitis. Etiology, demographics, risk factors, and management in 35 cases. *Oral Surg Oral Med Oral Pathol* 1992;74:149–154.
4. Marx RE, Johnson RP. Studies in the radiobiology of osteoradionecrosis and their clinical significance. *Oral Surg Oral Med Oral Pathol* 1987;64:379–390.
5. Epstein JB, Wong FL, Stevenson-Moore P. Osteoradionecrosis: clinical experience and a proposal for classification. *J Oral Maxillofac Surg* 1987;45:104–110.
6. Epstein JB, Rea G, Wong FL, et al. Osteonecrosis: study of the relationship of dental extractions in patients receiving radiotherapy. *Head Neck Surg* 1987;10:48–54.
7. Berger RP, Symington JM. Long-term clinical manifestation of osteoradionecrosis of the mandible: report of two cases. *J Oral Maxillofac Surg* 1990;48:82–84.
8. Friedman RB. Osteoradionecrosis: causes and prevention. *NCI Monogr* 1990;9:145–149.
9. Kluth EV, Jain PR, Stuchell RN, et al. A study of factors contributing to the development of osteoradionecrosis of the jaws. *J Prosthet Dent* 1988;59:194–201.
10. Van Merkesteyn JP, Groot RH, Bras J, et al. Diffuse sclerosing osteomyelitis of the mandible: clinical radiographic and histologic findings in twenty-seven patients. *J Oral Maxillofac Surg* 1988;46: 825–829.
11. Felsberg GJ, Gore RL, Schweitzer ME, et al. Sclerosing osteomyelitis of Garré (periostitis ossificans). *Oral Surg Oral Med Oral Pathol* 1990;70:117–120.
12. Suei Y, Taguchi A, Tanimoto K. Diffuse sclerosing osteomyelitis of the mandible: its characteristics and possible relationship to synovitis, acne, pustulosis, hyperostosis, osteitis (SAPHO) syndrome. *J Oral Maxillofac Surg* 1996;54:1194–1199 [Discussion 1199–1200].
13. Suei Y, Tanimoto K, Miyauchi M, et al. Partial resection of the mandible for the treatment of diffuse sclerosing osteomyelitis: report of four cases. *J Oral Maxillofac Surg* 1997;55:410–414 [Discussion 414–415].
14. Kahn MF, Hayem F, Hayem G, et al. Is diffuse sclerosing osteomyelitis of the mandible part of the synovitis, acne, pustulosis, hyperostosis, osteitis (SAPHO) syndrome? Analysis of seven cases. *Oral Surg Oral Med Oral Pathol* 1994;78:594–598.
15. Kahn AJ. The viral etiology of Paget's disease of bone: a new perspective [editorial] [see comments]. *Calcif Tissue Int* 1990;47:127–129.
16. Bataille R, Klein B. Etiology of Paget's disease of bone: a new perspective [Letter, Comment]. *Calcif Tissue Int* 1992;50:293–294.
17. Ralston SH, Helfrich MH. Are paramyxoviruses involved in Paget's disease? A negative view. *Bone* 1999;24(suppl):17–18.
18. Reddy SV, Menaa C, Singer FR, et al. Measles virus nucleocapsid transcript expression is not restricted to the osteoclast lineage in patients with Paget's disease of bone. *Exp Hematol* 1999;27:1528–1532.
19. Fraser WD. Paget's disease of bone. *Curr Opin Rheumatol* 1997; 9: 347–354.
20. Frame B, Marel GM. Paget disease: a review of current knowledge. *Radiology* 1981;141:21–24.
21. Merkow RL, Lane JM. Paget's disease of bone. *Orthop Clin North Am* 1990;21:171–189.
22. Dalinka MK, Aronchick JM, Haddad JG Jr. Paget's disease. *Orthop Clin North Am* 1983;14:3–19.
23. Fallon MD, Schwamm HA. Paget's disease of bone. An update on the pathogenesis, pathophysiology, and treatment of osteitis deformans. *Pathol Annu* 1989;24:115–159.
24. Drury BJ. Paget's disease of the skull and facial bones. *J Bone Joint Surg Am* 1962;44:174–179.
25. Gergely JM. Monostotic Paget's disease of the mandible. *Oral Surg Oral Med Oral Pathol* 1990;70:805–806.
26. Wheeler TT, Alberts MA, Dolan TA, et al. Dental, visual, auditory and olfactory complications in Paget's disease of bone. *J Am Geriatr Soc* 1995;43:1384–1391.
27. Woo TS, Schwartz HC. Unusual presentation of Paget's disease of the maxilla. *Br J Oral Maxillofac Surg* 1995;33:98–100.
28. Khetarpal U, Schuknecht HF. In search of pathologic correlates for hearing loss and vertigo in Paget's disease. A clinical and histopathologic study of 26 temporal bones. *Ann Otol Rhinol Laryngol Suppl* 1990;145:1–16.

29. Huvos AG, Butler A, Bretsky SS. Osteogenic sarcoma associated with Paget's disease of bone. A clinicopathologic study of 65 patients. *Cancer* 1983;52:1489–1495.
30. Huvos AG, Sundaresan N, Bretsky SS, et al. Osteogenic sarcoma of the skull. A clinicopathologic study of 19 patients. *Cancer* 1985;56: 1214–1221.
31. Salvati M, Ciappetta P, Raco A. Osteosarcomas of the skull. Clinical remarks on 19 cases. *Cancer* 1993;71:2210–2216.
32. Jacobs TP, Michelsen J, Polay JS, et al. Giant cell tumor in Paget's disease of bone: familial and geographic clustering. *Cancer* 1979; 44: 742–747.
33. Hutter RVP, Foote FW, Frazel EL, et al. Giant cell tumors complicating Paget's disease of bone. *Cancer* 1963;16:1044–1056.
34. Bhambhani M, Lamberty BG, Clements MR, et al. Giant cell tumours in mandible and spine: a rare complication of Paget's disease of bone. *Ann Rheum Dis* 1992;51:1335–1337.
35. Ankrom MA, Shapiro JR. Paget's disease of bone (osteitis deformans). *J Am Geriatr Soc* 1998;46:1025–1033.
36. Fox IH. Crystal induced synovitis. In: Kelley WN, ed. *Textbook of internal medicine,* 3rd ed. Philadelphia: Lippincott-Raven, 1996: 1130–1136.
37. Schumacher HR Jr. Pathology of crystal deposition diseases. *Rheum Dis Clin North Am* 1988;14:269–288.
38. Kleinman HZ, Ewbank RL. Gout of the temporomandibular joint. Report of three cases. *Oral Surg Oral Med Oral Pathol* 1969;27: 281–282.
39. Gross BD, Williams RB, DiCosimo CJ, et al. Gout and pseudogout of the temporomandibular joint. *Oral Surg Oral Med Oral Pathol* 1987;63:551–554.
40. Schumacher HR. Pathology of the synovial membrane in gout. Light and electron microscopic studies. Interpretation of crystals in electron micrographs. *Arthritis Rheum* 1975;18:771–782.
41. Fam AG, Topp JR, Stein HB, et al. Clinical and roentgenographic aspects of pseudogout: a study of 50 cases and a review. *Can Med Assoc J* 1981;124:545–551.
42. Ishikawa K, Masuda I, Ohira T, et al. A histological study of calcium pyrophosphate dihydrate crystal-deposition disease. *J Bone Joint Surg Am* 1989;71:875–886.
43. Keen CE, Crocker PR, Brady K, et al. Calcium pyrophosphate dihydrate deposition disease: morphological and microanalytical features. *Histopathology* 1991;19:529–536.
44. Beutler A, Rothfuss S, Clayburne G, et al. Calcium pyrophosphate dihydrate crystal deposition in synovium. Relationship to collagen fibers and chondrometaplasia. *Arthritis Rheum* 1993;36:704–715.
45. Chaplin AJ. Calcium pyrophosphate. Histological characterization of crystals in pseudogout. *Arch Pathol Lab Med* 1976;100:12–15.
46. Ishida T, Dorfman HD, Bullough PG. Tophaceous pseudogout (tumoral calcium pyrophosphate dihydrate crystal deposition disease). *Hum Pathol* 1995;26:587–593.
47. Haddad FS, Haddad GF, Zaatari G. Cranial osteomas: their classification and management. Report on a giant osteoma and review of the literature. *Surg Neurol* 1997;48:143–147.
48. Swanson KS, Guttu RL, Miller ME. Gigantic osteoma of the mandible: report of a case. *J Oral Maxillofac Surg* 1992;50:635–638.
49. Kaplan I, Calderon S, Buchner A. Peripheral osteoma of the mandible: a study of 10 new cases and analysis of the literature. *J Oral Maxillofac Surg* 1994;52:467–470.
50. Mirra JM, Picci P, Gold RH. *Bone tumors: clinical, radiologic and pathologic correlations.* Philadelphia: Lea & Febiger, 1989.
51. Fechner RE, Mills SE. *Tumors of the bone and joints.* Washington, DC: Armed Forces Institute of Pathology, 1993.
52. Earwaker J. Paranasal sinus osteomas: a review of 46 cases. *Skel Radiol* 1993;22:417–423.
53. Smith ME, Calcaterra TC. Frontal sinus osteoma. *Ann Otol Rhinol Laryngol* 1989;98:896–900.
54. Boysen M. Osteomas of the paranasal sinuses. *J Otolaryngol* 1978;7: 366–370.
55. Fu YS, Perzin KH. Non-epithelial tumors of the nasal cavity, paranasal sinuses, and nasopharynx. A clinicopathologic study. II. Osseous and fibro-osseous lesions, including osteoma, fibrous dysplasia, ossifying fibroma, osteoblastoma, giant cell tumor, and osteosarcoma. *Cancer* 1974;33:1289–1305.
56. Greenspan A. Benign bone-forming lesions: osteoma, osteoid osteoma, and osteoblastoma. Clinical, imaging, pathologic, and differential considerations. *Skel Radiol* 1993;22:485–500.
57. Whittet HB, Quiney RE. Middle turbinate osteoma: an unusual cause of nasal obstruction. *J Laryngol Otol* 1988;102:359–361.
58. Wilkes SR, Trautmann JC, DeSanto LW, et al. Osteoma: an unusual cause of amaurosis fugax. *Mayo Clin Proc* 1979;54:258–260.
59. Bartlett JR. Intracranial neurological complications of frontal and ethmoidal osteomas. *Br J Surg* 1971;58:607–613.
60. Schajowicz F. Bone-forming tumors. In: *Tumors and tumorlike lesions of bone. Pathology, radiology, and treatment.* New York: Springer-Verlag, 1994:30–35.
61. Lucas DR, Unni KK, McLeod RA, et al. Osteoblastoma: clinicopathologic study of 306 cases. *Hum Pathol* 1994;25:117–134.
62. Marsh BW, Bonfiglio M, Brady LP, et al. Benign osteoblastoma: range of manifestations. *J Bone Joint Surg Am* 1975;57:1–9.
63. Della Rocca C, Huvos AG. Osteoblastoma: varied histological presentations with a benign clinical course. An analysis of 55 cases. *Am J Surg Pathol* 1996;20:841–850.
64. Schajowicz F, Lemos C. Osteoid osteoma and osteoblastoma. Closely related entities of osteoblastic derivation. *Acta Orthop Scand* 1970;41:272–291.
65. Dorfman HD, Weiss SW. Borderline osteoblastic tumors: problems in the differential diagnosis of aggressive osteoblastoma and low-grade osteosarcoma. *Semin Diagn Pathol* 1984;1:215–234.
66. Bertoni F, Unni KK, Lucas DR, et al. Osteoblastoma with cartilaginous matrix. An unusual morphologic presentation in 18 cases. *Am J Surg Pathol* 1993;17:69–74.
67. Mirra JM, Kendrick RA, Kendrick RE. Pseudomalignant osteoblastoma versus arrested osteosarcoma: a case report. *Cancer* 1976;37: 2005–2014.
68. Cheung FM, Wu WC, Lam CK, et al. Diagnostic criteria for pseudomalignant osteoblastoma. *Histopathology* 1997;31:196–200.
69. Byers PD. Solitary benign osteoblastic lesions of bone. Osteoid osteoma and benign osteoblastoma. *Cancer* 1968;22:43–57.
70. Jackson RP, Reckling FW, Mants FA. Osteoid osteoma and osteoblastoma. Similar histologic lesions with different natural histories. *Clin Orthop* 1977:303–313.
71. Gitelis S, Schajowicz F. Osteoid osteoma and osteoblastoma. *Orthop Clin North Am* 1989;20:313–325.
72. Kirwan EO, Hutton PA, Pozo JL, et al. Osteoid osteoma and benign osteoblastoma of the spine. Clinical presentation and treatment. *J Bone Joint Surg Br* 1984;66:21–26.
73. Raskas DS, Graziano GP, Herzenberg JE, et al. Osteoid osteoma and osteoblastoma of the spine. *J Spinal Disord* 1992;5:204–211.
74. Loizaga JM, Calvo M, Lopez Barea F, et al. Osteoblastoma and osteoid osteoma. Clinical and morphological features of 162 cases. *Pathol Res Pract* 1993;189:33–41.
75. O'Connell JX, Nanthakumar SS, Nielsen GP, et al. Osteoid osteoma: the uniquely innervated bone tumor. *Mod Pathol* 1998;11:175–180.
76. Rosenthal DI, Hornicek FJ, Wolfe MW, et al. Percutaneous radiofrequency coagulation of osteoid osteoma compared with operative treatment [Comments]. *J Bone Joint Surg Am* 1998;80:815–821.
77. Garrington GE, Scofield HH, Cornyn J, et al. Osteosarcoma of the jaws. Analysis of 56 cases. *Cancer* 1967;20:377–391.
78. Bertoni F, Dallera P, Bacchini P, et al. The Istituto Rizzoli-Beretta experience with osteosarcoma of the jaw. *Cancer* 1991;68:1555–1563.
79. Clark JL, Unni KK, Dahlin DC, et al. Osteosarcoma of the jaw. *Cancer* 1983;51:2311–2316.
80. Unni K. *Dahlin's bone tumors. General aspects of data on 11,087 cases,* 5th ed. Philadelphia: Lippincott-Raven, 1996.
81. Zarbo RJ, Regezi JA, Baker SR. Periosteal osteogenic sarcoma of the mandible. *Oral Surg Oral Med Oral Pathol* 1984;57:643–647.
82. Newland JR, Ayala AG. Parosteal osteosarcoma of the maxilla. *Oral Surg Oral Med Oral Pathol* 1977;43:727–734.
83. Huvos. *Bone tumors. Diagnosis, treatment and prognosis.* WB Saunders, 1991:179–200.

84. Nora FE, Unni KK, Pritchard DJ, et al. Osteosarcoma of extragnathic craniofacial bones. *Mayo Clin Proc* 1983;58:268–272.
85. Munoz M, Goizueta C, Gil-Diez JL, et al. Osteocartilaginous exostosis of the mandibular condyle misdiagnosed as temporomandibular joint dysfunction [Letter]. *Oral Surg Oral Med Oral Pathol Oral Radiol Endod* 1998;85:494–495.
86. Kermer C, Rasse M, Undt G, et al. Cartilaginous exostoses of the mandible. *Int J Oral Maxillofac Surg* 1996;25:373–375.
87. Koole R, Steenks MH, Witkamp TD, et al. Osteochondroma of the mandibular condyle. A case report. *Int J Oral Maxillofac Surg* 1996;25:203–205.
88. Kerscher A, Piette E, Tideman H, et al. Osteochondroma of the coronoid process of the mandible. Report of a case and review of the literature. *Oral Surg Oral Med Oral Pathol* 1993;75:559–564.
89. Traub DJ, Marco WP, Eisenberg E, et al. Osteochondroma of the maxillary sinus: report of a case. *J Oral Maxillofac Surg* 1990;48: 752–755.
90. Brady FA, Sapp JP, Christensen RE. Extracondylar osteochondromas of the jaws. *Oral Surg Oral Med Oral Pathol* 1978;46:658–668.
91. Khosla A, Martin DS, Awwad EE. The solitary intraspinal vertebral osteochondroma. An unusual cause of compressive myelopathy: features and literature review. *Spine* 1999;24:77–81.
92. Arasil E, Erdem A, Yuceer N. Osteochondroma of the upper cervical spine. A case report. *Spine* 1996;21:516–518.
93. Cooke RS, Cumming WJ, Cowie RA. Osteochondroma of the cervical spine: case report and review of the literature. *Br J Neurosurg* 1994;8:359–363.
94. Tosios K, Laskaris G, Eveson J, et al. Benign cartilaginous tumor of the gingiva. A case report. *Int J Oral Maxillofac Surg* 1993;22: 231–233.
95. Snyder SR, Merkow LP. Benign chondroma of the palate: report of case. *J Oral Surg* 1973;31:873–875.
96. Dahlin DC, Ivins JC. Benign chondroblastoma. A study of 125 cases. *Cancer* 1972;30:401–413.
97. Turcotte RE, Kurt AM, Sim FH, et al. Chondroblastoma. *Hum Pathol* 1993;24:944–949.
98. Kurt AM, Unni KK, Sim FH, et al. Chondroblastoma of bone. *Hum Pathol* 1989;20:965–976.
99. Huvos AG, Marcove RC. Chondroblastoma of bone. A critical review. *Clin Orthop* 1973;95:300–312.
100. Varvares MA, Cheney ML, Goodman ML, et al. Chondroblastoma of the temporal bone. Case report and literature review. *Ann Otol Rhinol Laryngol* 1992;101:763–769.
101. Bertoni F, Unni KK, Beabout JW, et al. Chondroblastoma of the skull and facial bones. *Am J Clin Pathol* 1987;88:1–9.
102. Spahr J, Elzay RP, Kay S, et al. Chondroblastoma of the temporomandibular joint arising from articular cartilage: a previously unreported presentation of an uncommon neoplasm. *Oral Surg Oral Med Oral Pathol* 1982;54:430–435.
103. Bjornsson J, Unni KK, Dahlin DC, et al. Clear cell chondrosarcoma of bone. Observations in 47 cases. *Am J Surg Pathol* 1984;8:223–230.
104. Jaffe HL, Lichtenstein L. Chondromyxoid fibroma of bone. A distinctive benign tumor likely to be mistaken especially for chondrosarcoma. *Arch Pathol* 1948;45:541–551.
105. Wu CT, Inwards CY, O'Laughlin S, et al. Chondromyxoid fibroma of bone: a clinicopathologic review of 278 cases. *Hum Pathol* 1998; 29:438–446.
106. Zillmer DA, Dorfman HD. Chondromyxoid fibroma of bone: thirty-six cases with clinicopathologic correlation. *Hum Pathol* 1989;20: 952–964.
107. Koay CB, Freeland AP, Athanasou NA. Chondromyxoid fibroma of the nasal bone with extension into the frontal and ethmoidal sinuses. *J Laryngol Otol* 1995;109:258–261.
108. Lingen MW, Solt DB, Polverini PJ. Unusual presentation of a chondromyxoid fibroma of the mandible. Report of a case and review of the literature [Comments]. *Oral Surg Oral Med Oral Pathol* 1993; 75: 615–621.
109. Kitamura K, Nibu K, Asai M, et al. Chondromyxoid fibroma of the mastoid invading the occipital bone. *Arch Otolaryngol Head Neck Surg* 1989;115:384–386.
110. Carr NJ, Rosenberg AE, Yaremchuk MJ. Chondromyxoid fibroma of the zygoma. *J Craniofac Surg* 1992;3:217–222.
111. Frank E, Deruaz JP, de Tribolet N. Chondromyxoid fibroma of the petrous-sphenoid junction. *Surg Neurol* 1987;27:182–186.
112. Miyamoto E, Kuriyama T, Iwamoto M, et al. Cranial chondromyxoid fibroma. Case report. *J Neurosurg* 1981;55:1001–1003.
113. Wolf DA, Chaljub G, Maggio W, et al. Intracranial chondromyxoid fibroma. Report of a case and review of the literature. *Arch Pathol Lab Med* 1997;121:626–630.
114. Grotepass FW, Farman AG, Nortje CJ. Chondromyxoid fibroma of the mandible. *J Oral Surg* 1976;34:988–994.
115. Keel SB, Bhan AK, Liebsch NJ, et al. Chondromyxoid fibroma of the skull base: a tumor which may be confused with chordoma and chondrosarcoma. A report of three cases and review of the literature. *Am J Surg Pathol* 1997;21:577–582.
116. Patino-Cordoba JI, Turner J, McCarthy SW, et al. Chondromyxoid fibroma of the skull base. *Otolaryngol Head Neck Surg* 1998;118: 415–418.
117. Nielsen GP, Keel SB, Dickersin GR, et al. Chondromyxoid fibroma: a tumor showing myofibroblastic, myochondroblastic, and chondrocytic differentiation. *Mod Pathol* 1999;12:514–517.
118. Berkmen YM, Blatt ES. Cranial and intracranial cartilaginous tumours. *Clin Radiol* 1968;19:327–333.
119. Cianfriglia F, Pompili A, Occhipinti E. Intracranial malignant cartilaginous tumours. Report of two cases and review of literature. *Acta Neurochir* 1978;45:163–175.
120. Saito K, Unni KK, Wollan PC, et al. Chondrosarcoma of the jaw and facial bones. *Cancer* 1995;76:1550–1558.
121. Korten AG, ter Berg HJ, Spincemaille GH, et al. Intracranial chondrosarcoma: review of the literature and report of 15 cases. *J Neurol Neurosurg Psychiatry* 1998;65:88–92.
122. Rosenberg AE, Nielsen GP, Keel SB, et al. Chondrosarcoma of the base of the skull: a clinicopathologic study of 200 cases with emphasis on its distinction from chordoma. *Am J Surg Pathol* 1999;23: 1370–1378.
123. Rapidis AD, Archondakis G, Anteriotis D, et al. Chondrosarcomas of the skull base: review of the literature and report of two cases. *J Craniomaxillofac Surg* 1997;25:322–327.
124. Weber AL, Brown EW, Hug EB, et al. Cartilaginous tumors and chordomas of the cranial base. *Otolaryngol Clin North Am* 1995; 28: 453–471.
125. Rosenberg AE, Nielsen GP, Efrid JT, et al. Base of the skull chondrosarcomas. A clinicopathologic study of 130 cases [Abstract]. *Mod Pathol* 1997;9:12.
126. Semmelink HJ, Pruszczynski M, Wiersma-van Tilburg A, et al. Cytokeratin expression in chondroblastomas. *Histopathology* 1990; 16:257–263.
127. Walker WP, Landas SK, Bromley CM, et al. Immunohistochemical distinction of classic and chondroid chordomas. *Mod Pathol* 1991;4:661–666.
128. Huvos AG, Rosen G, Dabska M, et al. Mesenchymal chondrosarcoma. A clinicopathologic analysis of 35 patients with emphasis on treatment. *Cancer* 1983;51:1230–1237.
129. Nakashima Y, Unni KK, Shives TC, et al. Mesenchymal chondrosarcoma of bone and soft tissue. A review of 111 cases. *Cancer* 1986; 57:2444–2453.
130. Vencio EF, Reeve CM, Unni KK, et al. Mesenchymal chondrosarcoma of the jaw bones: clinicopathologic study of 19 cases. *Cancer* 1998;82:2350–2355.
131. Granter SR, Renshaw AA, Fletcher CD, et al. CD99 reactivity in mesenchymal chondrosarcoma. *Hum Pathol* 1996;27:1273–1276.
132. Okajima K, Honda I, Kitagawa T. Immunohistochemical distribution of S-100 protein in tumors and tumor-like lesions of bone and cartilage. *Cancer* 1988;61:792–799.
133. Salisbury JR, Isaacson PG. Distinguishing chordoma from chondrosarcoma by immunohistochemical techniques [Letter]. *J Pathol* 1986;148:251–252.
134. Sarasa JL, Fortes J. Ecchordosis physaliphora: an immunohistochemical study of two cases. *Histopathology* 1991;18:273–275.

135. Miettinen M, Lehto VP, Dahl D, et al. Differential diagnosis of chordoma, chondroid, and ependymal tumors as aided by anti-intermediate filament antibodies. *Am J Pathol* 1983;112:160–169.
136. Pardo-Mindan FJ, Guillen FJ, Villas C, Vazquez JJ. A comparative ultrastructural study of chondrosarcoma, chordoid sarcoma, and chordoma. *Cancer* 1981;47:2611–2619.
137. Wyatt RB, Schochet SS Jr, McCormick WF. Ecchordosis physaliphora. An electron microscopic study. *J Neurosurg* 1971;34: 672–677.
138. Abenoza P, Sibley RK. Chordoma: an immunohistologic study. *Hum Pathol* 1986;17:744–747.
139. Pena CE, Horvat BL, Fisher ER. The ultrastructure of chordoma. *Am J Clin Pathol* 1970;53:544–551.
140. Spjut HJ, Luse SA. Chordoma: an electron microscopic study. *Cancer* 1964;17:643–656.
141. Sibley RK, Day DL, Dehner LP, et al. Metastasizing chordoma in early childhood: a pathological and immunohistochemical study with review of the literature. *Pediatr Pathol* 1987;7:287–301.
142. Nielsen GP, Rosenberg AE, Liebsch NJ. Chordoma of the base of skull in children and adolescents. A clinicopathologic study of 35 cases. *Mod Pathol* 1996;9:11A.
143. Dorfman HD, Czerniak B. *Bone tumors,* 1st ed. St. Louis: CV Mosby, 1998.
144. Bottles K, Beckstead JH. Enzyme histochemical characterization of chordomas. *Am J Surg Pathol* 1984;8:443–447.
145. Heaton JM, Turner DR. Reflections on notochordal differentiation arising from a study of chordomas. *Histopathology* 1985;9:543–550.
146. Rutherfoord GS, Davies AG. Chordomas—ultrastructure and immunohistochemistry: a report based on the examination of six cases. *Histopathology* 1987;11:775–787.
147. Meis JM, Giraldo AA. Chordoma. An immunohistochemical study of 20 cases. *Arch Pathol Lab Med* 1988;112:553–556.
148. Rosenberg AE, Brown GA, Bhan AK, et al. Chondroid chordoma—a variant of chordoma. A morphologic and immunohistochemical study. *Am J Clin Pathol* 1994;101:36–41.
149. Ishida T, Dorfman HD. Chondroid chordoma versus low-grade chondrosarcoma of the base of the skull: can immunohistochemistry resolve the controversy? *J Neurooncol* 1994;18:199–206.
150. Jeffrey PB, Biava CG, Davis RL. Chondroid chordoma. A hyalinized chordoma without cartilaginous differentiation [Comments]. *Am J Clin Pathol* 1995;103:271–279.
151. Heffelfinger MJ, Dahlin DC, MacCarty CS, et al. Chordomas and cartilaginous tumors at the skull base. *Cancer* 1973;32:410–420.
152. Mitchell A, Scheithauer BW, Unni KK, et al. Chordoma and chondroid neoplasms of the spheno-occiput. An immunohistochemical study of 41 cases with prognostic and nosologic implications. *Cancer* 1993;72:2943–2949.
153. Marie PJ, de Pollak C, Chanson P, et al. Increased proliferation of osteoblastic cells expressing the activating Gs alpha mutation in monostotic and polyostotic fibrous dysplasia. *Am J Pathol* 1997;150: 1059–1069.
154. Weinstein LS, Shenker A, Gejman PV, et al. Activating mutations of the stimulatory G protein in the McCune-Albright syndrome [Comments]. *N Engl J Med* 1991;325:1688–1695.
155. Lichtenstein L. Polyostotic fibrous dysplasia. *Arch Surg* 1938;36: 874–898.
156. Lichtenstein L, Jaffe HL. Fibrous dysplasia of bone. *Arch Pathol Lab Med* 1942;33:777–816.
157. Albright F, Scoville WB, Sulkowitch HW. Syndrome characterized by osteitis fibrosa disseminata, areas of pigmentation and gonadal dysfunction. *Endocrinology* 1938;22:411–421.
158. Albright F, Butler AM, Hampton AO, et al. Syndrome characterized by osteitis fibrosa disseminata, areas of pigmentation and endocrine dysfunction with precocious puberty in females. *N Engl J Med* 1947;216:727–746.
159. Cabral CE, Guedes P, Fonseca T, et al. Polyostotic fibrous dysplasia associated with intramuscular myxomas: Mazabraud's syndrome. *Skel Radiol* 1998;27:278–282.
160. Waldron CA, Giansanti JS. Benign fibro-osseous lesions of the jaws: a clinical-radiologic-histologic review of sixty-five cases. *Oral Surg Oral Med Oral Pathol* 1973;35:190–201.
161. Slootweg PJ. Maxillofacial fibro-osseous lesions: classification and differential diagnosis. *Semin Diagn Pathol* 1996;13:104–112.
162. Yabut SM Jr, Kenan S, Sissons HA, et al. Malignant transformation of fibrous dysplasia. A case report and review of the literature. *Clin Orthop* 1988:281–289.
163. Ruggieri P, Sim FH, Bond JR, et al. Malignancies in fibrous dysplasia. *Cancer* 1994;73:1411–1424.
164. Waldron CA, Giansanti JS. Benign fibro-osseous lesions of the jaws: a clinical-radiologic-histologic review of sixty-five cases. II. Benign fibro-osseous lesions of periodontal ligament origin. *Oral Surg Oral Med Oral Pathol* 1973;35:340–350.
165. Eversole LR, Leider AS, Nelson K. Ossifying fibroma: a clinicopathologic study of sixty-four cases. *Oral Surg Oral Med Oral Pathol* 1985; 60:505–511.
166. Wenig BM, Vinh TN, Smirniotopoulos JG, et al. Aggressive psammomatoid ossifying fibromas of the sinonasal region: a clinicopathologic study of a distinct group of fibro-osseous lesions. *Cancer* 1995;76:1155–1165.
167. Margo CE, Ragsdale BD, Perman KI, et al. Psammomatoid (juvenile) ossifying fibroma of the orbit. *Ophthalmology* 1985;92:150–159.
168. Damjanov I, Maenza RM, Snyder GGD, et al. Juvenile ossifying fibroma: an ultrastructural study. *Cancer* 1978;42:2668–2674.
169. Margo CE, Weiss A, Habal MB. Psammomatoid ossifying fibroma. *Arch Ophthalmol* 1986;104:1347–1351.
170. Johnson LC, Yousefi M, Vinh TN, et al. Juvenile active ossifying fibroma. Its nature, dynamics and origin. *Acta Otolaryngol Suppl* 1991; 488:1–40.
171. Hirschl S, Katz A. Giant cell reparative granuloma outside the jaw bone. Diagnostic criteria and review of the literature with the first case described in the temporal bone. *Hum Pathol* 1974;5:171–181.
172. Bertoni F, Unni KK, Beabout JW, et al. Giant cell tumor of the skull. *Cancer* 1992;70:1124–1132.
173. Watkins LD, Uttley D, Archer DJ, et al. Giant cell tumors of the sphenoid bone. *Neurosurgery* 1992;30:576–581.
174. Wolfe JT 3d, Scheithauer BW, Dahlin DC. Giant-cell tumor of the sphenoid bone. Review of 10 cases. *J Neurosurg* 1983;59:322–327.
175. Yamamoto M, Fukushima T, Sakamoto S, et al. Giant cell tumor of the sphenoid bone: long-term follow-up of two cases after chemotherapy. *Surg Neurol* 1998;49:547–552.
176. Jaffe H. Giant cell reparative granuloma. Traumatic bone cyst and fibrous (fibro-osseous) dysplasia of the jawbones. *Oral Surg Oral Med Oral Pathol* 1953;6:159–175.
177. Whitaker SB, Waldron CA. Central giant cell lesions of the jaws. A clinical, radiologic, and histopathologic study. *Oral Surg Oral Med Oral Pathol* 1993;75:199–208.
178. Maruno M, Yoshimine T, Kubo T, et al. A case of giant cell reparative granuloma of the petrous bone: demonstration of the proliferative component. *Surg Neurol* 1997;48:64–68.
179. Mirabile R, Brown AS, Gisser S. Giant-cell granuloma of the jaw. *Plast Reconstr Surg* 1986;77:479–481.
180. Quick CA, Anderson R, Stool S. Giant cell tumors of the maxilla in children. *Laryngoscope* 1980;90:784–791.
181. Waldron CA, Shafer WG. The central giant cell reparative granuloma of the jaws. An analysis of 38 cases. *Am J Clin Pathol* 1966;45: 437–447.
182. Som PM, Lawson W, Cohen BA. Giant-cell lesions of the facial bones. *Radiology* 1983;147:129–134.
183. Abaza NA, el-Khashab MM, Fahim MS. Central giant cell reparative granuloma involving the mandible: report of case. *J Oral Surg* 1965;23:643–648.
184. Case records of the Massachusetts General Hospital. Weekly clinicopathological exercises. Case 10-1990. A 15-year-old girl with multiple radiolucent bony defects and multiple pulmonary nodules. *N Engl J Med* 1990;322:683–690.
185. Case records of the Massachusetts General Hospital. Weekly clinicopathological exercises. Case 20-1993. A 23-year-old woman with a

rapidly enlarging intraoral mass after a tooth extraction. *N Engl J Med* 1993;328:1478–1483.
186. Ciappetta P, Salvati M, Bernardi C, et al. Giant cell reparative granuloma of the skull base mimicking an intracranial tumor. Case report and review of the literature. *Surg Neurol* 1990;33:52–56.
187. Khosla VM, Korobkin M. Cherubism. *Am J Dis Child* 1970;120: 458–461.
188. Hamner JED, Ketcham AS. Cherubism: an analysis of treatment. *Cancer* 1969;23:1133–1143.
189. Wold LE, Swee RG, Sim FH. Vascular lesions of bone. *Pathol Annu* 1985;20:101–137.
190. Dorfman HD, Steiner GC, Jaffe HL. Vascular tumors of bone. *Hum Pathol* 1971;2:349–376.
191. Pinna V, Clauser L, Marchi M, et al. Haemangioma of the zygoma: case report. *Neuroradiology* 1997;39:216–218.
192. Palacios E, Valvassori G. Temporal bone hemangioma as a cause of facial paralysis. *Ear Nose Throat J* 1999;78:84.
193. Sweet C, Silbergleit R, Mehta B. Primary intraosseous hemangioma of the orbit: CT and MR appearance. *AJNR* 1997;18:379–381.
194. Moller G, Priemel M, Amling M, et al. The Gorham-Stout syndrome (Goram's massive osteolysis). A report of six cases with histopathological findings. *J Bone Joint Surg Br* 1999;91:501–506.
195. O'Connell JX, Kattapuram SV, Mankin HJ, et al. Epithelioid hemangioma of bone. A tumor often mistaken for low-grade angiosarcoma or malignant hemangioendothelioma [see comments]. *Am J Surg Pathol* 1993;17:610–617.
196. Lamovec J, Bracko M. Epithelioid hemangioma of small tubular bones: a report of three cases, two of them associated with pregnancy. *Mod Pathol* 1996;9:821–827.
197. Ben Romdhane K, Khattech R, Ben Othman M. Epithelioid hemangioma of bone [Letter, Comment]. *Am J Surg Pathol* 1994;18: 1270–1271.
198. Cone RO, Hudkins P, Nguyen V, et al. Histiocytoid hemangioma of bone: a benign lesion which may mimic angiosarcoma. Report of a case and review of literature. *Skel Radiol* 1983;10:165–169.
199. Tsuneyoshi M, Dorfman HD, Bauer TW. Epithelioid hemangioendothelioma of bone. A clinicopathologic, ultrastructural, and immunohistochemical study. *Am J Surg Pathol* 1986;10:754–764.
200. Kleer CG, Unni KK, McLeod RA. Epithelioid hemangioendothelioma of bone. *Am J Surg Pathol* 1996;20:1301–1311.
201. Boutin RD, Spaeth HJ, Mangalik A, et al. Epithelioid hemangioendothelioma of bone. *Skel Radiol* 1996;25:391–395.
202. Shin MS, Carpenter JT Jr, Ho KJ. Epithelioid hemangioendothelioma: CT manifestations and possible linkage to vinyl chloride exposure. *J Comput Assist Tomogr* 1991;15:505–507.
203. Abrahams TG, Bula W, Jones M. Epithelioid hemangioendothelioma of bone. A report of two cases and review of the literature. *Skel Radiol* 1992;21:509–513.
204. Wold LE, Unni KK, Beabout JW, et al. Hemangioendothelial sarcoma of bone. *Am J Surg Pathol* 1982;6:59–70.
205. Volpe R, Mazabraud A. Hemangioendothelioma (angiosarcoma) of bone: a distinct pathologic entity with an unpredictable course? *Cancer* 1982;49:727–736.
206. Campanacci M, Boriani S, Giunti A. Hemangioendothelioma of bone: a study of 29 cases. *Cancer* 1980;46:804–814.
207. Hartmann WH, Stewart FW. Hemangioendothelioma of bone: unusual tumor characterized by indolent course. *Cancer* 1962;15: 846–854.
208. Hopkins KM, Huttula CS, Kahn MA, Albright JE. Desmoplastic fibroma of the mandible: review and report of two cases. *J Oral Maxillofac Surg* 1996;54:1249–1254.
209. Nussbaum GB, Terz JJ, Joy ED Jr. Desmoplastic fibroma of the mandible in a 3-year-old child. *J Oral Surg* 1976;34:1117–1121.
210. Taguchi N, Kaneda T. Desmoplastic fibroma of the mandible: report of case. *J Oral Surg* 1980;38:441–444.
211. George DI Jr, Gould AR, Miller RL, et al. Desmoplastic fibroma of the maxilla. *J Oral Maxillofac Surg* 1985;43:718–725.
212. Pensak ML, Nestok BR, Van Loveren H, et al. Desmoplastic fibroma of the temporal bone. *Am J Otol* 1997;18:627–631.
213. Goldberg AN, Janecka IP, Sekhar LN. Desmoplastic fibroma of the skull: a case report. *Otolaryngol Head Neck Surg* 1995;112:589–591.
214. Hufnagel TJ, Artiles C, Piepmeier J, et al. Desmoplastic fibroma of parietal bone simulating eosinophilic granuloma. Case report. *J Neurosurg* 1987;67:449–451.
215. Sleeman DJ, Paterson A, Eveson JW. Desmoplastic fibroma of the maxillary alveolus. *Eur J Cancer* 1993;29B:151–152.
216. Selfa-Moreno S, Arana-Fernandez E, Fernandez-Latorre F, et al. Desmoplastic fibroma of the skull. Case report. *J Neurosurg* 1995; 82:119–120.
217. Fucci MJ, Lowry LD, Eriksen C, Kelly MF. Desmoplastic fibroma of the parapharyngeal space. *Otolaryngol Head Neck Surg* 1994; 110: 341–344.
218. Gnepp DR. *Pathology of the head and neck.* New York: Churchill Livingstone, 1988.
219. Stout AP. Juvenile fibromatoses. *Cancer* 1954;7:953–978.
220. Chung EB, Enzinger FM. Infantile myofibromatosis. *Cancer* 1981;48:1807–1818.
221. Kindblom LG, Angervall L. Congenital solitary fibromatosis of the skeleton: case report of a variant of congenital generalized fibromatosis. *Cancer* 1978;41:636–640.
222. Inwards CY, Unni KK, Beabout JW, et al. Solitary congenital fibromatosis (infantile myofibromatosis) of bone. *Am J Surg Pathol* 1991; 15:935–941.
223. Hasegawa T, Hirose T, Seki K, et al. Solitary infantile myofibromatosis of bone. An immunohistochemical and ultrastructural study. *Am J Surg Pathol* 1993;17:308–313.
224. Lingen MW, Mostofi RS, Solt DB. Myofibromas of the oral cavity. *Oral Surg Oral Med Oral Pathol Oral Radiol Endod* 1995;80:297–302.
225. Sugatani T, Inui M, Tagawa T, et al. Myofibroma of the mandible. Clinicopathologic study and review of the literature. *Oral Surg Oral Med Oral Pathol Oral Radiol Endod* 1995;80:303–309.
226. Tanaka H, Westesson PL, Emmings FG, et al. Simple bone cyst of the mandibular condyle: report a case. *J Oral Maxillofac Surg* 1996;54: 1454–1458.
227. Rubin MM, Murphy FJ. Simple bone cyst of the mandibular condyle. *J Oral Maxillofac Surg* 1989;47:1096–1098.
228. Matsumura S, Murakami S, Kakimoto N, et al. Histopathologic and radiographic findings of the simple bone cyst. *Oral Surg Oral Med Oral Pathol Oral Radiol Endod* 1998;85:619–625.
229. Hoffman S, Jacoway JR, Krolls SO. In: *Intraosseous and periosteal tumors of the jaw.* Series 2. Washington, DC: Armed Forces Institute of Pathology, 1985:165–169.
230. Bretschneider T, Dorenbeck U, Strotzer M, et al. Squamous cell carcinoma arising in an intradiploic epidermoid cyst. *Neuroradiology* 1999;41:570–572.
231. Kransdorf MJ, Sweet DE. Aneurysmal bone cyst: concept, controversy, clinical presentation, and imaging. *AJR* 1995;164:573–580.
232. Vergel De Dios AM, Bond JR, Shives TC, et al. Aneurysmal bone cyst. A clinicopathologic study of 238 cases. *Cancer* 1992;69: 2921–2931.
233. Martinez V, Sissons HA. Aneurysmal bone cyst. A review of 123 cases including primary lesions and those secondary to other bone pathology. *Cancer* 1988;61:2291–2304.
234. Ruiter DJ, van Rijssel TG, van der Velde EA. Aneurysmal bone cysts: a clinicopathological study of 105 cases. *Cancer* 1977;39:2231–2239.
235. Bataineh AB. Aneurysmal bone cysts of the maxilla: a clinicopathologic review. *J Oral Maxillofac Surg* 1997;55:1212–1216.
236. Leithner A, Windhager R, Lang S, et al. Aneurysmal bone cyst. A population based epidemiologic study and literature review. *Clin Orthop* 1999:176–179.
237. Braun J, Guilburd JN, Borovich B, et al. Occipital aneurysmal bone cyst: CT features. *J Comput Assist Tomogr* 1987;11:880–883.
238. Trent C, Byl FM. Aneurysmal bone cyst of the mandible. *Ann Otol Rhinol Laryngol* 1993;102:917–924.
239. Wojno KJ, McCarthy EF. Fibro-osseous lesions of the face and skull with aneurysmal bone cyst formation. *Skel Radiol* 1994;23:15–18.
240. Sanerkin NG, Mott MG, Roylance J. An unusual intraosseous lesion with fibroblastic, osteoclastic, osteoblastic, aneurysmal and fibromyx-

oid elements. "Solid" variant of aneurysmal bone cyst. *Cancer* 1983; 51:2278–2286.
241. Bertoni F, Bacchini P, Capanna R, et al. Solid variant of aneurysmal bone cyst. *Cancer* 1993;71:729–734.
242. Dehner LP, Sibley RK, Sauk JJ Jr, et al. Malignant melanotic neuroectodermal tumor of infancy: a clinical, pathologic, ultrastructural and tissue culture study. *Cancer* 1979;43:1389–1410.
243. Borello ED, Gorlin RJ. Melanotic neuroectodermal tumor of infancy—a neoplasm of neural crest origin. Report of a case associated with high urinary excretion of vanillylmandelic acid. *Cancer* 1966; 19:196–206.
244. Mosby EL, Lowe MW, Cobb CM, et al. Melanotic neuroectodermal tumor of infancy: review of the literature and report of a case. *J Oral Maxillofac Surg* 1992;50:886–894.
245. Cutler LS, Chaudhry AP, Topazian R. Melanotic neuroectodermal tumor of infancy: an ultrastructural study, literature review, and reevaluation. *Cancer* 1981;48:257–270.
246. Kapadia SB, Frisman DM, Hitchcock CL, et al. Melanotic neuroectodermal tumor of infancy. Clinicopathological, immunohistochemical, and flow cytometric study. *Am J Surg Pathol* 1993;17:566–573.
247. Young S, Gonzalez-Crussi F. Melanocytic neuroectodermal tumor of the foot. Report of a case with multicentric origin. *Am J Clin Pathol* 1985;84:371–378.
248. Pettinato G, Manivel JC, d'Amore ES, et al. Melanotic neuroectodermal tumor of infancy. A reexamination of a histogenetic problem based on immunohistochemical, flow cytometric, and ultrastructural study of 10 cases. *Am J Surg Pathol* 1991;15:233–245.
249. Johnson RE, Scheithauer BW, Dahlin DC. Melanotic neuroectodermal tumor of infancy. A review of seven cases. *Cancer* 1983;52: 661–666.
250. Ulbright TM, Amin MB, Young RH. *Tumors of the testis, adnexa, spermatic cord and scrotum.* Series 3. Washington, DC: Armed Forces Institute of Pathology, 1999.
251. Navas Palacios JJ. Malignant melanotic neuroectodermal tumor: light and electron microscopic study. *Cancer* 1980;46:529–536.
252. Lieberman PH, Jones CR, Steinman RM, et al. Langerhans cell (eosinophilic) granulomatosis. A clinicopathologic study encompassing 50 years [Comments]. *Am J Surg Pathol* 1996;20:519–552.
253. Willman CL, Busque L, Griffith BB, et al. Langerhans'-cell histiocytosis (histiocytosis X)—a clonal proliferative disease [Comments]. *N Engl J Med* 1994;331:154–160.
254. Howarth DM, Gilchrist GS, Mullan BP, et al. Langerhans cell histiocytosis: diagnosis, natural history, management, and outcome. *Cancer* 1999;85:2278–2290.
255. Kilpatrick SE, Wenger DE, Gilchrist GS, et al. Langerhans' cell histiocytosis (histiocytosis X) of bone. A clinicopathologic analysis of 263 pediatric and adult cases. *Cancer* 1995;76:2471–2484.
256. Giona F, Caruso R, Testi AM, et al. Langerhans' cell histiocytosis in adults: a clinical and therapeutic analysis of 11 patients from a single institution. *Cancer* 1997;80:1786–1791.
257. Emile JF, Wechsler J, Brousse N, et al. Langerhans' cell histiocytosis. Definitive diagnosis with the use of monoclonal antibody O10 on routinely paraffin-embedded samples. *Am J Surg Pathol* 1995;19: 636–641.
258. de la Monte SM, Dorfman HD, Chandra R, et al. Intraosseous schwannoma: histologic features, ultrastructure, and review of the literature. *Hum Pathol* 1984;15:551–558.
259. Habal MB. Malignant epithelioid schwannoma of the mandible and the skull base. *J Craniofac Surg* 1997;8:417–421.
260. Fawcett KJ, Dahlin DC. Neurilemmoma of bone. *Am J Clin Pathol* 1967;47:759–766.
261. Belli E, Becelli R, Matteini C, et al. Schwannoma of the mandible. *J Craniofac Surg* 1997;8:413–416.
262. Sadeghi EM, Koenig LJ, Clark D. Intrabony neurilemmoma: diagnosis and management. *J Am Dent Assoc* 1998;129:729–732.
263. Celli P, Cervoni L, Colonnese C. Intraosseous schwannoma of the vault of the skull. *Neurosurg Rev* 1998;21:158–160.
264. Minic AJ. Central schwannoma of the maxilla. *Int J Oral Maxillofac Surg* 1992;21:297–298.
265. Antonescu CR, Erlandson RA, Huvos AG. Primary leiomyosarcoma of bone: a clinicopathologic, immunohistochemical, and ultrastructural study of 33 patients and a literature review. *Am J Surg Pathol* 1997;21:1281–1294.
266. Nishida J, Sim FH, Wenger DE, et al. Malignant fibrous histiocytoma of bone. A clinicopathologic study of 81 patients [Comments]. *Cancer* 1997;79:482–493.
267. Sohail D, Kerr R, Simpson RH, et al. Malignant fibrous histiocytoma of the mandible: the importance of an accurate histopathological diagnosis. *Br J Oral Maxillofac Surg* 1995;33:166–168.
268. Anavi Y, Herman GE, Graybill S, et al. Malignant fibrous histiocytoma of the mandible. *Oral Surg Oral Med Oral Pathol* 1989;68: 436–443.
269. Akai M, Ohno T, Sugano I, et al. Case report 601: Malignant fibrous histiocytoma of skull and face presenting with massive osteolysis. *Skel Radiol* 1990;19:154–157.
270. Narvaez JA, Muntane A, Narvaez J, et al. Malignant fibrous histiocytoma of the mandible. *Skel Radiol* 1996;25:96–99.
271. Vaccani JP, Forte V, de Jong AL, et al. Ewing's sarcoma of the head and neck in children. *Int J Pediatr Otorhinolaryngol* 1999;48:209–216.
272. Siegal GP, Oliver WR, Reinus WR, et al. Primary Ewing's sarcoma involving the bones of the head and neck. *Cancer* 1987;60:2829–2840.
273. Villacin AB, Brigham LN, Bullough PG. Primary and secondary synovial chondrometaplasia: histopathologic and clinicoradiologic differences. *Hum Pathol* 1979;10:439–451.
274. Leu JZ, Matsubara T, Hirohata K. Ultrastructural morphology of early cellular changes in the synovium of primary synovial chondromatosis. *Clin Orthop* 1992:299–306.
275. Apte SS, Athanasou NA. An immunohistological study of cartilage and synovium in primary synovial chondromatosis. *J Pathol* 1992; 166:277–281.
276. Sciot R, Dal Cin P, Bellemans J, et al. Synovial chondromatosis: clonal chromosome changes provide further evidence for a neoplastic disorder. *Virchows Arch* 1998;433:189–191.
277. Sim FH, Dahlin DC, Ivins JC. Extra-articular synovial chondromatosis. *J Bone Joint Surg Am* 1977;59:492–495.
278. Sviland L, Malcolm AJ. Synovial chondromatosis presenting as painless soft tissue mass—a report of 19 cases. *Histopathology* 1995;27: 275–279.
279. Karlis V, Glickman RS, Zaslow M. Synovial chondromatosis of the temporomandibular joint with intracranial extension. *Oral Surg Oral Med Oral Pathol Oral Radiol Endod* 1998;86:664–666.
280. Davis RI, Hamilton A, Biggart JD. Primary synovial chondromatosis: a clinicopathologic review and assessment of malignant potential. *Hum Pathol* 1998;29:683–688.
281. Bertoni F, Unni KK, Beabout JW, et al. Chondrosarcomas of the synovium. *Cancer* 1991;67:155–162.
282. Ichikawa T, Miyauchi M, Nikai H, et al. Synovial chondrosarcoma arising in the temporomandibular joint. *J Oral Maxillofac Surg* 1998; 56:890–894.
283. Jaffe HL, Lichtenstein L, Sutro CJ. Pigmented villonodular synovitis, bursitis and tenosynovitis. *Arch Pathol* 1941;31:731–765.
284. Dorwart RH, Genant HK, Johnston WH, et al. Pigmented villonodular synovitis of synovial joints: clinical, pathologic, and radiologic features. *AJR* 1984;143:877–885.
285. Myers BW, Masi AT. Pigmented villonodular synovitis and tenosynovitis: a clinical epidemiologic study of 166 cases and literature review. *Medicine (Baltimore)* 1980;59:223–238.
286. Schwartz HS, Unni KK, Pritchard DJ. Pigmented villonodular synovitis. A retrospective review of affected large joints. *Clin Orthop* 1989:243–255.
287. Rao AS, Vigorita VJ. Pigmented villonodular synovitis (giant-cell tumor of the tendon sheath and synovial membrane). A review of eighty-one cases. *J Bone Joint Surg Am* 1984;66:76–94.
288. Tanaka K, Suzuki M, Nameki H, et al. Pigmented villonodular synovitis of the temporomandibular joint. *Arch Otolaryngol Head Neck Surg* 1997;123:536–539.
289. Omura S, Mizuki N, Bukawa H, et al. Diffuse variant tenosynovial giant cell tumor of the temporomandibular joint: report of a case. *J Oral Maxillofac Surg* 1998;56:991–996.

290. Sciot R, Rosai J, Dal Cin P, et al. Analysis of 35 cases of localized and diffuse tenosynovial giant cell tumor: a report from the Chromosomes and Morphology (CHAMP) study group. *Mod Pathol* 1999;12: 576–579.
291. Choong PF, Willen H, Nilbert M, et al. Pigmented villonodular synovitis. Monoclonality and metastasis—a case for neoplastic origin? *Acta Orthop Scand* 1995;66:64–68.
292. Ray RA, Morton CC, Lipinski KK, et al. Cytogenetic evidence of clonality in a case of pigmented villonodular synovitis. *Cancer* 1991; 67:121–125.
293. O'Connell JX, Fanburg JC, Rosenberg AE. Giant cell tumor of tendon sheath and pigmented villonodular synovitis: immunophenotype suggests a synovial cell origin [see comments]. *Hum Pathol* 1995;26: 771–775.

12

LYMPHOMA AND LYMPHOID HYPERPLASIA IN HEAD AND NECK SITES

JUDITH A. FERRY
NANCY LEE HARRIS

In this chapter, we discuss reactive lymphoid hyperplasias and lymphomas with a predilection for head and neck involvement. Many types of lymphoma can affect the cervical lymph nodes or extranodal sites in the head and neck. It is beyond the scope of this chapter to discuss systematically all types of lymphomas. In our discussion of lymph nodes, we focus on reactive lesions and discuss lymphoma to the extent that it is in the differential diagnosis of these reactive disorders. Conversely, in the sections on extranodal sites, we focus on the lymphomas that may involve these sites and the reactive lesions that are part of their differential diagnosis.

REACTIVE LESIONS OF CERVICAL LYMPH NODES

Lymph nodes can be involved by a seemingly endless variety of reactive processes; in this chapter, those that preferentially involve cervical lymph nodes are discussed (Table 1). Some of these reactive processes can affect extranodal lymphoid tissue of the head and neck, and this is also discussed below.

Infectious Mononucleosis

Viral infections of many types can be associated with lymphadenopathy. Although the diagnosis of infectious mononucleosis (IM), a symptomatic Epstein-Barr virus (EBV) infection, is usually established on clinical grounds, when enlarged lymph nodes are examined via biopsy, they frequently cause problems in the differential diagnosis. IM most often affects adolescents and young adults, although cases of IM in young children and in elderly adults have been reported. Manifestations of IM include fever, pharyngitis, cervical lymphadenopathy, rash, hepatosplenomegaly, atypical peripheral blood lymphocytosis, and a positive heterophile antibody (Monospot) test result. However, in young children with IM, the heterophile antibody test result is negative in the majority of cases (1,2). In more severe cases, there may be generalized lymphadenopathy, hepatic dysfunction, peripheral cytopenias and even a hemophagocytic syndrome. In most cases, the illness is self-limited, but rarely, intercurrent infection, Guillain-Barré syndrome, or splenic rupture with hemorrhage results in death (3–5).

The lymph nodal architecture is typically distorted but not effaced by an expanded paracortex containing a polymorphous population of lymphoid cells, including small lymphocytes, intermediate-sized lymphoid cells, immunoblasts, tingible body macrophages, and sometimes plasma cells (Fig. 1A and B). The immunoblasts may be atypical, with pleomorphic or lobulated nuclei; binucleated cells resembling Reed-Sternberg (RS) cells may be identified. Centrocytes (cleaved follicle center cells) should not be seen in the interfollicular region, however. Mitotic figures may be numerous. Individual cell necrosis and zonal necrosis are sometimes found. Reactive follicles may be present, but the follicular hyperplasia is usually an inconspicuous feature. Sinuses are patent in at least some areas, and frequently they are dilated. Sinuses contain histiocytes and a polymorphous population of lymphoid cells, including immunoblasts. Lymphoid cells sometimes infiltrate the capsule and extend into perinodal adipose tissue. Similar histologic features are found in the tonsils of patients with IM (4–7).

The small and intermediate-sized cells in the paracortex are predominantly T cells. The ratio of T-helper (CD4-positive) to T-suppressor (CD8-positive) cells may be normal or reversed. Most paracortical immunoblasts are B cells (Fig. 1C). The blasts typically show focal CD30 (Ki-1) staining; they are CD15 (Leu-M1) and epithelial membrane antigen (EMA) negative (1,6,8). A variable number of the B cells express EBV-associated latent antigens, including latent membrane protein (LMP) or Epstein-Barr nuclear antigen (EBNA), and some B cells express the replication-associated BZLF1 protein. The number of LMP-positive cells tends to be greater in involved tonsillar tissue, whereas in lymph nodes and spleen, LMP-positive cells are less commonly found (9). Using *in situ* hybridization, EBV-encoded RNA (EBER) can be detected in many of the paracortical immunoblasts (8).

The florid immunoblastic reaction occurring in IM gives rise to a lengthy differential diagnosis that includes reactive and neoplastic conditions. Obtaining adequate clinical information is

TABLE 1. LYMPHOID HYPERPLASIA AND LYMPHADENITIS IN CERVICAL LYMPH NODES

- Viral infections
  - Epstein-Barr virus (infectious mononucleosis)
  - Cytomegalovirus
  - Herpes simplex virus type I
  - Human immunodeficiency virus
- Bacterial infections
  - Pyogenic bacteria, especially *Staphylococcus* and *Streptococcus*
  - *Bartonella henselae* (cat scratch disease)
  - Mycobacteria
    - Tuberculosis
    - Atypical mycobacteria
- Protozoal infections
  - *Toxoplasma gondii*
- Autoimmune disease
  - Systemic lupus erythematosus
- Disorders of uncertain etiology
  - Kikuchi's disease
  - Kawasaki's disease
  - Sinus histiocytosis with massive lymphadenopathy
  - Kimura's disease

important in order to make the correct diagnosis, whether the differential includes lymphoma or other types of reactive hyperplasia. If the patient is known to have clinical or laboratory evidence of IM, a diagnosis of Hodgkin's disease or non-Hodgkin's lymphoma should be made with caution.

When immunoblasts and intermediate-sized lymphoid cells are numerous, the possibility of non-Hodgkin's lymphoma is often a consideration. In favor of IM are lack of architectural effacement, presence of areas readily recognizable as reactive hyperplasia, a polymorphous background of lymphoid cells without centrocytes, patent sinuses containing lymphoid cells (including immunoblasts), and lack of monotypic immunoglobulin expression on immunophenotyping (7). Because anaplastic large cell (Ki-1–positive) lymphoma sometimes partially involves lymph nodes, with preferential involvement of the paracortex and sinuses, anaplastic large cell lymphoma may enter the differential diagnosis. In IM, most blasts are B cells and some are CD30 positive, but they are typically EMA negative. Anaplastic large cell lymphoma is a T-cell or null cell lymphoma composed of cells that are usually larger and more pleomorphic, with more cytoplasm and a tendency for a more cohesive pattern of growth than the immunoblasts of IM. In addition, the neoplastic cells strongly and diffusely express CD30 and coexpress EMA (1). Genotyping studies may be helpful in problematic cases, because clonal immunoglobulin gene rearrangement is readily demonstrable in most B-cell lymphomas, and most cases of anaplastic large cell lymphoma show clonal T-cell receptor gene rearrangement. Recently, however, it has been demonstrated that the T-cell response to EBV is an antigen-driven, oligoclonal, or clonal expansion of CD8-positive T cells; the clonal populations regress with resolution of IM (10,11). Thus, results of genotyping should be interpreted with caution in cases in which IM is in the differential diagnosis.

Hodgkin's disease is often included in the differential diagnosis because RS-like cells are often seen in IM; however, they do

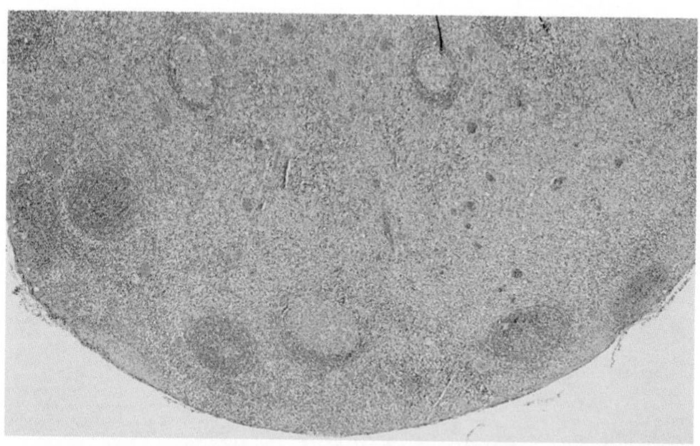
A

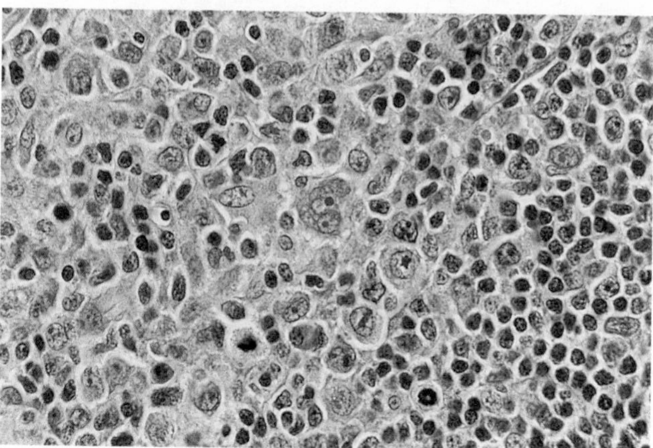
B

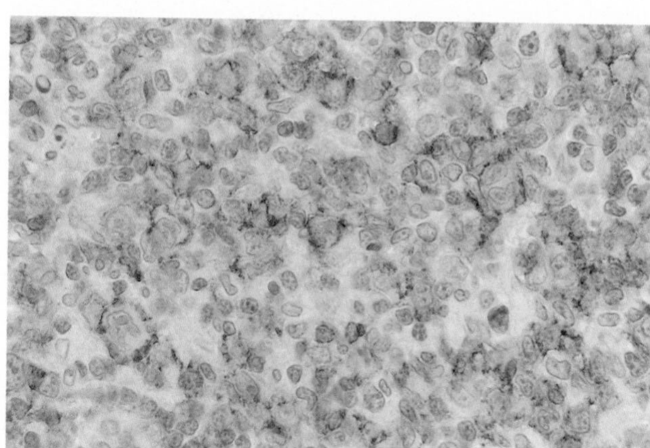
C

FIGURE 1. Tonsil in a patient with infectious mononucleosis. **A:** The tonsillar surface is eroded. Reactive follicles, although present, are not numerous. The interfollicular compartment is expanded. **B:** Higher power view of the interfollicular area shows a polymorphous population of cells, including small lymphocytes, immunoblasts and histiocytes. Occasional mitotic figures are seen. **C:** With antibodies to B cells (L26/CD20), there is staining of large cells, including cells with irregular nuclei and binucleated cells (immunoperoxidase technique on paraffin sections).

not usually meet strict morphologic criteria for RS cells. Hodgkin's disease is more often associated with obliteration of the lymph nodal architecture. The polymorphous background of lymphoid cells ranging from small to intermediate and large in the paracortex and sinuses seen in IM is very helpful in excluding Hodgkin's disease, in which background lymphocytes are all typically small (7). Immunoblasts in IM are CD15 negative, in contrast to the CD15 expression by RS cells that is found in most cases of Hodgkin's disease.

Other viral infections, vaccination, certain drugs and acute reaction to severe necrotizing processes can produce lymphadenopathy with histologic features similar to or indistinguishable from those of IM. Clinical information can be helpful in investigating the etiology of the lymphadenopathy. In IM, EBER-positive immunoblasts are typically present in large numbers, whereas in other conditions, EBER-positive cells are usually absent, although a few EBER-positive small lymphocytes may be seen (1,6,12). Because the Monospot test may be negative in some patients with IM, especially in young children, serologic testing for EBV-specific antibodies, such as those to viral capsular antigen, can be helpful in establishing a diagnosis.

Cytomegaloviral Infection

Cytomegalovirus (CMV) can cause localized or generalized lymphadenopathy (13,14). Lymph node enlargement due to CMV infection may be found in patients who are otherwise asymptomatic. It also may be seen in the setting of a heterophile-negative, IM-like illness. It accounts for 8% of cases with the clinical features of IM and for half of such illnesses that are heterophile negative (2). Compared with IM due to EBV, the mononucleosis-like syndrome due to CMV was more frequent among young children (<4 years old) and was associated with cervical lymphadenopathy slightly less often (75% of cases compared with 93% due to EBV) in a large pediatric series studied by Lajo and colleagues (2), although a predilection to affect younger children has not been uniformly observed in other studies (2). CMV can infect lymphoid tissues in patients who have or have had Hodgkin's disease, non-Hodgkin's lymphoma, or acquired or inherited immunodeficiency syndromes (15), or in patients with a normal immune system. For example, CMV infection is often seen in patients with common variable immunodeficiency (13,15,16).

On microscopic examination (Fig. 2), involved lymph nodes most often show florid follicular hyperplasia and monocytoid B-cell hyperplasia (see later section on Lymphoid Proliferations of the Salivary Glands for a discussion of monocytoid B cells, Table 10) (17). Paracortical hyperplasia also may be prominent; in such cases, paracortical immunoblasts are sometimes abundant (15). Infected cells contain a large eosinophilic intranuclear inclusion (mean size 9 μ), and often also contain multiple tiny eosinophilic to amphophilic cytoplasmic inclusions (15). Cells with inclusions are usually present focally in relatively small numbers, but occasionally they are numerous (14,15). Neutrophils and histiocytes are often scattered around the infected cells. Inclusions are typically found among monocytoid B cells; finding inclusions in the paracortex also has been described (13,15). The infected cells are sometimes recognizable as endothelial; in other instances, histiocytes appear to be infected (13–15).

Cytomegalovirus-infected cells can be identified in tissue sections using antibodies to CMV-associated antigens, or with *in situ* hybridization with probes for viral genetic material (14,15). Cells containing inclusions express CD15, usually with a Golgi region or diffuse cytoplasmic pattern of staining, but membrane staining is uncommon (15).

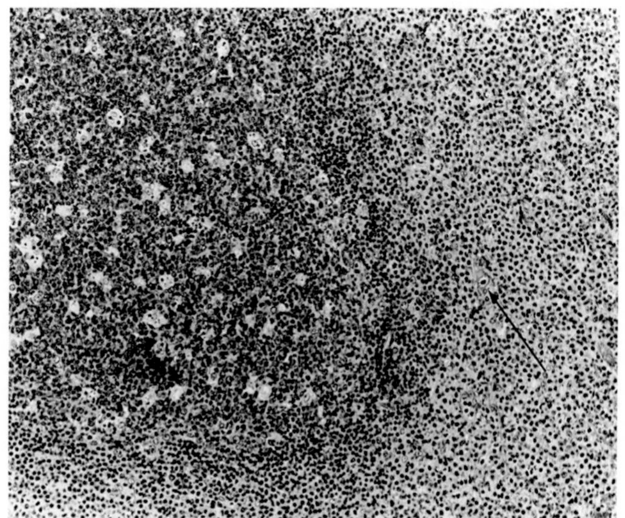

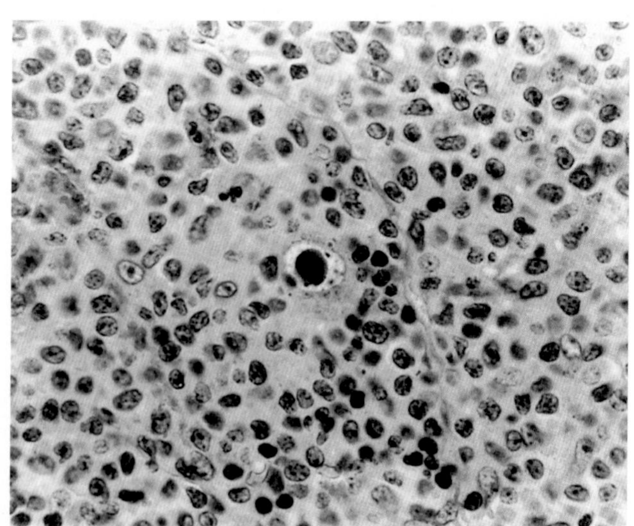

FIGURE 2. Cytomegaloviral lymphadenitis. **A:** Low power shows a large floridly reactive follicle with many tingible body macrophages (at left) and a parafollicular band of monocytoid B cells (at right). Within the monocytoid B cells, a cytomegaloviral inclusion is recognizable (*arrow*). **B:** High power shows a cytomegalovirus-infected cell with a large discrete nuclear inclusion in the midst of monocytoid B cells and rare granulocytes.

The two main entities that should be included in the differential diagnosis of CMV lymphadenitis are reactive hyperplasia due to some cause other than CMV and Hodgkin's disease. The overall appearance of the lymph node in CMV lymphadenitis is similar to that of *Toxoplasma* lymphadenitis. In most cases, however, the characteristic epithelioid cell aggregates of toxoplasmosis are not seen. Cells with nuclear viral inclusions may resemble RS cells and variants on routinely stained sections, raising the question of Hodgkin's disease. Further complicating the differential diagnosis is the fact that in early Hodgkin's disease, RS cells may be present in clusters of monocytoid B cells. In addition, CD15 expression by the virally infected cells heightens the resemblance to Hodgkin's disease. However, CMV lymphadenitis is much less likely than Hodgkin's disease to cause obliteration of the nodal architecture. More often, CMV-infected cells are found focally in a lymph node showing intact architecture. Cells harboring virus often contain numerous granular cytoplasmic inclusions, whereas the cytoplasm of RS cells is pale and agranular. Cells with inclusions may be identifiable as endothelial cells, excluding a diagnosis of Hodgkin's disease. Membrane staining by CD15 is more common in RS cells than in CMV-infected cells (15). Immunostaining with CMV-specific antibodies provides a definitive diagnosis of CMV lymphadenitis.

Herpes Simplex Viral Lymphadenitis

Infection by herpes simplex virus (type I or II) can cause localized or generalized lymphadenopathy, or involve lymph nodes in the setting of widespread visceral infection. When localized, the lymphadenopathy most often affects inguinal nodes (18–22), although cervical nodes and rarely tonsils also may be involved (19,23). Lymphadenopathy is usually painful. Typical mucocutaneous herpetic lesions are found in most patients, but they may be inconspicuous, or they may not appear until after a lymph node biopsy has been performed. Nearly half of patients who present with herpes simplex lymphadenitis (HSL) have a history of a hematolymphoid malignancy, or develop a malignancy shortly after the diagnosis of HSL. Although disseminated herpes simplex infection has a poor prognosis, isolated HSL is self-limited in most cases (18–22).

Lymph nodes show prominent paracortical hyperplasia, with areas of necrosis sometimes accompanied by follicular hyperplasia. Paracortical immunoblasts may be numerous. The necrotic areas contain neutrophils, karyorrhectic or amorphous eosinophilic debris, and a variable number of viral inclusions, ranging from rare to abundant. Most of the cells with viral inclusions are uninucleate, although a few multinucleated cells are seen. Intact neutrophils are most abundant in early lesions and may be absent in long-standing lymphadenitis. Histiocytes often surround the necrotic areas, but granulomas are absent. Inflammation may extend into perinodal soft tissue (18–22). Similar changes are found in the tonsils in herpetic tonsillitis (23). In some cases, the inclusions are thought to be in T-immunoblasts (20); in others, stromal cells, rather than lymphoid cells, may be infected.

The diagnosis can be confirmed using immunohistochemical stains, *in situ* hybridization, electron microscopy or viral culture. The differential diagnosis includes other types of necrotizing lymphadenitis and, in some cases, lymphoma. Varicella zoster virus rarely causes lymphadenitis; the histologic features are similar to those of HSL (19). Immunohistochemical staining for viral antigens and clinical information are helpful in differentiating HSL from lymphadenitis due to varicella. The lack of granulomatous inflammation with epithelioid or palisading histiocytes provides evidence against infections caused by mycobacteria, fungi, yersinia, cat scratch bacilli, and lymphogranuloma venereum (19). IM lacks viral inclusions and usually lacks prominent zonal necrosis. When there is pronounced paracortical expansion with numerous immunoblasts, the differential diagnosis should include diffuse large cell lymphoma. In HSL, the nodal architecture may be distorted, although it is not obliterated (i.e., sinuses remain patent), in contrast to most lymphomas. Discrete foci of necrosis are unusual, and herpes simplex virus inclusions are absent in lymphoma, except in the rare case in which both herpes simplex virus and lymphoma involve the same lymph node (22).

Human Immunodeficiency Virus–Associated Lymphadenopathy

Human immunodeficiency virus (HIV) infection is associated with lymphadenopathy due to a variety of reactive lesions and neoplasms. Acute symptomatic HIV infection may present as an IM-like illness with fever, pharyngitis, and cervical lymphadenopathy in approximately 16% of cases (24). Persistent generalized lymphadenopathy, defined as extrainguinal lymphadenopathy persisting for at least 3 months and involving at least two noncontiguous node groups, is common among HIV-positive patients. Persistent generalized lymphadenopathy mainly affects men, and is often accompanied by fever, weight loss, headaches, and malaise.

A range of changes is found in lymphadenopathy associated with HIV infection. Similar changes may be found in organized extranodal lymphoid tissue. When the lymphoid tissue of Waldeyer's ring is affected, patients may present with a large, obstructive nasopharyngeal mass, nasal stuffiness, nasal bleeding, hearing loss, or a combination of these findings. The hearing loss may result from obstruction of the eustachian tubes (25). Florid follicular hyperplasia, the most common pattern, is characterized by large, irregular germinal centers with a high mitotic rate, numerous blast cells, many tingible body macrophages, and ill-defined, attenuated, or effaced mantle zones (Fig. 3). There is often follicle lysis, (i.e., infiltration of and division or fragmentation of germinal centers by small lymphocytes of the mantle zone). The interfollicular region contains a mixture of immunoblasts, plasma cells, lymphocytes, and histiocytes with prominent vascularity. Monocytoid B cells are often prominent. Sinus histiocytosis, epithelioid histiocytes, polykaryocytes, erythrophagocytosis, and areas with features of dermatopathic lymphadenitis may be seen.

Lymphoid depletion is found in late stages of persistent generalized lymphadenopathy. Lymphoid follicles are decreased in number or absent. Residual follicles are burnt out or regressively transformed (Fig. 4). The interfollicular region contains scattered lymphocytes, immunoblasts, plasma cells, and many blood vessels. Amorphous eosinophilic material may be present, or

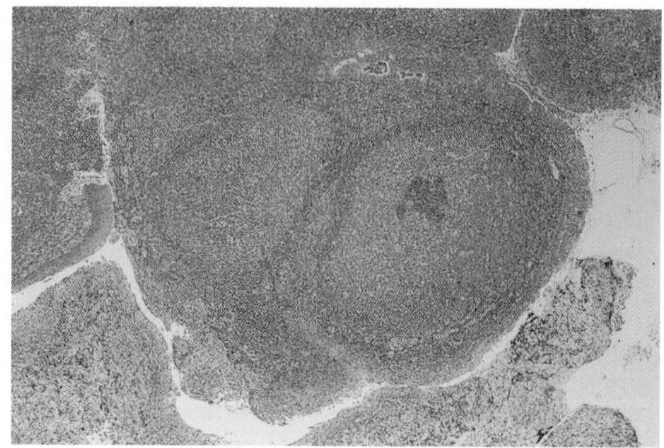

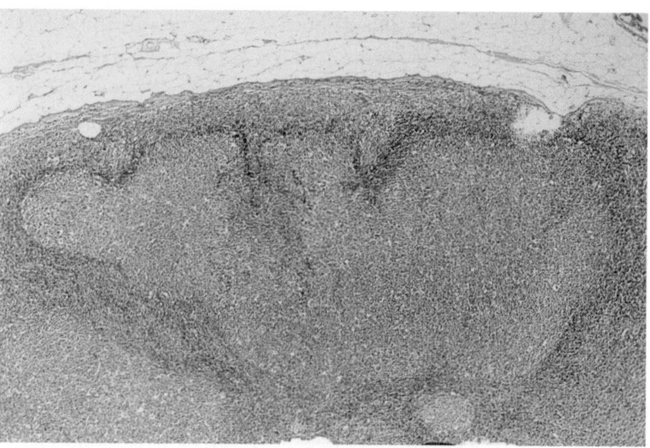

FIGURE 3. Florid follicular hyperplasia associated with HIV infection. **A:** In this patient with persistent generalized lymphadenopathy, the nasopharynx shows multiple large reactive follicles. **B:** A reactive follicle in this cervical lymph node is markedly enlarged and irregularly shaped, and has an attenuated mantle zone.

there may be fibrosis, and the node has a pale, depleted appearance. Lymph nodes with lymphoid depletion are indicative of an advanced stage of immunodeficiency, and these patients frequently develop opportunistic infections, Kaposi's sarcoma, or malignant lymphoma (26,27). In some cases, lymph nodes show changes intermediate between florid follicular hyperplasia and lymphoid depletion (26).

In HIV-associated lymphadenopathy, HIV-associated antigens are detected in follicular dendritic cells (FDCs) in germinal centers. Follicles contain polytypic B cells. The interfollicular region contains decreased numbers of CD4-positive cells, and the CD4:CD8 ratio is usually reversed. In occasional cases, EBV LMP is expressed by some cells. *In situ* hybridization reveals HIV RNA in germinal centers and, often, evidence of prior EBV infection (28). Lymph nodes showing more advanced lymphoid depletion may contain a large number of EBER-positive cells.

In some lymph nodes with depletion, there may be one or more features of Castleman's disease (angiofollicular lymphoid hyperplasia). Rarely, HIV-positive patients develop multicentric Castleman's disease; the histologic features of involved lymph nodes may be indistinguishable from those of Castleman's disease in the HIV-negative population. In a recent study of 20 HIV-positive patients with multicentric Castleman's disease, peripheral lymphadenopathy was found in 90%, and fever, splenomegaly, and anemia were found in all cases. Many patients also had hepatomegaly, severe weight loss, and respiratory symptoms. Fifteen patients also had Kaposi's sarcoma. Histologic examination revealed Castleman's disease of the plasma cell type or of the mixed plasma cell and hyaline-vascular type. On follow-up, 14 patients died, with a median survival of 14 months. Causes of death included Kaposi's sarcoma, progressive Castleman's disease, infection, and non-Hodgkin's lymphoma (29). In this series, patients more often had respiratory symptoms and Kaposi's sarcoma than is associated with multicentric Castleman's disease in the general population. Nearly all cases of multicentric Castleman's disease in HIV-positive patients and about half the cases of multicentric Castleman's disease in other patients contain Kaposi's sarcoma–associated herpes virus/human herpes virus type 8 (HHV-8) (30,31).

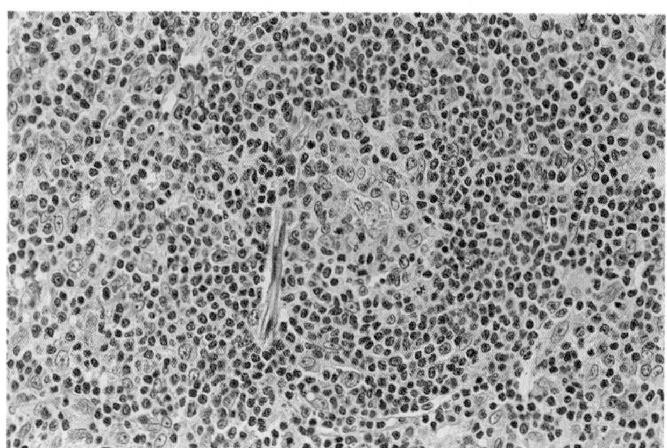

FIGURE 4. Follicular involution associated with HIV infection. The follicle is small and sclerotic, and depleted of lymphoid cells.

The differential diagnosis of HIV-associated lymphadenopathy includes nonspecific reactive hyperplasia in HIV-negative patients and malignant lymphoma. No one feature or constellation of histologic features allows definitive distinction between lymph nodes from HIV-positive and HIV-negative patients, although it has been suggested that polykaryocytes, epithelioid histiocytes and mantle zone effacement may be significantly more common in HIV-positive patients (27).

Non-Hodgkin's lymphoma enters the differential diagnosis in cases of florid follicular hyperplasia with follicles with attenuated mantle zones and an interfollicular region with numerous blasts, resulting in apparent obliteration of normal nodal architecture. Immunohistochemical stains for B- and T-cell antigens and immunoglobulin are helpful in delineating lymphoid follicles and paracortex and demonstrating that follicles are occupied by B cells expressing polytypic immunoglobulin.

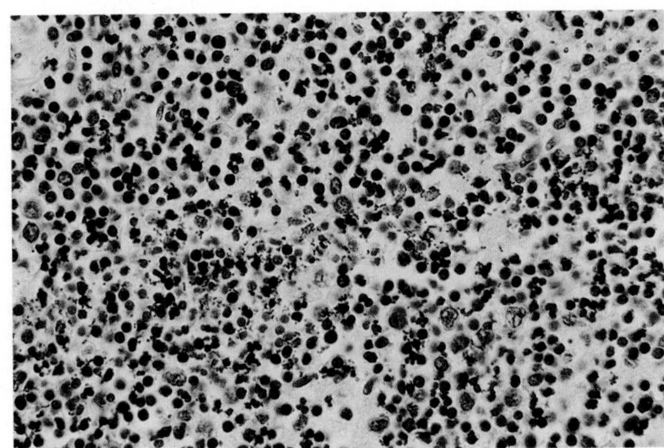

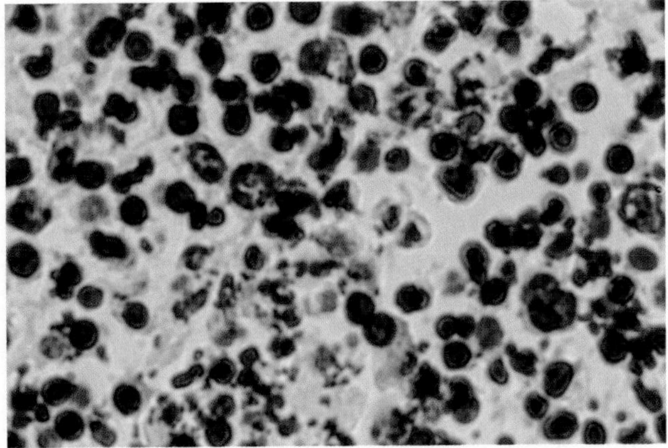

FIGURE 5. Streptococcal lymphadenitis in a 6-year-old boy. Numerous cocci are found among degenerated lymphoid cells and granulocytes in this lymph node that had been enlarged for 1 day. Cultures grew group A β-hemolytic *Streptococcus* (Brown-Hopps stain). **A:** Low power. **B:** Oil immersion.

Pyogenic Bacterial Lymphadenitis

Bacterial infections are a common cause of cervical lymphadenopathy. Acute lymphadenitis due to streptococcal or staphylococcal infection, although not often examined via biopsy, is probably the most common cause of bacterial cervical lymphadenopathy in children (Fig. 5). Microscopic examination of early lesions may show predominantly paracortical hyperplasia; later, follicular hyperplasia is prominent and there is a variably dense paracortical neutrophilic infiltrate (32,33).

Cat Scratch Disease

Cat scratch disease is the most common cause of chronic, benign lymphadenopathy in the United States, with about 24,000 cases occurring per year (34). For reasons that may be related to the breeding patterns of cats, it is more common between July and December than between January and June (35,36). Cat scratch disease is caused in a majority of cases by infection with *Bartonella* (formerly called *Rochalimaea*) *henselae,* and in a minority of cases by *Afipia felis* (35,37,38). *Bartonella henselae* is the same agent that causes many cases of acquired immunodeficiency syndrome (AIDS)-related bacillary angiomatosis (36). Although cat scratch disease can affect patients of any age, the majority are under 20 years of age. A history of exposure to a cat (typically a kitten with fleas) can be found in nearly all cases. The infectious agent has been found within the gastrointestinal tract of fleas, and it is possible that fleas act as vectors in transmission of the disease (36,38). Three to five days after exposure, a papule develops in the skin at the inoculation site; the papule typically becomes vesiculated and then crusted over during the next several days. Regional lymphadenopathy is usually found 1 to 2 weeks after recognition of the papule.

The lymphadenopathy, which is often tender, usually involves only one node, and although more than one lymph node in the same area may be affected, lymphadenopathy hardly ever involves more than one group of nodes. However, noncontiguous lymphadenopathy may develop if there is more than one inoculation site or if the inoculation is midline and organisms drain to lymph nodes bilaterally. The axilla is the single most common site for adenopathy (45%), but when all affected lymph nodes from the region of the head and neck are considered, they account for approximately 33% of cases. When the inoculation site is the eye, patients may develop the oculoglandular syndrome of Parinaud (granulomatous conjunctivitis and preauricular lymphadenopathy). More than half of patients have fever, but it is usually low grade (<39°C). Patients also may experience malaise, anorexia, or, rarely, nausea or abdominal pain. The disease is usually mild and self-limited, and some cases go unrecognized. Severe complications, occurring in up to 2% of cases, include involvement of the nervous system, bone, lung, liver, or spleen. Neurologic manifestations include encephalopathy, encephalitis, meningitis, myelitis, and involvement of cranial or peripheral nerves. The liver and spleen may be the sites of abscess formation. The skeleton is rarely involved by a necrotizing granulomatous osteomyelitis, sometimes via direct extension from an affected lymph node. Patients with lung involvement may have pneumonia or pleural effusions (34,36,39).

The tiny cat scratch bacilli may be difficult to recognize in histologic sections, and they are difficult to culture. Therefore, serologic studies may be helpful in establishing a definite diagnosis (40). In addition, probes for *Bartonella*-specific genetic sequences are available that can be used to detect cat scratch disease using the polymerase chain reaction (PCR) (35).

The histologic appearance of the infected lymph nodes changes over time. The earliest changes are follicular hyperplasia with a prominent proliferation of monocytoid B cells. Subsequently, within aggregates of monocytoid B cells, small foci of necrosis with a few neutrophils, and scant fibrin and cellular debris appear. These foci are usually close to, or encroach upon, germinal centers, or they may be adjacent to the subcapsular sinus. In some cases they are found in the vicinity of a small blood vessel. The paracortex is hyperplastic. Sinuses contain immunoblasts, neutrophils, and histiocytes. With time, the necrotic foci enlarge, extending deeper into the node. They contain pus, fibrin, and abundant cellular debris and acquire a rim of macrophages. The foci continue to enlarge and coalesce, and they are surrounded by palisading histiocytes, producing the

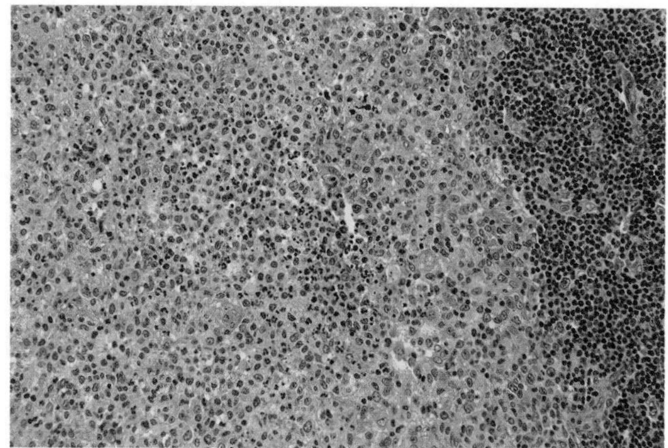
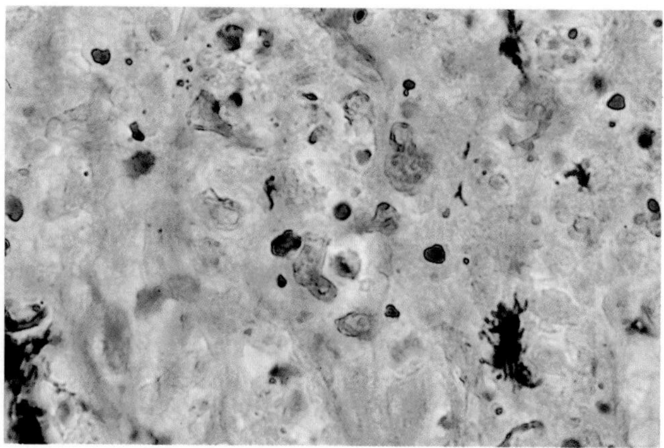

FIGURE 6. Cat scratch disease. **A:** Microabscess formation within an aggregate of monocytoid B cells. **B:** Multiple cat scratch bacilli—singly, in tiny clusters, and in larger clumps—are seen in this Warthin-Starry–stained section.

classic stellate microabscess or granuloma (Fig. 6A) (41). The cat scratch bacillus is a small, slender, pleomorphic, weakly gram-negative rod up to 3 μ long. Its small size makes it very difficult to see, but using a Warthin-Starry stain, the bacilli are coated with the black reaction product, making them appear larger and more readily visualized. Bacilli are present singly, in chains, or in large clumps (Fig. 6B). They may be found in the walls of blood vessels, in macrophages in necrotic areas, in sinus histiocytes, or in the extracellular space, but they are not found in neutrophils. Bacilli are most numerous in the stages of early necrosis within clusters of monocytoid B cells. When well-developed stellate abscesses have formed, the organisms can be difficult to detect (37,41). Immunophenotyping studies have shown that the granulomas contain a variable admixture of B and T cells, in addition to histiocytes (42).

A variety of microorganisms cause necrotizing lymphadenitis that can be considered in the differential diagnosis of cat scratch disease. Clinical features, including age, risk factors for different types of infection, anatomic distribution of lymphadenopathy, and severity of disease; special stains on tissue sections; serologic studies; and culture are helpful in establishing a definite diagnosis. Infection caused by certain bacteria, including *Chlamydia trachomatis* (lymphogranuloma venereum), *Francisella tularensis* (tularemia), *Hemophilus ducreyi* (chancroid), *Yersinia enterocolitica* (pseudotuberculous mesenteric lymphadenitis), *Listeria monocytogenes* (listeriosis), *Pseudomonas mallei* (glanders), and *Pseudomonas pseudomallei* (melioidosis) can be associated with a necrotizing lymphadenitis with histologic features that may be indistinguishable from those of cat scratch disease. In nearly all cases, the diseases listed above are associated with significantly greater morbidity than cat scratch disease. Early cat scratch disease also may resemble *Toxoplasma* lymphadenitis.

As noted above, infection by pyogenic cocci may be associated with an acute suppurative lymphadenitis with follicular hyperplasia that can suggest cat scratch disease. Unlike cat scratch disease, however, the pyogenic cocci typically do not elicit a rim of palisading histiocytes around areas of suppurative necrosis. One exception is in cases of chronic granulomatous disease of childhood, in which palisading granulomas with suppurative necrosis may be found in association with infection due to *Staphylococcus aureus* and a variety of gram-negative bacteria. The appearance can closely resemble that of cat scratch disease (43).

Mycobacteria (e.g., *Mycobacterium tuberculosis* and atypical mycobacteria) and fungi can produce lymphadenitis with granulomatous microabscesses that may resemble those of cat scratch disease, and the most important differential diagnosis may be between cat scratch disease and atypical mycobacterial infection of cervical lymph nodes in children. Young children in particular, whose immune systems may be immature, may develop a suppurative response to acid-fast bacilli thay may be similar to the microabscesses of cat scratch disease. Conversely, in some late-stage cases of cat scratch disease, the necrotic material acquires a pink, amorphous quality closely resembling the caseation necrosis characteristic of tuberculosis. Special stains for microorganisms may be helpful in establishing a diagnosis. The distinction is clinically relevant, because cat scratch disease does not usually require treatment, whereas infection by *M. tuberculosis* should be treated with antibiotics and infection by atypical mycobacteria with surgical excision of involved nodes.

Mycobacterial Lymphadenitis

Infection by *M. tuberculosis* is a serious global health problem, with approximately one third of the world's population harboring *M. tuberculosis.* In Central Africa, for example, tuberculous lymphadenitis is the most common finding among patients who undergo a superficial lymph node biopsy. Nearly all of them are HIV positive (44). Although tuberculosis is much less common among individuals in the United States than in other parts of the world, the number of cases has increased recently due to HIV infection, homelessness, and poor living conditions. Administration of incomplete courses of antibiotic treatment because of poor patient compliance also has led to the emergence of increased numbers of drug-resistant strains (45).

Mycobacterial lymphadenitis can occur in isolation, or in conjunction with pulmonary tuberculosis or disseminated infection. Involved nodes are usually slowly enlarging, nontender masses that may be associated with draining sinuses. Any lymph node can be involved, but the cervical nodes are most often affected (33,46). Mycobacterial lymphadenitis may be due to infection by *M. tuberculosis* or atypical mycobacteria (*M. scrofulaceum, M. kansasii,* or *M. avium* complex) (45,47,48). Patients with lymphadenitis due to *M. tuberculosis* are usually adults who present with constitutional symptoms (fever, fatigue, and weight loss) and have associated pulmonary tuberculosis. The peripheral lymph nodes involved tend to be in the supraclavicular fossa or posterior cervical triangle. Frequently, multiple lymph nodes are involved bilaterally, and there are draining sinuses. Results of the purified protein derivative (PPD) test are usually strongly positive. Patients with lymphadenitis due to atypical mycobacteria are usually young children without systemic symptoms, pulmonary tuberculosis, or a history of tuberculous exposure. The lymph nodes affected are usually preauricular or submandibular, and involvement is unilateral. Draining sinuses occur, but they are uncommon in the absence of surgical intervention. The PPD test result is negative or weakly positive (46). The distinction between tuberculous and atypical mycobacterial lymphadenitis is important, because tuberculosis must be treated with antibiotics and lymphadenitis due to atypical mycobacteria, which are often resistant to standard antituberculous antibiotic treatment, may be cured by complete surgical excision alone (46,49). In HIV-positive patients, atypical mycobacteria, especially *M. avium-intracellulare,* can be associated with disseminated infection.

Lymph nodes in immunocompetent patients show multiple, well-formed granulomas composed of epithelioid histiocytes and Langhans-type giant cells; caseation necrosis is present to a variable extent in the centers of the granulomas. In atypical mycobacterial infection, granulomas may contain neutrophils, with suppurative necrosis, rather than caseous necrosis. A Ziehl-Neelsen stain is used to identify the organisms, which are usually few in number in immunocompetent patients. Immunosuppressed patients sometimes fail to develop well-formed granulomas; involved tissues may contain only loose aggregates of histiocytes containing numerous microorganisms. Culture is needed to diagnose cases in which organisms cannot be identified in tissue sections, and to distinguish definitively between infections by *M. tuberculosis* and atypical mycobacteria (45). In contrast to the admixture of B and T cells found in the granulomas of cat scratch disease, in mycobacterial infection the lymphocytes associated with the granulomas are T cells, whereas B cells are virtually absent (42).

The differential diagnosis of mycobacterial lymphadenitis is broad. Cases with little or no necrosis resemble sarcoidosis. A Ziehl-Neelsen stain and culture are helpful in establishing a diagnosis; however, the Ziehl-Neelsen stain is often negative in cases of mycobacterial infection unless there is necrosis. A wide variety of microorganisms, including fungi, cat scratch bacilli, *Brucella* species, spirochetes, and *Leishmania,* can be associated with granulomatous lymphadenitis. Caseation necrosis is more common in mycobacterial infections, although necrosis resembling caseation may be seen in fungal infections and, less often, with other infections. In cases of primary or secondary syphilis, lymph nodes may show non-necrotizing or suppurative granulomas, but they are found in the setting of marked follicular hyperplasia and plasmacytosis. Cat scratch disease, a common cause of necrotizing granulomatous lymphadenitis in children, is more likely to be associated with exposure to a cat, a cutaneous inoculation site, and tender lymphadenopathy, compared with atypical mycobacterial lymphadenitis in immunocompetent children (49).

Granulomatous inflammation, often accompanied by extensive necrosis, may be found in tissues involved by Hodgkin's disease. Identification of RS cells, which tend to be found in greatest numbers at the periphery of necrotic areas, confirms the diagnosis of Hodgkin's disease. The presence of a polymorphous inflammatory cell infiltrate, with eosinophils and plasma cells, is more common in Hodgkin's disease than in mycobacterial infection. Non-Hodgkin's lymphomas also may occasionally be associated with granulomas, but this is much less common than in Hodgkin's disease.

Metastatic carcinoma can be associated with granulomas in lymph nodes. In cases of nasopharyngeal carcinoma metastatic to lymph nodes, there may be a marked necrotizing granulomatous lymphadenitis (50). The granulomatous inflammation may obscure the neoplastic population, and the carcinoma may be overlooked (Fig. 7). Granulomas also can be found in lymph nodes draining carcinoma but which are themselves free of metastases.

Toxoplasma (Piringer-Kuchinka) Lymphadenitis

Although lymphadenitis due to other types of protozoal infection has been reported, infection by *Toxoplasma gondii* is the only one encountered with any frequency. Toxoplasmosis is a common cause of lymphadenopathy, particularly in the cervical area. In one study, 15% of lymph nodes with reactive hyperplasia showed histologic features consistent with *Toxoplasma* lymphadenitis (51). This type of lymphadenopathy was first described by Piringer-Kuchinka in 1952 (52) and is thus sometimes called Piringer-Kuchinka lymphadenitis. The five modes of clinical presentation of toxoplasmosis are lymphadenopathy, as noted above, encephalitis, chorioretinitis, disseminated infection, and congenital infection (52). The most frequent clinical manifestation of *T. gondii* infection is enlargement of a single lymph node, most commonly in the cervical area. Patients are usually otherwise asymptomatic, or may have malaise, fever, or a sore throat (53). An atypical lymphocytosis may be seen. The disease is self-limited. Rarely, immunocompetent patients develop serious complications, such as myocarditis or encephalitis, which may be fatal. Immunodeficient patients may develop lymphadenopathy, but are at high risk for severe manifestations, especially encephalitis. Infection during pregnancy may be associated with fetal morbidity or mortality.

Lymph nodes show florid follicular hyperplasia, prominent bands of parasinusoidal and parafollicular monocytoid B cells, and many small, irregular paracortical clusters of epithelioid histiocytes, some of which encroach on germinal centers (Fig. 8). The microorganisms are identified in lymph nodes only rarely, even when cases are studied using the PCR (54). The diagnosis can be confirmed using serologic studies: in 95% of cases with the triad of histologic findings described above, results of serology show infection by *T. gondii* (51).

The differential diagnosis of *Toxoplasma* lymphadenitis in-

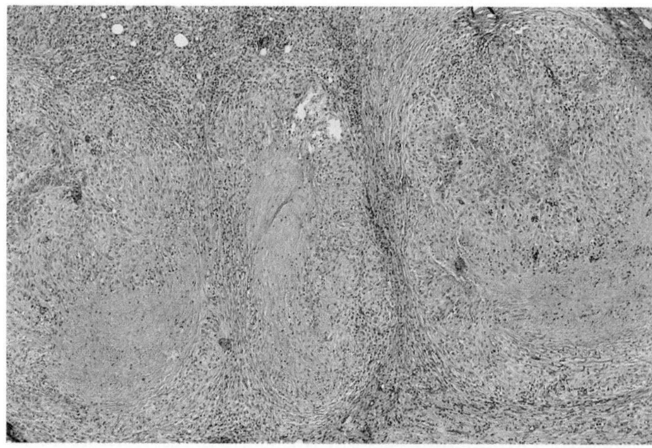

FIGURE 7. Necrotizing granulomatous lymphadenitis in association with metastatic carcinoma of probable nasopharyngeal origin. **A:** Large granulomas occupy much of this cervical lymph node. **B:** Higher power shows a necrotizing granuloma with epithelioid and palisading histiocytes. Also seen, at the periphery of the granulomas, are small cords of basophilic cells with a higher nuclear:cytoplasmic ratio than the histocytes. **C:** The basophilic cells with a high nuclear:cytoplasmic ratio represent subtle nodal involvement by metastatic carcinoma. The neoplastic cells are seen here in a loose cluster surrounded by histiocytes.

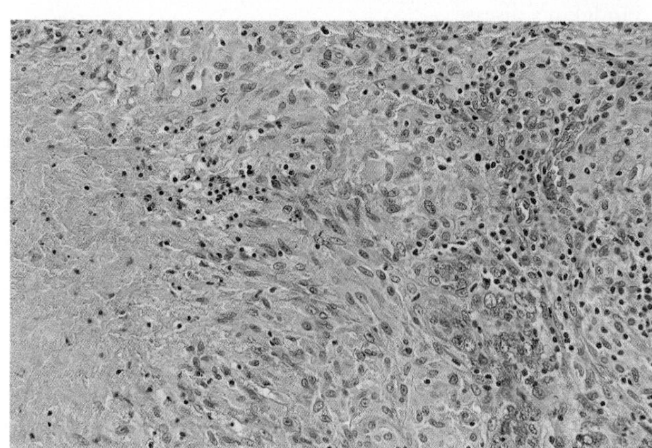

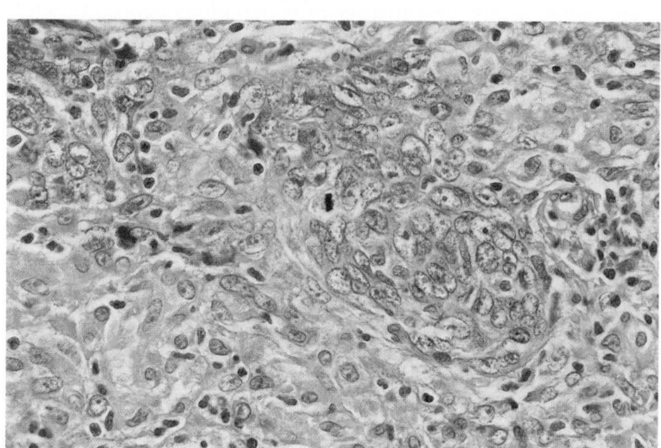

cludes other types of lymphadenitis associated with follicular hyperplasia or clusters of histiocytes. Early or partial nodal involvement by cat scratch disease, sarcoidosis or mycobacteria, or primary or secondary syphilis can result in an appearance that resembles *Toxoplasma* lymphadenitis, except that in none of these disorders is there a tendency for epithelioid histiocytes to encroach on lymphoid follicles. Significant areas of necrosis and true granuloma formation are unusual in toxoplasmosis and should lead to consideration of other infections. *Leishmania* can produce a lymphadenitis closely resembling that of *Toxoplasma*; it also can be associated with a necrotizing or non-necrotizing granulomatous lymphadenitis. With *Leishmania* infection, however, microorganisms are usually identifiable in epithelioid histiocytes.

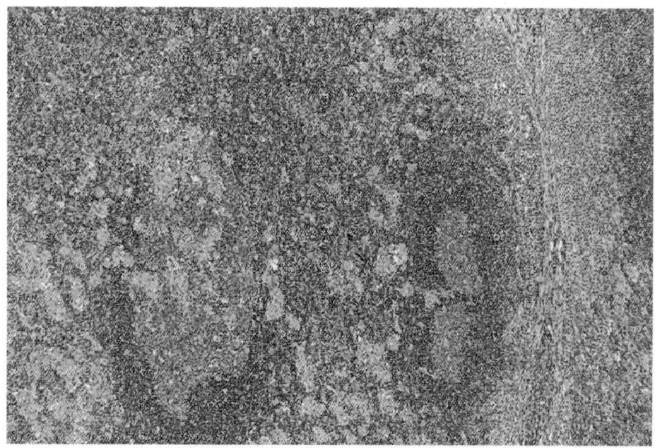

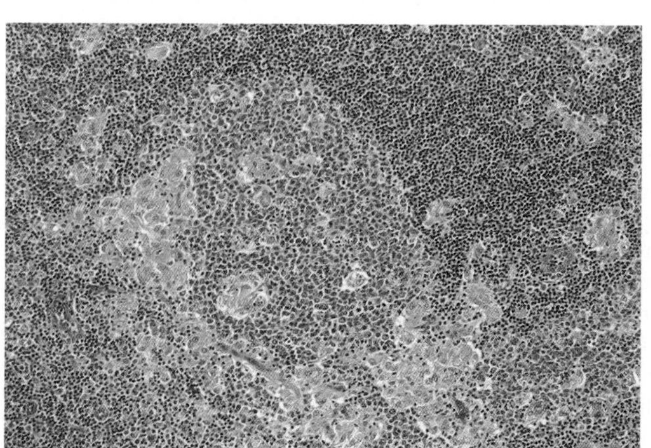

FIGURE 8. *Toxoplasma* lymphadenitis. **A:** Low-power examination shows reactive follicles, clusters of epithelioid histiocytes, and broad, parasinusoidal bands of pale monocytoid B cells. **B:** Higher power shows multiple aggregates of epithelioid histiocytes around and within follicles.

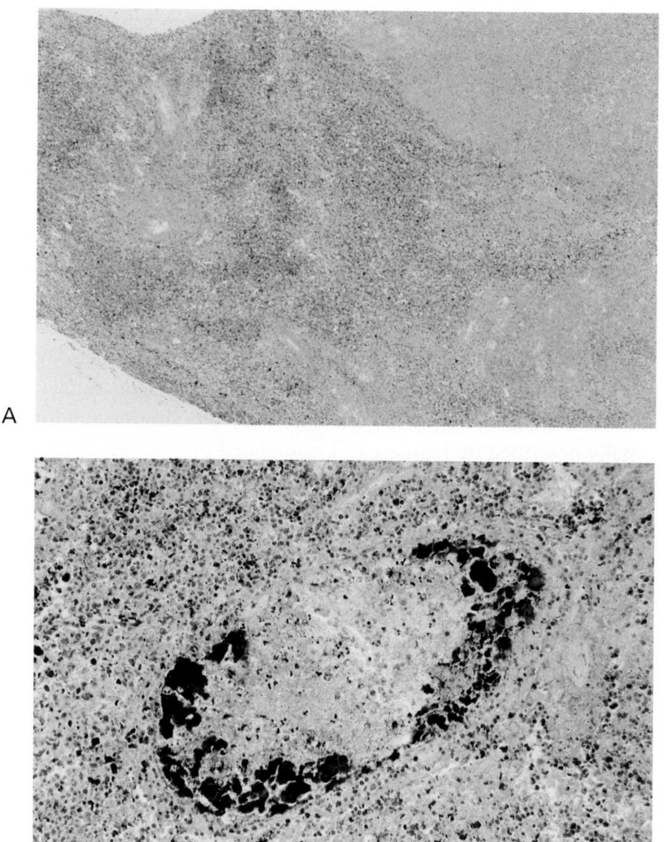

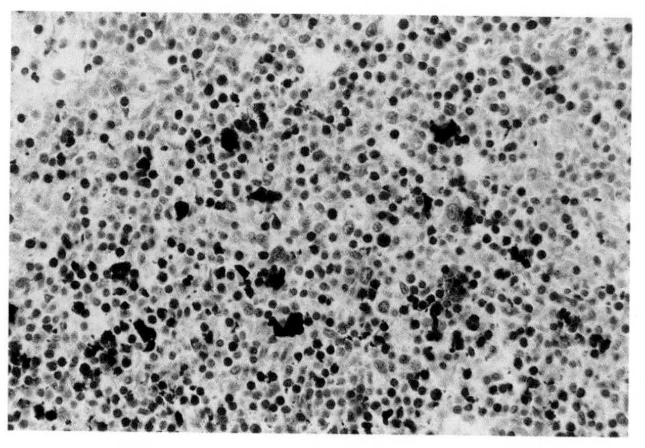

FIGURE 9. Lymphadenitis associated with systemic lupus erythematosus. **A:** Low power shows a lymph node with extensive necrosis; the necrotic material in most areas is amorphous and eosinophilic. **B:** In some areas, residual lymphocytes are recognizable, but most have undergone apoptosis. **C:** Deeply basophilic nuclear material is encrusted on the basement membrane of this blood vessel (Azzopardi phenomenon).

Lupus Lymphadenitis

Systemic lupus erythematosus is an autoimmune disorder that predominantly affects adolescents and young adults, with a female preponderance. It is characterized by a broad spectrum of clinical manifestations, including arthritis or arthralgias, fever, rash, renal disease, anorexia, nausea and vomiting, serositis, and neurologic manifestations. Up to two thirds of patients have lymphadenopathy (lupus lymphadenitis), the most common site of which is the cervical area (43% of cases). Less common sites of involvement are the mesenteric (21%), axillary (18%), and inguinal (17%) lymph nodes. In 12% of cases, there is generalized lymphadenopathy (55). Patients with lymphadenopathy tend to be slightly younger (mean 36 years with adenopathy vs. 45 years without adenopathy) and to have more complaints of fatigue, fever, and weight loss; more cutaneous abnormalities; more frequent hepatomegaly and splenomegaly; and higher titers of anti–double-stranded (ds) DNA antibodies than those without lymphadenopathy (56).

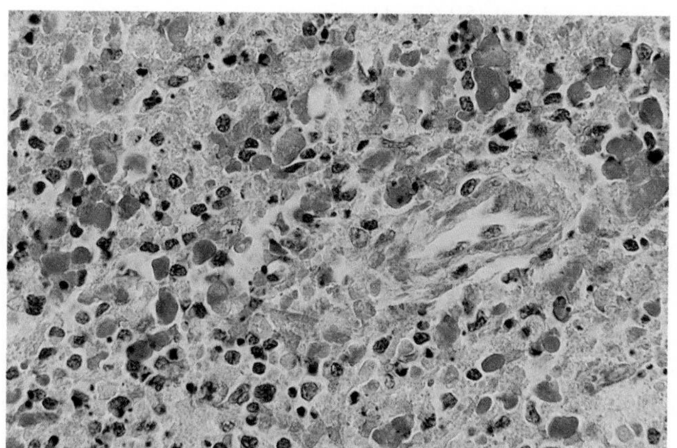

FIGURE 10. Lymphadenitis associated with systemic lupus erythematosus. In this example of lupus lymphadenitis, there are numerous hematoxylin bodies.

Lymph nodes in lupus lymphadenitis may be edematous, with areas of hemorrhage. The lymph node architecture may be distorted, but it is not obliterated. Follicles are hyperplastic or inconspicuous. The paracortex often contains foci of necrosis, with a central zone of amorphous pink material (Figs. 9 and 10). In early lesions, there may be little or no cellular reaction around the necrotic areas. In older lesions, large numbers of histiocytes, with admixed small and large lymphoid cells, surround the necrosis. Immunoblasts may form a prominent component of the infiltrate. Granulocytes are sparse or absent. Plasma cells are usually infrequent, but are found in large numbers in occasional cases. Hematoxylin bodies—ill-defined violet structures thought to represent degenerated nuclei that have reacted with antinuclear antibodies—are sometimes found in areas of necrosis; they are virtually pathognomonic of lupus. Blood vessels in the necrotic foci may show the Azzopardi phenomenon, in which dark blue nuclear material is deposited on the basement membrane of blood vessels. Periarterial and periarteriolar fibrosis also may be seen (55,57).

Little published information is available concerning the immunophenotypic findings in lupus lymphadenitis. In one reported case, however, cells in and around the necrotic areas were predominantly histiocytes and CD3-positive CD8-positive T cytotoxic suppressor cells. Outside of the necrotic areas, paracortical cells were predominantly CD4 positive. Lymphoid follicles expressed polytypic immunoglobulin (57).

Because in some cases of lupus lymphadenitis there are numerous large lymphoid cells, a diagnosis of non-Hodgkin's lymphoma may be entertained. In favor of lupus lymphadenitis are preservation of nodal architecture, characteristic necrotic areas, admixed histiocytes, and hematoxylin bodies. In difficult cases, immunophenotyping may be helpful in excluding lymphoma. Because of the extensive necrosis often found in lupus lymphadenitis, an infectious process may enter the differential diagnosis. However, neutrophils are sparse to absent in lupus and abundant in many different types of infectious lymphadenitis. The necrotic material in lupus lymphadenitis may resemble caseous necrosis, raising the possibility of tuberculous lymphadenitis, but epithelioid histiocytes, Langhans-type giant cells, and granulomas are not features of lupus lymphadenitis. Kikuchi's disease may be a difficult differential diagnostic problem.

Kikuchi's Disease

Kikuchi's disease, also known as histiocytic necrotizing lymphadenitis, Kikuchi's lymphadenitis, Kikuchi-Fujimoto disease, and subacute necrotizing lymphadenitis, seems to be more prevalent among Asians than Western populations. Most patients are young adults, with a female preponderance (58–61). The typical presentation is with unilateral, often painful, cervical lymphadenopathy. Other lymph nodes are affected much less often. Infrequently, there is generalized lymphadenopathy. Approximately half of patients have fever at presentation. Peripheral blood abnormalities that may be present include anemia and neutropenia; an atypical lymphocytosis is found in 25% of cases. Fewer than 5% of patients have a leukocytosis. Occasionally, patients have a rash. The disease is self-limited and most patients recover without therapy. Less than 5% develop recurrent lymphadenopathy (58–61). A viral etiology is suspected for most cases of Kikuchi's disease, but a definite etiology has not been demonstrated (60). A number of case reports have described Kikuchi's disease occurring in association with EBV, human herpesvirus-6 (HHV-6) (62), HHV-8 (63), HIV (64), human T-cell leukemia/T-lymphotropic virus type 1 (HTLV-1) (65), toxoplasmosis, parvovirus (66), and Hashimoto's thyroiditis (67). There is also a case report of Kikuchi's disease occurring in association with a ruptured silicone breast implant (68). Kikuchi's disease-like changes have been found in inguinal nodes of a patient with a malignant fibrous histiocytoma of the thigh (69), and we have seen changes of Kikuchi's disease in lymph nodes draining a colonic carcinoma and a breast carcinoma. Some aspects of Kikuchi's disease suggest it may represent a self-limited autoimmune disorder (58). It is possible that the histologic and immunohistologic features of Kikuchi's disease can be produced by a variety of stimuli.

Lymph nodes (Fig. 11) show prominent paracortical hyperplasia with one or more round or irregular, discrete or confluent eosinophilic areas in the cortex or paracortex containing histiocytes, lymphocytes, immunoblasts, plasmacytoid monocytes, and karyorrhectic and eosinophilic granular debris. The necrotic debris is most abundant in the centers of these areas, whereas immunoblasts are most numerous at the periphery. The histiocytes are of a variety of types, including phagocytic, nonphagocytic, and foamy histiocytes. Phagocytic histiocytes with eccentric sickle-shaped nuclei have been called crescentic histiocytes, whereas nonphagocytic histiocytes with eccentric nuclei are termed signet-ring histiocytes. Plasmacytoid monocytes (originally described by Lennert as T-associated plasma cells and plasmacytoid T cells) (70) are medium-sized cells with round nuclei, dispersed chromatin, small nucleoli, and a moderate amount of faintly amphophilic cytoplasm. They are seen in small clusters in the paracortex of reactive lymph nodes. Although they are situated in the T-cell region of lymph nodes and express some T cell–associated antigens (CD2, CD45RO, CD43), they lack T cell–specific antigens (CD3) and express monocyte-associated antigens (CD68). Their function is not known. In Kikuchi's lymphadenitis, aggregates of plasmacytoid monocytes are frequently seen in non-necrotizing areas; early foci of necrosis appear to begin within clusters of plasmacytoid monocytes. The necrosis is apoptotic rather than suppurative. Epithelioid histiocytes, plasma cells, eosinophils, and neutrophils are virtually absent. The characteristic foci may be relatively small and confined to the paracortex, or they may occupy the majority of the lymph node. The infiltrate may extend beyond the capsule into perinodal soft tissue. Follicular hyperplasia may be seen, but it is not a constant or prominent feature (58–61).

Kikuchi's disease can be subclassified into three histologic subtypes; these may represent different stages in the evolution of the disease. In the proliferative type, microscopic examination reveals the mixture of cells described above, with apoptosis, but without coagulative necrosis. In the necrotizing type, lymph nodes show large areas of necrosis in addition to the changes characteristic of the proliferative type. In the xanthomatous type, there is a predominance of foamy histiocytes, and necrosis can be present or absent (59,61,71).

Immunohistochemical analysis confirms the presence of a mixture of lymphoid cells, histiocytes, and plasmacytoid monocytes. The lymphoid cells express pan T-cell antigens CD3, CD43, and CD45RO; most of them are T-cytotoxic/suppressor (CD8 positive). The histiocytes are lysozyme, CD68, and Ki-M1P positive. (61,62) The plasmacytoid monocytes are Ki-M1P, CD68, and CD4 positive, and they express some T cell–associated, but not T cell–specific antigens, as noted above (62,72). Although B cells are found if reactive follicles are present, B cells are virtually absent in the areas of the node with histiocytes and cellular debris.

Descriptions of Kikuchi's disease have not been found in Western medical literature until relatively recently, which accounts for the lack of familiarity with the characteristic features among many pathologists. The information available is mainly found in pathology literature, so clinicians may be even less fa-

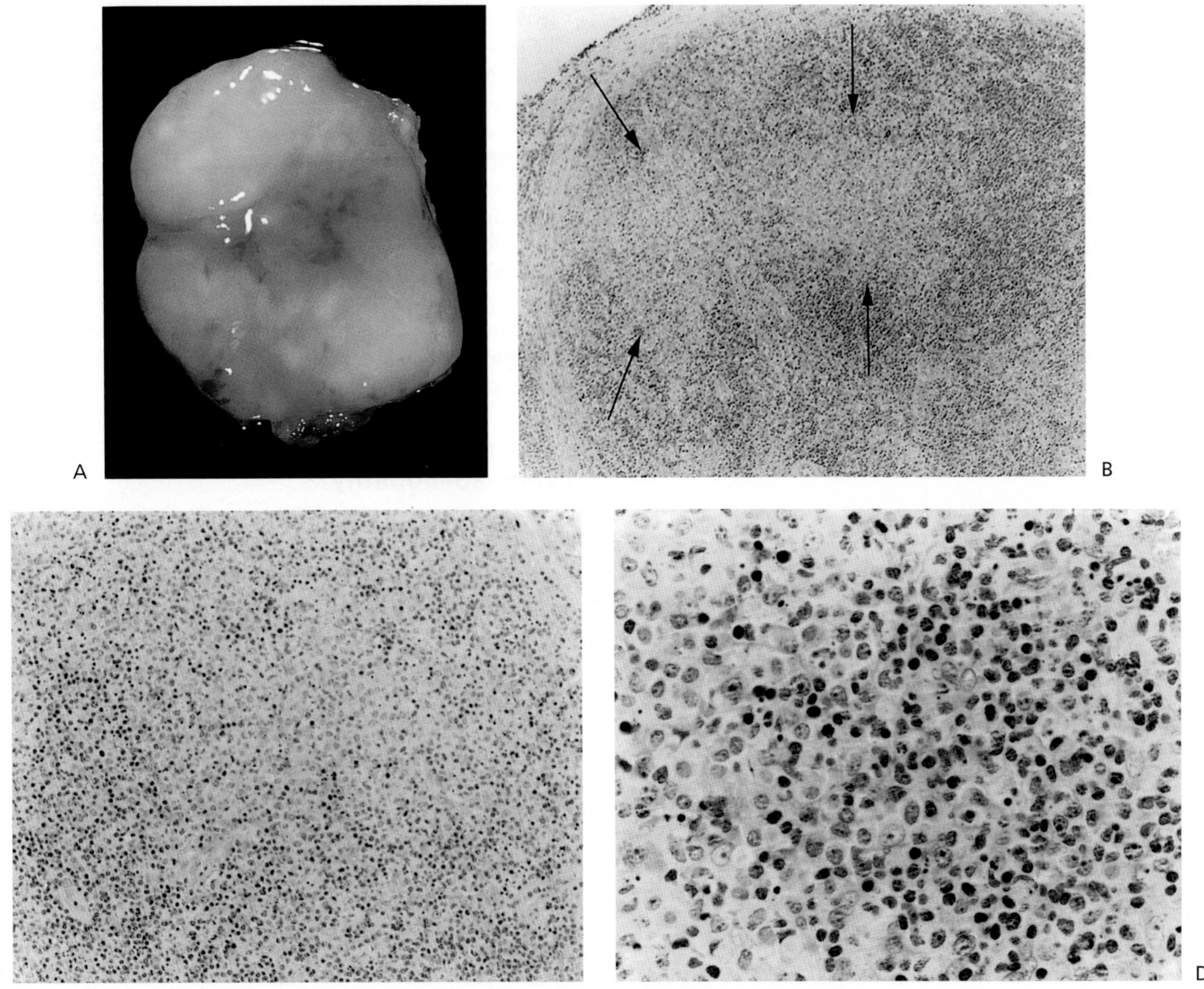

FIGURE 11. Kikuchi's disease in a cervical lymph node. **A:** Gross examination of a section of the node shows multiple small, oval, opaque yellow foci. **B:** Microscopic examination shows coalescent pale foci (*arrows*) characteristic of Kikuchi's disease, in a background of paracortical hyperplasia. **C:** Medium-power view of one of the pale foci shows a polymorphous population of cells with numerous histiocytes. **D:** High power shows a mix of histiocytes, lymphocytes, plasmacytoid monocytes, few immunoblasts and apoptotic debris.

miliar with Kikuchi's disease than their colleagues in pathology (73). Hence the problems in establishing a diagnosis, and depending on the composition of the infiltrate in the affected nodes, a variety of reactive and neoplastic disorders can enter the differential diagnosis.

Because necrosis is such a prominent component of Kikuchi's disease, infectious lymphadenitis is often a consideration. However, neutrophils, suppurative necrosis, and granulomas, features characteristic of many types of infectious lymphadenitis, are not found in Kikuchi's disease. HSL can resemble Kikuchi's disease, particularly in older lesions with few intact neutrophils. Although histiocytes may be prominent in herpetic lymphadenitis, the histiocytic infiltrate is generally even more pronounced in Kikuchi's disease, and viral inclusions are absent. When immunoblasts are abundant, non-Hodgkin's lymphoma enters the differential diagnosis. Familiarity with the spectrum of changes found in Kikuchi's disease, and identification of areas with the characteristic polymorphous infiltrate are essential to rendering the correct diagnosis. In addition, Kikuchi's disease more often shows partial nodal involvement than lymphoma. The vast majority of lymphomas in Western countries are B-cell lymphomas, whereas most immunoblasts in Kikuchi's disease are typically CD8-positive T cells, so that finding B-cell lineage antigens on the large lymphoid cells would tend to exclude Kikuchi's disease and lead to more serious consideration of the possibility of lymphoma. Monotypic immunoglobulin expression confirms a diagnosis of B-cell lymphoma. In especially problematic cases, molecular genetic analysis may be helpful in investigating the possibility of lymphoma.

When crescentic or signet ring-type histiocytes are prominent, metastatic carcinoma of the the signet ring cell type can be considered in the differential diagnosis. However, histiocytes in

Kikuchi's disease lack nuclear atypicality, may contain cellular debris but do not contain mucin, and express histiocyte-related antigens rather than keratins (59). In addition, the classic clinical setting for Kikuchi's disease—a young woman with isolated cervical lymphadenopathy—differs greatly from the scenario expected in a patient with signet ring cell carcinoma. Lymphadenitis in patients with systemic lupus erythematosus can closely resemble Kikuchi's disease (61). Finding hematoxylin bodies, plasma cells, or deposition of nuclear material on blood vessels (the Azzopardi phenomenon) supports a diagnosis of lupus lymphadenitis over Kikuchi's disease, but these features may not be found in every case of lupus lymphadenitis. Clinical features are sometimes helpful in making a definitive distinction. Because of the difficulty in definitively excluding lupus on microscopic examination, clinicians may consider performing a workup for autoimmune disease in some cases showing histologic features of Kikuchi's disease.

Kawasaki's Disease

Kawasaki's disease, also known as mucocutaneous lymph node syndrome and infantile polyarteritis nodosa, is an acute febrile disease of uncertain etiology that predominantly affects young children, with a slight male preponderance (male:female ratio 1.5:1) and a higher prevalence among Asians. The cause is uncertain, but most evidence suggests an infectious etiology. The requirements of the Centers for Disease Control and Prevention for the diagnosis of Kawasaki's disease include the finding of fever of 5 or more days, unresponsiveness to antibiotics, and at least four of the following five features: (a) bilateral conjunctival congestion; (b) abnormalities of lips and oral cavity including diffuse erythema, dry fissured lips, and prominent lingual papillae (strawberry tongue); (c) abnormalities of the skin of the distal extremities, including erythema of palms and soles with edema early on and desquamation of fingertips later in the course of the disease; (d) polymorphous, nonvesicular, primarily truncal rash; and (e) acute, nonsuppurative cervical lymphadenopathy, not due to any other identifiable cause (74,75). Other findings that may be present are cardiac abnormalities (e.g., electrocardiographic changes, cardiomegaly, murmurs), diarrhea, arthritis or arthralgia, proteinuria, sterile pyuria, neutrophilic leukocytosis with a leftward shift, anemia, thrombocytosis, elevated sedimentation rate, aseptic meningitis, mild jaundice, and elevated transaminases (75). Most patients recover after an illness of 3 to 4 weeks' duration, but in 1% to 3% of cases, patients die of complications of coronary arteritis (aneurysm with thrombosis). In fatal cases, postmortem examination often discloses a vasculitis involving large elastic and muscular arteries (74). Fatalities can occur at any time, from the acute phase of the disease until several years later (74–76). Prompt administration of intravenous gamma globulin reduces the risk of coronary arterial changes, emphasizing the importance of prompt diagnosis (77).

There are only a few published reports on the histologic features of lymph nodes in Kawasaki's disease. Reactive lymphoid hyperplasia, presumably with nonspecific features, has been described (76). In other cases, the features are more distinctive. Findings include paracortical expansion by lymphocytes and a variable number of immunoblasts, plasma cells, and histiocytes. The paracortex also may contain small to large areas of necrosis containing karyorrhectic debris. Blood vessels around the necrotic areas appear increased in number; they are lined by swollen endothelial cells and contain fibrin thrombi. Although the lymphoadenopathy is classically described as nonsuppurative, in some cases necrotic areas contain neutrophils. A concentric perivascular arrangement of lymphocytes and histiocytes may be found; however, true vasculitis is only rarely described in lymph nodes. Follicular hyperplasia is not usually conspicuous. Eosinophils and granulomas are not described (74,75). In one case, lymphoid depletion was found, but this may have been a consequence of high-dose steroid therapy rather than a result of Kawasaki's disease alone (75).

Sinus Histiocytosis with Massive Lymphadenopathy

Sinus histiocytosis with massive lymphadenopathy (SHML), first described in 1969 by Rosai and Dorfman, and thus also known as Rosai-Dorfman disease (78), is a disorder of uncertain etiology that mainly affects children and young adults. The classical clinical presentation is with massive, painless, bilateral cervical lymphadenopathy. Occasionally other node groups are involved, and infrequently there is generalized lymphadenopathy. In about one third of cases, extranodal sites, including skin, upper respiratory tract, bone, or central nervous system (CNS), are involved. Patients commonly have fever, leukocytosis, anemia, elevated erythrocyte sedimentation rate, and polyclonal hypergammaglobulinemia. In about 10% of cases, patients have associated immunologic abnormalities, including susceptibility to infection, autoantibody-induced cytopenias, glomerulonephritis, and arthritis.

The prognosis for most patients is excellent, although lymphadenopathy can persist for years (78–81). The prognosis is less favorable in patients with immunologic dysfunction or multiple sites of involvement (79,80). Fourteen (6.5%) of the patients listed in the Sinus Histiocytosis with Massive Lymphadenopathy Registry have died, although in only 2 of the 14 fatal cases was death directly attributable to SHML. In most cases death was due to infection or to complications of immunologically mediated diseases (80).

Gross examination reveals one or more enlarged lymph nodes, which may be matted together. Sectioning reveals bright yellow tissue that may resemble adipose tissue. On microscopic examination, there is marked dilatation of cortical and medullary sinuses by large histiocytes with round to oval vesicular nuclei, often with prominent nucleoli, and abundant, pale, vacuolated cytoplasm with ill-defined cell borders (Fig. 12A). The histiocytes contain intact-appearing lymphocytes, and less often, plasma cells, neutrophils, and erythrocytes, a phenomenon referred to as emperipolesis ("wandering about within") (Fig. 12B and C). The presence of emperipolesis is in contrast to the much more common finding (in other conditions) of phagocytosis, in which cells taken in by histiocytes appear degenerated. The intervening lymphoid tissue shows nonspecific changes; it may become quite compressed by the expanded sinuses. Medullary cords contain lymphocytes and plasma cells. Eosinophils are

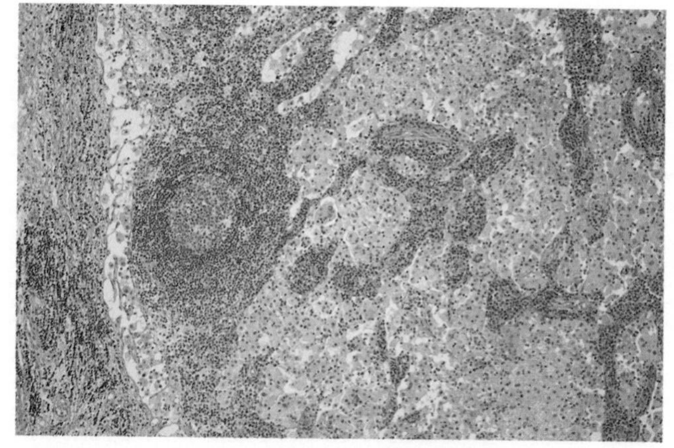

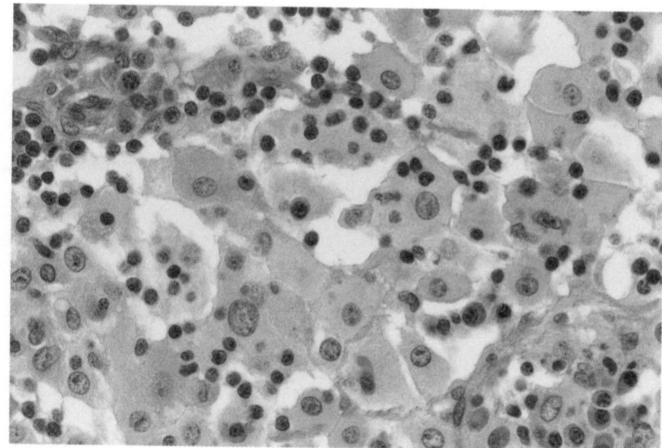

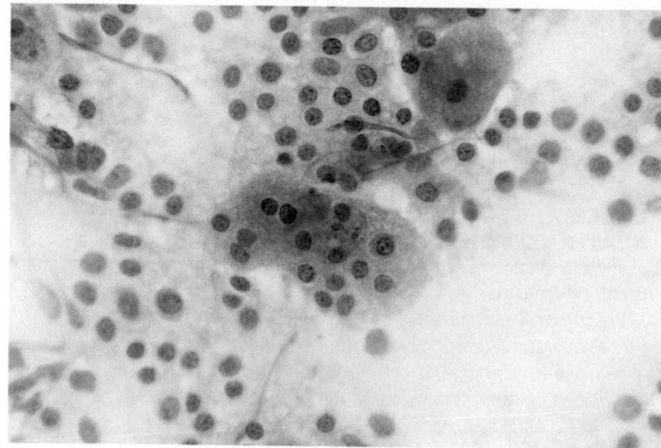

FIGURE 12. Sinus histiocytosis with massive lymphadenopathy. **A:** The lymph node shows marked dilatation of sinuses, which are filled by histiocytes. Also present are a reactive follicle and compressed cords of paracortex. **B:** High-power examination within the sinuses shows histiocytes with relatively large nuclei, sometimes with distinct nucleoli, and abundant granular eosinophilic cytoplasm. Several histiocytes contain intact-appearing lymphocytes within their cytoplasm (emperipolesis). **C:** A touch preparation shows a histiocyte with emperipolesis, in a background of small lymphocytes.

usually absent. The capsule and perinodal soft tissue are often fibrotic, and there may be areas of fibrosis within the node (78,81,82).

Immunohistochemical analysis has shown that the SHML histiocytes are positive for S-100 protein, α_1-antitrypsin, α_1-antichymotrypsin, CD11b, CD11c, CD14, CD33, CD68, and activation antigens (CD30, transferrin receptor, and interleukin 2 receptor) (78,81–83).

The histologic features of SHML in lymph nodes are so distinctive that making a diagnosis is generally straightforward. Nonspecific reactive hyperplasia with sinus histiocytosis is the entity most likely to be considered in the differential diagnosis of SHML. However, in nonspecific hyperplasia, lymph nodes are not as large, enlargement is not as persistent, sinuses are not as distended, and individual histiocytes are not as large as in SHML. Sinus histiocytes may show phagocytosis, but emperipolesis is not a feature. Most sinus histiocytes are S-100 negative. Examination of a touch preparation may be helpful in identifying the characteristic histiocytes of SHML.

Kimura's Disease

Kimura's disease is a chronic inflammatory disorder that mainly affects the area of the head and neck; it is associated with one or more large lesions (typically 2–5 cm) in subcutaneous tissue and major salivary glands, along with lymphadenopathy. Lymphadenopathy may be bilateral and is usually painless. Kimura's disease affecting the lacrimal gland has been described. Rarely, this disorder produces lesions away from the head and neck, including the groin, axilla, forearm, and popliteal area (84). Kimura's disease affects patients from childhood to middle age; most patients are young adults, with a male preponderance. The disease is more common among Asian populations. Patients may have peripheral eosinophilia and elevated serum immunoglobulin E (IgE) levels. Lesions may persist or recur over a period of months or years. When Kimura's disease was first described, it was thought to represent a neoplastic process, and was only later recognized as reactive. Accordingly, findings on physical examination often suggest a diagnosis of a salivary gland tumor or lymphoma (84). Kimura's disease is of uncertain etiology, but may represent an aberrant immune reaction to an unknown stimulus (84,85).

Lesions in salivary glands and subcutaneous tissue are poorly circumscribed and consist of a dense infiltrate of lymphocytes, eosinophils, mast cells, and plasma cells with many small blood vessels containing prominent endothelial cells. Numerous reactive follicles are present; their germinal centers may be pierced by blood vessels, or may be invaded and disrupted by eosinophils (Fig. 13). In about half of cases, there is deposition of homogeneous eosinophilic material in the interstitium of the germinal centers. Polykaryocytes may be present, most often in the follicles. Fibrosis is very common, but its extent is variable. It may be in the form of concentric perivascular or (in salivary glands) periductal rings of collagen, but over time it may progress to dif-

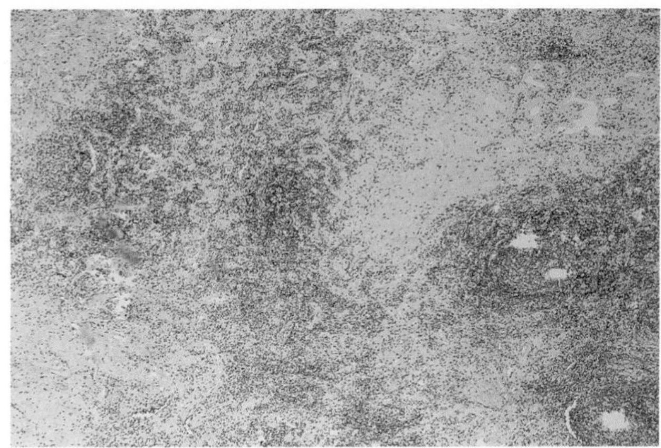
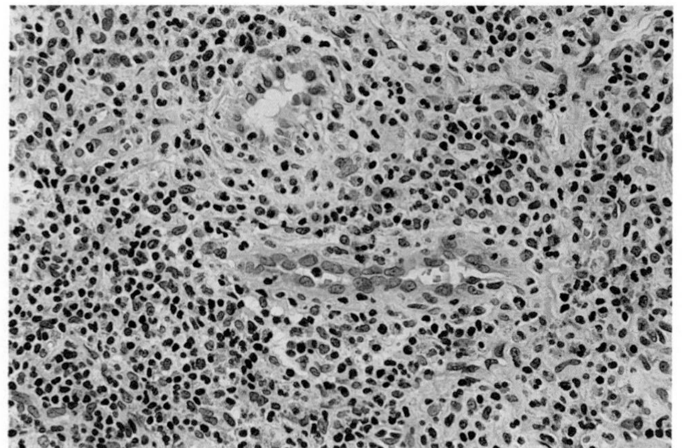

FIGURE 13. Kimura's disease. **A:** Low-power examination shows soft tissue with dense fibrosis and a patchy lymphoid infiltrate with reactive follicles. **B:** Higher power shows lymphocytes, eosinophils, and small blood vessels in a fibrotic background.

fuse, extensive hyalinization of the involved tissues with only scattered lymphocytes, plasma cells, eosinophils, and mast cells. Involved lymph nodes show follicular hyperplasia with increased numbers of eosinophils in the paracortex, sinuses, and perinodal soft tissue, as well as within follicles, sometimes with formation of eosinophilic microabscesses. Paracortical postcapillary venules are increased. Fibrosis tends to be less severe in lymph nodes than in subcutis or salivary glands.

Kimura's disease has the distinctive finding of IgE-positive dendritic networks in germinal centers. The prominence of eosinophils, the presence of mast cells, and the characteristic IgE deposition in germinal centers reinforce the idea that Kimura's disease may be a manifestation of an abnormal immunologic response (84).

The main entity in the differential diagnosis of Kimura's disease is angiolymphoid hyperplasia with eosinophilia or epithelioid hemangioma. In many early reports the two disorders were grouped together as one disease. Both angiolymphoid hyperplasia with eosinophilia and Kimura's disease tend to produce lesions with prominent blood vessels and eosinophils in the region of the head and neck. However, angiolymphoid hyperplasia with eosinophilia is associated with larger numbers of smaller lesions that are better circumscribed and more superficially located (i.e., in the dermis). Lymphoid follicles and fibrosis are not always seen in angiolymphoid hyperplasia with eosinophilia. Angiolymphoid hyperplasia with eosinophilia is not associated with lymphadenopathy or salivary gland involvement. The most distinctive feature of angiolymphoid hyperplasia with eosinophilia is prominent epithelioid, or histiocytoid, endothelial cells, larger than the endothelial cells seen in Kimura's disease. Angiolymphoid hyperplasia with eosinophilia may represent a benign vascular tumor rather than a type of lymphoid hyperplasia, and for this reason it also has been called epithelioid hemangioma (85) (see Chapter 13).

LYMPHOMAS OF THE HEAD AND NECK

Cervical lymph nodes may be involved by lymphomas of any type, and these will not be discussed in detail here. Extranodal

TABLE 2. LYMPHOID NEOPLASMS IN THE UPDATED REAL AND WHO CLASSIFICATIONS[a]

- B-cell neoplasms
  - Precursor B-cell neoplasm
    - *Precursor B-lymphoblastic leukemia/lymphoma (B-ALL/LBL)*
  - Mature (peripheral) B-cell neoplasms
    - *B-cell chronic lymphocytic leukemia/small lymphocytic lymphoma (B-CLL/SLL)*
    - B-cell prolymphocytic leukemia
    - Lymphoplasmacytic lymphoma
    - Splenic marginal zone B-cell lymphoma (with or without villous lymphocytes)
    - Hairy cell leukemia
    - *Plasma cell myeloma/plasmacytoma*
    - *Extranodal marginal zone B-cell lymphoma of MALT type*
    - Nodal marginal zone B-cell lymphoma (with or without monocytoid B cells)
      - *Follicular lymphoma*
      - *Mantle cell lymphoma*
      - *Diffuse large B-cell lymphoma*
      - *Burkitt's lymphoma*
- T and NK-cell neoplasms
  - Precursor T-cell neoplasm
    - *Precursor T-lymphoblastic lymphoma/leukemia (T-ALL/LBL)*
  - Mature (peripheral) T-cell neoplasms
    - T-cell prolymphocytic leukemia (T-PLL)
    - T-cell granular lymphocytic leukemia
    - Aggressive NK cell leukemia
    - Adult T-cell lymphoma/leukemia ($HTLV1^{+}$)
    - Extranodal NK/T-cell lymphoma, nasal type
    - Enteropathy-type T-cell lymphoma
    - Hepatosplenic $\gamma\delta$ T-cell lymphoma
    - Subcutaneous panniculitis-like T-cell lymphoma
    - *Mycosis fungoides/Sezary syndrome*
      - Anaplastic large T/null cell lymphoma (ALCL), primary cutaneous type
    - *Peripheral T-cell lymphoma, unspecified*
    - *Angioimmunoblastic T-cell lymphoma*
    - *Anaplastic large T/null cell lymphoma (ALCL), primary systemic type*

[a] More common entities are italicized.
NK, natural killer.

lymphomas can arise in a variety of head and neck sites. The most common is Waldeyer's ring, which, although extranodal, harbors lymphoid tissue under normal circumstances and is therefore not a true extralymphatic site. Waldeyer's ring accounts for at least half of head and neck lymphomas reported in most series; other sites include the nose and paranasal sinuses, salivary gland, oral cavity, and larynx in descending order of frequency. Lymphomas also may arise in the thyroid gland and in the eye and ocular adnexa.

Lymphomas are now classified using a combination of morphologic features, immunophenotype, and genetic characteristics. The primary subdivisions are B-cell lymphomas, T-cell and natural killer (NK)-cell lymphomas, and Hodgkin's disease. Hodgkin's disease, although common in cervical lymph nodes, is rare in non-nodal head and neck sites, and will not be discussed here. Within the categories of B-cell lymphomas and T/NK-cell lymphomas, many distinct entities have been defined, which have been summarized in the Revised European-American Classification of Lymphoid Neoplasms (REAL Classification) (86) and will form the basis of the upcoming World Health Organization (WHO) Classification (87). These diseases are summarized in Table 2. Immunologic and genetic features that are useful in the diagnosis and classification of lymphomas are summarized in Tables 3 and 4.

The various types of lymphomas occur with different frequencies in different head and neck sites (Table 5). For example, T/NK-cell lymphoma is common in the nasal cavity, but exceedingly rare elsewhere. Extranodal marginal zone B-cell lymphoma [mucosa-associated lymphoid tissue (MALT) lymphoma] is common in the thyroid and salivary glands and in the ocular adnexa, but rare in Waldeyer's ring. Diffuse large B-cell lymphoma is the most common lymphoma of Waldeyer's ring and paranasal sinuses but is rare in the ocular adnexa. The natural history of the lymphomas in the different sites is also distinctive: ocular lymphoma is likely to be associated with CNS involvement; MALT lymphomas of the salivary and thyroid glands are often associated with autoimmune disease (Sjögren's syndrome and Hashimoto's thyroiditis, respectively); MALT lymphomas of any site tend to relapse in other extranodal sites; and Waldeyer's ring lymphoma is often associated with gastrointestinal involvement.

LYMPHOMAS OF WALDEYER'S RING

Introduction and Classification

Waldeyer's ring is an intercommunicating network of lymphoid tissue located in the faucial, nasopharyngeal (adenoid), and lingual tonsils, which is part of the normal MALT system (see Chapter 5). In contrast to mucosal or epithelial sites that do not normally contain MALT, such as the stomach, lung, thyroid, and salivary gland, sites of normal MALT (Waldeyer's ring and the Peyer's patch region of the distal ileum) are rarely involved by MALT lymphoma (extranodal marginal zone B-cell lymphoma of the MALT type). Isaacson has suggested that this phenomenon can be explained by the hypothesis that "acquired MALT" in the course of an immunologic reaction constitutes the substrate for the development of MALT lymphoma (88).

In studies using the Rappaport classification and Working Formulation, the most common type of lymphoma is diffuse

TABLE 3. IMMUNOHISTOLOGIC AND GENETIC FEATURES OF COMMON B-CELL NEOPLASMS

Neoplasm	SIg; CIg	CD5	CD10	CD23	CD43[a]	CD103	Cyclin D1	Genetic Abnormality	Immunoglobulin Genes
B-CLL/SLL	+; −/+	+	−	+	+	−	−/+	trisomy 12; 13q	R, U
Lymphoplasmacytic lymphoma	+; +	−	−	−	−/+	−	−	t(9;14); del 6(q23)	R, M
Hairy cell leukemia	+; −	−	−	−	+	++	+/−	none known	R, M
Splenic marginal zone lymphoma	+; −/+	−	−	−	−	+	−	del 7q	R, M
Follicle center lymphoma	+; −	−	+/−	−/+	−	−	−	t(14;18); bcl-2	R, M, O
Mantle cell lymphoma	+; −	+	−	−	+	−	+	t(11;14); bcl-1	R, U
MALT lymphoma	+; +/−	−	−	−/+	−/+	−	−	trisomy 3 t(11;18)	R, M, O
Diffuse large B-cell lymphoma	+/−	−	−/+	NA	−/+	NA	−	t(14;18), t(8;14), t(3;v) (q 27;v); bcl-2, myc, bcl-6	R, M
Burkitt's lymphoma	+	−	+	−	−	NA	-	t(8;14), t(2;8), t(8;22); c-myc; EBV−/+	R,M

[a] Positivity may vary depending on antibody used.

F, frozen sections; P, paraffin sections; R, rearranged; G, germline; M, mutated; U, unmutated; O, ongoing mutations; TCR, T-cell receptor gene; Ig, immunoglobulin; S, surface; C, cytoplasmic; +, >90% positive; +/−, >50% positive; −/+, <50% positive; −, <10% positive; EBV, Epstein-Barr virus; NA, not applicable, *, mutations in the Ig gene V region indicate exposure to antigen; PTCL-NOS, peripheral T-cell lymphoma, unspecified; NPM/ALK, nucleophosmin-anaplastic lymphoma kinase; ALCL, anaplastic large cell lymphoma; B-CLL/SLL, B-cell chronic lymphocytic leukemia/small lymphocytic lymphoma; T-PLL, T-cell prolymphocytic leukemia; T-LGL, T-cell granular lymphocytic leukemia; NK-LGL, natural killer-cell granular lymphocytic leukemia; Cytotox. Granule, TIA-1, perforin, and/or granzyme B; IVDA, intravenous drug abuse; Ig, immunoglobulin; MoIg, monotypic immunoglobulin; MBC, monocytoid B cells.

TABLE 4. IMMUNOHISTOLOGIC AND GENETIC FEATURES OF COMMON T-CELL NEOPLASMS

Neoplasm	CD3 S;C	CD5	CD7	CD4	CD8	CD30	TCR	NK (16, 56)	Cytotox Granule	EBV	Genetic Abnormality	T-Receptor Genes
T-PLL	+	–	+	+/–	–/+	–	αβ	–/+	–	–	inv 14 trisomy 8q	R
T-LGL	+	–	+	–	+	–	αβ	+/–	+	–	none known	R
NK-LGL	–	–	+	–	+/–	–	–	–/+	+	+	none known	G
Extranodal NK/T-cell lymphoma	–; +	–	+	–	+/–	–	–	+	+	++	none known	G
Hepatosplenic γδ T-cell lymphoma	+	–	+	–	–	–	γδ	–/+	+	–	Iso 7q	R
Enteropathy-type T-cell lymphoma	+	+	+	–	+/–	+/–	αβ	–	+	–	none known	R
Subcutaneous panniculitis-like T-cell lymphoma	+	+	+	–	+	–/+	αβ	–	+	–	none known	R
PTCL-NOS	+/–	+/–	+/–	+/–	–/+	–/+	αβ > γδ	–/+	–/+	–/+	inv 14; complex	R
Angioimmunoblastic lymphoma	+	+	+	+/–	–	–	αβ	–	NA	+/–	none known	R
ALCL, primary systemic	+/–	+/–	NA	–/+	–/+	++	αβ	–	+	–	t(2;5); NPM/ALK	R
ALCL, cutaneous	+/–	+/–	+/–	+/–	–	++	αβ	–	–/+	–	none known	R

F, frozen sections; P, paraffin sections; R, rearranged; G, germline; M, mutated; U, unmutated; O, ongoing mutations; TCR, T-cell receptor gene; Ig, immunoglobulin; S, surface; C, cystoplasmic; +, >90% positive; +/–, >50% positive; –/+, <50% positive; –, <10% positive; EBV, Epstein-Barr virus; NA, not applicable, *, mutations in the Ig gene V region indicate exposure to antigen; PTCL-NOS, peripheral T-cell lymphoma, unspecified; NPM/ALK, nucleophosmin-anaplastic lymphoma kinase; ALCL, anaplastic large cell lymphoma; B-CLL/SLL, B-cell chronic lymphocytic leukemia/small lymphocytic lymphoma; T-PLL, T-cell prolymphocytic leukemia; T-LGL, T-cell granular lymphocytic leukemia; NK-LGL, natural killer-cell granular lymphocytic leukemia; Cytotox. Granule, TIA-1, perforin, and/or granzyme B; IVDA, intravenous drug abuse; Ig, immunoglobulin; MoIg, monotypic immunoglobulin; MBC, monocytoid B cells.

large cell or histiocytic lymphoma (50%), with follicular lymphoma accounting for 15% to 20%, and smaller numbers classified as diffuse small cleaved/poorly differentiated lymphocytic or small noncleaved/undifferentiated types (89,90).

In studies using the Kiel Classification, the most common type of lymphoma in this location is centroblastic (55%–80%), with smaller numbers of centroblastic/centrocytic (10%–20%), centrocytic (0–10%), and Burkitt's (5%) types (91,92). MALT and monocytoid B-cell lymphomas accounted for 4 of 79 cases in one series (91); in a study of 329 cases of low-grade lymphoma of Waldeyer's ring from Kiel, only 12 cases of MALT lymphoma were identified, 2 of which occurred in patients with a history of gastric lymphoma. Thus, MALT lymphoma appears to account for only about 4% of Waldeyer's ring lymphomas. In a study of

TABLE 5. DISTRIBUTION OF LYMPHOMAS IN HEAD AND NECK SITES

Site	Common Lymphomas	%	Associated Findings
Waldeyer's ring	Diffuse large B-cell lymphoma	50–60	Gastrointestinal lymphoma
	Follicular lymphoma	10	
	Burkitt's lymphoma	10	
	Mantle cell lymphoma	5	Disseminated disease
Nasal cavity	Extranodal NK/T-cell lymphoma, nasal type	70	Other extranodal sites Hemophagocytic syndrome
	Diffuse large B-cell lymphoma	30	
Paranasal sinuses	Diffuse large B-cell lymphoma	80	
Oral cavity	Diffuse large B-cell lymphoma	50	HIV infection
	Follicular lymphoma	15	
	MALT lymphoma	10	
Larynx	MALT lymphoma	50	
	Diffuse large B-cell lymphoma	50	
Salivary gland	MALT lymphoma	30	Sjögren's syndrome
	Follicular lymphoma	30	
	Diffuse large B-cell lymphoma	30	
Thyroid	Diffuse large B-cell lymphoma	50	
	MALT lymphoma	50	Hashimoto's thyroiditis
Ocular adnexa	MALT lymphoma	50	
	Follicular lymphoma	20	
Eye	Diffuse large B-cell lymphoma	>90	Central nervous system lymphoma

NK, natural killer; MALT, mucosa-associated lymphoid tissue.

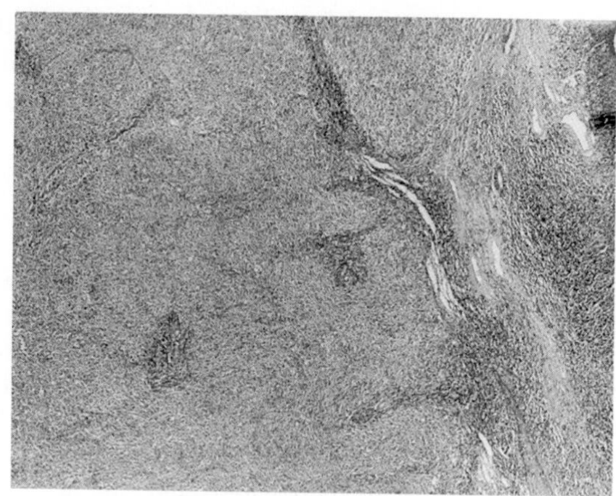
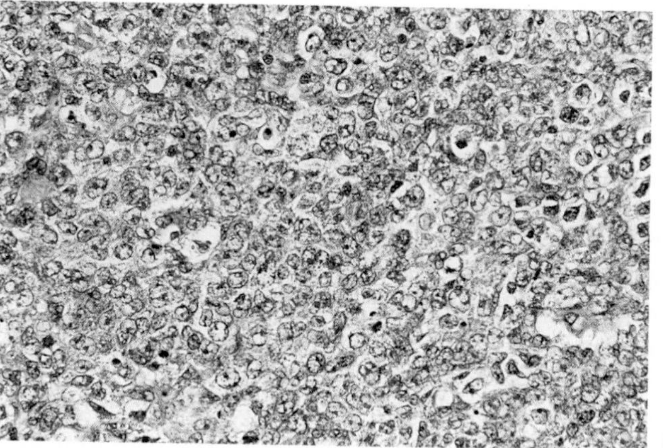

FIGURE 14. Diffuse large B-cell lymphoma of the tonsil. **A:** At low magnification, there is diffuse and patchy effacement of the architecture. **B:** The cells are large and round; many have peripheral nucleoli (centroblasts), whereas a few have central nucleoli (immunoblasts). Several mitotic figures are present.

MALT lymphomas of all sites, Thieblemont and colleagues found only 3 of 108 cases to involve Waldeyer's ring (93).

Pathologic Features of Waldeyer's Ring Lymphomas

The morphologic, immunophenotypic, and genetic features of lymphomas in Waldeyer's ring are similar to those of the specific lymphoma subtypes in other sites. The presence of lymphoid cells within the mucosal epithelium is not a reliable indicator of MALT-type lymphoma in this site, because both normal and neoplastic lymphoid cells may be seen within the epithelium in all types of lymphoma involving tonsillar tissue.

Diffuse Large B-cell Lymphoma

Diffuse large B-cell lymphoma is composed of a relatively monomorphous population of large cells with round to oval nuclei, one or more nucleoli, usually resembling centroblasts (large noncleaved follicle center cells) or immunoblasts, or a combination of the two (Fig. 14). Occasional cases are composed of multilobated cells or anaplastic large cells with abundant cytoplasm, resembling anaplastic large T-cell lymphoma. The cells are typically positive for CD45 (leukocyte common antigen) and pan B-cell antigens (CD20/L26, CD79a), may express immunoglobulin heavy and light chains (best detected on frozen sections), and are negative for cytokeratin and other epithelial markers. The differential diagnosis is mainly with poorly differentiated carcinoma, and a combination of morphologic features and immunohistochemistry is usually sufficient to establish the diagnosis.

Burkitt's Lymphoma

Burkitt's lymphoma presents with tonsillar involvement relatively rarely and is more common in children and immunosuppressed patients. Like diffuse large B-cell lymphoma, it produces a diffuse, destructive infiltrate (Fig. 15). At low magnification, a starry sky pattern is evident (i.e., the presence of abundant pale tingible body macrophages in a blue cellular background is rem-

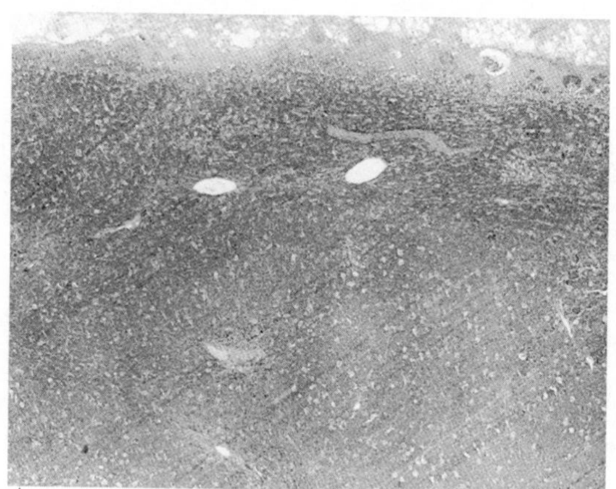
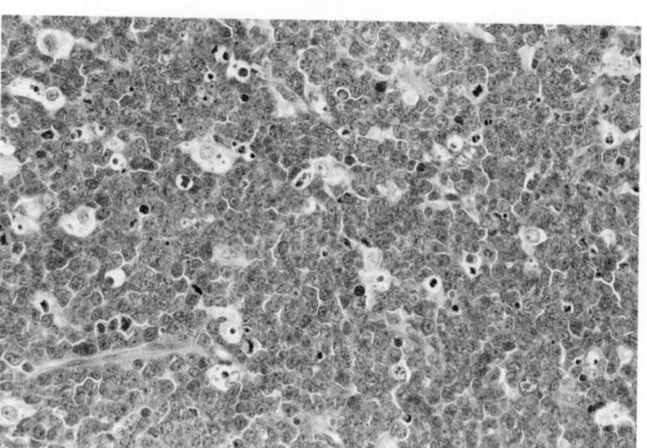

FIGURE 15. Burkitt's lymphoma of the tonsil. **A:** At low magnification, there is architectural effacement with infiltration of the overlying epithelium, and there is a prominent starry sky pattern. **B:** At high magnification, the cells are smaller than those of the large cell lymphoma, and there are numerous mitotic figures.

iniscent of many stars in the night sky). The cells are smaller and more uniform than those of diffuse large B-cell lymphoma, and there is typically a high mitotic rate (10 or more mitoses per high-power field) and a proliferation fraction (Ki-67) of greater than 99%.

Follicular Lymphoma

Follicular lymphoma involving the tonsil must be distinguished from follicular hyperplasia. Typically, the follicles are increased in number, poorly circumscribed, and closely packed (Fig. 16). Polarization into dark and light zones, which is typical of reactive tonsillar follicles, is absent, as is a starry sky pattern of phagocytic histiocytes or tingible body macrophages. The follicles tend to contain a monomorphous population of centrocytes (small or large cleaved cells), with a minority of centroblasts, although the proportion of these cells may vary, as in the different grades of nodal follicular cell lymphomas (see standard hematopathology texts). Staining for *bcl-2* and immunoglobulin light chains (best on frozen sections) can be useful in confirming the diagnosis. In equivocal cases, PCR analysis for immunoglobulin heavy chain or *bcl-2* gene rearrangement can be helpful.

Mantle Cell Lymphoma

Although it accounts for only a small fraction of Waldeyer's ring lymphomas, mantle cell lymphoma (MCL) frequently involves the tonsil, and this may be the site of the initial diagnostic biopsy (Fig. 17). The infiltrate may be diffuse or nodular, or may have a mantle zone pattern; thus, it may mimic follicular lymphoma or MALT lymphoma. Most cases are composed of a uniform population of small to medium-sized cells with irregular nuclei and scant cytoplasm. Occasional mitoses are seen, and there are typically single epithelioid histiocytes scattered throughout the infiltrate. In about 10% of the cases, the cell size is larger, with some pleomorphism, and a higher mitotic rate. These cases may be misdiagnosed as diffuse large B-cell lymphoma. The characteristic immunophenotype of MCL (CD5 positive and cyclin D1 positive) is helpful in the differential diagnosis, and distinguishes it from MALT, follicular, and diffuse large B-cell lymphomas.

Clinical Features of Waldeyer's Ring Lymphomas

Waldeyer's ring is the second most common site of extranodal lymphoma, after the gastrointestinal tract, and comprises about 10% of the cases in most series (94). It is the most common extranodal site of head and neck lymphoma, accounting for over 60% of the cases (89). The faucial tonsils are the most common location, followed by the nasopharynx and base of the tongue. The median age of occurrence is in the sixth decade of life, with a slight male predominance. The majority of patients with diffuse large B-cell lymphoma present with localized disease or with cervical lymph node involvement (stage I and II, 50%–70%) (89,91,95). Survival depends on stage and histologic type, with localized lymphomas associated with significantly better survival than those with nodal involvement, and follicular lymphoma associated with better overall survival than large B-cell or MCL (89–91). Menarguez and associates found that patients with lymphomas of Waldeyer's ring had a significantly better 5-year overall survival rate than an unselected contemporaneous series of nodal lymphomas (65% vs. 36%), and that this was explained by earlier clinical stage at diagnosis (91).

An association between Waldeyer's ring and gastrointestinal lymphomas has been reported by many investigators. Overall, approximately 10% of patients with Waldeyer's ring lymphoma are found to have gastrointestinal involvement, either at the time of the diagnosis or as a site of relapse (89,90,95). The most common site of gastrointestinal involvement is the stomach; however, both large and small bowel involvement have been reported. This association raises the possibility that at least some of the large cell lymphomas of both gastric and Waldeyer's ring locations are of MALT rather than nodal type. Support for this

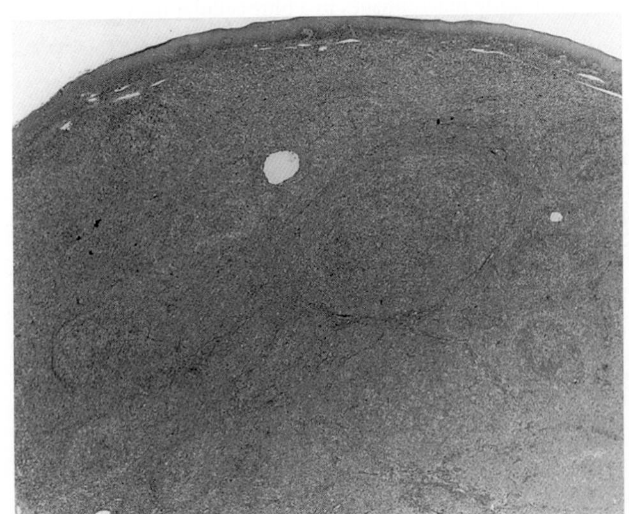
A

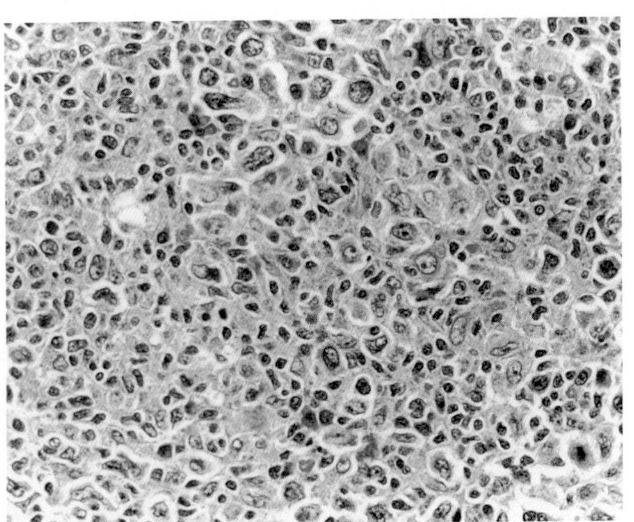
B

FIGURE 16. Follicular lymphoma of the tonsil. **A:** At low magnification the architecture is effaced by numerous large, closely packed follicles, which lack distinct mantle zones. **B:** At high magnification, the cells are a mixture of centrocytes (small cells with irregular cleaved nuclei and scant cytoplasm) and centroblasts (large oval noncleaved cells) with peripheral nucleoli and basophilic cytoplasm.

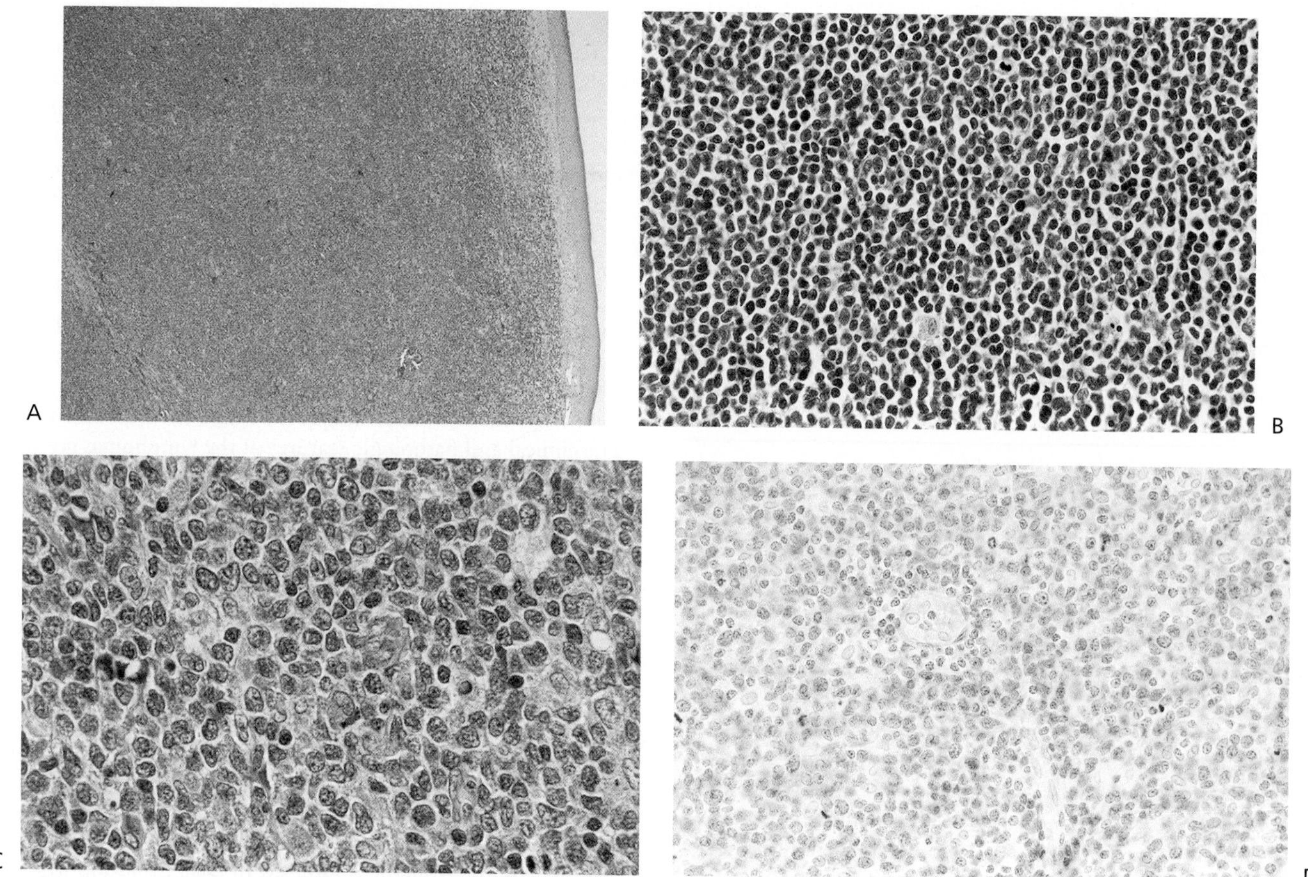

FIGURE 17. Mantle cell lymphoma of the tonsil. **A:** At low magnification, the architecture is effaced by a diffuse lymphoid infiltrate, with sparing of the epithelium. **B:** At high magnification, the cells are small, slightly irregular, and uniform, with chromatin that is uniformly distributed and slightly less dense than that of a small lymphocyte. Scattered epithelioid histiocytes are present. There are occasional mitotic figures. **C:** Blastoid/pleomorphic variant of mantle cell lymphoma, showing larger cells with more dispersed chromatin and nuclear pleomorphism, with increased mitotic activity, resembling large cell or lymphoblastic lymphoma. **D:** Immunohistochemical stain for cyclin D1, showing nuclear staining of about 80% of the neoplastic cells in the case of blastoid mantle cell lymphoma. Normal lymphocytes are unstained.

hypothesis comes from two cases reported by Paulsen and Lennert, in which gastric involvement preceded tonsillar involvement by MALT lymphoma, one of which had a large cell component in both the tonsil and stomach (96)

LYMPHOMAS OF THE NASAL CAVITY AND PARANASAL SINUSES

Lymphoma is the second most common type of malignant tumor to arise in the area of the nose and paranasal sinuses, following squamous cell carcinoma (97). In the United States and Western Europe, 0.44% to 2.2% of all extranodal non-Hodgkin's lymphomas and 6.4% to 13% of extranodal lymphomas of the head and neck arise in the nose and paranasal sinuses (98). The incidence of lymphoma in this anatomic site is higher in the Orient and in South America (99,100). In Japan, for example, 6.8% of lymphomas are estimated to arise in the sinonasal area (99). Two main types of lymphoma are found in the sinonasal tract: ordinary, monomorphous lymphoma of more common type, most of which are diffuse large B-cell lymphoma arising in paranasal sinuses, and extranodal NK/T-cell lymphoma of the nasal type, arising in the nose or other midline anatomic structures (99,101). In a recent study of 58 patients with paranasal sinus and nasal cavity lymphomas at Massachusetts General Hospital (Table 6), the most common type was diffuse large B-cell lymphoma (57%), followed by extranodal NK/T-cell lymphoma of the nasal type (29%). Patients with sinus involvement only were more likely to have diffuse large B-cell lymphoma, whereas those with nasal involvement only were more likely to have NK/T-cell lymphoma (p = 0.000125) (Table 7) (102,103). In the text that follows, we discuss first nasal cavity lymphoma, with emphasis on extranodal NK/T-cell lymphoma of the nasal type, as the prototype of lymphomas arising in the nasal cavity, and then review the features of paranasal sinus lymphomas.

Extranodal NK/T-cell Lymphoma of the Nasal Type

Cases of extranodal NK/T-cell lymphoma of the nasal type comprise a subset of the group of disorders known as *lethal midline granuloma,* which is a generic term for a clinical syndrome of progressive, relentless, ulcerative, necrotizing, destructive mid-

TABLE 6. SINONASAL LYMPHOMA AT MASSACHUSETTS GENERAL HOSPITAL, 1960–1998

	No. of Cases[a]	%
B-cell lymphomas	36	65
Marginal zone B-cell lymphoma	1	2
Diffuse large B-cell lymphoma	33	59
Burkitt's lymphoma	1	2
Burkitt-like lymphoma	1	2
T- or NK cell lymphomas	19	35
Peripheral T-cell lymphoma, not otherwise characterized	1	2
Extranodal NK/T-cell lymphoma, nasal type	17	31
Adult T-cell lymphoma (HTLV-1+)	1	2
Total	55[a]	100

[a] Omitting cases that could not be classified.
NK, natural killer.

facial disease. A variety of entities, including bacterial and fungal infection, carcinoma, Wegener's granulomatosis, monomorphous lymphoma, and nasal-type NK/T-cell lymphoma, can result in the clinical syndrome of lethal midline granuloma (104–106). In 1966, the term *polymorphic reticulosis* was first applied to cases of primary lymphoma of the nose, often associated with a clinical picture of lethal midline granuloma, in which there was a polymorphous inflammatory cell infiltrate in addition to atypical lymphoid cells (107). Subsequently, it was noted that such cases frequently showed angiocentric localization of the atypical cells, often associated with infiltration and destruction of blood vessels, and the designation *angiocentric lymphoma* came into use (108). However, angioinvasion and angiocentric growth cannot be identified in all cases, so the term *angiocentric lymphoma* is not always accurate. Characterization of the lymphoid infiltrate by immunohistochemistry showed expression of T cell–associated antigens, and the term *nasal T-cell lymphoma* was also suggested for this disorder (109). Additional studies suggested that many cases may be of NK-cell lineage, and that cases with similar clinicopathologic features can occur away from the nose; therefore, the term *nasal/nasal type NK/T-cell lymphoma* was adopted by a workshop on T-cell lymphomas (110,111), and modified to *extranodal NK/T-cell lymphoma of the nasal type* in the REAL and WHO classifications.

Clinical Features

Extranodal NK/T-cell lymphoma of the nasal type is much more common in Asian countries than in the United States or Europe where it is rare; it also appears to be common in Latin American countries such as Mexico and Peru, where it occurs in Indians. The clinical and pathologic features of the lymphomas are similar, independent of the ethnic background of the affected patient (111). Nasal lymphoma shows a male preponderence, with a male:female ratio of 2 to 3:1. This lymphoma can affect patients of any age, but most are adults. Occasionally, nasal/nasal-type lymphoma presents in childhood or adolescence. The median age of occurrence in most series is 45 to 50 years (104, 105,110,112–119).

Patients with extranodal NK/T-cell lymphoma of the nasal type most often present with nasal obstruction or with bloody or purulent rhinorrhea (104–106,114,119,120). Other common symptoms include local pain, nasal crusting, numbness, facial swelling, and changes due to extension into the orbit such as diplopia or proptosis (100,104,105,113,114,116,117,119,120). In some studies, systemic symptoms of fever or weight loss also have been common at presentation (104,105,112,117,120). Occasionally, patients have had relatively mild symptoms related to the sinonasal tract for many years prior to the diagnosis of lymphoma (106,113,120).

The majority of cases of extranodal NK/T-cell lymphoma of the nasal type, as indicated by the name of the lymphoma, arise

TABLE 7. SINONASAL LYMPHOMA: COMPARISON OF DIFFUSE LARGE B-CELL LYMPHOMA AND EXTRANODAL NK/T-CELL LYMPHOMA, NASAL TYPE

	Diffuse Large B-cell Lymphoma	Extranodal NK/T-cell Lymphoma, Nasal Type
Age of patients	Mostly older adults; rarely children	Young and middle-aged adults
Sex	M > F	M > F
Racial predisposition	None	Asians, Native Americans
Sites	Paranasal sinuses > nose	Nasal cavity > sinuses
Mid-facial destructive disease	Rare	Common
Ocular symptoms (tearing, proptosis, other)	Common	Less common
Orbital invasion	Common	Less common
EBV positivity	Rare (immunosuppression)	Most cases
Clinical behavior	Moderately aggressive; may respond to RT, CT	Aggressive; may respond to RT; localized cases may be cured; prognosis generally poor
Hemophagocytic syndrome	Not described	May occur; usually rapidly fatal

EBV, Epstein-Barr virus; RT, radiation therapy; CT, chemotherapy.

in the nasal cavity (86,104,119), but occasional cases primarily involve the palate (112,119), the nasopharynx (104,121), the ethmoid sinus (116,122), the larynx (104,105), and sites distant from the head and neck.

Examined from another viewpoint, in Asian populations most lymphomas arising in the nasal cavity are extranodal NK/T-cell lymphoma of the nasal type. In one large series from Hong Kong, 55% of lymphomas confined to the nasal cavity were classified as NK/T-cell lymphomas (consistent with nasal type), 16% were T-cell lymphomas (non-nasal type), and 29% were B-cell lymphomas (123). In another study from Hong Kong, 8 of 10 cases were classified as T-cell lymphoma, whereas only 2 of 10 were B-cell lymphoma (124). In a Japanese series, 35 nasal lymphomas were T-cell lymphomas, 8 were B-cell lymphomas, and 2 were not subclassified (125). Even in Western populations, where lymphomas of NK- and T-cell lineage are less common than in the Orient, a relatively high proportion of nasal lymphomas have been of T- or NK-cell origin in some studies. In a study from the Massachusetts General Hospital, 7 of 9 cases of lymphoma predominantly or exclusively involving the nasal cavity had an immunophenotype consistent with T-cell lymphoma; most had conspicuous angioinvasion and necrosis (120). In a more recent, larger series, a similar result was found: 8 of 11 cases of lymphoma confined to the nasal cavity were NK/T-cell type (102,103). This result has not been uniform, however. In a study from Kiel, 28 nasal cavity lymphomas were B-cell lineage tumors of a variety of histologic types, whereas only 5 were thought to be T-cell lymphomas (126).

Physical examination in cases of extranodal NK/T-cell lymphoma of the nasal type of recent onset reveals friable mucosa, frequently without an obvious mass. With progression of the disease, extensive destruction of tissue, including bone, cartilage, and soft tissue, occurs. If the nasal septum is involved, it may become perforated (104). These lesions may extend to involve adjacent structures, including paranasal sinuses, nasopharynx, oropharynx, hypopharynx, tonsil, palate, gingiva, orbit, and even the CNS or cranial nerves (105,112,113,116,120, 124,125).

Pathologic Features

Microscopic examination typically reveals an infiltrate of atypical, pleomorphic lymphoid cells, often ranging in size from small or medium-sized to large (Fig. 18A–E). The neoplastic cells have round, irregular, or lobated nuclei, and often, distinct rims of

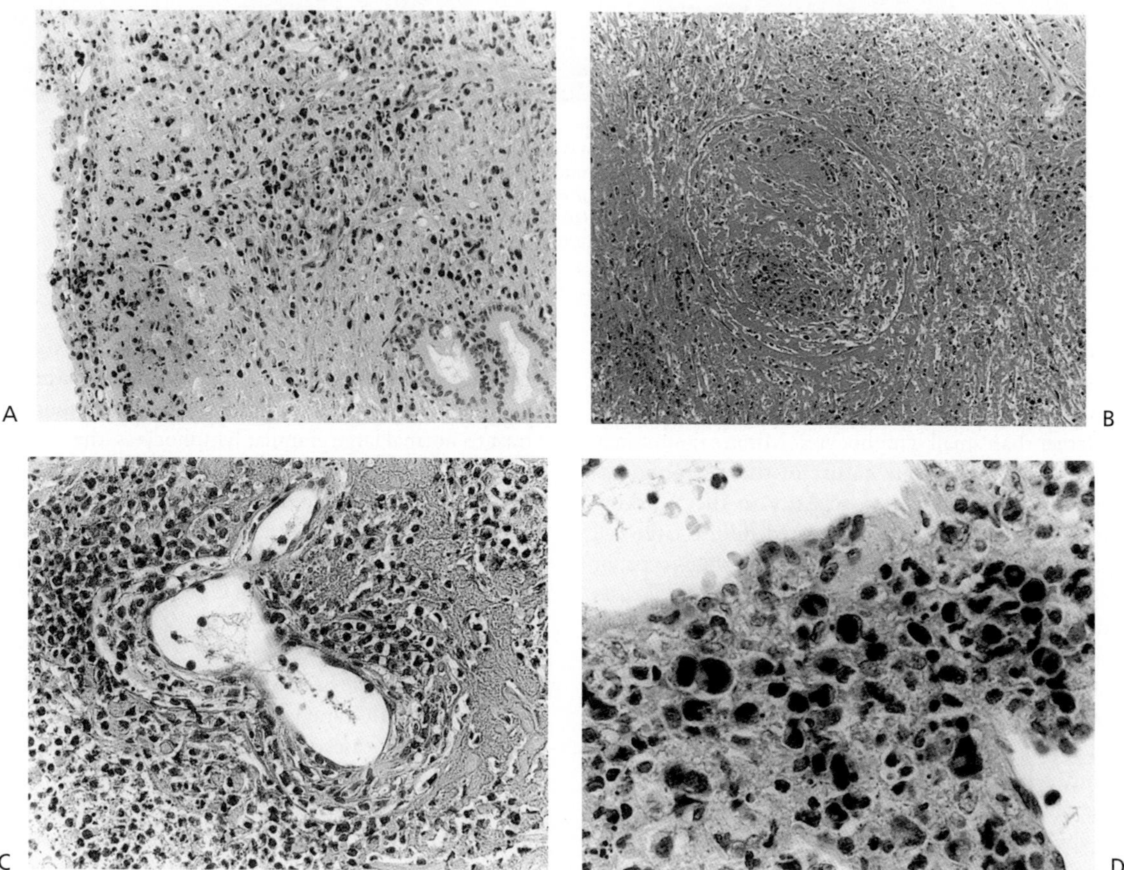

FIGURE 18. Nasal NK/T-cell lymphoma. **A:** The lymphoma consists of atypical lymphoid cells scattered in a background of fibrosis and necrotic debris. **B:** In this case, necrosis is particularly extensive. The ghost of a large blood vessel is seen in the center of the field. **C:** Atypical lymphoid cells infiltrate the wall of a small blood vessel. Cellular debris is seen around the periphery of the illustration. **D:** In this case, cytologic atypia is striking, with a predominance of medium and large cells with large, irregular, dark nuclei.

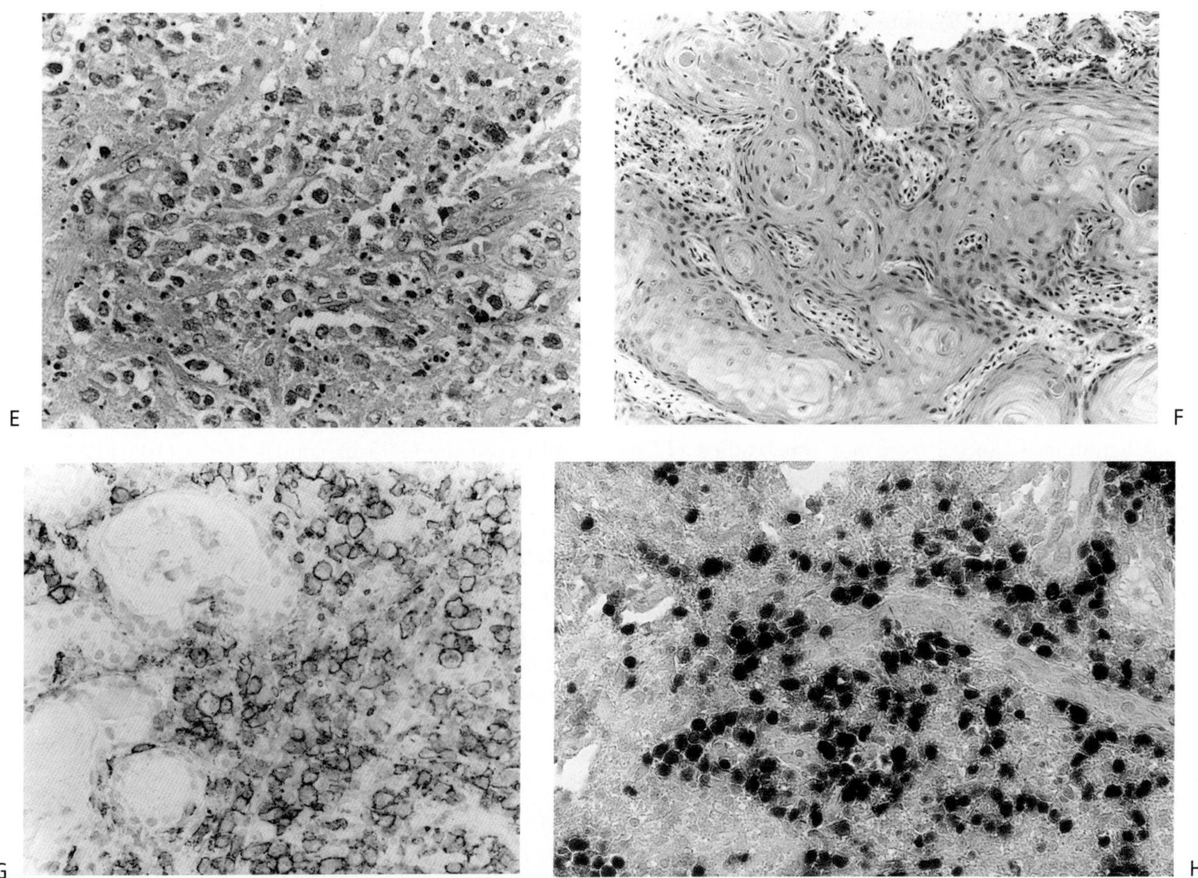

FIGURE 18. *(Continued)* **E:** In this case, cytologic atypia is less striking. Although some atypical lymphoid cells with irregular nuclei are present, there is a predominance of small lymphoid cells, histiocytes, and necrotic debris. **F:** Marked pseudoepitheliomatous hyperplasia was overlying this nasal lymphoma. **G:** Neoplastic cells are CD45RO positive (immunohistochemical technique on paraffin section). **H:** Neoplastic cells are Epstein-Barr virus–encoded RNA (EBER) positive, indicating the presence of Epstein-Barr virus (*in situ* hybridization on a paraffin section).

pale cytoplasm. Rare large cells resembling RS cells may be seen. In most cases, the neoplastic population shows overt cytologic atypia, but in others, atypia is subtle, and the neoplastic cells are only slightly larger than small lymphocytes. Mitotic figures may be frequent. The polymorphous nature of these lymphomas sometimes makes them difficult to classify in the Working Formulation, but most have been designated diffuse large cell lymphoma, often of the immunoblastic, polymorphous type, or diffuse mixed small and large cell lymphoma. Occasional cases are classified as diffuse small cleaved cell lymphoma. In many, but not all cases, atypical lymphoid cells surround and invade the walls of blood vessels, often with resultant mural necrosis and luminal thrombosis. The lymphomas are frequently associated with mucosal ulceration, coagulative necrosis, and an admixture of inflammatory cells, including neutrophils, histiocytes, plasma cells, and less often eosinophils. In some cases, inflammatory cells may be abundant, and necrosis extensive, and lymphoma may only be recognizable focally (98,104,105,113–116, 119,120,123). Squamous metaplasia of respiratory epithelium is common (107). Neoplastic cells may invade the overlying squamous epithelium and be associated with striking pseudoepitheliomatous hyperplasia (Fig. 18F) (113,120). Perineural invasion has been described (98). When touch preparations are examined, neoplastic cells usually are found to have cytoplasmic azurophilic granules, similar to those of large granular lymphocytes. In contrast to normal large granular lymphocytes, the nuclei may be enlarged with dispersed chromatin and distinct nucleoli (112,127).

Extranodal NK/T-cell lymphoma of the nasal type expresses antigens associated with T-cell or NK-cell lineage (86). Immunophenotyping on paraffin sections in nearly all cases tested has shown expression of CD45RO, CD43, or cytoplasmic CD3, and often of all three (Fig. 18G), whereas B-cell antigens are consistently absent (98,99,104,105,112–114,116,120,128). When frozen tissue has been available, expression of CD2, CD3, CD4, CD5, CD7, and CD8 has been demonstrated in a variable number of the cases tested, with the proportion of cases with these markers often varying widely from one series to another. Overall, CD2 is almost always expressed, CD3 and CD7 are expressed in approximately half of cases, CD8 is found in fewer than half of cases, and CD4 and CD5 are uncommonly expressed. CD56 is almost always found, whereas CD57 is almost always absent, and CD16 is variably present (98,99,105,113, 116,118–121,123,128). Relatively small numbers of cases have been tested with antibodies to the α/β T-cell receptor (βF1) and the γ/δ T-cell receptor (TCRδ1); only a minority of cases have tested positive with these markers (105,116,118,121). Granzyme B, TIA-1, and perforin, constituents of cytotoxic granules, can be detected in most cases (116,128).

Molecular genetic analysis has shown that T-cell receptor genes are in the germline configuration in the majority of cases, although in occasional cases, there is clonal rearrangement of the T-cell receptor β, γ, or δ chain genes, or of more than one of these genes. The immunoglobulin heavy chain gene in these cases is consistently germline (105,120,121,129). The absence of T-cell receptor gene rearrangement, together with the expression of CD56 and lack of T cell–specific antigens (sCD3, TCR αβ or γδ) led to the proposal of an NK-cell nature for most of these cases. Although there is general agreement that cases with clonal T-cell receptor genes are true T-cell lymphomas, and that those without clonal rearrangement are most likely of NK-cell lineage, there is controversy concerning the immunophenotype that defines and distinguishes NK- and T-cell lymphomas. However, T- and NK-cell types of nasal/nasal-type T/NK- cell lymphoma are indistinguishable on routine histologic examination, and have similar clinical features, so their separation is not of practical importance.

Extranodal NK/T-cell lymphomas of the nasal type also share a strong association with EBV. In nearly all cases, there is intense staining of nearly all neoplastic cells using *in situ* hybridization for EBER (Fig. 18H) (99,104,113,119,129). LMP is expressed in approximately half of cases, although staining may be faint, or may be in only a subset of tumor cells. EBNA type 1 may be expressed, but EBNA types 2 through 6 are generally absent (99,105,113,129). The EBV is in a clonal, episomal form, indicating that it infects the cell that gives rise to the lymphoma prior to initiation of cellular multiplication (129). Cytogenetic analysis has revealed some recurring abnormalities, including isochromosome 6p, isochromosome 1q, partial deletion of 6q, and abnormalities of 11q (115).

Because of their similarities, T cells and NK cells most likely are derived from a common precursor (127). It is possible that this precursor, or the immature or mature T cells and NK cells derived from it, may become infected by EBV and undergo neoplastic transformation to give rise to extranodal NK/T-cell lymphoma of the nasal type (121).

Staging, Treatment, and Outcome

At presentation, most patients have localized (Ann Arbor stage I or II) disease. A review of recently published series of extranodal NK/T-cell lymphomas of the nasal type shows that approximately 62% present with stage I disease, 19% with stage II disease, 3% with stage III disease, and 16% with stage IV disease. Sites of disease away from the nose include the lymph nodes, lung, CNS, testis, skin, liver, and other extranodal sites. Marrow involvement occurs, but it is relatively uncommon. Peripheral blood involvement is rare (105,113,116,118,120,123–125, 128). Presentation with systemic symptoms is associated with an increased risk of stage IV disease (119).

Most patients have been treated with radiation with or without chemotherapy. A minority have been treated with chemotherapy alone. In a few series, outcome has been favorable. For example, in a series from the Massachusetts General Hospital, 11 of 15 patients with extranodal NK/T-cell lymphoma of the nasal type (all but one with stage I disease) were free of disease at last follow-up (102,103,120). In one series from China, patients with disease limited to the nasal cavity had a 90% 5-year overall survival rate, whereas patients with more extensive local disease or disseminated disease had a significantly worse outcome (130). The first 9 patients diagnosed as having polymorphic reticulosis in Eichel's 1966 report all had stage I disease, and all survived more than 5 years following treatment with radiation alone (107). In most series, however, survival is poor. The 5-year overall survival rate ranges from 24% to 49% (113,123,124), and in one series the 3-year survival rate was only 9% (105). The median survival rate has ranged from less than 6 months to 25 months in several large series (105,119, 123,124,131). Patients succumb to persistent local or systemic disease (104).

In a minority of cases, the course is complicated by a systemic hemophagocytic syndrome, characterized by fever, hepatosplenomegaly, jaundice, pancytopenia, and coagulopathy (106,115,120,132), which is usually rapidly fatal. It is suggested that the neoplastic cells may be induced by the EBV that they harbor to secrete cytokines that activate histiocytes and promote hemophagocytosis. Although the interaction of multiple cytokines is probably required for the development of a full-blown hemophagocytic syndrome, tumor necrosis factor α (TNF-α) has been implicated as a major culprit in the pathogenesis of the process (132).

A better prognosis is associated with localized disease. Radiation therapy is an essential component of the treatment of extranodal NK/T-cell lymphoma of the nasal type, because these lymphomas are insensitive to chemotherapy. In one series, for example, 15 of 19 patients treated with radiation with or without chemotherapy achieved a complete remission, in contrast to only 1 of 8 treated with chemotherapy alone (113). It appears that a subset of patients with localized disease treated aggressively with radiation therapy may attain long-term survival, but if there is advanced stage disease, or if a relapse occurs, the prognosis is very poor (104,117). In a handful of cases, autologous bone marrow transplantation has been used successfully in the treatment of nasal lymphoma (115,125,127). The efficacy of this technique should be tested in a larger number of patients.

The prognosis of extranodal NK/T-cell lymphoma of the nasal type appears to be worse than that of B-cell lymphomas and of monomorphous (non-nasal type) T-cell lymphomas arising in the sinonasal tract and nasopharynx (122,123,131), and worse than that of lymphomas arising in lymph nodes in general (125).

Differential Diagnosis

The differential diagnosis of extranodal NK/T-cell lymphoma includes reactive lesions and other types of lymphomas (B-cell lymphomas and non-nasal type T-cell lymphomas). Problems in the distinction from reactive lesions derive from two sources: (a) necrosis is so extensive, and admixed inflammatory cells are so abundant that the neoplastic population is obscured; and (b) cytologic atypia is subtle, making it difficult to distinguish neoplastic cells from non-neoplastic lymphocytes. In the first instance, in cases in which lymphoma is a clinical possibility, the pathologist may have to inform the surgeon that the specimen is nondiagnostic and advise him to obtain additional tissue until viable, representative tissue is found. In the second instance, even when neoplastic cells are only slightly atypical, they are usually at least slightly larger, with slightly more irregular nuclei and somewhat more pale cytoplasm, with a higher mitotic rate than small lymphocytes in a chronic inflammatory cell infiltrate. Because the number of CD56-positive cells in reactive processes is virtually always small, and because CD56 is found in nearly all extranodal NK/T-cell lymphomas, the presence of numerous CD56-positive cells strongly favors lymphoma. The presence of many EBER-positive cells also favors lymphoma, although EBER can be found in other types of lymphoma and in nasopharyngeal carcinoma. An abnormal immunophenotype with loss of one or more pan T-cell antigens, or the finding of clonal EBV or clonal T-cell receptor genes would confirm a diagnosis of lymphoma.

B-cell lymphomas and non-nasal–type T-cell lymphomas in the sinonasal area usually lack angioinvasion and angiocentric localization, and they are usually without prominent necrosis, epitheliotropism, and pseudoepitheliomatous hyperplasia. B-cell lymphomas more commonly arise in paranasal sinuses and Waldeyer's ring, whereas nasal localization favors the T/NK-cell type (122,123). Compared with B-cell lymphoma, the incidence of extranodal NK/T-cell lymphoma of the nasal type is associated with a higher male:female ratio, a younger median age (63 vs. 53 years), and more frequent presentation with mid-facial destruction (21% of cases vs. 67%). Most B-cell lymphomas in this site are diffuse large cell type, so any other histologic type, especially diffuse mixed, should raise the question of T/NK-cell lymphoma or T-cell lymphoma (123,126). B-cell and T/NK-cell lymphomas can be distinguished easily with immunophenotyping. Most B-cell lymphomas lack EBV. The differential diagnosis with non-nasal–type T-cell lymphoma may be difficult in some cases, but angiocentric, necrotizing lymphomas with CD56 expression and EBV can be considered extranodal NK/T-cell lymphoma of the nasal type, whereas T-cell lineage lymphomas lacking angioinvasion, CD56, and EBV can be considered non-nasal–type peripheral T-cell lymphomas (Table 7) (101).

Paranasal Sinus Lymphoma

Clinical Features

Despite their proximity to the nose, the paranasal sinuses are affected by lymphomas with clinicopathologic features that differentiate them from those that tend to affect primarily the nose. Paranasal sinus lymphoma affects men slightly more often than women and predominantly affects middle aged to older adults (102,103,133–135), although a number of cases affecting children have been described (136–139). Most have no predisposing medical conditions, although several cases of paranasal sinus lymphoma have occurred in HIV-positive patients (102,103, 140–142), one presented in a patient who had received cyclosporine for severe psoriasis (143), and one occurred in an immunosuppressed renal transplant recipient (144).

The symptoms commonly associated with paranasal sinus lymphoma are similar to those of nasal lymphoma, and include nasal obstruction or discharge, facial swelling, pain or numbness, sinus pressure, toothache, and loosening of teeth or headache. When the lymphoma involves adjacent structures, patients may present with neurologic abnormalities, proptosis, diplopia, decreased visual acuity, and even blindness (89,100,102,103, 133–135,137–142,145–147). One patient had a syndrome of inappropriate antidiuretic hormone due to sellar extension. Only rarely do patients have constitutional symptoms at presentation, but fever and night sweats have been described (89,140,141). Several patients have had long-standing symptoms thought to be related to allergic rhinosinusitis prior to developing more severe symptoms attributed to lymphoma (146). Many of the symptoms of lymphoma mimic those of chronic sinusitis, however, which may be why these lymphomas have frequently attained a large, bulky size before a biopsy is performed and a diagnosis is established.

The maxillary sinus is the most common site of involvement, followed by the ethmoid sinus, sphenoid sinus, and frontal sinus. Frequently, multiple sinuses are involved simultaneously (102,103,126,133,135,137,139–142). The lymphomas are often associated with destruction of adjacent bone, and it is not unusual for them to invade locally to involve neighboring sites, especially the nasal cavity and orbit, but also the CNS, pterygopalatine fossa, base of the skull, nasopharynx, infratemporal fossa, soft tissue overlying the sinuses, cavernous sinus, and palate (138,139,141–143,148).

Pathologic Features

The most common histologic type of paranasal sinus lymphoma is diffuse large B-cell lymphoma, accounting for approximately two thirds of cases (Fig. 19). A minority of them have been subclassified as immunoblastic. Other types, in decreasing order of frequency, have been classified according to the Working Formulation as diffuse mixed small and large cell, small noncleaved (Burkitt's and Burkitt-like), diffuse small cleaved cell, and small lymphocytic, but they are all much less common. Follicular lymphoma is rare, accounting for fewer than 3% of cases (100,126,133–135,138–142,146,147,149). Rare cases of anaplastic large cell lymphoma (126), intravascular lymphoma (150,151), and adult T-cell leukemia/lymphoma (102,103,145) presenting with sinus involvement have been described.

Immunohistochemical studies have shown that more than three fourths of paranasal lymphomas are of B-cell lineage, with the remainder interpreted as T-cell or T/NK-cell lymphomas (100,126,133,134,141–143,145,147,149,151). Evidence based on small numbers of cases suggests that maxillary sinus lymphomas are nearly exclusively B-cell lineage tumors, whereas the ethmoid sinus, a midline structure like the nose, can be affected by either B- or T-cell lymphomas. In one Japanese study, all maxillary sinus lymphomas were B-cell lineage tumors, whereas ethmoid sinus and nasal lymphomas were more likely to be T-cell (or NK-cell) lymphomas, and the comparison was highly significant ($p = 0.005$) (133). We found a similar result in the Massachusetts General Hospital series (102,103). The lymphomas in HIV-positive patients have been diffuse large B-cell

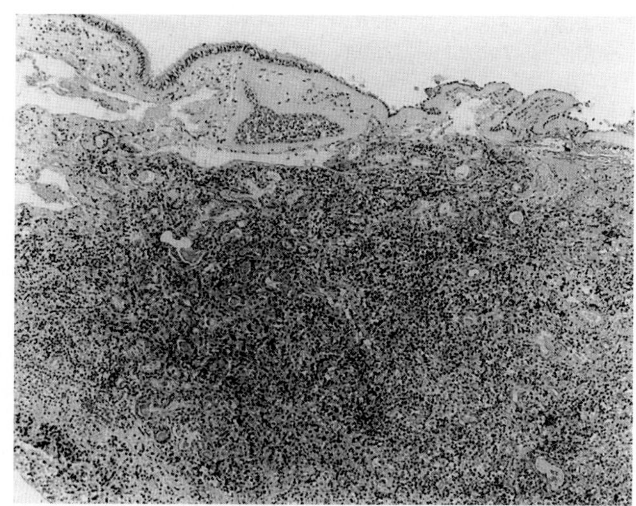

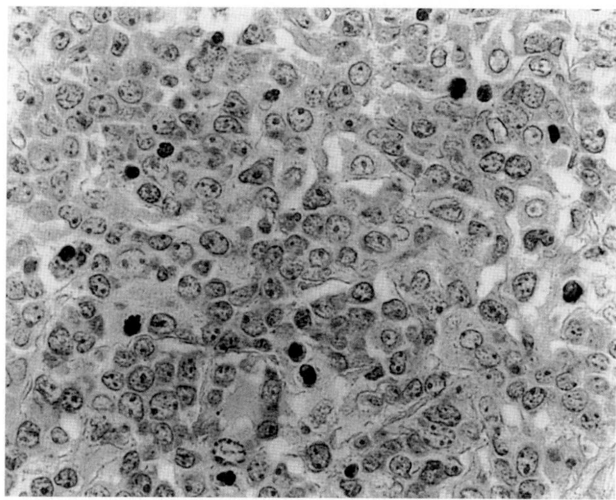

FIGURE 19. Paranasal sinus diffuse large B-cell lymphoma. **A:** Low power shows a dense, diffuse infiltrate of lymphoid cells beneath respiratory epithelium that is largely intact. **B:** High-power shows large transformed lymphoid cells and frequent mitotic figures.

lymphomas, diffuse mixed small and large cell lymphomas, and Burkitt's lymphoma (140–142). Paranasal sinus lymphomas in children are most often Burkitt's lymphoma, followed by diffuse large B-cell lymphoma; other types are less common (136). Unlike nasal T/NK-cell lymphoma, paranasal sinus B-cell lymphomas are not uniformly associated with EBV. In one Asian study, however, 40% of sinonasal B-cell lymphomas contained EBV (99). Only small numbers of Western sinonasal B-cell lymphomas have been tested for EBV, and the frequency has been similar to (152) or less than (134) that found in Asian cases. In the study from Massachusetts General Hospital, we found 2 of 11 cases of diffuse large B-cell lymphomas to be EBV positive; both were in immunosuppressed patients, one HIV positive and one on treatment for leukemia (102,103).

Staging, Treatment, and Outcome

The majority of cases are localized at presentation. A review of published cases shows that approximately 57% are Ann Arbor stage I, 23% are stage II, 2% are stage III, and 18% are stage IV (122,134,135,138–142,145–147,149,153). Sites involved in stage IV cases include the CNS, lung, bones, kidney, and gastrointestinal tract (122,135,138,139,141).

In early studies, patients were typically treated with radiation therapy alone (154). However, radiation alone was associated with a high proportion of treatment failures, and although radiation alone was thought acceptable for localized tumor, the addition of chemotherapy was frequently recommended for patients with widespread disease (153). Most patients currently receive radiation and chemotherapy. Some investigators have reported a high proportion of cases with progression of disease in the CNS, and for this reason suggest that CNS prophylaxis may be important in achieving long-term disease-free survival (89).

When sinus lymphomas relapse or progress, they often involve lymph nodes and may involve a variety of extranodal sites, including CNS (as noted above), lung, bone, ovary, testis, liver, spleen, and skin (102,103,134,148). Local failures are uncommon, especially when optimal radiation is included in their therapy (89). In contrast to relapses of nasal T/NK-cell lymphoma, some relapses of paranasal sinus lymphomas can be successfully treated.

Results of follow-up have varied from one study to another. Some have reported that lymphoma of the paranasal sinuses has a worse prognosis than lymphomas of other sites in the head and neck, with a 5-year survival rate of only 12% in one series in which most patients received radiation only (89). In another study in which most patients received chemotherapy and radiation, the 5-year survival rate was 80% (133). Adding chemotherapy is no guarantee of a favorable outcome however, because in another recent study in which all patients received combined modality therapy, the 5-year survival rate was only 29% (134).

Differential Diagnosis

The differential diagnosis of paranasal sinus lymphoma of B-cell lineage includes NK/T-cell lymphomas, as discussed previously, and other types of neoplasms. Occasionally chronic sinusitis may be considered in the differential diagnosis, but because most sinus lymphomas are composed of large cells, when well-preserved tissue is available for examination, this is not usually a difficult distinction.

OCULAR ADNEXAL LYMPHOID INFILTRATES

The ocular adnexa—the orbit (including the lacrimal gland), conjunctiva, and eyelids—may be involved by inflammatory processes as well as by malignant lymphomas of many types, either at presentation or at relapse. The orbit is the most common site of lymphoid infiltrates, followed by the conjunctiva; the eyelids are least often affected (155). A large proportion of ocular adnexal lymphoid infiltrates are composed of small lymphoid cells lacking cytologic atypia. It can be difficult or impossible to distinguish between reactive and neoplastic processes on routinely stained sections in such cases, especially because biopsy samples are often small, and in extranodal sites, criteria for architectural effacement are less well established than in lymph nodes. Furthermore, presenting symptoms and findings on physical examination are often similar. For years, investigators labored to identify histologic criteria that would predict which cases would be associated with systemic disease (156–158). With the advent of immunophenotyping, however, making the distinction between lymphoma and non-neoplastic infiltrates became relatively straightforward. With the help of immunophenotyping, lesions with ocular adnexal lymphoid infiltration can be divided into three major categories: (a) inflammatory pseudotumor, (b) reactive lymphoid hyperplasia, and (c) lymphoma.

Inflammatory pseudotumor is a non-neoplastic lesion with a variably cellular, polymorphous infiltrate of small lymphocytes, plasma cells, immunoblasts, and histiocytes in a stroma with areas that are hyalinized, edematous, or both. Blood vessels, often with hypertrophic endothelial cells, can be present in large numbers. Follicles with germinal centers are usually absent or scant. Eosinophils and neutrophils can be seen (159). Immunohistochemical studies in such cases show a mixture of T cells, B cells, and polytypic plasma cells.

Cases of reactive lymphoid hyperplasia show predominantly follicular hyperplasia without a prominent diffuse component. Immunophenotyping shows no evidence of a clonal population.

A lymphoid infiltrate can be classified as lymphoma if there is sufficient cytologic or architectural atypia for a histologic diagnosis of lymphoma, or if immunophenotyping or genetic analysis reveals a monoclonal population. Most cases with a dense and diffuse infiltrate of lymphoid cells are composed of monoclonal B cells and thus represent lymphoma (156,160,161). In a minority of cases in which there is a dense, predominantly diffuse infiltrate of small lymphoid cells, no monoclonal population can be identified. In these cases, molecular genetic analysis is often helpful in establishing clonality. If clonality cannot be demonstrated, a descriptive diagnosis, such as "dense lymphocytic infiltrate" or "dense lymphoplasmacytic infiltrate," is made.

The usefulness of immunophenotypic demonstration of clonality in predicting outcome has been evaluated in several studies, with some showing that monotypic immunoglobulin expression correlates with decreased survival ($p < 0.05$) and increased risk of disseminated lymphoma ($p < 0.001$) (162), whereas others find that patients with monoclonal and polyclonal lesions had similar outcomes (155,161). However, molecular genetic analysis has shown that the majority of ocular adnexal lymphoid infiltrates that do not fulfill histologic or immunohistologic criteria for lymphoma have had one or more variably sized clonal populations of B cells, suggesting that these infiltrates either represent lymphoma or a lymphoproliferative disorder that may eventually evolve into lymphoma (Fig. 20) (163–165). A high proportion of ocular adnexal lymphomas have features of MALT lymphomas (156,166–169). Marginal zone B-cell lymphomas of the MALT type can present in a variety of extranodal sites and tend to remain localized for long periods of time. This may account for the failure of some lymphomas to disseminate and thus to make less clear-cut the distinction between the prognosis of lymphoma and non-neoplastic lymphoid infiltrates in the ocular adnexa. Thus, with the exception of inflammatory pseudotumor and some reactive lymphoid hyperplasia, it appears that most orbital lymphoid infiltrates are indolent lymphoproliferative disorders that respond well to local therapy, but have some potential for recurrence and dissemination.

In summary, the distinction between benign and malignant ocular adnexal lymphoid infiltrates is based on a combination of

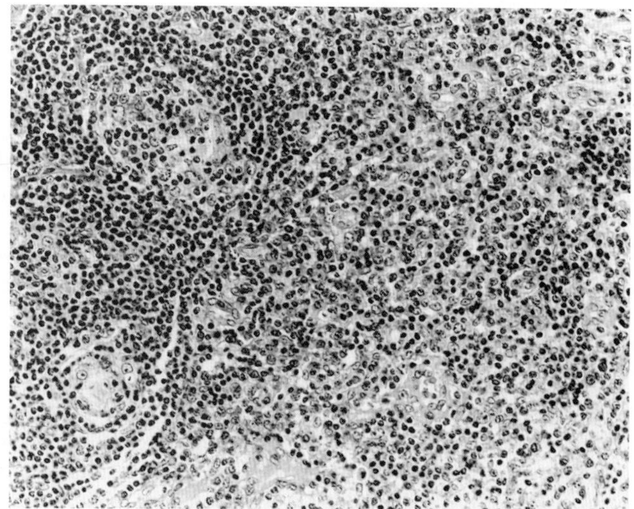

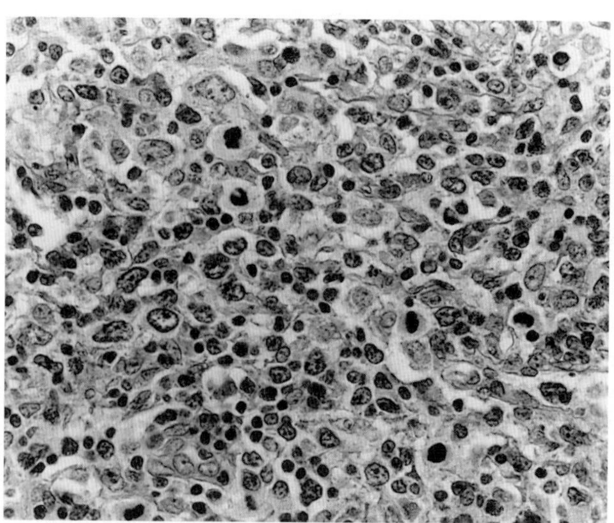

FIGURE 20. Dense lymphoplasmacytic infiltrate of the orbit, followed by lymphoma. **A:** The patient had an orbital lymphoid infiltrate with two small follicles (at left) and a diffuse infiltrate of small lymphocytes, mature plasma cells, and small blood vessels. No clonal population was found using immunohistochemistry. **B:** After having recurrent, bilateral orbital lymphoplasmacytic infiltrates for 16 years, the patient developed the large B-cell lymphoma shown here in a submandibular lymph node. The lymphoma disseminated and the patient eventually died of lymphoma.

morphologic and immunophenotypic features, as it is in other extranodal lymphoid infiltrates. In cases in which histology is indeterminate and immunophenotyping shows no monotypic population, molecular genetic studies can be done if clinically indicated. If there is no evidence of a clonal population (162) and if staging reveals no lymphoma in other sites (155), the patient's risk for dissemination is very low.

Ocular Adnexal Lymphoma

Clinical Features

Ocular adnexal lymphoma accounts for 1% to 2% of all lymphomas (170,171). The orbit is the second most common extranodal primary site for head and neck lymphoma, following Waldeyer's ring (172). Lymphoid tumors account for 10% of orbital mass lesions, and lymphoma is the most common orbital malignancy (170,173). Lymphomas in this site predominantly affect women (male:female ratio 2:3), with a median or mean age in the sixties or early seventies in most series (155,162, 167,174,175). Only rare cases have been described in children (176–178). Occasional patients have a prior history of Sjögren's syndrome, Hashimoto's thyroiditis (167,179,180), myoepithelial sialadenitis (MESA) without Sjögren's syndrome (181), rheumatoid arthritis (182), sarcoidosis (183), nonlymphoid malignancy (167), myasthenia gravis (167), or contact lens wear (168), and a few patients are HIV positive (184,185). Recently, one group of investigators described finding evidence of hepatitis C virus infection in 50% of patients with MALT lymphoma arising in a variety of sites (180). However, most patients with orbital lymphoma have no known systemic or ophthalmologic disease (174).

Patients with ocular adnexal lymphoma present with variable symptoms, including proptosis, ptosis, a palpable or visible mass, diplopia, tearing, or discomfort (155,158,171,174,186,187). A decrease in visual acuity is unusual. Systemic symptoms such as fever, weight loss, or night sweats have been reported in only rare cases (171). In cases in which lymphoma is confined to the conjunctiva, the usual finding is a raised, salmon-colored lesion that is mobile over the surface of the eye and that is not associated with ocular displacement, motility disturbance, or decreased visual acuity (158). The masses are typically described as slowly enlarging (171); they may be firm, rubbery, fleshy, or soft (155). In 10% (155,188,189) to 25% (171), there is bilateral involvement.

Pathologic Features

Lymphoma of any type can present with ocular adnexal involvement, but most of them are low-grade neoplasms composed of small lymphoid cells, often with plasmacytoid differentiation (156,190). In a series of cases classified according to the Working Formulation, there were 50% small lymphocytic lymphoma, 20% follicular small cleaved cell, 7.5% follicular mixed, 2.5% follicular large cell, 12.5% diffuse small cleaved cell, 2.5% diffuse mixed, 2.5% diffuse large cell, and 2.5% small noncleaved cell lymphoma (162). When subclassified according to the REAL Classification, in a series of 132 cases, 53% were extranodal marginal zone (MALT) lymphoma, 2% B-cell small lymphocytic lymphoma/B-cell chronic lymphocytic leukemia, 2% MCL, 20% follicle center, 8% large B-cell, 1% Burkitt's lymphoma, and 14% low grade, not subclassifiable (191). Thus, in this as in other subsequent series, the majority of ocular adnexal lymphomas appear to be extranodal marginal zone B-cell lymphomas (low-grade B-cell lymphoma of MALT) (Fig. 21) (174,175,189). The histologic and immunohistologic features of marginal zone lymphomas are described in more detail in the later section on Lymphomas of the Salivary Glands.

Organized MALT has been found in the conjunctiva in 31% of cases in an autopsy series of individuals with no prior history of ophthalmologic abnormalities (192). Such lymphoid tissue could be the substrate from which conjunctival MALT lymphomas arise. The origin of lymphomas in the orbit and eyelids is unknown, because these sites are thought to lack endogenous lymphoid tissue (158).

In certain groups, ocular adnexal lymphomas deviate from the predominance of low-grade B-cell lymphoma found in older adults in the general population. Of the rare cases reported in children, one was a Burkitt's lymphoma (176) and two were diffuse large cell lymphomas, one of which was an immunoblastic lymphoma of T-cell lineage (177,178). Orbital lymphoma occasionally affects HIV-positive patients, almost all of whom are young men with risk factors of homosexuality or intravenous drug use. In this group, most lymphomas are diffuse large B-cell lymphomas of immunoblastic type; Burkitt's lymphoma is the next most common (174,185,193). In a study from Hong Kong, a minority of orbital lymphomas were low-grade B-cell lymphomas presenting with localized disease, whereas a majority were intermediate or high-grade T-cell lymphomas predominantly affecting men and presenting with disseminated disease (187). The researchers noted that some of these may represent nasal lymphomas with invasion into the orbit, but it is possible that the clinicopathologic features of ocular adnexal lymphoma in Asian populations differ from those found in Western populations.

Immunophenotype

Nearly all ocular adnexal lymphomas are B-cell lineage non-Hodgkin's lymphomas that express monotypic immunoglobulin, usually IgM. Immunophenotyping using frozen tissue or cell suspensions in cases of marginal zone lymphoma reveals CD5- and CD10-negative B cells with surface immunoglobulin of one light chain type (kappa or lambda). In cases with plasmacytic differentiation, monotypic cytoplasmic immunoglobulin expression may be detected on paraffin sections (155,156,161, 166,167,173,188,190). Rare cases are immunoglobulin-negative B-cell lymphomas (156,190). Rare patients with T-cell lymphoma have had ocular adnexal lymphoma at presentation (187,194).

Genetic Features

Ocular adnexal B-cell lymphomas show clonal rearrangement of the immunoglobulin heavy chain gene. In the few cases of MALT type lymphoma that have been studied, the *bcl-1, bcl-2,* and *c-myc* genes have been germline (168,195). In patients with bilateral ocular adnexal lymphoma, molecular genetic features

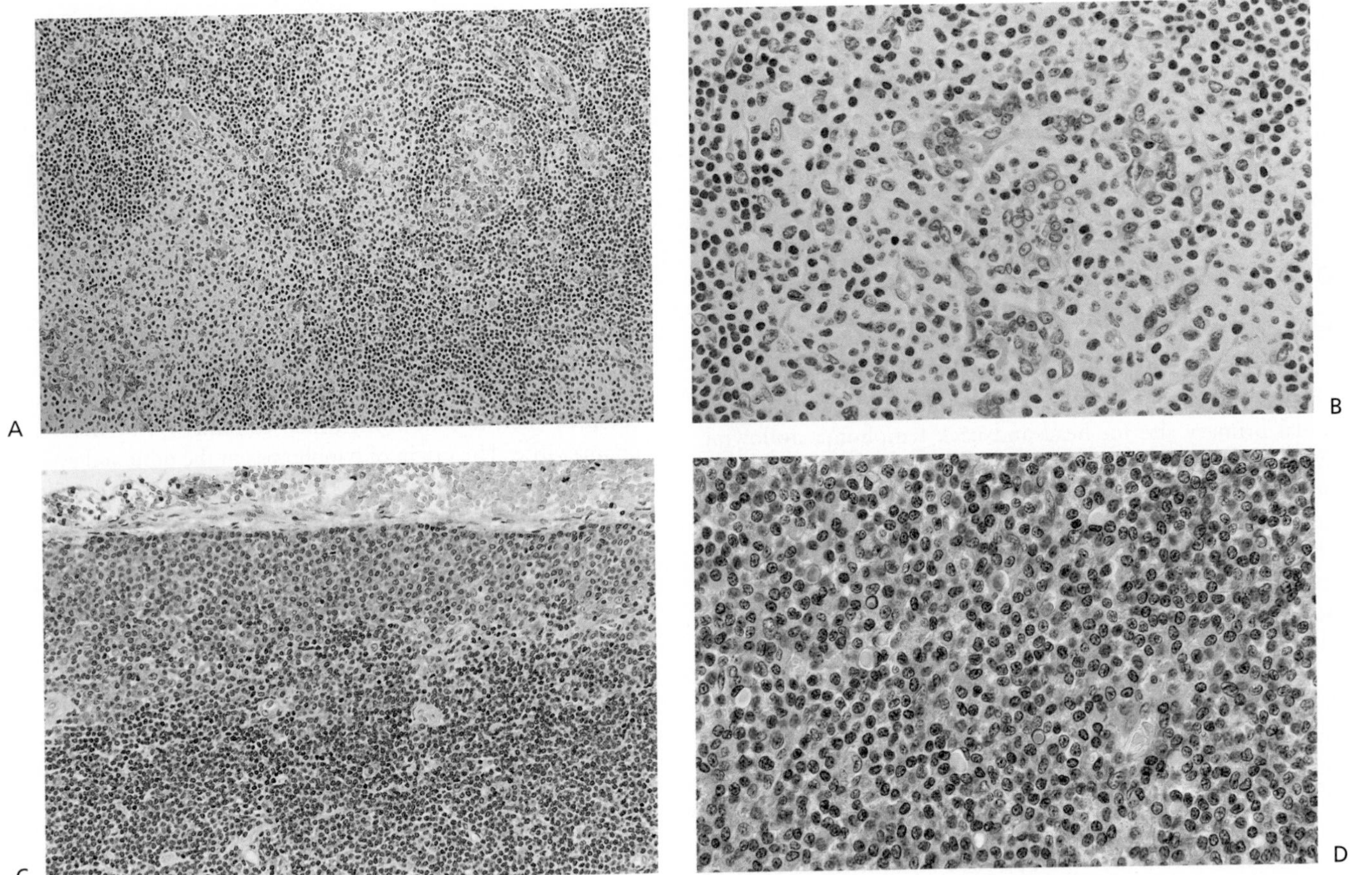

FIGURE 21. Marginal zone B-cell lymphoma of the ocular adnexa. **A:** There are irregular aggregates of pale monocytoid B cells in a background of small, dark lymphoid cells. Also seen is a reactive follicle (upper right). **B:** A well-formed lymphoepithelial lesion, composed of small cords and clusters of epithelial cells and monocytoid B cells is shown. Such lymphoepithelial lesions are uncommon in the ocular adnexa. **C:** This marginal zone lymphoma shows striking plasmacytic differentiation. A thick band of amphophilic plasma cells overlies a zone of basophilic small lymphocytes. **D:** In this case, Dutcher bodies are seen.

are reported to be identical, consistent with a single neoplastic clone involving both sites, rather than two distinct, unrelated primary tumors (163,168,196). Analysis of the immunoglobulin heavy chain gene mutation pattern in ocular adnexal marginal zone lymphomas has shown somatic mutations, consistent with a post–germinal center stage of development, similar to marginal zone lymphomas of other sites (197).

Differential Diagnosis of Ocular Adnexal Lymphoma

Reactive versus Neoplastic Lymphoid Infiltrates

The most important entity in the differential diagnosis of ocular adnexal lymphoma is a reactive lymphoid infiltrate. As noted above, immunophenotyping is the most definitive way to distinguish reactive from neoplastic infiltrates of small lymphoid cells. However, certain features are more common in lymphomas and may be helpful in differential diagnosis if immunophenotyping is unavailable. In a large series of ocular adnexal lymphoid infiltrates, Medeiros and co-workers found cytologic atypia and Dutcher bodies only in cases expressing monotypic immunoglobulin (lymphoma). Reactive germinal centers were more frequently found in polytypic (reactive) lesions ($p <$ 0.0001). When histologically indeterminate lesions alone were considered, germinal centers were still found more often in lesions expressing polytypic immunoglobulin ($p < 0.05$). Features not helpful in distinguishing between lesions with polytypic and monotypic immunoglobulin included infiltrative borders, muscle, vascular or neural invasion, nerve entrapment, polykaryocytes, zones of plasma cells and hemosiderin (156). Bilateral lesions and bony erosion are reported to be more frequent in lymphoma than in reactive lesions (159). Similarly, if staining for immunoglobulin is technically suboptimal, other immunohistologic clues may be used for a diagnosis of lymphoma. Frozen section immunohistochemical studies have shown that only lymphomas have a B- to T-cell ratio of 4 or greater; CD5, CD6, or CD43 coexpression by B cells; or loss of a pan B-cell antigen (188).

Subclassification of Low-grade B-Cell Lymphoma

Another problem in differential diagnosis is precise subclassification of the low-grade lymphomas. Most ocular adnexal lymphomas are classified as small lymphocytic or small lymphocytic plasmacytoid in the Working Formulation. However, these categories translate to several distinct REAL Classification entities that may be difficult to distinguish on a small biopsy specimen. Most are extranodal marginal zone B-cell lymphomas; these are lymphomas that usually present with localized disease, respond well to local therapy alone, and if they relapse typically do so as isolated extranodal lesions. Microscopic examination reveals a diffuse infiltrate of small lymphocytes, marginal zone B cells, or monocytoid B cells, with an admixture of a few centroblasts or immunoblasts. Plasma cells are often present and may be abundant, with a zonal distribution. Reactive germinal centers, with or without follicular colonization (infiltration of the germinal center by neoplastic small lymphocytes), may be scattered among the neoplastic cells. When the lymphoma involves the conjunctiva, neoplastic cells may invade the overlying epithelium, but in the orbital soft tissue apart from the lacrimal gland, which is devoid of epithelium, lymphoepithelial lesions are obviously not formed. Even when the lacrimal gland is involved, well-formed lymphoepithelial lesions are very unusual. The other low-grade B-cell lymphomas account for a minority of ocular adnexal lymphomas. They may show stage IV disease at presentation, with frequent marrow involvement (86), in contrast to MALT lymphoma. They include B-cell small lymphocytic lymphoma/B-cell chronic lymphocytic leukemia (B-SLL/CLL), MCL, lymphoplasmacytic lymphoma (immunocytoma), splenic marginal zone lymphoma, and follicle center lymphoma.

A diagnosis of B-SLL/CLL may be made if pseudofollicles containing medium-sized prolymphocytes and large paraimmunoblasts are found in a background of small round lymphocytes, and the diagnosis is confirmed by demonstrating CD5 and CD23 coexpression by neoplastic B cells. The orbit is rarely the presenting site of SLL/CLL, but orbital disease may occur secondarily.

Mantle cell lymphoma is composed of a monomorphous population of small irregular lymphoid cells with scant cytoplasm without admixed centroblasts or immunoblasts, often with more mitotic figures than are seen in MALT lymphoma. The neoplastic cells express CD5 and cyclin D1. MCL may occasionally present with extranodal disease localized to the orbit, but most patients have widespread disease on staging. This is an important diagnosis to make, because MCL is usually more aggressive than the other low-grade B-cell lymphomas.

Lymphoplasmacytic lymphoma by definition lacks the marginal zone or monocytoid B cells characteristic of MALT lymphomas, but recognizing these cells is fraught with difficulty on small, sometimes artifactually distorted orbital biopsies. We have seen a single case of splenic marginal zone B-cell lymphoma that secondarily involved the orbit (191); a correct diagnosis would not have been possible in this case without the clinical history (191).

There are a total of 13 low-grade orbital lymphomas with plasmacytic features reported in the literature that presented with widespread disease or developed widespread disease shortly thereafter. Many of the cases were associated with a serum paraprotein. These features are consistent with lymphoplasmacytic lymphoma (198–200), but in one series there was a female preponderance (198) and in two there was a tendency to home to MALT sites, such as subcutaneous tissue (198,199), features that suggest a relationship with marginal zone lymphoma. It may not be possible to distinguish the rare case of marginal zone B-cell lymphoma that presents with disseminated disease from the rare case of lymphoplasmacytic lymphoma presenting with orbital involvement. The biologic relationship between these two entities is not known.

The differential diagnosis of follicle center lymphoma with marginal zone lymphoma with admixed reactive follicles, particularly when the follicles are colonized by neoplastic cells, may be difficult. Follicle center lymphoma is also a relatively common type of ocular adnexal lymphoma, making up approximately 20% of cases (191). The presence of sheets of cells with oval to slightly irregular nuclei and abundant cytoplasm (monocytoid B cells) between and sometimes within follicles favors marginal zone lymphoma, whereas the presence of crowded follicles with a prominent component of small angulated (cleaved) cells with scant cytoplasm favors follicle center lymphoma. In diffuse areas of follicle center lymphoma there is often significant sclerosis. By immunophenotype, follicle center lymphoma cells may be CD10 positive; follicles will be *bcl-2* positive in contrast to the *bcl-2*-negative follicles of marginal zone lymphoma. Follicle center lymphomas are typically CD43 negative.

Staging, Treatment, and Outcome

Approximately 80% of patients have disease confined to the ocular adnexa, unilaterally or bilaterally. The remainder are roughly equally divided between Ann Arbor stage II and stage IV disease, with only rare cases with stage III disease (167,171,173,186,201). In a number of studies, marginal zone lymphomas, as well as cases classified using the Rappaport Classification or the Working Formulation as well differentiated lymphocytic lymphoma, small lymphocytic lymphoma (some with plasmacytoid features) and intermediate lymphocytic lymphoma—all of which could represent marginal zone lymphomas—have been more likely to present with stage I disease than other types of lymphoma (155,156,186,201,202).

In general, cases of localized low-grade lymphomas are treated with radiation. Cases of intermediate or high-grade lymphoma, whether localized or widespread, are usually treated with a combination of ocular adnexal radiation and chemotherapy. Chemotherapy is used in localized intermediate and high-grade lymphoma because of a reported 40% to 60% risk of distant relapse with radiation alone, and because such cases are frequently locally destructive, with invasion into paranasal sinuses or intracranial extension (171). Chemotherapy is also usually added to radiation in disseminated low-grade lymphoma (171,186,201). Radiation therapy achieves excellent local control of disease; freedom from local recurrence is close to 100% (171,175,186,196,202,203). Prevention and treatment of extraocular dissemination is not as successful, but the prognosis of ocular adnexal lymphoma overall is good. For example, in one study, the overall survival at 4 years was 90%, whereas the 4-year disease-free survival rate was 65% (201). In another, the disease-free survival rate at 5 years was 70% and the overall survival rate at 5 years was 93% (171). In a study that included only patients with localized disease, the 6-year disease-free survival rate was 77% and the overall survival rate was 89% (202).

When relapses occur, they may be in extraocular sites or in the opposite orbit (171). In one study, marginal zone lymphomas that relapsed tended to spread to other extranodal sites, distinct from the pattern of spread associated with other low-grade B-cell lymphomas (203). In one case, a patient with an ocular adnexal lymphoma developed an isolated relapse in the kidney (204).

Patients who present with disease localized to the ocular adnexa have a much better prognosis than those with more widespread disease (155,173,187,201). Interestingly, considering how strongly stage affects prognosis, isolated bilateral ocular adnexal disease does not have a worse prognosis than unilateral disease (162,171,174,196). In one study, cases of conjunctival lymphoid infiltrates were least likely to be associated with systemic spread (20% of cases) and cases involving the lids were most likely to be associated with systemic spread (67%), whereas orbital infiltrates carried an intermediate risk (35%) (155).

The histologic type of lymphoma is also important in defining outcome. Patients with marginal zone lymphoma, the most common type, have an excellent prognosis (189). In most reports patients with high-grade lymphoma have had a worse outcome (186,189,201). Although this may in part reflect the fact that more aggressive lymphomas may present with higher stage disease, in one report the Working Formulation grade was prognostically important even when only patients with localized disease were considered (171). Lymphomas with a high proliferation fraction and with p53 expression are also reported to have a less favorable outcome (174). Bony erosion also has been associated with a worse prognosis (201), but most lymphomas with bony erosion are large cell lymphomas (167,177,185). In one large series men had a worse survival than women ($p < 0.03$) (162).

Secondary Ocular Adnexal Lymphoma

The ocular adnexa also may be secondarily involved by lymphomas arising in other sites; an estimated 5.3% of non-Hodgkin's lymphoma patients develop ocular adnexal involvement during the course of their disease (170). The involvement may be in the form of relapse or progression of a lymphoma arising in lymph nodes or extranodal sites, or it may occur via direct extension from adjacent structures (167,205). Patients affected in this way are usually middle-aged to older adults with a similar to slightly younger mean age than those with primary ocular adnexal lymphoma (167,170). A variety of types of non-Hodgkin's lymphoma can be found in this setting, although the incidence of marginal zone lymphoma (167) or (using the Working Formulation) small lymphocytic lymphoma (156) is lower than it is among primary ocular adnexal lymphomas. The most common type of secondary lymphoma is follicle center lymphoma. In one study of 10 patients with lymphoma relapsing in the ocular adnexa, 6 had follicle center lymphoma, 2 had MCL, and one each had marginal zone lymphoma and diffuse large B-cell lymphoma (167).

The prognosis for patients with secondary ocular adnexal lymphomas is worse than for those with primary disease. Patients are more likely to have disseminated disease at presentation (156). Although the ocular adnexal lymphoma can usually be eradicated, the extraocular disease frequently persists or progresses (170). In one series of 10 patients, by the time of last follow-up, 5 had died of lymphoma, 3 were alive with disease, 1 had died free of lymphoma, and 1 had died with the disease status unknown (167).

OCULAR LYMPHOMA

Clinical Features

Ocular lymphoma (lymphoma involving the globe) is less common than ocular adnexal lymphoma. Over 100 cases have been reported, but most have been described in single case reports or small series, with only a few large series in the literature (206–208). However, the frequency of ocular lymphoma appears to have increased during recent years (206,209). Ocular lymphoma predominantly affects older adults, with a mean age in the sixth or seventh decade in most series (206–215), although occasionally young adults (208,213,216–218) and rarely children (206,219,220) are affected. Unlike the situation with most other types of lymphoma, and similarly to ocular adnexal lymphoma, ocular lymphoma shows a female preponderance, with women affected twice as often as men (206,207,209, 211–213,215–217,221,222). Most patients have no known predisposing conditions, but a number of cases in HIV-infected patients (223–225) and in iatrogenically immunosuppressed allograft recipients (219,226–228) have been described.

By far, the most common presenting complaints are related to unilateral or bilateral blurred vision, floating spots, or both (206,209,211). Pain, redness (209,212,222,229), and acute loss of vision (216) are unusual but have been described. Although symptoms are often unilateral, ophthalmologic examination reveals involvement of both eyes in about 80% of cases, but the severity of involvement may differ between the two eyes (211,214).

On ophthalmoscopic examination, in almost all cases there is a variable number of cells with a translucent gray appearance in sheets and clumps suspended in the vitreous. In some cases this cellular infiltrate is so dense that it precludes visualization of the fundus. In a minority of cases, abnormalities are confined to the vitreous. In a majority, the retina, the uveal tract (choroid, iris, and ciliary body), or both are affected. Whitish, yellow–white, or gray–white infiltrates or multifocal plaque-like lesions may be seen beneath the retinal pigment epithelium. There also may be areas of edema, hemorrhage, necrosis, or retinal detachment. The retinal artery may become occluded. Over time, areas of scarring and atrophy may develop. The optic nerve head may be infiltrated by tumor. The uvea also may be affected, sometimes with the formation of large masses. The posterior uvea (choroid) is more often involved than the anterior uvea (iris and ciliary body). As a result of these changes, visual acuity is usually diminished. Other manifestations include increased intraocular pressure, keratic precipitates (deposits of cells on the posterior surface of the cornea), and anterior chamber cells and flare [presence of increased protein causing the normally clear fluid of the anterior chamber to become cloudy (flare) with tiny particles (cells) suspended in the fluid] (206,207,209,211–215,230,231).

In many cases, there is a substantial delay between the onset of symptoms and establishing a diagnosis. The interval to diagnosis has occasionally been longer than 2 years (208) and is occasionally more than 10 years (207). Some cases are not diagnosed until autopsy (207,211,213), although in more recent reports it has usually been possible to render a diagnosis more expeditiously. Based on the findings described above, the clinical impression is often an inflammatory process. Ocular lymphoma can mimic a variety of non-neoplastic conditions, including chronic idiopathic uveitis, vitritis, retinal vasculitis (209), optic neuritis, amyloidosis, sarcoidosis, and infections, including toxoplasmosis, syphilis, tuberculosis, Whipple's disease, and CMV infection (207,213). Ocular lymphoma resembling choroidal melanoma also has been described (231). The entity most commonly considered in the differential diagnosis based on clinical findings is chronic posterior uveitis, and it may not be until the lesion has proven to be unresponsive or poorly responsive to steroid therapy that the possibility of lymphoma is considered. In some cases, the onset of neurologic symptoms due to CNS involvement provides the clue that leads to the diagnosis of lymphoma (209).

A variety of techniques have been used to document the presence of ocular lymphoma, including vitreous aspirate, vitrectomy, anterior chamber aspiration, and retinal or choroidal biopsy. In patients with a blind, painful eye, the diagnosis may be established in an ocular enucleation specimen. In patients with CNS disease, lymphoma may be first identified on a brain biopsy or on cytologic examination of cerebrospinal fluid (206–209,212,215,222). The mode most commonly used is microscopic examination of vitreous, but the sensitivity of this procedure may be limited by admixed inflammatory cells obscuring the neoplastic population or by prior steroid therapy, which may eliminate a variable number of tumor cells. Frequently two or even three vitreous specimens must be examined before a definite diagnosis is rendered (206,208,209,214,221).

At the Massachusetts General Hospital, the diagnosis of ocular lymphoma is most often made on a vitreous aspirate subjected to a combination of cytologic and flow cytometric examination. This is a sensitive method that permits identification of small populations of neoplastic cells (Fig. 22).

Pathologic Features

Nearly all cases of ocular lymphoma, including those occurring in HIV-positive patients and in allograft recipients, are diffuse large cell lymphomas (Fig. 22), although the older designation, reticulum cell sarcoma, is used in many reports (206,209, 214,223,224,226–228). A few cases have been described as poorly differentiated lymphocytic lymphoma and diffuse mixed lymphocytic and histiocytic lymphoma (211). Microscopic examination reveals a dense, diffuse infiltrate of large atypical lymphoid cells, sometimes with a perivascular pattern, especially at the periphery of the lesion or in the retina (211). A few cases of intravascular lymphoma (also known as angiotropic lymphoma or neoplastic angioendotheliomatosis) have involved the eye (232,233).

On cytologic examination, neoplastic cells frequently have irregularly shaped, sometimes lobated nuclei, coarse chromatin, and prominent nucleoli. Mitotic figures are often found. Necrotic debris and interspersed inflammatory cells may be seen (208,214,221).

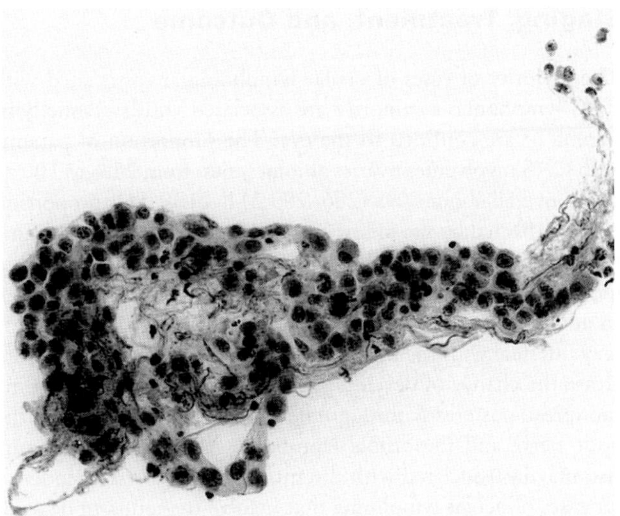

FIGURE 22. Ocular diffuse large B-cell lymphoma. In this vitreous aspirate, there are fragments of vitreous with a dense infiltrate of large, atypical lymphoid cells, some with the appearance of plasmacytoid immunoblasts (Papanicolaou stain).

Rarely, the eyes may be involved by low-grade lymphoma, a process that has been called inflammatory pseudotumor, lymphoid hyperplasia, and early stage lymphoid infiltrates of the uvea. This process produces slowly progressive choroidal thickening in one or, less often, both eyes. Microscopic examination discloses histologic features reminiscent of extranodal marginal zone B-cell (MALT) lymphoma, including diffuse infiltrates of lymphocytes, plasmacytoid lymphocytes, Dutcher bodies, interspersed reactive germinal centers, or a combination of these findings. Although the nature of this disorder was controversial, demonstration of monotypic immunoglobulin has shown that it is a low-grade lymphoma (234,235). In many cases, there is adjacent extraocular disease, the symptoms of which often precede the intraocular disease, suggesting that some of these lesions represent local spread from a MALT lymphoma arising in the ocular adnexa.

The vast majority of intraocular lymphomas have been B-cell types (209,210,215,224,227,228) (including all four cases in one series of intravascular lymphoma) (232). A few cases presenting with ocular involvement have been interpreted as peripheral T-cell lymphoma (212), including one associated with HTLV-1 (236), one associated with EBV, two angiocentric lymphomas (216), and one lymphoma composed of large granular lymphocytes (222). T-cell receptor gene rearrangement has been reported in one study (222). Of the few cases of T-cell lymphoma, it is interesting that three have presented with anterior uveitis, in contrast to the much more common finding of posterior uveitis in B-cell lymphoma (222,237). A few cases of Hodgkin's disease have been described in older reports (238) but we are not familiar with a convincing case of ocular Hodgkin's disease.

Staging, Treatment, and Outcome

The majority of cases of ocular lymphoma are associated with CNS lymphoma; a minority are associated with systemic lymphoma or are confined to the eye. The proportion of patients with CNS involvement varies among series, from 25% to 100%, and is overall about 70% (206–209,211–213). This proportion may be affected by the follow-up interval because the mean time to development of CNS disease is approximately 2 years, and in individual cases may be up to 9 or 10 years (206,207,209,211). In addition, aggressive treatment of isolated ocular lymphoma may interfere with the natural history of the disease and may decrease the chance of developing CNS involvement. Lymphoma can spread posteriorly through the lamina cribrosa to involve the optic nerve and the orbital leptomeninges. Ocular lymphoma also may be associated with distant spread. There is a tendency for cases of ocular lymphoma that involve the retina to be associated with spread into the CNS or to remain confined to the eye. Those involving the uvea tend to be associated with systemic spread, although this distinction is not absolute, and many exceptions to this rule occur (211,225). The association between CNS lymphoma and ocular lymphoma is so strong that some consider ocular lymphoma, in the absence of systemic disease, to be a subset of CNS lymphoma (209). Any portion of the CNS may be involved, but in one report of five cases of ocular lymphoma associated with CNS disease, the CNS involvement in all cases was ipsilateral to the first involved or more severely involved eye (211).

Patients with associated CNS lymphoma develop ocular involvement prior to, simultaneous with, or following documentation of CNS disease. The most common scenario is presentation with ocular symptoms, with development of neurologic symptoms later, whereas a minority of patients have ocular and neurologic symptoms simultaneously or present with neurologic symptoms and only later have ocular disease. Systemic spread can be to lymph nodes or to a variety of extranodal sites (207).

Patients with isolated ocular lymphoma who are not treated definitively generally develop increasingly extensive involvement of their eyes, sometimes over a period of many years, often resulting in blindness (207). Ocular lymphoma frequently responds very well to radiation therapy, although some patients achieve only a partial remission or have little response to radiation (207). Although lymphomatous infiltrates often regress with radiation, restoration of sight is not guaranteed, depending on the extent of damage to the retina (226). Patients treated with ocular radiation alone usually progress to CNS or, less often, systemic involvement. Although isolated ocular lymphoma is associated with little, if any, mortality, survival of patients with CNS lymphoma is poor.

Treatment with whole-brain radiation, in addition to ocular radiation, may decrease the chance of developing CNS lymphoma, or may result in regression of CNS disease in those who have already developed CNS involvement. However, the rate of relapse with radiation alone is high, with mortality rates as high as 80% (207). Patients receiving intravenous or intrathecal chemotherapy, or both, may have a slightly better outlook. However, there is no large series of uniformly treated patients with this uncommon tumor, so it is difficult to draw definite conclusions. Because radiation may be associated with ocular morbidity, including retinopathy and cataracts, intravitreal methotrexate has been suggested recently as a possible alternative therapy for ocular lymphoma (239).

Secondary Ocular Lymphoma

Approximately 25% of CNS lymphoma patients have ocular involvement (240). The eyes also may be secondarily involved by systemic lymphoma from nodal and extranodal primary sites (212,229). In one unusual case, a 4-year-old boy with a B-cell lymphoma of the sinuses and nasopharynx developed acute bilateral blindness due to involvement of both optic nerves. Prompt institution of combination chemotherapy yielded restoration of vision and a durable complete remission (220). The eyes have been involved in mycosis fungoides (230) and in disseminated adult T-cell lymphoma/leukemia (241). Rarely the eyes also have been the site of large cell transformation (Richter's syndrome) in patients with chronic lymphocytic leukemia (242,243).

ORAL CAVITY LYMPHOMA

Clinical Features

The oral cavity, including the palate, gingiva, tongue, buccal mucosa, floor of the mouth, and lips, is the primary site of approximately 2% of all extranodal lymphomas (94,244). In addition, lymphoma arising in the bones of the jaw may invade into adjacent soft tissues and present as an oral cavity mass (245,246). In recent years, there has been an increase in cases of lymphoma of the oral cavity, because of the tendency for patients with HIV infection to develop non-Hodgkin's lymphoma with involvement of the oral cavity (247,248). Nonimmunosuppressed patients of any age can be affected, with children as young as 3 years (245,249) and adults as old as 94 years (247) reported. However, most patients are middle-aged to older adults, with a mean or median age in the sixth or seventh decade in several large series, with a slight male preponderance (244,245,247,250–252). In contrast, HIV-infected patients with oral cavity lymphoma are almost all men who are overall younger, with an approximate median age of 40 years. Most acquire HIV through homosexual contact, whereas a few become infected by intravenous drug use or heterosexual contact (Table 8) (246–248,253–255).

Patients complain of localized or diffuse soft tissue swelling, pain that may be spontaneous or provoked by eating, mucosal ulceration or discoloration, paresthesias, anesthesia, and loosening of teeth (245,246,248,250,251,254,256–260). The lesion may be described as rapidly enlarging, especially in HIV-positive patients (248). A small minority have systemic symptoms of fever or weight loss (245,261). The sites most often affected, in both HIV-positive and HIV-negative patients, are the palate/maxilla and gingiva, with tongue, buccal mucosa, floor of the mouth, and lips affected less often (244–248,253, 255,260,262). Soft tissue involvement is more common than bony involvement (245). Physical examination reveals an exophytic, often polypoid mass in the majority of cases. In a minor-

TABLE 8. ORAL CAVITY LYMPHOMA IN HIV-POSITIVE AND HIV-NEGATIVE PATIENTS

	HIV Negative	HIV Positive
Age of patients	Middle-aged and older adults; rarely, children	Young and middle-aged adults
Male preponderance	Slight	Great
Risk factors	None known	Most: homosexual Minority: IVDA, heterosexual
Associated conditions	Not described	Oral candidiasis, oral hairy leukoplakia
Histologic types	Diffuse large B-cell lymphoma Follicle center lymphoma Mantle cell lymphoma Marginal zone B-cell lymphoma	Diffuse large B-cell lymphoma Burkitt-like lymphoma Plasmablastic lymphoma
EBV positivity	9%	76%
Outcome	Varies with grade and stage	Very poor

HIV, human immunodeficiency virus; IVDA, intravenous drug abuse; EBV, Epstein-Barr virus.

ity, the lymphoma is an infiltrative, ulcerated lesion with raised margins (244). The lymphomas range in size from 1 to 10 cm, with a mean size of 2.9 cm. Physical examination also reveals oral candidiasis, hairy leukoplakia, or both in some HIV-infected patients (248,254,262).

Pathologic Features

Lymphomas of a wide variety of types arise in the oral cavity. Among nonimmunosuppressed patients, approximately half of oral lymphomas are the diffuse large B-cell type. The next most common type is follicle center lymphoma (16%), followed by MCL (10%), marginal zone B-cell lymphoma (6%), Burkitt's lymphoma and Burkitt-like lymphoma (4%), lymphoblastic lymphoma of B- and T-cell types (7%), peripheral T-cell lymphoma (5%), and anaplastic large cell lymphoma (3%). A minority of the large cell lymphomas are composed of immunoblasts (245,247,251,252,257,259).

Marginal zone lymphomas may infiltrate the overlying surface epithelium or the epithelium of minor salivary glands, sometimes forming lymphoepithelial lesions; Dutcher bodies are found in some cases (244,247,256). In a study that focused on marginal zone B-cell lymphoma of the oral cavity, the authors found that some large cell lymphomas contained a population of neoplastic small lymphoid cells and plasma cells and suggested that such cases may represent high-grade transformation of low-grade marginal zone lymphomas rather than *de novo* large cell lymphomas (256).

Follicle center lymphoma of the oral cavity may be less frequent among Asians. In three Japanese series of a total of 59 cases, there were no cases of follicular lymphoma (251,259,263). When follicle center lymphomas do occur, their histologic features are similar to those of follicle center lymphomas in other sites. In contrast, large cell lymphomas seem to be more prevalent among Asians (259,263).

A few cases of peripheral T-cell lymphoma (unspecified type) also have been described; peripheral T-cell lymphomas may be more common in this site among Asian patients than among Western patients. In a study conducted in the United States, only 1 of 24 cases (4%) was a T-cell lymphoma (247), whereas in two studies from Japan, 6 of 54 patients (11%) and 8 of 25 patients (32%) had a T-cell lymphoma (252,259). In one of these Japanese studies, 5 cases (9%), and in one American series, 1 of 34 (3%) were classified as true histiocytic lymphomas, a highly unusual finding (250,252). A case of enteropathy-associated T-cell lymphoma first diagnosed in the oral cavity has been described in an elderly white woman (258). Cutaneous T-cell lymphoma (mycosis fungoides) rarely involves the oral cavity. The majority of these cases are found in the setting of long-standing, advanced disease, but in exceptional cases, the first manifestation of cutaneous T-cell lymphoma is seen in the oral cavity. It has been suggested that the uncommon CD8-positive type of cutaneous T-cell lymphoma may be more likely to involve the oral cavity than the more common CD4-positive type (264,265).

In one study, B-cell lymphomas were more likely to be exophytic masses, whereas T-cell lymphomas were more likely to be infiltrative, ulcerative lesions. In the same study, B-cell lymphomas were divided into high-grade and low-grade types. The high-grade B-cell lymphomas (diffuse large cell, Burkitt's, Burkitt-like, and lymphoblastic) tended to be twice as large, on average, as the low-grade B-cell lymphomas and the T-cell lymphomas (244).

Oral Cavity Lymphoma in HIV-positive Patients

Oral lymphomas in HIV-infected individuals are less heterogeneous than those found in the general population, and are virtually exclusively diffuse high-grade lymphomas of B-cell lineage in the vast majority of cases. Eighty-five percent are diffuse large B-cell type, 5% are Burkitt's or Burkitt-like, 2.5% are T-cell anaplastic large cell lymphoma, and 7.5% are peripheral T-cell lymphoma (unspecified type). Many of the large cell lymphomas have a predominance of immunoblasts (246–248,253,255, 260,262,266). Recently Delecluse and colleagues described a

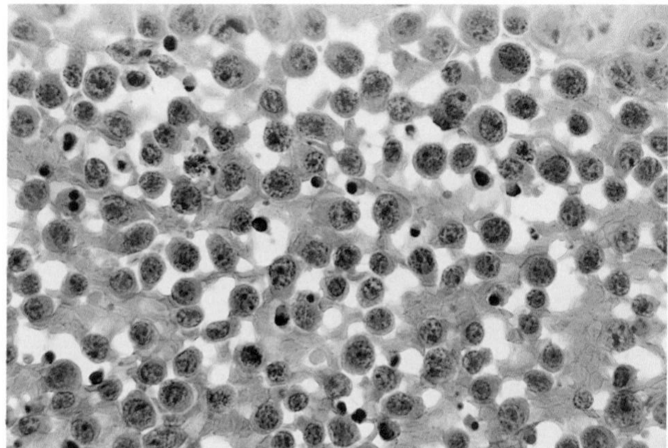

FIGURE 23. Plasmablastic lymphoma in an HIV-positive patient. An aspirate of a palatal lesion shows numerous large, atypical, immature plasmacytoid cells with prominent nucleoli (Papanicolaou stain).

distinctive subset of HIV-associated diffuse large B-cell lymphoma occurring in the oral cavity, which they called plasmablastic lymphoma. The neoplastic cells have the appearance of plasmacytoid immunoblasts or plasmablasts, with vesicular eccentrically placed nuclei, prominent nucleoli, and abundant cytoplasm with a paranuclear clear zone or hof (Fig. 23). These neoplasms have a high mitotic rate, frequent single cell necrosis, and scattered tingible body macrophages, giving a starry sky pattern. The immunophenotype of these tumors is their most distinctive feature. Unlike nearly all other B-cell lymphomas, they usually lack both the leukocyte common antigen (CD45) and the B-cell antigen (CD20). However, they are usually CD79a positive, often contain cytoplasmic immunoglobulin, and show clonal immunoglobulin heavy chain gene rearrangement; these features establish their B-cell lineage (253). The morphology and immunophenotype suggest that these may be anaplastic plasmacytomas.

Epstein-Barr virus is known to infect, and to persist in, oropharyngeal and nasopharyngeal epithelium and lymphoid tissue. Therefore, the question of the role of EBV in the pathogenesis of lymphomas in this area has been raised. The majority of HIV-associated oral lymphomas, both B- and T-cell types, contain EBV. Using *in situ* hybridization, usually with probes for EBER, approximately 76% of cases are positive (246–248, 253,255,260,262). Among cases classified as plasmablastic lymphoma, 60% are EBER positive, and 56% of the EBER-positive plasmablastic lymphomas express EBV LMP (253). In contrast, only about 9% of oral lymphomas in nonimmunosuppressed patients are EBER positive (247,251,258). This suggests that EBV may well play a role in the pathogenesis of the majority of HIV-associated lymphomas, but that it is not a major contributing factor in the development of oral cavity lymphoma in the general population (Table 8).

Staging, Treatment, and Outcome

At presentation most patients have localized disease, although a substantial minority have disseminated disease. Approximately 62% of patients have Ann Arbor stage I disease, 7% have stage II disease, 1% have stage III disease, and 30% have stage IV disease (245,246,251,253,257,263). The proportion with localized and disseminated disease is similar in HIV-positive and HIV-negative patients.

The prognosis differs substantially between HIV-positive and HIV-negative patients. Regarding HIV-negative patients, in one large series in which only one patient was noted to be HIV positive, for example, the mean disease-free survival was 31 months and the mean overall survival was 38 months. Stage and grade both affected the outcome. When cases in this study were stratified according to Working Formulation grade (low, intermediate, or high), there was a significant impact on prognosis ($p = 0.007$). Patients with low-grade lymphoma had 100% long-term disease-free survival, and patients with intermediate grade lymphoma had 60% long-term disease-free survival, but all patients with high-grade lymphoma had failed within approximately 2 years. Patients with localized disease (stage I/II) had better disease-free survival ($p = 0.0001$) and better overall survival ($p = 0.001$) than patients with advanced stage (III/IV) disease (245). Other studies have confirmed a relationship between stage and grade, as well as outcome (249–251,259), and have reported similar survival data (249,250).

Patients with AIDS have a much worse prognosis. In 75% of reported cases, the patients died, all within 18 months of the diagnosis of lymphoma. In some cases, causes other than lymphoma contributed to the patient's demise, however. Follow-up of the minority of patients who remain alive is often short (median, ~1 year), and some of them are alive with disease (245,246,253,255,260,262,266). In one remarkable case, a patient with a prior diagnosis of AIDS developed lymphoma in three different sites in the oral cavity at three different times. The lymphoma at each site regressed without specific therapy before it reappeared at a new site. The patient died of other causes 11 months after presentation (266).

Differential Diagnosis

The most important pitfall in the diagnosis of lymphoma of the oral cavity is failure to suspect lymphoma on physical examination. Lymphomas in this site can mimic a variety of common dental conditions, including periodontal disease, acute necrotizing gingivitis, and dental infections (248,257,258). The appearance of some lesions may suggest squamous cell carcinoma or salivary gland carcinoma (245). In HIV-positive patients, Kaposi's sarcoma, deep fungal infections, and HIV-associated periodontal disease also enter the clinical differential diagnosis (248,266). Once a biopsy is obtained, assuming tissue is well preserved and representative of the tumor, the diagnosis is usually straightforward. Occasionally problems in pathologic interpretation arise, however. In a case of anaplastic large cell lymphoma with many eosinophils, diagnoses of eosinophilic ulcer and eosinophilic granuloma were considered, and a diagnosis of lymphoma was not established until the patient developed a local recurrence 5 years later (257). The HIV-associated plasmablastic lymphomas may cause difficulty in diagnosis because of their characteristic failure to express leukocyte common antigen (CD45) and CD20 (pan B cell) (253). Familiarity with this entity is important to avoid inappropriate exclusion of a diagnosis of lymphoma after learning that such a tumor is CD45 and CD20 negative. Adding antibodies to CD79a and immunoglobulin to the panel used for analysis can be helpful in establishing a diagnosis. If uncertainty persists, genotyping can be obtained to demonstrate clonal immunoglobulin heavy or light chain gene rearrangement.

LARYNGEAL LYMPHOMA

Clinical Features

Malignant lymphoma only rarely involves the larynx, accounting for less than 1% of laryngeal neoplasms (267), but a number of well-documented cases of primary laryngeal lymphoma have been reported in the literature. Patients with primary lymphoma of the larynx have ranged in age from 4 to 86 years at the time of presentation, but most have been middle aged to older adults, with a slight male preponderance (approximately 1.5:1) (105,267–278). Several patients have had other malignancies, including concurrent laryngeal squamous cell carcinoma (269,270,278). Two patients were HIV positive (268,272).

Patients present with dysphonia (most often hoarseness), dyspnea, sometimes with acute laryngeal obstruction, sore throat, foreign body sensation, or dysphagia (104,267,269–271). Two children presented with progressive airway obstruction mimicking croup and epiglottitis (276). Systemic symptoms are very uncommon, except that a number of patients with dysphagia have experienced weight loss (274,279). The tumors are most often smooth-surfaced, submucosal, elevated, frequently polypoid lesions (269,274), although occasionally they are papillary (278) or ulcerated and fungating (272). The tumors may be pedunculated (270) and may prolapse into the airway (272). Their location is most often supraglottic, but there may be glottic or subglottic extension (267,269,271,273). Occasionally the lymphoma appears to arise from the true cords (278) or the subglottis (267,275). In a few cases the larynx has been one site of involvement in cases of multifocal lymphoma in the head and neck (280). In one case, for example, there was involvement of the larynx, nose, and soft palate (271). It has been suggested that laryngeal lymphomas arise from the lymphoid tissue that can be found in the larynx, mainly in the epiglottis and supraglottic larynx, correlating with the distribution of lymphomas of the larynx (274).

Pathologic Features

Histologic evaluation reveals two main types of lymphomas occurring with roughly equal frequency: diffuse large B-cell lymphoma and extranodal marginal zone B-cell lymphoma (MALT type), together accounting for approximately 80% of cases. Although the question of whether any of the large cell lymphomas represent high-grade transformation of a MALT lymphoma has been raised, this has not been demonstrated. The MALT lymphomas have shown classic histologic features, including the presence of centrocyte-like cells, lymphoepithelial lesions, and reactive follicles with follicular colonization (267,269,270,274,277,278,280). In addition, several cases classified as small lymphocytic lymphoma, lymphoplasmacytic lymphoma, or diffuse small cleaved cell lymphoma have been described (267,271,275); it is possible that they also represent MALT lymphomas. Rare cases of follicular lymphoma (267) and peripheral T-cell lymphoma (269) and several cases of angiocentric or nasal-type T/NK-cell lymphoma (104,105,113,272) also have been reported. In one study of extranodal NK/T-cell lymphoma, all nasal lymphomas were EBV positive, but the single laryngeal lymphoma in the study was EBV negative (105).

Staging, Treatment, and Outcome

Information on staging is available in only a few cases, but in approximately 72% of cases there is Ann Arbor stage I disease; in 20% stage II disease, and in 8% stage IV disease (105,113,267, 269,270,272,273,278,279,281,282). Three patients with multifocal head and neck involvement had MALT lymphoma or lymphoma classified as lymphoplasmacytic (271,280). Most patients can be successfully treated with a combination of surgery and radiation (275,279), although laryngeal lymphoma sometimes results in sudden death due to acute airway obstruction (274,281). When patients develop relapses, they tend to be isolated, extranodal tumors in the upper respiratory tract, stomach, orbit, and skin, and even when relapses occur, there may be long disease-free intervals (275,279). The behavior of these lymphomas is similar to that associated with MALT lymphomas in other sites (269). A review of published cases shows that 52% were alive and well at last follow-up, 17% had died of other causes (free of lymphoma), 3% were alive with lymphoma, and 28% had died of lymphoma, although 25% of the patients in the last category died of acute airway obstruction and cannot be considered to have failed therapy, and another 25% of those who died had nasal-type lymphoma, a category known to have a poor prognosis (105,113,267,269–275,278,279,281,282). B-cell lymphomas of the larynx, both low- and high-grade types, that can be treated with curative intent have a good prognosis.

Secondary Laryngeal Involvement by Lymphoma

On occasion, the larynx is secondarily involved by lymphoma. One patient with a cutaneous diffuse large B-cell lymphoma developed a unifocal relapse in the larynx 2 years after the initial diagnosis of lymphoma. One year following treatment of the relapse, the patient was alive and well (283). The larynx has been involved in the course of a peripheral T-cell lymphoma that presented in the oral cavity and resulted in the death of the patient (261). In some instances, patients with disseminated lymphoma of a variety of histologic types have symptomatic laryngeal involvement, or asymptomatic involvement that may not be identified until autopsy (113,284).

LYMPHOID PROLIFERATIONS OF THE SALIVARY GLANDS

Lymphoid proliferations of the salivary glands may be either reactive or neoplastic. The two major reactive lesions are the lym-

TABLE 9. LYMPHOID PROLIFERATIONS OF THE SALIVARY GLAND

Non-neoplastic
Simple lymphoepithelial cyst
Cystic lymphoid hyperplasia
Lymphoepithelial sialadenitis
Neoplastic
Extranodal marginal zone B-cell lymphoma of MALT type
Follicular lymphoma
Diffuse large B-cell lymphoma
Other nodal type lymphomas

MALT, mucosa-associated lymphoid tissue.

phoepithelial sialadenitis (LESA) associated with Sjögren's syndrome, variously known as benign lymphoepithelial lesion or MESA, and cystic lymphoid hyperplasia (cystic lymphoepithelial lesion) of HIV infection. Lymphomas of the salivary glands are predominantly B-cell types and include extranodal marginal zone B-cell lymphoma of the MALT type, follicular lymphoma, and large B-cell lymphoma (Table 9) (285).

Non-neoplastic Lymphoid Proliferations

Simple Lymphoepithelial Cyst

Benign lymphoepithelial cysts occur sporadically, predominantly in the parotid glands, unrelated to AIDS or Sjögren's syndrome. They are thought to arise from either intraparotid lymph nodes or branchial cleft remnants. They typically occur as unilateral, solitary lesions in middle-aged men, and do not recur after excision. Histologically, they consist typically of a unilocular cyst with a variable epithelial lining (squamous, respiratory, columnar, or a mixture), surrounded by reactive lymphoid tissue, often with germinal centers (Fig. 24) (285).

Cystic Lymphoid Hyperplasia of the Salivary Gland

Cystic lymphoid hyperplasia of the salivary gland is most commonly seen in patients with HIV infection or AIDS, but also can be seen in patients with other immune deficiencies or in normal individuals. The HIV-positive patients are more often intravenous drug abusers than homosexuals, who present with unilateral or bilateral salivary gland enlargement in the context of progressive generalized lymphadenopathy (286–288). The parotid gland is involved more often than the submandibular gland. Although the lesion histologically resembles extranodal marginal zone B-cell lymphoma of MALT, patients with cystic lymphoid hyperplasia do not appear to be at increased risk of lymphoma development (289). Morphologically identical lesions in HIV-positive and HIV-negative individuals have been postulated to result from ductal obstruction by exuberant lymphoid hyperplasia (290).

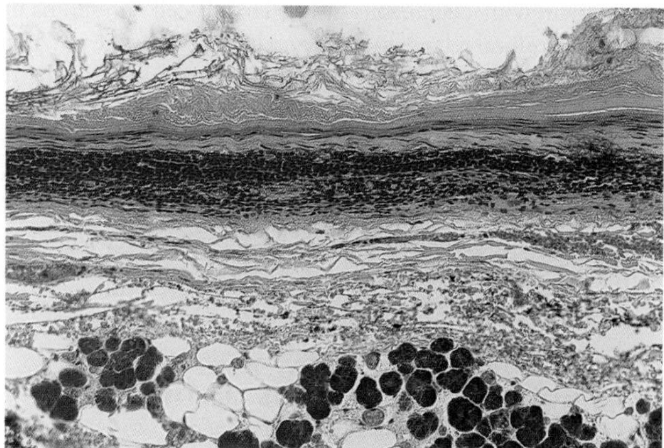

FIGURE 24. Simple lymphoepithelial cyst of the parotid gland. The cyst is lined by an attenuated layer of keratinizing squamous epithelium with lymphoid tissue external to it.

Morphologic Features

The glands show single or multiple cysts lined by a flattened columnar epithelium, similar to that seen in LESA, surrounded by a prominent lymphoid infiltrate, with florid follicular hyperplasia and prominent infiltration of the epithelium by lymphocytes (Fig. 25). The lesions may be well- or poorly circumscribed. The infiltrate is dominated by large, reactive follicles with germinal centers, which may show follicle lysis and diminished mantle zones, similar to the follicles in reactive lymph nodes in HIV-positive patients with progressive generalized lymphadenopathy. The interfollicular regions show a mixture of small lymphocytes, plasma cells, and immunoblasts. Lymphocytes, including monocytoid B cells, are present in the epithelium in small aggregates and may form lymphoepithelial lesions (defined as aggregates of three or more lymphoid cells in a nest within the epithelium). They also may be present focally around the epithelium or in the marginal zones of reactive follicles, but do not form broad sheets. Plasma cells are numerous but do not form broad sheets. There is morphologic overlap with LESA, and LESA also has been reported in patients with AIDS (291,292), suggesting that these lesions may be different morphologic manifestations of the same process.

The etiology of the lesion is not known. By immunohistochemistry, both the lymphoid cells and plasma cells express polytypic immunoglobulin light chains, and are therefore non-neoplastic. Staining and *in situ* hybridization for EBV proteins and RNA have revealed evidence of this agent in some cases (293). In one study (289), HIV protein and RNA were detected in the FDCs of the germinal centers in a case of cystic lymphoid hyperplasia of the salivary gland.

Differential Diagnosis

The major differential diagnosis of cystic lymphoid hyperplasia is with MALT lymphoma. The absence of interfollicular expanses of marginal zone (centrocyte-like or monocytoid B) cells is the most important histologic feature in this differential diagnosis, because MALT lymphomas may have virtually all the features described in the cystic lymphoepithelial lesion. In MALT lymphomas, the neoplastic cells are the small B cells and marginal zone cells in the interfollicular region, and evidence of expansion of this compartment is the most important morphologic clue to the diagnosis. The presence of broad sheets or zones

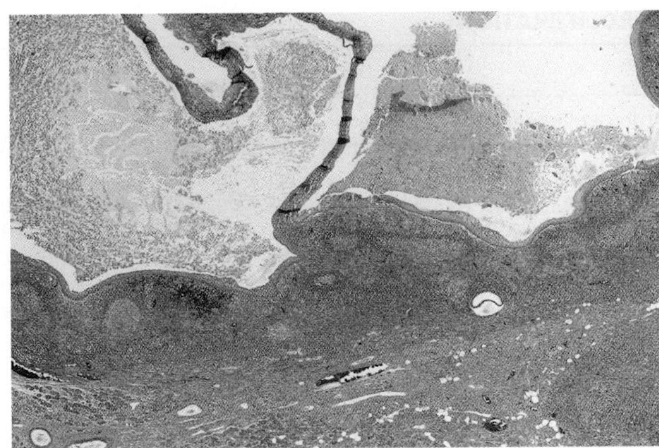

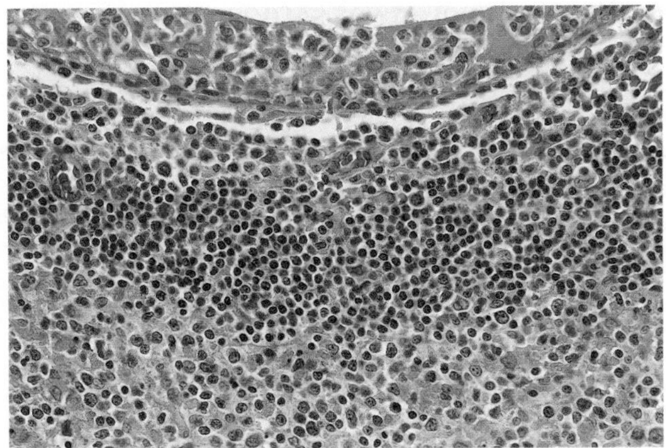

FIGURE 25. Cystic lymphoid hyperplasia of the salivary gland in a patient with HIV infection. **A:** There is dilatation of large salivary ducts, surrounded by prominent reactive follicles, but without expansion of marginal zones. **B:** There is infiltration of the ductal epithelium by lymphocytes.

of plasma cells also raises the suspicion of MALT lymphoma. If features suspicious for MALT lymphoma are present, immunophenotyping should be done; if both lymphocytes and plasma cells are polyclonal, particularly in the setting of HIV infection, the lesion may be considered benign.

Cystic lymphoid hyperplasia also must be distinguished from simple lymphoepithelial cysts (not associated with AIDS) and from Warthin's tumor. The former are unilocular, usually arising in an intraparotid lymph node, are lined by either columnar or squamous epithelium without infiltrating lymphocytes, and do not contain lymphoepithelial lesions. The latter shows characteristic bilayered oncocytic epithelium, with an inner columnar and outer basaloid layer, usually forming papillary, ductal, or slit-like structures, without lymphoid cells infiltrating the epithelium; again, lymphoepithelial lesions are not seen.

Lymphoepithelial Sialadenitis and Sjögren's Syndrome

Terminology and Clinical Features

This distinctive pathologic lesion of the salivary glands has a long history and has gone by many names (Table 10). Johann Mikulicz, in 1892, reported a 42-year-old man with symmetrical enlargement of the lacrimal and salivary glands [cited by Morgan and Castleman (294)]. Although he considered this as a benign disease of unknown etiology, excluding other specifically known causes of salivary or lacrimal gland enlargement, later investigators used the heading *Mikulicz's disease* or *Mikulicz's syndrome* for heterogeneous disorders producing salivary or lacrimal gland enlargement, including lymphoma and infectious diseases. In 1952, Godwin reported the pathologic features of 10 cases of lymphoid infiltrates of the salivary glands, consisting of both lymphoid hyperplasia and epithelial alterations, which he suggested was the pathologic lesion of what had come to be called *Mikulicz's disease.* He coined the term *benign lymphoepithelial lesion* (BLEL), and suggested that it replace the term *Mikulicz disease* (295).

In 1953, Morgan and Castleman, who failed to cite Godwin's report of the year before, described the histologic features of 18 additional cases, and suggested that this specific pathologic entity be called *Mikulicz's disease* (294). Morgan and Castleman found that a prominent component of this lesion was an alteration of the salivary ducts in the centers of the lobules, consisting of "an increase and piling up of nuclei with . . . loss of polarity in the position of the epithelial cells but also external to them, yet within the basement membrane, in a location which normally would be accorded to myoepithelial cells . . . resulting in a thickening of the layer of cells between the basement membrane and the lumen . . . and . . . narrowing of the lumen . . . This disorganization was . . . increased by the migration of lymphoid cells into the altered ducts . . . The involved ducts assumed the form of solid, branching, densely cellular cords lying in a stroma or sea of lymphoid tissue." They coined the term *epimyoepithelial islands* for these altered ducts, because of the belief that both epithelial and myoepithelial cells were present. They observed that 15 of their 18 patients were women, mostly middle aged, and questioned whether this disorder might be related to Hashimoto's thyroiditis, another lymphocytic infiltrate that affected older women. They were more impressed, however, by the similarities between their patients and those reported by Sjögren (296), and concluded that Mikulicz's disease was "merely one manifestation of a more generalized symptom complex known as Sjögren's syndrome." The clinical syndrome described by Sjögren as "keratoconjunctivitis sicca," and that has come to be known as Sjögren's syndrome, is characterized by dry eyes and dry mouth, variable enlargement of salivary and lacrimal glands, and the frequent presence of serum autoantibodies of various types and other connective tissue diseases, such as rheumatoid arthritis.

With the advent of immunophenotyping studies in the 1970s and 1980s and the recognition that many of these lymphoid proliferations were in fact low-grade lymphomas (297,298), and not benign, the term *benign lymphoepithelial lesion* has fallen out of favor. The term *myoepithelial sialadenitis* was later introduced for the histopathologic lesion (298). However, it is now known that the spindle-shaped cells involved in these lesions are not myoepithelial cells, but rather basal epithelial cells. The term *lymphoepithelial lesion* is now widely used to refer to the structures pro-

TABLE 10. TERMINOLOGY OF SALIVARY GLAND LYMPHOID PROLIFERATIONS

Term	Definition
Mikulicz's disease	Chronic enlargement of the lacrimal and/or salivary glands with a characteristic morphology (epimyoepithelial islands and lymphoid hyperplasia)
Mikulicz's syndrome	Enlargement of the salivary and/or lacrimal glands for any reason
Sjögren's syndrome (keratoconjunctivitis sicca, sicca syndrome, sicca complex)	A complex exocrinopathy with dry eyes, dry mouth, often with swelling of salivary and lacrimal glands; may be associated with rheumatoid arthritis; all patients have microscopic evidence of myoepithelial sialadenitis.
Benign lymphoepithelial lesion	Another term for the salivary gland lesion of Mikulicz's disease. The term *lymphoepithelial lesion* is also used for focal ductal or mucosal infiltrates of lymphoid cells in mucosa-associated lymphoid tissue (MALT) or in MALT type lymphomas.
Myoepithelial sialadenitis (MESA) Suggested new term: Lymphoepithelial sialadenitis (LESA)	Another term for the salivary gland infiltrate of Mikulicz's disease.
Epimyoephelial island Suggested new term: Lymphoepithelial lesion	A term given by Morgan and Castleman for the characteristic proliferative ductal lesion of Mikulicz's disease; initially thought to represent a mixed proliferation of epithelial and myoepithelial cells with infiltrating lymphocytes; now known to be predominantly epithelial.
Monocytoid B cell	A B cell with an irregular or folded nucleus and abundant, pale cytoplasm, resembling a monocyte, found in parafollicular and perisinusoidal aggregates in some cases of florid follicular hyperplasia of lymph nodes (toxoplasma lymphadenitis); often postulated to be a post-germinal center memory B cell.
Marginal zone B cell	A B cell found in the marginal zone of the spleen and Peyer's patch follicles; nucleus resembles that of a centrocyte, with a moderate amount of pale cytoplasm; resembles a monocytoid B cell, but typically smaller; rearranged and mutated Ig genes consistent with a postgerminal center, memory B cell.
Centrocyte-like cell	A B cell found in MALT type lymphomas; nucleus resembles that of a centrocyte, with a moderate amount of pale cytoplasm; resembles a monocytoid B cell, but typically smaller; thought to correspond to a marginal zone B cell of Peyer's patch. Now synonymous with marginal zone B cell.

duced by marginal zone or monocytoid B cells infiltrating the epithelium in normal MALT or in MALT lymphomas of other sites (299). Therefore, it seems reasonable at this time to drop the terms *epimyoepithelial island* and *myeoepithelial sialadenitis* in favor of the terms *lymphoepithelial lesion* and *lymphoepithelial sialadenitis.*

Virtually all patients who fit the clinical definition of Sjögren's syndrome have LESA; however, only 50% of patients with LESA have Sjögren's syndrome. Patients with other connective tissue diseases (particularly rheumatoid arthritis) may develop LESA, and it may occur as isolated salivary gland enlargement in patients without any other associated diseases. In this review, the term *LESA/Sjögren's syndrome* will be used to encompass both patients with Sjögren's syndrome, all of whom have LESA, and patients with LESA without Sjögren's syndrome.

Morphologic Features

Lymphoepithelial sialadenitis is characterized by a lymphoid infiltrate with follicular hyperplasia, surrounding and infiltrating salivary ducts, with disorganization and proliferation of the ductal epithelial cells to form lymphoepithelial lesions, and with corresponding atrophy of acinar tissue (Fig. 26). The lobular architecture of the gland is preserved. Lymphoepithelial lesions are most prominent in the parotid gland; they may be absent in submandibular and minor salivary glands and in the lacrimal glands. Although a number of studies suggested that the cells comprising these structures were predominantly myoepithelial (300,301), the weight of current evidence suggests that they are basal epithelial cells of large intrasalivary ducts (302–304). Cystically dilated salivary ducts may be present, but they are less striking than in HIV-related cystic lymphoid hyperplasia. Reactive follicles are prominent; they have large germinal centers, often irregular in outline, with a prominent starry sky pattern, and do not show expansion of the mantle or marginal zones. The interfollicular regions show small lymphocytes, scattered immunoblasts, and often numerous plasma cells, usually not in broad sheets. The process is typically diffuse or multifocal within the gland, but islands of normal acini are often preserved.

The lymphoepithelial islands contain lymphoid cells of monocytoid or marginal zone type. Monocytoid B cells are medium-sized cells with lobated or indented nuclei and abundant, pale cytoplasm, often with distinct cell borders, resembling peripheral blood monocytes (305). Marginal zone B cells resemble monocytoid B cells and are thought to be related to them (306–308); they are slightly smaller, with nuclei that resemble centrocytes (cleaved cells) of the germinal center, and pale cytoplasm that is less distinct than that of monocytoid B cells. These cells were called centrocyte-like cells by Isaacson and Wright (299,309). Lennert (310) and others have concluded that at least a subset of centrocyte-like cells may be identical to monocytoid B cells. Both types of cells are thought to be post–germinal center memory B cells with the capacity to differentiate into plasma cells, although this has not been proven except in the spleen (311). Although usage varies among experts, the term *monocytoid*

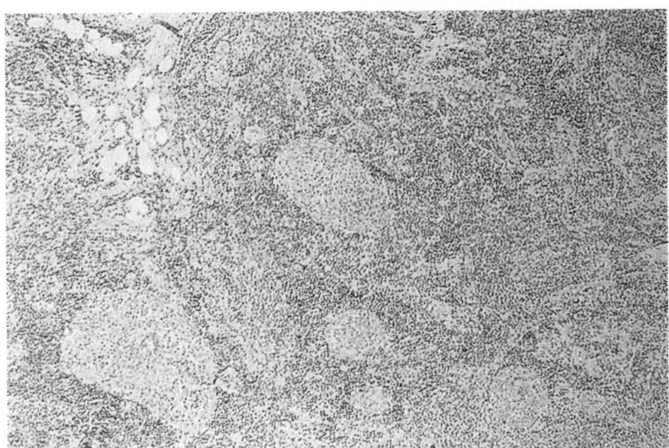

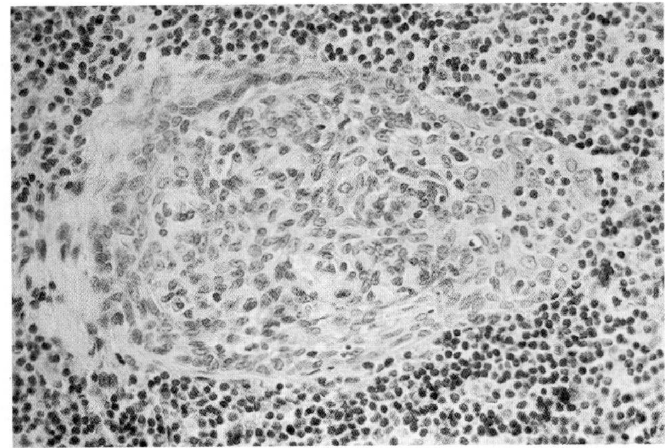

FIGURE 26. Lymphoepithelial sialadenitis. **A:** There is a prominent lymphoid infiltrate with obliteration of acini. **B:** Lymphoepithelial lesion showing rare monocytoid B cells within but not around the epithelium.

B cell is used here to refer to a cell identical to those seen in *Toxoplasma* lymphadenitis, and the term *marginal zone B cell* is used to refer to a smaller cell with less nuclear irregularity and less cytoplasm than a typical monocytoid cell, but larger and with more cytoplasm than a small lymphocyte.

Marginal zone B cells are seen in the majority of MALT lymphomas; monocytoid B cells are less universal, and both marginal zone and monocytoid B cells may be present in the same tumor. For this reason, the REAL Classification uses the term *extranodal marginal zone B-cell lymphoma of MALT type, with or without monocytoid B cells* to describe this disorder (86). Although MALT lymphomas of other sites may have only marginal zone cells with no typical monocytoid B cells, the salivary gland and lymph node lymphomas in patients with Sjögren's syndrome or LESA typically have prominent aggregates of typical monocytoid B cells (312,313).

In LESA uncomplicated by lymphoma, the monocytoid or marginal zone B cells are found in aggregates within the lymphoepithelial lesions, and they are typically restricted to this location (Fig. 26B) (314). A narrow rim of these cells may be present around the epithelium, but this is usually no more than one or two cells thick. Nests or aggregates of monocytoid B cells are not found within the diffuse lymphoid infiltrate; if they are present, they should raise the possibility of MALT lymphoma. Varying degrees of hyalinization may be present within the lymphoepithelial lesions, and in long-standing cases, they may be completely sclerotic (294).

Differential Diagnosis

The most important differential diagnosis of LESA is MALT lymphoma. The most important features in the differential diagnosis with MALT lymphoma are the number and distribution of monocytoid B cells. Monocytoid B cells in LESA are typically confined to the lymphepithelial lesions and are not found in large clusters or sheets. They are present in aggregates within the epithelial nests, and may form small rings or cuffs around them, but are not present in large aggregates, sheets, or strands outside of the epithelium. If monocytoid B cells are found outside of the lymphoepithelial lesions, either in the form of broad halos around lymphoepithelial lesions, or particularly as broad, anastomosing strands, a diagnosis of MALT lymphoma should be suspected (314–318). A second important feature is the presence of sheets of plasma cells, with or without Dutcher bodies. Either of these features should prompt the performance of immunophenotyping studies to determine whether either the lymphocytic or the plasma cell component expresses monotypic immunoglobulin.

Lymphoepithelial sialadenitis also must be distinguished from other types of chronic sialadenitis. The most important features defining LESA are the presence of ducts with infiltrating lymphocytes, lymphoepithelial lesions, and a dense lymphoid infiltrate with prominent germinal centers and destruction of acini.

Etiology

Lymphoepithelial sialadenitis is believed to be an autoimmune disease. Although EBV has been suggested as an etiologic agent, this has not been confirmed in the majority of cases (319). Hepatitis C virus has been associated with LESA in a small number of cases (320). This finding is intriguing, because hepatitis C has been associated with other conditions that overlap autoimmune disorders and low-grade B-cell lymphomas, such as Waldenstrom's macroglobulinemia and cryoglobulinemia (321). An increased incidence of LESA has been reported in patients with HIV infection (292).

Clinical Features and Relationship to MALT-type Lymphoma

Patients with LESA/Sjögren's syndrome are typically women (>80%), with a broad age range, but with a median in the sixth decade. They present with sicca syndrome (dry eyes and dry mouth), parotid swelling, or both. The parotid glands are usually most prominently involved, but the disease also affects submandibular and minor salivary glands.

Many studies have shown an association between LESA/Sjögren's syndrome and lymphoma. Most studies prior to

1980 considered only the risk of extrasalivary lymphoma or high-grade lymphoma of the salivary gland, because the possibility that the low-grade lymphoid infiltrates in the salivary gland were themselves neoplastic had not been recognized. Talal first reported the association in 1967 (322). In 1976, Kassan and associates provided the first estimate of the risk in a large group of patients: in 136 women they found 7 extrasalivary lymphomas, a relative risk of 44 compared with the normal population (323). The most important risk factor in that series was parotid irradiation, probably an indicator for symptomatic salivary gland enlargement and an underlying low-grade lymphoma. Overall, approximately 4% to 7% of patients with either Sjögren's syndrome or LESA will eventually develop overt extrasalivary lymphoma (297,324).

With the advent of immunophenotyping studies, it was recognized that many cases considered to be BLEL/MESA actually had monotypic immunoglobulin and were therefore probably neoplastic (297). It was then possible to examine the relative frequency of salivary versus extrasalivary and low- versus high-grade lymphomas in these patients. Overall, in salivary glands with LESA, various researchers have found that 25% to 80% have morphologic or immunophenotypic evidence of low-grade MALT lymphoma in the salivary gland (298,315,317,325). Of these, 10% to 45% developed extrasalivary lymphoma, often after very long intervals. The risk of developing extrasalivary lymphoma is closely related to the presence of either broad strands of monocytoid B cells between the lymphoepithelial lesions or the presence of monotypic immunoglobulin light chain expression by either lymphoid cells or plasma cells (298,315,317,325). Both broad strands and prominent halos of monocytoid B cells are highly correlated with monotypic Ig expression (Table 11).

In contrast to the detection of monoclonality by light chain expression, detection of B-cell clones in salivary gland lesions by Southern blot or PCR analysis of immunoglobulin gene rearrangement has not proven to be a reliable predictor of clinical behavior in LESA/Sjögren's syndrome. Fishleder and associates in 1987 (326) reported that Southern blot analysis of 10 salivary gland biopsy samples from patients with LESA/Sjögren's syndrome showed clonally rearranged immunoglobulin genes in all cases; however, this did not correlate with either morphologic or clinical evidence of lymphoma. Furthermore, one of two cases with sequential biopsies showed an unrelated clone in the second biopsy. This study led to the concept that LESA/Sjögren's syndrome may be a setting in which oligoclonal populations of B cells may arise, one of which may eventually become dominant, resulting in overt lymphoma. Subsequent studies, however, have shown a smaller proportion of cases to be monoclonal: in three studies, most using PCR, on over 100 patients, an average of 60% of the cases had clonal immunoglobulin gene rearrangements (315,319,325), and in patients with more than one biopsy, the majority have shown the same clone in sequential biopsies (319,325). Recently, however, Lasota and colleagues (327) documented the emergence of a second distinct clone over a 9-year period in a single patient with Sjögren's syndrome: one clone was found in two sequential biopsies, whereas a second, unrelated clone was found in a third. In addition, Bahler and Swerdlow (328) found three of seven (43%) patients to have different clones in sequential biopsies and one patient with emergence of a second clone together with the original clone. Taken together, these studies suggest that oligoclonality with outgrowth of sequential clones may occur early in LESA/Sjögren's syndrome, but that once an overt, monoclonal lymphoma develops, subsequent tumors are more often recurrences than second tumors.

Despite the detection of monoclonality in a high proportion of the cases, none of these studies showed a correlation between clonality as determined by immunoglobulin gene rearrangement and either morphologic or clinical evidence of lymphoma (315,325). Thus, it appears that molecular genetic analysis has little or no practical role in the clinical diagnosis of salivary gland lymphoma in a setting of LESA/Sjögren's syndrome (Table 12).

Lymphomas of the Salivary Glands

Lymphomas comprise 2% to 5% of salivary gland neoplasms. Approximately 20% are associated with Sjögren's syndrome or LESA. In one report, 35% were large cell lymphoma (usually diffuse large B-cell lymphoma), 35% were follicular lymphoma, and 30% were other low-grade lymphomas [50% associated with either Sjögren's syndrome or LESA (329)]. The parotid gland is most commonly involved, accounting for 70% of the cases, followed by the submandibular (25%), sublingual, and minor salivary glands (<10%). In the earlier literature, cases associated with LESA/Sjögren's syndrome were typically described as small lymphocytic or lymphoplasmacytoid lymphomas in the Working Formulation or Kiel Classification, whereas *de novo*

TABLE 11. LYMPHOEPITHELIAL SIALADENITIS/SJÖGREN'S SYNDROME: CORRELATION OF MORPHOLOGY, IMMUNOPHENOTYPE, AND OUTCOME

		Monocytoid B Cells		Monotypic Ig and Monocytoid B Cells		Extrasalivary Lymphoma		
	N	Halos	Strands	Halos	Strands	Total	MBC Strands	MoIg
Hyjek (1988)	17	NA	53%	NA	100%	10%	11%	11%
Hsi (1995)	23	22%	26%	36%	67%	17%	67%	100%
Quintana (1997)	46	18%	51%	22%	24%	15%	44%	33%

Ig, immunoglobulin; MoIg, monotypic immunoglobulin; MBC, monocytoid B cells.

TABLE 12. LYMPHOEPITHELIAL SIALADENITIS/SJÖGREN'S SYNDROME: MOLECULAR GENETIC ANALYSIS OF CLONALITY

	Method	Specimens (Patients)	Clonal	Sequential Biopsies	Same Clone	Correlation	
						Morphology	Outcome
Fishleder (1987)	Southern blot	10 (8)	100%	2	50%	No	No
Diss (1995)	PCR	62 (45)	56%	7	100%	Yes	No
Hsi (1996)	PCR	28 (22)	57%	6	NA	No	No
Quintana (1997)	PCR	52 (46)	63%	14	100%	No	No

PCR, polymerase chain reaction.

cases were more commonly follicular lymphomas or large cell lymphomas of the types usually found in lymph nodes (329,330).

Marginal Zone B-cell/MALT Lymphoma

Morphologic Features

Mucosa-associated lymphoid tissue lymphoma of the salivary gland typically produces a dense lymphoid infiltrate, with obliteration of acini (Fig. 27). The lesion may form a localized mass or diffusely involve the gland. Similarly to LESA, lymphoid follicles with reactive germinal centers are usually present; lymphoepithelial lesions are usually prominent and contain clusters of monocytoid B cells. In contrast to LESA, monocytoid B cells usually form broad halos around the epithelial cell nests, and extend away from them in broad strands, often linking together several lymphoepithelial lesions (317,318,325). Thus, in LESA, the low-power impression is predominantly that of follicular hyperplasia and lymphoepithelial lesions, whereas in MALT it is of broad, diffuse sheets of lymphoid cells expanding the interfollicular region. Reactive follicles are often present, but may in some cases be infiltrated or overrun by marginal zone/monocytoid B cells (follicular colonization), giving the appearance in some cases of a follicular lymphoma (331). Occasionally, the neoplastic cells appear to undergo blastic transformation within the reactive follicles. Aggregates of epithelioid histiocytes may be present. Scattered immunoblasts and plasma cells are typically present in the interfollicular region. Plasma cells are often nu-

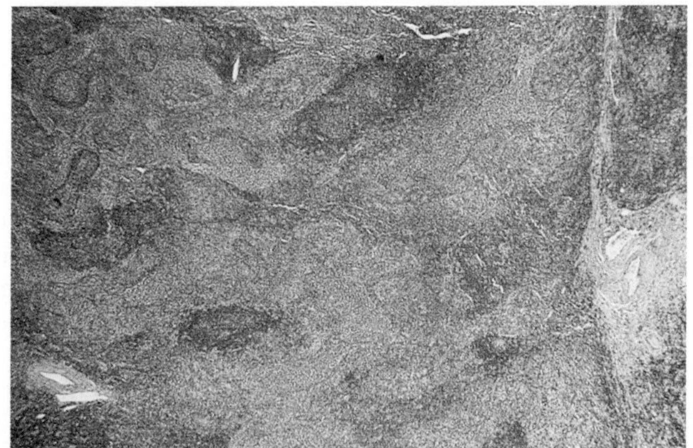
A

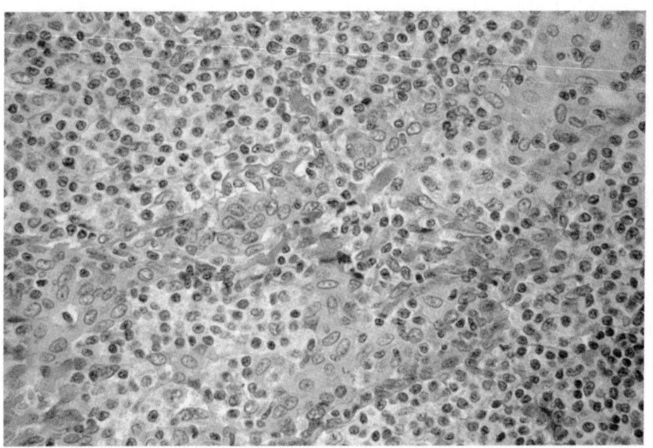
B

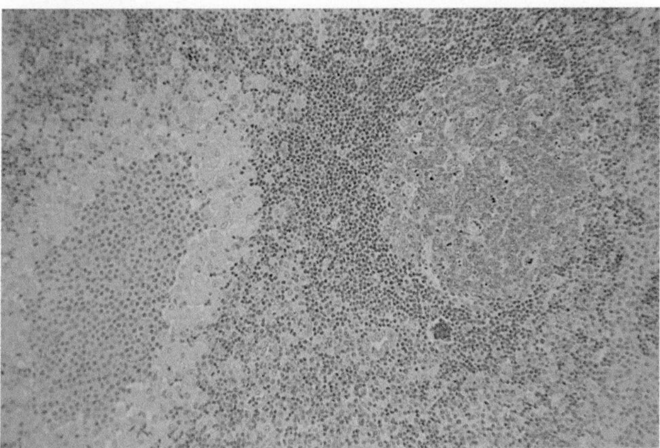
C

FIGURE 27. Extranodal marginal zone B-cell/mucosa-associated lymphoid tissue (MALT) lymphoma of the salivary gland. There is a dense, destructive lymphoid infiltrate with no preserved acini. **A:** At low magnification, there are broad strands of pale cells surrounding and extending away from lymphoepithelial lesions, alternating with dark areas containing small lymphocytes. **B:** At high magnification, monocytoid B cells are seen both within and around a lymphoepithelial lesion. **C:** Lymph node from a patient with Sjögren's syndrome and a MALT lymphoma of the salivary gland, showing a nest of monocytoid B cells surrounded by epithelioid histiocytes.

merous and may be scattered singly or may form confluent sheets.

Intraparotid or cervical nodes may be involved; these often show partial preservation of the architecture, with open sinuses and reactive follicles, with prominent clusters of monocytoid B cells in the perifollicular region. A feature that seems to be peculiar to lymph node involvement by the MALT lymphoma associated with LESA/Sjögren's syndrome is the presence of tight clusters of monocytoid B cells surrounded by epithelioid histiocytes (Fig. 27C).

Immunophenotype

Mucosa-associated lymphoid tissue lymphomas of the salivary glands express monotypic surface immunoglobulin (lymphocytes and monocytoid B cells), and in the majority of the cases plasma cells are also monoclonal. They express pan B-cell antigens (CD20, CD22) and lack CD5 and CD10. They are cyclin D1 negative. Expression of CD43 and CD23 is variable. Lack of CD5 is useful in distinguishing these tumors from B-cell small lymphocytic lymphoma and MCL, lack of CD10 in distinguishing them from follicular lymphoma. Absence of cyclin D1 is useful in ruling out MCL.

Staining with antibodies against FDCs reveals follicular aggregates of FDCs associated with reactive follicles or remnants of colonized follicles. In distinction from follicular lymphoma, staining with immunoglobulin light chains is useful in determining whether the follicles are neoplastic; *bcl-2* is also useful. However, MALT lymphomas with follicular colonization can present a problem in the differential diagnosis, because these may show light chain restriction in the follicles. Staining for *bcl-2* may still be useful, however, because neoplastic marginal zone cells within the follicles are reported to be *bcl-2* negative, even when the extrafollicular cells are positive (332–335).

Genetic Features

The majority of the cases have clonal rearrangements of the immunoglobulin genes. The variable (V) regions of the immunoglobulin genes show somatic mutation (336), indicating a post–germinal center stage of differentiation, consistent with a memory B cell. However, when the PCR products are cloned and sequenced, there is intraclonal variation, indicating ongoing somatic mutation (327,336); this property is thought to belong only to germinal center cells, but has been reported in MALT lymphomas of other sites as well (337,338). The germline variable region families used by the salivary MALT lymphomas resemble those seen in autoantibodies and in other neoplasms such as Waldenstrom's macroglobulinemia and B-SLL/CLL (339), consistent with an autoimmune-mediated process. An oncogene associated with MALT lymphoma has not been described. Trisomy 3 and translocation t(11;18)(q21;q21) have been reported in 60% to 80% and in 20% to 50% of salivary and gastric cases, respectively (340–344).

Clinical Features

As described above, MALT lymphomas of the salivary gland typically arise in a setting of LESA, with or without Sjögren's syndrome. The age and sex distribution is similar to that of Sjögren's syndrome, with a predominance of older women. MALT lymphomas of the salivary gland, like MALT lymphomas in other sites, are indolent lymphomas that may remain stable and minimally symptomatic for long periods. However, as noted above, there is a significant risk of both extrasalivary dissemination (20%–45% of the cases) and high-grade transformation.

The most common sites of extrasalivary spread are cervical lymph nodes, although other extranodal sites, such as the stomach, lung, and skin, are also common, and distant lymph node or bone marrow involvement may occur. For the most part, extrasalivary spread is also of the low-grade B-cell type (75%–80%), consistent with recurrent MALT lymphoma; of the 15% to 25% of high-grade lymphomas that have developed in the reported series, most were diffuse large B-cell lymphomas, presumed to represent high-grade transformation of the MALT lymphoma. Cases of Waldenstrom's macroglobulinemia also have been reported (323). There are also several reports of peripheral T-cell lymphomas developing in patients with Sjögren's syndrome or salivary gland MALT lymphoma, involving skin, lymph nodes, and other extranodal sites, most of which have behaved aggressively (314,345–347).

The majority of extrasalivary lymphomas in these patients do not result in significant morbidity or mortality, with or without treatment (298,314,315,317,318,346). Thus, the decision of whether or not and how to treat salivary MALT lymphoma in these patients is not straightforward. It appears that the most compelling reason to treat would be to prevent the development of high-grade lymphoma; however, there are no data that address the efficacy of treatment in preventing high-grade transformation.

Follicular Lymphoma

Occurrence

Thirty-five percent to 50% of salivary gland lymphomas are follicular lymphomas (329,330,348), usually involving intrasalivary lymph nodes. When follicular lymphoma does involve the salivary gland parenchyma, it is usually present in lymph nodes as well, and staging often reveals distant disease (348). Follicular lymphoma also has been reported arising in or involving Warthin's tumors of the parotid gland (349).

Morphology

Follicular lymphomas of the salivary gland most often produce a circumscribed mass, which can often be identified as a lymph node by virtue of some residual architecture, such as a subcapsular sinus. However, extensive parenchymal involvement also may occur (Fig. 28). In contrast to MALT lymphomas, ductal structures are inconspicuous, and when present, appear normal, without prominent lymphoid infiltration. However, occasional lymphoepithelial lesions can occur in salivary glands involved by follicular lymphoma. The histologic features are similar to those of follicular lymphoma in lymph nodes, with a uniform proliferation of follicles, often with little intervening lymphoid tissue (Fig. 28A). At high magnification, the follicles typically have a predominance of centrocytes, with rare centroblasts; lack a starry sky pattern, mitotic activity, and polarization; and often lack well-formed mantle zones (Figs. 16A,B and 28B).

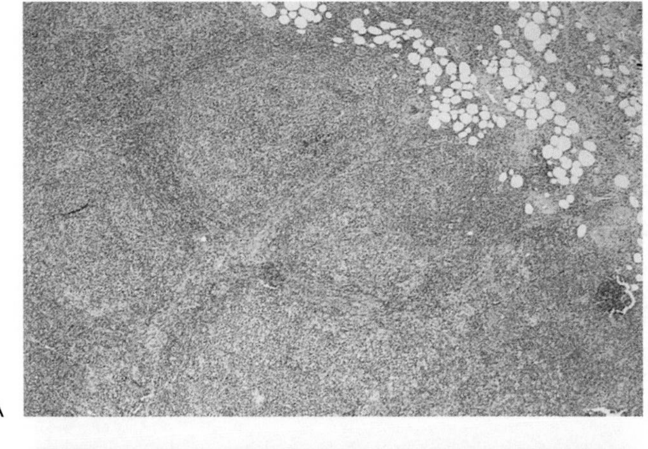
A

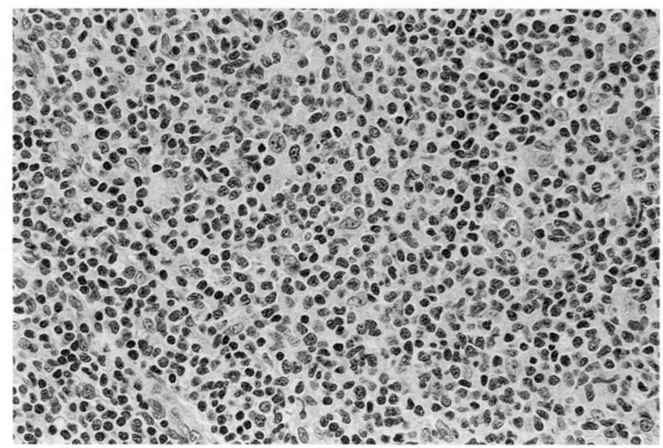
B

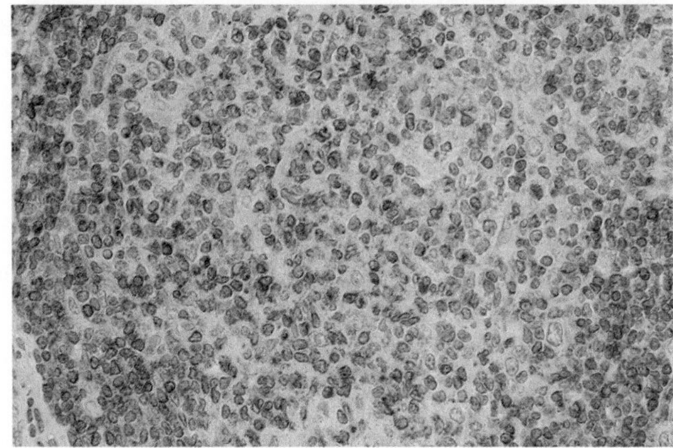
C

FIGURE 28. Follicular lymphoma of the salivary gland. **A:** At low magnification, there is an infiltrate of closely packed follicles. **B:** At high magnification, the follicles contain predominantly centrocytes, giving them a monomorphous appearance. **C:** Immunohistochemical stain for *Bcl-2* shows positive cells in the follicle, confirming the diagnosis of follicular lymphoma.

Immunophenotype and Genetic Features

Neoplastic follicles typically show immunoglobulin light chain restriction on frozen sections, and are usually *Bcl-2* positive on both frozen and paraffin sections (Fig. 28C). CD10 may be present in about 50% of the cases. CD43 is typically negative. Southern blot or PCR reveals *bcl-2* gene rearrangement in most cases.

Aggressive Lymphomas

Most aggressive lymphomas in the salivary glands are diffuse large B-cell lymphomas, but rare cases of peripheral T-cell lymphoma, lymphoblastic lymphoma, and Burkitt-like lymphoma have been reported. It is not known how many of the diffuse large B-cell lymphomas arise from preexisting MALT lymphomas and how many are of nodal type or represent transformation of follicular lymphoma. Diffuse large B-cell lymphoma produces a diffuse, destructive infiltrate, composed of cells that are typically at least two to three times the size of normal lymphocytes, with mitotic activity. The differential diagnosis includes other poorly differentiated malignant tumors, particularly lymphoepithelioma-like carcinoma and melanoma. Demonstration of leukocyte-associated antigens (CD45, CD20) and absence of cytokeratins and other nonlymphoid markers can be useful in the differential diagnosis.

LYMPHOID PROLIFERATIONS OF THE THYROID

The two major types of lymphoid proliferations found in the thyroid gland are Hashimoto's thyroiditis and lymphoma. As in the salivary gland, there is considerable evidence to suggest that many primary thyroid lymphomas arise in a background of acquired MALT associated with chronic inflammation. Thyroiditis is covered in Chapter 9. In this section, we will focus on the development and differential diagnosis of lymphoma.

Hashimoto's Thyroiditis

Lymphocytic (Hashimoto's) thyroiditis is an autoimmune disease of the thyroid, in which antibodies to thyroglobulin result in destruction of the thyroid epithelium and hypothyroidism (350). The thyroid gland is the major source of the autoantibodies (351). Hashimoto's thyroiditis is characterized by a lymphoid infiltrate that consists of reactive B-cell follicles with prominent germinal centers, interfollicular plasma cells, and scattered interfollicular T cells (Fig. 29) (352–354). The T cells are predominantly of the CD4-positive (helper) type (355). Plasma cells are present around and within the follicles, and immune complexes can be seen in the follicular basement membrane (353,354,356). Lymphoid cells may surround and infil-

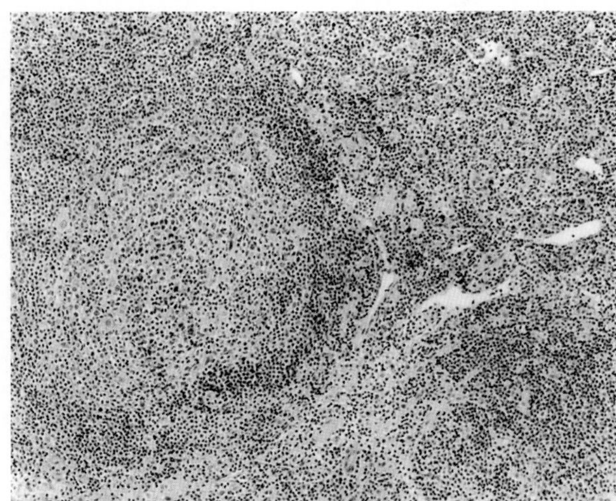
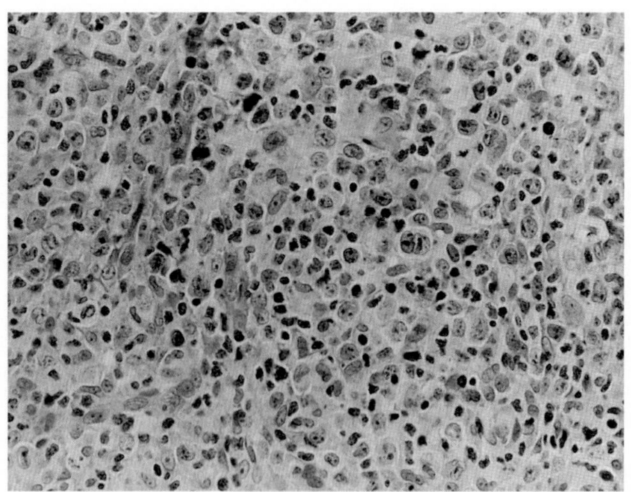

FIGURE 29. Diffuse large B-cell lymphoma of the thyroid associated with Hashimoto's thyroiditis. **A:** A reactive lymphoid follicle with a germinal center, surrounded by a diffuse infiltrate of small lymphocytes, with extensive destruction of the thyroid epithelium. **B:** Elsewhere in the thyroid, there was diffuse involvement by lymphoma. The neoplastic cells are predominantly large, resembling centroblasts and immunoblasts. There are admixed smaller cells as well as reactive histiocytes.

trate the thyroid follicles, producing so-called lymphoepithelial lesions (353,355); however, these are usually inconspicuous and consist predominantly of T cells (352). Thyroid follicular cells typically become eosinophilic (Hürthle cell or oxyphil change), and eventually thyroid follicles are destroyed and replaced by fibrous tissue. Thyroid epithelium in areas of dense lymphoid infiltration acquires HLA-Dr antigens, which are not found on normal thyroid epithelial cells and may be associated with immunologically mediated destruction of these cells (354). The acquired lymphoid tissue in the thyroid thus has morphologic features consistent with MALT (353).

Patients with Hashimoto's thyroiditis are at increased risk for development of lymphoma of the thyroid; the overall risk of lymphoma is greater than threefold, and that of thyroid lymphoma is estimated to be at least 70-fold greater than that for the normal population; if low-grade MALT-type lymphomas are considered, the risk may be even greater (357–359). The lymphomas that develop are typically primary in the thyroid. In some cases, the same immunoglobulin heavy and light chains have been recognized in both the low-grade and high-grade components, suggesting that apparently primary large cell lymphoma of the thyroid arises from a low-grade lymphoma in at least some of the cases (353,360). Studies assessing the status of the immunoglobulin gene in cases of Hashimoto's thyroiditis have failed to demonstrate evidence of clonal rearrangement (352,355), in contrast to studies on the lymphoid infiltrates in the salivary glands in Sjögren's syndrome (325,326,361).

Lymphomas of the Thyroid

Classification

Lymphoma comprises approximately 5% of thyroid neoplasms, and the thyroid accounted for 2.5% of extranodal lymphomas in the series of Freeman and associates (94). Most series in the earlier literature report a predominance of diffuse large-cell lymphoma (362–365); however, with the advent of immunophenotyping studies and recognition of lymphomas of small lymphoid cells in extranodal sites, a higher proportion of low-grade lymphomas has been recognized. Studies since 1977 have shown 30% to 80% of primary thyroid lymphomas to be of low-grade types (366–373). In studies using the Rappaport classification or Working Formulation, the low-grade types have been classified predominantly as follicular or diffuse small cleaved or mixed types, small lymphocytic, and intermediate lymphocytic (367). In studies using the Kiel Classification, most cases were initially classified as centroblastic/centrocytic, follicular, or diffuse, often with plasmacytoid differentiation (366), with a smaller number called lymphoplasmacytic or centrocytic (369,370,372). Ultimately, these lymphomas were recognized by Isaacson and colleagues as a distinctive lymphoma arising from and replicating many features of MALT (extranodal marginal zone B-cell lymphoma of the MALT type) (353,374). Although there has not been a recent reevaluation of a large series of unselected primary thyroid lymphomas, it is likely that most cases previously reported as centroblastic/centrocytic, centrocytic, follicular, intermediate lymphocytic, small lymphocytic, and lymphoplasmacytic lymphomas of the thyroid are actually examples of what is now known as extranodal marginal zone B-cell lymphoma of the MALT type (86).

Extranodal Marginal Zone (MALT) Lymphoma

Morphologic Features

The morphologic features of MALT lymphoma of the thyroid gland are similar to those of the salivary gland and other sites. Reactive follicles with germinal centers are often prominent, and the interfollicular region contains a polymorphous infiltrate of lymphocytes, marginal zone B cells with irregular nuclei and pale cytoplasm, and plasma cells. Both marginal zone B cells and plasma cells surround and infiltrate thyroid follicles, producing

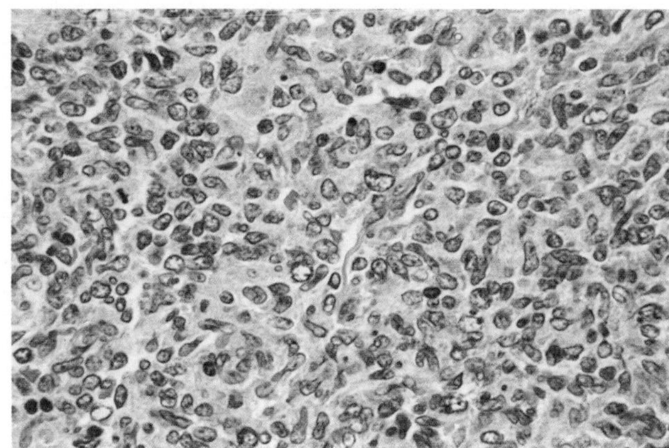

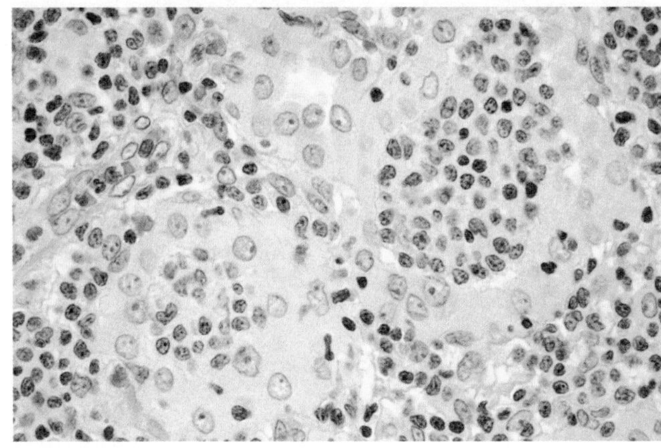

FIGURE 30. Extranodal marginal zone lymphoma of the mucosa-associated lymphoid tissue (MALT) type, involving the thyroid. **A:** At low magnification, there is destruction of the thyroid architecture; both large follicular structures and a diffuse infiltrate of pale cells are present. **B:** The follicle centers contain centroblasts and centroctes, consistent with reactive follicles, but there are increased numbers of small, centrocyte-like cells, which showed immunoglobulin light chain restriction. This is an example of follicular colonization. **C:** A thyroid follicle is infiltrated by small cells with irregular nuclei and abundant cytoplasm, consistent with marginal zone or monocytoid B cells.

lymphoepithelial lesions. Follicular colonization may be prominent, giving the process a follicular pattern, and demonstrating a similarity to follicular lymphoma (Fig. 30). In some cases, the neoplastic cells undergo blast transformation within the germinal centers; although this phenomenon can be seen in MALT lymphomas at any site, it appears to be relatively more common in thyroid lymphomas (331,374).

Immunophenotype and Genetic Features

These are identical to those of MALT lymphomas in other sites (340,343,344,374).

Diffuse Large B-cell Lymphoma

Diffuse large B-cell lymphoma accounted for 20% to 50% of primary thyroid lymphomas in recent series (366,369,371,372). Diffuse large B-cell lymphoma of the thyroid is morphologically and immunophenotypically similar to large B-cell lymphoma in other sites (Fig. 31). In reported series, most cases contain a predominance of centroblast-like cells (centroblastic or large noncleaved cell lymphoma), whereas 10% to 30% are reported to consist predominantly of immunoblasts. In both types, the cells are two to three times the size of a small lymphocyte, with vesicular chromatin, round to oval nuclei, and basophilic cytoplasm. Centroblasts have one to three peripherally located nucleoli and relatively scant cytoplasm, whereas immunoblasts have a prominent central nucleolus and more abundant cytoplasm and may appear plasmacytoid. In the vast majority of cases (70%–100%) in which evaluable uninvolved thyroid tissue is present, there is evidence of Hashimoto's thyroiditis. In an as yet unknown proportion of these, there is a component of marginal zone B-cell lymphoma of the MALT type (353,360).

Burkitt's and Burkitt-like Lymphoma

Many series of thyroid lymphomas contain one or more cases classified as "undifferentiated," "small noncleaved cell," or "lymphoblastic" types (the Kiel Classification equivalent of Burkitt's lymphoma). These account for less than 5% of the reported cases (363,364,366,369–372). Burkitt's lymphoma and Burkitt-like lymphoma of the thyroid are morphologically and immunophenotypically similar to those occurring elsewhere. The cells are smaller than centroblasts or immunoblasts, with round nuclei, rather dark chromatin, and multiple small nucleoli. The cytoplasm is relatively abundant and deeply basophilic, and the cells may have a cohesive growth pattern. A starry-sky pattern of phagocytic histiocytes is typically present. Mitotic activity is brisk and may exceed 10 per 10 high-power fields. The proliferation fraction using antibody to Ki-67 is greater than 99%.

Clinical data were available on only seven of the cases included in the reported series (363,364,366,370–372). The median age was 64 years, but two patients were only 20 years old (one man, one woman). All of the older patients were women.

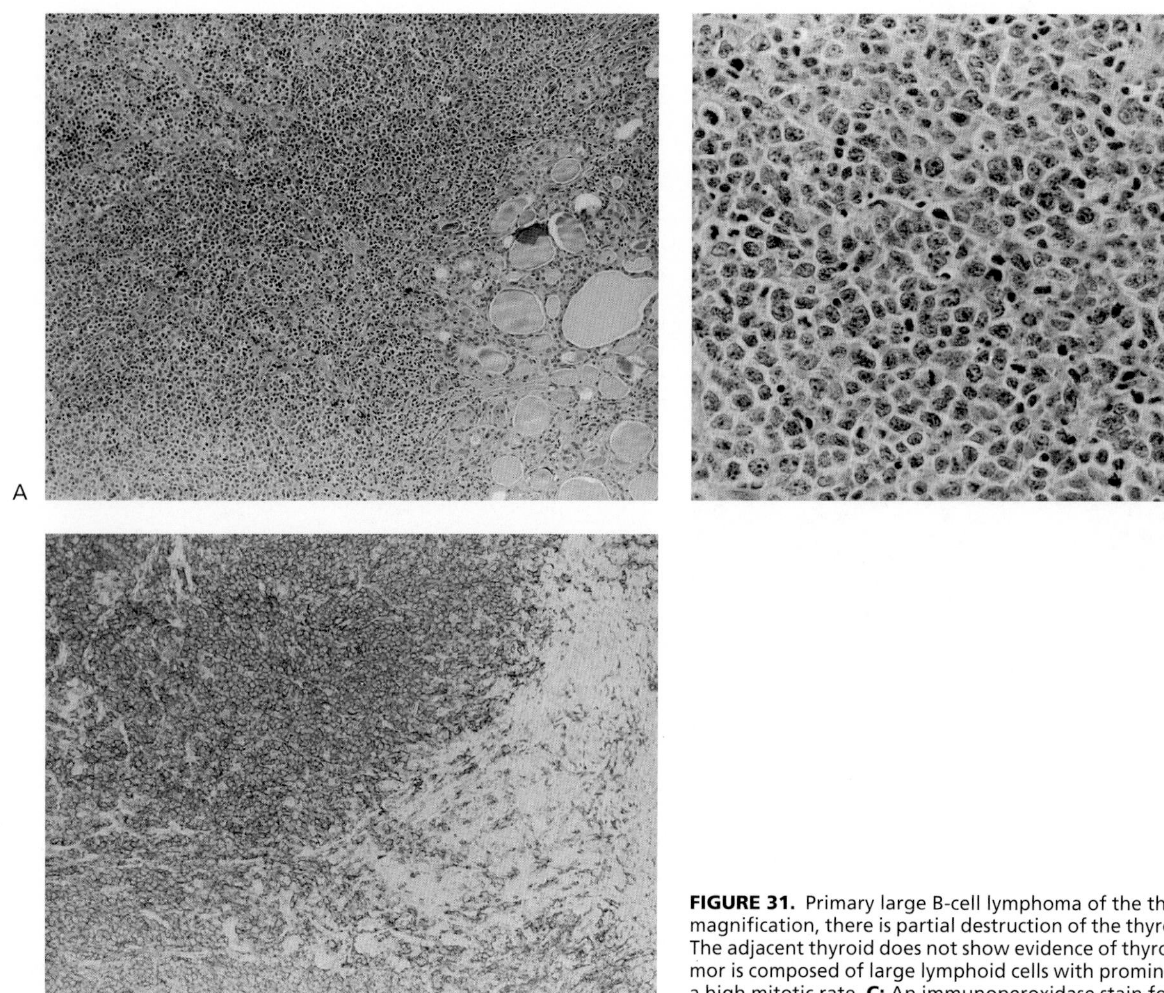

FIGURE 31. Primary large B-cell lymphoma of the thyroid. **A:** At low magnification, there is partial destruction of the thyroid architecture. The adjacent thyroid does not show evidence of thyroiditis. **B:** The tumor is composed of large lymphoid cells with prominent nucleoli and a high mitotic rate. **C:** An immunoperoxidase stain for CD20 confirms the B-cell nature of the neoplasm.

Most patients had disease outside of the thyroid (stage 3 or 4). All of the older patients were dead of disease in less than 1 year. The two younger patients received chemotherapy and radiation, and were both free of disease (at 2 and 3 years).

Plasmacytoma of the Thyroid

Most series of thyroid lymphomas include an occasional case of plasmacytoma; these appear to account for about 5% of thyroid hematologic malignancies (375,376). Association with Hashimoto's thyroiditis is similar to that found in thyroid lymphomas. Interestingly, in contrast to lymphomas, a male predominance was reported in one series, and the female preponderance seen in lymphoma is not seen in reported cases (375). Some plasmacytomas have been associated with a serum paraprotein, but only rarely with multiple myeloma (377). The clinical course of the reported cases has generally been indolent, with more than 50% being long-term survivors. The paraprotein has disappeared after local therapy in most cases.

The morphologic features of the reported cases are variable. Aozasa described prominent follicles in the majority of the cases, many with reactive germinal centers, surrounded by the dense plasma cell infiltrate (375), whereas others have described more solid infiltrates of plasma cells (377). In one reported case, plasma cells surrounded neoplastic follicles, consistent with follicular lymphoma, with a different immunoglobulin heavy and light chain from the plasma cells (378). It is tempting to speculate that these cases are simply MALT lymphomas with extreme plasmacytic differentiation. Against this interpretation is the fact that these tumors express predominantly IgG or IgA and are associated with a paraprotein, similar to plasmacytomas of other sites, and unlike most MALT lymphomas. However, several reports have shown that, in contrast to MALT lymphomas of other sites, those in the thyroid often express IgG or IgA (353,369). Thus, the relationship between what have been reported as plasmacytomas and true MALT-type lymphomas of the thyroid remains to be determined.

Clinical Features of Thyroid Lymphomas

From the reported literature, it is difficult to separate the clinical features of MALT-type lymphomas of the thyroid from those of diffuse large B-cell lymphoma; thus, they will be considered together here. As mentioned above, patients with clinical evidence of Hashimoto's thyroiditis have an increased risk of developing thyroid lymphoma. In the reported series of thyroid lymphomas, a clinical history of hypo- or hyperthyroidism has been reported in only a minority of the cases; however, of patients tested for antithyroglobulin antibodies, the majority of the patients in several series (70% to 80%) had them (366,367,371). In a population-based study from Denmark, Pedersen reported 3 of 50 patients to have a history of Hashimoto's thyroiditis (379). The male:female ratio is the lowest of any hematologic malignancy; in most series, over 80% of the patients are female (362,366, 367,371,379). The median age is in the seventh decade, and the disease rarely occurs before age 40.

Most patients have been treated with radiation therapy, with or without chemotherapy. The overall 5-year survival rate in most series is in the range of 40% to 60%. In many series, the stage of the disease at the time of the diagnosis was the most important predictor of outcome, with patients with stage 1 disease having a 70% to 80% 5-year survival rate (362–364,372,379). Cases without extrathyroidal extension have a very low recurrence rate, and it has been argued that they can be treated with surgery alone (380).

Histologic type is a less strong predictor of outcome in most series. Maurer and associates reported a better survival for cases with cleaved cell morphology than for those with noncleaved or immunoblastic cells; however, this was not statistically significant (364).

EXTRAMEDULLARY PLASMACYTOMA

Clinical Features

Neoplasms composed of plasma cells can present in several different ways: as multiple myeloma, as solitary plasmacytoma of bone, or as extramedullary plasmacytoma (EMP) (381). EMP is the least common of the three. The most common site for EMP is the head and neck, with approximately 80% of cases arising in this location (382,383). In most cases, EMP of the head and neck is an isolated lesion, but occasionally patients with multiple myeloma develop head and neck involvement (384). In addition, solitary plasmacytomas may affect bones in the region of the head and neck (385), but the discussion that follows focuses on isolated EMP.

Extramedullary plasmacytoma of the head and neck is virtually exclusively a disease of adults. Patients range from 20 (386) to 84 (382) years of age, with most patients being between 50 and 70, and 80% (385) to 95% (384) of patients being over age 40. Men are affected three to four times more often than women (381,384,385,387,388). EMP is most commonly found in the nasal cavity, nasopharynx, and paranasal sinuses, but occasionally involves the tonsils, pharynx, larynx, middle ear, palate, thyroid, parotid gland, and orbit (381–384,386–390). Rarely, multiple EMPs may be found, synchronously (388,391) or metachronously (392).

Pathologic Features

On gross examination, lesions in the upper respiratory tract or oral cavity are usually polypoid, pedunculated or sessile, fleshy, yellow–gray, or dark red submucosal lesions with a smooth or nodular surface that usually appears intact but may be ulcerated. In some cases, there is destruction of adjacent bone (381,382,384). In the rare case of plasmacytoma of the thyroid, the lesions may be as large as 10 cm, and may be associated with difficulty breathing (384).

On microscopic examination, the tumors are composed of sheets of plasma cells (Figs. 32 and 33). The neoplastic cells can closely resemble normal plasma cells or can be large and atypical. Plasmacytomas can be divided into low, intermediate, and high-grade tumors, in which low-grade tumors contain cells similar to normal plasma cells, intermediate grade tumors have a majority of cells with enlarged nuclei with prominent nucleoli, while retaining the abundant cytoplasm and paranuclear hof of a normal plasma cell, and high-grade tumors are composed of plasmablasts with large nuclei, prominent central nucleoli, scant cytoplasm, and an inconspicuous hof (382). The mitotic rate may be high, especially in poorly differentiated tumors. Rarely, there are tingible body macrophages, giving a starry sky pattern (382,384). Stroma is usually sparse, but in a small minority of cases, there is fibrosis or amyloid deposition; the latter is sometimes associated with a giant cell reaction. Stromal ectopic bone and pseudoangiomatoid change also have been described (382,384,387,393). Immunohistochemical studies typically demonstrate monotypic cytoplasmic immunoglobulin expression of IgG or IgA type. In some cases, only light chain is expressed (382,384). Rarely, EMPs express IgD (392). *In situ* hybridization for κ and λ messenger RNA also can be used to show light chain restriction. EBV is usually absent (394).

Staging, Treatment, and Outcome

Recommended staging procedures include careful physical examination, skeletal survey, bone marrow biopsy, and evaluation of serum for paraprotein. As noted earlier, in most cases, the EMP is an isolated lesion, but in a few cases, staging reveals multiple myeloma. Ten percent to 20% have spread to cervical lymph nodes (382,384). Approximately 25% of patients have a serum M component (382).

The standard treatment for EMP is radiation therapy. Most patients achieve local control of disease and have uneventful follow-up (382,386). In a minority, there is persistent or recurrent local disease that rarely leads to the death of the patient (382). In an estimated 8% to 32% of cases, there is progression to multiple myeloma (382,390), which is usually fatal. Multiple myeloma develops in most cases in the first 2 years after diagnosis, but rarely, myeloma appears after an interval of up to 15 years (382). We have seen a unique case in which a 53-year-old man presented with a nasal plasmacytoma, and over the course of 20 years developed a left testicular plasmacytoma, a right epididymal plasmacytoma, and multiple cutaneous plasmacytomas, all of which were treated with excision or local radiation therapy. After this period, new plasmacytomas apparently spontaneously failed to appear, and the patient was well and free of disease for the next 9 years (395).

The prognosis of EMP of the head and neck is better than that of osseous plasmacytoma, which almost always progresses to myeloma (382). A number of clinical and pathologic features

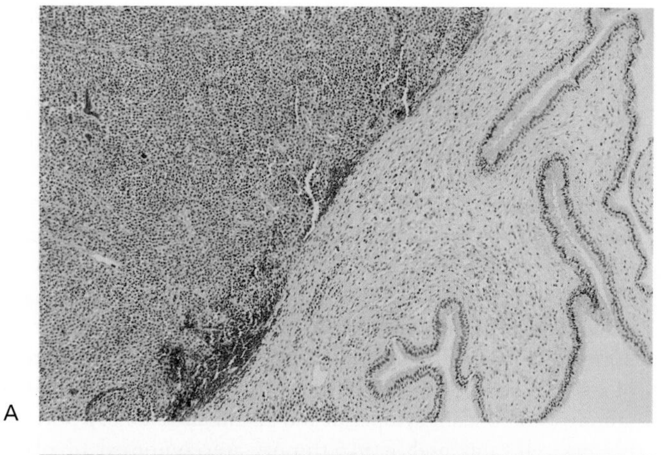

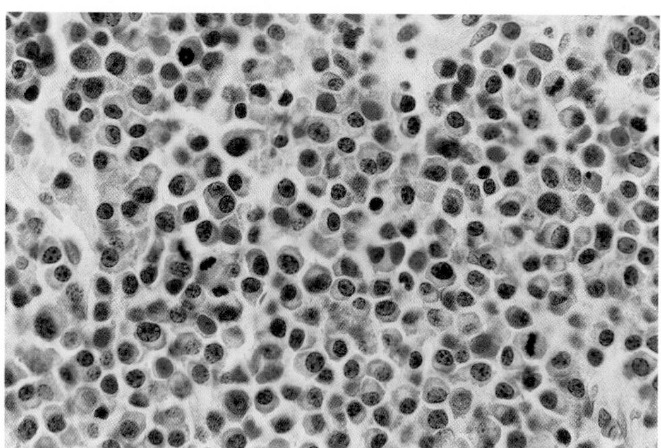

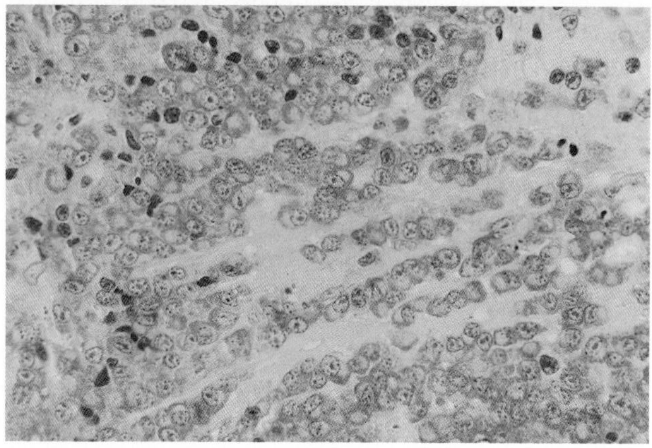

FIGURE 32. Plasmacytoma, maxillary antrum. **A:** Low power shows a dense cellular infiltrate beneath intact respiratory mucosa. **B:** High power shows a pure population of mature to slightly immature plasma cells with a few binucleated forms. **C:** With a Giemsa stain, the cytoplasm of the neoplastic cells is deep blue and the pale Golgi region is easily recognizable.

have been suggested to affect prognosis. One study suggested that younger patients were more likely to have widespread disease than older patients (381). The finding of a serum paraprotein may be a clue that the patient has myeloma (384,386), but if there is no evidence of myeloma on staging, and if the paraprotein disappears after the EMP is treated, it does not signify a worse prognosis (382,387). Several studies suggest that bony invasion is associated with more frequent progression to myeloma (381,387), although there is not complete agreement on this point (385). Grade is an important prognostic factor. In one study, low-grade tumors were much more often associated with local control of disease than intermediate or high-grade tumors ($p = 0.0019$) (382). In another study, patients with poorly differentiated tumors were more likely to die than those with well- or moderately differentiated tumors (384). In one study, local recurrences appeared in 7 of 16 cases with a κ-positive tumor, but in only 1 of 7 with a λ-positive tumor (382). This finding is unexpected but intriguing; however, others have not found a difference in prognosis for κ-positive and λ-positive tumors (388). Additional studies should be performed in an attempt to investigate the significance of the immunophenotype. It has been suggested that patients with a bad prognostic factor, such as high grade, be treated more aggressively, with a higher dose of radiation, or with the addition of chemotherapy (382).

FIGURE 33. Plasmacytoma in the nasopharynx. In this case, there is an unusually large number of Mott cells (plasma cells with multiple cytoplasmic inclusions of immunoglobulin).

Differential Diagnosis

The differential diagnosis of EMP includes a variety of reactive neoplastic conditions. On physical examination, other entities that may be considered include nasal polyp, squamous cell carcinoma, and, because these tumors may be deep red, hemangioma and paraganglioma. On microscopic examination, well-differentiated EMP may raise the question of plasma cell granuloma and other reactive lesions with a prominent component of plasma cells; a polymorphous cellular infiltrate, more abundant stroma and polytypic immunoglobulin expression are evidence against

TABLE 13. HEAD AND NECK PLASMACYTOMA VERSUS EXTRANODAL MARGINAL ZONE B-CELL LYMPHOMA (MALT-TYPE)

	Plasmacytoma	Marginal Zone Lymphoma
Common sites	Nasal cavity, nasopharynx, paranasal sinuses	Orbit, salivary gland, thyroid
Composition	Plasma cells, plasmablasts	Lymphocytes, marginal zone B cells, with or without plasma cells
Reactive follicles	Absent	Often present
Lymphoepithelial lesions	Absent	Often present (varies by site)
Immunoglobulin isotype	G, A, or light chain only	M > G > A
Pan-B antigens	Typically absent	Present on at least some cells

plasmacytoma. Extranodal marginal zone lymphomas with numerous plasma cells also can enter the differential diagnosis (Table 13). A component of neoplastic B-lymphocytes and IgM expression favor lymphoma. A pure population of plasma cells and IgG, IgA, or light chain only expression favor plasmacytoma. Poorly differentiated EMP may mimic immunoblastic lymphoma, granulocytic sarcoma, or melanoma. EMP in the nasopharynx may suggest a diagnosis of undifferentiated carcinoma. In the thyroid, anaplastic carcinoma may be a consideration (384). Careful histologic examination, special stains, and immunohistochemical studies are helpful in establishing a diagnosis.

ACKNOWLEDGMENT

We are grateful to Bernadette Vijayakanthan and Carol Ann Gould for secretarial assistance, to Steve Conley and Michelle Forrestall for photography, and to Dr. John F. Ferry for helpful comments concerning the text of the manuscript.

REFERENCES

1. Segal GH, Kjeldsberg CR, Smith GP, et al. CD30 antigen expression in florid immunoblastic proliferations. A clinicopathologic study of 14 cases. *Am J Clin Pathol* 1994;102:292–298.
2. Lajo A, Bourque C, del Castillo F, et al. Mononucleosis caused by Epstein-Barr virus and cytomegalovirus in children: a comparative study of 124 cases. *Pediatr Infect Dis J* 1994;13:56–60.
3. Bailey RE. Diagnosis and treatment of infectious mononucleosis [Review]. *Am Fam Physician* 1994;49:879–888.
4. Custer RP, Smith EB. The pathology of infectious mononucleosis. *Blood* 1948;3:830–857.
5. Mroczek EC, Weisenburger DD, Grierson HL, et al. Fatal infectious mononucleosis and virus-associated hemophagocytic syndrome. *Arch Pathol Lab Med* 1987;111:530–535.
6. Abbondanzo SL, Sato N, Straus SE, et al. Acute infectious mononucleosis. *Am J Clin Pathol* 1990;93:698–702.
7. Salvador AH, Harrison EGJ, Kyle RA. Lymphadenopathy due to infectious mononucleosis: its confusion with malignant lymphoma. *Cancer* 1971;27:1029–1040.
8. Niedobitek G, Herbst H, Young LS, et al. Patterns of Epstein Barr virus infection in non-neoplastic lymphoid tissue. *Blood* 1992; 790: 2520–2526.
9. Isaacson PG, Schmid C, Pan L, et al. Epstein Barr virus latent membrane protein expression by Hodgkin and Reed Sternberg-like cells in acute infectious mononucleosis. *J Pathol* 1992;167:267–271.
10. Malik U, Oleksowicz L, Dutcher J, et al. Atypical clonal T-cell proliferation in infectious mononucleosis. *Med Oncol* 1996;13:207–213.
11. Callan M, Steven N, Krausa P, et al. Large clonal expansions of $CD8^+$ T cells in acute infectious mononucleosis. *Nat Med* 1996;2:906–911.
12. Niedobitek G, Agathanggelou A, Herbst H, et al. Epstein-Barr virus (EBV) in infectious mononucleosis: virus latency, replication and phenotype of EBV-infected cells. *J Pathol* 1997;182:151–159.
13. Abramowitz A, Livni N, Morag A, Ravid Z. An immunoperoxidase study of cytomegalovirus lymphadenitis. *Arch Pathol Lab Med* 1982; 106:115–118.
14. Younes M, Podesta A, Helie M, et al. Infection of T but not B lymphocytes by cytomegalovirus in lymph node. *Am J Surg Pathol* 1991;15:75–80.
15. Rushin JM, Riordan GP, Heaton RB, et al. Cytomegalovirus-infected cells express Leu M1 antigen. A potential source of diagnostic error. *Am J Pathol* 1990;136:989–995.
16. Case Records of the Massachusetts General Hospital. Case 7-1995. *N Engl J Med* 1995;332:663–671.
17. Joubert M, Morin C, Moreau A, et al. Histopathologic features of cytomegalovirus lymphadenitis in the "immunocompetent" patient. *Ann Pathol* 1996;16:254–260.
18. Howat A, Campbell A, Stewart D, et al. Generalized lymphadenopathy due to herpes simplex virus type 1. *Histopathology* 1991;19: 563–564.
19. Miliauskas J, Leong A. Localized herpes simplex lymphadenitis: report of three cases and review of the literature [Review]. *Histopathology* 1991;19:355–360.
20. Tamaru J, Mikata A, Horie H, et al. Herpes simplex lymphadenitis: report of two cases with review of the literature. *Am J Surg Pathol* 1990;14:571–577.
21. Taxy J, Tillawi I, Goldman P. Herpes simplex lymphadenitis: an unusual presentation with necrosis and viral particles. *Arch Pathol Lab Med* 1985;109:1043–1044.
22. Epstein J, Ambinder R, Kuhajda F, et al. Localized herpes simplex lymphadenitis. *Am J Clin Pathol* 1986;86:444–448.
23. Wat P, Strickler J, Myers J, et al. Herpes simplex infection causing acute necrotizing tonsillitis. *Mayo Clin Proc* 1994;69:269–271.
24. Vanhems P, Allard R, Cooper D, et al. Acute human immunodeficiency virus type 1 disease as a mononucleosis-like illness: is the diagnosis too restrictive? *Clin Infect Dis* 1997;24:965–970.
25. Shahab I, Osborne B, Butler J. Nasopharyngeal lymphoid tissue masses in patients with human immunodeficiency virus-1. Histologic findings and clinical correlation. *Cancer* 1994;74:3083–3088.
26. Ioachim H, Gonin W, Roy M, et al. Persistent lymphadenopathies in people at high risk for HIV infection. Clinicopathologic correlations and long-term follow up in 79 cases. *Am J Clin Pathol* 1990;93:208.
27. O'Murchadha M, Wolf B, Neiman R. The histologic features of hyperplastic lymphadenopathy in AIDS-related complex are nonspecific. *Am J Surg Pathol* 1987;11:94–99.
28. Shibata D, Weiss L, Nathwani B, et al. Epstein-Barr virus in benign lymph node biopsies from individuals infected with the human immunodeficiency virus is associated with concurrent or subsequent development of non-Hodgkin's lymphoma. *Blood* 1993;77:1527–1533.

29. Oksenhendler E, Duarte M, Soulier J, et al. Multicentric Castleman's disease in HIV infection: a clinical and pathological study of 20 patients. *AIDS* 1996;10:61–67.
30. Cesarman E, Knowles D. Kaposi's sarcoma-associated herpesvirus: a lymphotropic human herpesvirus associated with Kaposi's sarcoma, primary effusion lymphoma, and multicentric Castleman's disease. *Semin Diagn Pathol* 1997;14:54–66.
31. Soulier J, Grollet L, Oksenhendler E, et al. Kaposi's sarcoma–like herpesvirus-like DNA sequences in multicentric Castleman's disease. *Blood* 1995;84:1276–1280.
32. Yamauchi T, Ferrieri P, Anthony B. The aetiology of acute cervical adenitis in children: serological and bacteriological studies. *J Med Microbiol* 1980;13:37–43.
33. Beiler H, Eckstein T, Roth H, et al. Specific and nonspecfic lymphadenitis in childhood: etiology, diagnosis, and therapy. *Pediatr Surg Int* 1997;12:108–112.
34. Adal KA, Cockerell CJ, Petri WA. Cat scratch disease, bacillary angiomatosis and other infections due to Rochalimaea. *N Engl J Med* 1994;330:1509–1515.
35. Bergmans AM, Groothedde JW, Schellekens JF, et al. Etiology of cat scratch disease: comparison of polymerase chain reaction detection of *Bartonella* (formerly *Rochalimaea*) and *Afipia felis* DNA with serology and skin tests. *J Infect Dis* 1995;171:916–923.
36. Anderson B, Neuman M. *Bartonella* spp. as emerging human pathogens. *Clin Microbiol Rev* 1997;10:203–219.
37. Wear D, Margileth A, Hadfield T, et al. Cat-scratch disease: a bacterial infection. *Science* 1983;221:1403–1404.
38. Spach DH, Koehler JE. *Bartonella*-associated infections. *Infect Dis Clin North Am* 1998;12:137–155.
39. Case Records of the Massachusetts General Hospital. Case 22-1992. *N Engl J Med* 1992;326:1480–1489.
40. Zangwill K, Hamilton D, Perkins B, et al. Cat Scratch disease in Connecticut. *N Engl J Med* 1993;329:8–13.
41. Miller-Catchpole R, Variakojis D, Vardiman JW, et al. Cat scratch disease. Identification of bacteria in seven cases of lymphadenitis. *Am J Surg Pathol* 1986;10:276–281.
42. Facchetti F, Agostini C, Chilosi M, et al. Suppurative granulomatous lymphadenitis. Immunohistochemical evidence for a B-cell–associated granuloma. *Am J Surg Pathol* 1992;16:955–961.
43. Case records of the Massachusetts General Hospital. *N Engl J Med* 1993;329:714–721.
44. Bem C, Patil PS, Bharucha H, et al. Importance of human immunodeficiency virus–associated lymphadenopathy and tuberculous lymphadenitis in patients undergoing lymph node biopsy in Zambia. *Br J Surg* 1996;83:75–78.
45. Simon HB. Infections due to mycobacteria. *Infect Dis* 1995;7:1–25.
46. Kanlikama M, Gokalp A. Management of mycobacterial cervical lymphadenitis. *World J Surg* 1997;21:516–519.
47. Dandapat MC, Mishra BM, Dash SP, et al. Peripheral lymph node tuberculosis: a review of 80 cases. *Br J Surg* 1990;77:911–912.
48. Subrahmanyam M. Role of surgery and chemotherapy for peripheral lymph node tuberculosis. *Br J Surg* 1993;80:1547–1548.
49. Suskind DL, Handler SD, Tom L, et al. Nontuberculous mycobacterial cervical adenitis. *Clin Pediatr (Phila)* 1997;36:403–409.
50. Wockel W, Wernert N. Excessive epithelioid cell granulomatous reaction associated with a lymphoepithelial carcinoma (Schmincke-Regaud). *Pathol Res Pract* 1986;181:349–352.
51. Tuzuner N, Dogusoy G, Demirkesen C, et al. Value of lymph node biopsy in the diagnosis of acquired toxoplasmosis. *J Laryngol Otol* 1996;110:348–352.
52. Rose I. Morphology and diagnostics of human toxoplasmosis. *Gen Diagn Pathol* 1997;142:257–270.
53. Montoya J, Remington J. Studies on the serodiagnosis of toxoplasmic lymphadenitis. *Clin Infect Dis* 1995;20:781–789.
54. Weiss L, Chen Y-Y, Berry G, et al. Infrequent detection of Toxoplasma gondii genome in toxoplasmic lymphadenitis: a polymerase chain reaction study. *Hum Pathol* 1992;23:154–158.
55. Fox RA, Rosahn PD. The lymph nodes in disseminated lupus erythematosus. *Am J Pathol* 1943;19:73–79.
56. Shapira Y, Weinberger A, Wysenbeek AJ. Lymphadenopathy in systemic lupus erythematosus. Prevalence and relation to disease manifestations. *Clin Rheumatol* 1996;15:335–338.
57. Medeiros LJ, Kaynor B, Harris NL. Lupus lymphadenitis: report of a case with immunohistologic studies on frozen sections. *Hum Pathol* 1989;20:295–299.
58. Dorfman R, Berry G. Kikuchi's histiocytic necrotizing lymphadenitis: an analysis of 108 cases with emphasis on differential diagnosis. *Semin Diagn Pathol* 1988;5:329–345.
59. Tsang W, Chan J, Ng C. Kikuchi's lymphadenitis. A morphologic analysis of 75 cases with special reference to unusual features. *Am J Surg Pathol* 1994;18:219–231.
60. Kikuchi M, Takeshita M, Eimoto T, et al. Histiocytic necrotizing lymphadenitis: clinicopathologic, immunologic and HLA typing study. In: Hanaoka M, Kadin M, Mikata A, eds. *Lymphoid malignancy: immunocytology and cytogenetics.* New York: Fields & Wood, 1990:251–257.
61. Kuo T. Kikuchi's disease (histiocytic necrotizing lymphadenitis). A clinicopathologic study of 79 cases with an analysis of histologic subtypes, immunohistology and DNA ploidy. *Am J Surg Pathol* 1995; 9: 798–809.
62. Sumiyoshi Y, Kikuchi M, Ohsima K, et al. Human herpesvirus-6 genomes in histiocytic necrotizing lymphadenitis (Kikuchi's disease) and other forms of lymphadenitis. *Am J Clin Pathol* 1993;99: 609–614.
63. Huh J, Kang G, Gong G, et al. HHV 8 DNA sequences in Kikuchi's disease [Abstract]. *Mod Pathol* 1998;11:131.
64. Pasquinucci S, Donisi P, Cavinato F, et al. Kikuchi's disease in a patient infected with AIDS. *AIDS* 1991;5:235.
65. Bataille V, Harland C, Behrens J, et al. Kikuchi disease (histiocytic necrotizing lymphadenitis) in association with HTLV-1. *Br J Dermatol* 1997;136:610–612.
66. Yufu Y, Matsumoto M, Miyamura T, et al. Parvovirus B19-associated haemophagocytic syndrome with lymphadenopathy resembling histiocytic necrotizing lymphadenitis (Kikuchi's disease). *Br J Haematol* 1997;96:868–871.
67. Rubio S, Plewinsky T, Sabatini M, et al. Kikuchi's disease associated with Hashimoto's thyroiditis. *J Endocrinol Invest* 1996;19:136–137.
68. Sever C, Leith C, Appenzeller J, et al. Kikuchi's histiocytic necrotizing lymphadenitis associated with ruptured silicone breast implant. *Arch Pathol Lab Med* 1996;120:380–385.
69. Chan J, Ng C. Kikuchi's histiocytic necrotizing lymphadenitis in the regional lymph nodes of malignant fibrous histiocytoma: causal or coincidental? *Histopathology* 1988;12:448–451.
70. Lennert K, Remmele W. Karyometrische untersuchungen an lymphknotenzellen des menschen: I. Mitt. germinoblasten, lymphoblasten und lymphozyten. *Acta Haematol* 1958;19:99–113.
71. Nathwani B. Kikuchi-Fujimoto disease. *Am J Surg Pathol* 1991;15: 196–197.
72. Facchetti F, deWolf-Peters C, Mason D, et al. Plasmacytoid T cells: immunohistochemical evidence for their monocyte/macrophage origin. *Am J Pathol* 1988;133:15–21.
73. Case Records of the Massachusetts General Hospital. Case 5-1997. *N Engl J Med* 1997;336:1904–1912.
74. Giesker D, Pastuszak W, Forouhar F, et al. Lymph node biopsy for early diagnosis in Kawasaki disease. *Am J Surg Pathol* 1982;6: 493–501.
75. Marsh W, Bishop J, Koenig H. Bone marrow and lymph node findings in a fatal case of Kawasaki's disease. *Arch Pathol Lab Med* 1980; 104:563–567.
76. Landing B, Larson E. Pathological features of Kawasaki disease (mucocutaneous lymph node syndrome). *Am J Cardiovasc Pathol* 1987; 1:218–229.
77. Park A, Batchra N, Rowler A, et al. Patterns of Kawasaki syndrome presentation. *Int J Pediatr Otorhinolaryngol* 1997;40:41–50.
78. Rosai J, Dorfman R. Sinus histiocytosis with massive lymphadenopathy. A newly recognized benign clinicopathologic entity. *Arch Pathol* 1969;87:63–70.
79. Rosai J. Sinus histiocytosis with massive lymphadenopathy. *Am J Surg Pathol* 1991;15:191–192.

80. Foucar E, Rosai J, Dorfman R. Sinus histiocytosis with massive lymphadenopathy. An analysis of 14 deaths occurring in a patient registry. *Cancer* 1984;54:1834–1840.
81. Sacchi S, Artusi T, Torelli U, et al. Sinus histiocytosis with massive lymphadenopathy [Review]. *Leuk Lymphoma* 1992;7:189–194.
82. Montgomery E, Meis J, Frizzera G. Rosai-Dorfman disease of soft tissue. *Am J Surg Pathol* 1992;16:122–129.
83. Paulli M, Rosso R, Kindl S, et al. Immunophenotypic characterization of the cell infiltrate in five cases of sinus histiocytosis with massive lymphadenopathy (Rosai-Dorfman disease). *Hum Pathol* 1992;23:647–654.
84. Li T, Chen X, Wang S, et al. Kimura's disease: a clinicopathologic study of 54 Chinese patients. *Oral Surg Oral Med Oral Pathol Oral Radiol Endod* 1996;82:549–555.
85. Googe P, Harris N, Mihm M. Kimura's disease and angiolymphoid hyperplasia with eosinophilia: two distinct histopathological entities. *J Cutan Pathol* 1987;14:263–271.
86. Harris NL, Jaffe ES, Stein H, et al. A revised European-American classification of lymphoid neoplasms: a proposal from the International Lymphoma Study Group. *Blood* 1994;84:1361–1392.
87. Jaffe ES, Harris NL, Diebold J, et al. World Health Organization classification of neoplastic diseases of the hematopoietic and lymphoid tissues. A progress report. *Am J Clin Pathol* 1999;111(suppl):8–12.
88. Isaacson PG, Spencer J. Malignant lymphoma of mucosa-associated lymphoid tissue. *Histopathology* 1987;11:445–462.
89. Jacobs C, Hoppe RT. Non-Hodgkin's lymphomas of head and neck extranodal sites. *Int J Radiat Oncol Biol Phys* 1985;11:357–364.
90. Shimm D, Dosoretz D, Harris NL, et al. Radiation therapy of Waldeyer's ring lymphoma. *Cancer* 1984;54:426–431.
91. Menarguez J, Mollejo M, Carion R, et al. Waldeyer ring lymphomas. A clinicopathological study of 79 cases. *Histopathology* 1994;24:13–22.
92. Chan JKC, Ng C, Lo S. Immunohistological characterization of malignant lymphomas of the Waldeyer's ring other than the nasopharynx. *Histopathology* 1987;11:885–889.
93. Thieblemont C, Bastion Y, Berger F, et al. Mucosa-associated lymphoid tissue gastrointestinal and nongastrointestinal lymphoma behavior: analysis of 108 patients. *J Clin Oncol* 1997;15:1624–1630.
94. Freeman C, Berg JW, Cutler SJ. Occurrence and prognosis of extranodal lymphomas. *Cancer* 1972;29:252–260.
95. Hoppe R, Burke J, Glatstein E, et al. Non-Hogdkin's lymphoma. Involvement of Waldeyer's ring. *Cancer* 1978;42:1096–1104.
96. Paulsen J, Lennert K. Low-grade B-cell lymphoma of mucosa-associated lymphoid tissue type in Waldeyer's ring. *Histopathology* 1994;24:1–11.
97. Harbo G, Grau C, Bundgaard T, et al. Cancer of the nasal cavity and paranasal sinuses. A clinico-pathological study of 277 patients. *Acta Oncol* 1997;36:45–50.
98. Campo E, Cardesa A, Alos L, et al. Non-Hodgkin's lymphomas of nasal cavity and paranasal sinuses. An immunohistochemical study. *Am J Clin Pathol* 1991;96:184–190.
99. Tomita Y, Ohsawa M, Mishiro Y, et al. The presence and subtype of Epstein-Barr virus in B and T cell lymphomas of the sino-nasal region from the Osaka and Okinawa districts of Japan. *Lab Invest* 1995;73:190–196.
100. Abbondanzo S, Wenig B. Non-Hodgkin's lymphoma of the sinonasal tract. A clinicopathologic and immunophenotypic study of 120 cases. *Cancer* 1995;75:1281–1291.
101. Tomita Y, Ohsawa M, Qiu K, et al. Epstein-Barr virus in lymphoproliferative diseases in the sino-nasal region: close association with $CD56^+$ immunophenotype and polymorphic-reticulosis morphology. *Int J Cancer* 1997;70:9–13.
102. Cuadra-Garcia I, Proulx G, Wu C, et al. Sinonasal lymphoma: a clinicopathologic analysis of 58 cases. *Am J Surg Pathol* 1999;23:1356–1369.
103. Cuadra-Garcia I, Harris N, Proulx G, et al. Sinonasal lymphoma: an analysis of 57 cases [Abstact]. *Mod Pathol* 1999;12:135.
104. Davison S, Habermann T, Strickler J, et al. Nasal and nasopharyngeal angiocentric T-cell lymphomas. *Laryngoscope* 1996;106:139–143.
105. Harabuchi Y, Imai S, Wakashima J, et al. Nasal T-cell lymphoma causally associated with Epstein-Barr virus. Clinicopathologic, phenotypic, and genotypic studies. *Cancer* 1996;77:2137–2149.
106. Michaels L, Gregory M. Pathology of "non-healing (midline) granuloma." *J Clin Pathol* 1977;30:317–327.
107. Eichel B, Harrison E Jr, Devine K, et al. Primary lymphoma of the nose including a relationship to lethal midline granuloma. *Am J Surg* 1966;112:597–605.
108. Jaffe E. Pathologic and clinical spectrum of post-thymic T-cell malignancies. *Cancer Invest* 1984;2:413–426.
109. Ishii Y, Yamanaka N, Ogawa K, et al. Nasal T-cell lymphoma as a type of so-called "lethal midline granuloma." *Cancer* 1982;50:2336–2344.
110. Jaffe ES, Chan JK, Su IJ, et al. Report of the Workshop on Nasal and Related Extranodal Angiocentric T/Natural Killer Cell Lymphomas. Definitions, differential diagnosis, and epidemiology. *Am J Surg Pathol* 1996;20:103–111.
111. Jaffe E. Nasal and nasal-type T/NK cell lymphoma: a unique form of lymphoma associated with the Epstein-Barr virus. *Histopathology* 1995;27:581–583.
112. Aozasa K, Ohsawa M, Tomita Y, et al. Polymorphic reticulosis is a neoplasm of large granular lymphocytes with $CD3^+$ phenotype. *Cancer* 1995;75:894–901.
113. Nakamura S, Katoh E, Koshikawa T, et al. Clinicopathologic study of nasal T/NK-cell lymphoma among the Japanese. *Pathol Int* 1997;47:38–53.
114. Mishima K, Horiuchi K, Kojya S, et al. Epstein-Barr virus in patients with polymorphic reticulosis (lethal midline granuloma) from China and Japan. *Cancer* 1994;73:3041–3046.
115. Tien H-F, Su I-J, Tang J-L, et al. Clonal chromosomal abnormalities as direct evidence for clonality in nasal T/natural killer cell lymphomas. *Br J Haematol* 1997;97:621–625.
116. van Gorp J, de Bruin P, Sie-Go D, et al. Nasal T-cell lymphoma: a clinicopathological and immunophenotypic analysis of 13 cases. *Histopathology* 1995;27:139–148.
117. Sakata K, Hareyama M, Ohochu A, et al. Treatment of lethal midline granuloma type nasal T-cell lymphoma. *Acta Oncol* 1997;36:307–311.
118. Yamaguchi M, Kita K, Miwa H, et al. Frequent expression of P-glycoprotein/MDR1 by nasal T-cell lymphoma cells. *Cancer* 1995;76:2351–2356.
119. Kwong Y, Chan A, Liang R, et al. $CD56^+$ NK lymphomas: clinicopathological features and prognosis. *Br J Haematol* 1997;97:821–829.
120. Ferry JA, Sklar J, Zukerberg LR, et al. Nasal lymphoma: a clinicopathologic study with immunophenotypic and genotypic analysis. *Am J Surg Pathol* 1991;15:268–279.
121. Chiang A, Srivastava G, Lau P, et al. Differences in T-cell–receptor gene rearrangement and transcription in nasal lymphomas of natural killer and T-cell types: implications on cellular origin. *Hum Pathol* 1996;27:701–707.
122. Nakamura K, Uehara S, Omagari J, et al. Primary non-Hodgkin lymphoma of the sinonasal cavities: correlation of CT evaluation with clinical outcome. *Radiology* 1997;204:431–435.
123. Cheung MM, Chan JK, Lau WH, et al. Primary non-Hodgkin's lymphoma of the nose and nasopharynx: clinical features, tumor immunophenotype, and treatment outcome in 113 patients. *J Clin Oncol* 1998;16:70–77.
124. Yu K, Yu S, Teo P, et al. Nasal lymphoma: results of local radiotherapy with or without chemotherapy. *Head Neck* 1997;19:251–259.
125. Liang R, Todd D, Chan TK, et al. Treatment outcome and prognostic factors for primary nasal lymphoma. *J Clin Oncol* 1995;13:666–670.
126. Fellbaum C, Hansmann M-L, Lennert K. Malignant lymphomas of the nasal cavity and paranasal sinuses. *Virchows Arch* 1989;414:399–405.
127. Kwong Y, Chan A, Liang R. Natural killer cell lymphoma/leukemia: pathology and treatment. *Hematol Oncol* 1997;15:71–79.
128. de Bruin P, Kummer J, van der Valk P, et al. Granzyme B-expressing peripheral T-cell lymphomas: neoplastic equivalents of activated cytotoxic T cells with preference for mucosa-associated lymphoid tissue localization. *Blood* 1994;84:3785–3791.

129. Chiang A, Tao Q, Srivastava G, et al. Nasal NK- and T-cell lymphomas share the same type of Epstein-Barr virus latency as nasopharyngeal carcinoma and Hodgkin's disease. *Int J Cancer* 1996;68: 285–290.
130. Li YX, Coucke PA, Li JY, et al. Primary non-Hodgkin's lymphoma of the nasal cavity: prognostic significance of paranasal extension and the role of radiotherapy and chemotherapy. *Cancer* 1998;83:449–456.
131. Aviles A, Rodriguez L, Guzman R, et al. Angiocentric T-cell lymphoma of the nose, paranasal sinuses and hard palate. *Hematol Oncol* 1992;10:141–147.
132. Su I-J, Wang C-H, Cheng A-L, Chen R-L. Hemophagocytic syndrome in Epstein-Barr virus-associated T-lymphoproliferative disorders: disease spectrum, pathogenesis, and management. *Leuk Lymphoma* 1995;19:401–406.
133. Nakamura K, Uehara S, Omagari K, et al. Primary non-Hodgkin's lymphoma of the maxillary sinus. *Am J Clin Oncol* 1997;20:272–275.
134. Hausdorff J, Davis E, Long G, et al. Non-Hodgkin's lymphoma of the paranasal sinuses: clinical and pathological features, and response to combined-modality therapy. *Cancer J Sci Am* 1997;3:303–311.
135. Makepeace A, Fermont D, Bennett M. Non-Hodgkin's lymphoma of the nasopharynx, paranasal sinus and palate. *Clin Radiol* 1989;40: 144–146.
136. Wollner N, Mandell L, Filippa D, et al. Primary nasal-paranasal oropharyngeal lymphoma in the pediatric age group. *Cancer* 1990; 65:1438–1444.
137. Weisberger EC, Davidson DD. Unusual presentations of lymphoma of the head and neck in childhood. *Laryngoscope* 1990;100:337–342.
138. Juman S, Robinson P, Balkissoon A, et al. B-cell non-Hodgkin's lymphoma of the paranasal sinuses. *J Laryngol Otol* 1994;108:263–265.
139. Bumpous J, Martin D, Curran P, et al. Non-Hodgkin's lymphomas of the nose and paranasal sinuses in the pediatric population. *Ann Otol Rhinol Laryngol* 1994;103:294–300.
140. Schoem S, Morton A. Paranasal sinus Burkitt's lymphoma in a human immunodeficiency virus (HIV) positive male. *Ear Nose Throat J* 1989;69:844–846.
141. Pomilla P, Morris A, Jaworek A. Sinonasal non-Hodgkin's lymphoma in patients infected with human immunodeficiency virus: report of three cases and review. *Clin Infect Dis* 1995;21:137–149.
142. Goldstein J, Rubin J, Becker N, et al. Lymphoma of the maxillary sinus in a patient infected with human immunodeficiency virus type 1. *Head Neck* 1991;13:355–358.
143. Koo J, Kadonaga J, Wintroub B, et al. The development of B-cell lymphoma in a patient with psoriasis treated with cyclosporine. *J Am Acad Dermatol* 1992;26:836–840.
144. Shiong Y, Lian J, Lin C, et al. Epstein-Barr virus–associated T-cell lymphoma of the maxillary sinus in a renal transplant recipient. *Transplant Proc* 1992;24:1929–1931.
145. Inaki S, Okamura H, Chikamori Y. Adult T-cell leukemia/lymphoma originating in the paranasal sinus. *Arch Otolaryngol Head Neck Surg* 1988;114:1471–1473.
146. Frierson H Jr, Mills S, Innes D Jr. Non-Hodgkin's lymphomas of the sinonasal region: histologic subtypes and their clinicopathologic features. *Am J Clin Pathol* 1984;81:721–727.
147. Cooper D, Ginsberg S. Brief chemotherapy, involved field radiation therapy, and central nervous system prophylaxis for paranasal sinus lymphoma. *Cancer* 1992;69:2888–2893.
148. Tran L, Mark R, Fu Y, et al. Primary non-Hodgkin's lymphomas of the paranasal sinuses and nasal cavity. A report of 18 cases with stage IE disease. *Am J Clin Oncol* 1992;15:222–225.
149. Yamanaka N, Harabuchi Y, Sambe S, et al. Non-Hodgkin's lymphoma of Waldeyer's ring and nasal cavity. Clinical and immunologic aspects. *Cancer* 1985;56:768–776.
150. Stroup R, Sheibani K, Moncada A, et al. Angiotropic (intravascular) large cell lymphoma. A clinicopathologic study of seven cases with unique clinical presentations. *Cancer* 1990;66:1781–1788.
151. Wake A, Kakinuma A, Mori N, et al. Angiotropic lymphoma of paranasal sinuses with initial symptoms of oculomotor nerve palsy. *Intern Med* 1993;32:237–242.
152. Weiss L, Gaffey M, Chen Y-Y, et al. Frequency of Epstein-Barr viral DNA in "Western" sinonasal and Waldeyer's ring non-Hodgkin's lymphomas. *Am J Surg Pathol* 1992;16:156–162.
153. Duncavage J, Campbell B, Hanson G, et al. Diagnosis of malignant lymphomas of the nasal cavity, paranasal sinuses and nasopharynx. *Laryngoscope* 1983;93:1276–1280.
154. Brugere J, Schlienger M, Gerard-Marchant R, et al. Non-Hodgkin's malignant lymphomata of upper digestive and respiratory tract: natural history and results of radiotherapy. *Br J Cancer* 1975;31:435–440.
155. Knowles D, Jakobiec F, McNally L, et al. Lymphoid hyperplasia and malignant lymphoma occurring in the ocular adnexa (orbit, conjunctiva, and eyelids): a prospective multiparametric analysis of 108 cases during 1977 to 1987. *Hum Pathol* 1990;21:959–973.
156. Medeiros L, Harris N. Lymphoid infiltrates of the orbit and conjunctiva. A morphologic and immunophenotypic study of 99 cases. *Am J Surg Pathol* 1989;13:459–471.
157. Morgan G. Lymphocytic tumours of the conjunctiva. *J Clin Pathol* 1971;24:585–595.
158. Jakobiec F, Iwamoto T, Patell M, et al. Ocular adnexal monoclonal lymphoid tumors with a favorable prognosis. *Ophthalmology* 1986;93:1547–1557.
159. Knowles D, Jakobiec F. Ocular adnexal lymphoid neoplasms: clinical, histopathologic, electron microscopic, and immunologic characteristics. *Hum Pathol* 1982;13:148–162.
160. Harris N, Pilch B, Bhan A, et al. Immunohistologic diagnosis of orbital lymphoid infiltrates. *Am J Surg Pathol* 1984;8:83–91.
161. Turner R, Egbert P, Warnke R. Lymphocytic infiltrates of the conjunctiva and orbit: immunohistochemical staining of 16 cases. *Am J Clin Pathol* 1984;81:447–452.
162. Medeiros L, Harmon D, Linggood R, et al. Immunohistologic features predict clinical behavior of orbital and conjunctival lymphoid infiltrates. *Blood* 1989;74:2121–2129.
163. Neri A, Jakobiec F, Pelicci P-G, et al. Immunoglobulin and T cell receptor β chain gene rearrangement analysis of ocular adnexal lymphoid neoplasms: clinical and biologic implications. *Blood* 1987; 70: 1519–1529.
164. Knowles D, Athan E, Ubriaco A, et al. Extranodal noncutaneous lymphoid hyperplasias represent a continuous spectrum of B-cell neoplasia: demonstration by molecular genetic analysis. *Blood* 1989; 73: 1635–1645.
165. Jakobiec F, Neri A, Knowles D. Genotypic monoclonality in immunophenotypically polyclonal orbital lymphoid tumors. A model of tumor progression in the lymphoid system. The 1986 Wendell Hughes lecture. *Ophthalmology* 1987;94:980–994.
166. Ferry J, White W, Grove A, et al. Malignant lymphoma of ocular adnexa: a spectrum of B-cell neoplasia including low grade B-cell lymphoma of MALT type [Abstract]. *Lab Invest* 1992;66:77.
167. White W, Ferry J, Harris N, et al. Ocular adnexal lymphoma: a clinicopathologic study with identification of lymphomas of mucosa-associated-lymphoid-tissue (MALT) type. *Opthalmology* 1995;102: 1994–2006.
168. Wotherspoon A, Diss T, Pan L, et al. Primary low-grade B-cell lymphoma of the conjunctiva: a mucosa-associated lymphoid tissue type lymphoma. *Histopathology* 1993;23:417–424.
169. Petrella T, Bron A, Foulet A, et al. Report of a primary lymphoma of the conjunctiva. A lymphoma of MALT origin? *Pathol Res Pract* 1991;187:78–84.
170. Bairey O, Kremer I, Rakowsky E, et al. Orbital and adnexal involvement in systemic non-Hodgkin's lymphoma. *Cancer* 1994;73: 2395–2399.
171. Smitt M, Donaldson S. Radiotherapy is successful treatment for orbital lymphoma. *Int J Radiat Oncol Biol Phys* 1993;26:59–66.
172. Artese L, Alberti L, Lombardo M, et al. Head and neck non-Hodgkin's lymphomas. *Oral Oncol Eur J Cancer* 1995;31B:299–300.
173. Snead M, James J, Snead D, Robson D, Rizk S. Orbital lymphomas and Castleman's disease. *Eye* 1993;7:84–88.
174. Coupland SE, Krause L, Delecluse HJ, et al. Lymphoproliferative lesions of the ocular adnexa. Analysis of 112 cases. *Ophthalmology* 1998;105:1430–1441.

175. Baldini L, Blini M, Guffanti A, et al. Treatment and prognosis in a series of primary extranodal lymphomas of the ocular adnexa. *Ann Oncol* 1998;9:779–781.
176. Weisenthal R, Streeten B, Dubansky A, et al. Burkitt lymphoma presenting as a conjunctival mass. *Ophthalmology* 1995;102:129–134.
177. Leidenix M, Mamalis N, Olson R, et al. Primary T-cell immunoblastic lymphoma of the orbit in a pediatric patient. *Ophthalmology* 1993; 100:998–1002.
178. Karadeniz C, Bilgic S, Ruacan S, et al. Primary subconjunctival lymphoma: an unusual presentation of childhood non-Hodgkin's lymphoma. *Med Pediatr Oncol* 1991;19:204–207.
179. Ko G, Chow C, Yeung V, et al. Hashimoto's thyroiditis, Sjögren's syndrome and orbital lymphoma. *Postgrad Med J* 1994;70:448–451.
180. Luppi M, Longo G, Ferrari M, et al. Additional neoplasms and HCV infection in low-grade lymphoma of MALT type. *Br J Haematol* 1996;94:373–375.
181. Font R, Laucirica R, Rosenbaum P, et al. Malignant lymphoma of the ocular adnexa associated with the benign lymphoepithelial lesion of the parotid glands. Report of two cases. *Ophthalmology* 1992;99: 1582–1587.
182. Nassif P, Feldon S. Orbital lymphoma in a patient with Felty's syndrome. *J Ophthalmol* 1992;76:173–174.
183. Polito E, Leccisotti A. Orbital lymphoma in systemic sarcoidosis [Letter]. *Br J Ophthalmol* 1995;79:1057.
184. Matzkin D, Slamovits T, Rosenbaum P. Simultaneous intraocular and orbital non-Hodgkin's lymphoma in the acquired immune deficiency syndrome. *Ophthalmology* 1994;101:850–855.
185. Rahhal F, Rosberger D, Heinemann M-H. Aggressive orbital lymphoma in AIDS. *Br J Ophthalmol* 1994;78:319–321.
186. Platanias L, Putterman A, Vijayakumar S, et al. Treatment and prognosis of orbital non-Hodgkin's lymphomas. *Am J Clin Oncol* 1992; 15:79–83.
187. Liang R, Loke S, Chiu E. A clinico-pathological analysis of seventeen cases of non-Hodgkin's lymphoma involving the orbit. *Acta Oncol* 1991;30:335–338.
188. Medeiros L, Harris N. Immunohistologic analysis of small lymphocytic infiltrates of the orbit and conjunctiva. *Hum Pathol* 1990; 21: 1126–1131.
189. Nakata M, Matsuno Y, Katsumata N, et al. Histology according to the Revised European-American Lymphoma Classification significantly predicts the prognosis of ocular adnexal lymphoma. *Leuk Lymphoma* 1999;32:533–543.
190. Jeffrey P, Cartwright D, Atwater S, et al. Lacrimal gland lymphoma: a cytomorphologic and immunophenotypic study. *Diagn Cytopathol* 1995;12:215–222.
191. Ferry JA, Zukerberg LR, Fung C, et al. Ocular adnexal lymphoma. A study of 157 cases with a high frequency of marginal zone B-cell lymphoma [Abstract]. *Mod Pathol* 1995;8:109.
192. Wotherspoon A, Hardman-Lea S, Isaacson P. Mucosa-associated lymphoid tissue (MALT) in the human conjunctiva. *J Pathol* 1994; 174: 33–37.
193. Font R, Laucirica R, Patrinely J. Immunoblastic B-cell malignant lymphoma involving the orbit and maxillary sinus in a patient with acquired immune deficiency syndrome. *Ophthalmology* 1993;199: 966–970.
194. Sherman M, Van Dalen J, Conrad K. Bilateral orbital infiltration as the initial sign of a peripheral T-cell lymphoma presenting in a leukemic phase. *Ann Ophthalmol* 1990;22:93–95.
195. Hardman-Lea S, Kerr-Muir M, Wotherspoon A, et al. Mucosal-associated lymphoid tissue lymphoma of the conjunctiva. *Arch Ophthalmol* 1994;112:1207–1212.
196. McNally L, Jakobiec F, Knowles D. Clinical, morphologic, immunophenotypic, and molecular genetic analysis of bilateral ocular adnexal lymphoid neoplasms in 17 patients. *Am J Ophthalmol* 1987; 103:555–568.
197. Coupland SE, Foss HD, Anagnostopoulos I, Hummel M, Stein H. Immunoglobulin VH gene expression among extranodal marginal zone B-cell lymphomas of the ocular adnexa. *Invest Ophthalmol Vis Sci* 1999;40:555–562.
198. Lazzarino M, Morra E, Rosso R, et al. Clinicopathologic and immunologic characteristics of non-Hodgkin's lymphomas presenting in the orbit. A report of eight cases. *Cancer* 1985;55:1907–1912.
199. Khalil H, de Keizer R, Kluin P, et al. Clinical course and pathologic features of conjunctival non-Hodgkin's lymphoma. A report of six cases. *Graefes Arch Clin Exp Ophthalmol* 1990;228:246–251.
200. Brisbane J, Lessell S, Finkel H, et al. Malignant lymphoma presenting in the orbit: a clinicopathologic study of a rare immunoglobulin-producing variant. *Cancer* 1981;47:548–553.
201. Bennett C, Putterman A, Bitran J, et al. Staging and therapy of orbital lymphomas. *Cancer* 1986;57:1204–1208.
202. Fung C, Ferry J, Linggood R, et al. Extranodal marginal zone (MALT type) lymphoma of the ocular adnexae: a localized tumor with favorable outcome after radiation therapy. Proceedings of ASTRO 37th Annual Meeting. *Int J Radiat Oncol Biol Phys* 1996;36:199.
203. Eulau S, Hildebrand R, Warnke R, et al. Primary radiotherapy is curative for CS 1E orbital MALT lymphoma. *Int J Radiat Oncol Biol Phys* 1997;39:176.
204. Imahori S. Low-grade B-cell lymphoma of mucosa-associated lymphoid tissue involving kidney [Letter]. *Arch Pathol Lab Med* 1994;118:111–112.
205. Ramesh K, Gahukamble L, Gahukamble D. Intracranial Burkitt's lymphoma with extension into orbital spaces resulting in bilateral blindness. *Cent Afr J Med* 1994;40:220–222.
206. Peterson K, Gordon K, Heinemann M-H, et al. The clinical spectrum of ocular lymphoma. *Cancer* 1993;72:843–849.
207. Freeman L, Schachat A, Knox D, et al. Clinical features, laboratory investigations, and survival in ocular reticulum cell sarcoma. *Ophthalmology* 1987;94:1631–1639.
208. Char D, Ljung B-M, Miller T, et al. Primary intraocular lymphoma (ocular reticulum cell sarcoma) diagnosis and management. *Ophthalmology* 1988;95:625–630.
209. Whitcup S, de Smet M, Rubin B, et al. Intraocular lymphoma. Clinical and histopathologic diagnosis. *Ophthalmology* 1993;100: 1399–1406.
210. Wilson D, Braziel R, Rosenbaum J. Intraocular lymphoma. Immunopathologic analysis of vitreous biopsy specimens. *Arch Ophthalmol* 1992;110:1455–1458.
211. Qualman S, Mendelsohn G, Mann R, et al. Intraocular lymphomas. Natural history based on a clinicopathologic study of eight cases and review of the literature. *Cancer* 1983;52:878–886.
212. Ridley M, McDonald H, Sternberg P Jr, et al. Retinal manifestations of ocular lymphoma (reticulum cell sarcoma). *Ophthalmology* 1992; 99:1153–1161.
213. Siegel M, Dalton J, Friedman A, et al. Ten-year experience with primary ocular 'reticulum cell sarcoma' (large cell non-Hodgkin's lymphoma). *Br J Ophthalmol* 1989;73:342–346.
214. Buettner H, Bolling J. Intravitreal large-cell lymphoma. *Mayo Clin Proc* 1993;68:1011–1015.
215. Dean J, Novak M, Chan C-C, et al. Tumor detachments of the retinal pigment epithelium in ocular/central nervous system lymphoma. *Retina* 1996;16:47–56.
216. Brown S, Jampol L, Cantrill H. Intraocular lymphoma presenting as retinal vasculitis. *Surv Ophthalmol* 1994;39:133–140.
217. Maiuri F. Visual involvement in primary non-Hodgkin's lymphomas. *Clin Neurol Neurosurg* 1990;92:119–124.
218. Apple D, Boniuk M. Orbital lymphoma associated with acquired immune deficiency syndrome (AIDS). *Surv Ophthalmol* 1994;38: 371–380.
219. Clark W, Scott I, Murray T, et al. Primary intraocular posttransplantation lymphoproliferative disorder. *Arch Ophthalmol* 1998;116: 1667–1669.
220. Maier W, Laubert A, Weinel P. Acute bilateral blindness in childhood caused by rhabdomyosarcoma and malignant lymphoma. *J Laryngol Otol* 1994;108:873–877.
221. Ljung B-M, Char D, Miller T, et al. Intraocular lymphoma. Cytologic diagnosis and the role of immunologic markers. *Acta Cytol* 1988; 32: 840–847.

222. Goldey S, Stern G, Oblon D, et al. Immunophenotypic characterization of an unusual T-cell lymphoma presenting as anterior uveitis. A clinicopathologic case report. *Arch Ophthalmol* 1989;107:1349–1353.
223. Schanzer M, Font R, O'Malley R. Primary ocular malignant lymphoma associated with the acquired immune deficiency syndrome. *Ophthalmology* 1991;98:88–91.
224. Stanton C, Sloan D, Slusher M, Greven C. Acquired immunodeficiency syndrome-related primary intraocular lymphoma. *Arch Ophthalmol* 1992;110:1614–1617.
225. Rivero ME, Kuppermann BD, Wiley CA, et al. Acquired immunodeficiency syndrome-related intraocular B-cell lymphoma. *Arch Ophthalmol* 1999;117:616–622.
226. Ziemianski M, Godfrey W, Lee K, et al. Lymphoma of the vitreous associated with renal transplantation and immunosuppressive therapy. *Ophthalmology* 1980;87:596–601.
227. Kheterpal S, Kirkby G, Neuberger J, et al. Intraocular lymphoma after liver transplantation. *Am J Ophthalmol* 1993;116:507–508.
228. Johnson B. Intraocular and central nervous system lymphoma in a cardiac transplant recipient. *Ophthalmology* 1992;99:987–992.
229. Stephenson P, Duffey R, Ferguson J Jr. Intraocular histiocytic lymphoma: a pediatric case presentation. *J Pediatr Ophthalmol Strabismus* 1989;26:296–298.
230. Keltner J, Fritsch E, Cykiert R, et al. Mycosis fungoides. Intraocular and central nervous system involvement. *Arch Ophthalmol* 1977; 95:645–650.
231. Fredrick DR, Char DH, Ljung BM, et al. Solitary intraocular lymphoma as an initial presentation of widespread disease. *Arch Ophthalmol* 1989;107:395–397.
232. Al-Hazzaa S, Green W, Mann R. Uveal involvement in systemic angiotropic large cell lymphoma. Microscopic and immunohistochemical studies. *Ophthalmology* 1993;100:961–965.
233. Elner VM, Hidayat AA, Charles NC, et al. Neoplastic angioendotheliomatosis. A variant of malignant lymphoma immunohistochemical and ultrastructural observations of three cases. *Ophthalmology* 1986;93:1237–1245.
234. Ben-Ezra D, Sahel J, Harris N, et al. Uveal lymphoid infiltrates: immunohistochemical evidence for a lymphoid neoplasia. *Br J Ophthalmol* 1989;73:846–851.
235. Jakobiec F, Sacks E, Kronish J, et al. Multifocal static creamy choroidal infiltrates. An early sign of lymphoid neoplasia. *Ophthalmology* 1987;94:397–406.
236. Kohno T, Uchida H, Inomata H, et al. Ocular manifestations of adult T-cell leukemia/lymphoma. A clinicopathologic study. *Ophthalmology* 1993;100:1794–1799.
237. Saga T, Ohno S, Matsuda H, et al. Ocular involvement by peripheral T-cell lymphoma. *Arch Ophthalmol* 1984;102:399–402.
238. Primbs G, Monsees W, Irvine A. Intraocular Hodgkin's disease. *Arch Ophthalmol* 1961;66:477–482.
239. Fishburne B, Wilson D, Rosenbaum J, et al. Intravitreal methotrexate as an adjunctive treatment of intraocular lymphoma. *Arch Ophthalmol* 1997;115:1152–1156.
240. Hochberg F, Miller D. Primary central nervous system lymphoma. *J Neurosurg* 1988;68:835–853.
241. Kumar S, Gill P, Wagner D, et al. Human T-cell lymphotropic virus type I-associated retinal lymphoma. A clinicopathologic report. *Arch Ophthalmol* 1994;112:954–959.
242. Kaplan HJ, Meredith TA, Aaberg TM, et al. Reclassification of intraocular reticulum cell sarcoma (histiocytic lymphoma). Immunologic characterization of vitreous cells. *Arch Ophthalmol* 1980;98:707–710.
243. Hattenhauer M, Pach J. Ocular lymphoma in a patient with chronic lymphocytic leukemia. *Am J Ophthalmol* 1996;122:266–268.
244. Takahashi H, Fujita S, Okabe H, et al. Immunophenotypic analysis of extranodal non-Hodgkin's lymphomas in the oral cavity. *Pathol Res Pract* 1993;189:300–311.
245. Wolvius E, van der Valk P, van der Wal J, et al. Primary extranodal non-Hodgkin's lymphoma of the oral cavity. An analysis of 34 cases. *Oral Oncol Eur J Cancer* 1994;30B:121–125.
246. Hicks M, Flaitz C, Nichols C, et al. Intraoral presentation of anaplastic large-cell Ki-1 lymphoma in association with HIV infection. *Oral Surg Oral Med Oral Pathol* 1993;76:73–81.
247. Gulley M, Sargeant K, Grider D, et al. Lymphomas of the oral soft tissues are not preferentially associated with latent or replicative Epstein-Barr virus. *Oral Surg Oral Med Oral Pathol Oral Radiol Endod* 1995;80:425–431.
248. Lozada-Nur F, de Sanz S, Silverman S Jr, et al. Intraoral non-Hodgkin's lymphoma in seven patients with acquired immunodeficiency syndrome. *Oral Surg Oral Med Oral Pathol Oral Radiol Endod* 1996;82:173–178.
249. Eisenbud L, Sciubba J, Mir R, Sachs S. Oral presentations in non-Hodgkin's lymphoma: a review of thirty-one cases. *Oral Surg Oral Med Oral Pathol* 1983;56:151–156.
250. Howell R, Handlers J, Abrams A, et al. Extranodal oral lymphoma. Part II. Relationships between clinical features and the Lukes-Collins classification of 34 cases. *Oral Surg Oral Med Oral Pathol* 1987; 64: 597–602.
251. Fukuda Y, Ishida T, Fujimoto M, et al. Malignant lymphoma of the oral cavity: clinicopathologic analysis of 20 cases. *J Oral Pathol* 1987; 16:8–12.
252. Takahashi H, Kawazoe K, Fujita S, et al. Expression of Bcl-2 oncogene product in primary non-Hodgkin's malignant lymphoma of the oral cavity. *Pathol Res Pract* 1996;192:44–53.
253. Delecluse H, Anagnostopoulos I, Dallenbach F, et al. Plasmablastic lymphomas of the oral cavity: a new entity associated with the human immunodeficiency virus infection. *Blood* 1997;89:1413–1420.
254. Nittayananta W, Chungpanich S, Pongpanich S, Mitarnun W. AIDS-related non-Hodgkin's lymphoma presenting as delayed healing of an extraction wound. *Br Dent J* 1996;181:102–104.
255. Piluso S, Di Lollo S, Baroni G, et al. Unusual clinical aspects of oral non-Hodgkin lymphomas in patients with HIV infection. *Oral Oncol Eur J Cancer* 1994;30B:61–64.
256. Nadimi H. Subclasses of extranodal oral B-cell lymphomas express cIgM, plasmacytoid, and monocytoid differentiation. A study of 10 cases. *Oral Surg Oral Med Oral Pathol* 1994;77:392–397.
257. Rosenburg A, Biesma D, Sie-Go D, et al. Primary extranodal CD30-positive T-cell non-Hodgkin's lymphoma of the oral mucosa. Report of two cases. *Int J Oral Maxillofac Surg* 1996;25:57–59.
258. Shiboski C, Greenspan D, Dodd C, et al. Oral T-cell lymphoma associated with celiac sprue. A case report. *Oral Surg Oral Med Oral Pathol* 1993;76:54–58.
259. Shindoh M, Takami T, Arisue M, et al. Comparison between submucosal (extra-nodal) and nodal non-Hodgkin's lymphoma (NHL) in the oral and maxillofacial region. *J Oral Pathol Med* 1997;26: 283–289.
260. Vazquez-Pineiro T, de Frias L, Cristobal E, et al. HIV-associated oral pleomorphic B-cell malignant lymphoma. *Oral Surg Oral Med Oral Pathol Oral Radiol Endod* 1997;84:142–145.
261. Scully C, Eveson J, Witherow H, et al. Oral presentation of lymphoma: case report of T-cell lymphoma masquerading as oral Crohn's disease, and review of the literature. *Oral Oncol Eur J Cancer* 1993;29B:225–229.
262. Thomas J, Cotter F, Hanby A, et al. Epstein-Barr virus-related oral T-cell lymphoma associated with human immunodeficiency virus immunosuppression. *Blood* 1993;81:3350–3356.
263. Hashimoto N, Kurihara K. Pathological characteristics of oral lymphomas. *J Oral Pathol* 1982;11:214–227.
264. Sirois D, Miller A, Harwick R, et al. Oral manifestations of cutaneous T-cell lymphoma. A report of eight cases. *Oral Surg Oral Med Oral Pathol* 1993;75:700–705.
265. Quarterman M, Lesher J Jr, Davis L, et al. Rapidly progressive CD8-positive cutaneous T-cell lymphoma with tongue involvement. *Am J Dermatol* 1995;17:287–291.
266. Dodd C, Greenspan D, Heinic G, et al. Multi-focal oral non-Hodgkin's lymphoma in an AIDS patient. *Br Dent J* 1993;175: 373–377.
267. Ansell S, Habermann T, Hoyer J, et al. Primary laryngeal lymphoma. *Laryngoscope* 1997;107:1502–1506.

268. Siegel RJ, Browning D, Schwartz DA, et al. Cytomegaloviral laryngitis and probable malignant lymphoma of the larynx in a patient with acquired immunodeficiency syndrome. *Arch Pathol Lab Med* 1992; 116:539–541.
269. Kato S, Sakura M, Takooda S, et al. Primary non-Hodgkin's lymphoma of the larynx. *J Laryngol Otol* 1997;111:571–574.
270. Kawaida M, Fukuda H, Shiotani A, et al. Isolated non-Hodgkin's malignant lymphoma of the larynx presenting as a large pedunculated tumor. *ORL* 1996;58:171–174.
271. Bickerton R, Brockbank M. Lymphoplasmacytic lymphoma of the larynx, soft palate and nasal cavity. *J Laryngol Otol* 1988;102: 468–470.
272. Smith M, Browne J, Teot L. A case of primary laryngeal T-cell lymphoma in a patient with acquired immunodeficiency syndrome. *Am J Otolaryngol* 1996;17:332–334.
273. Wang C-C. Malignant lymphoma of the larynx. *Laryngoscope* 1972;82:97–100.
274. Morgan K, MacLennan K, Narula A, et al. Non-Hodgkin's lymphoma of the larynx (stage 1E). *Cancer* 1989;64:1123–1127.
275. Swerdlow J, Merl S, Davey F, et al. Non-Hodgkin's lymphoma limited to the larynx. *Cancer* 1984;53:2546–2549.
276. Cohen S, Thompson J, Siegel S. Non-Hodgkin's lymphoma of the larynx in children. *Ann Otol Rhinol Laryngol* 1987;96:357–361.
277. Diebold J, Audouin J, Viry B, et al. Primary lymphoplasmacytic lymphoma of the larynx: a rare localization of MALT-type lymphoma [Review]. *Ann Otol Rhinol Laryngol* 1990;99:577–580.
278. Hisashi K, Komune S, Inque H, et al. Coexistence of MALT-type lymphoma and squamous cell carcinoma of the larynx. *J Laryngol Otol* 1994;108:995–997.
279. Dickson R. Lymphoma of the larynx. *Laryngoscope* 1971;81:578–585.
280. Horny H-P, Ferlito A, Carbone A. Clinicopathological consultation. Laryngeal lymphoma derived from mucosa-associated lymphoid tissue. *Ann Otol Rhinol Laryngol* 1996;105:577–583.
281. Donnelly S, Hogan J, Bredin C. Sudden death from primary B-cell non-Hodgkin's lymphoma of the larynx. *Respir Med* 1991;85:77–79.
282. Hessan H, Houck J, Harvey H. Airway obstruction due to lymphoma of the larynx and trachea. *Laryngoscope* 1988;98:176–180.
283. Wells P, Wotherspoon A, Burnet N, et al. Cutaneous B-cell lymphoma with subsequent laryngeal involvement. *Clin Oncol* 1995;7: 62–64.
284. Horny H-P, Kaiserling E. Involvement of the larynx by hemopoietic neoplasms. An investigation of autopsy cases and review of the literature. *Pathol Res Pract* 1995;191:130–138.
285. Simpson RHW, Sarsfield PTL. Benign and malignant lymphoid lesions of the salivary glands. *Curr Diagn Pathol* 1997;4:91–99.
286. Smith FB, Rajdeo H, Panesar N, et al. Benign lymphoepithelial lesion of the parotid gland in intravenous drug users. *Arch Pathol Lab Med* 1988;112:742–745.
287. Finfer MD, Schinella RA, Rothstein SG, et al. Cystic parotid lesions in patients at risk for the acquired immunodeficiency syndrome. *Arch Otolaryngol Head Neck Surg* 1988;114:1290–1294.
288. Elliott JN, Oertel YC. Lymphoepithelial cysts of the salivary glands: histologic and cytologic features. *Am J Clin Pathol* 1990;93:39–43.
289. Labouyrie E, Merlio JPH, Beylot-Barry M, et al. Human immunodeficiency virus type 1 replication within cystic lymphoepithelial lesion of the salivary gland. *Am J Clin Pathol* 1993;100:41–46.
290. Maiorano E, Favia G, Viale G. Lymphoepithelial cysts of salivary glands: an immunohistochemical study of HIV-related and HIV-unrelated lesions. *Hum Pathol* 1998;29:260–265.
291. Ulirsch RC, Jaffe ES. Sjögren's syndrome–like illness associated with the acquired immunodeficiency syndrome–related complex. *Hum Pathol* 1987;18:1063–1068.
292. Terry JH, Loree T, Thomas M, et al. Major salivary gland lymphoepithelial lesions and the acquired immunodeficiency syndrome. *Am J Surg* 1991;162:324–329.
293. Arber DA, Shibata D, Chen Y-Y, et al. Characterization of the topography of Epstein-Barr virus infection in human immunodeficiency virus–associated lymphoid tissues. *Mod Pathol* 1992;5:559–566.
294. Morgan WS, Castleman B. A clinicopathologic study of "Mikulicz's disease." *Am J Pathol* 1953;29:471–503.
295. Godwin JT. Benign lymphoepithelial lesion of the parotid gland. *Cancer* 1952;5:1089–1103.
296. Morgan WS. The probable systemic nature of Mikulicz's disease and its relation to Sjögren's syndrome. *N Engl J Med* 1954;251:5–10.
297. Zulman J, Jaffe R, Talal N. Evidence that the malignant lymphoma of Sjögren's syndrome is a monoclonal B-cell neoplasm. *N Engl J Med* 1978;299:1215–1220.
298. Schmid U, Helbron D, Lennert K. Development of malignant lymphoma in myoepithelial sialadenitis (Sjögren's syndrome). *Virchows Arch* 1982;395:11–43.
299. Isaacson P, Spencer J. Malignant lymphoma of mucosa-associated lymphoid tissue. *Histopathology* 1987;11:445–462.
300. Caselitz J, Osborn M, Wustrow J, et al. Immunohistochemical investigations on the epimyoepithelial islands in lymphoepithelial lesions. Use of monoclonal keratin antibodies. *Lab Invest* 1986;55:426–432.
301. Dardick I, van Nostrand P, Rippstein A, et al. Characterization of epimyoepithelial islands in benign lymphoepithelial lesions of major salivary gland: an immunohistochemical and ultrastructural study. *Head Neck Surg* 1988;10:168–178.
302. Palmer RM, Eveson JW, Gusterson BA. Epimyoepithelial islands in lymphoepithelial lesions. An immunocytochemical study. *Virchows Arch* 1986;408:603–609.
303. Yoshihara T, Morita M, Ishii T. Ultrastructure and three-dimensional imaging of epimyoepithelial islands in benign lymphoepithelial lesions. *Eur Arch Otorhinolaryngol* 1995;252:106–111.
304. Qin C, Pan Y, Hashimoto J, et al. Destructive processes of salivary gland parenchyma and development of epimyoepithelial islands assessed by immunohistochemistry. *Arch Anat Cytol Pathol* 1994; 42: 16–25.
305. Cardoso de Almeida P, Harris N, Bhan A. Characterization of immature sinus histiocytes (monocytoid cells) in reactive lymph nodes by use of monoclonal antibodies. *Hum Pathol* 1984;15:330–335.
306. van Krieken J, von Schilling C, Kluin P, et al. Splenic marginal zone lymphocytes and related cells in the lymph node: a morphologic and immunohistochemical study. *Hum Pathol* 1989;20:320–325.
307. Van den Oord J, De Wolf-Peeters C, Desmet V. The marginal zone in the human reactive lymph node. *Am J Clin Pathol* 1986;86: 475–479.
308. Piris M, Rivas C, Morente M, et al. Monocytoid B-cell lymphoma, a tumour related to the marginal zone. *Histopathology* 1988;12: 383–392.
309. Isaacson P, Wright D. Malignant lymphoma of mucosa associated lymphoid tissue. A distinctive B cell lymphoma. *Cancer* 1983; 52:1410–1416.
310. Nizze H, Cogliatti S, von Schilling C, et al. Monocytoid B-cell lymphoma: morphological variants and relationship to low-grade B-cell lymphoma of the mucosa-associated lymphoid tissue. *Histopathology* 1991;18:403–414.
311. MacLennan I, Liu Y, Oldfield S, et al. The evolution of B-cell clones. *Curr Top Microbiol Immunol* 1990;159:37–63.
312. Ngan B-Y, Warnke R, Wilson M, et al. Monocytoid B-cell lymphoma: a study of 36 cases. *Hum Pathol* 1991;22:409–421.
313. Shin S, Sheibani K, Fishleder A, et al. Monocytoid B-cell lymphoma in patients with Sjögren's syndrome: a clinicopathologic study of 13 patients. *Hum Pathol* 1991;22:422–430.
314. Hsi ED, Zukerberg LR, Schnitzer B, et al. Development of extrasalivary gland lymphoma in myoepithelial sialadenitis. *Mod Pathol* 1995;8:817–824.
315. Quintana PG, Kapadia SB, Bahler DW, et al. Salivary gland lymphoid infiltrates associated with lymphoepithelial lesions: a clinicopathologic, immunophenotypic, and genotypic study. *Hum Pathol* 1997; 28:850–861.
316. Isaacson PG, Hyjek E. Immunoglobulin-gene rearrangement in benign lymphoepithelial lesions [Letter]. *N Engl J Med* 1987;317: 1157–1158.
317. Hyjek E, Smith W, Isaacson P. Primary B cell lymphoma of salivary gland and its relationship to myoepithelial sialadenitis (MESA). *Hum Pathol* 1988;19:766–776.

318. Falzon M, Isaacson P. The natural history of benign lymphoepithelial lesion of the salivary gland in which there is a monoclonal population of B cells: a report of two cases. *Am J Surg Pathol* 1991;15:59–65.
319. Diss TC, Wotherspoon AC, Speight P, et al. B-cell monoclonality, Epstein-Barr virus, and t(14;18) in myoepithelial sialadenitis and low-grade B-cell MALT lymphoma of the parotid gland. *Am J Surg Pathol* 1995;19:531–536.
320. Haddad J, Deny P, Munz-Gotheil C, et al. Lymphocytic sialadenitis of Sjögren's syndrome associated with chronic hepatitis C virus liver disease. *Lancet* 1992;339:571–589.
321. Casato M, Agnello V, Pucillo LP, et al. Predictors of long-term response to high-dose interferon therapy in type II cryoglobulinemia associated with hepatitis C virus infection. *Blood* 1997;90:3865–3873.
322. Talal N, Sokoloff L, Bargh W. Extrasalivary lymphoid abnormalities in Sjögren's syndrome (reticulum cell sarcoma, "pseudolymphoma," macroglobulinemia). *Am J Med* 1967;43:50–65.
323. Kassan S, Thomas T, Moutsopoulos H, et al. Increased risk of lymphoma in sicca syndrome. *Ann Intern Med* 1979;89:888–892.
324. Anderson LG, Talal N. The spectrum of benign to malignant lymphoproliferation in Sjögren's syndrome. *Clin Exp Immunol* 1971;9: 199–221.
325. Hsi ED, Siddiqui J, Schnitzer B, et al. Analysis of immunoglobulin heavy chain gene rearrangement in myoepithelial sialadenitis by polymerase chain reaction. *Am J Clin Pathol* 1996;106:498–503.
326. Fishleder A, Tubbs R, Hesse B, et al. Uniform detection of immunoglobulin-gene rearrangement in benign lymphoepithelial lesions. *N Engl J Med* 1987;316:1118–1121.
327. Lasota J, Miettenen M. Coexistence of different B-cell clones in consecutive lesions of low-grade MALT lymphoma of the salivary gland in Sjögren's disease. *Mod Pathol* 1997;10:872–878.
328. Bahler D, Swerdlow S. Clonal salivary gland infiltrates associated with myoepithelial sialadenitis (Sjögren's syndrome) begin as nonmalignant antigen-selected expansions. *Blood* 1998;91:1864–1872.
329. Gleeson MJ, Bennett MH, Cawson RA. Lymphomas of salivary glands. *Cancer* 1986;58:699–704.
330. Schmid U, Helbron D, Lennert K. Primary malignant lymphomas localized in salivary glands. *Histopathology* 1982;6:673–687.
331. Isaacson P, Wotherspoon A, Diss T, et al. Follicular colonization in B cell lymphoma of mucosa associated lymphoid tissue. *Am J Surg Pathol* 1991;15:819–828.
332. Ashton-Key M, Biddolph S, Stein H, et al. Heterogeneity of bcl-2 expression in MALT lymphoma. *Histopathology* 1995;26:75–78.
333. Isaacson PG, Wotherspoon AC, Diss TC. Bcl-2 expression in lymphomas. *Lancet* 1991;337:175–176.
334. Chetty R, Gatter K. Bcl-2 immunoexpression in MALT-lymphomas [Letter]. *Hum Pathol* 1996;27:1246–1247.
335. Nakamura S, Tsuneyoshi M. Bcl-2 immunoexpression in MALT-lymphomas [Letter]. *Hum Pathol* 1996;27:1247.
336. Bahler DW, Miklos JA, Swerdlow SH. Ongoing Ig gene hypermutation in salivary gland mucosa-associated lymphoid tissue-type lymphomas. *Blood* 1997;89:3335–3344.
337. Du M, Diss T, Xu C, et al. Somatic mutations and intraclonal variations in MALT lymphoma immunoglobulin genes [Abstract]. *Blood* 1995;86(suppl):181.
338. Qin Y, Greiner A, Trunk MJF, et al. Somatic hypermutation in low-grade mucosa-associated lymphoid tissue-type B-cell lymphoma. *Blood* 1995;86:3528–3534.
339. Bahler DW, Miklos JA, Kapadia SB, et al. Preferential use of specific immunoglobulin VH, D, and JH genes by salivary gland MALT lymphomas [Abstract]. *Blood* 1996;88:375.
340. Finn T, Isaacson P, Wotherspoon A. Numerical abnormality of chromosomes 3, 7, 12, and 18 in low grade lymphomas of MALT-type and splenic marginal zone lymphomas detected by interphase cytogenetics on paraffin embedded tissue [Abstract]. *J Pathol* 1993;170:335.
341. Wotherspoon AC, Pan L, Diss T, et al. Cytogenetic study of B-cell lymphoma of mucosa-associated lymphoid tissue. *Cancer Genet Cytogenet* 1992;58:35–38.
342. Wotherspoon AC, Finn TM, Isaacson PG. Trisomy 3 in low-grade lymphomas of mucosa-associated lymphoid tissue. *Blood* 1995; 85: 2000–2004.
343. Brynes RK, Almaguer R, Leathery K, et al. Numerical cytogenetic abnormalities of chromosomes 3, 7, and 12 in marginal zone B-cell lymphomas. *Mod Pathol* 1996;9:995–1000.
344. Ott G, Katzenberger T, Greiner A, et al. The t(11;18)(q21;q21) chromosome translocation is a frequent and specific aberration in low-grade but not high-grade malignant non-Hodgkin's lymphomas of the mucosa-associated lymphoid tissue (MALT) type. *Cancer Res* 1997;57:3944–3948.
345. McCurley TL, Collins RD, Ball E, et al. Nodal and extranodal lymphoproliferative disorders in Sjögren's syndrome: a clinical and immunopathologic study. *Hum Pathol* 1990;21:482–492.
346. Royer B, Cazals-Hatem D, Sibilia J, et al. Lymphomas in patients with Sjögren's syndrome are marginal zone B-cell neoplasms, arise in diverse extranodal and nodal sites, and are not associated with viruses. *Blood* 1997;90:766–775.
347. van der Valk P, Hollema H, van Voorst V, et al. Sjögren's syndrome with specific cutaneous manifestations and multifocal clonal T-cell populations progressing to a cutaneous pleomorphic T-cell lymphoma. *Am J Clin Pathol* 1989;92:357–361.
348. Colby T, Dorfman R. Malignant lymphomas involving the salivary glands. *Pathol Annu* 1979;14:307–324.
349. Medeiros LJ, Rizzi R, Lardelli P, et al. Malignant lymphoma involving a Warthin's tumor: a case with immunophenotypic and gene rearrangement analysis. *Hum Pathol* 1989;21:974–977.
350. Rose NR. The thyroid gland as source and target of autoimmunity. *Lab Invest* 1985;52:117–119.
351. McLachlan SM, McGregor A, Smith BR, et al. Thyroid-autoantibody synthesis by Hashimoto thyroid lymphocytes [Letter]. *Lancet* 1979; 1:162–163.
352. Hsi ED, Singleton TP, Svoboda S, et al. Characterization of the lymphoid infiltrate in Hashimoto thyroiditis by immunohistochemistry and polymerase chain reaction for immunoglobulin heavy chain gene rearrangement. *Am J Clin Pathol* 1998;110:327–333.
353. Hyjek E, Isaacson P. Primary B cell lymphoma of the thyroid and its relationship to Hashimoto's thyroiditis. *Hum Pathol* 1988;19: 1315–1326.
354. Aichinger G, Fill H, Wick G. *In situ* immune complexes, lymphocyte subpopulations, and HLA-DR-positive epithelial cells in Hashimoto thyroiditis. *Lab Invest* 1985;52:132–140.
355. Ben-Ezra J, Wu A, Sheibani K. Hashimoto's thyroiditis lacks detectable clonal immunoglobulin and T cell receptor gene rearrangements. *Hum Pathol* 1988;19:1444–1448.
356. Allison AC. Self-tolerance and autoimmunity in the thyroid. *N Engl J Med* 1976;295:821–827.
357. Holm LE, Blomgren H, Lowhagen T. Cancer risks in patients with chronic lymphocytic thyroiditis. *N Engl J Med* 1985;312:601–604.
358. Kato I, Tajima K, Suchi T, et al. Chronic thyroiditis as a risk factor of B-cell lymphoma in the thyroid gland. *Jpn J Cancer Res* 1985; 76:1085–1090.
359. Aozasa K. Hashimoto's thyroiditis as a risk factor of thyroid lymphoma. *Acta Pathol Jpn* 1990;40:459–468.
360. Noguchi M, Mori N, Kojima M, et al. A case report of malignant lymphoma with Hashimoto's thyroiditis. *Am J Clin Pathol* 1985;83: 650–655.
361. Katzin WE, Fishleder AJ, Tubbs RR. Investigation of the clonality of lymphocytes in Hashimoto's thyroiditis using immunoglobulin and T-cell receptor gene probes. *Clin Immunol Immunopathol* 1989; 51: 264–274.
362. Burke JS, Butler JJ, Fuller LM. Malignant lymphomas of the thyroid: a clinical pathologic study of 35 patients including ultrastructural observations. *Cancer* 1977;39:1587–1602.
363. Chak LY, Hoppe RT, Burke JS, et al. Non-Hodgkin's lymphoma presenting as thyroid enlargement. *Cancer* 1981;48:2712–2716.
364. Maurer R, Taylor CR, Terry R, et al. Non-Hodgkin lymphomas of the thyroid. A clinico-pathological review of 29 cases applying the Lukes-Collins classification and an immunoperoxidase method. *Virchows Arch* 1979;383:293–317.
365. Woolner LB, McConahey WM, Beahrs OH, et al. Primary malignant lymphoma of the thyroid. Review of forty-six cases. *Am J Surg* 1966;111:502–523.

366. Anscombe AM, Wright DH. Primary malignant lymphoma of the thyroid—a tumour of mucosa-associated lymphoid tissue: review of seventy-six cases. *Histopathology* 1985;9:81–97.
367. Aozasa K, Inoue A, Tajima K, et al. Malignant lymphomas of the thyroid gland. Analysis of 79 patients with emphasis on histologic prognostic factors. *Cancer* 1986;58:100–104.
368. Compagno J, Oertel JE. Malignant lymphoma and other lymphoproliferative disorders of the thyroid gland. A clinicopathologic study of 245 cases. *Am J Clin Pathol* 1980;74:1–11.
369. Faure P, Chittal S, Woodman-Memeteau F, et al. Diagnostic features of primary malignant lymphomas of the thyroid with monoclonal antibodies. *Cancer* 1988;61:1852–1861.
370. Heimann R, Vannineuse A, De Sloover C, et al. Malignant lymphomas and undifferentiated small cell carcinoma of the thyroid: a clinicopathological review in the light of the Kiel classification for malignant lymphomas. *Histopathology* 1978;2:201–213.
371. Rasbach DA, Mondschein MS, Harris NL, et al. Malignant lymphoma of the thyroid gland: a clinical and pathologic study of twenty cases. *Surgery* 1985;98:1166–1170.
372. Logue JP, Hale RJ, Stewart AL, et al. Primary malignant lymphoma of the thyroid: a clinicopathological analysis. *Int J Radiat Oncol Biol Phys* 1992;22:929–933.
373. Mizukami Y, Michigishi T, Nonomura A, et al. Primary lymphoma of the thyroid: a clinical, histological and immunohistochemical study of 20 cases. *Histopathology* 1990;17:201–209.
374. Isaacson PG, Androulakis-Papachristou A, Diss TC, et al. Follicular colonization in thyroid lymphoma. *Am J Pathol* 1992;141:43–52.
375. Aozasa K, Inoue A, Yoshimura H, et al. Plasmacytoma of the thyroid gland. *Cancer* 1986;58:105–110.
376. Kovacs CS, Mant MJ, Nguyen GK, et al. Plasma cell lesions of the thyroid: report of a case of solitary plasmacytoma and a review of the literature. *Thyroid* 1994;4:65–71.
377. More JR, Dawson DW, Ralston AJ, et al. Plasmacytoma of the thyroid. *J Clin Pathol* 1968;21:661–667.
378. Aozasa K, Inoue A, Katagiri S, et al. Plasmacytoma and follicular lymphoma in a case of Hashimoto's thyroiditis. *Histopathology* 1986; 10:735–740.
379. Pedersen RK, Pedersen NT. Primary non-Hodgkin's lymphoma of the thyroid gland: a population based study. *Histopathology* 1996;28:25–32.
380. Friedberg MH, Coburn MC, Monchik JM. Role of surgery in stage IE non-Hodgkin's lymphoma of the thyroid. *Surgery* 1994;116: 1061–1066 [Discussion 1066–1067].
381. Poole A, Marchetta F. Extramedullary plasmacytoma of the head and neck. *Cancer* 1968;22:14–21.
382. Susnerwala S, Shanks J, Banerjee S, et al. Extramedullary plasmacytoma of the head and neck region: clinicopathological correlation in 25 cases. *Br J Cancer* 1997;75:921–927.
383. Dolin S, Dewar JP. Extramedullary plasmacytoma. *Am J Pathol* 1956;32:83–103.
384. Kapadia S, Desai U, Cheng V. Extramedullary plasmacytoma of the head and neck. A clinicopathologic study of 20 cases. *Medicine* 1982; 61:317–329.
385. Gaffney C, Dawes P, Jackson D. Plasmacytoma of the head and neck. *Clin Radiol* 1987;38:385–388.
386. Woodruff R, Whittle J, Malpas J. Solitary plasmacytoma. I: Extramedullary soft tissue plasmacytoma. *Cancer* 1979;43: 2340–2343.
387. Harwood A, Knowling M, Bergsagel D. Radiotherapy of extramedullary plasmacytoma of the head and neck. *Clin Radiol* 1981;32:31–36.
388. Luboinski B, Caillaud J, Leridant A, et al. The usefullness of the immunoglobulin P.A.P. method for the prognostic evaluation of head and neck plasmacytoma. *Pathol Res Pract* 1985;179:629–630.
389. Aihara H, Tsutsumi Y, Ishikawa H. Extramedullary plasmacytoma of the thyroid, associated with follicular colonization and stromal deposition of polytypic immunoglobulins and major histocompatibility antigens. Possible categorization in MALT lymphoma. *Acta Pathol Jpn* 1992;42:672–683.
390. Rubin J, Johnson J, Killeen R, et al. Extramedullary plasmacytoma of the thyroid associated with a serum monoclonal gammopathy. *Arch Otolaryngol Head Neck Surg* 1990;116:855–859.
391. Waldron J, Mitchell D. Unusual presentations of extramedullary plasmacytoma in the head and neck. *J Laryngol Otol* 1988;102:102–104.
392. Ferlito A, Carbone A, Volpe R, et al. Late occurrence of IgD myeloma in plasmacytoma of nasal cavity, cervical lymph node and larynx. *J Laryngol Otol* 1982;96:759–766.
393. Sadek S, Dogra T, Khan M, et al. Plasmacytoma of the nasopharynx. (A case report with a follow-up of twelve years). *J Laryngol Otol* 1985;99:1289–1292.
394. Aguilera N, Kapadia S, Nalesnik M, et al. Extramedullary plasmacytoma of the head and neck: use of paraffin sections to assess clonality with *in situ* hybridization, growth fraction, and the presence of Epstein-Barr virus. *Mod Pathol* 1995;8:503–508.
395. Ferry J, Young R, Scully R. Testicular and epididymal plasmacytoma: a report of 7 cases, including three that were the initial manifestation of plasma cell myeloma. *Am J Surg Pathol* 1997;21:590–598.

13

DERMATOPATHOLOGY OF THE HEAD AND NECK

LYN M. DUNCAN

NEOPLASTIC PROLIFERATIVE PROCESSES

Neoplastic Proliferative Processes of the Epidermis and Adnexae

Epidermal Proliferations

Seborrheic Keratosis

Seborrheic keratoses are very commonly occurring benign epidermal proliferations that increase in number and size with age. The earliest signs of seborrheic keratoses are focal hyperpigmentation and a loss of the reflectiveness of the skin surface. Longstanding seborrheic keratoses are pedunculated or have a stuck-on appearance with a pigmented greasy or waxy surface and prominent keratin plugs. The clinical differential diagnosis may include pigmented basal cell carcinoma, pigmented actinic keratosis, and melanoma.

The histologic features of seborrheic keratosis include hyperkeratosis, often with a characteristic whorled pattern of intraepidermal keratin pseudocysts and exophytic epidermal hyperplasia composed of keratinocytes with small round nuclei and basophilic cytoplasm (Fig. 1). The hyperplasia does not penetrate the dermis beyond the level of the adjacent uninvolved epidermis, creating a lesion lying above a "straight line" drawn from one edge to the other. Another commonly seen pattern is a thinly trabecular or "adenoid" pattern. The keratinocytes are often hyperpigmented and form intraepidermal cyst-like spaces containing keratin (so-called horn cysts). In irritated seborrheic keratosis, whorls of keratinocytes form "squamous eddies" composed of more differentiated keratinocytes with abundant eosinophilic cytoplasm. Occasionally, seborrheic keratoses may proliferate down a hair follicle, with numerous squamous eddies; this lesion is termed "inverted follicular keratosis" (Fig. 2). Small duct-like spaces may be present within the seborrheic keratosis; the differential diagnosis includes intraepidermal eccrine poroma (hidracanthoma simplex). The epithelium lining these duct-like spaces is carcinoembryonic antigen (CEA)$^+$ in eccrine poroma and CEA$^-$ in seborrheic keratosis.

Lentigo (Melanotic Macule)

A lentigo is a flat round area of brown pigmentation ranging from 2 to 5 mm in diameter. Lentigines may occur on cutaneous or mucosal surfaces and may increase in number during pregnancy. The lesions may occur early in childhood and are benign. When observed in great numbers without a history of extensive sun exposure, lentigines may be a component of the LEOPARD syndrome (Lentigines, ECG anomalies, Ocular anomalies, Pulmonary stenosis, Abnormal genitalia, Retardation of growth, and Deafness), the NAME syndrome (1), the LAMB syndrome (2), Peutz-Jeghers syndrome (3), or centrofacial lentiginosis. Only rarely is a transition from lentigo to junctional nevus observed. The histologic features of lentigines include mild epidermal hyperplasia with variably elongated epidermal rete, basal layer epithelial hyperpigmentation, variably dense "lentiginous" (i.e., nonnested) melanocytic hyperplasia, and dermal pigment-laden macrophages (Fig. 3).

Lentigines may also occur on the oral mucosa including the hard palate, where they are usually referred to as melanotic macules. The histologic features of mucosal lentigines include variably elongated rete with acanthosis and focal basal layer epithelial hyperpigmentation. A lentiginous, nonnested proliferation of melanocytes may be present, and the underlying submucosa may contain pigment-laden macrophages.

Solar Lentigo (Senile Lentigo, Liver Spot)

Solar lentigos appear as flat, pigmented lesions on sun-exposed sites that may become several centimeters in diameter. Their clinical appearance may mimic that of lentigo maligna. The histologic features of solar lentigo include epidermal changes of either elongation of epidermal rete or epidermal atrophy, basal layer keratinocyte hyperpigmentation, lentiginous melanocytic hyperplasia, and solar elastosis. The superficial dermis usually contains pigment-laden macrophages and a sparse mononuclear cell infiltrate.

Warty Dyskeratoma

Warty dyskeratoma is a benign acantholytic epithelial proliferation that presents as a papule or nodule. In the rare event that it occurs in the oral cavity, it arises as papule on the gingiva or palate. The histologic features of warty dyskeratoma include an exophytic and endophytic crateriform epidermal hyperplasia with marked hyperkeratosis and acantholysis; that is, the epidermal (or mucosal) cells lose their intercellular adherence and apposition, round up, and separate from one another (Fig. 4). These acantholytic cells characteristically are dyskeratotic, have abnormally abundant intercellular keratin, and form characteris-

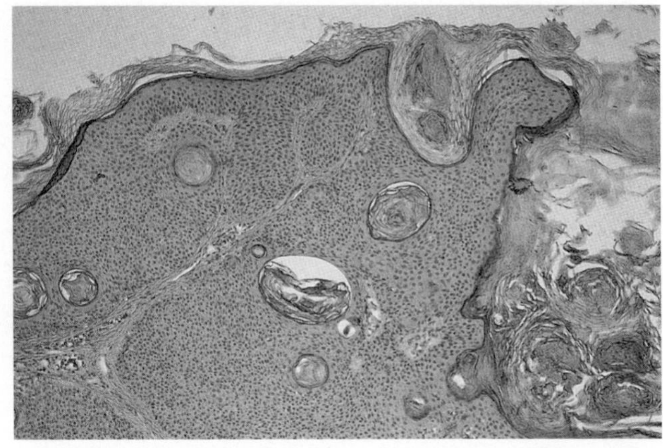

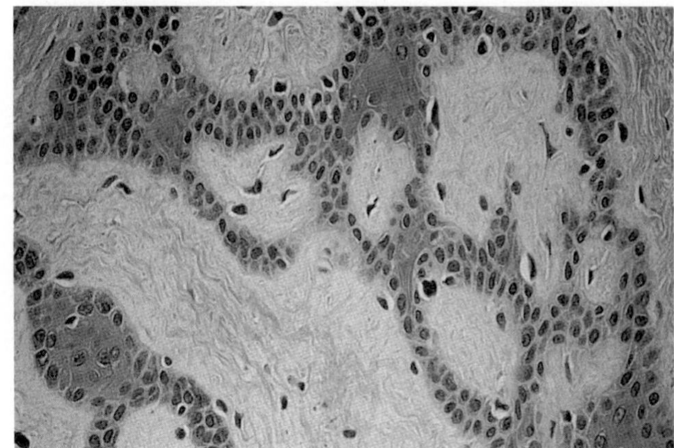

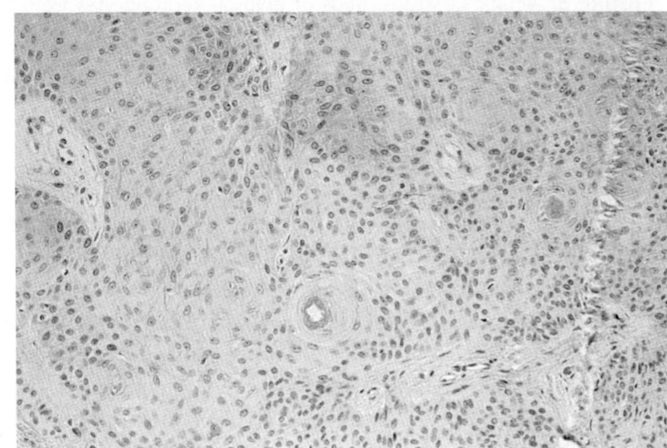

FIGURE 1. Seborrheic keratosis. **A:** Proliferation of relatively monomorphic basaloid keratinocytes with hyperkeratosis and horn cysts. **B:** Delicate interlacing trabeculae of pigmented keratinocytes in reticulated seborrheic keratosis. **C:** Whorls of keratinocytes form squamous eddies in irritated seborrheic keratosis.

tic structures known as corps ronds and grains. Villi of papillary dermis covered by a single layer of keratinocytes extend into the central crater. This pattern of acantholysis is similar to that observed in Darier's disease. The differential diagnosis in a biopsy of warty dyskeratoma may also include transient acantholytic dermatosis (Grover's disease).

Actinic Keratosis (Solar Keratosis)

Actinic keratoses commonly arise on the sun-exposed areas of the face and neck, particularly the cheeks, forehead, temples, and lower lip. They are often scaly and keratotic and may be clinically confused with squamous cell carcinoma or basal cell carcinoma. These premalignant epithelial lesions have a long latent period and only rarely are associated with the development of squamous cell carcinoma (4). Squamous cell carcinomas arising in solar keratoses are usually indolent and cured by local excision.

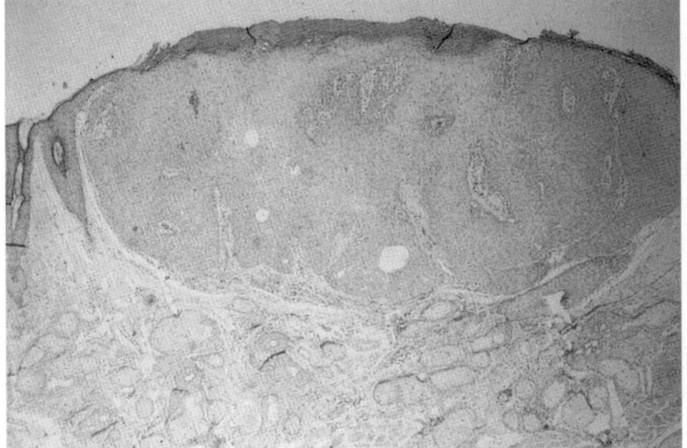

FIGURE 2. Inverted follicular keratosis (irritated seborrheic keratosis). Endophytic proliferation of basaloid keratinocytes with squamous eddies.

There are many histologic variants of actinic keratosis. The principal histologic findings are hyperkeratosis with parakeratosis, basal layer keratinocyte atypia (high nuclear-to-cytoplasmic ratio, nuclear and nucleolar enlargement, irregular chromatin distribution, nuclear pleomorphism), solar elastosis, and a superficial dermal mononuclear cell inflammatory infiltrate (Fig. 5). Buds of atypical basal layer keratinocytes extend into the papillary dermis, usually sparing the adnexal epithelium, but do not break off and invade the dermis as in carcinoma. Mitoses may be present and limited to the lower layers of the epidermis. Actinic keratoses can have significant atypia extending high up in the epidermis, but the full-thickness atypia of squamous cell carcinoma *in situ* is not seen.

Hypertrophic, lichenoid, acantholytic, atrophic, and spreading pigmented variants of actinic keratosis may have clinical findings that lead to a differential diagnosis including other neoplastic and inflammatory disorders. Hypertrophic actinic keratosis is marked by extensive epidermal hyperplasia. A lichenoid infiltrate is characteristic of lichenoid actinic keratosis. The histologic and clinical differential diagnosis may include lichen planus; however, keratinocytic atypia and parakeratosis are observed in lichenoid actinic keratosis but not in lichen planus.

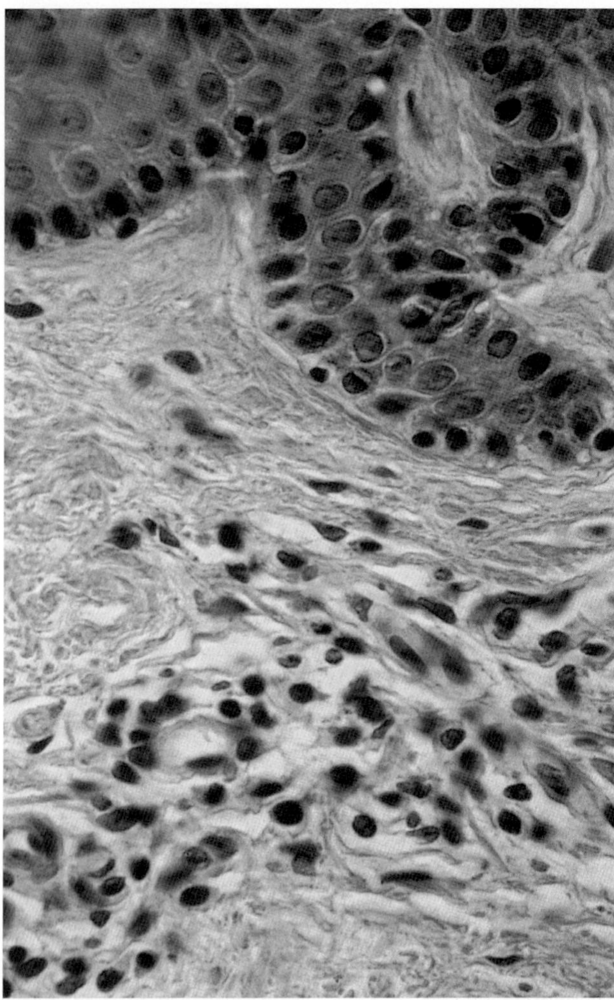

FIGURE 3. Lentigo. Hyperpigmentation of basal layer keratinocytes with slight epithelial hyperplasia forming buds of epithelium extending into the underlying stroma. Slight or absent lentiginous melanocytic hyperplasia.

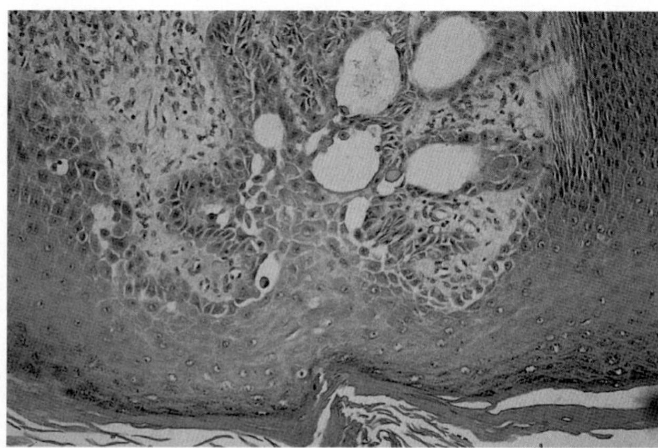

FIGURE 5. Actinic keratosis. Buds of atypical keratinocytes from the base of the epidermis protrude but do not invade into the papillary dermis with solar elastosis, a chronic inflammatory infiltrate, and parakeratosis. Acantholysis of the basal keratinocytes is occasionally present, as shown here.

Acantholytic and atrophic actinic keratosis show acantholysis (loss of intercellular adherence) and absence of the normal rete ridges, respectively. The histologic features of spreading pigmented actinic keratosis include hyperkeratosis, frequently without parakeratosis, atypia of basal layer keratinocytes, hyperpigmentation of basal layer keratinocytes, solar elastosis, and a variably dense dermal mononuclear cell inflammatory infiltrate (Fig. 6).

Squamous Cell Carcinoma *in Situ* (Bowen's Disease)

Squamous cell carcinoma *in situ* appears as an erythematous scaly area that may develop a granular moist surface. These lesions are usually flat but may become slightly elevated and rarely ulcerate.

The histologic features of squamous cell carcinoma *in situ* include full-thickness cytologic atypia of the epidermal ker-

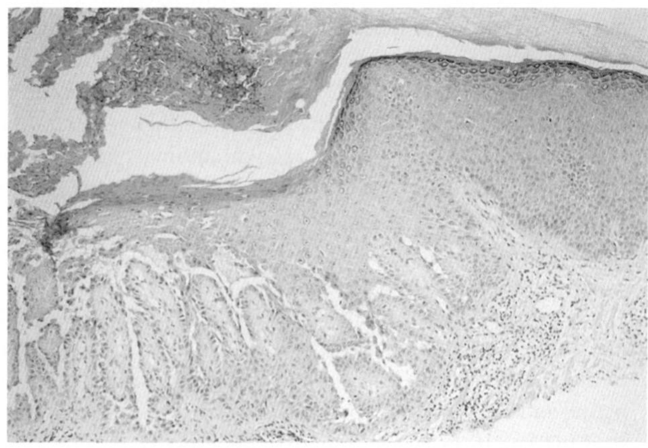

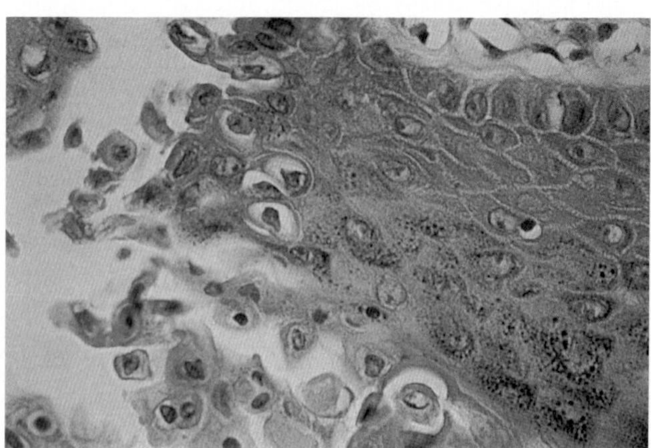

FIGURE 4. Warty dyskeratoma. **A:** Endophytic epithelial hyperplasia with villi of papillary dermis covered by a layer of acantholytic basaloid epithelium extending upward in the lesion center. **B:** Acantholytic dyskeratosis with corps ronds (anucleate keratinocytes with donut-shaped arrangement of eosinophilic cytoplasmic tonofilaments and basophilic keratohyaline granules) and grains (millet seed–like pyknotic parakeratotic nuclei).

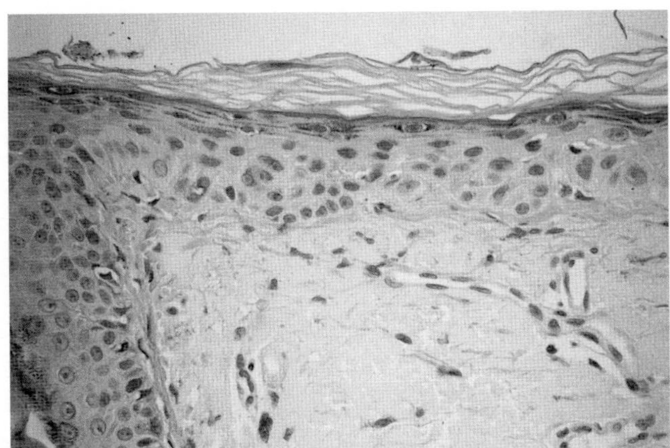

FIGURE 6. Spreading pigmented actinic keratosis. Atypical pigmented basal keratinocytes with marked basophilic homogeneous dermal solar elastosis and minimal hyperkeratosis.

atinocytes (Fig. 7), dyskeratosis, multinucleate keratinocytes, and mitoses at all levels of the epidermis, including the granular cell layer. Occasionally these tumors may have a nested growth pattern resembling mammary Paget's disease. Some forms of carcinoma *in situ* or Bowen's disease may be associated with the occurrence of visceral malignancies.

Squamous Cell Carcinoma, Invasive

Squamous cell carcinoma in the head and neck arises on the most sun-exposed sites, in particular the upper face and lower lip. The tumor initially appears as a firm indurated area, which may progress to form a papillomatous hyperkeratotic or ulcerated surface. Squamous cell carcinoma of the lip not infrequently presents as a nonhealing fissure or ulcer. Lesions of the vermilion of the lip and the ear metastasize with a higher frequency than squamous cell carcinomas arising elsewhere on the face or body. In addition to metastases to regional lymph nodes, as may be observed in squamous cell carcinoma arising in the lip, squamous cell carcinoma of the external ear and ear canal is often locally aggressive (5). Squamous cell carcinomas account for 45% of all tumors of the external and middle ear (6). When large tumors are allowed to persist in the external auditory canal, extension along the neurovascular bundles and perichondrial and periosteal tissue planes may lead to extensive destruction of the ear and surrounding structures.

The histologic features of cutaneous invasive squamous cell carcinoma are much the same as in other sites and include a proliferation of epidermal keratinocytes with variable keratinocyte atypia (less marked in well-differentiated tumors). Dyskeratosis, apoptosis, and numerous mitoses, frequently with atypical forms, are observed. Dermal invasion by individual cells or irregularly shaped nests of keratinocytes are present and often have

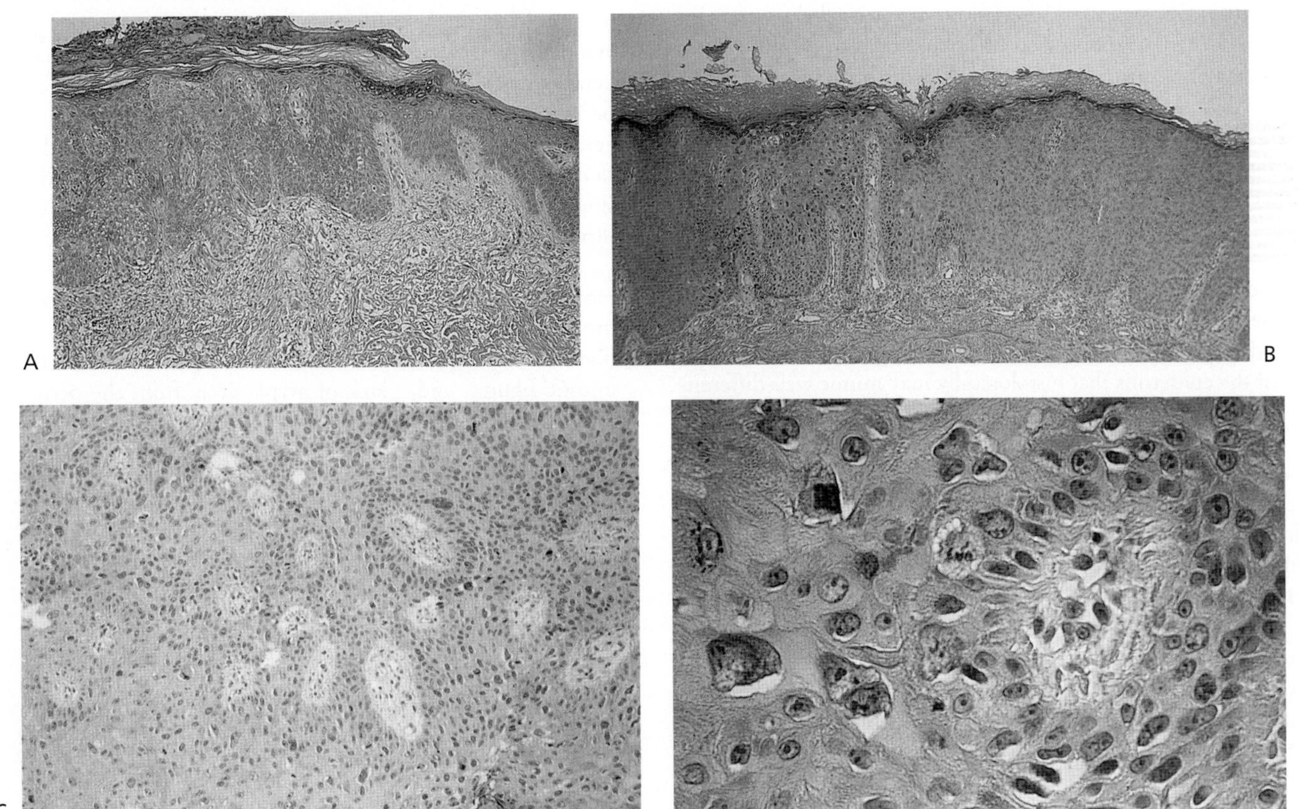

FIGURE 7. Squamous cell carcinoma *in situ.* **A:** Atypical keratinocytic proliferation at all levels of the epidermis, replacing and expanding the normal structure, with scale crust and a mild dermal mononuclear cell infiltrate. **B:** In contrast to the well-demarcated "clonal" pattern in **A,** more subtle full-thickness keratinocyte atypia. **C:** Loss of normal keratinocytic maturation from base to surface. **D:** Nuclear anaplasia, multinucleate cells, dyskeratosis, and mitoses.

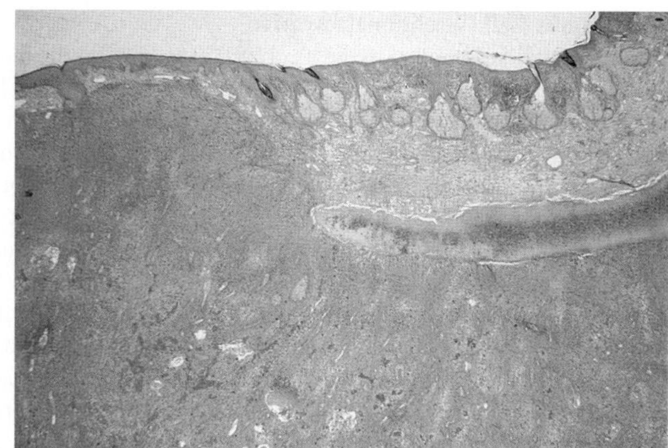

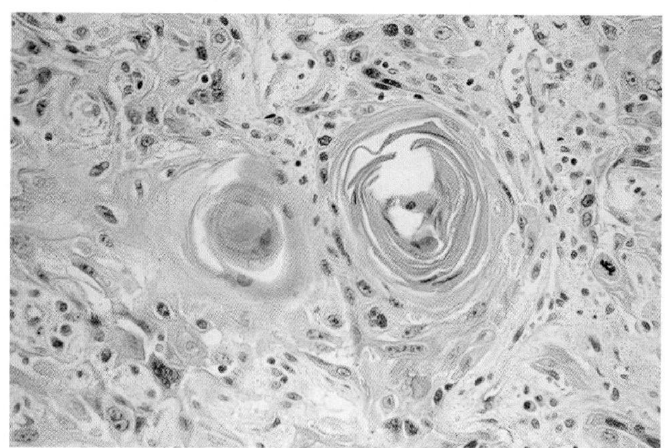

FIGURE 8. Squamous cell carcinoma, invasive. **A:** Endophytic proliferation of well-differentiated keratinocytes extends from the epidermal surface as a large mass of eosinophilic tumor cells that undermines the cartilage in this specimen from the ear. **B:** Keratinocytic atypia and keratinization with squamous pearls.

an associated desmoplastic stromal reaction (Fig. 8). Immunohistochemically, squamous cell carcinomas have a cytokeratin^{+}, vimentin^{-}, S-100 protein^{-}, HMB-45^{-}, CEA^{-}, epithelial membrane antigen (EMA)$^{\pm}$ phenotype (7).

Verrucous Carcinoma

An extensively verrucous lesion arising on the oral mucosa with a cauliflower-like appearance is characteristic of verrucous carcinoma (see Chapter 2). These lesions are so well differentiated histologically that a diagnosis of carcinoma is often difficult to render. Verrucous carcinoma displays a distinctive expansile, rather than infiltrative, growth pattern without significant cytologic atypia or atypical mitoses. These tumors may be extensively locally invasive but, in their pure form (i.e., not admixed with conventional squamous cell carcinoma), virtually never metastasize.

Pseudocarcinomatous Hyperplasia (Pseudoepitheliomatous Hyperplasia)

Pseudocarcinomatous hyperplasia is a benign reactive hyperplasia of the epidermis that histologically may mimic well-differentiated squamous cell carcinoma. Clinically this lesion may appear as a nodule with a verrucous surface or focal ulceration. Common settings for pseudocarcinomatous hyperplasia include deep fungal infections, lichen simplex chronicus, lichen planus, the margin of chronic ulcers, reactions to some drugs (halogenodermas), oral necrotizing sialometaplasia, and overlying some tumors including granular cell tumor.

The histologic features of pseudocarcinomatous hyperplasia include marked endophytic epidermal hyperplasia with hyperkeratosis and irregularly shaped dermal nests of squamous epithelium. There is an absence of marked nuclear anaplasia, extensive keratinization in the deep dermis, and desmoplastic stroma; when present, these findings favor a diagnosis of malignancy.

Keratoacanthoma

These keratinocytic proliferations are considered to be benign regressing tumors by some observers and a low-grade form of squamous cell carcinoma by others. Keratoacanthomas characteristically arise rapidly and often regress spontaneously. Their biological behavior is nonaggressive. They only rarely occur on the skin of the head and neck or the oral mucosa (8). A deep wedge biopsy or excision is necessary for histologic diagnosis because the features that aid in distinction from invasive squamous cell carcinoma are present at the deep margin of the tumor.

The histologic features of keratoacanthoma include an endophytic epidermal proliferation with a central keratin-filled crater. The proliferating keratinocytes have abundant clear to "glassy" cytoplasm with variable cytologic atypia of the peripheral layer of keratinocytes (Fig. 9). There may be dyskeratosis and colloid body formation (collections of extracellular homogeneous pink keratin-derived material). Intraepithelial eosinophil and polymorphonuclear cell microabscesses are often present, and occasionally the tumor is surrounded by a dense mononuclear cell infiltrate.

The main differential diagnosis of keratoacanthoma is squamous cell carcinoma. A variety of histologic features, including intraepithelial eosinophilic microabscesses, extrusion of elastic fibers into the epithelial layer, glassy cytoplasm, absent atypical mitotic figures, and a lack of atypia away from the peripheral

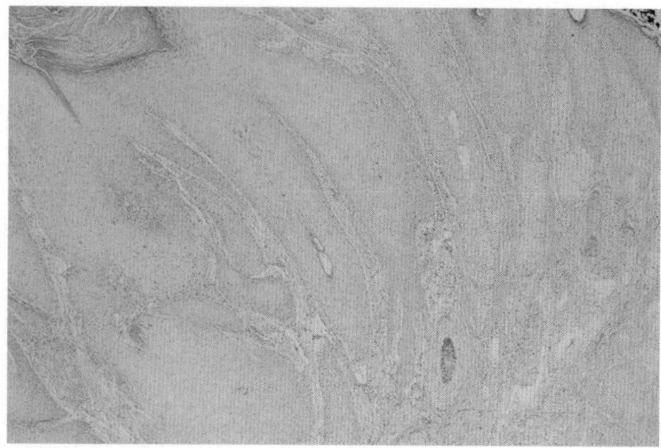

FIGURE 9. Keratoacanthoma. Crateriform endophytic proliferation of keratinocytes with abundant pale glassy cytoplasm.

portion of the lesions and in the surrounding epidermis have been described as favoring a diagnosis of keratoacanthoma. These criteria, however, are not universally accepted. Extension of the tumor into the dermis below the eccrine glands and keratinization with so-called "naked keratin" in the dermis at the deep aspect of the tumor are findings that support a diagnosis of invasive squamous cell carcinoma over that of keratoacanthoma. In addition, although keratinocytic atypia may be observed in keratoacanthoma, extensive nuclear anaplasia with the infiltration of the underlying dermis by individual anaplastic tumor cells also supports a diagnosis of malignancy.

Paget's Disease

The histologic features of Paget's disease are similar in mammary and extramammary sites; characteristically there is an intraepidermal proliferation of individual cells, and nests of cells, with tumor cells present at all epidermal levels (pagetoid spread) (Fig. 10). A layer of keratinocytes usually separates the tumor cells in Paget's disease from the basement membrane zone. The tumor cells in Paget's disease display abundant clear cytoplasm, occasionally with intracytoplasmic sialomucin that stains positively with alcian blue, mucicarmine, and PASD stains. Notably, the tumor cells of Paget's disease may also rarely contain melanin. Mitotic figures are rarely identified in extramammary Paget's disease. The tumor cells of Paget's disease have a cytokeratin$^+$, EMA$^+$, CEA$^+$, S-100$^-$, HMB-45$^-$ immunophenotype.

Basal Cell Carcinoma

Basal cell carcinoma typically appears as a translucent, pearly, pink papule with telangiectasia and occasionally focal pigmentation. This tumor may occasionally expand to form an erythematous plaque or develop into a nodule with focal ulceration (so called "rodent ulcer"). If allowed to persist, local invasion into the underlying soft tissues may occur. Tumors close to the eye, nose, and ear may be particularly destructive. The morpheic or morpheaform type of basal cell carcinoma may appear as a thickened yellow or gray sclerotic plaque or scar. Basal cell carcinomas are very common and usually occur on sun-exposed areas. They tend to invade locally but rarely metastasize. Rare large deeply invasive or metastatic basal cell carcinomas may be lethal (9). The nevoid basal cell carcinoma syndrome is a rare disorder characterized by the early onset of numerous, at times innumerable, basal cell carcinomas, ondontogenic keratocysts, palmar pitting, cutaneous cysts, calcification of the falx cerebri, and hypertelorism. The autosomal dominant gene responsible for this disorder is located on chromosome 9q.

There are many histologic types of basal cell carcinoma including superficial, nodular, metatypical, and morpheaform. The principal histologic features include a proliferation of basaloid epithelial cells extending from the epidermis into the underlying dermis with a characteristic palisading of the peripheral layer of basaloid cells (Fig. 11). The tumor cells have inconspicuous intercellular junctions and may display apoptosis and mitotic activity. Clefts containing mucin separate the tumor from the dermal stroma. Small buds of tumor extend from the epidermis in the superficial type of basal cell carcinoma, often highlighted by the characteristic separation from the surrounding mucin-rich stroma, whereas dermal nodules of basaloid cells, frequently with cystic necrosis or an adenoidal (or trabecular) pattern, are observed in the nodular variant. The term "metatypical basal cell carcinoma" is used when foci resembling squamous cell carcinoma are seen within a basal cell carcinoma. Individual tumor cells and strands of cells dissect through a densely fibrotic stroma in the morpheaform variant. Fibroepithelioma of Pinkus is a variant of basal cell carcinoma composed of anastomosing strands of epithelium extending from the epidermis with focal palisading of basaloid cells embedded in a fibrovascular dermal stroma with focal hyalinization. Basosquamous carcinoma is a collision tumor composed of a nodular basal cell carcinoma and an invasive squamous cell carcinoma. Excision with a narrow margin of uninvolved tissue is generally curative.

Lymphoepithelioma-like Carcinoma

This malignant epithelial tumor characteristically is surrounded by a dense reactive lymphoid infiltrate. It is not a lymphoma but may be mistaken for one (10). The histologic features include a dermal-based proliferation of mitotically active large atypical polygonal epithelial cells that stain immunohistochemically for

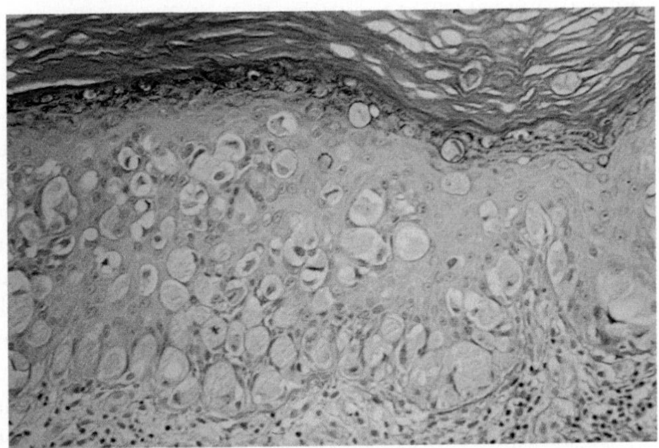

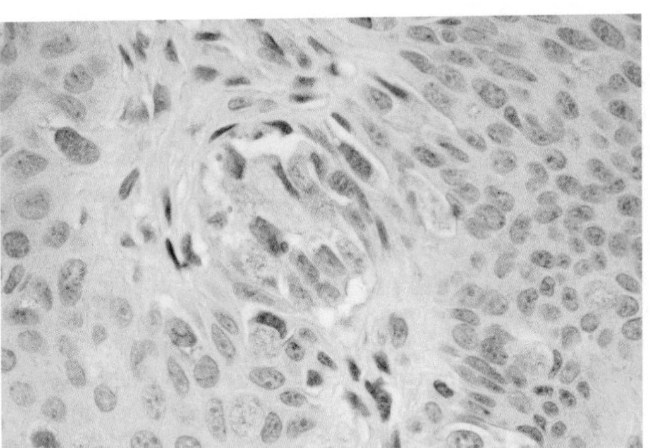

FIGURE 10. Paget's disease. **A:** Individual tumor cells with basophilic cytoplasm and pleomorphic nuclei scattered at all levels of the epidermis. **B:** Mucicarmine stain demonstrates rose-colored cytoplasmic mucin in the tumor cells.

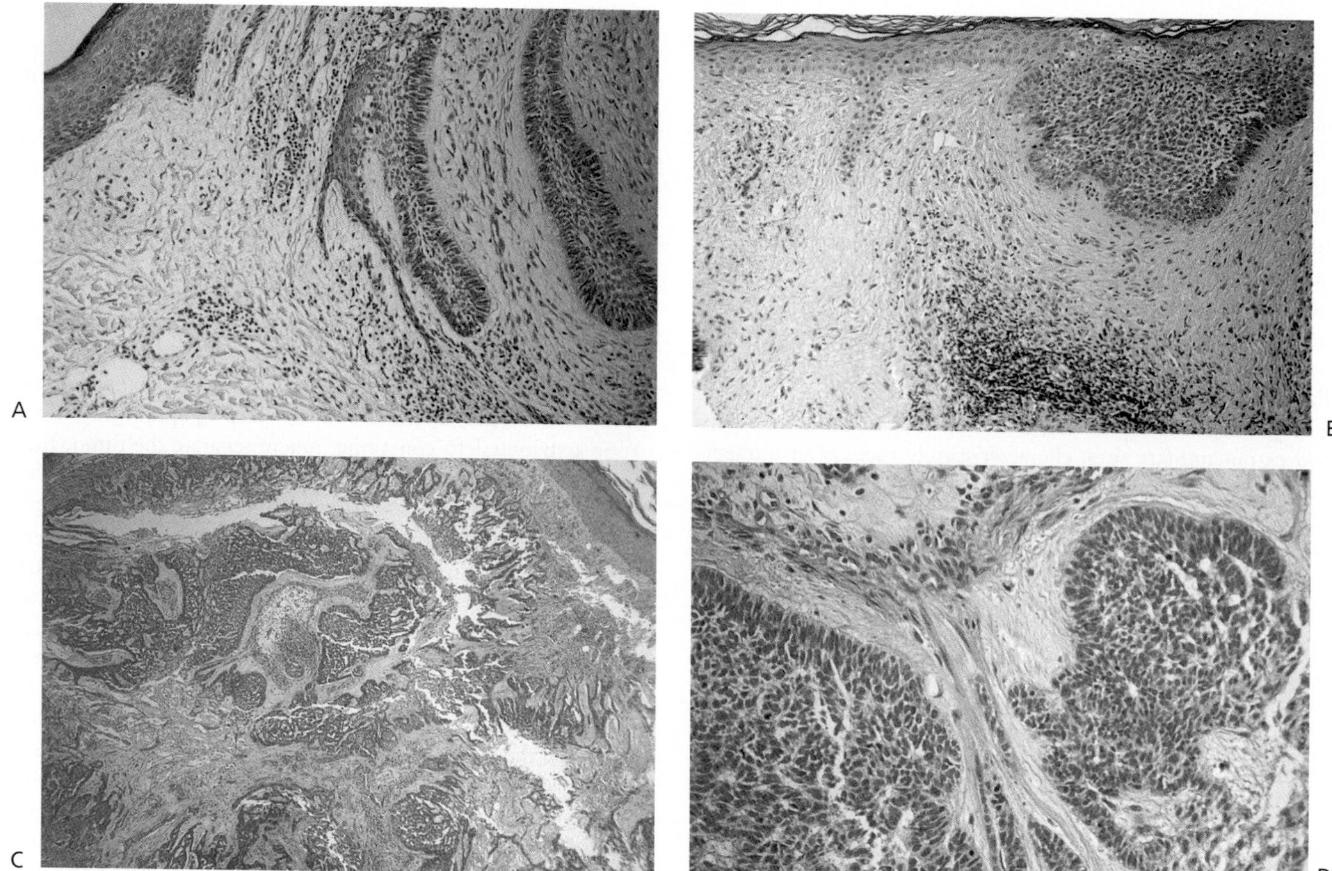

FIGURE 11. Basal cell carcinoma. **A:** Two elongated buds of basophilic tumor cells extend from the epidermis into a mucin-rich dermis in this superficial basal cell carcinoma. **B:** Proliferation of pigmented basaloid cells associated with a chronic inflammatory infiltrate in pigmented superficial basal cell carcinoma. **C:** Nodular basal cell carcinoma with a mucin-containing cleft separating tumor cells from the dermal stroma. **D:** Nodular basal cell carcinoma with an adenoidal growth pattern.

cytokeratins but not for leukocyte common antigen (LCA). The reactive inflammatory infiltrate is predominately lymphocytic with scattered plasma cells. This carcinoma with a very dense lymphoid infiltrate closely resembles the nonkeratinizing type of nasopharyngeal carcinoma (see Chapter 5).

Pilar Neoplasms (Neoplasms of Hair Appendages)

Trichoepithelioma

This benign tumor of germinative hair follicle epithelium presents as a slowly growing solitary nodule of the midface that may become several centimeters in diameter. These lesions rarely ulcerate and usually appear first early in life but are not recognized until adulthood. Multiple trichoepitheliomas may occur in a wide range of clinical settings, including (a) a familial autosomal dominantly inherited form, (b) Rombo syndrome (milia, hypotrichosis, trichoepithelioma, basal cell carcinoma, peripheral vasodilation with cyanosis, and vermiculate atrophoderma) (11), (c) Cowden's disease (trichilemmomas, visceral carcinoma, rarely trichoepitheliomas) (12), (d) systemic lupus erythematosus, and (e) myasthenia gravis.

Histologically, there is a circumscribed dermal proliferation of basaloid epithelium with basaloid cells arranged in small nests and nodules, occasionally with keratin cyst formation (Fig. 12). Pilar differentiation with papillary mesenchymal bodies resembling inverting tissue at the base of the hair bulb is a histologic hallmark of trichoepithelioma. Calcification and foreign body giant-cell reaction to keratin may also be present. As is characteristic of benign cutaneous adnexal tumors, the epithelial proliferation is embedded in a circumscribed fibrocellular stroma. The histologic differential diagnosis of trichoepithelioma most commonly includes basal cell carcinoma. Features that support a diagnosis of trichoepithelioma are the presence of keratin cysts, papillary mesenchymal bodies, and a hypocellular fibrous stroma. Findings that support a diagnosis of basal cell carcinoma include a fibromyxoid stroma, separation clefts between the basal epithelium and the stroma, and multifocal budding from the surface epidermis. In some cases, particularly small biopsy samples of large tumors, a definitive diagnosis may not be possible.

An even more challenging lesion from a diagnostic standpoint is desmoplastic trichoepithelioma. Desmoplastic trichoepithelioma presents as a solitary flesh-colored papule, usually on the face of a young woman. These lesions rarely become larger than 1 cm and have no known associated syndromes (13,14). In addition to a circumscribed dermal proliferation of basaloid cells arranged in small nests or strands with commonly

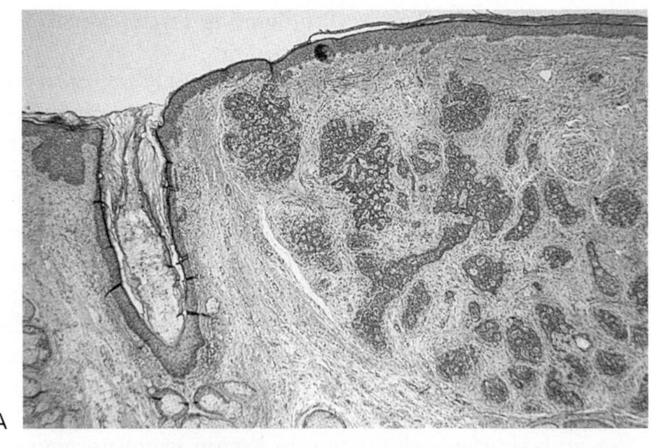

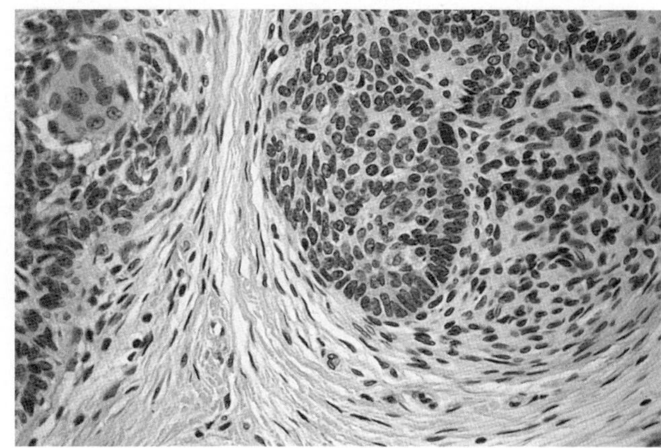

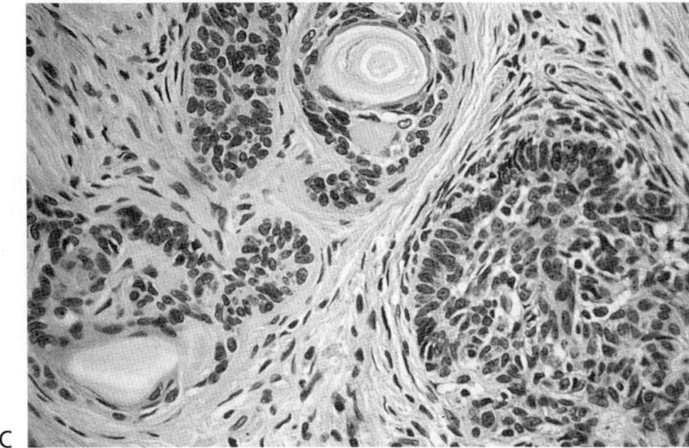

FIGURE 12. Trichoepithelioma. **A:** Well-circumscribed epithelial proliferation with a fibroblast-rich stroma; well-defined tumor stroma is a characteristic of benign adnexal tumors. **B:** Papillary mesenchymal bodies recapitulate the association of the primary hair germ epithelium with the dermal papilla in a claw-and-ball–like configuration. In contrast to basal cell carcinoma, the stroma in trichoepithelioma is fibroblastic without mucin or cleft formation at the epithelial–stromal junction. **C:** Proliferation of basaloid cells forming keratin cysts.

occurring keratotic cyst formation, desmoplastic trichoepithelioma is characterized by a densely sclerotic, hypocellular, well-circumscribed stroma (Fig. 13). The histologic differential diagnosis of this benign lesion includes two carcinomas: morpheaform basal cell carcinoma and microcystic adnexal carcinoma (15–19). Small clusters of basaloid cells, keratotic cysts with calcification, evidence of pilar differentiation, and extension only into the midreticular dermis support a diagnosis of desmoplastic trichoepithelioma (20). On the other hand, the presence of deep infiltration into the dermis, subcutaneous fat, or along neurovascular bundles, supports a diagnosis of carcinoma.

Immunohistochemical analysis of trichoepithelioma and desmoplastic trichoepithelioma reveals positive staining for cytokeratin 14, EMA, and LeuM1 but not CEA or cytokeratin 13. Microcystic adnexal carcinoma stains positively for all of these markers, including CEA and cytokeratin 13; these stains may be helpful in differentiating these tumors (21).

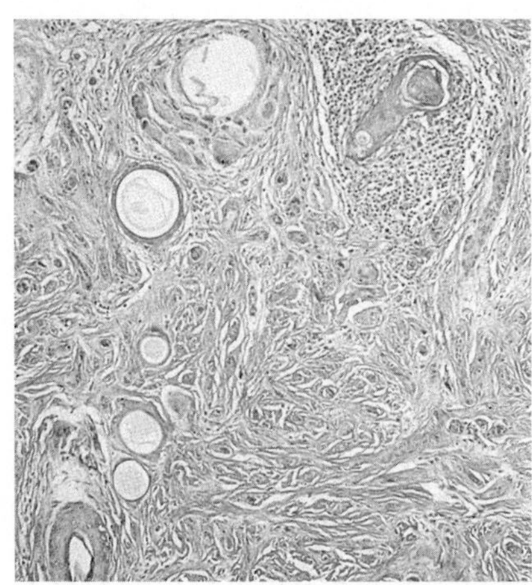

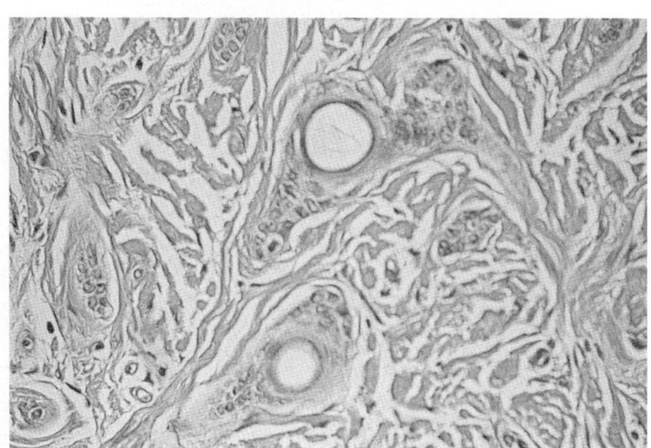

FIGURE 13. Desmoplastic trichoepithelioma. **A:** Proliferation of small cords and nests of basaloid cells with keratin cysts embedded in a densely fibrous stroma. **B:** Cords of tumor cells with small keratin cysts in desmoplastic trichoepithelioma mimic syringoma and microcystic adnexal carcinoma.

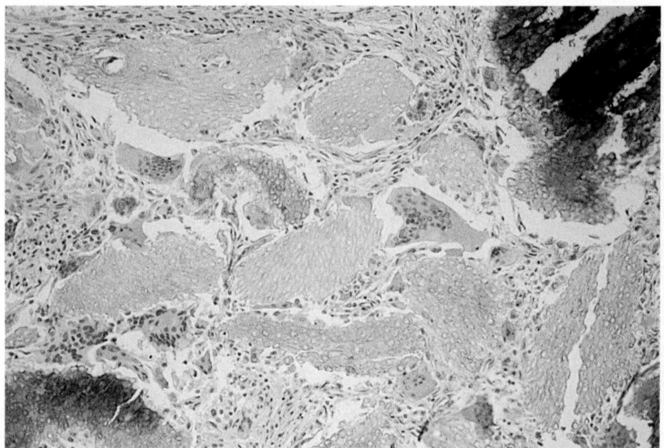

FIGURE 14. Pilomatrixoma. Sheets of shadow cells with focal calcification and foreign body giant-cell reaction.

Pilomatrixoma (Calcifying Epithelioma of Malherbe)

This relatively common lesion occurs mainly on the preauricular skin of children and young adults and usually presents as a firm deep dermal or subcutaneous nodule less than 4 cm in diameter with normal-appearing overlying epidermis. Complete excision is the treatment of choice (22). Pilomatrixoma is a tumor of germinative follicular epithelium composed of large dermal lobules of basaloid cells that surround cystic spaces containing keratin and sheets of eosinophilic shadow cells or ghost cells (cells containing the outline of a nucleus but without chromatin or nuclear basophilia) without an intervening granular cell layer (Fig. 14). Calcification is common, and ossification occurs in up to 20% of cases (23). An interesting observation has been the identification of extramedullary hematopoiesis in 5% of pilomatrixomas (24). A very rare malignant variant (pilomatrix carcinoma) has been reported (25).

Proliferating Pilar Tumor (Proliferating Trichilemmal Cyst)

Proliferating pilar tumor occurs most commonly as a solitary tumor on the scalp of adult women. These tumors are often deep and slowly growing, enlarging to several centimeters, not infrequently with the development of an ulcerated surface. Proliferating pilar tumor is a tumor of outer root sheath epithelium characterized by a solid and cystic epithelial proliferation extending from the epidermis into the dermis. The proliferation is composed of large, well-differentiated eosinophilic keratinocytes with a peripheral palisade of glycogenated epithelial cells, squamous eddies, and keratin cysts without a granular cell layer lining. Keratinization is of the more solid pilar type and is without the basket-weave appearance of epidermal keratin. A foreign body giant-cell reaction to keratin is not uncommon. Although the mitotic rate may be brisk, and some of the tumor cells may be pleomorphic, no significant nuclear anaplasia or necrosis is observed.

Because of the mitotic activity and the common finding of epithelial atypia, these tumors may be mistaken for squamous cell carcinoma or the very rare malignant counterpart of proliferating pilar tumor, pilar carcinoma (26,27). Features that support the diagnosis of a malignant tumor include significant nuclear anaplasia, extensive infiltration of surrounding structures, and tumoral necrosis; these features are not observed in proliferating pilar tumor. Complete excision of proliferating pilar tumor is recommended because these tumors have a high rate of recurrence.

Trichilemmoma

This tumor is common and occurs on the face and eyelids. Trichilemmoma is a benign tumor of outer root sheath epithelium composed of a lobule of epithelial cells with clear or pale glycogenated cytoplasm. The tumor protrudes from the epidermis or follicular infundibulum into the dermis. There is periph-

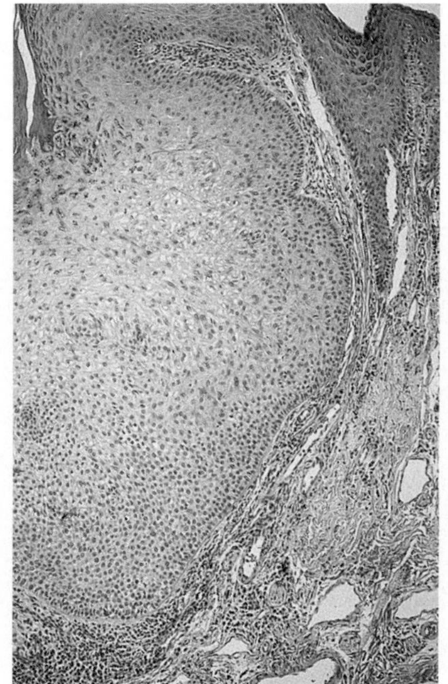

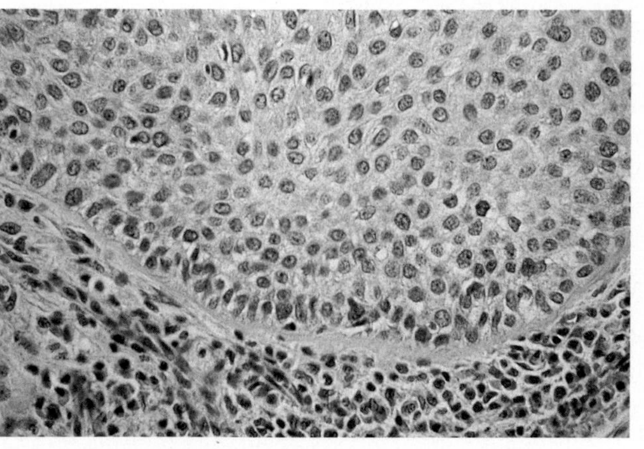

FIGURE 15. Trichilemmoma. **A:** Endophytic proliferation of keratinocytes with abundant clear cytoplasm. **B:** Homogeneous eosinophilic vitreous basement membrane separates the trichilemmal epithelium from the dermis.

eral palisading of basaloid epithelium separated from the dermis by a thickened PAS-positive basement membrane zone that resembles the outer follicular vitreous membrane (Fig. 15).

Trichofolliculoma

Trichofolliculoma is an uncommon benign tumor that usually occurs as a solitary papule or nodule on the face, scalp, or neck. There is a central pore containing a keratin plug and several fine hair shafts. Trichofolliculoma is a tumor of germinative follicular epithelium characterized by a dilated follicular infundibulum with multiple buds and lobules of squamous and basaloid epithelium resembling small abortive hair follicles extending from the follicular infundibulum into the dermis. The tumor epithelium is predominantly glycogenated with a palisaded peripheral layer of keratinocytes. Secondary hair follicles are often observed and may occasionally contain hair. When the histologic orientation of the specimen obscures the central hair follicle, the differential diagnosis may include basal cell carcinoma. In this case, absence of stromal mucinosis or separation clefts between the basal layer of keratinocytes and the stroma support a diagnosis of trichofolliculoma.

Dilated Pore of Winer

Dilated pore of Winer may occur as a solitary papule or as multiple lesions on the skin of the head and neck in adults (28). It is derived from the follicular outer root sheath and is closely related to pilar sheath acanthoma (29). Histologically, dilated pore of Winer is composed of a dilated follicular infundibulum containing a keratin plug with epithelial hyperplasia at the base of the pore. Occasionally, residual sebaceous glands or vellus hairs are observed at the base of the pore.

Fibrofolliculoma (Birt-Hogg-Dubé Syndrome)

Fibrofolliculoma usually manifests as multiple small papules on the face. These tumors are observed along with trichodiscomas, skin tags, and perifollicular fibromas in the Birt-Hogg-Dubé syndrome (30). Fibrofolliculoma is a mixed tumor of follicular epithelium and mesenchymal elements. It is characterized by anastomosing strands of epithelium extending from a hair follicle into a cellular fibrous stroma, often with abundant stromal mucin.

Folliculosebaceous Cystic Hamartoma

Folliculosebaceous cystic hamartoma usually occurs as an exophytic papule or nodule of the central face (31,32). The histologic features of folliculosebaceous cystic hamartoma include a dermal-based dilated follicular infundibulum or epithelial lined cyst with mature sebaceous glands radiating from the cyst (Fig. 16). The surrounding circumscribed mesenchymal component is composed of fat and densely fibrotic collagen. Varying degrees of follicular differentiation are observed.

Other follicular appendage tumors are rare curiosities and are described in more specialized texts (20).

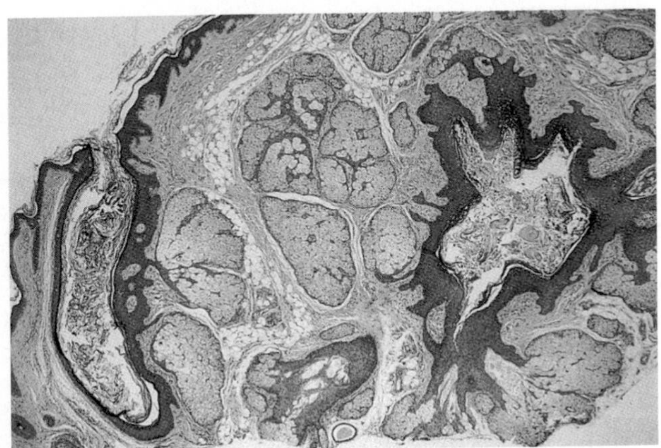

FIGURE 16. Folliculosebaceous cystic hamartoma. Mature and hyperplastic sebaceous glands extend into the dermis from widely patent hair follicle infundibulae, forming a circumscribed nodule of pilar and sebaceous elements.

Sebaceous Neoplasms and Proliferations

Nevus Sebaceus (Organoid Nevus, Nevus Sebaceus of Jadassohn)

Nevus sebaceus appears at birth as a solitary area of alopecia, usually on the scalp (33). These lesions usually go on to develop a verrucous surface during adolescence. Histologically, nevus sebaceus is a hamartoma of the pilosyringosebaceous apparatus. Early in childhood the proliferation of immature follicular structures and basaloid epidermal hyperplasia is striking. In adults, the immature follicles persist and are accompanied by apocrine glands (normally present only rarely in the scalp) and prominent sebaceous glands. Roughly a third of patients will develop an associated adnexal tumor, most commonly basal cell carcinoma or syringocystadenoma papilliferum (34–40). The characteristic histologic findings in nevus sebaceus are verrucous epidermal hyperplasia, immature or abortive hair follicles budding off the epidermis, sebaceous glands with ducts entering directly into the epidermis (as opposed to the usual case of sebaceous ducts emptying into the hair follicle), and ectatic apocrine glands (Fig. 17). Because of the association with the subsequent development of superimposed neoplasms, excision is often recommended.

Sebaceous Hyperplasia

Sebaceous hyperplasia is most commonly observed as one or more umbilicated yellow papules on the forehead of an elderly man. These benign proliferations may be clinically confused with basal cell carcinoma. The histologic findings in sebaceous hyperplasia are enlarged sebaceous lobules, generally completely encircling a central large follicular infundibulum (Fig. 18).

Sebaceous Adenoma

This solitary nonulcerated pale yellow nodular proliferation usually occurs on the face or neck of middle-aged or older patients. Histologically, sebaceous adenoma is composed of a circumscribed dermal nodule of sebaceous lobules with peripheral basaloid cells and central mature sebaceous cells (Fig. 19). In contrast to sebaceoma and sebaceous epithelioma, in sebaceous adenoma fewer than 50% of cells have a basaloid morphology, and most of the cells are mature lipidized sebocytes.

Sebaceous Adenoma with Atypia (Sebaceoma)

The literature regarding the terminology for sebaceous tumors with more atypia than a sebaceous adenoma but insufficient atypia for a diagnosis of sebaceous carcinoma is voluminous and without a general consensus. When the tumors that are clearly basal cell

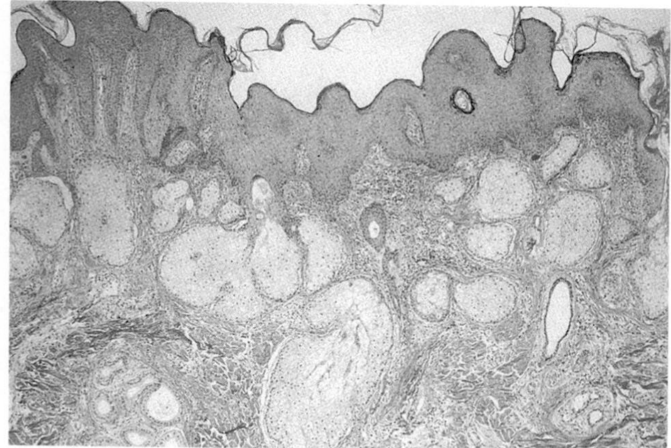

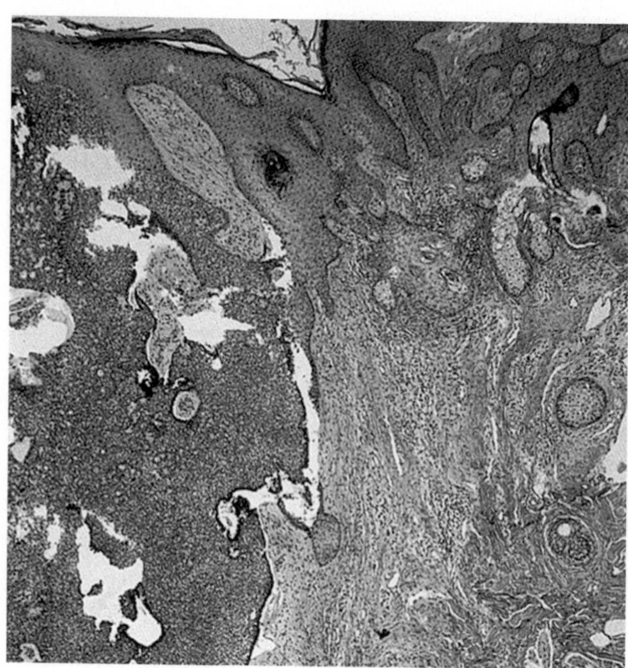

FIGURE 17. Nevus sebaceus. **A:** Epidermal hyperplasia, sebaceous glands entering into the epidermis and apocrine glands **(lower left corner). B:** Nodular basal cell carcinoma arising in nevus sebaceus **(left);** abortive sebaceous and follicular structures extend from the epidermis **(right).**

carcinomas with sebaceous differentiation (sebaceous epithelioma) are extracted from this group of lesions, the best diagnosis may be "sebaceous adenoma with atypia." The term sebaceoma has also been invoked to describe sebaceous proliferations that do not have sufficient histologic features to merit a diagnosis of sebaceous adenoma, basal cell carcinoma with sebaceous differentiation, or sebaceous carcinoma. The use of the term sebaceoma in this setting, however, may be confusing inasmuch as the literature describing sebaceoma refers to a very rare adnexal neoplasm with features of poroma and sebaceous adenoma. "Sebaceous adenoma with atypia" is used to describe a proliferation predominantly of basaloid sebaceous epithelium with histologic features that are atypical but insufficient for a diagnosis of basal cell carcinoma with sebaceous differentiation or sebaceous carcinoma. These atypical histologic features include a predominantly (>50%) basaloid proliferation with a minority of mature sebaceous elements, mitotic activity without atypical mitotic forms, and the formation of a relatively large tumor mass. These tumors are well circumscribed, without stromal desmoplasia or infiltrative margins. Such sebaceous proliferations with atypical features are commonly observed in the Muir-Torre (41,42) syndrome, in which cutaneous tumors with sebaceous differentiation and visceral malignancies occur in the same patient (43–49). The cutaneous manifestations of Muir-Torre syndrome include keratoacanthomas, sebaceous adenoma, sebaceous epithelioma, atypical sebaceous proliferations that are difficult to classify, and, rarely, sebaceous carcinoma. Many types of visceral malignancy have been reported in these patients, including gastrointestinal carcinoma (50% of cases), genitourinary cancers (25% of cases), breast carcinoma, laryngeal tumors, and lymphoma (50).

Sebaceous Epithelioma (Basosebaceous Epithelioma, Basal Cell Carcinoma with Sebaceous Differentiation)

As noted above, there is little consensus regarding the terminology for atypical sebaceous neoplasms. Nevertheless, most observers agree that the term sebaceous epithelioma refers to atypical sebaceous neoplasms that share many histologic features with basal cell carcinoma (51–56). These lesions usually are small, less than 1 cm in diameter, slow-growing papules that may have raised borders and ulcerated features very similar to basal cell car-

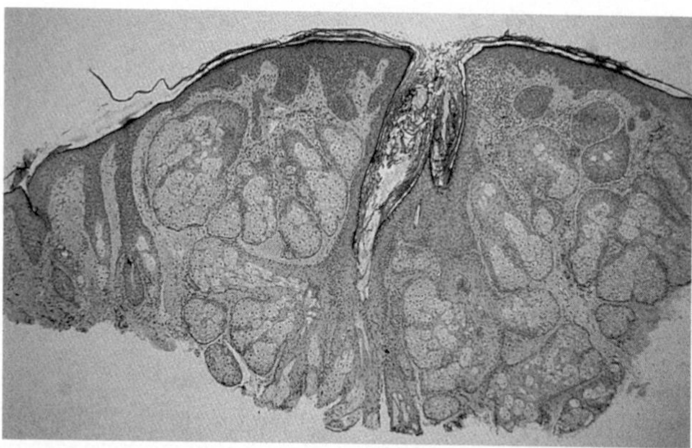

FIGURE 18. Sebaceous hyperplasia. Well-circumscribed nodule of mature sebaceous elements.

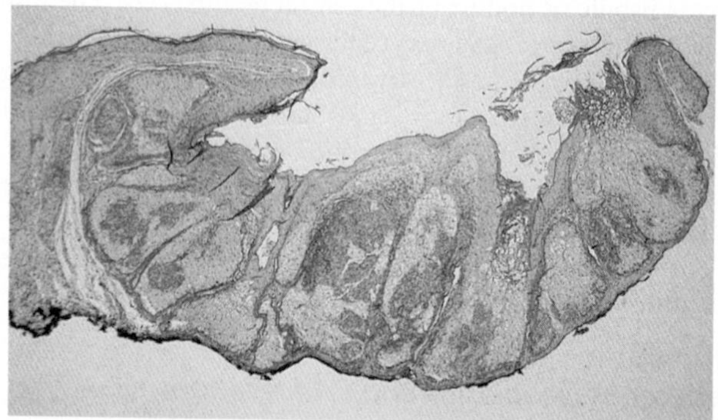

FIGURE 19. Sebaceous adenoma. Well-circumscribed nodule of basaloid and mature sebaceous epithelium surround an ectatic sebaceous duct. The basaloid cell component comprises fewer than 50% of the cells in this benign sebaceous tumor.

cinoma. These tumors also bear a histologic resemblance to basal cell carcinoma. Sebaceous epitheliomas lack the nuclear anaplasia and atypical mitotic figures characteristic of sebaceous carcinoma. Treatment is similar to that for basal cell carcinoma—complete excision. Histologically one observes a superficial ulcer with underlying dermal tumor nodules displaying sebaceous differentiation or a basaloid proliferation with cystic, solid, adenoid, and reticular growth patterns. Not infrequently one observes a palisade of basaloid cells with mucin-containing clefts separating the tumor epithelium from the stroma, similar to those observed in basal cell carcinoma. Usually more than 50% of the tumor cells display a basaloid morphology; occasionally there is connection of the tumor with the epidermis.

Sebaceous Carcinoma

Sebaceous carcinoma usually arises in the eyelids, either from the Meibomian glands or glands of Zeis. It may involve the conjunctiva diffusely and present as chronic blepharoconjunctivitis or as a chalazion. Approximately 30% of patients with chronic conjunctivitis refractory to treatment are subsequently diagnosed with conjunctival sebaceous carcinoma (57). A high index of suspicion and an early histopathologic examination are essential because early diagnosis and consequent surgical therapy of sebaceous carcinoma of the eyelid has been demonstrated to lead to a better outcome and higher survival rates than generally assumed. Thus, any "chalazion" persisting for more than a few months should be biopsied. Sebaceous carcinoma arises in men more frequently than in women, with a mean age of diagnosis of 60 years (58,59). Features that are associated with a high risk of metastasis and death include multifocal lesions, tumors of the upper lid, higher degree of invasion, and higher histologic grade (60). Sebaceous carcinoma necessitates mutilating orbital exenteration in 23% of patients (61), and metastasis is common, with a mortality rate approaching 15%.

Histologically, sebaceous carcinomas often have a prominent intraepithelial (often intraconjunctival) or pagetoid component (Fig. 20). This is manifested as an intraepidermal proliferation of atypical epithelial cells with variable degrees of sebaceous differentiation. Most often the atypical cells display a pagetoid growth pattern of single or small clusters of malignant cells; rarely small intraepidermal acini of atypical cells are observed. The process may at times, however, involve almost the entire epithelial thickness, resembling squamous cell carcinoma *in situ.* The differential diagnosis of pagetoid sebaceous carcinoma thus includes squamous cell carcinoma *in situ* as well as extramammary Paget's disease and melanoma *in situ* (Table 1). Histologically, the presence of sebaceous differentiation supports the diagnosis of pagetoid intraepithelial sebaceous carcinoma, as does the clinical history of a nonpigmented erythematous conjunctival lesion. Squamous cell carcinoma *in situ* often shows a transition from areas of actinic keratosis, and a precursor nevus or lentiginous melanocytic hyperplasia often accompanies melanoma *in situ.* A layer of keratinocytes usually separates the tumor cells in Paget's disease, pagetoid sebaceous carcinoma, as well as squamous cell carcinoma *in situ* of Bowenoid type from the basement membrane zone. Rather than sebaceous differentiation, the tumor cells in Paget's disease display abundant clear cytoplasm occasionally with intracytoplasmic sialomucin that stains positively with alcian blue, mucicarmine, and PASD stains.

A

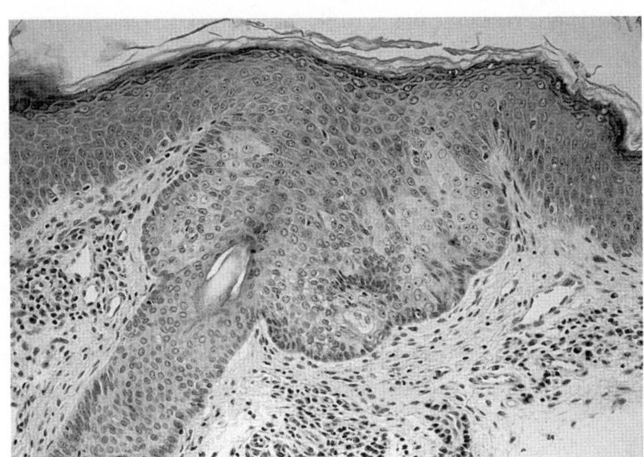

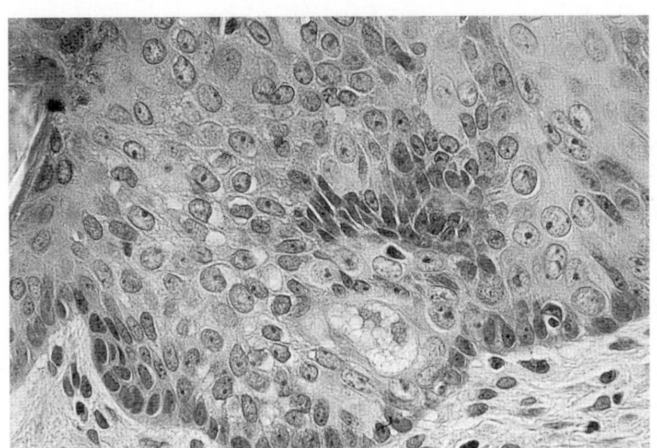

B

C

FIGURE 20. Sebaceous carcinoma. **A:** Atypical proliferation of sebaceous cells present at the junction of the hair follicle with the epidermis. **B:** Some atypical cells have intracytoplasmic lipid with scalloping of the tumor cell nuclei. **C:** Atypical cells at all levels of the epidermis with inconspicuous cytoplasmic lipid.

TABLE 1. HISTOLOGIC AND IMMUNOHISTOCHEMICAL FEATURES OF INTRAEPIDERMAL NEOPLASIA

	Extramammary Paget's Disease	Squamous Cell Carcinoma *in Situ*	Intraepithelial Sebaceous Carcinoma	Melanoma *in Situ*
Histologic features				
Pagetoid spread	+	+	+	+
Tumor cells disrupt basal keratinocytes	−	−	−	+
Nests	+	+/−	−/+	+
Gland formation	+	−	−	−
Mitotic activity	−	+	+	−
Dyskeratosis	−	+	−	−
Sebaceous differentiation	−	−	+	−
Histocytochemical findings				
Intracellular mucin	+/−	−	−	−
Intracellular melanin	−/+	−	−	+
Immunohistochemical findings				
Cytokeratin	+	+	+	−
EMA	+	−	+/−	−
CEA	+	−	−	−
S-100	−	−	−	+
HMB-45	−	−	−	+

Immunohistochemically, intraepithelial sebaceous carcinoma has a cytokeratin$^+$, EMA$^+$, CEA$^-$, S-100$^-$, HMB-45$^-$ phenotype, whereas squamous cell carcinomas have a cytokeratin$^+$, vimentin$^-$, S-100$^-$, HMB-45$^-$, CEA$^-$, EMA$^-$ phenotype, intraepidermal melanoma has an S-100$^+$, HMB-45$^+$, CEA$^-$, cytokeratin$^-$, EMA$^-$ immunophenotype, and the tumor cells of traditional glandular Paget's disease have a cytokeratin$^+$, EMA$^+$, CEA$^+$, S-100$^-$, HMB-45$^-$ immunophenotype (Table 1).

The histologic features of invasive sebaceous carcinoma include a poorly circumscribed dermal-based tumor with lobules of cytologically atypical epithelial cells showing varying degrees of sebaceous differentiation. Pagetoid involvement of overlying epidermis, as mentioned above, is a characteristic finding (62). Atypical mitoses and necrosis are occasionally observed. Prognostication and grading of sebaceous carcinoma is based on degree of differentiation and subepithelial infiltration. Grade 1 tumors display a lobular growth pattern with minimal stromal invasion. Grade 2 tumors are composed of irregularly shaped clusters and cords of tumor cells with infiltration of the stroma. Grade 3 tumors form solid sheets and irregular angulated groups of tumor cells with extensive infiltration, necrosis, and perineural, intravascular, or periadnexal invasion. Although the histologic grade is partially determined by extent of infiltrative growth, the degree of differentiation has some bearing on grade and prognosis. Well-differentiated tumors contain mature sebocytes with the characteristic clear cytoplasm packed with lipid droplets. The cells of poorly differentiated sebaceous carcinomas display only rare cytoplasmic lipids and have small pleomorphic, polygonal, and occasionally anaplastic nuclei. Necrosis is not uncommon in poorly differentiated tumors. Mitotic activity, including atypical mitotic figures, is observed in sebaceous carcinoma of all grades (63–65). It is noteworthy that sebaceous carcinoma of the eyelids and ocular adnexae are usually poorly differentiated, more so than is generally found elsewhere on the skin, where the tumor is decidedly uncommon. When evaluating a fat stain to aid in diagnosis, it is important to remember that dead cells of all types can imbibe fat, and thus, viable tumor cells must exhibit staining for the stain to be considered positive.

Sweat Gland Neoplasms

Syringocystadenoma Papilliferum

Syringocystadenoma usually occurs on the scalp or face at a young age as an alopecic region. The lesion eventually forms a plaque or nodule with a verrucous or crusted surface (66). This lesion represents the most common benign tumor to arise in association with nevus sebaceus (67). The histologic features of syringocystadenoma papilliferum include papillary epidermal hyperplasia with overlying scale crust and an underlying papillary epithelial proliferation, characteristically with invagination into a cystic space, frequently with epidermal contiguity (Fig. 21). One or a few layers of epithelium displaying focal apocrine decapitation secretion line fronds of stroma protruding into the space. There is also often a dense lymphocytic and plasma cell infiltrate in the surrounding dermis.

Cylindroma (Turban Tumor)

Cylindroma is a benign tumor that may occur as a single lesion or as multiple tumors on the scalp or face. The tumors arise in women more often than men and, when multiple, are frequently familial with an autosomal dominant inheritance. A striking presentation of multiple cylindromas (occasionally hundreds) on the scalp, appearing as though the patient is wearing a turban, is observed in the turban tumor syndrome (Ancell-Speigler) (68). In addition to multiple cylindromas, these patients also may have multiple trichoepitheliomas, and less commonly there is an association with spiradenomas. Clinically, cylindromas are firm nodules without apparent alteration of the skin surface. The histologic features of cylindroma include a circumscribed dermal-based epithe-

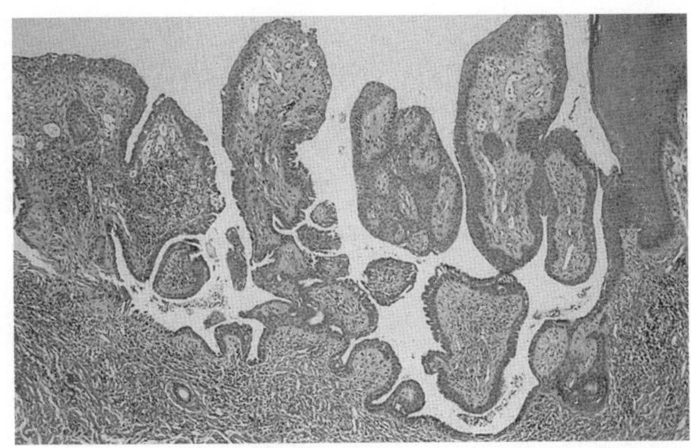
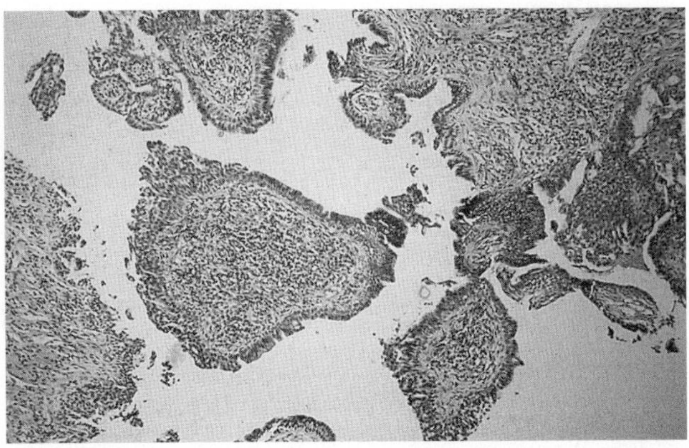

FIGURE 21. Syringocystadenoma papilliferum. **A:** Villi of papillary dermis are covered by apocrine epithelium contiguous with the epidermis. **B:** Apocrine decapitation secretion by the neoplastic epithelium lining papillary dermal fronds with an associated plasma cell–rich inflammatory infiltrate.

lial proliferation with a jigsaw-puzzle–like arrangement of closely packed tumor lobules, each surrounded by a thick eosinophilic membrane (Fig. 22). The tumor is composed of small basaloid cells and occasional larger cells with more abundant eosinophilic cytoplasm. Eosinophilic hyaline droplets are often observed within tumor lobules. Ductal differentiation is absent or inconspicuous, and necrosis and nuclear anaplasia are absent.

Apocrine Carcinoma

Primary carcinoma of Moll's gland is rare (69). These tumors arise in the eyelid and have a high rate of metastasis, particularly to regional lymph nodes, liver, lungs, and bone. Apocrine carcinomas may also rarely arise in the ceruminous glands of the external auditory canal. The histologic features of apocrine carcinoma include a poorly circumscribed dermal epithelial proliferation with focal apocrine differentiation displaying decapitation secretion and granular eosinophilic cytoplasm. The epithelial cells show varying degrees of cytologic atypia with prominent nucleoli and infiltrate through a desmoplastic stroma. The tumor cell cytoplasm often contains PAS$^+$ diastase-resistant, alcian blue$^+$, mucicarmine$^+$, and occasionally Perl's iron$^+$ material.

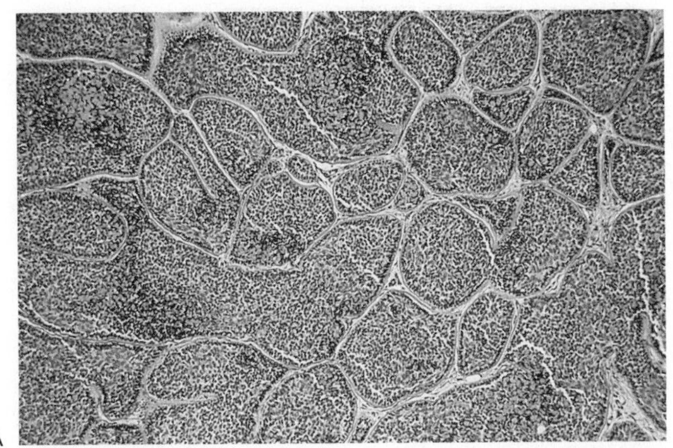
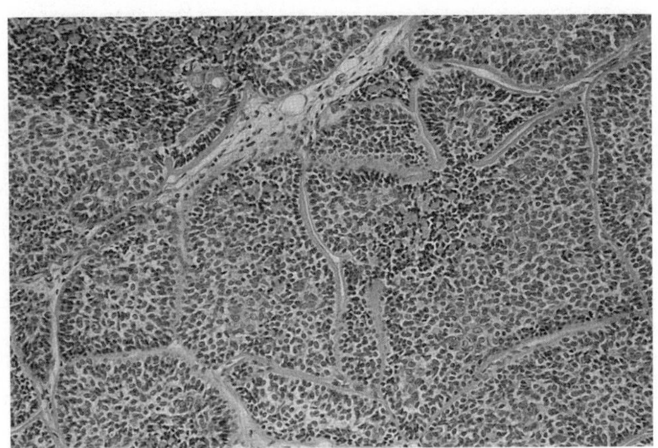
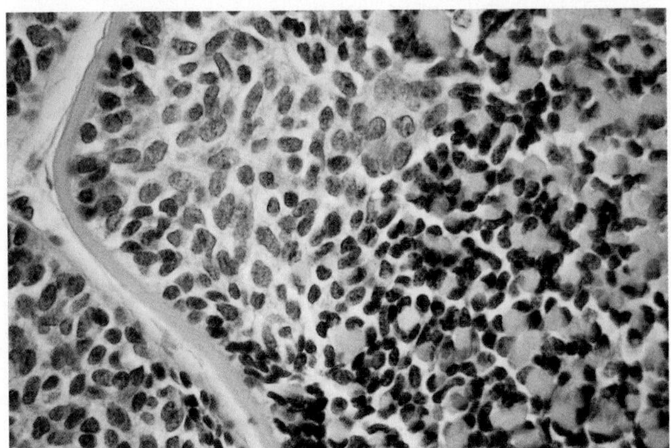

FIGURE 22. Cylindroma. **A:** Nests of basaloid tumor cells apposed to each other resembling pieces of a jigsaw puzzle. **B:** Thickened homogeneous ribbon of eosinophilic basement membrane material separates the epithelial nests. **C:** Proliferation of basaloid cells with homogeneous round eosinophilic deposits of basement membrane material characteristic of eccrine tumors.

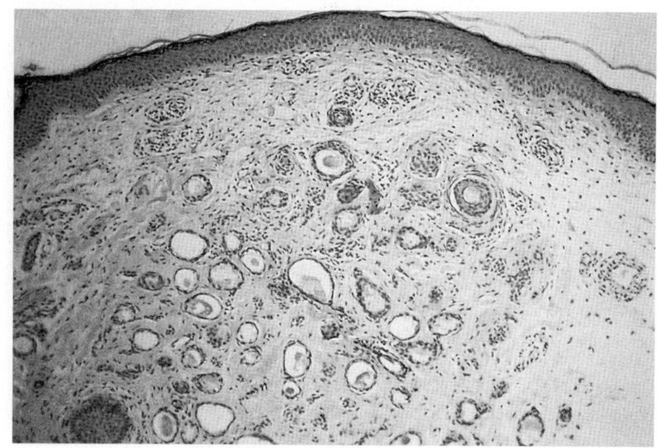
A

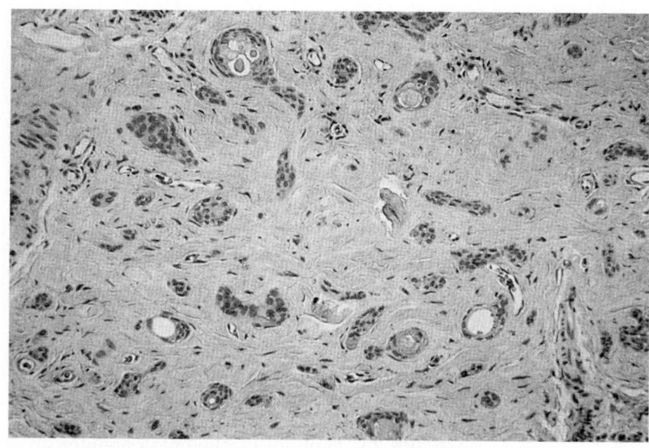
B

FIGURE 23. Syringoma. **A:** Circumscribed dermal epithelial proliferation forming small cysts and cords, embedded in an eosinophilic fibrocellular stroma. **B:** Tadpole-shaped and comma-shaped epithelial proliferations in a fibroblast-rich eosinophilic stroma.

Syringoma

Syringomas are benign tumors that often occur in a symmetric distribution around the eyelids and cheeks and may also present on the neck and anterior chest. They appear as multiple slightly yellow papules, usually less than 3 mm in diameter (70). The histologic features of syringoma include a circumscribed dermal proliferation of cuboidal epithelium forming small tadpole- or comma-shaped nests and tubules with a central eosinophilic cuticle lining a small space about the size of an eccrine sweat duct (Fig. 23). The tumor cells have small round nuclei without nuclear anaplasia.

Eccrine Poroma

In contrast to other adnexal tumors, which commonly occur on the skin of the head and neck, eccrine poroma is rare at these sites and is most often observed on the palms and soles (71,72). Based on differing patterns of growth, some observers use the terms hidracanthoma simplex, dermal duct tumor, and syringoacan-

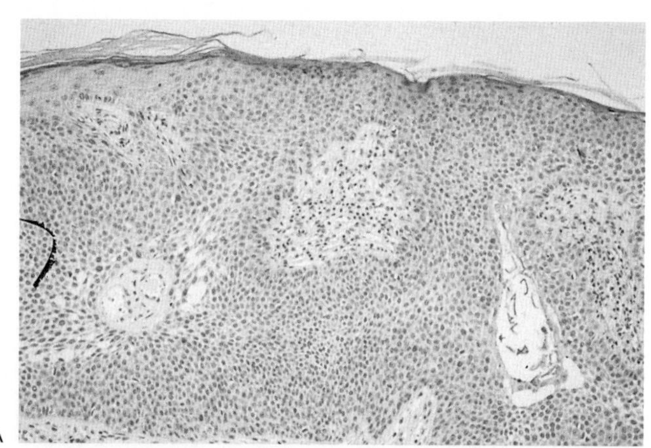
A

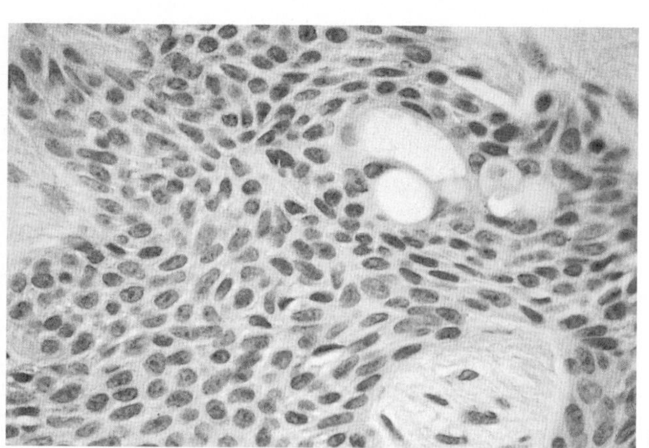
B

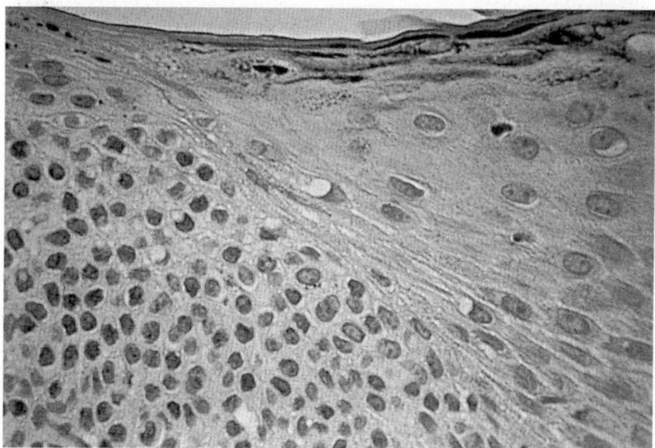
C

FIGURE 24. Eccrine poroma. **A:** Replacement of the epidermis by proliferation of monomorphic round keratinocytes, forming a pavement-like array in the acanthotic epidermis. **B:** Small cystic spaces contain a delicate eosinophilic cuticular lining. **C:** The proliferation of small monomorphic eccrine poroma cells is sharply demarcated from the normal keratinocytes.

thoma to describe variants of eccrine poroma displaying a predominantly intraepidermal pattern of growth, a dermally based tumor, and a proliferation with prominent overlying scale crust, respectively. The histologic features of the intraepidermal form of eccrine poroma include epidermal acanthosis with replacement of the epidermis by sheets of monomorphic cells with centrally placed round nuclei and eosinophilic cytoplasm (Fig. 24). There is an abrupt demarcation between tumor cells and the adjacent normal epidermis. Small sweat duct lumina are characteristically seen in the sheets of tumor cells. The histologic features of the dermally based eccrine poroma, termed dermal duct tumor, include an intraepidermal circumscribed nodular and cystic epithelial proliferation occasionally associated with an ectatic eccrine duct (Fig. 25). The tumor cells are monomorphic with round nuclei, even chromatin distribution, inconspicuous nucleoli, and eosinophilic cytoplasm. There is often evidence of ductal differentiation, and occasionally there is contiguity with the overlying epidermis.

Mixed Tumor (Chondroid Syringoma)

These benign tumors occur as large nodules on the scalp or face (73–76). In contrast, malignant chondroid syringoma more commonly occurs on the trunk (77–80). When it is present on the skin of the face, it is important to differentiate a cutaneous mixed tumor from involvement of the skin by pleomorphic adenoma of the salivary gland. The histologic features of the cutaneous mixed tumor are similar to those observed in pleomorphic adenoma (see Chapter 8) and include a circumscribed dermally based tumor composed of both mesenchymal and epithelial elements (Fig. 26). Nests and strands of tumor cells with ductal differentiation are embedded in a fibromyxochondroid stroma. No significant nuclear anaplasia, necrosis, or mitotic activity is observed.

Spiradenoma

This relatively uncommon tumor appears as a firm nodule ranging from 0.5 to 3 cm in diameter with a gray or blue hue (81,82). It usually occurs in young adults as a solitary, occasionally tender nodule on the anterior trunk or proximal extremities. Eccrine spiradenomas may occur in association with cylindromas. Rare malignant transformation has also been described (83–86). Complete excision is recommended because these tumors have a tendency to recur. Histologically, spiradenomas display dermally based nodules of basaloid epithelium appearing at scanning magnification as "blue balls" in the dermis (Fig. 27). The tumor is composed of cells with small round nuclei and scant cytoplasm and large cells with clear cytoplasm. Eosinophilic hyaline droplets are present within tumor nodules, as is a peripheral hyalinized eosinophilic basement membrane. Lymphangiectasia is a characteristic finding. Mitotic figures may be identified; however, atypical mitoses are absent. The lesion resembles cylindroma but has a less pronounced "jigsaw puzzle" appearance.

Clear Cell Hidradenoma (Eccrine Acrospiroma, Solid and Cystic Hidradenoma, Clear Cell Myoepithelioma)

Clear cell hidradenoma is an uncommon benign tumor that occurs on adult women as a firm nodule ranging from 0.5 to 3 cm in diameter with a hyperplastic or ulcerated epidermis (87–90).

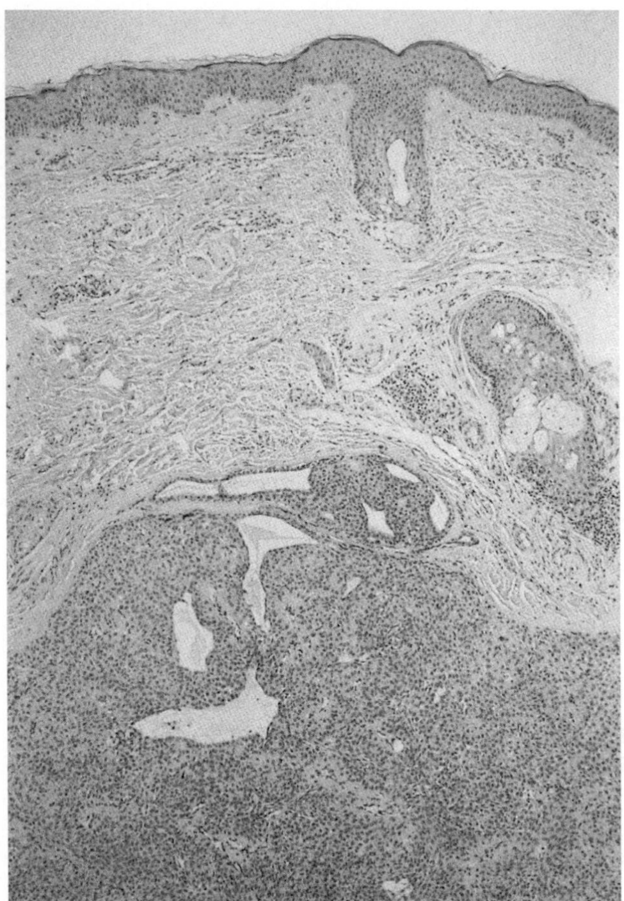

FIGURE 25. Eccrine poroma, dermal duct tumor variant. A tumor of the eccrine duct arising from the dermal portion of the duct as a nodular proliferation of monomorphic round keratinocytes with multiple foci of ductal differentiation.

These slowly growing tumors present as solitary lesions on the scalp, face, or anterior trunk. Surgical excision is curative. The histologic features of clear cell hidradenoma include a well-circumscribed dermally based epithelial proliferation forming large solid or partially cystic nodules composed of cells with round or oval nuclei and clear or eosinophilic cytoplasm. Tumor cells are often of different types, including rounded or polygonal cells and spindled or fusiform cells. Stromal deposits of eosinophilic basement membrane material and mitotic figures are present. No nuclear anaplasia, necrosis, or infiltrative pattern of growth is observed.

Eccrine Carcinoma, Ductal Type (Classic Eccrine Carcinoma, Malignant Acrospiroma)

Ductal eccrine carcinoma is the most common type of eccrine carcinoma and histologically resembles mammary ductal carcinoma. Eccrine carcinoma often clinically mimic basal cell carcinomas but are usually more biologically aggressive than the latter lesions. The histologic features include a dermally based epithelial proliferation displaying an infiltrate growth pattern at the periphery (Fig. 28). Nodules, nests, and cords of tumor cells with nuclear atypia and eosinophilic cytoplasm are observed. In foci of ductal differentiation the tumor cells have a CEA^+, gross

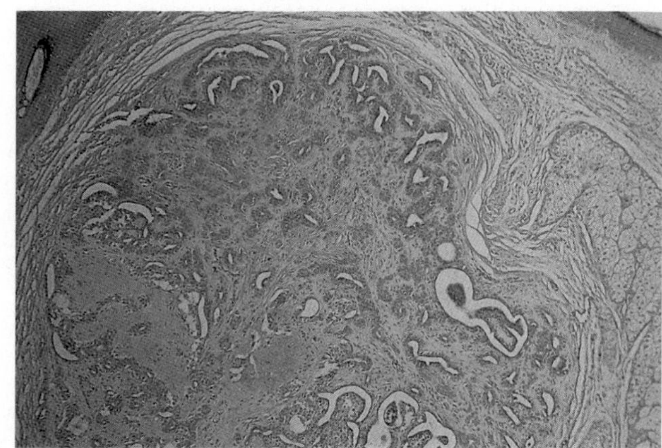
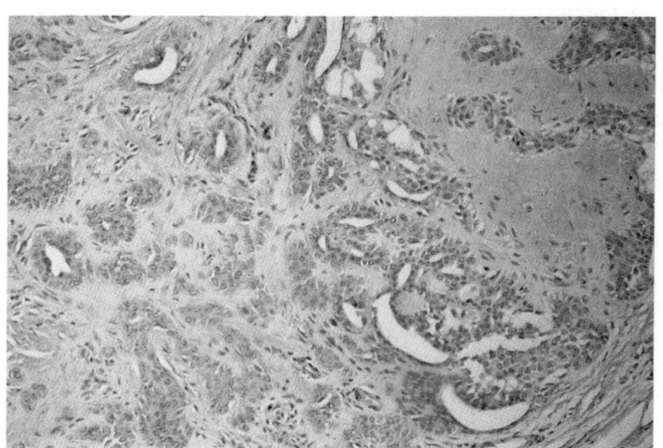

FIGURE 26. Mixed tumor. **A:** Proliferation of epithelium and stroma with myxochondroid stromal changes. **B:** Small basaloid epithelial cells and large epithelial cells with abundant cytoplasm form glands and cords embedded in a variably myxochondroid and fibrocellular stroma.

cystic disease fluid protein-15 $(GCDFP15)^{-}$ immunophenotype. Necrosis, ulceration, and numerous mitoses are characteristically present. Perineural and vascular invasion and atypical mitotic figures may also be observed.

Eccrine Carcinoma, Clear Cell Type (Clear Cell Hidradenocarcinoma)

Clear cell eccrine hidradenocarcinoma is a rare malignant form of clear cell hidradenoma that is characterized by poor circumscription, sheets of tumor cells, necrosis, perineural and vascular invasion, and variable cytologic atypia. Like its benign counterpart, these tumors are dermally based and show ductal differentiation, a proliferation of cells with clear cytoplasm, and stromal hyalinization (91).

Eccrine Carcinoma, Mucinous Type (Adenocystic Carcinoma)

Mucinous eccrine carcinoma is a rare tumor that occurs most commonly as a periorbital gray-pink nodule in elderly men. Wide surgical excision is the treatment of choice. The histologic features of mucinous eccrine carcinoma include a dermally based epithelial proliferation embedded in pools of stromal mucin. The epithelial cells form nests, cords, and ducts. Careful examination may lead to the identification of signet

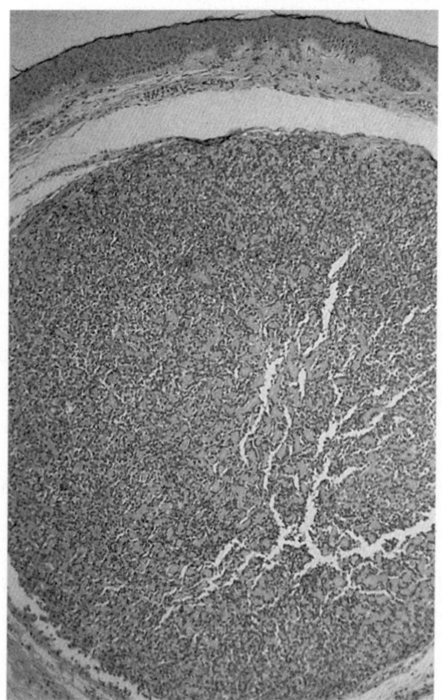
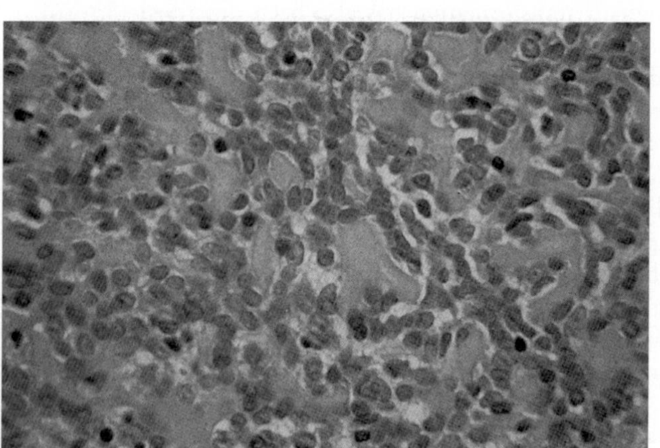

FIGURE 27. Spiradenoma. **A:** Forming a well-circumscribed "blue ball" in the dermis is a proliferation of small uniform basaloid keratinocytes. **B:** Two types of small basaloid cells form cords surrounding deposits of homogeneous eosinophilic basement membrane material.

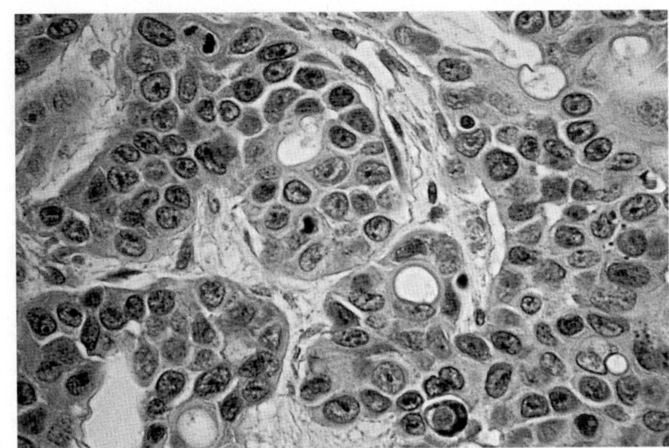
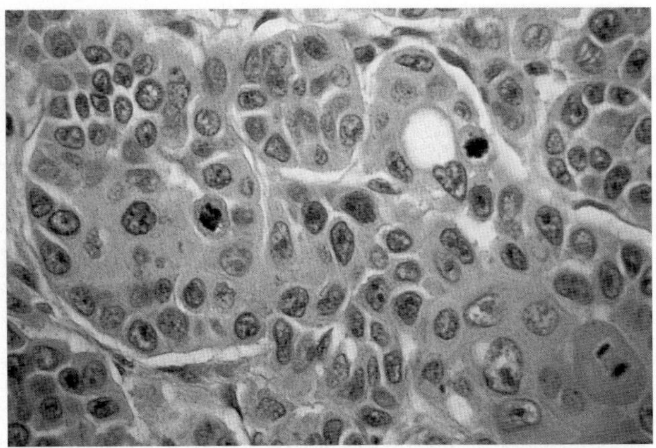

FIGURE 28. Eccrine carcinoma, ductal type. **A:** Proliferation of anaplastic keratinocytes forming small ducts. **B:** Mitotic activity, nuclear anaplasia, and duct formation.

ring cells. The differential diagnosis includes metastatic mucinous adenocarcinoma of extracutaneous origin. Eyelid tumors similar to these have been reported as "endocrine mucin-producing sweat gland carcinoma" (92). These latter tumors usually display less mucin and have neuroendocrine differentiation demonstrated immunohistochemically and ultrastructurally. Mucinous eccrine carcinoma should not be confused with mucoepidermoid carcinoma, which may rarely arise in the lacrimal sac (93).

Primary Cutaneous Adenoid Cystic Carcinoma

This is an exceedingly rare form of eccrine carcinoma that is histologically identical to adenoid cystic carcinoma of the salivary gland (see Chapter 8) and has been reported in the skin in only approximately 20 patients (94,95) and in the external auditory canal in 16 patients (96). These tumors may metastasize. Extension or metastasis from adenoid cystic carcinoma of the salivary gland should be excluded before a diagnosis of primary cutaneous adenoid cystic carcinoma is rendered.

Microcystic Adnexal Carcinoma (Sclerosing Sweat Duct Carcinoma, Malignant Syringoma, Syringoid Carcinoma)

This locally aggressive tumor occurs as a slow-growing plaque, usually of the central face, characteristically of the upper lip (15,21,97,98). Although microcystic adnexal carcinoma rarely metastasizes, the tumor may cause significant morbidity as a result of local recurrence and perineural invasion. Wide local excision is the treatment of choice; nevertheless, 50% of patients experience local recurrence (99).

Histologically, microcystic adnexal carcinoma is characterized by a dermal and subcutaneous epithelial proliferation, often with an associated poorly circumscribed eosinophilic hyalinized stroma (Fig. 29). The tumor is deeply invasive and composed of small keratinizing cysts, ducts, nests, and cords of cuboidal epithelium. Tadpole-like ductal structures similar to those observed in syringoma may be present. Characteristically, perineural invasion and infiltration into the underlying fat and muscle are observed. Notably, the epithelial cytology is usually deceptively banal, and the diagnosis often rests on the deeply infiltrative growth pattern. The differential diagnosis of microcystic adnexal carcinoma includes desmoplastic trichoepithelioma, syringoma, and infiltrative or morpheaform basal cell carcinoma. Making a specific diagnosis may be impossible on a superficial biopsy. In contrast to desmoplastic trichoepithelioma and syringoma, microcystic adnexal carcinoma is a poorly circumscribed tumor that extends deep into the reticular dermis and often involves the subcutaneous fat. Perineural invasion is characteristic of microcystic adnexal carcinoma and may also occur in basal cell carcinoma, but is not observed in desmoplastic trichoepithelioma and syringoma. Basal cell carcinoma will usually show a focus with characteristic clefts between the neoplastic basaloid epithelium and a mucin-rich stroma. These findings are not observed in microcystic adnexal carcinoma (17,20).

Cysts

There are several types of epithelial lined cysts that may arise on the skin of the head and neck (100). These cystic lesions are classified by the type of epithelial lining and the presence or absence of associated adnexal structures.

Epidermal Inclusion Cyst (Sebaceous Cyst, Wen)

Epidermal cysts may have origin in the epidermis or in the follicular infundibulum, as is evidenced by occasional contiguity of the cyst lining with the epidermal or hair follicle epithelium. Inclusion cysts are also common on the scalp, and they more commonly occur on other body sites than pilar cysts. Epidermal inclusion cysts (EIC) may arise following localized trauma or in the setting of Gardner's syndrome or nevoid basal cell carcinoma syndrome (101). Gardner's syndrome is characterized by desmoid tumors, osteomas, polyposis of the colon and multiple EICs (102,103).

The histologic features of epidermal inclusion cysts include a dermally based cyst lined by stratified squamous epithelium with a granular cell layer and loosely laminated keratinaceous cyst

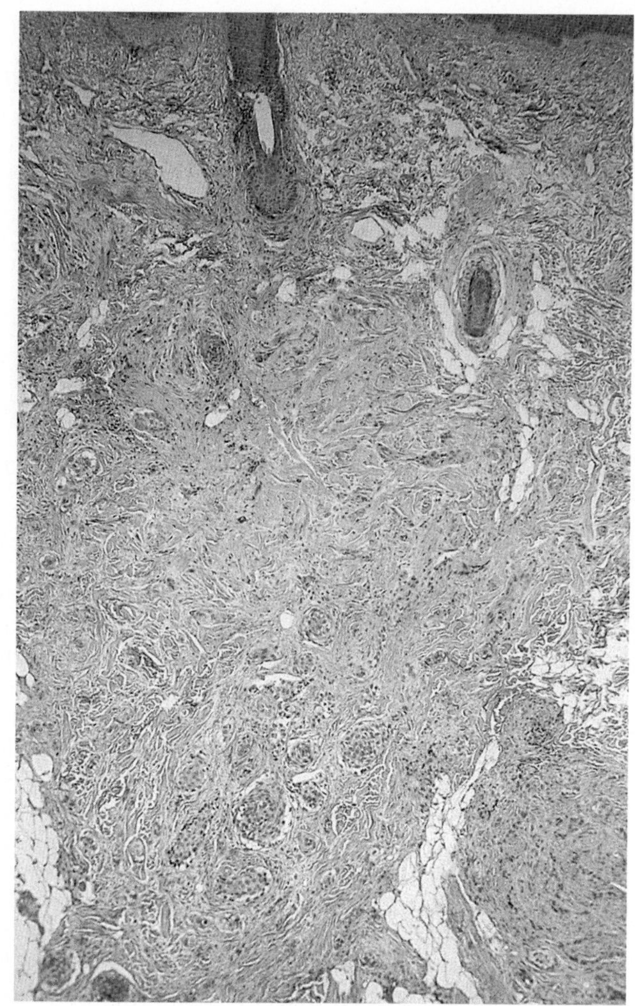

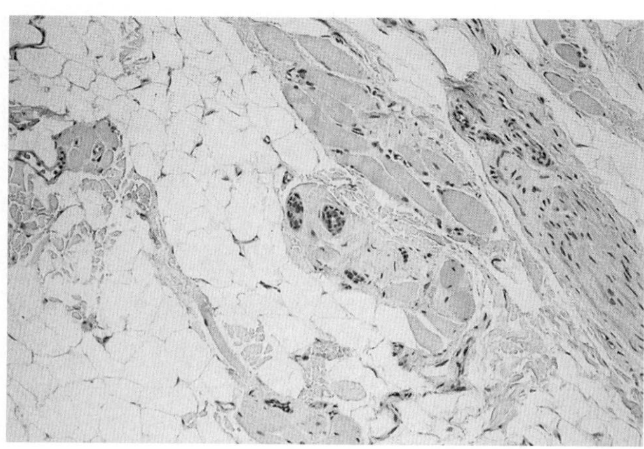

FIGURE 29. Microcystic adnexal carcinoma. **A:** Proliferation of small keratinocytes forming tubules and cords infiltrates through all levels of the dermis and into the subcutaneous fat. **B:** Tumor cells in a ductal arrangement infiltrate the fat and skeletal muscle.

contents ("basket-weave" keratin) (Fig. 30). Cyst rupture results in a foreign body giant-cell reaction, occasionally with cholesterol clefts and calcification. Multiple small (1–2 mm) EICs, often occurring on the face, are known as "milia."

Trichilemmal Cyst (Pilar cyst)

Perhaps the most common of these cysts to occur on the scalp is the trichilemmal cyst, so called because of the similarity of the cyst lining to the trichilemma or outer epithelial sheath of the hair follicle. Synonyms include pilar cyst, wen, and sebaceous cyst (104).

The histologic features of trichilemmal cyst include an epithelial-lined dermal-based cyst containing homogeneous compact eosinophilic keratin as opposed to the "basket-weave" keratin of epidermal inclusion cysts. The lining epithelium keratinizes without a granular cell layer (Fig. 31). In the event of previous cyst rupture, a foreign body giant-cell reaction is present. The epithelial proliferation is less extensive than in a proliferating pilar tumor (proliferating pilar cyst, pilar tumor; see above).

Steatocystoma

Unlike pilar cyst and epidermal cyst, steatocystoma is a true sebaceous cyst. These cysts arise from the sebaceous ductal epithelium and may be solitary or multiple. Steatocystoma multiplex is an autosomal dominantly inherited disorder that leads to multiple cysts most commonly arising on the anterior chest (105). When lanced the cysts express oily contents. The histologic features of steatocystoma include a dermally based cyst

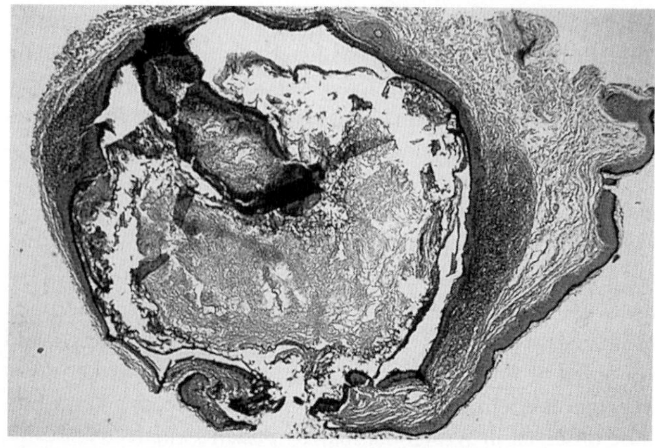

FIGURE 30. Epidermal inclusion cyst. Flattened layer of mature keratinocytes surround a cyst containing flaky eosinophilic keratin.

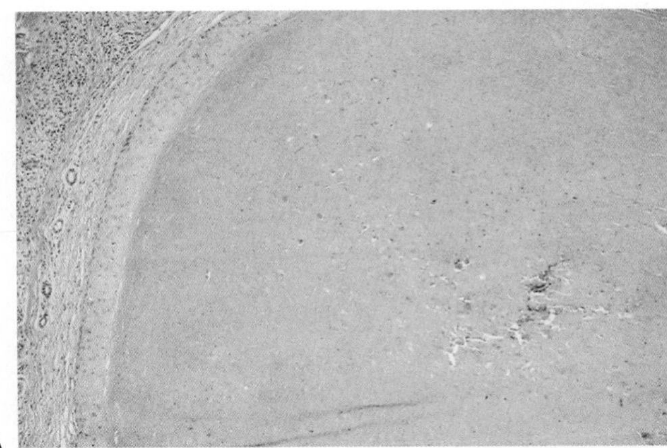

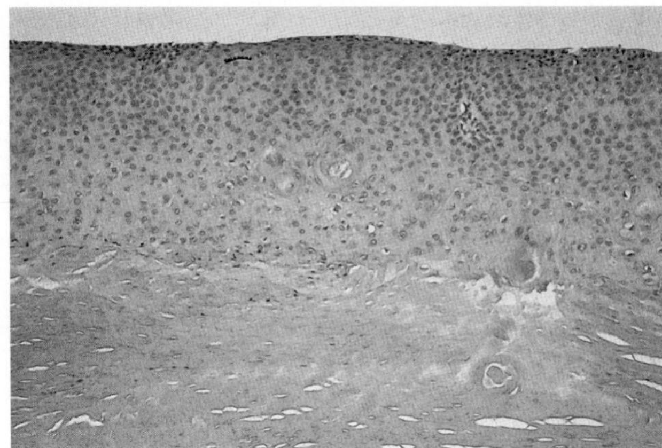

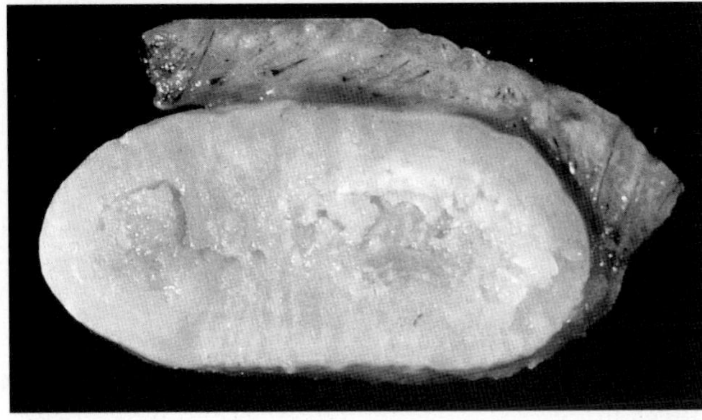

FIGURE 31. Pilar cyst. **A:** Keratinocytes with abundant clear cytoplasm and a palisaded peripheral layer surround homogeneous compact keratinaceous cyst contents. **B:** Pilar epithelium keratinizes without an intervening granular cell layer. **C:** Grossly, pilar cyst is a well-circumscribed dermal cyst with white to yellow compact keratin contents.

lined by attenuated squamous epithelium containing small foci of mature sebaceous epithelium and associated sebaceous glands (Fig. 32). There is a characteristic corrugated eosinophilic cuticle, and the cyst contains, not keratin, but proteinaceous material and vellus hairs.

Vellus Hair Cyst

Vellus hair cysts may occur as an eruption of asymptomatic papules on the face, neck, chest, or axillae (106,107). They may also arise in association with the autosomal dominant steatocystoma multiplex. The histologic features of vellus hair cyst include a thin-walled, epithelial-lined, dermal-based cyst lined by one or two layers of squamous epithelium with a granular cell layer. The cyst contains keratin and fragments of vellus hairs. The presence of keratin and a granular cell layer differentiate this cyst from steatocystoma.

Dermoid Cyst

Dermoid cyst is a rare ectodermal malformation that arises as a 1- to 4-cm in diameter nodule on the temporal scalp, forehead,

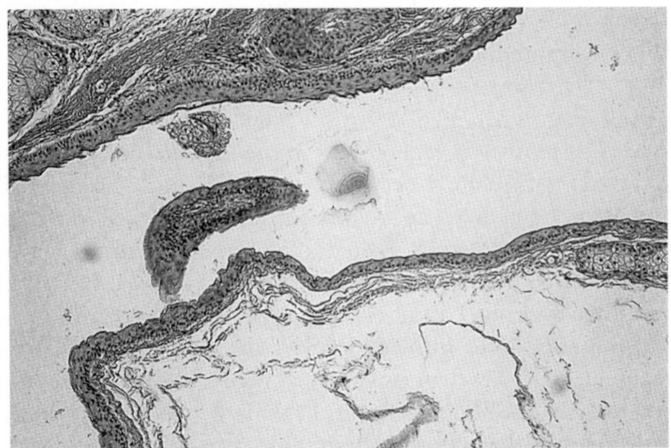

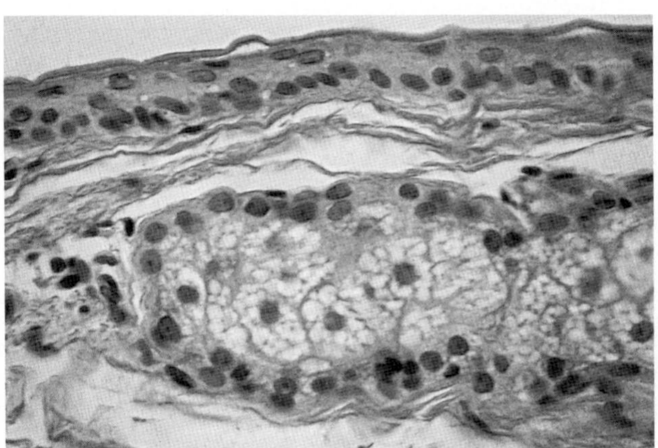

FIGURE 32. Steatocystoma. **A:** Cystic space lined by two or more layers of keratinocytes with a corrugated, wavy, eosinophilic cuticle. **B:** Sebaceous elements surround and attach to the cyst wall.

nasal dorsum, or the anterior-lateral neck. These lesions are usually noted at birth or early in childhood. The histologic features of dermoid cysts include an epithelial-lined dermally based cyst containing keratin, characteristically with adnexal structures incorporated into the cyst wall. Most commonly, the adnexal structures are immature or diminutive hair follicles and sebaceous glands.

The differential diagnosis of dermoid cyst may include cysts of the branchial cleft or thyroglossal duct, bronchogenic cyst, and thymic cyst. Branchial cleft cysts are lined by stratified squamous epithelium, keratinize with a granular cell layer, and are associated with a dense lymphoid infiltrate and occasionally cartilage or mucinous glands (108). Bronchogenic cysts have a pseudostratified lining epithelium that may be ciliated and contain goblet cells (109). Occasionally, the bronchogenic cyst has associated smooth muscle and mucous glands. Thyroglossal duct cysts are lined by pseudostratified or squamous epithelium that may be ciliated and contain goblet cells. Thyroid follicles are often present in the surrounding stroma. In general, the thyroglossal cyst wall does not have a smooth muscle component. Thymic cysts may have a stratified squamous, columnar, cuboidal, or pseudostratified epithelial lining. Occasionally no epithelial lining is identified. The presence of Hassall's corpuscles, lymphoid follicles, and cholesterol granulomas allows for the definitive diagnosis of thymic cyst (110). For a more thorough discussion of these developmental cysts, see Chapter 1.

Eccrine Hidrocystoma

These unilocular cysts arise as dome-shaped papules, most commonly around the eyelids or cheeks. They are almost always solitary and may be translucent or have a bluish hue. Enlargement in warm weather or following exercise is common. Histologically eccrine hidrocystomas are epithelial-lined, dermally based cysts lined by one or several layers of cuboidal epithelium (Fig. 33). The cyst may contain granular eosinophilic secretions.

Apocrine Hidrocystoma

These slowly enlarging cystic dome-shaped papules usually arise in the skin of the lateral canthus or lower eyelid. They may be translucent and have a bluish hue from a Tyndall effect. Their histologic features are similar to those of eccrine hidrocystoma; apocrine hidrocystomas display a dermally based cyst lined by one or several layers of cuboidal or columnar epithelium. When decapitation secretion is observed, the cyst is readily identified as apocrine rather than eccrine (Fig. 34). Occasionally the cyst contains granular eosinophilic or brown secretions.

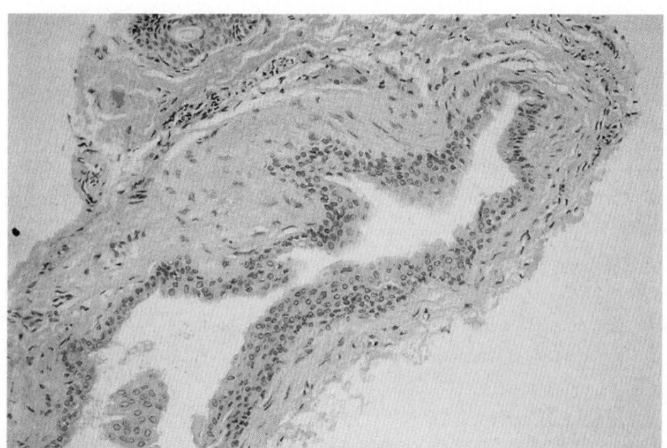

FIGURE 33. Eccrine hidrocystoma. Cystic space lined by cuboidal epithelium, occasionally with an eosinophilic cuticle. Rarely do more than three layers of epithelium form the cyst wall.

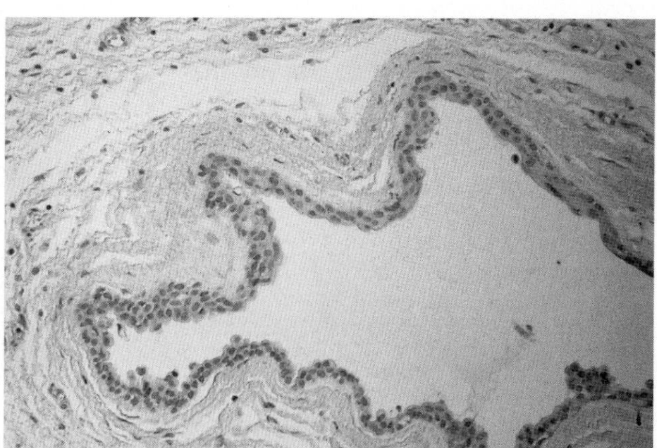

FIGURE 34. Apocrine hidrocystoma. Cystic space lined by eosinophilic epithelium with multiple foci of decapitation secretion.

Mesenchymal Neoplasms and Proliferations

This subject is also addressed in Chapter 10.

Fibroblastic and Fibrohistiocytic Proliferations

Cutaneous Angiofibroma (Fibrous Papule, Adenoma Sebaceum)

Cutaneous angiofibromas appear as small flesh-colored or pink papules that may simulate a dermal nevus, hemangioma, pyogenic granuloma, or basal cell carcinoma. Angiofibromas may occur as incidental lesions (fibrous papule of the nose) or in association with tuberous sclerosis (adenoma sebaceum). These lesions must not be confused with the angiofibromas of the nasopharynx. The histologic features of cutaneous angiofibroma include prominent superficial dermal vessels with vascular ectasia, papillary dermal and periadnexal fibrosis, and fibroblasts, focally with multiple stellate or triangular nuclei (Fig. 35).

Keloid

Keloids most noticeably occur on the earlobes but are also observed on the chin, neck, shoulders, upper trunk, and lower leg. Keloids result from an excessive proliferation of fibrous tissue following local trauma. Keloids may develop following very minor trauma or may arise in the setting of a surgical excision, localized infection, or an embedded foreign object. They most commonly occur in black individuals. Unlike keloids, hypertrophic scars have the potential to resolve. Some observers use the presence of homogeneous, hyalinized collagen in keloids to distinguish them from hypertrophic scars. The histologic features of keloid include thick hyalinized eosinophilic collagen fibers embedded in a fibrotic dermis, occasionally rich in connective tissue mucin.

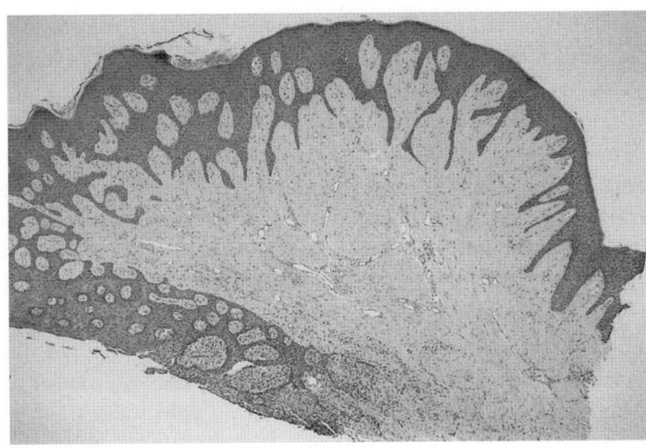
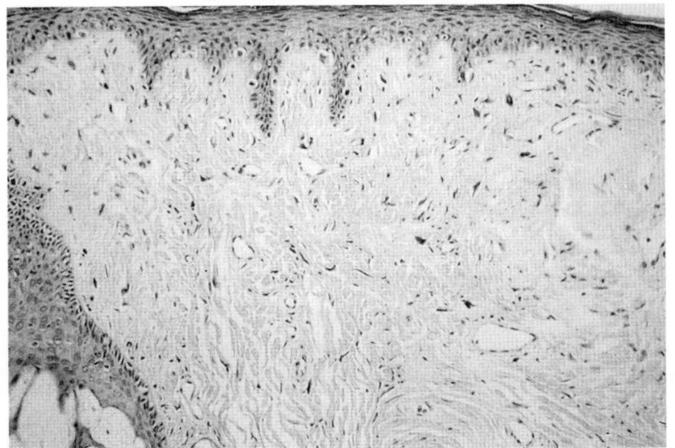

FIGURE 35. Cutaneous angiofibroma. **A:** Subepithelial proliferation of fibroblasts and small vessels forms a papule with overlying epidermal hyperplasia. **B:** Dermal fibrosis and scattered stellate multinucleate fibroblasts.

Atypical Fibroxanthoma (Malignant Fibrous Histiocytoma, Superficial Type)

Atypical fibroxanthoma (AFX) usually occurs as an erythematous nodule on the sun-damaged facial skin of elderly patients (111–113). This tumor is now more commonly diagnosed as a superficial form of malignant fibrous histiocytoma (114–116). Some consider AFX to be a superficial and benign form of malignant fibrous histiocytoma, but the author feels that the lesion is potentially malignant and that its favorable biological behavior results in no small part from its superficial location and consequent early discovery and treatment. An excisional specimen is needed to determine the depth of invasion of this atypical fibrous tumor, and complete surgical excision is the treatment of choice. Despite the marked nuclear anaplasia and mitotic activity observed in these tumors, they usually are indolent and only rarely recur or metastasize following complete local excision (113). The histologic features include a dermally based circumscribed, nonencapsulated, fibrohistiocytic proliferation composed of spindled cells and multinucleate cells that are often rounded or histiocytic-like and occasionally foamy (xanthomatous) with marked nuclear anaplasia, large irregularly shaped nuclei, and clumped chromatin (Fig. 36). Numerous atypical mitoses are observed. Characteristically, there is limited involvement of subcutaneous fat. Intracytoplasmic droplets of neutral fat or PAS^{+} diastase-resistant material are usually present. The tumors are immunohistochemically S-100^{-}, HMB-45^{-}, cytokeratin^{-}, and vimentin^{+} (113). A less atypical appearing spindle-cell nonpleomorphic variant of AFX has been described (117).

Dermatofibrosarcoma Protuberans

Dermatofibrosarcoma protuberans (DFSP) is a fibrohistiocytic neoplasm that usually occurs on the upper back or shoulder of middle-aged adults. Often presenting as an irregularly shaped indurated erythematous plaque, these tumors are associated with a high incidence of local recurrence. Interestingly, DFSP of the scalp has been associated with a higher incidence of recurrence than when these tumors arise at other sites (118). Approximately 10% of all DFSPs arise in the skin of the head and neck, most commonly on the forehead; more than 50% of these tumors recur locally (118–120). Periosteal attachment is not an uncommon finding in DFSP of the scalp. Treatment is complete surgical excision. Complete excision during the initial surgical procedure is important, as recurrence is associated with an in-

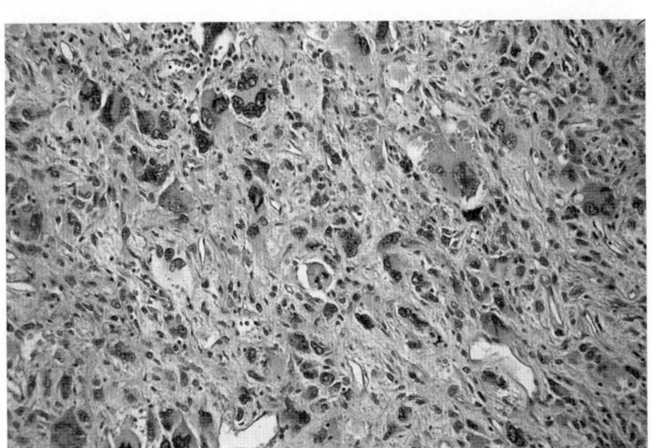
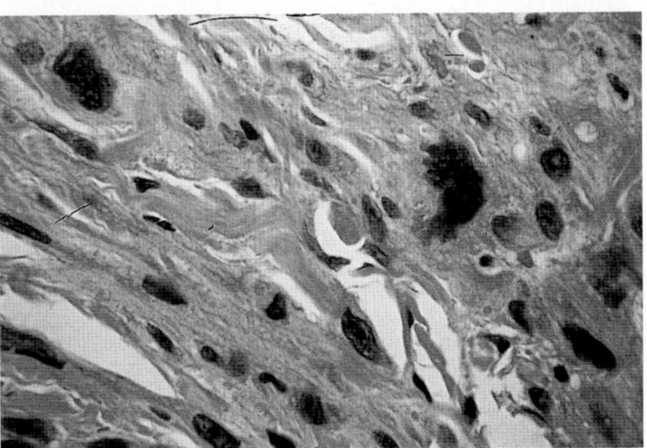

FIGURE 36. Atypical fibroxanthoma. **A:** Spindle cell proliferation with marked nuclear anaplasia and mitotic activity. **B:** Anaplastic tumor cells with large hyperchromatic irregularly shaped nuclei infiltrate through the dermal collagen.

creased risk of metastasis. Radiation therapy has been reported to be of variable use as an adjunctive therapy (121), although there is concern that in rare cases radiation may lead to the development of a more aggressive tumor (122).

Histologically, DFSP is a cellular proliferation of spindled cells with minimal cytologic pleomorphism and little mitotic activity (123,124). The spindled cells have a storiform or cartwheeled growth pattern and extend into the subcutaneous fat with a honeycomb pattern of infiltration (Fig. 37). Histologic variants of DFSP include pigmented (Bednar tumor), myxoid, myofibroblastic, and other rare types (125–128). Most notable are recent reports of DFSP with fibrosarcomatous areas (129–132).

The histologic differential diagnosis includes dermatofibroma and atypical fibroxanthoma (superficial malignant fibrous histiocytoma). Immunohistochemically, DFSP stains positively for vimentin and CD34; in contrast, dermatofibromas have few CD34-positive cells (133–138). Other fibrohistiocytic proliferations are discussed in Chapter 10.

Vascular Proliferations and Telangiectasias

This subject is also addressed in Chapter 10.

There are a wide variety of vascular lesions that may occur on the skin of the head and neck. These range from benign telangiectasias to high-grade angiosarcomas. Although the histologic appearance of the telangiectasias is similar, they may have a variety of clinical appearances including the Port-wine stain, "salmon" patch, "spider" angioma, Osler-Rendu-Weber disease lesion (hereditary hemorrhagic telangiectasia), ataxia telangiectasia (Louis-Bar syndrome), venous lake, and angiokeratoma. Only the latter two processes have a distinctive histologic appearance. Venous lakes frequently present on sun-damaged skin of the face, lips, and ears of elderly patients. These telangiectasias probably result from reduced integrity of the supporting connective tissue. The histologic features include ectasia of superficial dermal thin-walled vessels with flattened endothelial cells. Ectatic vascular spaces contain numerous erythrocytes.

Angiokeratoma

Angiokeratomas usually occur on the distal extremities or genitalia. In rare syndromes in which patients develop many of these lesions, they may be observed on the skin of the head and neck. Angiokeratoma may be observed in association with Fabry's disease, Klippel-Trenaunay syndrome, and Cobb's syndrome. The histologic features include epidermal hyperplasia with hyperkeratosis and marked ectasia of superficial dermal capillaries and venules. The vessels may appear to be present within the epidermis but actually have an intervening compressed rim of papillary dermis (Fig. 38).

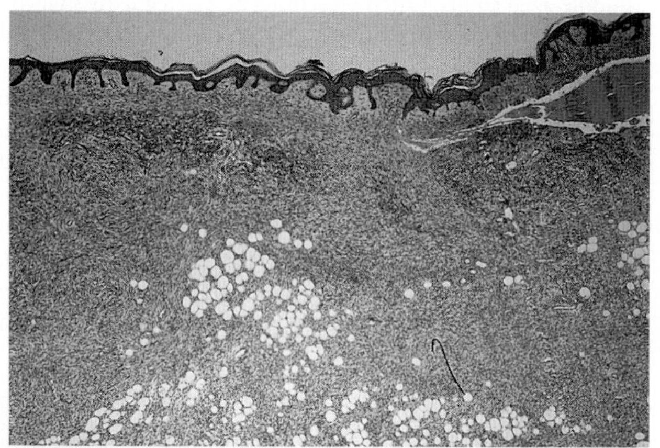
A

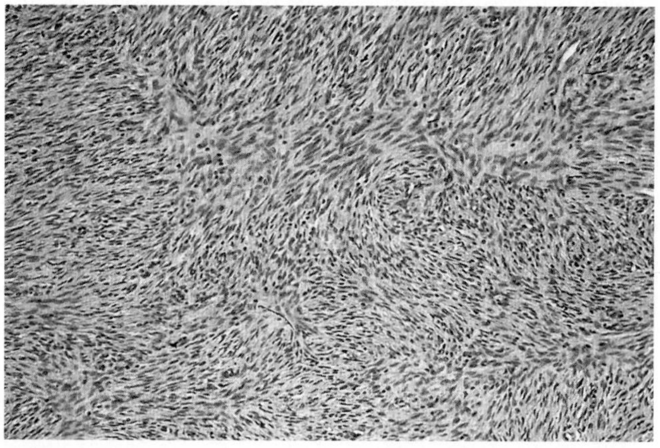
B

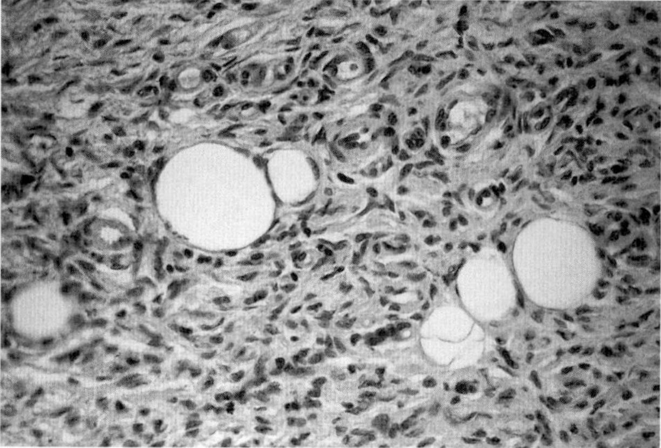
C

FIGURE 37. Dermatofibrosarcoma protuberans. **A:** A densely cellular proliferation of spindled cells infiltrates throughout the dermis and extends into the subcutis. **B:** Spindled cells with a whorled, storiform growth pattern. **C:** Tumor infiltrating the subcutaneous fat.

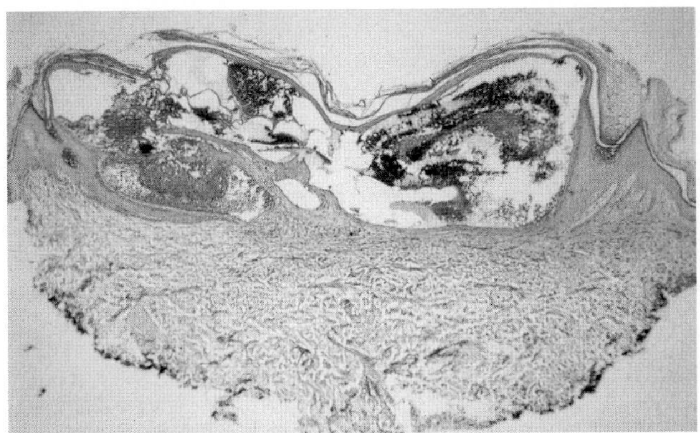

FIGURE 38. Angiokeratoma. Ectatic blood-filled vascular spaces in the superficial papillary dermis are closely engulfed by a collarette of epidermal hyperplasia.

Hemangioma, Capillary (Angiomatous Nevus)

Capillary hemangiomas occur frequently in children. These vascular malformations reach their maximum size by age 3 to 5 years and usually involute completely prior to puberty. Delaying surgical therapy until the peripubertal years is usually recommended. The histologic features include a dermal-based lobular proliferation of capillary-sized vessels with a single large "feeder" vessel for each vascular lobule. The vessels characteristically are lined by flattened endothelium.

Hemangioma, Juvenile (Cellular Hemangioma of Infancy, Strawberry Nevus)

Juvenile hemangioma represents an immature capillary hemangioma consisting of a dermal or subcutaneous nodular proliferation of small vessels lined by plump endothelia. Mitotic activity may be present. In early lesions the vascular lumina are inconspicuous; in late lesions fibrosis with regression and occasional thrombosis are observed. Although cellular and mitotically active, the lesions are benign. Angiosarcomas in children are extremely rare.

Hemangioma, Cavernous

Cavernous hemangiomas frequently occur in children as deeply situated lesions that are venous malformations rather than true neoplasms. As with many of the vascular abnormalities that appear in childhood, cavernous hemangiomas may be observed in association with a number of syndromes including Sturge-Weber syndrome (139,140), Kasabach-Merritt syndrome (141), Maffucci's syndrome (142,143), and blue rubber bleb nevus syndrome (144). The histologic features include a dermal or subcutaneous vascular proliferation composed of large ectatic thin-walled vascular spaces lined by a flattened endothelium and often containing erythrocytes. The vascular lumina may contain thrombi and focal calcification.

Sturge-Weber syndrome is characterized by the presence of a cavernous angioma of the ocular choroid with associated hemangiomas or a Port-wine stain involving the conjunctiva or the skin of the face in the region supplied by the trigeminal nerve, as well as leptomeningeal vascular lesions. Glaucoma is a complication in about 30% of cases.

Kasabach-Merritt syndrome is a consumptive coagulopathy that rarely occurs in association with congenital or acquired hemangiomas; the vascular lesion is thought to be the site of platelet sequestration and clotting factor consumption. Systemic corticosteroids are effective early on in the therapy of these lesions; this therapy both reduces the size of the angioma and helps to correct coagulation defects.

Maffucci's syndrome is characterized by multiple cavernous hemangiomas and enchondromas that become clinically apparent during childhood. Enchondromas and vascular lesions appearing as grape-like masses may disfigure the distal extremities. Patients with Maffucci's syndrome are also at increased risk for the development of sarcomas; chondrosarcomas arise in 15% of these patients. Carcinomas of the ovary and pancreas also show an increased incidence in Maffucci's syndrome.

Blue rubber bleb nevus syndrome is characterized by cavernous hemangiomas of the skin and gastrointestinal tract. These malformations may become quite large and are often sporadically painful.

Lymphangioma Circumscriptum

Lymphangioma circumscriptum is a superficial lymphangioma that rarely occurs on the skin of the neck and presents as a patch with multiple translucent vesicles. The histologic features include prominent ectasia of the superficial dermal lymphatics with overlying epidermal hyperplasia. Large ectatic vessels may appear to be present within the epidermis but are actually separated from the epidermis by a thin rim of papillary dermis (Fig. 39). Eosinophilic proteinaceous material and erythrocytes may be observed within the lymphatic lumina.

Angiolymphoid Hyperplasia with Eosinophilia (Epithelioid Hemangioma, Histiocytoid Hemangioma)

Angiolymphoid hyperplasia with eosinophilia usually occurs on the scalp, ears, or face of young or middle-aged women (145). Rare cases of oral mucosal involvement have also been described (146,147). These slowly growing red-brown nodules are usually asymptomatic. Histologically there is a dermal or subcutaneous vascular proliferation with associated lymphoid follicles and scattered eosinophils. Occasionally the eosinophilic infiltrate may be rather dense. Characteristically the vascular endothelial cells are hypertrophic with plump nuclei protruding into the vascular lumina; some of the endothelial cells contain prominent intracytoplasmic vacuoles. For further discussion see Chapter 10.

Kaposi's Sarcoma

Kaposi's sarcoma may occur as a patch, plaque, or tumor and has four clinically distinctive forms: (a) classic, (b) African, (c) immunosuppression associated, and (d) epidemic (AIDS associated). In contrast to the other three forms, epidemic Kaposi's sarcoma frequently involves the skin of the head and neck and the oral mucosa. These lesions have been observed as red-brown nodules but more commonly appear as subtle red-brown macules or patches that may resemble a bruise. Recent interest has been generated over the identification of human herpes virus type 8 (HHV-8) in lesions of epidemic Kaposi's sarcoma. Interestingly, HHV-8 has also been identified in a variety of other vascular proliferations including angiosarcoma and angiolymphoid hyperplasia (148,149). HHV-8 has also been re-

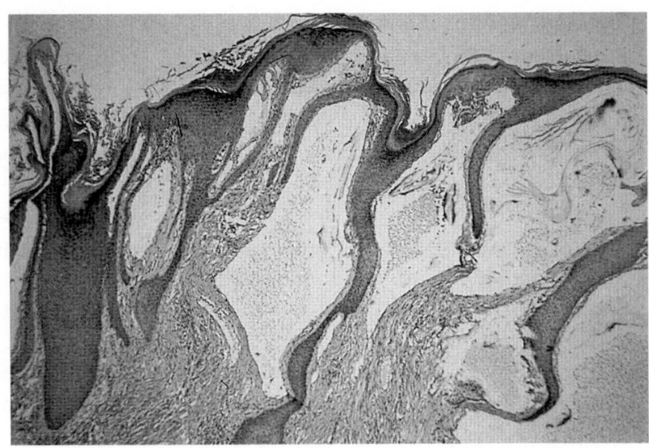
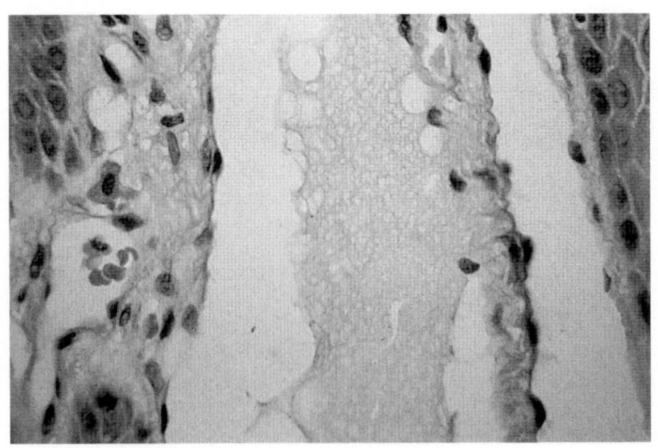

FIGURE 39. Lymphangioma circumscriptum. **A:** Ectatic vascular spaces in the superficial papillary dermis. **B:** Lymphatic spaces are lined by a solitary layer of endothelia and contain proteinaceous material.

ported in pemphigus, sarcoid, multiple myeloma, and Castleman's disease (150–153).

The histologic features of Kaposi's sarcoma include a superficial and deep dermal vascular proliferation with slit-like vascular spaces lined by plump endothelia (Fig. 40). A characteristic finding is the formation of new slit-like vessels around preexisting vessels. There is a variably dense spindle cell proliferation, which may be very inconspicuous in the early stages; in advanced lesions the spindled cells may appear to extend from vessel walls. Erythrocyte extravasation and hemosiderin deposition are usually present, and careful examination often reveals the presence of intracytoplasmic eosinophilic globules of erythrocyte remnants. Most cases display a lymphocytic and plasma cell infiltrate.

Angiosarcoma

This malignant tumor of endothelial cells characteristically arises on the scalp or face of elderly patients (154–156). It appears as an edematous dusky-red irregularly shaped plaque, occasionally with multiple associated nodules. Very rarely, angiosarcoma may

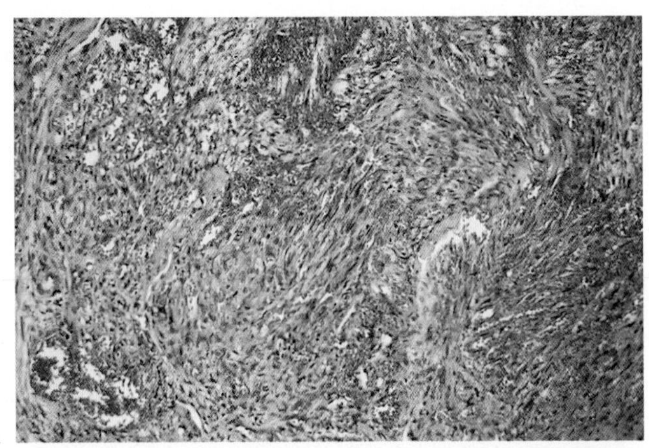
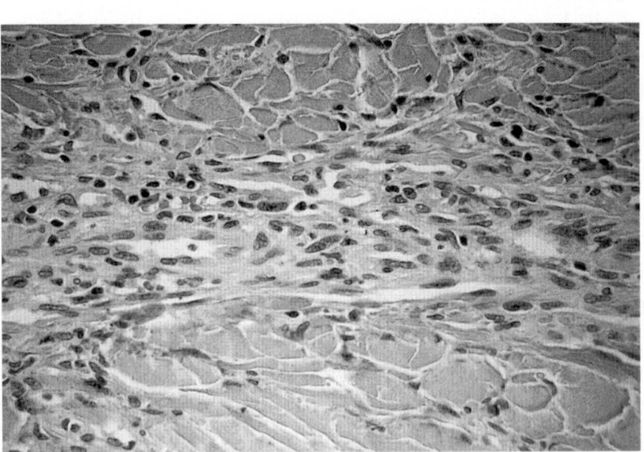
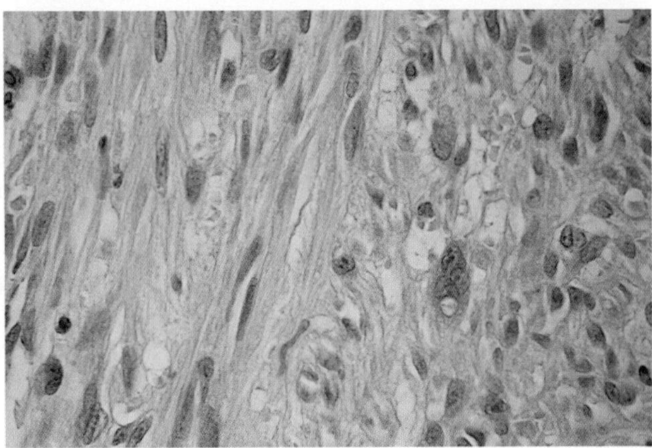

FIGURE 40. Kaposi's sarcoma. **A:** Intersecting fascicles of atypical spindled cells with extravasated erythrocytes. **B:** Preexisting vessels surrounded by tumor cells forming slit-like vascular spaces. **C:** Spindled tumor cells contain small homogeneous eosinophilic globules.

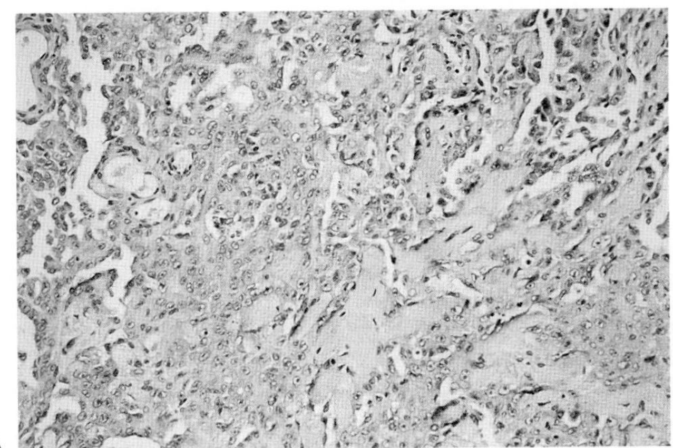

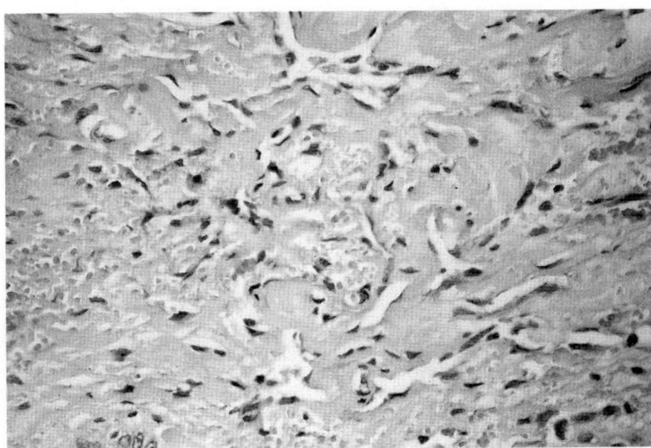

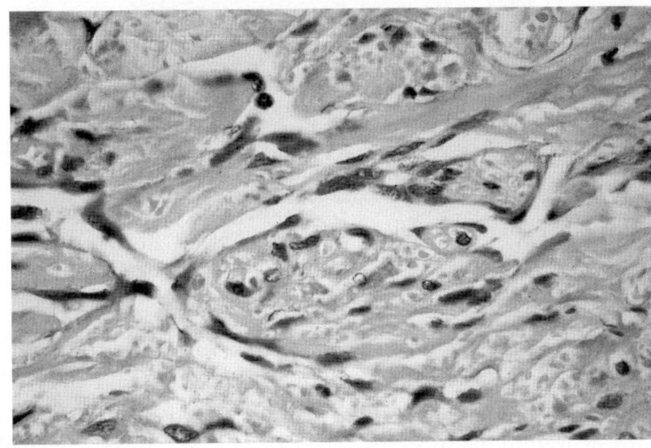

FIGURE 41. Angiosarcoma. **A:** High-grade angiosarcoma composed of poorly differentiated tumor cells forming sinusoidal vascular channels infiltrating along dermal collagen bundles. **B:** Well-differentiated angiosarcoma with atypical endothelial cells forming sinusoidal meshwork of vascular channels dissecting along reticular dermal collagen. **C:** Pleomorphic tumor cells with large densely chromatic nuclei line the spaces between collagen bundles.

arise in the paranasal soft tissues of children. These tumors have also been described following therapeutic radiation therapy for benign vascular tumors (157–159). The margins of the tumor are characteristically difficult to evaluate clinically and histologically. Although rare spontaneous regression has been reported, the 5-year mortality rate exceeds 80%. The histologic features include a proliferation of endothelial cells dissecting through dermal collagen with the formation of irregularly shaped anastamosing vascular channels (Fig. 41). The endothelial cells may pile up, forming tufts of epithelioid cells. In poorly differentiated tumors, marked nuclear anaplasia and sheets of epithelioid endothelial cells are present (see also Chapter 10).

Immunohistochemically these tumors have the following immunophenotype: $CD31^{+}$, $CD34^{+}$, *Ulex europaeus* $antigen^{+/-}$, factor $VIII^{-/+}$, $cytokeratin^{-}$, $S\text{-}100^{-}$. The differential diagnosis of poorly differentiated angiosarcoma includes malignant melanoma, carcinoma, and lymphoma. The immunohistochemical profile, in particular the $CD31^{+}$, $S\text{-}100^{-}$ phenotype, will help to differentiate this tumor from $CD31^{-}$, $S\text{-}100^{+}$ melanoma. In contrast to carcinomas, which will have a $cytokeratin^{+}$, $Ulex^{-}$, factor VIII^{-}, $CD31^{-}$ phenotype, angiosarcomas are $Ulex^{+}$, factor $VIII^{-/+}$, $CD31^{+}$ and almost always $cytokeratin^{-}$ (160). Other vascular proliferations are discussed in Chapter 10.

Lipomatous and Neural Proliferations

This subject is also addressed in Chapter 10.

Lipoma

Lipomas are common benign tumors of fat that present as soft, mobile, slowly growing masses. Although lipomas most commonly arise on the proximal extremities and upper trunk, a few clinically distinct disorders include lipomas involving the neck, scalp, and face. Benign symmetric lipomatosis occurs in middle-aged men as multiple symmetrically distributed lipomas of the neck and upper back in a horse-collar distribution (161–163). Multiple unilateral lipomas of the scalp and face with alopecia, scleral and corneal lesions, and cerebral calcification and cysts are observed in encephalocraniocutaneous lipomatosis (Fishman syndrome) (164,165). This may represent a limited form of the Proteus syndrome, which is characterized by multiple hamartomas including lipomas, epidermal nevi, hemangiomas, scoliosis, exostoses, and macrodactyly (166). It is likely that Joseph Merrick, the "Elephant Man," was affected by Proteus syndrome rather than by neurofibromatosis type 1 (167).

Intramuscular Lipoma (Infiltrating Lipoma)

Rarely, lipomas arising in the forehead may be mistaken clinically for an epidermal cyst. Lipomas in this location may be centered within the frontalis muscle or between the muscle and the underlying fascia. Complete excision requires a layered closure to repair the severed frontalis muscle (168,169). Similar to this lesion is the infiltrating lipoma of the face, which has been described as a congenital hamartoma (170). The histologic features of intramuscular lipoma include replacement of muscle by ma-

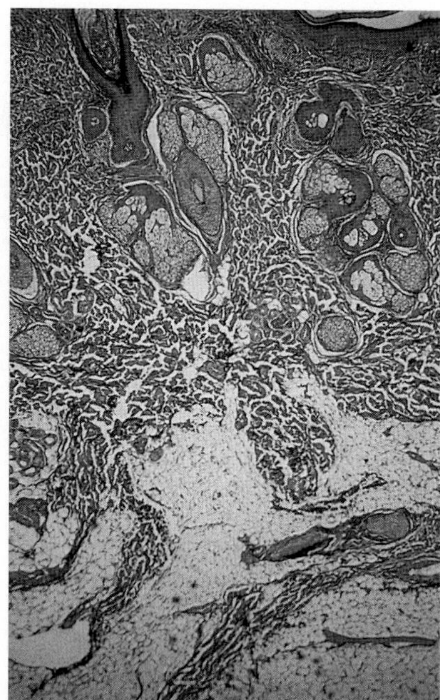

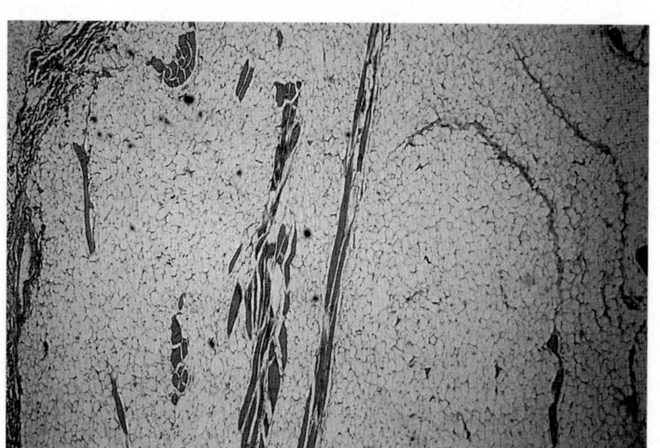

FIGURE 42. Intramuscular lipoma. **A:** The advancing edge of intramuscular lipoma merges imperceptively with the subcutaneous fat. **B:** Skeletal muscle fibers are observed enmeshed in the proliferation of mature adipose tissue.

ture fat with diffuse infiltration of muscle by lipocytes (Fig. 42). There is no nuclear anaplasia, nor are lipoblasts identified.

Neurofibroma

Neurofibromas and neurofibromatosis are described in more detail in Chapter 10. Clinically, solitary neurofibroma usually arises as a soft nodule or pedunculated lesion that is easily invaginated through the dermis with pressure; this is the "buttonhole sign." In contrast to these banal-appearing lesions, the plexiform neurofibromas of neurofibromatosis may be large and disfiguring (Fig. 43).

The histologic features of neurofibroma include a circumscribed dermal proliferation of spindled cells with narrow oval nuclei with tapered to pointed ends. The collagen fibers are delicate, wavy, and wispy. Mast cells are increased in number, and deposition of connective tissue mucin may be observed. Features of diffuse (extraneural) neurofibroma include replacement of the dermis and subcutis by neurofibroma and the formation of Meissner corpuscle–like structures termed tactoid bodies by some. Plexiform (intraneural) neurofibroma is pathognomonic for neurofibromatosis type 1 (NF-1, von Recklinghausen's disease). It arises from deeply located nerves and displays a proliferation of spindled cells with nuclei that taper to a point embedded in a fibromyxoid stroma. Small irregular nerve fascicles may be observed or highlighted with immunohistochemical stains. Perhaps the most characteristic finding in plexiform neurofibroma is the expansion of the nerve trunks, giving a plexiform appearance at low-power microscopy and the appearance of a tangle of worms or snakes grossly.

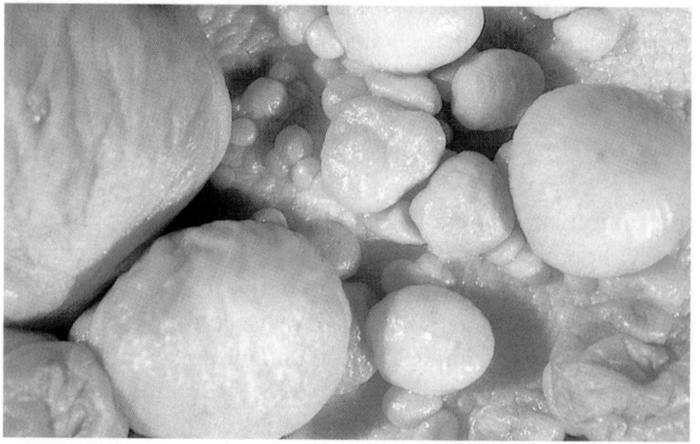

FIGURE 43. Neurofibroma. Multiple cutaneous neurofibromas in neurofibromatosis type 1.

Schwannoma (Neurilemmoma)

Schwannomas are discussed in more detail in Chapter 10. Although cutaneous schwannomas are uncommon and usually occur on the head, neck, and upper extremities, rare cases of schwannomas of the lip and tongue have been reported. These benign tumors are composed predominantly of Schwann cells and arise from the peripheral nerve sheath (171,172). The histologic features include an encapsulated dermal spindle cell proliferation and rarely a plexiform or multinodular growth pattern. Two characteristic growth patterns, termed Antoni A and Antoni B, are almost always observed. Antoni A areas are densely cellular and contain foci of palisaded nuclei surrounding acellular zones. These palisaded foci are termed Verocay bodies. Antoni B areas are hypocellular foci with loose, myxoid stroma, occasionally with hemorrhage and hemosiderin deposition.

Solitary Circumscribed Neuroma (Palisaded Encapsulated Neuroma)

Solitary circumscribed neuroma usually occurs as a solitary flesh-colored papule on the face, usually arising on the upper lip or

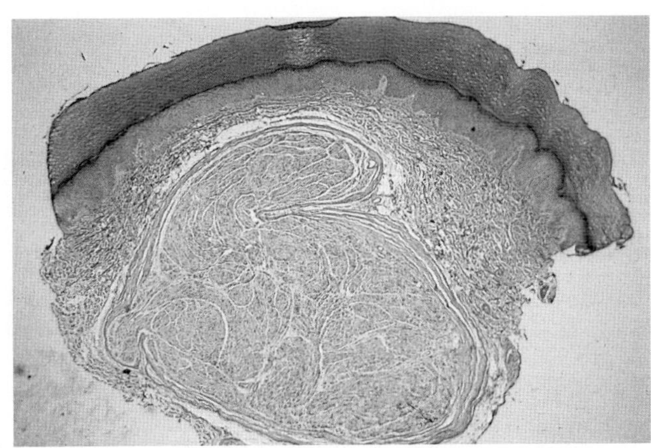
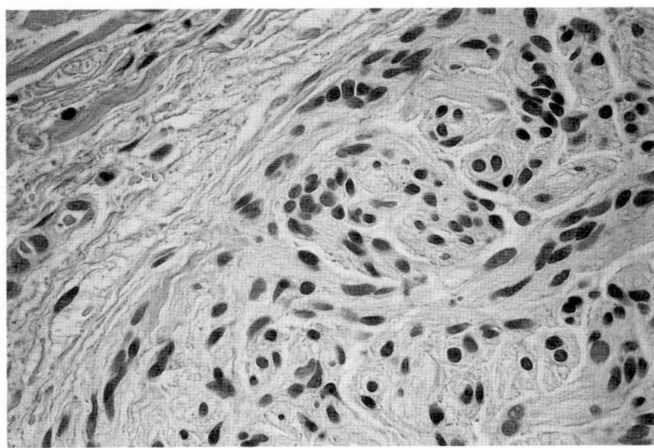

FIGURE 44. Solitary circumscribed neuroma. **A:** A circumscribed nodule composed of intersecting fascicles of spindled cells is present in the middermis. **B:** Spindled nuclei have tapered ends and eosinophilic wavy cytoplasm.

nose, areas near mucocutaneous junctions (173–177). Histologically there is a circumscribed or encapsulated dermal or subcutaneous spindle cell proliferation with atrophy or hyperplasia of the overlying epidermis (Fig. 44). The spindled cells have narrow tapered nuclei and are arranged in small irregularly shaped well-formed nerve fascicles. No significant stromal mucin or hemorrhage is present. This benign proliferation of $S\text{-}100^+$ Schwann cells is characterized by the presence of numerous interstitial axons staining positively for neurofilament proteins. The presence of axons and absence of a biphasic pattern help to distinguish solitary circumscribed neuroma from schwannoma.

Neurothekeoma (Nerve Sheath Myxoma)

Neurothekeoma usually arises as a 1- to 2-cm in diameter nodule on the scalp of a young adult. These tumors are histologically divided into two types: (a) myxoid or classic and (b) cellular (178,179). Histologically, neurothekeomas are characterized by the formation of multiple, nonencapsulated but circumscribed, dermal and subcutaneous lobules of spindled cells with plump nuclei (Fig. 45). Occasionally the spindled cells display a whorled and concentric growth pattern. Most neurothekeomas have a variable degree of nuclear atypia without significant mitotic activity. This proliferation is usually enmeshed in a myxoid dermal stroma. Notably, the cellular variant of neurothekeoma contains many cells with epithelioid cytology, mitotic activity, and nuclear atypia.

Whereas myxoid neurothekeomas stain positively for vimentin, S-100 protein, and occasionally epithelial membrane antigen (180,181), the cellular variant of neurothekeoma is S-100 protein negative but positive for vimentin and NK1/C3 (182).

Cutaneous Meningioma (Cutaneous Heterotopic Meningeal Nodule)

Cutaneous meningioma is a very rare tumor that arises in the skin of the scalp, forehead, and paravertebral skin (183–187). Histologically these lesions may appear as cords of meningothelial cells embedded in a collagenous stroma or display a cellular spindled and epithelioid cell proliferation with meningothelial whorls and psammoma bodies (Fig. 46). Immunohistochemical stains for S-100 protein, vimentin, and EMA are positive.

Merkel Cell Carcinoma (Primary Cutaneous Neuroendocrine Carcinoma)

Originally described as trabecular carcinoma in 1972 by Toker, this aggressive malignant tumor arises on the sun-exposed skin of elderly patients (188). The identification of neurosecretory granules with electron microscopy suggested that these tumors are of Merkel cell origin (189). In the absence of definitive evidence of a Merkel cell origin, the term primary cutaneous neuroendocrine carcinoma is favored by some pathologists (190). Complete excision is recommended; these tumors recur in approximately 30% of patients and metastasize to lymph nodes in over half of patients (191). Overall the mortality rate exceeds 30%. Merkel cell carcinoma is characterized histologically by a dermal proliferation of relatively small tumor cells arranged in trabeculae, cords, and sheets with an overlying grenz zone of uninvolved papillary dermis (Fig. 47). The tumor cells have oval nuclei with fine, evenly distributed chromatin and scant amphophilic cytoplasm. The nuclei contain multiple small inconspicuous basophilic nucleoli and commonly display a crush artifact with chromatin streaming. Frequent mitoses, tumor necrosis, and apoptosis are also usually present.

A punctate staining pattern for cytokeratins is characteristic of Merkel cell carcinoma (Fig. 47) but has also been observed in other small-cell carcinomas, particularly those arising in the lung (192). On the other hand, detection of cytokeratin 20 in a punctate pattern is observed in over 95% of Merkel cell carcinomas and is observed in small-cell carcinoma in fewer than 2% of cases (192). Occasionally, Merkel cell carcinoma may be epidermotropic. In these cases the differential diagnosis may include primary melanoma and cutaneous T-cell lymphoma. In contrast to the cytokeratin$^+$, EMA$^+$, neuron-specific enolase (NSE)$^+$, $S\text{-}100^-$, leukocyte common antigen (LCA)$^-$, CEA$^-$ immunophenotype of Merkel cell carcinoma, melanoma is $S\text{-}100^+$, EMA$^-$, cytokeratin$^-$, CEA$^-$, LCA$^-$; lymphomas are LCA$^+$ but negative for epithelial and neural markers (193,194). Electron microscopy reveals intracytoplasmic dense-core neurosecretory granules in Merkel cell carcinoma.

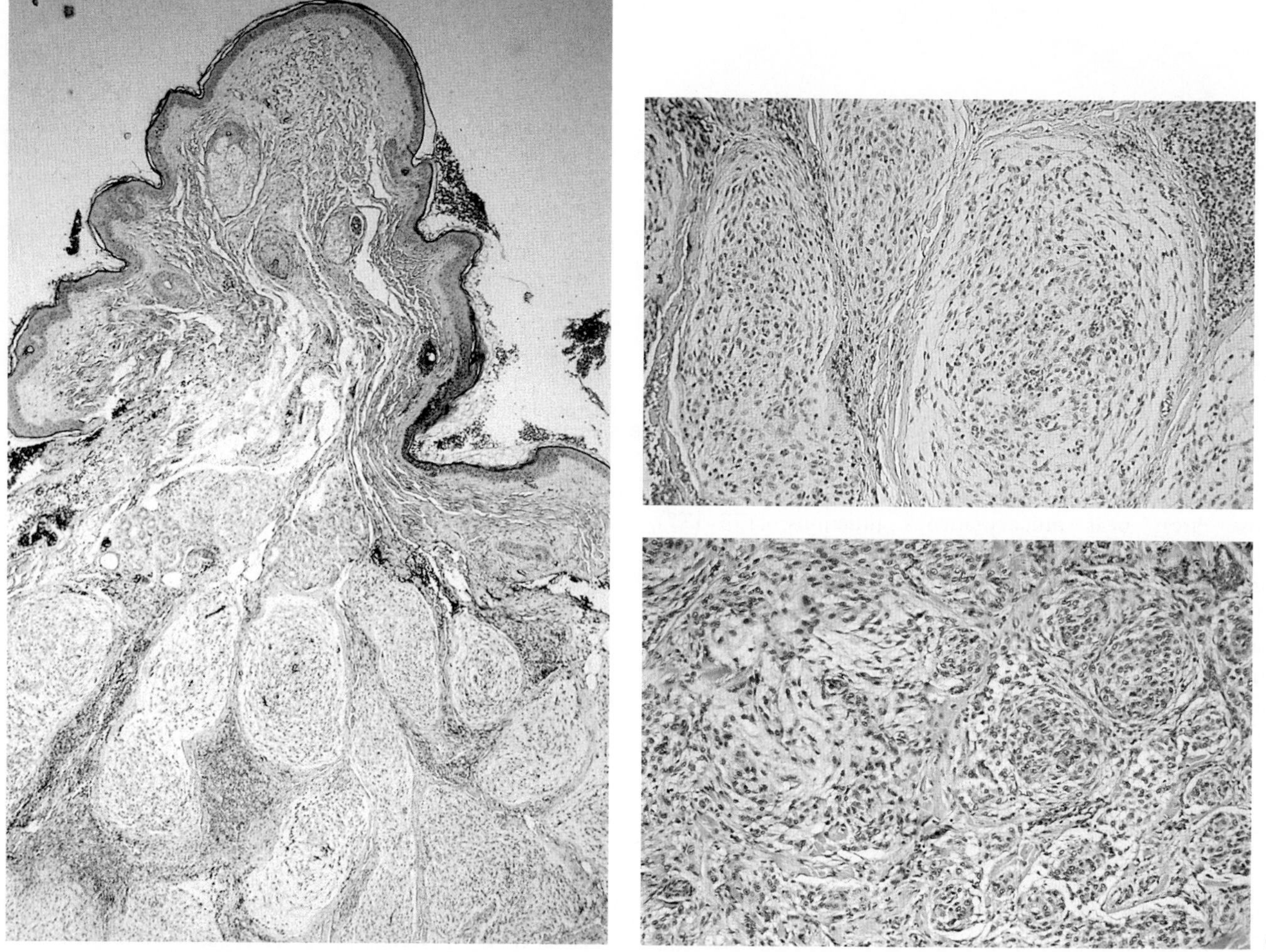

FIGURE 45. Neurothekeoma. **A:** Loosely formed nests of spindled cells are associated with a chronic inflammatory infiltrate. **B:** Small spindled cells forms whorls and nests with abundant myxoid stroma. **C:** Epithelioid and spindle cells in nests with abundant stromal mucin.

Melanocytic Neoplasms

Melanocytic proliferations in the skin usually involve both the epidermis and dermis. When benign, these intraepidermal and dermal melanocytic proliferations fall under the category of compound nevi. In contrast to compound nevi, junctional nevi are nested benign melanocytic proliferations limited to the epidermis, in the area of the dermal–epidermal junction. Dermal nevi occupy the dermis without a nested intraepidermal component. In addition to the classic extremely prevalent nested epithelioid dermal nevus, there are several distinctive forms of dermal melanocytic nevi; most common are those composed of pigmented dendritic melanocytes (cells with thin elongated processes). These dendritic melanocytoses are usually termed blue nevi because of the blue color observed clinically as a result of the Tyndall effect. There are a few specific types of pigmented dermal melanocytic proliferations that are notable because of their distinctive clinical presentations (nevus of Ota) or histologic features that may simulate malignant melanoma (cellular blue nevus, deep penetrating nevus, inverted type A nevus). Rarely, malignant melanoma arises in the setting of a benign blue nevus.

Dendritic Melanocytoses

Nevus of Ota (Nevus Fuscocaeruleus Ophthalmomaxillaris)

Nevus of Ota is a variant of blue nevus that affects the eyelids, conjunctiva, and sclera. It carries an increased risk of ocular melanoma and glaucoma. Nevus of Ota is one of several clinically distinctive dermal dendritic melanocytic proliferations, including nevus of Ito, occurring on the upper back, and Mongolian spot, which is found in the lumbosacral skin. These benign, hamartomatous, melanocytic proliferations are characterized histologically by the presence of a few pigmented dendritic melanocytes in the upper reticular dermis without significant alteration of the dermal stroma. The melanocytes may concentrate around vessels and adnexal structures. In contrast to the findings in classic blue nevi, few if any pigment-laden macrophages are observed in nevus of Ota.

Blue Nevus

Blue nevi may occur on the face or scalp but are most commonly observed on the hands and feet. They rarely occur in the oral cavity. These benign nevi are characteristically less than 1 cm in di-

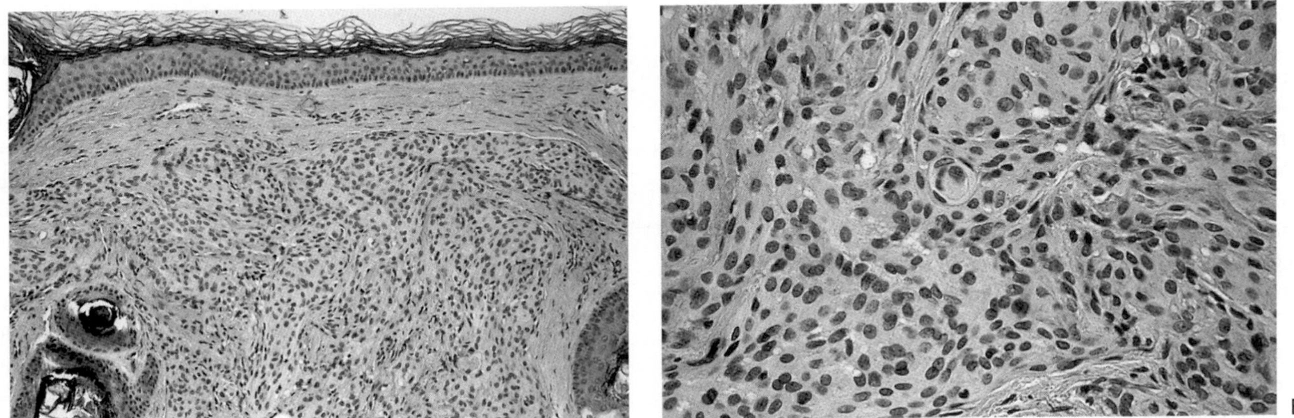

FIGURE 46. Cutaneous meningioma. **A:** Monomorphic epithelioid cells are arranged in the dermis in cohesive nests and sheets. **B:** Meningothelial cells with abundant amphophilic to eosinophilic cytoplasm form meningothelial whorls.

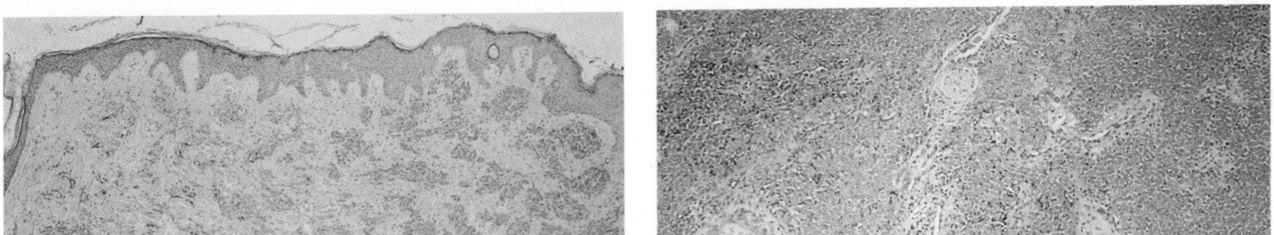

FIGURE 47. Merkel cell carcinoma. **A:** Trabeculae and cords of small blue cells dissect through the dermal collagen and focally display crush artifact. **B:** Sheets of tumor cells replace the dermal connective tissue and extend along nerves and around hair follicles. **C:** Nuclei with diffuse punctate chromatin characteristic of neuroendocrine tumors with apoptosis and mitotic figures. **D:** Punctate pattern of staining with antibodies for cytokeratins.

ameter, blue or blue-black, and flat or slightly elevated. The histologic features of blue nevus include a generally cellular symmetric dermal proliferation of pigmented dendritic cells (Fig. 48). The melanocytic dendritic processes are visible and contain numerous fine uniformly sized granules of cytoplasmic melanin. These pigmented dendritic melanocytes may infiltrate the adnexal adventia, nerves, and smooth muscle fascicles. Variable numbers of macrophages containing large irregular melanin granules are present and, in some cases, obscure the melanocytic proliferation. Some degree of dermal fibrosis or sclerosis is usually observed.

Cellular Blue Nevus

Cellular blue nevus presents as a 1- to 2-cm in diameter blue-gray or blue-black nodule usually on the sacrum, buttock, scalp, or face. Histologically, cellular blue nevus is composed of a well-circumscribed densely cellular nodular proliferation of nonpigmented spindled and epithelioid cells deeply situated in the dermis or subcutaneous fat (195). Careful examination will reveal pigmented dendritic melanocytes scattered throughout the tumor. The tumor cells often form a bulging nodule extending into the subcutaneous fat. This nodular proliferation is composed of nests and fascicles of fusiform cells with variably clear cytoplasm. The surrounding stroma is fibrotic and may contain pigment-laden macrophages. Cystic degeneration and vascular ectasia are also characteristic findings in cellular blue nevi (196). Rare reports of lymph node involvement by cellular blue nevi have been observed (197); the differential diagnosis of metastatic cellular blue nevus includes metastasis of a malignant blue nevus.

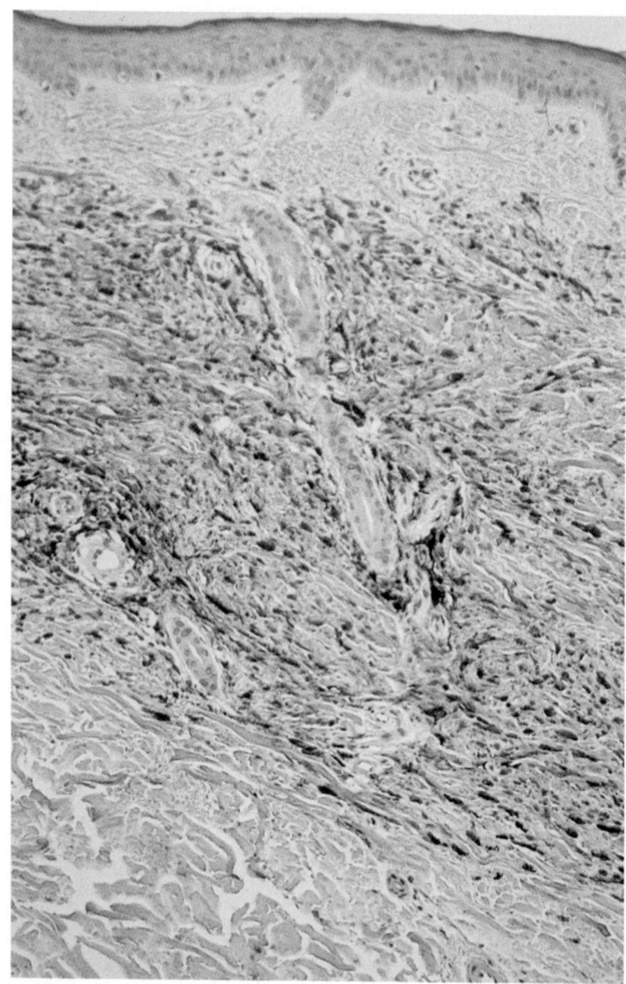

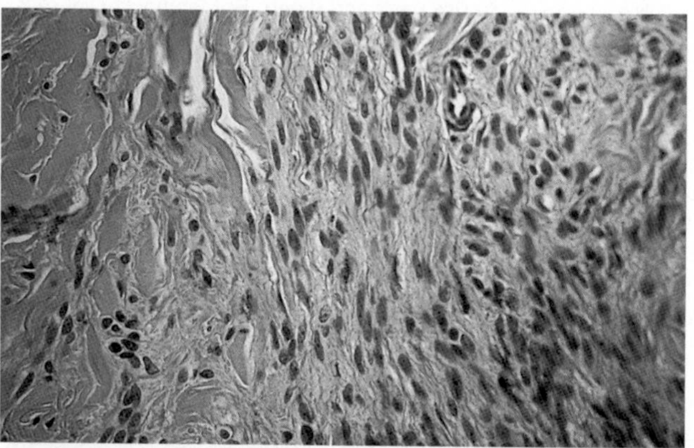

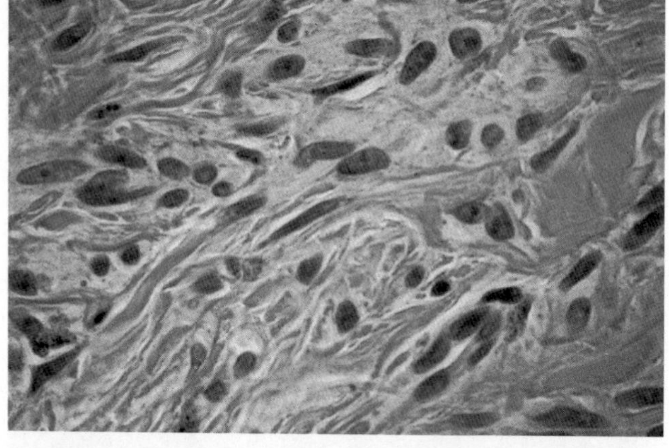

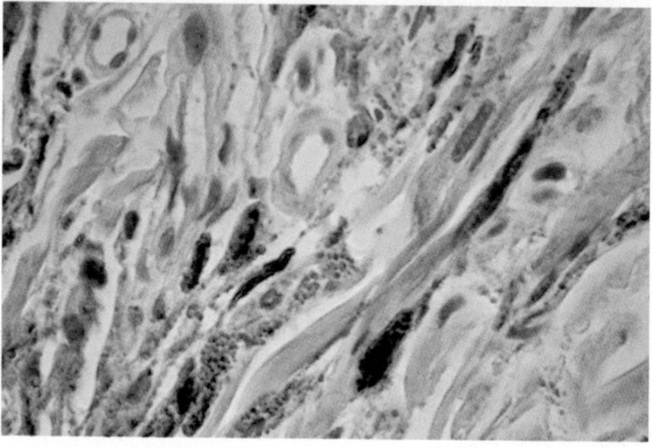

FIGURE 48. Blue nevus. **A:** Pigmented dendritic melanocytes dissect through the reticular dermal collagen. **B:** Spindled and dendritic melanocytes infiltrate the dermal connective tissue. **C:** Epithelioid melanocytes with sparse cytoplasmic pigment admixed with deeply pigmented dendritic melanocytes. **D:** Pigment-laden macrophages with coarse melanin granules admixed with finely pigmented dendritic melanocytes.

Although the distinction is usually quite challenging, in contrast to malignant blue nevi, atypical mitoses, necrosis, and nuclear anaplasia are not characteristic of cellular blue nevi. The cellular blue nevus should also be distinguished from blue nevus with hypercellularity, which is a benign blue nevus containing plump nonpigmented spindled melanocytes in the superficial dermis admixed with pigmented dendritic melanocytes. The bulging deep nodular melanocytic proliferation characteristic of cellular blue nevus is not observed in blue nevus with hypercellularity. Blue nevus with hypercellularity is a benign nevus that is treated identically to other blue nevi. In contrast, the risk of recurrence of cellular blue nevus is high; complete excision with a conservative resection margin is recommended.

Deep Penetrating Nevus

Deep penetrating nevi are deeply pigmented nevi found on the face, upper trunk, and proximal extremities. The histologic features of a deep penetrating nevus include a compound or dermal symmetric wedge-shaped melanocytic proliferation composed of pigmented spindled and epithelioid melanocytes (198–200). The melanocytes are arranged in nests and fascicles that extend into the deep dermis or subcutis. Pigment-laden macrophages are often present. Melanocytic atypia and mitotic activity are not characteristically observed in deep penetrating nevi. In contrast to blue nevi, deep penetrating nevi have less of a dendritic melanocytic component and a more prominent epithelioid melanocytic component. In addition, deep penetrating nevi usually display a nested intraepidermal melanocytic proliferation.

Inverted Type A Melanocytic Nevus (Combined Nevus, Clonal Nevus)

Inverted type A nevus is a histologically distinctive form of compound nevus that characteristically contains pigmented epithelioid cells at the deepest dermal aspect of the nevus, without pigmentation of the more superficially located melanocytes. The cytologic appearance of the pigmented epithelioid cells is similar to that of type A nevomelanocytes in the superficial dermis of the usual acquired compound nevi. The concentration of these cells at the deep aspect of the melanocytic proliferation is described by the term "inverted type A" because it appears as an inversion of the normal maturational phenomenon in which pigmented type A epithelioid cells are present superficially and nonpigmented type B and type C melanocytes are present more deeply (see below). Inverted type A nevus may have a dermal or compound melanocytic proliferation with the pigmented cells arranged in nests or nodules. There is a variable degree of dermal fibrosis and pigment-laden macrophages. No significant melanocytic atypia or mitotic activity is observed. Inverted type A nevi share many histologic features with deep penetrating nevi. In contrast to deep penetrating nevi, which are composed of pigmented spindled cells, the pigmented cells of inverted type A nevi have epithelioid cytology and are concentrated along the deep aspect of the lesion. These melanocytic proliferations may also have features similar to those observed in spindled and epithelioid cell nevi (201) (see below), or blue nevi, and in this setting are referred to as combined nevi (202).

Malignant Blue Nevus

Malignant blue nevus is an aggressive dermal melanocytic neoplasm that usually occurs on the scalp of men in their fifth decade of life. It appears as a blue or black nodule usually greater than 1.5 cm in diameter. These tumors metastasize to regional lymph nodes and may be fatal (203,204). Malignant blue nevi arise in the setting of benign blue nevi and are characterized by a multinodular proliferation of dermal spindle cells. An intraepidermal melanocytic proliferation is absent. Pigmentation and necrosis may be present but are often absent. There is often a background component of cellular blue nevus. The differential diagnosis includes cellular blue nevus and malignant melanoma. Cellular blue nevi are usually smaller and more uniform clinically than the large multinodular malignant blue nevi. The asymmetry, nuclear anaplasia, cellularity, mitotic activity, and necrosis often observed in malignant blue nevi are not characteristic of cellular blue nevi. The presence of a coexistent benign blue nevus helps to distinguish malignant blue nevus from metastatic melanoma and nodular malignant melanoma.

Benign Non-dendritic Melanocytic Proliferations

Melanocytic Nevus, Dermal (Intradermal Nevus)

As noted above, melanocytic nevi are termed "junctional" when the melanocytic proliferation is limited to the epidermis, "compound" when the melanocytic nests are located in both the epidermis and the underlying dermis, and "dermal" when they lack an intraepidermal component (Fig. 49). Other terms that are used in describing melanocytic proliferations include (a) lentiginous—a proliferation of melanocytes along the dermal epidermal junction as individual cells without significant nesting; (b) pagetoid—the presence of individual and nested melanocytes in the upper layers of the epidermis, similar to the changes observed in Paget's disease of the breast; and (c) maturation—a term used to describe the orderly progression of melanocytic cytology from the superficial dermal component to the deepest aspect of the nevus. In common acquired nevi, the cytologic appearance of melanocytes has been segregated into three types: (a) superficial type A cells, which have epithelioid morphology and pigmented cytoplasm; (b) midnevus type B cells, which are nonpigmented epithelioid or small cells with smaller nuclei and less cytoplasm than type A cells; and (c) at the nevus base, type C cells, which are nonpigmented cells with small round or spindled nuclei with inconspicuous cytoplasm that may be difficult to distinguish from lymphocytes or fibroblasts. Benign acquired nevi are the most common form of cutaneous melanocytic proliferation (Fig. 50). Histologically they have a symmetric appearance at scanning magnification and show some degree of cytologic maturation from the superficial to deep aspects of the nevus. Mitotic activity, ulceration, inflammation, ectatic vasculature, lack of cytologic maturation, and the appearance of several nests of cells that are cytologically atypical and distinct from the remainder of the melanocytic proliferation are findings that should prompt consideration of an unusual type of melanocytic nevus or malignant melanoma.

Melanocytic Nevus, Neurotized (Neural Nevus)

Neurotized nevi often occur on the skin of the face and probably represent age-related changes of a dermal nevus. The histologic

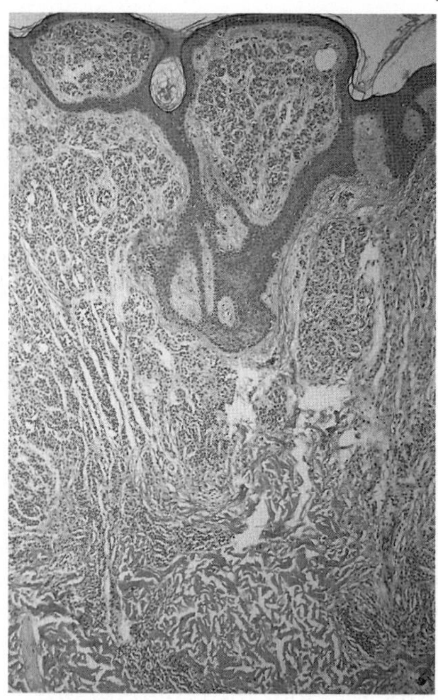

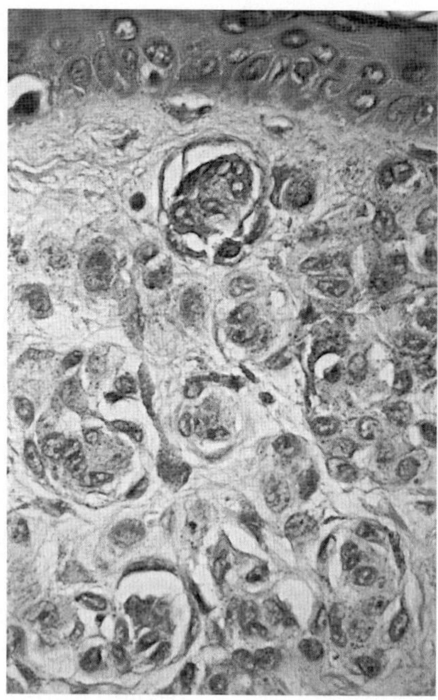

FIGURE 49. Dermal melanocytic nevus. **A:** Epithelioid melanocytes form nests in the superficial and middermis. **B:** Type A nevomelanocytes of epithelioid type with delicate cytoplasmic pigmentation are present at the surface of the nevus; deeper type B nevomelanocytes are nonpigmented and have less cytoplasm.

features of neurotized nevi include a predominance of type C nevomelanocytes, often with the formation of Meissner corpuscle–like structures. A common finding in neurotized nevi is a degenerative change that appears as fatty infiltration of the nevus. The differential diagnosis of neurotized dermal nevus includes neurofibroma. The presence of a residual nested component at the superficial dermal aspect of the nevus is helpful in confirming the diagnosis of neurotized nevus.

Melanocytic Nevus, Balloon Cell Type

Balloon cell nevus is rare; it usually occurs as a papule less than 5 mm in diameter on the skin of the head or neck. The "balloon" cells have small nuclei with prominent foamy or vesiculated cytoplasm and are observed in variable numbers admixed within an otherwise unremarkable dermal or compound nevus.

Melanocytic Nevus, Halo Type

The halo nevus clinically is a pigmented lesion less than 6 mm in diameter with a surrounding hypopigmented rim or "halo" (205). The histologic features are those of a compound or dermal nevus with a prominent lymphocytic inflammatory infiltrate (206–209). The inflammatory infiltrate is usually present in a lichenoid distribution in the superficial dermis, that is, concentrated at the dermal–epidermal interface or forming a subepithelial band of lymphocytes. The inflammatory infiltrate is often so dense that it obscures the underlying benign melanocytic proliferation. Pigment-laden macrophages and eosinophilic necrosis of nevus cells are often observed.

The differential diagnosis of halo nevus includes regression of a primary melanoma. In contrast to melanoma, the inflammatory infiltrate and melanocytic proliferation of halo nevi are

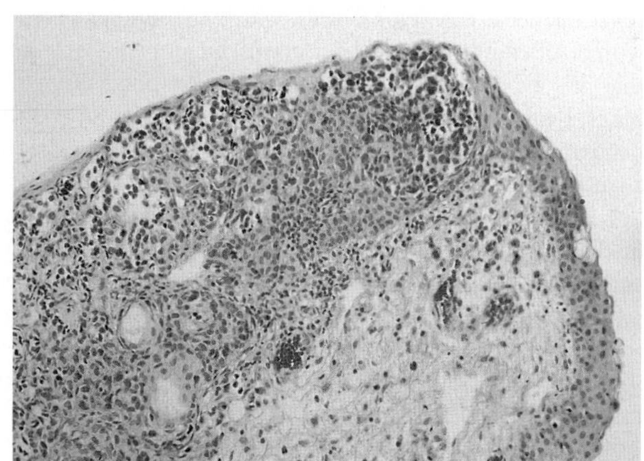

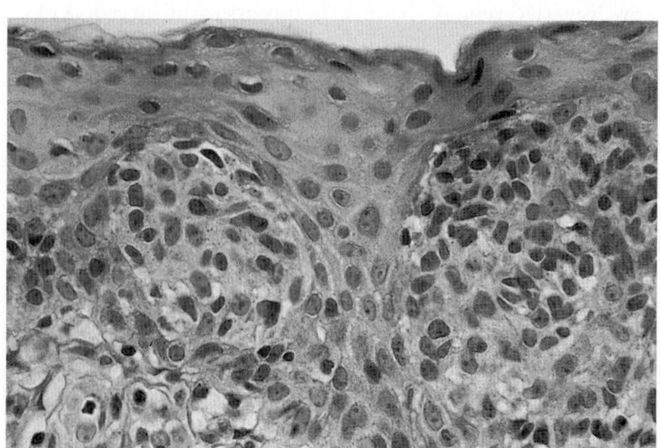

FIGURE 50. Conjunctival compound melanocytic nevus. **A:** Intraepithelial nests of melanocytes proliferate at the junction of the skin and conjunctival mucosa. **B:** Intraepithelial nests of delicately pigmented epithelioid nevomelanocytes.

symmetric with a well-defined base. On the other hand, atypical or numerous mitoses are not characteristic findings in halo nevi and should lead one to consider a diagnosis of melanoma.

Congenital Melanocytic Nevus

Congenital nevi are clinically classified according to size; those less than 1.5 cm are termed "small," those 1.5 to 20 cm "medium-sized," and those greater than 20 cm in diameter are termed "giant" (210). Because nevi may grow with age, the clinical category of the nevus may also change. The existence of divided nevi of the eyelids suggests that congenital nevi develop between 8 weeks of gestation, while the eyelids are still fused, and 24 weeks of gestation, when the eyelids first open (211). The associated risk of melanoma increases with the size of the congenital nevus (212).

The histologic features of congenital nevi include a few basic growth patterns (213): (a) plaque-like diffuse infiltration of the reticular dermis, (b) extension throughout the adventitial dermis and adnexal structures, including sebaceous glands and erector pili muscles, and (c) a perivascular distribution mimicking an inflammatory infiltrate. Maturation from superficial type A nevomelanocytes to deep type C nevomelanocytes is usually readily evident in congenital nevi. The two most common patterns observed in congenital nevi are extension around adnexal structures and involvement of the reticular dermis. Because of the increased number of adnexal structures on the skin of the face and scalp and the thin papillary dermis at these sites, many observers do not make the diagnosis of congenital nevus on the face or scalp based on these criteria. Nevertheless, in the presence of a perivascular distribution of nevomelanocytes, nesting within the epithelium of adnexal structures (particularly sebaceous glands), and with extension into the subcutaneous fat, a diagnosis of congenital nevus is warranted, even on the skin of the face and scalp (Fig. 51). Recognition of deep congenital nevi on the scalp is important because of the association with melanocytic proliferations involving the leptomeninges (214). Leptomeningeal melanocytosis is characterized by the presence of a banal proliferation of melanocytes in the subarachnoid cisterns. Associated clinical findings include hydrocephalus, seizures, and other neurologic signs. Melanoma may rarely arise in the setting of leptomeningeal melanocytosis.

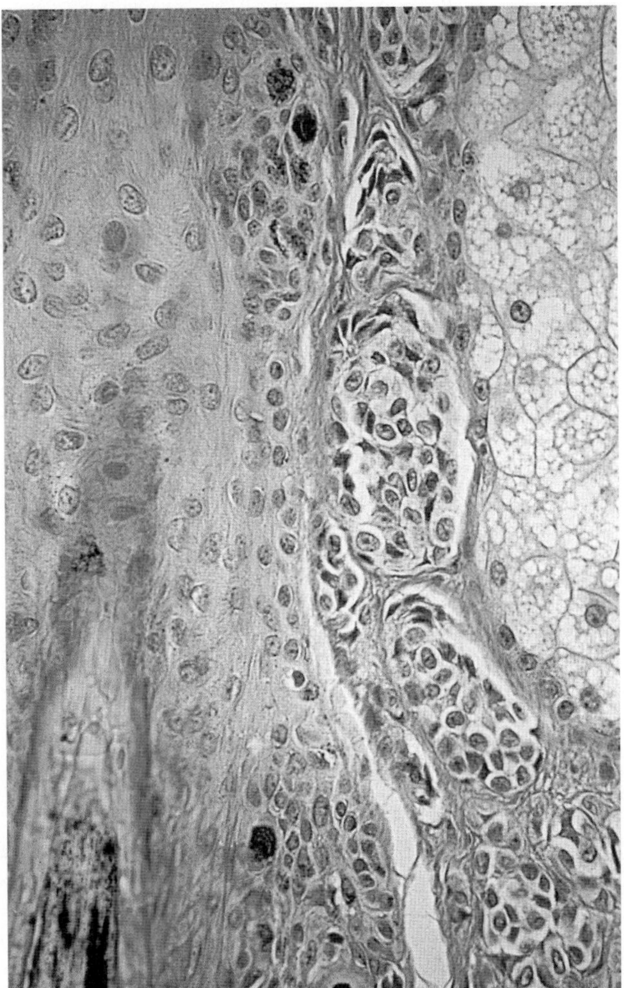

FIGURE 51. Congenital melanocytic nevus. Nests of benign nevomelanocytes infiltrate the hair follicle epithelium and dissect between the hair follicle and sebaceous glands.

Spindled and Epithelioid Cell Nevus (Spitz Nevus, Benign Juvenile Melanoma)

Spindled and epithelioid cell nevus most commonly appears in childhood as an erythematous papule or nodule on the face or leg, although it may occur at other sites (201,215–217). These lesions may grow rapidly to a diameter of 0.5 to 2 cm. Although they usually retain an intact surface epithelium, occasionally they may bleed or form a superficial crust. The erythema observed clinically correlates histologically with vascular ectasia of the superficial vascular plexus. Other histologic features of spindled and epithelioid cell nevi include a symmetric junctional, compound, or dermal melanocytic nevus composed of an admixture of cells with spindled and epithelioid cell morphology. The epithelioid cells of Spitz nevi have large nuclei with prominent eosinophilic nucleoli and abundant eosinophilic or amphophilic cytoplasm (Fig. 52). Characteristic findings include clefts overlying large intraepidermal nests, vertically oriented "raining down" intraepidermal nests containing spindled nevomelanocytes, and intraepidermal eosinophilic Kamino bodies. Kamino bodies are extracellular homogeneous eosinophilic aggregates of dyskeratotic debris and protein that are present more commonly in Spitz nevi than in melanoma (218). Individual epithelioid cells dissect through the reticular dermal collagen at the deep aspect of the nevus, and there is a variably dense inflammatory infiltrate, usually with telangiectasia. Not uncommonly, pagetoid growth and transepidermal elimination of nests are also observed.

Histologically, Spitz nevi may mimic melanoma (219–222). Indeed these nevi were described as childhood melanomas by Spitz in 1948 (201). Histologic features that favor a diagnosis of Spitz nevus include Kamino bodies (218), an overall symmetry at scanning magnification, and uniformity of nests from side to side at any given level of the dermis. Findings that support a diagnosis of melanoma include a brisk mitotic rate, mitoses close to the base of the lesion, abnormal mitoses, and the presence of nests of cells that are cytologically atypical and distinct from the

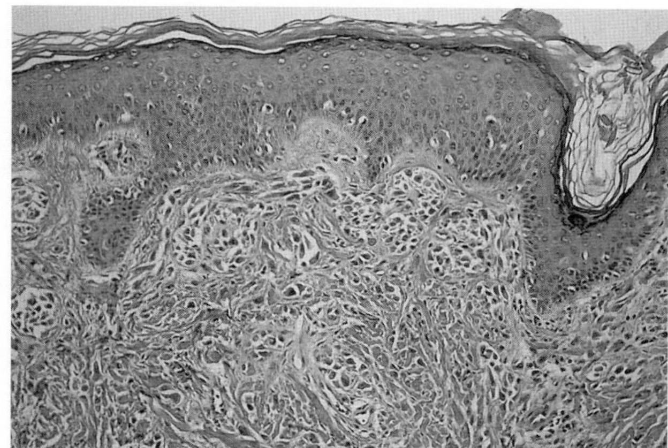

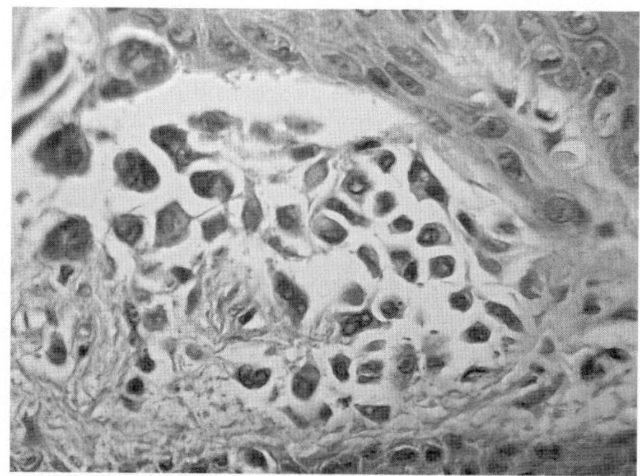

FIGURE 52. Spindled and epithelioid cell nevus. **A:** Plump spindled and epithelioid melanocytes proliferate as nests and individual cells in the superficial dermis. **B:** Clefting between the epidermal keratinocytes and a nest of epithelioid melanocytes.

remainder of the melanocytic proliferation, so-called *clonal atypia* (217,221). Complete excision with a narrow rim of normal tissue is recommended, as these lesions are even more difficult to distinguish from melanoma when they are recurrent lesions arising in a scar.

Dysplastic Nevus (Clark's Nevus, Nevus with Architectural Disorder and Cytologic Atypia)

Dysplastic melanocytic nevi are usually larger than 5 mm and display irregular pigmentation, jagged or irregular edges, and a degree of erythema or inflammation. Initially described by Elder as a sporadically occurring nevus in nonrelated patients, Clark and Lynch reported similar lesions that occurred in large numbers in patients with the familial atypical mole–malignant melanoma syndrome (FAMMS) (223). Whether arising in a familial or sporadic setting, dysplastic nevi are a risk factor for developing future melanoma, particularly in patients who have already had one melanoma. Although clinical features help to identify atypical nevi, the diagnosis of dysplastic nevus rests on the pathologic features (224). These tumors are graded based predominantly on cytologic atypia and somewhat on architectural features. Severely atypical dysplastic nevi are treated similarly to melanoma *in situ:* complete excision with a 0.5-cm margin of normal surrounding tissue.

The histologic features of dysplastic nevi remain controversial. A relatively reproducible approach has defined major and minor criteria (224). The presence of both major criteria and at least two of the four minor criteria allows the diagnosis of dysplastic nevus. The major criteria include (a) a lentiginous proliferation of cytologically atypical nevomelanocytes and (b) a "shoulder" of intraepidermal melanocytic nests extending 3 rete or more lateral to the underlying dermal melanocytic proliferation. The minor criteria include (a) enhanced vascularity of the superficial vascular plexus, (b) fibrosis, either concentric eosinophilic fibroplasia around the rete pegs or lamellar fibroplasia of the papillary dermis, (c) an inflammatory infiltrate, usually around the superficial venular plexus or in a lichenoid distribution, and (d) "bridging" of rete by expanded nests of melanocytes along the dermal–epidermal junction (Fig. 53). The dermal component of a dysplastic nevus usually does not show atypical features. In grading these lesions, pagetoid upward intraepidermal spread may be considered to be a severely atypical architectural feature; in the setting of dysplastic nevus, pagetoid spread does not necessarily indicate a diagnosis of melanoma *in situ* (see below). The principal differential diagnosis of dysplastic melanocytic nevi clinically and histologically is radial growth phase melanoma. Findings that favor a diagnosis of melanoma include a proliferation of cells in the epidermis or dermis that is cytologically distinct from the remainder of the melanocytic proliferation and dermal mitotic activity. One or a few nests of cells displaying nuclear hyperchromatism, dusty melanized cytoplasm, large nuclei with irregular nuclear contours, and prominent macronucleoli also support a diagnosis of melanoma. Likewise, the absence of maturation of the dermal melanocytic component suggests a diagnosis other than dysplastic nevus. As noted above, the dermal component of dysplastic nevi is usually banal and similar in appearance to that of benign acquired compound nevus.

Conjunctival Melanosis (Primary Acquired Melanosis, Benign Acquired Melanosis, Intraepithelial Melanocytic Hyperplasia)

Conjunctival melanosis appears clinically as a flat variably pigmented lesion in middle-aged or elderly Caucasian patients. The limbus or epibulbar interpalpebral region are the most common sites; however, the lesions may extend to involve the corneal epithelium. Approximately 25% of lesions clinically diagnosed as conjunctival melanosis progress to melanoma. Examination with a Woods lamp may aid in identifying the margins of the clinical lesion. The treatment of conjunctival melanosis with melanocytic atypia is complete excision. Cryotherapy has also been reported as an adjunctive therapy to local excision. Most importantly, the diagnosis of these lesions requires histologic examination (225,226).

Conjunctival melanosis can be separated into two categories of histologic lesions, those without melanocytic atypia (30%) and those with melanocytic atypia (70%) (227). The first category of lesions displays epithelial hyperpigmentation with or without a lentiginous melanocytic hyperplasia but without

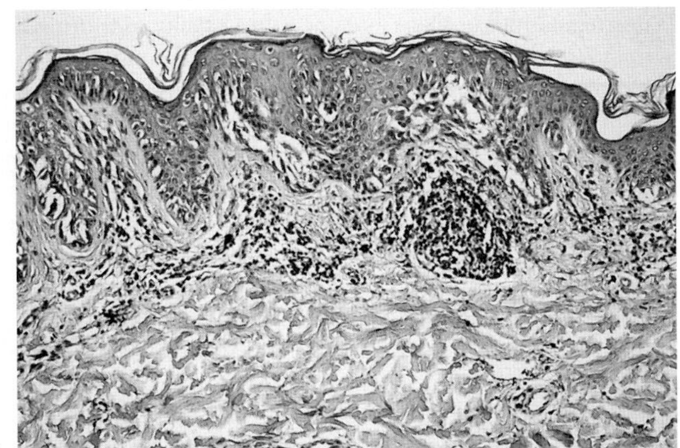

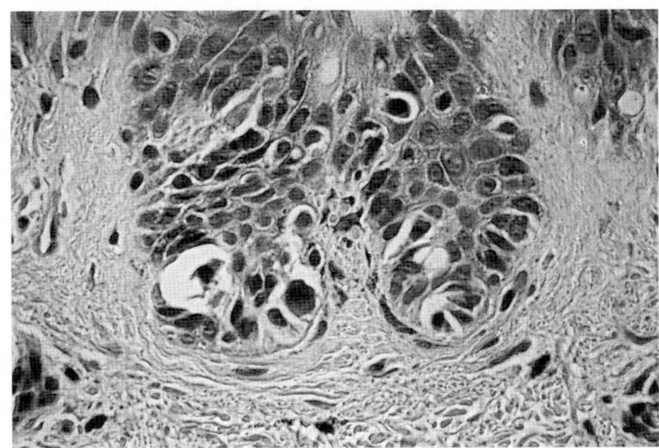

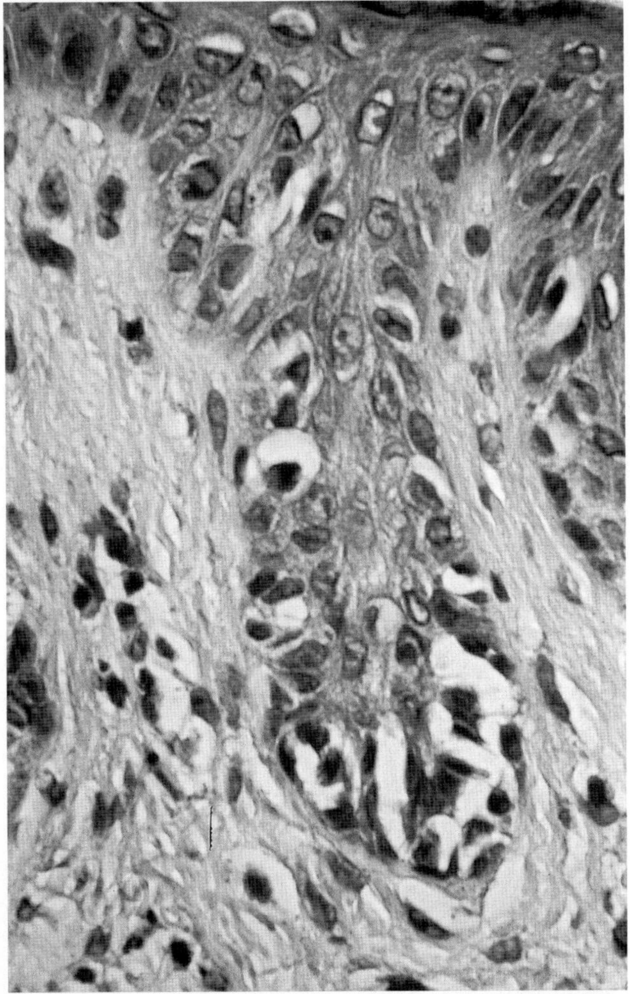

FIGURE 53. Dysplastic nevus. **A:** A lentiginous and nested proliferation of melanocytes extends along the base of the epidermis with an underlying dermal inflammatory infiltrate and slight dermal fibrosis. **B:** Slightly atypical junctional melanocytes with densely chromatic enlarged angulated nuclei and perinuclear clearing. **C:** Moderately atypical nevomelanocytes at the base of the epidermal rete have plump, densely chromatic nuclei and lightly pigmented or amphophilic cytoplasm.

melanocytic atypia. The second category of lesions displays atypical melanocytic hyperplasia and is a premalignant condition that evolves into melanoma in approximately 50% of patients. There are five principal growth patterns of atypical melanocytic hyperplasia in conjunctival melanosis: (a) basilar melanocytic hyperplasia (lentiginous melanocytic hyperplasia), (b) basilar nests (aggregates of three or more melanocytes), (c) intraepithelial nests above the basal layer epithelium, (d) pagetoid growth of individual cells (upward growth of melanocytes in the epithelium), and (e) replacement of the epithelium by atypical melanocytes. The histologic features that correlate with progression to melanoma include (a) a predominant growth pattern other than basilar melanocytic hyperplasia and (b) epithelioid melanocytic cytology (as opposed to spindled or small cell), with 90% and 75% of cases with these features progressing to invasive melanoma, respectively. In contrast, if the histologic lesion is composed of atypical basilar melanocytic hyperplasia only, the risk of evolution to melanoma is 22% (225).

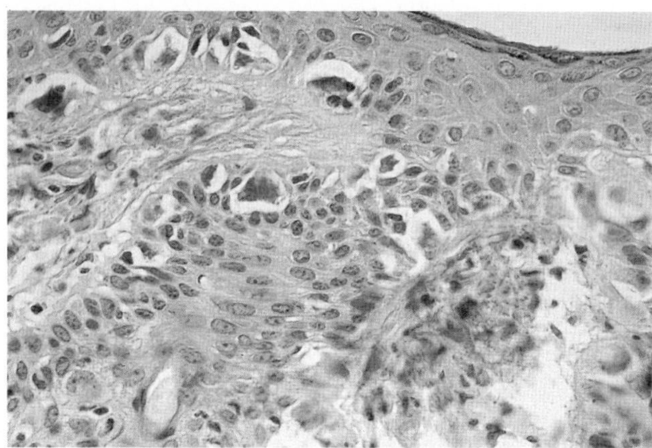

FIGURE 54. Lentigo maligna. Markedly atypical nevomelanocytes with large, densely chromatic pleomorphic nuclei extend as individual cells at the base of the epidermal and follicular epithelium. Dermal invasion is not present.

Lentigo Maligna

Lentigo maligna (Hutchinson's melanotic freckle) is the precursor lesion to lentigo maligna melanoma and is characterized by a long latent period. The lesion characteristically arises on extensively sun-damaged facial skin of elderly patients. Histologically, lentigo maligna is a cytologically atypical intraepidermal melanocytic proliferation characterized by a lentiginous proliferation with or without the formation of nests arising in the background of epidermal atrophy and marked solar elastosis (Fig. 54). Markedly atypical melanocytes with enlarged, angulated, densely chromatic nuclei are disposed as individual cells along the dermal–epidermal junction and extend down along pilosebaceous units. By definition there is no dermal melanocytic proliferation in lentigo maligna.

Malignant Melanoma

Melanoma

Melanoma is a malignant neoplasm of melanocytes. Clinically, melanoma is heralded by a pigmented lesion with recent change or irregularities in shape, size, or color, usually measuring more than 7 mm in diameter, with evidence or inflammation, oozing, bleeding, or itching. Over the past several years public awareness of melanoma has been heightened by a number of public health initiatives. The ABC method is a relatively easy way to remember the clinical features that are characteristic of melanoma: A, asymmetry; B, irregular border; C, color variation; D, diameter >6 mm; E, erythema. Approximately 10% of all melanomas occur on the head and neck (228–230). Approximately half of the melanomas arising on the head and neck are lentigo maligna type (LMM), followed by superficial spreading melanoma (SSM, 25%) and nodular melanoma (NMM, 23%) (231). LMM and NMM on average arise in older patients than do SSMs, with mean ages at diagnosis of 73 years, 69 years, and 57 years, respectively. LMMs most commonly occurs on the face, whereas NMM and SSM are more likely to be diagnosed on the scalp, neck, and ears (231).

Melanoma *in Situ*

The histologic features of melanoma *in situ* include an atypical intraepidermal melanocytic proliferation, often with a confluent lentiginous melanocytic proliferation along the dermal–epidermal junction and pagetoid spread (nests and individual tumor cells at all levels of the epidermis) (Fig. 55). By definition, melanoma *in situ* is melanoma limited to the epidermis without dermal melanoma. Characteristically there is marked cytologic atypia of the intraepidermal tumor cells, including nuclei larger than keratinocyte nuclei, nuclear hyperchromatism, irregular nuclear shapes, prominent eosinophilic nucleoli, and fine cytoplasmic melanin. In general, lentigo maligna melanoma *in situ* is characterized by a confluent lentiginous proliferation of melanocytes with densely chromatic rhomboidal and angulated nuclei, with formation of nests, dyscohesion, minimal pagetoid spread, epidermal atrophy, and marked solar elastosis. In contrast, superficial spreading melanoma *in situ* usually is composed of a nested and lentiginous proliferation of epithelioid melanocytes, usually with prominent pagetoid spread and with less epidermal atrophy than is usually observed in lentigo maligna melanoma *in situ.*

A 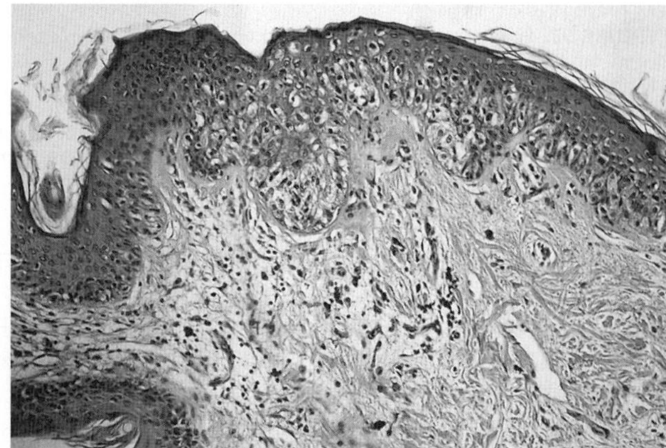

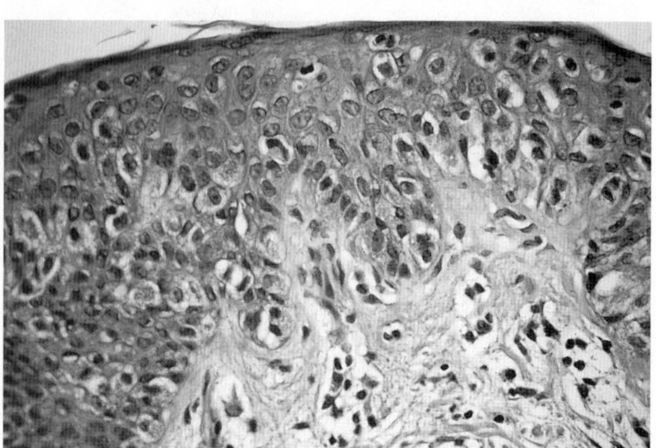 B

FIGURE 55. Superficial spreading malignant melanoma *in situ.* **A:** Lentiginous and nested intraepidermal melanocytic proliferation with individual melanocytes present at all levels of the epidermis (pagetoid spread). **B:** Pagetoid spread of cytologically atypical intraepidermal melanocytes.

There is some controversy regarding the term "melanoma *in situ*." In lesions that clinically appear as discrete nevi and histologically fulfill the criteria for dysplastic nevi, pagetoid spread and severe cytologic atypia may be interpreted as severe dysplasia. Lentigo maligna that demonstrates extensive intraepidermal nesting and pagetoid spread is usually referred to as lentigo maligna melanoma *in situ*. Indeed, a recent study shows that the intraepidermal component overlying invasive lentigo maligna melanoma always shows two or more of the following criteria: (a) confluence of junctional nests over three rete, (b) pagetoid spread, and (c) loss of cohesion between melanocytes of junctional nests (232). The authors propose that the term lentigo maligna melanoma *in situ* be applied to all cases of lentigo maligna that display two or more of these three atypical features (232). Finally, conjunctival acquired melanosis with severe melanocytic atypia and pagetoid spread but no nesting or subepithelial invasion may be termed conjunctival acquired melanosis with severe atypia.

The immunophenotype of intraepidermal melanoma is S-100^{+}, HMB45^{+}, CEA^{-}, cytokeratin^{-}, and EMA^{-}. The differential diagnosis of malignant melanoma *in situ* may include squamous cell carcinoma *in situ,* extramammary Paget's disease, and pagetoid sebaceous carcinoma (Table 1). Squamous cell carcinoma *in situ* often shows a transition from areas of actinic keratosis, and the pagetoid cells in squamous cell carcinoma *in situ* have a cytokeratin^{+}, EMA^{-}, CEA^{-}, S-100^{-}, HMB-45^{-} immunophenotype. The histologic features of Paget's disease are similar in mammary and extramammary sites; characteristically there is an intraepidermal proliferation of individual cells and nests of cells, with tumor cells present at all epidermal levels (pagetoid spread). A layer of keratinocytes usually separates the tumor cells in Paget's disease from the basement membrane zone. The tumor cells in Paget's disease display abundant clear cytoplasm, occasionally with intracytoplasmic sialomucin, which stains positively with alcian blue, mucicarmine, and PASD stains. Notably, the tumor cells of Paget's disease may also rarely contain melanin. Mitotic figures are rarely identified in extramammary Paget's disease. The tumor cells of Paget's disease have a cytokeratin^{+}, EMA^{+}, CEA^{+}, S-100^{-}, HMB-45^{-} immunophenotype.

Invasive Melanoma

Whereas *in situ* lesions are confined to the surface epithelium, invasive melanoma extends into the underlying dermis or submucosa. The invasive dermal component of melanoma may show a wide range of histologic features. Melanoma cells often are epithelioid with large atypical nuclei, prominent eosinophilic nucleoli, and abundant cytoplasm. Spindled melanoma cells have oval nuclei, clumped chromatin, prominent eosinophilic nucleoli, and spindled cytoplasm. Less commonly, melanomas may display a small-cell or plasmacytoid cytology. Mitotic activity is usually identified in the dermal component of melanoma. The dermal tumor cells may show a variety of growth patterns, including scattered individual cells and the formation of cords, nests, sheets, and expansile nodules of tumor cells. Although the nested pattern of melanoma is usually present, melanoma is known as the great imitator and may display cytologic and architectural features that closely resemble other malignant tumors including carcinoma and lymphoma.

Types of Invasive Melanoma

The growth patterns of malignant melanoma were described by Clark et al. as superficial spreading melanoma, lentigo maligna melanoma, acral lentiginous melanoma, and nodular melanoma (233). Invasive superficial spreading melanoma (SSM) accounts for more than 70% of all melanomas and 25% of melanomas arising on the head and neck (231). Histologically SSM is characterized by a cytologically atypical intraepidermal and dermal melanocytic tumor without evidence of cytologic maturation in the intradermal component. Dermal mitoses, a mononuclear cell inflammatory infiltrate, and dermal pigment-laden macrophages are often present (Fig. 56).

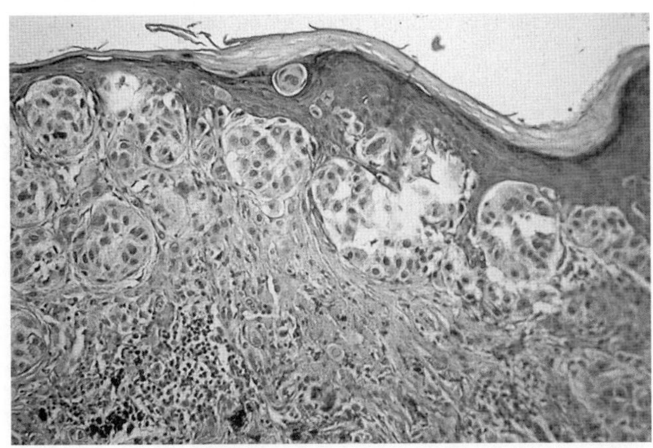

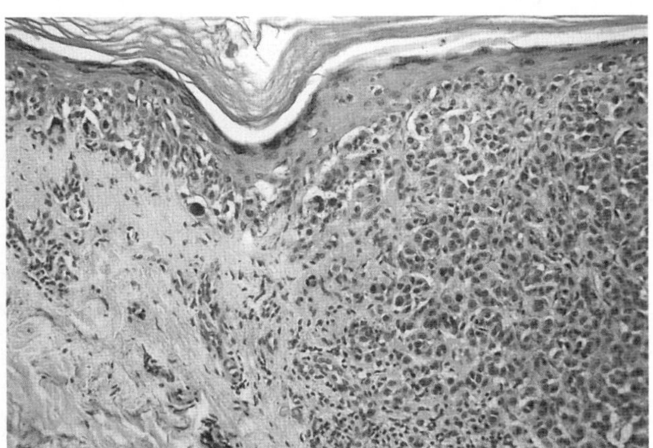

FIGURE 56. Superficial spreading malignant melanoma. **A:** Intraepidermal and superficial dermal nests (level II) of cytologically atypical melanocytes with focal pagetoid upward intraepidermal growth, dermal inflammation, and pigment-laden macrophages. **B:** Intraepidermal and dermal proliferation of atypical epithelioid melanocytes forming an expansile nodule in the superficial dermis (level III, vertical growth phase, right side of image); lateral to the dermal component an intraepidermal proliferation of individual and nested cytologically atypical melanocytes displays pagetoid spread (radial growth phase, left side of image).

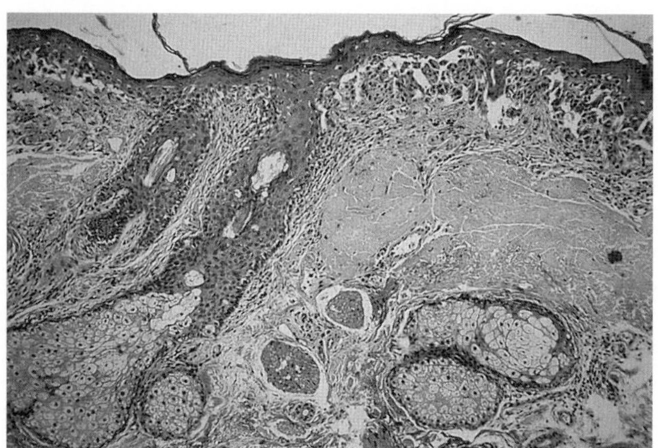

FIGURE 57. Lentigo maligna melanoma. Confluent nests of atypical nevomelanocytes with poor cellular cohesion extend along the base of the epidermis with focal invasion of the superficial dermis. Individual cytologically atypical melanocytes proliferate down the follicular epithelium.

Invasive lentigo maligna melanoma (LMM) accounts for fewer than 10% of all melanomas and usually occurs on the face and scalp, accounting for 50% of melanomas at these sites (231). Although the risk of metastasis following excision of early LMM is low, the risk of recurrence is high. The advancing margin of lentigo maligna melanoma may be subtle clinically and histologically. Because margins may be difficult to evaluate even in optimally processed tissue, evaluation of frozen section margins for lentigo maligna is not a recommended practice. Histologically LMM is characterized by an atypical intraepidermal and dermal melanocytic tumor, frequently with a spindle cell dermal component. As with lentigo maligna, extension of tumor along pilosebaceous units is often observed in LMM (Fig. 57). Features observed in LMM and common to all types of invasive melanoma include the absence of cytologic maturation of the dermal tumor and the presence of variable numbers of dermal mitoses.

Desmoplastic melanoma frequently occurs on the sun-exposed skin of the head and neck and usually arises in association with LMM. In addition to the features of lentigo maligna melanoma, the features of desmoplastic melanoma include dermal fibrosis or sclerosis and extension of individual atypical spindled melanoma cells throughout the dermis and into the subcutis (Fig. 58). Desmoplastic melanoma is frequently amelanotic and may display neurotropism. Patchy lymphoid infiltrates around deep dermal neurovascular bundles are a histologic clue to the presence of neurotropism (Fig. 59).

Acral lentiginous melanoma (ALM) is not discussed in this chapter. Aside from the site of occurrence, ALM shares many histologic features with mucosal lentiginous melanoma.

Mucosal lentiginous melanoma accounts for fewer than 5% of all melanomas. Mucosal lentiginous melanomas arise in the oral cavity. Melanomas in the head and neck may also arise in sinonasal or, rarely, laryngeal sites. The histologic features include the presence of a lentiginous, occasionally pagetoid, and nested radial growth phase, and, as with other forms of invasive melanoma, there is an absence of cytologic maturation of the dermal tumor and the presence of variable numbers of dermal mitoses.

Nodular melanoma (NMM) accounts for 10% to 15% of all melanomas. Histologically nodular melanomas are usually dome-shaped or polypoid, and often asymmetric at scanning magnification. By definition, vertical growth phase is present and radial growth phase is absent (see below). The intraepidermal melanoma is present overlying the dermal component but does not extend more than three epidermal rete lateral to the dermal component (Fig. 60). The invasive melanoma, displays an apparent lack of cytologic maturation of the dermal component, the formation of large expansile nests of tumor cells, loss of cohesion between tumor cells, and variable numbers of mitotic figures. A variably dense inflammatory infiltrate may be present and (as discussed below) has been shown to correlate with risk of metastasis. Rarely, nodular melanoma may resemble a dermal nevus at scanning magnification. The dermal component of these nevoid melanomas usually appears as two cytologically distinct populations, large atypical epithelioid cells and small cells. In this setting, the presence of individual epithelioid melanoma cells with prominent nucleoli dissecting through reticular dermal collagen fibers at the base of the lesion, and the identification of

A

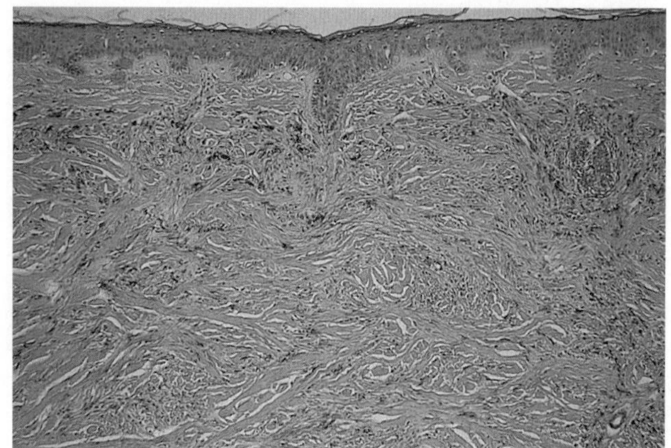

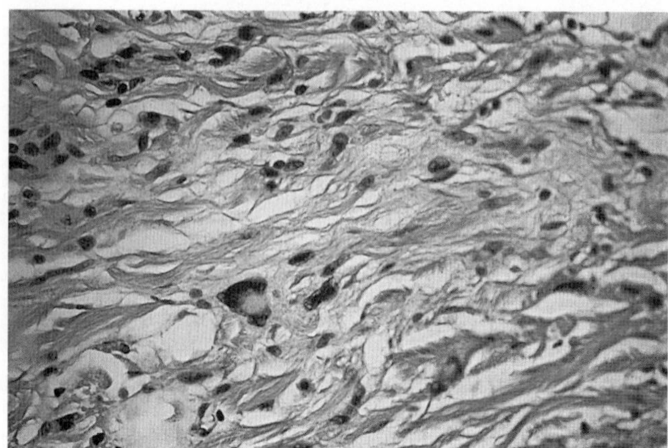

B

FIGURE 58. Desmoplastic malignant melanoma. **A:** Spindled melanoma cells dissect through a densely sclerotic, desmoplastic dermis. **B:** Melanoma cells with pleomorphic and anaplastic nuclei infiltrate through the dermal collagen.

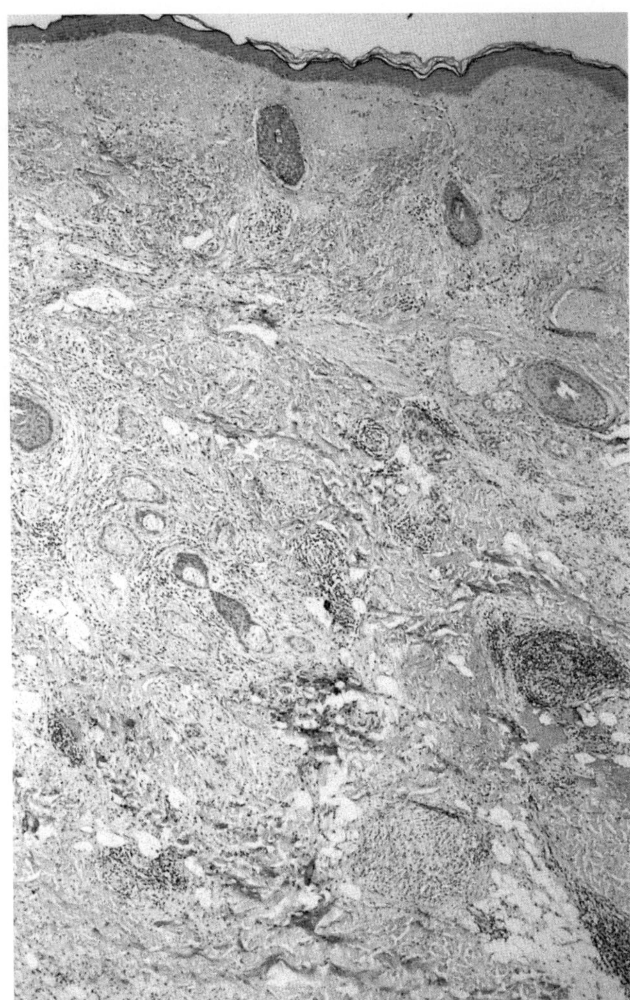

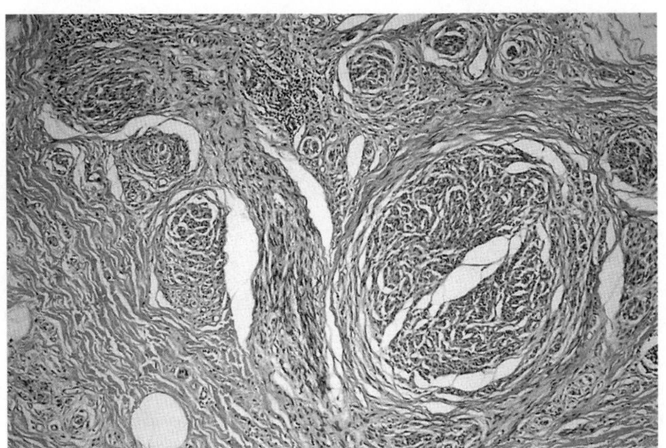

FIGURE 59. Neurotropic malignant melanoma. **A:** Inflammatory infiltrates about deep dermal neurovascular bundles at the site of neural involvement provide a clue to the presence of neurotropism. **B:** Extensively neurotropic melanoma invades and expands cutaneous nerves.

mitotic figures in the dermal component, support a diagnosis of melanoma.

The most common sites of extranodal melanoma metastases are skin, subcutaneous fat, and lung. Epidermotropic metastatic melanoma may mimic primary cutaneous melanoma. The histologic features of epidermotropic metastases include a collarette of acanthotic epidermis with central atrophy and a relatively inconspicuous intraepidermal component. The dermal component of metastatic melanoma often extends lateral to the intraepidermal component. The cells in melanoma metastases have uniform cytologic atypia devoid of maturation from the superficial to deep aspects of the proliferation.

Radial and Vertical Growth Phase

Subsequently to the description of different types of invasive melanoma, the intraepidermal proliferative patterns of malignant melanoma, melanoma *in situ,* and early microinvasive melanoma were described as the radial growth phase. The radial growth phase is significant because nearly 100% of patients with melanoma displaying only radial growth phase are cured by local surgical excision. The invasive radial growth phase is described as:

> isolated foci of melanoma cells present in the papillary dermis arrayed as single cells or as small clusters of cells, no more than 5 to 10 cells wide (234). Thickness is less than 0.76 mm in 97% of such tumors. No nest of dermal melanoma cells seems to have growth preference over other nests. All nests are similar in size. Cells are similar in form and pigment content to each other and to intraepidermal melanoma cells. Invasion is level II in 93% of these tumors. Mitotic figures are rare. (235)

On the other hand, vertical growth phase has been described as follows:

> melanoma cells in the dermis appear as a contiguous spherical or plaque-like aggregate larger than any nest of radial-growth-phase cells. Such aggregates are easily recognized when tumor thickness is >0.76 mm. When tumor thickness is <0.76 mm, the vertical growth phase appears as a cross-section of spherical aggregates of cells (15–25 cells wide) or as a plaque that fills and slightly widens the papillary dermis. Cells are different in form and in pigment from those of the radial growth phase. Invasion is level III, IV, or V in 90% of such tumors. Mitotic figures are usually seen. (235)

Table 2 shows the main histologic features that distinguish radial growth phase (RGP) melanoma from vertical growth phase (VGP) melanoma.

Melanoma, Prognostic Factors

By definition, superficial spreading melanoma, lentigo maligna melanoma, and acral or mucosal lentiginous melanoma all have

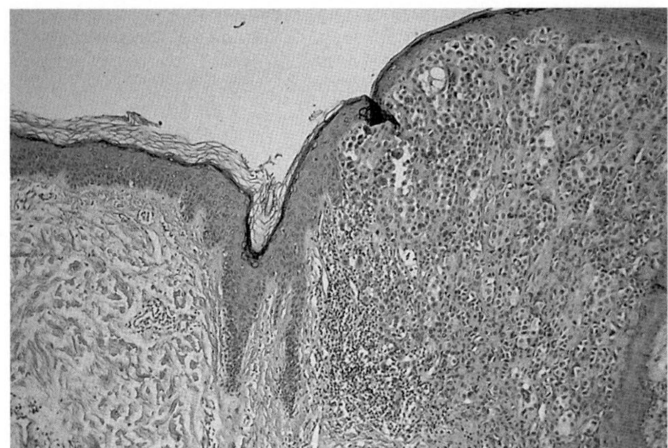
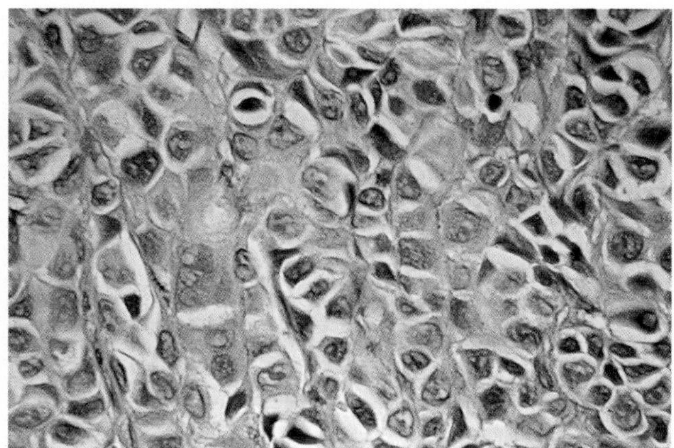
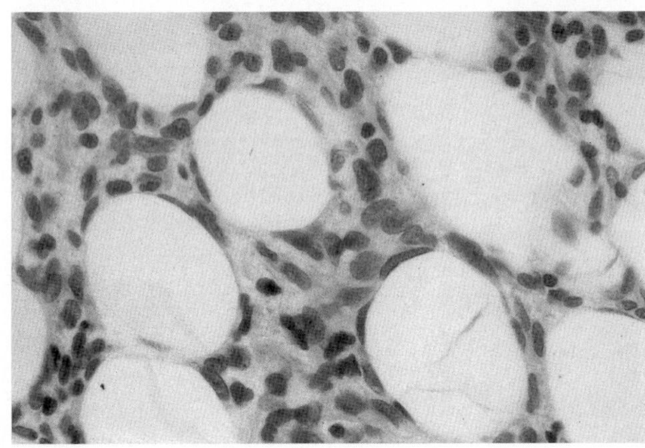

FIGURE 60. Nodular malignant melanoma. **A:** Markedly atypical epithelioid melanocytes proliferate as small nests in the epidermis and dermis to form a nodule of melanoma extending into the reticular dermis (level IV, vertical growth phase) without a lateral intraepidermal component. **B:** Epithelioid melanoma cells form compact nests and sheets of tumor cells with prominent macronucleoli and intranuclear inclusions. **C:** Melanoma extending into the subcutaneous fat (level V).

a radial growth phase component (Table 3). If these tumors present only in the RGP (VGP is absent), the chance of cure following complete excision approaches 100%. Nodular melanoma, on the other hand, presents in VGP and by definition does not have a RGP (Fig. 60). Because purely radial growth phase melanomas rarely metastasize, prognostic factors are reported only for melanomas with a vertical growth phase component (Table 4).

Thickness of the primary cutaneous tumor remains the gold standard in predicting prognosis and the initial treatment in patients with melanoma. Increased tumor thickness is associated with an increased risk of recurrence and metastasis. Thick melanomas are also associated with a poor chance of survival 5 years after diagnosis, in contrast to very thin tumors, which are usually cured by local excision (236).

TABLE 3. RADIAL GROWTH PHASE (RGP) AND VERTICAL GROWTH PHASE (VGP) IN CUTANEOUS MELANOMA[a] SUBTYPES

Melanoma Type	RGP	VGP
Superficial spreading melanoma (SSM)	+	+/−
Lentigo maligna melanoma (LMM)	+	+/−
Acral lentiginous melanoma (ALM)	+	+/−
Mucosal lentiginous melanoma	+	+/−
Nodular malignant melanoma (LMM)	−	+

[a] Superficial spreading melanoma, lentigo maligna melanoma, and acral (or mucosal) lentiginous melanoma, by definition, always have a radial growth phase component. In the event that a vertical growth phase develops in one of these three melanoma types, the tumor will display both RGP and VGP. On the other hand, nodular melanomas, by definition, do not have a radial growth phase. Nodular melanoma is a purely vertical growth phase tumor (436).

TABLE 2. HISTOLOGIC FEATURES THAT DISTINGUISH RADIAL GROWTH PHASE MELANOMA FROM VERTICAL GROWTH PHASE MELANOMA

	Radial Growth Phase	Vertical Growth Phase
Mitotic activity of the dermal component	Rare or none	Common
Nests of tumor cells in the dermis are larger than intraepidermal nests	No	Yes
Dermal expansile nodule of tumor cells	No	Yes
Cytologic appearance of the dermal melanoma distinct from the epidermal melanoma	No	Yes

TABLE 4. PROGNOSTIC FACTORS FOR CUTANEOUS MELANOMA

Tumor thickness (Breslow)[a]
Ulceration[a]
Anatomic level of invasion (Clark)[a]
Mitotic rate
Microscopic satellites[a]
Tumor infiltrating lymphocytes
Regression
Vascular invasion

[a] Factors required for AJCC staging.

Melanoma thickness (Breslow measurement) is measured with an ocular micrometer as the greatest distance perpendicular to the surface from the granular cell layer of the epidermis to the deepest melanoma cell in the dermis (Fig. 61). If an ulcer is present, the measurement is taken from the base of the ulcer to the deepest melanoma cell. There is a thin rim of papillary dermis that surrounds adnexal structures; a tongue of melanoma extending within or around a hair or eccrine duct should not be included in the measurement of tumor thickness. In the case of polypoidal tumors, the measurement is the thickest region of the tumor perpendicular to the surrounding skin surface, including the polypoidal excrescence (237). Tumor thickness should always be reported as a measurement in millimeters.

Ulceration has been described in many studies as an important prognostic factor in invasive melanoma (238–241). Ulcerated tumors are associated with decreased long-term survival and increased risk of metastasis compared to nonulcerated tumors, independent of tumor thickness. Ulceration is described as total absence of the epidermis overlying tumor with an overlying crust containing fibrin and cellular debris.

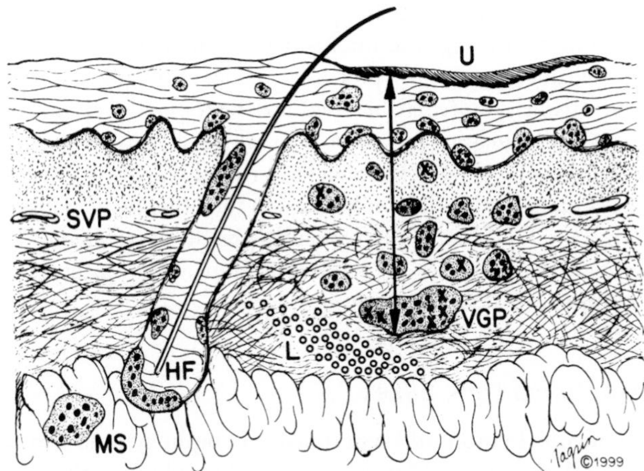

FIGURE 61. Diagrammatic representation of superficial spreading melanoma invasive into the reticular dermis (Clark level IV) below the superficial venular plexus (SVP) with extension down a hair follicle (HF), a microscopic satellite (MS), ulceration (U), mitoses (x) in the vertical growth phase (VGP) component, and a host response of lymphocytes (L) without infiltration of the tumor "TILs absent." The tumor thickness (Breslow) is the measurement shown by the *arrow.* (From Duncan LM. Prognostic indicators in melanoma. *Adv Dermatol* 1999;15:489–517, with permission.)

In 1969, Wallace Clark defined anatomic levels of invasion for melanoma that showed a strong correlation with potential for metastasis (Table 5). Although primary tumor thickness (Breslow) is the main prognostic parameter to be indicated in AJCC/UICC TNM staging, Clark's level of invasion should also be included in reports of thin melanomas because it adds significantly to the predictive value of staging in thin invasive tumors, particularly in the case of thin tumors invasive to anatomic level IV or V. Notably, level IV does not apply to a few tumor cells present in the superficial collagen fibers of the reticular dermis; rather, level IV tumors have a broad front of tumor cells extending more than four reticular dermal collagen fibers away from the papillary–reticular dermal junction.

The mitotic rate of the primary melanoma is reported as the number of mitotic figures per square millimeter or per 10 high-power fields. This measurement is made in the region of the vertical growth phase with the highest mitotic rate (235,242). Increased mitotic activity in the primary tumor is associated with a poor prognosis; patients with tumors that contained no mitoses, 1 to 6 mitoses/mm^2, and >6 mitoses/mm^2, had 8-year survival rates of 95%, 79.4%, and 38.2%, respectively, in a large series by Clark et al. (235).

Microscopic satellites are defined as a tumor nodule measuring more than 0.05 mm in diameter that is noncontiguous with the primary melanoma (243,244). By definition microscopic satellites are present in the section used for the Breslow measurement and occur only in tumors invasive to level IV or V. The microscopic satellite is distinguished from macroscopic satellitosis or in-transit metastases, which are grossly observable lesions less than or more than 5.0 cm from the primary tumor, respectively. The presence of microscopic satellites is an adverse prognostic finding and is associated with increased risk of metastasis.

When definitions of tumor-infiltrating lymphocytes (TILs) are strictly followed, the presence of TILs correlates strongly with survival (245) (Table 6). As described by Clark (235), the greater the density of lymphocytes infiltrating the vertical growth phase tumor, the greater the probability of survival 8 years after diagnosis.

The correlation of melanoma regression with survival has been controversial, in large part because of inconsistency in

TABLE 5. ANATOMIC LEVELS OF INVASIVE MELANOMA

Level I	Melanoma *in situ*, no invasion of the dermis
Level II	Individual cells and small nests are present in the papillary dermis, vertical growth phase is absent, and there is no tumor in the reticular dermis
Level III	Small and large tumor cell nests expand and fill the papillary dermis, pushing on the reticular dermis at the level of the superficial venular plexus; vertical growth phase is usually present; there is no tumor in the reticular dermis
Level IV	The tumor cells extend into the reticular dermis but do not involve the subcutaneous fat; vertical growth phase is present
Level V	Tumor extends into the subcutaneous fat; vertical growth phase is present

From Clark WH Jr, From L, Bernardino EA, et al. The histogenesis and biologic behavior of primary human malignant melanoma of the skin. *Cancer Res* 1969;29:705–727.

TABLE 6. TUMOR-INFILTRATING LYMPHOCYTES (TILs) IN CUTANEOUS MELANOMA: CRITERIA AND CORRELATION WITH PATIENT SURVIVAL

TILs	Criteria	10-Year Survival (245)
Brisk	TILs throughout the substance of the VGP[a] or present in the VGP and infiltrating across the entire base of the VGP	55%
Nonbrisk	TILs noted in one or more foci of the VGP	43%
Absent	Lymphocytes present but not infiltrating into the substance of the VGP *or* an absent lymphocytic infiltrate	27%

[a] VGP, vertical growth phase.

defining regression. Regression has historically been studied in the RGP component of a tumor that exhibits both RGP and VGP and is defined as focal complete absence of melanoma in the epidermis and the papillary dermis, flanked on either side by intraepidermal tumor. The papillary dermis at the site of regression is characterized by vascularity, fibrosis, and pigment-laden macrophages. Several recent studies have shown a correlation of extensive regression with adverse outcome in patients with thin melanomas (235,246).

In summary, there are a number of important prognostic indicators for cutaneous melanoma. Those factors listed in Table 4 should be included in pathologic reporting of all cutaneous melanomas in vertical growth phase. Tumor thickness, Clark level, the presence or absence of ulceration, and melanoma type should be reported in melanomas limited to radial growth phase (236).

Lymphoid Neoplasms and Lymphoma Look-alikes

General Features of Primary Cutaneous Lymphoma

Clinical Features

There are a number of clinically distinctive forms of cutaneous T-cell lymphomas. Their presentation may range from a solitary erythematous or violaceous nodule to multiple or occasionally solitary patches and infiltrated erythematous plaques to a markedly pruritic erythroderma. Whereas mycosis fungoides rarely involves the skin of the head and neck, $CD30^+$ anaplastic large-cell lymphoma, and NK/T-cell lymphoma more commonly involve the skin of the scalp and central face. In contrast to cutaneous T-cell lymphomas, most cutaneous B-cell lymphomas appear similar clinically, usually presenting as solitary or multiple erythematous papules or nodules that may coalesce to form plaques (247). Ulceration rarely occurs in cutaneous B-cell lymphomas. There is some regional predilection for various subtypes of tumors: follicle center lymphoma more commonly arises on the scalp, marginal zone lymphoma usually occurs on the trunk or extremities, benign cutaneous lymphoid hyperplasia is more commonly a truncal lesion, and the aggressive large B-cell lymphoma usually arises on the lower leg. Nevertheless, all types of cutaneous B-cell lymphoma can occur at any cutaneous site.

Histomorphology

Cutaneous T-cell lymphomas frequently show epidermotropism, in contrast to B-cell lymphomas, in which the tumor cells spare the epidermis and are usually separated from it by a grenz zone. Although T-cell lymphomas are usually diffuse and B-cell lymphomas are more frequently nodular, exceptions exist, especially in the skin. Finally, we now know that two features historically used by pathologists to support a diagnosis of cutaneous lymphoid hyperplasia are no longer valid: a dense superficial to middermal infiltrate that spares the subcutis ("top-heavy" infiltrate) and the presence of reactive lymphoid follicles are both commonly observed in cutaneous B-cell lymphomas.

Immunophenotype

An aberrant immunophenotype such as loss of one or more pan-T-cell antigens (CD2, CD3, CD5, or CD7) supports a diagnosis of cutaneous T-cell lymphoma. CD7 (Leu9) is the most common pan-T-cell antigen to be undetectable in cutaneous T-cell lymphoma; loss of a second T-cell antigen adds further support to the diagnosis of a neoplastic process. Loss of CD7 alone is not diagnostic, as CD7-negative T cells have occasionally been identified in reactive processes. As with T-cell lymphomas, an aberrant B-cell immunophenotype suggests a diagnosis of lymphoma. This is most commonly manifested as coexpression of CD43 and CD20. By definition, B-cell lymphoma is a monotypic proliferation of B lymphocytes; this can sometimes be demonstrated using immunohistochemical stains for κ and λ light chains in routinely processed tissue, although staining of frozen tissue is more reliable. Because the responder cell in cutaneous inflammatory processes is usually a T cell, an infiltrate composed of >75% B lymphocytes strongly supports a diagnosis of cutaneous B-cell lymphoma. On the other hand, dense reactive T-cell infiltrates are frequently present in cutaneous lymphoma; this should be kept in mind when interpreting immunohistochemical stains.

Lymphoma Look-alikes

Cutaneous Lymphoid Hyperplasia (Lymphocytoma Cutis, Pseudolymphoma of Spiegler-Fendt, Lymphadenosis Benigna Cutis)

Cutaneous lymphoid hyperplasia occurs as solitary or multiple persistent or self-healing nodules and is often a hypersensitivity reaction. Histologically atypical reactive lymphoid infiltrates may mimic B-cell lymphoma or T-cell lymphoma. Scanning magnification appearance varies from a dense perivascular infiltrate with inconspicuous germinal centers to a dense nodular follicular hyperplasia. In lesions resembling B-cell lymphoma there is a dense superficial and deep dermal infiltrate of B and T lymphocytes, often with epidermal hyperplasia, scale crust, parakeratosis, and interface dermatitis. Occasionally the infiltrate is separated from the epidermis by a grenz zone of uninvolved papillary dermis. Reactive follicles with germinal centers may be present but are often absent. In addition to a dense lymphoid infiltrate, there may be scattered eosinophils, plasma cells, and multinucleate giant cells. The lymphocyte cytology is usually not atypical; most of the lymphoid cells have round regular small nuclei and sparse cytoplasm. By definition, no light-chain restriction is identified immunohistochemically.

Reactive lymphoid infiltrates that mimic cutaneous T-cell lymphoma usually mimic mycosis fungoides and include lymphomatoid drug eruption and actinic reticuloid (chronic actinic dermatitis). Lymphomatoid drug eruption may display a lichenoid infiltrate with epidermotropism. The histologic distinction may be difficult. The presence of scale crust (parakeratosis with serum and nuclear debris), dyskeratosis, intraepidermal Langerhans' cell microabscesses and papillary dermal erythrocyte extravasation supports a diagnosis of a drug eruption. On the other hand, the presence of mounds of parakeratosis, Pautrier's microabscesses (intraepidermal nests of atypical T cells), atypical cells lining up like a string of pearls along the dermal epidermal junction and papillary dermal fibrosis all support a diagnosis of mycosis fungoides.

Actinic Reticuloid (Chronic Actinic Dermatitis)

Actinic reticuloid is a chronic photosensitivity dermatitis that often occurs on the sun-exposed facial skin of elderly men. In early lesions the histologic features include epidermal hyperplasia with spongiosis and focal parakeratosis. There is a lichenoid dermal mononuclear cell infiltrate with scattered eosinophils and plasma cells. Notably the infiltrating lymphocytes have enlarged convoluted densely chromatic nuclei. Well-developed lesions show similar changes but also display epidermotropism of atypical lymphocytes and mitotic activity in the dermal component. Stellate multinucleate fibroblasts in the superficial dermis and papillary dermal edema and fibrosis are common findings in late lesions. Immunophenotypically the lymphocytes usually are $CD8^+$, $CD4^-$, without loss of pan-T-cell antigens. This last finding is an important differentiating feature from cutaneous T-cell lymphoma. For further discussion see the section on photosensitivity reactions.

Cutaneous T-Cell Lymphoma

Mycosis Fungoides (Cutaneous T-Cell Lymphoma)

The histologic features of mycosis fungoides may be dramatic or subtle and include a lichenoid or nodular atypical T-cell infiltrate with epidermotropism and Pautrier's microabscesses (Fig. 62). Epidermotropism is defined as exocytosis through the epidermis of atypical T cells with enlarged densely chromatic convoluted nuclei, usually without significant spongiosis. The neo-

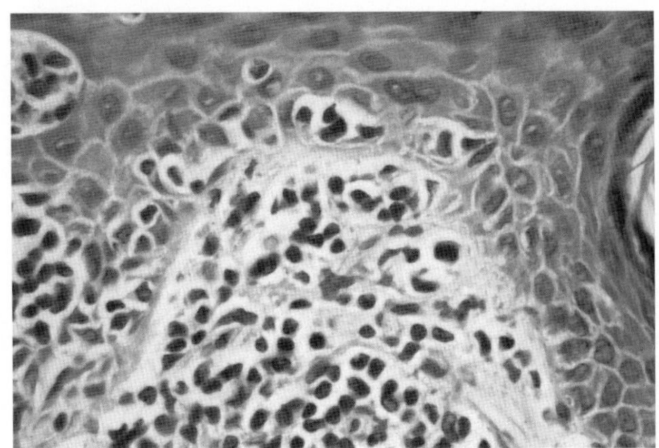

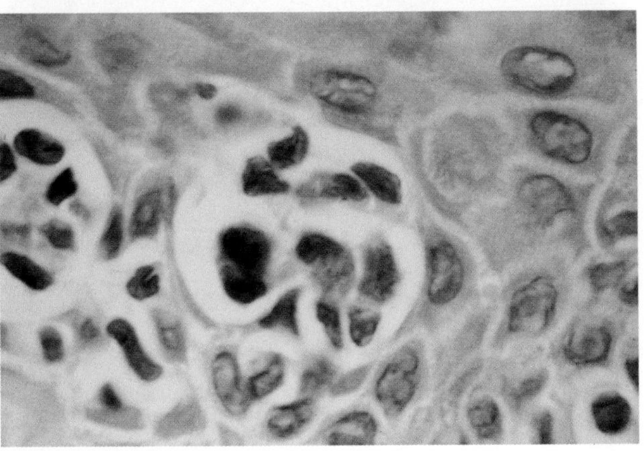

FIGURE 62. Mycosis fungoides. **A:** A dense lymphocytic infiltrate obscures the dermal–epidermal junction. **B:** Large lymphocytes with densely chromatic convoluted nuclei (Sezary cells) extend through the epidermis in aggregates (Pautrier microabscesses) and as individual cells (epidermotropism). **C:** Pautrier microabscess.

plastic T cells in mycosis fungoides characteristically have convoluted cerebriform nuclei (termed Sézary cells in the peripheral blood). Intraepidermal aggregates of atypical T cells are termed Pautrier's microabscesses. Other findings that are often observed in mycosis fungoides include the lining up of atypical lymphocytes along the dermal–epidermal junction, papillary dermal fibrosis, and, rarely, scattered large Reed-Sternberg–like cells (often $CD30^+$). Follicular mucinosis and eccrine gland hyperplasia may also be observed.

The neoplastic T cells in mycosis fungoides usually have a $CD4^+$, $CD8^-$ immunophenotype with loss of one or more of the pan-T-cell antigens CD2, CD5, and CD7.

Nasal or Nasal-type T/NK-Cell Lymphoma (Angiocentric Immunoproliferative Lesion, Polymorphic Reticulosis, Lethal Midline Granuloma)

Although T/NK-cell lymphoma may arise as a primary cutaneous tumor, when this lesion occurs on the skin of the face, it is often associated with nasal or nasal-type T/NK-cell lymphoma arising in the sinonasal tract. This process is described in detail in Chapter 12. These tumors often display an angiocentric growth pattern, as is reflected in their classification in the Revised European American lymphoma classification (REAL) and the European Organization for the Research and Treatment of Cancer (EORTC) lymphoma-staging schemes: in the REAL classification, angiocentric lymphoma (nasal-type T/NK-cell lymphoma); in the EORTC Cutaneous Lymphoma Classification, angiocentric lymphomas are included under the heading of pleomorphic small to medium-sized T-cell lymphoma. In addition to the above nomenclature, the terms angiocentric immunoproliferative lesion, lethal midline granuloma, nasal T-cell lymphoma, and lymphomatoid granulomatosis or polymorphic reticulosis have been used to describe angiocentric lymphomas. The nasal or nasal-type T/NK-cell lymphomas have been described predominantly as tumors of $CD56^+$ T/NK cells and are associated with Epstein-Barr virus (EBV) infection. On the other hand, most cases of pulmonary lymphomatoid granulomatosis have been identified as large B-cell lymphomas, also with an EBV association (248). Angiocentric lymphomas of both types have been observed in the skin, as well as angiocentric lymphomas that are composed of neither T/NK nor B cells.

Primary Cutaneous Anaplastic Large-Cell ($Ki\text{-}1^+$) Lymphoma

Primary cutaneous anaplastic large cell lymphoma (ALCL) usually presents as a solitary nodule in the seventh or eighth decade of life (249), rarely occurring in children (250,251). Dissemination occurs in fewer than 25% of patients; even with this spread beyond cutaneous sites, the 4-year survival exceeds 90% (252,253). Primary cutaneous ALCL has a much more favorable prognosis than does cutaneous ALCL arising in association with a primary ALCL of nodal origin (254,255).

This tumor histologically has a distinctively anaplastic appearance; hence, the inclusion of this terminology in the lymphoma classification schemes: in the REAL classification, anaplastic large cell lymphoma (ALCL); in the EORTC Cutaneous Lymphoma Classification, $CD30^+$ large T-cell lymphoma (anaplastic, pleomorphic, and immunoblastic types). Cutaneous ALCL is characterized by sheets of large anaplastic lymphocytes extending from the superficial dermis into the subcutaneous fat; more than 75% of the infiltrating cells display marked nuclear anaplasia. These Reed-Sternberg–like cells have one or more oval indented or irregularly shaped nuclei, prominent eosinophilic macronucleoli, and abundant cytoplasm (Fig. 63). Numerous mitoses are present, as is a moderately dense reactive inflammatory infiltrate at the periphery of the tumor. Small atypical lymphocytes are absent except in the rare case that has evolved from mycosis fungoides. The epidermis may be hyperplastic; however, epidermotropism is very rarely observed.

Immunophenotype The tumor cells stain strongly positive for CD30 (BerH2, Ki-1), with a characteristic punctate accentuation of stain in the perinuclear golgi region. Weak staining for the pan-T-cell antigens CD2, CD3, CD4, and CD5 may be observed. The tumor cells usually stain positively for the HLA-DR antigen, CD25, and CD45RO; EMA has been reported to be present in 33% of cases (249).

Genetic Studies Clonal rearrangement of the T-cell receptor genes is often present (256). In contrast to nodal $CD30^+$ lymphoma, t(2;5) (p23;q35) translocation and the resultant p80 NPM-ALK protein are usually not present (257–261). In contrast to their prognostic significance in primary nodal ALCL, when present, p80 expression and NPM-ALK transcripts resulting from t(2;5) (p23;q35) are not of diagnostic or prognostic significance in cutaneous $CD30^+$ lymphoid proliferations (255).

Cutaneous B-Cell Lymphoma

Follicle Center Lymphoma

Follicle center lymphoma is the most common primary cutaneous B-cell lymphoma. It presents as multiple or solitary cutaneous nodules or plaques, often on the scalp or trunk (262–264). The estimated 5-year survival is over 97% (265). This tumor is classified as follows: REAL classification, follicle center lymphoma; EORTC Cutaneous Lymphoma Classification, follicle center cell lymphoma (head and trunk).

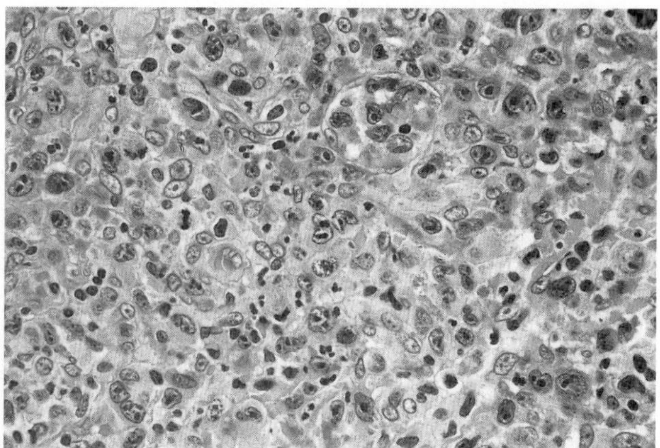

FIGURE 63. Anaplastic large-cell lymphoma, Ki-1 $(CD30)^+$. Large, occasionally multinucleate, anaplastic lymphoid cells with abundant eosinophilic cytoplasm and eosinophilic macronucleoli form a sheet of tumor in the reticular dermis with scattered apoptotic cells and mitotic figures.

Histologically, there is characteristically a middermal and subcuticular proliferation of centrocytes and centroblasts in a nodular pattern, simulating reactive lymphoid follicles (Fig. 64). The centrocytes usually outnumber the centroblasts, and there is an admixed benign T-cell infiltrate of variable density. Centrocytes have small cleaved nuclei with inconspicuous nucleoli, whereas centroblasts have large round nuclei with peripherally located basophilic nucleoli; centroblasts have a narrow rim of amphophilic to basophilic cytoplasm. A neoplastic proliferation of these cells often appears as large, irregularly shaped lymphoid follicles in the dermis. Occasionally, the neoplastic cells appear to spill out of the follicles and surround aggregates of benign small lymphocytes. This pattern is referred to as "inside-out follicles" by some observers and is also found in nodal follicle center lymphomas.

Immunophenotype There is light-chain restriction of the neoplastic follicle centers, and the follicle center cells have a $CD10^{+/-}$, $CD5^{-}$, $CD43^{-}$ immunophenotype. Cutaneous follicle center lymphomas express the bcl-2 protein in fewer than 30% of cases (266,267), in contrast to nodal follicle center lymphomas, which are almost all $bcl\text{-}2^{+}$. Because bcl-2 protein is normally present on most T cells and B cells, except B cells in reactive follicle centers, and follicle center lymphomas of the skin are often bcl-2-negative; a negative staining pattern of follicles with the remaining lymphocytes staining positively for bcl-2 does not allow for distinction between a reactive and neoplastic process.

Genetic Studies Primary cutaneous follicle center lymphoma typically does not have the association of t(14;18) observed in nodal follicle center lymphoma. Clonal rearrangement of immunoglobulin genes is often detected.

Marginal Zone B-Cell Lymphoma of MALT Type

Primary cutaneous marginal zone lymphoma is a low-grade B-cell lymphoma that shares features with extranodal lymphomas of mucosa-associated lymphoid tissue (MALT) type (268–274). Also known as monocytoid B-cell lymphoma, and lymphoma of skin-associated lymphoid tissue (SALT) (275), this tumor is classified as follows: REAL classification, extranodal marginal zone B-cell lymphoma (low-grade B-cell lymphoma of MALT type); EORTC Cutaneous Lymphoma Classification, marginal zone lymphoma (immunocytoma) (247,265,276,277). Marginal zone lymphoma probably represents the second most common form of primary cutaneous B-cell lymphoma after follicle center lymphoma (278,279). Primary cutaneous marginal zone lymphoma presents as a solitary nodule or as multiple erythematous nodules, often on the trunk or upper extremities of middle-aged women (273,274,280). It is rare in the head and neck, has an indolent behavior, and is associated with an excellent prognosis even in the event of dissemination (268,274,280).

Marginal zone lymphoma arising in the skin has histologic features similar to those described for marginal zone lymphoma arising in other sites. Primary cutaneous marginal zone lymphoma is characterized by a dermal proliferation of marginal zone (centrocyte-like) cells and/or monocytoid B cells, often with zones of plasma cells (Fig. 65). The neoplastic B cells surround reactive germinal centers, occasionally filling the interfollicular dermis (270,271,274,281). Marginal zone B cells have small, cleaved nuclei and variably abundant amphophilic cytoplasm. The foci with plasmacytic differentiation may contain plasma cells with intranuclear inclusions of immunoglobulin, termed Dutcher bodies. Marginal zone lymphomas that arise at other sites characteristically display infiltrations of glandular epithelium termed "lymphoepithelial lesions" (see Chapter 12). This finding is less commonly observed in cutaneous marginal zone lymphoma and when present is observed in the epithelium of the hair follicles. Invariably there is a reactive T-cell infiltrate admixed among the neoplastic B cells; in some cases the T cells outnumber the neoplastic B cells. These tumors share many histologic and clinical features with cutaneous lymphoid hyperplasia, a benign reactive proliferation of lymphocytes (see above). A few histologic features that support a diagnosis of lymphoma over a reactive process on routinely processed hematoxylin and eosin (H&E)-stained sections include the presence of a diffuse proliferation of marginal zone cells, reactive germinal centers, zones of plasma cells, the absence of epidermal change, and a diffuse pattern of infiltration. The density of the infiltrate, bottom-heavy or top-heavy distribution, presence of eosinophils, and a grenz zone are seen equally often in both disorders (281).

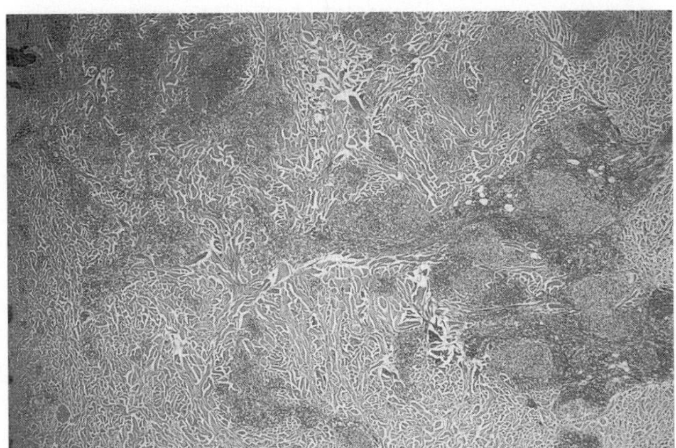

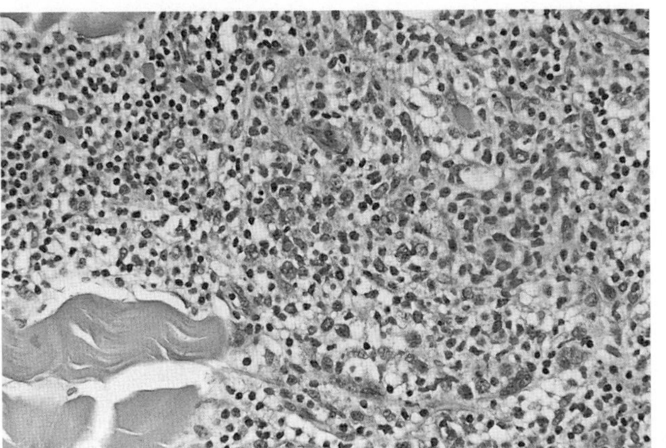

FIGURE 64. Follicle center lymphoma. **A:** Pale areas of irregularly shaped neoplastic lymphoid follicles in the superficial and deep dermis are surrounded by aggregates of small lymphocytes. **B:** Centroblasts and centrocytes dissect through the reticular dermal collagen.

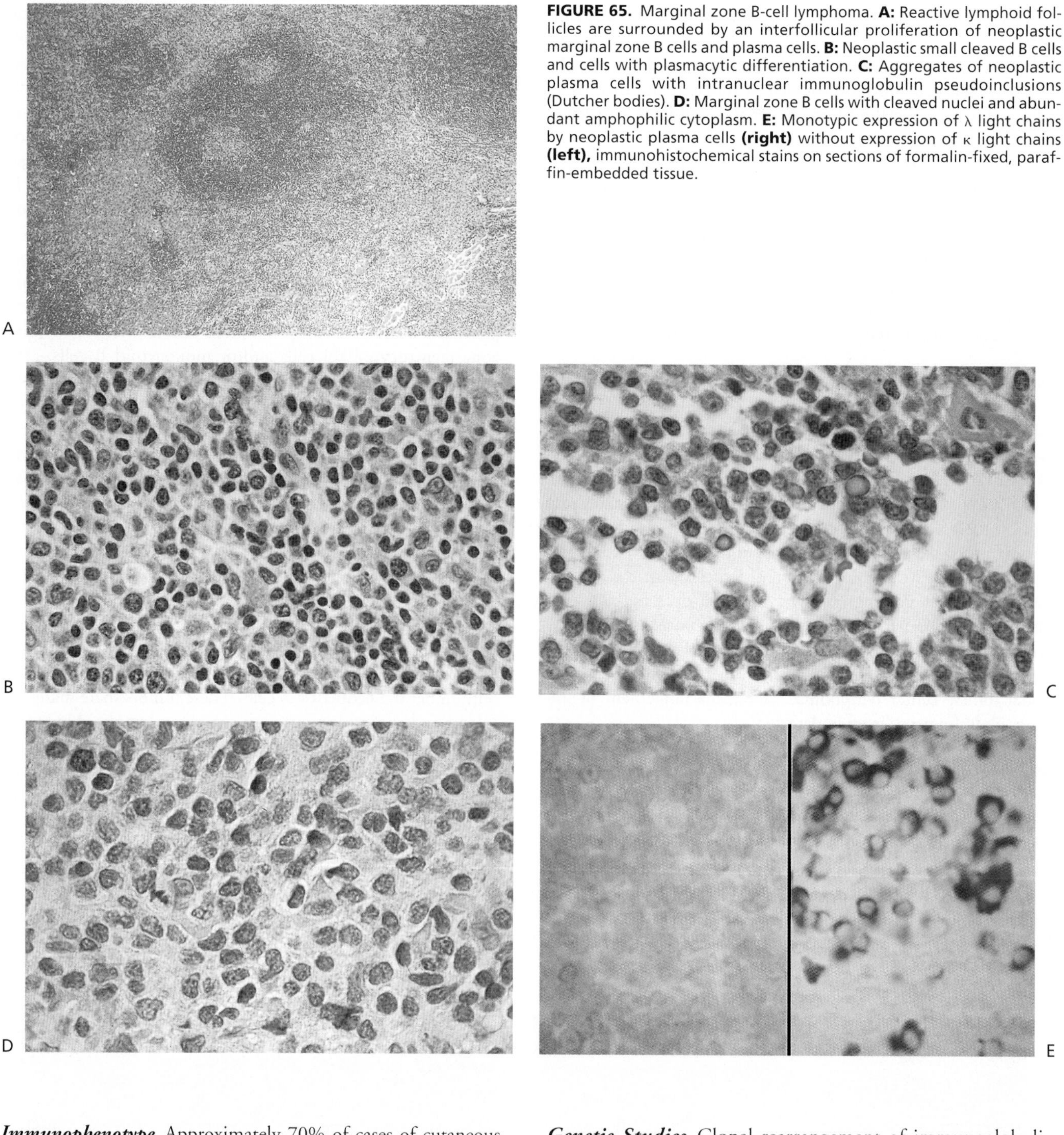

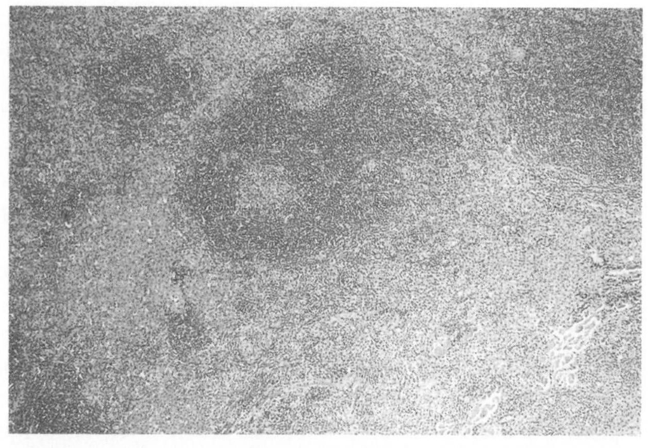

FIGURE 65. Marginal zone B-cell lymphoma. **A:** Reactive lymphoid follicles are surrounded by an interfollicular proliferation of neoplastic marginal zone B cells and plasma cells. **B:** Neoplastic small cleaved B cells and cells with plasmacytic differentiation. **C:** Aggregates of neoplastic plasma cells with intranuclear immunoglobulin pseudoinclusions (Dutcher bodies). **D:** Marginal zone B cells with cleaved nuclei and abundant amphophilic cytoplasm. **E:** Monotypic expression of λ light chains by neoplastic plasma cells **(right)** without expression of κ light chains **(left),** immunohistochemical stains on sections of formalin-fixed, paraffin-embedded tissue.

Immunophenotype Approximately 70% of cases of cutaneous marginal zone lymphoma contain neoplastic plasma cells; in these cases light-chain restriction is often identified with polyclonal antibodies against κ and λ light chains in formalin-fixed paraffin-embedded tissue (274,281). Characteristically in marginal zone lymphoma, one finds monotypic plasma cells and marginal zone cells in interfollicular regions, with polytypic follicle centers. The neoplastic marginal zone cells usually have a $CD20^+$, $CD22^+$, $CD5^-$, $CD10^-$, $CD23^-$ immunophenotype. It is important to note that the staining pattern when B- and T-cell stains are compared is deceptively benign with central zones of B cells and surrounding T cells.

Genetic Studies Clonal rearrangement of immunoglobulin heavy-chain genes has been detected using polymerase chain reaction (PCR)-based techniques in 70% of cutaneous marginal zone lymphomas (280).

Plasmacytoma (Plasma Cell Myeloma)

Cutaneous plasmacytoma usually occurs in the setting of disseminated multiple myeloma and may occur at any cutaneous site. The histologic features include a dense dermal infiltrate of light-chain–restricted plasma cells. Immature plasmablasts and mature plasma cells may be present. Mitotic activity and plasma cells with prominent eosinophilic nucleoli are atypical features

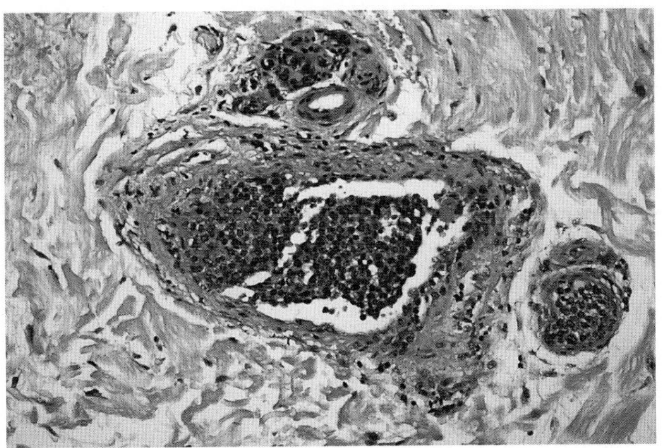

FIGURE 66. Intravascular lymphoma. Aggregates of large atypical B-cells occupy vascular lumina and focally extend into the perivascular connective tissue.

and should prompt analysis for light-chain restriction. Extramedullary plasmacytoma of skin is an unusual neoplastic proliferation of plasma cells that occurs without underlying myeloma. These tumors have been reported to progress to myeloma (282–285). Extramedullary plasmacytoma is discussed in further detail in Chapter 12.

Intravascular B-Cell Lymphoma (Angiotropic Lymphoma, Malignant Angioendotheliomatosis)

Classified in the REAL classification as diffuse large B-cell lymphoma and in the EORTC Cutaneous Lymphoma Classification as intravascular B-cell lymphoma, this tumor is characterized by an intravascular accumulation of large neoplastic B cells (Fig. 66) (286–288). These tumors most commonly appear as violaceous plaques on the trunk and lower extremities but may involve any cutaneous site including the skin of the head and neck. They may disseminate to involve extracutaneous sites. CNS involvement is not infrequently observed and is associated with a poor outcome. Patients with this disease have a poor prognosis and have been reported to have a 5-year survival less than 50%.

Immunophenotype These tumors express monotypic immunoglobulin and pan-B-cell antigens (CD19$^+$, CD20$^+$, CD22$^+$, CD79a$^+$).

NONINFECTIOUS INFLAMMATORY PROCESSES

Blistering Processes and Spongiotic Dermatitis

Disorders of the skin that cause blisters may be classified into those that are autoimmune-mediated diseases and those that are not. Most of the autoimmune-mediated blistering disorders that affect the skin of the head and neck, including pemphigoid, pemphigus, and linear IgA disease, have striking oral mucosal manifestations.

Pemphigus Vulgaris

More than half of the patients with pemphigus vulgaris present with oral lesions (289). These oral lesions are usually slowly healing painful erosions that precede the cutaneous lesions by several months. Conjunctival involvement is common, and lesions have been described in the vulvar mucosa, cervix, esophagus, and rectal mucosa. Although intact bullae are rarely seen in the mouth, cutaneous fluid-filled blisters arise on the face, trunk, groin, axillae, and sites of pressure.

Pemphigus vulgaris is characterized histologically by intraepithelial suprabasal layer acantholysis forming a blister lined along the base by a layer of keratinocytes resembling tombstones because of a lack of intercellular adhesion and retention of attachment to the epithelial basement membrane zone (Fig. 67). Acantholytic keratinocytes are observed within the suprabasal blister, as are villi of papillary dermis covered by a basal layer of keratinocytes. In addition to spongiosis (increased fluid between keratinocytes, accentuating the intercellular spinous connections), eosinophils may be present in the epithelium. These two findings together are termed "eosinophilic spongiosis." Eosinophilic spongiosis is a characteristic finding in pemphigus and is associated with an underlying superficial perivascular and interstitial mononuclear and eosinophilic infiltrate. The most

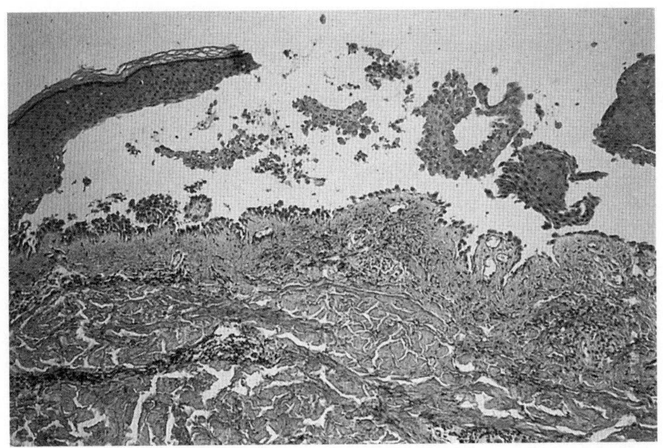

A

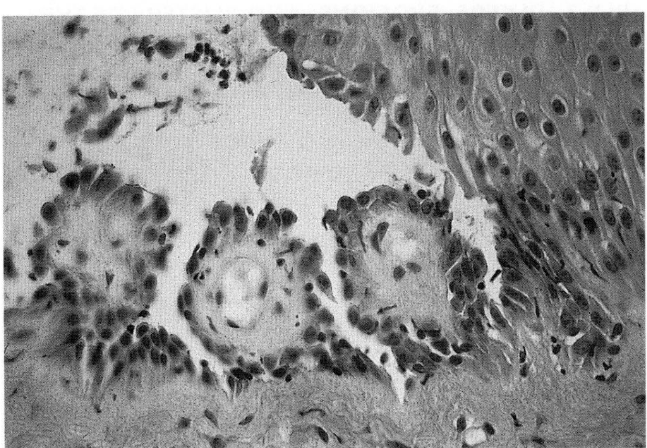

B

FIGURE 67. Pemphigus vulgaris. **A:** An intraepidermal blister contains acantholytic keratinocytes and eosinophils. **B:** Protruding upward into the blister cavity are villi of papillary dermis covered by a single layer of basal keratinocytes.

common processes that display eosinophilic spongiosis are pemphigus, pemphigoid, and hypersensitivity reactions (contact, drug, arthropod).

In pemphigus vulgaris, direct immunofluorescence shows intracellular IgG in a "chicken-wire" pattern in 80% to 90% of patients. C3 is present in almost all biopsies with acantholytic foci. Indirect immunofluorescence with the patient's serum is positive for IgG in 80% to 90% of patients with pemphigus vulgaris. The antibodies are directed against the desmosomal-associated 130-kDa desmoglein III and 80-kDa plakoglobin proteins.

The oral lesions of pemphigus may clinically resemble acute herpetic stomatitis, erythema multiforme, Behçet's disease, aphthous ulcers, and bullous lichen planus (Table 7). Although direct immunofluorescence is the most specific way of making the diagnosis of pemphigus in this setting, the histologic features may also be helpful (290). Herpetic stomatitis may show acantholysis; however, careful examination will reveal the characteristic viral cytopathic changes of herpes. The level of acantholysis in pemphigus is in the lower spinous layer of the epithelium, usually leading to a cleft just above the basal epithelial layer. In contrast, herpes shows full-thickness acantholysis with associated keratinocyte necrosis and serum-imbued parakeratotic crust. Erythema multiforme is also characterized by the presence of keratinocytic necrosis, but without acantholysis. A sparse submucosal inflammatory infiltrate and vacuolar change at the interface of the basal keratinocytes with the submucosa are also seen in erythema multiforme. In severe cases of erythema multiforme, such as Stevens-Johnson syndrome, full-thickness necrosis of the epithelium is observed. Like erythema multiforme, lichen planus shows changes at the interface of the epithelium with the submucosa. The normal basaloid appearance of the keratinocytes is often absent and replaced by more squamotized cells with abundant eosinophilic cytoplasm. When the band-like lichenoid infiltrate is particularly dense, the epidermal–submucosal junc-tion may be obscured by the infiltrate, or a subepithelial blister may appear. The presence of a granular cell layer and a lichenoid infiltrate in mucosal epithelium is strong evidence in favor of a diagnosis of lichen planus.

TABLE 7. ULCERS, EROSIONS, AND BLISTERS OF THE ORAL MUCOSA

Pemphigus
Pemphigoid
Dermatitis herpetiformis
Linear IgA disease
Lichen planus
Reiter's disease
Nutritional deficiency
Graft-versus-host disease
Herpes simplex
Erythema multiforme
Epidermolysis bullosa
Mucocele
Aphthae
Crohn's disease
Behçet's
Eosinophilic ulcer
Necrotizing sialometaplasia

Pemphigus Vegetans

In the early stages, pemphigus vegetans has a similar clinical presentation to pemphigus vulgaris. Well-developed cutaneous lesions of pemphigus vegetans have a vegetative surface studded with small pustules. Lesions have a particular predilection for the axillae and groin.

The histologic findings in pemphigus vegetans are similar to those of pemphigus vulgaris except that in the vegetans lesions there is marked epidermal hyperplasia with intraepidermal eosinophilic microabscesses (Fig. 68). These microabscesses probably correlate with the pustules observed clinically. Intraepidermal acantholysis leads to the formation of multifocal suprabasal clefts and bullae. These lesions also are associated with a dense dermal mononuclear and eosinophilic infiltrate. The immunofluorescence findings in pemphigus vegetans are similar to those found in pemphigus vulgaris.

Pemphigus Foliaceus

In pemphigus foliaceus patients present with small flaccid blisters that easily rupture to leave crusted erosions with surrounding erythema (291). Lesions usually first present on the face, scalp, chest, and back. Patients may become erythrodermic. Oral lesions are less common than in pemphigus vulgaris.

The level of acantholysis in the epidermis is more superficial in pemphigus foliaceus than in pemphigus vulgaris. There is a subcorneal intraepidermal cleft containing neutrophils and acantholytic keratinocytes with acantholysis and a superficial dermal mononuclear infiltrate with neutrophils and eosinophils. In pemphigus foliaceus, direct immunofluorescence shows intercellular deposition of IgG and C3 in 80% to 90% of biopsies. Indirect immunofluorescence is positive for IgG in 80% to 90% of patients. Antibodies are directed against the desmosomal-associated 160-kDa desmoglein I protein (292). Although occasionally the intercellular deposits are more concentrated in the superficial epidermis, often the immunofluorescent findings are indistinguishable from those observed in pemphigus vulgaris.

Paraneoplastic Pemphigus

Paraneoplastic pemphigus is an autoimmune blistering disorder that occurs in patients with hematologic neoplasms. The lymphoma invariably precedes the clinical presentation of pemphigus (293). All patients have developed both oral and cutaneous lesions (294,295), and although early diagnosis and treatment have provided some hope of controlling the disease, the development of paraneoplastic pemphigus is often associated with a fatal outcome.

The histologic findings in paraneoplastic pemphigus include a suprabasal or subepidermal cleft, acantholysis, dyskeratosis and vacuolization of basal layer keratinocytes, and exocytosis of mononuclear cells and eosinophils. Direct and indirect immunofluorescence show both intercellular and basement membrane zone deposition of IgG (Fig. 69) (296). These patients have antibodies directed against the following antigens: 250-kDa desmoplakin I; 230-kDa bullous pemphigoid Ag1; 210-kDa desmoplakin II; and 190-kDa proteins.

Bullous Pemphigoid

Bullous pemphigoid is usually a disease of the elderly; the average age of onset is 70 years. Pemphigoid commonly starts with a

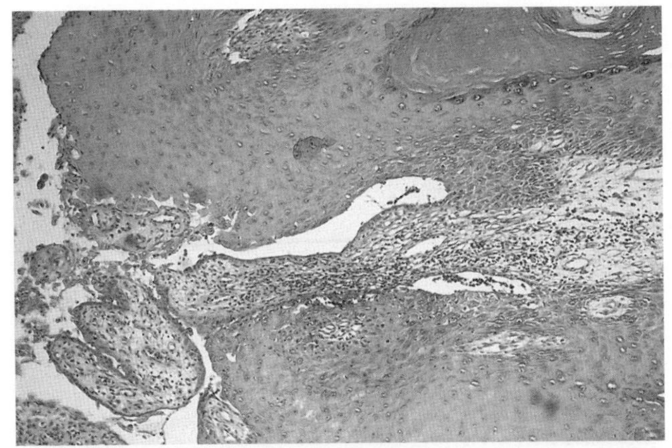

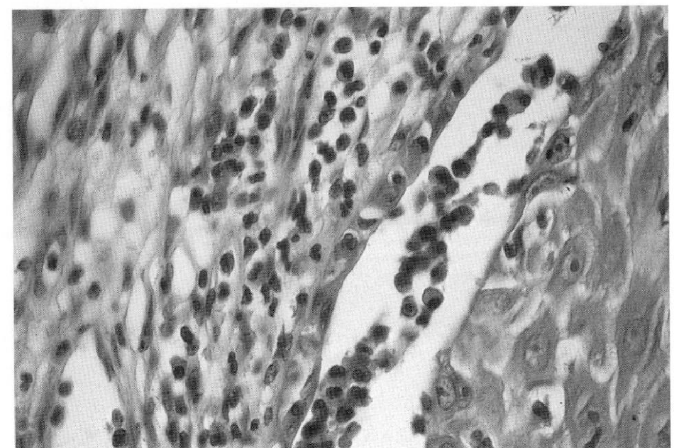

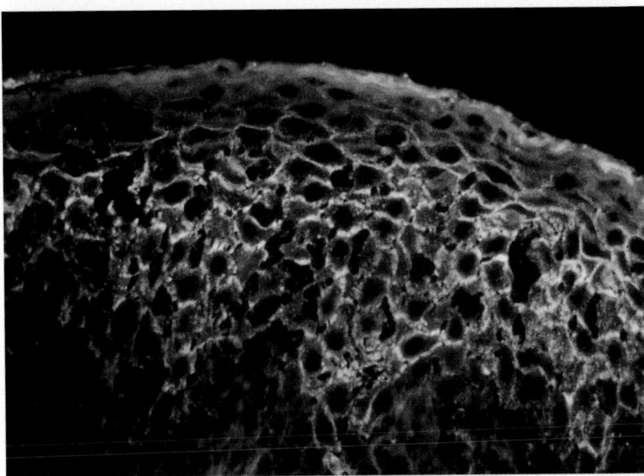

FIGURE 68. Pemphigus vegetans. **A:** Marked epidermal hyperplasia with intraepithelial eosinophilic microabscesses and a cleft above the basal layer keratinocytes. **B:** Intraepidermal suprabasal layer eosinophil microabscess. **C:** Intercellular "chicken-wire" pattern of IgG deposition observed with direct immunofluorescence.

nonspecific urticarial or eczematous rash on the upper extremities. Bullae may not develop for several months and appear mainly on the flexural aspects of extremities and on the central abdomen. These characteristically tense bullae are not easily ruptured but will extend laterally with applied pressure (Nikolsky's sign) and may reach diameters of 10 cm. Mucosal lesions rarely occur and are usually confined to the mouth.

Histologically, the early preeruptive stage of bullous pemphigoid shows basal layer vacuolization with the formation of small subepidermal clefts (Fig. 70). The site of the primary cleft is subepidermal, as opposed to the suprabasilar location of the clefts in the pemphigus group of lesions. Eosinophils may be observed along the dermal–epidermal junction with an underlying sparse superficial dermal mononuclear cell and eosinophilic infiltrate. Well-developed lesions of bullous pemphigoid are characterized by an eosinophil-containing subepidermal blister with eosinophilic spongiosis in the surrounding epidermis. Not uncommonly, the basal epidermis will regenerate, leading to a suprabasal location of the intraepidermal cleavage. There is an underlying superficial dermal mononuclear cell infiltrate with numerous eosinophils.

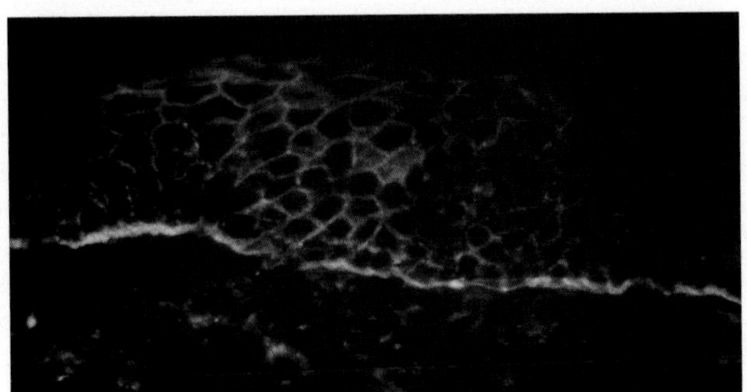

FIGURE 69. Paraneoplastic pemphigus. Direct immunofluorescence reveals both intercellular and basement membrane zone deposits of IgG.

Direct immunofluorescence staining reveals linear basement membrane zone deposition of C3 in more than 95% of patients and IgG in 90%. Indirect immunofluorescence staining of patients' serum against monkey or guinea pig esophagus or normal human skin reveals basement membrane zone deposition of IgG in 70% of patients with bullous pemphigoid. NaCl-split normal skin substrate may be useful in distinguishing bullous pemphigoid from epidermolysis bullosa acquisita. This technique differentiates between autoimmune disorders with immunoreactants directed above and below the lamina lucida of the basement membrane zone. The substrate is a frozen section of normal human skin previously split at the dermal–epidermal junction by incubation with 1 M NaCl (297). Indirect immunofluorescence staining is performed using the patient's serum. In bullous pemphigoid, reactants are deposited above the split, whereas in epidermolysis bullosa acquisita, reactants are deposited below the split.

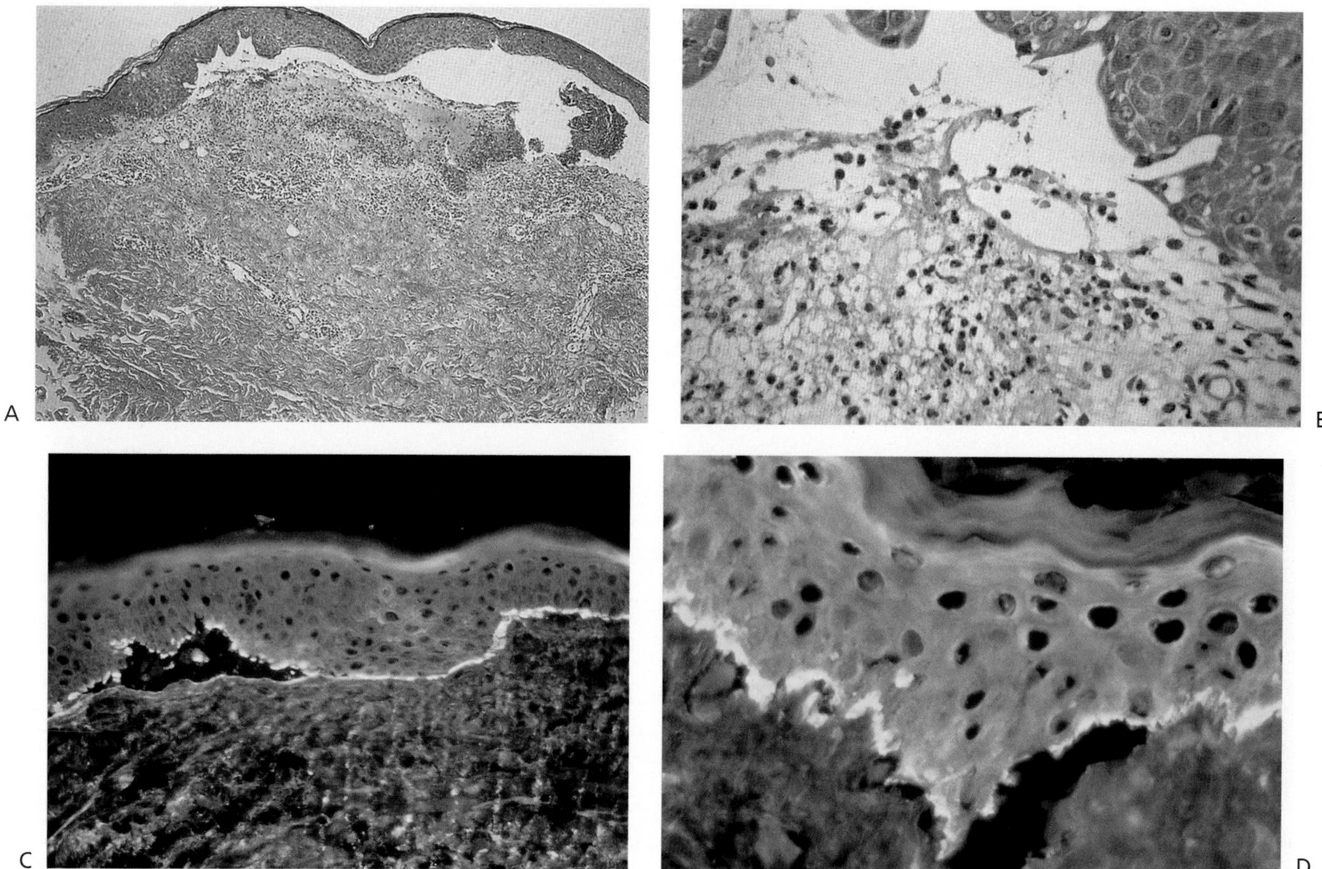

FIGURE 70. Bullous pemphigoid. **A:** Subepidermal blister with a superficial perivascular inflammatory infiltrate. **B:** Subepidermal blister with necrotic debris, fibrin deposition, and eosinophils. **C:** Direct immunofluorescence reveals linear deposition of IgG along the basement membrane zone. **D:** Indirect immunofluorescence of patient serum against NaCl split skin substrate reveals immunoreactants deposited along the basement membrane zone and along the roof of the subepidermal blister.

Cicatricial Pemphigoid

Cicatricial pemphigoid shares many histologic features with bullous pemphigoid and has a tendency to involve mucosal surfaces (298). Usually arising in elderly men, cicatricial pemphigoid has a chronic course, often with extensive scarring. Oral and ocular lesions occur in most patients with cicatricial pemphigoid, with other involved sites including the skin, larynx, trachea, esophagus, nasopharynx, and genital mucosa. Scarring is most commonly observed with conjunctival lesions and leads to blindness in up to 25% of patients. There are a few clinical variants of cicatricial pemphigoid; most clearly defined is the Brunsting-Perry variant in which patients develop blisters on the skin of the head and neck that heal as atrophic scars; no mucosal involvement is present (299,300).

The histologic findings of cicatricial pemphigoid include subepithelial cleavage with a somewhat lichenoid superficial mononuclear cell infiltrate with neutrophils and occasional eosinophils (Fig. 71). With advanced lesions epidermal atrophy and superficial dermal fibrosis are observed.

Direct immunofluorescence staining shows linear basement membrane zone deposition of IgG and C3 in 80% of patients (301,302). In contrast to bullous pemphigoid, in which indirect immunofluorescence staining (patient's serum) is positive in most patients, indirect immunofluorescence is positive in only 10% to 25% of patients with cicatricial pemphigoid.

Dermatitis Herpetiformis

Dermatitis herpetiformis is an intensely pruritic eruption that is distributed on the extensor surfaces of the extremities, particularly the knees and elbows. Lesions also frequently appear on the buttocks, axillae, trunk, face, and scalp. Oral lesions are present in up to 20% of patients and are usually asymptomatic. Rare reports of laryngeal involvement exist (303). Most patients have an associated gluten-sensitive enteropathy or celiac disease (304,305).

The characteristic histologic findings in dermatitis herpetiformis include vacuolar alteration of basal layer keratinocytes with fibrinoid degeneration of collagen and aggregates of neutrophils at the tips of the dermal papillae (Fig. 72). Multifocal small subepidermal clefts form and may coalesce to form bullae.

Direct immunofluorescence in dermatitis herpetiformis shows granular deposits of IgA in the dermal papillae in all patients (Fig. 72). A similar pattern of C3 deposition is observed in 70% of patients. Indirect immunofluorescence is negative using standard techniques; however, circulating antigluten antibodies and antireticulin antibodies may be detected in more than half of the patients with dermatitis herpetiformis.

Linear IgA Bullous Dermatosis

Linear IgA disease shares many features with dermatitis herpetiformis. Notably, there is a higher incidence of mucosal and con-

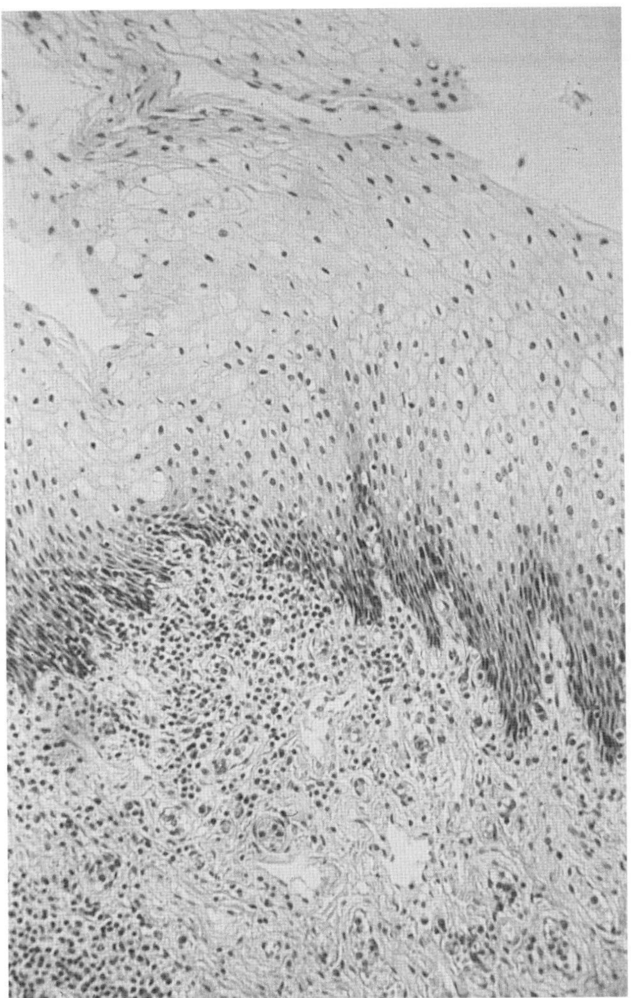

FIGURE 71. Cicatricial pemphigoid. Mucosal epithelium with a submucosal inflammatory infiltrate containing numerous eosinophils.

junctival involvement by linear IgA disease and less of an association with gluten-sensitive enteropathy. Also, by definition, direct immunofluorescence shows a linear deposition of IgA along the basement membrane zone in contrast to the scattered deposits observed in dermatitis herpetiformis. Indirect immunofluorescence is positive in 10% to 25% of cases. Antibodies are directed against 285-kDa and 97-kDa proteins.

Eosinophilic Ulcer

Although eosinophilic ulcer of the tongue is neither spongiotic nor a blistering process, it enters into both the clinical and histologic differential diagnosis of most of the processes discussed in this section. This benign self-limiting ulcer often affects the tongue (Table 7). It is thought possibly to be trauma related. Characteristically, the histologic findings include epithelial ulceration with acute and chronic inflammation, granulation tissue, and numerous eosinophils (306,307). Similar changes may be observed in eroded lesions of pemphigus, pemphigoid, and hypersensitivity reactions. No specific immunoreactants are detected with direct immunofluorescence. Direct immunofluorescence testing is useful in differentiating this lesion from pemphigoid and pemphigus.

Spongiotic Dermatitis, Acute and Subacute (Allergic Contact, Photoallergic)

Spongiosis is defined as an increase in the intercellular fluid in the epidermis. When spongiosis is mild, the "spinous" intercellular junctions are readily apparent; this is termed subacute spongiotic dermatitis. Examples of subacute spongiotic dermatitis include nummular eczema and atopic dermatitis (Fig. 73). In acute spongiotic dermatitis, such as poison ivy contact dermatitis, there is marked spongiosis with formation of intraepidermal vesicles.

The most common forms of spongiotic dermatitis to affect the skin of the face are seborrheic dermatitis and allergic contact dermatitis. Seborrheic dermatitis occurs in adults and presents as erythematous plaques and follicular papules with a characteristic greasy scale. The ears, scalp and face are preferred sites. In severe cases, lesions have a thick adherent greasy scale and may be associated with otitis externa or alopecia. Severe seborrheic dermatitis is one of the most common cutaneous manifestations of AIDS.

Histologically, seborrheic dermatitis is manifested by a mild or marked spongiosis, scale crust, perifollicular hyperkeratosis and parakeratosis, neutrophilic exocytosis, dermal edema, and a mild superficial perivascular mononuclear infiltrate with scat-

A

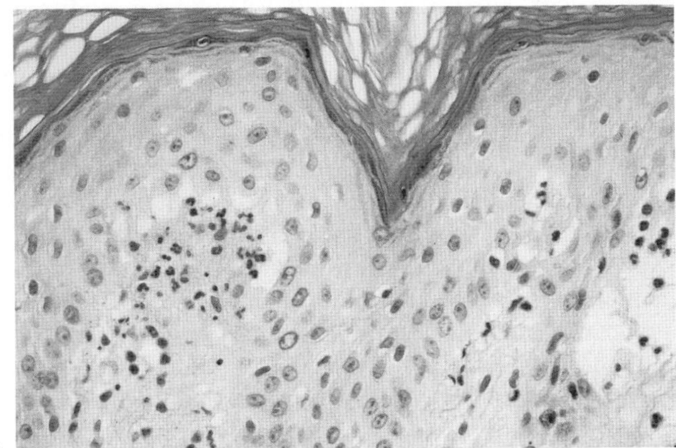

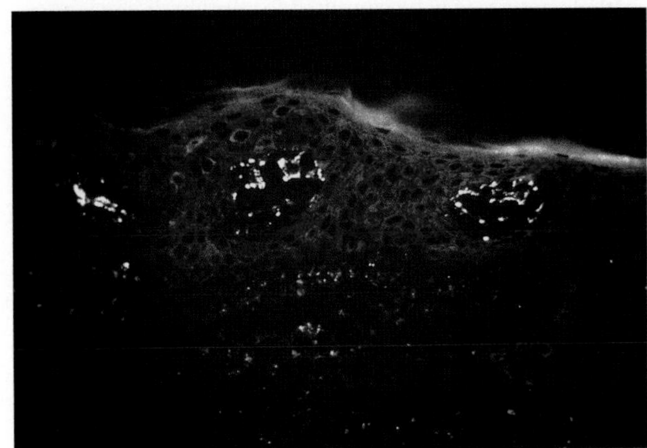

B

FIGURE 72. Dermatitis herpetiformis. **A:** Subepithelial neutrophilic microabscesses at the tips of the dermal papillae. **B:** Multifocal granular subepidermal deposition of IgA with direct immunofluorescence staining.

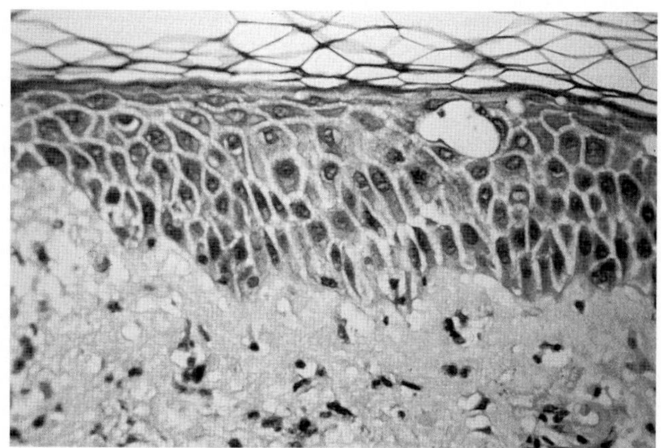

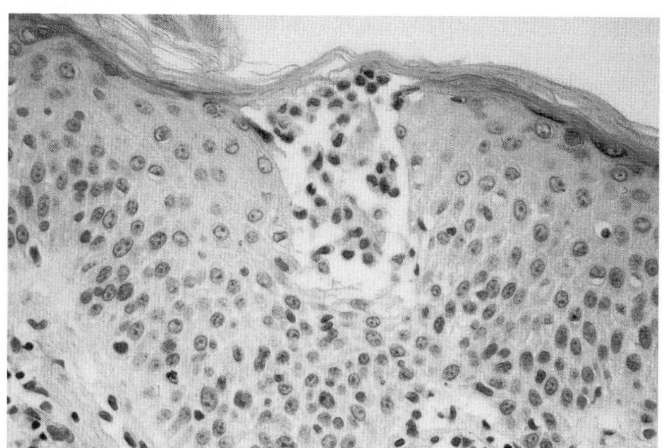

FIGURE 73. Acute spongiotic dermatitis. **A:** Prominent edema between keratinocytes (spongiosis) accentuates the intercellular bridges and focally leads to spongiotic microvesicles. **B:** Flask-shaped intraepidermal aggregates of Langerhans' cells are characteristic of contact hypersensitivity reactions.

tered histiocytes and neutrophils. As is characteristic of spongiotic dermatoses, in the acute stage there is prominent spongiosis; in chronic lesions there is a psoriasiform epidermal hyperplasia (see below) with slight spongiosis.

The differential diagnosis of chronic seborrheic dermatitis often includes psoriasis. The follicular accentuation of the hyperkeratotic scale and the presence of a serum- and neutrophil-imbued scale crust favor a diagnosis of seborrheic dermatitis. In addition to seborrheic dermatitis and psoriasis, superficial fungal infections are in the differential when neutrophilic exocytosis and parakeratosis are observed. The differential diagnosis of acute and subacute seborrheic dermatitis also includes hypersensitivity reactions. The presence of intraepidermal Langerhans' cell microabscesses is a characteristic finding in contact dermatitis. The composition of the dermal inflammatory infiltrate is also important. A hypersensitivity reaction to an ingested compound or contactant should be considered when the biopsy shows spongiotic dermatitis and eosinophils in the dermal inflammatory infiltrate. Eosinophilic spongiosis is the presence of eosinophils within a spongiotic epidermis. The differential diagnosis of eosinophilic spongiosis includes contact dermatitis, drug eruption, bite reaction, pemphigus, incontinentia pigmenti, and the early eczematous phase of bullous pemphigoid. Standard dermatopathology texts may be consulted for further discussion.

Papulosquamous Disorders

The papulosquamous disorders are inflammatory processes that involve the epidermis. In most cases of papulosquamous dermatitis the histologic findings are either predominantly psoriasiform or lichenoid. Psoriasiform dermatitis is characterized by a regular acanthosis of the epidermis; the term regular is used to indicate that a relatively straight line may be drawn along the base of the elongated and club-shaped epidermal rete. This regular pattern of hyperplasia is in contrast to the irregular epidermal hyperplasia that is observed in lichen planus. Parakeratosis is also a common finding in psoriasiform dermatitis. On the other hand, parakeratosis is rarely observed in lichenoid dermatitis, but rather, lichenoid dermatitis is characterized by a prominent epidermal granular cell layer. In addition to the hypergranulosis and irregular "sawtoothed" epithelial hyperplasia, a lichenoid inflammatory infiltrate is present. The lichenoid inflammatory pattern may be that of a dense lymphocytic inflammatory infiltrate along the dermal–epidermal junction, obscuring the basal layer keratinocytes, or it may occur as a linear band of lymphoid cells in the superficial dermis or submucosa. Normally a granular cell layer is not present in mucosal epithelium. The presence of basophilic keratohyaline granules in the superficial keratinocytes of mucosal epithelium is strong evidence in favor of a lichenoid process.

Psoriasiform Dermatitis

Psoriasis Vulgaris

The most common inflammatory papulosquamous disorder to involve the skin of the head and neck is psoriasis. Psoriasis is a chronic epidermal proliferative disease that characteristically presents as well-demarcated erythematous scaly plaques of the scalp and extensor surfaces of the extremities. In contrast to seborrheic dermatitis, which also is a scaly process involving the scalp, the plaques of psoriasis are more well demarcated and less commonly affect the eyelids, eyebrows, and face. There are a variety of therapies for psoriasis; one of the most effective is oral psoralen combined with ultraviolet light (PUVA). Recent studies have demonstrated an increased long-term risk of melanoma and nonmelanoma skin cancer in psoriasis patients treated with PUVA (308–310).

The histologic findings of psoriasis vulgaris vary significantly with the stage of the lesion. Characteristic features of early lesions include focal parakeratosis and underlying neutrophilic exocytosis into a slightly spongiotic epidermis, papillary dermal vascular ectasia and edema, and a sparse superficial perivascular lymphoid infiltrate (Fig. 74). The presence of neutrophils in the parakeratotic scale is a very characteristic finding in psoriasis and its variants. Later findings include a regular acanthosis of the epidermis, termed psoriasiform epidermal hyperplasia; the term "regular" is used to indicate that a relatively straight line may be drawn along the base of the club-shaped epidermal rete, in contrast to the irregular epidermal hyperplasia that is observed in lichen planus.

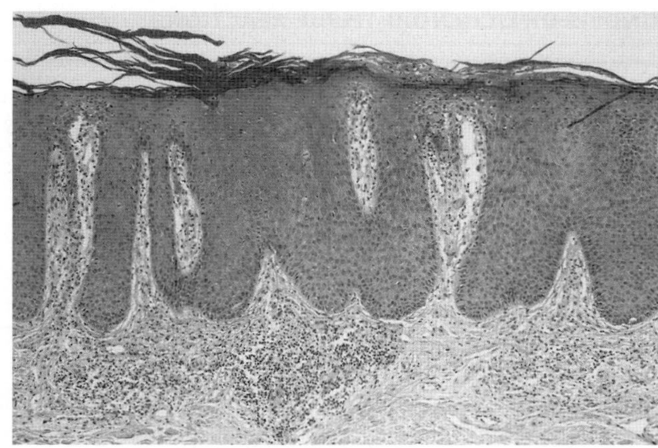

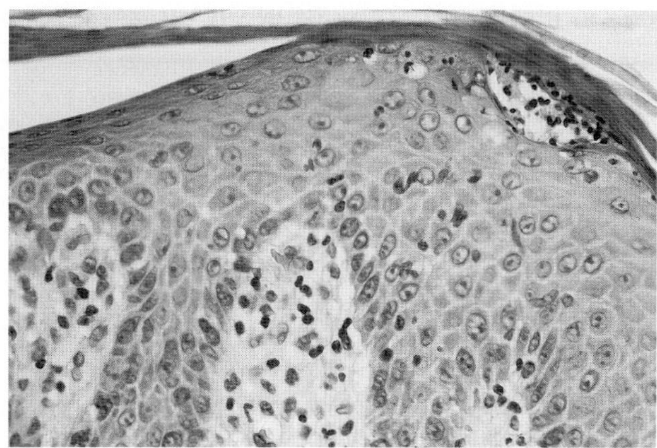

FIGURE 74. Psoriasis vulgaris. **A:** Parakeratosis, erythrocyte extravasation, and epidermal hyperplasia with a flat base, termed "regular" epidermal hyperplasia. **B:** Intracorneal neutrophilic microabscesses (Monro).

Although generally hyperplastic, the epidermis in psoriasis is attenuated or thinned overlying the papillary dermal pegs. There is loss of the epidermal granular cell layer and increased epidermal mitotic activity. The papillary dermal pegs are edematous and contain numerous ectatic vessels with erythrocyte extravasation and exocytosis of neutrophils through the overlying epidermis, hence the term "squirting papillae." Characteristic findings in psoriasis are intracorneal aggregates of neutrophils termed Munro microabscesses and epidermal spongiosis with neutrophils termed spongiform pustules of Kogoj. The dermis contains a superficial perivascular mononuclear cell infiltrate, usually devoid of eosinophils and neutrophils. In HIV-infected patients the infiltrate may also contain plasma cells (311,312). Treatment with high dose topical steroids may lead to reappearance of the granular cell layer.

Pustular Psoriasis (Acrodermatitis Continua, Impetigo Herpetiformis, Generalized Pustular Psoriasis of von Zumbusch)

A rare acute form of psoriasis, pustular psoriasis, is associated with a generalized eruption of sterile pustules often accompanied by fever, malaise, arthralgia, geographic tongue and lingual fissures. Precipitating factors include steroid withdrawal, stress, UV light exposure, extracutaneous malignancy, infection and drug reactions. The histologic features are those of acute psoriasis with numerous intraepidermal spongiform pustules of Kogoj and intracorneal Munro microabscesses. There is variable epidermal hyperplasia and a sparse superficial mononuclear cell infiltrate with scattered neutrophils. These changes are similar to those observed in geographic tongue and Reiter's disease.

Reiter's Disease

Reiter's disease occurs in young men as a triad of urethritis, arthritis, and conjunctivitis (313). By definition the arthritis is nonsuppurative and of at least 1 month's duration. One in three patients with reactive arthritis and approximately 1% with nongonococcal urethritis will develop Reiter's disease (314). There is also a close association between Reiter's disease and the HLA-B27 antigen and between Reiter's disease and AIDS (315,316).

The histologic features are identical to those of acute psoriasis. In particular, numerous intraepidermal spongiform pustules of Kogoj and intracorneal Munro microabscesses are present (Fig. 75). There is variable epidermal hyperplasia and a sparse superficial mononuclear cell infiltrate with scattered neutrophils. Leukocytoclastic vasculitis is also observed in some cases of Reiter's disease (317).

Prurigo Nodularis (Nodular Lichenification, Picker's Nodule)

Prurigo nodularis is a nodular, reactive, hyperkeratotic, epidermal hyperplasia that results from extensive scratching, picking, or rubbing. It may be considered to be an end-stage lesion of lichen simplex chronicus. Usually occurring in adults, the lesions are firm dermal nodules 1 to 2 cm in diameter, often with overlying verrucous hyperkeratosis and hyperpigmentation. Although usually pruritic, the lesions may ultimately become quite tender.

Histologically there is prominent epidermal hyperplasia that may be so extensive as to mimic well-differentiated squamous cell carcinoma, so-called pseudocarcinomatous hyperplasia.

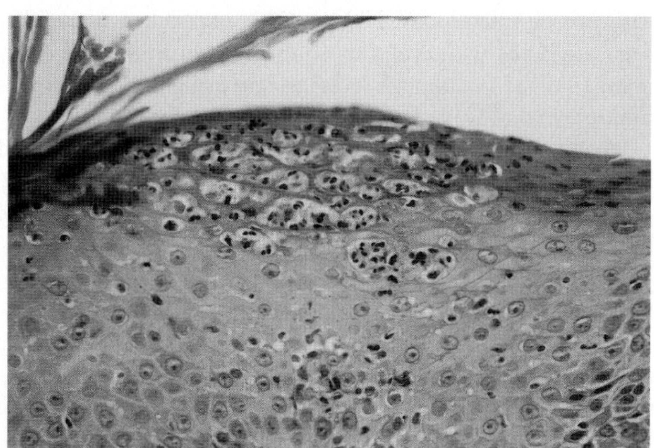

FIGURE 75. Reiter's disease. Loss of the granular cell layer of keratinocytes with intraepidermal neutrophilic microabscesses (Kogoj).

TABLE 8. HISTOLOGIC FINDINGS IN THE DIFFERENTIAL DIAGNOSIS OF LICHENOID TISSUE REACTIONS

Diagnosis	Irregular Epidermal Hyperplasia	Thickened Granular Cell Layer	Pigment Incontinence	Civatte Bodies, Colloid Bodies	Vacuolar Interface Change	Satellite-Cell Necrosis	Follicular Plugging
Lichen planus	+	+	+	+	−	−	−
Fixed drug eruption	−	−	+	−/+	+	+	−
Erythema multiforme	−	−	−/+	−	+	+	−
Lupus erythematosus	−	−	−/+	−/+	+	−	+
Paraneoplastic pemphigus	−/+	−	−/+	+	+	+	−
Lichenoid drug eruption	+	+	+	+	+	+	−

Other characteristic findings include orthohyperkeratosis, focal parakeratosis, dermal fibrosis with vertically oriented, thickened, brightly eosinophilic collagen bundles, occasional multinucleate stellate fibroblasts, variable hypertrophy of dermal nerves, and a mild lymphoid infiltrate with scattered histiocytes, eosinophils, plasma cells, and increased numbers of mast cells.

Lichenoid Processes

Table 8 summarizes some of the properties of these lesions.

Lichen Planus

Lichen planus presents as flat-topped, polygonal, violaceous shiny papules ranging from barely visible to a centimeter in diameter. Wickham's striae are characteristic lacey white lines observed in oral mucosal lesions and moistened cutaneous lesions in patients with lichen planus (318). Cutaneous lesions may appear in a linear array along scars or scratches (Koebner's phenomenon). Lichen planopilaris may involve the scalp, presenting as perifollicular spines and leading to alopecia. Lesions of the lower extremities, lower back, and wrists are most common; however, lichen planus can affect any cutaneous site. Mucosal lesions are common in patients with cutaneous lichen planus and may also be observed in the absence of cutaneous disease. The buccal mucosa is most commonly involved; however, lichen planus of the larynx and tympanic membrane have also been described. On the tongue, lichen planus appears as a slightly depressed white plaque (Table 9). Lingual involvement has been associated with candidiasis and diabetes. Oral lichen planus may form bullae and ulcerate, leading to a burning pain, particularly with hot or spicy foods. Hypertrophic oral lichen planus has been associated with evolution to invasive squamous cell carcinoma (319–321), although its being a premalignant condition is somewhat controversial.

Histologically, lichen planus is the prototype of a lichenoid tissue reaction. A lichenoid tissue reaction is characterized by an inflammatory infiltrate involving the basal keratinocytes of the epidermis, leading to keratinocyte necrosis and pigment deposition in the superficial dermis (Fig. 76). Remnants of apoptotic keratinocytes form eosinophilic Civatte bodies in the epidermis. When extruded into the papillary dermis, these tonofilament-rich aggregates of cellular material trap immunoglobulins and form eosinophilic colloid bodies that are PAS positive and resistant to digestion with diastase. Other histologic findings characteristic of lichen planus include an irregular epidermal hyperplasia in which the epidermal rete extend into the papillary dermis with jagged points, termed "saw-toothed" because of a similarity to the teeth of a serrated-edged saw. Orthohyperkeratosis and hypergranulosis are present. The basal layer keratinocytes have a squamotized appearance, resembling the cells of the more superficial layers of the epidermis. Scattered basal layer keratinocyte necrosis with Civatte bodies and colloid bodies are often present. A lichenoid or band-like lymphoid infiltrate may obscure the junction of the epidermis and dermis, and pigment-laden macrophages are often observed in the underlying dermis. In other foci, dissolution of the epidermal dermal junction may lead to the formation of subepidermal clefts known as Max-Joseph spaces. This subepidermal cleavage is extensive in bullous lichen planus and can lead to ulceration. Erosive lichen planus (lichen planus

TABLE 9. PIGMENTED, ERYTHEMATOUS, AND WHITE (LEUKOPLAKIC) LESIONS OF THE ORAL MUCOSA

Pigmented lesions of the oral mucosa
- Amalgam tattoo
- Fixed drug reaction
- Addison's disease
- Drug-induced (amiodarone, minocine)
- Kaposi's sarcoma
- Labial melanotic macule
- Melanoma

Erythematous lesions of the oral mucosa
- Herpes simplex stomatitis
- Candidiasis
- Lupus erythematosus
- Lichen planus
- Pemphigoid
- Pemphigus
- Allergic
- Hemangioma
- Kaposi's sarcoma
- Carcinoma, SIN (squamous intraepithelial neoplasia)
- Wegener's granulomatosis

White lesions of the oral mucosa (leukoplakia)
- Smokers hyperkeratosis
- Lip chewing
- Hairy leukoplakia
- Candidiasis
- Lichen planus
- Lupus erythematosus
- Graft-versus-host disease
- Syphilis
- White sponge nevus
- Geographic tongue
- Carcinoma
- Fordyce lesions (oral mucosal sebaceous glands)

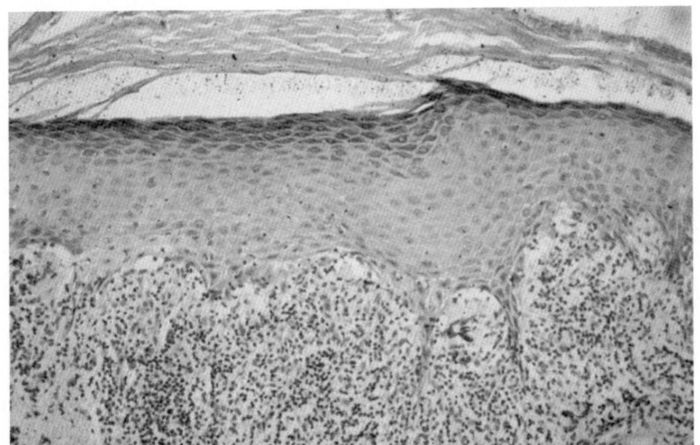

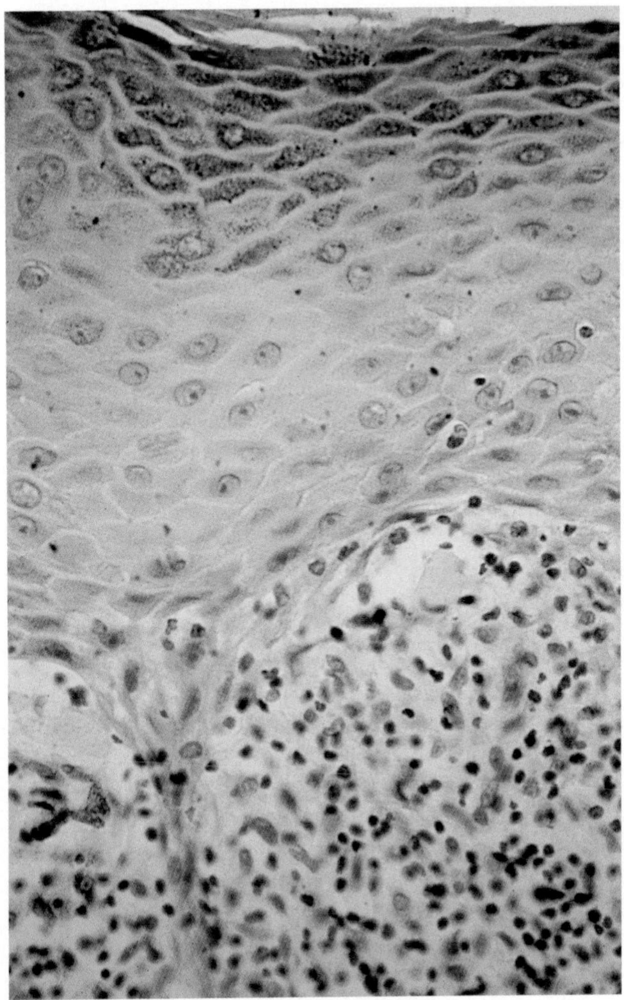

FIGURE 76. Lichen planus. **A:** Irregular sawtooth-like epidermal hyperplasia with a dense superficial dermal lymphoid infiltrate. **B:** Squamotization of basal layer keratinocytes with superficial dermal homogeneous eosinophilic globules (Civatte bodies) and pigment-laden macrophages.

with ulceration) of the oral mucosa and lower extremities has been associated with thymoma, hepatitis C, Castleman's tumor, and a variety of pharmaceutical agents (322–329). Lesions resembling erosive lichen planus have also been observed in paraneoplastic pemphigus associated with Castleman's tumor (330).

Erythema Dyschromicum Perstans (Ashy Dermatosis)

First described in South America, ashy dermatosis most commonly is seen in Hispanic patients. Macular ashy blue-gray pigmented lesions appear on the sun-exposed areas of the face, trunk, and extremities. They vary in size and appear in a background of hypomelanosis or hypermelanosis. This disorder is asymptomatic and persistent. Some have likened it to postinflammatory hyperpigmentation or lichen planus (331).

The histologic features of ashy dermatosis are similar to those of postinflammatory hyperpigmentation and characteristically show vacuolization of basal layer keratinocytes, with papillary dermal pigment-laden macrophages and a sparse superficial perivascular mononuclear infiltrate (Fig. 77). Occasionally, exo-

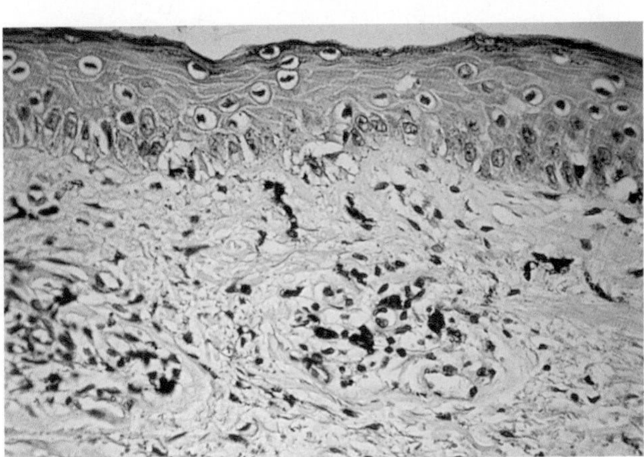

FIGURE 77. Erythema dyschromicum perstans. Vacuolar change of the basal keratinocytes with numerous papillary dermal pigment-laden macrophages.

cytosis of inflammatory cells and colloid bodies are present. In very late lesions, papillary dermal melanophages may be the only histologic abnormality.

Acute Graft-versus-Host Disease

The histologic features of acute graft-versus-host disease in bone marrow transplant or blood transfusion recipients may be subtle and include vacuolar alteration of the basal layer keratinocytes, dyskeratotic keratinocytes surrounded by lymphocytes, so-called "satellite cell necrosis," and dyskeratosis of the hair follicle epithelium. There is usually a sparse superficial perivascular mononuclear infiltrate with prominent exocytosis (migration of inflammatory cells through the epidermis) and a perieccrine and perineural mononuclear infiltrate (Fig. 78). The maturation disarray of the epithelium often observed in biopsies from patients with graft-versus-host disease is believed to result from the effect of chemotherapeutic agents.

Erythema Multiforme

Erythema multiforme is an immunologically mediated reaction pattern to many different stimuli. A variety of agents are known to precipitate attacks, including pharmaceuticals and infectious organisms. The cutaneous lesions begin as erythematous macules that increase in size to form the characteristic targetoid erythematous lesions with purpuric centers. The lesions appear in crops for a few days and then fade in a few weeks, often with residual postinflammatory hyperpigmentation. Lesions often present on the distal extremities and less commonly involve the face, neck and trunk. Occasionally, bullae and erosions may arise on the buccal mucosa (Table 7). In the Stevens-Johnson variant of erythema multiforme, patients have prominent mucosal erosions and hemorrhagic crusted lesions. The histologic changes are similar to those of erythema multiforme.

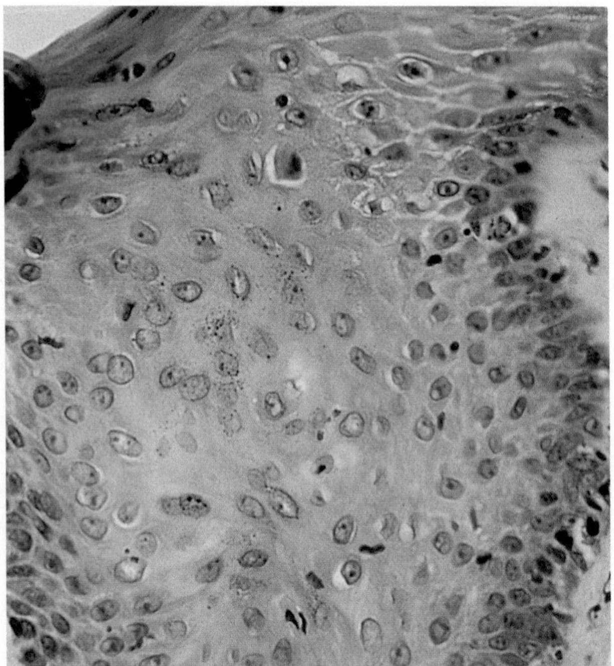

FIGURE 78. Acute graft-versus-host disease. Dyskeratosis of the hair follicle epithelium with keratinocytic maturation disarray.

The histologic features of erythema multiforme include keratinocyte dyskeratosis with satellite-cell necrosis, zones of epidermal necrosis, basal layer keratinocyte vacuolization, and, occasionally, bulla formation (Fig. 79). There is an interface dermatitis of mononuclear cells, often with colloid bodies (Civatte bodies) present in the papillary dermis as a result of keratinocytic damage. Also present are prominent papillary dermal edema and a perivascular mononuclear infiltrate, occasionally with eosinophils (particularly in those cases that are drug induced). "Satellite-cell necrosis" is the apposition of lymphocytes to necrotic keratinocytes and colloid bodies that is characteristic of erythema multiforme but may also be observed in other processes, including fixed-drug eruptions and graft-versus-host disease.

Toxic Epidermal Necrolysis

In toxic epidermal necrolysis, a variant of erythema multiforme, there is full-thickness necrosis of the epidermis, characterized clinically by sloughing of the epidermis in large sheets. In addition to full-thickness epidermal necrosis, full-thickness necrosis of follicular epithelium, satellite-cell necrosis (lymphocytes surrounding necrotic keratinocytes), and a sparse superficial perivascular mononuclear infiltrate are characteristically observed in toxic epidermal necrolysis (Fig. 80).

Vasculitis

Although most vasculitides are not localized to the skin of the head and neck, two forms of localized vasculitis involve the vessels of the face and temple, granuloma faciale and temporal arteritis. In addition, Behçet's disease may present with oral ulcerative lesions in the absence of documented vasculitis elsewhere (Table 7).

Granuloma Faciale

Granuloma faciale is a localized leukocytoclastic vasculitis that presents as brown or purple sharply circumscribed plaques or nodules on the nose, forehead, or cheeks. Lesions may be solitary or multiple, are asymptomatic, and have no associations with systemic disease or predisposition for systemic vasculitis. Histologically, granuloma faciale is a leukocytoclastic vasculitis with eosinophils (332–334). There is a dense polymorphous infiltrate composed of lymphocytes, histiocytes, neutrophils, eosinophils, plasma cells, and mast cells. Characteristically a neutrophilic infiltrate with nuclear dust (leukocytoclasia), fibrinoid necrosis of vessel walls in the superficial venular plexus, and a prominence of interstitial neutrophils, eosinophils, and histiocytes are present. A grenz zone of uninvolved papillary dermis separates the dermis from the epidermis, and erythrocyte extravasation with hemosiderin deposition is often observed.

The differential diagnosis of leukocytoclastic vasculitis in the skin is broad and includes mixed cryoglobulinemia, Henoch-Schönlein purpura, erythema elevatum diutinum, urticarial vasculitis, rheumatoid vasculitis, septic vasculitis, and drug-induced vasculitis. Nevertheless, the clinical presentation of granuloma

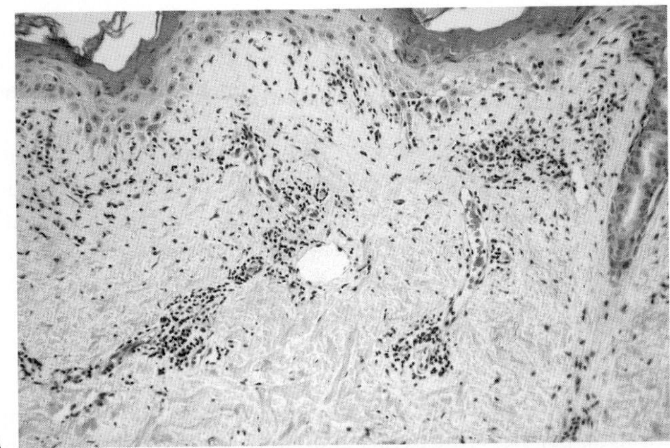

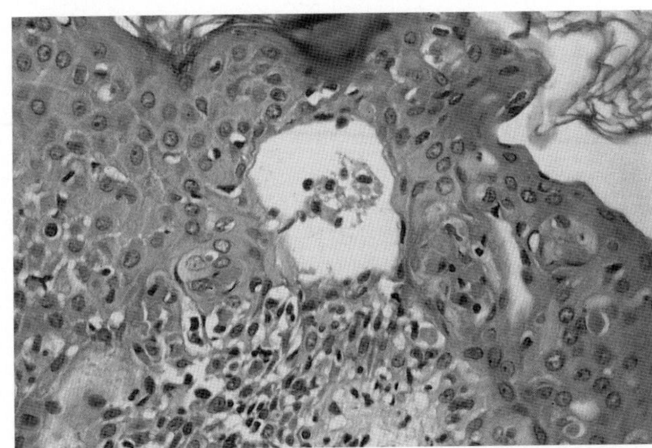

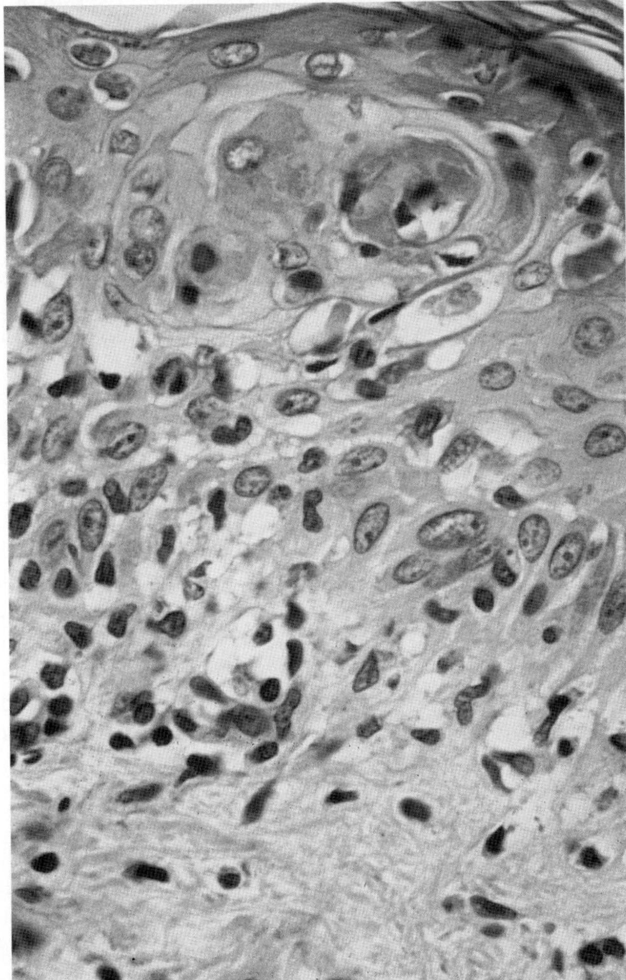

FIGURE 79. Erythema multiforme. **A:** Epidermal dyskeratosis with vacuolar change of the basal keratinocytes and inflammatory cells at the interface of the epidermis and dermis (vacuolar interface dermatitis) and a superficial perivascular inflammatory infiltrate. **B:** Dyskeratotic epidermal keratinocytes surrounded by lymphocytes (satellite cell necrosis). **C:** Satellite cell necrosis and vacuolar interface dermatitis.

faciale as soft well-demarcated plaques localized to the face is distinctive and allows for differentiation from these other forms of vasculitis.

Temporal Arteritis (Giant-Cell Arteritis)

The presence of tender nodules over the temporal or facial arteries with severe headache is the classical clinical presentation of temporal arteritis. Unilateral loss of vision may occur as a result of involvement of the ophthalmic artery or the central retinal artery.

Temporal arteritis is a vasculitis of medium-sized elastic arteries that most commonly involves the temporal artery, ophthalmic artery, retinal artery or branches of the carotid arteries (335,336). Characteristically the involved artery has skip lesions; thorough sectioning through the biopsied segment of vessel is often needed

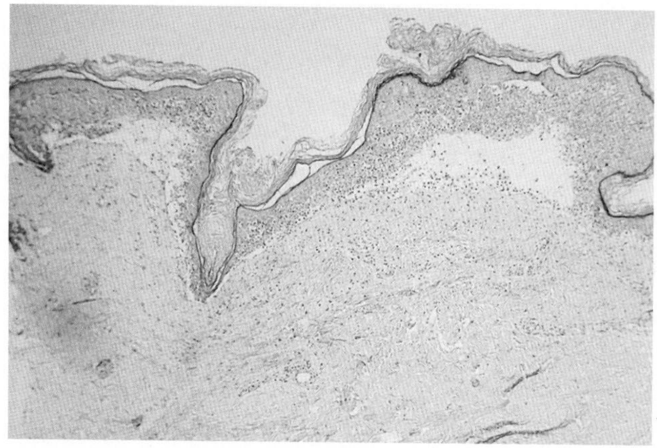

FIGURE 80. Toxic epidermal necrolysis. Full-thickness epidermal and follicular epithelial necrosis with sloughing epithelium from the underlying dermis.

to find the involved focus (337,338). Histologically there is a granulomatous vasculitis with focal destruction of the vascular wall and multinucleate giant cells containing fragments of internal elastic lamina. An elastic tissue stain will demonstrate discontinuity of the internal elastic lamina.

Behçet's Disease

Behçet's disease usually affects adult men and is characterized by the triad of recurrent aphthous stomatitis, painful genital ulcers, and iridocyclitis (339,340). Aphthous stomatitis occurs in more than 95% of patients and is the presenting complaint in approximately 50%. Ocular manifestations occur in approximately 90% of patients and include iridocyclitis, uveitis, and retinal vasculitis. Associated cutaneous findings include erythema nodosum-like lesions, sterile pustules at the site of venopuncture (pathergic reaction), thrombophlebitis, and a broad spectrum of acneiform papules, nodules, and pustular lesions (341). Other associated findings in Behçet's disease include arthralgias, pneumonitis, gastrointestinal ulcers, and central nervous system involvement. An association with the HLA antigens B5, BW51, B12, and DR7 has recently been described (340,342,343).

The histologic findings of the aphthae in Behçet's syndrome include ulceration and superficial mucosal necrosis with an underlying leukocytoclastic or lymphocytic vasculitis and a subepithelial lymphocytic infiltrate.

Noninfectious Granulomatous Processes and Histiocytic Proliferations

Epithelioid Cells, Histiocytes, and Giant Cells

Granulomatous Chelitis (Miescher-Melkersson-Rosenthal Syndrome; Oral Facial Granulomatosis)

Granulomatous cheilitis is manifest as a sudden angioedema-like swelling of the lip, often accompanied by fever and headache (344,345). The upper lip is most commonly involved, followed by the lower lip, cheek, forehead, eyelids, or scalp. The swelling waxes and wanes and with each episode returns slightly lower and progressively becomes less soft and more rubbery. Lymphadenopathy occurs in approximately 50% of patients, and facial nerve palsy in 30% (344,345). Granulomatous cheilitis is occasionally the presenting finding in Crohn's disease (346,347).

The histologic features of granulomatous cheilitis include marked dermal edema, lymphangiectasia, and a lymphohistiocytic infiltrate containing scattered plasma cells, occasionally with tuberculoid or epithelioid granulomas. Special stains do not reveal acid-fast bacilli or fungi. Not uncommonly the inflammatory infiltrate involves the underlying muscle.

Rosacea

Rosacea characteristically appears as erythematous, telangiectatic papules with edema and rarely follicular pustules. This ruddy erythematous eruption usually occurs on the skin of the cheeks, nose, chin, and forehead. Acute exacerbation may occur following sun exposure or alcohol ingestion. An association with HIV infection has been reported in some patients, particularly those of a younger age than is characteristic of rosacea (348,349). The histologic features of rosacea range from those of a perivascular and periadnexal lymphoid infiltrate to an extensive granulomatous dermatitis with acute folliculitis. Characteristically the changes include a perivascular and periadnexal mononuclear cell infiltrate with plasma cells and few giant cells, sebaceous gland hyperplasia, and tuberculoid granuloma formation with variable degrees of necrosis. Extensive caseation necrosis is rarely observed and, when present, should prompt a consideration of the diagnosis of lupus vulgaris (cutaneous tuberculous infection) and lupus miliaris disseminatus faciei.

Lupus Miliaris Disseminatus Faciei (Acne Agminata)

Lupus miliaris disseminatus faciei usually occurs on the upper lip but may also effect the chin, eyelids, eyebrows, and cheeks. Multiple yellow-brown papules arise in a somewhat symmetric distribution and persist for a year or so before resolving; scarring is common. The histologic findings include discrete epithelioid granulomas with caseation necrosis, occasional giant cells and a variable chronic inflammatory infiltrate (Fig. 81). Organisms are not seen on acid-fast or fungal stains.

Foreign Body Giant-Cell Reaction

A granulomatous tissue reaction may occur in response to a wide variety of foreign materials being introduced into the skin. Fragments of keratin, tattoo pigments, silica, and zirconium are well-known causes of granulomatous inflammation. A foreign body giant-cell reaction to keratin occurs with disruption of follicular epithelium or epithelial cyst walls, including ruptured epidermal or pilar cysts, pilonidal sinus, trichotillomania, and benign adnexal tumors including trichoepithelioma.

Cutaneous Crohn's Disease

Ulcerated oral mucosal lesions in Crohn's disease may represent aphthous stomatitis secondary to malabsorption or primary Crohn's disease (350). Linear ulcers often involve the buccal sulcus and may be associated with a "cobblestone" appearance of the mucosa. Fissures, splitting of the lips, and angular stom-

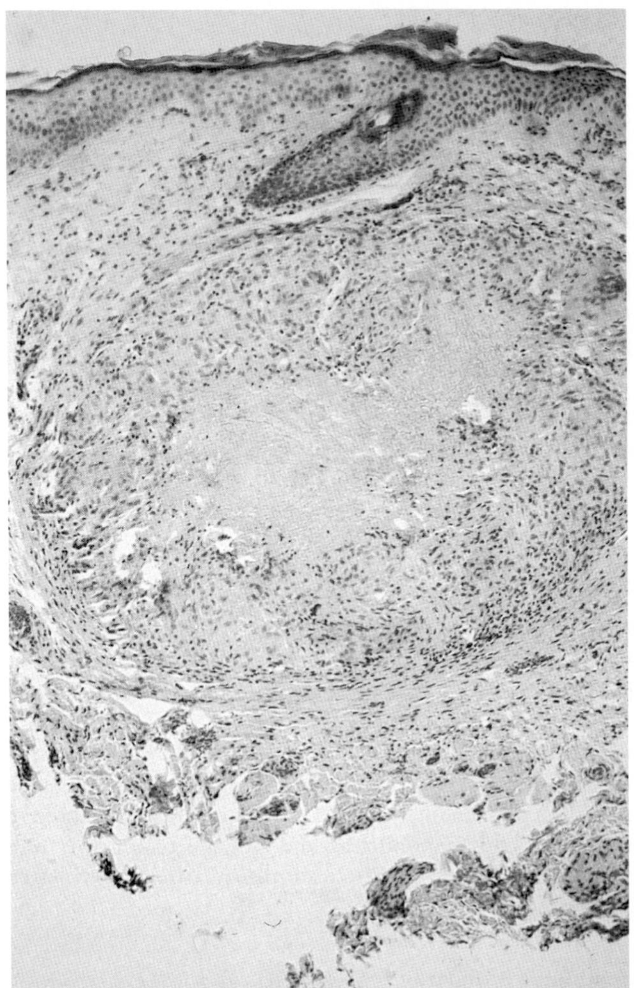

FIGURE 81. Lupus miliaris disseminatus faciei. Superficial dermal necrotizing granuloma composed of epithelioid cells and giant cells.

atitis are also findings in Crohn's disease (351). Rarely, metastatic Crohn's disease may occur on the skin of the face (352). The histologic findings in primary and metastatic Crohn's disease are similar and include a granulomatous inflammatory infiltrate with epithelioid granulomas similar to those observed in sarcoidosis, rarely with focal caseation, necrosis, and multinucleate giant cells that may contain asteroid bodies (353).

Sarcoid

Lupus pernio is a clinical form of sarcoidosis that presents as violaceous nodules on the nose, cheeks, and ears (354,355). Lupus pernio is associated with bone cysts and involvement of the upper respiratory tract, lacrimal gland, and kidney. Rarely lesions may occur in the oral mucosa (356). Lupus pernio is more refractory to treatment than sarcoidosis at other sites; involvement of the nasal mucosa and upper respiratory tract may lead to significant morbidity. Classic sarcoidal granulomas are well-demarcated, usually nonnecrotizing collections of epithelioid histiocytes and giant cells with a peripheral rim of lymphocytes. The absence of lymphocytes in the central areas of the granulomas has led some observers to describe sarcoidal granulomas as "naked." The giant cells may contain asteroid bodies (stellate aggregates of entrapped collagen and proteins) or Schaumann bodies (targetoid calcium containing deposits). Polarizable material and infectious organisms are typically absent (357–359). In cutaneous sarcoidosis the granulomas are present in the reticular dermis and may extend into the subcutaneous fat.

Xanthomatous

Sclerosing Lipogranuloma (Paraffinoma; Factitial Panniculitis)

Sclerosing lipogranuloma is a chronic foreign body reaction to injected material containing oils. The lesions develop a characteristic firm, rubbery appearance. One of the most characteristic histologic findings in sclerosing lipogranuloma is a low-power "Swiss cheese" appearance of the lower dermis and subcutis caused by the presence of numerous variably sized vacuoles (Fig. 82). The vacuoles contain lipid that stains positively in frozen tissue sections with the Sudan black and oil red O stains. There is also a granulomatous infiltrate containing lipid-laden macrophages, multinucleate giant cells with lipidized cytoplasm, and a variable mononuclear and polymorphonuclear inflammatory infiltrate with marked dermal fibrosis.

Xanthelasma

Xanthelasma usually involves the upper eyelids and the inner canthi as symmetric soft yellow coalescing papules. They may indicate the presence of hypercholesterolemia, although serum lipid levels are normal in over 50% of cases (360,361). Nevertheless, low-density lipoprotein (LDL) levels may be elevated in the absence of hyperlipidemia. Less commonly, xanthelasma is associated with chronic biliary obstruction. Histologically there is a superficial dermal infiltrate of histiocytes with finely vacuolated cytoplasm, termed foam cells or xanthoma cells (Fig. 83). The intracytoplasmic lipid indents nuclei,

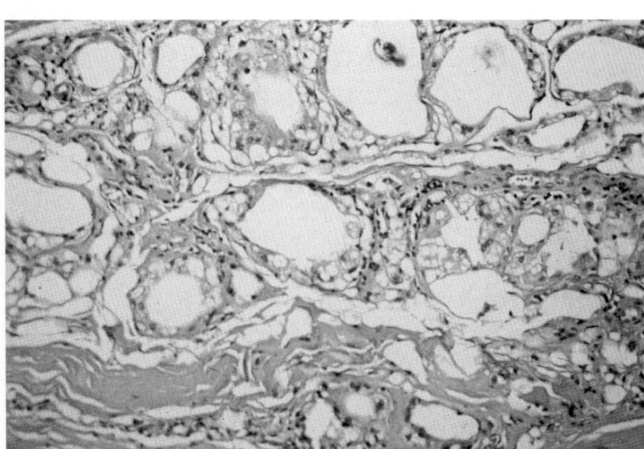

FIGURE 82. Sclerosing lipogranuloma. Granulomatous reaction with lipid-filled histiocytes and variable sized empty spaces embedded in a fibrotic reticular dermis.

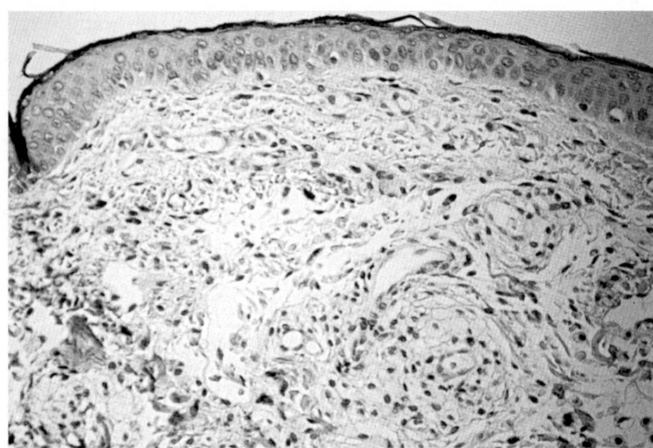

FIGURE 83. Xanthelasma. Perivascular and interstitial distribution of histiocytes with finely lipidized cytoplasm (xanthoma cells).

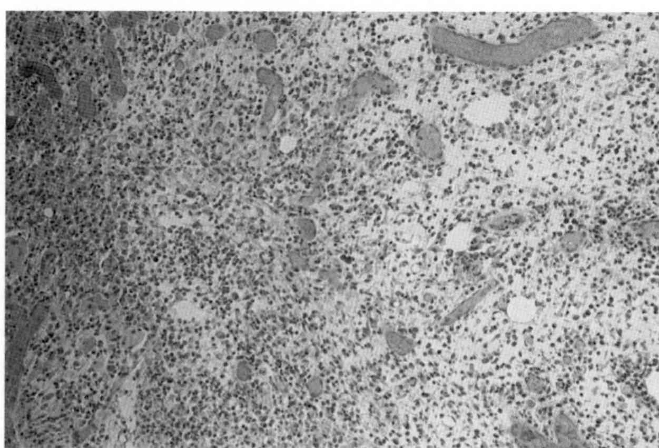

FIGURE 84. Chalazion. Xanthogranuloma with multinucleate giant cells, neutrophilic abscess, and fat droplets lined by neutrophils.

creating a scalloped appearance. No significant inflammatory infiltrate or epidermal changes are present.

Chalazion

Chalazion is a painless red swelling on the conjunctival surface of the eyelid caused by a granulomatous reaction in a Meibomian gland (a modified sebaceous gland). There is usually extravasation of the fatty Meibomian gland secretion with a lipogranulomatous reaction containing multinucleate giant cells with an associated neutrophilic infiltrate or microabscess (Fig. 84).

Verruciform Xanthoma

Verruciform xanthoma appears as an asymptomatic solitary erythematous or hyperkeratotic lesion most commonly arising on the gingiva. Histologically one characteristically observes verrucous epithelial hyperplasia with aggregates of histiocytes with foam cells or xanthoma cells in the subepithelial papillae (Fig. 85). The intracytoplasmic lipid indents nuclei, creating a scalloped appearance. A significant inflammatory infiltrate is usually absent.

Histiocytic and Necrobiotic

Pseudorheumatoid Nodule (Subcutaneous Granuloma Annulare)

These subcutaneous nodules may arise on the scalp or lower extremities of otherwise healthy children (i.e., children without rheumatoid arthritis) (362–366). The histologic features of pseudorheumatoid nodules are similar to those observed in rheumatoid nodules. There is a characteristic palisade of histiocytes and mononuclear and polymorphonuclear cells surrounding zones of fibrinoid degeneration of collagen (Fig. 86).

Granuloma Annulare

Granuloma annulare predominantly affects children and young adults but may occur at any age. Asymptomatic, nonpruritic erythematous papules coalesce to form a ring of lesions 1 to 5 cm in diameter. The papules are not hyperkeratotic and only rarely ulcerate. These annular lesions usually arise on the dorsum of the hands and feet, the fingers, the extensor aspects of the extremi-

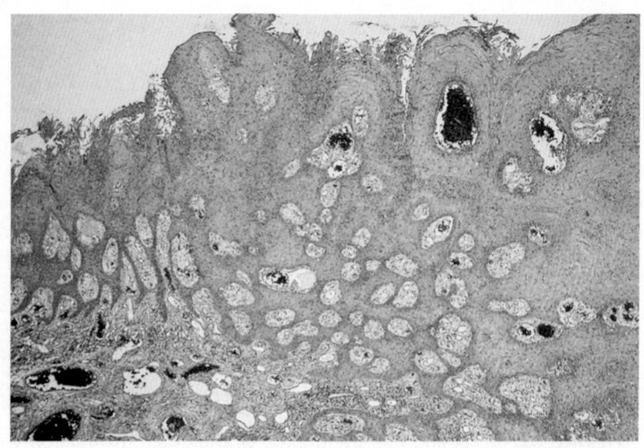

A

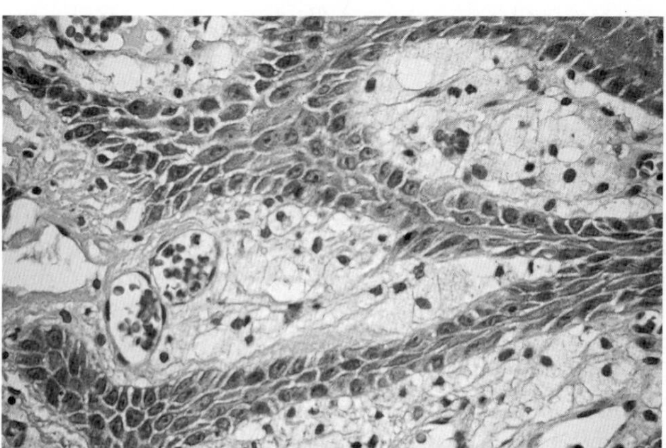

B

FIGURE 85. Verruciform xanthoma. **A:** Verrucous epidermal hyperplasia with xanthoma cells filling the papillary dermal pegs. **B:** The papillary dermal protrusions between the epidermal rete contain numerous finely lipidized histiocytes (xanthoma cells).

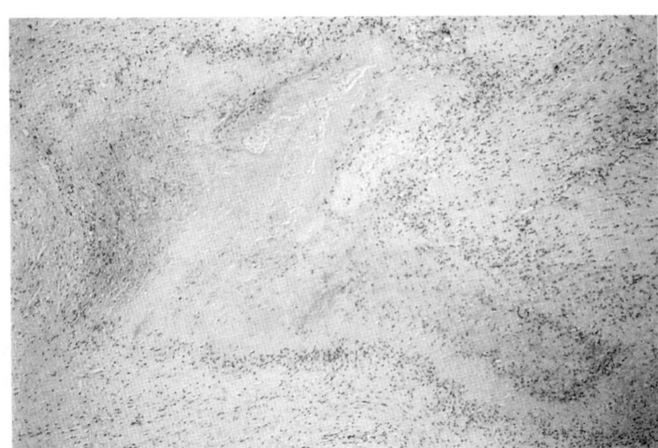
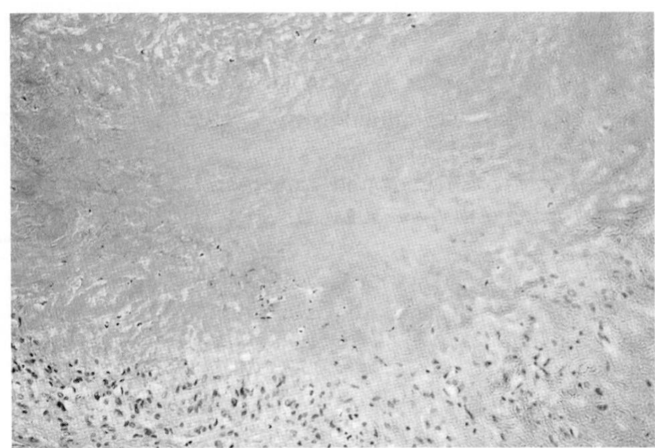

FIGURE 86. Pseudorheumatoid nodule. **A:** Palisaded granulomatous inflammation with central fibrinoid necrosis surrounded by a rim of nuclear debris. **B:** Fibrinoid necrosis with a rim of nuclear debris and a surrounding zone of epithelioid histiocytes.

ties, and the scalp and ears (367,368) but not the mucosa. Granuloma annulare usually resolves spontaneously but will recur in almost half of patients (369).

The characteristic histologic features are those of palisaded epithelioid histiocytes surrounding a loose-appearing dermis rich in connective tissue mucin (hyaluronic acid), a so-called "palisading granuloma" (Fig. 87). The dermal mucin appears on hematoxylin–eosin stain as threads of finely beaded basophilic material between collagen bundles and stains positively with colloidal iron and alcian blue stains. There is usually a sparse su-

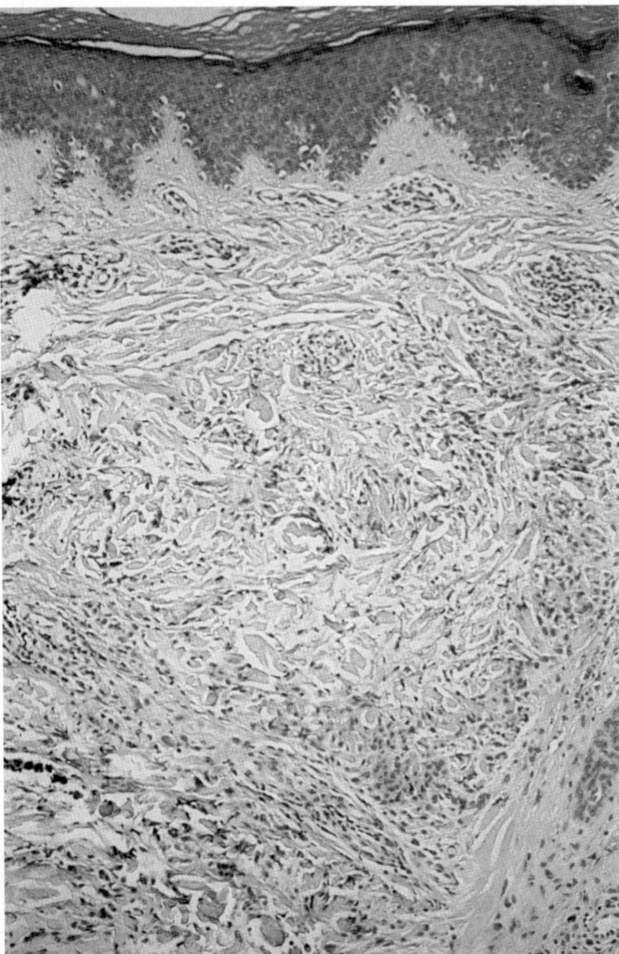
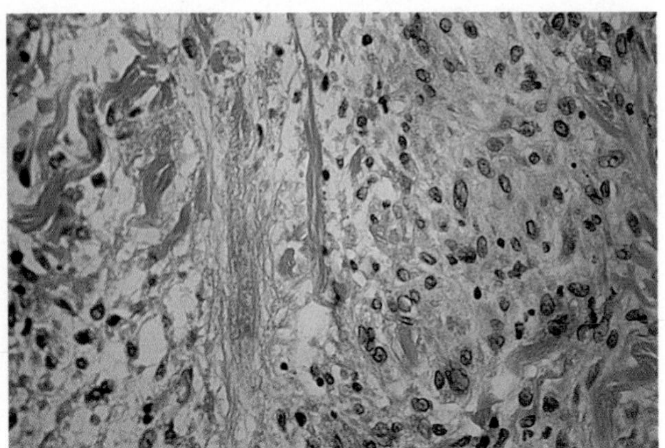

FIGURE 87. Granuloma annulare. **A:** Superficial dermal palisaded epithelioid cell granuloma with central basophilic mucin deposition. **B:** Epithelioid histiocytes surround a cell-poor, mucin-rich zone.

perficial perivascular lymphoid infiltrate. Giant cells are rarely present, and no significant vascular abnormalities are observed.

Annular Elastolytic Granuloma

Annular elastolytic granuloma is a descriptive term used for an annular arrangement of erythematous papules arising in the sun-exposed skin of adults that contain a granulomatous infiltrate with giant cells containing fragments of elastic fibers. Several variants of annular elastolytic granuloma have been described, including actinic granuloma, necrobiosis lipoidica of the face, and Meischer's granuloma (370,371). Whether these processes represent the same pathologic entity remains unclear (372–374). In general, these lesions heal without scarring or alopecia. The histologic features of the active border of annular elastolytic granuloma include a superficial and deep interstitial lymphohistiocytic infiltrate with multinucleate giant cells containing fragments of refractile elastic fibers. The central "burnt-out" region of these lesions is remarkable for a reduced number of elastic fibers.

Benign Cephalic Histiocytosis

This very rare asymptomatic papular eruption on the face of young children may spread to involve the ears, neck, scalp, trunk, and upper extremities but is in the end self-limiting. The histologic findings include a histiocytic proliferation with variable numbers of xanthoma cells and multinucleate cells, features similar to those observed in juvenile xanthogranuloma (see below) (375,376). Electron microscopy shows that up to 30% of the histiocytes contain intracytoplasmic comma-shaped bodies and coated vesicles (377); Birbeck granules (seen in Langerhans' histiocytes) are absent. The histiocytes have a $CD68^{+}$, factor $XIIIa^{+}$, $CD11b^{+}$, $S\text{-}100^{-}$, $CD1a^{-}$ immunophenotype.

Juvenile Xanthogranuloma

This normolipemic non-Langerhans'-cell xanthoma often presents in childhood as a red-brown papule or nodule on the face or neck; adults may less often be affected. Although usually sporadic, rare associations with systemic disease syndromes have been described (378–380). Occasional deep lesions, including orbital ones, occur. Histologically there is a nodular dermal proliferation of histiocytes with varying numbers of xanthoma cells and Touton giant cells (381–383), that is, giant cells characteristically containing multiple nuclei arranged in a circular wreath with a surrounding mantle of intracytoplasmic vacuoles (Fig. 88). Lymphocytes, neutrophils, plasma cells, and eosinophils may also be present. The histiocytes have a $CD68^{+}$, factor $XIIIa^{+}$, $lysozyme^{+}$, α_1-$antichymotrypsin^{+}$, $CD34^{-}$, $S\text{-}100^{-}$, $CD1a^{-}$ immunophenotype (381,383).

Langerhans' Cell Histiocytosis (Histiocytosis X)

Langerhans' cell histiocytosis, previously termed histiocytosis X, is a possibly neoplastic proliferation of Langerhans' cells that may involve the skin, bone, spleen, lung, central nervous system, and lymph nodes. Lesions may resolve spontaneously in some patients, but in other patients they may progress to lethal disease. Although predicting prognosis is difficult, onset late in life and the absence of visceral involvement are prognostically favorable findings (384–387). Mucocutaneous disease is found in more than 50% of patients (388). Rarely this tumor presents in the periorbital skin (389,390). The histologic features of Langerhans' cell histiocytosis include a variably dense dermal infiltrate or nodule of Langerhans' cells with deeply cleaved "reniform" nuclei and scattered eosinophils and lymphocytes. Also present are histiocytes with vacuolated cytoplasm (foam cells, xanthoma cells) and multinucleate giant cells (rarely of Touton type). Characteristically there is exocytosis of Langerhans' cells through the epidermis, sometimes with the formation of intraepidermal aggregates. The Langerhans' cells have an $S\text{-}100^{+}$, $CD1a^{+}$, $lysozyme^{-}$, $CD34^{-}$, $Mac\text{-}387^{-}$ immunophenotype (391,392). CD1a is an important marker that is positive in Langerhans' cells but not in other types of histiocytes. With electron microscopy, Birbeck granules are observed (393).

Systemic Reactions and Reactions to Foreign Substances

Drug Reactions

Phototoxic and Photoallergic Drug Eruptions

Pharmaceutical agents may sensitize patients to develop photoallergic or phototoxic hypersensitivity reactions. Photoallergic re-

A 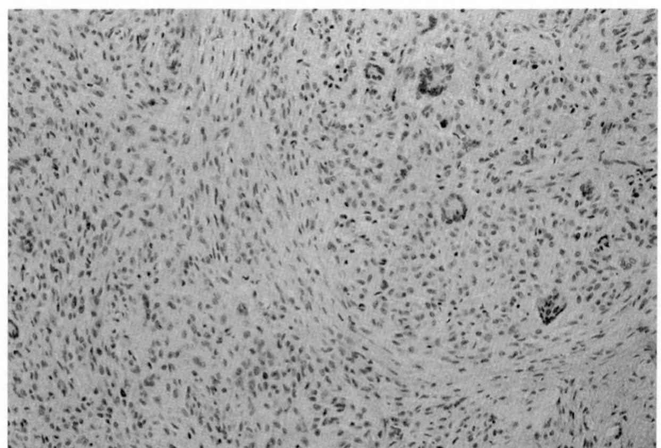

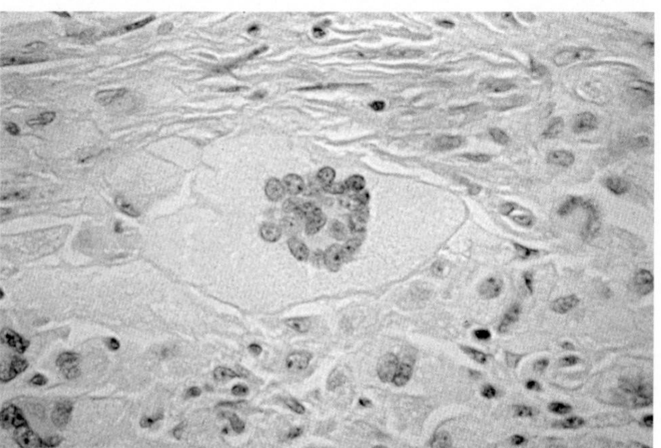 B

FIGURE 88. Juvenile xanthogranuloma. **A:** Nodular dermal proliferation of epithelioid histiocytes, multinucleate giant cells, and xanthoma cells. **B:** Multinucleate giant cells with a circular wreath of nuclei surrounded by a halo of cytoplasmic vacuoles (Touton giant cell).

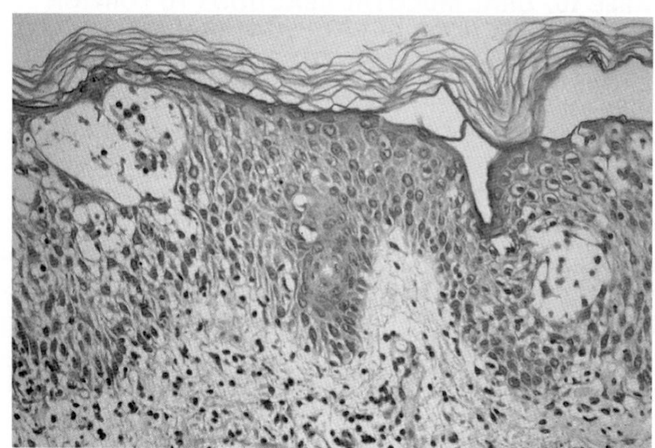

FIGURE 89. Photoallergic drug eruption. Marked intercellular edema (spongiosis) with a neutrophil-containing spongiotic microvesicle and normal basket-weave stratum corneum.

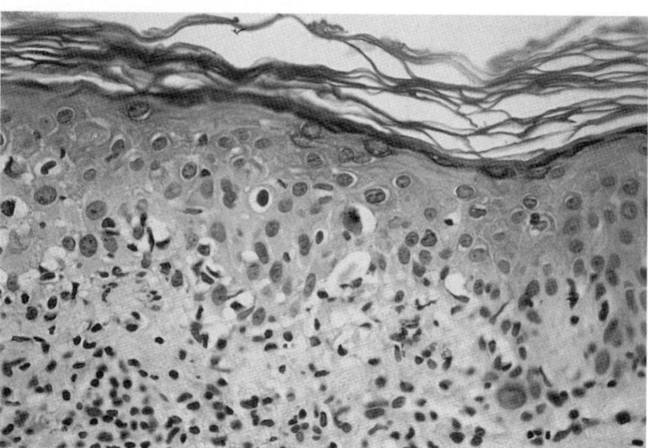

FIGURE 91. Fixed drug eruption. Epidermal keratinocyte dyskeratosis with a vacuolar change of the basal keratinocytes, inflammation at the interface of the epidermis and dermis (vacuolar interface dermatitis), and papillary dermal pigment-laden macrophages.

actions resemble allergic contact dermatitis histologically (Fig. 89), whereas phototoxic reactions resemble a severe sunburn and display a distinctive pattern of dyskeratosis without spongiosis or acanthosis but with a sparse superficial perivascular mononuclear infiltrate containing lymphocytes and scattered eosinophils (Fig. 90).

Fixed Drug Eruption

A fixed drug eruption is an erythematous or hyperpigmented macular lesion that arises shortly following exposure to an ingested antigen. This lesion reappears at the same site with repeated ingestion of the agent. These lesions may occur at any cutaneous site but have a predilection for the skin of the face and the oral and genital mucosa (Table 9). With complete withdrawal of the agent, a hyperpigmented or hypopigmented lesion usually persists.

The histologic features of fixed drug eruption include keratinocyte dyskeratosis at all levels of the epidermis, occasionally with clumped dyskeratotic cells and extensive epidermal necrosis (Fig. 91). There is focal interface dermatitis with vacuolization of basal layer keratinocytes, sometimes with formation of a subepidermal bulla. Pigment-laden macrophages may be numerous in recurrent lesions (Table 8).

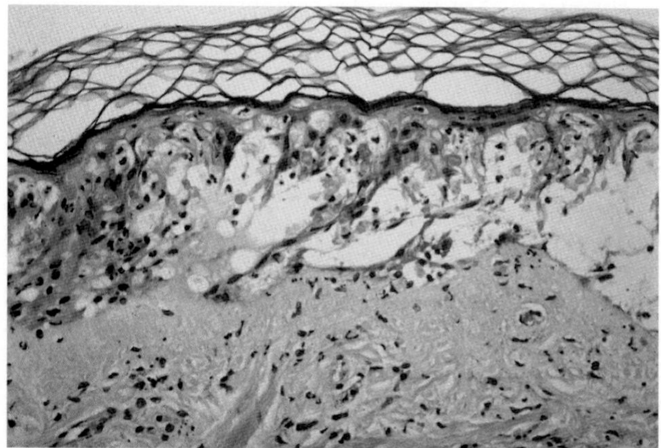

FIGURE 90. Phototoxic drug eruption. Multifocal epidermal keratinocyte dyskeratosis with a sparse inflammatory infiltrate and normal basket-weave stratum corneum.

Hyperpigmentation, Minocycline-Induced

Minocycline, an antibiotic related to tetracycline, may induce a slate gray or muddy brown discoloration of the skin or mucosa, in particular the gingival mucosa, as well as the thyroid gland (Table 9). The histologic findings include variable hyperpigmentation of basal-layer melanocytes with numerous dermal pigment-laden macrophages. The pigment may stain as melanin (black with Fontana-Masson stain) or as heme (blue with Perl's iron stain) or stain as both melanin and heme. Other agents that can cause similar clinical and histologic features of hyperpigmentation include amiodarone and antimalarial medications.

Argyria

Argyria is a slate blue discoloration of the skin that may follow prolonged ingestion of silver salts. The diagnostic histologic finding in argyria is the deposition of uniformly small round black granules in the perieccrine gland basement membrane zone. Granules may also be observed in other adnexal adventitia, capillary walls, and scattered diffusely along the dermal collagen and elastic fibers (Fig. 92). There is also basal-layer hyperpigmentation, and occasionally melanophages are observed.

Exogenous Ochronosis

Exogenous ochronosis is most commonly observed following the topical application of hydroxyquinone-containing bleaching compounds, usually to the face. The histologic findings are identical to those observed in alkaptonuria (endogenous ochronosis). Enlarged, tortuous, superficial papillary dermal elastic fibers are coated with ochre-colored deposits. Pigment-laden macrophages are also present.

Elastosis Perforans Serpiginosa

Elastosis perforans serpiginosa may occur as an incidental finding or after prolonged treatment with penicillamine. Grouped keratotic papules, often in an arcuate distribution, present on the face,

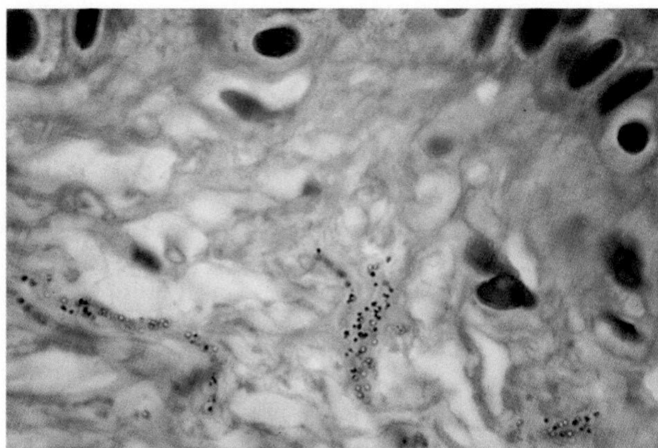

FIGURE 92. Argyria. Delicate uniformly sized black granules of silver are deposited along the dermal collagen fibers.

extremities, or upper trunk. Histologically, there is epidermal hyperplasia, often with a ball-like aggregate of degenerating dermal elastic fibers entrapped by a claw-like conformation of hyperplastic epidermis. Intraepidermal basophilic debris and degenerated elastic fibers are present in foci where the dermal contents are extruded through the epidermis. An elastic tissue stain confirms the presence of aggregates of coarse fragmented elastic fibers in the dermis and migrating through the epidermis. There is also an accompanying mononuclear infiltrate with scattered giant cells. Notably, jagged "bramble bush-like" elastic fibers are observed in penicillamine-associated elastosis perforans serpiginosa.

Amalgam Tattoo

Amalgam tattoos are characterized histologically by the presence of black silver pigment in macrophages or extracellularly in the buccal or gingival submucosa (Fig. 93) (Tables 9 and 10). The silver characteristically comes from dental amalgam fillings.

Light Reactions

Polymorphous Light Eruption

Polymorphous light eruption presents as pruritic erythematous papules and urticarial plaques on the neck, face, and upper extremities. The eruption arises within hours of an exposure and most commonly occurs in young women. Complete resolution within a week or so is common if light exposure does not continue. The histologic features of polymorphous light eruption include vacuolar alteration of basal-layer keratinocytes, marked papillary dermal edema, vacuolization of endothelial cells, and a patchy superficial and deep dermal, perivascular, and occasionally interstitial, mononuclear cell infiltrate (Fig. 94). Many of these histologic features are observed in discoid lupus erythematosus, which also may have a clinical history of photosensitivity. In contrast to the findings in lupus, polymorphous light eruption does not display a thickened epidermal basement membrane zone and will have negative serologic and lupus band tests.

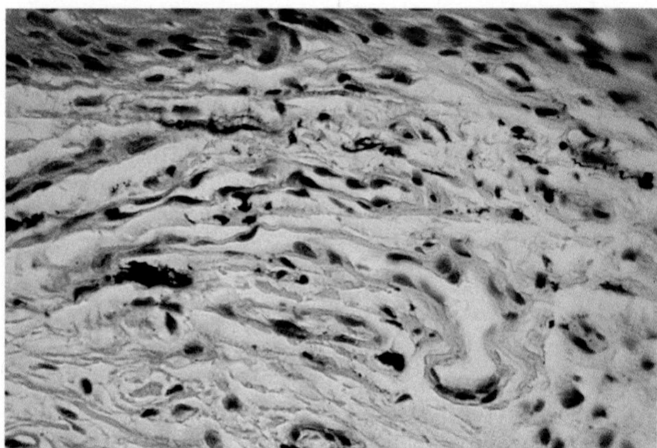

FIGURE 93. Amalgam tattoo. Irregularly shaped black particles are deposited in the superficial submucosa.

TABLE 10. ORAL MUCOSAL REACTIONS TO FOREIGN AGENTS, INFECTIOUS AGENTS, AND TRAUMA

Amalgam tattoo
Fixed drug reaction
Drug reactions with pigment deposits (amiodarone, minocine)
Smokers hyperkeratosis
Lip chewing
Hairy leukoplakia
Candidiasis
Herpes

Radiation Dermatitis

The earliest histologic features of radiation dermatitis include intracellular edema of epidermal keratinocytes with underlying dermal edema, vascular ectasia, and occasional subepidermal bullae. Chronic radiation dermatitis is characterized by epidermal atrophy or irregular epidermal hyperplasia, with hyperkeratosis, dyskeratosis, vascular ectasia, hyalinized dermal collagen, and, most notably, prominent, stellate, multinucleate fibroblasts (so-called "radiation fibroblasts").

Actinic Reticuloid (Chronic Actinic Dermatitis)

Actinic reticuloid is a chronic photosensitive dermatitis with cytologically atypical T cells. Patients present with a long history of light sensitivity with resultant dusky red-brown plaques on their face and upper extremities. These patients may develop leonine faces similar to that observed in porphyria. Actinic reticuloid may represent one end of a spectrum of persistent light reactions. Although some patients with actinic reticuloid have been described to develop cutaneous T-cell lymphoma, a clear relationship between actinic reticuloid and lymphoma has not been established.

Histologically, many of the features mimic those of mycosis fungoides (see section on mimics of cutaneous lymphoma). In early lesions the findings are not specific and include spongiosis, parakeratosis, epidermal hyperplasia, and a dense dermal mononuclear cell infiltrate with scattered eosinophils, plasma cells, and rare lymphocytes with large convoluted hyperchromatic nuclei. In addition to the findings above, late lesions display epidermotropism of atypical convoluted T cells, papillary dermal edema, and fibrosis with stellate multinucleate fibroblasts. Immunohistochemically, the atypical lymphocytes often have a $CD8^+$, $CD4^-$ phenotype without loss of pan-T-cell antigens.

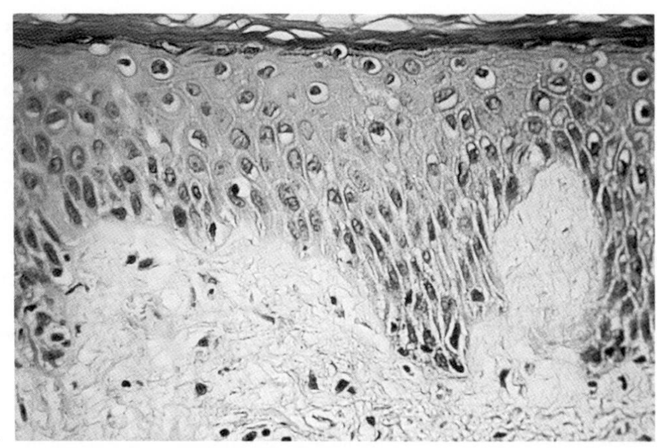

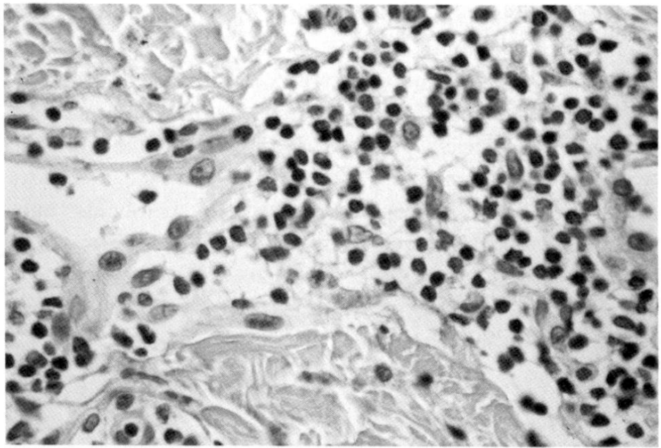

FIGURE 94. Polymorphous light eruption. **A:** Mild epidermal spongiosis and prominent subepidermal edema. **B:** Perivascular lymphoid infiltrate with endothelial cell hypertrophy and cytoplasmic vacuolization.

Reactions to the Cold

Cold Temperature–Induced Paniculitis (Popsicle Panniculitis)

Newborn infants and adults with chilblain may be susceptible to developing fat necrosis after extended exposure to cold temperatures. In infants who have been eating popsicles, cold panniculitis may arise at the angle of the mouth or on the cheeks. The indurated plaques soften and resolve after several weeks without scarring. Histologically, there is lobular panniculitis (inflammation of subcutaneous fat) with a perivascular mononuclear infiltrate.

Mucosal Keratotic Reactions

Hyperkeratotic lesions may develop on the oral mucosa as a response to trauma along the buccal mucosal occlusal line or on the dental ridges in edentulous patients who do not wear dentures. Smoker's keratosis may occur on the palate in pipe-smoking patients; characteristically there is diffuse hyperkeratosis of the palate with erythematous punctae at the orifices of inflamed salivary glands.

Degenerative Disorders and Connective Tissue Disease

Lipoatrophy and Lipodystrophy

Lipoatrophy refers to secondary loss of the subcutaneous fat following lupus panniculitis, morphea, or other connective tissue panniculitides. On the other hand, lipodystrophy is used to describe idiopathic forms of lipoatrophy including forms of partial and localized lipoatrophy as in hemifacial atrophy (394,395). Notably, some of the idiopathic lipodystrophies show an association with membranoproliferative glomerlonephritis, thyroid disease, and infections. Histologically, early lesions may show a perivascular lymphoplasmacytic infiltrate and an inflammatory lobular panniculitis with foam cells, and lymphocytes. More progressed lesions show myxoid or hyaline changes of the subcutaneous fat with replacement of the fat by collagen.

Lupus Erythematosus

As opposed to systemic lupus erythematosus, discoid lupus erythematosus is a benign skin disease that usually presents on the face as erythematous, well-demarcated plaques with follicular plugging. Ultimately the lesions become atrophic and leave variably pigmented scars. More than half of patients with discoid lupus will have positive serologic tests for lupus, most commonly anti-Ro/SSA antibodies (396,397). Approximately 10% to 20% of patients with discoid lupus will ultimately develop systemic lupus. This is particularly common among patients with very high levels of antinuclear antibodies (ANA) at presentation (398,399). Systemic lupus erythematosus (SLE) is defined as a multisystem autoimmune disease in which over 80% of patients develop cutaneous manifestations, arthralgias, arthritis, and fever, and over half of patients have renal involvement and lymphadenopathy (400,401). The erythematous malar rash of SLE is composed of erythematous plaques on the face and anterior chest that are less well defined than those of discoid lupus. In severe cases, patients may die from renal failure, infection, or complications of vasculitis, particularly when the vasculitis involves the central nervous system (402). The diagnosis of systemic lupus is made when a patient exhibits four or more of the 11 criteria set forth by the American Rheumatism Association (403). These criteria are (a) malar rash, (b) discoid rash, (c) photosensitivity, (d) oral ulcers, (e) nonerosive arthritis involving two or more peripheral joints, (f) serositis (pleurisy or pericarditis), (g) renal disease (casts or proteinuria), (h) neurologic disorder (seizures or psychosis), (i) hematologic disorder (hemolytic anemia, leukopenia, lymphopenia, or thrombocytopenia), (j) immunologic disorder (positive LE-cell preparation, anti-DNA antibodies, anti–smooth muscle nuclear antigen antibodies, false positive test for syphilis), and (k) antinuclear antibody. A diagnosis of systemic lupus is also made if any three of the following four findings are present: (a) cutaneous lesions consistent with lupus, (b) renal involvement, (c) serositis, and (d) joint involvement. Finally, in the presence of the above criteria, confirmation of the diagnosis with laboratory tests is required.

Histologically, the early changes of systemic lupus are nonspecific. Better-developed lesions have histologic features of subacute cutaneous lupus, lupus profundus, bullous lupus, and, less commonly, discoid lupus.

The characteristic histologic features in discoid lupus erythematosus include follicular hyperkeratosis, with carpet tack–like plugging of hair follicles, epidermal atrophy, an interface dermatitis with vacuolar degeneration of basal layer keratinocytes, thickening of the PAS-positive epidermal basement membrane zone, and a patchy, moderately dense, superficial and deep perivascular and periadnexal mononuclear cell infiltrate (Fig. 95). A colloidal iron stain or alcian blue stain often reveals increased dermal hyaluronic acid, also referred to as connective tissue mucin.

Direct immunofluorescence testing of frozen sections of a cutaneous or conjunctival biopsy may reveal deposition of immunoreactants along the epidermal basement membrane zone (404). This detection of immunoreactants, most commonly IgG and IgM in a granular continuous pattern along the basement membrane zone, is characterized as a positive lupus band test. The approximate frequency of a positive lupus band test with direct immunofluorescence may be influenced by sun exposure. In discoid lupus erythematosus, the incidence of a positive lupus band test is more than 90% in lesional skin and less than 1% in sun-exposed or non–sun-exposed clinically normal skin. On

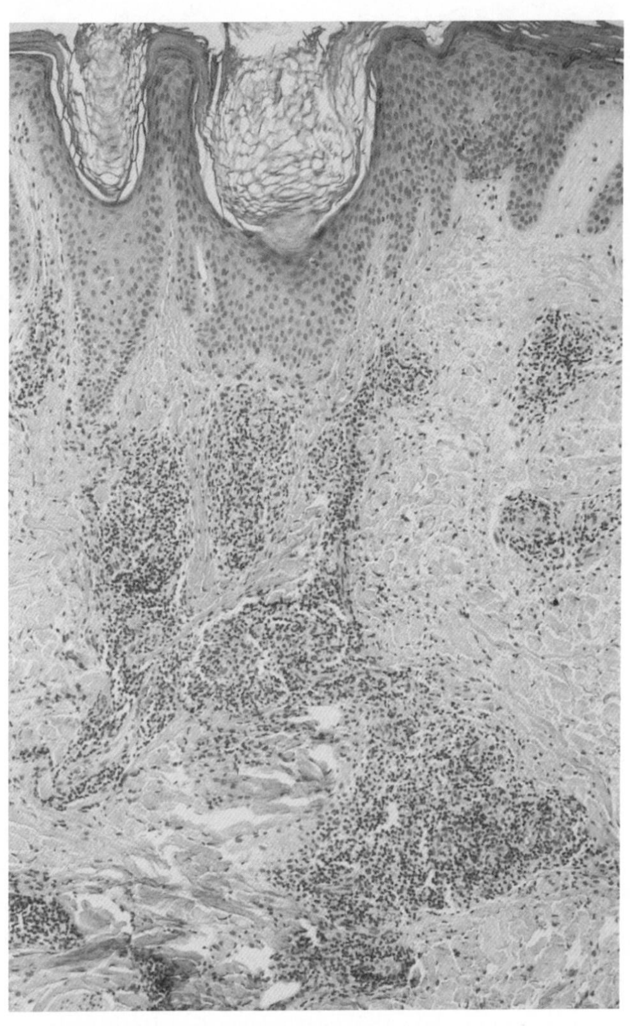

A

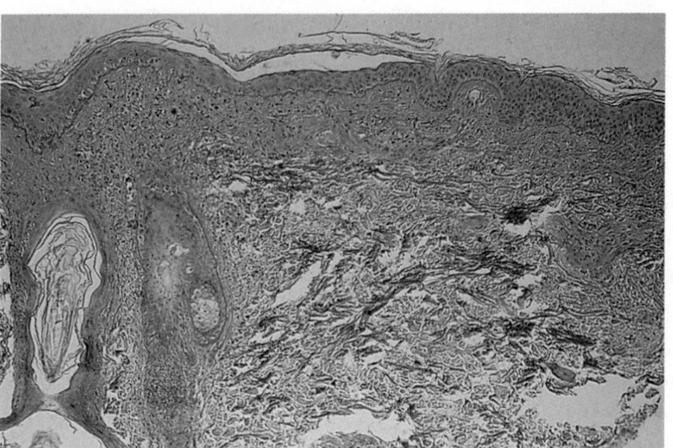

B

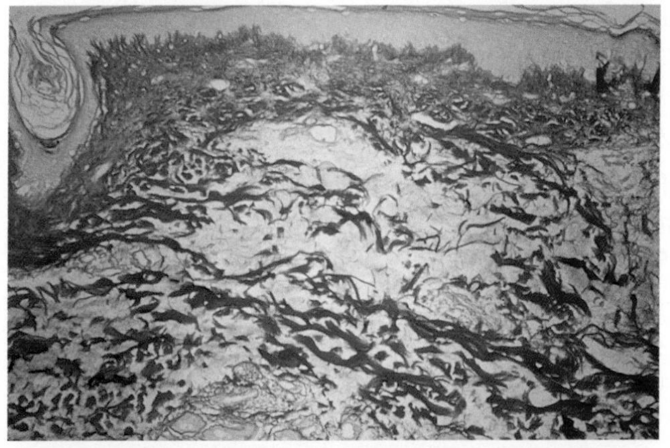

C

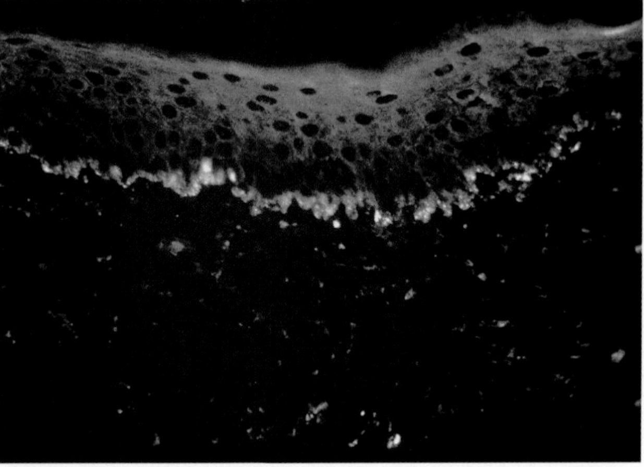

D

FIGURE 95. Lupus erythematosus. **A:** Follicular hyperkeratosis with a superficial and deep dermal perivascular and periadnexal lymphoid infiltrate in discoid lupus. **B:** Feathery thickened epidermal basement membrane zone stained magenta with PAS and diastase stain. **C:** Increased dermal hyaluronic acid (connective tissue mucin) stains blue with colloidal iron stain. **D:** Granular deposits of IgM along the epidermal basement membrane zone with direct immunofluorescence (positive lupus band test).

the other hand, the incidence of a positive lupus band test in SLE is over 90% in lesional skin and approximately 80% and 50% in sun-exposed and non–sun-exposed clinically normal skin, respectively.

Subacute Cutaneous Lupus Erythematosus

Subacute cutaneous lupus erythematosus (SCLE) is a variant of lupus that presents as annular plaques or papules on the sun-exposed areas of the face, neck, upper trunk, and extremities. This recurrent photosensitive eruption heals without scarring. Patients often have high serologic titers of anti-Ro/SSA antibodies and more commonly have a negative ANA than patients with other forms of lupus. The histologic features of SCLE are similar to those of discoid lupus except that SCLE shows more marked basal layer vacuolization, often with numerous colloid bodies, marked dermal edema and hyaluronic acid deposition, erythrocyte extravasation, dermal fibrin deposits, and less prominent hyperkeratosis and inflammatory infiltration than discoid lupus.

Lupus Profundus (Lupus Panniculitis)

Lupus profundus is a form of panniculitis that may present as tender nodules on the neck or scalp. The histologic features of lupus panniculitis include epidermal dyskeratosis, follicular plugging, basal-layer vacuolization, thickening of the epidermal basement membrane zone, and a superficial and deep perivascular and periadnexal infiltrate that extends into the interlobular septae of the subcutaneous fat. Marked septal fibrosis with perivascular hyalinization and occasional thrombosis of septal vessels is observed. There may be extensive hyaluronic acid deposition in the dermis and subcutaneous fat. Findings that are characteristic of lupus panniculitis that may aid in differentiating it from other forms of panniculitis include lymphoid follicles within the subcutaneous fat lobules and hyalinizing fat necrosis, occasionally with calcification (Fig. 96).

Dermatomyositis

The most characteristic cutaneous findings in dermatomyositis are a purple hued erythema of the eyelids, upper cheeks, forehead, and the temples, often with periorbital edema. An erythematous rash of the upper extremities and back may also be observed along with scaly plaques around the bases of the fingernails. When healing of the cutaneous lesions occurs, atrophy, telangiectasia, scarring, and hyperpigmentation or hypopigmentation are observed; these changes are described as poikiloderma atrophicans vasculare-like.

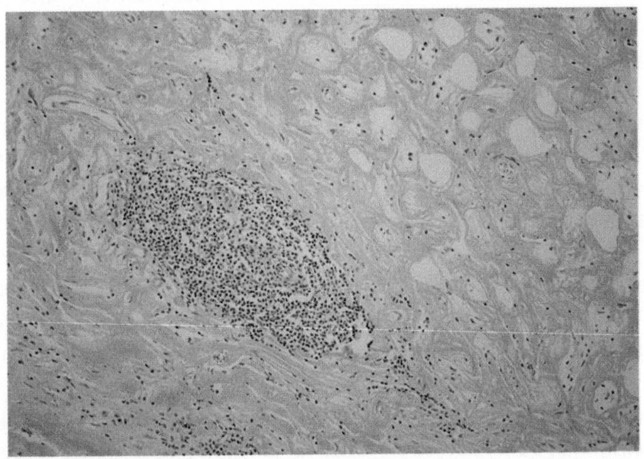

FIGURE 96. Lupus profundus. Eosinophilic hyalinized change of the subcutaneous fat and a small reactive lymphoid follicle.

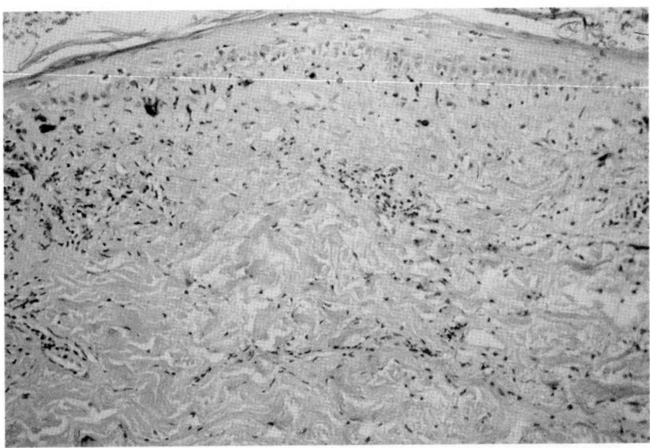

FIGURE 97. Dermatomyositis. Epidermal atrophy, vacuolar alteration of the basal layer epidermal keratinocytes, a sparse superficial dermal lymphoid infiltrate, and papillary dermal pigment-laden macrophages.

The histologic features of dermatomyositis depend on the clinical appearance of the cutaneous lesions. Erythematous lesions display epidermal atrophy with vacuolar degeneration of basal layer keratinocytes, papillary dermal edema, and a patchy perivascular and interstitial mononuclear cell infiltrate (Fig. 97). PAS-positive thickening of the basement membrane zone may be observed. These findings are similar to those of discoid lupus except that follicular plugging is less common in dermatomyositis. The poikiloderma atrophicans vasculare-like lesions also show epidermal atrophy with vacuolar degeneration of basal layer keratinocytes. The inflammatory infiltrate is more lichenoid than in early lesions and is accompanied by ectasia of the superficial venular plexus. There is usually an increase in dermal and subcutaneous hyaluronic acid and calcification of the subcutaneous fat.

Morphea (Localized Scleroderma)

Localized scleroderma may occur as circumscribed plaques, linear morphea, and unilateral linear frontoparietal lesions *(en coup de sabre),* occasionally with hemiatrophy of the face. The histologic findings in morphea include a mononuclear cell infiltrate at the junction of the subcutaneous fat and reticular dermis with replacement of subcutaneous fat by newly formed collagen (Fig. 98). The reticular dermal collagen bundles are thickened and homogenized and entrap the eccrine glands. Few fibroblast nuclei are observed within the sclerotic collagen. Perhaps because of the altered collagen, biopsies of morphea display a square rather than a tapered base.

Inflammatory Processes Involving Adnexae

Rhinophyma

Known in layman's terms as "whisky nose" or "grog blossom," this disorder has been traditionally associated with alcoholism.

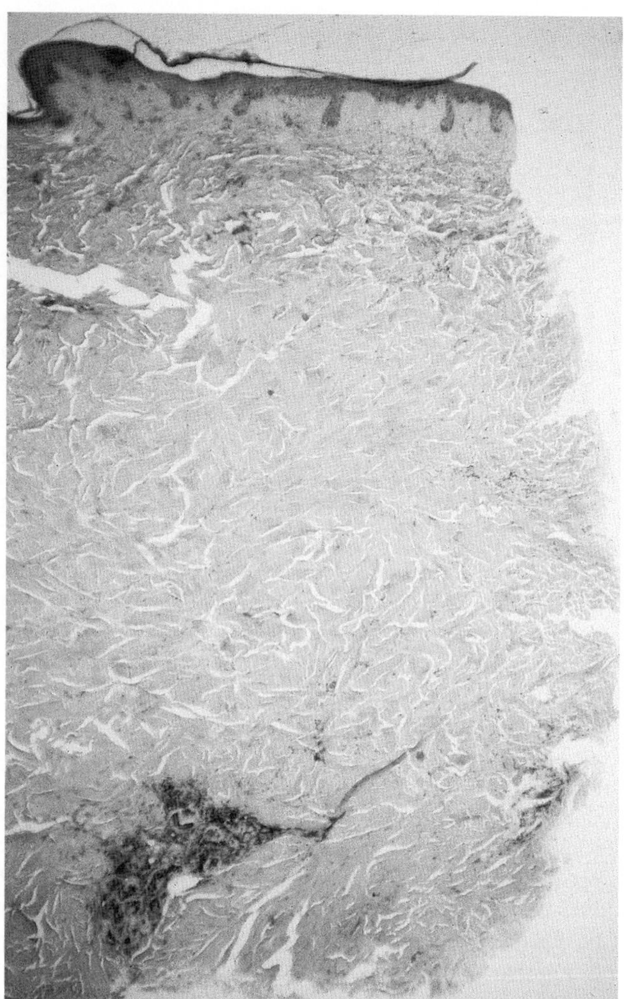

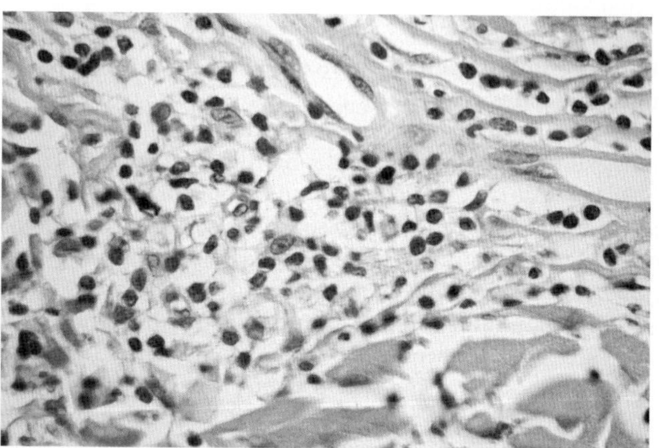

FIGURE 98. Morphea. **A:** Aggregates of lymphocytes at the junction of the reticular dermal collagen and perieccrine subcutaneous fat with a squared-off rather than tapered biopsy base. **B:** Perivascular lymphocytic infiltrate.

However, there is no evidence to support this association. The tip of the nose is commonly involved with extension to involve the paranasal areas in some patients. There is irregular swelling of the skin with widely patent follicular pores. The tip of the chin and earlobes may also be affected.

Histologically there is diffuse hypertrophy of the sebaceous glands and ducts with prominent sebaceous duct hyperkeratosis and periadnexal chronic inflammation (Fig. 99). The differential diagnosis includes sebaceous hyperplasia.

Pseudofolliculitis of the Beard

Pseudofolliculitis of the beard is a foreign body reaction to hair that occurs following shaving in patients with course curly hair. After having been shorn closely, the hair regrows and curls into the skin, invaginating into the epidermis and entering the dermis. A foreign body giant-cell reaction to the hair results and is often associated with abscess formation (405).

Eosinophilic Pustular Folliculitis

Eosinophilic pustular folliculitis may occur as an incidental finding of Ofuji's disease (406) or as an eruption in children (407) in association with HIV infection (408). The histologic features include eosinophilic spongiosis of follicular epithelium with a perifollicular mononuclear and eosinophilic infiltrate and, occasionally, intrafollicular eosinophil microabscesses (Fig. 100) (409).

Trichotillomania

Trichotillomania is a compulsive disorder manifested by the unrelenting plucking or pulling of hair. The characteristic histologic features of trichotillomania include increased numbers of follicles with keratinizing epithelium (catagen hairs), unlike the basaloid epithelium of anagen hair follicles, evidence of trauma to the hair bulb, and pigmentary casts (globules of melanin and hemosiderin) (410). The trauma-induced changes of the hair bulb are perhaps the easiest of the histologic findings to identify. These include the presence of clefts within the hair matrix, separating it from the vitreous basement membrane, erythrocyte extravasation, and numerous peribulbar pigment-laden macrophages. Trichotillomania is not associated with diminutive or miniaturized hair follicles, and there is a sparse or absent inflammatory infiltrate. This helps in distinguishing trichotillomania from two common forms of alopecia, androgenic (hereditary) alopecia and alopecia areata, which both show diminutive hair follicles.

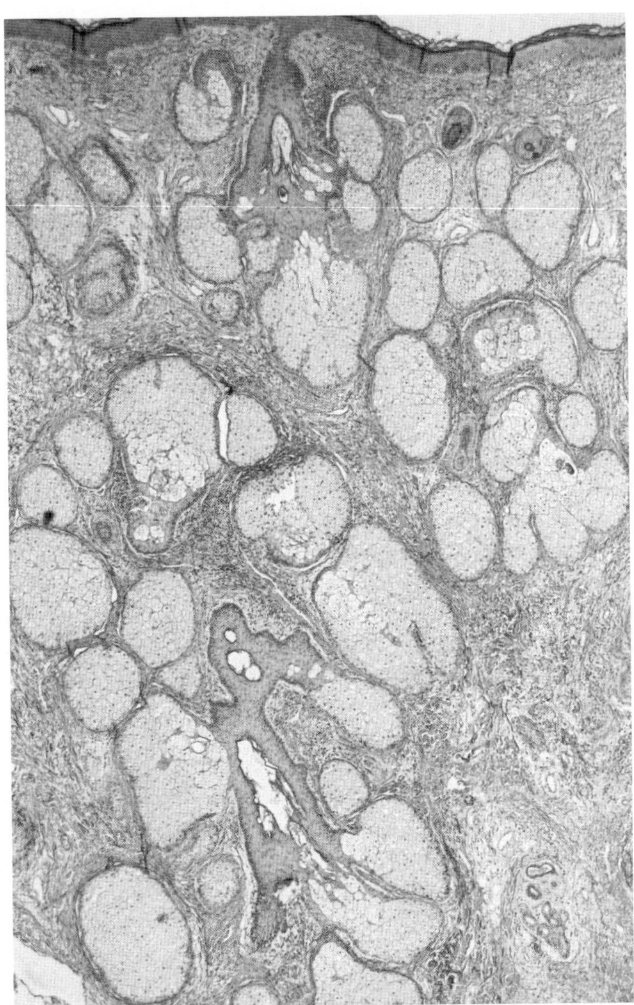

FIGURE 99. Rhinophyma. Hypertrophic sebaceous glands with prominent sebaceous duct hyperkeratosis and periadnexal chronic inflammation.

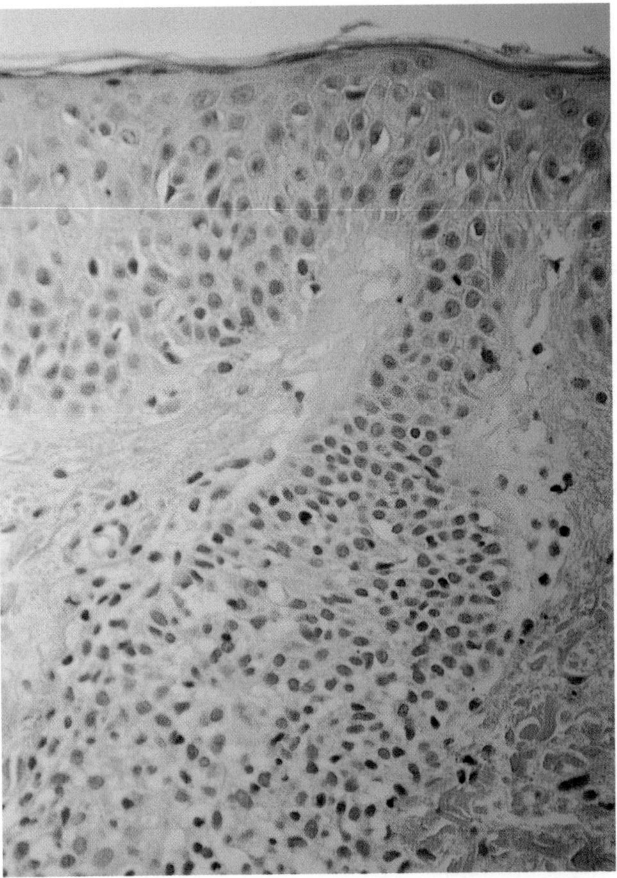

FIGURE 100. Eosinophilic pustular folliculitis. Intercellular edema of the hair follicle epithelium (follicular spongiosis) and eosinophils within the spongiotic foci.

Alopecia Mucinosa (Follicular Mucinosis)

Alopecia mucinosa may occur in an idiopathic form and in association with mycosis fungoides (a form of cutaneous T-cell lymphoma, see above). The benign idiopathic form most commonly affects children and young adults. The cutaneous lesions arise as grouped erythematous papules or indurated plaques, usually confined to the head and neck. The lymphoma-associated type of alopecia mucinosa is a disease of adults and is often more widely disseminated than the idiopathic form (411–413). The most striking histologic feature of alopecia mucinosa is the accumulation of hyaluronic acid within the outer root sheath epithelium of the hair follicles (follicular mucinosis) (Fig. 101). It is accompanied by reticular degeneration or spongiosis of the hair follicle epithelium. The mucin forms intrafollicular cystic spaces containing weakly basophilic mucin that stains positively with PAS, toluidine blue, alcian blue, and colloidal iron stains. In addition to the follicular changes, there is a variably dense lymphohistiocytic infiltrate with scattered eosinophils. Associated changes may include hyperplasia and infiltration of the eccrine glands, termed syringolymphoid hy-

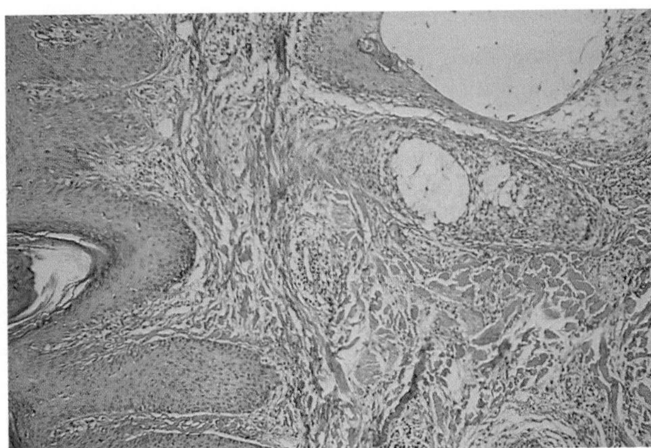

FIGURE 101. Alopecia mucinosa. Basophilic mucin is deposited between the keratinocytes of the hair follicle epithelium, forming intrafollicular mucin-containing microvesicles (follicular mucinosis). Also present is a perivascular infiltrate of lymphocytes with scattered eosinophils.

perplasia (414–416). Distinguishing the idiopathic from the paraneoplastic form of alopecia mucinosa is often difficult (417). Although there is some controversy as to which histologic features are most helpful, the presence of a markedly atypical lymphoid infiltrate with epidermotropism of atypical cells strongly favors the diagnosis of mycosis fungoides–associated follicular mucinosis (418,419).

Follicular Occlusion Triad

The follicular occlusion triad includes acne conglobata, hidradenitis suppurativa, and perifolliculitis capitis abscedens et suffodiens. These three processes with a primary pathogenesis of follicular hyperkeratosis occur on the buttocks and chest, axillae and groin, and scalp, respectively. The histologic findings include follicular hyperkeratosis with plugging and ectasia of the follicular infundibulum. Follicular rupture with associated granulomatous inflammation and abscess formation is usually present. Apocrine glands are often secondarily involved. Indeed, the predilection of hidradenitis suppurativa at sites where apocrine glands are numerous (axillae and groin) led to the original hypothesis that this is a disorder of apocrine glands, hence the term hidradenitis. It is now believed that follicular hyperkeratosis leads to plugging of the hair follicle. The apocrine duct normally empties apocrine secretions into the hair follicle; thus plugging of the hair follicle leads to secondary changes of the apocrine unit.

Herpes Folliculitis

Herpes folliculitis is a manifestation of herpes simplex virus infection that is particularly prevalent in patients with acquired immune deficiency syndrome (AIDS). The histologic findings in herpes folliculitis include hyperplasia of the follicular epithelium with squamotization of the basal layer epithelium. The characteristic cytopathic changes of herpes viral infection (multinucleate cells, "ground glass" appearance of nuclei with chromatin margination, eosinophilic intranuclear inclusions) are observed in the keratinocytes of the hair follicle outer root sheath. There is usually a surrounding dense mononuclear inflammatory infiltrate.

Lichen Planopilaris (Follicular Lichen Planus)

Lichen planopilaris predominantly affects the scalp and presents as erythematous hyperkeratotic follicular papules, which ultimately may develop into scarring alopecia. Typical cutaneous or mucosal lesions of lichen planus may also be present in patients with lichen planopilaris.

The histologic features of lichen planopilaris are similar to those of lichen planus but are centered around the epithelium of hair follicles rather than the interfollicular epidermis. In addition to prominent keratotic plugging of follicular infundibulae, there is a dense mononuclear cell infiltrate along the interface of the hair follicle epithelium and the dermis. Squamotization of the basal layer follicular epithelium and formation of spaces between the follicular epithelium and the dermis are characteristic findings. In addition, the adventitial dermis immediately surrounding the follicle shows a characteristic pattern of fibrosis.

INFECTIOUS DISEASES

Bacterial

Impetigo (Impetigo Contagiosa, Nonbullous Impetigo)

Impetigo contagiosa is a disease of school-aged children that presents as vesicles and pustules that develop thick yellow crusts. *Staphylococcus aureus* is the most common associated organism; group A streptococci may be the pathogenic organism in some cases. Rarely impetigo is associated with acute glomerulonephritis. The histologic findings in impetigo include an intraepidermal vesicle containing numerous neutrophils, occasionally with gram-positive cocci. There is an overlying scale crust with serous exudate and nuclear debris.

Ecthyma (Ecthyma gangrenosum)

Ecthyma gangrenosum is a cutaneous manifestation of *Pseudomonas* sepsis and presents as punched-out ulcers with hemorrhagic borders or erythematous nodules. The histologic features of ecthyma are similar to those of impetigo with more prominent ulceration and include intraepidermal neutrophilic pustules with epidermal ulceration associated with extensive scale crust and gram-negative bacilli within the superficial epidermis.

Furuncle (Acute Deep Folliculitis)

Furuncles present as fluctuant nodules, commonly on the scalp, and are sequelae of acute folliculitis. The histologic features of a furuncle include a deep dermal perifollicular neutrophilic abscess with multinucleate giant cells, keratinaceous debris, fragments of hair shaft, and, occasionally, colonies of bacterial cocci.

Leprosy

Leprosy is a chronic infection that usually involves the nasal mucosa and skin and is caused by *Mycobacterium leprae.* There are a number of clinical forms of leprosy ranging from lepromatous to tuberculoid (420). In addition, there is an indeterminate form as well as several acute reactional states that may interrupt the usual chronic course of leprosy. A thorough discussion of leprosy is beyond the scope of this text; only the histologic findings of lepromatous and tuberculoid leprosy are described. The characteristic features of lepromatous leprosy include a superficial and deep dermal lymphohistiocytic infiltrate separated from the epidermis by a grenz zone of uninvolved papillary dermis (Fig. 102). There is often a linear extension of foamy histiocytes along neurovascular bundles observed at scanning magnification. These linear granulomas are helpful in distinguishing leprosy from other forms of granulomatous inflammation. Histiocytes with foamy cytoplasm containing numerous acid-fast lepra bacilli are termed lepra cells or Virchow cells. The acid-fast bacilli are best demonstrated with a modified Ziehl-Neelsen or Fite stain. In tuberculoid leprosy, epithelioid granulomas are observed, and there are fewer detectable organisms. For treatment purposes, the lesions are termed paucibacillary (no detectable organisms) or multibacillary (one or many organisms) (421,422).

Rhinoscleroma

Rhinoscleroma, caused by *Klebsiella rhinoscleromatis* (Frisch bacilli), involves the upper respiratory tract and skin of the nose and upper lip (also see Chapter 4). The histologic features of

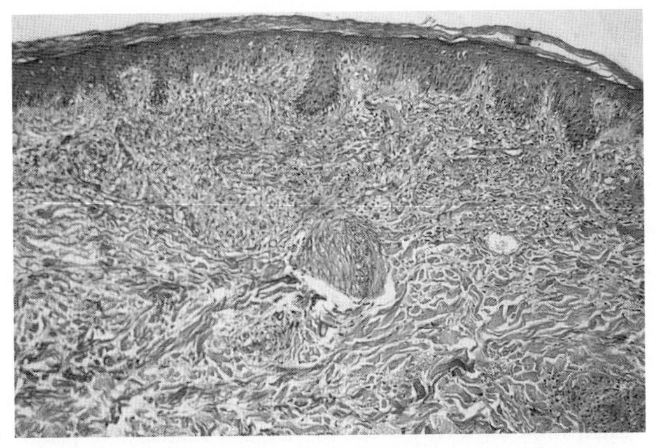
A

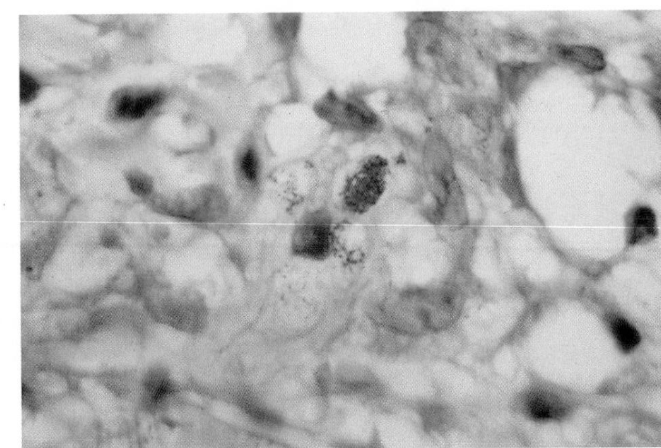
C

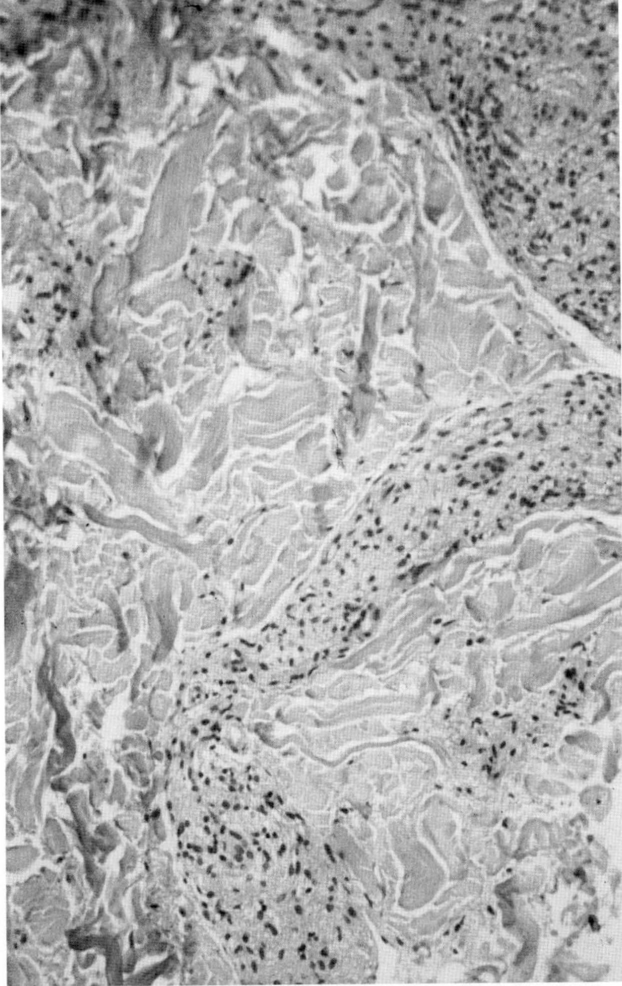
B

FIGURE 102. Leprosy. **A:** Superficial perivascular lymphohistiocytic infiltrate separated from the epidermis by a grenz zone of uninvolved papillary dermis. **B:** Linear extension of foamy histiocytes along neurovascular bundles. **C:** Foamy histiocytes containing numerous microorganisms (lepra cells, Virchow cells). Intracellular acid-fast bacilli stain fuchsia with a modified Ziehl-Neelsen (Fite) stain.

rhinoscleroma include variable epidermal hyperplasia with a dense dermal chronic inflammatory infiltrate composed of histiocytes, lymphocytes, and numerous plasma cells. In the full-blown active stage of the disease, the histiocytes (Mikulicz cells) contain numerous Frisch bacilli. Gram-negative Frisch bacilli are 2 to 3 μm in diameter and are best seen with a Warthin-Starry stain. Many of the plasma cells contain homogeneous intracytoplasmic eosinophilic globules termed Russell bodies. Russell bodies are PAS positive, diastase resistant, and represent aggregates of immunoglobulin. When lesions persist, they may develop a striking pseudoepitheliomatous hyperplasia with underlying dermal fibrosis and may be mistaken for well-differentiated squamous cell carcinoma.

Bacillary Angiomatosis (Bartonellosis)

Bacillary angiomatosis is most often associated with AIDS and presents as erythematous or brownish papules at any site including the mucosa. This disorder is caused by *Bartonella henselae*

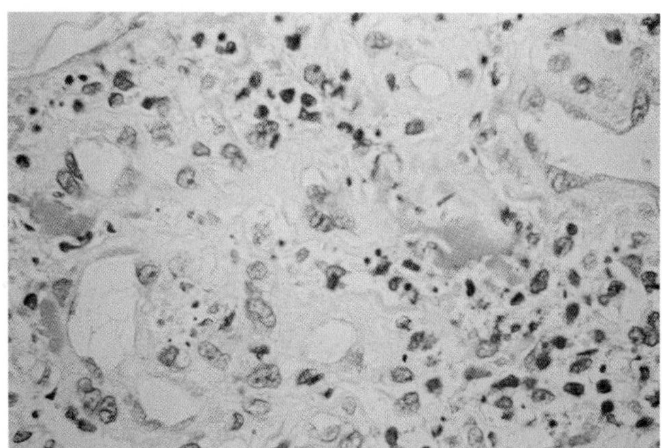

FIGURE 103. Bacillary angiomatosis. A proliferation of small capillaries with stromal edema, nuclear debris, and aggregates of amphophilic, finely granular, interstitial material representing clumps of bacterial organisms.

and *Bartonella quintana* and is histologically similar to the lesions of bartonellosis caused by *Bartonella bacilliformis* (423,424). The histologic features of bacillary angiomatosis include epidermal hyperplasia with a collarette of epidermis engulfing a vascular proliferation histologically resembling pyogenic granuloma. In addition to a proliferation of small capillaries and venules, there is prominent stromal edema with nuclear debris and aggregates of amphophilic, finely granular, interstitial material (Fig. 103). This amphophilic material represents clumps of bacterial organisms that may be observed with Warthin-Starry or Dieterle stains.

Fungal and Protozoal

Dermatophytes

Dermatophytes are keratinophilic fungi that cause ringworm and tinea. There are three genera of dermatophytes: *Trichophyton, Microsporum,* and *Epidermophyton.* Cutaneous dermatophyte infections are usually separated based on the site of involvement: tinea capitis (head), tinea faciei (face), tinea barbae (beard), tinea cruris (groin), tinea pedis (feet), onychomycosis (nails), and tinea corporis (body). Clinically the lesions may have a variety of appearances (425). Tinea capitis presents as a pustular folliculitis and occasionally progresses to form a suppurative boggy nodule termed a kerion or an alopecic lesion with yellow crust termed favus (426). Tinea faciei is rare and presents as scaling and erythema. Tinea pedis, or athlete's foot, presents as sharply demarcated erythematous fissured and scaling lesions on the soles. Majocchi's granuloma is a deep dermatophyte infection that occurs on the lower extremity and scalp (427). Tinea barbae, tinea corporis, and tinea cruris have similar clinical features; most commonly an erythematous annular centrifugally expanding lesion is observed.

Histologically the changes observed in dermatophyte infection are also quite varied. The epidermis usually displays some degree of spongiosis (intercellular edema accentuating the spinous connections between keratinocytes). The stratum corneum often contains neutrophils but may display septate hyphae sandwiched between layers of noninflamed compact orthohyperkeratosis keratin without nuclei, in contrast to parakeratosis, which has retained keratinocyte nuclei (428,429). Dermatophytes are septate hyphal organisms that may invade the dermis and lead to granulomatous inflammation as in Majocchi's granuloma. Invasion of the hair shaft may be observed in tinea capitis, and when organisms are limited to the hair shaft, they are termed endothrix. Dermatophytes stain positively with the PAS stain and are resistant to diastase digestion (Fig. 104).

Candidiasis

Monilial infections of the head and neck are most commonly located at the angles of the mouth (angular stomatitis or perlesch), in the oral mucosa (thrush), or on the tongue (median rhomboid glossitis) (430). In some patients oral candidiasis is the initial manifestation of AIDS (431). *Candida* is a budding yeast that forms chains of elongated yeasts resembling hyphae, termed pseudohyphae. The histologic features of candidiasis include intraepithelial aggregates of neutrophils with variable hyperkeratosis, epithelial hyperplasia, and spongiosis. There is usually an underlying mononuclear cell infiltrate with stromal edema. The yeasts and pseudohyphae are observed in the hyperkeratotic stratum corneum and stain positively with Gomori methenamine silver (GMS) stain and PAS stain and are resistant to diastase digestion.

Viral Infections

Verruca Vulgaris

Human papilloma virus causes a variety of cutaneous lesions including verruca vulgaris, the common wart (432). Children are most often affected, developing verrucous keratotic papules on the fingers and distal extremities. Warts may also occur in adults and may be extensive in size and number in immunosuppressed patients. Verruca vulgaris may occur at sites of trauma, particularly on the face following shaving.

Histologically there is marked epithelial hyperplasia with acanthosis and hyperkeratosis. The lower tips of the epithelial rete curve inward toward the center of the lesion, and the su-

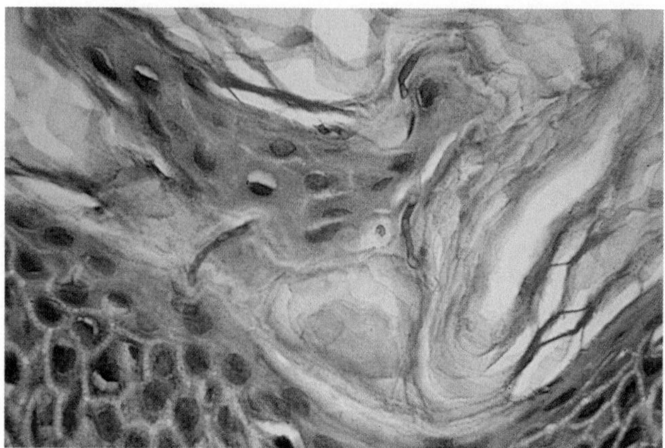

FIGURE 104. Dermatophyte. Septate hyphae in the stratum corneum stain magenta with PAS and diastase stain.

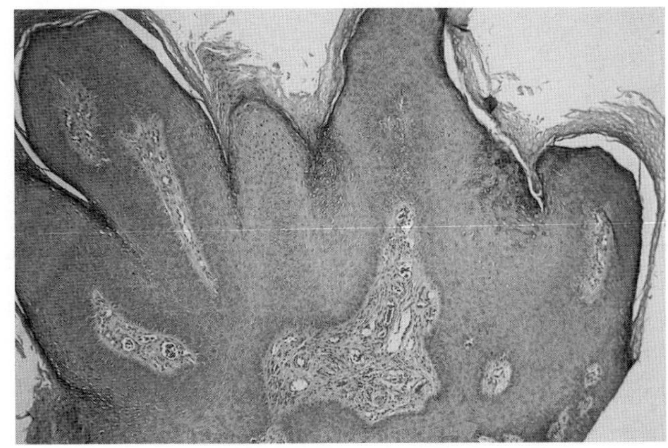

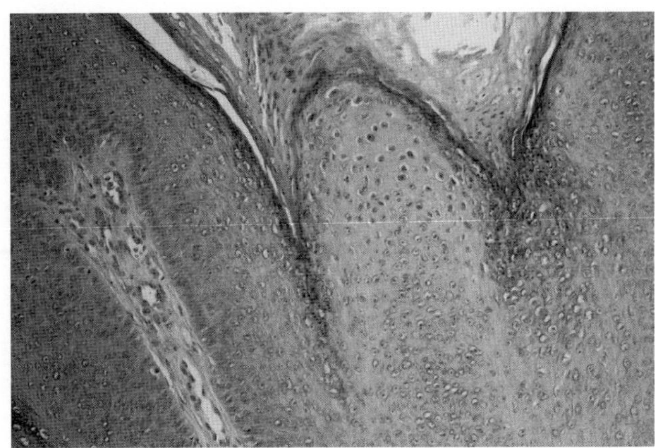

FIGURE 105. Verruca vulgaris. **A:** Epithelial hyperplasia with acanthosis and hyperkeratosis and curving of the epithelial rete toward the center of the lesion; tiers of parakeratosis alternate with valleys of superficial epidermal hypergranulosis. **B:** Ectatic blood-filled capillaries in the dermal papillae, parakeratosis overlying the epidermal rete ridges with keratohyaline granule clumping, nuclear hyperchromatism, crinkling of the keratinocytic nuclei, and perinuclear vacuole formation in the valleys between epidermal rete ridges.

perficial rete ridges form peaks and spires (Fig. 105). There may be erythrocyte extravasation into the stratum corneum, orthohyperkeratosis is observed in the valleys of stratum corneum, and tiers of parakeratosis cap the rete ridges. The epidermal granular cell layer may be absent at the tips of the rete underlying the parakeratosis; however, there is usually a prominent and thickened granular cell layer in the valleys of the epidermal rete. Occasionally koilocytic atypia with keratohyaline granule clumping, nuclear hyperchromatism, crinkling of the nuclear outline, and perinuclear vacuole formation are observed. These latter cytologic changes are not required, however, for a diagnosis of verruca. Usually the dermal changes are minimal and may include a mild perivascular mononuclear infiltrate.

Herpes Simplex

Herpes simplex virus, type 1 (HSV-1) and herpes simplex virus, type 2 (HSV-2) are the two main types of herpes simplex virus. HSV-1 causes most of the lesions of herpes to affect the skin and mucosa of the head and neck. In addition to the common perioral lesions known as cold sores, HSV-1 may cause lesions of the oral cavity, esophagus, eye, and pharynx. HSV causes a chronic infection of the sensory ganglia; lesions can be precipitated by a variety of factors including sunlight, fever, and stress. The cutaneous lesions present as crops of vesicles that ultimately rupture and develop serous crusts and may heal with scarring.

The histologic features of herpes simplex virus infection include epithelial acantholysis and ballooning degeneration. Ballooning degeneration causes a reticular or fenestrated appearance of the epithelium because of retained keratinocyte plasma membranes and cytoplasmic tonofilaments in the setting of intracellular keratinocytic edema with nuclear dropout. This is a characteristic histologic change observed in a variety of viral infections including viral exanthem. In HSV infection there is usually also epithelial necrosis and an overlying scale crust. The keratinocytic nuclei show a number of characteristic cytologic changes including the formation of multinucleate cells with closely packed or "molded" nuclei (Fig. 106). The nuclei often

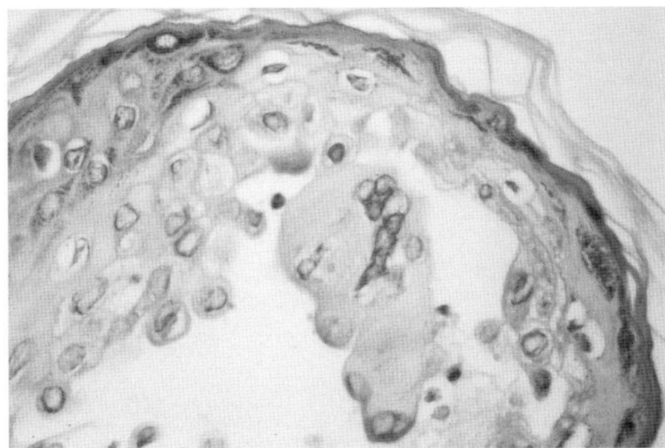

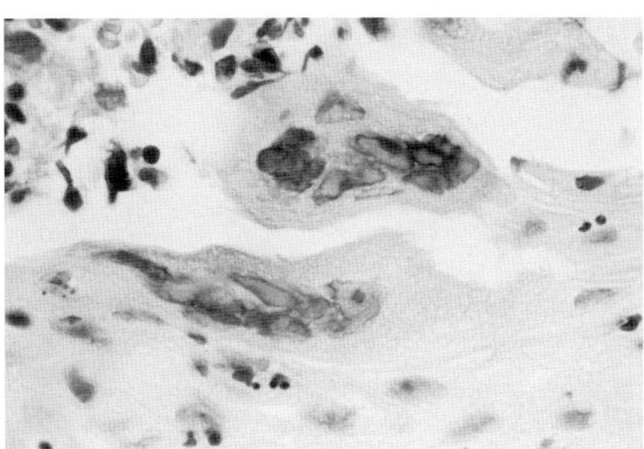

FIGURE 106. Herpes simplex. **A:** Epithelial necrosis with acantholysis, multinucleate cells with nuclear molding, and a delicate "ground-glass" chromatin pattern. **B:** Multinucleate cells with nuclear molding "ground-glass" chromatin and intranuclear eosinophilic inclusions.

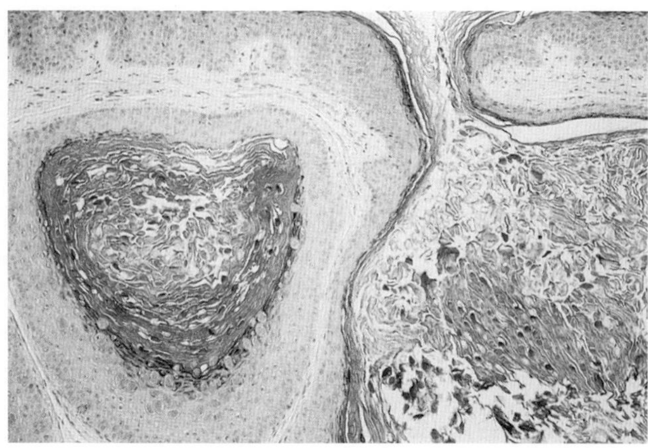

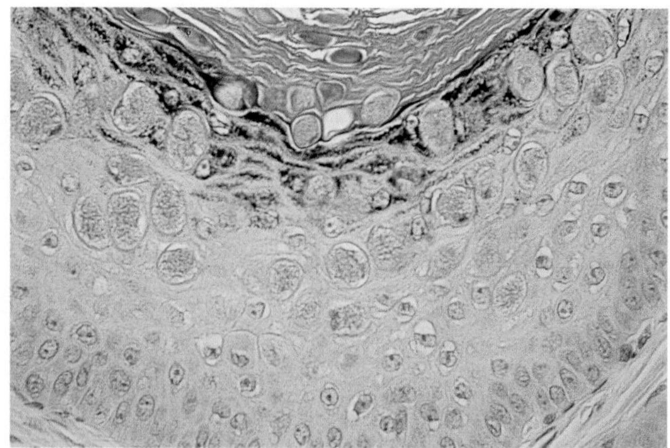

FIGURE 107. Molluscum contagiosum. **A:** Endophytic epidermal hyperplasia forms a central crater containing keratin and molluscum bodies (Henderson-Patterson bodies). **B:** Intracytoplasmic granular eosinophilic molluscum bodies compress the keratinocyte nuclei. Molluscum bodies are more solid and homogeneous in the stratum corneum.

display a delicate "ground-glass" chromatin pattern. Cowdry type A eosinophilic intranuclear inclusions are also frequently present (433). Involvement of the hair follicle epithelium is termed herpetic folliculitis and is particularly prevalent in patients with AIDS.

Molluscum Contagiosum

Molluscum contagiosum occurs as a dome-shaped papule with a central umbilication measuring up to a centimeter in diameter. Waxy material is usually easily expressed from the papule. Lesions are usually multiple and may be extensive in immunosuppressed patients and patients with AIDS. The lesions are caused by a poxvirus (434).

Histologically there is prominent endophytic volcano-like hyperplasia of the epidermis with a central crater containing keratin and molluscum bodies (Henderson-Patterson bodies) (Fig. 107). Molluscum bodies are intracytoplasmic homogeneous or slightly granular eosinophilic inclusion bodies. The molluscum bodies are largest at the epidermal surface and compress the keratinocyte nuclei. The inclusion bodies become more homogeneous and basophilic when they traverse the stratum granulosum.

Oral Hairy Leukoplakia

Oral hairy leukoplakia is caused by Epstein-Barr virus (EBV) and occurs on the lateral tongue, usually in HIV-positive patients (435) (Table 9). Delicate epithelial hyperplasia and hyperkeratosis lead to the development of projections from the tongue, giving it a hairy appearance clinically.

Histologically there is epithelial hyperplasia with parakeratosis, hair-like projections of keratin, and ballooning degeneration of keratinocytes. Perinuclear cytoplasmic clearing and nuclear pyknosis (koilocytosis) with intranuclear eosinophilic inclusions and chromatin margination are diagnostic findings (Fig. 108). The intranuclear inclusions are often of ground-glass type as in herpetic infection (EBV is a herpes virus), and the nuclear chromatin characteristically encircles the inclusion near the nuclear membrane like a wreath. Epstein-Barr viral-encoded RNA (EBER) may be detected by *in situ* hybridization or polymerase chain reaction techniques.

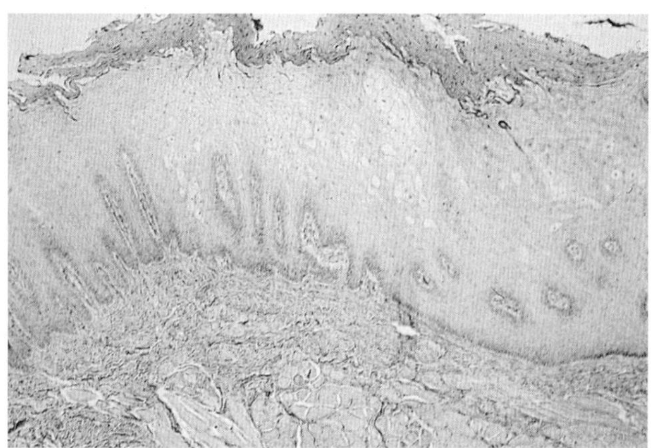

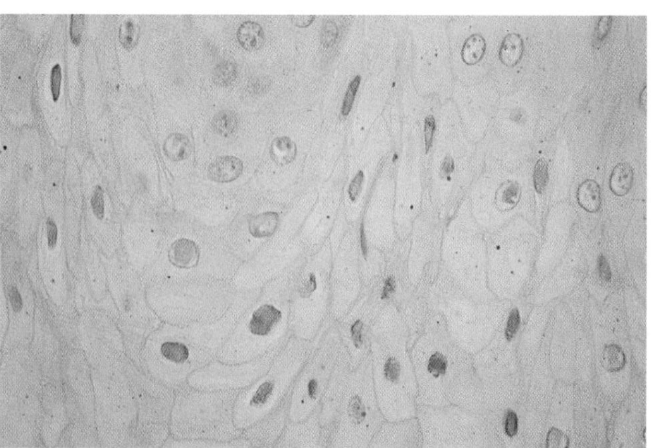

FIGURE 108. Hairy leukoplakia. **A:** Epithelial hyperplasia with parakeratosis, hair-like projections of keratin, and ballooning degeneration of keratinocytes. **B:** Keratinocytes display perinuclear cytoplasmic clearing and nuclear pyknosis with intranuclear eosinophilic inclusions and chromatin margination. Ground-glass–like amphophilic intranuclear inclusions are encircled by a wreath of nuclear chromatin.

REFERENCES

1. Atherton DJ, Pitcher DW, Wells RS, et al. A syndrome of various cutaneous pigmented lesions, myxoid neurofibromata and atrial myxoma: the NAME syndrome. *Br J Dermatol* 1980;103:421–429.
2. Rhodes AR, Silverman RA, Harrist TJ, et al. Mucocutaneous lentigines, cardiomucocutaneous myxomas, and multiple blue nevi: the "LAMB" syndrome. *J Am Acad Dermatol* 1984;10:72–82.
3. Jeghers H, McKusick VA, Katz KH. Generalized intestinal polyposis and melanin spots of the oral mucosa, lip and digits. A syndrome of diagnostic significance. *New Engl J Med* 1949;241:1031–1036.
4. Pinkus H. Keratosis senilis. A biologic concept of its pathogenesis and diagnosis based on the study of normal epidermis and 1730 seborrhoeic and senile keratoses. *Am J Clin Pathol* 1958;29:193–207.
5. Bailin PL, Levine HL, Wood BG, et al. Cutaneous carcinoma of the auricular and periauricular region. *Arch Otolaryngol* 1980;106: 692–696.
6. Chen KT, Dehner LP. Primary tumors of the external and middle ear. I. Introduction and clinicopathologic study of squamous cell carcinoma. *Arch Otolaryngol* 1978;104:247–252.
7. Shi SR, Bhan AK, Pilch BZ, et al. Immunohistochemical localization of keratin in head and neck neoplasms and normal tissues. *J Otolaryngol* 1985;14:323–329.
8. Whyte AM, Hansen LS, Lee C. The intraoral keratoacanthoma: a diagnostic problem. *Br J Oral Surg* 1986;24:438–441.
9. Cotran RS. Metastasizing basal cell carcinomas. *Cancer* 1961;14: 1036.
10. Swanson SA, Cooper PH, Mills SE, et al. Lymphoepithelioma-like carcinoma of the skin. *Mod Pathol* 1988;1:359–365.
11. Michaelsson G, Olsson E, Westermark P. The Rombo syndrome: a familial disorder with vermiculate atrophoderma, milia, hypotrichosis, trichoepitheliomas, basal cell carcinomas and peripheral vasodilation with cyanosis. *Acta Derm Venereol* 1981;61:497–503.
12. Brownstein MH, Wolf M, Bikowski JB. Cowden's disease: a cutaneous marker of breast cancer. *Cancer* 1978;41:2393–2398.
13. Brownstein MH, Shapiro L. Desmoplastic trichoepithelioma. *Cancer* 1977;40:2979–2986.
14. Zuccati G, Massi D, Mastrolorenzo A, et al. Desmoplastic trichoepithelioma. *Australas J Dermatol* 1998;39:273–274.
15. Goldstein DJ, Barr RJ, Santa Cruz DJ. Microcystic adnexal carcinoma: a distinct clinicopathologic entity. *Cancer* 1982;50:566–572.
16. Imber MJ. Benign cutaneous lesions potentially misdiagnosed as malignant neoplasms. *Semin Diagn Pathol* 1990;7:139–145.
17. Takei Y, Fukushiro S, Ackerman AB. Criteria for histologic differentiation of desmoplastic trichoepithelioma (sclerosing epithelial hamartoma) from morphea-like basal-cell carcinoma. *Am J Dermatopathol* 1985;7:207–221.
18. Triantafyllou A, Scott J, Blacklock A. Desmoplastic trichoepithelioma of the upper lip. A case report with histochemical features and observations on its histogenesis. *Oral Surg Oral Med Oral Pathol Oral Radiol Endod* 1995;80:445–450.
19. West AJ, Hunt SJ, Goltz RW. Solitary facial plaque of long duration. Desmoplastic trichoepithelioma. *Arch Dermatol* 1995;131:213.
20. Wick MR, Swanson PE. *Cutaneous adnexal tumors: a guide to pathological diagnosis.* Chicago: ASCP Press, 1991:238.
21. Wick MR, Cooper PH, Swanson PE, et al. Microcystic adnexal carcinoma. An immunohistochemical comparison with other cutaneous appendage tumors. *Arch Dermatol* 1990;126:189–194.
22. Yoshimura Y, Obara S, Mikami T, et al. Calcifying epithelioma (pilomatrixoma) of the head and neck: analysis of 37 cases. *Br J Oral Maxillofac Surg* 1997;35:429–432.
23. Kumasa S, Mori H, Tsujimura T, et al. Calcifying epithelioma of Malherbe with ossification. Special reference to lectin binding and immunohistochemistry of ossified sites. *J Cutan Pathol* 1987;14: 181–187.
24. Kaddu S, Beham-Schmid C, Soyer HP, et al. Extramedullary hematopoiesis in pilomatricomas. *Am J Dermatopathol* 1995;17: 126–130.
25. Lopansri S, Mihm MC Jr. Pilomatrix carcinoma or calcifying epitheliocarcinoma of Malherbe: a case report and review of literature. *Cancer* 1980;45:2368–2373.
26. Brownstein MH, Arluk DJ. Proliferating trichilemmal cyst: a simulant of squamous cell carcinoma. *Cancer* 1981;48:1207–1214.
27. Laing V, Knipe RC, Flowers FP, et al. Proliferating trichilemmal tumor: report of a case and review of the literature. *J Dermatol Surg Oncol* 1991;17:295–298.
28. Winer LH. The dilated pore, a trichoepithelioma. *J Invest Dermatol* 1954;23:181–188.
29. Mehregan AH, Brownstein MH. Pilar sheath acanthoma. *Arch Dermatol* 1978;114:1495–1497.
30. Birt AR, Hogg GR, Dube WJ. Hereditary multiple fibrofolliculomas with trichodiscomas and acrochordons. *Arch Dermatol* 1977;113: 1674–1677.
31. Templeton SF. Folliculosebaceous cystic hamartoma: a clinical pathologic study. *J Am Acad Dermatol* 1996;34:77–81.
32. Kimura T, Miyazawa H, Aoyagi T, et al. Folliculosebaceous cystic hamartoma. A distinctive malformation of the skin. *Am J Dermatopathol* 1991;13:213–220.
33. Hagan WE. Nevus sebaceus of Jadassohn: the head and neck manifestations. *Laryngoscope* 1987;97:909–914.
34. Jones EW, Heyl T. Naevus sebaceus. A report of 140 cases with special regard to the development of secondary malignant tumours. *Br J Dermatol* 1970;82:99–117.
35. Lentz CL, Altman J, Mopper C. Nevus sebaceus of Jadassohn. Report of a case with multiple and extensive lesions and an unusual linear distribution. *Arch Dermatol* 1968;97:294–296.
36. Lantis S, Leyden J, Thew M, et al. Nevus sebaceus of Jadassohn. Part of a new neurocutaneous syndrome? *Arch Dermatol* 1968;98: 117–123.
37. Domingo J, Helwig EB. Malignant neoplasms associated with nevus sebaceus of Jadassohn. *J Am Acad Dermatol* 1979;1:545–556.
38. Chun K, Vazquez M, Sanchez JL. Nevus sebaceus: clinical outcome and considerations for prophylactic excision. *Int J Dermatol* 1995;34:538–541.
39. Alessi E, Wong SN, Advani HH, et al. Nevus sebaceus is associated with unusual neoplasms. An atlas. *Am J Dermatopathol* 1988;10: 116–127.
40. Alessi E, Sala F. Nevus sebaceus. A clinicopathologic study of its evolution. *Am J Dermatopathol* 1986;8:27–31.
41. Torre D. Multiple sebaceous tumors. *Arch Dermatol* 1968;98: 549–550.
42. Muir EG, Yates-Bell AJ, Barlow KA. Multiple primary carcinomata of the colon, duodenum, and larynx associated with kerato-acanthoma of the face. *Br J Surg* 1967;54:191–195.
43. Burgdorf WH, Pitha J, Fahmy A. Muir-Torre syndrome. Histologic spectrum of sebaceous proliferations. *Am J Dermatopathol* 1986; 8:202–208.
44. Cohen PR, Kohn SR, Kurzrock R. Association of sebaceous gland tumors and internal malignancy: the Muir-Torre syndrome. *Am J Med* 1991;90:606–613.
45. Hall NR, Murday VA, Chapman P, et al. Genetic linkage in Muir-Torre syndrome to the same chromosomal region as cancer family syndrome. *Eur J Cancer* 1994;30A:180–182.
46. Cohen PR, Kohn SR, Davis DA, et al. Muir-Torre syndrome. *Dermatol Clin* 1995;13:79–89.
47. Bapat B, Xia L, Madlensky L, et al. The genetic basis of Muir-Torre syndrome includes the hMLH1 locus. *Am J Hum Genet* 1996;59: 736–739.
48. Suspiro A, Fidalgo P, Cravo M, et al. The Muir-Torre syndrome: a rare variant of hereditary nonpolyposis colorectal cancer associated with hMSH2 mutation. *Am J Gastroenterol* 1998;93: 1572–1574.
49. Lynch HT, Leibowitz R, Smyrk T, et al. Colorectal cancer and the Muir-Torre syndrome in a Gypsy family: a review. *Am J Gastroenterol* 1999;94:575–580.
50. Cohen PR. Muir-Torre syndrome in patients with hematologic malignancies. *Am J Hematol* 1992;40:64–65.

51. Zackheim HS. The sebaceous epithelioma. *Arch Dermatol* 1964;89: 711–724.
52. McMullan FH. Sebaceous epithelioma. *Arch Dermatol* 1955;71: 725–727.
53. Lasser A, Carter DM. Multiple basal cell epitheliomas with sebaceous differentiation. *Arch Dermatol* 1973;107:91–93.
54. Urban FH, Winkelmann RK. Sebaceous malignancy. *Arch Dermatol* 1961;84:113–122.
55. Rothko K, Farmer ER, Zeligman I. Superficial epithelioma with sebaceous differentiation. *Arch Dermatol* 1980;116:329–331.
56. Brownstein MH, Shapiro L. The pilosebaceous tumors. *Int J Dermatol* 1977;16:340–352.
57. Akpek EK, Polcharoen W, Chan R, et al. Ocular surface neoplasia masquerading as chronic blepharoconjunctivitis. *Cornea* 1999;18: 282–288.
58. Rao NA, Hidayat AA, McLean IW, et al. Sebaceous carcinomas of the ocular adnexa: A clinicopathologic study of 104 cases, with five-year follow-up data. *Hum Pathol* 1982;13:113–122.
59. Ni C, Kuo PK. Meibomian gland carcinoma: a clinicopathological study of 156 cases with long-period follow-up of 100 cases. *Jpn J Ophthalmol* 1979;23:388–401.
60. Wolfe JTD, Yeatts RP, Wick MR, et al. Sebaceous carcinoma of the eyelid. Errors in clinical and pathologic diagnosis. *Am J Surg Pathol* 1984;8:597–606.
61. Zurcher M, Hintschich CR, Garner A, et al. Sebaceous carcinoma of the eyelid: a clinicopathological study. *Br J Ophthalmol* 1998;82: 1049–1055.
62. Russell WG, Page DL, Hough AJ, et al. Sebaceous carcinoma of meibomian gland origin. The diagnostic importance of pagetoid spread of neoplastic cells. *Am J Clin Pathol* 1980;73:504–511.
63. Awan KJ. Sebaceous carcinoma of the eyelid. *Ann Ophthalmol* 1977;9:608–610.
64. Boniuk M, Zimmerman LE. Sebaceous carcinoma of the eyelid, eyebrow, caruncle, and orbit. *Trans Am Acad Ophthalmol Otolaryngol* 1968;72:619–642.
65. Foster CS, Allansmith MR. Chronic unilateral blepharoconjunctivitis caused by sebaceous carcinoma. *Am J Ophthalmol* 1978;86:218–220.
66. Helwig EB, Hackney VC. Syringocystadenoma papilliferum. *Arch Dermatol* 1955;71:361–372.
67. Grund JL. Syringocystadenoma papilliferum and nevus sebaceus (Jadassohn) occuring as a single tumor. *Arch Dermatol* 1952;65: 340–347.
68. Welch JP, Wells RS, Kerr CB. Ancell-Spiegler cylindromas (turban tumours) and Brooke-Fordyce trichoepitheliomas: evidence for a single genetic entity. *J Med Genet* 1968;5:29–35.
69. Aurora AL, Luxenberg MN. Case report of adenocarcinoma of glands of Moll. *Am J Ophthalmol* 1970;70:984–990.
70. Hashimoto K, DiBella RJ, Borsuk GM, et al. Eruptive hidradenoma and syringoma. Histological, histochemical, and electron microscopic studies. *Arch Dermatol* 1967;96:500–519.
71. Pinkus H, Rogin JR, Goldman P. Eccrine poroma. *Arch Dermatol* 1956;74:511–521.
72. Hu CH, Marques AS, Winkelmann RK. Dermal duct tumor: a histochemical and electron microscopic study. *Arch Dermatol* 1978;114: 1659–1664.
73. Hassab-el-Naby HM, Tam S, White WL, et al. Mixed tumors of the skin. A histological and immunohistochemical study. *Am J Dermatopathol* 1989;11:413–428. [Published erratum appears in *Am J Dermatopathol* 1990;12:108.]
74. Hirsch P, Helwig EB. Chondroid syringoma. *Arch Dermatol* 1961;84: 835–847.
75. Headington JT. Mixed tumors of the skin. *Arch Dermatol* 1961;84: 989–996.
76. Fernandez RJ. Mixed tumors of the skin of the salivary gland type. *J Invest Dermatol* 1976;60:49–58.
77. Harrist TJ, Aretz TH, Mihm MC Jr, et al. Cutaneous malignant mixed tumor. *Arch Dermatol* 1981;117:719–724.
78. Rosborough D. Malignant mixed tumours of the skin. *Br J Surg* 1963; 50:697–699.
79. Metzler G, Schaumburg-Lever G, Hornstein O, et al. Malignant chondroid syringoma: immunohistopathology. *Am J Dermatopathol* 1996;18:83–89.
80. Trown K, Heenan PJ. Malignant mixed tumor of the skin (malignant chondroid syringoma). *Pathology* 1994;26:237–243.
81. Kersting DW, Helwig EB. Eccrine spiradenoma. *Arch Dermatol* 1956;73:199–227.
82. Mambo NC. Eccrine spiradenoma: clinical and pathologic study of 49 tumors. *J Cutan Pathol* 1983;10:312–320.
83. Wick MR, Swanson PE, Kaye VN, et al. Sweat gland carcinoma *ex* eccrine spiradenoma. *Am J Dermatopathol* 1987;9:90–98.
84. McKee PH, Fletcher CD, Stavrinos P, et al. Carcinosarcoma arising in eccrine spiradenoma. A clinicopathologic and immunohistochemical study of two cases. *Am J Dermatopathol* 1990;12:335–343.
85. Evans HL, Su D, Smith JL, et al. Carcinoma arising in eccrine spiradenoma. *Cancer* 1979;43:1881–1884.
86. Cooper PH, Frierson HF Jr, Morrison AG. Malignant transformation of eccrine spiradenoma. *Arch Dermatol* 1985;121:1445–1448.
87. Winkelmann RK, Wolff K. Solid-cystic hidradenoma of the skin. Clinical and histopathologic study. *Arch Dermatol* 1968;97:651–661.
88. Kersting DW. Clear cell hidradenoma and hidradenocarcinoma. *Arch Dermatol* 1963;87:323–333.
89. O'Hara JM, Bensch K, Ioannides G, et al. Eccrine sweat gland adenoma, clear cell type. A histochemical study. *Cancer* 1966;19: 1438–1450.
90. Lever WF, Castleman B. Clear cell myo-epithelioma of the skin. Report of ten cases. *Am J Pathol* 1952;28:691–699.
91. Wong TY, Suster S, Nogita T, et al. Clear cell eccrine carcinomas of the skin. A clinicopathologic study of nine patients. *Cancer* 1994;73: 1631–1643.
92. Flieder A, Koerner FC, Pilch BZ, et al. Endocrine mucin-producing sweat gland carcinoma: a cutaneous neoplasm analogous to solid papillary carcinoma of breast. *Am J Surg Pathol* 1997;21:1501–1506.
93. Khan JA, Sutula FC, Pilch BZ, et al. Mucoepidermoid carcinoma involving the lacrimal sac. *Ophthal Plast Reconstr Surg* 1988;4:153–157.
94. Santa Cruz DJ. Sweat gland carcinomas: a comprehensive review. *Semin Diagn Pathol* 1987;4:38–74.
95. Seab JA, Graham JH. Primary cutaneous adenoid cystic carcinoma. *J Am Acad Dermatol* 1987;17:113–118.
96. Perzin KH, Gullane P, Conley J. Adenoid cystic carcinoma involving the external auditory canal. A clinicopathologic study of 16 cases. *Cancer* 1982;50:2873–2883.
97. Cooper PH, Mills SE, Leonard DD, et al. Sclerosing sweat duct (syringomatous) carcinoma. *Am J Surg Pathol* 1985;9:422–433.
98. Nickoloff BJ, Fleischmann HE, Carmel J, et al. Microcystic adnexal carcinoma. Immunohistologic observations suggesting dual (pilar and eccrine) differentiation. *Arch Dermatol* 1986;122:290–294.
99. Cooper PH. Sclerosing carcinomas of sweat ducts (microcystic adnexal carcinoma). *Arch Dermatol* 1986;122:261–264.
100. Massa MC, Medenica M. Cutaneous adnexal tumors and cysts: a review. Part II—Tumors with apocrine and eccrine glandular differentiation and miscellaneous cutaneous cysts. *Pathol Annu* 1987;22(Pt 1):225–276.
101. Barr RJ, Headley JL, Jensen JL, et al. Cutaneous keratocysts of nevoid basal cell carcinoma syndrome. *J Am Acad Dermatol* 1986;14: 572–576.
102. Leppard B, Bussey HJ. Epidermoid cysts, polyposis coli and Gardner's syndrome. *Br J Surg* 1975;62:387–393.
103. Narisawa Y, Kohda H. Cutaneous cysts of Gardner's syndrome are similar to follicular stem cells. *J Cutan Pathol* 1995;22:115–121.
104. Pinkus H. "Sebaceous cysts" are trichilemmal cysts. *Arch Dermatol* 1969;99:544–555.
105. Egbert BM, Price NM, Segal RJ. Steatocystoma multiplex. Report of a florid case and a review. *Arch Dermatol* 1979;115:334–335.
106. Esterly NB, Fretzin DF, Pinkus H. Eruptive vellus hair cysts. *Arch Dermatol* 1977;113:500–503.
107. Grimalt R, Gelmetti C. Eruptive vellus hair cysts: case report and review of the literature. *Pediatr Dermatol* 1992;9:98–102.

108. Betti R, Lodi A, Palvarini M, et al. Branchial cyst of the neck [letter]. *Br J Dermatol* 1992;127:195.
109. van der Putte SC, Toonstra J. Cutaneous "bronchogenic" cyst. *J Cutan Pathol* 1985;12:404–409.
110. Sanusi ID, Carrington PR, Adams DN. Cervical thymic cyst. *Arch Dermatol* 1982;118:122–124.
111. Fretzin DF, Helwig EB. Atypical fibroxanthoma of the skin. A clinicopathologic study of 140 cases. *Cancer* 1973;31:1541–1552.
112. Helwig EB. Atypical fibroxanthoma. *Texas J Med* 1963;59:664–667.
113. Helwig EB, May D. Atypical fibroxanthoma of the skin with metastasis. *Cancer* 1986;57:368–376.
114. Silvis NG, Swanson PE, Manivel JC, et al. Spindle-cell and pleomorphic neoplasms of the skin. A clinicopathologic and immunohistochemical study of 30 cases, with emphasis on "atypical fibroxanthomas." *Am J Dermatopathol* 1988;10:9–19.
115. Dehner LP. Malignant fibrous histiocytoma. Nonspecific morphologic pattern, specific pathologic entity, or both? [editorial]. *Arch Pathol Lab Med* 1988;112:236–237.
116. Wick MR, Fitzgibbon J, Swanson PE. Cutaneous sarcomas and sarcomatoid neoplasms of the skin. *Semin Diagn Pathol* 1993;10:148–158.
117. Calonje E, Wadden C, Wilson-Jones E, et al. Spindle-cell non-pleomorphic atypical fibroxanthoma: analysis of a series and delineation of a distinctive variant. *Histopathology* 1993;22:247–254.
118. Barnes L, Coleman JA Jr, Johnson JT. Dermatofibrosarcoma protuberans of the head and neck. *Arch Otolaryngol* 1984;110:398–404.
119. Mark RJ, Bailet JW, Tran LM, et al. Dermatofibrosarcoma protuberans of the head and neck. A report of 16 cases. *Arch Otolaryngol Head Neck Surg* 1993;119:891–896.
120. Rockley PF, Robinson JK, Magid M, et al. Dermatofibrosarcoma protuberans of the scalp: a series of cases. *J Am Acad Dermatol* 1989;21:278–283.
121. Suit H, Spiro I, Mankin HJ, et al. Radiation in management of patients with dermatofibrosarcoma protuberans. *J Clin Oncol* 1996;14:2365–2369.
122. Argiris A, Dardoufas C, Aroni K. Radiotherapy induced soft tissue sarcoma: an unusual case of a dermatofibrosarcoma protuberans. *Clin Oncol (R Coll Radiol)* 1995;7:59–61.
123. Fletcher CD, Evans BJ, MacArtney JC, et al. Dermatofibrosarcoma protuberans: a clinicopathological and immunohistochemical study with a review of the literature. *Histopathology* 1985;9:921–938.
124. Taylor HB, Helwig E. Dermatofibrosarcoma protuberans. A study of 115 cases. *Cancer* 1962;15:717–725.
125. Calonje E, Fletcher CD. Myoid differentiation in dermatofibrosarcoma protuberans and its fibrosarcomatous variant: clinicopathologic analysis of 5 cases. *J Cutan Pathol* 1996;23:30–36.
126. Dupree WB, Langloss JM, Weiss SW. Pigmented dermatofibrosarcoma protuberans (Bednar tumor). A pathologic, ultrastructural, and immunohistochemical study. *Am J Surg Pathol* 1985;9:630–639.
127. Fletcher CD, Theaker JM, Flanagan A, et al. Pigmented dermatofibrosarcoma protuberans (Bednar tumour): melanocytic colonization or neuroectodermal differentiation? A clinicopathological and immunohistochemical study. *Histopathology* 1988;13:631–643.
128. Frierson HF, Cooper PH. Myxoid variant of dermatofibrosarcoma protuberans. *Am J Surg Pathol* 1983;7:445–450.
129. Ding J, Hashimoto H, Enjoji M. Dermatofibrosarcoma protuberans with fibrosarcomatous areas. A clinicopathologic study of nine cases and a comparison with allied tumors. *Cancer* 1989;64:721–729.
130. O'Connell JX, Trotter MJ. Fibrosarcomatous dermatofibrosarcoma protuberans: a variant. *Mod Pathol* 1996;9:273–278.
131. Sato N, Kimura K, Tomita Y. Recurrent dermatofibrosarcoma protuberans with myxoid and fibrosarcomatous changes paralleled by loss of CD 34 expression. *J Dermatol* 1995;22:665–672.
132. Mentzel T, Beham A, Katenkamp D, et al. Fibrosarcomatous ("high-grade") dermatofibrosarcoma protuberans: clinicopathologic and immunohistochemical study of a series of 41 cases with emphasis on prognostic significance. *Am J Surg Pathol* 1998;22:576–587.
133. Weiss SW, Nickoloff BJ. CD-34 is expressed by a distinctive cell population in peripheral nerve, nerve sheath tumors, and related lesions. *Am J Surg Pathol* 1993;17:1039–1045.
134. Aiba S, Tabata N, Ishii H, et al. Dermatofibrosarcoma protuberans is a unique fibrohistiocytic tumour expressing CD34. *Br J Dermatol* 1992;127:79–84.
135. Kutzner H. Expression of the human progenitor cell antigen CD34 (HPCA-1) distinguishes dermatofibrosarcoma protuberans from fibrous histiocytoma in formalin-fixed, paraffin-embedded tissue. *J Am Acad Dermatol* 1993;28:613–617.
136. Ma CK, Zarbo RJ, Gown AM. Immunohistochemical characterization of atypical fibroxanthoma and dermatofibrosarcoma protuberans. *Am J Clin Pathol* 1992;97:478–483.
137. Haycox CL, Odland PB, Olbricht SM, et al. Immunohistochemical characterization of dermatofibrosarcoma protuberans with practical applications for diagnosis and treatment [see comments]. *J Am Acad Dermatol* 1997;37:438–444.
138. Goldblum JR, Tuthill RJ. CD34 and factor-XIIIa immunoreactivity in dermatofibrosarcoma protuberans and dermatofibroma. *Am J Dermatopathol* 1997;19:147–153.
139. Peterman AF, Hayes AB, Dockerty MB, et al. Encephalo-trigeminal angiomatosis (Sturge-Weber disease): clinical study of thirty-five cases. *JAMA* 1958;167:2169.
140. Royle HE, Lapp R, Ferrara ED, et al. The Sturge-Weber syndrome. *Oral Surg* 1966;22:490.
141. Straub PW, Kessler S, Schreiber A, et al. Chronic intravascular coagulation in Kasabach-Merritt syndrome. Preferential accumulation of fibrinogen ^{131}I in a giant hemangioma. *Arch Intern Med* 1972;129:475–478.
142. Kaplan RP, Wang JT, Amron NM, et al. Maffucci's syndrome: two case reports with a literature review. *J Am Acad Dermatol* 1993;29:894–899.
143. Loewinger RJ, Lichtenstein JR, Dodson WE, et al. Maffucci's syndrome: amesenchymal dysplasia and multiple tumour syndrome. *Br J Dermatol* 1977;96:317–322.
144. Ishii T, Asuwa N, Suzuki S, et al. Blue rubber bleb naevus syndrome. *Virchows Arch A Pathol Anat Histopathol* 1988;413:485–490.
145. Rosai J. Angiolymphoid hyperplasia with eosinophilia of the skin. Its nosological position in the spectrum of histiocytoid hemangioma. *Am J Dermatopathol* 1982;4:175–184.
146. Misselvish I, Podoshin L, Fradis M, et al. Angiolymphoid hyperplasia with eosinophilia of the oral mucous membrane. *Ear Nose Throat J* 1995;74:122–125.
147. Lopez JI, Battaglino SB. Angiolymphoid hyperplasia with eosinophilia of the lower lip. *Int J Dermatol* 1993;32:361–362.
148. Gyulai R, Kemeny L, Kiss M, et al. Herpesvirus-like DNA sequence in angiosarcoma in a patient without HIV infection. *N Engl J Med* 1996;334:540–541.
149. Gyulai R, Kemeny L, Adam E, et al. HHV8 DNA in angiolymphoid hyperplasia of the skin. *Lancet* 1996;347:1837.
150. Memar OM, Rady PL, Goldblum RM, et al. Human herpesvirus 8 DNA sequences in blistering skin from patients with pemphigus. *Arch Dermatol* 1997;133:1247–1251.
151. Di Alberti L, Piattelli A, Artese L, et al. Human herpesvirus 8 variants in sarcoid tissues. *Lancet* 1997;350:1655–1661.
152. Rettig MB, Ma HJ, Vescio RA, et al. Kaposi's sarcoma-associated herpesvirus infection of bone marrow dendritic cells from multiple myeloma patients. *Science* 1997;276:1851–1854.
153. Soulier J, Grollet L, Oksenhendler E, et al. Kaposi's sarcoma-associated herpesvirus-like DNA sequences in multicentric Castleman's disease. *Blood* 1995;86:1276–1280.
154. Cooper PH. Angiosarcomas of the skin. *Semin Diagn Pathol* 1987;4:2–17.
155. Holden CA, Spittle MF, Jones EW. Angiosarcoma of the face and scalp, prognosis and treatment. *Cancer* 1987;59:1046–1057.
156. Holden CA, Spaull J, Das AK, et al. The histogenesis of angiosarcoma of the face and scalp: an immunohistochemical and ultrastructural study. *Histopathology* 1987;11:37–51.
157. Handfield-Jones SE, Kennedy CT, Bradfield JB. Angiosarcoma arising in an angiomatous naevus following irradiation in childhood. *Br J Dermatol* 1988;118:109–112.

158. Caldwell JB, Ryan MT, Benson PM, et al. Cutaneous angiosarcoma arising in the radiation site of a congenital hemangioma. *J Am Acad Dermatol* 1995;33:865–870.
159. Goette DK, Detlefs RL. Postirradiation angiosarcoma. *J Am Acad Dermatol* 1985;12:922–926.
160. Hitchcock MG, Hurt MA, Santa Cruz DJ. Cutaneous granular cell angiosarcoma. *J Cutan Pathol* 1994;21:256–262.
161. Uhlin SR. Benign symmetric lipomatosis. *Arch Dermatol* 1979;115: 94–95.
162. Ruzicka T, Vieluf D, Landthaler M, et al. Benign symmetric lipomatosis Launois-Bensaude. Report of ten cases and review of the literature. *J Am Acad Dermatol* 1987;17:663–674.
163. Ross M, Goodman MM. Multiple symmetric lipomatosis (Launois-Bensaude syndrome). *Int J Dermatol* 1992;31:80–82.
164. Haberland C, Perou M. Encephalocraniocutaneous lipomatosis. A new example of ectomesodermal dysgenesis. *Arch Neurol* 1970;22: 144–155.
165. Fishman MA. Encephalocraniocutaneous lipomatosis. *J Child Neurol* 1987;2:186–193.
166. McCall S, Ramzy MI, Cure JK, et al. Encephalocraniocutaneous lipomatosis and the Proteus syndrome: distinct entities with overlapping manifestations. *Am J Med Genet* 1992;43:662–668.
167. Cohen MM Jr. Proteus syndrome: clinical evidence for somatic mosaicism and selective review. *Am J Med Genet* 1993;47:645–652.
168. Grosshams E, Fersing J, Marescaux J. Le lipome sous-aponevrotique frontal. *Ann Derm Venereol* 1987;114:335–340.
169. Salasche SJ, McCollough ML, Angeloni VL, et al. Frontalis-associated lipoma of the forehead. *J Am Acad Dermatol* 1989;20:462–468.
170. Slavin SA, Baker DC, McCarthy JG, et al. Congenital infiltrating lipomatosis of the face: clinicopathologic evaluation and treatment. *Plast Reconstr Surg* 1983;72:158–164.
171. Das Gupta TK, Brasfield RD, Strong EW, et al. Benign solitary Schwannomas (neurilemomas). *Cancer* 1969;24:355–366.
172. Dahl I, Hagmar B, Idvall I. Benign solitary neurilemmoma (schwannoma). A correlative cytological histologic study of 28 cases. *Acta Pathol Microbiol Scand [A]* 1984;92:91–101.
173. Reed RJ, Fine RM, Meltzer HD. Palisaded, encapsulated neuromas of the skin. *Arch Dermatol* 1972;106:865–870.
174. Fletcher CD. Solitary circumscribed neuroma of the skin (so-called palisaded, encapsulated neuroma). A clinicopathologic and immunohistochemical study. *Am J Surg Pathol* 1989;13:574–580.
175. Dover JS, From L, Lewis A. Palisaded encapsulated neuromas. A clinicopathologic study. *Arch Dermatol* 1989;125:386–389.
176. Megahed M. Palisaded encapsulated neuroma (solitary circumscribed neuroma). A clinicopathologic and immunohistochemical study. *Am J Dermatopathol* 1994;16:120–125.
177. Argenyi ZB. Immunohistochemical characterization of palisaded, encapsulated neuroma. *J Cutan Pathol* 1990;17:329–335.
178. Gallagher RL, Helwig EB. Neurothekeoma—a benign cutaneous tumor of neural origin. *Am J Clin Pathol* 1980;74:759–764.
179. Barnhill RL, Mihm MC Jr. Cellular neurothekeoma. A distinctive variant of neurothekeoma mimicking nevomelanocytic tumors. *Am J Surg Pathol* 1990;14:113–120.
180. Argenyi ZB, LeBoit PE, Santa Cruz D, et al. Nerve sheath myxoma (neurothekeoma) of the skin: light microscopic and immunohistochemical reappraisal of the cellular variant. *J Cutan Pathol* 1993; 20:294–303.
181. Husain S, Silvers DN, Halperin AJ, et al. Histologic spectrum of neurothekeoma and the value of immunoperoxidase staining for S-100 protein in distinguishing it from melanoma. *Am J Dermatopathol* 1994;16:496–503.
182. Barnhill RL. Nerve sheath myxoma (neurothekeoma). *J Cutan Pathol* 1994;21:91–93.
183. Argenyi ZB. Cutaneous neural heterotopias and related tumors relevant for the dermatopathologist. *Semin Diagn Pathol* 1996;13:60–71.
184. Theaker JM, Fletcher CD, Tudway AJ. Cutaneous heterotopic meningeal nodules. *Histopathology* 1990;16:475–479.
185. Penas PF, Jones-Caballero M, Garcia-Diez A. Cutaneous heterotopic meningeal nodules. *Arch Dermatol* 1995;131:731.
186. Suster S, Rosai J. Hamartoma of the scalp with ectopic meningothelial elements. A distinctive benign soft tissue lesion that may simulate angiosarcoma. *Am J Surg Pathol* 1990;14:1–11.
187. Barr RJ, Yi ES, Jensen JL, et al. Meningioma-like tumor of the skin. An ultrastructural and immunohistochemical study. *Am J Surg Pathol* 1993;17:779–787.
188. Toker C. Trabecular carcinoma of the skin. *Arch Dermatol* 1972;105: 107–110.
189. Tang CK, Toker C. Trabecular carcinoma of the skin: an ultrastructural study. *Cancer* 1978;42:2311–2321.
190. Sibley RK, Dehner LP, Rosai J. Primary neuroendocrine (Merkel cell?) carcinoma of the skin. I. A clinicopathologic and ultrastructural study of 43 cases. *Am J Surg Pathol* 1985;9:95–108.
191. Raaf JH, Urmacher C, Knapper WK, et al. Trabecular (Merkel cell) carcinoma of the skin. Treatment of primary, recurrent, and metastatic disease. *Cancer* 1986;57:178–182.
192. Chan JK, Suster S, Wenig BM, et al. Cytokeratin 20 immunoreactivity distinguishes Merkel cell (primary cutaneous neuroendocrine) carcinomas and salivary gland small cell carcinomas from small cell carcinomas of various sites. *Am J Surg Pathol* 1997;21:226–234.
193. LeBoit PE, Crutcher WA, Shapiro PE. Pagetoid intraepidermal spread in Merkel cell (primary neuroendocrine) carcinoma of the skin. *Am J Surg Pathol* 1992;16:584–592.
194. Gillham SL, Morrison RG, Hurt MA. Epidermotropic neuroendocrine carcinoma. Immunohistochemical differentiation from simulators, including malignant melanoma. *J Cutan Pathol* 1991;18: 120–127.
195. Rodriguez HA, Ackerman LV. Cellular blue nevus. Clinicopathologic study of forty-five cases. *Cancer* 1968;21:393–405.
196. Michal M, Baumruk L, Skalova A. Myxoid change within cellular blue naevi: a diagnostic pitfall. *Histopathology* 1992;20:527–530.
197. Temple-Camp CR, Saxe N, King H. Benign and malignant cellular blue nevus. A clinicopathological study of 30 cases. *Am J Dermatopathol* 1988;10:289–296.
198. Seab JA Jr, Graham JH, Helwig EB. Deep penetrating nevus. *Am J Surg Pathol* 1989;13:39–44.
199. Mehregan DA, Mehregan AH. Deep penetrating nevus. *Arch Dermatol* 1993;129:328–331.
200. Mehregan DR, Mehregan DA, Mehregan AH. Proliferating cell nuclear antigen staining in deep-penetrating nevi. *J Am Acad Dermatol* 1995;33:685–687.
201. Spitz S. Melanomas of childhood. *Am J Pathol* 1948;24:591–609.
202. Ball NJ, Golitz LE. Melanocytic nevi with focal atypical epithelioid cell components: a review of seventy-three cases. *J Am Acad Dermatol* 1994;30:724–729.
203. English JC 3rd, McCollough ML, Grabski WJ. A pigmented scalp nodule: malignant blue nevus. *Cutis* 1996;58:40–42.
204. Connelly J, Smith JL Jr. Malignant blue nevus. *Cancer* 1991;67: 2653–2657.
205. Frank SB, Cohen HJ. The halo nevus. *Arch Dermatol* 1964;89: 367–373.
206. Wayte DM, Helwig EB. Halo nevus. *Cancer* 1968;22:69–90.
207. Brownstein MH, Kazam BB, Hashimoto K. Halo congenital nevus. *Arch Dermatol* 1977;113:1572–1575.
208. Mooney MA, Barr RJ, Buxton MG. Halo nevus or halo phenomenon? A study of 142 cases. *J Cutan Pathol* 1995;22:342–348.
209. Penneys NS, Mayoral F, Barnhill R, et al. Delineation of nevus cell nests in inflammatory infiltrates by immunohistochemical staining for the presence of S-100 protein. *J Cutan Pathol* 1985;12:28–32.
210. Kopf AW, Bart RS, Hennessey P. Congenital nevocytic nevi and malignant melanomas. *J Am Acad Dermatol* 1979;1:123–130.
211. Hamming N. Anatomy and embryology of the eyelids: a review with special reference to the development of divided nevi. *Pediatr Dermatol* 1983;1:51–58.
212. Rhodes AR, Wood WC, Sober AJ, et al. Nonepidermal origin of malignant melanoma associated with a giant congenital nevocellular nevus. *Plast Reconstr Surg* 1981;67:782–790.
213. Rhodes AR, Sober AJ, Day CL, et al. The malignant potential of small congenital nevocellular nevi. An estimate of association based on a histologic study of 234 primary cutaneous melanomas. *J Am Acad Dermatol* 1982;6:230–241.

214. Reed WB, Becker SW Sr, Becker SW Jr, et al. Giant pigmented nevi, melanoma, and leptomeningeal melanocytosis. *Arch Dermatol* 1965;91:100–118.
215. Allen AC. Juvenile melanomas of children and adults and melano-carcinomas of children. *Arch Dermatol* 1960;82:325–335.
216. Filo V, Galbavy S, Pec J. Dome-shaped partly umbilicated tumor on the ear. Spitz nevus (SN). *Arch Dermatol* 1998;134:1629–1632.
217. Weedon D, Little JH. Spindle and epithelioid cell nevi in children and adults. A review of 211 cases of the Spitz nevus. *Cancer* 1977; 40:217–225.
218. Kamino H, Flotte TJ, Misheloff E, et al. Eosinophilic globules in Spitz's nevi. New findings and a diagnostic sign. *Am J Dermatopathol* 1979;1:319–324.
219. Bachaud JM, Shubinski R, Boussin G, et al. Stage I cutaneous malignant melanoma: risk factors of loco-regional recurrence after wide local excision and clinical perspectives. *Eur J Surg Oncol* 1992;18: 442–448.
220. Barnhill RL, Flotte TJ, Fleischli M, et al. Cutaneous melanoma and atypical Spitz tumors in childhood. *Cancer* 1995;76:1833–1845.
221. Walsh N, Crotty K, Palmer A, et al. Spitz nevus versus spitzoid malignant melanoma: an evaluation of the current distinguishing histopathologic criteria. *Hum Pathol* 1998;29:1105–1112.
222. Wong TY, Suster S, Duncan LM, et al. Nevoid melanoma: A clinicopathological study of seven cases of malignant melanoma mimicking spindle and epithelioid cell nevus and verrucous dermal nevus. *Hum Pathol* 1995;26:171–179.
223. Lynch HT, Frichot BC, Lynch JF. Familial atypical multiple mole—melanoma syndrome. *J Med Genet* 1978;15:352–356.
224. Clemente C, Cochran AJ, Elder DE, et al. Histopathologic diagnosis of dysplastic nevi: concordance among pathologists convened by the World Health Organization Melanoma Programme. *Hum Pathol* 1991;22:313–319.
225. Jakobiec FA, Folberg R, Iwamoto T. Clinicopathologic characteristics of premalignant and malignant melanocytic lesions of the conjunctiva. *Ophthalmology* 1989;96:147–166.
226. Farber M, Schutzer P, Mihm MC Jr. Pigmented lesions of the conjunctiva. *J Am Acad Dermatol* 1998;38:971–978.
227. Folberg R, McLean IW, Zimmerman LE. Conjunctival melanosis and melanoma. *Ophthalmology* 1984;91:673–678.
228. Sober AJ, Fitzpatrick TB, Mihm MC Jr. Primary melanoma of the skin: recognition and management. *J Am Acad Dermatol* 1980;2: 179–197.
229. O'Brien CJ, Coates AS, Petersen-Schaefer K, et al. Experience with 998 cutaneous melanomas of the head and neck over 30 years. *Am J Surg* 1991;162:310–314.
230. Donellan MJ, Seemayer T, Huvos AG, et al. Clinicopathologic study of cutaneous melanoma of the head and neck. *Am J Surg* 1972;124: 450–455.
231. Cox NH, Aitchison TC, Sirel JM, et al. Comparison between lentigo maligna melanoma and other histogenetic types of malignant melanoma of the head and neck. *Br J Cancer* 1996;73:940–944.
232. Tannous ZS, Lerner LH, Duncan LM, et al. Progression to invasive melanoma from malignant melanoma *in situ,* lentigo maligna type. *Hum Pathol* 2000;31:705–708.
233. Clark WH Jr, Elder DE, Van Horn M. The biologic forms of malignant melanoma. *Hum Pathol* 1986;17:443–450.
234. Elder DE, Van Belle P, Elenitsas R, et al. Neoplastic progression and prognosis in melanoma. *Semin Cutan Med Surg* 1996;15:336–348.
235. Clark WH Jr, Elder DE, Guerry D IV, et al. Model predicting survival in stage I melanoma based on tumor progression. *J Natl Cancer Inst* 1989;81:1893–1904.
236. Duncan LM. Prognostic indicators in melanoma. *Adv Dermatol* 1999;15:489–517.
237. McGovern VJ, Shaw HM, Milton GW. Prognostic significance of a polypoid configuration in malignant melanoma. *Histopathology* 1983;7:663–672.
238. Balch CM. Cutaneous melanoma: prognosis and treatment results worldwide. *Semin Surg Oncol* 1992;8:400–414.
239. Buzaid AC, Ross MI, Balch CM, et al. Critical analysis of the current American Joint Committee on Cancer staging system for cutaneous melanoma and proposal of a new staging system [see comments]. *J Clin Oncol* 1997;15:1039–1051.
240. Corona R, Mele A, Amini M, et al. Interobserver variability on the histopathologic diagnosis of cutaneous melanoma and other pigmented skin lesions. *J Clin Oncol* 1996;14:1218–1223.
241. Cochran AJ. Surgical pathology remains pivotal in the evaluation of "sentinal" lymph nodes. *Am J Surg Pathol* 1999;23:1169–1172.
242. Eldh J, Boeryd B, Peterson LE. Prognostic factors in cutaneous malignant melanoma in stage I. A clinical, morphological and multivariate analysis. *Scand J Plast Reconstr Surg* 1978;12:243–255.
243. Leon P, Daly JM, Synnestvedt M, et al. The prognostic implications of microscopic satellites in patients with clinical stage I melanoma. *Arch Surg* 1991;126:1461–1468.
244. Day CL Jr, Harrist TJ, Gorstein F, et al. Malignant melanoma. Prognostic significance of "microscopic satellites" in the reticular dermis and subcutaneous fat. *Ann Surg* 1981;194:108–112.
245. Clemente CG, Mihm MC Jr, Bufalino R, et al. Prognostic value of tumor infiltrating lymphocytes in the vertical growth phase of primary cutaneous melanoma. *Cancer* 1996;77:1303–1310.
246. Sondergaard K, Hou-Jensen K. Partial regression in thin primary cutaneous malignant melanomas clinical stage I. A study of 486 cases. *Virchows Arch [A]* 1985;408:241–247.
247. Santucci M, Pimpinelli N, Arganini L. Primary cutaneous B-cell lymphoma: a unique type of low-grade lymphoma. Clinicopathologic and immunologic study of 83 cases. *Cancer* 1991;67:2311–2326.
248. Guinee D, Jaffe E, Kingma D, et al. Pulmonary lymphomatoid granulomatosis: evidence for a proliferation of Epstein-Barr virus infected B-lymphocytes with a prominent T-cell component and vasculitis. *Am J Surg Pathol* 1994;18:753–764.
249. Krishnan J, Tomaszewski M, Kao G. Primary cutaneous CD30-positive anaplastic large-cell lymphoma. Report of 27 cases. *J Cutan Pathol* 1992;20:193–202.
250. De Bruin PC, Beljaards RC, Van Heerde P, et al. Differences in clinical behavior and immunophenotype between primary cutaneous and primary nodal anaplastic large cell lymphoma of T-cell or null cell phenotype. *Histopathology* 1993;23:127–135.
251. Sandlund JT, Pui C-H, Santana VM, et al. Clinical features and treatment outcome for children with $CD30^+$ large cell non-Hodgkin's lymphoma. *J Clin Oncol* 1994;12:895–898.
252. Willemze R, Beljaards RC. Spectrum of primary cutaneous CD30 (Ki-1)-positive lymphoproliferative disorders. A proposal for classification and guidelines for management and treatment. *J Am Acad Dermatol* 1993;28:973–980.
253. Beljaards RC, Kaudewitz P, Berti E, et al. Primary cutaneous CD30-positive large cell lymphoma: definition of a new type of cutaneous lymphoma with a favorable prognosis. A European multicenter study of 47 patients. *Cancer* 1993;71:2097–2104.
254. Paulli M, Berti E, Rosso R, et al. CD30/Ki-1–positive lymphoproliferative disorders of the skin—clinicopathologic correlation and statistical analysis of 86 cases: a multicentric study from the European Organization for Research and Treatment of Cancer Cutaneous Lymphoma Project Group. *J Clin Oncol* 1995;13:1343–1354.
255. Vergier B, Beylot-Barry M, Pulford K, et al. Statistical evaluation of diagnostic and prognostic features of $CD30^+$ cutaneous lymphoproliferative disorders: a clinicopathologic study of 65 cases. *Am J Surg Pathol* 1998;22:1192–1202.
256. MacGrogan G, Vergier B, Dubus P, et al. CD30 positive cutaneous large cell lymphomas. A comparative study of clinicopathologic and molecular features of 16 cases. *Am J Clin Pathol* 1996;105:440–450.
257. DeCoteau JF, Butmarc JR, Kinney MC, et al. The t(2;5) chromosomal translocation is not a common feature of primary cutaneous $CD30^+$ lymphoproliferative disorders: comparison with anaplastic large-cell lymphoma of nodal origin. *Blood* 1996;87:3437–3441.
258. Wood GS, Salvekar A, Schaffer J, et al. Evidence against a role for human T-cell lymphotrophic virus type I (HTLV-I) in the pathogenesis of American cutaneous T-cell lymphoma. *J Invest Dermatol* 1996;107:301–307.
259. Beylot-Barry M, Lamant L, Vergier B, et al. Detection of t(2;5) (p23;q35) translocation by reverse transcriptase polymerase chain reaction and *in situ* hybridization in CD30-positive primary cutaneous

lymphoma and lymphomatoid papulosis. *Am J Pathol* 1996;149:483–492.

260. Pulford K, Lamant L, Morris SW, et al. Detection of anaplastic lymphoma kinase (ALK) and nucleolar protein nucleophosmin (NPM)-ALK proteins in normal and neoplastic cells with the monoclonal antibody ALK1. *Blood* 1997;89:1394–1404.
261. Ott G, Katzenberger T, Siebert R, et al. Chromosomal abnormalities in nodal and extranodal CD30$^+$ anaplastic large cell lymphomas: infrequent detection of the t(2;5) in extranodal lymphomas. *Genes Chromosomes Cancer* 1998;22:114–121.
262. Garcia CF, Weiss LM, Warnke RA, et al. Cutaneous follicular lymphoma. *Am J Surg Pathol* 1986;10:454.
263. Nagatani T, Miyazawa M, Matsuzaki T, et al. Cutaneous B-cell lymphoma—a clinical, pathological and immunohistochemical study. *Clin Exp Dermatol* 1993;18:530–536.
264. Willemze R, Meijer CJLM, Sentis HJ, et al. Primary cutaneous large cell lymphomas of follicular center cell origin. *J Am Acad Dermatol* 1987;16:518.
265. Willemze R, Kerl H, Sterry W, et al. EORTC classification for primary cutaneous lymphomas: a proposal from the cutaneous lymphoma study group of the European Organization for the Research and Treatment of Cancer. *Blood* 1997;90:354–371.
266. Cerroni L, Volkenandt M, Rieger E, et al. Bcl-2 protein expression and correlation with the interchromosomal 14;18 translocation in cutaneous lymphomas and pseudolymphomas. *J Invest Dermatol* 1994;102:231–235.
267. Triscott JA, Ritter JH, Swanson PE, et al. Immunoreactivity for bcl-2 protein in cutaneous lymphomas and pseudolymphomas. *J Cutan Pathol* 1995;22:2.
268. Mattia AR, Ferry JA, Harris NL. Breast lymphoma. A B-cell spectrum including the low grade B-cell lymphoma of mucosa associated lymphoid tissue. *Am J Surg Pathol* 1993;17:574–587.
269. Pelstring RJ, Essel JH, Kurtin PJ, et al. Diversity of organ site involvement among malignant lymphomas of mucosa-associated tissues. *Am J Clin Pathol* 1991;96:738–745.
270. Isaacson P, Wright DH. Malignant lymphoma of mucosa-associated lymphoid tissue. A distinctive type of B-cell lymphoma. *Cancer* 1983;52:1410–1416.
271. Harris NL. Extranodal lymphoid infiltrates and mucosa-associated lymphoid tissue (MALT). A unifying concept [editorial]. *Am J Surg Pathol* 1991;15:879–884.
272. Harris NL. Low-grade B-cell lymphoma of mucosa-associated lymphoid tissue and monocytoid B-cell lymphoma. Related entities that are distinct from other low-grade B-cell lymphomas [editorial; comment]. *Arch Pathol Lab Med* 1993;117:771–775.
273. Bailey EM, Ferry JA, Harris NL, et al. Primary low-grade B-cell lymphoma of skin and soft tissue resembling lymphoma of mucosa-associated lymphoid tissue type. *J Cutan Pathol* 1993;20:532.
274. Bailey EM, Ferry JA, Harris NL, et al. Marginal zone lymphoma (low-grade B-cell lymphoma of mucosa-associated lymphoid tissue type) of skin and subcutaneous tissue. *Am J Surg Pathol* 1996;8:1011–1023.
275. Gianotti B, Santucci M. Skin-associated lymphoid tissue (SALT)-related B-cell lymphoma (primary cutaneous B-cell lymphoma). A concept and a clinicopathologic entity. *Arch Dermatol* 1993;129:353–355.
276. Duncan L, LeBoit P. Are primary cutaneous immunocytoma and marginal zone lymphoma the same disease? (editorial). *Am J Surg Pathol* 1997;21:1368–1372.
277. LeBoit PE, McNutt NS, Reed JA, et al. Primary cutaneous immunocytoma: a B-cell lymphoma that can easily be mistaken for cutaneous lymphoid hyperplasia. *Am J Surg Pathol* 1994;18:969–978.
278. Pimpinelli N, Santucci M, Mori M, et al. Primary cutaneous B-cell lymphoma: a clinically homogeneous entity? *J Am Acad Dermatol* 1997;37:1012–1016.
279. Bailey EM, Harris NL, Ferry JA, et al. Cutaneous B-cell lymphoma at the Massachusetts General Hospital, 1972–1994 [abstract]. *Lab Invest* 1996;74:39A.
280. Cerroni L, Signoretti S, Hofler G, et al. Primary cutaneous marginal zone B-cell lymphoma: a recently described entity of low-grade malignant cutaneous B-cell lymphoma. *Am J Surg Pathol* 1997;21:1307–1315.
281. Baldassano M, Bailey E, Ferry J, et al. Cutaneous lymphoid hyperplasia and cutaneous marginal zone lymphoma: Comparison of morphologic and immunophenotypic features. *Am J Surg Pathol* 1999;23:88–96.
282. Wong KF, Chan JK, Li LP, et al. Primary cutaneous plasmacytoma—report of two cases and review of the literature. *Am J Dermatopathol* 1994;16:392–397.
283. Chang YT, Wong CK. Primary cutaneous plasmacytomas. *Clin Exp Dermatol* 1994;19:177–180.
284. Llamas-Martin R, Postigo-Llorente C, Vanaclocha-Sebastian F, et al. Primary cutaneous extramedullary plasmacytoma secreting lambda IgG. *Clin Exp Dermatol* 1993;18:351–355.
285. Tuting T, Bork K. Primary plasmacytoma of the skin. *J Am Acad Dermatol* 1996;34:386–390.
286. DiGiuseppe JA, Nelson WG, Seifter EJ, et al. Intravascular lymphomatosis: a clinicopathologic study of 10 cases and assessment of response to chemotherapy. *J Clin Oncol* 1994;12:2573–2579.
287. Chang A, Zic JA, Boyd AS. Intravascular large cell lymphoma: a patient with asymptomatic purpuric patches and a chronic clinical course. *J Am Acad Dermatol* 1998;39:318–321.
288. Ferry JA, Harris NL, Picker LJ, et al. Intravascular lymphomatosis (malignant angioendotheliomatosis). A B-cell neoplasm expressing surface homing receptors. *Mod Pathol* 1988;1:444–452.
289. Robinson ND, Hashimoto T, Amagai M, et al. The new pemphigus variants [see comments]. *J Am Acad Dermatol* 1999;40:649–671.
290. Nousari HC, Anhalt GJ. Pemphigus and bullous pemphigoid. *Lancet* 1999;354:667–672.
291. Hans-Filho G, Aoki V, Rivitti E, et al. Endemic pemphigus foliaceus (fogo selvagem)—1998. The Cooperative Group on Fogo Selvagem Research. *Clin Dermatol* 1999;17:225–235.
292. Wu H, Wang ZH, Yan A, et al. Protection against pemphigus foliaceus by desmoglein 3 in neonates. *N Engl J Med* 2000;343:31–35.
293. Anhalt GJ. Paraneoplastic pemphigus. *Adv Dermatol* 1997;12:77–96 [discussion 97].
294. Robinson ND, Hashimoto T, Amagai M, et al. The new pemphigus variants. *J Am Acad Dermatol* 1999;40:649–671.
295. Sklavounou A, Laskaris G. Paraneoplastic pemphigus: a review. *Oral Oncol* 1998;34:437–440.
296. Anhalt GJ, Kim SC, Stanley J, et al. Paraneoplastic pemphigus. An autoimmune mucocutaneous disease associated with neoplasia. *N Engl J Med* 1990;323:1729–1735.
297. Gammon WB, Briggaman RA, Inman AO, et al. Differentiating anti-lamina lucida and anti-sublamina densa anti-BMZ antibodies by indirect immunofluorescence on 1.0 M sodium chloride-separated skin. *J Invest Dermatol* 1984;82:139–144.
298. Person JR, Rogers RSD. Bullous and cicatricial pemphigoid. Clinical, histopathologic, and immunopathologic correlations. *Mayo Clin Proc* 1977;52:54–66.
299. Brunsting LA, Perry HO. Benign pemphigoid? A report of seven cases with chronic scarring, herpetiform plaques about the head and neck. *Arch Dermatol* 1957;75:489.
300. Ahmed AR, Salm M, Larson R, et al. Localized cicatricial pemphigoid (Brunsting-Perry). A transplantation experiment. *Arch Dermatol* 1984;120:932–935.
301. Leonard JN, Hobday CM, Haffenden GP, et al. Immunofluorescent studies in ocular cicatricial pemphigoid. *Br J Dermatol* 1988;118:209–217.
302. Fine JD, Neises GR, Katz SI. Immunofluorescence and immunoelectron microscopic studies in cicatricial pemphigoid. *J Invest Dermatol* 1984;82:39–43.
303. Pegum JS, Mares A. Dermatitis herpetiformis with laryngeal involvement. *Br J Dermatol* 1963;75:123–124.
304. Katz SI, Strober W. The pathogenesis of dermatitis herpetiformis. *J Invest Dermatol* 1978;70:63–75.
305. Lahteenoja H, Irjala K, Viander M, et al. Oral mucosa is frequently affected in patients with dermatitis herpetiformis [letter]. *Arch Dermatol* 1998;134:756–758.

306. Doyle JL, Geary W, Baden E. Eosinophilic ulcer. *J Oral Maxillofac Surg* 1989;47:349–352.
307. Sklavounou A, Laskaris G. Eosinophilic ulcer of the oral mucosa. *Oral Surg Oral Med Oral Pathol* 1984;58:431–436.
308. Stern RS. Psoriasis. *Lancet* 1997;350:349–353.
309. Stern RS, Nichols KT, Vakeva LH. Malignant melanoma in patients treated for psoriasis with methoxsalen (Psoralen) and ultraviolet A radiation (PUVA). The PUVA Follow-Up Study. *N Engl J Med* 1997; 336:1041–1045.
310. Stern RS, Liebman EJ, Vakeva L. Oral psoralen and ultraviolet-A light (PUVA) treatment of psoriasis and persistent risk of nonmelanoma skin cancer. PUVA Follow-up Study. *J Natl Cancer Inst* 1998;90: 1278–1284.
311. Horn TD, Herzberg GZ, Hood AF. Characterization of the dermal infiltrate in human immunodeficiency virus-infected patients with psoriasis. *Arch Dermatol* 1990;126:1462–1465.
312. Weitzul S, Duvic M. HIV-related psoriasis and Reiter's syndrome. *Semin Cutan Med Surg* 1997;16:213–218.
313. Callen JP, Mahl CF. Oculocutaneous manifestations observed in multisystem disorders. *Dermatol Clin* 1992;10:709–716.
314. Keat A. Reiter's syndrome and reactive arthritis in perspective. *N Engl J Med* 1983;309:1606–1615.
315. Leirisalo M, Skylv G, Kousa M, et al. Followup study on patients with Reiter's disease and reactive arthritis, with special reference to HLA-B27. *Arthritis Rheum* 1982;25:249–259.
316. Brancato L, Itescu S, Skovron ML, et al. Aspects of the spectrum, prevalence and disease susceptibility determinants of Reiter's syndrome and related disorders associated with HIV infection. *Rheumatol Int* 1989;9:137–141.
317. Magro CM, Crowson AN, Peeling R. Vasculitis as the basis of cutaneous lesions in Reiter's disease. *Hum Pathol* 1995;26:633–638.
318. Rivers JK, Jackson R, Orizaga M. Who was Wickham and what are his striae? *Int J Dermatol* 1986;25:611–613.
319. Kaplan B, Barnes L. Oral lichen planus and squamous carcinoma. Case report and update of the literature. *Arch Otolaryngol* 1985;111: 543–547.
320. Reisman RJ, Schwartz AE, Friedman EW, et al. The malignant potential of oral lichen planus—diagnostic pitfalls. *Oral Surg Oral Med Oral Pathol* 1974;38:227–232.
321. Barnard NA, Scully C, Eveson JW, et al. Oral cancer development in patients with oral lichen planus. *J Oral Pathol Med* 1993;22:421–424.
322. Hogan DJ, Murphy F, Burgess WR, et al. Lichenoid stomatitis associated with lithium carbonate. *J Am Acad Dermatol* 1985;13: 243–246.
323. Gange RW, Jones EW. Bullous lichen planus caused by labetalol. *Br Med J* 1978;1:816–817.
324. Mobacken H, Nilsson LA, Olsson R, et al. Incidence of liver disease in chronic lichen planus of the mouth. *Acta Derm Venereol* 1984;64: 70–73.
325. Ashinoff R, Cohen R, Lipkin G. Castleman's tumor and erosive lichen planus: coincidence or association? Report of a case. *J Am Acad Dermatol* 1989;21:1076–1080.
326. Aronson IK, Soltani K, Paik KI, et al. Triad of lichen planus, myasthenia gravis, and thymoma. *Arch Dermatol* 1978;114:255–258.
327. Cribier B, Garnier C, Laustriat D, et al. Lichen planus and hepatitis C virus infection: an epidemiologic study. *J Am Acad Dermatol* 1994;31: 1070–1072.
328. Ellgehausen P, Elsner P, Burg G. Drug-induced lichen planus. *Clin Dermatol* 1998;16:325–332.
329. Cervoni E. Hepatitis C [letter; comment]. *Lancet* 1998;351: 1209–1210.
330. Jansen T, Plewig G, Anhalt GJ. Paraneoplastic pemphigus with clinical features of erosive lichen planus associated with Castleman's tumor. *Dermatology* 1995;190:245–250.
331. Bhutani LK. Ashy dermatosis or lichen planus pigmentosus: what is in a name? *Arch Dermatol* 1986;122:133.
332. Pedace FJ, Perry HO. Granuloma faciale. A clinical and histopathologic review. *Arch Dermatol* 1966;94:387–395.
333. Frost FA, Heenan PJ. Facial granuloma. *Australas J Dermatol* 1984;25: 121–124.
334. Johnson WC, Higdon RS, Helwig EB. Granuloma faciale. *Arch Dermatol* 1959;79:42–52.
335. Baum EW, Sams WM Jr, Payne RR. Giant cell arteritis: a systemic disease with rare cutaneous manifestations. *J Am Acad Dermatol* 1982;6:1081–1088.
336. Kinmont PDC, McCallum DI. Skin manifestations of giant-cell arteritis. *Br J Dermatol* 1964;76:299–308.
337. Allsop CJ, Gallagher PJ. Temporal artery biopsy in giant-cell arteritis. A reappraisal. *Am J Surg Pathol* 1981;5:317–323.
338. Klein RG, Campbell RJ, Hunder GG, et al. Skip lesions in temporal arteritis. *Mayo Clin Proc* 1976;51:504–510.
339. Jorizzo JL, Abernethy JL, White WL, et al. Mucocutaneous criteria for the diagnosis of Behçet's disease: an analysis of clinicopathologic data from multiple international centers. *J Am Acad Dermatol* 1995;32: 968–976.
340. Arbesfeld SJ, Kurban AK. Behçet's disease. New perspectives on an enigmatic syndrome [see comments]. *J Am Acad Dermatol* 1988;19: 767–779.
341. King R, Crowson AN, Murray E, et al. Acral purpuric papulonodular lesions as a manifestation of Behçet's disease. *Int J Dermatol* 1995;34:190–192.
342. Ota M, Mizuki N, Katsuyama Y, et al. The critical region for Behçet disease in the human major histocompatibility complex is reduced to a 46-kb segment centromeric of HLA-B, by association analysis using refined microsatellite mapping. *Am J Hum Genet* 1999;64: 1406–1410.
343. Falk K, Rotzschke O, Takiguchi M, et al. Peptide motifs of HLA-B51, -B52 and -B78 molecules, and implications for Behçet's disease. *Int Immunol* 1995;7:223–228.
344. Hornstein OP. Melkersson-Rosenthal syndrome. A neuro-muco-cutaneous disease of complex origin. *Curr Prob Dermatol* 1973;5: 117–156.
345. Worsaae N, Christensen KC, Schiodt M, et al. Melkersson-Rosenthal syndrome and cheilitis granulomatosa. A clinicopathological study of thirty-three patients with special reference to their oral lesions. *Oral Surg Oral Med Oral Pathol* 1982;54:404–413.
346. Levenson MJ, Ingerman M, Grimes C, et al. Melkersson-Rosenthal syndrome. *Arch Otolaryngol* 1984;110:540–542.
347. Carr D. Granulomatous cheilitis in Crohn's disease. *Br Med J* 1974; 4:636.
348. Helm KF, Menz J, Gibson LE, et al. A clinical and histopathologic study of granulomatous rosacea. *J Am Acad Dermatol* 1991;25: 1038–1043.
349. Vin-Christian K, Maurer TA, Berger TG. Acne rosacea as a cutaneous manifestation of HIV infection. *J Am Acad Dermatol* 1994;30: 139–140.
350. Croft CB, Wilkinson AR. Ulceration of the mouth, pharynx, and larynx in Crohn's disease of the intestine. *Br J Surg* 1972;59:249–252.
351. Burgdorf W. Cutaneous manifestations of Crohn's disease. *J Am Acad Dermatol* 1981;5:689–695.
352. Kolansky G, Kimbrough-Green C, Dubin HV. Metastatic Crohn's disease of the face: an uncommon presentation. *Arch Dermatol* 1993;129:1348–1349.
353. Eveson JW. Granulomatous disorders of the oral mucosa. *Semin Diagn Pathol* 1996;13:118–127.
354. Spiteri MA, Matthey F, Gordon T, et al. Lupus pernio: a clinicopathological study of thirty-five cases. *Br J Dermatol* 1985;112: 315–322.
355. Neville E, Mills RG, Jash DK, et al. Sarcoidosis of the upper respiratory tract and its association with lupus pernio. *Thorax* 1976;31: 660–664.
356. Gold RS, Sager E. Oral sarcoidosis: review of the literature. *J Oral Surg* 1976;34:237–244.
357. Li N, Bajoghli A, Kubba A, et al. Identification of mycobacterial DNA in cutaneous lesions of sarcoidosis. *J Cutan Pathol* 1999;26:271–278.
358. Ishige I, Usui Y, Takemura T, et al. Quantitative PCR of mycobacterial and propionibacterial DNA in lymph nodes of Japanese patients with sarcoidosis. *Lancet* 1999;354:120–123.
359. Popper HH, Klemen H, Hoefler G, et al. Presence of mycobacterial DNA in sarcoidosis. *Hum Pathol* 1997;28:796–800.

360. Tosti A, Varotti C, Tosti G, et al. Bilateral extensive xanthelasma palpebrarum. *Cutis* 1988;41:113–114.
361. Watanabe A, Yoshimura A, Wakasugi T, et al. Serum lipids, lipoprotein lipids and coronary heart disease in patients with xanthelasma palpebrarum. *Atherosclerosis* 1981;38:283–290.
362. Felner EI, Steinberg JB, Weinberg AG. Subcutaneous granuloma annulare: a review of 47 cases. *Pediatrics* 1997;100:965–967.
363. Trobs RB, Borte M, Voppmann A, et al. Granuloma annulare, nodular type—a subcutaneous pseudorheumatoid lesion in children. *Eur J Pediatr Surg* 1997;7:349–352.
364. Medlock MD, McComb JG, Raffel C, et al. Subcutaneous palisading granuloma of the scalp in childhood. *Pediatr Neurosurg* 1994;21: 113–116.
365. Evans MJ, Blessing K, Gray ES. Pseudorheumatoid nodule (deep granuloma annulare) of childhood: clinicopathologic features of twenty patients. *Pediatr Dermatol* 1994;11:6–9.
366. Moegelin A, Thalmann U, Haas N. Subcutaneous granuloma annulare of the eyelid. A case report. *Int J Oral Maxillofac Surg* 1995;24: 236–238.
367. Mills A, Chetty R. Auricular granuloma annulare. A consequence of trauma? *Am J Dermatopathol* 1992;14:431–433.
368. Cousin GC. Granuloma annulare of the supra-orbital region. A case report. *Br J Oral Maxillofac Surg* 1991;29:347–349.
369. Wells RS, Smith MA. The natural history of granuloma annulare. *Br J Dermatol* 1963;75:199–205.
370. Revenga F, Rovira I, Pimentel J, et al. Annular elastolytic giant cell granuloma—actinic granuloma? *Clin Exp Dermatol* 1996;21:51–53.
371. O'Brien JP. Actinic granuloma. An annular connective tissue disorder affecting sun- and heat-damaged (elastotic) skin. *Arch Dermatol* 1975;111:460–466.
372. Wilson Jones E. Actinic granuloma. *Am J Dermatopathol* 1980;2: 89–90.
373. Weedon D. Actinic granuloma: the controversy continues. *Am J Dermatopathol* 1980;2:90–91.
374. Barnhill RL, Goldenhersh MA. Elastophagocytosis: a non-specific reaction pattern associated with inflammatory processes in sun-protected skin. *J Cutan Pathol* 1989;16:199–202.
375. Zelger BG, Zelger B, Steiner H, Mikuz G. Solitary giant xanthogranuloma and benign cephalic histiocytosis—variants of juvenile xanthogranuloma. *Br J Dermatol* 1995;133:598–604.
376. Ayala F, Balato N, Iandoli R, et al. Benign cephalic histiocytosis. *Acta Derm Venereol* 1988;68:264–266.
377. Gianotti F, Caputo R, Ermacora E, Gianni E. Benign cephalic histiocytosis. *Arch Dermatol* 1986;122:1038–1043.
378. Zvulunov A, Barak Y, Metzker A. Juvenile xanthogranuloma, neurofibromatosis, and juvenile chronic myelogenous leukemia. World statistical analysis. *Arch Dermatol* 1995;131:904–908.
379. Ackerman CD, Cohen BA. Juvenile xanthogranuloma and neurofibromatosis. *Pediatr Dermatol* 1991;8:339–340.
380. Mann RE, Friedman KJ, Milgraum SS. Urticaria pigmentosa and juvenile xanthogranuloma: case report and brief review of the literature. *Pediatr Dermatol* 1996;13:122–126.
381. Sangueza OP, Salmon JK, White CR Jr, et al. Juvenile xanthogranuloma: a clinical, histopathologic and immunohistochemical study. *J Cutan Pathol* 1995;22:327–335.
382. Janney CG, Hurt MA, Santa Cruz DJ. Deep juvenile xanthogranuloma. Subcutaneous and intramuscular forms. *Am J Surg Pathol* 1991; 15:150–159.
383. Zelger B, Cerio R, Orchard G, et al. Juvenile and adult xanthogranuloma. A histological and immunohistochemical comparison. *Am J Surg Pathol* 1994;18:126–135.
384. Herzog KM, Tubbs RR. Langerhans cell histiocytosis. *Adv Anat Pathol* 1998;5:347–358.
385. Howarth DM, Gilchrist GS, Mullan BP, et al. Langerhans cell histiocytosis: diagnosis, natural history, management, and outcome. *Cancer* 1999;85:2278–2290.
386. Willman CL, McClain KL. An update on clonality, cytokines, and viral etiology in Langerhans cell histiocytosis. *Hematol Oncol Clin North Am* 1998;12:407–416.
387. Munn S, Chu AC. Langerhans cell histiocytosis of the skin. *Hematol Oncol Clin North Am* 1998;12:269–286.
388. Arico M, Egeler RM. Clinical aspects of Langerhans cell histiocytosis. *Hematol Oncol Clin North Am* 1998;12:247–258.
389. Chikama T, Yoshino H, Nishida T, et al. Langerhans cell histiocytosis localized to the eyelid. *Arch Ophthalmol* 1998;116:1375–1377.
390. Kumar S, Krenacs L, Raffeld M, et al. Subcutaneous panniculitis-like T-cell lymphoma is a tumor of cytotoxic T lymphocytes. *Lab Invest* 1997;76:129a.
391. Risdall RJ, Dehner LP, Duray P, et al. Histiocytosis X (Langerhans' cell histiocytosis). Prognostic role of histopathology. *Arch Pathol Lab Med* 1983;107:59–63.
392. Harrist TJ, Bhan AK, Murphy GF, et al. Histiocytosis-X: *in situ* characterization of cutaneous infiltrates with monoclonal antibodies. *Am J Clin Pathol* 1983;79:294–300.
393. Hashimoto K, Kagetsu N, Taniguchi Y, et al. Immunohistochemistry and electron microscopy in Langerhans cell histiocytosis confined to the skin. *J Am Acad Dermatol* 1991;25:1044–1053.
394. Hagari Y, Sasaoka R, Nishiura S, et al. Centrifugal lipodystrophy of the face mimicking progressive lipodystrophy. *Br J Dermatol* 1992; 127:407–410.
395. Gurbuz O, Yucelten D, Ergun T, et al. Partial lipodystrophy. *Int J Dermatol* 1995;34:36–37.
396. Lee LA, Roberts CM, Frank MB, et al. The autoantibody response to Ro/SSA in cutaneous lupus erythematosus. *Arch Dermatol* 1994;130: 1262–1268.
397. Callen JP, Fowler JF, Kulick KB. Serologic and clinical features of patients with discoid lupus erythematosus: relationship of antibodies to single-stranded deoxyribonucleic acid and of other antinuclear antibody subsets to clinical manifestations. *J Am Acad Dermatol* 1985;13:748–755.
398. Callen JP. Systemic lupus erythematosus in patients with chronic cutaneous (discoid) lupus erythematosus. Clinical and laboratory findings in seventeen patients. *J Am Acad Dermatol* 1985;12:278–288.
399. Provost TT. The relationship between discoid and systemic lupus erythematosus. *Arch Dermatol* 1994;130:1308–1310.
400. Pisetsky DS, Gilkeson G, St Clair EW. Systemic lupus erythematosus. Diagnosis and treatment. *Med Clin North Am* 1997;81:113–128.
401. Shen GQ, Shoenfeld Y, Peter JB. Anti-DNA, antihistone, and antinucleosome antibodies in systemic lupus erythematosus and drug-induced lupus. *Clin Rev Allergy Immunol* 1998;16:321–334.
402. Callen JP, Kingman J. Cutaneous vasculitis in systemic lupus erythematosus. A poor prognostic indicator. *Cutis* 1983;32:433–436.
403. Tan EM, Cohen AS, Fries JF, et al. The 1982 revised criteria for the classification of systemic lupus erythematosus. *Arthritis Rheum* 1982; 25:1271–1277.
404. Heiligenhaus A, Dutt JE, Foster CS. Histology and immunopathology of systemic lupus erythematosus affecting the conjunctiva. *Eye* 1996;10:425–432.
405. Strauss JS, Kligman AM. Pseudofolliculitis of the beard. *Arch Dermatol* 1956;74:533.
406. Ofuji S, Ogino A, Horio T, et al. Eosinophilic pustular folliculitis. *Acta Derm Venereol* 1970;50:195–203.
407. Duarte AM, Kramer J, Yusk JW, et al. Eosinophilic pustular folliculitis in infancy and childhood. *Am J Dis Child* 1993;147:197–200.
408. Rosenthal D, LeBoit PE, Klumpp L, et al. Human immunodeficiency virus-associated eosinophilic folliculitis. A unique dermatosis associated with advanced human immunodeficiency virus infection. *Arch Dermatol* 1991;127:206–209.
409. McCalmont TH, Altemus D, Maurer T, et al. Eosinophilic folliculitis. The histologic spectrum. *Am J Dermatopathol* 1995;17:439–446.
410. Muller SA. Trichotillomania: a histopathologic study in sixty-six patients. *J Am Acad Dermatol* 1990;23:56–62.
411. Binnick AN, Wax FD, Clendenning WE. Alopecia mucinosa of the face associated with mycosis fungoides. *Arch Dermatol* 1978;114: 791–792.
412. Gilliam AC, Lessin SR, Wilson DM, et al. Folliculotropic mycosis fungoides with large-cell transformation presenting as dissecting cellulitis of the scalp. *J Cutan Pathol* 1997;24:169–175.

413. Wilkinson JD, Black MM, Chu A. Follicular mucinosis associated with mycosis fungoides presenting with gross cystic changes on the face. *Clin Exp Dermatol* 1982;7:333–339.
414. Tomaszewski MM, Lupton GP, Krishnan J, et al. Syringolymphoid hyperplasia with alopecia. *J Cutan Pathol* 1994;21:520–526.
415. Tannous Z, Baldassano MF, Li VW, et al. Syringolymphoid hyperplasia and follicular mucinosis in a patient with cutaneous T-cell lymphoma. *J Am Acad Dermatol* 1999;41:303–308.
416. DaCosta-Bonta M, Tannous ZS, Demierre MF, et al. Rapidly progressing mycosis fungoides presenting as follicular mucinosis. *J Am Acad Dermatol* (in press).
417. Gibson LE, Muller SA, Leiferman KM, et al. Follicular mucinosis: clinical and histopathologic study. *J Am Acad Dermatol* 1989;20: 441–446.
418. Lancer HA, Bronstein BR, Nakagawa H, et al. Follicular mucinosis: a detailed morphologic and immunopathologic study. *J Am Acad Dermatol* 1984;10:760–768.
419. Mehregan DA, Gibson LE, Muller SA. Follicular mucinosis: histopathologic review of 33 cases. *Mayo Clin Proc* 1991;66:387–390.
420. Ridley DS. Histological classification and the immunological spectrum of leprosy. *Bull World Health Org* 1974;51:451–465.
421. Van Brakel WH, de Soldenhoff R, McDougall AC. The allocation of leprosy patients into paucibacillary and multibacillary groups for multidrug therapy, taking into account the number of body areas affected by skin, or skin and nerve lesions [see comments]. *Lepr Rev* 1992;63:231–246.
422. Elder D. *Lever's histopathology of the skin, 8th ed.* Philadelphia: Lippincott-Raven, 1997.
423. Adal KA, Cockerell CJ, Petri WA Jr. Cat scratch disease, bacillary angiomatosis, and other infections due to Rochalimaea. *N Engl J Med* 1994;330:1509–1515.
424. Cottell SL, Noskin GA. Bacillary angiomatosis: Clinical and histologic features, diagnosis and treatment. *Arch Intern Med* 1994; 154:524.
425. Hay RJ. Chronic dermatophyte infections. I. Clinical and mycological features. *Br J Dermatol* 1982;106:1–7.
426. Frieden IJ, Howard R. Tinea capitis: epidemiology, diagnosis, treatment, and control. *J Am Acad Dermatol* 1994;31:S42–S46.
427. Smith KJ, Neafie RC, Skelton HGD, et al. Majocchi's granuloma. *J Cutan Pathol* 1991;18:28–35.
428. Ackerman AB. Neutrophils within the cornified layer as clues to infection by superficial fungi. *Am J Dermatopathol* 1979;1:69–75.
429. Gottlieb GJ, Ackerman AB. The "sandwich sign" of dermatophytosis. *Am J Dermatopathol* 1986;8:347–350.
430. Mooney MA, Thomas I, Sirois D. Oral candidosis. *Int J Dermatol* 1995;34:759–765.
431. Klein RS, Harris CA, Small CB, et al. Oral candidiasis in high-risk patients as the initial manifestation of the aquired immunodeficiency syndrome. *N Engl J Med* 1984;311:354–358.
432. Laurent R, Kienzler J-L. Epidemiology of HPV infections. *Clin Dermatol* 1985;3:64–70.
433. Nahass GT, Goldstein BA, Zhu WY, et al. Comparison of Tzanck smear, viral culture, and DNA diagnostic methods in detection of herpes simplex and varicella-zoster infection. *JAMA* 1992;268: 2541–2544.
434. Smith KJ, Skelton HGD, Yeager J, et al. Molluscum contagiosum. Ultrastructural evidence for its presence in skin adjacent to clinical lesions in patients infected with human immunodeficiency virus type 1. Military Medical Consortium for Applied Retroviral Research [see comments]. *Arch Dermatol* 1992;128:223–227.
435. Lupton GP, James WD, Redfield RR, et al. Oral hairy leukoplakia. A distinctive marker of human T-cell lymphotropic virus type III (HTLV-III) infection. *Arch Dermatol* 1987;123:624–628.
436. McGovern VJ, Mihm MC Jr, Bailly C, et al. The classification of malignant melanoma and its histologic reporting. *Cancer* 1973;32: 1446–1457.
437. Clark WH Jr, From L, Bernardino EA, et al. The histogenesis and biologic behavior of primary human malignant melanoma of the skin. *Cancer Res* 1969;29:705–727.

14

CYTOPATHOLOGY OF THE HEAD AND NECK

14A

CYTOPATHOLOGY OF THE SALIVARY GLANDS, NECK, SOFT TISSUE, AND SKIN

TERI L. COOPER

SALIVARY GLANDS

Accurate interpretation of a fine-needle aspirate (FNA) of a mass in or near a salivary gland may be more difficult than for any other body site. The reasons are numerous. Multiple tissue types are confined to a small anatomic area. Several primary salivary gland malignancies exhibit only subtle (if any) malignant nuclear features. Considerable overlap exists in architectural patterns of benign and malignant neoplasms. Squamous, glandular, oncocytic, and sebaceous differentiations are common in many lesions. The rarity of many salivary gland neoplasms impedes acquisition of requisite experience. Many neoplasms are often cystic or accompanied by a dense lymphocytic infiltrate which can be misleading on FNA.

Because of these factors, accurate interpretation of these aspirates demands not only a familiarity with the cytomorphology but also a thorough understanding of the clinical and radiologic findings, to serve as a "double check" of the morphology. To this end, this discussion emphasizes clinical and radiologic characteristics as well as morphology.

Diagnostic Approach

Requisites for diagnostic accuracy include (a) an experienced aspirator, (b) a pathologist with extensive experience in salivary gland histology, cytomorphology and diagnostic pitfalls, and (c) access to all relevant clinical, laboratory, and radiologic data. This is best accomplished if the cytopathologist interpreting the specimen also performs the biopsy (1); however, excellent results can also be obtained if there is a team approach, with free flow of communication between the clinician and pathologist.

The aspirator must extensively sample the lesion by three or more biopsies with a 23- or 25-gauge needle and prepare multiple cellular well-preserved thin smears (2,3). (Smears provide greater diagnostic information than liquid-based preparations and are the preferred preparation method.) A combination of air-dried, Romanovsky-stained, and alcohol-fixed, Papanicolaou-stained smears offers the most diagnostic information (1,4,5) because the former highlights cytoplasmic differentiation and extracellular products (stroma/mucin), whereas alcohol preservation is superlative for evaluation of nuclear detail, identification of keratin, and extrapolation from formalin-fixed histomorphology in rare lesions. Because many salivary gland neoplasms are cystic, the aspirator should drain all fluid from a cystic lesion and perform multiple biopsies of any residual mass. In addition, the aspirator should know when to acquire additional material for special studies such as lymphocyte markers, cultures, and immunocytochemical stains.

The cytopathologist must thoroughly understand salivary gland histopathology and cytopathology and synthesize the clinical and radiologic features into a diagnostic whole. Definitive diagnoses never should be rendered on marginal material or in a clinical and radiologic vacuum. Pertinent clinical information includes exact tissue plane of the lesion, nerve symptoms, severe pain on FNA, and the presence of a residual mass in a cystic lesion. In addition, history of a prior malignancy, radiotherapy, and duration of the mass is essential. Important radiologic findings include the character of the lesional margins (circumscribed versus infiltrative) and any associated masses in the region.

The most fundamental question salivary gland FNA should answer is: can the patient be spared superficial parotidectomy? In aspirates with ambiguous morphology, an attempt should be made to classify the lesion as neoplastic or nonneoplastic, salivary or other origin, benign or malignant (6), and a differential diagnosis given if possible. This provides useful triage information to the surgeon. Properly utilized, up to one third of patients can be spared surgery by FNA (2,6–8).

Normal Salivary Gland

FNA of normal salivary gland yields a polymorphous population of very cohesive cells. A triad of acinar cells, ductal cells, and adipose tissue is commonly identified. Acinar cells form cohesive,

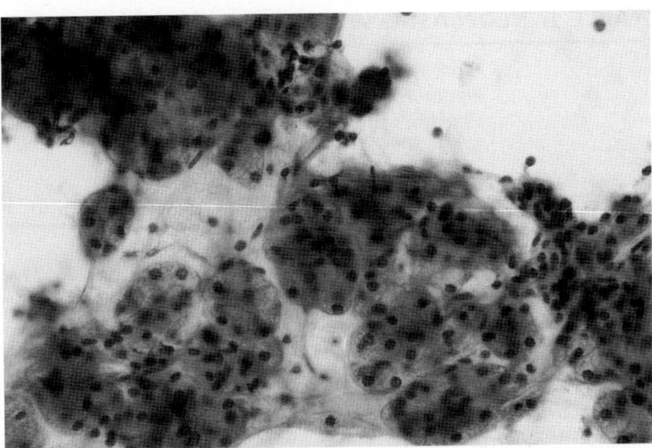

FIGURE 1. Normal salivary gland. Cohesive acini formed by cells with finely vacuolated cytoplasm. Ductal cells and fat not evident in this view (Papanicolaou stain, 400×).

spherical, "grape-like" formations composed of triangular cells with abundant, vacuolated to granular cytoplasm and round, uniform nuclei (Fig. 1).

Ductal cells form cohesive, flat "honeycomb" sheets of polygonal cells with small, uniform nuclei. Frequently, whole lobules are present with adipose tissue interspersed among the acini.

The differential diagnosis of normal salivary gland includes a geographic miss of the lesion, normal but prominent submandibular gland, sialadenosis, and lipoma.

Normal salivary gland is most often obtained when the needle *has not sampled the lesion;* therefore, whenever it is the sole finding, it must be ascertained if the sample is representative. If clinical or radiographic studies reveal a mass lesion, the sample should be called unsatisfactory, or a note made on the cytopathology report that the findings may not be representative. One exception is the use of FNA to distinguish a prominent submandibular gland from a neoplasm. The finding of normal salivary gland in the setting of normal radiologic findings can be clinically reassuring. Such patients should receive ongoing clinical follow-up.

Sialadenosis should be suspected when there is bilateral, diffuse, progressive parotid gland swelling in a patient with a history of diabetes, malnutrition, alcoholic cirrhosis, bulimia, endocrinopathy, antihypertensive therapy, or excessive use of sympathomimetic drugs (9,10). FNA yields thick, cohesive, arborizing aggregates of acinar cells with extreme crowding, such that the acini appear fused. Unlike normal salivary gland, adipose tissue may be absent. On high power, the acinar cells appear swollen to up to 30% larger than normal (9), with vacuolated, clear, or granular cytoplasm exhibiting well-defined cell borders (9,11). Bilaterality and absence of a dominant mass by physical or radiologic examination are requisite before sialadenosis can be rendered as a diagnosis (10,11).

Lipomas in the salivary gland occur as a defined soft mass. FNA yields abundant mature adipose tissue (12). These findings alone are never diagnostic and require computerized tomography or magnetic resonance imaging (CT/MRI) correlation. If the clinical, radiologic, and FNA findings are consistent with lipoma, the patient may be spared surgery.

Key Features of Normal Salivary Gland

1. Cohesive cells with "grape-like" acini
2. Fat, acinar, and ductal cells
3. Absent mass on x-ray

Cystic Lesions

Mucus Retention Cyst

A variety of inflammatory, developmental, and neoplastic lesions give rise to cysts in the salivary gland. Most common are mucus retention cysts and salivary duct cysts, which are often caused by lithiasis. Clinically, the patient reports waxing and waning salivary gland swelling with or without pain. FNA yields a scantly cellular specimen composed of mucus, rare lymphocytes, histiocytes, and, on occasion, rare squamous cells, glandular cells, or oncocytes (11) (Fig. 2). No residual mass persists after the cyst fluid is completely drained.

The most significant lesion to distinguish from a mucus retention cyst is an inadequately sampled *low-grade mucoepidermoid carcinoma* (MECA). These lesions are frequently cystic, and failure to adequately sample the lesion can yield smears morphologically identical to a mucus retention cyst. The aspirator must completely drain all cyst fluid, carefully reexamine the patient, and perform multiple biopsies of any residual mass (6,11,13–15) (see also mucoepidermoid carcinoma in this chapter).

Occasionally duct obstruction results from a neoplasm that is obscured by secondary mucus retention. If clinical or radiographic findings are inconsistent with an inflammatory process, or a residual mass persists, the report should include a morphologic description with a differential diagnosis (10).

Branchial Cleft Cyst

These commonly occur anterior to the ear or along the anterior border of the sternocleidomastoid muscle. FNA reveals benign

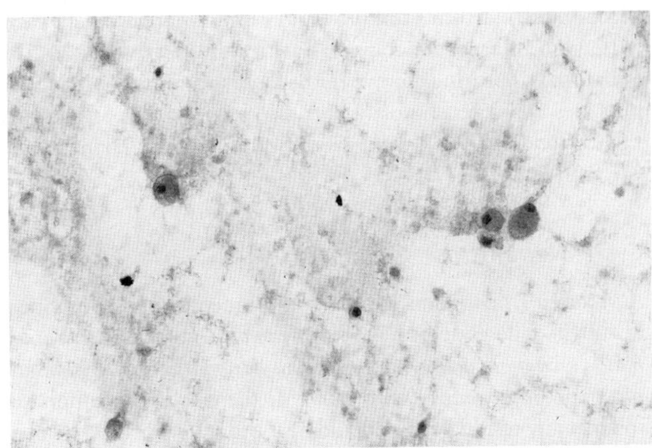

FIGURE 2. Mucus retention cyst. Mucin and admixed foamy histiocytes. If a clinical mass persists, further evaluation is warranted (Papanicolaou stain, 320×).

squamous cells with or without occasional lymphocytes. In the setting of acute inflammation with reparative atypia, a significant differential diagnosis occurs with metastatic squamous cell carcinoma. Therefore, caution is warranted if a squamous cyst exhibits acute inflammation or lacks well-preserved cells with classic malignant nuclear chromatin abnormalities (see Neck, branchial cleft cyst in this chapter).

Human Immunodeficiency Virus (HIV)-Associated Lymphoepithelial Cyst

With the advent of the HIV epidemic, the number of lymphoepithelial cysts (LEC) sampled by FNA has increased (11,14,16–19). Clinically, these lesions present as multiple bilateral parotid cysts associated with diffuse cervical lymphadenopathy; however, some patients will have only a single, unilateral mass on physical examination (20). The CT scan is characteristic, exhibiting multifocal cysts with peripheral enhancement along with cervical lymphadenopathy (17,20).

The FNA morphology is characterized by a triad of (a) a heterogeneous population of reactive lymphocytes, (b) foamy histiocytes, and (c) scant squamous cells, which may be anucleate or exhibit superficial or intermediate cell morphology (17). Because florid lymphocytic follicular hyperplasia is the major feature of this lesion, the smears are dominated by a variety of small and large lymphocytes, immunoblasts, plasma cells, follicular dendritic cells, and tingible body macrophages. The scant squamous component consists predominantly of anucleate squames (17,20). Less frequent findings include a granular, proteinaceous background, multinucleated histiocytes, hemosiderin-laden macrophages, and granuloma-like histiocytic aggregates (18). Glandular cells with delicate pale cytoplasm are not a feature of this lesion. When these findings are identified in an FNA of a patient with characteristic radiologic findings, an HIV test is warranted.

The differential diagnosis of benign LEC associated with HIV includes *branchial cleft cyst, Warthin's tumor, mucoepidermoid carcinoma* (MECA) (16), and *myoepithelial sialadenitis* (MESA). The scant epithelial component and dominant, polymorphous lymphocytic population characteristic of LEC would be unusual in all other lesions in the differential diagnosis. MECA and Warthin's tumor would exhibit more epithelial cells with glandular or oncocytic features, respectively (16,20). Squamoid-appearing epimyoepithelial islands infiltrated by lymphocytes characteristic of MESA are not found in aspirates of LEC. None of these lesions would exhibit LEC's characteristic CT scan image.

Cystic Neoplasms

A variety of neoplasms exhibit a prominent cystic component (Table 1). These include *Warthin's tumor, low-grade mucoepidermoid carcinoma, acinic cell carcinoma, pleomorphic adenoma,* and *metastatic squamous cell carcinoma.* It therefore bears emphasizing that any residual mass should be thoroughly sampled by multiple FNA passes. In institutions in which the cytopathologist does not perform the FNA, the clinicians must be carefully educated regarding this point because false-negative diagnoses will result from inadequate sampling. If only limited clinical data are available, it is wise to refrain from a definitive negative diagnosis on aspirates consisting of cyst contents only.

TABLE 1. NEOPLASMS WITH CYSTIC CHANGE

Mucoepidermoid carcinoma
Pleomorphic adenoma
Warthin's tumor
Acinic cell carcinoma
Metastatic squamous cell carcinoma

Axioms for Cysts

1. Any residual mass must be explained
2. Contents of cystic MECA and retention cysts may be identical
3. Cystic salivary gland neoplasms are common
4. Inflamed benign squamous cysts can mimic SCCA

Inflammatory Lesions

Sialadenitis

Acute sialadenitis is usually a clinical diagnosis and is rarely sampled by FNA (Fig. 3). Possible etiologies include viruses (including mumps), bacteria (from duct obstruction or stasis of secretions), and actinomyces. One case of florid cytomegalovirus sialadenitis in an HIV-positive patient led to a false-positive diagnosis of carcinoma as a result of difficulty recognizing the characteristic viral inclusions on air-dried Romanovsky smears (21).

In contrast, *chronic sialadenitis* may cause a discrete salivary gland mass through scarring. The resultant, ill-defined, sometimes painful mass may cause clinical suspicion of malignancy and is thus a frequent target of FNA. Common etiologies of chronic sialadenitis include sialolithiasis (in which the patient reports waxing and waning swelling or pain) and radiation therapy for squamous cell carcinoma of the head and neck. In the latter

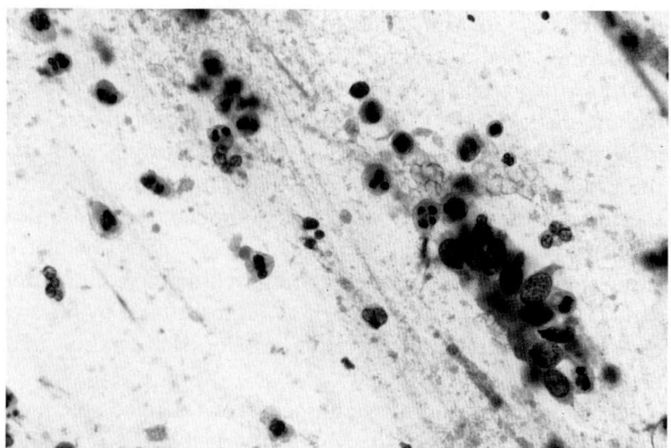

FIGURE 3. Acute sialadenitis. Ciliated columnar cells admixed with background mucin and neutrophils (Papanicolaou stain, 640×).

setting, FNA can be particularly helpful in distinguishing a benign, secondary phenomenon from metastatic squamous cell carcinoma.

Chronic inflammation results in fibrosis and acinar atrophy; therefore, the two FNA hallmarks of this lesion are scant cellularity and small, markedly cohesive spherical clusters of uniform duct-like cells (representing ducts and atrophic acini) (6,11,14,19). These may be embedded within, or associated with, fibrous tissue fragments (Fig. 4). Acinar cells are scant to absent, and few if any single epithelial cells are seen. Lymphocytes are usually scant to moderate and are predominantly small and mature (19). Histiocytes, atypical squamous metaplasia (5,6,11,22), and/or a mucoid background may be present. Marked nuclear atypia may be seen in aspirates of radiated glands (8,11). Unusual findings include psammoma bodies (23), ciliated columnar cells (10), and small square, rectangular, or needle-shaped crystals (24,25), which suggest lithiasis.

The differential diagnosis of chronic sialadenitis includes a low-grade neoplasm, low-grade mucoepidermoid carcinoma (MECA), myoepithelial sialadenitis (MESA), and squamous cell carcinoma.

The uniform small, tightly cohesive, cuboidal epithelial cells in acinar-like clusters result in a monomorphic cell population that can suggest a *low-grade neoplasm* to the unwary. The scant cellularity, fibrosis, lymphocytes, and lack of resemblance to known salivary gland neoplasms favor sialadenitis.

The presence of background mucus, foamy histiocytes, and lymphocytes, with or without squamous metaplasia, may resemble low-grade *MECA* (6,10,11). However, if adequately sampled, MECA yields a moderately to abundantly cellular aspirate of loosely cohesive sheets and clusters of glandular and intermediate cells (26), in contrast to the scant cellularity and tightly cohesive ducts of chronic sialadenitis (see MECA).

Myoepithelial sialadenitis (MESA) only superficially enters into the differential diagnosis. The cohesive spherical clusters typical of chronic sialadenitis in no way resemble the large, squamoid sheets of MESA.

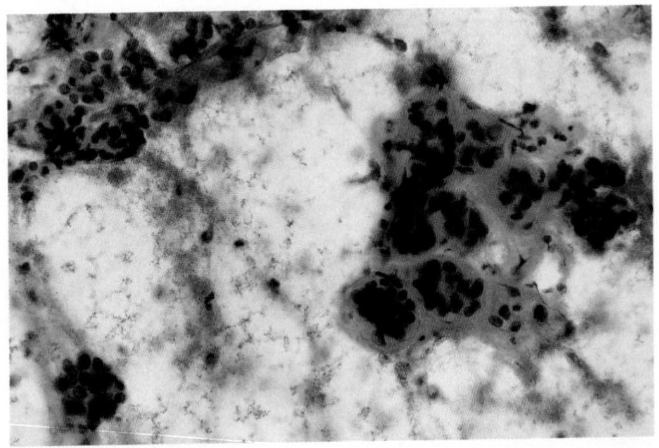

FIGURE 4. Chronic sialadenitis. Atrophic acini with periacinar fibrosis and background lymphocytes. The cellular monomorphism from atrophy can be mistaken for a neoplasm (Papanicolaou stain, 250×).

Atypical squamous metaplasia, particularly in a patient who has had radiation therapy for squamous cell carcinoma, is another potential pitfall. Scant cellularity and cohesive epithelial clusters typify radiation effect on FNA (6,8,11,13), in contrast to the moderate to abundant cellularity with many single, mitotically active abnormal cells in aspirates of *squamous cell carcinoma* (see Neck, SCCA).

Key Features of Chronic Sialadenitis

1. Scantly cellular
2. Monomorphic, cohesive clusters of duct-like cells
3. Fibrous tissue
4. Scant to moderate lymphocytes
5. Ciliated cells, crystalloids, or psammoma bodies rarely present

Granulomatous Disease

Salivary glands may be primarily involved by granulomatous inflammation or may be an innocent bystander to granulomatous lymphadenitis. Sarcoidosis is bilateral in approximately 50% of patients and frequently involves the lymph nodes as well as parotid gland parenchyma.

Smears exhibit aggregates of epithelioid histiocytes. These are large cells with abundant pink cytoplasm, ill-defined cell borders, uniform, pale oval to "boomerang"-shaped nuclei, finely dispersed chromatin, and consistent small nucleoli (27). Associated findings may include lymphocytes, neutrophils, or granular background necrosis. If granulomas are identified on FNA, repeat biopsies for cultures are indicated (see the section on lymph nodes in this chapter).

The most significant diagnostic pitfalls are *Hodgkin's disease* and *T-cell lymphoma,* which may be associated with granulomas or aggregates of epithelioid histiocytes. If atypical background lymphocytes are identified, material should be submitted for lymphocyte marker studies.

Key Features of Granulomatous Disease

1. Aggregates of large, pale histiocytes with oval to elongate nuclei
2. Variable lymphocytes, neutrophils, or necrosis
3. Cultures indicated
4. Exclude lymphoma

Myoepithelial Sialadenitis (Benign Lymphoepithelial Lesion)

Myoepithelial sialadenitis (MESA) may be unilateral or bilateral, cystic or solid. Diffuse parotid gland enlargement in a 40- to 60-year-old woman is the most common clinical presentation. Clinical associations include Sjögren's syndrome and lymphoma.

The abundantly cellular smears exhibit a mixed lymphocytic population along with plasma cells, histiocytes, and tingible

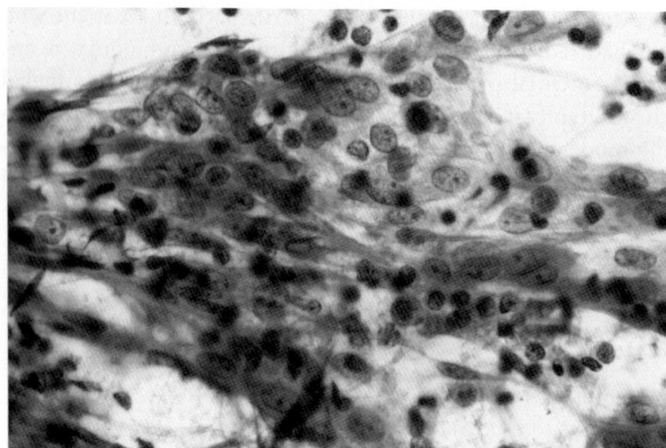

FIGURE 5. Myeloepithelial sialadenitis. Cohesive sheets of squamoid epithelial cells with reactive nuclei and lymphocytic infiltrate. If lymphocytic population is predominant, lymphoid immunophenotyping may be indicated to exclude a mucosa-associated lymphoid tissue (MALT) lymphoma (Papanicolaou stain, 500×).

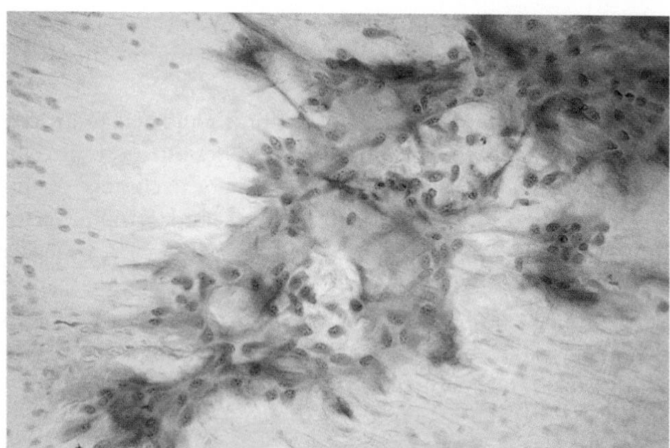

FIGURE 6. Pleomorphic adenoma. Dyshesive plasmacytoid myoepithelial cells with ample cytoplasm, intimately admixed with fibrillar, chondromyxoid stroma (Papanicolaou stain, 250×).

body macrophages. Large, cohesive sheets of ductal or squamous epithelium with pale cytoplasm and overlapping, repair-like nuclei (19) are infiltrated by numerous lymphocytes (Fig. 5). These correspond to epimyoepithelial islands. Acini are conspicuously absent (5,11,14,28). Calcifications have been reported (29).

The differential diagnosis includes chronic sialadenitis, Warthin's tumor, and lymphoma. MESA lacks the scant cellularity and tightly cohesive spherical epithelial clusters of *chronic sialadenitis.*

Careful attention to the cell cytoplasm and organization should readily distinguish *Warthin's tumor* from MESA. The densely granular cytoplasm, sharp cell borders, and honeycomb sheets typical of the former contrast with the less organized sheets of pale cells in MESA. In addition, lymphocytes do not infiltrate Warthin's tumor epithelium.

Low-grade lymphoma of mucosa-associated lymphoid tissue (MALT) type is associated with MESA. Six percent of patients with Sjögren's syndrome develop malignant lymphoma [30(p. 387)]. Aspirates of MALT lymphoma may be polymorphous but are composed predominantly of intermediate-sized lymphocytes (one and a half times the size of a mature lymphocyte) with moderate pale cytoplasm, round to irregular nuclei, clumped chromatin, and small nucleoli (31). If a background of typical MESA is present, the admixture of reactive and malignant lymphocytes may be polymorphous and difficult, if not impossible, to recognize as malignant (31). Additional biopsies are indicated to procure material for immunophenotyping if MESA is identified on FNA or the patient has a known history of Sjögren's syndrome (5).

Key Features of Myoepithelial Sialadenitis

1. Highly cellular with mixed, predominantly lymphoid, inflammation and tingible body macrophages (TBMs)
2. Cohesive epithelial sheets infiltrated by lymphocytes
3. Overlapping, repair-like epithelial nuclei
4. Immunophenotyping indicated to exclude MALT lymphoma

Benign Neoplasms

Pleomorphic Adenoma

Pleomorphic adenoma (PA) is the most common salivary gland neoplasm in adults and children, comprising up to 75% of all salivary gland tumors [30(p. 39)]. It therefore behooves the cytopathologist to be well acquainted with its broad morphologic spectrum. It presents as a firm, mobile, circumscribed, painless mass in the tail of the parotid, superficial or deep to the angle of the mandible, typically in 20- to 50-year-old women. The submandibular gland and minor salivary glands of the lateral palate are also common locations [30(p. 39)].

Grossly, FNA yields moderate mucoid to firm translucent material that may resist smearing. Microscopy reveals a triad of stroma, myoepithelial cells, and epithelial cells in varying proportions.

Fibromyxoid stroma stains translucent gray-green on Pap stain and magenta on Romanovsky stains. The presence of numerous collagen fibrils and spindle or epithelial cells enmeshed within the stroma is virtually diagnostic of PA (32,33) (Fig. 6). Acellular stromal globules that can mimic adenoid cystic carcinoma may be seen in a minority of PAs (33,34) (Fig. 7).

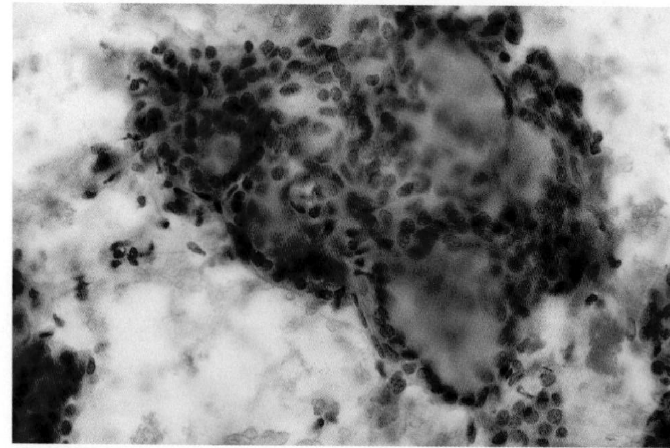

FIGURE 7. Pleomorphic adenoma mimicking adenoid cystic carcinoma. Spheres of acellular stroma surrounded by basaloid cells. Typical chondromyxoid stroma admixed with myoepithelial cells was present elsewhere on the smear (hematoxylin and eosin stain, 640×).

Approximately 30% of PAs are cellular, with scant to absent stroma (34,35). Therefore, familiarity with the cell morphology is essential for diagnostic accuracy. Myoepithelial cells form loosely cohesive arborizing sheets of haphazardly arranged spindle, plasmacytoid, or clear cells [11,14,30(p. 44)] showing indistinct cell borders (35), and numerous background single spindle and plasmacytoid cells are easily identified (32,35,36). The oval nuclei of the stubby spindle cells are smooth and uniform, with fine chromatin and scant bipolar cytoplasm. Plasmacytoid ("hyaline") cells exhibit round nuclei with powdery chromatin, eccentrically placed within moderate, dense, often "glassy" cytoplasm. Lacy pale cytoplasm characterizes clear cells.

Uniform cuboidal cells with scant to moderate cytoplasm, smooth nuclei, fine chromatin, and absent nucleoli, arranged as sheets and branching ducts typify the epithelial component. It is often possible to identify transition areas in which the epithelial cells blend into the spindle myoepithelial cells (11).

Squamous, oncocytic, sebaceous, or mucinous (37) metaplasia occurs and may be a prominent feature (34). Other incidental findings include the presence of tyrosine crystals (38), calcifications resembling psammoma bodies (2), intranuclear cytoplasmic inclusions (39), and abundant extracellular mucin (37). Scattered cells with mild to moderate nuclear atypia are seen in 5% to 10% of aspirates (33,34,40) (Fig. 8).

The FNA diagnosis of PA is usually straightforward (34,35). Specificity for the diagnosis of pleomorphic adenoma ranges from 91.3% to 98.4% in experienced hands (33,35).

Significant diagnostic difficulties may arise when only one of the components is present, and PA is a frequent source of false-positive and false-negative diagnoses (33–35). Its differential diagnosis includes adenoid cystic carcinoma, basal cell adenoma, carcinoma *ex* pleomorphic adenoma, low-grade MECA, a benign cyst, polymorphous low-grade adenocarcinoma, and epithelial–myoepithelial carcinoma.

Because of major differences in surgical approach and prognosis, *adenoid cystic carcinoma* (ADCC) is the most significant lesion to distinguish from PA. The three most reliable features favoring PA over ADCC are (a) fibromyxoid stroma containing intimately admixed collagen fibrils and spindle cells (30,32,33), (b) polymorphous cells with ample cytoplasm (41) (particularly single plasmacytoid cells) (35,36), and (c) the absence of nerve symptoms (15,42). (Detailed differential features are described under adenoid cystic carcinoma.) It bears emphasizing that occasional aspirates of PA may be virtually identical to ADCC (32). A diagnosis of PA should be questioned if there is evidence of nerve dysfunction or infiltrative growth. A differential diagnosis is recommended if ambiguous morphology is present.

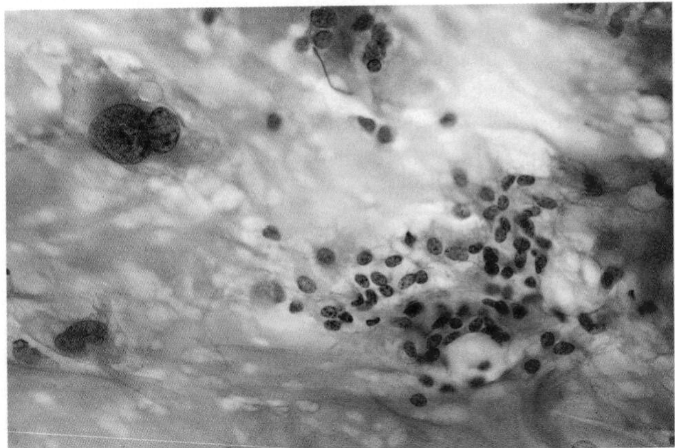

FIGURE 8. Atypical cells in pleomorphic adenoma. Rare, large, bizarre cells admixed with otherwise typical pleomorphic adenoma elements (hematoxylin and eosin stain, 400×). Case courtesy of Dr. Essam Ahmed.

Extracellular and intracellular mucin (originating from dilated ducts or glandular metaplasia, respectively) may be identified in FNA of PA (37), resulting in diagnostic confusion with *low-grade MECA.* To further confuse the issue, bland intermediate cells of MECA often resemble the epithelial cells of PA. Elsheikh (35) emphasized the fibrillar nature of PA stroma with enmeshed spindle cells as distinct from stringy, acellular mucin admixed with foamy macrophages in MECA. Although squamous and glandular metaplasia may be a prominent feature of pleomorphic adenoma, spindle and plasmacytoid myoepithelial cells are not seen in MECA. If the morphology is ambiguous, a differential diagnosis and excision are warranted.

Differentiation of a cellular PA from a *basal cell adenoma* (BCA) may be exceedingly difficult; however, the point is moot because both neoplasms are benign, and the therapy is the same. The heterogeneity of the cell population, amount of stroma, and the degree of cohesion are the primary differentiating features. BCA is composed of smaller, more monomorphic cells with tighter cohesion and a more orderly architecture than PA (35). BCA's usually extremely scant stroma consists of minute, hyaline globules or peripheral wraps around cohesive cellular clusters (43–45). Many naked nuclei may be present in the background of BCA aspirates; however, the single, plasmacytoid cells of PA are not seen (35).

The presence of mild to moderate nuclear atypia in 5% to 10% of PA (33,34,40) may cause confusion with *carcinoma* ex *pleomorphic adenoma* (CEPA). Clinical history, nuclear morphology, and predominance of typical PA help distinguish these two lesions. The clinical history of a longstanding mass with sudden, rapid growth, pain, or facial nerve symptoms is typical of malignant transformation in CEPA. In addition, carcinoma should be suspected when there is a predominance of abnormal cells with classic malignant nuclear features present with only scant or absent stroma (40). Scattered cells with mild to moderate nuclear atypia in the setting of an otherwise typical pleomorphic adenoma should be tolerated (14,33,34,40). If the morphology or history is indefinite, a diagnosis of "pleomorphic adenoma with atypia" (33) is warranted, followed by frozen section at the time of surgery.

Cystic degeneration occurs in 7% of PAs, and failure to sample the lesion adequately can result in an erroneous diagnosis of *benign cyst not otherwise specified* (NOS) or *mucus retention cyst.* Proper FNA technique and knowledge of a residual mass will prevent this pitfall.

Epithelial–myoepithelial carcinoma has been misdiagnosed as PA. Recognition of a dimorphic pattern of basaloid and clear cells with nuclear atypia and the absence of fibromyxoid stroma (46,47) in the former will prevent misdiagnosis.

Polymorphous low-grade adenocarcinoma may be difficult if not impossible to distinguish from PA. Location outside the palate, or in a young individual, statistically favors PA.

Pleomorphic Adenoma

- Fibromyxoid stroma with enmeshed cells, collagen fibrils
- Spindle and plasmacytoid cells with glassy cytoplasm
- Loose cohesion, background single cells
- Stroma, myoepithelial cells, epithelial cells

Pitfalls (Differential Diagnosis)

1. Hyaline globules (ADCC)
2. Nuclear atypia 5–10% (CEPA)
3. Mucin (intra- and extracellular) (MECA)
4. Cystic change (mucocele, MECA)
5. No or scant stroma; cellular PA (BCA, ADCC)
6. Squamous or glandular metaplasia (MECA)

Warthin's Tumor

Warthin's tumor (WT) accounts for 4% to 11% of all salivary gland neoplasms and 10% of all benign salivary gland neoplasms [30(pp. 68–69)]. The location is almost always the parotid gland because of its origin from unique ductal inclusions within parotid lymph nodes. Up to 10% may be bilateral or multifocal [30(p. 69)]. Unlike most salivary gland neoplasms, men are more commonly affected than women, with an average age of 60 years. A doughy, circumscribed mass in the tail of the parotid is the typical presentation. Aspiration often yields abundant, mucoid or turbid, white or dark brown ("motor oil") fluid.

The diagnostic triad of WT includes flat sheets of oncocytes, lymphocytes, and granular background debris (48). Oncocytes are polygonal cells with ample, dense, finely granular cytoplasm, uniform, smooth nuclei with even chromatin, and prominent, off-center nucleoli, arranged as flat, "honeycomb" sheets with sharp cell borders (26) (Fig. 9). The cytoplasm is red or green on Pap stain, gray-blue on Romanovsky stain, with obvious granularity at high power. Masson's trichrome will highlight the cytoplasmic granules (11,14).

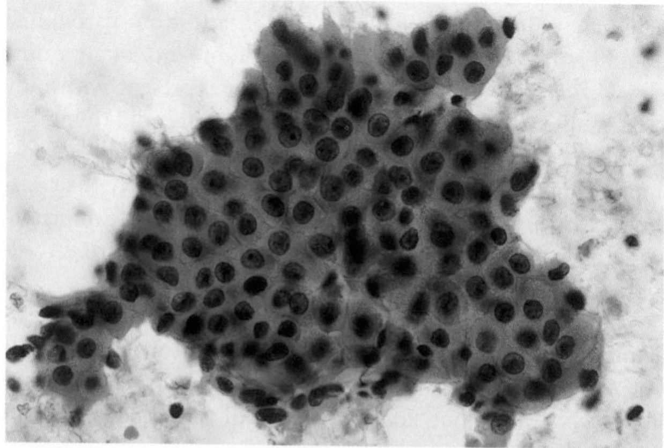

FIGURE 9. Warthin's tumor. Flat sheets of cells with ample granular cytoplasm, sharp cell borders, and orderly placement of nuclei, in a background of lymphocytes and cyanophilic debris (Papanicolaou stain, 640×).

The lymphoid component may be small, mature lymphocytes (28) or a mixture of small and reactive lymphocytes along with tingible body macrophages and germinal center fragments (48). Mast cells may be prominent but are nonspecific (48,49). Infarction (occurring in up to 6% of Warthin's tumors) (50) or inflammation can cause markedly atypical squamous metaplasia in a necrotic background (51–53).

Background debris, if present, is amorphous, granular (green on Pap stain), with admixed karyorrhectic debris and occasional small, diamond-shaped, brightly eosinophilic cell ghosts resembling small anucleate keratinized squames. Occasionally the background is mucoid (48).

Definite diagnosis of Warthin's tumor requires the presence of oncocytes and lymphocytes (48). Accurate diagnosis is important because FNA may be used to avoid surgery in elderly patients who are poor operative risks. Problems in interpretation arise when only one of the three components is present or when there is inflammation with reactive changes. The differential diagnosis includes squamous cell carcinoma, low-grade mucoepidermoid carcinoma (MECA), acinic cell carcinoma, oncocytoma, and myoepithelial sialadenitis.

Several false-positive diagnoses of *squamous cell carcinoma* have been reported because of markedly atypical squamous metaplasia in inflamed or partially infarcted WTs (51–53). Smears from these lesions exhibit scant, frequently keratinized, "tadpole" and spindled squamous cells with markedly irregular, but very degenerate ("India ink"), atypical nuclei present in a background of necrotic debris and acute inflammation (51–53). Occasional preserved, nonkeratinized squamous cells exhibit enlarged, smooth, vesicular nuclei with prominent nucleoli, typical of repair (51). These cells originate from reactive metaplastic, squamous epithelium adjacent to inflammatory erosions in the lining of cystic tumors. An awareness of this phenomenon is the most important factor in avoiding misdiagnosis. The abnormal cells in WT are scant, degenerate, and lack definitive malignant nuclear features in contrast to the numerous well-preserved single cells with classic malignant nuclear chromatin irregularities of squamous cell carcinoma (22,51–54). Background sheets of benign oncocytes favor WT (14,22,48,54). Extreme caution should always be used in the setting of acute inflammation on FNA, and some authors recommend entertaining a definite diagnosis of cystic squamous cell carcinoma only when many well-preserved cells exhibit classic nuclear malignant features (54) (see the section on the neck in this chapter).

The combination of mucoid background (14,48), sheets of polygonal epithelial cells, and lymphocytes can be mistaken for low-grade *MECA* (11,55) (Fig. 10). The distinction is based on the architecture of the epithelial sheets. Cohen (5) emphasized disorganized three-dimensional sheets of cells with overlapping nuclei and ill-defined cell borders as characteristic of MECA, in contrast to the orderly, flat, honeycomb sheets with sharp cell borders of Warthin's tumor. Location outside the parotid favors MECA. Oncocytes, lymphocytes, mast cells, squamous, and glandular cells can be prominent in both lesions.

On low power, *acinic cell carcinoma* (ACC) may resemble WT (11) because it has sheets of polygonal cells with dense cytoplasm

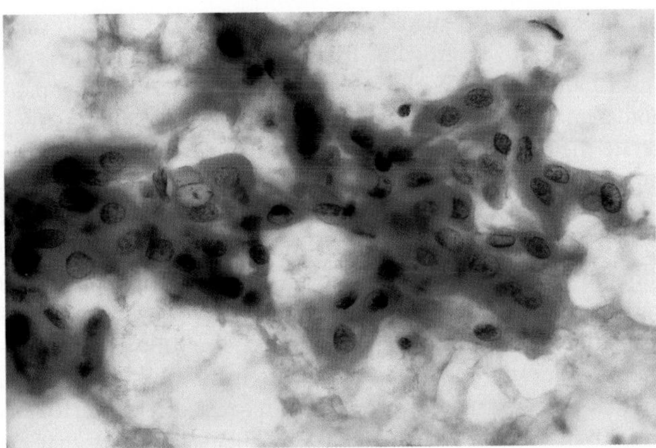

FIGURE 10. Warthin's tumor with focal glandular metaplasia (left of center). The remainder of the smear showed typical features of Warthin's tumor (Papanicolaou stain, 640×).

and uniform nuclei present in a background of lymphocytes and stripped epithelial nuclei mimicking lymphocytes. Vascular supporting stroma, finely vacuolated cytoplasm, lack of architectural polarity, and numerous stripped ("naked") epithelial nuclei favor ACC (14). Densely granular oncocytes are not seen in ACC.

Oncocytomas have denser cytoplasmic granularity and lack the lymphocytes or granular cyst debris of Warthin's tumor (11,14). The distinction is significant because oncocytomas may be multifocal or recur (30,56), and rare malignant oncocytomas have been reported (56,57).

Architectural and cytoplasmic features distinguish myoepithelial sialadenitis (MESA) from Warthin's tumor (28). MESA lacks an orderly arrangement of granular cells with sharp cell borders, and oncocytes are absent. Lymphocytes do not infiltrate Warthin's tumor epithelium.

Warthin's Tumor

- Parotid gland, elderly men
- Granular oncocytes
- Flat sheets; sharp cell borders
- Lymphocytes
- Granular background debris

Pitfalls (Differential Diagnosis)

1. Keratinizing reactive squamous metaplasia in inflamed or infarcted WT (Met SCCA)
2. Mucoid background (MECA)
3. Cyst contents only on sample (mucocele, MECA)
4. Confusion of oncocytes with squamous/acinar cells (MECA, ACC)
5. 6% infarct (SCCA)

Basal Cell Adenoma

Seventy-five percent of basal cell adenomas (BCA) arise in the parotid gland. The submandibular gland and upper lip are other common locations [30(p. 81)]. This tumor affects a slightly older age group (mean age 58 years) than PA and presents as a circumscribed, mobile, painless nodule. Multiple skin adnexal tumors, particularly cylindromas, may be associated with one or multiple basal cell adenomas (dermal analogue subtype) [30(p. 82),58].

Although BCA accounts for only 2% [30(p. 81)] of salivary gland neoplasms, familiarity with its morphology is important because these benign lesions can be indistinguishable from adenoid cystic carcinoma on FNA (43,59–61).

Cytologic hallmarks of BCA include (a) bland, basaloid cells, (b) cohesive architecture, and (c) scant to absent stroma. On low power, the sample is abundantly cellular, composed of sheets and branching three-dimensional trabeculae of small, uniform cells with basophilic nuclei and scant cytoplasm (2,11,14,43–45,62) in a background of abundant "naked" basaloid nuclei (35,43,63,64) (Fig. 11). The bland nuclei exhibit smooth contours, and even chromatin, without hyperchromasia or nucleoli. Basosquamous whorls, if present, are a characteristic feature (2,11,14,60). Stroma varies with the subtype of BCA but is usually scant (even absent), consisting of acellular homogeneous wisps or bands, often surrounding the periphery of the cell clusters (43–45,60). In addition, small basophilic stromal globules, which are smaller and stain more eosinophilic on Pap stain (more basophilic on air-dried preparations) than those of adenoid cystic carcinoma, may be present (6,59–61,65).

The differential diagnosis of BCA includes adenoid cystic carcinoma (foremost), cellular pleomorphic adenoma, metastatic basal cell carcinoma, the rare basal cell adenocarcinoma, and skin appendage tumors.

Distinction from *adenoid cystic carcinoma* (ADCC) is based primarily on (a) architecture of the cell clusters, (b) amount, size, and staining characteristics of the stroma, and (c) clinical presence of pain or nerve palsy. Stroma is scant, difficult to find, and often wrapped around the periphery of cell groups in BCA in contrast to the usually obvious globules and cylinders of cribriform ADCC (60,64). The large globules of ADCC are pale gray on Pap stain and bright magenta on Romanovsky stain, as opposed to the small, eosinophilic (Pap) or basophilic (Romanovsky) globules of BCA (11,14,44,61,62).

ADCC is characterized by hollow cell balls, tubes, and sieve-like sheets formed by orderly displacement of cells by transpar-

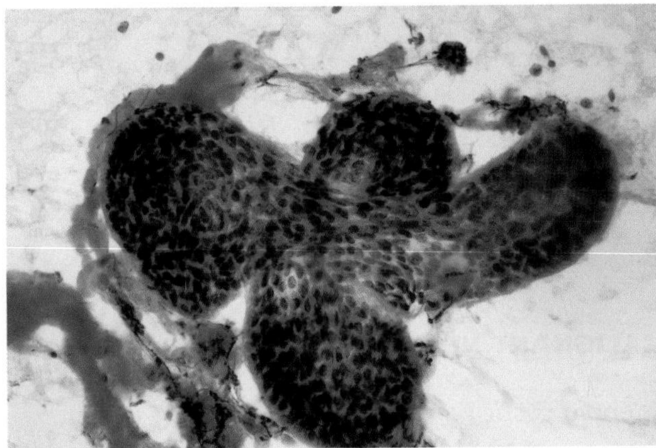

FIGURE 11. Basal cell adenoma, membranous type. Interanastomosing clusters and trabeculae of uniform basaloid cells surrounded by a thin band of homogeneous, cyanophilic stroma (Papanicolaou stain, 400×).

ent (Pap) stroma, compared to the dense, chaotic cell clusters of BCA (60). Finally, basosquamous whorls are not a feature of ADCC (2,11,14,32).

It may not be possible to distinguish solid ADCC from BCA reliably by individual cell morphology (59,60). Nuclear pleomorphism, irregular, granular chromatin, and hyperchromasia favor ADCC (11,14,44,65) but are not always present (59). Clinical history and radiologic findings are essential in such cases (59). One should be wary of a diagnosis of ADCC in the setting of a circumscribed, painless, mobile mass. Likewise, a benign diagnosis should be viewed with suspicion in lesions of the palate or if nerve symptoms are present. Given the degree of morphologic overlap, a descriptive signout with a differential diagnosis is warranted if the morphology is borderline.

Cellular pleomorphic adenoma (PA) may be confused with BCA. The cells of PA are less cohesive, more polymorphous, and exhibit more cytoplasm than BCA. Spindle and plasmacytoid cells are not a feature of BCA, and PA stroma is usually more abundant.

Cutaneous basal cell carcinoma (BCCA) rarely metastasizes to parotid lymph nodes and may mimic BCA because of the character of the cells and metachromatic desmoplastic tumor stroma. BCCA exhibits moderate nuclear atypia, apoptotic necrosis, and keratinization (66). Accurate history is essential.

The rare *basal cell adenocarcinoma* is distinguished from BCA by the presence of many mitoses, prominent small nucleoli, and moderate cytoplasm in the former (63,64,67), although the two neoplasms may be strikingly cytologically similar.

Because of the morphologic similarity of dermal appendage tumors such as *eccrine spiradenoma* (68) and *cylindroma* (69), and the coexistence of these lesions in some patients, detailed history, including the tissue plane of the lesion, is essential for an accurate diagnosis.

Basal Cell Adenoma

- Parotid gland (75%)
- Basaloid cells
- Cohesive, branching clusters, trabeculae
- Scant to absent stroma
  - Wrapped around periphery of clusters
  - Tiny globules
- No nerve symptoms
- Mobile, circumscribed mass
- ± Associated skin appendage tumors

Pitfalls (Differential Diagnosis)

1. Basement membrane–like stromal balls (ADCC)
2. Can be identical to solid ADCC

MALIGNANT NEOPLASMS

Adenoid Cystic Carcinoma

Adenoid cystic carcinoma (ADCC) accounts for 7.5% of all malignant salivary gland neoplasms, 4% of all salivary gland neoplasms, and is most commonly found in the parotid gland and palate of 30- to 50-year-old women [30(p. 203)]. Clinically these tumors are slowly growing masses that may be mobile when small [30(p. 204)]. With time, fixation to adjacent tissue, pain, and cranial nerve palsy frequently develop. Oral lesions often ulcerate the overlying mucosa. Despite its name, cystic change is rare. Three histologic types are recognized: tubular (cylindromatous), cribriform, and solid.

ADCC is defined cytologically by (a) tight cohesion, (b) monomorphic basaloid cells with virtually no cytoplasm, and (c) variable acellular hyaline stroma in globular or cylindromatous formations. FNA of the tubular or cribriform subtype yields numerous thick three-dimensional, tightly cohesive clusters, branching trabeculae, or small aggregates of epithelial cells (41,70). In alcohol-fixed material, large tissue fragments may exhibit a "sieve-like" or mosaic pattern as a result of the virtually transparent stroma displacing the cells (60,70) (Fig. 12).

Individual cells exhibit virtually absent cytoplasm (11,14,35,41,65), indistinct cell borders, and oval to angulated nuclei with coarse chromatin and variably present small nucleoli (41,65,70). Mitoses are rare. Variable numbers of single cells or cells with appreciable cytoplasm are present (70), but are usually fewer in number than PA or BCA. Spindle cells and plasmacytoid cells are not seen (35,36).

The cribriform and tubular subtypes exhibit classic hyaline stromal globules ("gumballs") (11,41,59,70) or cylinders consisting of sharply circumscribed, completely acellular spheres, cords, or tubes, alone or surrounded by cells. These stain bright magenta (Romanovsky stains) or gray to transparent (Papanicolaou stain). Characteristically, a sharp epithelial cell–stroma interface exists with the cell nuclei arranged parallel to the stroma's long axis, giving the cells a "stuck on" appearance (32,41,59,71). Epithelial cells and collagen fibrils are usually not enmeshed within the stroma; however, fibrillar stroma is present in a minority of aspirates (36). Although easily identified, and esthetically pleasing, hyaline globules are not specific for ADCC, and reliance on these as a sole diagnostic criterion will result in false-positive or otherwise erroneous diagnoses (Table 2).

In solid ADCC, the characteristic stroma is absent, and the presence of small hyperchromatic cells may make this variant dif-

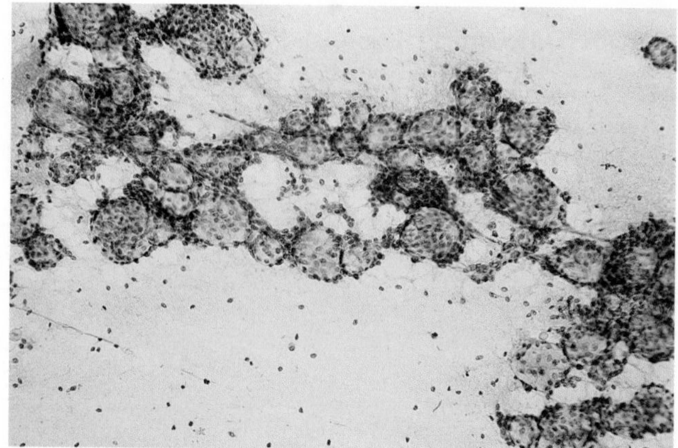

FIGURE 12. Adenoid cystic carcinoma. Mosaic pattern caused by translucent stromal spheres displacing the uniform "naked" nuclei. Cohesive epithelial cluster with clean background (Papanicolaou stain, 150×).

TABLE 2. NEOPLASMS WITH HYALINE STROMAL BALLS

Adenoid cystic carcinoma
Pleomorphic adenoma
Basal cell adenoma
Epithelial–myoepithelial carcinoma
Polymorphous low-grade carcinoma
Skin appendage tumors

ficult to discern from other basaloid neoplasms (Fig. 13). The cells of this subtype resemble those described above; however, some authors report decreased cohesion, greater nuclear pleomorphism, coarser chromatin, conspicuous nucleoli, and variably present mitoses or necrosis (59,65,72). Some aspirates of solid ADCC lack these features and are indistinguishable from BCA (43,59,72).

The diagnosis of ADCC should be based on careful assessment of the cell morphology with exclusion of known mimics and attention to clinical findings such as a poorly defined, fixed lesion, severe pain on aspiration, or facial nerve symptoms. Because of the number of false-positive diagnoses of ADCC (33,34), and the potentially disastrous consequences of radical surgery with sacrifice of the facial nerve, some authors (15,42) (including me) require the presence of nerve symptoms or infiltrative growth in addition to characteristic cytomorphology for a definitive ADCC diagnosis. Although these features strongly support a malignant diagnosis, facial nerve symptoms rarely have been reported in unusually located or infarcted benign salivary gland neoplasms (50,73). Therefore, correlation with the radiographic appearance of an infiltrative versus circumscribed mass is advised.

The differential diagnosis of ADCC includes basal cell adenoma, pleomorphic adenoma, polymorphous low-grade adenocarcinoma, epithelial–myoepithelial carcinoma, small-cell carcinoma, and a variety of basaloid neoplasms that do not originate in the salivary gland, such as metastatic basal cell carcinoma and benign skin appendage tumors.

Basal cell adenoma (BCA) lacks the organized, tightly cohesive, ball-like or mosaic cell clusters of ADCC and, instead, forms arborizing trabeculae with a chaotic cellular arrangement in a background of single cells (60). More importantly, stroma is usually extremely scant in BCA and limited to small globular or thin wraps at the periphery of cell groups. Basosquamous whorls are not seen in ADCC (32,72). Differences in the staining quality of the stroma, cell–stromal interface, and hyperchromasia and granularity of the nuclei have been proposed as criteria to distinguish ADCC from BCA (6,60,61,65); however, these features are subtle, inconsistently identified, and, therefore, not entirely reliable (59).

Numerous stromal fragments readily distinguish the cylindromatous type of ADCC from BCA (60); however, solid ADCC lacks stroma. Marked nuclear membrane and chromatin abnormalities, mitoses, or necrosis favors solid ADCC (11,14,44,65). However, not all ADCC aspirates will exhibit these features, and BCA may be indistinguishable from this lesion (43,59,72). The presence of nerve symptoms and location outside the parotid support ADCC.

Approximately 5% of *pleomorphic adenomas* (PA) may exhibit a cylindromatous stroma, and smears of these lesions may contain fields that are indistinguishable from ADCC. Careful attention to (a) amount of cytoplasm, (b) cell cohesion, (c) nature of the background, (d) stromal cellularity, (e) cell–stroma interface, and (f) clinical symptoms should permit accurate distinction between these lesions. On low power, PA exhibits loosely cohesive, arborizing sheets and trabeculae of haphazardly arranged cells in a background of numerous single spindle and plasmacytoid cells, in contrast to the tightly cohesive balls, cylinders, and mosaic sheets of ADCC (32,35,36,41,70). The polymorphous cuboidal, spindle, and plasmacytoid cells of PA exhibit more cytoplasm than the "naked nuclei" of ADCC (36,41). Most importantly, ADCC stroma consists of hyaline, acellular tubes, and spheres with a sharp cell–stromal interface as opposed to the more amorphous chondromyxoid PA stroma, which contains numerous, intimately admixed spindle cells and collagen fibrils (32,33,41) (Fig. 14).

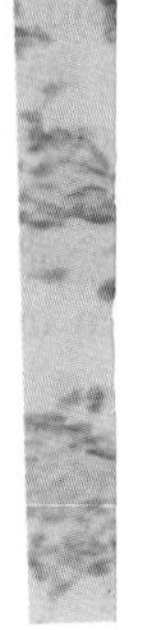

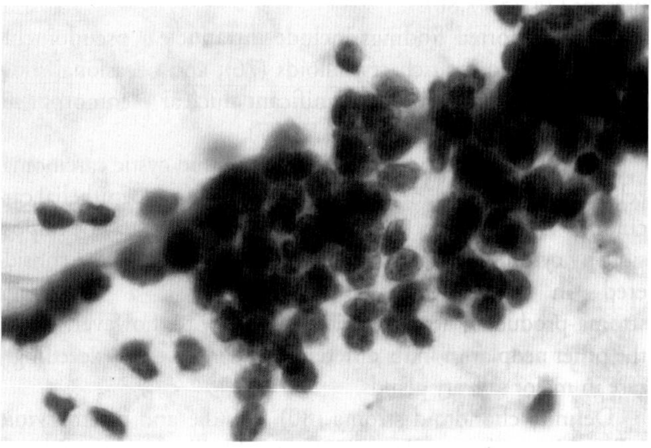

FIGURE 13. Solid adenoid cystic carcinoma. Angulated basaloid cells in cohesive clusters lacking stroma. Although significant nuclear atypia is present in this instance, the nuclei may be bland enough to mimic a basal cell adenoma (hematoxylin and eosin, 640×).

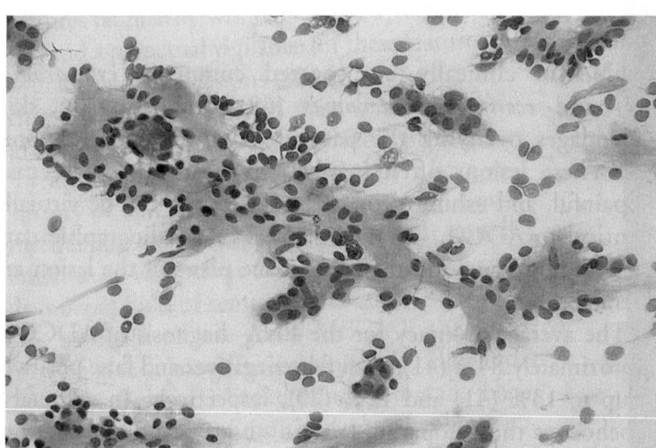

FIGURE 14. Adenoid cystic carcinoma mimicking pleomorphic adenoma. This lesion exhibits a cylindromatous stromal pattern with "naked" nuclei "stuck on" to perimeter of stroma. Compare with Fig. 6 (Papanicolaou stain, 320×).

resort because the standard of care in the treatment of head and neck carcinoma is *en bloc* removal of neck nodes (133,143).

The differential diagnosis of well-differentiated and cystic SCC includes inflamed branchial cleft or epidermal inclusion cyst, papillary thyroid carcinoma, pilomatrixoma, and cystic Warthin's tumor.

Inflamed lymphoepithelial (branchial cleft) cyst with reactive atypia may be impossible to separate from well-differentiated or cystic SCC (149,150). Clinically, branchial cleft cysts usually occur in a younger population, whereas SCC affects elderly men; however, there is significant age overlap (147). Large "intermediate"-type squamous cells of branchial cleft cysts are not a feature of carcinoma (148). Keratin pearls, necrotic epithelial cells, and miniature, atypical parakeratotic cells with increased N/C ratios or angulated nuclei are rarely found in benign lesions (143,144,146,147) and, if present, constitute a minor population admixed with numerous benign elements. The atypical cells of benign lesions typically form flat, cohesive, polarized sheets of cells with uniform pale nuclei, smooth nuclear borders, evenly dispersed chromatin, and prominent nucleoli typical of repair (143,147) (see also discussions of branchial cleft cyst in this chapter).

Inflamed or irradiated epidermal inclusion cysts (EIC) are predominantly composed of large (superficial cell sized) anucleate squames and lack the high N/C ratio, hyperchromasia, and nuclear membrane and chromatin irregularities of carcinoma (148). Ruptured epidermal inclusion cysts with granulomatous inflammation yield very cellular aspirates in which reactive histiocytes may be mistaken for carcinoma; however, the former exhibit small nuclei (neutrophil sized), fine chromatin, prominent nucleoli, and cell-to-cell uniformity (148). Aggregates of histiocytes can be seen engulfing keratin, further confirming their histiocytic origin. A history of radiation therapy and knowledge of the tissue plane of the lesion are also useful in preventing misdagnosis (see also discussions of EIC in this chapter).

Papillary thyroid carcinoma may yield a cystic aspirate with clusters of polygonal cells with dense, "metaplastic"-appearing cytoplasm (141,145). The resemblance to SCC is only superficial, for papillary carcinoma lacks keratinization and exhibits the typical pale grooved nuclei with or without occasional intranuclear pseudoinclusions as contrasted to the usually hyperchromatic pyknotic nuclei of SCC.

Pilomatrixoma exhibits a mixture of small uniform basaloid cells in tight clusters with aggregates of glassy, amorphous, orangeophilic to pink debris (ghost cells), with or without giant cells and calcification. Necrosis and malignant nuclear irregularities are not seen (144,151).

Reactive changes in cystic Warthin's tumors usually consist of a few abnormal orangeophilic cells with degenerate nuclei in a background of typical oncocytes and granular or mucoid debris (148). Well-preserved cells with malignant nuclear features are not present (see discussions of Warthin's tumor in this chapter).

In summary, to avoid misdiagnosis in cystic or well-differentiated squamous lesions, the wary cytopathologist should (a) require classic malignant nuclear membrane or chromatin abnormalities for a definitive diagnosis of carcinoma, especially in the setting of acute inflammation, (b) check the background for any evidence of a second cell population representing a benign lesion, (c) perform multiple passes to insure adequate sampling, and (d) know the history and radiologic appearance of the lesion including the tissue plane and history of radiation therapy (148).

Squamous Cell Carcinoma

1. Polygonal cells with hard, "glassy" cytoplasm
2. Often obvious malignant nuclear features
3. Well-differentiated SCC: miniature, abnormally shaped, keratinized cells with high N/C ratios
4. Cystic SCC with scant, abnormally shaped keratinized cells ± pearls in a histiocytic background
5. Preserved cells with definite nuclear membrane or chromatin irregularities required for definitive diagnosis

Other Variants of Squamous Cell Carcinoma

These lesions (see Chapters 2 and 7) are usually readily identified as malignant; however, their unusual morphology may result in failure to recognize the upper aerodigestive tract as the site of origin.

Spindle cell (sarcomatoid) squamous cell carcinoma yields sheets and syncytia of monotonous spindle cells with mild to moderate hyperchromasia and nuclear membrane irregularities. Usually mitoses are absent (144). These lesions can be misdiagnosed as melanoma or a soft-tissue lesion. Immunocytochemical stains for pankeratin, S-100 protein, and HMB45 and mesenchymal markers may be useful in ambiguous cases.

Small, rounded groups of cells, along with smaller aggregates of polygonal cells arrayed as single files or bent chains in aspirates of *adenoid (acantholytic) squamous cell carcinoma* may suggest adenocarcinoma to the unwary (152). However, closer inspection reveals definite squamous features including polygonal cells with dense, circumscribed cytoplasm, keratinization, and frequent single dyskeratotic cells (152). This variant of SCC most frequently arises in the oral cavity, tongue, nasopharynx, and skin of the head and neck (152).

Basaloid squamous cell carcinoma may be confused with metastatic small-cell carcinoma, adenoid cystic carcinoma, and nasopharyngeal carcinoma. FNA yields a mixture of large, cohesive cell nests and cords as well as many single cells. The cells are small, with scant cytoplasm, mildly pleomorphic nuclei, fine chromatin, and small but consistent nucleoli (153,154). Necrosis and mitoses are frequently present, but molding is uncommon (153,154). Pseudoglandular spaces surrounded by eosinophilic (Pap stain), PAS with diastase–positive hyaline material is present in approximately 50% of cases (153,154). Rare single keratinized cells or foci of typical SCC may or may not be present (153,154). Alcian blue stain reveals stromal mucin within the cell groups.

Basaloid SCC may be very difficult to distinguish from metastatic *small-cell carcinoma;* however, the presence of large tissue fragments, fine nuclear chromatin, minimal molding, and focal squamous differentiation favors the former. It may be impossible to distinguish the two without immunocytochemical

TABLE 2. NEOPLASMS WITH HYALINE STROMAL BALLS

Adenoid cystic carcinoma
Pleomorphic adenoma
Basal cell adenoma
Epithelial–myoepithelial carcinoma
Polymorphous low-grade carcinoma
Skin appendage tumors

ficult to discern from other basaloid neoplasms (Fig. 13). The cells of this subtype resemble those described above; however, some authors report decreased cohesion, greater nuclear pleomorphism, coarser chromatin, conspicuous nucleoli, and variably present mitoses or necrosis (59,65,72). Some aspirates of solid ADCC lack these features and are indistinguishable from BCA (43,59,72).

The diagnosis of ADCC should be based on careful assessment of the cell morphology with exclusion of known mimics and attention to clinical findings such as a poorly defined, fixed lesion, severe pain on aspiration, or facial nerve symptoms. Because of the number of false-positive diagnoses of ADCC (33,34), and the potentially disastrous consequences of radical surgery with sacrifice of the facial nerve, some authors (15,42) (including me) require the presence of nerve symptoms or infiltrative growth in addition to characteristic cytomorphology for a definitive ADCC diagnosis. Although these features strongly support a malignant diagnosis, facial nerve symptoms rarely have been reported in unusually located or infarcted benign salivary gland neoplasms (50,73). Therefore, correlation with the radiographic appearance of an infiltrative versus circumscribed mass is advised.

The differential diagnosis of ADCC includes basal cell adenoma, pleomorphic adenoma, polymorphous low-grade adenocarcinoma, epithelial–myoepithelial carcinoma, small-cell carcinoma, and a variety of basaloid neoplasms that do not originate in the salivary gland, such as metastatic basal cell carcinoma and benign skin appendage tumors.

Basal cell adenoma (BCA) lacks the organized, tightly cohesive, ball-like or mosaic cell clusters of ADCC and, instead, forms arborizing trabeculae with a chaotic cellular arrangement in a background of single cells (60). More importantly, stroma is usually extremely scant in BCA and limited to small globular or thin wraps at the periphery of cell groups. Basosquamous whorls are not seen in ADCC (32,72). Differences in the staining quality of the stroma, cell–stromal interface, and hyperchromasia and granularity of the nuclei have been proposed as criteria to distinguish ADCC from BCA (6,60,61,65); however, these features are subtle, inconsistently identified, and, therefore, not entirely reliable (59).

Numerous stromal fragments readily distinguish the cylindromatous type of ADCC from BCA (60); however, solid ADCC lacks stroma. Marked nuclear membrane and chromatin abnormalities, mitoses, or necrosis favors solid ADCC (11,14,44,65). However, not all ADCC aspirates will exhibit these features, and BCA may be indistinguishable from this lesion (43,59,72). The presence of nerve symptoms and location outside the parotid support ADCC.

Approximately 5% of *pleomorphic adenomas* (PA) may exhibit a cylindromatous stroma, and smears of these lesions may contain fields that are indistinguishable from ADCC. Careful attention to (a) amount of cytoplasm, (b) cell cohesion, (c) nature of the background, (d) stromal cellularity, (e) cell–stroma interface, and (f) clinical symptoms should permit accurate distinction between these lesions. On low power, PA exhibits loosely cohesive, arborizing sheets and trabeculae of haphazardly arranged cells in a background of numerous single spindle and plasmacytoid cells, in contrast to the tightly cohesive balls, cylinders, and mosaic sheets of ADCC (32,35,36,41,70). The polymorphous cuboidal, spindle, and plasmacytoid cells of PA exhibit more cytoplasm than the "naked nuclei" of ADCC (36,41). Most importantly, ADCC stroma consists of hyaline, acellular tubes, and spheres with a sharp cell–stromal interface as opposed to the more amorphous chondromyxoid PA stroma, which contains numerous, intimately admixed spindle cells and collagen fibrils (32,33,41) (Fig. 14).

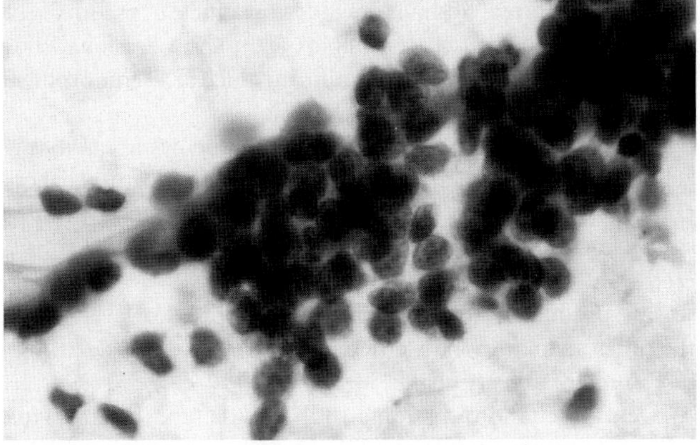

FIGURE 13. Solid adenoid cystic carcinoma. Angulated basaloid cells in cohesive clusters lacking stroma. Although significant nuclear atypia is present in this instance, the nuclei may be bland enough to mimic a basal cell adenoma (hematoxylin and eosin, 640×).

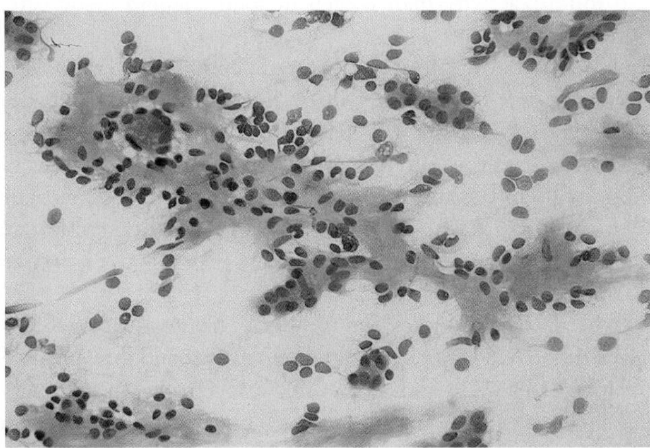

FIGURE 14. Adenoid cystic carcinoma mimicking pleomorphic adenoma. This lesion exhibits a cylindromatous stromal pattern with "naked" nuclei "stuck on" to perimeter of stroma. Compare with Fig. 6 (Papanicolaou stain, 320×).

Because distinction of ADCC from cellular pleomorphic adenoma can be difficult, the wise cytopathologist should carefully scan the background of all slides for any features of pleomorphic adenoma (32) and check the clinical history for signs of nerve symptoms before rendering a definitive diagnosis. If clinical, radiologic, and morphologic features are not absolutely definitive, descriptive signout with a differential diagnosis is indicated (see also Pleomorphic Adenoma in this chapter).

Polymorphous low-grade adenocarcinoma (PLGA) resembles ADCC by frequently involving the palate and exhibiting hyaline globules and tightly cohesive cell balls and clusters composed of bland cells (74). Unlike ADCC, the cells of PLGA exhibit moderate cytoplasm, with cuboidal to columnar forms (11,14,75,76). Nucleoli are present (74), chromatin is fine, not clumped, and the nuclei are rounder, larger, and more uniform in PLGA (77). Significant morphologic overlap exists, and it may be impossible to distinguish the two by cytomorphology alone (74,75). This may not be significant because the treatment is the same. For palate lesions it is wise always to consider PLGA in the differential diagnosis, particularly in elderly patients (35,41,75).

Epithelial–myoepithelial carcinoma (EMC) exhibits hyaline globules and three-dimensional balls of uniform basaloid cells (13,41,77). However, EMC is a biphasic tumor, and recognition of a second population of cells with clear cytoplasm and atypical nuclei, frequently located at the periphery of the basaloid cell aggregates, excludes ADCC (14,46,47). This feature is most evident on Pap-stained material and may not be seen on air-dried preparations (77). In addition, acellular hyaline material frequently surrounds the epithelial clusters in a ring-like fashion in EMC (47), unlike ADCC.

FNA of *metastatic basal cell carcinoma* (BCCA) yields tightly cohesive clusters of small basaloid cells (66) with or without nuclear palisading. Metachromatically staining stroma has been described in BCCA (66); however, stromal globules are not characteristic. Apoptotic cell necrosis, mitoses, and squamous differentiation with keratinization favor BCCA (66).

Small-cell undifferentiated carcinoma, whether primary or metastatic, typically exhibits greater nuclear anaplasia, necrosis, and mitotic activity than is seen in solid adenoid cystic carcinoma (78).

FNA of clinically unsuspected cutaneous *cylindromas* (69) and *eccrine spiradenomas* (68) originating in skin appendages overlying the parotid gland have been reported. These lesions often involve the head and neck, may be painful, and exhibit cytologic features that can be virtually identical to ADCC. Detailed clinical and radiographic data regarding duration and the exact tissue plane of the lesion are essential.

The average accuracy for the FNA diagnosis of ADCC is approximately 84% (41), with false negatives and false positives of up to 13% (41) and 12% (70), respectively. In summary, it behooves the cytopathologist to observe caution, caution, and more caution with careful synthesis of the cytomorphology and clinical and radiographic findings before rendering a diagnosis of ADCC. It is an uncommon lesion that is frequently mimicked on FNA by more common, benign lesions (11,14,41,79).

Adenoid Cystic Carcinoma

- Nerve symptoms
- Ill-defined fixed mass
- Tightly cohesive clusters, sheets, and cords (single cells)
- "Naked" basaloid cells
- Stroma
  - Acellular hyaline globules, cylinders
  - 11% fibromyxoid stroma
  - Nuclei "stuck on" parallel to long axis of stroma

Pitfalls (Differential Diagnosis)

1. Stromal balls not specific (PA, BCA, PLGA, etc.)
2. Basaloid cells (PLGA, BCA, BCC, skin appendage)
3. Solid variant, no stroma (BCA, sm cell CA)
4. Resemble skin appendage tumors
5. Nerve symptoms requisite for diagnosis

Polymorphous Low-Grade Adenocarcinoma

Polymorphous low grade adenocarcinoma (PLGA) comprises approximately 7% of all minor salivary gland tumors [30(p. 216)]. At the Armed Forces Institute of Pathology (AFIP), PLGA was identified as twice as common as adenoid cystic carcinoma and the third most common neoplasm of salivary gland origin [30(p. 216)]. It occurs almost exclusively in minor salivary glands, particularly the palate but also throughout the oral cavity [30(p. 216)]. Women and African Americans over 50 years of age are most commonly affected [30(p. 217)]. Clinically, the lesion appears as a circumscribed, asymptomatic nodule.

Aspirates are highly cellular and composed of clusters, papillae, and sheets of small cuboidal to columnar cells with uniform, round or oval nuclei and scant to moderate cytoplasm (74,75,77,80). Papillae with a central stromal core are characteristic (77). Hyaline stromal globules, with or without associated palisaded cells or dispersed myxohyaline matrix, are frequently present (74,75,77,80).

Other reported findings include intranuclear pseudoinclusions (74), tyrosine-rich crystalloids (76), and occasional short spindle cells (80). Mitoses, significant nuclear pleomorphism, and necrosis are not present (74,75,77).

The differential diagnosis includes adenoid cystic carcinoma, cellular pleomorphic adenoma, and epithelial–myoepithelial carcinoma. Distinction of these lesions from PLGA may be impossible by cytomorphology alone. PLGA should always be considered in the differential diagnosis of a low-grade stroma-producing neoplasm of the oral cavity; however, unlike the other neoplasms in its differential diagnosis, it is exceedingly rare in major salivary glands.

Definite chondroid stroma (80), spindle and plasmacytoid cells with ample cytoplasm (77), or a fibrillar matrix with enmeshed cells (74) favors *pleomorphic adenoma* over PLGA. *Epithelial–myoepithelial carcinoma* (EMC) occurs predominantly in major salivary glands and is distinguished by its biphasic composition of basaloid epithelial cells surrounded by clear to vacuolated myoepithelial cells (best seen on Papanicolaou stain) (77). If this feature is not appreciated, the two lesions may appear virtually identical. *Adenoid cystic carcinoma* lacks papillary formations (77) and exhibits smaller, more angulated and hyperchromatic nuclei with frequent nucleoli (74,77).

Accuracy for a malignant diagnosis of PLGA is approximately 86% (77).

Polymorphous Low-Grade Adenocarcinoma

- Palate or oral cavity in the elderly
- Papillae with central stroma
- Acini and sheets
- Cuboidal or columnar cells with bland nuclei
- Hyaline stromal globules
- Absent mitoses, anaplasia, necrosis

Pitfalls (Differential Diagnosis)

1. Hyaline globules (ADCC, EMC)
2. Extracellular stroma (PA)
3. Polymorphous cells (PA)

Epithelial–Myoepithelial Carcinoma

Epithelial–myoepithelial carcinoma (EMC) accounts for approximately 1% of salivary gland neoplasms, and up to 90% involve the major salivary glands [30(p. 268)]. Women in the seventh decade are most commonly affected. Clinically, EMC presents as a firm, circumscribed, painless mass [30(pp. 268–269)].

The cytologic hallmark of EMC is the presence of spherical cell aggregates formed by a core of acellular hyaline matrix, surrounded by a midlayer of uniform basaloid epithelial cells, which in turn is covered by a peripheral rim of clear or vacuolated myoepithelial cells (46,47,81,82). The proportion of clear to basaloid cells in the clusters varies from a predominance of one or the other to an even mixture (46). Oval hyperchromatic nuclei with clumped chromatin and frequent nucleoli characterize the basal cells, whereas the clear cells frequently exhibit pink (Romanovsky) or pale gray (Papanicolaou) (46) vacuolated cytoplasm and mild nuclear pleomorphism. The stroma is readily visible as acellular, pink hyaline globules (46,47,83) but also as amorphous rings surrounding the periphery of the cell clusters (47).

The differential diagnoses include *adenoid cystic carcinoma, polymorphous low-grade adenocarcinoma,* and *pleomorphic adenoma.* The biphasic cell population, particularly clear vacuolated cells, coupled with characteristic stroma, favors the diagnosis of EMC (46,47,83) (see also differential diagnostic discussion under these tumor headings).

Epithelial–Myoepithelial Carcinoma

- Major salivary glands (90%), elderly women
- Biphasic cell population
  - Central basaloid cells
  - Peripheral clear cells
- Hyaline stromal globules
- Mild nuclear atypia

Pitfalls (Differential Diagnosis)

1. Hyaline globules (ADCC, PLGA)
2. Polymorphous cells (PA, PLGA)

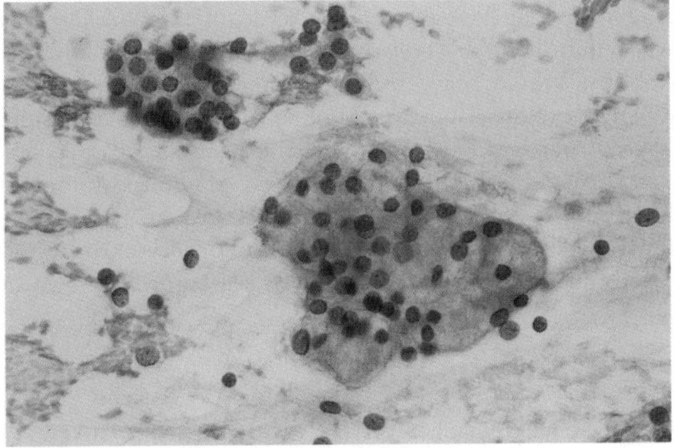

FIGURE 15. Low-grade mucoepidermoid carcinoma. A cluster of frothy glandular cells with bland, overlapping nuclei below a smaller cluster of intermediate cells with scant, homogeneous cytoplasm. Note background mucus and resemblance of glandular cells to foamy histiocytes (Papanicolaou stain, 400×).

Mucoepidermoid Carcinoma

Mucoepidermoid carcinoma (MECA) is the most common malignant neoplasm of salivary glands [84(p. 271)], the second most common salivary gland tumor in children [84(p. 272)], and is one of the most frequent sources of false-negative diagnoses in FNA cytology (5,6,8,13,54,55,85–87). In a meta-analysis of the literature, Klijanienko (88) noted up to one third of MECAs were underdiagnosed; however, diagnostic accuracy increases with experience (88,89). The recognition of this neoplasm on FNA requires familiarity with its various cytomorphologic idiosyncracies and a perpetual vigilance for these features in all cystic and low-grade epithelial lesions (88).

MECA presents as a solitary, painless mass in the parotid, submandibular gland, palate, or buccal mucosa and is present for an average of 1.5 years [84(p. 156)]. These tumors have been associated with a history of ionizing radiation [84(p. 155)]. Low-grade MECA is frequently cystic; however, in most but not all cases (87), a residual mass will persist after drainage of the cyst fluid. FNA yields mucoid fluid or semisolid material.

The diagnostic hallmark of low-grade MECA is the synchronous presence of glandular cells, intermediate cells, and squamous cells, with or without a background of mucin. The glandular component may consist of multivacuolated columnar to polygonal cells with numerous intracytoplasmic mucin vacuoles and bland nuclei (14,87–90). When these are shed into a fluid medium, they may “round up” and mimic foamy macrophages. Goblet cells may be present (11,90) (Fig. 15).

Intermediate cells form cohesive but disorganized multilayered sheets of overlapping, small, polygonal cells with uniform vesicular nuclei, small nucleoli, and blue-green (Papanicolaou) or pink to purple (Romanovsky) cytoplasm (26,88,89) (Fig. 16). Single cells may be present. Their morphology is reminiscent of immature squamous metaplasia seen in exfoliative cytology of the female genital tract.

Squamous cells occur singly and in sheets with centrally placed, uniform, vesicular nuclei, prominent nucleoli, and distinct cell borders (88,89). Glandular cells and intermediate cells predominate in low-grade MECA, whereas squamous cells dominate high-grade lesions.

The background mucin stains translucent gray-blue (Papanicolaou) or magenta-blue (Romanovsky) and may be watery with admixed inflammatory cells and foamy glandular cells or dense and "stringy" resembling stroma (26,91). In a statistical analysis of MECA, Cohen (5) found that the combined presence of (a) overlapping groups, (b) intermediate cells, and (c) squamous cells was 97% sensitive and 100% specific for MECA.

Other features that may be encountered in aspirates of MECA are dense lymphocytic infiltrate (24% of cases) (88) (Fig. 16), crystalloids (88), intranuclear cytoplasmic pseudoinclusions (92), mast cells (10% of cases) (49), clear cells (88), sebaceous differentiation (90), and oncocytes.

High-grade MECA is usually readily recognized as malignant but may be difficult to distinguish from undifferentiated or squamous cell carcinoma of primary or metastatic origin (8,11,14,88,89). The aspirates are abundantly cellular and composed of polygonal cells with irregular nuclear membranes, clumped chromatin, and prominent nucleoli (8,11,14,88,89) (Fig. 17). Prominent squamous differentiation in the form of polygonal cells with discrete cell borders and dense cytoplasm may be present, as may necrosis and mitoses. Glandular differentiation may be scant to absent and frequently requires mucin stains for identification (8,11). The presence of abundant keratinization with pearl formation is more commonly seen in squamous cell carcinoma of primary or metastatic origin (8,11,89).

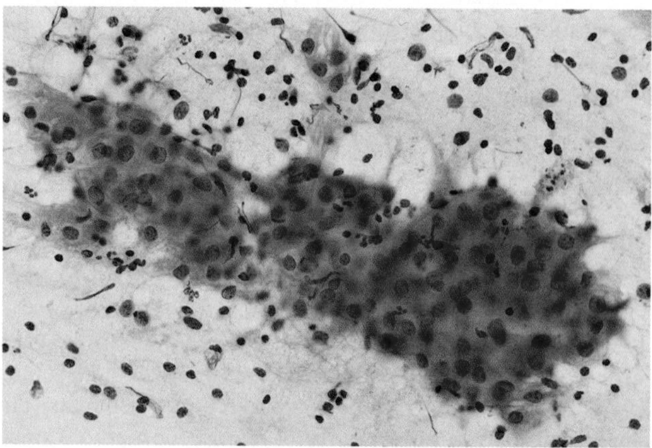

FIGURE 16. Intermediate-grade mucoepidermoid carcinoma. Cluster of intermediate cells with uniform, overlapping nuclei present in a background of lymphocytes and mucin. A prominent lymphocytic infiltrate may be seen in up to 24% of mucoepidermoid carcinoma aspirates. Compare with Warthin's tumor (Fig. 9) (hematoxylin and eosin stain, 400×).

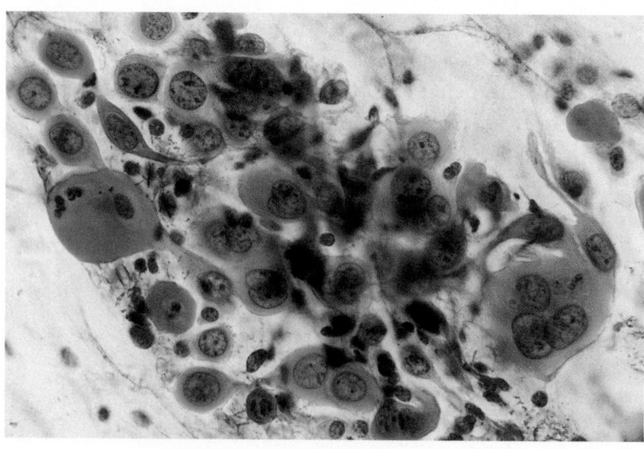

FIGURE 17. High-grade mucoepidermoid carcinoma. Polygonal to spindled cells with dense, "glassy" cytoplasm and obvious malignant nuclear features. Glandular differentiation not evident in this field; however, rare cells with vacuolated cytoplasm were present elsewhere in smear (Papanicolaou stain, 640×).

Because high-grade MECA may be treated with radical surgical excision and sacrifice of the facial nerve, the distinction between a metastasis and high-grade MECA is important but may not be possible by cytomorphology alone. Ancillary studies such as panendoscopy of the upper aerodigestive tract and radiologic studies may be required for this distinction.

The differential diagnosis of low-grade MECA is broad and includes mucus retention cyst, chronic sialadenitis, Warthin's tumor, acinic cell carcinoma, pleomorphic adenoma, and clear-cell neoplasms.

If epithelium is present in an aspirate from a *mucus retention cyst,* it will be scant and composed of ductal cells and squamous cells arranged in flat, orderly sheets, unlike the overlapping groups of MECA (11,26). FNA diagnosis of a mucus retention cyst warrants careful follow-up, with further evaluation of any persistent or recurrent mass.

Twenty-four percent of low-grade MECAs may be accompanied by a dense lymphocytic infiltrate (Table 3) (93), and the combination of lymphocytes and sheets of intermediate cells may mimic *Warthin's tumor* (WT). To further compound the problem, MECA may exhibit oncocytic metaplasia, whereas WT may exhibit glandular and/or squamous metaplasia and a thin mucoid background. Architectural and cytoplasmic features distinguish these lesions. MECA is composed of disorganized sheets of cells with significant nuclear overlap and three-dimensionality (26), whereas flat sheets of oncocytes with good architectural polarity and well-defined cell borders are seen in

TABLE 3. NEOPLASMS WITH LYMPHOID INFILTRATE

Warthin's tumor
Mucoepidermoid carcinoma (24%)
Acinic cell carcinoma (10%)
Pleomorphic adenoma
Metastases to lymph node

WT (26,89). If glandular or squamous metaplasia is present in WT, it will be a minor component in a background of typical oncocytic sheets and lymphocytes (11,28,89). A report conveying a differential diagnosis is warranted for borderline morphology.

Pleomorphic adenoma enters the differential diagnosis when its aspirate yields background mucin or focal glandular or squamous metaplasia (37). Typical fibromyxoid stroma and loosely cohesive cuboidal, spindle, and plasmacytoid cells favor pleomorphic adenoma, as opposed to the sheets of overlapping intermediate and glandular cells of MECA (37).

Occasional diagnostic difficulties arise with *acinic cell carcinoma* (14) because of the vacuolated cells in acinic cell carcinoma mimicking the glandular cells of MECA. Large cytoplasmic vacuoles favor acinic cell carcinoma, whereas MECA cytoplasm is finely vacuolated (79). Review of all material will usually show background mucin or squamous or intermediate cells in low-grade MECA (94) and typical acinar-type cells in a background of naked nuclei, with or without a capillary stromal meshwork in acinic cell carcinoma (79).

If clear-cell change is present, MECA may be difficult to distinguish from other primary and metastatic *clear-cell neoplasms* of salivary gland. Mucin stains are positive in MECA (95).

Accuracy for the diagnosis of malignancy in MECA is approximately 78%, but only 38% for an exact diagnosis of MECA.

Low-Grade Mucoepidermoid Carcinoma

- Polymorphous cell population
  - Glandular: goblet, foamy, columnar
  - Intermediate: immature squamous metaplasia
  - Squamous (no keratin)
- Sheets with overlapping nuclei
- Mucin background (often cystic)
- 24% lymphoid background

Pitfalls (Differential Diagnosis)

1. Mucinous cyst contents sampled only (mucocele)
2. Bland nuclei (PA)
3. Intermediate cells confused with oncocytes (WT)
4. Intermediate cells confused with epithelial–myoepithelial cells (cellular PA)
5. Background mucin confused with stroma (PA)
6. Lymphoid background and intermediate cells confused with WT

High-Grade MECA

- Anaplastic nuclei
- ± Necrosis
- Predominantly squamous
  - Glandular differentiation often scant to absent
  - Keratinization rare

Pitfalls

1. Confusion with SDC, SCCA, or metastatic carcinoma
2. Keratinization favors metastasis

Acinic Cell Carcinoma

Acinic cell carcinoma (ACC) accounts for 17% of salivary gland malignancies, 6% of all salivary gland neoplasms, is the third most common salivary gland neoplasm in children, and is bilateral in approximately 3% of cases [30(pp. 183,185)]. Eighty-three percent arise in the parotid gland [30(p. 183)]. Women with a mean age of 44 years are most commonly affected [30(p. 184)]. Clinically the lesion presents as a circumscribed, mobile, slowly growing mass with pain or tenderness present in over one third of patients [30(p. 185)].

Because malignant nuclear features are rare in ACC, the FNA diagnosis rests on architecture and the recognition of acinar-type cytoplasmic differentiation (96,97). Histologically acinar cells, intercalated ductal cells, vacuolated cells, clear cells, and nonspecific glandular cells in a variety of cystic and solid patterns define ACC [30(p. 185–197)]. FNA features include a monotonous population of large, vacuolated or granular, polygonal cells with prominent dyshesion, numerous stripped epithelial nuclei, and a prominent supporting stromal capillary network.

The FNA sample is abundantly cellular, composed of sheets and solid three-dimensional clusters of very dyshesive, large, acinar-type cells with finely vacuolated cytoplasm and indistinct cell borders (11,14,79,96,97) (Fig. 18). The cells are larger than normal acinar cells (97). Fine cytoplasmic granules (blue on Pap; red on Romanovsky stain) may be present; however, these are fewer in number and more basophilic on Papanicolaou stain than those of oncocytes (79). Highly vacuolated cells may also be seen (79). The nuclei are deceptively uniform and bland, with occasional small nucleoli (79,96,97). The background may be finely granular, consisting of cytoplasmic fragments (79), and almost always exhibits abundant stripped epithelial nuclei (96). Frequently, the tumor cells are loosely adherent to a prominent meshwork of delicate capillaries.

Higher-grade carcinomas exhibit greater nuclear and chromatin irregularities; however, they also exhibit less obvious acinar differentiation (96). Clear cells can be prominent in 1% of tumors (95). Ancillary findings in ACC aspirates include a dense

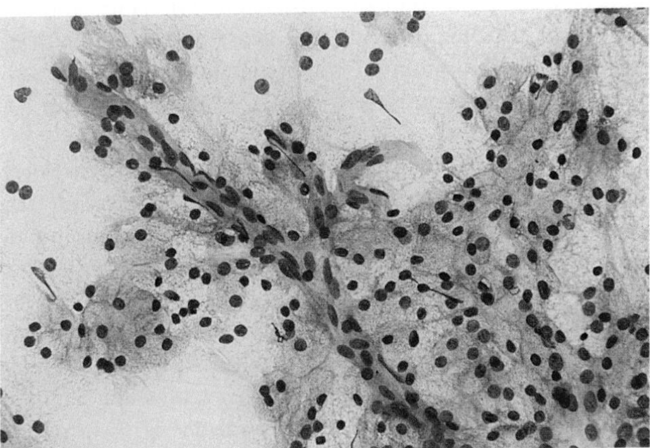

FIGURE 18. Acinic cell carcinoma. Dyshesive sheets of cells with frothy to finely granular cytoplasm and uniform overlapping nuclei surrounding a capillary. Note stripped epithelial cell nuclei in background (Diff-Quik stain, 500×).

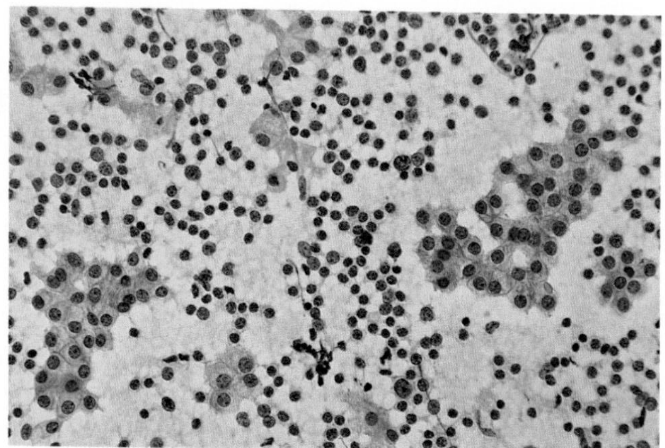

FIGURE 19. Acinic cell carcinoma with lymphocytic infiltrate. Dyshesive, disorderly sheets of cells with vacuolated to finely granular cytoplasm in a lymphoid background. Note vacuolated cells singly and in small clusters. Typical acinic cell carcinoma morphology was present elsewhere on smear. Compare with Warthin's tumor (Fig. 9) (Papanicolaou stain, 400×).

lymphoid infiltrate in up to 10% of aspirates (41,79) (Fig. 19) and occasional psammoma bodies (98). The papillary cystic variant of ACC exhibits greater cohesion with large monolayer epithelial sheets, many cells with large cytoplasmic vacuoles, and no stripped nuclei (94).

The differential diagnosis includes normal parotid gland, Warthin's tumor, mucoepidermoid carcinoma, benign cyst, and lesions with clear-cell or sebaceous differentiation.

Architecture and cell polymorphism readily distinguish ACC from *normal salivary gland.* The tightly cohesive grape-like clusters of acinar cells admixed with ducts and fat in the latter contrast sharply with the disorganized monomorphic sheets of dyshesive acinic cells supported by a capillary meshwork in ACC (41,96).

Stripped background nuclei and the not infrequent lymphoid infiltrate, coupled with sheets of acinic cells, may mimic *Warthin's tumor.* True oncocytes are densely granular as opposed to finely vacuolated or scantly granular acinic cells. In addition, Warthin's oncocytes are tightly cohesive with sharp cell borders, lacking the dyshesion, three-dimensionality, and delicate vascular stroma of ACC. The dense granular cystic background of Warthin's tumor is not present in ACC. If there is any doubt as to the diagnosis, cells of ACC stain positively for PAS with diastase.

The differential diagnosis with *mucoepidermoid carcinoma* (MECA) is usually not difficult; however, in occasional aspirates of ACC, clear cells or vacuolated cells will predominate, mimicking glandular cells. Mucin positivity distinguishes these lesions.

Cystic degeneration is not uncommon in ACC (96), and therefore the cyst contents from an inadequately sampled lesion may be virtually indistinguishable from a *benign cyst.* Sampling of any residual mass should prevent misdiagnosis.

An aspirate of the rare *sebaceous lymphadenoma* could closely mimic ACC with lymphoid stroma. Sebaceous cells, in contrast to acinar cells, are smaller, with less cytoplasm, more uniformly sized vacuoles, and absent cytoplasmic granularity (90). A PAS with diastase stain will be negative, and a fat stain positive, in sebaceous lesions.

The diagnostic accuracy for malignancy in aspirates of ACC ranges from 76.7% to 91%; however, the accuracy for exact diagnosis of ACC ranges from 13.7% to 67.5% (41,79).

ACINIC CELL CARCINOMA

- Dyshesive sheets and aggregates of foamy to granular cells with bland nuclei
- Capillary meshwork
- Naked round background nuclei
- 10% with lymphoid background
- ± clear-cell change

Pitfalls (Differential Diagnosis)

1. Bland nuclei (normal salivary gland, WT, MECA)
2. Cystic change (mucocele, MECA, WT)
3. Clear or granular cells misdiagnosed (MECA, WT, metastatic renal cell carcinoma)
4. Lymphoid background (WT)

Carcinoma ex Pleomorphic Adenoma

Carcinoma *ex* pleomorphic adenoma (CEPA) occurs in fewer than 9% of pleomorphic adenomas (PA) and accounts for approximately 5% of all malignant salivary gland neoplasms [30(p. 229)]. The mean age of onset is 60 years, reflecting the average of 15 to 20 years required for malignant transformation of a pleomorphic adenoma [30(p. 229)]. Clinically, the lesion is often fixed and painless at presentation [30(p. 229)]. A clinical history of sudden rapid growth in a longstanding mass, with or without facial nerve symptoms, is classic for CEPA and is an extremely important aid in the diagnosis because residual PA may be absent in FNA samples (93,99). Adenocarcinoma not otherwise specified (NOS) or salivary duct carcinoma is the most common malignancy to arise from a pleomorphic adenoma [30(p. 229)]. However, a diverse array of malignant components have been described, including squamous cell carcinoma, undifferentiated carcinoma, MECA, ACC, or virtually any subtype of salivary gland carcinoma [30(p. 229),93,99,100].

The hallmark of CEPA on FNA is the presence of numerous, unequivocally malignant cells with obvious nuclear membrane and chromatin abnormalities (40), admixed with foci of typical PA, in a patient with a classic clinical history. Because the residual pleomorphic adenoma may be small, multiple samples should be obtained when malignant transformation is suspected, with a diligent search for evidence of benign PA stroma or cellular elements.

The differential diagnosis includes focal atypia in a PA, a high-grade salivary gland, or metastatic carcinoma, and true carcinosarcoma.

Scattered moderately atypical cells in an otherwise classic background occur in up to 10% of *pleomorphic adenomas* (33,40) in contrast to a predominance of malignant cells with scant or absent benign PA in true CEPA (14,15,40). Clinical history of rapid growth or nerve symptoms supports CEPA. In ambiguous aspirates, a signout of "PA with atypical features" and excision with frozen section is warranted.

Aspirates of *carcinosarcoma* exhibit a malignant mesenchymal component (chondrosarcoma, osteosarcoma, or undifferentiated sarcoma) (101) in addition to the malignant epithelial component.

Other *primary and metastatic carcinomas* are in the differential diagnosis if background features of residual PA are not identified on FNA. The clinical history of a significant change in a long-standing mass would not likely be present in those conditions.

Salivary Duct Carcinoma

Salivary duct carcinoma (SDC) presents as a rapidly growing, painless mass, with or without nerve symptoms in the parotid (86%) or submandibular gland (7%) of elderly men [30(p. 325)]. It is rare, representing 0.2% of salivary gland neoplasms [30(p. 325)].

On FNA, the lesion can be partially cystic because of necrosis (102). Characteristic FNA features include (a) large polygonal cells with finely granular or dense (squamoid) cytoplasm; (b) cribriform pattern; and (c) necrosis (91,103,104). Aspirates are highly cellular, yielding clusters, sheets, and rare papillae of medium to large, polygonal to cuboidal cells with moderate to marked nuclear irregularity and hyperchromasia, clumped chromatin, and variably prominent nucleoli (91,102–106) (Fig. 20). Occasionally, only mild nuclear atypia is seen (104). Flat, focally cribriform sheets are characteristic, if present (91,102,103). The eosinophilic cytoplasm is characteristically finely granular; however, dense "glassy" squamoid cells with mucin-negative intracytoplasmic vacuoles may be prominent.

Necrosis is a feature in most aspirates (103), and occasionally background mucin is seen (104). Other reported findings include keratin (102), psammoma bodies (102), intranuclear pseudoinclusions (106), metachromatic stroma (104), and eccentric nuclei (106). The cells stain positively for PAS, cytokeratin, and B72.3 but are usually negative for mucin.

Oncocytic neoplasms, high grade MECA, metastatic adenocarcinoma (particularly breast), and other high-grade primary carcinomas must be distinguished from this lesion. Although granular, the cells exhibit higher nuclear-to-cytoplasmic ratios, less granularity, and greater nuclear anaplasia than oncocytes (91,103). Intracytoplasmic mucin favors MECA. Because distinction from these lesions may not be possible by cytomorphology alone, SDC should be considered in any FNA of a rapidly growing parotid mass in an elderly man, particularly if there are cells with ample eosinophilic cytoplasm.

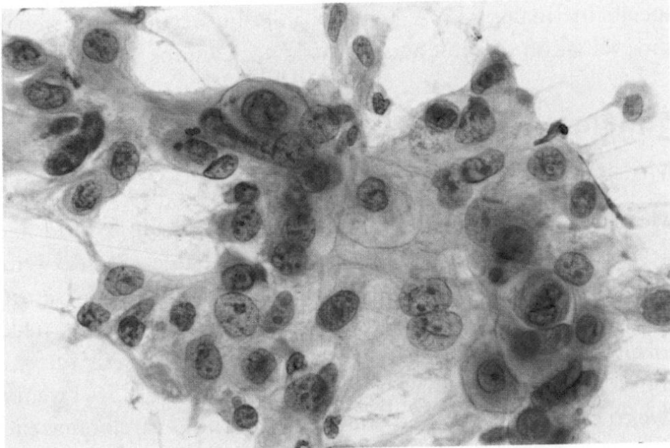

FIGURE 20. Salivary duct carcinoma. Sheets of large polygonal cells with finely granular cytoplasm, obvious malignant nuclear features, and prominent nucleoli. Note rounded space left of center suggestive of cribriform space (hematoxylin and eosin stain, 640×).

Salivary Duct Carcinoma

- Major salivary glands in elderly men
- Polygonal, finely granular cytoplasm
- Pleomorphic nuclei
- ± Prominent nucleoli
- Sheets, clusters, ± cribriform sheets
- Necrosis

Pitfalls (Differential Diagnosis)

1. Granular cytoplasm (WT, oncocytoma)
2. Cribriform sheets (metastatic breast carcinoma)
3. Polygonal, pleomorphic cells (MECA)

LESIONS OF INTRAPAROTID LYMPH NODES

A wide array of lymph node pathology may occur in or around a salivary gland (11,14,107,108). *Reactive lymphoid hyperplasia* is a significant FNA diagnosis because it can obviate the need for open biopsy (108). Smears are abundantly cellular, exhibiting a polymorphous population of small, intermediate, and large lymphocytes with scattered tingible body macrophages and germinal center fragments. Confirmatory lymphocyte marker studies by immunocytochemical stains or flow cytometry may be required to make the subtle distinction from low-grade lymphoma (11,108) (see also additional discussion in neck section of this chapter).

Malignant lymphoma has been a classic source of false-negative diagnoses on salivary gland FNA (5,6,8,54,55,86,87). The cytologic diagnosis rests on identification of a monomorphic population of lymphocytes with abnormal nuclear morphology. Tingible body macrophages are generally absent; however, their presence should not be used as the sole benign diagnostic criterion because they may be present in high-grade or necrotic lymphomas. Low-grade lymphoma, particularly marginal zone (MALT) type, frequently involves the parotid or adjacent lymph nodes and may yield polymorphous lymphocytes. Concurrent lymphocyte marker studies by flow cytometry or immunocytochemistry have significantly decreased false-negative diagnoses (31,108) and are required for the correct interpretation of benign and malignant lymphoid lesions (109) (see detailed discussion in myoepithelial sialadenitis and neck sections in this chapter).

Metastatic Disease

Metastases comprise approximately 10% of malignant neoplasms in the major salivary glands [30(p. 403)]. Typical primary sites of origin include the skin and upper aerodigestive tract, and therefore, metastatic squamous cell carcinoma and melanoma are most common. Lung, kidney, breast, prostate, and colon carcinomas represent the most common distant sites of origin [30(p. 405)]. Metastatic renal cell carcinoma may be difficult to distinguish from primary clear-cell carcinoma of salivary gland origin (95).

Although a clinical history of a known carcinoma is the single most important factor permitting correct diagnosis, many clinicians fail to provide this information, and several patients present with an unknown primary. A high index of suspicion is requisite for diagnostic accuracy. When unusual cytomorphology is encountered, metastases should be considered, and ancillary endoscopic or radiologic studies recommended.

Aspirates of the rare primary salivary gland lymphoepithelial carcinoma yield an admixture of undifferentiated cells and lymphocytes that may be misdiagnosed as a metastasis. Smears of this lesion are characterized by syncytial sheets of large cohesive cells with marked nuclear pleomorphism, vesicular nuclei, prominent nucleoli, high N/C ratios, and obvious mitotic activity (110). The clinical history is characteristic. This lesion has a dramatic prevalence among Eskimos and Chinese and, like undifferentiated nasopharyngeal carcinoma, is strongly associated with Epstein-Barr virus. It is not possible to distinguish primary lymphoepithelial carcinoma of salivary gland origin from metastatic nasopharyngeal carcinoma by cytomorphology alone.

Lymphoepithelial Carcinoma

- Eskimos and Chinese; EBV association
- Syncytial sheets
- Pleomorphic, vesicular nuclei
- Prominent nucleoli
- Lymphoid background

Pitfall

1. Rule out metastatic nasopharyngeal carcinoma

Sensitivity and Specificity

Numerous studies have proven FNA a safe, reliable, accurate, and economical method to evaluate masses in or near a salivary gland (2–4,6–8,13–15,28,54,85–87,111–117). The sensitivity ranges from 73% to 95% (2,3,6,28,54,85,87,111–115,117), specificity from 94% to 100% (2–4,6,28,54,85,87,111–115), and diagnostic accuracy from 66.4% to 100% (2,13,85,86,111,113,114,117). The positive and negative predictive values can be as high as 98% and 96%, respectively (6,28). In general, accuracy is significantly better for the diagnosis of benign than malignant disease (5,6,116–119) because of difficulty in detecting primary salivary gland carcinoma of low nuclear grade such as MECA, ACC, and lymphoma. Several authors (5,15,118–120) have reported that accuracy of FNA approaches that of frozen section. In these studies, FNA was often complementary to frozen section, and some authors (120,121) suggest that the combination of FNA and frozen section improves the accuracy for both methods.

Because of significant differences in the way these studies define sensitivity, specificity, false positives, and false negatives, variation in the numbers of cases reported, number of cases with histologic follow-up, and experience of the individuals procuring and interpreting the biopsies, it is difficult to extrapolate from this literature to an individual practice of cytopathology. However, certain observations appear constant. Diagnostic accuracy is highly dependent on the experience of the aspirator and the interpreting pathologist (5,6,11,15,28,54,113,114,117, 122–124). In addition, a definite diagnosis cannot always be rendered on FNA of a salivary gland. When ambiguous morphology is encountered, a descriptive signout with a differential diagnosis is advised (6). Because accuracy is high for assessing whether the lesion is of salivary gland or other origin, as well as whether the lesion is neoplastic or nonneoplastic (i.e., determining the need for surgical intervention) (2,13,111,113,114), FNA has an extremely important role in the triage of patients with swelling in the region of a salivary gland (2,6–8). In the hands of highly experienced individuals, it can also provide a definitive classification of salivary gland neoplasms in the majority of aspirates (2–4,6,8,87,112).

THE NECK

Fine-needle aspiration biopsy (FNA) is perfectly suited for the initial evaluation of a neck mass. First, masses are easily identified and readily accessible to FNA. Second, some feel that open biopsy of suspected metastatic squamous cell carcinoma from head and neck primaries is contraindicated. Third, reactive lymph nodes, benign cysts, and soft tissue lesions account for a large proportion of neck lesions, and FNA can readily allay patient anxiety, as well as spare many patients the morbidity of open biopsy. Fourth, the overwhelming majority of neck lesions in children are benign, and FNA can provide reliable, accurate diagnostic information without subjecting this population to open biopsy (125,126).

Indications for further evaluation include any mass greater than 1.5 cm, fixation to adjacent tissue (127), or persistance for 2 to 3 weeks without response to antibiotic therapy (128). Various authors (4,127–140) have reported high sensitivity and specificity, making FNA a safe, reliable, and accurate first step in the evaluation of adult and pediatric neck lesions.

Squamous Lesions

Metastatic Squamous Cell Carcinoma

Metastatic squamous cell carcinoma (SCC) from a head and neck primary is a frequent cause of palpable cervical lymphadenopathy (140). FNA is particularly useful in this setting because open biopsy can obscure clinical TNM staging, make formal neck dissection more difficult, and may possibly increase the risk of local recurrence or distant metastases (133). Twenty-five to fifty percent of head and neck squamous carcinomas present as a neck mass (128,133,140), particularly those arising from the tongue, pharynx, and tonsil (127,129).

Clinically, metastatic SCC produces a hard, circumscribed, nontender mobile mass along the border of the sternocleidomastoid muscle, most frequently along the upper internal jugular vein (129). The more cephalad the mass, the more likely the metastasis originated from the upper aerodigestive tract (133). Middle-aged to elderly men with a history of smoking or ethanol use are most commonly affected. However, there is a subpopulation of 20- to 40-year-old patients who develop oral or tonsillar carcinomas without a history of classic risk factors (141).

FNA of a solid metastasis yields a few drops of semisolid material. Approximately one sixth of squamous metastases are cystic, and FNA of these lesions yields several milliliters of thick, turbid or clear, yellow fluid, often resembling pus (142). Diagnostic cells can be very difficult to identify in the cyst contents only; therefore, multiple passes focusing on the lesion's periphery are indicated to insure adequate sampling.

The cytomorphology depends on whether the lesion is cystic or not, as well as the histologic grade. *Moderately or poorly differentiated squamous cell carcinoma* is usually a straightforward FNA diagnosis. Aspirates are cellular and composed of loose, disorganized sheets and many single cells. The cells are polygonal with dense, well-defined cytoplasm and a centrally placed, hyperchromatic nucleus with obvious malignant nuclear membrane and chromatin irregularities (Fig. 21). Keratin is often present, staining orangeophilic (Papanicolaou stain) or "robin's egg blue" (Romanovsky stain) (143).

The differential diagnosis of poorly differentiated SCC includes mucoepidermoid carcinoma, squamous cell carcinoma from other primary sites (such as lung), and other high-grade carcinomas of various origins.

Well-differentiated squamous cell carcinoma may pose diagnostic difficulty because of its deceptively bland nuclei. On low power, aspirates are cellular, with disorganized sheets, clusters, and single keratinized cells. The FNA hallmark of this lesion is numerous miniature, keratinized ("pumpkin orange" on Pap) cells with unusual shapes, high N/C ratios, irregular nuclear contours, and keratin pearls (143,144). These may be oval, spindled, or polygonal and resemble dysplastic parakeratotic cells seen in exfoliative cytology of the female genital tract. Because most of the nuclei are pyknotic (from keratinization), diagnostic well-preserved cells may be difficult to find. In very well-differentiated carcinomas, significant nuclear atypia or pleomorphism may be absent (143,144). Other features often present in aspirates of metastatic, well-differentiated SCC include many small anucleated squames, necrosis, calcification, and a giant-cell or histiocytic reaction to keratin plaques (143,144).

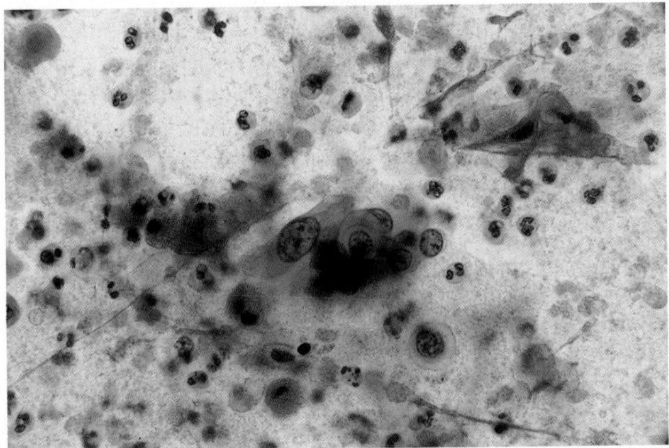

FIGURE 21. High-grade squamous cell carcinoma. Well-preserved cells with dense "hyaline" cytoplasm, marked parachromatin clearing, irregular nuclear outlines, and pearl formation. Necrosis and degenerate keratinized cells present in background (Papanicolaou stain, 500×).

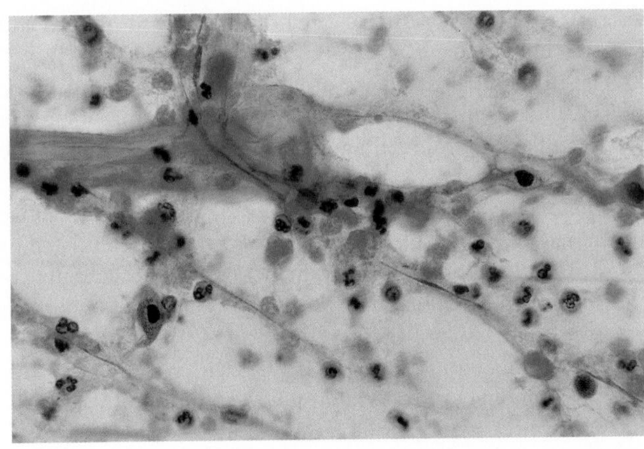

FIGURE 22. Cystic squamous cell carcinoma. Miniature, abnormally shaped keratininzed squamous cells with high N/C ratios and irregular nuclear membranes. Although these cells are suspicious for well-differentiated squamous cell carcinoma, well-preserved cells with classic nuclear irregularities of malignancy are required for a definitive diagnosis (Papanicolaou stain, 400×).

The presence of unusually shaped, miniature, keratinizing squamous cells with high N/C ratios is suspicious for malignancy. Because inflammatory change in inflamed squamous cysts enters into the differential diagnosis, at least a few, well-preserved cells with definitive malignant nuclear and chromatin irregularities should be identified before rendering a definite positive diagnosis.

Cystic metastases of squamous cell carcinoma often arise from a clinically silent primary in the tonsil, base of tongue, or oropharynx (141,143). On FNA, these lesions yield relatively scant squamous cells admixed with histiocytes in a proteinaceous or clean background (141,144–146) (Fig. 22). Acute inflammation is usually scant to absent (145). Keratin debris in the form of small, abnormally shaped, anucleate squames, often with pearl formation, is frequently present. Abnormally shaped orangeophilic keratinized cells with increased N/C ratios and pyknotic nuclei, with irregular nuclear outlines, are present in variable numbers (146,147). A careful search may reveal rare sheets or single cells with preserved nuclei and classic malignant nuclear features sufficient to permit a definitive malignant diagnosis (141,143).

Occasionally, the nuclear features may be so bland as to suggest a benign lesion. However, any lesion with atypical parakeratotic cells should be regarded with suspicion. Multiple biopsies of the lesion's periphery should be performed in an attempt to sample a more solid area (148). If well-preserved cells with unequivocal malignant nuclear features are not identified, the FNA should be considered suspicious (141,143,147,148), and panendoscopy of the upper airway with multiple biopsies of the tonsil and oropharynx may be indicated (133). Repeat FNA by the cytopathologist with rapid interpretation may also yield a diagnostic sample. Open biopsy should be viewed as a procedure of last resort because the standard of care in the treatment of head and neck carcinoma is *en bloc* removal of neck nodes (133,143).

The differential diagnosis of well-differentiated and cystic SCC includes inflamed branchial cleft or epidermal inclusion cyst, papillary thyroid carcinoma, pilomatrixoma, and cystic Warthin's tumor.

Inflamed lymphoepithelial (branchial cleft) cyst with reactive atypia may be impossible to separate from well-differentiated or cystic SCC (149,150). Clinically, branchial cleft cysts usually occur in a younger population, whereas SCC affects elderly men; however, there is significant age overlap (147). Large "intermediate"-type squamous cells of branchial cleft cysts are not a feature of carcinoma (148). Keratin pearls, necrotic epithelial cells, and miniature, atypical parakeratotic cells with increased N/C ratios or angulated nuclei are rarely found in benign lesions (143,144,146,147) and, if present, constitute a minor population admixed with numerous benign elements. The atypical cells of benign lesions typically form flat, cohesive, polarized sheets of cells with uniform pale nuclei, smooth nuclear borders, evenly dispersed chromatin, and prominent nucleoli typical of repair (143,147) (see also discussions of branchial cleft cyst in this chapter).

Inflamed or irradiated epidermal inclusion cysts (EIC) are predominantly composed of large (superficial cell sized) anucleate squames and lack the high N/C ratio, hyperchromasia, and nuclear membrane and chromatin irregularities of carcinoma (148). Ruptured epidermal inclusion cysts with granulomatous inflammation yield very cellular aspirates in which reactive histiocytes may be mistaken for carcinoma; however, the former exhibit small nuclei (neutrophil sized), fine chromatin, prominent nucleoli, and cell-to-cell uniformity (148). Aggregates of histiocytes can be seen engulfing keratin, further confirming their histiocytic origin. A history of radiation therapy and knowledge of the tissue plane of the lesion are also useful in preventing misdiagnosis (see also discussions of EIC in this chapter).

Papillary thyroid carcinoma may yield a cystic aspirate with clusters of polygonal cells with dense, "metaplastic"-appearing cytoplasm (141,145). The resemblance to SCC is only superficial, for papillary carcinoma lacks keratinization and exhibits the typical pale grooved nuclei with or without occasional intranuclear pseudoinclusions as contrasted to the usually hyperchromatic pyknotic nuclei of SCC.

Pilomatrixoma exhibits a mixture of small uniform basaloid cells in tight clusters with aggregates of glassy, amorphous, orangeophilic to pink debris (ghost cells), with or without giant cells and calcification. Necrosis and malignant nuclear irregularities are not seen (144,151).

Reactive changes in cystic Warthin's tumors usually consist of a few abnormal orangeophilic cells with degenerate nuclei in a background of typical oncocytes and granular or mucoid debris (148). Well-preserved cells with malignant nuclear features are not present (see discussions of Warthin's tumor in this chapter).

In summary, to avoid misdiagnosis in cystic or well-differentiated squamous lesions, the wary cytopathologist should (a) require classic malignant nuclear membrane or chromatin abnormalities for a definitive diagnosis of carcinoma, especially in the setting of acute inflammation, (b) check the background for any evidence of a second cell population representing a benign lesion, (c) perform multiple passes to insure adequate sampling, and (d) know the history and radiologic appearance of the lesion including the tissue plane and history of radiation therapy (148).

Squamous Cell Carcinoma

1. Polygonal cells with hard, "glassy" cytoplasm
2. Often obvious malignant nuclear features
3. Well-differentiated SCC: miniature, abnormally shaped, keratinized cells with high N/C ratios
4. Cystic SCC with scant, abnormally shaped keratinized cells ± pearls in a histiocytic background
5. Preserved cells with definite nuclear membrane or chromatin irregularities required for definitive diagnosis

Other Variants of Squamous Cell Carcinoma

These lesions (see Chapters 2 and 7) are usually readily identified as malignant; however, their unusual morphology may result in failure to recognize the upper aerodigestive tract as the site of origin.

Spindle cell (sarcomatoid) squamous cell carcinoma yields sheets and syncytia of monotonous spindle cells with mild to moderate hyperchromasia and nuclear membrane irregularities. Usually mitoses are absent (144). These lesions can be misdiagnosed as melanoma or a soft-tissue lesion. Immunocytochemical stains for pankeratin, S-100 protein, and HMB45 and mesenchymal markers may be useful in ambiguous cases.

Small, rounded groups of cells, along with smaller aggregates of polygonal cells arrayed as single files or bent chains in aspirates of *adenoid (acantholytic) squamous cell carcinoma* may suggest adenocarcinoma to the unwary (152). However, closer inspection reveals definite squamous features including polygonal cells with dense, circumscribed cytoplasm, keratinization, and frequent single dyskeratotic cells (152). This variant of SCC most frequently arises in the oral cavity, tongue, nasopharynx, and skin of the head and neck (152).

Basaloid squamous cell carcinoma may be confused with metastatic small-cell carcinoma, adenoid cystic carcinoma, and nasopharyngeal carcinoma. FNA yields a mixture of large, cohesive cell nests and cords as well as many single cells. The cells are small, with scant cytoplasm, mildly pleomorphic nuclei, fine chromatin, and small but consistent nucleoli (153,154). Necrosis and mitoses are frequently present, but molding is uncommon (153,154). Pseudoglandular spaces surrounded by eosinophilic (Pap stain), PAS with diastase–positive hyaline material is present in approximately 50% of cases (153,154). Rare single keratinized cells or foci of typical SCC may or may not be present (153,154). Alcian blue stain reveals stromal mucin within the cell groups.

Basaloid SCC may be very difficult to distinguish from metastatic *small-cell carcinoma;* however, the presence of large tissue fragments, fine nuclear chromatin, minimal molding, and focal squamous differentiation favors the former. It may be impossible to distinguish the two without immunocytochemical stains for neuroendocrine markers and clinical and radiographic (particularly chest x-ray) findings. Likewise, it may not be possible to reliably distinguish solid adenoid cystic carcinoma from basaloid SCC; however, adenoid cystic carcinoma rarely metastasizes to lymph nodes (153,154).

Other Variants of Squamous Cell Carcinoma

1. Spindle cell SCC: Syncytia of hyperchromatic spindle cells; keratin positive
2. Adenoid SCC: Rounded groups with single files or bent chains but typical squamous cytoplasm or keratinization
3. Basaloid SCC: Large nests, cords, and single cells with necrosis, mitoses, PAS-positive stroma, and absent molding

Lymphoepithelial (Branchial Cleft) Cyst

Branchial cleft cyst presents as a soft, doughy swelling at the level of the hyoid bone, often partially covered by the sternocleidomastoid muscle (155). Two thirds of patients are younger than 30; however, these lesions may present at any age (155). If inflamed, the lesion can be tender and fixed, with pain on movement of the neck (149). FNA yields several milliliters of turbid to clear yellow fluid (142).

Morphologically, aspirates of branchial cleft cysts are moderately cellular and composed predominantly of large polygonal superficial and intermediate-type squamous cells reminiscent of a vaginal Pap smear (143,148,150,155) (Fig. 23). Anucleate squames may be present, with or without scant background lymphocytes or histiocytes. Keratinization is not a characteristic feature of this lesion. On high power, the N/C ratio is very low, and the nuclei are approximately the size of a neutrophil. The chromatin is fine, and the nuclear membranes are smooth (143,155).

If the aspirate exhibits the characteristic morphology, and the lesion completely disappears after drainage, the findings are diagnostic of branchial cleft cyst (155). When acute inflammation and reactive changes are present, a differential diagnosis arises with cystic metastatic squamous cell carcinoma (144,148). Aspirates of inflamed branchial cleft cysts yield abundant acute inflammation with many keratinized cells (143,149). The squamous cells are round to polyhedral; however, occasional tadpole or unusual shapes are identified (143,149) (Fig. 24). The nuclei may be enlarged and hyperchromatic with irregular lobulation (149).

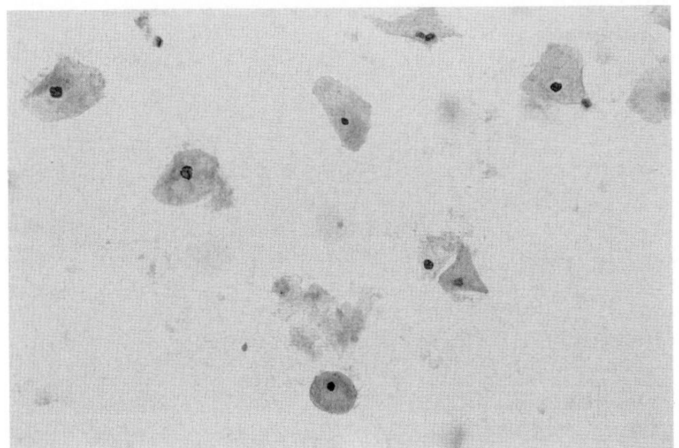

FIGURE 23. Branchial cleft cyst. Superficial and intermediate-type squamous cells in a clean background (Papanicolaou stain, 250×).

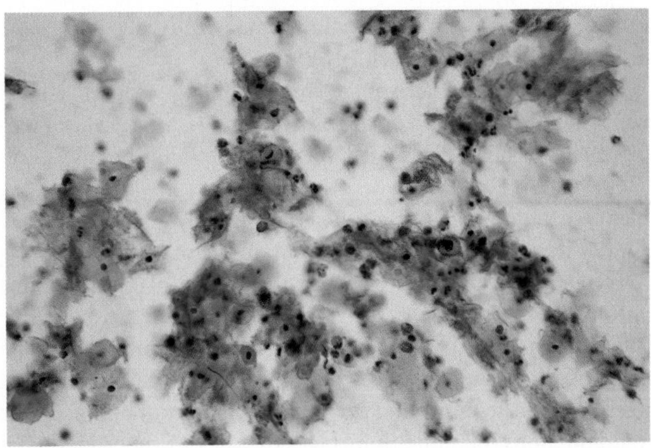

FIGURE 24. Branchial cleft cyst with reactive changes. Scattered small keratinized squamous cells present in a background of superficial and intermediate-type squamous cells and acute inflammation. Compare with Fig. 22 (Papanicolaou stain, 250×).

Caution should always be exercised when interpreting aspirates with acute inflammation, particularly in young patients with a characteristic physical exam or in whom the mass has completely disappeared after the FNA (147). Similarly, because some SCCs can exhibit deceptively bland nuclei, caution should be used for a benign diagnosis in an elderly male smoker with a persistent mass (147). A predominant population of large, "intermediate"-type squamous cells, and/or the lack of well-preserved cells with definitive malignant nuclear features favors a branchial cleft cyst. Conversely, SCC should be suspected when there is a persistent mass or a monomorphic population of keratinized cells with high N/C ratios or abnormal shapes (143,144,146,147). Any atypical squamous lesion that does not exhibit definitive diagnostic criteria should be described, and further evaluation recommended (143,155).

Branchial Cleft Cyst

1. Intermediate and superficial cells similar to vaginal Pap smear
2. Scant lymphocytes and histiocytes
3. With inflammation, rare, bizarre keratinized cells or sheets of reparative epithelium possible
4. Young patient, no residual mass after FNA

Epidermal Inclusion Cyst or Pilar Cyst

FNA of an epidermal inclusion cyst (EIC) or pilar cyst is often occasioned when a mass becomes apparent after weight loss or alopecia is seen in a patient undergoing therapy for a known malignancy. Clinically, the lesion is a circumscribed, doughy, partially mobile nodule within the dermis or subcutis. Grossly, FNA yields scant pasty white material that may exude a characteristic foul odor when smeared (143,148).

Microscopically, the aspirate consists of large (superficial cell size) anucleate keratinized squames that may exhibit central pallor (nuclear ghosts), arranged singly and as amorphous aggregates (Fig. 25) (148). Rare cells may exhibit tiny pyknotic nuclei. Pilar cysts cannot be distinguished from EIC by cytomorphology alone. The former are more common on the scalp.

Diagnostic difficulties occur in the setting of acute inflammation, rupture, or when the cyst has been in the field of prior radiation therapy. With inflammation, sheets of repair-type squamous cells with enlarged round nuclei, fine chromatin, and prominent nucleoli may be evident in a background of acute or granulomatous inflammation (Fig. 26). Lack of single epithelial cells with nuclear chromatin irregularity or hyperchromasia, as well as the lack of atypical or miniature keratinized cells, coupled with the clinical findings should lead to a correct diagnosis (143,148). Hyperchromasia, malignant nuclear features, and single cells with high N/C ratios are usually absent (148).

With rupture, histiocytes with enlarged reactive nuclei and prominent nucleoli, arranged in sheets and clusters surrounding keratin, may be mistaken for carcinoma. The striking nuclear uniformity, similarity to nuclei of multinucleated giant cells, engulfment of keratin, and the lack of malignant nuclear features favor inflammatory changes.

Radiation therapy can result in clusters of cells with nuclear and cytoplasmic vacuoles, cytoplasmic polychromasia, but normal N/C ratios and smooth nuclei (148). Lack of classic features of malignancy, coupled with location and clinical history, should prevent misdiagnosis.

Epidermal Inclusion Cyst or Pilar Cyst

1. Often foul odor when smeared
2. Aggregates of large, anucleate, keratinized squames
3. With acute inflammation, sheets of repair-type squamous cells or histiocytes possible
4. Expect radiation changes if cyst present in therapeutic field

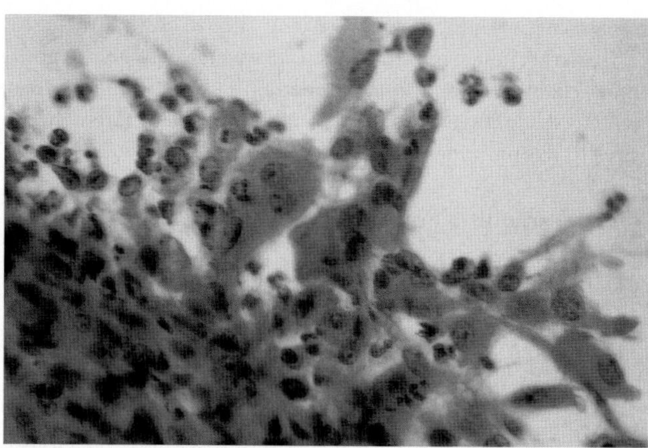

FIGURE 26. Reactive changes in an epidermal inclusion cyst. Sheets of squamous cells with uniform, repair-type nuclei admixed with acute inflammation. Compare with Fig. 21 (Papanicolaou stain, 400×).

Pilomatrixoma

Pilomatrixoma may be misdiagnosed as metastatic squamous cell carcinoma (see skin section in this chapter).

Thyroglossal Duct Cyst

Thyroglossal duct cysts present as a circumscribed, firm, painless swelling in the midline of the neck, close or attached to the hyoid bone (155). Occasionally a lateral location is present (156). The lesion moves with deglutition or protrusion of the tongue. Children are primarily affected; however, it has been reported in all age groups. Women are more commonly affected than men. Accurate FNA diagnosis is important so the hyoid bone can be removed when the lesion is excised.

FNA yields variable amounts of yellow cloudy mucoid fluid (142,156). On low power, the aspirate is sparsely cellular, with histiocytes and inflammatory cells predominating over epithelial cells (Fig. 27). A mucoid to granular background is present (143,150,155,156). Polygonal "intermediate"-type or metaplas-

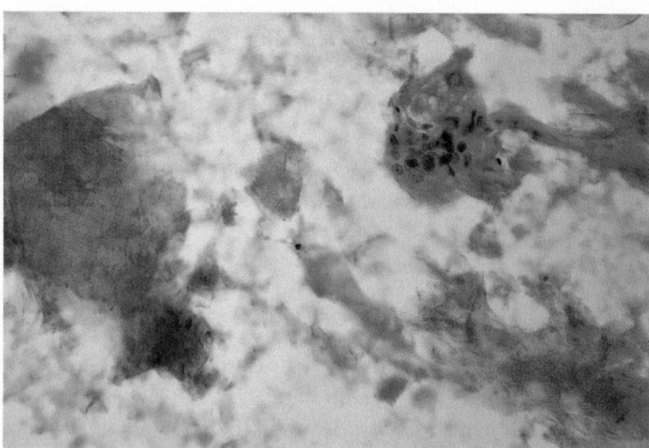

FIGURE 25. Epidermal inclusion cyst or pilar cyst. Large, anucleate, keratinized squames present singly and in plaques. Single giant cell engulfing keratin (Papanicolaou stain, 200×).

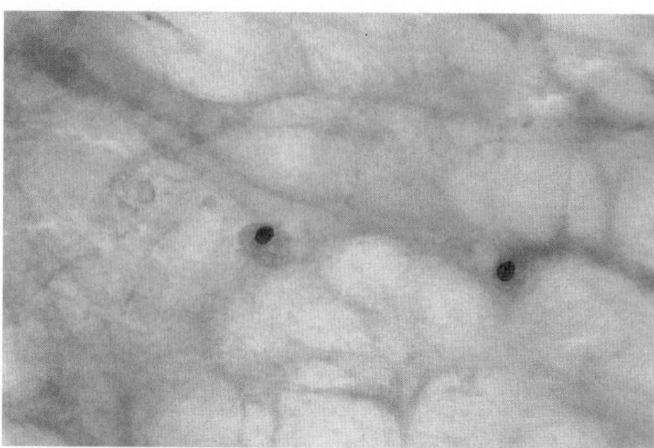

FIGURE 27. Thyroglossal duct cyst. Foamy histiocytes present in a mucoid background. Although not present here, superficial-type squamous or ciliated columnar cells may be present (Papanicolaou stain, 400×).

tic squamous cells are the predominant epithelial cell in all cases (150,155). Ciliated columnar cells are seen in approximately 20% of cases (156), and thyroid follicular cells are rare (143,156).

Because metastatic squamous cell carcinoma is less of a concern in midline lesions, the presence of squamous cells (155) or ciliated cells (156) in an aspirate of a cystic midline neck lesion without a residual mass is diagnostic.

The differential diagnosis includes a thyroid goiter with cystic degeneration, branchial cleft cyst, and metastatic squamous cell carcinoma.

Thyroid goiter with cystic degeneration lacks squamous or ciliated cells and exhibits greater numbers of hemosiderin-laden macrophages. Colloid is absent in a thyroglossal duct cyst (156). *Branchial cleft cyst* is distinguished by a more lateral location and greater numbers of squamous cells. *Metastatic squamous cell carcinoma* is commonly lateral, and small keratinized cells with variable nuclear atypia are present (156).

Carcinoma arises in approximately 1% of thyroglossal duct cysts (157). Eighty-five percent are papillary carcinoma, and the remainder are squamous (150) or anaplastic carcinoma (157). Medullary carcinoma has not been reported. Clinically suspicious findings include the presence of a hard, fixed midline mass that has increased in size (150) or the persistence of a mass after drainage of cyst contents. Papillary carcinoma should be suspected when, in addition to cyst contents, FNA yields papillary clusters with large, pale grooved nuclei, with or without psammoma bodies (157).

Thyroglossal Duct Cyst

1. Predominantly histiocytes with rare "intermediate"-type squamous or ciliated columnar cells
2. No residual mass after FNA
3. Children primarily affected

Other Lymph Node Metastases

Although squamous cell carcinoma of the upper aerodigestive tract is the most common origin of metastases involving the head and neck, origin from other sites, such as melanoma and thyroid, is not uncommon. The site of the metastatic deposit may provide a clue to the primary site of origin. Metastases to the posterior triangle of the neck commonly originate from the nasopharynx, scalp, and, rarely, sinuses (133). Primaries from breast and lung metastasize to bilateral supraclavicular lymph nodes; however, because of the anatomy of the thoracic duct, metastases to the left supraclavicular ("Virchow's") node may also originate in the abdomen or pelvis (158). Malignant lymphoma, melanoma, thyroid carcinoma, and salivary gland carcinomas (133) commonly cause malignant cervical adenopathy in young adults and women.

Nasopharyngeal Carcinoma

Undifferentiated nasopharyngeal carcinoma (NPC) is endemic in southern China and has a strong association with Epstein-Barr virus (see Chapter 5). Up to 75% of patients initially present with a neck mass (133). Accurate FNA diagnosis is important because this lesion is treated with radiation and chemotherapy rather than radical surgery (159), and a primary lesion is never identified in approximately 5% of patients, even after careful search of the nasopharynx.

Aspirates of NPC are cellular with a predominance of cohesive sheets and clumps of large cells with moderately pleomorphic, oval, vesicular nuclei and one to three prominent nucleoli (143,159) (Fig. 28). Single cells and numerous stripped nuclei are frequently present, as are mitoses and scattered spindled nuclei (143,159). Mature lymphocytes are often at admixed with the epithelium.

The differential diagnosis includes malignant lymphoma and metastatic poorly differentiated squamous cell carcinoma from other aerodigestive tract primary sites.

The dispersed single cells of *malignant lymphoma* contrast sharply with NPC's marked cohesion. If the findings are equivocal, immunocytochemical stains for keratin and leukocyte common antigen will usually result in a definitive diagnosis.

Metastatic poorly differentiated *squamous cell carcinoma* of the head and neck shows clear evidence of squamous differentiation, such as dense cytoplasm with sharp cell borders or keratinization (see squamous cell carcinoma). Pacchioni (160) has reported in-situ hybridization for Epstein-Barr encoded RNA (EBER-1) of the Epstein-Barr virus on cell block material as a useful adjunct for the FNA diagnosis of undifferentiated NPC.

Nasopharyngeal carcinoma

1. Endemic in southern China
2. Cohesive sheets of large cells
3. Vesicular nuclei with one to three prominent nucleoli
4. Mature lymphocytes in background and admixed with epithelium

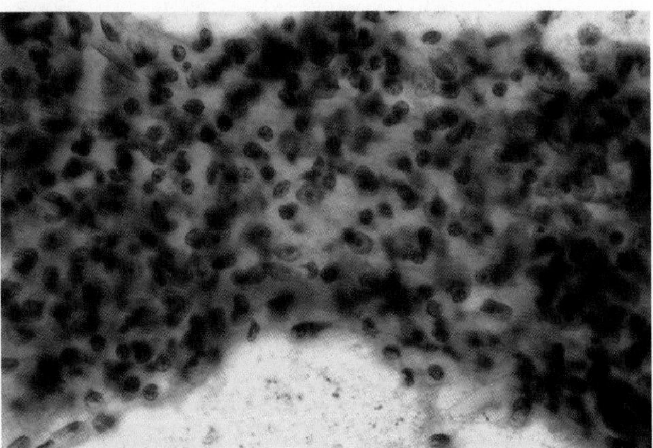

FIGURE 28. Nasopharyngeal carcinoma. Tightly cohesive syncytial sheets of epithelial cells with large, round, vesicular nuclei and prominent nucleoli, extensively obscured by mature lymphocytes (Papanicolaou stain, 400×).

Melanoma

The cytomorphology of melanoma has been described on material derived from scrapes and FNA of primary lesions (151,161) and metastases to skin and lymph nodes (162). On low power, aspirates of melanoma are abundantly cellular and composed of variably pleomorphic dispersed cells with occasional clusters. A variety of cell types may be present, either as the sole component or in combination (143,151,161,162) (Fig. 29).

The majority of melanomas are composed of epithelioid cells that are large, round to "plasmacytoid" cells with sharp cell borders, variable cytoplasm, and round eccentric nuclei. Intranuclear cytoplasmic pseudoinclusions and bi- and multinucleation are seen in most lesions; however, in some aspirates, only rare cells display these features. The nuclei can be deceptively bland, often exhibiting smooth contours and variably fine or coarse chromatin. One to three macronucleoli are present in most cells (143,161,162).

Aspirates of a small number of melanomas yield only bipolar spindle cells with thin cytoplasmic processes and oval, elongate nuclei with rounded ends (161,162). Intranuclear pseudoinclusions are rare in this cell type (161).

Many melanomas exhibit a mixture of spindle and epithelioid cells. Other findings that may be present in aspirates of some melanomas include giant, bizarre cells, small, round, uniform cells (resembling large lymphocytes), mitoses, cell wrapping, necrosis, and nuclear lobulation (161,162).

Although melanin is highly specific for melanoma, it is present in only 40% to 50% of aspirates (161,162). Finely granular, "dusty," nonrefractile melanin should be carefully distinguished from larger, refractile globules of hemosiderin. Additionally, melanin should be identified in tumor cells (rather than histiocytes), for a definitive diagnosis (143).

The most reliable features discriminating melanoma from other neoplasms include the presence of melanin, dyshesion, "plasmacytoid" epithelioid cells with variable nuclear atypia, bi- or multinucleation, macronucleoli, intranuclear cytoplasmic pseudoinclusions, and a mixture of epithelioid and spindle cells (143,161,162). These features may be prominent or may be identified in only rare cells. In addition, none is specific for melanoma, nor are any of these features present in all aspirates (143,161,162).

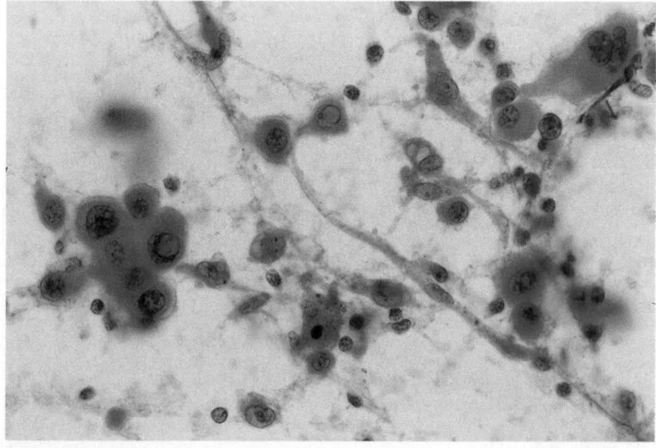

FIGURE 29. Malignant melanoma, morphologic spectrum. Pigmented spindle cells with bland nuclei. Dyshesive epithelioid cells with eccentric nuclei, dense cytoplasm, intranuclear cytoplasmic pseudoinclusions, and occasional multinucleation. Marked range in size from histiocyte-like to gigantic. Background of melanophages and lymphocytes (Papanicolaou stain, 500× or 640×).

The differential diagnosis of melanoma varies with the predominant cell type and the degree of nuclear anaplasia. Epithelioid malignant melanoma must be differentiated from *reactive macrophages, adenocarcinoma, pheochromocytoma,* and *pleomorphic sarcomas.* As a rule, malignant melanoma is less cohesive than carcinoma, and its clusters are arranged in a haphazard fashion as contrasted with the often three-dimensional aggregates with sharp cell borders seen in metastatic adenocarcinoma (162). *Spindle cell sarcomas, schwannoma,* and *nodular fasciitis* may resemble spindle cell melanoma. Small-cell predominant melanoma may mimic *malignant lymphoma* and *metastatic seminoma* (162). Because of significant morphologic overlap in these diagnostic categories, electron microscopy or immunocytochemical stains for S-100, HMB45, MART-1, keratin, leukocyte common antigen, and mesenchymal markers may be required for a definite diagnosis.

Melanoma

1. Dyshesive
2. Large "plasmacytoid" or spindle cells, or mixture of both
3. Macronucleoli
4. Intranuclear cytoplasmic pseudoinclusions
5. Multinucleate cells
6. Melanin present in 40–50%

Metastatic Renal Cell Carcinoma

Renal cell carcinoma (RCC) is one of the more common carcinomas metastatic to thyroid and salivary gland and occasionally presents as a lump in the head and neck. Approximately 10% of RCC present as a metastasis, and therefore, a history of neoplasia may not be present (163). Clinically, metastatic RCC is a circumscribed, mobile, often pulsatile mass that may be within skin, lymph nodes, or salivary gland.

Because of RCC's vascularity, aspirates are frequently hemodilute and scant. The cells are loosely cohesive, with ample vacuolated or granular cytoplasm (Fig. 30). The finely vacuolated lacy cytoplasm of clear cells is best seen on air-dried Romanovsky smears (163). The degree of nuclear pleomorphism varies with grade; however, low-grade lesions may exhibit deceptively bland oval to round nuclei with finely granular chromatin and minimal irregularity (163). Prominent nucleoli are a consistent feature but may be inconspicuous in well-differentiated lesions. Because of the fragility of the cytoplasm, often only stripped nuclei with prominent nucleoli are present in a background of blood or enmeshed in fibrin strands.

The differential diagnosis of metastatic RCC in the head and neck includes *histiocytes, fat necrosis, large cell malignant lymphoma (if only stripped nuclei are present), sebaceous carcinoma,* and *clear cell neoplasms* of salivary gland origin (95,163). RCC is cytokeratin-, vimentin-, and epithelial membrane antigen

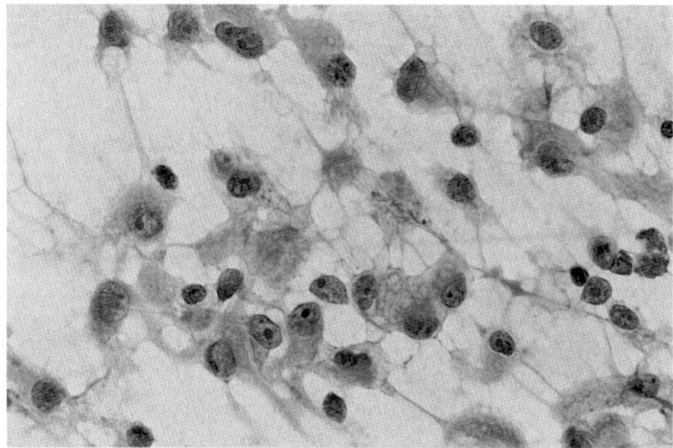

FIGURE 30. Metastatic renal cell carcinoma. Dispersed cells with delicate cytoplasm, round, vesicular nuclei, and prominent nucleoli. Typical bloody background is not evident in this aspirate (Papanicolaou stain, 640×).

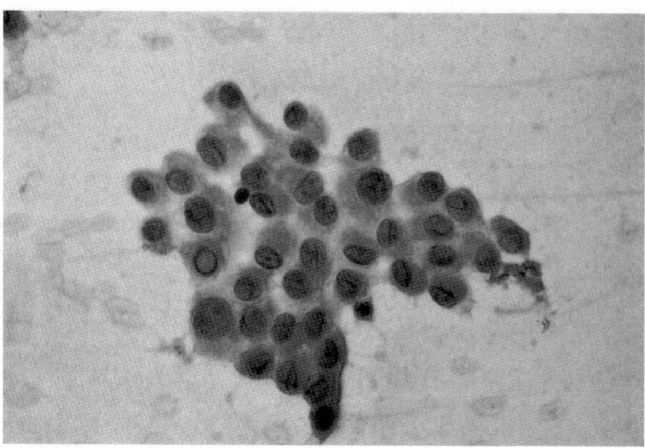

FIGURE 31. Papillary thyroid carcinoma. Flat sheets of cuboidal cells with focally dense, "glassy" cytoplasm, and round nuclei with frequent grooves and inclusions (Papanicolaou stain, 400×).

(EMA)–positive by immunocytochemical stains, PAS-positive, diastase-sensitive, oil red O–positive, and mucicarmine-negative. Awareness of renal cell carcinoma as a frequent source of metastatic carcinoma to the head and neck is the single most useful tool in recognizing this entity (163).

Renal Cell Carcinoma

1. Often hemodilute with scant stripped nuclei enmeshed in fibrin
2. Cohesive cells with vacuolated (clear) or granular cytoplasm
3. Round nuclei with finely granular chromatin
4. Usually prominent nucleoli (may be absent in well-differentiated lesions)

Metastatic Papillary Thyroid Carcinoma

An occult papillary thyroid carcinoma may present as palpable lymph node metastases. In particular, cystic metastases may result in erroneous diagnoses if not considered in the differential diagnosis.

Aspirates of papillary carcinoma are highly cellular and composed of disorganized sheets, papillary syncytial fragments, or microfollicular clusters of cells with enlarged, pale nuclei and evenly dispersed chromatin (164). Typical features of papillary carcinoma such as intranuclear cytoplasmic pseudoinclusions and grooves are present, as are small nucleoli (Fig. 31). Colloid may be present in the background or within follicular-type aggregates (164). Occasionally, the cells may exhibit moderate dense, well-defined, glassy, "metaplastic-type" cytoplasm.

Metastatic *squamous cell carcinoma, carotid body tumor,* and *benign cysts* enter into the differential diagnosis of papillary carcinoma; however, the characteristic nuclear features coupled with a papillary or follicular architecture and/or the presence of colloid, usually lead to a straightforward diagnosis. Intranuclear cytoplasmic pseudoinclusions are totally nonspecific and may be seen in malignant melanoma, pleomorphic adenoma, metastatic lung carcinoma, paragangliomas, and other lesions primary in the head and neck. In equivocal cases, immunocytochemical studies for thyroglobulin are useful in confirming the diagnosis.

Papillary Thyroid Carcinoma

1. Highly cellular with sheets, papillae, or microfollicles
2. Large, pale nuclei with grooves or inclusions
3. ± Colloid
4. Metaplastic cytoplasm
5. Often cystic (with residual mass)

Metastatic Medullary Thyroid Carcinoma

Medullary thyroid carcinoma may present as a lymph node metastasis from an occult primary. This neoplasm exhibits a wide array of morphologies on FNA and therefore can be easily misdiagnosed if not considered in the differential diagnosis.

Aspirates are cellular and composed of predominantly single cells with occasional cell fragments (165,166). Bose described four patterns: "microfollicular," with empty or amyloid-filled lumina; "papilla-like," with finger-like projections; "dispersed," with predominantly single plasmacytoid cells; and "anaplastic," with large, pleomorphic, dissociated cells (165). The four described cell types include plasmacytoid (small cells with eccentric nuclei and moderate, well-defined cytoplasm), small round cell ("lymphocyte- or carcinoid-like" with round nuclei and scant cytoplasm) (165), spindle cell (short, "stubby" cells with oval nuclei and scant bipolar cytoplasm), and large, anaplastic cells (abundant cytoplasm, eccentric nuclei, and variable nucleoli) (165,166) (Fig. 32). The nuclei of the various cell types are uniform, round to oval, with coarse chromatin and variable pleomorphism. Occasionally, marked atypia with giant and multinucleated cells may be present (165,166). Amyloid is present in 60% to 70% of aspirates (165) and consists of amorphous extracellular matrix, which may appear identical to colloid (165,166).

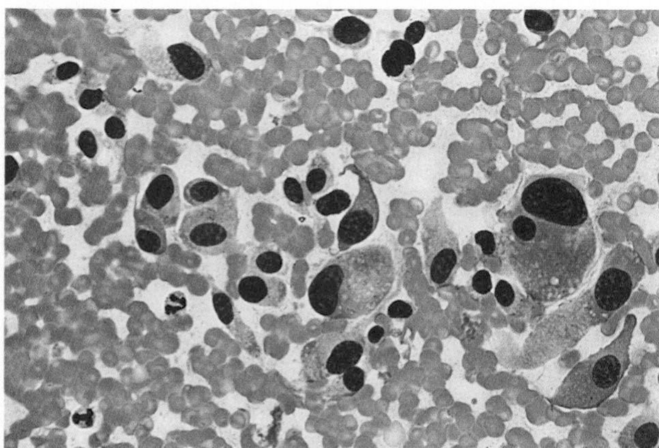

FIGURE 32. Medullary carcinoma, morphologic spectrum. Small, lymphocyte-like cells with eccentric cytoplasm, spindle cells, and large, pleomorphic cells with eccentric nuclei. Any cell type may dominate the morphology (Diff-Quik stain, 500×).

Additional findings include intranuclear cytoplasmic pseudoinclusions, calcifications resembling psammoma bodies, and red cytoplasmic granules on Romanovsky stains (165). The latter vary from fine and dust-like to coarse and obvious and may be present in only rare cells (165,166).

The differential diagnosis includes *papillary, anaplastic, and follicular carcinomas* of thyroid origin, *melanoma,* and *carotid body tumor.* Medullary carcinoma should always be considered when a neck aspirate exhibits a dissociated population of plasmacytoid or short spindle cells. Positive immunocytochemical stains for calcitonin and chromogranin or elevated serum calcitonin may be required for a definitive diagnosis.

Medullary Thyroid Carcinoma

1. Usually markedly dyshesive
2. Plasmacytoid, lymphocyte-like, spindle cell, or large anaplastic cells
3. Uniform nuclei with "salt and pepper" chromatin
4. Amyloid in 60–70%
5. Variably present red granules on air-dried smear
6. Intranuclear cytoplasmic pseudoinclusions

Primary Lymphoid Processes

See Chapter 12 for more information on these subjects.

Reactive Lymphadenopathy

Reactive lymphadenopathy frequently involves the head and neck. Clinical features favoring a reactive process include recent history of pharyngitis, generalized viral infection, or dental infection. A history of cat exposure should be sought because cat-scratch disease and toxoplasmosis frequently involve cervical lymph nodes. Small size of nodes, short duration of symptoms, tenderness, and mobility are additional clinical features favoring a benign process.

Because some types of malignant lymphoma may be difficult to distinguish from reactive processes by cytomorphology alone, material from all lymph node aspirates should be submitted for immunophenotyping (167). In addition, any clinically suspicious or abnormally persistent lymph node should be excised, especially if confirmatory lymphocyte marker studies were not submitted with the original aspirate.

Morphology

Cell polymorphism, although not specific, is the hallmark of a reactive lymph node. FNA yields large numbers of dispersed lymphocytes, which vary in size, shape, nuclear characteristics, mitotic activity, and amount of cytoplasm (168) (Fig. 33). These include small, round lymphocytes, small and large cleaved lymphocytes, immunoblasts, and plasma cells.

Markers of germinal center formation include tingible body macrophages (TBMs), dendritic reticulum cells, and mixed lymphoid aggregates. TBMs exhibit round to reniform smooth nuclei with fine chromatin, small nucleoli, and moderate vacuolated cytoplasm containing abundant basophilic, karyorrhectic debris (168). These are dispersed singly and in germinal center fragments. Dendritic cells resemble histiocytes; however, they lack cytoplasmic debris, and are usually found in aggregates (representing germinal center fragments) admixed with lymphocytes and TBMs (168).

Although follicular lymphoid hyperplasia is the most common cause of reactive lymphadenopathy, it should be borne in mind that lymph nodes enlarged by paracortical hyperplasia (typical of dermatopathic lymphadenitis or some viral infections) or unstimulated lymph nodes will not exhibit the above features (168). Therefore, neither monomorphism nor the absence of germinal centers automatically implies a malignant lymphoid process.

Conversely, occasional lymphomas or Hodgkin's disease may exhibit a polymorphous cell population. A benign diagnosis should be based on the lymphocyte morphology. Benign lymphoid nuclei lack protrusions, angulation, irregular nuclear

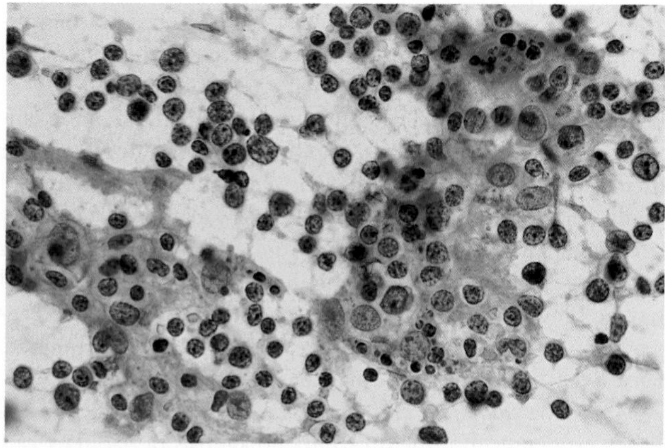

FIGURE 33. Follicular lymphoid hyperplasia. Aggregates of pale follicular dendritic cells (pale vesicular nuclei, small nucleoli, and ill-defined cyanophilic cytoplasm), tingible body macrophages, and a spectrum of small and large lymphocytes. The cohesive fragments represent germinal centers (Papanicolau stain, 640×).

membranes and chromatin distribution, or abnormally large nucleoli (168). Immunophenotyping is recommended to confirm the polyclonal nature of the process and to exclude abnormal T-cell phenotypes (167).

Differential Diagnosis of Reactive Lymphadenopathy

1. *Follicular lymphoma* (small cleaved, and mixed small- and large-cell malignant lymphoma). Aspirates of this lymphoma are more biphasic than truly polymorphous and lack tingible body macrophages or a broad spectrum of lymphocytes. Indeed, the absence of tingible body macrophages in an aspirate from an enlarged node should be a warning to examine the lymphocytes carefully for abnormal nuclear features or lack of a broad range of polymorphism. Immunophenotyping may be required for a correct diagnosis (109).
2. *Non-Hodgkin's lymphoma with tingible body macrophages.* These include some follicular center cell lymphomas, Burkitt's or Burkitt-like lymphoma, and partial involvement of a node by lymphoma. A monomorphic lymphoid population with abnormal nuclear morphology and immunophenotype should lead to a correct diagnosis (168) (see also the discussion of malignant lymphoma in this chapter).
3. *T-cell malignant lymphoma or Hodgkin's disease.* Prominent epithelioid histiocytes, eosinophils, and capillary fragments are not typical of reactive lymphoid hyperplasia (168) and should alert one to the possibility of T-cell malignant lymphoma or Hodgkin's disease. The presence of abnormal lymphocytes with irregular nuclei in a wide range of sizes, or atypical large lymphocytes with abundant cytoplasm, should raise a suspicion of T-cell lymphoma (169). Likewise, the presence of scattered large abnormal cells with prominent nucleoli is suspicious for Hodgkin's disease. Immunophenotyping may reveal an abnormal T-cell population in the case of T-cell malignant lymphoma (167,169) but may not be helpful in Hodgkin's disease.
4. *Paracortical hyperplasia or dermatopathic lymphadenopathy.* If the expected morphology of benign lymphoid hyperplasia is limited to follicular hyperplasia, aspirates of paracortical hyperplasia (such as dermatopathic lymphadenopathy) could result in a misdiagnosis of lymphoma or even metastatic melanoma. These aspirates are polymorphous and often exhibit a dense network of interdigitating reticulum cells (168). Pigment-laden histiocytes are often present; however, tingible body macrophages and germinal center fragments are not prominent. The bland nuclear morphology and intimate relationship of the interdigitating reticulum cells with the lymphocytes should prevent a misdiagnosis of lymphoma (168). Immunophenotype and clinical history of dermatitis or cutaneous trauma in the region help support the diagnosis.
5. *Unstimulated lymph node.* See the discussion of malignant lymphoma differential diagnosis in this chapter.
6. *Small clonal population of lymphoma.* These aspirates may appear morphologically benign and frequently require immunophenotyping (particularly by flow cytometry) to prevent false-negative diagnosis (167,170). See also the discussion of lymphoma in this chapter.
7. *Infectious agents.* See next section.

Reactive Lymphadenopathy

1. Polymorphous population
2. Tingible body macrophages and germinal center fragments with dendritic reticulum cells
3. Absence of nuclear or chromatin irregularities
4. Polymorphism or tingible body macrophages present in some lymphomas
5. Confirmatory immunophenotyping usually indicated

Infectious Lymphadenopathy

Mycobacterial Infections

Infections with *Mycobacterium tuberculosis* as well as atypical mycobacteria commonly affect cervical lymph nodes. *M. tuberculosis* may present as a unilateral cervical mass with multiple enlarged, firm to fluctuant, matted nodes. Systemic symptoms may or may not be present, and a chest x-ray is abnormal in only 55% of patients (171). Atypical mycobacterial infection is more frequent in the United States and usually presents as a rapidly enlarging upper cervical or preauricular mass with overlying skin erythema in a child less than 5 years old. The organisms are frequently present in soil, house dust, and water and are thought to enter via the oral cavity, possibly related to thumb sucking (172). There are no systemic symptoms, and chest x-ray is normal (172).

FNA reveals typical nodular aggregates of epithelioid histiocytes, often in a background of necrosis and lymphocytes (172). Acute inflammation may be present in either type of mycobacterial infection but is more common with atypical mycobacteria. Aspirate material should be sent for cultures; however, *Mycobacterium avium* complex grows in only 50% to 60% of cultures submitted from surgical material (173).

The differential diagnosis includes other necrotizing granulomatous infections such as fungi and cat-scratch disease. A positive tuberculin skin test may be of help in selected cases (172). In addition, the cytopathologist should always be aware that granulomas are a nonspecific finding that can also be associated with malignant lymphoma, Hodgkin's disease, and metastatic squamous cell carcinoma (144).

Mycobacterial Lymphadenitis

1. Nodular aggregates of epithelioid histiocytes
2. Lymphocytes and necrosis
3. Acute inflammation (more common in atypical mycobacteria)
4. Atypical mycobacteria more common in children
5. Correlate with cultures

Cat-Scratch Disease

This infectious lymphadenitis commonly affects children and young adults. Ninety percent have a history of exposure to cats, and 70% report an actual cat scratch (174). Unilateral, frequently matted, regional lymphadenopathy develops 1 to 3 weeks after exposure. Cervical nodes are the third most commonly affected site, after the axilla and epitrochlear nodes (174). Fifty percent of lesions will suppurate.

Findings on FNA vary with the stage of the lesion. Aspirates of early lesions will reveal only nonspecific follicular hyperplasia (174). However, aspirates of intermediate to late-stage lesions exhibit aggregates of confluent elongated epithelioid histiocytes with spindled, frequently wavy nuclei (174). Some aggregates exhibit a suggestion of peripheral palisading (174). Many neutrophils are present; however, necrosis is not seen (174). Scattered giant cells with polyengulfment and/or a mixed reactive lymphoid population may be present. Stains for fungi and acid-fast bacilli (AFB) are negative. Warthin-Starry stains are usually negative on aspirates with a characteristic morphology because the bacteria are not usually found in granulomas (174). The FNA findings can be suggestive of cat-scratch disease in the setting of appropriate history and the exclusion of other possible causes of suppurative granulomas (174).

Cat-Scratch Disease

1. History of exposure
2. Early lesion—follicular hyperplasia only
3. Mid- to late lesions—confluent epithelioid histiocyte aggregates, many neutrophils, and scattered giant cells
4. Necrosis not prominent
5. Fungal, AFB stains negative; Warthin-Starry stain often negative
6. Exclude other causes of suppurative granulomas

Toxoplasmosis

Toxoplasmosis is a benign, self-limited infection caused by the protozoan *Toxoplasma gondii* and acquired by exposure to cats or uncooked meat. Cervical lymph nodes are most commonly involved. Although serologies are diagnostic, FNA or excisional biopsy is occasioned by clinicians who have not considered the diagnosis, or when persistent lymphadenopathy raises a suspicion of malignancy. Indeed, approximately 15% of unexplained cervical lymphadenopathy is thought to be caused by toxoplasmosis (175).

FNA yields an abundantly cellular polymorphous lymphoid population including immunoblasts, plasma cells, and germinal center fragments (175,176). Tingible body macrophages and mitoses may be prominent. Epithelioid histiocytes with abundant cytoplasm, indistinct cell borders, oval or elongate vesicular nuclei, and small nucleoli are present singly and in aggregates. Characteristic of toxoplasmosis, these cells lack evidence of phagocytosis (175). Giant cells and necrosis are absent (175,176).

The differential diagnosis includes granulomatous infectious disease, Hodgkin's disease, and malignant lymphoma. In granulomatous infections, epithelioid and giant cells predominate, in contrast to the lymphoid predominance with absent giant cells in toxoplasmosis (175,176). Bacteriologic cultures are negative in toxoplasmosis.

Hodgkin's disease and T-cell lymphoma lack the background of follicular hyperplasia with germinal center fragments (175). Before a diagnosis of toxoplasmosis is suggested, the background lymphocytes should be carefully studied and correlated with immunophenotyping to exclude an abnormal lymphoid population. Finally, the diagnosis should be confirmed by *Toxoplasma* serologies (175,176).

Toxoplasmosis

1. Lymphocytes predominate
2. Polymorphous lymphocytes including immunoblasts, TBMs, and germinal center fragments
3. Epithelioid histiocytes, singly and in small aggregates, without evidence of phagocytosis
4. Absent giant cells and necrosis
5. Exclude lymphoma and Hodgkin's disease

Infectious Mononucleosis

Young adults with classic clinical features of mononucleosis including severe pharyngitis, bilateral lymphadenopathy, fever, splenomegaly, atypical lymphocytosis on peripheral blood smear, and positive heterophil antibody are rarely, if ever, subjected to lymph node FNA. However, atypical presentations including illness in middle-aged patients, heterophile-negative patients, or massive (up to 4 cm) unilateral lymphadenopathy may be biopsied to exclude malignancy (177).

The FNA hallmark of mononucleosis is a broad spectrum of immunoblasts ranging from small plasmacytoid lymphocytes with abundant eccentric blue cytoplasm, perinuclear hof, absent nucleoli, and condensed, clumped chromatin, to large immunoblasts characterized by large, round nuclei with smooth membranes, open chromatin, prominent nucleoli, and scant to moderate basophilic to pale cytoplasm (177). Occasional binucleate forms are present. A variety of intermediate forms will be present and are best appreciated on air-dried preparations (177). These cells appear very active and eye-catching; however, recognition of the spectrum of reactive changes, cellular polymorphism, and background germinal center formation should suggest the correct diagnosis (177).

Although transformed immunoblasts are characteristic of mononucleosis, some aspirates will yield only nonspecific follicular hyperplasia or a mixture of follicular hyperplasia and less exuberant immunoblastic transformation (177).

Binucleate immunoblasts do not mimic Reed-Sternberg cells sufficiently to cause confusion with Hodgkin's disease (177). A significant differential diagnosis exists with non-Hodgkin's lymphoma (NHL) because of the large number of activated lymphocytes (177). Careful analysis of the background small lymphocytes reveals typical benign lymphocytes in mononucleosis, whereas in NHL the small lymphocytes are commonly folded, twisted, or angulated (177). Immunophenotyping and confirmatory Epstein-Barr virus serologies are useful in confirming the benign nature of the process (177).

Infectious Mononucleosis

1. Prominent spectrum of immunoblasts ranging from small plasmacytoid lymphocytes to large immunoblasts; occasional binucleate forms
2. Polymorphous population
3. Background germinal center fragments
4. Exclude non-Hodgkin's lymphoma
5. Polyclonal phenotype; positive EBV serology

Actinomycosis

This infection affects lymph nodes and soft tissues of the head and neck; however, its incidence has decreased in the United States as a result of improved oral hygiene (178). Craniofacial actinomycosis usually follows a dental extraction or jaw injury (179). The palate, cheek, parotid, maxilla, and submandibular regions are most commonly affected (178). Clinically, actinomyces can mimic malignancy by forming an indurated, "woody" lesion with dense fibrosis, with or without draining sinuses (178,179).

Acute inflammation predominates in aspirates. Scattered histiocytes and occasional lymphocytes may also be present. Careful search will reveal balls of filamentous bacteria surrounded by neutrophils (so-called "sulfur granules") (178,179) (Fig. 34). The gram positive, branching, filamentous bacteria stain positively for methenamine silver and are acid-fast negative. Cultures are positive in fewer than 60% of cases (178). The bacteria may be easily overlooked and, therefore, should always be searched for in acute inflammatory lesions of the head and neck (178).

Actinomycosis

1. History of periodontal disease, dental extraction, or jaw injury
2. Neutrophilic inflammation predominates
3. Scant balls of filamentous bacteria
4. Gram-positive, methenamine silver–positive, AFB-negative
5. Cultures often negative

Sarcoidosis

Sarcoidosis commonly involves the head and neck, particularly the parotid gland or cervical lymph nodes. Aspirates yield granulomas characterized by nodular aggregates of polygonal to spindled epithelioid histiocytes with round or reniform to "boomerang"-shaped nuclei, pale chromatin, and small but distinct nucleoli within ill-defined, delicate pale cytoplasm (27) (Fig. 35). Occasional cuffing by mature lymphocytes may be present, and giant cells may be seen (27).

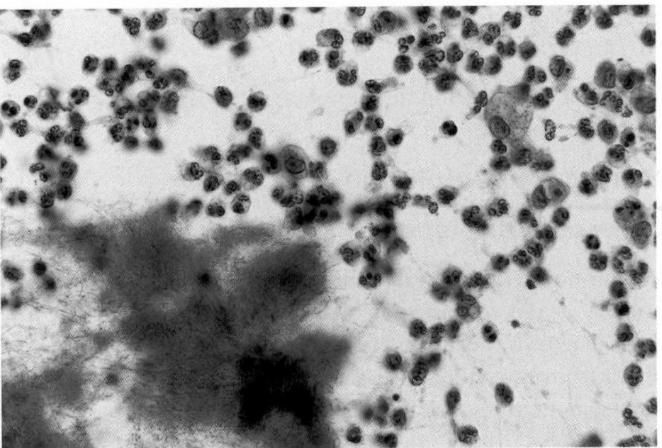

FIGURE 34. Actinomyces. Characteristic "cotton wool" aggregates of filamentous bacteria in a background of abundant acute inflammation (Papanicolau stain, 640×).

Granulomas are nonspecific; therefore, infectious processes must be excluded by appropriate microbiological studies. Aspirates should always be carefully evaluated for the presence of an abnormal background lymphoid population to exclude the possibility of Hodgkin's, or non-Hodgkin's lymphoma and correlated with immunophenotype, if indicated. Finally, the presence of characteristic clinical and radiographic findings, positive serum angiotensin-converting enzyme (ACE), and negative PPD, support the diagnosis of sarcoidosis.

Sarcoidosis

1. Nodular epithelioid histiocyte aggregates
2. Polygonal to spindled pale cells with fine chromatin
3. Elongate to "boomerang"-shaped nuclei
4. ± Lymphocytes and giant cells
5. Exclude lymphoma; correlate with cultures, and serum ACE

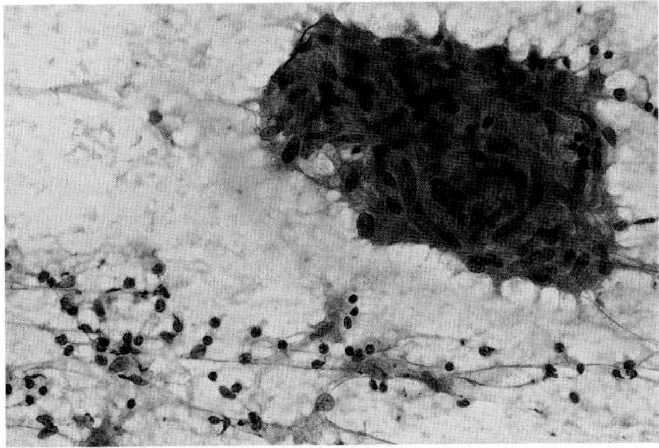

FIGURE 35. Sarcoidosis. Nodular aggregate of spindled to polygonal epithelioid histiocytes with oval to spindled nuclei, pale chromatin, and small nucleoli, admixed with background lymphocytes (hematoxylin and eosin stain, 400×).

Eosinophilic Granuloma and Langerhans' Histiocytosis

This topic is covered in depth in Chapter 14B under Orbit.

Malignant Lymphoma

General Considerations

Lymph nodes in the head and neck are frequently involved by primary or recurrent malignant lymphoma. In addition to primary diagnosis, documenting malignancy, and separating lymphoid from nonlymphoid lesions, FNA of lymphoma is useful for staging, rapidly documenting recurrence, obtaining material for additional marker studies, and documenting disease in a mass left *in situ* to gauge therapeutic response.

Approach

Accurate FNA diagnosis of lymphoma requires expertise on the part of the cytopathologist as well as the availability of ancillary studies. If these are not available, FNA should not be performed on lymphoid lesions (109). To achieve diagnostic accuracy, material must be procured for air-dried and alcohol-fixed smears and immunophenotyping. Proliferation markers assessed by flow cytometry are useful for lymphoma subclassification (109,180). Finally, cytogenetics may be useful when cytomorphology and immunophenotyping yield ambiguous results (181). Three to five passes with vigorous oscillation technique are required to obtain enough material for all diagnostic studies (109). The Zedjalea technique, in which no suction is applied to the needle, minimizes peripheral blood contamination and is ideal for lymph node FNA (182). Rapid interpretation at the time of FNA is extremely useful to insure that enough diagnostic material is obtained. The ultimate goal is not only to distinguish malignant from benign lymphoid proliferations but also to accurately grade and subtype the lymphoma.

If leukemia or granulocytic sarcoma is suspected, ancillary studies including immunophenotyping, histochemical stains, nucleic acid flow cytometry, cytogenetics, and gene rearrangement studies may be indicated (109,167,170).

Immunophenotyping

Depending on the number of cells available, immunophenotyping can demonstrate whether there is immunoglobulin light chain restriction, aid in subtyping B-cell neoplasms, and demonstrate aberrant T-cell antigen expression or deleted pan-T-cell antigens (109,167,170). The assay may be performed on acetone-fixed cytospins (167) or by flow cytometry (183–185), with results of approximately equal quality (183). Cytospins have the advantage of requiring fewer cells and permitting concurrent evaluation of morphology and immunophenotype without use of special machinery (167,183); however, they are labor intensive, require interpretive expertise, do not permit evaluation for coexpression of antigens, and permit only a limited panel (183). Flow cytometry requires additional equipment and greater numbers of cells, and abnormal T-cell populations may be masked by peripheral blood contamination (183). Its advantages include fast, reproducible, automated results, lower cost per biopsy, analysis of antigen coexpression (183), and assessment of ploidy and S-phase (109,167).

Although many lymphomas may be diagnosed as malignant by morphology alone, marker studies should always be performed on lymph node aspirates. They are required in monomorphic lesions that are suspicious for low-grade malignant lymphoma and for all polymorphous lymphoid processes (109). Markers help identify subtle abnormal cell populations; however, normal markers do not exclude Hodgkin's disease, T-cell malignant lymphoma, and small clonal lymphoid populations; therefore, all clinically suspicious lymph nodes with negative FNA results should be excised.

Gene Rearrangement Studies

Although not necessary for the standard evaluation of B-cell monotypic malignant lymphomas, gene rearrangement studies may prove useful in the following instances: (a) aspirates with atypical lymphoid morphology and polyclonal or equivocal clonality; (b) aspirates with an aberrant T-cell phenotype, loss of pan-T-cell antigens, or in which T cells predominate with low-grade morphologic atypia; (c) morphologically malignant lymphocytes with equivocal light chain expression (null cell or unsatisfactory marker studies) (181). Katz identified these features in approximately 25% of lymphoma aspirates (181).

Because the presence of gene rearrangement is not synonymous with malignancy, it must be correlated with clinical and morphologic features before a definite malignant diagnosis can be rendered (181). This is especially important in a setting of the adult immunodeficiency syndrome (AIDS) and cutaneous lymphoid hyperplasias (181). Because gene rearrangement studies are not indicated in the majority of aspirates, material can be procured, spun down into a pellet, and saved frozen until results of morphologic analysis and immunophenotyping are known (181).

Morphology

A detailed discussion of the various morphologic and immunophenotypic features of the more than 20 subtypes of malignant lymphoma has been well provided elsewhere (109), and is beyond the scope of this chapter. Instead, the focus will be on general diagnostic criteria for malignant lymphoma and potential pitfalls which may result in false-negative or false-positive diagnoses.

Whenever an aspirate yields a monomorphic population of lymphocytes, lymphoma should be strongly suspected. The markedly cellular smears are composed of monotonous lymphocytes devoid of germinal center fragments. Although tingible body macrophages are a marker for germinal center formation (and therefore benignancy), they may be present, even expected, in some high grade lymphomas.

On high power, nuclear size, configuration, chromatin pattern, and degree of atypia vary with the subtype of lymphoma. Lymphomas of small or intermediate cells exhibit banal nuclei (CLL or small B cell) or only subtle nuclear protrusions or clefts (low-grade follicular center cell) and are more easily suspected by

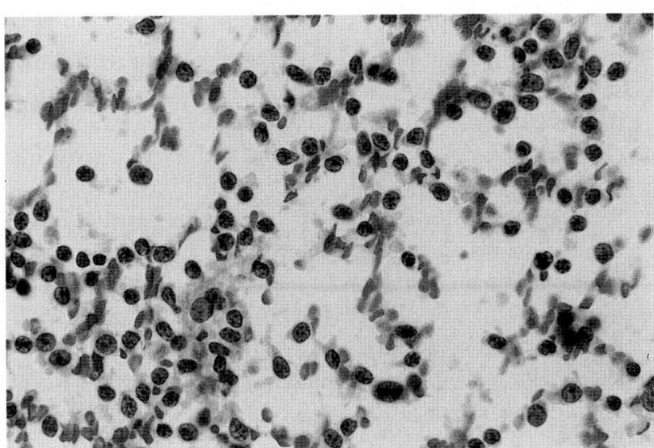

FIGURE 38. Follicle center lymphoma. Dimorphic population of small and large lymphocytes with angulated or convoluted nuclei, more open chromatin pattern than mature lymphocytes, and occasional small nucleoli. Occasional follicular dendritic cells (upper left of center) admixed. Tingible body macrophages absent (Papanicolaou stain, 640×).

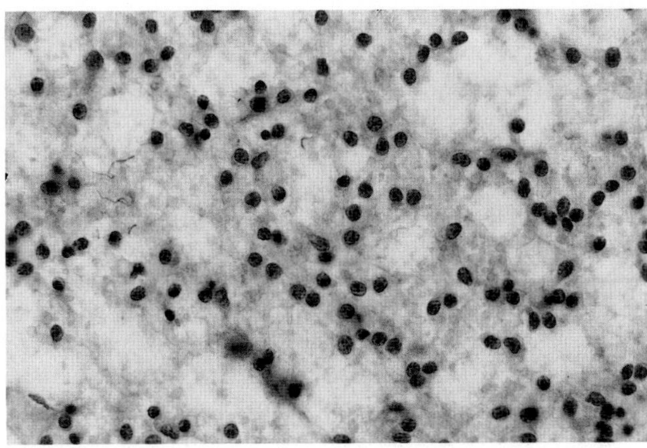

FIGURE 40. Unstimulated lymph node. Monomorphic mature lymphocytes with condensed chromatin. Tingible body macrophages absent. Use of clinical features and immunophenotyping may be required to exclude small lymphocytic lymphoma (Papanicolaou stain, 640×).

(Fig. 40). Clinical features such as a longstanding, small (<1 cm), localized lymph node, younger age, and the absence of peripheral blood lymphocytosis favors an unstimulated node over low grade lymphoma. Lymphocyte marker studies in this setting are essential to confirm or exclude an abnormal B- or T-cell population.

2. *Tingible body macrophages* (TBMs). Although TBMs are commonly used as a marker for germinal center formation, and therefore a benign process, they may be a frequent, even expected, feature of high-grade or necrotic lymphomas such as Burkitt's or Burkitt-like lymphoma (Fig. 41). The diagnosis of a benign, reactive process must be based on the lymphocyte morphology and immunophenotype, not ancillary cells. Conversely, the absence of TBMs in the setting of a clinically enlarged lymph node should raise suspicion of the possibility of a low-grade lymphoma because numerous TBMs should be present in a lymph node enlarged by benign follicular hyperplasia. In such cases, lymphocyte markers are essential because follicular center cell lymphoma, grade 2 (mixed small- and large-cell lymphoma) can be easily overlooked, and is a frequent cause of false negatives.
3. *Small clonal populations of malignant cells* (partial nodal replacement by lymphoma and "T-cell–rich B-cell" lymphoma). In some instances, these aspirates yield truly benign cells, and false negatives are caused by sampling error. At other times, a small population of malignant lymphocytes is masked by the greater numbers of benign reactive cells. In these cases, immunophenotyping, particularly by flow cytometry, may identify the abnormal lymphoid population (167,170). Any clinically suspicious or persistent node with a benign FNA diagnosis should be excised (109,170).
4. *Paracortical hyperplasia.* It is generally not difficult to distinguish classic follicular lymphoid hyperplasia from non-Hodgkin's lymphoma. However, in certain settings such as viral infections or dermatopathic lymphadenopathy, the presence of increased numbers of activated lymphocytes may oc-

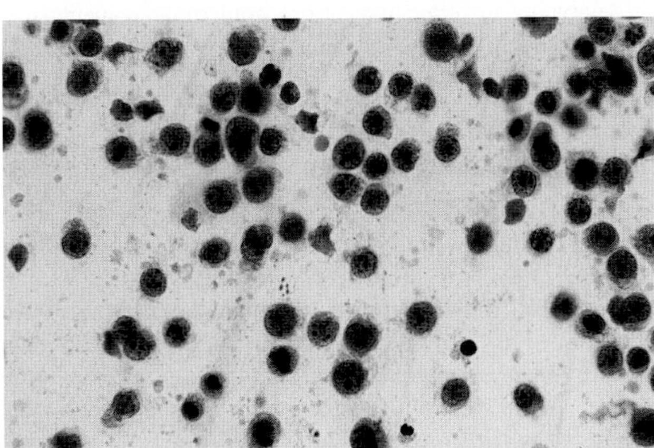

FIGURE 39. Large B-cell malignant lymphoma. Monomorphic large lymphocytes with irregular nuclear contours and multiple, often membrane-bound nucleoli (Papanicolaou stain, 640×).

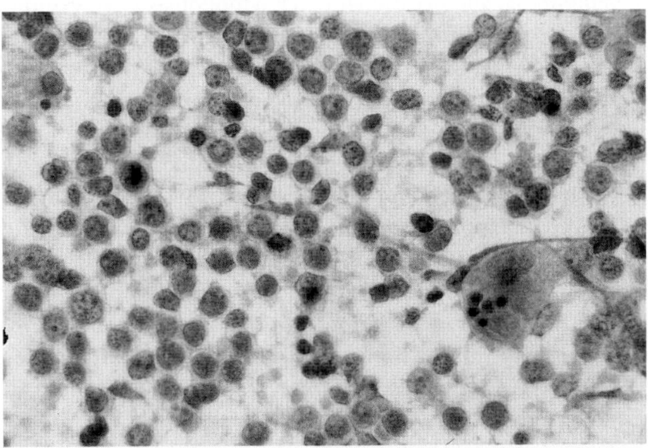

FIGURE 41. Burkitt's lymphoma. Monomorphic intermediate to large lymphocytes with open chromatin, multiple nucleoli, and scant cytoplasm, admixed with tingible body macrophages. Compare with Fig. 33.

casionally generate suspicion of malignancy (168,177). The recognition of a spectrum of reactive lymphocytes, benign immunophenotype, and the clinical confirmation of a specific etiology are useful in discriminating benign from malignant lesions (177). The node should be excised if the diagnosis is uncertain or if it fails to regress after resolution of systemic symptoms (177).

5. *Peripheral T-cell lymphoma* (PTL). Most non-Hodgkin's lymphomas in the United States are of B-cell origin, and therefore, most of the criteria for the FNA diagnosis of lymphoma are geared toward B-cell lesions. Although peripheral T-cell lymphoma (PTL) is less common, it accounts for approximately 30% of all aggressive lymphomas (169). Because its FNA morphology is considerably different than the average B-cell lymphoma, familiarity with its FNA findings is important to prevent false-negative diagnoses.

   Aspirates of PTL are polymorphous, with abundant epithelioid histiocytes, plasma cells, and eosinophils.Careful evaluation of the lymphocytes will reveal either a spectrum of abnormal small, intermediate, and large lymphocytes with nuclear protrusions, irregularities, and grooves as well as chromatin clumping and clearing, or a subpopulation of abnormal small or large lymphocytes with nuclear atypia (169). Occasionally large atypical lymphocytes may exhibit abundant cytoplasm or multilobated nuclei. Mononuclear Reed-Sternberg–like cells with giant nucleoli may be present (169).

   Clues to the recognition of PTL include cell polymorphism (particularly epithelioid histiocytes and eosinophils) and a spectrum of abnormal lymphocytes ranging from small through intermediate to large (169). Phenotypic features include a single dominant T-cell phenotype, loss of one or more pan-T-cell antigens, predominance of a CD4 phenotype, or aberrant phenotype (such as coexpression of CD4 and CD8) (169). The routine use of a broad panel of markers is essential to recognize these lesions (169). Gene rearrangement studies may be useful to confirm the diagnosis (181).
6. *Granulomatous or polymorphous morphology.* Although monomorphism is an important FNA feature of many lymphomas, polymorphism, even numerous granulomas, does not exclude lymphoma. Indeed, Hodgkin's disease, T-cell lymphoma, and occasional B-cell lymphomas often exhibit a mixture of neutrophils, eosinophils, plasma cells, and, in particular, epithelioid histiocytes. It is therefore critical that the final diagnosis rest on the lymphoid morphology, not on ancillary background cells. The presence of ample epithelioid histiocytes or eosinophils is not a typical feature of reactive lymphadenopathy, and should precipitate a careful search for a subpopulation of lymphocytes with abnormal nuclear or chromatin features, or Reed-Sternberg–like variants. This is particularly important because a limited panel of markers may not identify Hodgkin's cells or T-cell lymphoma. In this setting especially, it is imperative to excise the lymph node if the FNA is not clearly diagnostic of a benign entity or if the node persists.
7. *Granulocytic sarcoma.* As in histopathology, granulocytic sarcoma may be misdiagnosed as non-Hodgkin's lymphoma. If present, basophil or eosinophil precursors or myelomonocytic-type blasts are useful in morphologically distinguishing these entities (109,186,187). Myeloid cytoplasmic granules may be easily identified on Romanovsky stains. In addition, stains for lysozyme, NASD chloracetate esterase (186), or myeloperoxidase and Sudan black B (109,187) are useful in confirming myeloid origin. Clinical and bone marrow findings are often helpful.
8. *Nonlymphoid malignancy.* Some lymphomas, particularly T-cell and anaplastic large-cell lymphoma, can mimic nonlymphoid malignancies (Fig. 42). Conversely, melanoma, carcinoma, sarcoma, and Hodgkin's disease can mimic non-Hodgkin's lymphomas. In this setting, immunocytochemical stains or electron microscopy may be required for a definitive diagnosis (188).

Accuracy in FNA Diagnosis of Malignant Lymphoma

FNA of lymph nodes is 90% to 95% accurate for the diagnosis of metastatic disease, 10% to greater than 90% accurate in the diagnosis of non-Hodgkin's lymphoma, and 56% to 89% for Hodgkin's disease (109). In experienced hands, with ancillary studies, the accuracy for the diagnosis of non-Hodgkin's lymphoma is 91% for palpable lesions (positive predictive value 98%) (109). Frequent causes of unsatisfactory specimens include necrosis, bad technique (170), and small size or difficult location of the lesion.

Non-Hodgkin's Lymphoma

1. Monomorphic lymphocytes
2. Nuclear angulations and protrusions ("noses")—low-grade lymphoma
3. Large, irregular, vesicular nuclei with clumped chromatin —high-grade lymphoma
4. Immunophenotyping usually required
5. TBMs, epithelioid histiocytes, or eosinophils may be present
6. Peripheral T-cell lymphoma exhibits a range of abnormal lymphocytes from small to large
7. Granulomas or cell polymorphism does not exclude Hodgkin's or T-cell lymphoma
8. Some high-grade lymphomas may require immunophenotyping to differentiate from nonlymphoid malignancies

Hodgkin's Disease

A diagnosis of Hodgkin's disease (HD) should be entertained whenever there is a randomly distributed subpopulation of large abnormal single or multinucleated cells with or without macronucleoli, in a background of benign-appearing small lymphocytes. The benign component usually predominates (109,189–191). The presence of an admixture of eosinophils, plasma cells, neutrophils, epithelioid histiocytes, or granulomas should always raise a suspicion of HD.

Aspirates of HD are usually scant to moderately cellular, in contrast to the high cellularity of non-Hodgkin's lymphoma and reactive lymph nodes. Background cells predominate over the

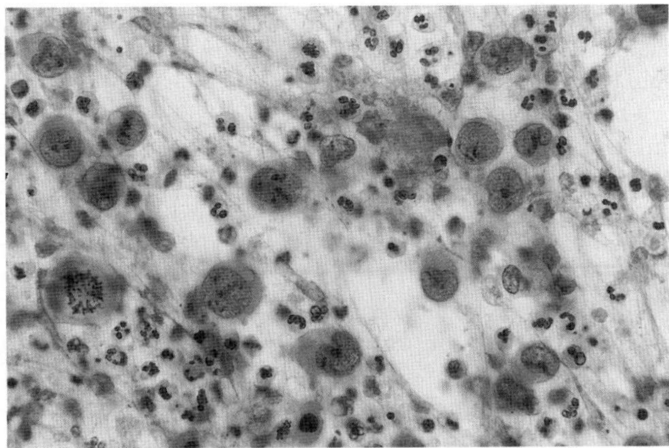

FIGURE 42. Anaplastic large-cell lymphoma. Large, pleomorphic mitotically active lymphocytes with ample cytoplasm. Immunophenotyping or immunocytochemistry may be required to exclude carcinoma or melanoma (Papanicolaou stain, 640×).

abnormal cells (189) and may consist entirely of small lymphocytes or a mixture of eosinophils, plasma cells, epithelioid histiocytes, and granulomas. As in surgical pathology, the polymorphism of the benign reactive cells is often the first clue to search for the numerically fewer, and occasionally obscured, malignant Hodgkin's cells.

Diagnostic Reed-Sternberg (R-S) cells are usually of giant size (40–100 μm), typically with two or multiple nuclei, finely reticular chromatin, 2 to 4 macronucleoli, and pale cytoplasm with variable vacuolation (192) (Fig. 43). These may be infrequent or absent. Hodgkin's cells are large mononuclear cells (25–50 μm) with reticulated chromatin and one or two nucleoli (109,192). These considerably outnumber R-S cells and may be the only diagnostic malignant cell present. Lacunar cells are large (20–50 μm) and display lobulated or convoluted nuclei with overlapping segments and moderate clear to pale cytoplasm (109,192).

Other findings in HD aspirates include granulomas, necrosis, metachromatic, slightly fibrillar stroma, and large, bizarre, polypoid cells that lack nucleoli (189).

Classic R-S cells in a characteristic background are diagnostic of HD (191). In addition, some authors propose that the presence of Hodgkin's cells in the appropriate background is diagnostic, even in the absence of classic R-S cells (109). At minimum the presence of these cells should elicit a suspicious diagnosis.

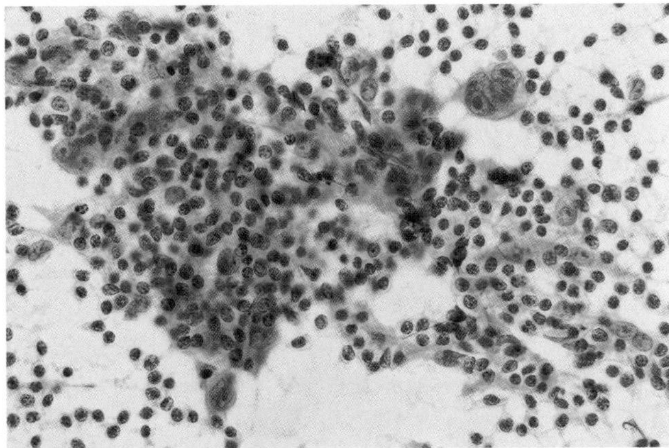

FIGURE 43. Hodgkin's lymphoma. Small, mature lymphocytes predominate with only occasional large mononuclear and binucleate Reed-Sternberg cells showing macronucleoli approaching the size of a mature lymphocyte (Papanicolaou stain, 500×).

Although some authors have shown that the number of Hodgkin's R-S cells increases with progression from lymphocyte-predominant to mixed-cellularity HD, an attempt at subtyping by FNA is generally considered not worthwhile (191) because accuracy approaches only 70% (192).

Hodgkin's cells may be positive for CD15 and CD30; however, this is an inconsistent and nonspecific finding. Therefore, accurate diagnosis rests primarily on cytomorphology alone.

The accuracy of the diagnosis of Hodgkin's disease ranges from 88% to 98% (189) with a positive predictive value of 93.5% (191). Diagnostic errors are usually errant subclassification as non-Hodgkin's malignancy rather than failure to recognize the process as malignant (191,192).

Pitfalls in the diagnosis of Hodgkin's disease include an increased number of unsatisfactory specimens because of fibrosis or necrosis, failure to recognize the small number of background Hodgkin's cells, resulting in misdiagnosis as an inflammatory or granulomatous process, and misinterpretation of reactive, virally stimulated benign lymphocytes as Hodgkin's cells (189,191).

Differential Diagnosis

The differential diagnosis of Hodgkin's disease includes:

1. *Peripheral T-cell lymphoma.* It may be exceptionally difficult to distinguish peripheral T-cell lymphoma (PTL) from HD by FNA morphology alone (169,170). Both lesions may exhibit large abnormal cells; however, in PTL a spectrum of atypical small, intermediate, and large lymphocytes is present in the background, as opposed to HD's benign, mixed inflammatory background (169). Large, immunoblast-like malignant cells are present in some PTL; however, true binucleate "owl's eye" R-S cells are not seen (169). Both lesions may stain positively for CD15 and CD30 (170). The presence of many R-S cells with low proliferative activity that are positive for CD15 and negative for CD45 favors HD (109), whereas a dominant T-cell phenotype, loss of pan-T-cell antigens, and abnormal gene rearrangement studies support PTL (109,167).
2. *Granulomatous disease.* Nonnecrotizing granulomas on FNA warrant a high index of suspicion. Their presence should precipitate a diligent search of the background for atypical lymphocytes before a benign diagnosis is rendered. In addition, if numerous, granulomas may cause sampling errors in which the abnormal cells are not present in the smear. Therefore, if the clinical context is not compatible with an infectious process or sarcoidosis, excision is warranted.
3. *Other malignancies.* Carcinoma, melanoma, and non-Hodgkin's lymphoma (NHL) may mimic HD. In particular, nasopharyngeal, breast, and lung carcinoma may exhibit R-S–like cells (192). The presence of cohesion, and a predominance of abnormal over mixed inflammatory cells favors metastatic carcinoma. Melanoma yields a dyshesive cell population; however, the presence of intranuclear inclusions or pigment (189) is a useful distinguishing feature. As discussed

above, some B- and T-cell NHLs may be confused with HD. Atypical small background lymphocytes or a lack of the typical mixed inflammatory background, coupled with the immunophenotype, should permit an accurate diagnosis of NHL. Immunocytochemical studies for cytokeratin, S-100 protein or HMB45, CD45 and CD15 or CD30, are also useful.

4. *Reactive lymphoid hyperplasia.* Because the background, reactive cells predominate over Hodgkin's cells, failure to recognize the smaller number of large atypical cells may result in a false-negative diagnosis. Careful evaluation of the entire sample should reveal a population of large abnormal cells in HD.
5. *Unsatisfactory Specimen.* FNAs of lymph nodes are usually abundantly cellular. Because fibrosis is common in Hodgkin's disease, aspirates are commonly less cellular than in typical reactive or malignant lymphoid processes. Scantly cellular aspirates of clinically suspicious lymph nodes should be followed by repeat FNA or excision.

Hodgkin's Disease

1. Scant to moderately cellular
2. Characteristic pattern of mixed inflammatory cells predominating, with scant, randomly distributed large abnormal cells
3. Classic Reed-Sternberg cells scant to absent
4. Large mononuclear cells with giant nucleoli (Hodgkin's cells) often diagnostic
5. Granulomas, necrosis, and metachromatic stroma may be present
6. CD15 or CD30 positivity helpful if present

FNA OF SOFT TISSUE

A detailed description of the array of soft tissue lesions affecting the head and neck is beyond the scope of this chapter (see Chapter 10). Therefore, this discussion focuses on the most common soft tissue lesions and those that may lead to erroneous diagnoses. Because accurate diagnosis of soft tissue lesions by FNA can be extremely difficult, there are several prerequisites: (a) an experienced aspirator, (b) access to all clinical and radiologic data, (c) a cytopathologist with broad experience with the diagnostic criteria and pitfalls of interpreting soft tissue FNA (193,194), and (d) rapid interpretation performed at the time of biopsy to ensure enough material is obtained for electron microscopy, immunocytochemistry, and genetic studies (usually three to five passes are required) (195,196).

Benign Nerve Sheath Tumors

Up to one third of solitary schwannomas occur in the head and neck (197). The lateral upper neck near the carotid artery is a common location (71,143), and frequently, the clinical differential diagnosis is between schwannoma and carotid body tumor. A characteristic clinical finding is pain on insertion of the needle, often of an "electric" type, which radiates in the distribution of a nerve (143,198).

The FNA morphology varies depending on the cellularity of the lesion and whether degenerative (ancient) or cystic (199) changes are present. Schwannoma usually cannot be distinguished from neurofibroma by FNA (143).

On low power, there are large irregular clusters composed of interlacing or swirling spindle cells, at times associated with blood vessels (71). These represent Antoni A regions. Less cellular fragments with a myxoid background correspond to Antoni B regions (71). The tissue fragments exhibit loose, vague cellular palisading blending into compact fascicles with no evidence of storiform or herringbone patterns (197) (Fig. 44). Rarely, clumps of cells with fibrillary cytoplasm and nuclear palisading at one edge, consistent with Verocay bodies, may be seen (199).

On high power, the spindle cells exhibit wavy, fibrillar cytoplasm and mildly pleomorphic, plump, elongate nuclei with occasional bends and grooves (143). The chromatin is finely granular without clumps, clearing, or nucleoli (71). Characteristic of neural lesions, fine cytoplasmic processes form a delicate fibrillar meshwork background in the tissue fragments (71,198). Myxoid change may or may not be present, and necrosis and mitoses are absent. Ancient change manifests as scattered, enlarged, pleomorphic, hyperchromatic nuclei with smudgy chromatin in a predominant population of uniform spindle cells (199,200).

The differential diagnosis of benign nerve sheath tumors includes reactive fibroblastic proliferations such as nodular fasciitis or hypertrophic scar, low-grade malignant nerve sheath tumor, and other low-grade spindle cell sarcomas. Reactive fibroblastic lesions exhibit plumper oval nuclei and lack the radiating pain (198), the background delicate fibrillar meshwork, suggestion of nuclear palisading, and the mild nuclear pleomorphism of benign nerve sheath tumors (71).

Benign Nerve Sheath Tumors

1. Clusters of interlacing spindle cells ± blood vessels or myxoid background
2. Variably pleomorphic, plump, elongate nuclei with occasional bends and grooves
3. Fibrillar background meshwork in tissue fragments
4. Scattered enlarged, pleomorphic, hyperchromatic nuclei present in ancient lesions
5. Absent fascicular or storiform pattern

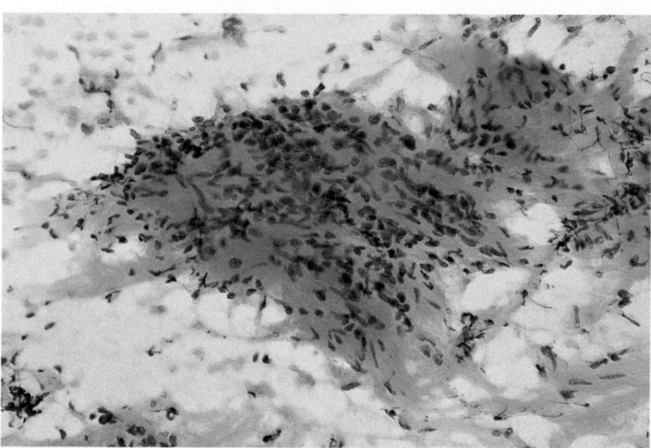

FIGURE 44. Schwannoma. Spindle cells with bent nuclei and focal nuclear palisading enmeshed in a fibrillar background (Papanicolaou stain, 200×).

Malignant peripheral nerve sheath tumors are more cellular and exhibit less architectural organization than their benign counterparts. The component cells are smaller, less spindled, and have a higher N/C ratio because of nuclear enlargement and hyperchromasia, resulting in densely cellular fragments with little ground substance (71,143,200). On high power, the nuclei often exhibit comma or "twisted pear" shapes (200) (Fig. 45). In contrast to the scattered degenerate pleomorphic cells of benign nerve sheath tumors with ancient change, malignant lesions exhibit diffuse nuclear enlargement, hyperchromasia, and coarse chromatin with parachromatin clearing (71,143,200) in the majority of cells. Necrosis may be present in high-grade lesions. Definite diagnosis of sarcoma may not be possible in low-grade lesions (198). Although high-grade lesions are easily recognized as sarcoma, electron microscopy (EM) and positive S-100 protein staining by immunocytochemistry may be required to subclassify them as neural (71).

Low-grade neural sarcomas must be distinguished from their benign counterparts and sarcomas of other mesenchymal origin. In general, benign lesions are less cellular, exhibit only rare pleomorphic cells in an overall population of uniform, benign cells, and lack definitive malignant nuclear features (71,143,199,200). Distinction from other spindle cell sarcomas, such as leiomyosarcoma and fibrosarcoma, may require EM and immunocytochemistry studies (71,200).

Malignant Nerve Sheath Tumors

1. Densely cellular tissue fragments
2. Small, hyperchromatic spindle cells with high N/C ratio
3. ± Necrosis or mitoses

Synovial Sarcoma

Synovial sarcoma involving the head and neck most commonly arises from the parapharynx, anterior neck, cheek, or tongue of young adults. The most characteristic presentation is a mass high in the neck or just inferior to the jaw (201).

On low power the aspirate is highly cellular, composed predominantly of densely cellular fragments admixed with scattered single cells (143,201,202). Two types of medium-sized cells may be identified (201). The first are stubby, plump spindle cells with scant bipolar cytoplasm and blunt hyperchromatic nuclei, which frequently exhibit longitudinal folds (Fig. 46). The second is polygonal and mesothelial-like and arranged in clumps, sheets, or duct-like structures. These exhibit round, regular nuclei with fine chromatin, smooth borders, and occasional nucleoli (143,201,202). Rare mitoses may be present.

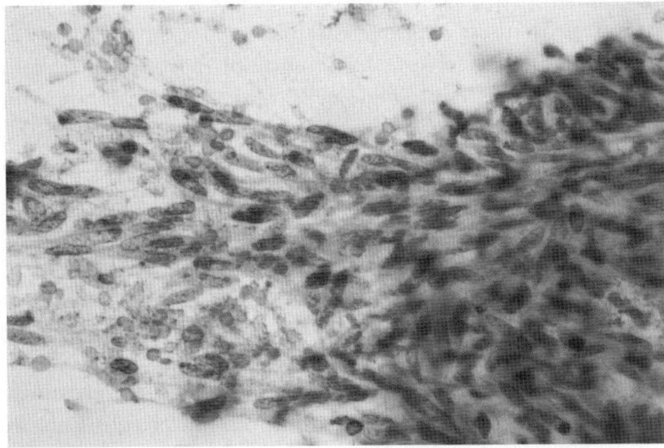

FIGURE 45. Malignant peripheral nerve sheath tumor. Tissue fragments displaying greater cellularity, crowding, hyperchromasia, and higher N/C ratio than Schwannoma (Papanicolaou stain, 400×).

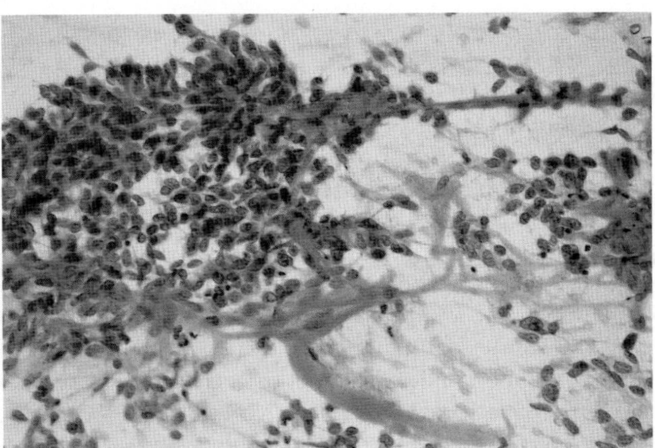

FIGURE 46. Synovial sarcoma. Densely cellular specimen composed of plump, "stubby" spindle cells, focally admixed with hyalinized collagen (Papanicolaou stain, 200×).

A biphasic pattern is highly suggestive of synovial sarcoma; however, mesothelioma or an epithelial neoplasm occasionally enter into the differential diagnosis. The monomorphic subtype of synovial sarcoma must be distinguished from fibrosarcoma, and benign and malignant nerve sheath tumors. High-grade synovial sarcoma often exhibits round or oval cells and must be distinguished from round-cell liposarcoma and hemangiopericytoma. Full evaluation of the clinical and radiographic findings, coupled with electron microscopy and immunocytochemical stains for cytokeratin and mesenchymal markers, are often required for a definitive diagnosis.

Synovial Sarcoma

1. Highly cellular
2. Densely cellular tissue fragments
3. Stubby, plump spindle cells with hyperchromatic nuclei, ± longitudinal folds
4. Polygonal, mesothelial-like cells in sheets or ducts, if biphasic

Rhabdomyosarcoma

This condition is described in Chapter 14B, in the section on the orbit.

Tumors of Adipose Tissue

Lipomas are common subcutaneous neoplasms but are difficult to definitively diagnose on FNA because of their morphologic identity with subcutaneous fat (193). Aspirates yield aggregates of large adipocytes with a single, uniformly sized lipid vacuole and small round peripheral nuclei with fine chromatin. In larger tissue fragments, delicate capillaries are admixed with the adipocytes (203–205).

Occasionally, regressive changes are evidenced by clusters of vacuolated macrophages with fine chromatin and small nucleoli. These may cause concern about well-differentiated liposarcoma; however, the vacuoles in regressive changes do not indent the nuclei, and nuclear atypia is absent (203). In addition, subcutaneous (i.e., superficial) liposarcomas are extremely rare. An aspirate composed of only adipose tissue is usually caused by a geographic miss of a more significant lesion; therefore, the diagnosis of lipoma cannot be rendered without strict clinical and radiologic correlation to ensure the specimen is representative (193).

Two variants of lipoma common in the head and neck may lead to cytologic misinterpretation. Awareness of the characteristic clinical and morphologic findings should prevent misdiagnosis.

Pleomorphic lipoma typically presents as a circumscribed subcutaneous mass that has been present for years in the neck or upper back of a 45- to 65-year-old man (205,206). FNA yields pleomorphic cells with irregular, round or oval, hyperchromatic nuclei and coarse chromatin surrounded by wispy, vacuolated, eosinophilic cytoplasm (204,206). Many giant cells with multiple (more than four) bizarre, degenerate nuclei overlapping in a characteristic wreath-like fashion (florette-type giant cells) are present (204,206), as are occasional large intranuclear vacuoles (204).

The unusual appearance of this lesion has led to misdiagnosis as anaplastic carcinoma (206). The longstanding history and typical florette-type giant cells, coupled with the absence of well-preserved, definitively malignant nuclei should prevent misdiagnosis. Florette cells have been rarely identified in liposarcoma, and therefore, their presence alone is not diagnostic of a benign lesion (206).

Spindle cell lipoma characteristically is a longstanding lesion in the posterior neck of middle-aged to elderly men. Aspirates yield adipose tissue with features similar to lipoma, admixed with a variable number of cellular spindle cell fragments composed of mildly pleomorphic, hyperchromatic, nuclei with occasionally prominent nucleoli and no mitoses. Lipoblasts are not present (143,205,207).

If the spindle cell component is prominent, knowledge of the location and long duration without change is essential to prevent overdiagnosis as a malignant spindle cell neoplasm (205).

Lipoma

1. Clusters of large adipocytes with single, uniform size lipid vacuoles
2. Clinicoradiographic correlation required to exclude geographic miss
3. Pleomorphic lipoma—neck/upper back, middle aged man; longstanding history
   - Florette-type giant cells
   - Absent lipoblasts
4. Spindle cell lipoma—posterior neck, elderly men, longstanding duration
   - Typical adipose tissue fragments
   - Cellular spindle cell fragments
   - Absent lipoblasts

Nodular Fasciitis

This condition is described in Chapter 14B, in the section on the orbit.

Granular Cell Tumor

This condition is described in Chapter 14B, in the section on the oral cavity.

Carotid Body Tumor (Paraganglioma)

The role of FNA in the evaluation of a suspected carotid body tumor is controversial (208–210). Noninvasive studies such as CT scan and Doppler flow color imaging yield results highly suggestive of carotid body tumor (210,211), and MRI (210) or arteriogram (208,210) is definitively diagnostic. These tumors can surround the carotid artery, and there is one case report of embolic cerebrovascular accident and death 6 days following an FNA (208). Because noninvasive studies are diagnostic, and significant complications may occur, some authors (including me) believe FNA is contraindicated for these lesions (208). Conversely, Fleming reported no complications using 22- and 25-gauge needles and concluded FNA was useful in the preoperative evaluation of these lesions (209). Regardless of this controversy, the majority of carotid body tumors undergo FNA because the lesion was never considered in the clinical diagnosis. Most are clinically suspected to be an abnormal lymph node (209) or schwannoma. Familiarity with the clinical presentation is important so that biopsy may be undertaken with caution, or not at all.

Carotid body tumors occur most commonly in the fifth decade, and both sexes are equally affected. Incidence is increased in populations subjected to chronic hypoxia (209). Ninety percent are sporadic. The remainder are familial, and, of these, 30% will be bilateral (210). These tumors present as a slowly growing 3- to 6-cm painless neck mass at the mandibular angle. Typical signs on physical examination include a bruit and transmitted pulsations; however, the majority of "pulsatile" lesions in this area are lymph nodes adjacent to the carotid artery, rather than carotid body tumors (133). A characteristic feature is lateral mobility but vertical fixation (208,209).

Cellularity is dependent on the degree of hemodilution in aspirates of these highly vascular neoplasms (209,212). Adequate samples consist of a mixture of sheets, clusters, follicle-like structures, and single cells. Three cell types are commonly present (208). The first are uniform round or oval cells with abundant, finely granular, pale (green on Pap, pink on Romanovsky) (208,209) cytoplasm, indistinct cell borders, and smooth, bland, eccentric round to oval nuclei with fine chromatin (Fig. 47). Cohesive three-dimensional clusters may strongly resemble microfollicles of follicular thyroid lesions. On Romanovsky stain, characteristic red cytoplasmic granules may be visible (208).

Variable numbers of large cells with irregular to bizarre nuclei and frequent stripped large pleomorphic nuclei constitute the second cell type (143,208,209,212,213). The final cell type con-

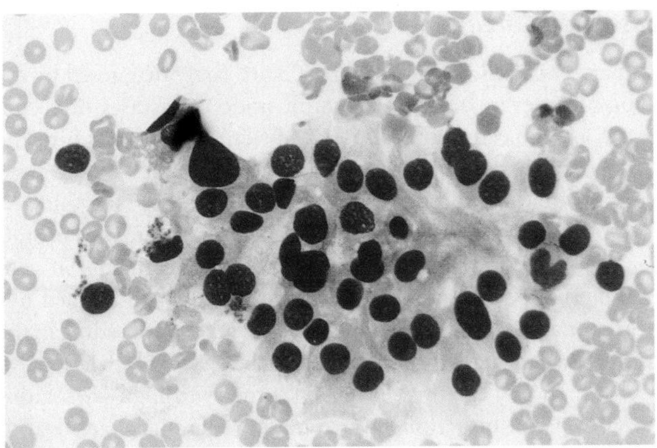

FIGURE 47. Carotid body tumor. Small, plasmacytoid cells with delicate cytoplasm admixed with occasional cells with large nuclei. Suggestion of follicular arrangement **(right).** Although red cytoplasmic granules may be present in the cytoplasm, they are not a feature of this aspirate (Diff-Quik stain, 640×).

sists of uniform spindle cells which may be scarce (143,208,209,212,213). Additional findings include rare intranuclear cytoplasmic pseudoinclusions, large, irregular nucleoli, and the absence of necrosis (209).

When the diagnosis of paraganglioma is considered in the differential diagnosis, the constellation of clinical and morphologic features leads to a straightforward diagnosis. Failure to consider carotid body tumor, however, may result in a variety of misdiagnoses, including thyroid neoplasms, nerve sheath tumors, metastatic carcinoma, and vascular neoplasms.

If the rosette or follicular pattern is well developed, paragangliomas strongly resemble *follicular thyroid neoplasms.* However, the latter usually exhibit uniform nuclei with dense, coarse chromatin and lack spindle cells or red cytoplasmic granules. The presence of spindle cells, abundant vacuolated cytoplasm, and bizarre nuclei favor paraganglioma over *papillary thyroid carcinoma* (143,209,212). Immunocytochemical stains for thyroglobulin, chromogranin, and S-100 protein are helpful in difficult cases.

Nerve sheath tumors exhibit a combination of spindle cells and occasional pleomorphic elongate nuclei and occur in the same anatomic location. However, they lack follicle-like structures and uniform, round to oval cells with eccentrically placed round nuclei (206,208,213). *Vascular neoplasms* such as hemangiopericytoma may be considered if spindle cells predominate. The presence of large pleomorphic cells and the polymorphous cell composition would be unusual for a primary vascular neoplasm (209).

Because of the nuclear pleomorphism, nucleoli, intranuclear pseudoinclusions, and cellularity, carotid body tumors can easily be misdiagnosed as malignant. A high index of suspicion and awareness of the characteristic clinical findings are important to avoid misdiagnoses. Immunocytochemistry and/or radiographic studies are indicated when the diagnosis is uncertain (143,206,210).

Carotid Body Tumor

1. Pulsatile mass
2. Mixture of uniform plasmacytoid, large pleomorphic, and spindle cells
3. Follicle-like structures frequently present
4. Red cytoplasmic granules
5. Rare intranuclear cytoplasmic pseudoinclusions
6. Large irregular nucleoli
7. Chromogranin- and S-100 protein–positive

FNA OF CUTANEOUS LESIONS

Although primary cutaneous neoplasms are seldom biopsied by FNA, the head and neck is the primary site of origin of several malignant skin tumors that may metastasize to regional lymph nodes or recur without an epidermal origin. In addition, a variety of benign skin appendage tumors present as subcutaneous nodules, and their cytomorphology is easily confused with a variety of salivary gland neoplasms. The most common and those that may cause diagnostic errors are discussed.

Pilomatrixoma

Pilomatrixoma (calcifying epithelioma of Malherbe) presents as a longstanding, hard, relatively deep, 1- to 3-cm mass most often in the skin of the head and neck (214). Children and young adults are most frequently affected; however, it is not uncommon in adults (214). If not suspected clinically or recognized morphologically, it can be a source of positive malignant diagnoses (215).

Aspirates are cellular and polymorphous. Three epithelial cell types are characteristically present: basaloid, squamous, and ghost cells (143,151,215–217).

Basaloid cells often predominate and are small cells with uniform round vesicular nuclei, with or without nucleoli, arranged in thick, tight clusters, loose sheets, and singly. Scattered clusters may show squamous differentiation (216) (Fig. 48).

Ghost cells are most easily identified on Romanovsky stain as polygonal squames with pale, gray-blue cytoplasm and central pallor (217). Occasionally, only the outline of the cell is visible, and aggregates of ghost cells may form a lattice-like structure (215–217) reminiscent of the cell walls of plant material. On alcohol-fixed material, the ghost cells may appear as brightly eosinophilic or orangeophilic amorphous debris that is easily overlooked (217). Often, calcifications are associated with this element.

Squamous cells with bland nuclei, with or without keratinization, are present in most aspirates (143,215,217). Ancillary findings that may or may not be present include giant cells, calcification, inflammatory cells, and debris (143,215–217).

Recognition of the synchronous presence of basaloid, ghost, and squamous cells, coupled with the lack of true malignant nuclear features, should permit an accurate diagnosis (143, 151,215–217). In addition, the clinical findings and history of a

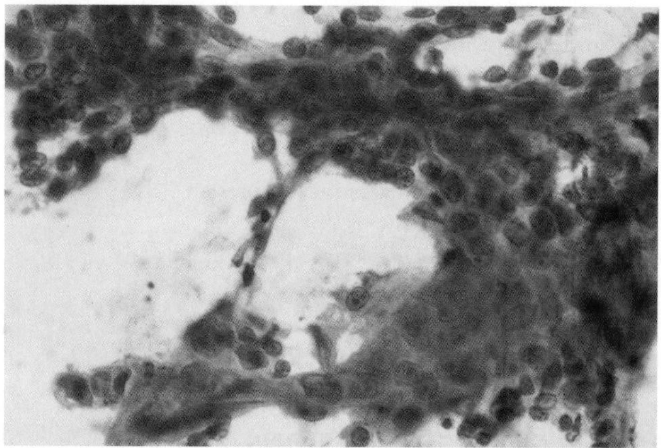

FIGURE 48. Pilomatrixoma. Clusters of basaloid and squamous cells with uniform nuclei and focally prominent nucleoli. Ghost cells not present in this field (hematoxylin and eosin, 400×).

longstanding mass are often helpful in preventing misdiagnosis (215).

Because clinicians often misdiagnose this lesion as a pathologic lymph node, the most fundamental requirement for an accurate diagnosis is a high index of suspicion. If, however, pilomatrixoma is not considered in the differential diagnosis, a wide variety of misdiagnoses may ensue. In a review of the literature, Wong found only 4 of 16 aspirates of pilomatrixoma were correctly diagnosed (217). Overdiagnosis of the basaloid and squamous cells leads to a misdiagnosis of *squamous cell carcinoma, basal cell carcinoma,* and *Merkel cell carcinoma.* The nuclei of pilomatrixoma are smooth, with uniform chromatin, and do not exhibit diagnostic criteria of malignancy. The small abnormal keratinized cells of squamous cell carcinoma (144) are not a feature of this lesion, nor are the tightly cohesive clusters of basaloid cells with prominent nucleoli and peripheral palisading characteristic of basal cell carcinoma (218). Neither Merkel cell carcinoma nor squamous cell carcinoma would exhibit ghost cells or the polymorphism of cell types evident in pilomatrixoma (217), nor would they present as a longstanding mass without change.

Because of the young age of the patients, *small round-cell tumors of childhood* enter into the differential diagnosis; however, these lack the uniform nuclear membrane and chromatin and polymorphism of cell types evident in pilomatrixoma (215).

Skin overlying the parotid gland is a frequent site for pilomatrixoma, and in this location it misdiagnosed as *basaloid salivary gland neoplasms* including pleomorphic adenoma, basal cell adenoma, and adenoid cystic carcinoma. The presence of ghost cells and knowledge of the tissue plane of the lesion should permit an accurate diagnosis (215–217).

Pilomatrixoma

1. Longstanding mass, often in cheek of young adults
2. Uniform basaloid cells with bland chromatin
3. Lattice-like ghost cells (Romanovsky) or amorphous eosinophilic debris (Pap)
4. Bland squamous cells
5. ± Calcification, giant cells, inflammation

Basal Cell Carcinoma

Primary basal cell carcinomas (BCC) are rarely diagnosed by cytology; however, occasional lymph node metastases or recurrences are subjected to FNA. In addition, BCC enters into the differential diagnosis of many basaloid neoplasms of the head and neck, and familiarity with its cytomorphology is of value.

On low power, aspirates are moderately cellular, with prominent cell cohesion evidenced by tight tissue fragments in geographic shapes with sharply delineated borders and marked nuclear overlap (143,151,218) (Fig. 49). Peripheral palisading in the clusters is characteristic but inconsistently present (143,151,218).

On high power, the cells are uniform, with high N/C ratios and a thin rim of peripheral cytoplasm. The nuclei are oval to spindle shaped but rarely round. Chromatin is evenly distributed, and nucleoli are usually present but rarely prominent. Other features that may be present include focal keratinization or squamous differentiation and scant metachromatic stroma.

The differential diagnosis includes all basaloid neoplasms of the head and neck, and therefore, careful clinical correlation and attention to diagnostic criteria are imperative. Prominent cohesion with sharply defined tissue fragments and focal peripheral palisading are the most characteristic features of BCC (143, 151,218). Among the most significant lesions to distinguish is the solid variant of adenoid cystic carcinoma and basal cell adenoma, which show marked cohesion but lack sharp group borders and peripheral palisading (218). Pilomatrixoma exhibits a more polymorphous cell population with amorphous shadow cells. Greater nuclear anaplasia and necrosis are present in sebaceous carcinoma.

Basal Cell Carcinoma

1. Tightly cohesive fragments with geographic shapes
2. ± Peripheral palisading
3. Oval to spindled nuclei, even chromatin, and scant cytoplasm
4. ± Squamous differentiation
5. ± Metachromatic stroma

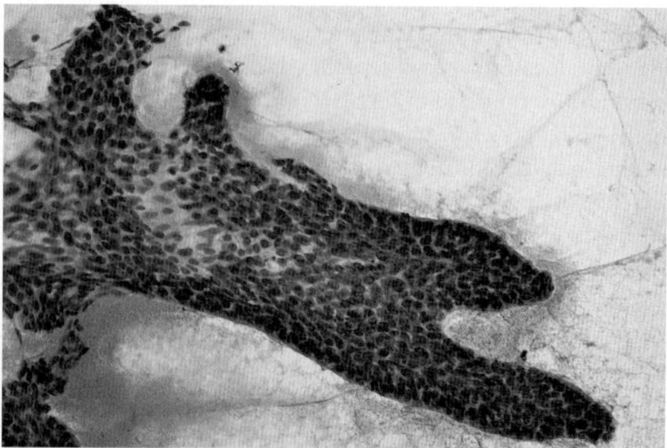

FIGURE 49. Basal cell carcinoma. Tightly cohesive, geographically shaped clusters of basaloid cells with peripheral palisading (hematoxylin and eosin, 200×).

Merkel Cell Carcinoma

Merkel cell carcinoma has a predilection for the subepidermal skin of the face and upper extremities of elderly individuals and frequently metastasizes early to cervical lymph nodes and parotid glands.

Aspirates are often cellular and monotonous, composed predominantly of single cells with occasional clusters and sheets (143,151,219) (Fig. 50). On high power, the nuclei are round and surrounded by a thin rim of cytoplasm. The chromatin is fine to dark with one or more inconspicuous nucleoli. Little or no molding is present, and numerous mitoses are seen (143,151,219). Some authors (219,220) have described "paranuclear button-like inclusions" consisting of 2- to 3-μm crescentic shaped or discoid globules located in the cytoplasm adjacent to the nucleus. These are best seen in hematoxylin and eosin preparations but will appear as clear or unstained on Romanovsky stains (219,220) and correspond to the clumps of intermediate filaments identified on immunocytochemical stains.

The differential diagnosis includes metastatic small-cell undifferentiated carcinoma, which exhibits greater molding and lacks characteristic immunocytochemical findings (151). Because of the dispersed nature of the cells, malignant lymphoma may enter into the differential diagnosis; however, Merkel cell carcinomas are CD45-negative and exhibit focal cohesion. Electron microscopy or immunocytochemical stains for cytokeratin, neurofilament, and neuron-specific enolase (NSE) with characteristic perinuclear staining are helpful in confirming the diagnosis.

Merkel Cell Carcinoma

1. Predominantly single cells
2. Round, vesicular nuclei; scant cytoplasm
3. Scant to absent molding
4. Numerous mitoses
5. "Perinuclear button-like inclusions"
6. Positive cytokeratin, neurofilament, and NSE

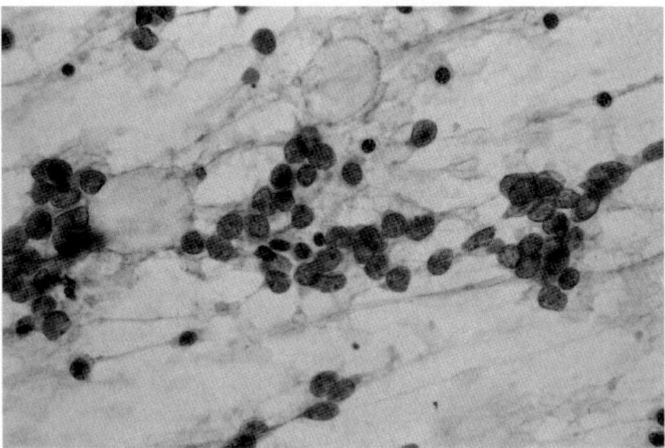

FIGURE 50. Merkel cell carcinoma. Dyshesive small cells with round to oval nuclei, stippled chromatin, and absent nucleoli, arranged singly and as rosettes (Papanicolaou stain, 400×).

Melanoma

See the section on lymph node metastases.

Sebaceous Carcinoma

This rare carcinoma usually arises from the Mebomian glands of the eyelid and often gives rise to lymph node or visceral metastases. Clinically, they are often misdiagnosed as a chalazion (143,221).

Aspirates are highly cellular and composed of irregular clumps, whole lobules, or loose aggregates of closely packed cells. Single cells are present, and their number depends on the carcinoma's degree of differentiation. Abundant necrosis is often seen, including individual cell necrosis within lobules (143,221).

On high power, the cells are large, with foamy, finely reticulated, eosinophilic cytoplasm. Variable numbers of cytoplasmic vacuoles result in bubbly cytoplasm; however, this feature is decreased in less well-differentiated lesions. The N/C ratio is high with coarse nuclear chromatin, prominent nucleoli, and significant anaplasia. Mitoses are frequent (143,221). A second population of basaloid (143) or squamous cells (151) may be present. If sebaceous carcinoma is suspected, air-dried smears should be prepared for oil red O stains (143,221).

The differential diagnosis includes basal cell carcinoma, chalazion, and adenocarcinoma. Basal cell carcinomas may exhibit variably vacuolated cells consistent with sebaceous differentiation; however, these are a minor component, and basal cell carcinoma lacks the anaplasia of sebaceous carcinoma (221). Aspirates of chalazion yield lipid-laden macrophages, debris, and inflammatory cells without evidence of nuclear anaplasia or mitotic activity. Adenocarcinoma may be mimicked by the three-dimensional clusters of sebaceous carcinoma. Careful attention to the clinical features, presence of squamous differentiation or oil red O positivity favors a diagnosis of sebaceous carcinoma.

Sebaceous Carcinoma

1. Clumps, lobules, and loose aggregates
2. Foamy, eosinophilic cytoplasm; high N/C ratio
3. Coarse chromatin, prominent nucleoli, anaplasia
4. Mitoses and necrosis
5. ± Basaloid or squamous cells
6. Oil red O^+

Skin Appendage Tumors

Some appendage tumors, notably eccrine spiradenoma (68), eccrine cylindroma (69), proliferating trichilemmal cyst (222), chondroid syringoma (223), and pilomatrixomas (215–217), have a propensity for the skin of the head and neck. These may be easily confused with salivary gland neoplasms or squamous carcinoma on FNA and are discussed elsewhere in this chapter. Three useful parameters in distinguishing these from more ominous parenchymal neoplasms are long duration with minimal change of the lesion, superficial location, and circumscription. A high index of suspicion is the single most important factor in avoiding misdiagnosis.

Clinical Features of Skin Appendage Tumors

1. Long duration with minimal change
2. Superficial location
3. Circumscription
4. High index of suspicion

Metastases to the Skin

Cutaneous metastases occur in 1.5% to 2% of malignancies (224,225) and portend an ominous prognosis. The scalp skin is the third most common site affected, after abdomen and chest wall (225). Skin metastases most commonly originate from melanoma, renal cell carcinoma, and adenocarcinomas of the lung and breast (225). Plasmacytoma, small cell carcinoma, oropharyngeal, and sinonasal carcnomas are also frequent sources of scalp metastases (224). Because of the prevalence of metastases to this area, any scalp mass should be considered for FNA (224).

The differential diagnosis includes skin adnexal tumors (particularly proliferating trichilemmal cyst) (222), nodular and clear cell hidradenoma (226), and sebaceous carcinoma.

REFERENCES

1. Rollins SD. Editorial comments: a prescription for reducing diagnostic pitfalls. *Diagn Cytopathol* 1994;10(2):172–173.
2. Qizilbash AH, Sianos J, Young JEM, et al. Fine needle aspiration biopsy cytology of major salivary glands. *Acta Cytol* 1985;29(4): 503–512.
3. Oertel YC, Zorsky PE. Fine needle aspiration as a means to cost-effective health care. *South Med J* 1993;86:282–284.
4. Frable WJ. Fine-needle aspiration biopsy: a review. *Hum Pathol* 1983;14:9–28.
5. Cohen MB, Reznicek MJ, Miller TR. Fine-needle aspiration biopsy of the salivary glands. *Pathol Annu* 1992;27:213–245.
6. Orell SR. Diagnostic difficulties in the interpretation of fine needle aspirates of salivary gland lesions: the problem revisited. *Cytopathology* 1995;6:285–300.
7. Heller KS, Dubner S, Chess Q, et al. Value of fine needle aspiration biopsy of salivary gland masses in clinical decision-making. *Am J Surg* 1992;164:667–670.
8. Layfield LJ, Glasgow BJ. Diagnosis of salivary gland tumors by fine-needle aspiration cytology: a review of clinical utility and pitfalls. *Diagn Cytopathol* 1991;7(3):267–272.
9. Ascoli V, Albedi FM, De Blasiis R. Sialadenosis of the parotid gland: report of four cases diagnosed by fine-needle aspiration cytology. *Diagn Cytopathol* 1993;9(2):151–155.
10. Stanley MW, Bardales RH, Beneke J, et al. Sialolithiasis. Differential diagnostic problems in fine-needle aspiration cytology. *Am J Clin Pathol* 1996;106:229–233.
11. Zarka MA. Fine-needle aspiration of the salivary glands. *Pathology* 1996;4:287–318.
12. Layfield LJ, Glasgow BJ, Goldstein N, et al. Lipomatous lesions of the parotid gland. Potential pitfalls in fine needle aspiration biopsy diagnosis. *Acta Cytol* 1991;35(5):553–556.
13. Bhatia A. Fine needle aspiration cytology in the diagnosis of mass lesions of the salivary gland. *Indian J Cancer* 1993;30(1):26–30.
14. Cramer H, Layfield L, Lampe H. Fine needle aspiration of salivary gland lesions. In: Schmidt WA, Miller TR, Katz RL, et al, eds. *Cytopathology annual.* Baltimore: Williams & Wilkins, 1993:181–206.
15. Young JA. Diagnostic problems in fine needle aspiration cytopathology of the salivary glands. *J Clin Pathol* 1994;47:193–198.
16. Weidner N, Geisinger KR, Sterling RT, et al. Benign lymphoepithelial cysts of the parotid gland. A histologic, cytologic, and ultrastructural study. *Am J Clin Pathol* 1986;85:395–401.
17. Finfer MD, Gallo L, Perchick A, et al. Fine needle aspiration biopsy of cystic benign lymphoepithelial lesion of the parotid gland in patients at risk for the acquired immune deficiency syndrome. *Acta Cytol* 1990;34(6):821–826.
18. Elliott JN, Oertel YC. Lymphoepithelial cysts of the salivary glands. Histologic and cytologic features. *Am J Clin Pathol* 1990;93: 39–43.
19. Chai C, Dodd LG, Glasgow BJ, et al. Salivary gland lesions with a prominent lymphoid component: cytologic findings and differential diagnosis by fine-needle aspiration biopsy. *Diagn Cytopathol* 1997; 17(3):183–190.
20. Tao L-C, Gullane PJ. HIV infection-associated lymphoepithelial lesions of the parotid gland: aspiration biopsy cytology, histology, and pathogenesis. *Diagn Cytopathol* 1991;7(2):158–162.
21. Wax TD, Layfield LJ, Zaleski S, et al. Cytomegalovirus sialadenitis in patients with the acquired immunodeficiency syndrome: a potential diagnostic pitfall with fine-needle aspiration cytology. *Diagn Cytopathol* 1994;10(2):169–174.
22. Mooney EE, Dodd LG, Layfiend LJ. Squamous cells in fine-needle aspiration biopsies of salivary gland lesions: potential pitfalls in cytologic diagnosis. *Diagn Cytopathol* 1996;15:447–452.
23. Frierson HF, Fechner RE. Chronic sialadenitis with psammoma bodies mimicking neoplasia in a fine-needle aspiration specimen from the submandibular gland. *Am J Clin Pathol* 1991;95:884–888.
24. Gupta RK. Fine needle aspiration cytodiagnosis of sialadenitis with crystalloid formation. *Pathology* 1997;29:102–103.
25. Jayaram G, Khurana N, Basu S. Crystalloids in a cystic lesion of parotid salivary gland: diagnosis by fine-needle aspiration. *Diagn Cytopathol* 1993;9:70–71.
26. Cohen MB, Fisher PE, Holly EA, et al. Fine needle aspiration biopsy diagnosis of mucoepidermoid carcinoma. Statistical analysis. *Acta Cytol* 1990;34(1):43–49.
27. Frable MA, Frable WJ. Fine needle aspiration biopsy in the diagnosis of sarcoid of the head and neck. *Acta Cytol* 1984;28:175–177.
28. MacLeod CB, Frable WJ. Fine-needle aspiration biopsy of the salivary gland: problem cases. *Diagn Cytopathol* 1993;9(2):216–225.
29. Günhan O, Celasun B, Dogan N, et al. Fine needle aspiration cytology findings in a benign lymphoepithelial lesion with microcalcifications. A case report. *Acta Cytol* 1992;36:744–747.
30. Ellis GL, Auclair PL. Tumors of the salivary glands. In: Rosai J, Sobin LH, eds. *Atlas of tumor pathology, 17th ed.* Washington, DC: Armed Forces Institute of Pathology, 1996.
31. Cha I, Long SR, Ljung B-ME, et al. Low-grade lymphoma of mucosa-associated tissue in the parotid gland: a case report of fine-needle aspiration cytology diagnosis using flow cytometric immunophenotyping. *Diagn Cytopathol* 1997;16(4):345–349.
32. Kapadia SB, Dusenbery D, Dekker A. Fine needle aspiration of pleomorphic adenoma and adenoid cystic carcinoma of salivary gland origin. *Acta Cytol* 1997;41:487–492.
33. Viguer JM, Vicandi B, Jiménez-Heffernan JA, et al. Fine needle aspiration cytology of pleomorphic adenoma. *Acta Cytol* 1997;41: 786–794.
34. Klijanienko J, Vielh P. Fine-needle sampling of salivary gland lesions I. Cytology and histology correlation of 412 cases of pleomorphic adenoma. *Diagn Cytopathol* 1996;14(3):195–200.
35. Elsheikh TM, Bernacki EG. Fine needle aspiration cytology of cellular pleomorphic adenoma. *Acta Cytol* 1996;40:1165–1175.
36. Lee S-S, Cho K-J, Jang J-J. Differential diagnosis of adenoid cystic carcinoma from pleomorphic adenoma of the salivary gland on fine needle aspiration cytology. *Acta Cytol* 1996;40:1246–1252.

37. Stanley MW, Lowhagen T. Mucin production by pleomorphic adenomas of the parotid gland: a cytologic spectrum. *Diagn Cytopathol* 1990;6(1):49–52.
38. Bottles K, Ferrell LD, Miller TR. Tyrosine crystals in fine needle aspirates of a pleomorphic adenoma of the parotid gland. *Acta Cytol* 1984;28(4):490–492.
39. Murty DA, Sodhani P. Intranuclear inclusions in pleomorphic adenoma of salivary gland: a case report. *Diagn Cytopathol* 1993;9(2): 194–196.
40. Eneroth C-M, Zajicek J. Aspiration biopsy of salivary gland tumors III. Morphologic studies on smears and histologic sections from 368 mixed tumors. *Acta Cytol* 1966;10(6):440–454.
41. Klijanienko J, Vielh P. Fine-needle sampling of salivary gland lesions III. Cytologic and histologic correlation of 75 cases of adenoid cystic carcinoma: review and experience at the Institut Curie with emphasis on cytologic pitfalls. *Diagn Cytopathol* 1997;17(1):36–41.
42. Löwhagen T, Tani EM, Skoog L. Salivary glands and rare head and neck lesions. In: Bibbo M, ed. *Comprehensive cytopathology.* Philadelphia: WB Saunders, 1991:621–648.
43. Stanley MW, Horwitz CA, Henry MJ, et al. Basal-cell adenoma of the salivary gland: a benign adenoma that cytologically mimics adenoid cystic carcinoma. *Diagn Cytopathol* 1988;4(4):342–346.
44. Sparrow SA, Frost FA. Salivary monomorphic adenomas of dermal analogue type: report of two cases. *Diagn Cytopathol* 1993;9(3): 300–303.
45. Gupta RK. Aspiration cytodiagnosis of dermal analogue tumor, a rare subtype of salivary gland monomorphic adenoma. A case report. *Acta Cytol* 1996;40:331–334.
46. Arora VK, Misra K, Bhatia A. Cytomorphologic features of the rare epithelial–myoepithelial carcinoma of the salivary gland. *Acta Cytol* 1990;34(2):239–242.
47. Carrillo R, Poblet E, Rocamora A, et al. Epithelial–myoepithelial carcinoma of the salivary gland. Fine needle aspiration cytologic findings. *Acta Cytol* 1990;34(2):243–247.
48. Klijanienko J, Vielh P. Fine-needle sampling of salivary gland lesions II. Cytology and histology correlation of 71 cases of Warthin's tumor (adenolymphoma). *Diagn Cytopathol* 1996;16(3):221–225.
49. Bottles K, Löwhagen T, Miller TR. Mast cells in the aspiration cytology differential diagnosis of adenolymphoma. *Acta Cytol* 1985;29 (4):513–515.
50. Allen CM, Damm D, Neville B, et al. Necrosis in benign salivary gland neoplasms. Not necessarily a sign of malignant transformation. *Oral Surg Oral Med Oral Pathol* 1994;78(4):455–461.
51. Laucirica R, Farnum JB, Leopold SK, et al. False-positive diagnosis in fine-needle aspiration of an atypical Warthin's tumor: histochemical differential stains for cytodiagnosis. *Diagn Cytopathol* 1989;5(4): 412–415.
52. Chen KTK. Aspiration cytology of metaplastic Warthin's tumor mimicking squamous-cell carcinoma (letter to the editor). *Diagn Cytopathol* 1991;7(3):330–331.
53. van den Brekel MWM, Risse EKJ, Tiwari RM, et al. False-positive fine needle aspiration cytologic diagnosis of a Warthin's tumor with squamous metaplasia as a squamous-cell carcinoma (letter to the editor). *Acta Cytol* 1991;35:477–478.
54. Layfield LJ, Tan P, Glasgow BJ. Fine-needle aspiration of salivary gland lesions. Comparison with frozen sections and histologic findings. *Arch Pathol Lab Med* 1987;111:346–353.
55. Sauer T, Freng A, Djupesland P. Immediate interpretation of FNA smears from the head and neck region. *Diagn Cytopathol* 1992;8(2): 116–118.
56. Chang A, Harawi SJ. Oncocytes, oncocytosis, and oncocytic tumors. In: Rosen PP, Fechner RE, eds. *Pathology annual, vol 27.* Norwalk, CT: Appleton & Lange, 1992:263–304.
57. Laforga JB, Aranda FI. Oncocytic carcinoma of parotid gland: fine-needle aspiration and histologic findings. *Diagn Cytopathol* 1994; 11(3):376–379.
58. Herbst EW, Utz W. Multifocal dermal-type basal cell adenomas of parotid glands with co-existing dermal cylindromas. *Virchows Arch Pathol Anat* 1984;403:95–102.
59. Stanley MW, Horwitz CA, Rollins SD, et al. Basal cell (monomorphic) and minimally pleomorphic adenomas of the salivary glands. Distinction from the solid (anaplastic) type of adenoid cystic carcinoma in fine-needle aspiration. *Am J Clin Pathol* 1996;106: 35–41.
60. Hood IC, Qizilbash AH, Salama SSS, et al. Basal-cell adenoma of parotid. Difficulty of differentiation from adenoid cystic carcinoma on aspiration biopsy. *Acta Cytol* 1983;27(5):515–520.
61. Layfield LJ. Fine needle aspiration cytology of a trabecular adenoma of the parotid gland. *Acta Cytol* 1985;29(6):999–1002.
62. Hruban RH, Erozan YS, Zinreich SJ, et al. Fine-needle aspiration cytology of monomorphic adenomas. *Am J Clin Pathol* 1988;90:46–51.
63. Tawfik O, Tsue T, Pantazis C, et al. Salivary gland neoplasms with basaloid cell features: report of two cases diagnosed by fine-needle aspiration cytology. *Diagn Cytopathol* 1999;21:46–50.
64. Klijanienko J, El-Naggar AK, Vielh P. Comparative cytologic and histologic study of fifteen salivary basal-cell tumors: differential diagnostic considerations. *Diagn Cytopathol* 1999;21:30–34.
65. Eneroth C-M, Zajicek J. Aspiration biopsy of salivary gland tumors IV. Morphologic studies on smears and histologic sections from 45 cases of adenoid cystic carcinoma. *Acta Cytol* 1969;13(2):59–63.
66. Stanley MW, Horwitz CA, Bardales RH, et al. Basal cell carcinoma metastatic to the salivary glands: differential diagnosis in fine-needle aspiration cytology. *Diagn Cytopathol* 1997;16(3):247–252.
67. Pisharodi LR. Basal cell adenocarcinoma of the salivary gland. Diagnosis by fine-needle aspiration cytology. *Am J Clin Pathol* 1995; 103:603–608.
68. Kolda TF, Ardaman T-DT, Schwartz MR. Eccrine spiradenoma mimicking adenoid cystic carcinoma on fine needle aspiration. A case report. *Acta Cytol* 1997;41:852–858.
69. Bondeson L, Lindholm K, Thorstenson S. Benign dermal eccrine cylindroma. A pitfall in the cytologic diagnosis of adenoid cystic carcinoma. *Acta Cytol* 1983;27(3):326–328.
70. Nagel H, Jotze HJ, Laskawi R, et al. Cytologic diagnosis of adenoid cystic carcinoma of salivary glands. *Diagn Cytopathol* 1999;20: 358–366.
71. Hood IC, Qizilbash AH, Young JEM, et al. Needle aspiration cytology of a benign and a malignant schwannoma. *Acta Cytol* 1984;28(2): 157–164.
72. Yu GH, Caraway NP. Poorly-differentiated adenoid cystic carcinoma: cytologic appearance in fine-needle aspirates of distant metastases. *Diagn Cytopathol* 1996;15(4):296–300.
73. Layfield LJ, Reznicek M, Lowe M, et al. Spontaneous infarction of a parotid gland pleomorphic adenoma. Report of a case with cytologic and radiographic overlap with a primary salivary gland malignancy. *Acta Cytol* 1992;36(3):381–386.
74. Gibbons D, Saboorian MH, Vuitch F, et al. Fine-needle aspiration findings in patients with polymorphous low grade adenocarcinoma of the salivary glands. *Cancer* 1999;87:31–36.
75. Frierson HF, Covell JL, Mills SE. Fine-needle aspiration cytology of terminal duct carcinoma of minor salivary gland. *Diagn Cytopathol* 1987;3(2):159–162.
76. Cleveland DB, Cosgrove MM, Martin SE. Tyrosine-rich crystalloids in a fine needle aspirate of a polymorphous low grade adenocarcinoma of a minor salivary gland. A case report. *Acta Cytol* 1994;38(2): 247–251.
77. Klijanienko J, Vielh P. Salivary carcinomas with papillae: cytology and histology analysis of polymorphous low-grade adenocarcinoma and papillary cystadenocarcinoma. *Diagn Cytopathol* 1998;19: 244–249.
78. Koss LJ. Diagnostic cytology seminar. *Acta Cytol* 1979;23(1):1–29.
79. Nagy H, Laskawi R, Büter JJ, et al. Cytologic diagnosis of acinic-cell carcinoma of salivary glands. *Diagn Cytopathol* 1997;16(5):402–412.
80. Watanabe K, Ono N, Saito K, et al. Fine-needle aspiration cytology of polymorphous low-grade adenocarcinoma of the tongue. *Diagn Cytopathol* 1999;20:167–169.
81. Kocjan G, Milroy C, Fisher EW, et al. Cytological features of epithelial–myoepithelial carcinoma of salivary gland: potential pitfalls in diagnosis. *Cytopathology* 1993;4:173–180.

82. Klijanienko J, Vielh P. Fine-needle sampling of salivary gland lesions VII. Cytology and histology correlation of five cases of epithelial–myoepithelial carcinoma. *Diagn Cytopathol* 1998;19:405–409.
83. Klijanienko J, Vielh P. Fine-needle sampling of salivary gland lesions VI. Cytological review of 44 cases of primary salivary squamous-cell carcinoma with histological correlation. *Diagn Cytopathol* 1998;18(3):174–178.
84. Ellis GL, Auclair PL, Gnepp DR. *Major problems in pathology, vol 25: Surgical pathology of the salivary glands.* Philadelphia: WB Saunders, 1991.
85. Jayaram N, Ashim D, Rajwanshi A, et al. The value of fine-needle aspiration biopsy in the cytodiagnosis of salivary gland lesions. *Diagn Cytopathol* 1989;5(4):349–354.
86. Zurrida S, Alasio L, Tradati N, et al. Fine-needle aspiration of parotid masses. *Cancer* 1993;72:2306–2311.
87. Frable MS, Frable WJ. Fine-needle aspiration biopsy of salivary glands. *Laryngoscope* 1991;101:245–249.
88. Klijanienko J, Vielh P. Fine-needle sampling of salivary gland lesions IV. Review of 50 cases of mucoepidermoid carcinoma with histologic correlation. *Diagn Cytopathol* 1997;17(2):92–98.
89. Zajicek J, Eneroth C-M, Jakobsson P. Aspiration biopsy of salivary gland tumors VI. Morphologic studies on smears and histologic sections from mucoepidermoid carcinoma. *Acta Cytol* 1976;20(1):35–41.
90. Hayes MMM, Cameron RD, Jones EA. Sebaceous variant of mucoepidermoid carcinoma of the salivary gland. A case report with cytohistologic correlation. *Acta Cytol* 1993;37(2):237–241.
91. Elsheikh TM, Bernacki EGJ, Pisharodi L. Fine-needle aspiration cytology of salivary duct carcinoma. *Diagn Cytopathol* 1994;11(1):47–51.
92. Dβvila RM. Nuclear pseudoinclusions in a case of parotid mucoepidermoid carcinoma. *Diagn Cytopathol* 1996;14(1):72–74.
93. Klijanienko J, El-Naggar AK, Servois V, et al. Mucoepidermoid carcinoma *ex* pleomorphic adenoma. Nonspecific preoperative cytologic findings in six cases. *Cancer Cytopathol* 1998;84:231–234.
94. Sauer T, Jebsen PW, Olsholt R. Cytologic features of papillary-cystic variant of acinic-cell adenocarcinoma: a case report. *Diagn Cytopathol* 1994;10(1):30–32.
95. Layfield LJ, Glasgow BJ. Aspiration cytology of clear-cell lesions of the parotid gland: morphologic features and differential diagnosis. *Diagn Cytopathol* 1993;9(6):705–712.
96. Eneroth C-M, Jakobsson P, Zajicek J. Aspiration biopsy of salivary gland tumors V. Morphologic investigations on smears and histologic sections of acinic cell carcinoma. *Acta Radiol Suppl* 1971;310:85–93.
97. Klijanienko J, Vielh P. Fine-needle sampling of salivary gland lesions V: Cytology of 22 cases of acinic cell carcinoma with histologic correlation. *Diagn Cytopathol* 1997;17:347–352.
98. Bottles K, Löwhagen T. Psammoma bodies in the aspiration cytology smears of an acinic-cell tumor. *Acta Cytol* 1985;29(2):191–192.
99. Geisinger KR, Reynolds GD, Vance RP, et al. Adenoid cystic carcinoma arising in a pleomorphic adenoma of the parotid gland. An aspiration cytology and ultrastructural study. *Acta Cytol* 1985;29(4):522–526.
100. Jacobs JC. Low grade mucoepidermoid carcinoma *ex* pleomorphic adenoma. A diagnostic problem in fine needle aspiration biopsy. *Acta Cytol* 1994;38(1):93–97.
101. Granger JK, Houn H-Y. Malignant mixed tumor (carcinosarcoma) of parotid gland diagnosed by fine-needle aspiration biopsy. *Diagn Cytopathol* 1991;7:427–432.
102. Dee S, Masood S, Issacs JHJ, et al. Cytomorphologic features of salivary duct carcinoma on fine needle aspiration biopsy. A case report. *Acta Cytol* 1993;37(4):539–542.
103. Fyrat P, Cramer H, Feczko JD, et al. Fine-needle aspiration biopsy of salivary duct carcinoma: report of five cases. *Diagn Cytopathol* 1997;16(6):526–530.
104. Khurana KK, Pitman MB, Powers CN, et al. Diagnostic pitfalls of aspiration cytology of salivary duct carcinoma. *Cancer Cytopathol* 1997;81:373–378.
105. Colecchia M, Frigo B, Leopardi OM. Salivary duct carcinoma of the parotid gland. Report of a case with cytologic and immunocytochemical findings on fine needle aspiration biopsy. *Acta Cytol* 1997;41(2):593–597.
106. Gal R, Strauss M, Zohar Y, et al. Salivary duct carcinoma of the parotid gland. Cytologic and histopathologic study. *Acta Cytol* 1985;29(3):454–456.
107. Chan MKM, McGujire LJ. Cytodiagnosis of lesions presenting as salivary gland swellings: a report of seven cases. *Diagn Cytopathol* 1992;8(5):439–443.
108. MacCallum PL, Lampe HB, Cramer H, et al. Fine-needle aspiration cytology of lymphoid lesions of the salivary gland: a review of 35 cases. *J Otolaryngol* 1996;25(5):300–304.
109. Katz RL. Cytologic diagnosis of leukemia and lymphoma. Values and limitations. *Clin Lab Med* 1991;11(2):469–499.
110. Gunhan O, Celasun B, Safali M, et al. Fine needle aspiration cytology of malignant lymphoepithelial lesion of the salivary gland. A report of two cases. *Acta Cytol* 1994;38(5):751–754.
111. Jayaram G, Verma AK, Sood N, et al. Fine needle aspiration cytology of salivary gland lesions. *J Oral Pathol Med* 1994;23(6):256–261.
112. Frable MS, Frable WJ. Fine-needle aspiration biopsy revisited. *Laryngoscope* 1982;92:1414–1418.
113. Candel A, Gattuso P, Reddy V, et al. Is fine needle aspiration biopsy of salivary gland masses really necessary? *ENT J* 1993;72:485–489.
114. O'Dwyer P, Farrar WB, James AG, et al. Needle aspiration biopsy of major salivary gland tumors. Its value. *Cancer* 1986;57:554–557.
115. McGurk M, Hussain K. Role of fine needle aspiration cytology in the management of the discrete parotid lump. *Ann R Coll Surg Engl* 1997;79:198–202.
116. Deans GT, Spence RAJ, Briggs K. An audit of surgery of the parotid gland. *Ann R Coll Surg Engl* 1995;77:188–192.
117. Pitts DB, Hilsinger RL, Karandy E, et al. Fine-needle aspiration in the diagnosis of salivary gland disorders in the community hospital setting. *Arch Otolaryngol Head Neck Surg* 1992;118:479–482.
118. Cross DL, Gansler TS, Morris RC. Fine needle aspiration and frozen section of salivary gland lesions. *South Med J* 1990;83(3):283–286.
119. Cohen MB, Ljung BE, Boles R. Salivary gland tumors. Fine-needle aspiration vs frozen-section diagnosis. *Arch Otolaryngol Head Neck Surg* 1986;112:867–869.
120. Megerian CA, Maniglia AJ. Parotidectomy: a ten year experience with fine needle aspiration and frozen section biopsy correlation. *ENT J* 1994;73(6):377–380.
121. Hillel AD, Fee WEJ. Evaluation of frozen section in parotid gland surgery. *Arch Otolaryngol* 1983;109:230–232.
122. Stern SJ, Suen JY. Salivary gland tumors. *Curr Opin Oncol* 1993;5:518–525.
123. Eneroth CM, Franzen S, Zajicek J. Cytologic diagnosis on aspirate from 1000 salivary-gland tumours. *Acta Otolaryngol* 1966;224(Suppl):168–172.
124. Eisele DW, Sherman ME, Koch WM, et al. Utility of immediate onsite cytopathological procurement and evaluation in fine needle aspiration biopsy of head and neck masses. *Laryngoscope* 1992;102:1328–1330.
125. Connolly AAP, MacKenzie K. Paediatric neck masses—a diagnostic dilemma. *J Laryngol Otol* 1997;111:541–545.
126. Eisenhut CC, King DE, Nelson WA, et al. Fine-needle biopsy of pediatric lesions: a three-year study in an outpatient biopsy clinic. *Diagn Cytopathol* 1996;14:43–50.
127. Hilal EY. Advances in otolaryngology—head and neck surgery. Diagnosis of head and neck cancer. *Lebanese Med J* 1994;42:212–215.
128. Patt BS, Schaefer SD, Buitch F. Role of fine-needle aspiration in the evaluation of neck masses. *Med Clin North Am* 1993;77:611–623.
129. Mixon T, Gianoli G. Fine needle aspiration in head and neck surgery. *J Louisiana State Med Soc* 1992;145:505–508.
130. Crosby JH. The role of fine-needle aspiration biopsy in the diagnosis and management of palpable masses. *J Med Assoc Georgia* 1996;85:33–36.
131. Donahue BJ, Cruickshank JC, Bishop JW. The diagnostic value of fine needle aspiration biopsy of head and neck masses. *ENT J* 1995;74:483–486.
132. Atula TS, Grenman R, Varpula M, et al. Palpation, ultrasound, and ultrasound-guided fine-needle aspiration cytology in the assessment of

cervical lymph node status in head and neck cancer patients. *Head Neck* 1996;18:545–551.

133. Kleid S, Millar HS. The case against open neck biopsy. *Aust NZ J Surg* 1993;63:678–681.
134. Jones AS, Cook JA, Phillips DE, et al. Squamous carcinoma presenting as an enlarged cervical lymph node. *Cancer* 1993;72:1756–1761.
135. Abram AC, Nabizadeh S, Feldman PS, et al. Fine needle aspiration (FNA) in diagnosing recurrent squamous cell carcinoma of the head and neck: truth or consequences? *Laryngoscope* 1993;103: 1073–1075.
136. Platt JD, Davidson D, Nelson CL, et al. Fine-needle aspiration biopsy: an analysis of 89 head and neck cases. *J Oral Maxillofac Surg* 1990;48:702–706.
137. Young JEM, Archibald SD, Shier KJ. Needle aspiration cytologic biopsy in head and neck masses. *Am J Surg* 1981;142:484–489.
138. Barnard NA, Paterson AW, Irvine GH, et al. Fine needle aspiration cytology in maxillofacial surgery—experience in a district general hospital. *Br J Oral Maxillofac Surg* 1993;31:223–226.
139. Kaur A, Chew CT, Lim-Tan SK. Fine needle aspiration of 123 head and neck masses—an initial experience. *Ann Acad Med Singapore* 1993;22:303–306.
140. Engzell U, Jakobsson PA, Sigurdson Å, et al. Aspiration biopsy of metastatic carcinoma in lymph nodes of the neck. A review of 1101 consecutive cases. *Acta Otolaryngol* 1971;72:138–147.
141. Thompson HY, Fulmer RP, Schnadig VJ. Metastatic squamous cell carcinoma of the tonsil presenting as multiple cystic neck masses. Report of a case with fine needle aspiration findings. *Acta Cytol* 1994;38:605–607.
142. Roy M, Bhattacharyya A, Sanyal S, et al. Study of benign superficial cysts by fine needle aspiration cytology. *J Indian Med Assoc* 1995;93: 8–9,13.
143. Layfield LJ. Fine-needle aspiration of the head and neck. *Pathology* 1996;4:409–438.
144. Pisharodi LR. False-negative diagnosis in fine-needle aspirations of squamous-cell carcinoma of head and neck. *Diagn Cytopathol* 1997; 17:70–73.
145. Verma K, Mandal S, Kapila K. Cystic change in lymph nodes with metastatic squamous cell carcinoma. *Acta Cytol* 1995;39:478–480.
146. Bernacki EGJ, Schulz R. Fine needle aspiration cytology of low grade cystic necrotic squamous cell carcinoma of the head and neck: a diagnostic pitfall. *Acta Cytol* 1994;38:854.
147. Burgess KL, Hartwick RWJ, Bedard YC. Metastatic squamous carcinoma presenting as a neck cyst. Differential diagnosis from inflamed branchial cleft cyst in fine needle aspirates. *Acta Cytol* 1993;37: 494–498.
148. Ramzy I, Rone R, Schantz HD. Squamous cells in needle aspirates of subcutaneous lesions: a diagnostic problem. *Am J Clin Pathol* 1986; 85:319–324.
149. Warson F, Blommaert D, De Roy G. Inflamed branchial cyst: a potential pitfall in aspiration cytology (letter to the editor). *Acta Cytol* 1986;30:201–202.
150. Frierson HF. Cysts of the head and neck sampled by fine-needle aspiration. Sources of diagnostic difficulty (editorial). *Am J Clin Pathol* 1996;106:559–560.
151. Layfield LJ, Glasgow BJ. Aspiration biopsy cytology of primary cutaneous tumors. *Acta Cytol* 1993;37:679–688.
152. Dodd LG. Fine-needle aspiration cytology of adenoid (acantholytic) squamous-cell carcinoma. *Diagn Cytopathol* 1995;12:168–172.
153. Banks ER, Frierson HF, Covell JL. Fine needle aspiration cytologic fidnings in metastatic basaloid squamous cell carcinoma of the head and neck. *Acta Cytol* 1992;36:126–131.
154. Ma TK-F. Fine needle aspiration cytodiagnosis of basaloid-squamous cell carcinoma metastatic to a cervical lymph node (letter to the editor). *Acta Cytol* 1993;37:977–979.
155. Engzell U, Zajicek J. Aspiration biopsy of tumors of the neck I. Aspiration biopsy and cytologic findings in 100 cases of congenital cysts. *Acta Cytol* 1970;14(2):51–57.
156. Shaffer MM, Oertel YC, Oertel JE. Thyroglossal duct cysts. Diagnostic criteria by fine-needle aspiration. *Arch Pathol Lab Med* 1996;120:1039–1043.
157. Chen KTK. Cytology of thyroglossal cyst papillary carcinoma. *Diagn Cytopathol* 1993;9:318–321.
158. Cervin JR, Silverman JF, Loggie BW, et al. Virchow's node revisited. Analysis with clinicopathologic corrleation of 152 fine-needle aspiration biopsies of supraclavicular lymph nodes. *Arch Pathol Lab Med* 1995;119:727–730.
159. Chan MKM, McGuire LJ, Lee JCK. Fine needle aspiration cytodiagnosis of nasopharyngeal carcinoma in cervical lymph nodes. A study of 40 cases. *Acta Cytol* 1989;33(3):344–350.
160. Pacchioni D, Negro F, Valente G, et al. Epstein-Barr virus detection by *in situ* hybridization in fine-needle aspiration biopsies. *Diagn Mol Pathol* 1994;3:100–104.
161. Woyke S, Domagala W, Czerniak B, et al. Fine needle aspiration cytology of malignant melanoma of the skin. *Acta Cytol* 1980;24(6): 529–538.
162. Perry MD, Gore M, Seigler HF, et al. Fine needle aspiration biopsy of metastatic melanoma. A morphologic analysis of 174 cases. *Acta Cytol* 1986;30:385–396.
163. Saleh H, Masood S, Wynn G, et al. Unsuspected metastatic renal cell carcinoma diagnosed by fine needle aspiration biopsy. A report of four cases with immunocytochemical contributions. *Acta Cytol* 1994;38: 554–561.
164. Matsuda M, Nagumo S, Koyama H, et al. Occult thyroid cancer discovered by fine-needle aspiration cytology of cervical lymph node: a report of three cases. *Diagn Cytopathol* 1991;7:299–303.
165. Bose S, Kapila K, Verma K. Medullary carcinoma of the thyroid: a cytological, immunocytochemical, and ultrastructural study. *Diagn Cytopathol* 1992;8:28–32.
166. Kini SR, Miller M, Hamburger JI, et al. Cytopathologic features of medullary carcinoma of the thyroid. *Arch Pathol Lab Med* 1984; 108:156–159.
167. Sneige N. Diagnosis of lymphoma and reactive lymphoid hyperplasia by immunocytochemical analysis of fine-needle aspiration biopsy. *Diagn Cytopathol* 1990;6:39–43.
168. Stani J. Cytologic diagnosis of reactive lymphadenopathy in fine needle aspiration biopsy specimens. *Acta Cytol* 1987;31:8–13.
169. Katz RL, Gritsman A, Cabanillas F, et al. Fine-needle aspiration cytology of peripheral T-cell lymphoma. A cytologic, immunologic, and cytometric study. *Am J Clin Pathol* 1989;91:120–131.
170. Sneige N, Dekmezian RH, Katz RL, et al. Morphologic and immunocytochemical evaluation of 220 fine needle aspirates of malignant lymphoma and lymphoid hyperplasia. *Acta Cytol* 1990;34: 311–322.
171. Penfold CN, Revington PJ. A review of 23 patients with tuberculosis of the head and neck. *Br J Oral Maxillofac Surg* 1996;34:508–510.
172. Cox HJ, Brightwell AP, Riordan T. Non-tuberculous mycobacterial infections presenting as salivary gland masses in children: investigation and conservative management. *J Laryngol Otol* 1995;109: 525–530.
173. Tunkel DE, Romaneschi KB. Surgical treatment of cervicofacial nontuberculous mycobacterial adenitis in children. *Laryngoscope* 1995; 105:1024–1028.
174. Silverman JF. Fine needle aspiration cytology of cat scratch disease. *Acta Cytol* 1985;29:542–547.
175. Christ ML, Feltes-Kennedy M. Fine needle aspiration cytology of toxoplasmic lymphadenitis. *Acta Cytol* 1982;26:425–428.
176. Macey-Dare LV, Kocjan G, Goodman JR. Acquired toxoplasmosis of a submandibular lymph node in a 9-year-old boy diagnosed by fine-needle aspiration cytology. *Int J Paediatr Dent* 1996;6:265–269.
177. Stanley MW, Steeper TA, Horwitz CA, et al. Fine-needle aspiration of lymph nodes in patients with acute infectious mononucleosis. *Diagn Cytopathol* 1990;6:323–329.
178. Das DK, Gulati A, Bhatt NC, et al. Fine needle aspiration cytology of oral and pharyngeal lesions. A study of 45 cases. *Acta Cytol* 1993;37: 333–342.
179. Hong IS, Mezghebe HM, Gaiter TE, et al. Actinomycosis of the neck: diagnosis by fine-needle aspiration biopsy. *J Natl Med Assoc* 1993;85: 145–146.
180. Katz RL, Caraway NP. FNA lymphoproliferative diseases: myths and legends. *Diagn Cytopathol* 1995;12:99–100.

181. Katz RL, Hirsch-Ginsberg C, Childs C, et al. The role of gene rearrangements for antigen receptors in the diagnosis of lymphoma obtained by fine-needle aspiration. A study of 63 cases with concomitant immunophenotyping. *Am J Clin Pathol* 1991;96:479–490.
182. Hamaker RA, Moriarty AT, Hamaker RC. Fine-needle biopsy techniques of aspiration versus capillary in head and neck masses. *Laryngoscope* 1995;105:1311–1314.
183. Robins DB, Katz RL, Swan FJ, et al. Immunotyping of lymphoma by fine-needle aspiration. A comparative study of cytospin preparations and flow cytometry. *Am J Clin Pathol* 1994;101:569–576.
184. Zander DS, Iturraspe JA, Everett ET, et al. Flow cytometry. *In vitro* assessment of its potential application for diagnosis and classification of lymphoid processes in cytologic preparations from fine-needle aspirates. *Am J Clin Pathol* 1994;101:577–586.
185. Moriarty AT, Wiersema L, Snyder W, et al. Immunophenotyping of cytologic specimens by flow cytometry. *Diagn Cytopathol* 1993;9:252–258.
186. Bizzaro N, Briani G. Myelosarcoma preceding acute leukemia diagnosed by fine needle lymph node aspiration: report of two cases. *Leukemia Lymphoma* 1993;10:395–399.
187. Dey P, Radhika S, Rajwanshi A, et al. Fine needle aspiration biopsy of orbital and eyelid lesions. *Acta Cytol* 1993;37:903–907.
188. Papadimitriou JC, Abruzzo LV, Bourquin PM, et al. Correlation of light microscopic, immunocytochemical and ultrastructural cytomorphology of anaplastic large cell Ki-1 lymphoma, an activated lymphocyte phenotype. A case report. *Acta Cytol* 1996;40:1283–1288.
189. Kardos TF, Vinson JH, Behm FG, et al. Hodgkin's disease: diagnosis by fine-needle aspiration biopsy. Analysis of cytologic criteria from a selected series. *Am J Clin Pathol* 1986;86:286–291.
190. Das DK, Gupta SK, Datta BN, et al. Fine needle aspiration cytodiagnosis of Hodgkin's disease and its subtypes I. Scope and limitations. *Acta Cytol* 1990;34:329–336.
191. Fulciniti F, Vetrani A, Zeppa P, et al. Hodgkin's disease: diagnostic accuracy of fine needle aspiration; a report based on 62 consecutive cases. *Cytopathology* 1994;5:226–233.
192. Das DK, Gupta SK. Fine needle aspiration cytodiagnosis of Hodgkin's disease and its subtypes. II. Scope and limitations. *Acta Cytol* 1990;34:337–341.
193. Layfield LJ, Anders KH, Glasgow BJ, et al. Fine-needle aspiration of primary soft-tissue lesions. *Arch Pathol Lab Med* 1986;110:420–424.
194. James LP. Cytopathology of mesenchymal repair. *Diagn Cytopathol* 1985;1:91–104.
195. Silverman JF, Joshi VV. FNA biopsy of small round cell tumors of childhood: cytomorphologic features and the role of ancillary studies. *Diagn Cytopathol* 1994;10:245–255.
196. Nguyen G-K. What is the value of fine-needle aspiration biopsy in the cytodiagnosis of soft-tissue tumors? *Diagn Cytopathol* 1988;4:352–355.
197. Stastny JF, Frable WJ. Diagnosis of primary nerve sheath tumor of the sphenoid sinus by fine needle aspiration biopsy. A case report. *Acta Cytol* 1993;37(2):242–246.
198. Neifer R, Nguyen G-K. Aspiration cytology of solitary schwannoma. *Acta Cytol* 1985;29:12–14.
199. Ramzy I. Benign schwannoma: demonstration of verocay bodies using fine needle aspiration. *Acta Cytol* 1977;21:316–319.
200. Vendraminelli R, Cavazzana AO, Poletti A, et al. Fine-needle aspiration cytology of malignant nerve sheath tumors. *Diagn Cytopathol* 1992;8:559–562.
201. Koivuniemi A, Nickels J. Synovial sarcoma diagnosed by fine-needle aspiration biopsy. A case report. *Acta Cytol* 1978;22:6.
202. Sápi Z, Bodó M, Megyesi J, et al. Fine needle aspiration cytology of biphasic synovial sarcoma of soft tissue. Report of a case with ultrastructural, immunohistologic and cytophotometric studies. *Acta Cytol* 1990;34(1):69–73.
203. Walaas L, Kindblom L-G. Lipomatous tumors: a correlative cytologic and histologic study of 27 tumors examined by fine needle aspiration cytology. *Hum Pathol* 1985;16:6–18.
204. Åkerman M, Rydholm A. Aspiration cytology of lipomatous tumors: a 10-year experience at an orthopedic oncology center. *Diagn Cytopathol* 1987;3:295–301.
205. Cohen MB, Layfield LJ. Fine needle aspiration biopsy of soft tissue tumors. In: Schmidt W, Miller T, Katz R, et al, eds. *Cytopathology annual, vol 3.* Chicago: ASCP Press, 1994:101–132.
206. Dundas KE, Wong MP, Suen KC. Two unusual benign lesions of the neck masquerading as malignancy on fine-needle aspiration cytology. *Diagn Cytopathol* 1995;12:272–279.
207. Lew WYC. Spindle cell lipoma of the breast: a case report and literature review. *Diagn Cytopathol* 1993;9:434–437.
208. Engzell U, Franzén S, Zajicek J. Aspiration biopsy of tumors of the neck II. Cytologic findings in 13 cases of carotid body tumor. *Acta Cytol* 1971;15(1):25–30.
209. Fleming MV, Oertel YC, Rodriguez ER, et al. Fine-needle aspiration of six carotid body paragangliomas. *Diagn Cytopathol* 1993;9:510–515.
210. Leonetti JP, Donzelli JJ, Littooy FN, et al. Perioperative strategies in the management of carotid body tumors. *Otolaryngol Head Neck Surg* 1997;117:111–115.
211. Takeuchi Y, Numata T, Konno A, et al. Differential diagnosis of pulsatile neck masses by Doppler color flow imaging. *Ann Otol Rhinol Laryngol* 1995;104:633–638.
212. Jacobs DM, Waisman J. Cervical paraganglioma with intranuclear vacuoles in a fine needle aspirate. *Acta Cytol* 1987;31(1):29–32.
213. González-Cámpora R, Otal-Salaverri C, Panea-Flores P, et al. Fine needle aspiration cytology of paraganglionic tumors. *Acta Cytol* 1988;32(3):386–390.
214. Lever WF, Schaumburg-Lever G. *Histopathology of the skin, 7th ed.* Philadelphia: JB Lippincott, 1990.
215. Sánchez CS. Mimics of pilomatrixomas in fine-needle aspirates. *Diagn Cytopathol* 1996;14:75–83.
216. Domanski HA, Domanski AM. Cytology of pilomatrixoma (calcifying epithelioma of Malherbe) in fine needle aspirates. *Acta Cytol* 1997;41:771–777.
217. Wong MP, Yuen ST, Collins RJ. Fine-needle aspiration biopsy of pilomatrixoma: still a diagnostic trap for the unwary. *Diagn Cytopathol* 1994;10:365–370.
218. Malberger E, Tillinger R, Lichtig C. Diagnosis of basal-cell carcinoma with aspiration cytology. *Acta Cytol* 1984;28(3):301–304.
219. Gherardi G, Marveggio C, Stiglich F. Parotid metastasis of Merkel cell carcinoma in a young patient with ectodermal dysplasia. Diagnosis by fine needle aspiration cytology and immunocytochemistry. *Acta Cytol* 1990;34:831–836.
220. Pettinato G, De Chiara A, Insabato L. Diagnostic significance of intermediate filament buttons in fine needle aspirates of neuroendocrine (Merkel cell) carcinoma of the skin (letter to the editor). *Acta Cytol* 1989;33:420–421.
221. Hood IC, Qizilbash AH, Salama SS, et al. Needle aspiration cytology of sebaceous carcinoma. *Acta Cytol* 1984;28:305–312.
222. Biernat W, Kordek R. Proliferating tricholemmal cyst: a possible pitfall in cytological diagnosis. *Diagn Cytopathol* 1996;15:73–75.
223. Masood S, Hardy NM. Fine needle aspiration cytology of chondroid synringoma. Report of a case. *Acta Cytol* 1988;32(4):482–484.
224. Bardales RH, Stanley MW. Subcutaneous masses of the scalp and forehead: diagnosis by fine-needle aspiration. *Diagn Cytopathol* 1995;12:131–134.
225. Srinivasan R, Ray R, Nijhawan R. Metastatic cutaneous and subcutaneous deposits from internal carcinoma. An analysis of cases diagnosed by fine needle aspiration. *Acta Cytol* 1993;37:894–898.
226. Kumar N, Verma K. Clear cell hidradenoma simulating breast carcinoma: a diagnostic pitfall in fine-needle aspiration of breast. *Diagn Cytopathol* 1996;15:70–72.

14B

CYTOPATHOLOGY OF THE EYE, ORBIT, JAWS, ORAL CAVITY, AND SINONASAL TRACT

MICHELE M. WEIR

THE EYE

The cytologic examination of intraocular material obtained from the anterior chamber or the vitreous is a useful procedure that can confirm a variety of clinical conditions (1–31). Some examples include phacolytic and ghost cell glaucomas, certain infections, diabetic proliferative retinopathy, and intraocular neoplasms (1–31). Unfortunately, most cytopathology personnel have limited experience with intraocular specimens. In addition, significant diagnostic material may be present in only a small number of intraocular fluid specimens (10%), compounding the problem of inexperience (1). In this section, the cytologic features of common and some unusual conditions of the globe are described.

The Glaucomas

Blood-Induced (Ghost Cell) Glaucoma

Blood-induced glaucoma is secondary to blockage of the aqueous flow through the trabecular meshwork in the anterior chamber by degenerated red blood cells, called "ghost cells" because of their loss of hemoglobin (1,6). Ghost cells develop after hemorrhage secondary to trauma, surgery, or primary retinal disease (6). Anterior chamber or vitreous fluids in this condition show pale staining, spherical ghost cells with denatured hemoglobin (Heinz bodies) clumped to their inner surface membranes (Fig. 1). In addition, hemosiderin and histiocytes with engulfed red blood cells ("hemolytic cells") may be seen (1,6). Neutrophils and lymphoid cells are typically absent (6). Uveitis-induced glaucoma must be distinguished from blood-induced glaucoma. Inflammation is absent in the latter condition. Misinterpretation of ghost cells as degenerated inflammatory cells is an important pitfall (6).

Blood-Induced (Ghost Cell) Glaucoma

1. Ghost cells (degenerated red blood cells) with Heinz body formation
2. Hemolytic cells (histiocytes containing red blood cells)
3. Hemosiderin
4. Paucity of inflammation
5. No lens material
6. History of trauma, surgery, or primary retinal disease

Phacolytic Glaucoma

Phacolysis is the dissolution and extraction of the crystalline lens (32). Phacolytic glaucoma occurs secondary to mechanical blockage of the flow of aqueous fluid out of the anterior chamber by protein debris and lens-containing macrophages, which may follow extracapsular cataract extraction (1). An inflammatory host response ensues (phacoanaphylactic reaction) to the unmasked, previously sequestered lens proteins. Anterior chamber and vitreous fluids show lens fragments, mixed acute and chronic inflammation, and debris. Lens fragments appear as striated parallel lamellated structures, which may have nuclei (1). The anterior chamber can also show phacolytic cells, which are lens-containing macrophages (1,7). Phacolytic glaucoma must be distinguished from *bacterial endophthalmitis* because the latter requires antibiotic treatment. Endophthalmitis typically shows abundant inflammation composed of neutrophils, macrophages, multinucleated histiocytes and lymphoid cells, without lens material (1,8).

Phacolytic Glaucoma

1. Phacolytic cells (lens-containing histiocytes)
2. Lens material
3. Mixed acute and chronic inflammation
4. Recent cataract removal or lens trauma

Uveitis Glaucoma

1. Mixed inflammation, depending on cause
2. No ghost cells, hemolytic cells
3. No lens material

Diabetic Proliferative Retinopathy

Proliferative retinopathy associated with diabetes consists of fibrovascular tissue growth posterior to the vitreous and anterior to the retina, which can pull on the retina and lead to retinal or vitreous hemorrhage or to retinal detachment (1,9). Cytologic examination of the vitreous fluid shows fibrovascular membrane fragments composed of proliferating spindle fibroblasts and delicate blood vessels (1) (Fig. 2). If hemorrhage has occurred, then red blood cells may be present. Retinal pigment epithelium can also be seen if retinal tears are present but are not specific for diabetic retinopathy (1,8). They appear as small cuboidal cells with

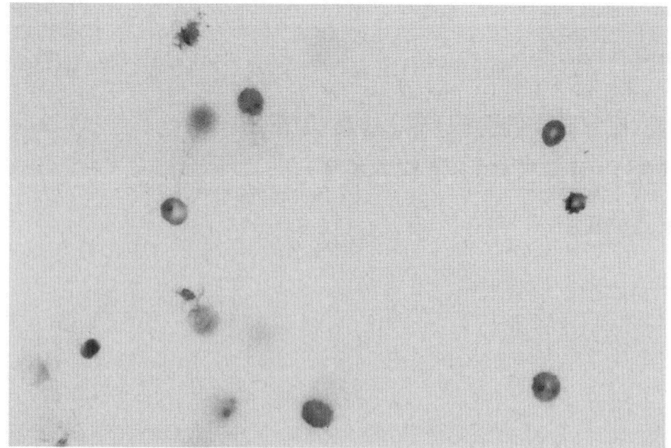

FIGURE 1. Ghost cell glaucoma. Basophilic red blood cells with membrane-based clumps of denatured hemoglobin (Heinz bodies) (Diff-Quik stain, 640×).

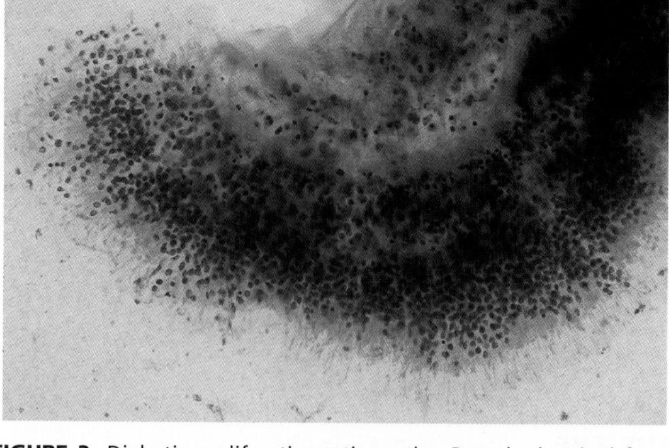

FIGURE 3. Diabetic proliferative retinopathy. Detached retinal fragments are often present (Papanicolaou stain, 200×).

central, sometimes pyknotic, nuclei and granular cytoplasmic melanin (1,8). Detached retinal fragments may also be found, composed of elongated bipolar or unipolar cells arranged in pseudostratified groups, or small lymphocyte-like cells (1) (Fig. 3).

Diabetic Proliferative Retinopathy

1. Fibrovascular membrane fragments
2. Retinal pigment epithelium
3. Detached retinal fragments
4. Recent or old hemorrhage

Inflammations and Infections

Bacterial Endophthalmitis

Bacterial endophthalmitis is an acute bacterial infection of the eye, usually occurring postoperatively, that requires immediate antibiotic treatment. The cytologic findings in the vitreous fluid include abundant acute inflammation (neutrophils) admixed with chronic inflammation (lymphocytes, macrophages, and multinucleated histiocytes) (1,8,10). It must be differentiated from *phacoanaphylactic reaction* or *phacolytic glaucoma,* as previously discussed. The latter condition would show lens fragments and lens-containing histiocytes along with an inflammatory component.

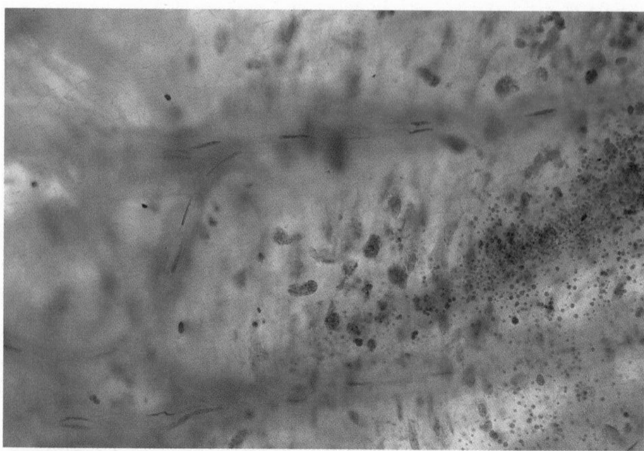

FIGURE 2. Diabetic proliferative retinopathy. Fibrovascular membrane consisting of capillaries, retinal pigment epithelium **(center),** and recent hemorrhage **(right center)** (Papanicolaou stain, 400×).

Bacterial Endophthalmitis

1. Abundant acute inflammation
2. Admixed chronic inflammation
3. Multinucleated histiocytes
4. No lens material
5. History of recent surgery or trauma

Other Infections and Inflammation

Intraocular fluid samples may be submitted frequently to exclude infectious etiologies for ocular disease. Yield is low for the identification of viral inclusions, *Toxoplasma,* and *Propionibacterium* in intraocular fluid specimens, possibly as a result of sampling error (11). Many intraocular specimens from patients with suspected infections (even with fungal infections) may show nonspecific acute or chronic inflammation or both (11,12,14) (Figs. 4 and 5). Fungal organisms reported in intraocular samples have included *Candida* species, *Aspergillus,* and *Coccidioidomycosis* (1,8,10,11). Vitreous specimens from patients with *Toxoplasma* chorioretinitis may show only multinucleated giant cells (10). In Whipple's disease, vitreous fluid may show periodic acid–Schiff (PAS)-positive material within macrophages. In toxocariasis, prominent eosinophils may be seen, usually without identification of the organism (14,15). In sarcoidosis, only mature lymphoid cells may be present in intraocular specimens, without granulomas (11).

The important differential diagnosis is *malignant lymphoma.* In reactive inflammatory processes, there is usually a mixed population of small and slightly larger lymphoid cells with neutrophils, and sometimes plasma cells and histiocytes. Malignant

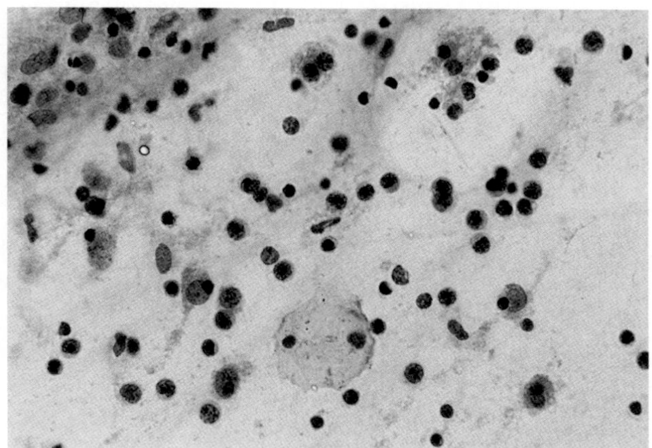

FIGURE 4. Chronic uveitis. Large and small lymphocytes admixed with macrophages (Papanicolaou stain, 640×).

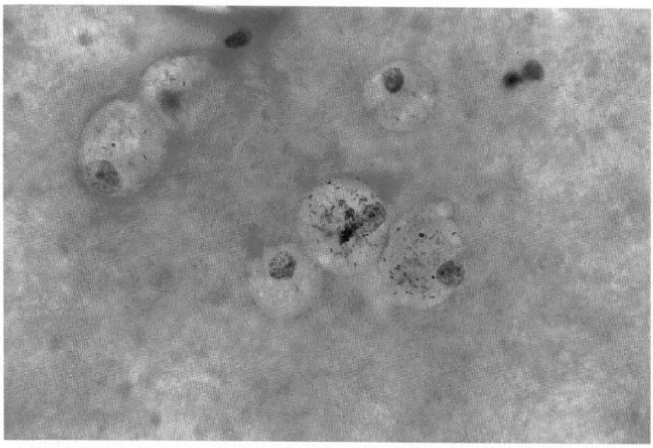

FIGURE 6. Coats' disease. Melanin-containing foamy histiocytes embedded in proteinaceous exudate (Papanicolaou stain, 500×).

lymphoma (diffuse large B-cell type) shows large lymphoid cells with nuclear atypia, including nuclear irregularity and protrusions (2,4). Reactive small lymphocytes may be in the background. Immunophenotyping (immunocytochemical stains or flow cytometry) can clarify this matter (see Malignant Lymphoma section).

Coats' Disease

Coats' disease is a condition of exudative retinal detachment in young men that can mimic retinoblastoma clinically (14). Vitreous fluids show numerous foamy macrophages with engulfed melanin pigment (Figs. 6 and 7) in a background of lymphocytes and red blood cells (14). Many of the macrophages contain lipid, which can be highlighted with an oil red O stain on air-dried material (15). An important cytologic pitfall is melanoma, in which intracytoplasmic melanin pigment can also be identified. However, the distinction of melanoma from Coats' disease can usually be made clinically (i.e., presence of a mass lesion, adult patient for melanoma). Morphologically, melanoma cells are spindled to ovoid with mild nuclear pleomorphism, small distinct nucleoli, and longitudinal nuclear grooves in contrast to the foamy macrophages of Coats' disease, which have eccentric nuclei and vacuolated cytoplasm (2–4). Retinal pigment epithelium is distinguished from pigmented histiocytes by their being small cuboidal cells with pyknotic central nuclei (see Diabetic Proliferative Retinopathy) (1,8).

Coats' Disease

1. Appropriate clinical situation: young man, exudative retinal detachment
2. Foamy histiocytes containing melanin pigment and lipid
3. Lymphoid cells in background
4. Lack of nuclear atypia in pigmented cells

Intraocular Neoplasms

Not all intraocular neoplasms require, or are amenable to, intraocular sampling by vitreous removal or FNA. Usually, cytologic examination is employed in specific clinical situations to

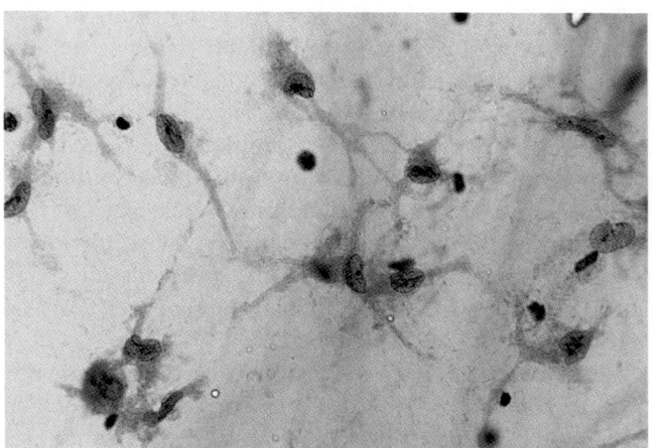

FIGURE 5. Chronic uveitis. Dendritic-appearing fibroblasts and histiocytes often seen in chronic inflammatory processes. Compare with malignant melanoma (Fig. 9) (Papanicolaou stain, 640×).

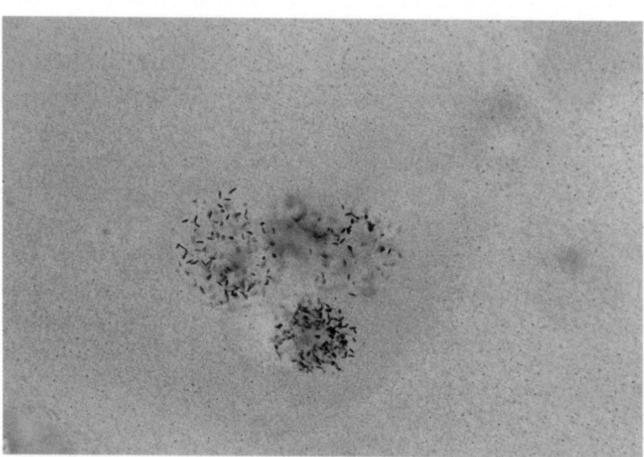

FIGURE 7. Coats' disease. Stain confirming melanin. The histiocytes also stain positively for oil red O (Fontana-Masson stain, 500×).

distinguish an inflammatory process from a neoplasm (most commonly malignant lymphoma), to document metastatic disease, or to make a definitive diagnosis that cannot be made by noninvasive methods (2,11,12,14–16). In a small series (17 cases), a positive predictive value of 92% for diagnosing malignancy by intraocular fluid cytology has been reported (2). For pediatric orbital malignancies, a positive predictive value of 100% and an overall accuracy of 95% have been reported (14).

Pediatric Neoplasms

Medulloepithelioma

Medulloepithelioma, a neuroepithelial tumor of the ciliary body, is more common in children (3). Cytologic examination shows a small cell population with round to oval hyperchromatic nuclei, high nuclear-to-cytoplasmic ratios, even nuclear chromatin, and occasional nuclear indentations, small nucleoli, and nuclear molding (14). Specimens are less cellular than for retinoblastoma cases (14). Cell arrangements include small groups, cords, and single cells (3,14,15). Necrosis is usually absent (14). Background hyaluronic acid may be seen (3).

Rosette formation and heterologous elements (skeletal muscle, cartilage, brain) seen by histology are unusual in cytology specimens (3). Malignant potential cannot be predicted by cytologic examination (3). Important differential diagnoses include other small cell tumors (see Retinoblastoma section).

Medulloepithelioma

1. Small cell tumor
2. Cord arrangement
3. Rarely rosettes, heterologous elements (skeletal muscle, cartilage, brain)
4. Absent necrosis
5. Background hyaluronic acid

Retinoblastoma

Retinoblastoma is the most common intraocular tumor in children and is usually diagnosed by noninvasive methods (18). However, in some specific cases, intraocular cytology is used to confirm the diagnosis. The cytologic findings of intraocular retinoblastoma include a hypercellular specimen composed of small cells on low power with background necrosis and degenerated nuclear fragments (3,14,18,19). Higher magnification shows single or clustered small cells, two to three times larger than a mature lymphocyte, with high nuclear-to-cytoplasmic ratios, round irregular nuclei, nuclear molding, scant cytoplasm, even chromatin, and occasional Flexner-Wintersteiner rosettes (palisaded cells around a central lumen) (14,18,19). Nucleoli are not prominent (14,18,19). Immunocytochemical markers are usually positive for neuron-specific enolase (NSE) and negative for desmin and leukocyte common antigen (20).

Important differential diagnoses include other small-cell intraocular tumors such as medulloepithelioma and metastatic neuroblastoma. Clinical features (age, site of mass) may be useful in distinguishing these lesions, given their similar morphologic appearances. *Medulloepitheliomas* arise in the ciliary body, are associated with a hyaluronic acid matrix, may show striated muscle or cartilaginous differentiation, and lack the distinctive retinoblastoma Flexner-Wintersteiner rosettes (3). *Metastatic neuroblastoma* may be indistinguishable from retinoblastoma by cytology (Fig. 8) and immunohistochemistry alone, and the clinical history of neuroblastoma elsewhere is crucial in the distinction.

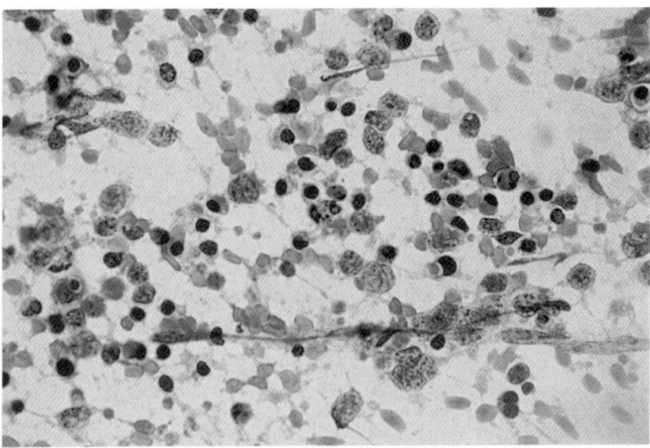

FIGURE 8. Neuroblastoma. Necrotic small-cell neoplasm with nuclear molding, crush artifact, and coarse chromatin. Rosettes not present in this example. Clinical features are required to discriminate metastatic neuroblastoma from primary retinoblastoma (Papanicolaou stain, 400×).

Retinoblastoma

1. Small-cell tumor with scant cytoplasm
2. Nuclear molding
3. Crushed nuclear fragments
4. Rosettes
5. NSE positive

Adult Neoplasms

Adenoma

Fuchs' adenoma, or coronal adenoma, arises from the ciliary body as a benign, slow-growing, possibly hyperplastic lesion (3,5). It may encroach on the iris as a pigmented mass and be confused with, and overtreated as, a malignant melanoma (22). Aspirates may be acellular but, if successfully obtained, show bland polygonal epithelial cells in groups and sheets surrounded by dense PAS-positive extracellular matrix material (3,22,23). Round nuclei with inconspicuous nucleoli are surrounded by abundant cytoplasm (22,23). Normal pigmented and nonpigmented ciliary epithelium may also be present in a bilayer arrangement without matrix material (23).

The differential diagnoses include melanoma arising from the iris or ciliary body, ciliary body adenocarcinoma, leiomyoma and neurofibroma. The latter two lesions would contain spindle cells without matrix material. *Ciliary body adenocarcinoma* shows nuclear atypia and decreased cellular cohesion (3). *Melanomas* are usually pigmented and consist of spindle or epithelioid cells, with mild nuclear pleomorphism, longitudinal nuclear grooves and small or prominent nucleoli (2–4,23).

Adenoma

1. Bland nonpigmented epithelium with round nuclei
2. Cohesive groups
3. Extracellular PAS$^+$ matrix material
4. Associated normal ciliary epithelium

Leiomyoma

Leiomyomas usually occur in young women in the ciliary body or anterior uvea (3,21). Aspirates show cohesive spindle cells with elongated cytoplasm and blunt-ended nuclei typical of smooth muscle tumors from other body sites (3). Some nuclei are round to oval, and nucleoli are absent (3). Differential diagnoses include nonpigmented melanomas and neurogenic tumors. The presence of nuclear atypia and distinct nucleoli in *melanoma* are helpful distinguishing features (2–4). *Neurogenic tumors* typically show elongated bent nuclei with pointed ends (23). Immunocytochemical markers for actins and desmin should identify leiomyomas in challenging cases.

Leiomyoma

1. Spindle cell tumor
2. Blunt-ended nuclei without nucleoli
3. Absent pigmentation
4. Cohesive groups
5. Actin and desmin positive

Malignant Melanoma

Malignant melanoma, the most common primary intraocular malignancy in adults, is usually uveal or choroidal in origin when seen as cytologic specimens (3,22). In intraocular cytology specimens, ocular melanoma commonly appears as loosely cohesive spindle cells with small, distinctive nucleoli, longitudinal nuclear grooves, mild nuclear atypia, fine nuclear chromatin, and bipolar cytoplasmic processes (2–4,22) (Fig. 9). In addition, an epithelioid morphology can be seen alone or in combination with the spindle cell form (22). Epithelioid cells are more dyshesive and larger (because of abundant cytoplasm) than the spindle cells (22). They show enlarged nuclei with more prominent nucleoli (sometimes multiple), and increased nuclear atypia (irregular contours and dispersed chromatin) (2–4,22). Sometimes, ciliary body melanomas are composed of smaller rounder cells (twice the size of red blood cells) with round nuclei and small distinct nucleoli (3). Intracytoplasmic melanin is usually identified in many of the cells of ocular melanomas. Amelanotic melanomas do occur, however, and immunocytochemistry can confirm a diagnosis of melanoma (vimentin, S-100 protein, and HMB-45 immunoreactivity) (3,4).

Differential diagnostic considerations for pigmented cells include *retinal pigment epithelium* and *melanin-containing histiocytes,* as previously described. Other spindle cell lesions such as uveal nevus, leiomyomas and neural tumors can pose problems. The uveal nevus is smaller, with slower growth, and lacks the nuclear atypia and nucleoli of melanoma (2). The *leiomyoma* and *neural tumors* similarly lack the nuclear changes of melanoma (3). The epithelioid melanoma may be difficult to distinguish from *metastatic carcinoma,* and immunocytochemistry is helpful in the distinction (cytokeratin immunoreactivity in carcinoma) (2).

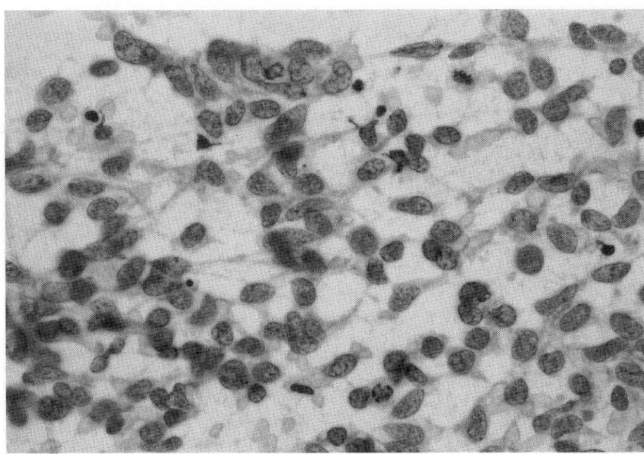

FIGURE 9. Malignant melanoma. Spindle cells with oval nuclei, small nucleoli, and delicate cytoplasmic processes. Compare with reactive fibroblasts (Fig. 5) (Papanicolaou stain, 400×).

Melanoma

1. Dyshesive cellular sample
2. Spindle cells with longitudinal nuclear grooves
3. Epithelioid cells with prominent nucleoli and nuclear atypia
4. Intracytoplasmic melanin pigment
5. Vimentin, S-100 protein, and HMB-45 positive; cytokeratin negative

Metastatic Carcinoma

Metastatic carcinoma is the most common intraocular malignancy, of which breast and lung are frequent sites of origin (3,24). Other primary sites reported include colon, nasopharynx, endometrium, and thyroid (2,3,11,12). The cytologic appearance is comparable to that of the primary (Fig. 10). Adenocarcinoma shows cells with vacuolated cytoplasm and multiple nucleoli arranged in papillary fragments or as single cells (4,12). An important differential diagnosis is *epithelioid malignant melanoma* (see above).

Metastatic Carcinoma

1. Dyshesive cell groups
2. Malignant nuclear features
3. Lack of pigmentation
4. Primary tumor elsewhere
5. Cytokeratin positive; S-100, HMB-45 negative

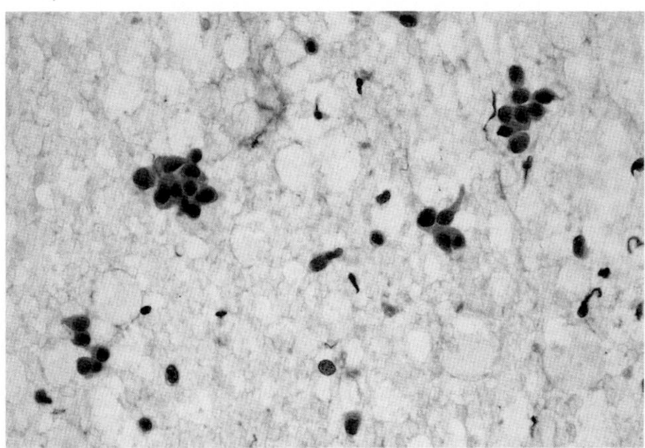

FIGURE 10. Ductal carcinoma of the breast. Monomorphic, small columnar, and plasmacytoid cells arranged singly and as dyshesive clusters. Breast carcinoma is a frequent source of intraocular metastatic carcinoma (Papanicolaou stain, 320×).

Malignant Lymphoma

Intraocular lymphomas are rare and usually occur in patients with systemic or primary central nervous system lymphomas. Most are diffuse large B-cell lymphomas and, less commonly, grade 1 or 2 follicle-center lymphomas (International Working Formulation, IWF: follicular predominantly small cleaved or mixed cell) (2,25,26). Aspirates of diffuse large B-cell lymphoma show large, dyshesive lymphoid cells with noticeable nuclear atypia, including irregular nuclear contours, nuclear protrusions, irregular coarse chromatin, and prominent nuclear membrane-based nucleoli (2,4,26,27,29,30) (Fig. 11). Small reactive lymphocytes and nonlymphoid inflammatory cells can be seen in the background (26,27). The distinction from an inflammatory process can be difficult, especially when the sample is scant or there are only a few large, malignant cells in a background of small reactive lymphocytes (2,26). A mixed spectrum of small and slightly larger lymphocytes and the absence of significant nuclear atypia favor a reactive process.

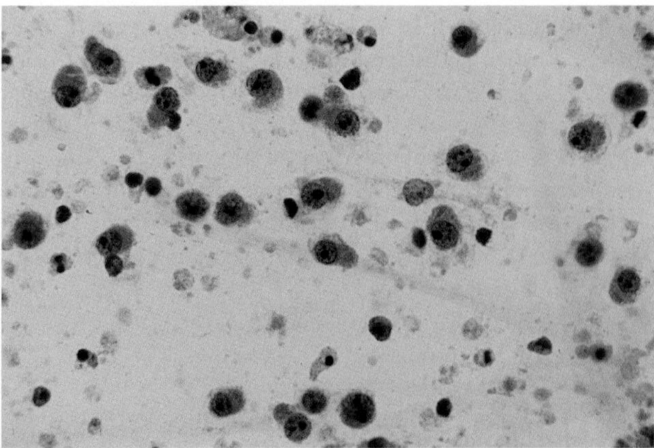

FIGURE 11. Large B-cell lymphoma (immunoblastic lymphoma). Monomorphic large lymphocytes with ample eccentric cytoplasm, vesicular nuclei, and prominent nucleoli (Papanicolaou stain, 640×).

The use of immunocytochemical markers or immunophenotyping by flow cytometry may help in this distinction. *Uveitis* typically consists of T-cell lymphocytes, in contrast to diffuse large B-cell lymphoma, which often shows immunoglobulin light chain restriction (29,31). Repeat sampling may be necessary in scant samples, or in cases which lack definitive features of malignant lymphoma, but the clinical suspicion for lymphoma is high (27,28,30).

Aspirates of follicle center cell lymphomas (grades 1 and 2) show small atypical lymphocytes intermixed with a variable number of larger atypical lymphocytes (similar to the cells of large B-cell lymphoma), depending on the grade. Immunophenotyping is essential in distinguishing grade 1 follicle center cell lymphomas from reactive processes (see also Lymphoma of Neck).

Malignant Lymphoma, Diffuse Large B-Cell Type

1. Monomorphic cell population composed of large dyshesive cells
2. Nuclear irregularity and protrusions
3. Prominent nucleoli, nuclear membrane based
4. Lack of mixed spectrum of lymphocytes and plasma cells
5. Immunocytochemistry is helpful

THE ORBIT

Fine-needle aspiration biopsy (FNA) is a reliable, simple technique for the rapid diagnosis of orbital masses (33–45). A wide spectrum of lesions may be encountered, including inflammatory pseudotumors, infections, and a variety of neoplasms, which can be challenging to cytopathology personnel with limited exposure to orbital cytology. In this section, the cytologic findings of common and unusual orbital lesions are discussed.

Nonneoplastic Conditions: Cysts

Dermoid Cyst

Dermoid cysts typically arise in children but can be seen in adults (3,23,39,44). They are located in the superolateral orbit and are derived from embryonic remnants (3). With rupture, an enlarging mass forms. On FNA, anucleated keratinized squamous cells and keratin debris are seen (23,33,39,41,44) (Fig. 12). If ruptured, granulomas and multinucleated histiocytes can be identified (3,23,39). Rarely, smears may show hair shaft material, although usually adnexal structures are seen only on histology (3,44).

Differential diagnoses include *epidermal inclusion cyst* and *pilar cyst,* which lack adnexal structures. Care must be taken not to overcall a ruptured dermoid cyst as malignant (*squamous cell carcinoma* or *sebaceous carcinoma*). Attention to the lack of malignant nuclear features in dermoid cyst contents is crucial in the distinction (see Squamous Lesions of Neck).

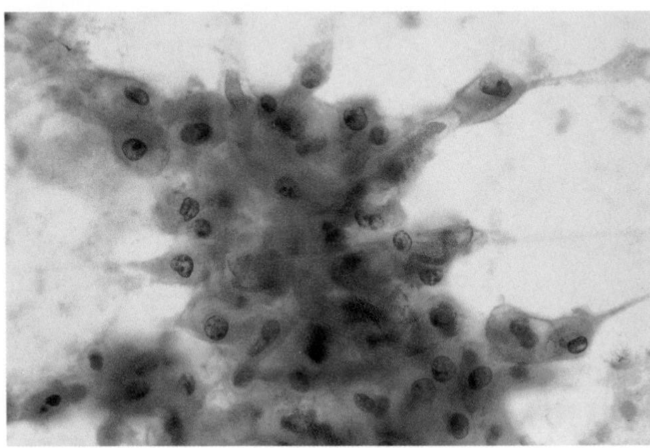

FIGURE 12. Ruptured keratinized squamous cyst. Histiocytic reaction to anucleate keratinized squames consistent with cyst rupture (Papanicolaou stain, 400×).

Dermoid Cyst

1. Anucleated keratinized squamous cells
2. Keratin debris
3. Rare adnexal structures
4. Granulomas, giant cells if ruptured
5. Benign nuclear cytologic features

Enterogenous Cyst

Enterogenous cysts are derived from misplaced embryonic endodermal epithelial remnants and are usually located on the anterior surface of the spinal cord or rarely intracranially (46). FNA yields benign cuboidal glandular cells and mucinous columnar cells (mucicarmine positive) with bland uniform nuclei in a background of debris, lymphocytes, and histiocytes (46) (Fig. 13). Carcinoembryonic antigen (CEA) cyst fluid levels are high (46). The differential diagnosis includes *metastatic adenocarcinoma,* which would show malignant nuclear features.

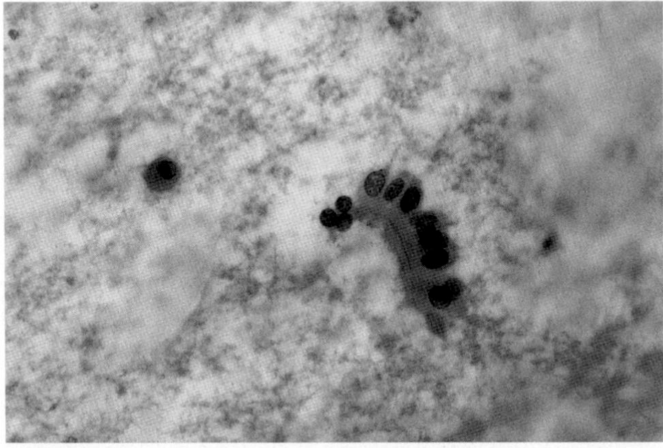

FIGURE 13. Enterogenous cyst. Ciliated columnar cells and histiocytes in a proteinaceous background. Cuboidal or mucin-containing columnar cells may also line such cysts (Papanicolaou stain, 400×).

Enterogenous Cyst

1. Cuboidal and columnar cells
2. Bland nuclei
3. Intracytoplasmic mucin
4. Cyst contents
5. High CEA levels (cyst fluid)

Inflammatory Lesions

Sarcoidosis

Sarcoidosis can involve the lacrimal gland, optic nerve, or extraocular muscles and may be unilateral or bilateral. FNA smears show granulomas consisting of aggregates of epithelioid histiocytes with spindle or ovoid reniform nuclei and abundant cytoplasm (3,44). Multinucleated giant cells and lymphocytes are also present (44). The differential diagnoses include other causes of granulomas, including ruptured dermoid cyst, mycobacterial or fungal infection, and Wegener's granulomatosis. Correlation with microbiologic cultures and antineutrophil cytoplasmic antibodies (ANCA) is necessary because sarcoidosis is a diagnosis of exclusion.

Wegener's Granulomatosis

Wegener's granulomatosis is a granulomatous vasculitis that commonly involves the lung, kidney, and paranasal sinuses. Sometimes the orbit or lacrimal gland shows a rapidly expanding mass, which can be difficult to aspirate (3). Aspirated smears show granulomas, necrosis (or fibrinoid degeneration of collagen), pyknotic nuclei, and multinucleated giant cells (3). Demonstration of vasculitis by cytology is not possible. Other granulomatous processes must be excluded (mycobacteria, fungi, sarcoidosis), and correlation with microbiologic cultures, clinical findings, and ANCA results is essential.

Infections

Mycobacterial and fungal infections may present as orbital masses amenable to FNA, which can also obtain material for microbiological studies (38,39). Aspiration smears show granulomas, multinucleated giant cells, and a variable background of lymphocytes, neutrophils, eosinophils, and granular necrotic material (38,39) (Fig. 14). Samples from immunosuppressed hosts may lack inflammation. *Aspergillus* and *Mucor* species can be identified in FNA smears (38) (Fig. 15).

Granulomatous Inflammation

1. Epithelioid histiocytes
2. Multinucleated giant cells
3. Background mixed inflammation
4. Necrosis with infections, Wegener's granulomatosis
5. Fungi (if infectious)

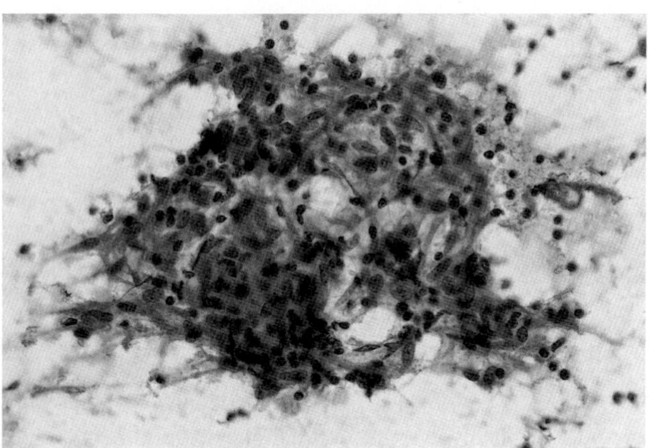

FIGURE 14. Tuberculosis. Nodular aggregate of spindled epithelioid histiocytes with oval to indented spindled nuclei in a background of lymphocytes and granular necrosis. Material submitted for culture grew *M. tuberculosis* (hematoxylin and eosin stain, 400×).

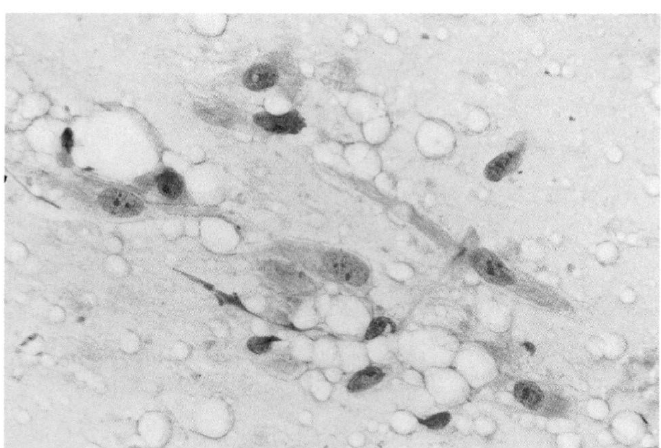

FIGURE 16. Nodular fasciitis. Reactive spindled to ganglion-like fibroblasts in a mucoid matrix (hematoxylin and eosin stain, 640×).

Nodular Fasciitis

Nodular fasciitis is a rapidly growing, tender, subcutaneous lesion composed of benign myofibroblasts located most commonly in the extremities of adults and the head and neck of children (47). It can present as a rapidly growing orbital mass (47,48). Aspiration smears show fibrovascular fragments with attached and dispersed, variably sized, plump, oval to spindle fibroblasts, with oval to round nuclei, smooth nuclear contours, small nucleoli, and long wavy cytoplasmic processes (47,49) (Fig. 16). The nuclei may be eccentric and enlarged, associated with abundant cytoplasm, resembling ganglion cells (47). Characteristic extracellular mucoid fibrillar material (blue to red-purple) may be seen in air-dried smears (47) (proliferative fasciitis; see Chapter 10). Mitoses can be seen but are not atypical. Background elements include red blood cells, neutrophils, lymphocytes, and macrophages (47).

Differential diagnoses include fibromatosis, granulation tissue, and spindle cell tumors (neuroma, leiomyoma, fibrosarcoma, myxofibrosarcoma, and myxoid liposarcoma). *Fibromatosis* shows bland spindle cell groups and collagen without an inflammatory component on aspiration smears. *Granulation tissue* can closely mimic nodular fasciitis because of vascular fragments, but instead of a predominant population of fibroblasts, it shows many more neutrophils clinging to small blood vessels. *Sarcomas,* important diagnostic considerations, show greater nuclear atypia, more uniform cell population, background necrosis, cellular dyshesion, and absent background inflammation (49).

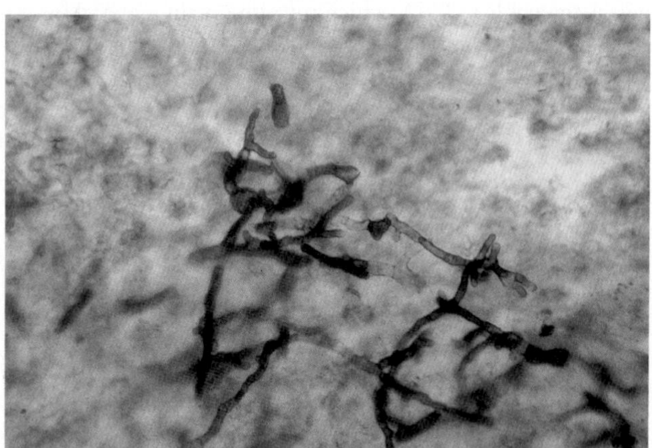

FIGURE 15. Aspergillosis. Narrow, acutely branching, septate fungal hyphae with parallel walls (methenamine silver stain, 400×).

Nodular Fasciitis

1. Fibrovascular fragments
2. Reactive, enlarged, or ganglion-like fibroblasts
3. Mucoid matrix
4. Background inflammation

Inflammatory Pseudotumor

Inflammatory pseudotumor, or reactive lymphoid hyperplasia of the orbit (see Chapter 12), may present as an orbital mass at times involving the lacrimal gland (38). Aspirates show mixed populations of small and large lymphocytes, macrophages, plasma cells, and eosinophils (3,38,39,44). The lesion must be differentiated from malignant lymphoma, particularly extranodal marginal zone B-cell lymphoma of mucosa-associated lymphoid tissue (MALT) type (Fig. 17) (see Chapter 12). Immunophenotyping of aspirate material by flow cytometry or by immunohistochemical markers on needle core biopsy specimens or touch imprints is essential (50). As a rule, reactive lesions show a more heterogeneous mixed lymphocyte and nonlymphocyte population than malignant lymphoma. Immunophenotyping of a reactive process shows predominantly T-cell lymphocytes, with or without polyclonal B cells (51).

Inflammatory Pseudotumor

1. Mixed population of small and large lymphoid and nonlymphoid cells
2. Polyclonal B cells, predominance of T cells

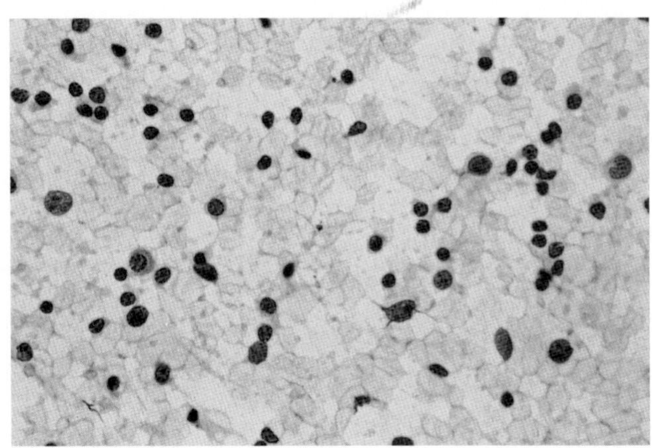

FIGURE 17. Mucosa-associated lymphoid tissue (MALT) lymphoma. Mixed lymphoid population with occasional plasma cells and a predominance of small lymphocytes. Immunophenotyping is often required to distinguish this lymphoma from inflammatory pseudotumor (Papanicolaou stain, 400×).

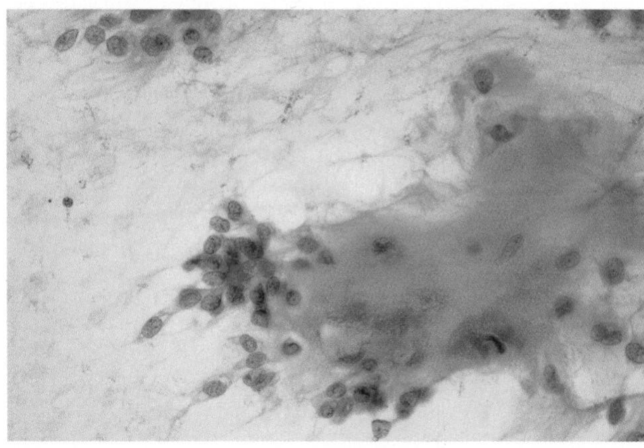

FIGURE 19. Pleomorphic adenoma. Spindled to plasmacytoid myoepithelial cells enmeshed in chondromyxoid stroma (Papanicolaou stain, 400×).

Neoplasms

Lacrimal Gland

Pleomorphic Adenoma

Pleomorphic adenoma (benign mixed tumor) comprises about 50% of lacrimal gland tumors, affects primarily middle-aged men, and presents as a painless superotemporal orbital mass (3,39). Aspiration smears are biphasic, showing epithelial–myoepithelial and stromal elements (Figs. 18 and 19). The epithelial–myoepithelial cells are present singly and in sheets and show even nuclear chromatin, round to oval eccentric nuclei, and rare small nucleoli (3,33,35,39). These cells can merge with and become enmeshed within the typical chondromyxoid matrix of this tumor, which is a characteristic purple-magenta in air-dried smears (Romanovsky or Diff-Quik stained) and bluish-green in alcohol-fixed smears (Papanicolaou stain) (3,33,35,39). Other elements may include squamous metaplastic cells, keratin, glandular epithelium, and adipose tissue (3). Some tumors can undergo cystic change, hampering accurate cytologic diagnosis. An important pitfall is *adenoid cystic carcinoma,* which also has purple-magenta extracellular material on Romanovsky or Diff-Quik–stained air-dried material. However, in this tumor, careful inspection will reveal a uniform population of small basaloid cells with atypical angular nuclei and high nuclear-to-cytoplasmic ratios, which are not intermingled with the extracellular material but form a rim around it (see Salivary Gland Neoplasms).

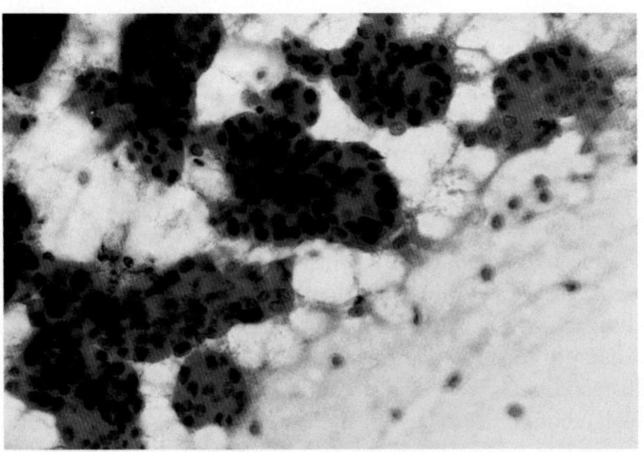

FIGURE 18. Normal lacrimal gland. Tightly cohesive acini formed by cells with granular cytoplasm and uniform nuclei. Monomorphism of the epithelial cells could lead to misdiagnosis as a neoplasm (Papanicolaou stain, 500×).

Pleomorphic Adenoma

1. Biphasic tumor
2. Bland epithelial–myoepithelial cell sheets
3. Chondromyxoid matrix (best seen with Romanovsky or Diff-Quik stain)
4. Merging of matrix with cells
5. Cystic change possible

Adenoid Cystic Carcinoma

Adenoid cystic carcinoma can present as a painful or painless lacrimal gland mass in young to middle-aged groups (3,39). This tumor may show perineural invasion and tends to recur. Aspirates are cellular and composed of dyshesive small uniform cells with round to oval nuclei, coarse chromatin, irregular nucleoli, and scant cytoplasm arranged singly or in crowded groups (3,35,39). Mitotic figures and necrosis may be apparent (3). In the cribriform variant, globules, balls, and finger-like structures of pale translucent (Papanicolaou stain) or magenta (Diff-Quik or Romanovsky stain) extracellular basement membrane material are surrounded by tumor cells (3,35,39) (Fig. 20). In the solid or basaloid variant, solid sheets of small cells without extracellular material are identified (3,39).

Differential diagnoses include pleomorphic adenoma as previously discussed and metastatic small-cell carcinoma, which lacks extracellular material and cell ball formation.

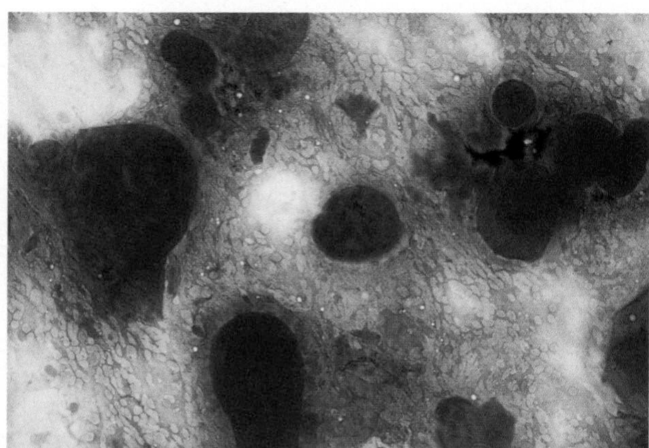

FIGURE 20. Adenoid cystic carcinoma. Stromal balls and finger-like structures surrounded by "naked" basaloid nuclei (Diff-Quik stain, 200×).

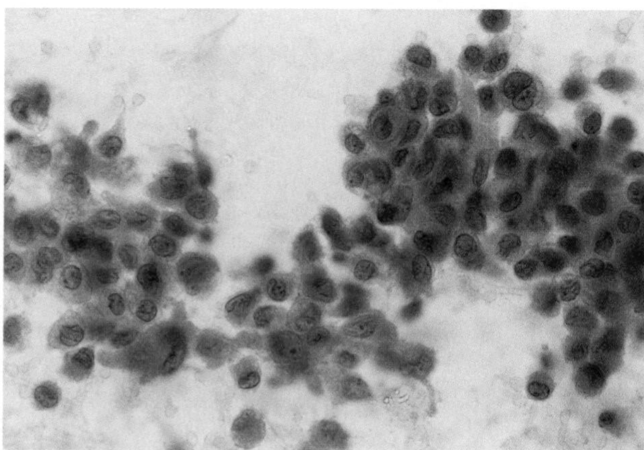

FIGURE 21. Eosinophilic granuloma. Dispersed small histiocytes with convoluted, grooved, or twisted nuclei. Eosinophils not prominent in this example (hematoxylin and eosin stain, 640×).

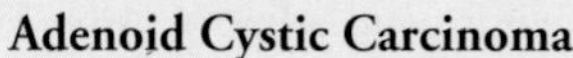

Adenoid Cystic Carcinoma

1. Cellular smear
2. Small cells with angulated nuclei and scant cytoplasm
3. Acellular extracellular balls and finger-like structures
4. Cell rosettes, balls, sheets
5. Necrosis at times

Adenocarcinoma

Primary adenocarcinoma of the lacrimal gland is an uncommon, usually high-grade lesion. Aspiration smears show clusters and acini composed of mucin-containing cells with significant nuclear atypia and mitotic activity (3). Numerous dyshesive tumor cells and necrosis are present (3). Metastatic adenocarcinoma must be excluded on clinical grounds.

Adenocarcinoma

1. Malignant glandular cells
2. Necrosis
3. Acinar formation
4. Mucicarmine positive cells

Malignant Lymphoma

See later section on lymphoma.

Pediatric Neoplasms

Eosinophilic Granuloma

Eosinophilic granuloma is a proliferation of Langerhans' histiocytes that occurs in children and young adults. The orbital lesion can present as a lytic area of bone or as a soft tissue mass. Aspirates show small histiocytes (Langerhans' cells) with pale, vesicular, indented, grooved, or twisted nuclei, absent to tiny nucleoli, and abundant, ill-defined, pale cytoplasm (3,23,34,52,53) (Fig. 21). The background shows a variable number of eosinophils with some neutrophils and large multinucleated histiocytes with nuclei resembling those of the Langerhans' cells (3,23,34,38,53). Immunocytochemical markers for CD1a and S-100 protein highlight the histiocytes. Electron microscopy (EM) shows the distinctive pentalaminar racquet-shaped Birbeck granules.

The diagnostic pitfalls include granulomatous inflammation, lymphoma, osteomyelitis, rhabdomyosarcoma, and Ewing's sarcoma. Attention to the prominent eosinophil population and characteristic histiocytes is important in recognizing eosinophilic granuloma. Neutrophils usually predominate in aspirates of *osteomyelitis* (53). Correlation with microbiology cultures can identify the cause of *granulomatous inflammation* and exclude eosinophilic granuloma. *Diffuse large B-cell lymphoma cells* show prominent nucleoli, high nuclear-to-cytoplasmic ratios, and open chromatin (53). Both *rhabdomyosarcoma* and *Ewing's sarcoma* can be distinguished from eosinophilic granuloma by their monotonous small round cell population with high nuclear-to-cytoplasmic ratios and absence of eosinophils and histiocytes (52).

Eosinophilic Granuloma

1. Single small histiocytic cells with vesicular grooved nuclei
2. Eosinophils
3. CD1a, S-100 protein immunophenotype
4. Birbeck granules on EM

Rhabdomyosarcoma

Rhabdomyosarcoma is the most common primary malignant neoplasm of the orbit in children and can also be seen in young adults (3,39). The embryonal subtype (see Chapter 10) is most frequently encountered at this site. Aspirates are cellular and show clusters, loose sheets, and predominantly single cells, which are small (about twice as large as mature lymphocytes), oval to round to spindled (tadpole, triangular, ribbon-shaped) (3,35,39) (Fig. 22). A myxoid or tigroid background may be evident on Romanovsky stains (54). Nuclei are round to oval, eccentric, and may show prominent nucleoli (39). In a small number of cases,

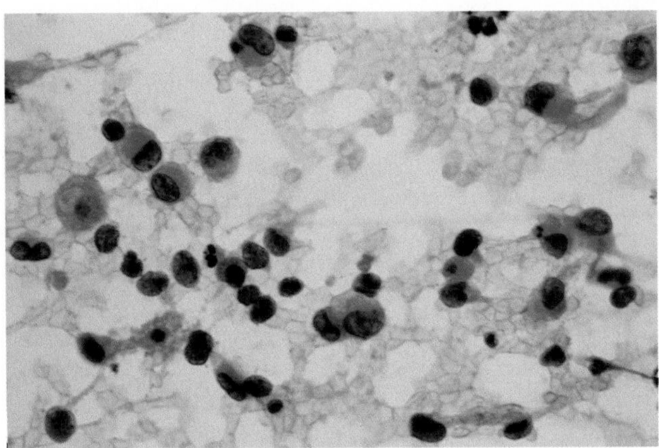

FIGURE 22. Rhabdomyosarcoma. Small round cells, some of which exhibit eccentric, dense cytoplasm. Occasional "strap-like" cells present **(lower right)** (Papanicolaou stain, 400×).

rhabdomyoblasts, binucleated cells, and true cross striations are seen (3,39). The cytoplasm of elongate cells can be filamentous or dense (pink-red on Papanicolaou stain, gray-blue on Romanovsky stain) (52). Muscle differentiation should be confirmed with immunocytochemical markers (desmin, actins, myoglobin) or by electron microscopy (myofilaments, Z-band material).

Differential diagnostic considerations include eosinophilic granuloma, and other orbital small round-cell neoplasms of childhood, namely, *retinoblastoma* and metastatic neuroblastoma. The clinical finding of an intraocular mass (retinoblastoma), or of an abdominal mass (neuroblastoma) is helpful in making the distinction. Retinoblastoma and neuroblastoma cells show higher nuclear-to-cytoplasmic ratios compared to rhabdomyosarcoma cells because of smaller amounts of cytoplasm. Nuclear molding, crushed nuclear fragments, and rosette formation favor retinoblastoma or neuroblastoma. *Eosinophilic granuloma* can be overcalled as rhabdomyosarcoma because of its dyshesive small oval histiocytic cells (52). Careful attention to the nuclear grooves, cleaves, and folds, in association with eosinophils, distinguishes eosinophilic granuloma (52).

Rhabdomyosarcoma

1. Small oval to round to spindled cells
2. Eccentric nuclei
3. Rhabdomyoblasts and cross-striations
4. Lack of nuclear molding, rosettes, nuclear fragments
5. Muscle differentiation (electron microscopy, immunohistochemical markers)

Retinoblastoma

Intraocular retinoblastoma may uncommonly involve the orbit as it spreads from the optic nerve, or an orbital mass may be the first sign of a recurrent retinoblastoma (39). The cytomorphology has been previously described (see Intraocular Cytology).

Metastatic Neuroblastoma

Neuroblastoma may spread to the orbit from a primary in the adrenal gland. Smears show a small round-cell tumor with a cytomorphologic appearance comparable to the primary lesion (3,42,52). The cells show high nuclear-to-cytoplasmic ratios, scant cytoplasm, nuclear molding, and finely granular cytoplasm (42,52). A necrotic background is apparent (52). Rosettes may be seen (42,52) (Fig. 23). Immunocytochemical markers (neuron-specific enolase, NSE) and electron microscopy (EM) studies (dense-core secretory granules, neurotubules) can be helpful (46,52). The morphology and immunohistochemical profile are identical to retinoblastoma, and the clinical information may be the only distinguishing feature. Other orbital small round-cell neoplasms such as rhabdomyosarcoma must also be considered, as previously described.

Neuroblastoma

1. Small round-cell tumor with rosette formation
2. Nuclear molding
3. Background necrosis
4. NSE positive
5. Neurotubules, dense-core granules on EM
6. Adrenal or retroperitoneal mass

Meningeal, Neural, and Glial Tumors

Meningioma

Meningiomas of the orbit may arise from the optic nerve meninges or may represent extension from an intracranial site. In aspirate smears, the cells form tight clusters with a characteristic whorling pattern, which may be associated with psammoma bodies (33,35,42,44,45,55). The cuboidal to round cells can be admixed with some elongated cells, may show intranuclear pseudoinclusions, and have bland round nuclei with fine chromatin (3,33,35,55,56) (Fig. 24). Meningioma cells are usually positive for epithelial membrane antigen (EMA) and negative for glial fibrillary acidic protein (GFAP).

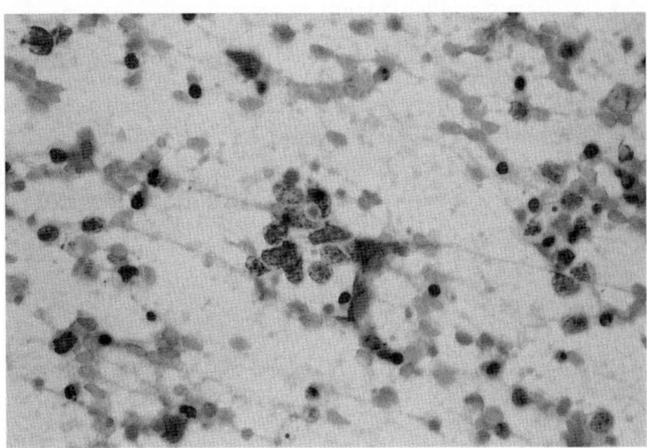

FIGURE 23. Neuroblastoma. Rosette of small, molded nuclei with stippled chromatin in a background of necrosis (Papanicolaou stain, 400×).

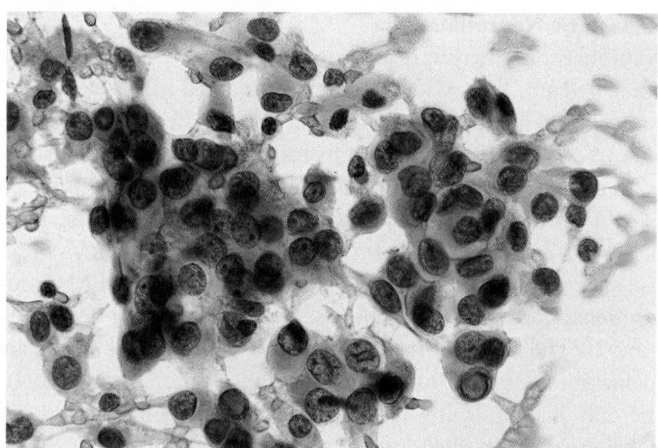

FIGURE 24. Meningioma. Cuboidal cells with dense cytoplasm, focal whorling pattern, and intranuclear cytoplasmic pseudoinclusions (Papanicolaou stain, 640×).

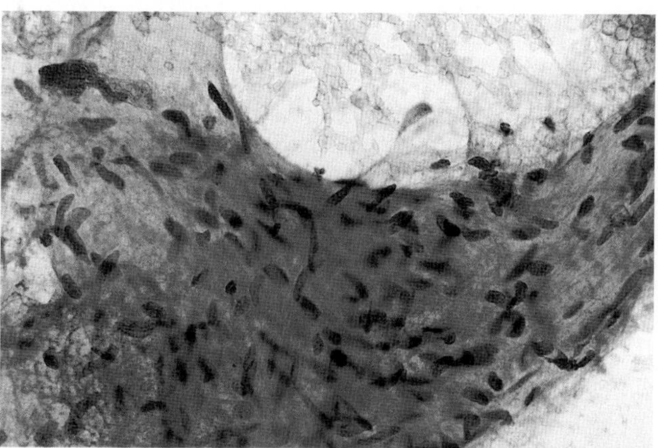

FIGURE 25. Schwannoma with ancient changes. Spindle cells with elongate, bent nuclei enmeshed within a background of delicate cytoplasmic fibrils. Occasional large, pleomorphic cells with smudgy chromatin present **(upper left)** (Papanicolaou stain, 500×).

Possible pitfalls include glial, nerve sheath, and smooth muscle tumors. Smears of glial tumors show more elongated cells in a fibrillary background, in contrast to meningioma. The cells are positive for GFAP. Smooth muscle tumors show spindled cells with blunt-ended nuclei, whereas nerve sheath tumors show spindle cells with tapered angulated nuclei (35).

Meningioma

1. Round to cuboidal, sometimes elongated cells
2. Whorling pattern without fibrillary background
3. Intranuclear pseudoinclusions
4. Psammoma bodies
5. EMA positive, GFAP negative

Schwannoma

Schwannoma may present as an orbital mass and can be associated with neurofibromatosis (3,23). Aspirate smears may be scant and difficult to interpret. If material is found, spindle cells with bent, tapered nuclei without prominent nucleoli are seen arranged in loose groups (3,23,35,56). The cytoplasm may become stripped away, and myxoid material can be seen (3,23). Nuclear atypia must be interpreted with caution, as it can be seen as a degenerative phenomenon in ancient schwannomas (Fig. 25). Immunocytochemical stains are positive for S-100 protein but negative for GFAP.

Pitfalls include other spindle cell neoplasms, such as smooth muscle tumors and meningiomas, as previously discussed. Differentiation from neurofibroma may be nearly impossible by cytology, but smears show thin fiber-like cells with elongated nuclei and fibrillar cytoplasm (33).

Schwannoma

1. Spindle cell tumor
2. Tapered bent nuclei
3. Atypical nuclei in "ancient" tumors
4. Stripped cytoplasm
5. Myxoid material
6. S-100 protein positive, GFAP negative

Pilocytic Astrocytoma

Pilocytic astrocytomas can arise from the optic nerve and may be associated with neurofibromatosis. The patients are usually children or young adults. Aspirate smears may be scant and show spindle cells in tightly cohesive clusters with bland nuclei, lightly stippled chromatin, and few small nucleoli (3,33). A fibrillary background is present (3). Immunohistochemical markers are positive for glial fibrillary acidic protein (GFAP) and negative for epithelial membrane antigen (EMA), in contrast to meningioma. Differential diagnostic considerations include *meningioma, schwannoma,* and *smooth muscle tumors* as previously described.

Pilocytic Astrocytoma

1. Spindle cell tumor
2. Fibrillary background
3. Bland nuclei
4. GFAP positive, EMA negative

Lymphoplasmacytic Proliferations

Plasmacytoma and Myeloma

Plasmacytoma and multiple myeloma rarely can produce an orbital mass and may be the presenting problem (3,38,57). On aspirate smears, mature plasma cells with eccentric nuclei and cartwheel chromatin can be seen along with binucleate and immature plasma cells (3,38,57) (Fig. 26). Amyloid is identified as extracellular irregularly shaped fragments of material, often associated with multinucleated giant cells (57). Multiple bone lesions, elevated serum calcium, and an M component on immunoelectrophoresis can distinguish multiple myeloma. Cytologic pitfalls include reactive processes with abundant plasma cells and malignant lymphomas with plasmacytoid differentiation or reactive plasma cells. Generally, *reactive lesions* show plasma cells, without nuclear atypia, in association with a mixed population of lymphocytes and histiocytes. *Malignant lymphomas* with plasmacytoid differentiation or reactive plasma cells have a monotonous atypical lymphoid population.

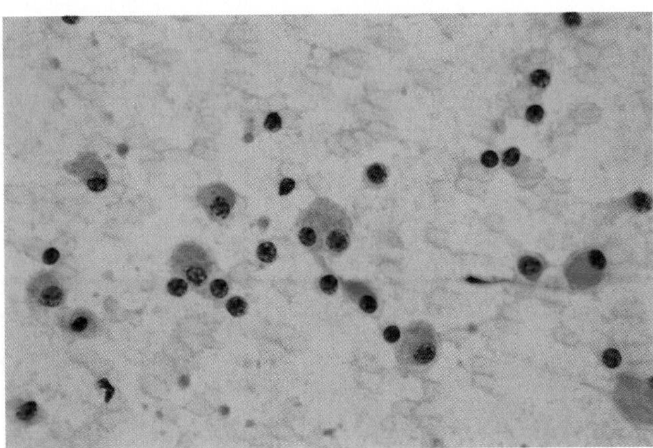

FIGURE 26. Multiple myeloma. Monomorphic, dispersed plasma cells with focal binucleation (Papanicolaou stain, 400×).

Plasmacytoma and Myeloma

1. Dyshesive single cells
2. Pure single-cell population
3. Mature and immature plasma cells
4. Bi- and multinucleation
5. Rare amyloid

Malignant Lymphoma

Identification of malignant lymphomas of the orbit and lacrimal gland may be difficult because of the predominance of lymphomas composed of small cells with minimal atypia and the presence of extranodal monoclonal B-cell populations in patients with Sjögren's syndrome (51,58–60). The most common orbital subtypes are extranodal marginal zone B-cell lymphoma of low-grade MALT type (IWF: B-cell small lymphocytic lymphoma, SLL) and follicle center cell lymphomas (IWF: follicular lymphomas) (58) (Fig. 27). The smears of low-grade MALT lymphoma show a uniform population of small lymphocytes with regular nuclei, coarse chromatin, and scant cytoplasm (58). However, a polymorphous population including intermediate-sized lymphocytes with slightly irregular nuclei, and plasmacytoid cells with eccentric nuclei and tags of cytoplasm, can be seen (58). In large B-cell lymphoma, large cells with irregular nuclei, showing coarse chromatin and prominent nucleoli, may be seen with a variable number of small to intermediate-sized lymphocytes with prominent nuclear folds and clefts (58). Immunoglobulin light-chain restriction or aberrant B-cell phenotype is identified by flow cytometry (58).

Extensive work has shown that the benign polyclonal inflammatory pseudotumors are less common than was thought in the preimmunophenotyping era (27% of ocular adnexal lymphoid proliferations) and that the majority of extranodal small lymphocytic proliferations are monoclonal B-cell neoplasms (61–63). Ocular adnexal low-grade MALT lymphoma (IWF: B-cell SLL) and mantle cell lymphoma (IWF: intermediate lymphocytic lymphoma) are less often associated with extraocular lymphoma compared to other subtypes (27% vs. 46%) (61). The majority of patients have an indolent clinical course with clinical stage 1E ocular adnexal lymphoid proliferations, regardless of subtype (61).

Metastatic Carcinoma

Metastatic carcinoma involves the orbit as an extraocular mass and may comprise 10% to 33% of orbital masses (36,40–42). FNA plays an important diagnostic role, at times sparing the patient surgery. The most common sites of origin are breast, lung, and prostate (Fig. 28), with other sites including kidney, urinary bladder, salivary gland, skin, esophagus, and stomach, among others (3,23,35,36,40–43,64–66).

THE MANDIBLE AND MAXILLOFACIAL AREAS

The popularity of preoperative evaluation by fine-needle aspiration biopsy (FNA) of mandibular and maxillofacial lesions has lagged behind the use of FNA at other sites. Recently, it has proven useful in confirming or establishing benign and malignant diagnoses and in identifying recurrences in certain clinical

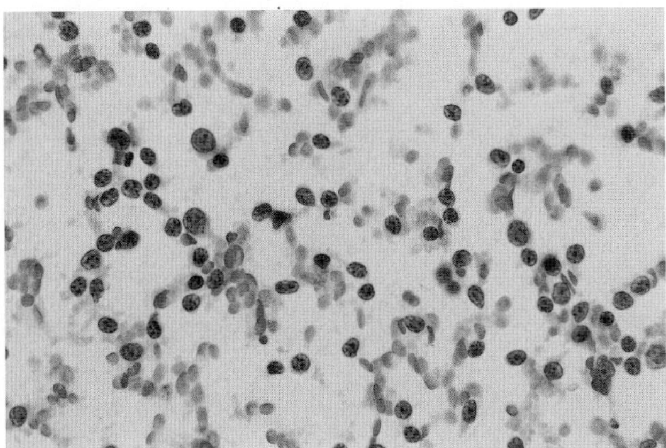

FIGURE 27. Follicle center malignant lymphoma. Dimorphic population of small and large lymphocytes with irregular nuclear indentations and protrusions as well as open chromatin and small nucleoli (Papanicolaou stain, 640×).

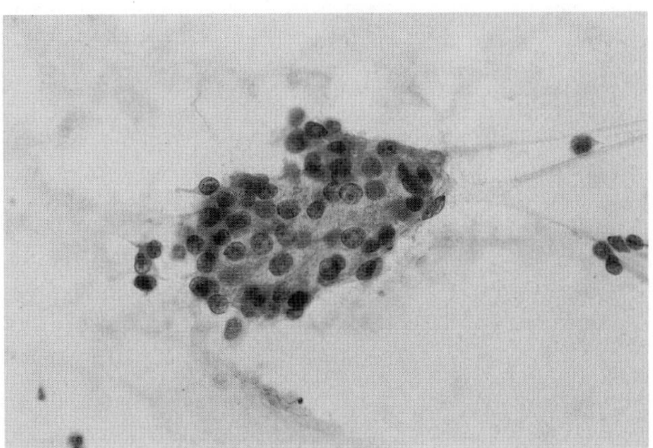

FIGURE 28. Metastatic prostate carcinoma to orbit. Acinar arrangement of cells with delicate cytoplasm, round, vesicular nuclei, and prominent nucleoli (Papanicolaou stain, 400×).

circumstances (67–75). Cytopathology personnel will undoubtedly encounter more fine-needle aspiration biopsy specimens from the jaw and facial region, and the following section describes odontogenic cysts and tumors as well as osseous lesions that may be sampled by FNA.

Odontogenic Cysts

Odontogenic cysts are derived from tooth-forming elements and are often difficult to aspirate because of a rim of intact bone. The use of an 18-gauge cutting needle to provide a pathway through the bone to the cyst has been helpful in obtaining diagnostic material in my experience. Only a few cases of odontogenic cysts diagnosed by needle aspiration have been described in the literature (70,72).

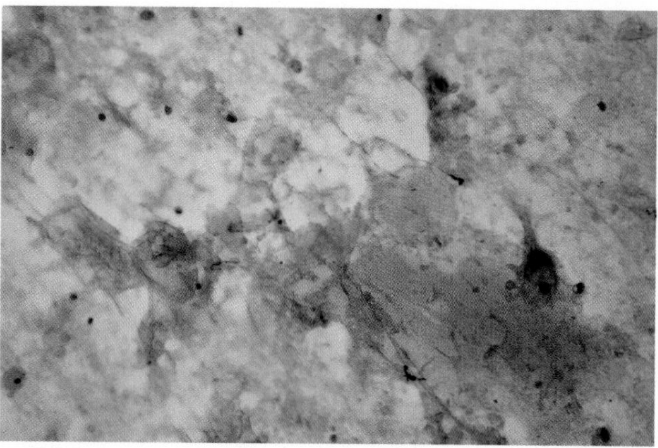

FIGURE 30. Odontogenic keratocyst. Clumps of anucleate keratin debris in a proteinaceous background (Papanicolaou stain, 200×).

Radicular (Periapical) Cyst

The radicular cyst is the most common jaw cyst and develops secondary to apical extension of pulp inflammation and proliferation of epithelial rests (72). Aspirates from this unilocular lucent cyst show a mixture of benign mature squamous, columnar, and cuboidal epithelial cells, with background keratin and inflammation (70) (Fig. 29). It must be distinguished from the odontogenic keratocyst, which shows keratinizing squamous cells with abundant background keratin but a paucity of inflammation (70).

Radicular (Periapical) Cyst

1. Mixed benign epithelium (squamous, columnar)
2. Keratin debris, generally scant
3. Inflammation

Odonotogenic Keratocyst

The odontogenic keratocyst is a unilocular or multilocular radiolucent cyst that arises from dental lamina and is located in the tooth-bearing jaw, most commonly at the mandibular third molar (72). Aspirated material shows anucleated and nucleated keratinized squamous cells and abundant keratin debris, which can be mineralized (70,72,74) (Fig. 30). Other diagnostic considerations include squamous cell carcinoma, cystic acanthomatous ameloblastoma, and keratinized follicular cyst (dentigerous cyst). The keratocyst should show more abundant anucleated and superficial squamous cells than the *follicular cyst* (74). Attention to a second basaloid cell population is important in identifying *ameloblastoma* (76). In some situations, the clinical and radiologic findings play a significant role in the distinction. *Squamous cell carcinoma* shows atypical nuclei and atypical cell shapes.

Dentigerous (Follicular) Cyst

The dentigerous cyst is a radiolucent lesion representing an accumulation of fluid, usually found in the region of the mandibular or maxillary third molar, surrounding the crown of an unerupted tooth (72). Aspiration removes a straw-colored fluid containing a few squamous cells and histiocytes (74) (Fig. 31).

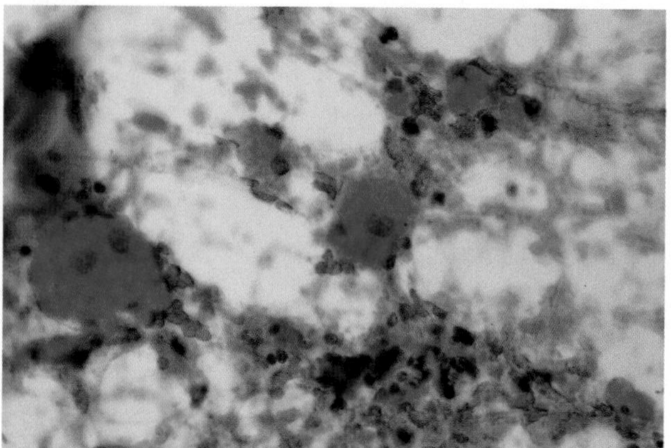

FIGURE 29. Radicular cyst. Inflammatory cells and foamy hemosiderin-laden histiocytes (Papanicolaou stain, 400×).

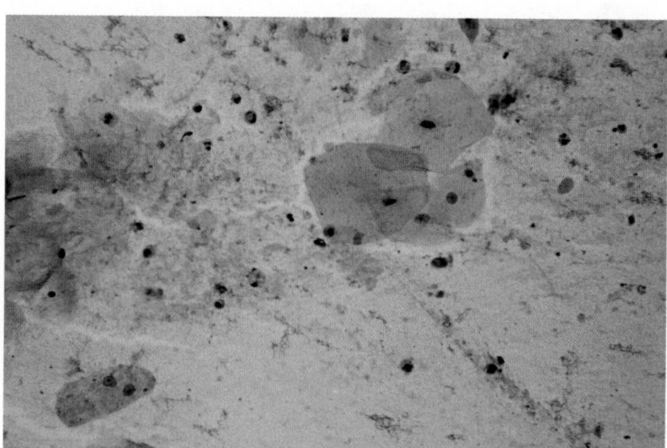

FIGURE 31. Dentigerous cyst. Superficial and intermediate squamous cells in a proteinaceous background (Papanicolaou stain, 200×).

The distinction from an *odontogenic keratocyst* and a *cystic acanthomatous ameloblastoma* may be difficult by cytology alone, as previously discussed.

Dentigerous (Follicular) Cyst

1. Specific location—unerupted third molar
2. Few squamous cells, without nuclear atypia
3. Histiocytes
4. Scant or absent keratin

Odontogenic Ghost Cell Tumor

The rare solid neoplastic form of the calcifying odontogenic cyst is called the odontogenic ghost cell tumor. It is found in older patients in contrast to the calcifying odontogenic cyst and is located in the central jaw or gingiva (72,73). One case report describes the cytologic findings of this solid variant (73). The aspiration smears show syncytial fragments composed of basaloid cells resembling ameloblastoma epithelium with round to oval uniform nuclei, granular chromatin, and small nucleoli (73). Ghost cells (anucleated cells with dense cytoplasm) are seen alone, or intermixed with the basaloid cells (73). Background findings include multinucleated histiocytes, calcified material, and hyalinized dentinoid admixed with the basaloid cells (73). Pitfalls include ameloblastoma and its related lesions, and squamous cell carcinoma. *Ameloblastoma* lacks the ghost cells and dentinoid material of the ghost cell tumor. *Squamous cell carcinoma* demonstrates noticeable nuclear atypia.

Odontogenic Ghost Cell Tumor

1. Basaloid cells without nuclear atypia
2. Ghost cells
3. Dentinoid material
4. Calcified debris

Odontogenic Tumors

Ameloblastoma

Ameloblastoma is a locally aggressive tumor that arises from odontogenic epithelial remnants, usually in the mandible (80%) but also in the maxilla (20%) (72). It can be unilocular or multilocular and destructive (72). It has a propensity for recurrence, and cases of metastatic (malignant) ameloblastoma have been described with cytologic appearances identical to the primary lesion (77–85). Aspirated material shows small dyshesive basaloid to columnar cells with round to oval nuclei showing fine chromatin, smooth to cleft contours, some grooving, single or multiple small nucleoli, and sometimes a teardrop shape (76,84–88) (Fig. 32). Cytoplasm is scant to absent (83,84). The basaloid cells show nuclear molding, crowding, and a central location compared to the peripheral palisading columnar cells (3,83,87). Tumor cells may cling to fibrovascular stromal fragments or can palisade around central fibrillary material (83). Squamous cells and keratin debris can be seen in the background of acanthomatous ameloblastomas (76,83,86). The cytologic appearance of ameloblastoma does not predict metastatic potential, although most ameloblastomas are benign (see Chapter 6) (Fig. 33).

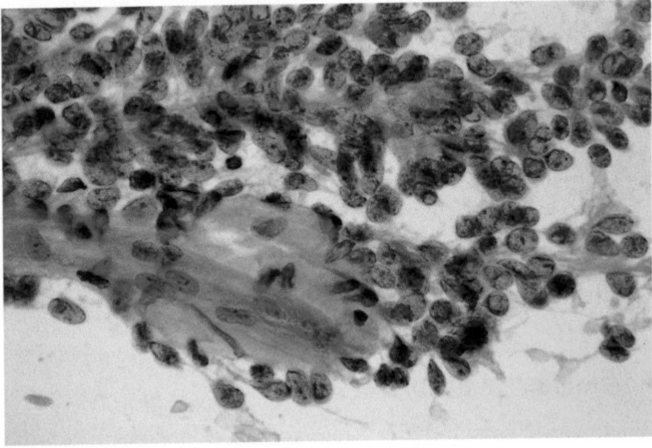

FIGURE 32. Ameloblastoma. Round to teardrop-shaped basaloid cells with focal nuclear molding and palisading surrounding a capillary **(left)** (Papanicolaou stain, 400×).

Differential diagnoses include adenoid cystic carcinoma, poorly differentiated squamous cell carcinoma, small-cell carcinoma, and other odontogenic tumors, including the ameloblastic fibroma. Ameloblastoma lacks the extracellular basement membrane material and the monomorphic population of uniform basaloid tumor cells of *adenoid cystic carcinoma.* The overtly malignant nuclei with necrosis and mitotic activity of *small-cell carcinoma* and *squamous cell carcinoma* help distinguish these entities from ameloblastoma (76). *Ameloblastic fibroma* shows a biphasic population of small basaloid cells and prominent mesenchymal spindle cells (89). The absence of dentin and cementum in ameloblastoma excludes some other *odontogenic tumors.*

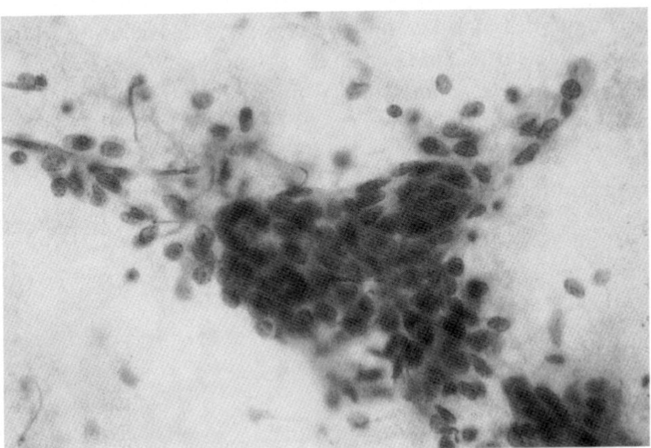

FIGURE 33. Metastatic ameloblastoma. Small cells with oval, vesicular nuclei, prominent nucleoli, focally exhibiting a whorled pattern. Compare with Fig. 32 (Papanicolaou stain, 400×).

Ameloblastoma

1. Heterogeneous cell population
2. Basaloid cells with nuclear molding, scant cytoplasm
3. Columnar cells with peripheral palisading
4. Squamous cells and keratin debris (acanthomatous variant)
5. Absent dentin, cementum, nuclear atypia, and mesenchymal component

Ameloblastic Carcinoma

Ameloblastic carcinoma is a rare aggressive malignant odontogenic carcinoma of the jaw (90). Aspiration smears can be hypercellular and show dyshesive cells with crowding, molding, and stripped cytoplasm, which cling to a fibrovascular network (91). The nuclei are hyperchromatic, grooved, and cleaved, with small nucleoli (91). Differential diagnostic considerations are the same as for ameloblastoma. *Small-cell carcinoma* may be difficult to distinguish by morphology alone, and the clinical history along with a positive neuron-specific enolase stain may be helpful. For *adenoid cystic carcinoma,* attention to extracellular basement membrane material is important in the distinction. *Poorly differentiated squamous carcinoma* can be a pitfall. However, some authors classify ameloblastic carcinoma as an intraosseous squamous cell carcinoma with peripheral features of ameloblastoma (72).

Ameloblastic Carcinoma

1. Dyshesive small cells
2. Nuclear crowding, molding
3. Atypical nuclear features

Ameloblastic Fibroma

Ameloblastic fibroma is an odontogenic tumor of children and young adults that appears radiologically identical to ameloblastoma (72). Aspirated material shows a biphasic tumor composed of hypercellular spindled stromal fragments and the typical palisading epithelial groups as described for ameloblastoma (89,92). Squamous cells and keratin may be seen (92). Necrosis, mitotic figures, cementum, and dentin are absent (87,90). As previously discussed, *ameloblastoma* lacks a prominent stromal mesenchymal component.

Ameloblastic Fibroma

1. Biphasic tumor
2. Spindle cell stroma
3. Typical ameloblastic epithelium

Odontogenic Myxoma

Myxoma of the facial bones is a rare locally invasive neoplasm that arises from the dental papilla (72,93). On aspiration, thick mucoid material can be removed (93). On low-power magnification, a fibrillary myxoid matrix with some capillaries is seen, admixed with scant spindle and stellate cells showing uniform round to oval nuclei (93) (Fig. 34). Pitfalls include other myxoid lesions that could invade or involve bone, such as *myxoid chondrosarcoma, chordoma,* and, less likely, *low-grade fibromyxosarcoma.* A prominent vascular network is typical of sarcomas, whereas the chordoma shows characteristic large, bubbly physaliferous cells.

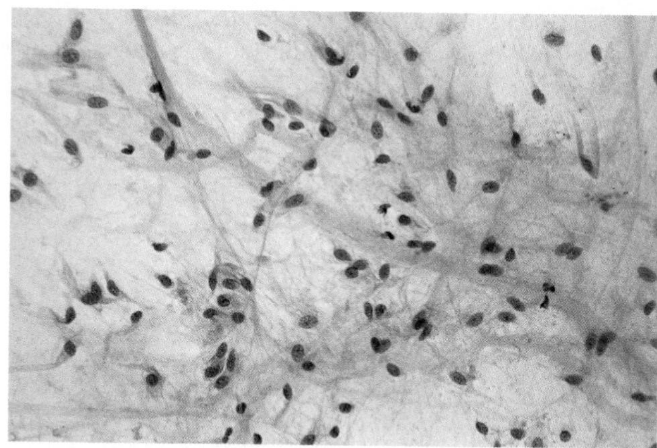

FIGURE 34. Myxoma. Uniform oval to spindle nuclei embedded in a background of myxoid ground substance and collagen fibrils. Blood vessels are absent (hematoxylin and eosin stain, 200×).

Odontogenic Myxoma

1. Myxoid extracellular material
2. Absent to minimal development of blood vessels
3. Spindle or stellate cells

Calcifying Epithelial Odontogenic Tumor (Pindborg's Tumor)

This tumor is an uncommon, locally invasive epithelial neoplasm usually located in the mandible at the molar area but also seen at extraosseous sites (72). Aspirated material shows clusters and sheets of epithelial cells with orangeophilic dense cytoplasm and central, round to oval nuclei showing coarse chromatin, prominent nucleoli, and intranuclear inclusions (75). Binucleation, multinucleation, and mucin-negative cytoplasmic vacuolization may be seen (75). Extracellular amorphous debris (amyloid-like material) and calcification (psammoma bodies) are prominent (75). Pitfalls include acanthomatous ameloblastoma, squamous cell carcinoma, and mucoepidermoid carcinoma. Attention to a second population of basaloid cells in addition to keratin debris and squamous cells identifies *ameloblastoma. Squamous cell carcinoma* shows atypical cell shapes, necrosis, and mitotic figures. The presence of intermediate cells and mucin-positive glandular cells help identify *mucoepidermoid carcinoma.*

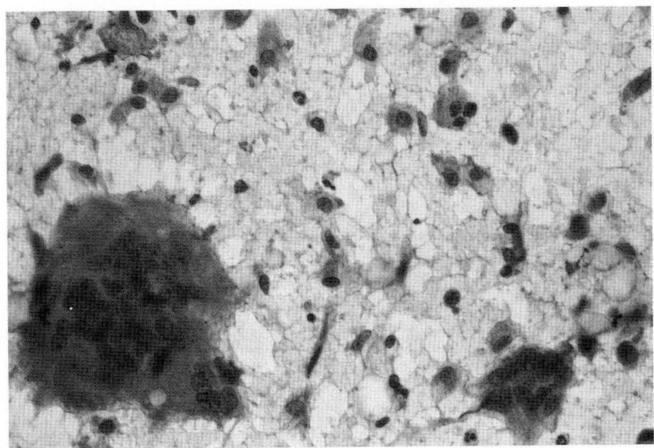

FIGURE 35. Giant-cell reparative granuloma. Bland spindled to epithelioid cells and multinucleated giant cells. Clinical and radiographic correlation is required to exclude other giant-cell lesions (hematoxylin and eosin stain, 200×).

Calcifying Epithelial Odontogenic Tumor (Pindborg's Tumor)

1. Squamoid cells with bi- and multinucleation
2. Amyloid-like extracellular material
3. Psammoma bodies
4. Mucin-negative vacuolated cells
5. Absent necrosis, mitotic figures

Osseous Tumors

Giant-Cell Reparative Granuloma

This lesion can be mucosal (peripheral) or intraosseous (central) in the jaw (67). Aspirates show sheets of plump to spindled stromal cells admixed with multinucleated giant cells (69,70, 74,94,95) (Fig. 35). Nuclear atypia is absent. The distinction from other giant-cell lesions (hyperparathyroidism, giant-cell tumor, and aneurysmal bone cyst) may be impossible on cytology alone, requiring clinical correlation and open biopsy in some situations (67,70,76). *Osteosarcoma* with giant cells is an important pitfall, but attention to the nuclear atypia within the spindle cell component distinguishes osteosarcoma.

Giant-Cell Reparative Granuloma

1. Spindled stromal cells without nuclear atypia
2. Multinucleated histiocytes
3. Clinical information essential

Aneurysmal Bone Cyst

Aneurysmal bone cyst is a nonneoplastic lesion that may mimic a neoplasm radiologically. It may be primary, secondary to a fracture, or form within a neoplasm (96). Aspirate material shows abundant blood with scant stromal spindle cells and giant cells (67,70). Distinction from other giant-cell lesions may be difficult, as previously outlined.

Cementifying Fibroma (Cementoossifying Fibroma)

The cementifying fibroma, a rare benign neoplasm, is a well-defined lesion located in the premolar–molar area of the mandible (72,97). Aspirate smears show spindled fibroblastic cells with even chromatin, indistinct nucleoli, and scant cytoplasm, arranged in clusters or as single cells (70,97). Psammomatous laminated calcifications (cementum) are charcteristic (70,97). The findings may overlap with *fibrous dysplasia.* However, the latter is not a circumscribed lesion radiographically and shows metaplastic bone without cementum material (72).

Cementifying Fibroma

1. Spindled fibroblastic cells
2. Lack of nuclear atypia
3. Lack of epithelial cells
4. Calcified material (cementum)

Chordoma

Chordoma is a malignant tumor that arises from notochord rests most commonly in the clivus, base of the skull, and cervical spine (96). Aspirates are cellular with strands of myxoid matrix encircling the cells (56,96). Small polygonal cells with moderate cytoplasm and small round to oval nuclei appear singly or clustered and are admixed with the characteristic physaliferous cells (large cells with bubbly cytoplasm and irregular nuclear contours) (98) (Fig. 36). Pitfalls include chondrosarcoma and metastatic adenocarcinoma with extracellular mucin. Careful attention to the dual-cell population and the encircling matrix material (highlighted well in air-dried Romanovsky-stained material) distinguishes chordoma from *chondrosarcoma.* Further, chordomas are cytokeratin positive, as

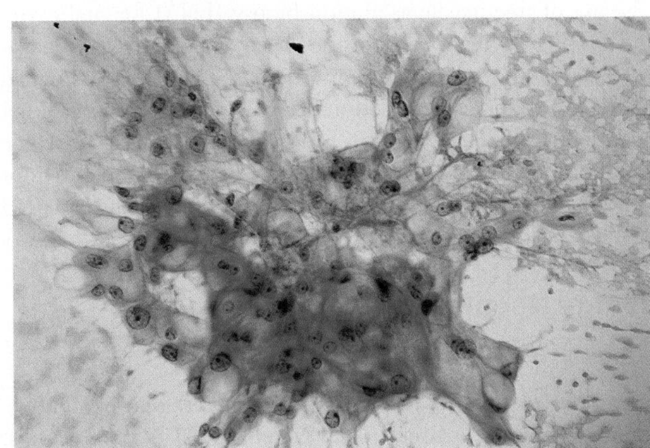

FIGURE 36. Chordoma. Cohesive sheets of highly vacuolated polygonal cells in a myxoid background. Note large, vacuolated physaliferous cell, upper right of center (Papanicolaou stain, 200×).

opposed to chondrosarcomas. Gland and/or cell ball formation are typical of adenocarcinomas.

Chordoma

1. Myxoid extracellular material encircling tumor cells
2. Physaliferous cells (large with bubbly cytoplasm)
3. Small polygonal cells
4. Nests and cords

Osteosarcoma

Osteosarcoma can uncommonly originate in the mandibular, maxillofacial, and skull bones. Jaw lesions may show chondroblastic differentiation (67). The aspirates show oval plasmacytoid or spindle cells with atypical nuclei, which may be markedly abnormal (67,98,99). Multinucleated pleomorphic giant tumor cells and mitotic figures with abnormal forms may be identified (67,98). Osteoid (red-pink on Romanovsky stain) appears as acellular clumps or as amorphous material alone or associated with tumor cells (67,98). Benign multinucleated giant osteoclast cells can be seen as well (67,98). Smears of chondroblastic osteosarcoma may show chondroid matrix (pink to magenta, Romanovsky stain; gray-green, Papanicolaou stain) with trapped neoplastic cells, which may be confused with chondrosarcoma on FNA, if osteoid is not identified (98). *Giant-cell lesions,* as previously discussed, may be confused with giant-cell–rich osteosarcoma. If osteoid matrix is absent or not recognized, osteosarcoma can be confused with other sarcomas.

Osteosarcoma

1. Osteoid
2. Atypical plasmacytoid or spindle cells
3. Pleomorphic single and giant cells

THE ORAL CAVITY AND OROPHARYNX

The use of fine-needle aspiration biopsy (FNA) for oral cavity and oropharyngeal lesions has not been as popular as its use at other sites. However, the diagnostic accuracy of FNA for oral cavity and oropharyngeal lesions is comparable to that at other body sites (68,70,71,100–102). This section focuses on some common and unusual lesions that may be encountered. Minor salivary gland lesions are not discussed, and the reader is referred to the Salivary Gland section.

Benign Neoplasms

Squamous Papilloma

Squamous papilloma, the most common intraoral benign epithelial neoplasm, is usually located on the palate, tongue, lips, and gingiva as an exophytic growth. FNA is not usually the diagnostic technique of preference. Cytomorphology is not specific and may show benign squamous cells, fibroblasts, and inflammation (101). An important pitfall is *squamous cell carcinoma,* which should show nuclear atypia and abnormal cell shapes if adequately sampled.

Squamous Papilloma

1. Benign squamous cells
2. Spindled fibroblasts
3. Inflammation

Granular Cell Tumor

Granular cell tumor, most examples of which are thought to be of schwann cell origin, is found most commonly in the tongue, followed by the chest wall and upper limbs, as a painless, solitary, less than 3-cm nodule (103,104). Aspirates show predominantly dissociated cells and small clusters, with eccentric round to oval small nuclei and abundant periodic acid–Schiff (PAS)-positive diastase-resistant granular cytoplasm (101,103) (Fig. 37). The basophilic granules are coarse, variably sized, and can obscure the nucleus (104). Rarely, a pseudofollicular pattern can be seen (105). Malignant potential cannot be predicted by cytology alone. Immunocytochemical markers are positive for S-100 protein and neuron-specific enolase (NSE) (103). Distinction from *histiocytes* may be difficult, but careful attention to the presence of clustering, lack of cytoplasmic vacuolization and a negative CD68 stain (histiocytic marker) helps to identify granular cell tumor. The absence of cross-striations and smaller cell size distinguishes granular cell tumor from *rhabdomyoma.* Background cytoplasmic debris in granular cell tumor aspirates should not be mistaken for a tumor diathesis (106).

Granular Cell Tumor

1. Clusters and single cells
2. Eccentric round to oval small nuclei
3. Abundant granular nonvacuolated PAS-positive cytoplasm
4. NSE, S-100 protein positive, CD68 negative

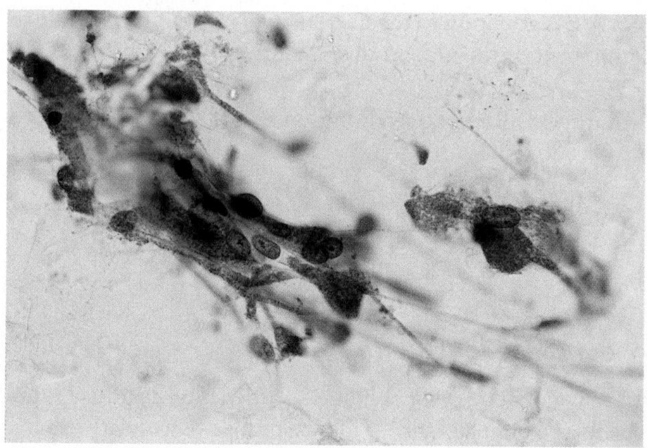

FIGURE 37. Granular cell tumor. Spindled to polygonal cells with abundant coarse cytoplasmic granules focally obscuring the uniform oval nucleus (Papanicolaou stain, 640×).

Rhabdomyoma

The adult type of rhabdomyoma is a rare slow-growing neoplasm usually identified in the larynx, pharynx, base of tongue, or floor of the mouth (103). Aspirates show isolated oval to polygonal to elongate large cells with abundant, well-demarcated, slightly granular, sometimes vacuolated cytoplasm and demonstrating intracytoplasmic cross striations or whorled structures (107,108). The uniform round nuclei show granular chromatin and a prominent nucleolus (107,108). Multinucleated tumor cells may be identified (107,108). Typically, the cells contain glycogen and show positive staining for myoglobin, desmin, and α smooth muscle actin (103). Electron microscopy shows thin and thick myofilaments with Z-band formation (108). Other diagnostic considerations include granular cell tumor, paraganglioma, and normal skeletal muscle. Granular cell tumor aspirates show smaller cells without multinucleation that tend to cluster and show coarsely granular cytoplasm without cross striations or vacuoles. Paraganglioma cells have central round to spindle nuclei demonstrating nuclear pleomorphism and are arranged in loose follicles (56). *Normal skeletal muscle* shows larger rectangular cells with cross striations (108). *Rhabdomyosarcoma* would be an unusual diagnostic consideration in this location and age group.

Rhabdomyoma

1. Large cells, some multinucleated, without nuclear atypia
2. No cell clustering
3. Abundant cytoplasm with cross-striations, whorls, vacuoles
4. Glycogen in cytoplasm

Malignant Neoplasms

Squamous Cell Carcinoma

Squamous cell carcinoma (SCC) comprises more than 90% of intraoral malignancies and is seen most commonly in the lip, tongue, and floor of the mouth (96). Aspirates show malignant squamous cells, either isolated or in groups, with nuclear atypia (irregular nuclear contours, parachromatin clearing, chromatin coarseness, irregular nucleoli) and variable keratinization (71,101) (Fig. 38). Keratin is orangeophilic with Papanicolaou stain and robin's egg blue on Romanovsky stain. Background necrosis, inflammation, and multinucleated histiocytic giant cells may be identified (101).

False-positive results can be seen after previous *radiation* or in *tissue repair,* where reactive nuclear atypia may be misinterpreted as malignant (68). With radiation, the atypical cells show a low nuclear-to-cytoplasmic ratio. False-negative results occur from sampling error (68,70,100,102). Other diagnostic considerations for well-differentiated SCC include squamous papilloma and mucoepidermoid carcinoma. *Squamous papilloma* lacks the nuclear atypia and the abnormal keratinized cells and cell shapes of SCC. However, some well-differentiated SCCs may be indistinguishable from squamous papilloma, necessitating biopsy. *Mucoepidermoid carcinoma* shows intermediate cells, glandular cells, and intracellular mucin.

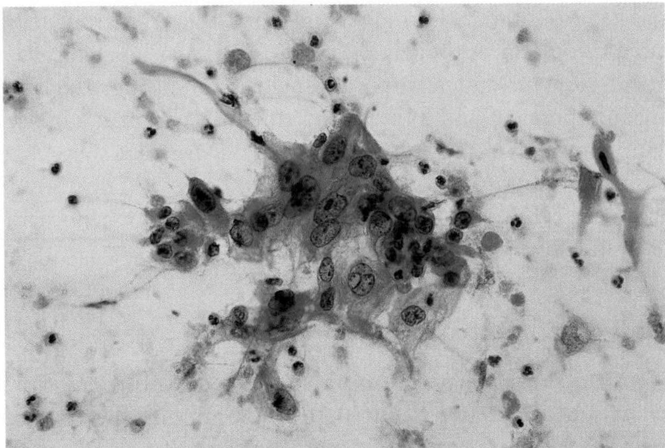

FIGURE 38. Squamous cell carcinoma. Three-dimensional sheet of polygonal cells with distinct cell borders and markedly abnormal nuclei. Tadpole-like cell to right of cluster and small keratinized cell to left (Papanicolaou stain, 500×).

Poorly differentiated SCC must be distinguished from *melanoma* and *metastatic carcinoma.* Melanoma shows dyshesive tumor cells and variable intracytoplasmic melanin. Immunohistochemical markers (vimentin, S-100 protein, HMB-45, possibly CEA) and the clinical circumstances are helpful in challenging cases.

Squamous Cell Carcinoma

1. Keratinized or nonkeratinized squamous cells, isolated or clustered
2. Range of nuclear atypia depending on differentiation
3. Abnormal cell shapes (fiber, caudate, spindle)
4. Background necrosis
5. Absent mucin, pigment

Malignant Lymphoma

Malignant lymphoma of the oral cavity is uncommon, and adequate biopsy material may be difficult to obtain because of its submucosal location (109). The use of FNA in conjunction with immunophenotyping by flow cytometry, or with immunocytochemistry, has proven useful in the diagnosis and subclassification of oral malignant lymphomas (101,109). Case series have described the morphologic appearances of non-Hodgkin's lymphomas including follicle center cell lymphoma (IWF: follicular lymphoma); diffuse large B-cell lymphoma; lymphoblastic lymphoma (IWF: lymphoblastic lymphoma); T-cell (Sézary) lymphoma and Burkitt-like lymphoma (IWF: small non–cleaved cell, non-Burkitt type lymphoma) (68,71,101,109). Large B-cell lymphoma aspirates typically show large dyshesive single lymphoid cells with scant cytoplasm, abnormal nuclei with open chromatin, and multiple nucleoli often located close to the nuclear membrane (101). In immunoblastic lymphoma, prominent single nucleoli, eccentric nuclei and more abundant cytoplasm are seen (101). Pitfalls include poorly differentiated squamous cell carcinoma, melanoma, and plasma cell dyscrasias. Smears of *squamous cell carcinoma* show variable cell cohesion and keratinization, with more abundant refractile sharply delineated cytoplasm. Although *melanoma* appears as isolated cells, a search for intranuclear pseudoinclusions, intracytoplasmic melanin pigment and more abundant cytoplasm than large-cell lymphoma aids in the diagnosis. *Plasma cell dyscrasias* show characteristic cells with clockface chromatin, eccentric nuclei, and abundant cytoplasm. In challenging cases, immunophenotyping or immunocytochemistry is valuable.

Metastatic Neoplasms

Metastatic tumors have uncommonly been described in the oral cavity and oropharynx (68,70,101). Common types include melanoma, anaplastic thyroid carcinoma, squamous cell carcinoma, and adenocarcinoma (lung, kidney, breast) (68,70,101). Morphology is typical of the primary lesion.

NASAL CAVITY, PARANASAL SINUSES, NASOPHARYNX

Malignant Neoplasms

Squamous Cell Carcinoma

Sinonasal squamous cell carcinoma (SCC), most commonly seen in the maxillary antrum, nasal cavity, and ethmoid sinuses, may be keratinizing or, less commonly, nonkeratinizing (67,96). Aspirates from well-differentiated SCC show squamous cells with keratinized dense cytoplasm, abnormal cell shapes (spindle, tadpole), and atypical, often pyknotic nuclei (67). Squamous pearls, cannibalization, and anucleate keratin may be seen (67). Keratin is robin's egg blue with Diff-Quik stain and orange-pink with Papanicolaou stain.

In poorly differentiated SCC, keratinization may be absent. Smears show poorly differentiated malignant cells isolated or in dyshesive clusters, with marked nuclear atypia (irregular contours, large nucleoli, and coarse chromatin). Pitfalls include squamous papilloma, melanoma, anaplastic large-cell lymphoma, and metastatic carcinoma, as previously discussed.

Squamous Cell Carcinoma

1. Nuclear atypia (most marked with poor differentiation)
2. Abnormal cell shapes, keratinization, squamous pearls (well differentiated)
3. Absent intracytoplasmic pigment and vacuoles

Nasopharyngeal Carcinoma

Nasopharyngeal carcinoma (see Chapter 5) may be a keratinizing or nonkeratinizing squamous cell carcinoma or an undifferentiated carcinoma (lymphoepithelioma). The morphology has been discussed under lymph node metastases. In addition, undifferentiated nasopharyngeal carcinoma may show background lymphocytes. FNA can obtain enough material for Epstein-Barr virus genome analysis by DNA amplification (110). In the nasopharynx, primary carcinoma must be distinguished from malignant lymphoma, particularly *anaplastic large cell lymphoma,* which shows small and large dispersed cells with some multinucleation (68,111). Cytoplasmic vacuolization, round to oval nuclei with prominent nucleoli, and a ropy chromatin pattern are identified (111). Expression of CD30 with variable EMA positivity supports a diagnosis of anaplastic large-cell lymphoma.

Olfactory Neuroblastoma

Olfactory neuroblastoma (see Chapter 4), an uncommon malignant neoplasm, arises as a polypoid mass from the nasal olfactory mucosa (96,112). Aspirates show small cells isolated and in clusters, with rare nuclear molding, rare rosettes surrounding a central empty space, and pseudorosettes surrounding fibrillary centers (112,113) (Fig. 39). Nuclei are round to oval, with small single or multiple nucleoli, thickened nuclear membranes and coarsely granular chromatin (112,113). Cytoplasmic processes or fibrils can be seen, or the cytoplasm is scant (112,113). Immunohistochemical stains are positive for neuron specific enolase (NSE) and chromogranin (114). Electron microscopy (EM) shows dense-core granules, neurotubules, and neurofilaments (114).

Differential diagnoses include other small-cell tumors, including small-cell carcinoma, carcinoid, metastatic neuroblastoma, poorly differentiated squamous cell carcinoma, lymphoma, melanoma, and rhabdomyosarcoma. *Small-cell carcinoma* shows more necrosis, nuclear molding, and nuclear atypia. The presence of rosettes and fibrillary processes excludes most other small-cell tumors except for metastatic neuroblastoma, which may show extensive true rosettes and pseudorosettes. Greater nuclear atypia is seen in *melanoma, rhabdomyosarcoma,* and *squamous cell carcinoma. Lymphomas* composed of small cells lack nuclear molding and usually show nuclear protrusions or cleaves.

Olfactory Neuroblastoma

1. Small-cell tumor
2. Rosettes, pseudorosettes, clusters
3. Cytoplasmic processes or fibrils
4. Uniform nuclei with nuclear molding
5. NSE-positive, dense-core granules on EM

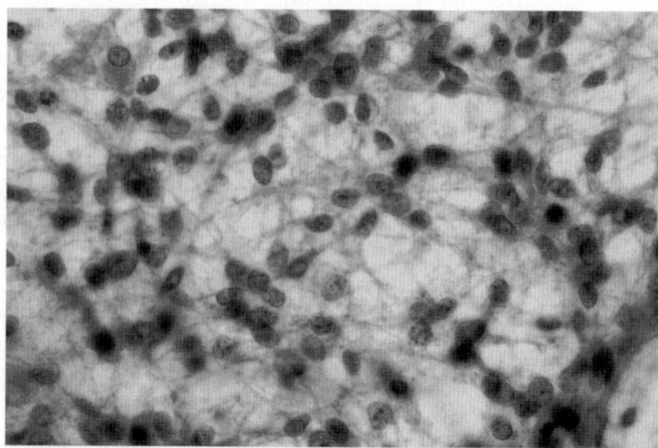

FIGURE 39. Peripheral neuroectodermal tumor. Small, oval nuclei with slight tendency to rosette formation **(midright)** dispersed in a fibrillar background. This pattern resembles olfactory neuroblastoma (Papanicolaou stain, 400×).

Malignant Melanoma

Malignant melanoma rarely arises from the nasal cavity and sinuses and may show a variety of patterns: small cell, spindle cell, epithelioid (plasmacytoid), and pleomorphic (96). Aspirates may show a wide range of appearances (67). Small cells with scant cytoplasm and rare to absent pigmentation can be confused with other small-cell tumors (Fig. 40). Dyshesive plasmacytoid cells with eccentric nuclei, binucleation and multinucleation, intranuclear pseudoinclusions, macronucleoli and variable dusty intracytoplasmic melanin pigment favor melanoma. Immunohistochemical markers are usually positive for vimentin, S-100 protein, HMB-45, and MART-1 in melanoma.

Malignant Melanoma

1. Dyshesive cells
2. Intracytoplasmic dusty melanin pigment
3. Variable cell shape: small, spindle, plasmacytoid, pleomorphic
4. S-100 protein, HMB-45, MART-1 positive

Malignant Lymphoma

Sinonasal lymphomas are usually diffuse large B-cell type. Many show immunoblastic features, and only a minority are of grade 1 and 2 follicle center cell origin (IWF: follicular predominantly small cleaved or mixed cell lymphomas) (96). Large B-cell malignant lymphoma appears similar to its counterpart at intraocular and orbital sites, as previously discussed. Pitfalls include *nasopharyngeal carcinoma,* poorly differentiated *squamous cell carcinoma,* and *malignant melanoma.* The lack of cohesion, with absent to scant cytoplasm, nuclear membrane-based nucleoli, and an open chromatin pattern favors *large-cell lymphoma.* (Fig. 41). Intracytoplasmic pigmentation, binucleation, and multinucleation identifies *malignant melanoma.* Immunocytochemical marker studies and flow cytometry immunophenotyping may aid in difficult cases. Malignant lymphomas composed of small cells may be difficult to discern from reactive processes and other small-cell tumors (melanoma, olfactory neuroblastoma, poorly differentiated squamous cell carcinomas) as previously outlined.

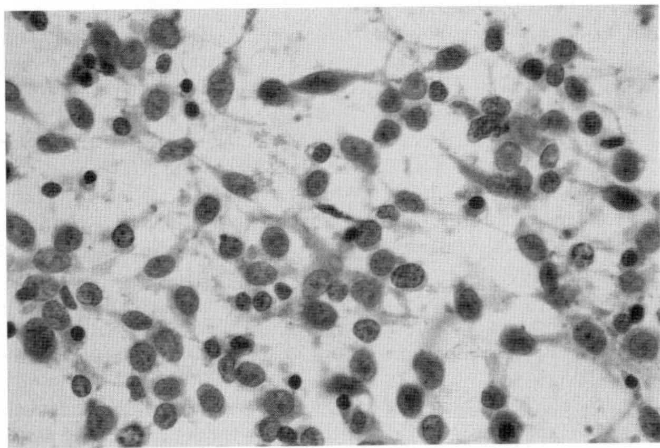

FIGURE 40. Malignant melanoma. Dispersed round to spindled cells with oval nuclei, coarse chromatin, and focal nucleoli. If the round cells predominate, distinction from malignant lymphoma may be difficult (hematoxylin and eosin stain, 400×).

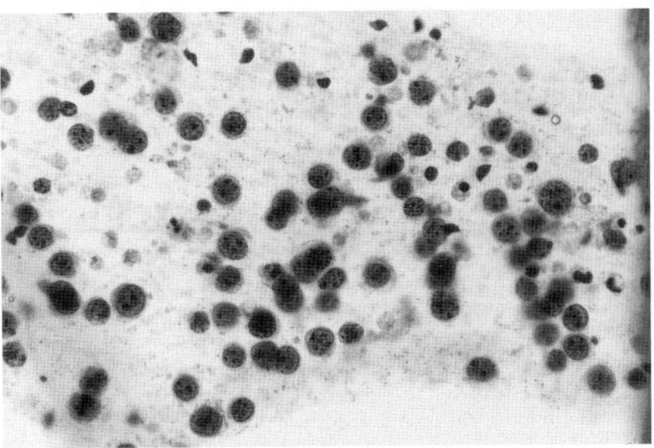

FIGURE 41. Large B-cell lymphoma. Monomorphic large lymphocytes with irregular nuclei and multiple membrane-bound nucleoli (Papanicolaou stain, 640×).

In Asia, T-cell lymphomas of the sinonasal area are more common (67,96). NK/T-cell lymphoma of nasal type (previously midline malignant reticulosis), a necrotizing angiocentric lymphoproliferative disorder, may be difficult to diagnose by cytology even with immunophenotyping because of its polymorphous appearance and difficulty in demonstrating an abnormal T-cell phenotype in some cases (96) (see Chapter 12).

REFERENCES

1. Mandell DB, Levy JJ, Rosenthal DL. Preparation and cytologic evaluation of intraocular fluids. *Acta Cytol* 1987;31:150–158.
2. Dávila RM, Miranda MC, Smith ME. Role of cytopathology in the diagnosis of ocular malignancies. *Acta Cytol* 1998;42:362–366.
3. Glasgow BJ. Orbit, Eye. In: Johnston W, ed. *ASCP theory and practice of cytopathology, vol 7, Cytopathology of the head and neck.* Chicago: ASCP Press, 1997: 373–381,397–403.
4. Scroggs MW, Johnston WW, Klintworth GK. Intraocular tumors. A cytopathologic study. *Acta Cytol* 1990;34:401–408.
5. Glasgow BJ. Intraocular fine-needle aspiration biopsy of coronal adenomas. *Diagn Cytopathol* 1991;7:230–242.
6. Campbell DG, Shields MB, Liebmann JM. Ghost cell glaucoma. In: Ritch R, Shields MB, Kriepin T, eds. *The glaucomas.* St Louis: CV Mosby, 1989:1230–1247.
7. Goldberg MF. Cytological diagnosis of phacolytic glaucoma utilizing millipore filtration of the aqueous. *Br J Ophthalmol* 1967;51:847–853.
8. Naib ZM, Clepper AS, Elliott SR. Exfoliative cytology as an aid in the diagnosis of ophthalmic lesions. *Acta Cytol* 1967;4:295–303.
9. Michels RG. Vitrectomy for complications of diabetic retinopathy. *Arch Ophthalmol* 1978;96:237–246.
10. Caya JG, Clowry LJ, Wollenberg NJ, et al. The clinicopathologic significance of vitreous fluid cytology examinations in a series of 38 patients. *Diagn Cytopathol* 1985;1:267–271.
11. Fischler DF, Prayson RA. Cytologic specimens from the eye: a clinicopathologic study of 33 patients. *Diagn Cytopathol* 1997;17:262–266.
12. Sanderson TL, Pustai W, Shelley L, et al. Cytologic evaluation of ocular lesions. *Acta Cytol* 1980;5:391–400.
13. Selsky EJ, Knox DL, Maumenee AE, et al. Ocular involvement in Whipple's disease. *Retina* 1984;4:103–106.
14. O'Hara BJ, Ehya H, Shields JA, et al. Fine needle aspiration biopsy in pediatric ophthalmic tumors and pseudotumors. *Acta Cytol* 1993;37:125–130.

15. Shields JA, Shields CL, Ehya H, et al. Fine-needle aspiration biopsy of suspected intraocular tumors. The 1992 Urwick Lecture. *Ophthalmology* 1993;100:1677–1684.
16. Augsburger JJ, Shields JA, Folberg R, et al. Fine needle aspiration biopsy in the diagnosis of intraocular cancer. Cytologic–histologic correlations. *Ophthalmology* 1985;92:39–49.
17. Palma O, Canali N, Scaroni P, et al. Fine needle aspiration biopsy: its use in the management of orbital and intraocular tumors. *Tumori* 1989;75:580–593.
18. Decaussin M, Boran MD-S, Salle M, et al. Cytological aspiration of intraocular retinoblastoma in an 11-year-old boy. *Diagn Cytopathol* 1998;19:190–193.
19. Char DH, Miller TR. Fine needle biopsy in retinoblastoma. *Am J Ophthalmol* 1984;97:686–690.
20. Arora R, Betharia SM. Fine needle aspiration biopsy of pediatric orbital tumors. An immunocytochemical study. *Acta Cytol* 1994;38: 511–516.
21. Shields JA, Shields CL, Eagle RC, et al. Observations on seven cases of intraocular leiomyoma. The 1993 Byron Demorest Lecture. *Arch Ophthalmol* 1994;112:521–528.
22. Char DH, Miller TR, Ljung B-M, et al. Fine needle aspiration biopsy in uveal melanoma. *Acta Cytol* 1989;33:590–605.
23. Glasgow BJ, Layfield LJ. Fine-needle aspiration biopsy of orbital and periorbital masses. *Diagn Cytopathol* 1991;7:132–141.
24. Font RL, Ferry AP. Carcinoma metastatic to the eye and orbit III. A clinicopathologic study of 28 cases metastatic to the orbit. *Cancer* 1976;38:1326–1335.
25. Qualman SJ, Mendelsohn G, Mann RB, et al. Intraocular lymphomas. Natural history based on a clinicopathologic study of eight cases and review of the literature. *Cancer* 1983;52:878–886.
26. Buettner H, Bolling JP. Intravitreal large-cell lymphoma. *Mayo Clin Proc* 1993;68:1011–1015.
27. Ljung B-M, Char D, Miller TR, et al. Intraocular lymphoma. Cytologic diagnosis and the role of immunologic markers. *Acta Cytol* 1988;32:840–847.
28. Blumenkranz MS, Ward T, Murphy S, et al. Applications and limitations of vitreoretinal biopsy techniques in intraocular large cell lymphoma. *Retina* 1992;12(3 Suppl):S64–S67.
29. Davis JL, Solomon D, Nussenblatt RB, et al. Immunocytochemical staining of vitreous cells. Indications, techniques and results. *Ophthalmology* 1992;99:250–256.
30. Char DH, Ljung B-M, Miller T, et al. Primary intraocular lymphoma (ocular reticulum cell sarcoma) diagnosis and management. *Ophthalmology* 1988;95:625–630.
31. Wilson DJ, Braziel R, Rosenbaum JT. Intraocular lymphoma. Immunopathologic analysis of vitreous biopsy specimens. *Arch Ophthalmol* 1992;110:1455–1458.
32. Dorland. *Dorland's illustrated medical dictionary, 26th ed.* Philadelphia: WB Saunders, 1985:998.
33. Das DK, Das J, Bhatt NC, et al. Orbital lesions. Diagnosis by fine needle aspiration cytology. *Acta Cytol* 1994;38:158–164.
34. Zajdela A, de Maublanc MA, Schlienger P, et al. Cytologic diagnosis of orbital and periorbital palpable tumors using fine-needle sampling without aspiration. *Diagn Cytopathol* 1986;2:17–20.
35. Font RL, Laucirica R, Ramzy I. Cytologic evaluation of tumors of the orbit and ocular adnexa: an analysis of 84 cases studied by the "squash technique." *Diagn Cytopathol* 1994;10:135–142.
36. Cangiarella JF, Cajigas A, Savala E, et al. Fine needle aspiration cytology of orbital masses. *Acta Cytol* 1996;40:1205–1211.
37. Krzystolik Z, Rosiawska A, Bedner E. The cytological, immunocytochemical and molecular genetic analysis in diagnosis of the neoplasms of the eye, eye adnexa and orbit. *Doc Ophthalmol* 1994;88: 155–163.
38. Dey P, Radhika S, Rajwanshi A, et al. Fine needle aspiration biopsy of orbital and eyelid lesions. *Acta Cytol* 1993;37:903–907.
39. Arora R, Rewari R, Betharia SM. Fine needle aspiration cytology of orbital and adnexal masses. *Acta Cytol* 1992;36:483–491.
40. Zajdela A, Vielh P, Schlienger P, et al. Fine-needle cytology of 292 palpable orbital and eyelid tumors. *Am J Clin Pathol* 1990;93:100–104.
41. Kennerdell JS, Slamovits TL, Dekker A, et al. Orbital fine-needle aspiration biopsy. *Am J Ophthalmol* 1985;99:547–551.
42. Czerniak B, Woyke S, Daniel B, et al. Diagnosis of orbital tumors by aspiration biopsy guided by computerized tomography. *Cancer* 1984;54:2385–2389.
43. Spoor TC, Kennerdell JS, Dekker A, et al. Orbital fine needle aspiration biopsy with B-scan guidance. *Am J Ophthalmol* 1980;89:274–277.
44. Kennerdell JS, Dekker A, Johnson BL, et al. Fine-needle aspiration biopsy. Its use in orbital tumors. *Arch Ophthalmol* 1979;97:1315–1317.
45. Dubois PJ, Kennerdell JS, Rosenbaum AE, et al. Computed tomographic localization for fine needle aspiration biopsy of orbital tumors. *Radiology* 1979;131:149–152.
46. Ballesteros E, Greenebaum E, Merriam JC. Fine-needle aspiration diagnosis of enterogenous cyst of the orbit: a case report. *Diagn Cytopathol* 1997;16:450–453.
47. Kaw YT, Cuesta RA. Nodular fasciitis of the orbit diagnosed by fine needle aspiration cytology. A case report. *Acta Cytol* 1993;37:957–960.
48. Meffert JJ, Kennard CD, Davis TL, et al. Intradermal nodular fasciitis presenting as an eyelid mass. *Int J Dermatol* 1996;35:548–552.
49. Dahl I, Åkerman M. Nodular fasciitis. A correlative cytologic and histologic study of 13 cases. *Acta Cytol* 1981;25:215–223.
50. Laucirica R, Font RL. Cytologic evaluation of lymphoproliferative lesions of the orbit/ocular adnexa: an analysis of 46 cases. *Diagn Cytopathol* 1996;15:241–245.
51. Harris NL, Pilch BZ, Bhan AK, et al. Immunohistologic diagnosis of orbital lymphoid infiltrates. *Am J Surg Pathol* 1984;8:83–91.
52. Layfield LJ, Glasgow B, Ostrzega N, et al. Fine-needle aspiration cytology and the diagnosis of neoplasms in the pediatric age group. *Diagn Cytopathol* 1991;7:451–461.
53. Katz RL, Silva EG, DeSantos LA, et al. Diagnosis of eosinophilic granuloma of bone by cytology, histology, and electron microscopy of transcutaneous bone-aspiration biopsy. *J Bone Joint Surg* 1980;62: 1284–1290.
54. Silverman JF, Joshi VV. FNA biopsy of small round cell tumors of childhood: cytomorphologic features and the role of ancillary studies. *Diagn Cytopathol* 1994;10:245–255.
55. Cristallini EG, Bolis GB, Ottaviano P. Fine needle aspiration biopsy of orbital meningioma. Report of a case. *Acta Cytol* 1990;34:236–238.
56. Orell SR, Sterret GF, Walters MN, et al. *Manual and atlas of fine needle aspiration cytology, 2nd ed.* New York: Churchill Livingstone, 1992:44,319, 329–331.
57. Yakulis R, Dawson RR, Wang SE, et al. Fine needle aspiration diagnosis of orbital plasmacytoma with amyloidosis. A case report. *Acta Cytol* 1995;39:104–110.
58. Jeffrey PB, Cartwright D, Atwater SK, et al. Lacrimal gland lymphoma: a cytomorphologic and immunophenotypic study. *Diagn Cytopathol* 1995;12:215–222.
59. Bahler DW, Swerdlow SH. Clonal salivary gland infiltrates associated with myoepithelial sialadenitis (Sjögren's syndrome) begin as nonmalignant antigen-selected expansions. *Blood* 1998;91:1864–1872.
60. Lasota J, Miettinen MM. Coexistence of different B-cell clones in consecutive lesions of low-grade MALT lymphomas of the salivary gland in Sjögren's disease. *Mod Pathol* 1997;10:872–878.
61. Knowles DM, Jakobiec FA, McNally L, et al. Lymphoid hyperplasia and malignant lymphoma occurring in the ocular adnexa (orbit, conjunctiva, and eyelids): a prospective multiparametric analysis of 108 cases during 1977 to 1987. *Hum Pathol* 1990;21:950–973.
62. McNally L, Jakobiec FA, Knowles DM. Clinical, morphologic, immunophenotypic, and molecular genetic analysis of bilateral ocular adnexal lymphoid neoplasms in 17 patients. *Am J Ophthalmol* 1987; 103:555–568.
63. Knowles DM, Jakobiec FA. Cell marker analysis of extranodal lymphoid infiltrates: to what extent does the determination of mono- or polyclonality resolve the diagnostic dilemma of malignant lymphoma v pseudolymphoma in an extranodal site? *Semin Diagn Pathol* 1985; 2:163–168.

64. Capone A, Slamovits TL. Discrete metastasis of solid tumors to extraocular muscles. *Arch Ophthalmol* 1990;108:237–243.
65. Singer MA, Warren F, Accardi F, et al. Adenocarcinoma of the stomach confirmed by orbital biopsy in a patient seropositive for human immunodeficiency virus. *Am J Ophthalmol* 1990;110:707–709.
66. Reifler DM, Kini SR, Liu D, et al. Orbital metastasis from prostatic carcinoma. Identification by immunocytology. *Arch Ophthalmol* 1984;102:292–295.
67. Layfield LJ. Nasal cavity, paranasal sinuses, jaw, and facial bones. In: Johnston W, ed. *ASCP theory and practice of cytopathology, vol 7, Cytopathology of the head and neck.* Chicago: ASCP Press, 1997: 112–121.
68. Daskalopoulou D, Rapidis AD, Maounis N, et al. Fine-needle aspiration cytology in tumors and tumor-like conditions of the oral and maxillofacial region. Diagnostic reliability and limitations. *Cancer Cytopathol* 1997;81:238–252.
69. Platt JC, Rodgers SF, Davidson D, et al. Fine-needle aspiration biopsy in oral and maxillofacial surgery. *Oral Surg Oral Med Oral Pathol* 1993;75:152–155.
70. Günhan O, Dogan N, Celasun B, et al. Fine needle aspiration cytology of oral cavity and jaw bone lesions. A report of 102 cases. *Acta Cytol* 1993;37:135–141.
71. Das DK, Gulati A, Bhatt NC, et al. Fine needle aspiration cytology of oral and pharyngeal lesions. A study of 45 cases. *Acta Cytol* 1993; 37:333–342.
72. Kramer IRH, Pindborg JJ, Shear M. *Histological typing of odontogenic tumours, 2nd ed.* New York: Springer-Verlag, 1992.
73. Stone CH, Gaba AR, Benninger MS, et al. Odontogenic ghost cell tumor: a case report with cytologic findings. *Diagn Cytopathol* 1998; 18:199–203.
74. Ramzy I, Aufdemorte TB, Duncan DL. Diagnosis of radiolucent lesions of the jaw by fine needle aspiration biopsy. *Acta Cytol* 1985; 29:419–424.
75. Fulciniti F, Vetrani A, Zeppa P, et al. Calcifying epithelial odontogenic tumor (Pindborg's tumor) on fine-needle aspiration biopsy smears: a case report. *Diagn Cytopathol* 1995;12:71–75.
76. Ramzy I, Rone R, Schantz HD. Squamous cells in needle aspirates of subcutaneous lesions: a diagnostic problem. *Am J Clin Pathol* 1986; 85:319–324.
77. Houston G, Davenport W, Keaton W, et al. Malignant (metastatic) ameloblastoma: report of a case. *J Oral Maxillofac Surg* 1993;51: 1152–1155.
78. Laughlin EH. Metastasizing ameloblastoma. *Cancer* 1989;64:776–780.
79. Inoue N, Shimojyo M, Iwai H, et al. Malignant ameloblastoma with pulmonary metastasis and hypercalcemia. Report of an autopsy case and review of the literature. *Am J Clin Pathol* 1988;90: 474–481.
80. Ikemura K, Tashiro H, Fujino H, et al. Ameloblastoma of the mandible with metastasis to the lungs and lymph nodes. *Cancer* 1972;29:930–940.
81. Harada K, Suda S, Kayano T, et al. Ameloblastoma with metastasis to the lung and associated hypercalcemia. *J Oral Maxillofac Surg* 1989; 47:1083–1087.
82. Ueda M, Kaneda T, Imaizumi M, et al. Mandibular ameloblastoma with metastasis to the lungs and lymph nodes: a case report and review of the literature. *J Oral Maxillofac Surg* 1989;47:623–628.
83. Weir MM, Centeno BA, Szyfelbein WM. Cytological features of malignant metastatic ameloblastoma: a case report and differential diagnosis. *Diagn Cytopathol* 1998;18:125–131.
84. Levine SE, Mossler JA, Johnston WW. The cytologic appearance of metastatic ameloblastoma. *Acta Cytol* 1981;25:295–298.
85. Sharma S, Misra K, Dev G. Malignant ameloblastoma. A case report. *Acta Cytol* 1993;37:543–546.
86. Radhika S, Nijhawan R, Das A, et al. Ameloblastoma of the mandible: diagnosis by fine-needle aspiration cytology. *Diagn Cytopathol* 1993; 9:310–313.
87. Stamatakos MD, Houston GD, Fowler CB, et al. Diagnosis of ameloblastoma of the maxilla by fine needle aspiration. A case report. *Acta Cytol* 1995;39:817–820.
88. Günhan O. Fine needle aspiration cytology of ameloblastoma. A report of 10 cases. *Acta Cytol* 1996;40:967–969.
89. Carrillo R, Cuesta C, Rodríguez-Peralto JL, et al. Ameloblastic fibroma. Report of a case with fine needle aspiration cytologic findings. *Acta Cytol* 1992;36:537–540.
90. Bruce RA, Jackson IT. Ameloblastic carcinoma. Report of an aggressive case and review of the literature. *J Cranio-Maxillary-Facial Surg* 1991;19:267–271.
91. Ingram EA, Evans ML, Zitsch RP. Fine-needle aspiration cytology of ameloblastic carcinoma of the maxilla: a rare tumor. *Diagn Cytopathol* 1996;14:249–252.
92. Bocklage TJ, Ardeman T, Schaffner D. Ameloblastic fibroma: a fine-needle aspiration case report. *Diagn Cytopathol* 1997;17:280–286.
93. Verma AK, Tandon R, Saxena S, et al. Aspiration cytology of maxillary myxoma. *Diagn Cytopathol* 1993;9:202–204.
94. Minkowitz G, Fernandez G. Aspirate cytology of giant cell tumors of the bone, giant cell reparative granulomas and pigmented villonodular synovitis: a comparative study (abstract). *Acta Cytol* 1994;38: 837.
95. Kaw YT. Fine needle aspiration cytology of central giant cell granuloma of the jaw. A report of two cases. *Acta Cytol* 1994;38:475–478.
96. Sternberg SS, Antonioli DA, Mills SE, et al, eds. *Diagnostic surgical pathology, 2nd ed, vol 1.* New York: Raven Press, 1994:304–309, 763–767,861–874.
97. Günhan O, Demirel D, Sengün O, et al. Cementifying fibroma diagnosed by fine needle aspiration cytology. A case report. *Acta Cytol* 1992;36:98–100.
98. Layfield LJ, Glasgow BJ, Anders KH, et al. Fine needle aspiration cytology of primary bone lesions. *Acta Cytol* 1987;31:177–184.
99. Agarwal PK, Wahal KM. Cytopathologic study of primary tumors of bones and joints. *Acta Cytol* 1983;27:23–27.
100. Scher RL, Oostingh PE, Levine PA, et al. Role of fine needle aspiration in the diagnosis of lesions of the oral cavity, oropharynx, and nasopharynx. *Cancer* 1988;62:2602–2606.
101. Domanski HA, Åkerman M. Fine-needle aspiration cytology of tongue swellings: a study of 75 cases. *Diagn Cytopathol* 1998;18: 387–392.
102. Castelli M, Gattuso P, Reyes C, et al. Fine needle aspiration biopsy of intraoral and pharyngeal lesions. *Acta Cytol* 1993;37:448–450.
103. Enzinger FM, Weiss SW. *Soft tissue tumors, 3rd ed.* St Louis: Mosby-Year Book, 1995.
104. Löwhagen T, Rubio CA. The cytology of the granular cell myoblastoma of the breast. Report of a case. *Acta Cytol* 1977;21:314–315.
105. Layfield LJ. Fine-needle aspiration of the head and neck. *Pathology* 1996;4:409–438.
106. Layfield LJ, Glasgow BJ. Aspiration biopsy cytology of primary cutaneous tumors. *Acta Cytol* 1993;37:679–688.
107. Bondeson L, Andreasson L. Aspiration cytology of adult rhabdomyoma. *Acta Cytol* 1986;30:679–682.
108. Eigenbrodt ML, Cunningham LF. Fine needle aspiration cytology of a rhabdomyoma of the pharynx. *Acta Cytol* 1986;30:528–532.
109. Liliemark J, Tani E, Mellstedt H, et al. Fine-needle aspiration cytology and immunocytochemistry of malignant non-Hodgkin's lymphoma in the oral cavity. *Oral Surg Oral Med Oral Pathol* 1989;68: 599–603.
110. Feinmesser R, Miyazaki I, Cheung R, et al. Diagnosis of nasopharyngeal carcinoma by DNA amplification of tissue obtained by fine-needle aspiration. *N Engl J Med* 1992;326:17–21.
111. Sgrignoli A, Abati A. Cytologic diagnosis of anaplastic large cell lymphoma. *Acta Cytol* 1997;41:1048–1052.
112. Fagan MF, Rone R. Esthesioneuroblastoma: cytologic features with differential diagnostic considerations. *Diagn Cytopathol* 1985;1:322–326.
113. Jelen M, Wozniak Z, Rak J. Cytologic appearance of esthesioneuroblastoma in a fine needle aspirate. *Acta Cytol* 1988;32:377–380.
114. Ferris CA, Schnadig VJ, Quinn FB, et al. Olfactory neuroblastoma. Cytodiagnostic features in a case with ultrastructural and immunohistochemical correlation. *Acta Cytol* 1988;32:381–385.

14C

CYTOPATHOLOGY OF THE THYROID GLAND

WILLIAM C. FAQUIN

Nodules of the thyroid gland are very common. In fact, it is estimated that as many as 4% to 7% of the adult population has a palpable thyroid enlargement, and up to 10 times this number of individuals may have subclinical nodules that can be detected only by ultrasound or at autopsy (1–5). Thyroid nodules are more common in women at an older age, with a history of radiation exposure, or with certain diets rich in goitrogens or deficient in iodine (6–8). The vast majority of thyroid nodules are benign, with only a small fraction representing malignant disease; malignant thyroid lesions account for approximately 1.1% of all cancers annually (9,10). This extremely large number of benign thyroid lesions and the small number of admixed malignant ones creates a clinical dilemma: how to manage patients with a detectable thyroid enlargement that statistically is more likely to be benign. Over the past two decades, fine-needle aspiration (FNA) has developed as the most reliable method for detecting clinically significant thyroid lesions and for guiding the clinical management of patients by helping to select out those individuals more likely to have a malignancy (11–14).

From the cytopathologist's point of view, thyroid lesions to be evaluated by FNA can be divided into two groups: (a) those lesions for which FNA is primarily a screening procedure and (b) those lesions for which FNA is a diagnostic test. The first group, where FNA is a screening procedure, consists of follicular and oncocytic lesions of the thyroid including multinodular goiter, follicular adenoma, follicular carcinoma, and oncocytic neoplasms. For this group of lesions, FNA is able to identify a majority that are almost certainly benign and that, in many instances, can be managed without direct surgical intervention. The remainder of the cases fall into a category of follicular neoplasms where histologic evaluation is necessary to distinguish a benign follicular lesion from a malignant one. The second group of thyroid lesions is that for which FNA is a diagnostic test and includes inflammatory lesions as well as malignancies (papillary thyroid carcinoma, insular carcinoma, anaplastic carcinoma, medullary carcinoma, malignant lymphoma, and metastatic disease).

ACCURACY OF THYROID FNA

Thyroid FNA is widely accepted as a highly cost-effective and accurate means of evaluating a thyroid nodule (14). It is considered by many to be the most sensitive and most specific nonsurgical thyroid cancer test available (3,15,16). Results from several groups indicate that thyroid FNA is at least as accurate as frozen section, and for papillary thyroid carcinomas, the most common thyroid malignancy, the accuracy of FNA is superior to that of frozen section (17–21). False-negative and false-positive FNA diagnoses occur, but they are uncommon, averaging less than 5% and 1%, respectively (3). In experienced hands, the diagnostic accuracy of thyroid FNA for technically satisfactory specimens is greater than 95%, with positive predictive values of 89% to 98% and negative predictive values of 94% to 99% (6,22–25). Approximately 5% to 10% of thyroid aspirates are considered "unsatisfactory" (fewer than six groups of follicular cells each containing 10 or more cells) (11); however, very few (1.1%) of these patients are subsequently found to have a malignancy (2,3,16,26,27).

NORMAL THYROID ELEMENTS DETECTED BY FNA

The two principal components of a normal thyroid aspirate are the thyroid hormone-producing follicular cells and colloid. C cells are generally too few to be recognized by FNA under normal conditions, and scant inflammatory cells may be present but are generally associated with benign inflammatory conditions (11). Aspirated follicular cells are uniform, low cuboidal-type cells forming flat cohesive sheets with a honeycomb arrangement and without significant crowding, microfollicles, or papillary formations (6,28,29). The normal follicles obtained during thyroid aspiration are macrofollicles, generally comprised of more than 12 follicular cells per follicle, and surrounding spheres of colloid (30). Often, the follicular epithelium may appear as a flat sheet because of fragmentation of macrofollicles or as spherical structures as a result of collapse of the macrofollicle with extrusion of the colloid during smear preparation (Fig. 1). Single intact follicular cells are scant in benign aspirates, although scattered follicular cell naked nuclei resembling lymphoctyes are frequently observed (31). The nuclei of normal follicular cells are round to oval, somewhat variable in size, with a smooth nuclear membrane and a granular and mildly hyperchromatic chromatin pattern and inconspicuous nucleoli. The cytoplasm of the follicular cell is pale and delicate with poorly defined cell borders, whereas a dense waxy cytoplasm, a feature of papillary thyroid carcinomas, is considered abnormal (32–34). When reactive or reparative changes occur, follicular cells can show enlarged nuclei with prominent nucleoli; however, the chromatin pattern remains fine, and the cells maintain their cohesiveness and orderly arrangement.

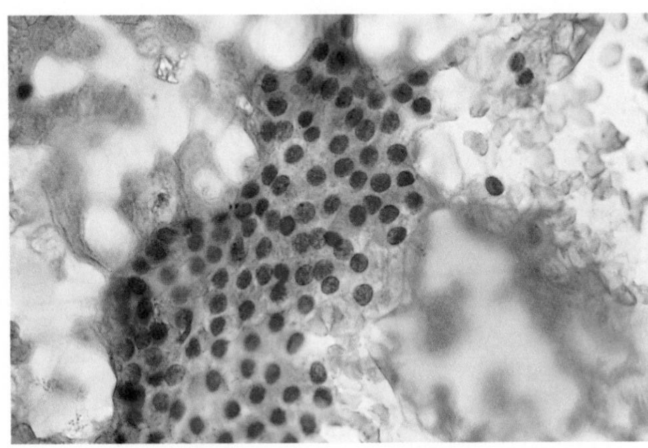
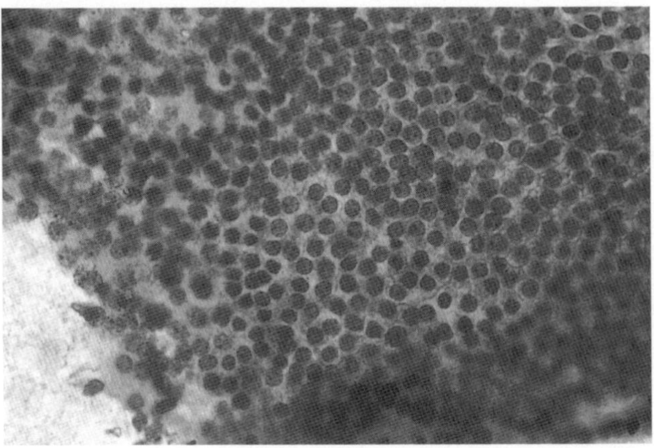

FIGURE 1. Normal follicular cells in flat sheets with an orderly honeycomb arrangement **(A)** and in collapsed macrofollicles **(B).** (Papanicolaou stain.)

Under conditions in which the thyroid is hyperfunctional, the follicular cells may develop a highly vacuolated cytoplasm, an appearance often referred to as a flame cell (6,35). Flame cells are commonly seen in toxic goiter (Graves' disease), and when numerous, their presence suggests the diagnosis. However, flame cells can also be seen in a variety of other conditions, including multinodular goiter and Hashimoto's thyroiditis (36).

Oncocytic changes in follicular cells occur in a variety of nonneoplastic and neoplastic disorders of the thyroid. These cells are known by several different names, including Hurthle cells, oncocytes, Askanazy cells, and oxyphilic cells (6). Microscopically, Hurthle cells are characterized by the presence of abundant finely granular cytoplasm that stains blue to eosinophilic using the Papanicolaou stain. Hurthle cells typically have a plasmacytoid appearance because of their eccentrically placed enlarged nuclei. Nucleoli may be very prominent or inconspicuous, and nuclear atypia is widely variable (37,38).

Scant chronic inflammatory cells may be present normally or may be abundant in cases of thyroiditis. Occasionally, however, naked nuclei of normal follicular cells may mimic lymphocytes. Generally, lymphocytes are distinguished from naked follicular nuclei by their thin rim of intact cytoplasm, more heterogeneous chromatin, and less prominent nuclear membranes (6). Other features supporting a lymphoid origin include the presence of background lymphoglandular bodies (small detached fragments of lymphocyte cytoplasm) as well as a spectrum of nuclear sizes reflecting the range of maturation of the lymphoid population.

Colloid, the storage site of thyroid hormone, changes in form depending on the functional state of the thyroid, with pale, watery colloid being produced by more active thyroid glands. In general, the presence of abundant colloid in fine-needle aspirates of the thyroid tends to be a feature of benign thyroid lesions, as abundant colloid correlates with the presence of many macrofollicles, whereas scant colloid and abundant cells correlate with microfollicular or neoplastic thyroid lesions (39). Microscopically, colloid has two forms, watery and dense (Fig. 2). Watery colloid is often easier to appreciate in air-dried Diff-Quik–stained smears, where it is recognized by its characteristic linear cracking artifact (6,11). In contrast to watery colloid, which can be difficult to identify in Papanicoulaou-stained smears, dense colloid is easy to appreciate in both air-dried and alcohol-fixed prepara-

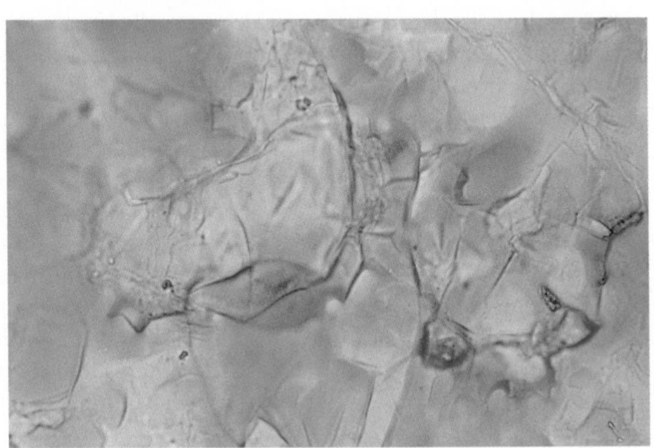
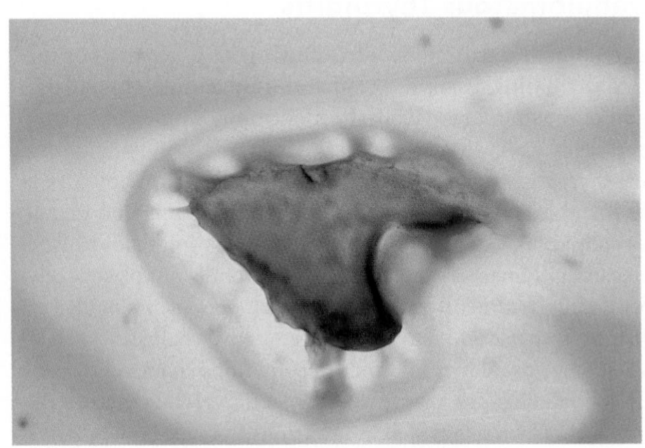

FIGURE 2. Colloid. Abundant watery colloid showing a characteristic linear cracking pattern **(A)** and dense colloid with irregular, sharp edges **(B).** (Papanicolaou stain.)

tions. It appears as irregular collections of sharp-edged homogeneous material staining green or orange in Pap and deep purple using Diff-Quik (11).

Normal Thyroid Elements Detected by FNA

1. Follicular cells in flat sheets and macrofollicles
2. Orderly honeycomb arrangement of cells
3. Watery or dense colloid
4. Scant chronic inflammatory cells
5. Rare Hurthle cells
6. Blood

NONNEOPLASTIC CONDITIONS

Acute Thyroiditis

Acute thyroiditis is a rare condition, usually bacterial in origin, that typically is a clinical diagnosis and, therefore, infrequently aspirated (40,41). Occasionally, however, acute thyroiditis may present as a focal thyroid nodule mimicking a thyroid neoplasm (e.g., an inflamed anaplastic thyroid carcinoma) and leading to FNA (6). Microscopically, the aspirated material consists of an abundance of neutrophils along with histiocytes and necrotic debris (41). Associated follicular epithelium may show reparative changes such as nuclear enlargement, abundant cytoplasm, and prominent nucleoli. Bacteria or other organisms may be identified in smears, and often the most clinically useful information will be obtained from culture and sensitivity testing of the aspirated material.

Cytologic Features of Acute Thyroiditis

1. Abundant neutrophils
2. Histiocytes
3. Necrotic debris
4. Scant follicular cells with reparative changes

Granulomatous Thyroiditis

Granulomatous thyroiditis, also known as DeQuervain's or subacute thyroiditis, is an uncommon diffuse and painful enlargement of the thyroid typically affecting young women (42). In its later stages, it may have a nodular character. FNA of granulomatous thyroiditis tends to yield a scantily cellular specimen (43). Microscopically, giant cells, especially surrounding and engulfing colloid, as well as nodular aggregates of epithelioid histiocytes (granulomas) are seen (Fig. 3). Lymphocytes, plasma cells, eosinophils, and neutrophils may also be present. Follicular epithelium is sparse and may show degenerative changes with reactive atypia (44). Thyroid aspirates containing giant cells raise a differential diagnosis that includes systemic granulomatous diseases such as sarcoid as well as infections, foreign bodies, palpation thyroiditis, Hashimoto's thyroiditis, and papillary thyroid carcinoma (6,45).

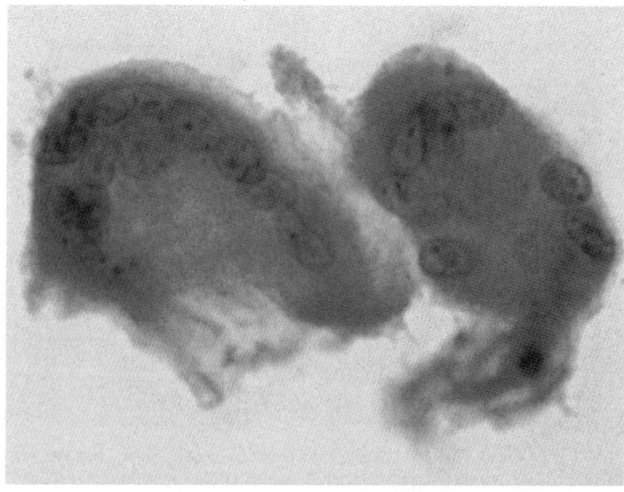

FIGURE 3. Granulomatous thyroiditis. Giant cells present in a scantily cellular thyroid aspirate. (Papanicolaou stain.)

Cytologic Features of Granulomatous Thyroiditis

1. Scant cellularity
2. Giant cells
3. Clusters of epithelioid histiocytes
4. Chronic inflammation
5. Follicular cells with degenerative changes

Chronic Lymphocytic Thyroiditis (Hashimoto's Thyroiditis)

Hashimoto's thyroiditis is an autoimmune disorder clinically presenting in middle-aged white women as hypothyroidism and a diffuse thyroid enlargement (7,42). In a small proportion of cases (fewer than 10%), a dominant thyroid nodule may be present (46). Microscopically, the thyroid aspirate shows the characteristic combination of two features: lymphocytes and oncocytic follicular epithelium (Fig. 4) (43). The smear background typically contains a combination of abundant lymphocytes, plasma cells, lymphohistiocytic aggregates, fragments of germinal centers, and tingible body macrophages (47,48). In over 75% of cases, the follicular epithelium, which is usually less abundant than the inflammatory component of the aspirate, shows a prominent oncocytic metaplasia (Hurthle cells) as evidenced by abundant finely granular cytoplasm (49). Occasional follicular cells may display marked atypia. Nononcocytic follicular epithelium is also usually present, and colloid is scant. Other features that may be seen include flame cells, squamous metaplasia, occasional microfollicles, and giant cells (6,43). In most cases, the diagnosis of Hashimoto's thyroiditis is straightforward in thyroid aspirates, although in a small subset of cases, the atypical features of the nonneoplastic Hurthle cells (including pleomorphic bizarre nuclei and prominent nucleoli) can mimic an oncocytic neoplasm. The latter, however, lacks a significant lymphoid population.

Another thyroid disorder containing increased numbers of lymphocytes is chronic nonspecific thyroiditis. In this condition,

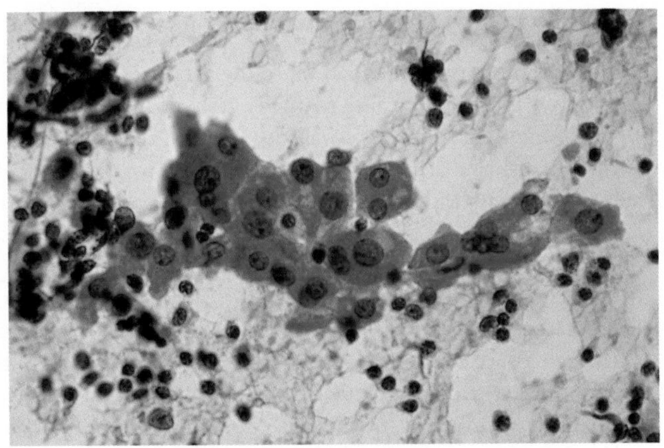
A

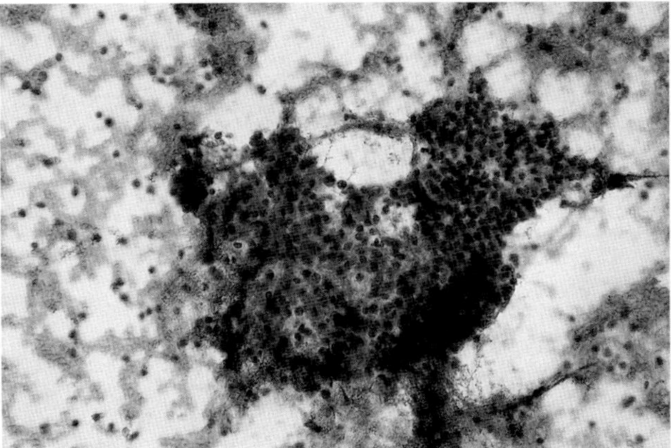
B

FIGURE 4. Hashimoto's thyroiditis. **A:** Hurthle cells in a background of abundant lymphocytes. **B:** Germinal center fragments. (Papanicolaou stain.)

Hurthle cells are rare, and, unlike Hashimoto's thyroiditis, antithyroid antibodies are negative or low in titer (6). Hashimoto's thyroiditis is known to be associated with an increased incidence of malignant lymphoma (50), but the usual features of a reactive lymphoid process including the presence of a mixed population of lymphocytes with many small mature lymphocytes and occasional tingible body macrophages support a benign process. Flow cytometry can be a useful ancillary technique for those cases where an involvement by malignant lymphoma is suspected.

Cytologic Features of Hashimoto's Thyroiditis

1. Abundant lymphocytes and plasma cells
2. Germinal center fragments
3. Follicular cells with oncocytic changes (Hurthle cells)

Riedel's Thryoiditis

Riedel's thryoiditis is an extremely rare sclerosing thyroid condition primarily affecting middle-aged women (7). FNAs of this lesion are frequently scantily cellular and often may be technically unsatisfactory (31,51). Microscopically, fragments of collagenous fibrous tissue, scattered spindle cells, and chronic inflammatory cells are seen. The clinical findings of a hard thyroid mass with extension outside of the thyroid into surrounding structures of the neck may suggest a malignant process, but the absence of malignant tumor cells in the fine-needle aspirate rules this out. Cytologically, the main differential diagnosis is with the fibrosing variant of Hashimoto's thyroiditis, which in most cases is distinguished from Riedel's thyroiditis by the presence of Hurthle cells as well as numerous lymphocytes and germinal center fragments, features not found in Riedel's thyroiditis (6,51).

Toxic Goiter (Graves' Disease)

Toxic goiter or Graves' disease is a diffuse hyperfunctional thyroid disorder of middle-aged women. It is usually diagnosed clinically and thus is seldom sampled by FNA. When it is encountered, the cytologic features include a cellular and often bloody smear with watery colloid and with atypical follicular cells (nuclear enlargement, mild pleomorphism, and conspicuous nucleoli) (52). The cytoplasm of the follicular cells is highly vacuolated, and in air-dried preparations stained with Romanowsky-type stains, the vacuoles contain a homogeneous metachromatic material that stains darker at the edges of the cell. Cells with these characteristics are often referred to as flame cells (6). Other features seen in Graves' disease include focal Hurthle cell change as well as occasional epithelioid cell granulomas, multinucleated giant cells, and scant lymphocytes (52,53). Although the cytologic features of Graves' disease are fairly characteristic, there is some overlap with two other entities, Hashimoto's thyroiditis and subacute thyroiditis: these thyroid disorders are distinguished from Graves' disease by their abundant rather than scant Hurthle cells and giant cells, respectively.

Cytologic Features of Graves' Disease

1. Cellular smear
2. Flame cells
3. Abundant vacuolated cytoplasm
4. Metachromatic vacuolar material using Romanowsky stains

Amyloid Goiter

Amyloid goiter is a condition characterized by either focal or diffuse infiltration of the thyroid by amyloid (11). It occurs in approximately 80% of patients with secondary amyloidosis and in up to 50% of patients with primary amyloidosis (54). Thyroid aspirates show a scantily cellular smear with abundant amorphous material that stains pink or orange with the Papanicolaou stain (Fig. 5). Amyloid may be difficult to distinguish from colloid in fine-needle aspirates, but its identity as amyloid can be confirmed by demonstrating the characteristic apple-green dichroism using the Congo-red stain (11,54). Follicular cells are usually scant in amyloid goiter, and occasional multinucleated

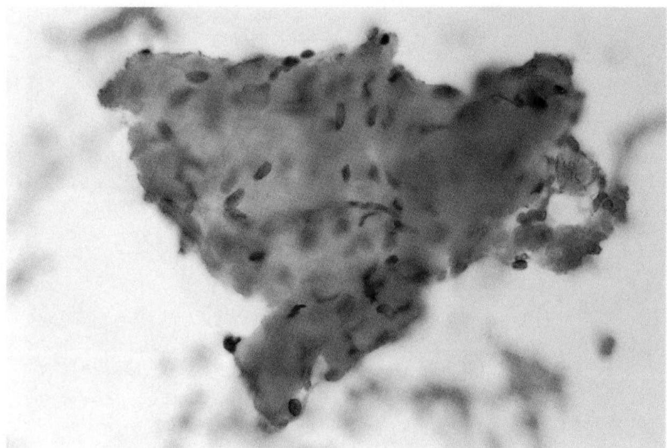

FIGURE 5. Amyloid goiter. Amorphous opaque, eosinophilic-staining amyloid in a Papanicolaou-stained thyroid aspirate. (Courtesy of Dr. Edmund Cibas, Brigham and Women's Hospital, Boston, MA.)

giant cells may be present. The main differential diagnosis of amyloid goiter is with amyloid-rich medullary carcinoma, which may also present as a scantily cellular aspirate with abundant amyloid. Medullary carcinoma can be ruled out, however, by carefully searching to exclude the presence of diagnostic malignant neuroendocrine tumor cells.

Black Thyroid

Black thyroid is a condition among patients chronically taking antibiotics of the tetracycline group such as minocycline, and resulting in grossly detectable dark-brown pigmentation of the thyroid (55,56). It is usually an incidental finding on FNA. Aspirates of black thyroid show follicular cells with otherwise normal cytologic features except for the presence of numerous dark, course granules within the cytoplasm (Fig. 6). The granules often stain for melanin. Although uncommon in a thyroid aspirate, recognition of this unusual feature as a benign condition may prevent unnecessary surgery in these patients (11,55).

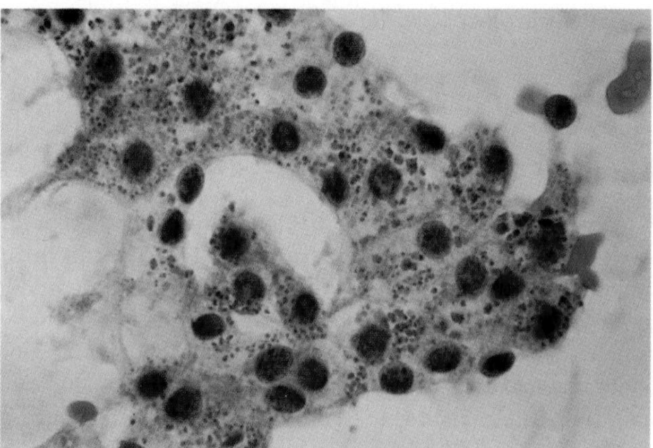

FIGURE 6. Black thyroid. Papanicolaou-stained thyroid aspirate showing follicular cells containing abundant coarse brown cytoplasmic granules (Courtesy of Dr. Edmund Cibas, Brigham and Women's Hospital, Boston, MA.)

Radiation-Related Changes

Radiation, both external radiation to the neck as well as systemic radioactive iodine, can cause marked cytologic atypia in thyroid FNAs, potentially leading to a false-positive diagnosis (6,57). Although usually arranged in flat sheets, occasional follicular cells affected by radiation may be markedly enlarged (giant), highly pleomorphic, or bizarre (58). Nuclear atypia includes dark and coarsely granular chromatin, prominent nucleoli, and intranuclear pseudoinclusions (59). The cytoplasm of radiated follicular cells is generally abundant and often vacuolated. Although there may be significant nuclear enlargement, the overall nuclear-to-cytoplasmic ratio will usually remain relatively unchanged. Because of the presence of the sometimes markedly atypical or bizarre cells, the differential diagnosis of radiation-related changes includes follicular carcinoma and anaplastic carcinoma (11). However, the lack of a predominant microfollicular pattern as seen in many follicular carcinomas, and the absence of the dyshesive single cell pattern and abundant frankly malignant cells of anaplastic carcinoma help to rule out these two malignancies.

Cytologic Features of Radiation-Related Changes

1. Cell enlargement with preservation of a normal N/C ratio
2. Flat sheets of orderly cells
3. Occasional pleomorphic or bizarre cells
4. Abundant vacuolated cytoplasm
5. Intranuclear pseudoinclusions

FOLLICULAR AND ONCOCYTIC LESIONS: FNA AS A SCREENING TEST

Follicular lesions including multinodular goiter, follicular adenomas, follicular carcinomas, and oncocytic neoplasms comprise a majority of the lesions sampled by FNA of the thyroid gland (32). This large group of thyroid lesions is diagnosed histologically based primarily on architectural features such as capsular or vascular invasion rather than on cytologic criteria (7,60,61). For this reason, it is not possible to use cytologic principles to distinguish each of these histologic entities. Instead, the role of FNA in evaluating follicular and oncocytic lesions of the thyroid is to function as a screening test (11,61). Thus, although a specific diagnosis may not be given, it is possible to subcategorize these lesions into two groups: those that are almost certainly benign (including most multinodular goiters and some adenomas) and those that are suspicious for a follicular neoplasm and possibly malignant (including all carcinomas and some adenomas) (Table 1). This subcategorization identifies a majority of patients with benign lesions for whom surgical intervention can usually be avoided (11,12,62).

The cytologic criteria used to distinguish benign from suspicious thyroid lesions include the follicular group architecture, smear cellularity, amount of colloid, and cytologic atypia (11). By far, the most important of these criteria is follicular architecture, specifically whether the lesion is composed predominantly

TABLE 1. FNA OF FOLLICULAR LESIONS OF THE THYROID

Cytologic Feature	FNA Diagnosis	Histologic Diagnosis
Predominantly macrofollicular	Benign	Multinodular goiter and some follicular adenomas
Predominantly microfollicular or trabecular	Suspicious for a follicular neoplasm	Follicular carcinomas and some follicular adenomas

of macrofollicles or microfollicles, trabeculae, and crowded groups. This approach works because follicular carcinomas are virtually never composed of macrofollicles (61). In smears of thyroid aspirates, macrofollicles are recognized as colloid-filled spheres, usually with far more than 12 follicular cells, or as flat sheets of evenly spaced follicular cells. The flat sheets result from fragmentation of macrofollicles with extrusion of colloid during the smear preparation. Smears with a predominance of macrofollicles and flat orderly honeycomb sheets of follicular cells are diagnosed as benign thyroid nodules by FNA. In contrast, thyroid aspirates composed of microfollicles (small follicular groups of 6–12 follicular cells in a ring with or without a small amount of central colloid) or crowded trabeculae and groups of overlapping follicular cells are a feature of follicular carcinomas as well as some adenomas (2). These aspirates are diagnosed as suspicious for a follicular neoplasm, and it is this group of patients for whom surgical removal of the lesion is generally considered warranted (16).

Benign Follicular Lesions

Follicular lesions of the thyroid gland diagnosed as benign by FNA include multinodular goiters and follicular adenomas with a predominant macrofollicular pattern (see above) (Fig. 7). The aspirates of these lesions are hypo- to moderately cellular with moderate to abundant colloid (63). Follicular cells are generally cytologically bland with nuclei of uniform size with evenly dispersed granular chromatin and inconspicuous nucleoli. Often foam cells may be present, particularly in cases with cystic degeneration (Fig. 8). Problems may arise in diagnosing these lesions when the aspirates are hypercellular, when occasional microfollicles or Hurthle cells are present, or when spindle-shaped cells are found. All of these features may be seen in aspirates of benign thyroid conditions, and when focally present in a background of macrofollicles and flat uncrowded orderly follicular sheets, the smear should be diagnosed as benign even if the specimen is hypercellular (11). In fact, the presence of different cell types including normal follicular cells, Hurthle cells, flame cells, and foam cells favors a multinodular goiter (63).

Suspicious Follicular Lesions

The majority of follicular lesions diagnosed by FNA as suspicious for a follicular neoplasm are adenomas with a microfollicular or trabecular architecture, and a minority are actually follicular carcinomas (64–66). Most suspicious aspirates are hypercellular, contain scant colloid (reflecting the abundance of microfollicles), and some may show prominent nuclear atypia (enlarged pleomorphic nuclei, uneven clumped chromatin, prominent nucleoli, and grooves) (Fig. 9) (6). The key feature, however, in identifying this group of lesions is the finding of a significant proportion of microfollicles, trabeculae, or crowded overlapping clusters of follicular cells (Fig. 10).

One follicular neoplasm that is particularly important to recognize because of its resemblance to papillary thyroid carcinoma is the hyalinizing trabecular adenoma (67,68). Cytologic features of this lesion include follicular cells in aggregates and as single cells associated with amorphous hyaline material that is not amyloid. The atypical nuclei of these cells have nuclear grooves and intranuclear pseudoinclusions mimicking papillary carcinoma, but the finding of stromal material, which may be scant, is useful in suggesting the correct diagnosis (see below) (68,69).

A

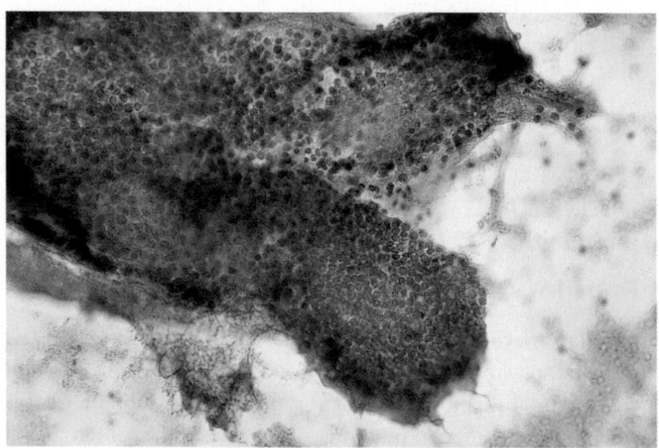

B

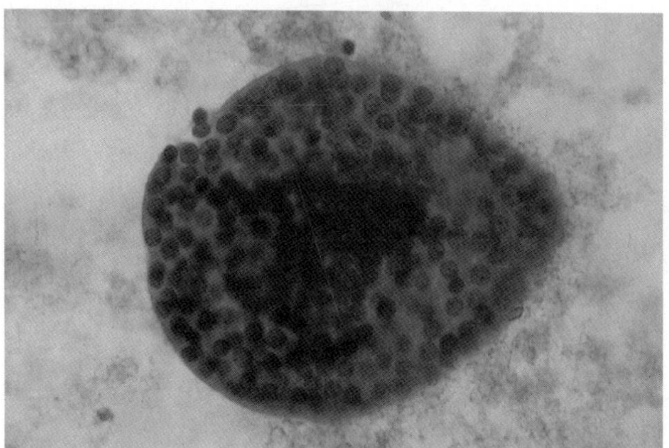

FIGURE 7. Macrofollicular adenoma. Papanicolaou-stained smear showing collapsed macrofollicles from a thyroid aspirate (**A** and **B**).

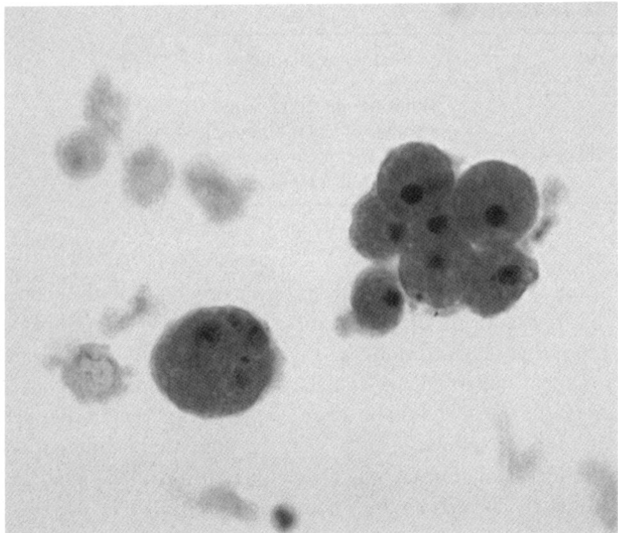

FIGURE 8. Hemosiderin-laden macrophages. These cells with abundant foamy cytoplasm are a feature of cystic degeneration and can be seen in both benign and malignant thyroid lesions. (Papanicolaou stain.)

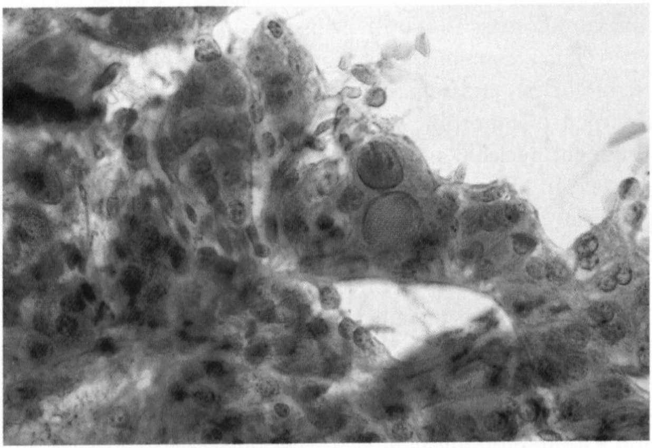

FIGURE 9. Follicular neoplasm (microfollicular adenoma). Cellular aspirate with scant colloid and atypical follicular cells forming microfollicles. (Papanicolaou stain.)

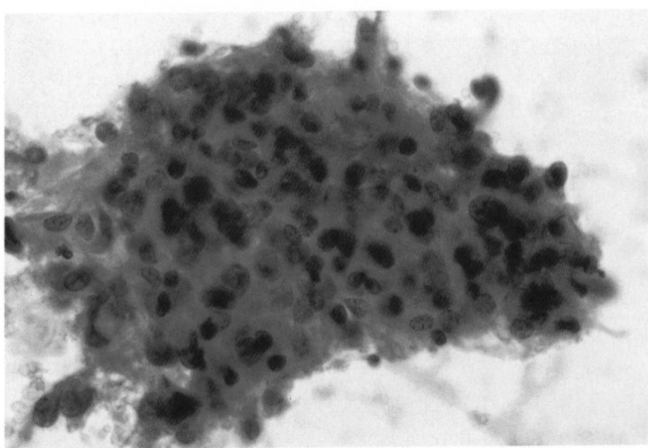

FIGURE 10. Follicular neoplasm (follicular carcinoma). Crowded clusters of follicular cells and absence of a follicular architecture. (Papanicolaou stain.)

ONCOCYTIC (HURTHLE CELL) NEOPLASMS

A significant proportion of follicular neoplasms of the thyroid are those with oncocytic (Hurthle cell) features and include both Hurthle cell adenomas and Hurthle cell carcinomas (Fig. 11) (7,70–72). These two neoplasms cannot be distinguished by FNA because, like other follicular lesions of the thyroid, their histologic diagnosis depends on recognizing the presence or absence of capsular and/or vascular invasion (73). Therefore, both of these neoplasms are diagnosed by FNA as suspicious for an oncocytic (Hurthle cell) neoplasm. FNA correctly identifies the vast majority of Hurthle cell neoplasms as neoplastic (38). In addition, FNA is important in distinguishing between true Hurthle cell neoplasms and other benign conditions with Hurthle cell changes such as Hashimoto's thyroiditis or multinodular goiter.

The typical cytologic features of Hurthle cell neoplasms include a cellular smear with a uniform population of dyshesive cells with abundant granular cytoplasm, small red nucleoli, and finely granular chromatin (38,74,75). Nuclei are usually eccentrically placed, giving a plasmacytoid appearance, and binucleation is common. Colloid tends to be scant, and chronic inflammation is absent or sparse. The cells can appear bland and often form crowded three-dimensional aggregates as well as occasional sheets with well-defined cell borders and follicles (38). In Hashimoto's thyroiditis and multinodular goiter, Hurthle cells tend to represent a minor cellular component, and the Hurthle cells often lack the prominent nucleoli characteristic of true Hurthle cell neoplasms (11). Another important thyroid lesion that should be excluded when evaluating a Hurthle cell neoplasm is medullary carcinoma because both are characterized by a population of dyshesive plasmacytoid cells. In contrast to Hurthle cell neoplasms, medullary carcinomas have a "salt-and-pepper" chromatin pattern, lack nucleoli, and contain red cytoplasmic granules in Diff-Quik–stained smears. When in doubt, however, immunocytchemical stains for calcitonin and thyroglobulin can be used to differentiate these two neoplasms.

Cytologic Features of Oncocytic (Hurthle Cell) Neoplasms

1. Uniform population of dyshesive cells
2. Abundant oncocytic cytoplasm
3. Plasmacytoid appearance
4. Prominent red nucleoli

MALIGNANT THYROID LESIONS: FNA AS A DIAGNOSTIC TEST

Papillary Thyroid Carcinoma

Papillary thyroid carcinoma is by far the most common malignant neoplasm of the thyroid, accounting for up to 80% of all thyroid malignancies (7). It is typically an indolent neoplasm that is more common in young to middle-aged women as well as in patients with a history of prior radiation exposure (76). FNA is highly accurate in the diagnosis of papillary thyroid carcinoma

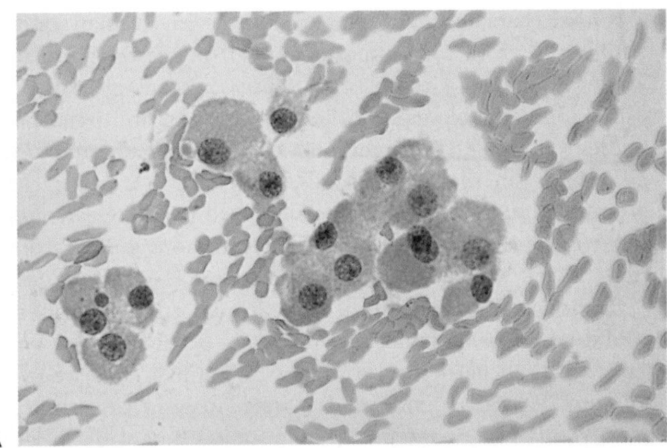
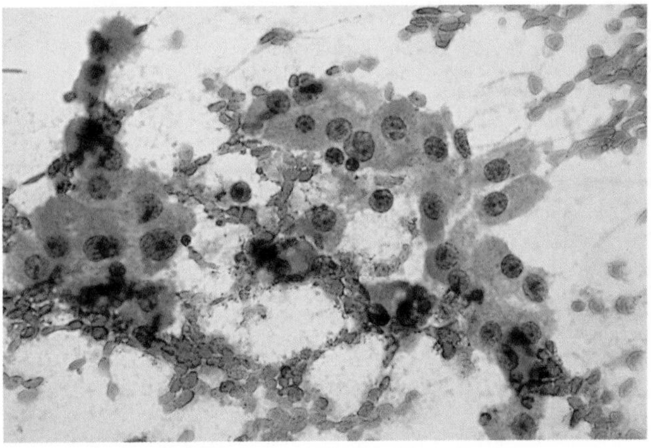

FIGURE 11. Hurthle cell neoplasms. Papanicolaou-stained smears containing dyshesive cells with abundant granular cytoplasm. Architectural features, not present in cytologic smears, are required to distinguish between a Hurthle cell adenoma **(A)** and a Hurthle cell carcinoma **(B).**

(77) because the classic diagnostic criteria are principally cytologic characteristics. Over 90% of papillary thyroid carcinomas are correctly diagnosed as positive or suspicious on FNA (11,32).

Aspirates of this neoplasm are usually cellular with mildly enlarged epithelial cells in flat sheets and crowded clusters that have lost the orderly honeycomb arrangement typical of benign lesions. The cytoplasm of papillary carcinoma can vary from scant to abundant and densely granular or eosinophilic, but the character of the cytoplasm is not considered a primary diagnostic feature. Instead, it is the nucleus that holds the cytologic key to diagnosing this thyroid cancer.

The nuclei of papillary thyroid carcinoma are enlarged and oval with mild pleomorphism, a pale finely granular "powdery" chromatin pattern, and one or more small but prominent marginated nucleoli (33,34,78). Nuclear hyperchromasia, necrosis, mitoses, and bizarre nuclei are not typically seen. The most sensitive, diagnostically important feature of papillary thyroid carcinomas is the presence of longitudinal nuclear grooving (Fig. 12) (79,80). Nuclear grooves are seen in almost all cases of papillary thyroid carcinoma, although they may be sparse in up to 25% of cases. The nuclear grooves are more easily appreciated in cytologic preparations than in histologic sections. Grooved nuclei are not specific for papillary thyroid carcinoma because they may be seen at least focally in a variety of other benign and malignant thyroid conditions, including chronic thyroiditis, multinodular goiter, follicular adenomas, and carcinomas (79,80). However, when diffusely present, this feature is highly suggestive of papillary thyroid carcinoma.

Another important cytologic feature of papillary thyroid carcinomas is the presence of intranuclear cytoplasmic pseudoinclusions, found in over 90% of cases (Fig. 13) (34,78). True intranuclear pseudoinclusions are characterized by a sharply defined membrane and homogeneous contents with cytoplasmic staining qualities. They represent invaginations of cytoplasm into the nucleus, explaining their designation as "pseudoinclusions." Although intranuclear pseudoinclusions can be found in many other primary thyroid as well as nonthyroid neoplasms, their presence in aspirated follicular epithelial cells of the thyroid

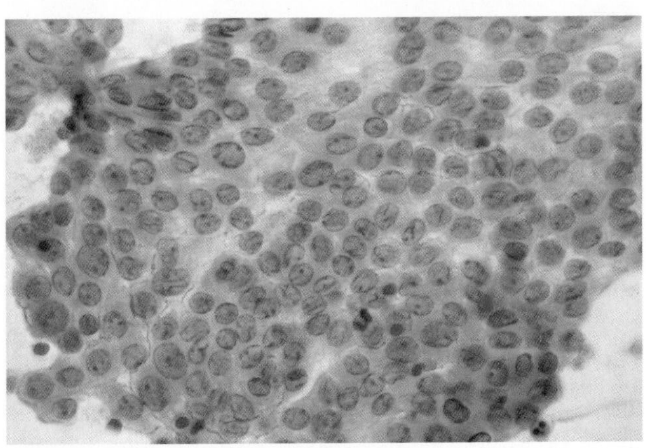

FIGURE 12. Papillary thyroid carcinoma. Flat sheet of cells with pale chromatin and longitudinal nuclear grooves. (Papanicolaou stain.)

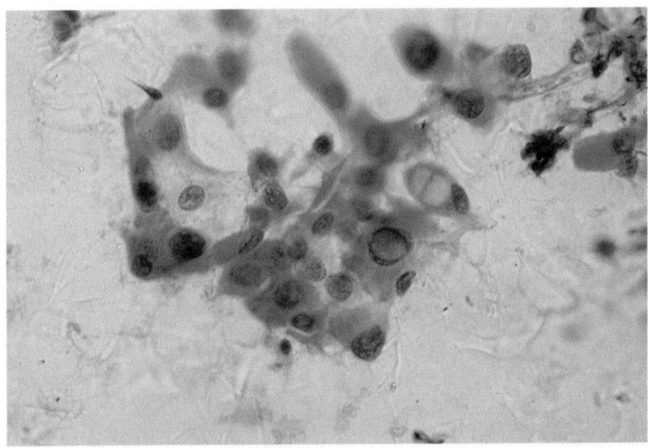

FIGURE 13. Papillary thyroid carcinoma. Carcinoma cells with dense cytoplasm, and atypical nuclei with grooves; a prominent intranuclear pseudoinclusion is present. (Papanicolaou stain.)

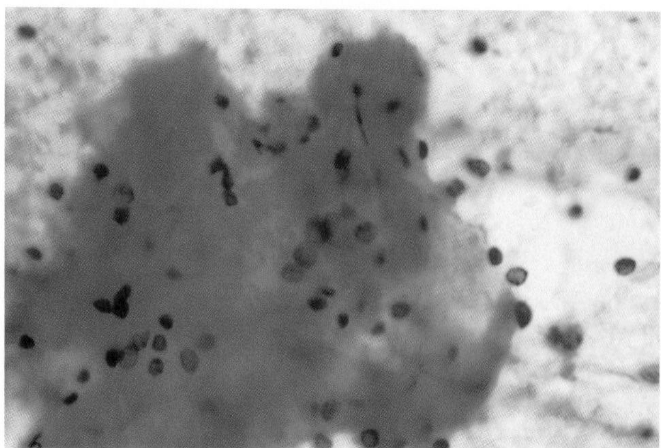

FIGURE 14. Hyalinizing trabecular adenoma. Papanicolaou-stained smear showing dense hyaline stromal material with scattered small uniform follicular cells.

in combination with one or more other nuclear features such as pale chromatin and nuclear grooves is virtually diagnostic of papillary thyroid carcinoma (6,34,78). A key thyroid neoplasm that needs to be included in the differential diagnosis of papillary thyroid carcinoma is hyalinizing trabecular adenoma (Fig. 14). This uncommon lesion is frequently mistaken for papillary thyroid carcinoma in thyroid aspirates (69,81). Although the nuclei contain nuclear grooves and intranuclear pseudoinclusions, a clue to the diagnosis of hyalinizing trabecular adenoma is the presence of metachromatic basement membrane–like material irregularly deposited between cells (82,83).

Papillary structures of various types are found in more than 90% of papillary thyroid carcinomas, and their presence (recognizable microscopically at low power) suggests the possibility of a papillary thyroid carcinoma (Fig. 15) (33). The various papillary structures that may be encountered include three-dimensional, branching papillae with fibrovascular cores; avascular dome-shaped cell aggregates; and two-dimensional flat sheets of cells with finger-like projections (6). Papillary structures may also be seen in hyperplastic disorders, but the nuclear features of papillary carcinoma are not present.

Other characteristic cytologic features seen in many cases of papillary thyroid carcinoma include an increased granular or waxy ("squamoid") cytoplasmic density, viscous often hypereosinophilic "bubble gum" colloid, giant cells, and psammoma bodies (53,78,84,85). Psammoma bodies (laminated round calcifications) in thyroid aspirates, especially in a cystic background, strongly suggest the possibility of papillary carcinoma; however, they must be distinguished from nonspecific calcifications as well as laminated inspissated colloid (Fig. 16).

Although FNA is highly accurate for detecting papillary thyroid carcinomas, false-negative diagnoses occur in about 5% of cases (34). In particular, papillary carcinomas that are cystic (about 17% of cases) may yield aspirated material consisting primarily of cyst contents (foam cells, hemosiderin-laden macrophages, and acellular debris), with only rare epithelial cells (86). Special caution, including a careful search for epithelial cells with nuclear features of papillary thyroid carcinoma, is recommended whenever one is dealing with an aspirate of a thyroid cyst (11). In addition to false-negative cases, occasional thyroid aspirates may lack the classic features of papillary thyroid carcinoma, thus resulting in a suggestive but indeterminate diagnosis. Few ancillary studies have been described to assist the cytopathologist in diagnosing aspirates of papillary thyroid carcinoma; however, several groups have used immunoreactivity to cytokeratin 19 in histologic preparations, and its application may prove useful in cytologic preparations as well (Fig. 17) (87,88).

In addition to the usual type of papillary carcinoma, several variants such as the follicular variant (89) and tall-cell and columnar cell variants may be detected by FNA (90,91). The follicular variant of papillary thyroid carcinoma is not uncommon, but it may pose a diagnostic challenge because of the lack of papillarity and the abundance of microfollicles mimicking a follicular neoplasm. Up to 85% of papillary carcinomas have been found to have variable numbers of follicular structures, with the greatest proportion being found in the follicular variant of papillary thyroid carcinoma (92). In contrast to the mildly to moderately hyperchromatic chromatin seen in follicular neoplasms, the follicular variant of papillary thyroid carcinoma exhibits the

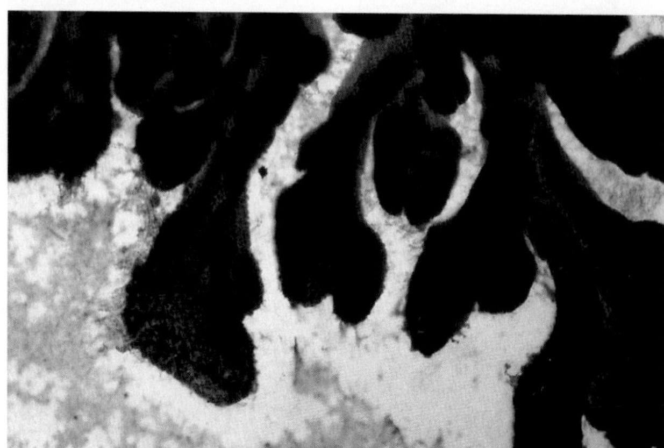

FIGURE 15. Papillary thyroid carcinoma. Papanicolaou-stained smear showing classic papillary architectural features of papillary carcinoma.

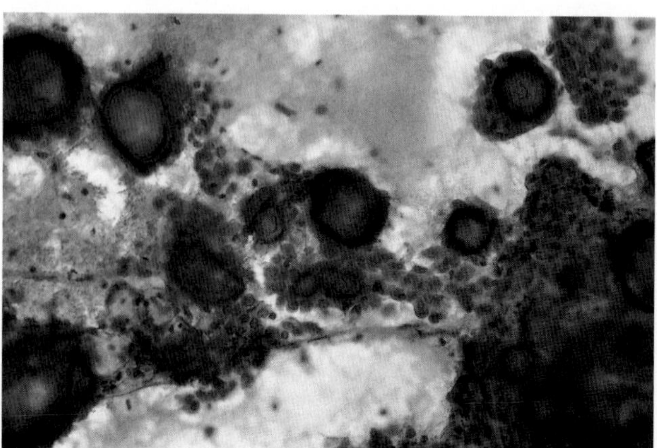

FIGURE 16. Papillary thyroid carcinoma. Clusters of cells surrounding psammoma bodies with their characteristic concentric laminations. (Papanicolaou stain.)

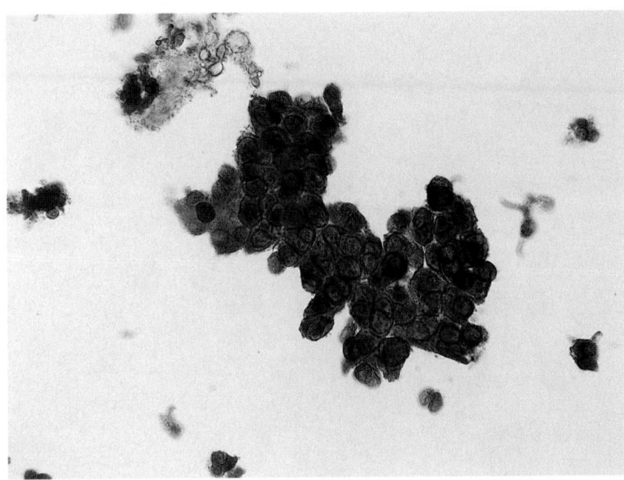

FIGURE 17. Papillary thyroid carcinoma showing positive immunocytochemical reactivity for cytokeratin 19.

typical pale, powdery chromatin along with nuclear grooves and intranuclear pseudoinclusions of papillary carcinoma (92). The tall-cell variant of papillary thyroid carcinoma also has the classic nuclear features but is characterized by abundant granular cytoplasm resembling that of Hurthle cells (90,93). In fact, this variant is sometimes misdiagnosed as a Hurthle cell neoplasm by FNA. Another rare variant of papillary carcinoma is the columnar cell variant, which also has the nuclear features of papillary carcinoma, but the cells are elongate and lack abundant cytoplasm (91). Cells of this variant tend to show crowded, stratified clusters of cells resembling cells from a colonic adenoma. Both the tall-cell and columnar cell variants of papillary thyroid carcinoma are important to recognize because they carry a worse prognosis for the patient than the usual type (7).

Cytologic Features of Papillary Thyroid Carcinoma

1. Nuclear grooves, intranuclear pseudoinclusions, and pale "powdery" chromatin
2. Disordered or overlapping epithelial cells
3. Dense waxy cytoplasm
4. Papillary groups
5. "Bubble-gum" colloid
6. Psammoma bodies
7. Giant cells

Poorly Differentiated Thyroid Carcinoma (Insular Carcinoma)

Insular carcinoma of the thyroid represents approximately 4% to 7% of thyroid carcinomas (94) and is associated with a prognosis intermediate between that of well-differentiated follicular carcinoma and anaplastic carcinoma (95,96). Aspirates of this lesion are cellular with many single cells as well as crowded clusters, trabeculae, and microfollicles with scant colloid (Fig. 18). The malignant cells are small and monomorphic (sometimes with a plasmacytoid appearance), with delicate cytoplasm and a high nuclear-to-cytoplasmic ratio. Nuclei are generally round, mildly hyperchromatic, and cytologically bland, although some cells may have nuclear grooves and prominent nucleoli, and occasional cells are highly pleomorphic (94,96,97). Necrosis can often be identified within the smear background. Although a cytologic diagnosis of malignancy is sometimes possible, especially if highly pleomorphic cells are present, the differential diagnosis includes a follicular neoplasm, anaplastic carcinoma, papillary carcinoma, and medullary carcinoma (6). Insular carcinoma does not contain the large number of bizarre giant cells seen in anaplastic carcinoma, nor does it have the abundant nuclear grooves of papillary carcinoma, nor the "salt-and-pepper" chromatin of medullary carcinoma. For diagnostically difficult cases, immuncytochemistry can be used because insular carcinomas are thyroglobulin positive and calcitonin negative.

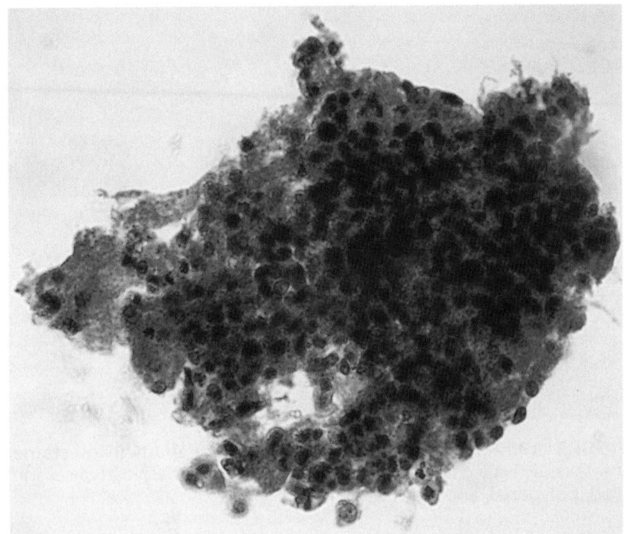

FIGURE 18. Insular carcinoma. Crowded and overlapping group of small, dark cells with scant finely granular cytoplasm. Papanicolaou stain.) (Courtesy of Dr. Edmund Cibas, Brigham and Women's Hospital, Boston, MA.)

Anaplastic Thyroid Carcinoma

Anaplastic thyroid carcinoma accounts for approximately 5% to 10% of all thyroid cancers and is associated in almost all cases with a rapidly fatal prognosis (7,98,99). The cytologic appearance of this highly aggressive carcinoma includes a cellular smear with malignant-appearing, sometimes bizarre, spindled and multinucleated tumor giant cells in groups and as single cells in a background of tumor diathesis (blood, fibrin, inflammation, necrotic cells, and debris) (Fig. 19) (100). The nuclei of anaplastic thyroid carcinoma are highly pleomorphic, with dark, irregular chromatin clumping, macronucleoli, and occasional intranuclear pseudoinclusions (99). Numerous mitotes and abnormal mitotic figures may be seen. In some cases, a variable degree of squamous differentiation may be present, raising the possibility of a poorly differentiated squamous cell carcinoma (99).

The differential diagnosis of anaplastic carcinoma includes metastatic carcinoma, particularly squamous cell carcinoma, and medullary carcinoma. Most anaplastic carcinomas are positive for cytokeratins, but the majority of cases are negative for thy-

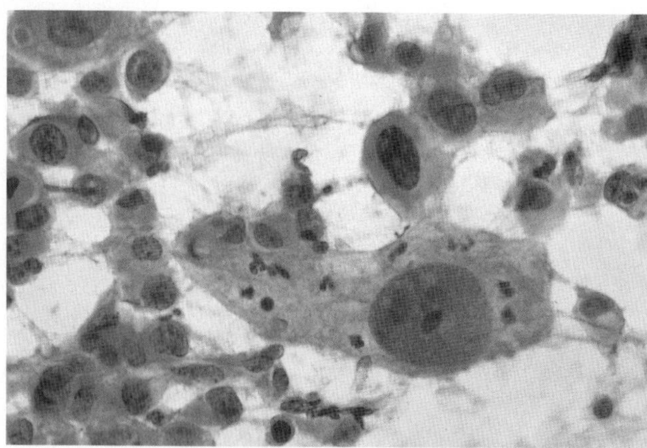

FIGURE 19. Anaplastic thyroid carcinoma. Papanicolaou-stained smear showing a characteristic combination of dyshesive atypical spindled, polygonal, and giant cells.

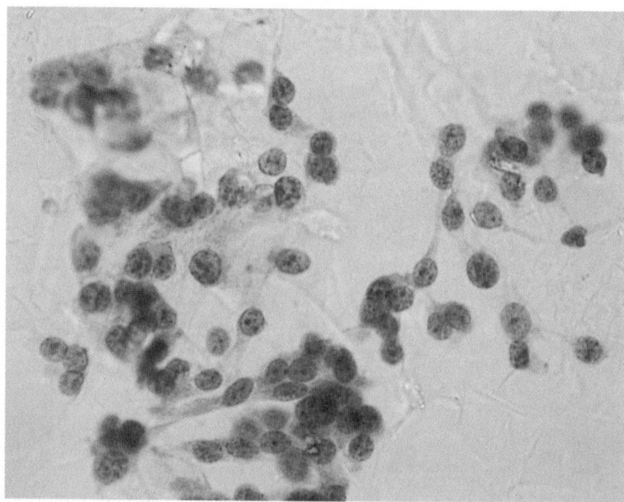

FIGURE 20. Medullary carcinoma. Dispersed population of neuroendocrine cells, many of which have a plasmacytoid appearance. (Modified hematoxylin and eosin.)

roglobulin and calcitonin. Because a significant proportion of anaplastic carcinomas arise from preexisting follicular or papillary carcinomas, a clinical history of a prior thyroid carcinoma can in some cases be very helpful in arriving at a definitive diagnosis.

Cytologic Features of Anaplastic Thyroid Carcinoma

1. Markedly pleomorphic spindle cells and/or tumor giant cells
2. Macronucleoli
3. Numerous mitoses and atypical mitotic figures
4. Background tumor diathesis
5. Squamous differentiation

Medullary Thyroid Carcinoma

Medullary thyroid carcinoma is a neuroendocrine carcinoma arising from the C cell of the thyroid and accounting for approximately 5% of all thyroid cancers (7,101). Whereas the majority (80–90%) of medullary carcinomas are sporadic, approximately 10% to 20% are familial, arising in association with the multiple endocrine neoplasia (MEN) syndrome (102). Sporadic tumors tend to be solitary, but familial ones are often bilateral or multiple. Approximately 75% of medullary carcinomas are correctly diagnosed in FNA specimens; the rest are misdiagnosed as other thyroid neoplasms (11,32).

Cytologically, medullary thyroid carcinoma is characterized by fairly uniform, predominantly dispersed, neuroendocrine cells and amyloid (Fig. 20) (103,104). Some loose cell clusters or even follicles may be present. Depending on the case, a variable combination of any of three cell types occurs: plasmacytoid, spindle, and granular (6,105). Nuclei tend to be eccentrically placed, and the chromatin shows a typical neuroendocrine "salt-and-pepper" texture with inconspicuous nucleoli (104). The malignant cells have a moderate to abundant amount of finely granular cytoplasm, which shows characteristic red cytoplasmic granules using Romanowsky-type stains (11,106). Multinucleation and intranuclear pseudoinclusions are common (Fig. 21) (104). Because, in some cases, the cells may show a marked spindled appearance, medullary thyroid carcinoma should be considered in the differential diagnosis of any FNA of a spindle cell lesion of the head and neck region. Up to 80% of cases of medullary thyroid carcinoma contain some degree of amyloid, which appears as amorphous dense pink material that is indistinguishable from dense colloid in Papanicolaou-stained smears; its presence can be confirmed using the Congo red stain (104).

The differential diagnosis of medullary thyroid carcinoma includes Hurthle cell neoplasms, anaplastic carcinoma, and papillary thyroid carcinoma. The "salt-and-pepper" chromatin of medullary carcinoma helps to distinguish it from both papillary carcinoma with its pale "powdery" chromatin and Hurthle cell neoplasms with their prominent nucleoli and hyperchromatic

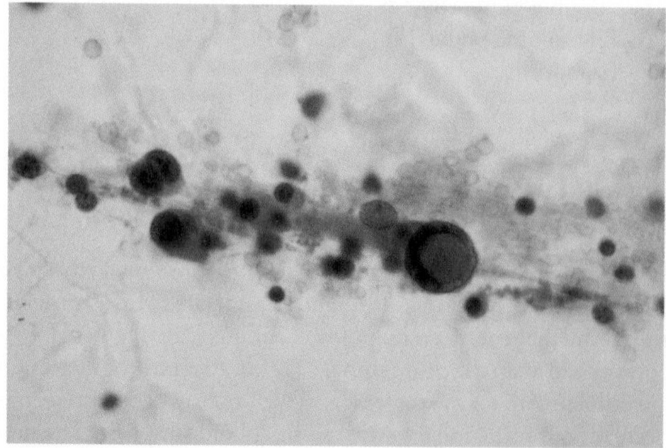

FIGURE 21. Medullary carcinoma. Intranuclear pseudoinclusions are a feature of this neoplasm. (Modified hematoxylin and eosin.)

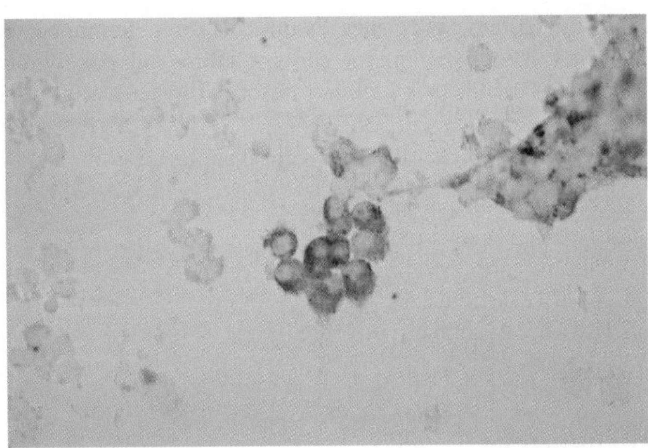

FIGURE 22. Positive immunocytochemical reactivity of medullary carcinoma for calcitonin.

chromatin. In cases with a predominant spindle cell pattern, anaplastic carcinoma may be considered in the differential diagnosis, but giant cells and marked nuclear atypia are usually absent. For difficult cases, positive immunocytochemical staining for calcitonin and carcinoembryonic antigen (CEA) is helpful (Fig. 22) (104). In addition, the tumor cells of medullary carcinoma are immunocytochemically negative for thyroglobulin.

Cytologic Features of Medullary Carcinoma

1. Uniform population of dispersed plasmacytoid or spindle cells
2. "Salt-and-pepper" chromatin
3. Intranuclear pseudoinclusions
4. Multinucleation
5. Red cytoplasmic granules with Romanowsky stains
6. Amyloid

Malignant Lymphoma

Malignant lymphoma, particularly non-Hodgkin's lymphoma, accounts for approximately 1% to 2% of primary thyroid malignancies and is most common in the setting of Hashimoto's thyroiditis (107,108). Other primary thyroid lymphoproliferative disorders, including Hodgkin's disease, plasmacytoma, and T-cell lymphomas, have been reported but are rare (108,109). Malignant lymphoma of the thyroid is more common in older women, most often presenting as either sudden enlargement of a longstanding diffuse goiter or as a dominant unilateral thyroid mass (107). Diffuse large B-cell lymphomas account for more than 75% of cases and appear as cellular aspirates of uniform large, highly atypical immature lymphocytes in a background of scant to absent follicular cells (11,108). The dispersed large lymphocytes often have irregular nuclear membranes and contain prominent nucleoli; lymphoglandular bodies are identifiable in the smear background (108). The primary differential diagnosis of malignant lymphoma involving the thyroid is with Hashimoto's thyroiditis because of the abundance of lymphoid cells. Although a diffuse large B-cell lymphoma can usually be distinguished from the mixed lymphoid population seen in Hashimoto's thyroiditis, involvement by other lymphomas composed of small or mixed small and large lymphocytes may be difficult to distinguish from Hashimoto's. Features favoring Hashimoto's thyroiditis include a combination of mature and immature lymphocytes in all stages of maturation with a prominent population of small mature lymphocytes and some plasma cells; tingible body macrophages are not a useful feature because they may be seen in both benign and malignant conditions (11). When the possibility of involvement by a lymphoproliferative disorder is suspected, ancillary marker studies such as flow cytometry or immunocytochemistry (using air-dried cytospins) are useful.

Metastatic Neoplasms

Metastatic tumors to the thyroid may present as a solitary nodule, but they are uncommonly encountered, being detected in approximately 0.1% of thyroid FNAs (110,111). The most frequent metastatic tumors to the thyroid include kidney, colorectal, lung, breast, melanoma, lymphoma, and head and neck squamous cell carcinoma (110,112). The possibility of a metastatic tumor should be considered whenever there is a history of a primary cancer elsewhere in the body, and especially whenever the cytologic features of the malignant cells do not match those of standard thyroid neoplasms (papillary carcinoma, follicular carcinoma, medullary carcinoma, and anaplastic carcinoma) (11). Approximately 25% to 50% of metastatic tumors to the thyroid do not have a prior history (110,111); however, even in a patient with a known extrathyroidal malignancy, most thyroid nodules are benign (6). Although infrequent, one of the most difficult thyroid metastases to diagnoses is renal cell carcinoma, which can mimic the cytologic features of a follicular neoplasm (Fig. 23) (110). Immunocytochemistry for thyroglobulin on smears or cell block material can be very helpful in evaluating

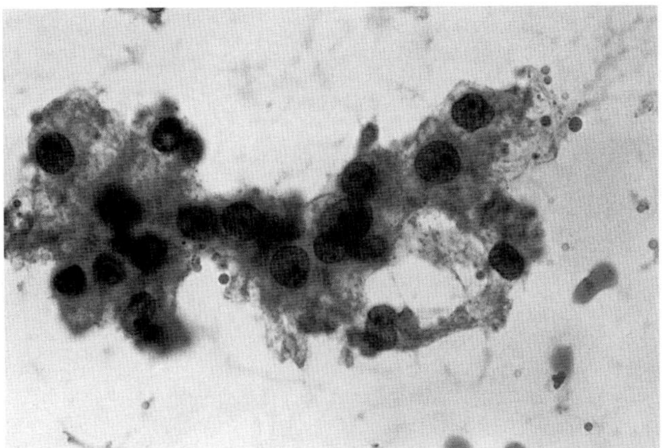

FIGURE 23. Metastatic renal cell carcinoma. Thyroid aspirate showing a cluster of mildly atypical cells with a low N/C ratio. This carcinoma can be difficult to distinguish from a follicular neoplasm. (Papanicolaou stain.) (Courtesy of Dr. Edmund Cibas, Brigham and Women's Hospital, Boston, MA.)

such challenging cases. When assessing a thyroid malignancy, neither mucin nor keratin can be taken as evidence supporting an extrathyroidal origin for the malignant cells, as both of these are known to occur in a subset of primary tumors of the thyroid (6).

Metastatic Tumors to the Thyroid

1. Kidney
2. Colorectal
3. Breast
4. Lung
5. Lymphoma
6. Melanoma
7. Head and neck squamous cell carcinoma

PARATHYROID TUMORS

Palpable but clinically silent parathyroid nodules are occasionally mistaken for nodules involving the thyroid and thus aspirated (29,113). The cytologic features of parathyroid neoplasms overlap with those of follicular lesions of the thyroid, making them difficult to diagnose. Aspirates are generally cellular, with a monomorphic population of small cells in sheets, crowded clusters, and microfollicles (Fig. 24) (11,29). Unlike thyroid neoplasms, colloid is not present. Nuclei of parathyroid cells resemble those of follicular cells: round with coarsely granular chromatin, small inconspicuous to prominent nucleoli, and minimal pleomorphism (29). Cytologic features that are useful in distinguishing parathyroid neoplasms from thyroid are the uniformity and small size of the cells, the tight cohesion of the cell clusters, and many naked nuclei (113). Occasionally, parathyroid neoplasms are cystic, yielding a characteristic water-clear fluid on FNA, a feature that, in an FNA of the neck, should strongly suggest a parathyroid origin (113). In contrast, the fluid obtained from cystic lesions of the thyroid is generally blood-tinged, tan, or brown. In difficult cases, immunocytochemistry for thyroglobulin, chronogranin, and parathyroid hormone is useful, as is a clinical history of hypercalcemia.

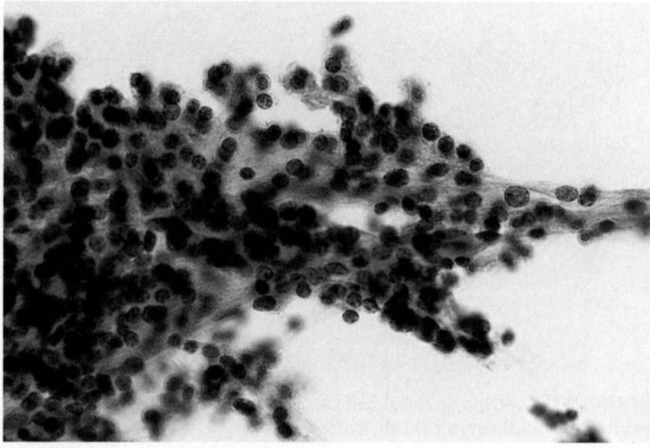

FIGURE 24. Parathyroid adenoma. Papanicolaou-stained smear showing uniform small cells with scant cytoplasm in crowded clusters.

Cytologic Features of Parathyroid Neoplasms

1. Monomorphic population of small cells
2. Tightly cohesive cell clusters
3. Sheets, cords, and microacini
4. Many naked nuclei
5. Absence of colloid

REFERENCES

1. Vander JB, Gaston EA, Dawber TR. The significance of nontoxic thyroid nodules. Final report of a 15-year study of the incidence of thyroid malignancy. *Ann Intern Med* 1968;69:537–540.
2. Gharib H, Goellner JR, Johnson DA. Fine-needle aspiration cytology of the thyroid. A 12-year experience with 11,000 biopsies. *Clin Lab Med* 1993;13:699–709.
3. Gharib H, Goellner JR. Fine-needle aspiration biopsy of the thyroid: an appraisal [see comments]. *Ann Intern Med* 1993;118:282–289.
4. Rojeski MT, Gharib H. Nodular thyroid disease. Evaluation and management. *N Engl J Med* 1985;313:428–436.
5. Christensen SB, Ericsson UB, Janzon L, et al. The prevalence of thyroid disorders in a middle-aged female population, with special reference to the solitary thyroid nodule. *Acta Chir Scand* 1984;150:13–19.
6. DeMay R. Thyroid. In: DeMay R, ed. *The art and science of cytopathology.* Chicago: ASCP Press, 1996;704–778.
7. Rosai J, Carcangiu M, DeLellis R. *Atlas of tumor pathology: tumors of the thyroid gland.* Washington, DC: Armed Forces Institute of Pathology, 1992.
8. Belfiore A, La Rosa GL, La Porta GA, et al. Cancer risk in patients with cold thyroid nodules: relevance of iodine intake, sex, age, and multinodularity [see comments]. *Am J Med* 1992;93:363–369.
9. Wingo PA, Tong T, Bolden S. Cancer statistics, 1995. *CA Cancer J Clin* 1995;45:8–30. (Published erratum appears in *CA Cancer J Clin* 1995;45(2):127–128.)
10. Belfiore A, Rosa GL, Giuffrida D, et al. The management of thyroid nodules. *J Endocrinol Invest* 1995;18:155–158.
11. Cibas ES. Thyroid gland. In: Cibas ES, Ducatman BS, eds. *Cytology: diagnostic principles and clinical correlates.* Philadelphia: WB Saunders, 1996:217–242.
12. Suen KC. How does one separate cellular follicular lesions of the thyroid by fine-needle aspiration biopsy? *Diagn Cytopathol* 1988;4:78–81.
13. Galloway JW, Sardi A, DeConti RW, et al. Changing trends in thyroid surgery. 38 years' experience. *Am Surg* 1991;57:18–20.
14. Rimm DL, Stastny JF, Rimm EB, et al. Comparison of the costs of fine-needle aspiration and open surgical biopsy as methods for obtaining a pathologic diagnosis. *Cancer* 1997;81:51–56.
15. Campbell JP, Pillsbury HCD. Management of the thyroid nodule. *Head Neck* 1989;11:414–425.
16. Gharib H. Fine-needle aspiration biopsy of thyroid nodules: advantages, limitations, and effect. *Mayo Clin Proc* 1994;69:44–49.
17. Rodriguez JM, Parrilla P, Sola J, et al. Comparison between preoperative cytology and intraoperative frozen-section biopsy in the diagnosis of thyroid nodules. *Br J Surg* 1994;81:1151–1154.
18. Mazzaferri EL, de los Santos ET, Rofagha-Keyhani S. Solitary thyroid nodule: diagnosis and management. *Med Clin North Am* 1988;72:1177–1211.
19. Kopald KH, Layfield LJ, Mohrmann R, et al. Clarifying the role of fine-needle aspiration cytologic evaluation and frozen section exami-

nation in the operative management of thyroid cancer. *Arch Surg* 1989;124:1201–1204. (Discussion *Arch Surg* 1989;124:1204–1205).

20. Klemi PJ, Joensuu H, Nylamo E. Fine needle aspiration biopsy in the diagnosis of thyroid nodules. *Acta Cytol* 1991;35:434–438.
21. Layfield LJ, Mohrmann RL, Kopald KH, et al. Use of aspiration cytology and frozen section examination for management of benign and malignant thyroid nodules [see comments]. *Cancer* 1991;68:130–134.
22. Gharib H, Goellner JR. Evaluation of nodular thyroid disease. *Endocrinol Metab Clin North Am* 1988;17:511–526.
23. Frable MA, Frable WJ. Thin needle aspiration biopsy of the thyroid gland. *Laryngoscope* 1980;90:1619–1625.
24. Frable WJ. The treatment of thyroid cancer. The role of fine-needle aspiration cytology. *Arch Otolaryngol Head Neck Surg* 1986;112:1200–1203.
25. La Rosa GL, Belfiore A, Giuffrida D, et al. Evaluation of the fine needle aspiration biopsy in the preoperative selection of cold thyroid nodules. *Cancer* 1991;67:2137–2141.
26. Ashcraft MW, Van Herle AJ. Management of thyroid nodules. II: Scanning techniques, thyroid suppressive therapy, and fine needle aspiration. *Head Neck Surg* 1981;3:297–322.
27. Nathan AR, Raines KB, Lee YT, et al. Fine-needle aspiration biopsy of cold thyroid nodules. *Cancer* 1988;62:1337–1342.
28. Kini SR, Miller JM, Hamburger JI. Cytopathology of thyroid nodules. *Henry Ford Hosp Med J* 1982;30:17–24.
29. Kini S. Thyroid. In: Kini S, ed. *Color atlas of differential diagnosis in exfoliative and aspiration cytopathology.* Baltimore: Williams & Wilkins, 1999:249–254.
30. Hamburger JI, Husain M. Semiquantitative criteria for fine-needle biopsy diagnosis: reduced false-negative diagnoses. *Diagn Cytopathol* 1988;4:14–17.
31. Atkinson BF. Fine needle aspiration of the thyroid. *Monogr Pathol* 1993;35:166–199.
32. Kini S. Thyroid. In: Klines T, ed. *Guides to clinical aspiration biopsy series.* New York: Igaku-Shoin, 1996.
33. Akhtar M, Ali MA, Huq M, et al. Fine-needle aspiration biopsy of papillary thyroid carcinoma: cytologic, histologic, and ultrastructural correlations. *Diagn Cytopathol* 1991;7:373–379.
34. Kini SR, Miller JM, Hamburger JI, et al. Cytopathology of papillary carcinoma of the thyroid by fine needle aspiration. *Acta Cytol* 1980;24:511–521.
35. Soderstrom N, Nilsson G. Cytologic diagnosis of thyrotoxicosis. *Acta Med Scand* 1979;205:263–265.
36. Friedman M, Shimaoka K, Getaz P. Needle aspiration of 310 thyroid lesions. *Acta Cytol* 1979;23:194–203.
37. Heimann A, Moll U. Spinal metastasis of a thyroglobulin-rich Hurthle cell carcinoma detected by fine needle aspiration. Light and electron microscopic study of an unusual case. *Acta Cytol* 1989;33:639–644.
38. Gonzalez JL, Wang HH, Ducatman BS. Fine-needle aspiration of Hurthle cell lesions. A cytomorphologic approach to diagnosis. *Am J Clin Pathol* 1993;100:231–235.
39. Biscotti CV, Hollow JA, Toddy SM, et al. ThinPrep versus conventional smear cytologic preparations in the analysis of thyroid fine-needle aspiration specimens. *Am J Clin Pathol* 1995;104:150–153.
40. Berger SA, Zonszein J, Villamena P, et al. Infectious diseases of the thyroid gland. *Rev Infect Dis* 1983;5:108–122.
41. Singh SK, Agrawal JK, Kumar M, et al. Fine needle aspiration cytology in the management of acute suppurative thyroiditis. *Ear Nose Throat J* 1994;73:415–417.
42. Hopwood NJ, Kelch RP. Thyroid masses: approach to diagnosis and management in childhood and adolescence. *Pediatr Rev* 1993;14:481–487.
43. Jayaram G, Marwaha RK, Gupta RK, et al. Cytomorphologic aspects of thyroiditis. A study of 51 cases with functional, immunologic and ultrasonographic data. *Acta Cytol* 1987;31:687–693.
44. Guarda LA, Baskin HJ. Inflammatory and lymphoid lesions of the thyroid gland. Cytopathology by fine-needle aspiration. *Am J Clin Pathol* 1987;87:14–22.
45. Carney JA, Moore SB, Northcutt RC, et al. Palpation thyroiditis (multifocal granulomatous folliculitis). *Am J Clin Pathol* 1975;64:639–647.
46. Friedman M, Shimaoka K, Rao U, et al. Diagnosis of chronic lymphocytic thyroiditis (nodular presentation) by needle aspiration. *Acta Cytol* 1981;25:513–522.
47. Tani E, Skoog L. Fine needle aspiration cytology and immunocytochemistry in the diagnosis of lymphoid lesions of the thyroid gland. *Acta Cytol* 1989;33:48–52.
48. Poropatich C, Marcus D, Oertel YC. Hashimoto's thyroiditis: fine-needle aspirations of 50 asymptomatic cases. *Diagn Cytopathol* 1994;11:141–145.
49. Tseleni-Balafouta S, Kyroudi-Voulgari A, Paizi-Biza P, et al. Lymphocytic thyroiditis in fine-needle aspirates: differential diagnostic aspects. *Diagn Cytopathol* 1989;5:362–365.
50. Holm LE, Blomgren H, Lowhagen T. Cancer risks in patients with chronic lymphocytic thyroiditis. *N Engl J Med* 1985;312:601–604.
51. Schwaegerle SM, Bauer TW, Esselstyn CB Jr. Riedel's thyroiditis. *Am J Clin Pathol* 1988;90:715–722.
52. Jayaram G, Singh B, Marwaha RK. Graves' disease. Appearance in cytologic smears from fine needle aspirates of the thyroid gland. *Acta Cytol* 1989;33:36–40.
53. Basu D, Jayaram G. A logistic model for thyroid lesions. *Diagn Cytopathol* 1992;8:23–27.
54. Kapila K, Verma K. Amyloid goiter in fine needle aspirates. *Acta Cytol* 1993;37:257–258.
55. Keyhani-Rofagha S, Kooner DS, Landas SK, et al. Black thyroid: a pitfall for aspiration cytology. *Diagn Cytopathol* 1991;7:640–643.
56. Wajda KJ, Wilson MS, Lucas J, et al. Fine needle aspiration cytologic findings in the black thyroid syndrome. *Acta Cytol* 1988;32:862–865.
57. Block MA, Dailey GE, Robb JA. Thyroid nodules indeterminate by needle biopsy. *Am J Surg* 1983;146:72–78.
58. Murphy E, Cervantes QF. Atypical changes in thyroid follicular cells secondary to radioiodine. *Am J Roentgenol Radium Ther Nucl Med* 1970;109:724–728.
59. Carr RF, LiVolsi VA. Morphologic changes in the thyroid after irradiation for Hodgkin's and non-Hodgkin's lymphoma. *Cancer* 1989;64:825–829.
60. Kini SR, Miller JM, Hamburger JI, et al. Cytopathology of follicular lesions of the thyroid gland. *Diagn Cytopathol* 1985;1:123–132.
61. Gardner HA, Ducatman BS, Wang HH. Predictive value of fine-needle aspiration of the thyroid in the classification of follicular lesions. *Cancer* 1993;71:2598–2603.
62. Hamberger B, Gharib H, Melton LJD, et al. Fine-needle aspiration biopsy of thyroid nodules. Impact on thyroid practice and cost of care. *Am J Med* 1982;73:381–383.
63. Harach HR, Zusman SB, Saravia Day E. Nodular goiter: a histo-cytological study with some emphasis on pitfalls of fine-needle aspiration cytology. *Diagn Cytopathol* 1992;8:409–419.
64. Altavilla G, Pascale M, Nenci I. Fine needle aspiration cytology of thyroid gland diseases. *Acta Cytol* 1990;34:251–256.
65. Caraway NP, Sneige N, Samaan NA. Diagnostic pitfalls in thyroid fine-needle aspiration: a review of 394 cases. *Diagn Cytopathol* 1993;9:345–350.
66. Layfield LJ, Reichman A, Bottles K, et al. Clinical determinants for the management of thyroid nodules by fine-needle aspiration cytology. *Arch Otolaryngol Head Neck Surg* 1992;118:717–721.
67. Jayaram G. Fine needle aspiration cytology of hyalinizing trabecular adenoma of the thyroid [letter]. *Acta Cytol* 1999;43:978–980.
68. LiVolsi VA, Gupta PK. Thyroid fine-needle aspiration: intranuclear inclusions, nuclear grooves and psammoma bodies—paraganglioma-like adenoma of the thyroid. *Diagn Cytopathol* 1992;8:82–83.
69. Goellner JR, Carney JA. Cytologic features of fine-needle aspirates of hyalinizing trabecular adenoma of the thyroid. *Am J Clin Pathol* 1989;91:115–119.
70. Gonzalez-Campora R, Herrero-Zapatero A, Lerma E, et al. Hurthle cell and mitochondrion-rich cell tumors. A clinicopathologic study. *Cancer* 1986;57:1154–1163.

71. Marzano LA, Finelli L, Marranzini A, et al. Hurthle cell neoplasm. *Int Surg* 1989;74:97–98.
72. Bondeson L, Bondeson AG, Ljungberg O, et al. Oxyphil tumors of the thyroid: follow-up of 42 surgical cases. *Ann Surg* 1981;194: 677–680.
73. Flint A, Lloyd RV. Hurthle-cell neoplasms of the thyroid gland. *Pathol Annu* 1990;25:37–52.
74. Vodanovic S, Crepinko I, Smoje J. Morphologic diagnosis of Hurthle cell tumors of the thyroid gland. *Acta Cytol* 1993;37:317–322.
75. Kini SR, Miller JM, Hamburger JI. Cytopathology of Hurthle cell lesions of the thyroid gland by fine needle aspiration. *Acta Cytol* 1981; 25:647–652.
76. LiVolsi VA. Papillary neoplasms of the thyroid. Pathologic and prognostic features. *Am J Clin Pathol* 1992;97:426–434.
77. Cady B. Papillary carcinoma of the thyroid. *Semin Surg Oncol* 1991; 7:81–86.
78. Kaur A, Jayaram G. Thyroid tumors: cytomorphology of papillary carcinoma. *Diagn Cytopathol* 1991;7:462–468.
79. Rupp M, Ehya H. Nuclear grooves in the aspiration cytology of papillary carcinoma of the thyroid. *Acta Cytol* 1989;33:21–26.
80. Francis IM, Das DK, Sheikh ZA, et al. Role of nuclear grooves in the diagnosis of papillary thyroid carcinoma. A quantitative assessment on fine needle aspiration smears. *Acta Cytol* 1995;39:409–415.
81. Carney JA, Ryan J, Goellner JR. Hyalinizing trabecular adenoma of the thyroid gland. *Am J Surg Pathol* 1987;11:583–591.
82. Bondeson L, Bondeson AG. Clue helping to distinguish hyalinizing trabecular adenoma from carcinoma of the thyroid in fine-needle aspirates. *Diagn Cytopathol* 1994;10:25–29.
83. Cerasoli S, Tabarri B, Farabegoli P, et al. Hyalinizing trabecular adenoma of the thyroid. Report of two cases, with cytologic, immunohistochemical and ultrastructural studies. *Tumori* 1992;78:274–279.
84. Leung CS, Hartwick RW, Bedard YC. Correlation of cytologic and histologic features in variants of papillary carcinoma of the thyroid. *Acta Cytol* 1993;37:645–650.
85. Miller TR, Bottles K, Holly EA, et al. A step-wise logistic regression analysis of papillary carcinoma of the thyroid. *Acta Cytol* 1986; 30:285–293.
86. Muller N, Cooperberg PL, Suen KC, et al. Needle aspiration biopsy in cystic papillary carcinoma of the thyroid. *Am J Roentgenol* 1985; 144:251–253.
87. Baloch ZW, Abraham S, Roberts S, et al. Differential expression of cytokeratins in follicular variant of papillary carcinoma: an immunohistochemical study and its diagnostic utility. *Hum Pathol* 1999;30: 1166–1171.
88. Schelfhout LJ, Van Muijen GN, Fleuren GJ. Expression of keratin 19 distinguishes papillary thyroid carcinoma from follicular carcinomas and follicular thyroid adenoma. *Am J Clin Pathol* 1989;92:654–658.
89. Baloch ZW, Gupta PK, Yu GH, et al. Follicular variant of papillary carcinoma. Cytologic and histologic correlation. *Am J Clin Pathol* 1999;111:216–222.
90. Johnson TL, Lloyd RV, Thompson NW, et al. Prognostic implications of the tall cell variant of papillary thyroid carcinoma. *Am J Surg Pathol* 1988;12:22–27.
91. Evans HL. Columnar-cell carcinoma of the thyroid. A report of two cases of an aggressive variant of thyroid carcinoma. *Am J Clin Pathol* 1986;85:77–80.
92. Harach HR, Zusman SB. Cytologic findings in the follicular variant of papillary carcinoma of the thyroid. *Acta Cytol* 1992;36:142–146.
93. Harach HR, Zusman SB. Cytopathology of the tall cell variant of thyroid papillary carcinoma. *Acta Cytol* 1992;36:895–899.
94. Pietribiasi F, Sapino A, Papotti M, et al. Cytologic features of poorly differentiated "insular" carcinoma of the thyroid, as revealed by fine-needle aspiration biopsy. *Am J Clin Pathol* 1990;94:687–692.
95. Bal C, Padhy AK, Panda S, et al. "Insular" carcinoma of thyroid. A subset of anaplastic thyroid malignancy with a less aggressive clinical course. *Clin Nucl Med* 1993;18:1056–1058.
96. Flynn SD, Forman BH, Stewart AF, et al. Poorly differentiated ("insular") carcinoma of the thyroid gland: an aggressive subset of differentiated thyroid neoplasms. *Surgery* 1988;104:963–970.
97. Sironi M, Collini P, Cantaboni A. Fine needle aspiration cytology of insular thyroid carcinoma. A report of four cases. *Acta Cytol* 1992;36: 435–439.
98. Venkatesh YS, Ordonez NG, Schultz PN, et al. Anaplastic carcinoma of the thyroid. A clinicopathologic study of 121 cases. *Cancer* 1990; 66:321–330.
99. Brooke PK, Hameed M, Zakowski MF. Fine-needle aspiration of anaplastic thyroid carcinoma with varied cytologic and histologic patterns: a case report. *Diagn Cytopathol* 1994;11:60–63.
100. Guarda LA, Peterson CE, Hall W, et al. Anaplastic thyroid carcinoma: cytomorphology and clinical implications of fine-needle aspiration. *Diagn Cytopathol* 1991;7:63–67.
101. Harach HR, Bergholm U. Medullary carcinoma of the thyroid with carcinoid-like features [see comments]. *J Clin Pathol* 1993;46:113–117.
102. Saad MF, Ordonez NG, Rashid RK, et al. Medullary carcinoma of the thyroid. A study of the clinical features and prognostic factors in 161 patients. *Medicine (Baltimore)* 1984;63:319–342.
103. Kaur A, Jayaram G. Thyroid tumors: cytomorphology of medullary, clinically anaplastic, and miscellaneous thyroid neoplasms [see comments]. *Diagn Cytopathol* 1990;6:383–389.
104. Bose S, Kapila K, Verma K. Medullary carcinoma of the thyroid: a cytological, immunocytochemical, and ultrastructural study. *Diagn Cytopathol* 1992;8:28–32.
105. Kini SR, Miller JM, Hamburger JI, et al. Cytopathologic features of medullary carcinoma of the thyroid. *Arch Pathol Lab Med* 1984; 108:156–159.
106. Das A, Gupta SK, Banerjee AK, et al. Atypical cytologic features of medullary carcinoma of the thyroid. A review of 12 cases. *Acta Cytol* 1992;36:137–141.
107. Matsuzuka F, Miyauchi A, Katayama S, et al. Clinical aspects of primary thyroid lymphoma: diagnosis and treatment based on our experience of 119 cases. *Thyroid* 1993;3:93–99.
108. Jayaram G, Rani S, Raina V, et al. B cell lymphoma of the thyroid in Hashimoto's thyroiditis monitored by fine-needle aspiration cytology. *Diagn Cytopathol* 1990;6:130–133.
109. Jayaram G. Hodgkin's disease beginning as a thyroid nodule [letter, comment]. *Acta Cytol* 1993;37:256–257.
110. Schmid KW, Hittmair A, Ofner C, et al. Metastatic tumors in fine needle aspiration biopsy of the thyroid. *Acta Cytol* 1991;35:722–724.
111. Smith SA, Gharib H, Goellner JR. Fine-needle aspiration. Usefulness for diagnosis and management of metastatic carcinoma to the thyroid. *Arch Intern Med* 1987;147:311–312.
112. Ivy HK. Cancer metastatic to the thyroid: a diagnostic problem. *Mayo Clin Proc* 1984;59:856–859.
113. Layfield LJ. Fine needle aspiration cytology of cystic parathyroid lesions. A cytomorphologic overlap with cystic lesions of the thyroid. *Acta Cytol* 1991;35:447–450.

INDEX

A

Acantholytic squamous cell carcinoma, laryngeal, 258, 259f
Acanthoma, spectacle frame, 56
Acinic cell carcinoma, 318–320, 319f
  salivary, 117, 620, 620t
    in children, 337
    cytopathology of, 631–632, 631f, 632f
Acne agminata, 592
Acoustic neuromas, 72–73, 72f, 73f
  bilateral, 73, 73f
Acral lentiginous melanoma (ALM), 572, 573f
Acrodermatitis continua, 587
Acrospiroma
  eccrine, 303, 303f, 549–550
  malignant, 550, 551f
Actinic dermatitis, chronic, 577
Actinic keratosis, 535–536, 536f, 537f
Actinic reticuloid, 577, 598
Actinomycosis, 63
  cytopathology of, 645, 645f
  laryngeal, 232
  nasopharyngeal, with abscess, 166
Adamantinoma. *See* Ameloblastoma(s)
Adenocarcinoma(s). *See also* specific types, e.g., Hidradenocarcinoma, Lymphadenocarcinoma
  lacrimal gland, 672
  laryngeal and hypopharyngeal, 269–270, 270f
  middle ear, papillary, 71
  nasopharyngeal, 175–177, 175f–176f
  salivary gland, 116–117, 329t, 331
    basal cell, 315–317, 315f, 316f
    polymorphous low-grade, 117, 329–331, 330f
      cytopathology of, 628–629
    terminal duct, 329–331, 330f
  sinonasal, 117–119, 119f
    colonic type, 119, 119f
    low-grade, 117–119, 118f, 119f
    mixed, 119
    mucinous, 119, 119f
    papillary, 119
    solid, 119
Adenocystic hidradenocarcinoma, 550–551
Adenoid cystic carcinoma (ACC), 320–323, 321f
  clinical behavior and treatment of, 322–323
  clinical data on, 320–321
  cutaneous primary, 551
  cytopathology of, 67t, 626–628, 626f, 627f
  definition of, 320
  differential diagnosis of, 322
  gross appearance of, 321
  histologic features of, 321–322, 321f
  immunohistochemistry of, 322
  lacrimal gland, 671–672, 672f
  laryngeal, 269–270, 270f
  salivary-type, 115–116, 116f
  studies of, special, 322
  ultrastructure of, 322
Adenoids, with follicular lymphoid hyperplasia, 160–161, 161f
Adenolymphoma, 308–310, 309f, 310f
Adenoma(s)
  basal cell, 312–315, 313f, 314f, 314t (*See also* Basal cell adenoma)
    congenital, 22
    cytopathology of, 625–626, 625f
  canalicular, 317–318, 317f
  carcinoma ex pleomorphic, salivary, 117
  ceruminal gland, 58, 58f
  ear
    low-grade, of probable endolymphatic sac origin, 73–74, 74f
    middle, 67–68, 68f
  follicular, 356–357, 356f
    atypical, 357
  Hurthle cell, 364, 365f
  hyalinizing trabecular, 357, 357f
    cytopathology of, 694, 694f
  ocular, 666–667
  oncocytic cell, 382
  parathyroid, 380–381, 380f
    cytopathology of, 698, 698f
  pituitary, 147–148, 147f
  pleomorphic (*See* Pleomorphic adenoma)
  sebaceous, 311, 312f, 543, 544f
Adenoma sebaceum, 554, 555f
Adenomatoid odontogenic tumor (AOT), 144–145, 215–216, 216f
Adenomatous (nodular) goiter, 355–356, 355f
Adenosquamous carcinoma, laryngeal, 270, 271f
Adipocytic tumors, 397–401
  angiolipoma, 397, 397f
  hibernoma, 398–399, 399f
  laryngeal and hypopharyngeal, 274, 275f
  lipoblastoma, 398, 398f
  lipoma, 397 (*See also* Angiolipoma; Lipoma(s))
    chondroid, 399, 399f
    cytopathology of, 653–654
    pleomorphic, 398, 398f
    spindle cell, 397–398, 397f
  liposarcoma, 399–401, 400f
    dedifferentiated, 401
    myxoid, 400, 400f
    pleomorphic, 401, 401f
    round cell, 400–401, 400f
    well-differentiated, 400, 400f
Adnexal carcinoma, microcystic, 551, 552f
Aerodigestive tract, upper. *See* Upper Aerodigestive tract
Afipia felis infection, 481–482, 482f
Alcohol, in upper aerodigestive tract neoplasia, 34–35
Alkaptonuria, ear in, 55
Allergic contact dermatitis, 585–586, 586f
Alopecia mucinosa, 603–604, 603f
Alveolar rhabdomyosarcoma, salivary gland, 334, 335f
Alveolar soft part sarcoma (ASPS), 426
Amalgam tattoo, 588t, 598, 598f, 598t
Ameloblastic carcinoma, 226, 226f
  mandibular and maxillary, 678
Ameloblastic fibroma, 223–225, 224f
  mandibular and maxillary, 678
Ameloblastic fibroodontoma, 225
Ameloblastic fibrosarcoma, 227
Ameloblastic odontoma, 225
Ameloblastoma(s), 208–215
  acanthomatous, 210, 210f
  basal cell, 210
  cystic, 209
  desmoplastic, 211, 212f
  follicular, 209–210, 210f
  ghost-cell, 210–211, 218
    dentinogenic, 210–211
  granular cell, 210, 211f
  intraosseous, classical, 209, 211f
  malignant, 225–226
  multicystic, 209–212, 210f–212f
  odontogenic mandibular and maxillary, 677–678, 677f
  peripheral, 214–215, 214f
  plexiform, 210, 211f
  sinonasal, 143–144, 143f
  solid, 209–212, 210f–212f
  spindle cell, 210, 211f
  unicystic, 212–214, 213f
Amyloid deposition
  laryngeal, 241–242, 241f
  nasopharyngeal, 165–166, 166f
  in Waldeyer's ring, 184–185
Amyloid goiter, 689–690, 690f
Anaplastic carcinoma
  sinonasal, 131–132, 131f
  thyroid, 365–366, 366f
    cytopathology of, 695–696, 696f
Anaplastic large-cell (Ki-1^{+}) lymphoma, primary cutaneous, 578, 578f
Ancient change, 417
Aneurysmal bone cyst, 462–463, 462f, 463f
  mandibular and maxillofacial, 679
Angiocentric immunoproliferative lesion, 578
Angiocentric lymphoma, 496

Angioendotheliomatosis, malignant, 581, 581f
Angiofibroma
cutaneous, 554, 555f
giant cell, 406–407, 406f
nasopharyngeal, juvenile, 167–170, 168f–170f
Angiokeratoma, 556, 557f
Angiolipoma, 397, 397f
Angiolymphoid hyperplasia with eosinophilia, 558
Angiomatous nevus, 556–557
Angiosarcoma(s)
cutaneous, 558–559, 559f
pericytic and vascular, 415, 415f
skeletal, 460
thyroid, 372
Angiotropic lymphoma, 581, 581f
Annular elastolytic granuloma, 596
Antrochoanal polyps, 84–86
Apex of petrous temporal bone tumors, 73–74
Apical scar, 198, 198f
Apocrine carcinoma, 547
Apocrine hidrocystoma, 554
Appendix of the ventricle, 237
Argyria, 597, 598f
Arteriovenous hemangioma, 412, 412f
Arteriovenous malformations, 412, 412f
Arteritis, temporal (giant-cell), cutaneous, 591–592
Arthritis, rheumatoid, laryngeal, 242
Ashy dermatosis, 589–590, 589f
Aspergillosis
laryngeal, 232
orbital, 669, 670f
Astrocytoma, pilocytic, orbital, 674
Athyrosis, 350–351
Auditory canal tumors, internal, 71
Auricle, petrified, 57

B

B cell
marginal zone, 514t
monocytoid, 514t
B-cell lymphoma. *See* Lymphoma(s), B-cell
Bacillary angiomatosis (BA), 389, 390f
bartonellosis, 605–606, 606f
Bacterial endophthalmitis, 664
Bacterial infections
cutaneous, 604–606, 605f, 606f
endophthalmitis, 664
pyogenic bacterial lymphadenitis, 481, 481f
Bartonella henselae infection, 481–482, 482f
Bartonellosis, 605–606, 606f
Basal cell adenocarcinoma, salivary gland, 315–317, 315f, 316f
Basal cell adenoma, 312–315
clinical behavior and treatment of, 315
clinical data on, 312–313
congenital, 22
cytopathology of, 625–626, 625f
definition of, 312
differential diagnosis of, 314–315
gross appearance of, 313, 313f
histologic features of, 313–314, 313f, 314f, 314t
ultrastructure of, 314
Basal cell carcinoma (BCC)
cutaneous, 539, 540f
cytopathology of, 656, 656f
of ear, 57
with sebaceous differentiation, 545
Basal cell nevus syndrome, 205–206
Basaloid squamous cell carcinoma, 262–264, 263f, 264f
cytopathology of, 636–637
sinonasal, 123–124, 123f
of upper aerodigestive tract, 48–49, 48f–49f
Basosebaceous epithelioma, 545
Behçet's disease, cutaneous, 592
Benign cephalic histiocytosis, 596
Benign lymphoepithelial lesion (BLEL), 513, 514t
Benign mixed tumor, salivary, 114–115, 115f
Betel quid (betel nuts), neoplasia from, 34
Black thyroid, 690, 690f
Blastomycosis, laryngeal, 231–232
Blistering processes, 581–586
allergic contact, photoallergic, 585–586, 586f
bullous pemphigoid, 582–583, 584f
cicatricial pemphigoid, 584, 585f
dermatitis herpetiformis, 584, 585f
eosinophilic ulcer, 582t, 585
linear IgA bullous dermatosis, 584–585
paraneoplastic pemphigus, 582, 583f
pemphigus foliaceus, 582
pemphigus vegetans, 582, 583f
pemphigus vulgaris, 581–582, 581f, 582t
Blood-induced (ghost cell) glaucoma, 663, 664f
Blue nevus, 563–564, 564f
cellular, 564–565
malignant, 565
Boeck's sarcoid, 352
Bone and joint diseases, 438–469
eosinophilic granuloma of bone, 464–466, 465f
Ewing's sarcoma, 467
fibroosseous lesions, 453–456
fibrous dysplasia, 453–454, 453f
ossifying fibroma, 454, 454f, 455f
psammomatoid ossifying fibroma, 454–456, 455f
fibrous tumors, 460–461
desmoplastic fibroma, 460
myofibroma and myofibromatosis, 460–461, 461f
giant cell–rich lesions, 456–458
giant cell reparative granuloma, 457–458, 457f, 458f
giant cell tumor, 456, 456f
Langerhans' cell histiocytosis of bone, 464–466, 465f
leiomyosarcoma, 466–467
malignant fibrous histiocytoma, 467
melanotic neuroectodermal tumor of infancy, 463–464, 463f, 464f
non-neoplastic lesions, 438–443
inflammatory and ischemic, 438–440
osteomyelitis, 438
infectious, 438–439, 439f
sclerosing, diffuse, 439–440, 440f
sclerosing, of Garré, 439–440, 440f
osteoradionecrosis, 439, 439f
metabolic, 440–443
calcium pyrophosphate dihydrate crystal deposition disease (pseudogout), 442–443, 443f
crystal-induced synovial and joint diseases, 441
monosodium urate crystal deposition disease (gout), 441–442, 442f
Paget's disease of bone, 440–441, 440f, 441f
non–bone-forming lesions, 447–453
primitive neuroectodermal tumor, 467
schwannoma, 466
tumors and tumorlike lesions of bone, 443–467
bone-forming lesions, 443–447
osteoblastoma, 444–445, 444f
osteoid osteoma, 445–446, 445f, 446f
osteoma, 443–444, 443f, 444f
osteosarcoma, 446–447, 447f
primitive neuroectodermal tumor, 445–446, 445f, 446f
cartilage-forming lesions, 447–453
chondroblastoma, 447–448, 448f
chondromyxoid fibroma, 448–449, 449f
chondrosarcoma, 449–451, 450f
chordoma, 451–453, 452f
enchondroma and osteochondroma, 447
mesenchymal chondrosarcoma, 451, 451f
cystic lesions, 461–463
aneurysmal, 462–463, 462f, 463f
epidermoid, 461, 462f
simple, 461
in ear, 59
tumors and tumorlike lesions of joints, 467–469
pigmented villonodular synovitis, 468–469, 469f
primary synovial chondromatosis, 467–468, 468f
vascular tumors, 458–460
angiosarcoma, 460
epithelioid hemangioendothelioma, 459–460
hemangioma, 458–459, 459f
malignant, 459–460
Bone cyst(s)
aneurysmal, 462–463, 462f, 463f
mandibular and maxillofacial, 679
epidermoid, 461, 462f
simple, 461
Bowen's disease, 536–537, 537f
Branchial cleft cysts, 1, 2f, 8–11, 9f–11f
cytopathology of, 637, 637f
in salivary gland, 619–620
first, 10, 10f, 11f
third and fourth, 11
of thyroid, 11, 11f
Branchial cleft fistulas, 8
Branchial cleft sinuses, 8
Branchial cysts, 162
nasopharyngeal, 160
Branchiogenic carcinoma, 9
Breast carcinoma, intraocular metastasis of, 667, 668f
Bullous pemphigoid, 582–583, 584f
Burkitt's and Burkitt-like lymphomas
cytopathology of, 648f, 648t, 649, 649f
thyroid, 521–522
tonsillar, 493–494, 493f

C

Calcifying epithelial odontogenic tumor (CEOT), 144, 144f, 216–218, 217f
cytopathology of, 678–679
Calcifying epithelioma of Malherbe, 542, 542f
cytopathology of, 638, 655–656, 656f
Calcifying odontogenic cyst (COC), 207, 218, 219f

Calcium pyrophosphate dihydrate crystal deposition disease (pseudogout), 442–443, 443f
Canalicular adenoma, 317–318, 317f. *See also* Basal cell adenoma
Candidiasis, laryngeal, 232
Capillary hemangioma, 412, 412f, 556–557
Carcinoid tumor, 265–266, 266f
  atypical, 266–267, 267f
Carcinoma. *See also* specific sites and types, e.g., Upper aerodigestive tract, squamous neoplasia of
  branchiogenic, 9
  embryonal, 22
Carcinoma ex pleomorphic adenoma (CEPA, malignant mixed tumor), 299–301, 300f, 301f
  salivary, 117
    cytopathology of, 632–633
Carcinoma showing thymuslike differentiation (CASTLE), 370–371, 370f
Carcinosarcoma, of salivary gland, 301–302, 301f
Carotid body tumor. *See* Paraganglioma
Cartilage-forming lesions, 447–453
  chondroblastoma, 447–448, 448f
  chondromyxoid fibroma, 448–449, 449f
  chondrosarcoma, 449–451, 450f
  chordoma, 451–453, 452f
  enchondroma, 447
  mesenchymal chondrosarcoma, 451, 451f
  osteochondroma, 447
Cartilaginous tumors, laryngeal, 270–274, 272f, 273f
CASTLE (carcinoma showing thymuslike differentiation), 370–371, 370f
Cat scratch disease, 481–482, 482f
  cytopathology of, 643–644
Cavernous hemangioma, 412, 557
Cellular hemangioma of infancy, 557
Cementifying fibroma, 454, 454f, 455f
  mandibular and maxillofacial, 679
Cementoblastoma, 222, 223f
Cementoma, true, 222, 223f
Cementoossifying fibroma, 454, 454f, 455f
  mandibular and maxillofacial, 679
Cementum, *vs.* bone, 222
Centocyte-like cell, 514t
Cephalic histiocytosis, benign, 596
Cerebellopontine angle tumors, 71, 73–74
Ceruminal gland adenoma, 58, 58f
Ceruminal gland neoplasms
  benign, 58, 58f
  malignant, 58–59, 59f
Ceruminoma, 58, 58f
Cervical thymic cyst, 14–15, 14f
Cervicothyroidal teratomas, 17–19, 17f–19f
Chalazion, 594, 594f
Cherubism, 22
Choanal atresia, 158
Cholesteatoma (epidermoid cyst), 87–88
  of ear, 74
  of middle ear, 63
    acquired, 63–67, 64f, 65f, 66t, 67f
Cholesterol granuloma
  of ear, 74, 74f
  sinonasal, 87–88
Chondroblastoma, 447–448, 448f
Chondrodermatitis nodularis chronica helicis, 56
Chondroid lipoma, 399, 399f
Chondroid syringoma, 549, 550f
  cytopathology of, 657–658
Chondroma, 429, 429f
Chondromalacia, idiopathic cystic, of ear, 57, 57f
Chondromatosis, primary synovial, 467–468, 468f
Chondromesenchymal hamartoma, 22, 22f, 23f
Chondromyxoid fibroma, 448–449, 449f
Chondrosarcoma(s), 449–451, 450f
  with additional malignant component, 272, 273f
  of larynx, 270–274, 272f, 273f
  mesenchymal, 451, 451f
  of thyroid cartilage, 271–272, 272f
Chordoma(s), 451–453, 452f
  mandibular and maxillofacial, 679–680, 679f
  nasopharyngeal, 177–178, 178f
Choristoma(s), 1, 67, 67f, 429, 429f
  phakomatous, 15–16, 16f
  salivary gland, 20
Cicatricial pemphigoid, 584, 585f
  laryngeal, 243
Clark's nevus, 568, 569f
Classical intraosseous ameloblastoma, 209
Clear cell hidradenocarcinoma, 550
Clear cell hidradenoma, 549–550
Clear cell myoepithelioma, 303, 303f, 549–550
Clear cell odontogenic carcinoma, 227, 227f
Clonal nevus, 565
Coats' disease, 665, 665f
Cocaine abuse, sinonasal lesions from, 100–101
Coccidioidomycosis, laryngeal, 231–232
Cold reactions, cutaneous, 599
Cold temperature–induced panniculitis, 599
Collagenous fibroma, 403–404, 404f
Colonic type adenocarcinoma, sinonasal, 119, 119f
Combined nevus, 565
Congenital anomalies, 1–24
  diagnosis of, 2, 2f
  embryonal rhabdomyosarcoma, 24
  fetal rhabdomyoma, 24, 24f
  hemangioma, 24
  heterotopias, 15–17
    ectopic hamartomatous thymoma, 16–17, 16f
    phakomatous choristoma, 15–16, 16f
    salivary gland, 15
  lymphangioma, 24
  of neuroectoderm and surface ectoderm, 2–8
    dermoid cyst and dermoid, 6–8, 7f, 8f
    encephalocele, 3
    extranasal heterotopic neuroglial tissue, 5
    nasal glial heterotopia, 3–5, 4f, 4t, 5f
    rudimentary meningocele, 5–6, 6f, 7f
  pathogenesis and pathology of, 1–2, 2t
  persistent embryonic remnants, 8–15
    branchial cleft cysts and sinuses, 1, 2f, 8–11, 9f–11f
    cervical thymic cyst, 14–15, 14f
    ectopic thymus, 15, 15f
    ectopic thyroid, 13–14
    heterotopic parathyroid, 15
    lateral aberrant thyroid, 14
    persistent thymopharyngeal duct cyst, 15
    thymic cysts, 14
    thymopharyngeal duct cysts, 14
    thyroglossal duct cyst, 1, 8, 11–13, 12f, 13f, 351
      cytopathology of, 638–639, 638f
  soft tissue lesions, 24
  tissue overgrowth, 17–22
    cherubism, 22
    chondromesenchymal hamartoma, 22, 22f, 23f
    congenital basal cell adenoma, 22
    embryonal carcinoma, 22
    fibrous dysplasia, 22
    giant cell granuloma, 22
    hamartoma, 22
    juvenile pleomorphic adenoma, 22
    polycystic (dysgenetic) disease, 22
    salivary gland anlage tumor, 20, 21f, 166–167, 166f, 167f, 337
    salivary gland choristoma, 20
    sialoblastoma (embryoma), 20, 20f
    teratomas, 17–20, 17f–19f
  tumors, 1, 2t
Congenital basal cell adenoma, 22
Congenital epulis, 416
Congenital fibrosarcoma (CFS), 408–409, 408f, 409f
Congenital pleomorphic adenoma, 20, 21f
Congenital stapes fixation, 75–76
Conjunctival melanosis, 568–569
Connective tissue disease, cutaneous. *See* Cutaneous degenerative disorders and connective tissue disease
Connective tissue neoplasms, in ear, 59
Contact ulcers, vocal cord, 236–237, 237f
Craig's paradental cyst, 201–202
Cranial fasciitis (CF), 392
Craniofacial development, 2
Crohn's disease
  cutaneous, 592–593
  laryngeal, 234–235, 235f
Cryptococcosis, laryngeal, 231–232
Crystal-induced synovial and joint diseases, 441
Cutaneous. *See also* Dermatopathology
Cutaneous adenoid cystic carcinoma, primary, 551
Cutaneous anaplastic large-cell (Ki-1^{+}) lymphoma, primary, 578, 578f
Cutaneous angiofibroma, 554, 555f
Cutaneous B-cell lymphoma, 578–581. *See also under* Lymphoma(s), B-cell
Cutaneous Crohn's disease, 592–593
Cutaneous degenerative disorders and connective tissue disease, 599–601
  dermatomyositis, 601, 601f
  lipoatrophy and lipodystrophy, 599
  lupus erythematosus, 599–601, 600f
    subacute cutaneous, 601
  lupus profundus, 601, 601f
  morphea, 601, 602f
Cutaneous heterotopic meningeal nodule, 561, 563f
Cutaneous infections. *See also* Dermatopathology, infectious diseases
  bacterial, 604–606, 605f, 606f
  fungal, 606, 606f
  protozoal, 606, 606f
  viral, 606–609, 607f, 608f
Cutaneous lymphoid hyperplasia, 576–577
Cutaneous lymphoid neoplasms and lymphoma look-alikes, 576–581. *See also* Lymphoid hyperplasia; Lymphoma(s)
Cutaneous lymphoma, primary, 576
Cutaneous meningioma, 561, 563f

Cutaneous metastases, 658
Cutaneous neuroendocrine carcinoma, primary, 561, 563f
Cutaneous papulosquamous disorders, 586–590. *See also* Dermatopathology, noninfectious inflammatory processes
  lichenoid processes, 588–590, 588t
  psoriasiform dermatitis, 586–588
Cutaneous T-cell lymphoma, 577–581. *See also under* Lymphoma(s), T-cell
Cutaneous vascular proliferations and telangiectasias, 556–559
  angiokeratoma, 556, 557f
  angiolymphoid hyperplasia with eosinophilia, 558
  angiosarcoma, 558–559, 559f
  hemangioma
    capillary, 556–557
    cavernous, 557
    epithelioid, 558
    juvenile, 557
  Kaposi's sarcoma, 558, 558f
  lymphangioma circumscriptum, 557, 557f
  strawberry nevus, 557
Cylindroma (turban tumor), 547–548, 547f
  of ear, 58, 58f
  eccrine, 657–658
Cyst(s)
  bone, 461–463
    aneurysmal, 462–463, 462f, 463f
      mandibular and maxillofacial, 679
    epidermoid, 461, 462f
    simple, 461
  branchial, 162
    nasopharyngeal, 160
  branchial cleft, 1, 2f, 8–11, 9f–11f
    cytopathology of, 10, 10f, 11f
    first, 10, 10f, 11f
    in salivary gland, 619–620
    third and fourth, 11
    of thyroid, 11, 11f
  calcifying odontogenic, 207, 218, 219f
  cervical thymic, 14–15, 14f
  Craig's paradental, 201–202
  dentigerous, 202–203, 202f–204f, 676–677, 676f
  dermoid, 553–554
    congenital, 6–8, 7f, 8f
    orbital, 668–669, 669f
  developmental lateral periodontal, 202f, 206, 206f–207f
  duct retention, 163, 163f
  enteric (enterogenous), 11
    orbital, 669, 669f
  epidermal, 551–554
    apocrine hidrocystoma, 554
    dermoid, 553–554
    eccrine hidrocystoma, 554, 554f
    inclusion, 551–552, 552f
    steatocystoma, 552–553, 553f
    trichilemmal, 552, 553f
    vellus hair, 553
  epidermal inclusion, 551–552, 552f
    cytopathology of, 637–638, 638f
  epidermoid, 461, 462f
    of ear, 74
  eruption, 202f, 204
  fissural, jaw, 195, 196f
  follicular, 202–203, 202f–204f, 676–677, 676f
  foregut duplication, 11
  gingival, 202f, 206, 206f–207f
  glandular odontogenic, 207, 207f
  glandular retention, 163, 163f
  globulomaxillary, 195, 196f
  HIV-associated lymphoepithelial, 620
  incisive canal, 199–200, 199f–200f
  inflammatory lateral periodontal, 201, 202f
  of jaws, 195, 196f
    fissural, 195, 196f
    globulomaxillary, 195, 196f
    nonodontogenic developmental, 199–201
      nasolabial, 200–201, 200f–201f
      nasopalatine duct, 199–200, 199f–200f
    odontogenic, histologic typing of, 201, 201t
  lymphoepithelial, 288, 288f
    cytopathology of, 637, 637f
    HIV-associated, 620
    salivary gland, simple, 512, 512f
    simple, 512, 512f
    tonsillar, 183, 184f
  mucus retention, 619, 619f
  nasoalveolar, 200–201, 200f–201f
  nasolabial, 104, 200–201, 200f–201f
  nasopalatine duct, 199–200, 199f–200f
  nasopharyngeal, 162–163
  odontogenic, 201–207
    calcifying, 207, 218, 219f
    carcinomas arising in, 226–227
    dentigerous, 676–677, 676f
    developmental, 202–207
      calcifying, 207
      dentigerous, 202–203, 202f–204f
      eruption, 202f, 204
      gingival, 202f, 206, 206f–207f
      glandular, 207, 207f
      keratocyst, 204–205, 204f–205f
      lateral periodontal, 202f, 206, 206f–207f
      nevoid basal cell carcinoma syndrome, 205–206
    histologic typing of, 201, 201t
    inflammatory, 201–202
      Craig's paradental, 201–202
      lateral periodontal, 201, 202t
      paradental, 201–202
    keratocyst, 204–205, 204f–205f, 676, 676f
    periapical, 676, 676f
    radicular, 676, 676f
  oncocytic, 163, 163f
    laryngeal, 243, 243f
  oral cavity, 195, 196f
  parathyroid, 15, 382
    heterotopic, 15
  periapical, 197, 197f–198f, 676, 676f
  periodontal, lateral
    developmental, 206, 206f–207f
    inflammatory, 201, 202f
  pilar, 552, 553f
    cytopathology of, 551–552, 552f, 637–638, 638f
  proliferating trichilemmal, 542
    cytopathology of, 657–658
  radicular, 197–198, 197f–198f
    lateral, 198
  Rathke's cleft, 163
  residual, 197–198
  saccular, laryngeal, 238, 238f, 239f
  salivary duct, 287, 287f
  salivary gland, 286–288, 287f, 287t, 288f
  sebaceous, 551–552, 552f
    cytopathology of, 637–638, 638f
  thymic, 14
    cervical, 14–15, 14f
  thymopharyngeal duct, 14
    persistent, 15
  thyroglossal duct, 1, 8, 11–13, 12f, 13f, 351
    cytopathology of, 638–639, 638f
  Tornwaldt's, 162, 162f, 163f
  trichilemmal, 552, 553f
    proliferating, 542
      cytopathology of, 657–658
  vellus hair, 553
Cystic ameloblastoma, 209
Cystic chondromalacia, idiopathic, 57, 57f
Cystic lymphoid hyperplasia, of salivary gland, 512–513, 513f
  with HIV, 291–292, 292f
Cytomegalovirus infection, lymphadenopathy in, 478–479, 478f
Cytopathology, 618–698
  of cutaneous lesions, 655–658
  of eye, 663–668
  of lymph nodes
    intraparotid, 633–634
    metastases to, 639–642 (*See also* specific cancers, e.g., Nasopharyngeal carcinoma)
  of lymphoid processes, primary, 642–643, 642f
  of malignant lymphoma, 633, 646–652, 675, 675f, 681–682, 683, 683f (*See also* Lymphoma(s), malignant)
  of mandible and maxillofacial areas, 675–680 (*See also* Mandible and maxillofacial areas)
  of nasal cavity, paranasal sinuses, and nasopharynx, 682–683
  of neck, 634–639 (*See also* specific disorders, e.g., Squamous cell carcinoma)
  of oral cavity and oropharynx, 680–682
  of orbit, 668–675 (*See also* Orbital diseases)
  of salivary glands, 618–633 (*See also under* Salivary gland(s))
  of soft tissue, 652–655
  of thyroid, 686–698 (*See also* Thyroid)

D

de Quervain's disease, 352–353
de Quervain's thyroiditis, 352–353
  cytopathology of, 688, 688f
Deep penetrating nevus, 565
Dendritic melanocytoses, 562–565. *See also under* Melanocytic neoplasms, cutaneous
Dental follicles, 195–196, 196f
Dentigerous (follicular) cyst, 202–203, 202f–204f, 676–677, 676f
Dentinogenic ghost-cell tumor, 210–211, 218
Dermatitis
  actinic, chronic, 577, 598
  allergic contact, 585–586, 586f
  photoallergic, 585–586, 586f
  psoriasiform, 586–588
    generalized pustular psoriasis of von Zumbusch, 587
    prurigo nodularis, 587–588
    psoriasis vulgaris, 586–587, 587f
    pustular psoriasis, 587
    Reiter's disease, 587, 587f

radiation, 598
spongiotic, 585–586, 586f
Dermatitis herpetiformis, 584, 585f
Dermatofibrosarcoma protuberans, 555–556, 556f
Dermatomyositis, 601, 601f
Dermatopathology, 534–608
infectious diseases, 604–608
bacillary angiomatosis, 605–606, 606f
bacterial, 604–606, 605f, 606f
dermatophytes, 606, 606f
ecthyma, 604
fungal, 606, 606f
furuncle, 604
herpes simplex, 607–608, 607f
impetigo, 604
leprosy, 604, 605f
molluscum contagiosum, 608, 608f
oral hairy leukoplakia, 608, 608f
protozoal, 606, 606f
rhinoscleroma, 604–605
verruca vulgaris, 606–607, 607f
viral, 606–609, 607f, 608f
neoplastic proliferative processes, 534–581
of epidermis and adnexae, 534–554 (*See also* Epidermal neoplasms)
lymphoid neoplasms and lymphoma look-alikes, 576–581 (*See also* Lymphoid hyperplasia; Lymphoma(s))
melanocytic, 561–576 (*See also* Melanocytic neoplasms, cutaneous)
mesenchymal, 554–561 (*See also* Soft tissue pathology)
fibroblastic and fibroproliferative, 554–559
atypical fibroxanthoma, 554–555, 555f
cutaneous angiofibroma, 554, 555f
dermatofibrosarcoma protuberans, 555–556, 556f
fibrous papule, 554, 555f
keloid, 554
malignant fibrous histiocytoma, superficial type, 554–555, 555f
lipomatous and neural proliferations, 559–561
cutaneous heterotopic meningeal nodule, 561, 563f
cutaneous meningioma, 561, 563f
cutaneous neuroendocrine carcinoma, primary, 561, 563f
lipoma, 559
lipoma, intramuscular, 559, 560f
Merkel cell carcinoma, 561, 563f, 657, 657f
neurofibroma, 559–560, 560f
neurothekeoma, 560–561, 562f
palisaded encapsulated neuroma, 560, 561f
schwannoma, 560
solitary circumscribed neuroma, 560, 561f
vascular proliferations and telangiectasias, 556–559 (*See also* Vascular proliferations and telangiectasias, cutaneous)
metastases, 658
noninfectious inflammatory processes, 581–604
blistering processes, 581–585 (*See also* Blistering processes)
degenerative disorders and connective tissue disease, 599–601
dermatomyositis, 601, 601f
lipoatrophy and lipodystrophy, 599
lupus erythematosus, 599–601, 600f
subacute cutaneous, 601
lupus profundus, 601, 601f
morphea, 601, 602f
granulomatous processes and histiocytic proliferations, 592–596
epithelioid cells, histiocytes, and giant cells, 592–593, 593f
acne agminata, 592
cutaneous Crohn's disease, 592–593
foreign body giant-cell reaction, 592
granulomatous cheilitis, 592
lupus miliaris disseminatus faciei, 592
Miescher-Melkersson-Rosenthal syndrome, 592
oral facial granulomatosis, 592
rosacea, 592
sarcoid, 593
histiocytic and necrobiotic, 594–596, 595f, 596f
annular elastolytic granuloma, 596
benign cephalic histiocytosis, 596
granuloma annulare, 594–596, 595f
juvenile xanthogranuloma, 596, 596f
Langerhans' cell histiocytosis, 596
pseudorheumatoid nodule, 594, 595f
xanthomatous, 593–594, 593f, 594f
chalazion, 594, 594f
paraffinoma, 593, 593f
sclerosing lipogranuloma, 593, 593f
verruciform xanthoma, 594, 594f
xanthelasma, 593–594, 594f
inflammatory processes involving adnexae, 601–604
alopecia mucinosa, 603–604, 603f
eosinophilic pustular folliculitis, 602, 603f
follicular occlusion triad, 604
herpes folliculitis, 604
lichen planopilaris, 604
pseudofolliculitis of the beard, 602
rhinophyma, 601–602, 603f
trichotillomania, 602
papulosquamous disorders, 586–590
lichenoid processes, 588–590, 588t
acute graft-*versus*-host disease, 590, 590f
erythema dyschromicum perstans, 589–590, 589f
erythema multiforme, 590, 591f
lichen planus, 588–589, 588t, 589f
toxic epidermal necrolysis, 590, 592f
psoriasiform dermatitis, 586–588
generalized pustular psoriasis of von Zumbusch, 587
prurigo nodularis, 587–588
psoriasis vulgaris, 586–587, 587f
pustular psoriasis, 587
Reiter's disease, 587, 587f
spongiotic dermatitis, 585–586, 586f
systemic and foreign substance reactions, 596–601
cold reactions, 599
cold temperature–induced panniculitis, 599
drug reactions, 596–598
amalgam tattoo, 588t, 598, 598f, 598t
argyria, 597, 598f
elastosis perforans serpiginosa, 597–598
exogenous ochronosis, 597
fixed drug eruption, 597, 597f
hyperpigmentation, minocycline-induced, 597
phototoxic and photoallergic drug eruptions, 596–597, 597f
light reactions, 598
actinic reticuloid, 598
polymorphous light eruption, 598, 599f
radiation dermatitis, 598
mucosal keratotic reactions, 599
vasculitis, 582t, 590–592
Behçet's disease, 592
granuloma faciale, 590–591
temporal arteritis, 591–592
Dermatophytes, 606, 606f
Dermatosis
ashy, 589–590, 589f
linear IgA bullous, 584–585
Dermoid(s)
congenital, 6–8, 7f, 8f
hairy, 7–8, 7f, 8f
nasopharyngeal, 158–159, 159f
of oropharynx, 184
sinonasal, 104–105
Dermoid cysts, 553–554
congenital, 6–8, 7f, 8f
orbital, 668–669, 669f
Desmoplastic fibroblastoma (collagenous fibroma), 403–404, 404f, 460
Desmoplastic melanoma, 572, 572f, 573f
Developmental lateral periodontal cyst, 206, 206f–207f
Diabetic proliferative retinopathy, 663–664, 664f
Diffuse large B-cell lymphoma
vs. extranodal NK/T-cell, nasal type, 495, 500t
intraocular, 668, 668f
thyroid, 521, 522f, 697
tonsillar, 493, 493f
Diffuse sclerosing osteomyelitis, 439–440, 440f
Digestive tract, upper. *See* Upper Aerodigestive tract
Dilated pore of Winer, 543
Diphtheria
laryngeal, 233, 234f
tonsils in, 181, 181f
Drug eruptions. *See also* Drug reactions
fixed, 597, 597f
phototoxic and photoallergic, 596–597, 597f
Drug reactions, cutaneous, 596–598
amalgam tattoo, 588t, 598, 598f, 598t
argyria, 597, 598f
elastosis perforans serpiginosa, 597–598
exogenous ochronosis, 597
fixed drug eruption, 597, 597f
hyperpigmentation, minocycline-induced, 597
phototoxic and photoallergic drug eruptions, 596–597, 597f
Duct retention cyst, 163, 163f

Ductal carcinoma of the breast, intraocular metastasis of, 667, 668f
Dysgenetic disease, 22
of parotid glands, 287, 287f
Dysplastic nevus (Clark's nevus), 568, 569f

E

Ear, 53–76
benign fibroosseous lesion, 59
biopsy of, 53
external and ear canal, 53–59
neoplasms of, 57–59
epithelial, 57–59, 58f, 59f
adenoma of ceruminal glands, 58, 58f
basal cell carcinoma, 57
ceruminal gland, benign, 58, 58f
ceruminal gland, malignant, 58–59, 59f
connective tissue and bone, 59
cylindroma, 58, 58f
exostosis, 59
melanotic, 58–59, 59f
monostotic fibrous dysplasia, 59
myxoma, 59
ossifying fibroma, 59
osteoma, 59
pleomorphic adenoma, 58
squamous cell carcinoma, 57
squamous cell carcinoma, verrucous, 57–58
syringocystadenoma papilliferum, 58
reticuloendothelial
Langerhans' cell histiocytosis, 59
malignant lymphoma, 59
non-neoplastic lesions of, 53–57
chondrodermatitis nodularis chronica helicis, 56
difficult to classify, 55–56, 56f
epithelioid hemangioma, 56–57, 56f
gout, 55, 55f
idiopathic cystic chondromalacia, 57, 57f
inflammatory, 53–55
infections, 53–54
keratin implantation granuloma, 55
keratosis obturans, 54–55
keratosis of tympanic membrane, 55
malignant otitis externa, 53
noninfectious, 54
relapsing polychondritis, 54, 54f
unknown origin, 54–55, 54f
keloid, 57
Kimura's disease, 57
malakoplakia, 55–56, 56f
metabolic conditions, 55, 55f
ochronosis, 55
petrified auricle, 57
spectacle frame acanthoma, 56
xanthoma with hyperlipoproteinemia, 55
inner and temporal bone, 71–74
congenital stapes fixation in, 75–76
Kaposi's sarcoma in (metastatic), 74
metastatic cancer in, 74
neoplasms of, 71–74
apex of petrous temporal bone tumors, 73–74
cerebellopontine angle tumors, 71, 73–74
cholesteatoma, 74
cholesterol granuloma, 74, 74f
internal auditory canal tumors, 71
lipoma, 73
low-grade adenoma of probable endolymphatic sac origin, 73–74, 74f
neurofibromatosis 2, 73, 73f
vestibular schwannoma, 72–73, 72f, 73f
osteogenesis imperfecta in, 76
otosclerosis of, 74–75, 75f
middle and mastoid, 60–71
neoplasms of, true
extending from other sites, 71, 71f
jugular paraganglioma, 71
locally arising, 67–71, 68f–70f
adenoma, 67–68, 68f
neural, 71
papillary adenocarcinoma, 71
paraganglioma, 68–70, 69f, 70f
rhabdomyosarcoma, 71
Schneiderian-type mucosal papilloma, 70–71
squamous cell carcinoma, 70, 70f
meningioma, 71, 71f
metastatic, 71
yolk sac tumor, 71
non-neoplastic lesions of, 60–67
cholesteatoma, 63
acquired, 63–67, 64f, 65f, 66t, 67f (*See also* Cholesteatoma)
choristoma, 67, 67f
developmental, tumor-like, 67, 67f
difficult to classify, 63–67
hamartoma, 67
inflammatory, 60–63, 60f–63f
actinomycosis, 63
otitis media, 60–62, 60f–62f
otitis media, AIDS, 63, 63f
otitis media, mycobacterial (TB), 62–63, 62f
otitis media, with effusion, 62, 62f
sarcoidosis, 63
Wegener's granulomatosis, 63
Eccrine acrospiroma, 303, 303f, 549–550
Eccrine carcinoma
clear cell type, 550
ductal type (classic), 550, 551f
mucinous type, 550–551
Eccrine cylindroma, 657–658
Eccrine hidrocystoma, 554, 554f
Eccrine poroma, 548f, 549, 549f
Eccrine spiradenoma, 657–658
Ecthyma, 604
Ecthyma gangrenosum, 604
Ectoderm anomalies, 2–8. *See also* Neuroectoderm and surface ectoderm anomalies
Ectomesenchymal chondromyxoid tumor (ECT), 429–430, 429f
Ectopic hamartomatous thymoma, 16–17, 16f
Ectopic thymus, 15, 15f
Ectopic thyroid, 13–14
Elastosis perforans serpiginosa, 597–598
Embryoma (sialoblastoma), 20, 20f
salivary gland, in children, 336–337, 337f
Embryonal carcinoma, 22
Embryonal rhabdomyosarcoma, 24
Embryonic remnants, persistent, 8–15. *See also under* Congenital anomalies
Encephalocele, 3
nasopharyngeal, 163
sinonasal, 146, 146f
Enchondroma, 447
Endodermal sinus tumor, 20
Endophthalmitis, bacterial, 664
Enteric (enterogenous) cysts, 11
orbital, 669, 669f
Eosinophilic angiocentric fibrosis
laryngeal, 247
sinonasal, 137
Eosinophilic granuloma
of bone, 464–466, 465f
of orbit, pediatric, 672, 672f
Eosinophilic pustular folliculitis, 602, 603f
Eosinophilic ulcer, 582t, 585
Epidermal cysts, 551–554
apocrine hidrocystoma, 554
dermoid, 553–554
eccrine hidrocystoma, 554, 554f
epidermal inclusion, 551–552, 552f
pilar, 552, 553f, 657–658
steatocystoma, 552–553, 553f
trichilemmal, 552, 553f, 657–658
vellus hair, 553
Epidermal inclusion cyst (sebaceous cyst, wen), 551–552, 552f
cytopathology of, 637–638, 638f
Epidermal neoplasms
intraepidermal, 546, 546t
pilar, 540–543 (*See also* Pilar neoplasms)
cytopathology of, 637–638, 638f
sebaceous, 543–546 (*See also* Sebaceous neoplasms and proliferations)
sweat gland, 546–551 (*See also* Sweat gland neoplasms)
Epidermal proliferations, 534–540
actinic keratosis, 535–536, 536f, 537f
basal cell carcinoma, 539, 540f
keratoacanthoma, 538–539, 538f
lentigo, 534, 536f
lymphoepithelioma-like carcinoma, 539–540
Paget's disease, 539, 539f
pseudocarcinomatous hyperplasia, 538
pseudoepitheliomatous hyperplasia, 538
seborrheic keratosis, 534, 535f
solar lentigo, 534
squamous cell carcinoma
invasive, 537–538, 538f
in situ (Bowen's disease), 536–537, 537f
verrucous carcinoma, 538
warty dyskeratoma, 534–535, 536f
Epidermoid cyst, 461, 462f
of ear, 74
Epidermolysis bullosa dystrophica, laryngeal, 243
Epiglottitis, acute, 232–233, 233f
Epignathus, 19
Epimyoepithelial island, 513, 514, 514t
Epithelial tumors, salivary gland. *See under* Salivary gland(s)
Epithelial–myoepithelial carcinoma, salivary gland, 328–329, 328f, 329t
cytopathology of, 629
Epithelioid cell nevus, 567–568, 568f
Epithelioid hemangioendothelioma (EHE), 413–414, 413f, 459–460
Epithelioid hemangioma (EH, histiocytoid hemangioma), 412–413, 413f, 558
of ear, 56–57, 56f

Epithelioid sarcoma (ES), 426–427, 426f
Epithelioma(s). *See also* specific types, e.g., Myoepithelioma
  basosebaceous, 545
  calcifying, of Malherbe, 542, 542f
    cytopathology of, 638, 655–656, 656f
  sebaceous, 545
Epulis, congenital, 416
Eruption cyst, 202f, 204
Erythema dyschromicum perstans (ashy dermatosis), 589–590, 589f
Erythema multiforme, 590, 591f
Ewing's sarcoma
  extraskeletal, 428–429, 428f
  skeletal, 467
Exogenous ochronosis, 597
Exostosis, of ear, 59
Extraabdominal desmoid tumor, 401–402, 401f. *See also* Fibromatosis
Extramedullary plasmacytoma (EMP), 523–525, 524f
  clinical features of, 523
  differential diagnosis of, 524–525, 525t
  laryngeal, 275
  nasopharyngeal, 178–179, 179f
  pathologic features of, 523, 524f
  staging, treatment, and outcome of, 523–524
Extranasal heterotopic neuroglial tissue, 5
Extranodal marginal zone (MALT) lymphoma
  B-cell, 515
  of thyroid, 520–521, 521f
Extranodal NK/T-cell lymphoma, nasal type, 495–500
  clinical features of, 496–497
  differential diagnosis of, 499–500
  vs. diffuse large B-cell lymphoma, 495, 500t
  pathologic features of, 497–499, 497f–498f
  staging, treatment, and outcome of, 499
Extraoccipital encephaloceles, 3
Extraskeletal Ewing's sarcoma, 428–429, 428f
Extravasation mucoceles, salivary gland, 288, 288f
Eye diseases, 663–668
  bacterial endophthalmitis, 664
  Coats' disease, 665, 665f
  diabetic proliferative retinopathy, 663–664, 664f
  glaucomas, 663, 664f
  inflammations and infections, 664–665, 665f
  neoplasms
    adult, 666–668
      adenoma, 666–667
      leiomyoma, 667
      malignant lymphoma, 668, 668f
      malignant melanoma, 667, 667f
      metastatic carcinoma, 667, 668f
    intraocular, 665–666
    pediatric, 666, 666f
      medulloepithelioma, 666
      neuroblastoma, 666, 666f
      retinoblastoma, 666, 666f
  of orbit, 668–675 (*See also* Orbital diseases)
  uveitis, chronic, 664, 665f

F

Factitial panniculitis, 593, 593f
Familial fibrous dysplasia, 22
Familial hypocalciuric hypercalcemia (FHH), 385
Fasciitis
  cranial, 392
  nodular, 392, 392f
  ossifying, 392
  periosteal, 392
  proliferative, 393
Fetal rhabdomyoma, 24, 24f
Fibroblastic and fibroproliferative processes, 391–395, 401–410. *See also* Fibroblastoma(s); Fibroma(s); Fibromatosis
  collagenous fibroma, 403–404, 404f
  cutaneous, 554–559
    atypical fibroxanthoma, 554–555, 555f
    cutaneous angiofibroma, 554, 555f
    dermatofibrosarcoma protuberans, 555–556, 556f
    fibrous papule, 554, 555f
    keloid, 554
    malignant fibrous histiocytoma, superficial type, 554–555, 555f
  fibromatosis, 401–402, 401f
    infantile, 402
  fibromatosis colli, 402, 402f
  fibrosarcoma, 407–408, 408f
    congenital, 408–409, 408f, 409f
    sclerosing epithelioid, 409
  Gardner's syndrome, 402
  giant cell angiofibroma, 406–407, 406f
  giant cell fibroblastoma, 407, 407f
  head-bangers tumor, 393
  hereditary gingival fibromatosis, 403
  intranodal myofibroblastoma, 405
  juvenile hyalin fibromatosis, 402–403, 402f, 403f
  myofibroma, solitary, 404–405
  myofibromatosis, 404–405
  myofibrosarcoma, 409
  nodular fasciitis and variants, 392, 392f
  nuchal fibrocartilagenous pseudotumor, 393–394, 394f
  nuchal fibroma, 403, 403f
  peripheral ossifying fibroma, 394–395, 394f
  posttraumatic spindle cell nodule, 391–392, 391f
  proliferative fasciitis, 393
  proliferative myositis, 393, 393f
  sinonasal, 137–143
    fibrohistiocytic tumors, 140–141, 140f
    fibrosarcoma, 139–140, 139f
    myxoma, 138–139
    peripheral nerve sheath tumors, 141–142, 141f
    rhabdomyosarcoma, 142–143
    solitary fibrous tumor, 138, 138f
  solitary fibrous tumor, 405–406, 405f, 406f
Fibroblastoma(s)
  desmoplastic, 403–404, 404f, 460
  giant cell, 407, 407f
Fibrofolliculoma (Birt-Hogg-Dubé syndrome), 543
Fibrohistiocytic tumors, sinonasal, 140–141, 140f
Fibroma(s), 460–461. *See also* Angiofibroma; Neurofibroma
  ameloblastic, 223–225, 224f, 678
  cementifying, 454, 454f, 455f
  chondromyxoid, 448–449, 449f
  collagenous, 403–404, 404f
  desmoplastic, 403–404, 404f, 460
  granular cell ameloblastic, 221–222, 222f
  laryngeal, 274–275
  myo-, 460–461, 461f
    solitary, 404–405
  myxo-, 220, 221f
  nuchal, 403, 403f
  odontogenic, 220–221, 220f, 221f
  ossifying
    cement-, 454, 454f, 455f
    of ear, 59
    juvenile, 454–456, 455f
    peripheral, 394–395, 394f
    psammomatoid, 454–456, 455f
  sinonasal, 136
    solitary, 138, 138f
  storiform perineurial, 416–417, 416f
Fibromatosis, 401–402, 401f. *See also* Myofibromatosis; Neurofibromatosis
  aggressive, 401–402, 401f
  hereditary gingival, 403
  infantile, 402
  juvenile hyalin, 402–403, 402f, 403f
Fibromatosis colli (FC), 402, 402f
Fibroosseous dysplasia, 453–454, 453f
Fibroosseous lesions, 453–456
  of ear, benign, 59
  fibrous dysplasia, 453–454, 453f
  ossifying fibroma, 454, 454f, 455f
  psammomatoid ossifying fibroma, 454–456, 455f
Fibrosarcoma(s)
  ameloblastic, 227
  congenital, 408–409, 408f, 409f
  myo-, 409
  sclerosing epithelioid, 409
  sinonasal, 139–140, 139f
Fibrous dysplasia, 22, 453–454, 453f
  familial, 22
Fibrous papule (adenoma sebaceum), 554, 555f
Fibrous tumors. *See* Fibroma(s)
Fibroxanthoma, atypical, 554–555, 555f
Field cancerization, 256
Field effect, 35, 256
Fine-needle aspiration (FNA) biopsy, 2, 2f. *See also* Cytopathology; specific cites, e.g., Salivary glands
Fine-needle aspiration–induced histologic changes, in salivary glands, 292, 292f
Fixed drug eruption, 597, 597f
Follicle center lymphoma, 578–579, 579f
  cytopathology of, 647f, 647t, 649f
  orbital, 675, 675f
Follicular adenomas, 356–357, 356f
  atypical, 357
Follicular carcinoma, of thyroid, 363–364, 363f
  with medullary thyroid carcinoma, 369
Follicular cyst, 676–677, 676f
  dentigerous, 202–203, 202f–204f
Follicular lichen planus, 604
Follicular lymphoid hyperplasia, adenoid, 160–161, 161f
Follicular lymphoma(s)
  salivary gland, 518–519, 519f
  tonsillar, 494, 494f
Follicular mucinosis, 603–604, 603f
Follicular occlusion triad, 604

Folliculitis
acute deep, 604
eosinophilic pustular, 602, 603f
herpes, 604
pseudo-, of the beard, 602
Folliculosebaceous cystic hamartoma, 543, 543f
Foregut duplication cysts, 11
Foreign body giant-cell reaction, 592
Foreign body reactions, cutaneous, 596–601. *See also under* Dermatopathology, noninfectious inflammatory processes
Fulminant invasive fungal sinusitis, 91–92, 92f
Fungal infections
of external ear and ear canal, 53
of eye, 664
of orbit, 669
of sinonasal tract, 88–92
chronic, 88–91, 90f
fulminant invasive sinusitis, 91–92, 92f
of skin, 606, 606f
Fungiform papilloma, 108–109, 108f
Fungus ball, 88–91, 90f
Furuncle (acute deep folliculitis), 604

G

Gardner's syndrome, 402
Generalized pustular psoriasis of von Zumbusch, 587
Ghost cell ameloblastoma, 218
Ghost cell glaucoma, 663, 664f
Ghost cell tumor, odontogenic, 218, 677
Giant cell angiofibroma (GCA), 406–407, 406f
Giant cell arteritis, cutaneous, 591–592
Giant cell fibroblastoma (GCF), 407, 407f
Giant cell granuloma, 22, 457–458, 457f, 458f
peripheral, 395, 395f
Giant cell reparative granuloma (GCRG), 457–458, 457f, 458f
mandibular and maxillofacial, 679, 679f
Giant cell tumor (GCT), 456, 456f
Gingival cysts, 202f, 206, 206f–207f
Gingival fibromatosis (GF), hereditary, 403
Gingival granular cell tumor of infants, 416
Gingivitis, 199
plasma cell, 199
Glandular neoplasms
metastatic, 120, 120f
non–salivary-type, 117–120
colonic, 119, 119f
mixed, 119
mucinous, 119, 119f
papillary, 119
sinonasal, 117–119, 119f
low-grade adenocarcinoma, 117–119, 118f, 119f
solid, 119
salivary-type
acinic cell carcinoma, 117 (*See also* Acinic cell carcinoma)
cytopathology of, 631–632, 631f, 632f
adenocarcinoma not otherwise specified, 116–117
adenoid cystic carcinoma, 115–116, 116f
carcinoma ex pleomorphic adenoma, 117
cytopathology of, 632–633
mucoepidermoid carcinoma, 117 (*See also* Mucoepidermoid carcinoma (MEC, MECA))
cytopathology of, 629–631, 629f, 630f, 630t
oncocytic neoplasms, 117
pleomorphic adenoma, 114–115, 115f
polymorphous low-grade adenocarcinoma, 117
cytopathology of, 628–629
sinonasal, 114–120
salivary-type, 114–117
Glandular odontogenic cyst, 207, 207f
Glandular retention cysts, 163, 163f
Glaucomas, 663, 664f
Glioma, nasal, 3–5, 4f, 4t, 5f
Globe lymphoma, 506–508, 507f
secondary, 508
Glomangioma, 411, 411f
Glomus tumor, 411, 411f
Glottic carcinomas, 255–256, 255f. *See also* Squamous cell carcinoma, of larynx and hypopharynx
Goiter
amyloid, 689–690, 690f
multinodular, with adenomatous change, 356–357, 356f
nodular (adenomatous), 355–356, 355f
toxic (Graves' disease), 354–355, 355f
cytopathology of, 689
Gout, 441
ear in, 55, 55f
laryngeal, 243
Graft-*versus*-host disease, acute, 590, 590f
Granular cell ameloblastic fibroma, 221–222, 222f
Granular cell odontogenic tumor, 221–222, 222f
Granular cell tumor(s) (GCT), 415–416, 415f, 416f
cytopathology of, 680–682, 681f
gingival, of infants, 416
of jaws, 221–222, 222f
laryngeal, 251–253, 252f
Granulocytic sarcoma, laryngeal, 275
Granuloma(s). *See also* Lipogranuloma; Xanthogranuloma
annular elastolytic, 596
cholesterol
of ear, 74, 74f
sinonasal, 87–88
eosinophilic
of bone, 464–466, 465f
orbital pediatric, 672, 672f
giant cell, 22, 457–458, 457f, 458f
peripheral, 395, 395f
giant cell reparative, 457–458, 457f, 458f
mandibular and maxillofacial, 679, 679f
hair, in ear and ear canal, 54
intravenous pyogenic, 390
keratin implantation, 55
lateral, 198
lethal midline, 495–496, 578
periapical, 197, 197f
peripheral giant cell, 395, 395f
pyogenic, 389–390, 390f
sinonasal, 134–135, 135f
sinonasal cholesterol, 87–88
starch, in ear and ear canal, 54
Teflon, 238–239, 239f
in tonsils, 183, 183f
vocal cord, 236–237, 237f
Granuloma annulare, 594–596, 595f
Granuloma faciale, cutaneous, 590–591
Granuloma fissuratum, 56
Granuloma gravidarum, 390
Granulomatosis, oral facial, 592
Granulomatous chelitis, 592
Granulomatous inflammation, in salivary tissue, 289
cytopathology of, 621
Granulomatous thyroiditis, 352–353
cytopathology of, 688, 688f
Graves' disease, 354–355, 355f
cytopathology of, 689
"Grog blossom," 601–602, 603f

H

Haemophilus influenzae type B (HIB), epiglottitis from, 232–233, 233f
Hair appendages, neoplasms of, 540–543. *See also* Pilar neoplasms
Hair granuloma, in ear and ear canal, 54
Hairy leukoplakia, oral, 608, 608f
Hairy polyp
oropharyngeal, 184
sinonasal, 104–105
teratoid, 7–8, 7f, 8f
Hamartoma(s), 1
congenital, 22
chondromesenchymal, 22, 22f, 23f
meningothelial, 5–6, 6f, 7f
folliculosebaceous cystic, 543, 543f
laryngeal, 246f, 247
of middle ear, 67
nasal, 22
nasolabial, 104
nasopharyngeal, 164–165, 164f–165f
sinonasal, 103–104, 104f
Hashimoto's thyroiditis, 353–354, 353f, 354f, 519–520, 520f
cytopathology of, 688–689, 689f
papillary carcinoma and, 358
sclerosing mucoepidermoid carcinoma with eosinophilia and, 369
Head-bangers tumor, 393
Heerfordt's disease, 289
Hemangioameloblastoma, 210
Hemangioendothelioma, 413–414, 413f
epithelioid, 413–414, 413f, 459–460
spindle cell, 414, 414f
Hemangioma(s), 412–413, 412f, 413f
arteriovenous, 412, 412f
capillary, 412, 412f, 556–557
cavernous, 412, 557
cellular, of infancy, 557
congenital, 24
epithelioid, 412–413, 413f, 558
of ear, 56–57, 56f
histiocytoid, 558
juvenile, 557
parotid gland, pediatric, 336, 336f
sinonasal, lobular capillary, 134–135, 135f
subglottic, 249–250, 249f
vascular, 458–459, 459f
venous, 412, 412f
Hemangiopericytoma, 410–411, 410f, 411f
infantile, 410–411, 411f
sinonasal, 135–136, 136f
Hereditary gingival fibromatosis, 403
Herpes folliculitis, 604
Herpes simplex viral infection, 607–608, 607f
of external ear and ear canal, 53–54
Herpes simplex viral lymphadenitis, 479
Herpes zoster infection, of external ear and ear canal, 54

Heterotopia(s), 1, 2t, 15–17
CNS, 145–148
nasal glial, 145–146, 145f
ectopic hamartomatous thymoma, 16–17, 16f
nasal glial, 3–5, 4f, 4t, 5f
phakomatous choristoma, 15–16, 16f
salivary gland, 15
Heterotopic brain, 158
Heterotopic meningeal nodule, cutaneous, 561, 563f
Heterotopic parathyroid cyst, 15
Hibernoma, 398–399, 399f
Hidradenocarcinoma
adenocystic, 550–551
clear cell, 550
Hidradenoma
clear cell, 549–550
solid and cystic, 549–550
Hidrocystoma
apocrine, 554
eccrine, 554, 554f
Histiocytic necrotizing lymphadenitis (Kikuchi's disease), 486–488, 487f
Histiocytoid hemangioma, 558
Histiocytosis
benign cephalic, 596
sinus, with massive lymphadenopathy, 246–247, 488–489, 489f
Histiocytosis X, 596
of bone, 464–466, 465f
in ear, 59
Histoplasmosis, laryngeal, 231–232
HIV-associated lymphadenopathy, 479–480, 480f
HIV-associated lymphoepithelial cyst, 620
HIV infection, tonsillitis with, 181–182, 182f–183f
Hodgkin's disease (HD), diagnosis of, 650–652, 651f
Human immunodeficiency virus. *See* HIV entries
Hurthle cell adenoma, 364, 365f
cytopathology of, 692, 693f
Hurthle cell carcinoma, 364–365, 365f
cytopathology of, 692, 693f
Hutchinson's melanotic freckle, 570, 570f. *See also* Lentigo maligna melanoma (LMM)
Hyalin fibromatosis, juvenile, 402–403, 402f, 403f
Hyaline myoepithelioma, 303, 303f
Hyaline stromal balls, neoplasms with, 627t
Hyalinizing trabecular adenoma, 357, 357f
cytopathology of, 694, 694f
Hypercalcemia, familial hypocalciuric, 385
Hyperlipoproteinemia, xanthoma with, ear in, 55
Hyperparathyroidism, secondary, 385
Hyperparathyroidism–jaw tumor syndrome, 382
Hyperpigmentation, minocycline-induced, 597
Hypoparathyroidism, 379
Hypopharyngeal carcinomas, 256, 256f. *See also* Squamous cell carcinoma, of larynx and hypopharynx
Hypopharyngeal diverticulum, 239
Hypopharynx, anatomy of, 230

I

Idiopathic cystic chondromalacia (pseudocysts), 57, 57f
Idiopathic (subglottic) laryngotracheal stenosis, 244, 245f
Impetigo, 604
Impetigo contagiosa, 604
Impetigo herpetiformis, 587
Incisive canal cyst, 199–200, 199f–200f
Infantile fibromatosis (IF), 402
Infantile hemangiopericytoma (IH), 410–411, 411f
Infantile myofibromatosis, 460–461, 461f
Infantile polyarteritis nodosa, 488
Infections. *See also* specific types, e.g., Bacterial infections, Herpes simplex virus infection
of ear, 53–54
of orbit, 669, 670f
of skin, 604–608 (*See also* Dermatopathology, infectious diseases)
Infectious mononucleosis (IM)
cytopathology of, 644–645
lymph nodes in, 476–478, 477f
nasopharynx in, 161, 161f
tonsillitis with, 182–183
Inflammatory lateral periodontal cyst, 201, 202f
Inflammatory myofibroblastic tumor (IMT), laryngeal, 244–246, 246f
Inflammatory pseudotumor
orbital, 670, 671f
parotid gland, 292, 292f
sinonasal, 136–137, 137f
tonsillar, 185
Insular carcinoma, of thyroid, 365, 366f
cytopathology of, 695, 695f
Internal auditory canal tumors, 71
Intraepidermal neoplasia, 546, 546t
Intraepithelial melanocytic hyperplasia, 568–569
Intranodal myofibroblastoma (IMF), 405
Intraocular neoplasms, 665–666
Intravascular B-cell lymphoma, 581, 581f
Intravenous pyogenic granuloma, 390
Inverted type A melanocytic nevus (combined nevus, clonal nevus), 565

J

Jaws. *See also* Oral cavity and jaws
fissural cysts of, 195, 196f
globulomaxillary cyst of, 195, 196f
granular cell tumor of, 221–222, 222f
nonodontogenic developmental cysts of, 199–201
nasolabial, 200–201, 200f–201f
nasopalatine duct, 199–200, 199f–200f
odontogenic cysts of, histologic typing of, 201, 201t
Joints. *See also* Bone and joint diseases
crystal-induced diseases of, 441
tumors and tumorlike lesions of, 467–469
pigmented villonodular synovitis, 468–469, 469f
primary synovial chondromatosis, 467–468, 468f
Jugular paraganglioma, 71
Juvenile hemangioma, 557
Juvenile hyalin fibromatosis (JHF), 402–403, 402f, 403f
Juvenile nasopharyngeal angiofibroma, 167–170, 168f–170f
Juvenile ossifying fibroma, 454–456, 455f
Juvenile pleomorphic adenoma, 22
Juvenile xanthogranuloma, 596, 596f

K

Kaposi's sarcoma (KS), 414, 414f, 558, 558f
in ear (metastatic), 74
laryngeal, 274, 274f
Kawasaki's disease, 488
Keloids
cutaneous, 554
in ear, 57
Keratin implantation granuloma, 55
Keratinizing squamous cell carcinoma, sinonasal, 121, 121f
Keratoacanthoma, 538–539, 538f
Keratocysts, odontogenic, 204–205, 204f–205f, 676, 676f
Keratosis
actinic (solar), 535–536, 536f, 537f
seborrheic, 534, 535f
tympanic membrane, 55
Keratosis obturans, 54–55
Keratotic reactions, cutaneous mucosal, 599
Kikuchi-Fujimoto disease, 486–488, 487f
Kikuchi's disease, 486–488, 487f
Kikuchi's lymphadenitis, 486–488, 487f
Kimura's disease
in ear, 57
in larynx, 235
lymph nodes in, 489–490, 490f
Kuttner's tumor, 289, 289f

L

Lacrimal gland neoplasms, 671–672
adenocarcinoma, 672
adenoid cystic carcinoma, 671–672, 672f
pleomorphic adenoma, 671, 671f
Langerhans' cell histiocytosis (histiocytosis X), 596
of bone, 464–466, 465f
of ear, 59
Large-cell carcinoma, salivary, 333, 333f
Laryngeal cancer. *See* Squamous cell carcinoma, of larynx and hypopharynx
Laryngeal chondromas, 270–271
Laryngeal chondrosarcomas, 270–274, 272f, 273f
Laryngeal lymphoma, 511
secondary, 511
Laryngeal paragangliomas, 265
Laryngeal saccule, 237
Laryngeal sarcomas, 270
Laryngoceles, 237–238, 237f, 238f
Laryngopharynx. *See also* Hypopharynx; Larynx and hypopharynx
anatomy of, 230
Laryngotracheal stenosis, idiopathic (subglottic), 244, 245f
Laryngotracheobronchopathia chondroosteoplastica, 243–244, 244f
Larynx and hypopharynx, 230–276
anatomy of, 230, 231f
degenerative, autoimmune, and metabolic diseases of, 240–243
amyloid, 241–242, 241f
cicatricial pemphigoid, 243
epidermolysis bullosa dystrophica, 243
gout, 243
pemphigus vulgaris, 242–243

Larynx and hypopharynx (*contd.*)
relapsing polychondritis, 242
rheumatoid arthritis, 242
Wegener's granulomatosis, 240, 240f
histologic dysplasia and squamous intraepithelial neoplasia in, 40t
idiopathic conditions of, 243–247
hamartomas, 246f, 247
inflammatory myofibroblastic tumor, 244–246, 246f
oculopharyngeal muscular dystrophy, 244, 245f
oncocytic cyst, 243, 243f
sinus histiocytosis with massive lymphadenopathy, 246–247
subglottic laryngotracheal stenosis, 244, 245f
tracheopathia osteoplastica, 243–244, 244f
inflammatory lesions of, 230–235
infectious, 230–233
acute, 232–233, 233f
diphtheria, 233, 234f
fungal, 231–232, 232f
rarities, 232
Trichinella spiralis, 232, 232f
tuberculosis, 231, 232f
noninfectious, 233–235
Crohn's disease, 234–235, 235f
necrotizing sialometaplasia, 234
sarcoidosis, 233–234, 235f
mechanical and chemical lesions of, 235–240
contact ulcers and "granulomas," 236–237, 237f
laryngoceles and saccular cysts, 237–238, 237f–239f
Teflon granuloma, 238–239, 239f
vocal cord polyps, 235–236, 236f
Zenker's diverticulum, 239–240
neoplasms of, 247–276
benign, 247–253
granular cell, 251–253, 252f, 680–682, 681f
others, 253, 253f, 254f
paraganglioma, 250–251, 250f
rhabdomyoma, 253, 253f, 681
salivary gland-type, 249
schwannomas, 253, 253f
squamous cell carcinoma, papillary and exophytic, 247–248
squamous papilloma, 247–249, 248f, 680
subglottic hemangioma, 249–250, 249f
verrucous, 248
malignant, 253–276
adenocarcinoma, 269–270, 270f, 271f
cartilaginous, 270–274, 272f, 273f
extramedullary plasmacytoma, 275
fibrosarcomas, 274–275
granulocytic sarcoma, 275
Kaposi's sarcoma, 274, 274f
liposarcomas, 274, 275f
lymphoepitheliomatous carcinoma (nasopharyngeal-type), 264
lymphoma, 275, 681–682
malignant fibrous histiocytoma, 274
mast cell sarcoma, 275
melanoma, 275–276, 276f
mycosis fungoides, 275
neuroendocrine, 264–269 (*See also* Neuroendocrine carcinoma(s), laryngeal)
rhabdomyosarcoma, 274
sarcomas, rare, 275
squamous cell carcinoma, 253–264 (*See also* Squamous cell carcinoma, of larynx and hypopharynx)
synovial sarcomas, 274
Lateral aberrant thyroid, 14, 351
Lateral periodontal cyst
developmental, 206, 206f–207f
inflammatory, 201, 202f
Leiomyoma, 424, 424f, 667
Leiomyosarcoma (LMS), 424, 424f
of bone, 466–467
Lentigo (melanotic macule), 534, 536f
solar (senile), 534
Lentigo maligna melanoma (LMM), 570, 570f, 572, 572f
invasive, 572, 572f
Leprosy, 97–98, 604, 605f
laryngeal, 232
Lethal midline granuloma, 495–496, 578
Lichen planopilaris (follicular lichen planus), 604
Lichen planus, 588–589, 588t, 589f
follicular, 604
Lichenoid processes, cutaneous, 588–590, 588t
acute graft-*versus*-host disease, 590, 590f
erythema dyschromicum perstans, 589–590, 589f
erythema multiforme, 590, 591f
lichen planus, 588–589, 588t, 589f
toxic epidermal necrolysis, 590, 592f
Light eruption, polymorphous, 598, 599f
Light reactions, cutaneous, 598
actinic reticuloid, 598
polymorphous light eruption, 598, 599f
radiation dermatitis, 598
Linear IgA bullous dermatosis, 584–585
Lipadenoma, 382
Lipoatrophy, 599
Lipoblastoma, 398, 398f
Lipodystrophy, 599
Lipogranuloma, sclerosing, 593, 593f
Lipoma(s), 397
angio-, 397, 397f
chondroid, 399, 399f
cutaneous, 559
intramuscular (infiltrating), 559, 560f
cytopathology of, 653–654
of ear, 73
pleomorphic, 398, 398f
of salivary gland, 619
spindle cell, 397–398, 397f
Lipomatous proliferations, cutaneous, 559–561. *See also* Dermatopathology, neoplastic proliferative processes
Liposarcoma(s), 399–401, 400f
dedifferentiated, 401
laryngeal and hypopharyngeal, 274, 275f
myxoid, 400, 400f
pleomorphic, 401, 401f
round cell, 400–401, 400f
well-differentiated, 400, 400f
Liver spot (solar lentigo), 534
Lobular capillary hemangioma, sinonasal, 134–135, 135f
Low-grade adenoma of probable endolymphatic sac origin, in ear, 73–74, 74f
Lupus erythematosus, 599–601, 600f
subacute cutaneous, 601
Lupus lymphadenitis, 485–486, 485f
Lupus miliaris disseminatus faciei, 592
Lupus panniculitis, 601, 601f
Lupus profundus, 601, 601f
Lymph nodes
intraparotid, 633–634
metastases to, 639–642 (*See also* specific cancers, e.g., Nasopharyngeal carcinoma)
Lymphadenitis
cervical lymph node, 477t
cytomegaloviral, 478–479, 478f
herpes simplex viral, 479
histiocytic necrotizing, 486–488, 487f
lupus, 485–486, 485f
mycobacterial, 482–483, 484f
Piringer-Kuchinka, 483–484, 484f
pyogenic bacterial, 481, 481f
toxoplasma, 483–484, 484f
Lymphadenocarcinoma, sebaceous, 312
Lymphadenoma, sebaceous, 311, 311f
Lymphadenopathy
HIV–associated, 479–480, 480f
infectious, 643–646
actinomycosis, 645, 645f
cat-scratch disease, 643–644
mononucleosis, 644–645
mycobacterial, 643
sarcoidosis, 645, 645f
toxoplasmosis, 644
massive, sinus histiocytosis with, 246–247, 488–489, 489f
reactive, 633
cytopathology of, 642–643, 642f
Lymphadenosis benigna cutis, 576–577
Lymphangioma, 411–412, 411f
congenital, 24
Lymphangioma circumscriptum, 557, 557f
Lymphoangiomatous tonsillar polyps, 183–184, 184f
Lymphoblastic lymphoma, pediatric salivary, 337
Lymphocytic (Hashimoto's) thyroiditis, 353–354, 353f, 354f, 519–520, 520f
cytopathology of, 688–689, 689f
papillary carcinoma and, 358
sclerosing mucoepidermoid carcinoma with eosinophilia and, 369
Lymphocytoma cutis, 576–577
Lymphoepithelial carcinoma, salivary, 333–334, 334f
Lymphoepithelial cysts, 288, 288f
cytopathology of, 637, 637f
salivary gland, simple, 512, 512f
simple, 512, 512f
tonsillar, 183, 184f
Lymphoepithelial lesion, 513–514, 514t
benign, 513, 514t
of salivary glands, 291, 291f
Lymphoepithelial sialadenitis (LESA), 513–516, 514t
clinical features of, 513–514
and MALT-type lymphoma, 515–516, 516t, 517t
differential diagnosis of, 515

etiology of, 515
morphologic features of, 514–515, 515f
terminology of, 513–514, 514t
Lymphoepithelioma, 50, 50f
Lymphoepithelioma-like carcinoma, 539–540
Lymphoepitheliomatous (nasopharyngeal-type) carcinoma, 264
Lymphoid hyperplasia. *See also* Lymphoma(s)
cutaneous (lymphocytoma cutis), 576–577
actinic reticuloid, 577
pseudolymphoma of Spiegler-Fendt, 576–577
reactive, 633
of orbit, 670
reactive lesions of cervical lymph nodes, 476–491, 477t
cytomegaloviral infection, 478–479, 478f
cytopathology of, 642–643, 642f
herpes simplex viral lymphadenitis, 479
HIV-associated lymphadenopathy, 479–480, 480f
infectious mononucleosis, 476–478, 477f
cytopathology of, 644–645
Kawasaki's disease, 488
Kikuchi's disease, 486–488, 487f
Kimura's disease, 489–490, 490f
lupus lymphadenitis, 485–486, 485f
mycobacterial lymphadenitis, 482–483, 484f
cytopathology of, 643
pyogenic bacterial lymphadenitis, 481, 481f
sinus histiocytosis with massive lymphadenopathy, 488–489, 489f
toxoplasma lymphadenitis, 483–484, 484f
reactive lymphadenopathy, 642–643, 642f
Lymphoid infiltrate, neoplasms with, 630t
Lymphoid papillary hyperplasia of tonsils, 184
Lymphoid proliferations
of salivary glands, 511–519 (*See also* Salivary gland, lymphoid proliferations of)
of thyroid, 519–523 (*See also* Thyroid, lymphoid proliferations of)
Hashimoto's thyroiditis, 353–354, 353f, 354f, 519–520, 520f (*See also* Hashimoto's thyroiditis)
cytopathology of, 688–689, 689f
Lymphoma(s), 490–491
angiocentric, 496
B-cell
cutaneous, 578–581
angiotrophic, 581, 581f
follicle center, 578–579, 579f
intravascular B-cell, 581, 581f
malignant angioendotheliomatosis, 581, 581f
marginal zone, of MALT type, 579–580, 580f
plasmacytoma, 580–581
diffuse large
vs. extranodal NK/T-cell, nasal type, 495, 500t
of thyroid, 521, 522f, 697
in Waldeyer's ring, 493, 493f
immunohistologic and genetic features of, 491, 491t
intraocular, 668, 668f
large, 648f, 648t
small, 647f, 647t
classifications of, 490t, 491
REAL and WHO, 490t, 491
cutaneous, primary, 576
distribution of, 491, 492t
Hodgkin's, diagnosis of, 650–652, 651f
of larynx, 511
secondary, 511
lymphoblastic, pediatric salivary, 337
malignant
approach to, 646
cytopathology of, 646–652, 681–682, 683, 683f
of ear, 59
of eye, 668, 668f
gene arrangement studies of, 646
general considerations in, 646
immunophenotyping of, 646
of larynx, 275
morphology of, 646–648
with large or intermediate lymphocytes, 647–648, 648f, 648t, 649f
with small lymphocytes, 646–647, 647f, 647t, 649f
non-Hodgkin's, 648–650, 649f, 651f
of oral cavity and oropharynx, 681–682
of orbit, 675, 675f
of salivary gland, 334–335
in children, 337
cytopathology of, 633
sinonasal, 101–103, 102f, 683, 683f
of thyroid, 371–372, 371f, 697
of Waldeyer's ring, 187–189, 188f
MALT, 670, 671f
of nasal cavity and paranasal sinuses, 495–501 (*See also* Nasal cavity and paranasal sinuses, lymphomas of)
nasal T-cell, 496
non-Hodgkin's, diagnosis of, 648–650, 649f, 651f
ocular, 506–508, 507f
secondary, 508
ocular adnexal, 503–506, 504f
clinical features of, 503
differential diagnosis of, 504–505
pathologic features of, 503–504, 504f
secondary, 506
staging, treatment, and outcome of, 505–506
ocular adnexal lymphoid infiltrates in, 501–506
diagnosis of, 502–503, 502f
of oral cavity, 508–511
clinical features of, 508–509, 509t
differential diagnosis of, 510–511
in HIV-positive patients, 509–510, 509t, 510f
pathologic features of, 509
staging, treatment, and outcome of, 510
plasmacytoma, extramedullary, 523–525, 524f
of salivary gland, 516–519
aggressive, 519
follicular, 518–519, 519f
marginal zone B-cell/MALT, 517–518, 517f
T-cell
cutaneous, 577–581
angiocentric immunoproliferative lesion, 578
cutaneous anaplastic large-cell (Ki-1$^+$) lymphoma, primary, 578, 578f
lethal midline granuloma, 578
mycosis fungoides, 577–578, 577f
nasal or nasal-type T/NK-cell lymphoma, 578
polymorphic reticulosis, 578
cytopathology of, 648f, 648t
immunohistologic and genetic features of, 491, 492t
nasal, 496
T/NK-cell, nasal or nasal type, 496, 578
extranodal, 495–500 (*See also* Extranodal NK/T-cell lymphoma, nasal type)
of thyroid, 520–523
Burkitt's and Burkitt-like, 521–522
classification of, 520
cytopathology of, 697
diffuse large B-cell, 521, 522f, 697
extranodal marginal zone (MALT), 520–521, 521f
plasmacytoma, 522–523, 697
of Waldeyer's ring, 491–495 (*See also* Waldeyer's ring, lymphomas of)

M

Malakoplakia, 55–56, 56f
Malignant acrospiroma, 550, 551f
Malignant angioendotheliomatosis, 581, 581f
Malignant fibrous histiocytoma (MFH), 409–410
bone, 467
laryngeal, 274
myxoid, 409–410, 410f
storiform–pleomorphic, 409, 410f
superficial type, 554–555, 555f
Malignant lymphoma(s). *See* Lymphoma(s), malignant
Malignant melanoma. *See* Melanoma(s), malignant
Malignant otitis externa, 53
Malignant peripheral nerve sheath tumors (MPNST), 420–421, 420f
cytopathology of, 653, 653f
Malignant syringoma (syringoid carcinoma), 551, 552f
MALT (mucosa-associated lymphoid tissue) lymphoma, 670, 671f
extranodal marginal zone, of thyroid, 520–521, 521f
lymphoepithelial sialadenitis and Sjögren's syndrome and, 515–516, 516t, 517t
marginal zone B-cell
cutaneous, 579–580, 580f
extranodal, 515
of salivary gland, 517–518, 517f
Mandible and maxillofacial areas, 675–680
odontogenic cysts in, 676–677
dentigerous, 676–677, 676f
ghost cell tumor, 677
keratocyst, 676, 676f
radicular, 676, 676f
odontogenic tumors in, 677–679
ameloblastic carcinoma, 678
ameloblastic fibroma, 678
ameloblastoma, 677–678, 677f
calcifying epithelial, 678–679
myxoma, 678, 678f

Mandible and maxillofacial areas (*contd.*)
  osseous tumors in, 679–680
    aneurysmal bone cyst, 679
    cementifying fibroma, 679
    chordoma, 679–680, 679f
    giant-cell reparative granuloma, 679, 679f
    osteosarcoma, 680
Mantle cell lymphoma (MCL)
  cytopathology of, 647t
  of Waldeyer's ring, 494, 495f
Marginal zone B cell, 514t
Marginal zone lymphoma of MALT type
  B-cell, 579–580, 580f
    extranodal, 515
    plasmacytoma *vs.*, 525, 525t
    of salivary glands, 517–518, 517f
  extranodal, of thyroid, 520–521, 521f
Mast cell sarcoma, laryngeal, 275
Maxillary sinus, squamous cell carcinoma of, 123
Maxillofacial areas. *See* Mandible and maxillofacial areas
Meckel-Gruber syndrome, 3
Medullary thyroid carcinoma, 367–369, 368f
  cytopathology of, 696–697, 696f, 697f
    lymph node metastases in, 641–642, 642f
  with follicular thyroid carcinoma, 369
Medulloepithelioma, 666
Melanocytic neoplasms, cutaneous, 561–576
  benign proliferations, 565–570
    conjunctival melanosis, 568–569
    dysplastic nevus, 568, 569f
    intraepithelial melanocytic hyperplasia, 568–569
    lentigo maligna, 570, 570f
    melanocytic nevus, 565–567 (*See also* Melanocytic nevus)
    nevus with architectural disorder and cytologic atypia, 568, 569f
    spindled and epithelioid cell nevus, 567–568, 568f
    Spitz nevus, 567–568, 568f
  dendritic melanocytoses, 562–565
    blue nevus, 563–564, 564f
      cellular, 564–565
      malignant, 565
    deep penetrating nevus, 565
    inverted type A melanocytic nevus, 565
    nevus of Ota, 562–563
  malignant melanoma, 570–576 (*See also* Melanoma(s), malignant)
Melanocytic nevus, 565–567
  balloon cell type, 566
  congenital, 567, 567f
  dermal, 565, 566f
  halo type, 566–567
  neurotized, 565–566
Melanoma(s)
  acral lentiginous, 572, 573f
  benign juvenile, 567–568, 568f
  cytopathology of, 640, 640f
  desmoplastic, 572, 572f, 573f
  lentigo maligna, 570, 570f, 572, 572f
    invasive, 572, 572f
  lymph node metastases of, 640, 640f
  malignant, 570–576
    cytopathology of, 640, 640f, 683, 683f
    growth phases of, 573, 574t
    invasive, 571
      acral lentiginous, 572, 573f
      anatomic levels of, 575, 575t
      desmoplastic, 572, 572f, 573f
      lentigo maligna melanoma, 572, 572f
      mucosal, 572
      nodular, 572–573, 574f
      superficial spreading, 571, 571f, 575f
      types of, 571–573, 571f–574f
    laryngeal, 275–276, 276f
    nasal cavity, 683, 683f
    ocular, 667, 667f
    prognostic factors in, 573–576, 574t, 575f, 575t, 576t
    sinonasal, 133–134, 133f
    in situ, 570–571, 570f
    thickness of, 575, 575f
    tumor-infiltrating lymphocytes in, 575, 576t
  mucosal lentiginous, 572
  superficial spreading, invasive, 571, 571f, 575f
Melanosis, conjunctival, 568–569
Melanotic macule, 534, 536f
Melanotic neoplasms, of ear (ceruminal gland), 58–59, 59f
Melanotic neuroectodermal tumor of infancy (MNTI), 463–464, 463f, 464f
Meningeal nodule, cutaneous heterotopic, 561, 563f
Meningioma(s)
  cutaneous, 561, 563f
  middle ear, 71, 71f
  orbital, 673–674, 674f
  sinonasal, 146–147, 146f
Meningocele(s), 3
  rudimentary, 5–6, 6f, 7f
  sinonasal, 146
Meningoencephalocele, sinonasal, 146, 146f
Meningothelial hamartoma, 5–6, 6f, 7f
Merkel cell carcinoma, 561, 563f
  cytopathology of, 657, 657f
Mesenchymal chondrosarcoma, 451, 451f
Metastatic tumors. *See* specific sites, e.g., Nasal cavity and paranasal sinuses, metastatic tumors
Microcarcinoma, 360
Microcystic adnexal carcinoma, 551, 552f
Microinvasive carcinoma, of upper aerodigestive tract, 41–42, 41f
Miescher-Melkersson-Rosenthal syndrome, 592
Mikulicz's disease (syndrome), 513, 514t
Minocycline-induced hyperpigmentation, 597
Mixed tumor. *See also* Pleomorphic adenoma
  recurrent, 299, 299f
  of salivary gland, 296–299
    benign, 114–115, 115f
    malignant, 117, 299–302, 300f–302f
      carcinoma ex pleomorphic adenoma, 299–301, 300f, 301f
        cytopathology of, 632–633
      incidence of, 299
  of sweat gland (chondroid syringoma), 549, 550f
    cytopathology of, 657–658
Moderately differentiated neuroendocrine carcinoma (MDNEC), 266–267, 267f
Molluscum contagiosum, 608, 608f
Monocytoid B cell, 514t
Mononucleosis, infectious
  cytopathology of, 644–645
  lymph nodes in, 476–478, 477f
  nasopharynx in, 161, 161f
  tonsillitis with, 182–183
Monosodium urate crystal deposition disease (gout), 441–442, 442f
Monostotic fibrous dysplasia, 59
Morphea (localized scleroderma), 601, 602f
Mucin, allergic, 89–90, 90f
Mucinous adenocarcinoma, sinonasal, 119, 119f
Mucocele(s), 86–87, 86f
  salivary gland, 288, 288f
Mucocutaneous lymph node syndrome, 488
Mucoepidermoid carcinoma (MEC, MECA)
  of larynx and hypopharynx, 270, 270f
  of salivary gland, 117, 323–326, 324f, 620, 620t
    in children, 337
    clinical behavior and treatment of, 325–326
    clinical data on, 323
    cytopathology of, 629–631, 629f, 630f, 630t
    definition of, 323
    differential diagnosis of, 325
    grades of, 324–325
    gross appearance of, 324
    histologic features of, 324, 324f
    immunohistochemistry of, 325
    low-grade, 619, 619f
    special studies on, 325
Mucormycosis, 91–92, 92f
Mucosa-associated lymphoid tissue (MALT) lymphoma. *See* MALT
Mucosal keratotic reactions, cutaneous, 599
Mucosal lentiginous melanoma, 572
Mucus retention cyst, 619, 619f
Multifocal idiopathic fibrosclerosis, tonsillar, 185
Multinodular goiter with adenomatous change, 356–357, 356f
Multiple endocrine neoplasia (MEN), 384–385
Multiple myeloma, orbital, 674–675, 675f
Mycobacterial infections, orbital, 669, 670f
Mycobacterial lymphadenitis, 482–483, 484f
Mycobacterial lymphadenopathy, 643
Mycosis fungoides, 577–578, 577f
  laryngeal, 275
Myeloma(s)
  multiple, orbital, 674–675, 675f
  plasma cell, 580–581 (*See also* Plasmacytoma)
    extramedullary, 523–525, 524f
Myoepithelial carcinoma, of salivary glands, 305, 305f
Myoepithelial sialadenitis (MESA), 513, 514, 514t
  cytopathology of, 621–622, 622f
Myoepithelioma, 302
  clear cell, 549–550
  hyaline, 303, 303f
  plasmacytoid, 303, 303f
  of salivary gland, 302–305, 303f, 304f
    clinical behavior and treatment of, 305
    clinical data on, 303
    definition of, 302
    differential diagnosis of, 304
    flow cytometry of, 304
    gross appearance of, 303
    histologic features of, 303–304, 303f, 304f

immunohistochemistry of, 304
ultrastructure of, 304, 304f
Myofibroblastoma, intranodal, 405
Myofibroma, 460–461, 461f
solitary, 404–405
Myofibromatosis, 404–405
infantile, 460–461, 461f
Myofibrosarcoma, 409
Myogenetic tumors, 421–424
leiomyoma, 424, 424f, 667
leiomyosarcoma, 424, 424f, 466–467
rhabdomyoma, 421–422, 421f, 422f
cytopathology of, 681
fetal, 24, 24f
laryngeal, 253, 253f
rhabdomyosarcoma, 422–424, 422f, 423f (*See also* Rhabdomyosarcoma)
Myositis. *See also* Dermatomyositis
proliferative, 393, 393f
Myositis ossificans (MO), 395–396, 396f
Myospherulosis, 87, 87f
Myxofibroma, 220, 221f
Myxofibrosarcoma, 409–410, 410f
Myxoid liposarcoma, 400, 400f
Myxoid malignant fibrous histiocytoma, 409–410, 410f
Myxoid polyp, vocal cord, 235–236, 236f
Myxoma(s)
ear, 59
nerve sheath, 560–561, 562f
odontogenic, 218–220, 219f
mandibular and maxillary, 678, 678f
sinonasal, 138–139

N

Nasal cavity and paranasal sinuses, 80–148
anatomy of, 80
clinical relevance of, 81
cholesteatoma in, 87–88
CNS heterotopias and related lesions of, 145–148
encephalocele, 146, 146f
meningioma, 146–147, 146f
nasal glial heterotopia, 145–146, 145f
pituitary adenoma, 147–148, 147f
cytopathology of, 682–683, 682f, 683f
dermoids and hairy polyp in, 104–105
embryology of, 80
fungal diseases of, 88–92
chronic, 88–91, 90f
fulminant invasive sinusitis, 91–92, 92f
glandular neoplasms of, 114–120
metastatic, 120, 120f
non–salivary-type, 117–120
colonic, 119, 119f
mixed, 119
mucinous, 119, 119f
papillary, 119
sinonasal, 117–119, 119f
sinonasal low-grade adenocarcinoma, 117–119, 118f, 119f
solid, 119
salivary-type, 114–117
acinic cell carcinoma, 117
cytopathology of, 631–632, 631f, 632f
adenocarcinoma not otherwise specified, 116–117
adenoid cystic carcinoma, 115–116, 116f
carcinoma ex pleomorphic adenoma, 117
cytopathology of, 632–633
mucoepidermoid carcinoma, 117 (*See also* Mucoepidermoid carcinoma)
oncocytic neoplasms, 117
pleomorphic adenoma, 114–115, 115f
polymorphous low-grade adenocarcinoma, 117
cytopathology of, 628–629
hamartomas in, 103–104, 104f
histology of, 81–82, 82f
lymphatic drainage of, 80–81
lymphomas of, 495–501
extranodal NK/T-cell, nasal type, 495–500
clinical features of, 496–497
differential diagnosis of, 499–500
vs. diffuse large B-cell, 495, 500t
pathologic features of, 497–499, 497f–498f
staging, treatment, and outcome of, 499
incidence of, 495, 496t
malignant, 683, 683f
paranasal sinus, 500–501, 501f
malignant melanoma in, 683, 683f
metastatic tumors in, 148
mid-facial necrotizing lesions of, 92–103
clinical presentation of, 92–93
cocaine abuse, 100–101
histology of, 92, 93t
leprosy, 97–98
lymphomas, malignant, 101–103, 102f
rhinoscleroma, 98–99, 98f, 99f
rhinosporidiosis, 99–100, 99f
sarcoidosis, 95–96, 96f
tuberculosis, 96–97
Wegener's granulomatosis, 93–95, 94f
mucocele in, 86–87, 86f
myospherulosis in, 87, 87f
nasolabial cyst-hamartoma in, 104
nasopharyngeal carcinoma of (*See* Nasopharyngeal carcinoma)
neoplasms of,
from adjacent structures, 143–145, 143f, 144f
ameloblastoma, 143–144, 143f
malignant melanoma, 133–134, 133f, 683, 683f (*See also* Melanoma(s), malignant)
mesenchymal, 134–143
eosinophilic angiocentric fibrosis, 137
fibrohistiocytic, 140–141, 140f
fibroma, 136
fibromatosis, 137–143
fibrosarcoma, 139–140, 139f
fibrous, 136–137, 137f
hemangiopericytoma, 135–136, 136f
inflammatory pseudotumor, 136–137, 137f
lobular capillary hemangioma, 134–135, 135f
myxoma, 138–139
peripheral nerve sheath, 141–142, 141f
pyogenic granuloma, 134–135, 135f
rhabdomyosarcoma, 142–143
solitary fibrous, 138, 138f
tumefactive fibroinflammatory lesion, 136–137, 137f
vascular, 134–136, 135f, 136f
odontogenic, 143–144, 143f
adenomatoid, 144–145
calcifying epithelial, 144, 144f
neuroendocrine, neural and neuroectodermal tumors of, 124–134
olfactory neuroblastomas in, 124–129, 682, 682f (*See also* Olfactory neuroblastomas)
paraganglioma in, 132–133
small cell carcinoma and allied tumors in, 129–131, 130f
undifferentiated (anaplastic), 131–132, 131f
olfactory neuroblastoma of, 682, 682f
rhinitis caseosa in, 87–88
Schneiderian papillomas of, 106–108, 107f
columnar, 111–113, 112f
dysplasia and malignancy in, 113–114
fungiform, 108–109, 108f
inverted, 109–111, 109f–111f
sinonasal cholesterol granuloma in, 87–88
sinusitis in, 82–88 (*See also* Sinusitis)
squamous cell carcinoma of, 120–124, 123
basaloid, 123–124, 123f
clinical data on, 120–121
histopathologic features of, 121
keratinizing, 121, 121f
of nasal vestibule, 123
nonkeratinizing, 121–123, 122f, 123f
sinonasal, 682
of maxillary sinus, 123
of nasal cavity, 123
of nasal vestibule, 123
teratocarcinosarcoma in, 106
teratoma in, 105–106
Nasal glial heterotopia, 3–5, 4f, 4t, 5f, 145–146, 145f
Nasal glioma, 3–5, 4f, 4t, 5f
Nasal lesions, congenital, 3, 4t
Nasal/nasal type NK/T-cell lymphoma, 496, 578
extranodal, 495–500 (*See also* Extranodal NK/T-cell lymphoma, nasal type)
Nasal polyps, inflammatory, 84–86, 84f, 85f
Nasal T-cell lymphoma, 496
Nasal vestibule, squamous cell carcinoma of, 123
Nasoalveolar cyst, 200–201, 200f–201f
Nasolabial cyst, 104, 200–201, 200f–201f
Nasolabial hamartoma, 104
Nasopalatine duct cyst, 199–200, 199f–200f
Nasopharyngeal carcinoma (NPC), 49–50, 170–174
biological behavior and therapy of, 174
clinical data on, 170–171
cytopathology of, 639–640, 639f, 682
differential diagnosis of, 174
epidemiology and etiology of, 170
histopathology of, 171, 171t
lymph node metastases of, 639–640, 639f
nonkeratinizing, 171–174, 171t, 172f–173f
squamous cell, 171, 171f, 171t
Nasopharyngeal-type carcinoma, 264
Nasopharynx, 157–179. *See also* Waldeyer's ring
anatomy of, 157
benign neoplasms of, 166–170
juvenile angiofibroma, 167–170, 168f–170f

Nasopharynx (*contd.*)
rarities, 170
salivary gland anlage tumor, 20, 21f, 166–167, 166f, 167f, 337
congenital anomalies of, 157–160
branchial cyst, 160
choanal atresia, 158
dermoids, 158–159, 159f
heterotopic brain, 158
pharyngeal stenosis, 158
teratomas, 159–160, 160f
inflammatory lesions of, 160–161, 161f
malignant tumors of, 170–179
adenocarcinoma, 175–177, 175f–176f
chordomas, 177–178, 178f
extramedullary plasmacytomas, 178–179, 179f
lymphoma, 179
metastases, 178, 178f
nasopharyngeal carcinoma, 49–50, 170–174 (*See also* Nasopharyngeal carcinoma)
cytopathology of, 639–640, 639f, 682
rarities, 179
sarcomas, 177, 177f
non-neoplastic tumorous conditions of, 162–166
actinomycosis with abscess, 166
amyloid deposition, 165–166, 166f
cysts, 162–163
branchial, 162
encephalocele, 163
glandular retention, 163, 163f
Rathke's cleft, 163
Tornwaldt's, 162, 162f, 163f
hamartomas, 164–165, 164f–165f
Necrotizing sialometaplasia, 234, 290, 290f
Neoplasia. *See* specific sites, e.g., Dermatopathology, neoplastic proliferative processes; specific types, e.g., Papillary squamous cell neoplasia
Nerve sheath myxoma, 560–561, 562f
Nerve sheath tumors, 415–421
benign, 652, 652f
cytopathology of, 652–653, 652f, 653f
granular cell, 415–416, 415f, 416f
malignant, 653, 653f
peripheral, 420–421, 420f
cytopathology of, 653, 653f
neurofibroma, 417–419
localized, 418–419, 418f, 419f
neurofibromatosis, 418
solitary, 417–418, 417f
palisaded encapsulated neuroma, 417
perineurioma, 416–417, 416f
schwannoma, 419–420, 419f, 420f
cytopathology of, 652, 652f
solitary circumscribed neuroma, 417
Neural neoplasms, of middle ear, 71
Neural proliferations, cutaneous, 559–561. *See also* Dermatopathology, neoplastic proliferative processes
Neurilemmoma, 560
Neuroblastoma(s)
metastatic, orbital pediatric, 673, 673f
olfactory, 124–129, 682, 682f (*See also* Olfactory neuroblastomas)
pediatric, 666, 666f
Neuroectoderm and surface ectoderm anomalies, 2–8
dermoid cyst and dermoid, 6–8, 7f, 8f
encephalocele, 3
extranasal heterotopic neuroglial tissue, 5
nasal glial heterotopia, 3–5, 4f, 4t, 5f
rudimentary meningocele, 5–6, 6f, 7f
Neuroendocrine carcinoma(s)
cutaneous primary, 561, 563f
laryngeal, 264–269
moderately differentiated, 266–267, 267f
poorly differentiated, 267–269, 268f, 269f
well-differentiated, 265–266, 266f
Neurofibroma(s), 417–419, 559–560, 560f
diffuse, 418–419, 418f
localized, 418–419, 418f, 419f
neurofibromatosis, 418, 419
plexiform, 418, 418f
solitary, 417–418, 417f
Neurofibromatosis, 418, 419
type 1, 418
type 2, 418
bilateral acoustic neuromas, 73, 73f
Neuroglial heterotopia, extranasal, 5
Neuroma(s)
acoustic, 72–73, 72f, 73f
bilateral, 73, 73f
palisaded encapsulated, 417, 560, 561f
solitary circumscribed, 417, 560, 561f
traumatic, 396–397, 396f
Neurothekeoma (nerve sheath myxoma), 560–561, 562f
Nevoid basal cell carcinoma syndrome, 205–206
Nevus(i)
angiomatous, 556–557
with architectural disorder and cytologic atypia, 568, 569f
basal cell nevus syndrome, 205–206
blue, 563–564, 564f
cellular, 564–565
malignant, 565
Clark's, 568, 569f
clonal, 565
combined, 565
deep penetrating, 565
dysplastic, 568, 569f
epithelioid cell, 567–568, 568f
intradermal, 565, 566f
melanocytic
balloon cell type, 566
congenital, 567, 567f
dermal, 565, 566f
halo type, 566–567
inverted type A, 565
neurotized, 565–566
neural, 565–566
organoid, 543, 544f
spindled, 567–568, 568f
Spitz, 567–568, 568f
strawberry, 557
Nevus fuscocaeruleus ophthalmomaxillaris, 562–563
Nevus of Ota (nevus fuscocaeruleus ophthalmomaxillaris), 562–563
Nevus sebaceus, 543, 544f
Nevus sebaceus of Jadassohn, 543, 544f
NK/T-cell lymphoma, nasal or nasal type, 496, 578
extranodal, 495–500 (*See also* Extranodal NK/T-cell lymphoma, nasal type)
Nodular (adenomatous) goiter, 355–356, 355f
Nodular fasciitis (NF), 392, 392f
orbital, 670, 670f
Nodular lichenification, 587–588
Nodular malignant melanoma (NMM), 572–573, 574f. *See also* Melanoma(s), malignant
Nodules. *See* specific types, e.g., Papillary hyperplastic nodule
Non-Hodgkin's lymphoma, diagnosis of, 648–650, 649f, 651f
Nonbullous impetigo, 604
Nonkeratinizing squamous cell carcinoma, sinonasal, 121–123, 122f, 123f
Nose
histology of, 81
lymphatic drainage of, 80–81
Nuchal fibrocartilagenous pseudotumor (NFP), 393–394, 394f
Nuchal fibroma, 403, 403f

O

Occipital encephaloceles, 3
Occult-type papillary carcinoma, 360, 360f
Ochronosis (alkaptonuria), 55
ear in, 55
exogenous, 597
Ocular adnexa, 501
Ocular adnexal lymphoid infiltrates, 501–506. *See also* Ocular adnexal lymphoma; Ocular lymphoma
diagnosis of, 502–503, 502f
Ocular adnexal lymphoma, 503–506
clinical features of, 503
differential diagnosis of, 504–505
pathologic features of, 503–504, 504f
secondary, 506
staging, treatment, and outcome of, 505–506
Ocular inflammations and infections, 664–665, 665f
Ocular lymphoma, 506–508, 507f, 664–665
secondary, 508
Oculopharyngeal muscular dystrophy, 244, 245f
Odontoameloblastoma, 225
Odontodysplasia, regional, 196, 196f
Odontogenic carcinoma, 225–227. *See also* Odontogenic tumors
ameloblastic carcinoma, 226, 226f
ameloblastoma, malignant, 225–226
clear-cell, 227, 227f
ghost cell, 227, 677
intraosseous carcinoma, primary, 226
in odontogenic cysts, 226–227
Odontogenic cysts, 201–207
carcinomas arising in, 226–227
dentigerous, 676–677, 676f
developmental, 202–207
calcifying, 207
dentigerous, 202–203, 202f–204f
eruption, 202f, 204
gingival, 202f, 206, 206f–207f
glandular, 207, 207f
keratocyst, 204–205, 204f–205f
lateral periodontal, 202f, 206, 206f–207f
nevoid basal cell carcinoma syndrome, 205–206
histologic typing of, 201, 201t
inflammatory, 201–202
Craig's paradental, 201–202
lateral periodontal, 201, 202t
keratocyst, 676, 676f
radicular, 676, 676f
Odontogenic fibroma, 220–221, 220f, 221f

Odontogenic ghost cell carcinoma (tumor), 218, 227, 677
Odontogenic keratocyst, 204–205, 204f–205f, 676, 676f
Odontogenic myxoma, 218–220, 219f
Odontogenic tumors, 208–227, 677–679
  adenomatoid, 144–145, 215–216, 216f
  ameloblastic fibroma, 223–225, 224f
  ameloblastic fibroodontoma, 225
  ameloblastic fibrosarcoma, 227
  ameloblastoma, 208–215, 677–678, 677f (*See also* Ameloblastoma)
  calcifying epithelial, 144, 144f, 216–218, 217f, 678–679
  calcifying odontogenic cyst, 207, 218, 219f
  cementoblastoma, 222, 223f
  cementum *vs.* bone in, 222
  classification of, 208, 208t
    WHO, 208, 209t
  granular cell, 221–222, 222f
  mandibular and maxillary
    ameloblastic carcinoma, 678
    ameloblastic fibroma, 678
    ameloblastoma, 677–678, 677f
    calcifying epithelial, 678–679
    myxoma, 678, 678f
  myxoma, 218–220, 219f
  odontoameloblastoma, 225
  odontogenic carcinoma, 225–227
    ameloblastic, 226, 226f
    malignant ameloblastoma, 225–226
    in odontogenic cysts, 226–227
    primary intraosseous, 226
  odontogenic fibroma, 220–221, 220f–221f
  odontoma, 223, 224f
  sinonasal, 143–144, 143f
  squamous, 215, 215f
Odontoma, 223, 224f
Olfactory neuroblastomas, 124–129
  biologic behavior of, 127–128
  clinical data on, 124
  cytopathology of, 682, 682f
  differential diagnosis of, 127
  electron microscopy of, 127, 129f
  grade I, 125, 125f, 125t
  grade II, 125–126, 125t, 126f
  grade III, 125t, 126, 126f
  grade IV, 125t, 126
  gross appearance of, 125
  histologic features of, 125–126, 125f–126f, 125t
    unusual, 126
  immunohistochemistry of, 127, 128t
  phenotypic spectrum of, 124, 124f
  radiologic studies on, 124
Oncocytic carcinoma, 308, 308f
Oncocytic cell adenoma, 382
Oncocytic cyst(s), 163, 163f
  laryngeal, 243, 243f
Oncocytic neoplasms
  laryngeal, 249
  salivary, 117
Oncocytoma, 305–308, 306f, 307f
  clinical behavior and treatment of, 308
  clinical data on, 306
  definition of, 305–306
  differential diagnosis of, 307–308
  gross appearance of, 306, 306f
  histochemistry of, 307
  histologic features of, 306–307, 306f
  ultrastructure of, 307, 307f
Oral cavity and jaws, 195–227
  cysts in, 195, 196f
  dental follicles in, 195–196, 196f
  gingivitis in, 199
  nonodontogenic developmental cysts of, 199–201
    nasolabial, 200–201, 200f–201f
    nasopalatine duct, 199–200, 199f–200f
  odontogenic cysts of, 201–207
    developmental, 202–207 (*See also under* Odontogenic cysts)
    histologic typing of, 201, 201t
    inflammatory, 201–202
      Craig's paradental, 201–202
      lateral periodontal, 201, 202t
  odontogenic tumors of, 208–227 (*See also* Odontogenic tumors)
  parulis in, 199, 199f
  periapical lesions in, 196–199
    apical scar, 198, 198f
    granuloma, 197, 197f
    radicular cyst, 197–198, 197f–198f
      lateral, 198
    residual cyst, 197–198
  pericoronitis in, 198–199, 198f
  periodontitis in, 199
Oral cavity and oropharynx, 680–682
  benign neoplasms of
    granular cell tumor, 680, 680f
    rhabdomyoma, 681
    squamous papilloma, 680
  malignant neoplasms of, 681–682
    malignant lymphoma, 681–682
    metastatic neoplasms, 682
    squamous cell carcinoma, 681, 681f
Oral cavity lymphomas, 508–511
  clinical features of, 508–509, 509t
  differential diagnosis of, 510–511
  in HIV-positive patients, 509–510, 509t, 510f
  pathologic features of, 509
  staging, treatment, and outcome of, 510
Oral facial granulomatosis, 592
Oral hairy leukoplakia, 608, 608f
Orbital diseases, 668–675
  cysts, 668–669
    dermoid, 668–669, 669f
    enterogenous, 669, 669f
  inflammatory lesions, 669–670
    infections, 669, 670f
    inflammatory pseudotumor, 670, 671f
    nodular fasciitis, 670, 670f
    sarcoidosis, 669
    Wegener's granulomatosis, 669
  neoplasms, 671–675
    lacrimal gland, 671–672
      adenocarcinoma, 672
      adenoid cystic carcinoma, 671–672, 672f
      pleomorphic adenoma, 671, 671f
    malignant lymphoma, 675, 675f
    meningioma, 673–674, 674f
    metastatic carcinoma, 675
    myeloma, 674–675, 675f
    pediatric, 672–673
      eosinophilic granuloma, 672, 672f
      neuroblastoma, metastatic, 673, 673f
      retinoblastoma, 673
      rhabdomyosarcoma, 672–673, 673f
    pilocytic astrocytoma, 674
    plasmacytoma, 674–675
    schwannoma, 674, 674f
Orbital teratoma, 19–20
Organoid nevus, 543, 544f
Oronasopharyngeal teratomas, 19
Osseous tumors, mandibular and maxillofacial, 679–680, 679f
  aneurysmal bone cyst, 679
  cementifying fibroma, 679
  chordoma, 679–680, 679f
  giant-cell reparative granuloma, 679, 679f
  osteosarcoma, 680
Ossifying fasciitis, 392
Ossifying fibroma, 454, 454f, 455f
  of ear, 59
  juvenile, 454–456, 455f
  mandibular and maxillofacial, 679
Osteoblastoma, 444–445, 444f
Osteochondroma, 447
Osteogenesis imperfecta, of ear, 76
Osteoid osteoma, 445–446, 445f, 446f
Osteoma, 429, 429f, 443–444, 443f, 444f
  of ear, 59
  osteoid, 445–446, 445f, 446f
Osteomyelitis, 438
  infectious, 438–439, 439f
  sclerosing
    diffuse, 439–440, 440f
    of Garré, 439–440, 440f
Osteoradionecrosis, 439, 439f
Osteosarcoma, 446–447, 447f
  mandibular and maxillofacial, 680
Otitis externa, malignant, 53
Otitis media, 60–62, 60f–62f
  AIDS, 63, 63f
  with effusion, 62, 62f
  mycobacterial (tuberculous), 62–63, 62f
Otosclerosis, of ear, 74–75, 75f

P

Paget's disease
  of bone, 440–441, 440f, 441f
  cutaneous, 539, 539f
Palisaded encapsulated neuroma, 417, 560, 561f
Palpation thyroiditis, 353
Panniculitis
  cold temperature–induced, 599
  factitial, 593, 593f
  lupus, 601, 601f
  popsicle, 599
Papillary adenocarcinoma
  of middle ear, 71
  sinonasal, 119
Papillary and exophytic squamous cell carcinoma of the larynx, 247–248
Papillary cystadenoma lymphomatosum (adenolymphoma), 308–310, 309f, 310f
Papillary endothelial hyperplasia (PEH), 390–391, 392f
Papillary hyperplastic nodule, 357
Papillary squamous cell carcinoma, 264, 264f, 265f
  of upper aerodigestive tract, 46–47, 46f, 47f
Papillary thyroid carcinoma, 358–363, 358t, 359f
  columnar cell, 362
  cytopathology of, 641, 641f, 692–695, 693f–695f
  diagnosis of, 358–360, 359f
  diffuse sclerosing, 361–362, 361f, 362

Papillary thyroid carcinoma (*contd.*)
encapsulated, 361, 361f
epidemiology of, 358
etiology of, 358
follicular variant of, 360–361, 360f
cytopathology of, 694–695
Hashimoto's thyroiditis and, 358
histology of, 359, 359f
immunohistochemistry of, 360
lymph node metastases of, 641, 641f
microcarcinoma in, 360, 360f
molecular genetics of, 360
occult-type, 360, 360f
prognosis of, 362
solid variant of, 361
tall cell variant of, 362, 362f
cytopathology of, 695
treatment of, 363
variants of
with aggressive behavior, 361–362, 361f, 362f
with favorable prognosis, 360–361, 360f, 361f
Papilloma(s)
Schneiderian (sinonasal), 106–108, 107f
columnar, 111–113, 112f
dysplasia and malignancy in, 113–114
fungiform, 108–109, 108f
inverted, 109–111, 109f–111f
Schneiderian-type mucosal, of middle ear, 70–71
squamous
laryngeal, 247–249, 248f
tonsillar, 185, 185f
in upper aerodigestive tract, 46–47, 46f, 47f
Papulosquamous disorders, cutaneous, 586–590
lichenoid processes, 588–590, 588t (*See also* Lichenoid processes, cutaneous)
psoriasiform dermatitis, 586–588 (*See also* Psoriasiform dermatitis)
Paradental cyst, 201–202
Paraffinoma (factitial panniculitis), 593, 593f
Paraganglioma, 68–70, 69f, 70f, 427–428, 427f, 428f
cytopathology of, 654–655, 655f
jugular, 71
laryngeal, 250–251, 250f
sinonasal, 132–133
Paranasal sinus(es), 80–148. *See also* Nasal cavity and paranasal sinuses
lymphatic drainage of, 81
Paranasal sinus lymphoma, 500–501, 501f
Paraneoplastic pemphigus, 582, 583f
Parasialadenoma, 293
Parasialoma, 293
Parathyroid adenoma, 380–381, 380f
cytopathology of, 698, 698f
Parathyroid cysts, 15, 382
Parathyroid glands, 379–385
adenoma of, 380–381, 380f
cytopathology of, 698, 698f
anatomy of, 379
carcinoma of, 382–383, 383f
cytopathology of, 698
familial hypocalciuric hypercalcemia and, 385
frozen sectioning of, 384
function of, 379
heterotopic, 15
hyperparathyroidism and, secondary, 385
hyperparathyroidism–jaw tumor syndrome and, 382
hypoparathyroidism and, 379
lipadenoma of, 382
multiple endocrine neoplasia in, 384–385
oncocytic cell adenoma in, 382
parathyromatosis in, 381–382
primary hyperplasia of, 383–384, 383f
water clear cell hyperplasia of, 384
Parathyromatosis, 381–382
Parotid glands. *See also* Salivary gland(s)
inflammatory pseudotumor of, 292, 292f
polycystic disease of, 287, 287f
Parulis, 199, 199f
Pemphigoid
bullous, 582–583, 584f
cicatricial, 584, 585f
Pemphigus, paraneoplastic, 582, 583f
Pemphigus foliaceus, 582
Pemphigus vegetans, 582, 583f
Pemphigus vulgaris, 581–582, 581f, 582t
laryngeal, 242–243
Periapical granuloma, 197, 197f
Periapical lesions, 196–199
apical scar, 198, 198f
granuloma, 197, 197f
radicular cyst, 197–198, 197f–198f
lateral, 198
residual cyst, 197–198
Pericoronitis, 198–199, 198f
Pericytic and vascular tumors, 410–415
angiosarcoma, 415, 415f
glomus tumor, 411, 411f
hemangioendothelioma, 413–414, 413f
epithelioid, 413–414, 413f
spindle cell, 414, 414f
hemangioma, 412–413, 412f, 413f
hemangiopericytoma, 410–411, 410f, 411f
Kaposi's sarcoma, 414, 414f
lymphangioma, 411–412, 411f
Perineurioma, 416–417, 416f
Periodontal cyst, lateral
developmental, 206, 206f–207f
inflammatory, 201, 202f
Periodontitis, 199
Periosteal fasciitis, 392
Peripheral giant cell granuloma (PGG), 395, 395f
Peripheral nerve sheath tumors, sinonasal, 141–142, 141f
Peripheral ossifying fibroma (POF), 394–395, 394f
Peritonsillar abscess, 180, 180f
Persistent embryonic remnants, 8–15. *See also under* Congenital anomalies
Persistent thymopharyngeal duct cyst, 15
Petrified auricle, 57
Petrosectomy, 53
Petrous temporal bone tumors, apex of, 73–74
Phacolytic glaucoma, 663
Phakomatous choristoma, 15–16, 16f
Pharyngeal stenosis, 158
Photoallergic dermatitis, 585–586, 586f
Photoallergic drug eruptions, 596–597, 597f
Phototoxic drug eruptions, 596–597, 597f
Picker's nodule, 587–588
Pigmented villonodular synovitis (PVNS), 468–469, 469f
Pilar cyst, 552, 553f
cytopathology of, 551–552, 552f, 637–638, 638f
Pilar neoplasms (hair appendages)
cytopathology of, 657–658
dilated pore of Winer, 543
fibrofolliculoma, 543
folliculosebaceous cystic hamartoma, 543, 543f
pilomatrixoma, 542, 542f
cytopathology of, 638, 655–656, 656f, 657–658
proliferating pilar tumor, 542
proliferating trichilemmal cyst, 542, 657–658
trichilemmoma, 542, 542f
trichoepithelioma, 540–541, 541f
trichofolliculoma, 542–543
Pilar tumor, proliferating, 542
Pilocytic astrocytoma, orbital, 674
Pilomatrixoma (calcifying epithelioma of Malherbe), 542, 542f
cytopathology of, 638, 655–656, 656f, 657–658
Pindborg tumor, 144, 144f
mandibular and maxillary, 678–679
Piringer-Kuchinka lymphadenitis, 483–484, 484f
Pituitary adenoma, 147–148, 147f
Plasma cell gingivitis, 199
Plasma cell myeloma, 580–581
Plasmacytoid myoepithelioma, 303, 303f
Plasmacytoma (plasma cell myeloma), 580–581
extramedullary, 523–525, 524f
clinical features of, 523
differential diagnosis of, 524–525, 525t
laryngeal, 275
pathologic features of, 523, 524f
staging, treatment, and outcome of, 523–524
orbital, 674–675
of thyroid, 522–523
Pleomorphic adenoma (PA, mixed tumor), 296–299
in children, 337
congenital, 20, 21f
of ear, 58
juvenile, 22
of lacrimal gland, 671, 671f
of larynx, 249
of salivary gland, 114–115, 115f, 296–299, 620, 620t
clinical data on, 296
cytogenetics of, 298
cytopathology of, 622–624, 622f, 623f
definition of, 296
differential diagnosis of, 298–299
gross appearance of, 297, 297f
histologic features of, 297–298, 297f, 298f
immunohistochemistry of, 298
metastasizing, 302, 302f
radiologic studies of, 296
recurrent, 299, 299f
treatment and clinical behavior of, 299
ultrastructural studies of, 298
Pleomorphic lipoma, 398, 398f
Pleomorphic liposarcoma (PLS), 401, 401f
Plexiform neurofibroma, 418, 418f
Polyarteritis nodosa, infantile, 488
Polychondritis, relapsing, 54, 54f

Polycystic (dysgenetic) disease, 22
of parotid glands, 287, 287f
Polymorphic reticulosis, 496, 578
Polymorphous light eruption, 598, 599f
Polymorphous low-grade adenocarcinoma, salivary gland, 117, 329–331, 330f
cytopathology of, 628–629
Polyp(s)
antrochoanal, 84–86
hairy, 7–8, 7f, 8f
oropharyngeal, 184
sinonasal, 104–105
inflammatory nasal, 84–86, 84f, 85f
lymphoangiomatous tonsillar, 183–184, 184f
Poorly differentiated neuroendocrine carcinoma (PDNEC), 266–267, 267f
Popsicle panniculitis, 599
Poroma, eccrine, 548f, 549, 549f
Posttraumatic spindle cell nodule (PSCN), 391–392, 391f
Primary intraosseous carcinoma (PIOC), 226
Primary synovial chondromatosis, 467–468, 468f
Primitive neuroectodermal tumor (PNET), 445–446, 445f, 446f
of bone, 467
of soft tissue, 428–429, 428f
Proliferating pilar tumor, 542
Proliferating trichilemmal cyst, 542
cytopathology of, 542, 657–658
Proliferative fasciitis, 393
Proliferative myositis, 393, 393f
Prostate carcinoma, orbital metastasis of, 675
Protozoal cutaneous infections, 606, 606f
Prurigo nodularis (nodular lichenification, picker's nodule), 587–588
Psammomatoid (juvenile) ossifying fibroma, 454–456, 455f
Pseudocarcinomatous hyperplasia, 538
Pseudocysts, in ear, 57, 57f
Pseudoepitheliomatous hyperplasia, 538
Pseudofolliculitis of the beard, 602
Pseudogout, 442–443, 443f
Pseudolymphoma of Spiegler-Fendt, 576–577
Pseudorheumatoid nodule, 594, 595f
Pseudotumor, inflammatory sinonasal, 136–137, 137f
Pseudovascular adenoid squamous cell carcinoma, laryngeal, 258, 259f
Psoriasiform dermatitis, 586–588
generalized pustular psoriasis of von Zumbusch, 587
prurigo nodularis, 587–588
psoriasis vulgaris, 586–587, 587f
pustular psoriasis, 587
Reiter's disease, 587, 587f
Psoriasis
generalized pustular, of von Zumbusch, 587
pustular, 587
Psoriasis vulgaris, 586–587, 587f
Pustular psoriasis, 587
Pyogenic bacterial lymphadenitis, 481, 481f
Pyogenic granuloma (PG), 389–390, 390f
sinonasal, 134–135, 135f
Pyriform sinus, carcinomas of, 256

R

Radiation dermatitis, 598
Radicular cysts, 197–198, 197f–198f
lateral, 198
odontogenic, 676, 676f
Ranula, 288
Rathke's cleft cyst, 163
Reactive lymphadenopathy, 633
cytopathology of, 642–643, 642f
Reactive lymphoid hyperplasia, 633
of orbit, 670
Recurrent mixed tumor, 299, 299f
Regional odontodysplasia, 196, 196f
Reidel's thyroiditis, 689
Reinke's edema, 235–236
Reiter's disease, 587, 587f
Relapsing polychondritis, 54, 54f
laryngeal, 242
Renal cell carcinoma (RCC)
lymph node metastases in, 640–641, 641f
thyroid metastases in, 697–698, 697f
Residual (radicular) cyst, 197–198
Retention mucoceles, 288
Retinoblastoma, 666, 666f
pediatric, 673
Retinopathy, diabetic proliferative, 663–664, 664f
Rhabdomyoma, 421–422, 421f, 422f
cytopathology of, 681
fetal, 24, 24f
laryngeal, 253, 253f
Rhabdomyosarcoma (RMS), 422–424, 422f, 423f
cytopathology of, 672–673, 673f
embryonal, 24
of larynx, 274
of middle ear, 71
of salivary gland
alveolar, 334, 335f
in children, 337
sinonasal, 142–143
Rheumatoid arthritis, laryngeal, 242
Rhinitis caseosa, 87–88
Rhinophyma, 601–602, 603f
Rhinoscleroma, 98–99, 98f, 99f, 604–605
laryngeal, 232
Rhinosporidiosis, 99–100, 99f
Riedel's disease, 355
Rosacea, 592
Rosai-Dorfman disease, 246–247, 488–489, 489f
Round cell liposarcoma, 400–401, 400f
Rudimentary meningocele, 5–6, 6f, 7f

S

Saccular cysts, laryngeal, 238, 238f, 239f
Salivary duct carcinoma, 326–327, 326f, 327f
cytopathology of, 633, 633f
Salivary duct cysts, 287, 287f
Salivary gland(s), 284–337
accessory, 286
congenital anomalies of, 286
cytopathology of, 618–633
diagnostic approach to, 618
diseases of, 287t
embryogenesis of, 284
heterotopia of, 286
histology of, 284–285, 284f–286f
inflammatory and non-neoplastic lesions of, 286–293
cystic lymphoid hyperplasia with HIV, 291–292, 292f
cysts, 286–288, 287f, 287t, 288f
cytopathology of, 619–620
branchial cleft, 619–620
cystic neoplasms, 620, 620t
HIV-associated lymphoepithelial, 620
mucus retention, 619, 619f
cytopathology of, 620–622
fine-needle aspiration–induced histologic changes, 292, 292f
granulomatous disease, 621
inflammatory pseudotumors, 292, 292f
irradiation effects, 289, 290f
lymphoepithelial lesions, 291, 291f
necrotizing sialometaplasia, 290, 290f
other, 293
sialadenitis, 289, 289f
cytopathology of, 620–621, 620f, 621f
myoepithelial, 513, 514, 514t
cytopathology of, 621–622, 622f
sialadenosis, 289–290
sialolithiasis, 288–289, 289f
Sjögren's syndrome, 291
lipomas in, 619
lymphoid proliferations of, 511–519
classification of, 512, 512t
cystic lymphoid hyperplasia, 512–513, 513f
lymphoepithelial, simple, 512, 512f
lymphoepithelial sialadenitis and Sjögren's syndrome, 513–516
clinical features of, 513–514
and MALT-type lymphoma, 515–516, 516t, 517t
differential diagnosis of, 515
etiology of, 515
morphologic features of, 514–515, 515f
terminology of, 513–514, 514t
lymphomas, 516–519
aggressive, 519
follicular, 518–519, 519f
marginal zone B-cell/MALT, 517–518, 517f
non-neoplastic, 512–513, 512f, 513f
terminology of, 513, 514t
metastasis to, 335
mucoepidermoid carcinoma of, low-grade, 619, 619f
neoplastic lesions of, 293–337
adenocarcinomas, 329t
alveolar rhabdomyosarcoma, 334, 335f
biopsy of, 294–295
in children, 335–337
benign epithelial, 337
embryoma or sialoblastoma, 336–337, 337f
hemangioma, 336, 336f
lymphomas and sarcomas, 337
malignant epithelial, 337
clinical findings in, 294
clinical staging of, 296
cytogenetics of, 296
cytopathology of, 622–633
benign, 622–626
malignant, 626–633
distribution of, 294
electron microscopy of, 296
epithelial neoplasms, 296–334
acinic cell carcinoma, 318–320, 319f
cytopathology of, 631–632, 631f, 632f

Salivary gland(s) (*contd.*)
adenocarcinomas, other, 331
adenoid cystic carcinoma, 320–323, 321f (*See also* Adenoid cystic carcinoma)
cytopathology of, 626–628, 626f, 627f, 627t
basal cell adenocarcinoma, 315–317, 315f, 316f
benign, other, 318
canalicular adenoma, 317–318, 317f
epithelial–myoepithelial carcinoma, 328–329, 328f, 329t
cytopathology of, 629
large-cell carcinoma, 333, 333f
lymphoepithelial carcinoma, 333–334, 334f
malignant mixed tumor, 299–302, 300f–302f
carcinoma ex pleomorphic adenoma, 299–301, 300f, 301f, 632–633
carcinosarcoma, 301–302, 301f
metastasizing pleomorphic adenoma, 302, 302f
mucoepidermoid carcinoma, 323–326, 324f (*See also* Mucoepidermoid carcinoma)
cytopathology of, 629–631, 629f, 630f, 630t
myoepithelial carcinoma, 305, 305f
myoepithelioma, 302–305, 303f, 304f (*See also* Myoepithelioma)
oncocytic carcinoma, 308, 308f
oncocytoma, 305–308, 306f, 307f (*See also* Oncocytoma)
pleomorphic adenoma (mixed tumor), 296–299, 297f, 298f (*See also* Pleomorphic adenoma, of salivary gland)
in children, 337
cytopathology of, 622–624, 622f, 623f
recurrent, 299
salivary duct carcinoma, 326–327, 326f, 327f
cytopathology of, 633, 633f
sebaceous adenoma, 311, 312f
sebaceous carcinoma, 312, 312f
sebaceous lymphadenocarcinoma, 312
sebaceous lymphadenoma, 311, 311f
small-cell carcinoma, 332–333, 333f
squamous cell carcinoma, primary, 331–332, 332f
terminal duct adenocarcinoma, 329–331, 330f
undifferentiated carcinomas, 332–334, 333f
Warthin's tumor, 308–310, 309f, 310f
carcinoma in, 310–311, 310f
cytopathology of, 624–625, 624f, 625f
etiology of, 294
histochemistry of, 295–296
histogenesis and classification of, 293–294, 293t
histologic diagnostic methods for, ancillary, 295–296
immunohistochemistry of, 296
incidence of, 294
malignant lymphomas, primary, 334–335
cytopathology of, 633
oncogenes in, 296
oropharyngeal, minor, 187
unilateral *vs.* bilateral, 294
normal, 618–619, 619f
sialadenosis of, 619
Salivary gland anlage tumor (SGAT), 20, 21f, 166–167, 166f, 167f, 337
Salivary gland choristoma, 20
Salivary gland heterotopias, 15
Salivary gland-type tumors, 249
SAPHO syndrome, 439
Sarcoid, 593
Sarcoidosis, 95–96, 96f
cytopathology of, 645, 645f
of larynx, 233–234, 235f
of middle ear, 63
of orbit, 669
of thyroid, 352
Sarcomas. *See* specific types, e.g., Fibrosarcomas
Sarcomatoid carcinoma, of larynx and hypopharynx, 260–262, 261f–262f
Schneiderian carcinoma–endodermal sinus tumor, mixed, 20
Schneiderian (sinonasal) papillomas, 106–108, 107f
columnar, 111–113, 112f
dysplasia and malignancy in, 113–114
fungiform, 108–109, 108f
inverted, 109–111, 109f–111f
Schneiderian-type mucosal papilloma, of middle ear, 70–71
Schwannoma(s), 419–420, 419f, 420f
of bone, 466
cellular, 419, 420f
cutaneous, 560
cytopathology of, 652, 652f
laryngeal, 253, 253f
orbital, 674, 674f
plexiform, 420
vestibular, 72–73, 72f, 73f
Scleroderma, localized, 601, 602f
Sclerosing epithelioid fibrosarcoma, 409
Sclerosing lipogranuloma, 593, 593f
Sclerosing mucoepidermoid carcinoma with eosinophilia, 369
Sclerosing osteomyelitis of Garré, 439–440, 440f
Sclerosing sweat duct carcinoma, 551, 552f
Sebaceoma, 543–545
Sebaceous adenoma, 311, 312f, 543, 544f
with atypia, 543–545
Sebaceous carcinoma, 312, 312f, 545–546, 545f, 546t
cytopathology of, 657
Sebaceous cells, 311
Sebaceous cyst, 551–552, 552f
cytopathology of, 637–638, 638f
Sebaceous epithelioma, 545
Sebaceous hyperplasia, 543, 544f
Sebaceous lymphadenocarcinoma, 312
Sebaceous lymphadenoma, 311, 311f
Sebaceous neoplasms and proliferations, 543–546
basal cell carcinoma with sebaceous differentiation, 545
basosebaceous epithelioma, 545
nevus sebaceus, 543, 544f
sebaceous adenoma, 543, 544f
with atypia, 543–545
sebaceous carcinoma, 312, 312f, 545–546, 545f, 546t
cytopathology of, 657
sebaceous epithelioma, 545
sebaceous hyperplasia, 543, 544f
Seborrheic keratosis, 534, 535f
Senile lentigo, 534
SETTLE (spindle epithelial tumor with thymuslike differentiation), 369–370, 370f
Severe combined immunodeficiency disease (SCID), tonsils in, 189
Sialadenitis, 289, 289f
acute, 620, 620f
chronic, 620–621, 621f
chronic sclerosing, of submandibular gland, 289, 289f
lymphoepithelial, 513–516, 514t (*See also* Lymphoepithelial sialadenitis)
myoepithelial, 513, 514, 514t
cytopathology of, 621–622, 622f
Sialadenoma, 293
Sialadenosis, 289–290, 619
Sialoblastoma (embryoma), 20, 20f
salivary gland, in children, 336–337, 337f
Sialolithiasis, 288–289, 289f
Sialoma, 293
Sialometaplasia, necrotizing, 234, 290, 290f
Simple bone cyst (SBC), 461
Sinonasal cholesterol granuloma, 87–88
Sinonasal diseases. *See* Nasal cavity and paranasal sinuses
Sinonasal fibromatosis. *See* Fibromatosis, sinonasal
Sinonasal low-grade adenocarcinoma, 117–119, 118f, 119f
Sinonasal (Schneiderian) papillomas, 106–108, 107f
columnar, 111–113, 112f
dysplasia and malignancy in, 113–114
fungiform, 108–109, 108f
inverted, 109–111, 109f–111f
Sinus histiocytosis with massive lymphadenopathy (SHML), 246–247, 488–489, 489f
Sinusitis, 82–88
acute, 82
chronic, 82–84, 83f
fulminant invasive fungal, 91–92, 92f
inflammatory nasal and antrochoanal polyps in, 84–86, 84f, 85f
Sjögren's syndrome, 513–516, 514t
clinical features of, 513–514
and MALT-type lymphoma, 515–516, 516t, 517t
differential diagnosis of, 515
etiology of, 515
morphologic features of, 514–515, 515f
in salivary glands, 291
terminology of, 513–514, 514t
Skin. *See* Cutaneous; Dermatopathology
Skin appendage tumors, 657–658
Small-cell carcinoma, 266–267, 267f
salivary, 332–333, 333f
sinonasal, 129–131, 130f
thyroid, 369
Small-cell neuroendocrine carcinoma, 266–267, 267f
Soft tissue pathology, 389–430
congenital lesions, 24
neoplasms, 397–430

adipocytic tumors, 397–401 (*See also* Adipocytic tumors)
alveolar soft part sarcoma, 426
chondroma, 429
ectomesenchymal chondromyxoid tumor, 429–430, 429f
epithelioid sarcoma, 426–427, 426f
extraskeletal Ewing's sarcoma, 428–429, 428f
fibroblastic and myofibroblastic tumors, 401–410 (*See also* Fibroblastic and fibroproliferative processes)
myogenetic tumors, 421–424
leiomyoma, 424, 424f
leiomyosarcoma, 424, 424f
rhabdomyoma, 421–422, 421f, 422f
rhabdomyosarcoma, 422–424, 422f, 423f
nerve sheath tumors, 415–421 (*See also* Nerve sheath tumors)
osteoma, 429, 429f
paraganglioma, 427–428, 427f, 428f (*See also* Paraganglioma)
cytopathology of, 654–655, 655f
pericytic and vascular tumors, 410–415 (*See also* Pericytic and vascular tumors)
primitive neuroectodermal tumor, 428–429, 428f
synovial sarcoma, 424–426, 425f, 426f
cytopathology of, 653, 653f
non-neoplastic lesions, 389–397
fibroblastic proliferations, 391–395 (*See also* Fibroblastic and fibroproliferative processes)
others, 395–397
myositis ossificans, 395–396, 396f
peripheral giant cell granuloma, 395, 395f
traumatic neuroma, 396–397, 396f
vascular proliferations, 389–391
bacillary angiomatosis, 389, 390f
papillary endothelial hyperplasia, 390–391, 391f
pyogenic granuloma, 389–390, 390f
Solar keratosis, 535–536, 536f, 537f
Solar lentigo, 534
Solid adenocarcinoma, sinonasal, 119
Solitary circumscribed neuroma (SCN), 417, 560, 561f
Solitary fibrous tumor (SFT), 405–406, 405f, 406f
sinonasal, 138, 138f
Spectacle frame acanthoma (granuloma fissuratum), 56
Spindle cell carcinoma (SpCC)
of head and neck, 260–262, 261f–262f
of upper aerodigestive tract, 47–48, 47f
Spindle cell hemangioendothelioma (SCH), 414, 414f
Spindle cell lipoma, 397–398, 397f
Spindle cell tumors, 303, 303f
Spindle epithelial tumor with thymuslike differentiation (SETTLE), 369–370, 370f
Spindled nevus, 567–568, 568f
Spiradenoma, 549, 550f
eccrine, 657–658
Spitz nevus (benign juvenile melanoma), 567–568, 568f
Spongiosis, 585
Spongiotic dermatitis, 581–586. *See also under* Dermatopathology, noninfectious inflammatory processes
acute and subacute, 585–586, 586f
Squamous cell carcinoma (SCC), 34
acantholytic (adenoid)
cytopathology of, 636
laryngeal, 258, 259f
of aerodigestive tract, upper, 44–50, 256 (*See also under* Upper aerodigestive tract, squamous neoplasia of)
field cancerization (effect) in, 256
invasive, 41–44 (*See also under* Upper aerodigestive tract, squamous neoplasia of)
basaloid, 262–264, 263f, 264f
cytopathology of, 636–637
sinonasal, 123–124, 123f
of upper aerodigestive tract, 48–49, 48f–49f
cutaneous, invasive, 537–538, 538f
of ear, 57
middle, 70, 70f
verrucous, 57–58
exophytic, of larynx and hypopharynx, 247–248
grading of, 42–43, 42f, 43f
keratinizing, sinonasal, 121, 121f
of larynx and hypopharynx, 253–264
acantholytic, 258, 259f
basaloid-squamous, 262–264, 263f, 264f
exophytic, 247–248
invasive, 254–259
clinical findings in, 255–257, 255f, 256f
epidemiology of, 254–255
pathologic findings in, 257–259, 257f–259f
treatment and biological behavior of, 259
malignant, 253–264
papillary, 247–248, 264, 264f, 265f
preinvasive lesions in, 253–254, 254f
pseudovascular adenoid, 258, 259f
spindle cell, 260–262, 261f–262f
cytopathology of, 636
verrucous, 259–260, 260f, 261f
of maxillary sinus, 123
metastatic, 634
cytopathology of, 634–636, 635f
of nasal cavity and paranasal sinuses, 120–124
cytopathology of, 682
of nasal vestibule, 123
in odontogenic cysts, 226–227
of oral cavity and oropharynx, 681, 681f
papillary, 264, 264f, 265f
of larynx and hypopharynx, 247–248
pharyngeal, 185–187, 187f, 188f
pseudovascular adenoid, 258, 259f
laryngeal, 258, 259f
of salivary glands, 331–332, 332f
metastatic, 620, 620t
sinonasal, 120–124
basaloid, 123–124, 123f
clinical data on, 120–121
histopathology of, 121
keratinizing, 121, 121f
of maxillary sinus, 123
of nasal cavity, 123
of nasal vestibule, 123
nonkeratinizing, 121–123, 122f, 123f
spindle cell, 636
of thyroid, 366–367, 367f
of tonsils, 185–187, 187f, 188f
ventriculosaccular, 257, 257f
verrucous, of ear, 57–58
Squamous cell carcinoma in situ (Bowen's disease), cutaneous, 536–537, 537f
Squamous intraepithelial neoplasia (SIN)
high-grade, 40f
histologic grading of, 39–40, 39f, 40f, 40t
histology of, 36–40, 36f–40f, 40t
keratinizing, 38, 38f
laryngeal, 253–254, 254f
nonkeratinizing, 38–39, 38f
Squamous neoplasia, of upper aerodigestive tract, 34–50. *See also* Upper aerodigestive tract, squamous neoplasia of
Squamous odontogenic tumor (SOT), 215, 215f
Squamous papilloma(s)
cytopathology of, 680
laryngeal, 247–249, 248f
tonsillar, 185, 185f, 186f
in upper aerodigestive tract, 46–47, 46f, 47f
Stapes fixation, congenital, 75–76
Starch granuloma, in ear and ear canal, 54
Steatocystoma, 552–553, 553f
Storiform perineurial fibroma, 416–417, 416f
Storiform–pleomorphic malignant fibrous histiocytoma, 409, 410f
Strawberry nevus, 557
Subglottic hemangioma, 249–250, 249f
Subglottic laryngotracheal stenosis, 244, 245f
Submandibular gland, chronic sclerosing sialadenitis of, 289, 289f
Sulfur granules, in tonsils, 179, 179f
Superficial spreading melanoma (SSM), invasive, 571, 571f, 575f
Supraglottic carcinomas, 255–256, 255f. *See also* Squamous cell carcinoma, of larynx and hypopharynx
Supraglottitis, 232–233, 233f
Sweat duct carcinoma, sclerosing, 551, 552f
Sweat gland neoplasms, 546–551
acrospiroma, malignant, 550, 551f
adenocystic hidradenocarcinoma, 550–551
apocrine carcinoma, 548–549
clear cell hidradenocarcinoma, 550
clear cell hidradenoma, 549–550
clear cell myoepithelioma, 549–550
cutaneous adenoid cystic carcinoma, primary, 551
cylindroma, 547–548, 547f
eccrine carcinoma
clear cell type, 550
ductal type (classic), 550, 551f
mucinous type, 550–551
eccrine poroma, 548f, 549, 549f
microcystic adnexal carcinoma, 551, 552f
mixed tumor, 549, 550f
cytopathology of, 657–658
sclerosing sweat duct carcinoma, 551, 552f
spiradenoma, 549, 550f
syringocystadenoma papilliferum, 546–547, 547f
syringoma, 548f, 549
malignant, 551, 552f
Synovial chondromatosis, primary, 467–468, 468f

Synovial sarcoma(s), 274, 424–426, 425f, 426f
cytopathology of, 653, 653f
of larynx and hypopharynx, 274, 274f
Synovitis, pigmented villonodular, 468–469, 469f
Synsialadenoma, 293
Synsialoma, 293
Syphilis, laryngeal, 232
Syringocystadenoma papilliferum, 546–547, 547f
of ear, 58
Syringoid carcinoma, 551, 552f
Syringoma, 548f, 549
chondroid, 549, 550f
cytopathology of, 657–658
malignant, 551, 552f
Systemic lupus erythematosus (SLE), lymphadenitis with, 485–486, 485f
Systemic reactions, cutaneous, 596–601. *See also under* Dermatopathology, noninfectious inflammatory processes

T

T-cell lymphoma. *See* Lymphoma(s), T-cell
T/NK-cell lymphoma, nasal or nasal type, 496, 578
extranodal, 495–500 (*See also* Extranodal NK/T-cell lymphoma, nasal type)
Tall cell papillary carcinoma, 362, 362f
Tangier's disease, 189
Teflon granuloma, 238–239, 239f
Telangiectasias. *See* Cutaneous vascular proliferations and telangiectasias
Temporal arteritis (giant-cell arteritis), cutaneous, 591–592
Temporal bone. *See also under* Ear
apex of petrous tumors of, 73–74
Teratocarcinosarcoma, 20
sinonasal, 106
Teratoid polyp, 7–8, 7f, 8f
Teratoma(s)
cervicothyroidal, 17–19, 17f–19f
congenital, 17–20, 17f–19f
nasopharyngeal, 159–160, 160f
orbital, 19–20
oronasopharyngeal, 19
sinonasal, 105–106
thyroid, 372
Terminal duct adenocarcinoma (TDC), 329–331, 330f
Thymic cysts, 14
cervical, 14–15, 14f
Thymoma, ectopic hamartomatous, 16–17, 16f
Thymopharyngeal duct cysts, 14
persistent, 15
Thymus, ectopic, 15, 15f
Thyroglossal duct cyst (TDC), 1, 8, 11–13, 12f, 13f, 351
cytopathology of, 638–639, 638f
Thyroid, 350–373
anatomy of, 350, 351f
athyrosis and, 350–351
autoimmune processes in, 353–355, 353f–355f
diffuse thyroid hyperplasia, 354–355, 355f
Hashimoto's thyroiditis, 353–354, 353f, 354f
Riedel's disease, 355
black, 690, 690f
cytopathology of, 686–698
accuracy of FNA in, 686
colloid in, 687, 687f
follicular cells in, 686, 687f
follicular lesions in, 690–691, 691f, 691t, 692f
malignant lesions in, 692–698, 693f–698f
non-neoplastic conditions in, 688–690, 688f–690f
normal, 686–688, 687f
oncocytic neoplasms in, 692, 692f
ectopic, 13–14, 350
follicular lesions of
benign, 691, 691f, 692f
FNA screening of, 690–692, 691f, 691t, 692f
suspicious, 691, 692f
inflammation and infection of, 351–353
sarcoidosis, 352
thyroiditis (*See also* Thyroiditis)
acute, 351–352, 352f
cytopathology of, 688
palpation, 353
subacute, 352–353
cytopathology of, 688, 688f
tuberculous, 351–352, 352f
intrathoracic, 350
lateral aberrant, 14, 351
lingual, 350
lymphoid proliferations of, 519–523
Hashimoto's thyroiditis, 353–354, 353f, 354f, 519–520, 520f
lymphomas
Burkitt's and Burkitt-like, 521–522
classification of, 520
diffuse large B-cell, 521, 522f, 697
extranodal marginal zone (MALT), 520–521, 521f
plasmacytoma of, 522–523
radiation-related changes to, 690
substernal, 350
thyroglossal duct cysts, 351 (*See also* Thyroglossal duct cyst)
tumors of, benign, 355–357, 355f, 356f
follicular adenomas, 356–357, 356f
atypical, 357
Hurthle cell tumors, 364, 692, 693f
hyalinizing trabecular adenoma, 357, 357f
cytopathology of, 694, 694f
nodular goiter, 355–356, 355f
papillary hyperplastic nodule, 357
tumors of, malignant, 357–373
anaplastic carcinoma, 365–366, 366f
cytopathology of, 695–696, 696f
angiosarcoma, 372
classification of, 358, 358t
with clear cells, 367
FNA of, 692–698
follicular carcinoma, 363–364, 363f
with medullary carcinoma, 369
frozen sectioning in surgery for, 372–373
Hurthle cell tumors, 364–365, 365f, 692, 693f
lymphoma, 371–372, 371f, 697
medullary carcinoma, 367–369, 368f
cytopathology of, 696–697, 696f, 697f
lymph node metastases in, 641–642, 642f
with follicular carcinoma, 369
metastases, 373, 373f, 697–698, 697f
papillary carcinoma (*See* Papillary thyroid carcinoma)
poorly differentiated carcinoma, 365, 366f
cytopathology of, 695, 695f
of probable thymic/branchial origin, 369–371
carcinoma showing thymuslike differentiation, 370–371, 370f
spindle epithelial tumor with thymuslike differentiation, 369–370, 370f
sclerosing mucoepidermoid carcinoma with eosinophilia, 369
small cell carcinoma, 369
squamous cell carcinoma, 366–367, 367f
teratomas, 372
Thyroid cancer. *See* Thyroid; specific types, e.g., Papillary thyroid carcinoma
Thyroid cartilage, chondrosarcoma of, 271–272, 272f
Thyroid hyperplasia, diffuse, 354–355, 355f
Thyroiditis
acute, 351–352, 352f
cytopathology of, 688
granulomatous, 352–353
cytopathology of, 688, 688f
Hashimoto's, 353–354, 353f, 354f, 519–520, 520f
cytopathology of, 688–689, 689f
papillary carcinoma and, 358
sclerosing mucoepidermoid carcinoma with eosinophilia and, 369
nonsuppurative, 352–353
palpation, 353
Reidel's, 689
subacute, 352–353
cytopathology of, 688, 688f
tuberculous, 351–352, 352f
Tingle body macrophages (TBMs), 649, 649f
Tissue overgrowth, 17–22. *See also* Congenital anomalies, tissue overgrowth; specific types, e.g., Teratomas
Tobacco, in upper aerodigestive tract neoplasia, 34–35
Tonsil(s), 179. *See also* Waldeyer's ring
sulfur granules in, 179, 179f
Tonsillitis, 180–183
etiology of, 180
gross appearance of, 181, 181f
histologic features of, 181–183, 181f–183f
peritonsillar abscess in, 180, 180f
Tornwaldt's cyst, 162, 162f, 163f
Toxic epidermal necrolysis, 590, 592f
Toxic goiter, diffuse (Graves' disease), 354–355, 355f
cytopathology of, 689
Toxoplasma lymphadenitis, 483–484, 484f
Toxoplasmosis, 644
Tracheopathia osteoplastica, laryngeal, 243–244, 244f
Traumatic neuroma (TN), 396–397, 396f
Trichilemmal cyst, 552, 553f
proliferating, 542, 657–658
Trichilemmoma, 542, 542f
Trichoepithelioma, 540–541, 541f
Trichofolliculoma, 542–543
Trichotillomania, 602
Tuberculosis, 96–97
laryngeal, 231, 232f
orbital, 669, 670f

Tuberculous thyroiditis, 351–352, 352f
Tumefactive fibroinflammatory lesion, sinonasal, 136–137, 137f
Tumors. *See also* specific types, e.g., Adipocytic tumors
  congenital, 1, 2t
Turban tumor, 547–548, 547f
  of ear, 58, 58f
  eccrine, 657–658
Tympanic membrane, keratosis of, 55

U

Ulcers
  eosinophilic, 582t, 585
  vocal cord, contact, 236–237, 237f
Undifferentiated carcinoma. *See also* Anaplastic carcinoma
  sinonasal, 131–132, 131f
Upper aerodigestive tract
  dysplasia of, histologic grading of, 39–40, 39f, 40f, 40t
  squamous neoplasia of, 34–50
    clinical presentation of, 35–36, 36t
    epidemiology of, 34–35
    histologic grading of, 39–40, 39f, 40f, 40t
    histology of, 36–40, 36f–40f, 40t
    multicentricity of, 35
    squamous cell carcinoma, invasive, histology of, 41–44
      grading of, 42–43, 42f, 43f
      microinvasive, 41–42, 41f
      pattern of invasion of, 43, 43f, 44f
      vascular invasion of, 43–44, 44f
    squamous cell carcinoma, special subtypes of, 44–50
      basaloid, 48–49, 48f–49f
      lymphoepithelioma, 50, 50f
      nasopharyngeal, 49–50, 170–174 (*See also* Nasopharyngeal carcinoma (NPC))
        cytopathology of, 639–640, 639f
      papillary, 46–47, 46f, 47f
      spindle cell, 47–48, 47f
        cytopathology of, 636
      verrucous, 44–46, 45f, 46t
Uveitis, chronic, 664, 665f

V

Vallecula, 183, 184f
Vascular proliferations and telangiectasias, cutaneous, 556–559. *See also* Cutaneous vascular proliferations and telangiectasias
Vascular tumors, 458–460
  hemangioma, 458–459, 459f
  malignant, 459–460
    angiosarcoma, 460
    epithelioid hemangioendothelioma, 459–460
Vasculitis, cutaneous, 582t, 590–592
  Behçet's disease, 592
  granuloma faciale, 590–591
  temporal arteritis, 591–592
Vellus hair cyst, 553
Venous hemangioma, 412, 412f
Ventriculosaccular squamous cell carcinoma, 257, 257f
Verruca vulgaris, 606–607, 607f
Verrucous carcinoma(s), 538
  laryngeal, 248, 259–260, 260f, 261f
  of upper aerodigestive tract, 44–46, 45f, 46t
Verrucous squamous cell carcinoma, of ear, 57–58
Vestibular schwannoma (acoustic neuroma), 72–73, 72f, 73f
Viral infections
  of external ear and ear canal, 53–54
  of skin, 606–609, 607f, 608f
Vocal cord nodules, 235–236, 236f
Vocal cord polyps, 235–236, 236f
Vocal cord ulcers, contact, 236–237, 237f

W

Waldeyer's ring, 179–189, 491
  anatomy of, 179–180, 179f, 180f
  lymphomas of, 187–189, 188f, 491–495
    clinical features of, 494–495
    introduction and classification of, 491–493
    pathologic features of, 493–494
      with Burkitt's lymphoma, 493–494, 493f
      with diffuse large B-cell lymphoma, 493, 493f
      with follicular lymphoma, 494, 494f
      with mantle cell lymphoma, 494, 495f
  neoplasms in
    benign, 185, 185f–186f
    malignant, 185–189
      lymphomas, 187–189, 188f
      metastatic, 189, 189f
      squamous cell carcinoma, 185–187, 187f, 188f
  non-neoplastic masses in, 183–185, 184f
  severe combined immunodeficiency disease and, 189
  Tangier's disease and, 189
  tonsillitis in, 180–183
    etiology of, 180
    gross appearance of, 181, 181f
    histologic features of, 181–183, 181f–183f
    peritonsillar abscess in, 180, 180f
Warthin's tumor, 308–310, 309f, 310f, 620, 620t
  carcinoma in, 310–311, 310f
Warty dyskeratoma, 534–535, 536f
Water clear cell hyperplasia, 384
Wegener's granulomatosis, 93–95, 94f
  in larynx, 240, 240f
  in middle ear, 63
  in orbit, 669
Well-differentiated neuroendocrine carcinoma (WDNEC), 265–266, 266f
Wen (epidermal inclusion cyst), 551–552, 552f
  cytopathology of, 637–638, 638f
"Whisky nose," 601–602, 603f

X

Xanthelasma, 593–594, 594f
Xanthogranuloma, juvenile, 596, 596f
Xanthoma. *See also under* Dermatopathology, noninfectious inflammatory processes
  with hyperlipoproteinemia, of ear, 55
  verruciform, 594, 594f

Y

Yolk sac tumor, of ear, middle, 71

Z

Zellballen, 266, 267
  in paraganglioma, 250–251, 250f, 427
Zenker's (hypopharyngeal) diverticulum, 239